Handbook of Models for Human Aging

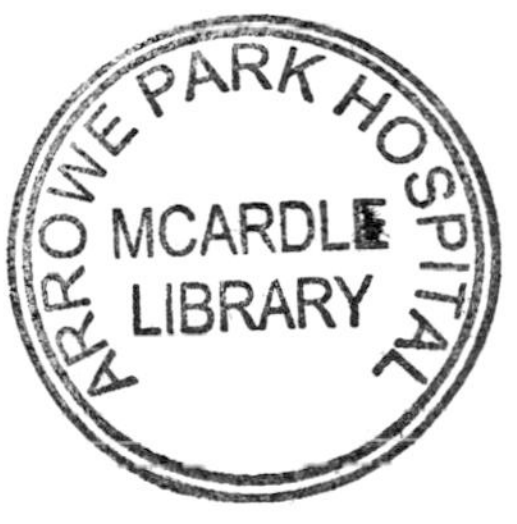

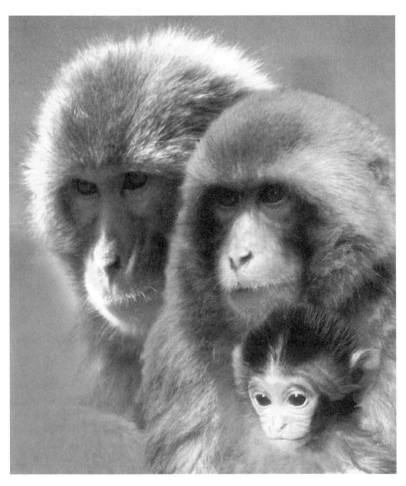

Images of young, middle aged, and old macaque monkeys. From the archive of the Oregon National Primate Research Center, Beaverton, OR. Used with permission. (See the color plate section.)

Handbook of Models for Human Aging

EDITOR

P. Michael Conn

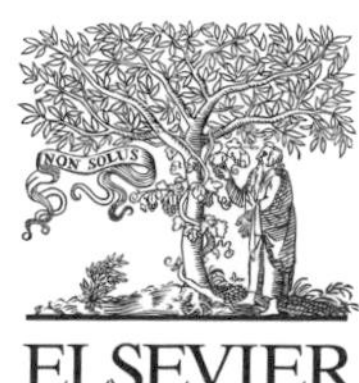

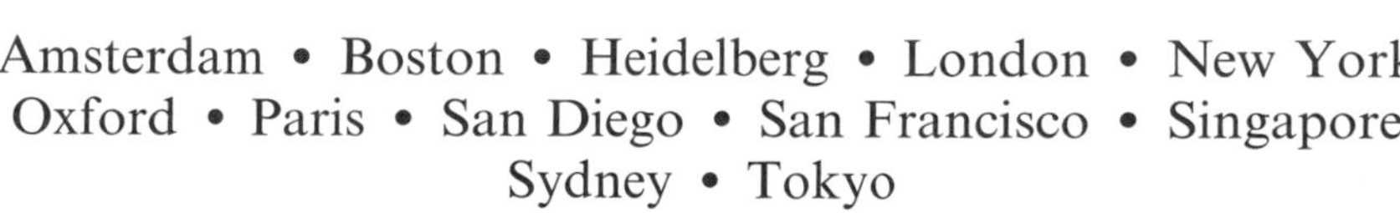
Amsterdam • Boston • Heidelberg • London • New York
Oxford • Paris • San Diego • San Francisco • Singapore
Sydney • Tokyo

Elsevier Academic Press
30 Corporate Drive, Suite 400, Burlington, MA 01803, USA
525 B Street, Suite 1900, San Diego, California 92101-4495, USA
84 Theobald's Road, London WC1X 8RR, UK

This book is printed on acid-free paper. ♾

Library of Congress Cataloging-in-Publication Data
Handbook of models for human aging / editor, P. Michael Conn.
p. cm.
Includes bibliographical references and indes.
ISBN-13: 978-0-12-369391-4 (casebound : alk. paper)
ISBN-10: 0-12-369391-8 (casebound : alk. paper)
1. Aging--Handbooks, manuals, etc. I. Conn, P. Michael.
[DNLM: 1. Aging. 2. Models, Biological. 3. Models, Animal.
WT 104 H2346 2006]
QP86.H347 2006
612.6′7--dc22 2005026227

British Library Cataloguing-in-Publication Data
A catalogue record for this book is available from the British Library.

ISBN 13: 978-0-12-369391-4
ISBN 10: 0-12-369391-8

For all information on all Elsevier Academic Press publications
visit our Web site at www.books.elsevier.com

Printed in the United States of America

06 07 08 09 10 9 8 7 6 5 4 3 2 1

ADVISORY BOARD

Contents

III. Animal Models

A. Non-mammalian Systems

B. Mammalian Systems

IV. Comparative Models

V. Disease-States and Normal Aging

A. Disease States

B. Health Issues Affecting the Elderly

C. Approaches to Treatment and Models

Contributors

The number in parentheses indicates the chapter to which the author contributed.

Claude Alain (64)
Rotman Research Institute, Baycrest Centre for Care, Toronto, Ontario; Department of Psychology, University of Toronto, Ontario, Canada

Mikhail F. Alexeyev (41)
Department Cell Biology and Neuroscience, University of South Alabama, Mobile, Alabama

David B. Allison (14)
Section on Statistical Genetics, Department of Biostatistics and Clinical Nutrition Research Center, Department of Nutrition Sciences, University of Alabama at Birmingham, Birmingham, Alabama

Gro V. Amdam (23)
School of Life Sciences, Arizona State University, Tempe, Arizona

Thomas P. Andriacchi (77)
Department of Mechanical Engineering, Stanford University, Stanford, California

Robert Arking (25)
Department of Biological Sciences, Wayne State University, Detroit, Michigan

Volker Arndt (13)
Division of Clinical Epidemiology and Aging Research, German Cancer Research Center, Heidelberg, Germany

Thiruma V. Arumugam (79)
Laboratory of Neurosciences, National Institute of Aging Intramural Research Program, Baltimore, Maryland

Ragnar Asplund (71)
Research and Development Unit, Family Medicine Stockholm, Ostersund, Sweden

Steven N. Austad (1)
Department of Cellular and Structural Biology, Barship Institute for Longevity and Aging Studies, University of Texas Health Science Center, San Antonio, Texas

Gustavo Barja (16)
Department of Animal Biology-II (Animal Physiology), Complutense University, Madrid, Spain

Yvonne Barnett (66)
College of Science and Technology, Nottingham Trent University, Nottingham, United Kingdom

Andrzej Bartke (34)
Departments of Physiology and Internal Medicine, Southern Illinois University School of Medicine, Springfield, Illinois

Barry D. Bavister (39)
Department of Biological Sciences, University of New Orleans, New Orleans, Louisiana

Stephen A. Benjamin
Department of Microbiology, Immunology and Pathology, Colorado State University, Fort Collins, Colorado

Carlo Bertoni-Freddari (40)
Neurobiology of Aging Laboratory, INRCA Research Department, Ancona, Italy

Jennifer L. Bizon (32)
Behavioral and Cellular Neuroscience, Department of Psychology, Texas A&M University, College Station, Texas

Klaus Bobacz (70)
Department of Internal Medicine III, Division of Rheumatology, Medical University of Vienna, Vienna, Austria

Carol A. Brenner (39)
Department of Biological Sciences, University of New Orleans, New Orleans, Louisiana

Hermann Brenner (13)
Division of Clinical Epidemiology and Aging Research, German Cancer Research Center, Heidelberg, Germany

Anja Brunet-Rossinni (36)
Department of Biology, University of Wisconsin, La Crosse, Wisconsin

André C. Carpentier (55)
Department of Medicine, University of Sherbrooke, Quebec, Canada

Tiziana Casoli (40)
Neurobiology of Aging Laboratory, INRCA Research Department, Ancona, Italy

Carlo Cavallotti (67)
Section of Anatomy, Department of Cardiovascular, Respiratory and Morphological Sciences, University "La Sapienza," Rome, Italy

Peter Celec (52)
Biomed Research and Publishing Group, Institute of Pathophysiology, Department of Molecular Biology, Comenius University, Bratislava, Slovakia

Christiane Charriaut-Marlangue (42)
Groupe Hypoxie et Ischémie Cérébrale Développementale UMR-CNRS 7102, Pierre and Marie Curie University, Paris, France

Andrew Chin (78)
Department of Medicine, Division of Cardiology, Weill Medical College of Cornell University, New York, New York

Alan Cohen (22)
Department of Biology, University of Missouri–St. Louis, St. Louis, Missouri

Klaus-Günter Collatz (21)
Institut Biologie I (Zoologie), University of Freiburg, Freiburg, Germany

P. Michael Conn
Oregon National Primate Research Center, Beaverton, Oregon; Oregon Health and Science University, Portland, Oregon

Judith Corr (62)
Department of Anthropology, Grand Valley State University, Allendale, Michigan

Glen R. Cunningham (63)
St. Luke's Episcopal Hospital, Houston, Texas

R. John Davenport (8)
Brain Science Program, Brown University, Providence, Rhode Island

Mary E. Delany (29)
Department of Animal Science, University of California, Davis, California

Olga Dela Rosa (66)
Department of Cellular Biology, Physiology and Immunology, Faculty of Medicine, University of Cordoba, Cordoba, Spain

João Pedro de Magalhães (2)
Department of Genetics, Harvard Medical School, Boston, Massachusetts

Giuseppina Di Stefano (40)
Neurobiology of Aging Laboratory, INRCA Research Department, Ancona, Italy

Inga J. Duignan (78)
Department of Medicine, Division of Cardiology, Weill Medical College of Cornell University, New York, New York

Benjamin J. Dyson (64)
Department of Psychology, University of Sussex, Brighton, United Kingdom

Jay M. Edelberg (78)
Department of Medicine, Division of Cardiology, Weill Medical College of Cornell University, New York, New York

Rita B. Effros (4)
Department of Pathology and Laboratory Medicine, David Geffen School of Medicine, University of California, Los Angeles, California

Paola Fabrizio (19)
Andrus Gerontology Center, Division of Biogerontology, University of Southern California, Los Angeles, California

Patrizia Fattoretti (40)
Neurobiology of Aging Laboratory, INRCA Research Department, Ancona, Italy

Caleb E. Finch
Ethel Percy Andrus Gerontology, Center University of Southern California, Los Angeles, California

Harry Fisch (51)
College of Physicians and Surgeons, Columbia University, New York, New York

Alfred L. Fisher (81)
Department of Medicine, Division of Geriatrics, University of California, San Francisco; San Francisco VA Medical Center, San Francisco, California

Kevin R. Fontaine (14)
Johns Hopkins University School of Medicine, Baltimore, Maryland

Rosalyn Forsey (66)
Cell Biology and Physiology Unit, Unilever Research Colworth, Unilever, United Kingdom Central Resources Ltd. Sharnbrook, Bedford, United Kingdom

Lourdes A. Fortepiani (83)
Department of Physiology and Biophysics, University of Mississippi Medical Center, Jackson, Mississippi

D. Robert Frisina (76)
International Center for Hearing and Speech Research, National Technical Institute for the Deaf, Rochester Institute of Technology, Rochester, New York; Otolaryngology Department, University of Rochester School of Medicine and Dentistry, Rochester, New York

Robert D. Frisina (76)
Otolaryngology, Biomedical Engineering and Neurobiology and Anatomy Departments, University of Rochester School of Medicine and Dentistry, Rochester, New York; International Center for Hearing and Speech Research, National Technical Institute for the Deaf, Rochester Institute of Technology, Rochester, New York

Tamas Fülöp (55, 66)
Research Center on Aging,
University of Sherbrooke, Sherbrooke,
Quebec, Canada

Michael P. Gardner (20)
School of Biological Sciences,
University of Bristol, Bristol,
United Kingdom

Leonid A. Gavrilov (5)
Center on Aging, NORC and the
University of Chicago, Chicago, Illinois

Natalia S. Gavrilova (5)
Center on Aging, NORC and the
University of Chicago, Chicago, Illinois

David Gems (20)
Department of Biology,
University College London, London,
United Kingdom

Paolo U. Giacomoni (82)
Clinique Laboratories, Melville, New York

Gavin Gillespie (27)
University of Michigan, Ann Arbor, Michigan

Andrea C. Gore (43)
Division of Pharmacology/Toxicology,
Institute for Cellular and Molecular Biology,
and Institute for Neuroscience, The University
of Texas at Austin, Austin, Texas

Adalsteinn Gudmundsson (61)
University Hospital of Iceland-Reykjavik,
Reykjavik, Iceland

John C. Guerin
Ageless Animals, Centenarian Species and
Rockfish Project, Portland, Oregon

Paul Hasty (49)
Department of Molecular Medicine,
University of Texas Health Science Center,
San Antonio, Texas

J. Fielding Hejtmancik (68)
Ophthalmic Genetics Section,
Ophthalmic Genetics and Visual
Function Branch, National Eye Institute,
National Institutes of Health, Bethesda,
Maryland

Kevin P. High (53)
Sections of Infectious Diseases and Hematology/Oncology and Molecular Medicine,
Wake Forest University Health Sciences,
Winston Salem, North Carolina

Rabih Hijazi (63)
Department of Medicine, Division of Endocrinology, Baylor College of Medicine;
Michael E. DeBakey VA Medical Center,
Houston, Texas

David B. Hogan (50)
Professor and Brenda Strafford Foundation
Chair in Geriatric Medicine, University of
Calgary, Calgary, Alberta, Canada

Jacquelyne M. Holm (78)
Department of Medicine, Division of Cardiology, Weill Medical College of Cornell
University, New York, New York

Donna J. Holmes (30)
Department of Biological Sciences,
University of Idaho, Moscow, Idaho

C. Christopher Hook (7)
Division of Hematology, Mayo Clinic,
Rochester, Minnesota

Radu Iliescu (83)
Department of Physiology and Biophysics,
University of Mississippi Medical Center,
Jackson, Mississippi

Donald K. Ingram (38)
Laboratory of Experimental Gerontology,
Intramural Research Program, Gerontology
Research Center, National Institute on Aging,
National Institutes of Health, Baltimore,
Maryland

Takeshi Iwata (68)
Laboratory of Cellular and Molecular Biology, National Institute of Sensory Organs, National Hospital Organization Tokyo Medical Center, Tokyo, Japan

Pudur Jagadeeswaran (26)
Department of Biological Sciences, University of North Texas, Denton, Texas

Jean-Paul Janssens (54)
Division of Pulmonary Diseases, Geneva University Hospital, Geneva, Switzerland

Christopher A. Jolly (65)
Division of Nutritional Sciences, University of Texas at Austin, Austin, Texas

Palmi V. Jonsson (61)
University Hospital of Iceland-Reykjavik, Reykjavik, Iceland

Matt Kaeberlein (18)
Department of Genome Sciences, University of Washington, Seattle, Washington

Mark Kantorow (68)
Department of Biomedical Science, Florida Atlantic University, Boca Raton, Florida

Scott W. Keith (14)
Section on Statistical Genetics, Department of Biostatistics, University of Alabama at Birmingham, Birmingham, Alabama

Evan T. Keller (27)
University of Michigan, Ann Arbor, Michigan

Jill M. Keller (27)
University of Michigan, Ann Arbor, Michigan

R. Lee Kennedy (69)
Department of Medicine, James Cook University, Douglas, Queensland, Australia

E.Y.H. Khoo (69)
Department of Diabetes, Queen's Medical Centre, Nottingham, United Kingdom

Shuji Kishi (27)
Department of Cancer Biology, Dana-Farber Cancer Institute and Department of Pathology, Harvard Medical School, Boston, Massachusetts

Steven G. Kohama (38)
Division of Reproductive Sciences, Oregon National Primate Center, Beaverton, Oregon

Jens Krøll (44)
Hafnia Unit of Biogerontology, Frederiksberg, Denmark

Dolores J. Lamb (45)
Department of Molecular and Cell Biology, Scott Department of Urology, Baylor College of Medicine, Houston, Texas

Sarah M. Lambert (51)
Department of Urology, Columbia University Medical Center, New York, New York

Mark A. Lane (38)
Laboratory of Experimental Gerontology, Intramural Research Program, Gerontology Research Center, National Institute on Aging, National Institutes of Health, Baltimore, Maryland

Frieder R. Lang (74)
Department of Psychology, Martin–Luthur–University of Halle–Wittenberg, Halle/Saale, Germany

Anis Larbi (55, 66)
Center on Aging Research, University Institute on Geriatrics, University of Sherbrooke, Québec, Canada

Keith E. Latham (46)
The Fels Institute for Cancer Research and Molecular Biology and the Department of Biochemistry, Temple University School of Medicine, Philadelphia, Pennsylvania

Susan P. LeDoux (41)
Department Cell Biology and Neuroscience, University of South Alabama, Mobile, Alabama

Harry LeVine, III (11)
Sanders-Brown Center on Aging, University of Kentucky, Lexington, Kentucky

Kirk C. Lo (45)
Mt. Sinai Hospital, University of Toronto School of Medicine, Toronto, Canada

Valter D. Longo (19)
Andrus Gerontology Center, Division of Biogerontology, University of Southern California, Los Angeles, California

Jacqueline A. Maffucci (43)
Institute for Neuroscience, University of Texas at Austin, Austin, Texas

Erminia Mariani (66)
Laboratorio di Immunologia e Genetica, Instituto di Ricerca Codivilla–Putti, IOR, Bologna; Departimento di Medicina Interna e Gastroenterologia, University of Bologna, Italy

Puneet Masson (51)
College of Physicians and Surgeons, Columbia University, New York, New York

Julie A. Mattison (38)
Laboratory of Experimental Gerontology, Intramural Research Program, Gerontology Research Center, National Institute on Aging, National Institutes of Health, Baltimore, Maryland

Mark P. Mattson (79)
Laboratory of Neurosciences, National Institute of Aging Intramural Research Program, Baltimore, Maryland

Samy I. McFarlane (58)
Division of Endocrinology, Diabetes and Hypertension, Osteoporosis Diagnostic Center, State University New York–Downstate Health Science Center at Brooklyn, Brooklyn, New York

William Meier-Ruge (40)
Institute of Pathology, University of Basel, Basel, Switzerland

Keith C. Meyer (60)
Section of Allergy, Pulmonary, and Critical Care Medicine, Department of Medicine, University of Wisconsin Medical School and Public Health, Madison, Wisconsin

Richard A. Miller (3)
Pathology Department and Geriatrics Center, University of Michigan School of Medicine, Ann Arbor VA Medial Center, Ann Arbor, Michigan

Satomi Miwa (22)
Institute for Aging and Health, Henry Wellcome Laboratory for Biogerontology Research, University of Newcastle, Newcastle-upon-Tyne, United Kingdom

Raymond J. Monnat, Jr. (80)
Departments of Pathology and Genome Sciences, University of Washington, Seattle, Washington

Arshag D. Mooradian (56)
Division of Endocrinology, Diabetes and Metabolism, St. Louis University, St. Louis, Missouri

Paul S. Mueller (7)
Division of General Internal Medicine, Mayo Clinic, Rochester, Minnesota

Annegret Mündermann (77)
Department of Mechanical Engineering, Stanford University, Stanford, California

Ranganath Muniyappa (58)
Endocrine Section Laboratory of Clinical Investigation, National Center for Complementary and Alternative Medicine, National Institutes of Health, Bethesda, Maryland

Nancy L. Nadon (33)
National Institute on Aging, Bethesda, Maryland

J.O. Nehlin (44)
Novo Nordisk and Odense University Hospital, Odense, Denmark

James F. Nelson
Department of Physiology, University of Texas Health Science Center, San Antonio, Texas

Simone Neri (66)
Laboratorio di Immunologia e Genetica, Instituto di Ricerca Codivilla–Putti, IOR, Bologna; Departimento di Medicina Interna e Gastroenterologia, University of Bologna, Italy

John Nicasio (58)
State University New York–Downstate, Brooklyn, New York

Michelle Nicolle (32)
Kulynych Center for Memory and Cognition Research, Departments of Gerontology and Physiology/Pharmacology, Wake Forest University School of Medicine, Winston-Salem, North Carolina

S. Jay Olshansky
School of Public Health, University of Illinois, Chicago, Illinois

Mary Ann Ottinger (30, 38)
Department of Animal and Avian Sciences, University of Maryland, College Park, Maryland; Laboratory of Experimental Gerontology, Intramural Research Program, Gerontology Research Center, National Institute on Aging, National Institutes of Health, Baltimore, Maryland

Joel D. Parker (24)
School of Biological Sciences, University of Southampton, Southampton, United Kingdom

Karen M. Parker (24)
Formerly of the Department of Ecology and Evolution, University of Lausanne, Lausanne, Switzerland

Cam Patterson (72)
Carolina Cardiovascular Biology Center, University of North Carolina at Chapel Hill, Chapel Hill, North Carolina

Graham Pawelec (66)
Center for Medical Research, University of Tübingen Medical School, Tübingen, Germany

Thomas Perls (46)
Department of Geriatrics, Boston University Medical Center, Boston, Massachusetts

Nicola Pescosolido (67)
Section of Ophthalmology, Department of Sciences of Aging, University "La Sapienza," Rome, Italy

Kiran Rabheru (59)
Department of Psychiatry, University of British Columbia, Vancouver General Hospital, Vancouver, British Columbia, Canada

Jane F. Reckelhoff (83)
Department of Physiology and Biophysics, University of Mississippi Medical Center, Jackson, Mississippi

Sylvain Renolleau (42)
Groupe Hypoxie et Ischémie Cérébrale Développementale UMR-CNRS 7102, Pierre and Marie Curie University, Paris, France

Rocco Rossinni (36)
Department of Biology, University of Wisconsin, La Crosse, Wisconsin

George S. Roth (38)
Laboratory of Experimental Gerontology, Intramural Research Program, Gerontology Research Center, National Institute on Aging, National Institutes of Health, Baltimore, Maryland

Mary Ellen Rousseau (73)
Nurse-Midwifery Specialty, Yale University School of Nursing, New Haven, Connecticut

Olav Rueppell (23)
Department of Biology, University of North Carolina at Greensboro, Greensboro, North Carolina

Kurt W. Runge (17)
Department of Molecular Genetics, Cleveland Clinic Lerner College of Medicine, Cleveland, Ohio

David C. Samuels (48)
Virginia Bioinformatics Institute, Virginia Polytechnic Institute and State University, Blacksburg, Virginia

Alberto Sanz (16)
Department of Animal Biology-II (Animal Physiology), Complutense University, Madrid, Spain

Peter N. Schlegel (51)
Department of Urology, Weill Medical College of Cornell University, New York, New York

Christian Schöneich (9)
Department of Pharmaceutical Chemistry, University of Kansas, Lawrence, Kansas

Isao Shimokawa (31)
Investigative Pathology, Nagasaki University Graduate School of Biomedical Sciences, Nagasaki City, Japan

Christina T. Siwak (35)
Institute for Brain Aging and Dementia, University of California, Irvine, California

Scott A. Small (12)
Taub Institute for Research on Alzheimer's Disease and the Aging Brain; Department of Neurology and Department of Pathology, Center for Neurobiology and Behavior, Columbia University College of Physicians and Surgeons, New York, New York

Michael D. Smith (6)
College of Public Health, University of Kentucky, Lexington, Kentucky

Roy G. Smith
Huffington Center on Aging, Baylor College of Medicine, Houston, Texas

Joel S. Snyder (64)
Rotman Research Institute, Baycrest Centre for Geriatric Care, Toronto, Ontario, Canada

Rafael Solana (66)
Department of Cellular Biology, Physiology and Immunology, Faculty of Medicine, University of Cordoba, Cordoba, Spain

Richard L. Sprott (1)
Barship Institute for Longevity and Aging Studies, Department of Cellular and Structural Biology, University of Texas Health Science Center, San Antonio, Texas

Evelyn Strauss (8)
American Association for the Advancement of Science, Washington, District of Columbia

Ilse-Gerlinde Sunk (70)
Department of Internal Medicine III, Division of Rheumatology, Medical University of Vienna, Vienna, Austria

Susan E. Swanberg (29)
Department of Animal Science, University of California, Davis, California

P. Dwight Tapp (35)
John Tu and Thomas Yuen Center for Functional Onco-Imaging, College of Medicine, University of California, Irvine, California

Loraine Tarou (62)
Department of Psychology, Grand Valley State University, Allendale, Michigan

Daniel Tessier (55)
Center on Aging Research, University Institute on Geriatrics, University of Sherbrooke, Québec, Canada

Jon Tolson (66)
Center for Medical Research, University of Tübingen Medical School, Tübingen, Germany

Jan Vijg (49)
Department of Physiology and Barshop Institute for Longevity and Aging Studies, University of Texas Health Science Center; Geriatric Research Education and Clinical Center, South Texas Veterans Health Care System, San Antonio, Texas

Mark E. Viney (20)
School of Biological Sciences, University of Bristol, Bristol, United Kingdom

Hans-Werner Wahl (74)
Department of Social and Environmental Gerontology, University of Heidelberg, Heidelberg, Germany

Lary C. Walker (11)
Yerkes National Primate Research Center and Department of Neurology, Emory University, Atlanta, Georgia

Jeremy D. Walston (57)
Johns Hopkins University School of Medicine, Baltimore, Maryland

Chenxi Wang (14)
Department of Epidemiology and Clinical Investigation Sciences, University of Louisville, Louisville, Kentucky

Lawrence J. Whalley (75)
Department of Mental Health, University of Aberdeen, Aberdeen, United Kingdom

Shannon Whirledge (45)
Department of Molecular and Cell Biology, Baylor College of Medicine, Houston, Texas

John R. Williams (15)
Department of Infectious Disease Epidemiology, Faculty of Medicine, Imperial College London, London, United Kingdom

Glenn L. Wilson (41)
Department Cell Biology and Neuroscience, University of South Alabama, Mobile, Alabama

Iain A. Wilson (37)
Department of Neuroscience and Neurology, University of Kuopio, Kuopio, Finland

Julie M. Wu (38)
Department of Animal and Avian Sciences, University of Maryland, College Park, Maryland; Laboratory of Experimental Gerontology, Intramural Research Program, Gerontology Research Center, National Institute on Aging, National Institutes of Health, Baltimore, Maryland

Zhun Xu (65)
Division of Nutritional Sciences, University of Texas at Austin, Austin, Texas

Licy Yanes (83)
Department of Physiology and Biophysics, University of Mississippi Medical Center, Jackson, Mississippi

Mary B. Zelinski (38)
Division of Reproductive Sciences, Oregon National Primate Center, Beaverton, Oregon

Preface

Aging research crosses all areas of physiology and also relies upon biological, mathematical, and chemical tools for its study. Accordingly, putting together a volume that aims to cover all models of human aging was a daunting task. The effort was made to cast a large net, but invariably some areas have been overlooked and not every viewpoint has been included. Despite its shortcomings, we hope the *Handbook* will serve as a useful broad-based overview for anyone involved in research on aging and age-related disease.

The editor thanks the authors, selected for their expertise and prominence in the field, for timely submission of well-circumscribed overviews, as well as their inclusion of previously unpublished "insider tips" from their respective disciplines.

I also appreciate the efforts of colleagues at Elsevier for embracing the significance of the project. Finally, I wish to thank Jo Ann Binkerd for assisting in the record keeping associated with this volume.

P. Michael Conn

1

Historical Development of Animal Models of Aging

Richard L. Sprott and Steven N. Austad

The use of animal models for research parallels the rise of modern science, beginning in the late 19th century with relatively primitive experiments and increasing in sophistication as relevant science progressed. The science of aging (gerontology) was relatively late in development, and its rise both parallels and is the result of the development of new, effective animal models. Many models, including inbred strains of mice and diet restricted mice and rats, were first developed for cancer research. As investigators began to explore the underpinnings of cancer reductions and cancer biology in these models, their utility for aging was soon apparent. The creation of the NIA in 1975 provided a powerful boost to the development of models. The NIA developed a deliberate, rational strategy for animal model development, then funded the endeavor. NIA continues to be central to model development through its contract colonies and grant programs. Rodent models now number in the hundreds ranging from strains to "designer" individual genotypes. At the same time, models from a wide variety of other species have been developed and are becoming more generally available. Particular interest is being paid to the development of new, suitable nonhuman primate models.

Introduction

The history of animal model development in the United States is inextricably tied to the history of the National Institute on Aging (NIA). The rapid rise of biological, biomedical and behavioral research on aging beginning in the 1970s was a response to the growing realization of both the scientific and political establishments that the American population was aging and that the Baby Boomers would reach retirement in less than 50 years, an eternity for politicians and a moment for scientists. Even before NIA was created, scientists interested in aging began searching for animal models for their study. From the time of Clive McKay's calorie restriction (CR) studies in the 1930s through Morris Ross's CR studies in the late 1960s and early 1970s, most aging models resulted from studies actually developed to study cancer. With the advent of the NIA, the field began to develop rational strategies for selection and provision of animal models. Over the ensuing 3½ decades the variety of animal models developed and available for aging research has grown enormously in quality and sophistication. At the same time, most investigators still make too many choices based on convenience rather than on the basis of a real knowledge of the available models and their suitability for any specific research question.

This chapter treats the historical development of vertebrate models only. We have made no attempt to present the history of invertebrate models or the thousands of "designer" mouse mutants and special stocks which are well covered in subsequent chapters.

Caloric Restriction (CR)

For a complete history of this topic, see Edward Masoro's summary in his SAGE KE article "Subfield History: Caloric restriction, slowing aging, and extending life" (Masoro, 2003).

The modern history of the use of animal (at least rodent) models for research on aging begins with the research of Clive McKay, a noted nutritionist in the 1930s. In the course of research on cancer, McKay and his colleagues (McKay *et al.*, 1935) discovered that severe calorie restriction (to 60% of *ad libitum* levels) resulted in significant increases in the lifespan of rats. Interestingly, since McKay was primarily interested in cancer, the increased longevity effects were not followed up until the work of Morris Ross in the 1960s using Sprague–Dawley rats (Ross, 1961). Ross, too, was primarily interested in the impact of CR on tumor incidence and age of occurrence in his rat models. Ross's very careful studies through the 1960s and early 1970s brought caloric restriction's effects on longevity to the attention of gerontologists just at the time that gerontological research was receiving an influx of interest and funding in anticipation of the creation of the NIA.

Following the interest created by Ross and others, two major research programs exploring CR's effects on lifespan using rodent models arose in the 1970s.

One group based in the laboratory of Roy Walford at UCLA began studies of immune function in C57BL/6J mice under CR conditions (M. Gerbasse-Delima *et al.*, 1975). Over a period of years, Walford and his colleagues, most notably Richard Weindruch, studied the effects of CR on models ranging from mouse to rhesus monkeys and humans. These studies are ongoing and provide a lively subtext to the lifespan extension literature, as CR is to date the only intervention that reliably increases lifespan in mammals (Weindruch *et al.*, 1982; Yu *et al.*, 1985; Walford *et al.*, 1992).

At the same time the Walford group was engaged in its program with the objective of developing a human CR research agenda, another rigorous program of rodent CR research was developed by Edward Masoro and B.P. Yu at the University of Texas, Health Science Center, San Antonio using specific pathogen-free (SPF) F344 rats (Masoro *et al.*, 1982). The Masoro group concentrated on F344 rats. The evolution of that group's research has favored the development of more sophisticated rodent models, rather than progressing toward human research. Roger McCarter, now at Penn State, has worked to understand the physiological basis of the CR effect using F344 rats and the involvement of energy metabolism in the mechanism of action of CR using transgenic and nontransgenic C57BL/6 mice (McCarter *et al.*, 1997; McCarter *et al.*, 2002). As will be seen in the rest of this chapter, CR has a central place in the development of animal models for all of basic gerontology, not just in connection with lifespan extension.

The National Institute on Aging (NIA)

Even before it was formally created, the NIA played a pivotal role in the development of animal models for aging. For a more complete discussion of this topic, see (Sprott, 1991; Sprott and Austad, 1996). In 1970, aging research was the province of a small branch of the National Institute of Child Health and Human Development (NICHHD). But it was obvious that a new institute focused on aging was likely to be authorized as the political system was beginning to consider the consequences of the aging of the baby boom cohort. In the very earliest meetings to consider what an institute focused on research on aging might need, it was quickly apparent that the development of readily available, affordable models for basic research would be crucial to development of a robust research enterprise. A small task force was convened and asked to recommend "the best animal model for aging." The task force had no trouble quickly agreeing that no single model would suffice, as different research questions would demand different models, and providing a very detailed set of recommendations for "Development of the Rodent as a model system of aging" (Gibson, 1972). That recommendation was accepted by the research administrators responsible for planning the resources of a new institute. Not only was the recommendation accepted; to everyone's great surprise, it was actually acted upon. Those recommendations are presented in: Development of the Rodent as a Model System of Aging Book II (Gibson, *et al.*, 1979).

In response to the recommendations of the task force, the Aging Branch created the first central colony of aging rodents for use by gerontologists under contract to Charles River Breeding Laboratories in 1974. The NIA was formally established in 1974 and began to function in 1975. The initial rodent colony contained two rat genotypes (F344 and Sprague–Dawley) and three mouse genotypes (C57BL/6J, DBA/2J, and the F_1 hybrid B6D2F1). The first aged animals were available for use by investigators by 1977. A key observation quickly became apparent as these animals were incorporated into aging research programs. By selecting these genotypes and making them broadly and easily available, the NIA had, in effect, seriously channeled the directions in which aging research could go, since the colony soon became the sole source of aged animals in the United States. In addition, it soon became apparent that Sprague–Dawley rats were susceptible to multiple pathologies that shortened lifespan, and that the F44 rats fed normal diets had a high incidence of renal pathology in the environments that were then prevalent. The solutions were twofold. First, there was agreement that the number of mouse and rat genotypes needed to be expanded and that more F_1 hybrids, with hybrid vigor, needed to be made available. In 1978, the number of mouse genotypes was increased to nine (and later reduced to seven). Second, intercurrent diseases in NIA-supported contract facilities and to an even greater extent in the colony spaces utilized by grantees were clearly resulting in much research being conducted on sick and dying animals or on unrepresentative survivors. These environments ranged from what could be charitably called "maintenance" to "clean conventional." In 1980, the institute began to address this disease problem. SPF facilities were just beginning to come into use. In a very controversial move at the time, the institute decided that providing "clean conventional" animals allowed the existing disease problems to persist. NIA decided to provide only SPF animals even though this meant that animals coming from an NIA facility would likely get sick upon arrival in a grantee facility that had an intercurrent disease problem. Nevertheless, this policy was implemented in 1982 in the hope that the result would be a broad improvement in the facilities receiving animals. That decision was in our opinion one of the major factors in the rapid improvement in the quality of animal research being supported by the NIA. Today, SPF barrier facilities are the norm. In subsequent years, the NIA has refined the array of mice and rats available. Current information on available animal resources from NIA is available at http://www.nia.nih.gov/ResearchInformation/Scientific Resources/AgedRodentColoniesHandbook.

The National Academy of Sciences (NAS)

In December 1976, NIA held a workshop to address the question of whether an array of species might be needed to serve as models for various human conditions and processes. The outcome of that conference was a recommendation to commission a National Academy of Sciences study of the issues and the state of knowledge about all known mammalian models. The study was carried out by the Institute of Laboratory Animal Resources (ILAR) of the NAS, which created a "Committee on Animal Models for Research on Aging" for that purpose. The report of that committee was issued in book form (Mammalian Models for Research on Aging, NAS, 1981).

Subcommittees on carnivores, lagomorphs and rodents other than rats and mice, mice, rats, and nonhuman primates, reviewed the world's literature in the areas of nervous system and behavior, visual system, auditory system, skeletal system, respiratory system, cardiovascular system, endocrine system, reproductive system and obesity. That review, done nearly 25 years ago, remains the only major assessment of model systems for the broad range of questions of importance to investigators of aging. Given the tremendous advances in model development that have occurred since then, it is surely time for a new assessment. While such an assessment is expensive, it would be expected to more than pay for itself in increased efficiency of agency planning for provision of model animals and investigator choice of suitable models.

The Search for Biomarkers of Aging (NIA)

As soon as gerontologists began to be interested in interventions that might lengthen life, the question of how to test such interventions arose. The problem is trivial in very short-lived animals such as yeast, nematodes, fruit flies, and mice, since many generations of animals can be tested in the course of a single three-year experiment (NIH grant). However, the problem is far from trivial in longer lived species like dogs, monkeys, and humans. The best solution would be to develop a set of measures that could be used to assess the life-lengthening effects of an intervention in significantly less than the full lifespan of the organism. Such measures are called biomarkers of aging. For a full discussion of the issues see the special issue of *Experimental Gerontology; Biomarkers of Aging* (Sprott and Baker, 1988).

The need for biomarkers of aging also arises from the observation that chronological age and "biological" age are not synonymous. Obviously species age at different rates, but the question of whether individuals within a species do so as well has generated much controversy in the aging literature. If one assumes that aging is the net result of environmental damage (oxidative damage to DNA for example), then the question is moot. If, on the other hand, one assumes that there are basic aging processes that determine the rate at which organisms age (as there clearly are in annual plants), then assessing the rate of aging becomes a necessary part of the assessment of interventions designed to change that rate. Only in the case of a pure wear and tear or DNA damage theory would biomarkers of aging be an irrelevant concept. Since different species have different, but very predictable, lifespans (fruit flies 2 months; mice 2 to 3 years; chimpanzees as long as 60 years; and humans as long as 120 years), the question of how to compare the biological age status of individuals across species in order to make animal models useful became a primary rational for the development of biomarkers of aging.

In 1987 the NIA together with the National Center for Toxicological Research (NCTR) established colonies of mice and rats to be used in a ten-year, 18-laboratory effort to develop biomarkers of aging that could eventually be used to test interventions in humans. Since CR was then the only intervention that had ever been reliably been shown to increase longevity (slow the rate of aging?) in any organism, the NIA/NCTR colonies provided both *ad libitum* and calorie-restricted mice and rats on the assumption that any useful biomarker would have to be sensitive to CR as a longevity promoting intervention. These colonies were the first to make CR mice and rats available for widespread use. NIA continues to make CR rats of three genotypes available; see http://www.nia.nih.gov/ResearchInformation/ScientificResources/Aged RodentColoniesHandbook for details and current availability.

Twenty percent of all of the animals produced in the biomarker colonies were set aside for pathological assessment (10% cross-sectional and 10% longitudinal). These studies provided the most complete characterization of the pathology of three rat genotypes (Brown Norway, F344, Brown Norway, Brown Norway × F344 F_1) hybrid and four mouse genotypes (C57BL/6N, DBA/2J, C57BL/6N × DBA2/J F1 hybrid, and C57BL/6N × C3H hybrid) ever accomplished (Bronson, 1990; Lipman *et al.*, 1999 A and B; Turturo *et al.*, 1999). One of the questions to arise from these studies was whether the *ad libitum* feeding regimen is the optimum regimen or an abnormal one for rodents. While the issue is not yet resolved, interest in some level of CR as the "normal" diet is growing. Differences in diet content and amount between laboratories contribute a great deal of variability to studies of everything from biomarkers to pathology. The NIA Biomarkers Program controlled for this variability by rearing all test animals and shipping them to investigators in the program. In the absence of such control, it is often difficult to make cross-laboratory comparisons. See Hart *et al.* (1995) for a very thorough treatment of this issue.

The Senescence Accelerated Mouse

The Senescence Accelerated Mouse (SAM) strains of mice were developed by Toshio Takeda at the Chest Disease Research Institute, Kyoto University, as the result of an accidental outcrossing of AKR/J mice and another unknown albino mouse strain in 1968. After receiving several pairs of AKR/J mice Takeda began brother–sister mating to provide animals for his research. He soon began to notice that in some litters of the offspring most of the mice "showed a moderate to severe degree of loss of activity, hair loss and lack of glossiness, periopthalmic lesions, increased lordosis, and early death" (Takeda, 2004). Beginning in 1975 five litters of mice showing the accelerated senescence phenotype were selected to become the progenitors of lines of senescence-prone (P series) mice, while three litters of mice that were resistant to accelerated aging were selected as progenitors of the senescence resistant (R series). Lines from these progenitor litters were then maintained as inbred lines to create three lines of resistant and five prone lines. These lines can be considered a set of recombinant inbred mice resulting from a cross between AKR and at least one (possibly two) unknown albino strains. Genotyping studies are ongoing to determine the genotype of the outcross animals.

Over the ensuing three decades Takeda and his colleagues have characterized these mice for an extraordinary range of characteristics including behavior, pathology, reproductive capacity, lifespan, response to husbandry, and physiology. For the most current exploration of this set of mouse strains, see Nomura *et al.* (2004). This approach to development of models for aging research is very different from that used in the United States. American investigators are very resistant to the use of models of "accelerated" aging, as they believe that it is impossible to distinguish between accelerated aging and the life-shortening effects of disease or environmental insult. Only recently have any investigators in the United States and Europe begun to use these mice. One of the factors in the slight shift in attitude has been the fact that the differences in lifespan among SAM lines have persisted after the mice were moved to SPF facilities (Suzuki *et al.*, 2004). SAM mice are widely used in Asia for pharmacologic and neurodegenerative research, and are obtained in Asia from the SAM Research Council. SAM mice are available in the United States and Western Europe from the International Biogerontology Resource Institute (IBRI) through an arrangement with Harlan Sprague Dawley.

The International Biogerontology Resources Institute (IBRI)

An international resource development institute (IBRI) was begun at San Pietro al Natisone, Friuli, Italy in 1998. The mission of IBRI is to foster international collaboration on the biological resources needed to conduct aging research including cells, tissues, organs, and whole organisms, from *C. elegans* to nonhuman primates. Early emphasis has been placed on rats (*Rattus norvegicus*) and mice (*Mus domesticus*) to provide for the shared development of biological resources and for the development of research methods to utilize these resources; provide space, core shared research resources, and a core staff of research scientists with maximum opportunities for international collaboration with visiting scientists and fellows; provide an international education effort regarding the use of animal models in gerontological research; provide maximum barrier facilities to house defined pedigreed stocks and strains of rats, mice, and other animals in one location accessible to the worldwide scientific community; provide guidance, worldwide, for the efficient, cost-effective, and reliable production and distribution of animal models for aging research; and provide a facility for holding international conferences and symposia on biogerontologic resources. This fledgling organization is made up of a consortium of universities from the United States and Europe and its corporate partner, Harlan Sprague Dawley. The SAM Council maintains an active role in the provision and certification of SAM lines maintained by IBRI.

The major objective of IBRI is to collect and maintain all of the major animal models for aging research in one place and make them available to investigators at that facility for pilot experiments, and by shipment to an investigator's laboratory for more extensive experiments. IBRI hopes to soon develop new rodent and nonhuman primate models as well. Further information about IBRI can be obtained by contacting the first author of this chapter.

Other Rodents

Laboratory rodents are among the shortest-lived mammals known, which defines in a certain sense their value for life-span studies. Their already short lives may have been further shortened by hundreds of generations of inadvertent selection for rapid growth and high reproductive rate that mass breeding entails. In the 1960s, George Sacher began searching for a longer lived rodent species, similar in size and basic biology to the laboratory mouse, to investigate what it exactly is that longer lived species do better in the "protection-stabilization, and repair of its essential molecules" when compared with a mouse (Sacher and Hart, 1978). In 1962, Sacher began laboratory breeding of wild-caught house mice (*Mus musculus*) and white-footed mice (*Peromyscus leucopus*) trapped near the Argonne Laboratory site in northeast Illinois. The white-footed mouse was abundant near Argonne and had already been used in a variety of biomedical research contexts (King, 1968). Although he noticed that wild-caught house mice lived somewhat longer than laboratory mice, he did not pursue this line of inquiry. The white-footed mouse turned out to live more than twice as long as either wild-caught or laboratory house mice—more than 3.75 years on average with the longest-lived individuals surpassing 8 years. Sacher's laboratory published about a dozen papers comparing house and white-footed mice, as did Ron Hart's laboratory at the National Center for Toxicological Research. In the 1980s and early 1990s George Smith of UCLA began to inbreed *Peromyscus leucopus*. Although Dr. Smith is now retired, the strains he produced have now been inbred for more than 30 generations. They, along with various subspecies of seven species of *Peromyscus* and a variety of mutants, are currently available from the Peromyscus Genetics Stock Center (http://stkctr.biol.sc.edu) at the University of South Carolina in Columbus, South Carolina.

Although George Sacher did not follow up his observation that wild-caught house mice lived longer than domesticated laboratory mice, he alerted researchers to the possibility that wild populations of house mice might contain longevity-associated genes that had been lost in laboratory mice. Austad (1996) observed that the wide range of mouse body sizes in geographically diverse populations suggested that many wild mouse populations might bear local adaptations that would make them of considerable gerontological interest. Miller and colleagues (1999) pointed out that the history of laboratory mice from their initial derivation from "fancy mice" to their inadvertent selection for rapid growth, high fecundity and cancer-prone genotypes to the extensive inbreeding that had made them so valuable in one sense may have led to shortening of life as well. Mice captured from three field locales (Idaho; Majuro in the Marshall Islands; and Pohnpei in Micronesia) were compared for body size, developmental rate, various hormone parameters, and longevity with a synthetic laboratory stock bred from crossing four inbred strains (Miller *et al.*, 2000, 2002). Mice derived from the wild remained smaller than the laboratory stock even given unlimited food. They also grew more slowly, matured later, and had smaller litters compared with the laboratory mice. Mice from Idaho and Majuro lived somewhat longer than the laboratory stock whereas the Pohnpei mice did not. Associated with their longer life, Idaho mice exhibited reduced serum levels of IGF-1, leptin, and glycosylated hemoglobin compared with laboratory mice. Surprisingly, Majuro mice were hyperglycemic compared to laboratory mice despite their longer lives (Harper *et al.*, 2005). Genes present in these long-lived mice may be valuable tools for the analysis of the physiology and biochemistry of aging mice. Moreover, wild-derived mice have exceptional levels of physical performance, e.g., running speed, endurance, agility, compared with laboratory mice (Dohm *et al.*, 1994) and may be useful in dissecting the genetics of muscle physiology and coordination.

In recent years, a novel rodent species of exceptional gerontological interest has been discovered, the naked mole-rat (*Heterocephalus glaber*). This mouse-sized African species had been studied since the 1970s, mainly for its unique social system that resembles the eusocial colony organization of bees and ants (Sherman *et al.*, 1991). However, as captive colonies were maintained for longer and longer, it became clear that naked mole-rats were equally interesting for their very long lives. The current captive longevity record is more than 28 years, and many individuals live into their teens and twenties (O'Connor *et al.*, 2002; Buffenstein and Jarvis, 2002) and continue to function at a high level. The longevity record-holding male successfully inseminated a female shortly before his death. Rochelle Buffenstein's laboratory along with her many collaborators are now seriously pursuing mechanistic studies to elucidate how this species can live nearly 10 times longer than the similar-sized laboratory mouse.

Nonhuman Primates

Nonhuman primates have been employed in medical research since the second millennium BC in ancient Egypt; however, their modern medical use began in the late 19th century when they were used mainly to investigate infectious diseases such as syphilis (Fridman, 2002). Elie Metchnikov, the Nobel Prize–winning bacteriologist, was probably the first investigator to consider the study of nonhuman primates for the insights they might offer into human aging. On the occasion of his 70th birthday in 1915, he suggested that primate nurseries be constructed for the captive rearing of monkeys and apes, thus laying the conceptual groundwork for the primate research centers that exist today (Fridman, 2002). In a somewhat embarrassing first direct use of primates to address human aging, S.A. Voronoff developed a colony of baboons and chimpanzees in southern France to provide testicular tissue for transplantation into humans to achieve their "rejuvenation." This facility also provided primates to other researchers, such as I.P. Pavlov. The first major primate center specifically dedicated to research in the United States was established in Florida by Robert Yerkes in 1930.

The advantage of primates for aging research is their close evolutionary affinity with humans and consequent similarity (compared with rodents) in such traits as complex cognitive abilities, and similarity of response to drugs and vaccines.

Maintaining primates in good physical and mental health in captivity has always presented complex problems. Because of these complex husbandry issues, even defining what is an "aged" individual of a given species has not been easy. For instance, the maximum lifespan of rhesus macaques, capuchin monkeys, and marmosets reported in a 1979 review was 33, 43, and 9 years, respectively (Bowden and Jones, 1979). With improved husbandry, we now know that these three primates can live at least 40–44 years, 55 years, and 16 years, respectively, some 25–75% longer than previously thought (Roth *et al.*, 2004; Nowak, 1999; Smucny *et al.*, 2004). Their long lives and complex social needs make primate aging research difficult and expensive. However, the human relevance of health problems associated with aging in nonhuman primates is unparalleled. They must be studied.

The NIA has sought to help make aged rhesus macaques available to the research community by supporting their maintenance at several primate research facilities around the United States. Currently, about 150 macaques between 18 and 35 years of age are available for noninvasive research (http://www.nia.nih.gov/ResearchInformation/ScientificResources/). The Institute keeps a repository of stored primate tissue as well, also mostly from rhesus macaques.

The most serious and systematic studies of nonhuman primate aging have developed as a consequence of an attempt to determine whether caloric restriction extends life and prevents disease in primates as it does in laboratory rodents. Two such ongoing studies exist. In 1987, the intramural program of the NIA initiated an investigation of long-term caloric restriction in male rhesus macaques and squirrel monkeys. In both species, restriction was imposed at several ages by reducing food intake by 30% relative to age- and size-matched controls. Five years later, female rhesus were added to the study. In the intervening years, various short-term restriction experiments were also added, so that about 200 monkeys in sum are being investigated (Lane *et al.*, 2002; Mattison *et al.*, 2003). Similarly, at the Wisconsin Regional Primate Research Center, a caloric restriction study of 30 rhesus males (15 restricted, 15 controls) was initiated in 1989. Five years later, 30 females and an additional 16 males were added to the study. As in the NIA studies, the experimental animals are restricted to 70% of the control diet (Ramsey *et al.*, 2000). Due to the long life of monkeys (mean thought to be 25–26 years for rhesus, and maximum at least 40 years), definitive results are not yet available for either study. However, a side benefit of these studies is to characterize more thoroughly than ever before, the life- and health-span of very well cared for primates. For instance, squirrel monkeys were chosen as one species for the NIA study, because it was thought that their maximum longevity was less than 20 years. However the oldest animals in that study are now in their mid-to late 20s (J. Mattison, personal communication, 2005). Thus with excellent care, longevity increased fairly dramatically. It will be interesting to see whether there is also such an increase in longevity in the rhesus population.

One approach to making primate aging research less costly and time consuming would be the development of a small primate model (Austad, 1997). Advantages of a small model (rat-sized or smaller) are (1) lower per capita housing and maintenance costs; (2) the potential to maintain the animals in SPF conditions in standard laboratory animal facilities as is now standard for aging mouse and rat research; and (3) their accelerated life history, being that they reach sexual maturity earlier and are shorter-lived than larger primates. The most promising candidate species for a small primate model for aging research is the common marmoset (*Callithrix jacchus*). This species is native to eastern Brazil and has been used in biomedical research since the early 1960s (Ludlage and Mansfield, 2003). One major advantage of common marmosets compared with other small primates is that they are not listed in Appendix I of the Convention on International Trade in Endangered Species (CITES). Listing in CITES Appendix I severely limits availability of animals for research and prohibits commercial trade in a species. Marmosets are rat-sized, 300–400 g, reach sexual maturity at 12–18 months of age, typically produce twin births, have a mean longevity of 6–7 years (are considered "old" by 8–10 years) (Tardif, personal communication, 2004), and have a record maximum longevity of 16 years (Smucny *et al.*, 2004). Their captive husbandry and clinical care are well-developed (Ludlage and Mansfield, 2003), and they are currently maintained at five major research facilities (Smucny *et al.*, 2004). It is quite possible that the mean and maximum longevity reported for marmosets would creep upward as they begin to be maintained in SPF conditions, but even a 50% increase would still make them an exceptionally attractive primate aging model. Because of their high reproductive rate relative to larger primates, colonies can be expanded comparatively rapidly. Their habit of twinning would also allow littermates to be randomly assigned to treatment and control groups, giving some measure of genetic control in experimental protocols. A further advantage is that as of March 1, 2005 common marmosets have joined the official species queue for complete genome sequencing by the NIH/National Human Genome Research Institute.

Summary and Conclusions

Modern animal model use for aging research began with the calorie restriction studies of Clive McKay and Morris Ross. This research, initially for cancer, led to studies to understand the CR effect and eventually to the development of special colonies of mice and rats for that purpose. Beginning in the mid-1970s the NIA created central colonies of aged rodents, centrally raised by contract, fed uniform diets, and maintained in barrier facilities. These animals became the models of choice for almost all biological research on aging for a decade. Subsequently, many more rodent models were created and supplied by NIA. Nonhuman primate resources began to be developed and are now just beginning to become available. Currently primate research is conducted in a small number of laboratories at DRR supported primate centers and at the NIA intramural facilities.

Other animal models such as nematodes and fruit flies are being used for basic studies of many aging phenomena. These models are discussed in later chapters.

The history of animal model development for aging research is in many ways the history of biological research on aging. Without widely available and suitable animal models for research, the astonishing developments that have occurred in the last 4 or 5 decades in our understanding of aging could not have occurred. It should be obvious that support for models development is absolutely required for the continued development of this field of knowledge.

REFERENCES

Austad, S.N. (1996). The uses of intraspecific variation in aging research. *Experimental Gerontology 31*, 453–463.

Austad, S.N. (1997). Small nonhuman primates as potential models of human aging. *ILAR Journal 38(3)*, 142–147.

Baker, George T. III, and Sprott, R.L. (1988). Biomarkers of aging. In Sprott, R.L., and Baker, George T. III (Eds.) *Biomarkers of Aging*, pp. 233–438. Special Issue, *Experimental Gerontology 23(4/5)*.

Bowden, D.M., and Jones, M.L. (1979). Aging research in nonhuman primates. In Bowden, D.M. (Ed.), *Aging in Nonhuman Primates*, pp. 1–13. New York: Van Nostrand Reinhold.

Bronson, R.T. (1990). Rate of occurrence of lesions in 20 inbred and hybrid genotypes of rats and mice sacrificed at 6 month intervals during the last years of life. In Harrison, D.E. (Ed.), *Genetic Effects on Aging II*, pp. 279–258. Caldwell, NJ: Telford Press.

Buffenstein, R., and Jarvis, J.U. (2002). The naked mole-rat—A new record for the oldest living rodent. *AAAS Science of Aging Knowledge Environment. May 29*, (21):pe7.

Dohm, M.R., Richardson, C.S., and Garland, T. Jr. (1994). Exercise physiology of wild and random-bred laboratory house mice and their reciprocal hybrids. *Am. J. Physiol. 267*, R1098–R1108.

Fridman, E.P. (Nadler, R.D., Ed.) (2002). *Medical Primatology: History, Biological Foundations, and Applications*. London: Taylor and Francis.

Gerbasse-Delima, M., Liu, R. K., Cheney, K. E., Mickey, R., and Walford, R. L. (1975). Immune function and survival in long-lived mouse strain subjected to undernutrition. *Gerontologia* (Basel), *21*, 184–193.

Gibson, D.C. (1972). Development of the Rodent as a Model System of Aging. DHEW Publication No. (NIH)72-121, Vol. 1.

Gibson, D.C., Adelman, R.C., and Finch, C. (1979). Development of the Rodent as a Model System of Aging. DHEW Publication No. (NIH) 79-161. Book II.

Harper, J.M., Durkee, S.J., Smith-Wheelock, M., and Miller, R.A. (2005). Hyperglycemia, impaired glucose tolerance and elevated glycated hemoglobin levels in a long-lived mouse stock. *Exp. Gerontol. 40*, 303–314.

Hart, R.W., Neumann, D.A., and Robertson, R.T. (Eds.) (1995). *Dietary Restriction: Implications for the Design and Interpretation of Toxicity and Carcinogenicity Studies*. Washington, DC: ILSI Press.

King, J.A. (1968). *Biology of Peromyscus (Rodentia)*. Stillwater, OK: Oklahoma State University Press.

Lane, J.A., Mattison, J., Ingram, D.K., and Roth, G.S. (2002). Caloric restriction and aging in primates: Relevance to humans and possible CR mimetics. *Microsc. Res. Tech. 59*, 335–338.

Lipman, R.D., Dallal, G.E., and Bronson, R.T. (1999A). Lesion biomarkers of aging in B6C3F1 Hybrid Mice, *J. Gerontol. Biol. Sci. 54A* (11), B466–B477.

Lipman, R.D., Dallal, G.E., and Bronson, R.T. (1999B). Effects of genotype and diet on age-related lesions in Ad libitum fed and calorie-restricted F344, BN, and BNF3F1 rats, *J. Gerontol. Biol. Sci. 54A*, (11), B478–B491.

Ludlage, E., and Mansfield, K. (2003). Clincal care and diseases of the common marmoset (*Callithrix jacchus*). *Comp. Med. 53*, 369–382.

Masoro, E.J. (2003). Subfield history: Caloric restriction, slowing aging, and extending life. *AAAS, Sage KE*, Feb 26, 2003.

Masoro, E.J., Yu, B.P. and Bertrand H.A. (1982). Action of food restriction in delaying the aging process. *Proc. Natl. Acad. Sci. USA 79*, 4239–4241.

Mattison, J.A., Lane, M.A., Roth, G.S., and Ingram, D.K. (2003). Caloric restriction in rhesus monkeys. *Exp. Gerontol. 38*, 35–46.

McCarter, R., Shimokawa, A., Ikeno, Y., Higami, Y., Hubbard, G., Yu, B.P., and McMahan,C. (1997). Physical activity as a factor in the action of dietary restriction on aging: Effects in Fischer 344 Rats. *Aging Clin. Exp. Res. 9*, 73–79.

McCarter, R., Strong, R., Mejia, W., Goei, K., and Gibbs, M. (2002). Plasma glucose and body temperature as mediators of aging in caloric restriction. *Biogerontology 3:* Suppl 1, 11–12.

McKay, C.M., Crowell, M.F., and Maynard, L.A. (1935). The effect of retarded growth upon the length of life and upon the ultimate body size. *J. Nutr. 10*, 63–79.

Miller, R.A., Austad, S.N., Burke, D., Chrisp, C., Dysko, R., Galecki, A., Jackson, A., and Monnier, V. (1999). Exotic mice as models for aging research: Polemic and prospectus. *Neurobiology of Aging 20*, 217–231.

Miller, R.A., Dysko, R., Chrisp, C., Seguin, R., Linsalata, L., Buehner, G., Harper, J.M., and Austad, S.N. (2000). Mouse stocks derived from tropical islands: New models for genetic analysis of life history traits. *Journal of Zoology 250*, 95–104.

Miller, R.A., Harper, J.M., Dysko, R.C., Durkee, S.J., and Austad, S.N. (2002). Longer life spans and delayed maturation in wild-derived mice. *Experiment Biology and Medicine 227*, 500–508.

National Academy of Sciences. (1981). *Mammalian Models for Research on Aging*. Washington, DC: National Academy Press.

Nomura, Y., Takeda, T., and Okuma, Y. (Eds.) (2004). *The Senescence-Accelerated Mouse (SAM): An Animal Model of Senescence*. Amsterdam: Elsevier.

Nowak, R.M. (1999). *Walker's Mammals of the World*, 6th ed. Baltimore: Johns Hopkins University Press.

O'Connor, T.P., Lee, A., Jarvis, J.U., and Buffenstein, R. (2002). Prolonged longevity in naked mole-rats: Age-related changes in metabolism, body composition and gastrointestinal function. *Com. Biochem. Physiol. A. Mol. Integr. Physiol. 133*, 835–842.

Ramsey, J.J., Colman, R.J., Binkley, N.C., Christensen, J.D., Gresl, T.A., Kemnitz, J.W., and Weindruch, R. (2000).

Dietary restriction and aging in rhesus monkeys: The University of Wisconsin study. *Exp. Gerontol. 35*, 1131–1149.

Ross, M.H. (1961). Length of life and nutrition in the rat. *J. Nutr. 75*, 197–210.

Roth, G.S., Mattison, J.A., Ottinger, M.A., Chachich, M.E., Lane, M.A., and Ingram, D.A. (2004). Aging in rhesus monkeys: Relevance to human health interventions. *Science 305*, 1423–1426.

Sacher, G.A., and Hart, R.W. (1978). Longevity, aging and comparative cellular and molecular biology of the house mouse, *Mus musculus*, and the white-footed mouse, *Peromyscus leucopus*. *Birth Defects: Original Article Series 14*, 71–96.

Sherman, P.W., Jarvis, J.U.M., and Alexander, R.D., (Eds.) (1991). *The Biology of the Naked Mole-rat*. Princeton, NJ: Princeton University Press.

Smucny, D.A., Abbott, D.H., Mansfield, K.G., Schultz-Darken, N.J., Yamamoto, M.E., Alencar, A.I., and Tardif, S.D. (2004). Reproductive output, maternal age, and survivorship in captive common marmoset females (*Callithrix jacchus*). *Am. J. Primatol. 64*, 107–121.

Sprott, R.L. (1991). Development of animal models of aging at the National Institute on Aging. *Neurobiology of Aging 12*, 635–638.

Sprott, R.L., and Austad, S.N. (1996). Animal models for aging research. In Schneider, E.L., and Rowe, J.W. (Eds.), *Handbook of the Biology of Aging*, 4th ed., pp. 3–23. New York: Academic Press.

Sprott, R.L., and Baker, G.T. III (Eds.) (1988). *Biomarkers of Aging* Special Issue, *Experimental Gerontology 23(4/5)*, 233–438.

Suzuki, T., Iida, M., Masui, N., Okudaira S., Shimizu, M., Takagi, S., and Asai. H. (2004). Breeding system and background data for SAM mice at Japan SLC. In Nomura, Y., Takeda, T., and Okuma, Y. (Eds.), *The Senescence-Accelerated Mouse (SAM): An Animal Model of Senescence*, pp. 153–160. Amsterdam: Elsevier.

Takeda, T. (2004). Effects of environment on life span and pathobiological phenotypes in senescence-accelerated mice. In Nomura, Y., Takeda, T., and Okuma, Y. (Eds.) *The Senescence-Accelerated Mouse (SAM): An Animal Model of Senescence*, pp. 3–12. Amsterdam: Elsevier.

Turturo, A., Witt, W.W., Lewis, S., Hass, B.S., Lipman, R.D., and Hart, R. W. (1999). Growth curves and survival characteristics of the animals used in the Biomarkers of Aging Program. *J. Gerontol. Biol. Sci. 54A(11)*, B492–B501.

Walford, R.L., Harris, S.B., and Gunion, M.W. (1992). The calorically restricted low-fat nutrient-rich diet in Biosphere-2 significantly lowers blood glucose, total leukocyte count, cholesterol, and blood pressure in humans. *Proc. Natl. Acad. Sci. USA 89*, 11533–11537.

Weindruch, R., and Walford, R. L. (1982). Dietary restriction in mice beginning at 1 year of age: Effects on lifespan and spontaneous cancer incidence. *Science 215*, 1415–1418.

Yu, B.P., Masoro, E.J., and McMahan, C.A. (1985). Nutritional influences on aging of Fischer 344 rats: Physical, metabolic, and longevity characteristics. *J. Gerontol. 40*, 671–688.

2

Species Selection in Comparative Studies of Aging and Antiaging Research

João Pedro de Magalhães

A great range of life histories are observed among mammals. Understanding why different species age at different rates may provide clues about the mechanistic and genetic basis of aging. This work focuses on animal species and their use in comparative studies of aging. Firstly, I debate how to compare aging across different species, including physiological parameters and statistical analyses. Afterwards, a selection of species for use in the comparative biology of aging is suggested. Taking into account that the ultimate aim of research on aging is to benefit people, my selection is largely based on primates. Primates feature such a vast range of aging phenotypes that comparative studies of aging need not employ other more distant species, except perhaps a few rodents. A number of animal species that may serve as models of antiaging strategies are also presented. Examples include species that appear not to age, such as some turtles, and animals featuring regenerative mechanisms absent from humans. Studying the genetic and molecular basis of these traits may have potential implications for antiaging research. Sequencing the genome of these species should then be a priority.

Introduction

Different species of animals age at radically different paces. A salmon will degenerate and die within days after spawning while some turtles, studied for decades, do not show signs of aging. Among mammals too a great range of life histories are observed. Even under the best laboratory conditions a mouse (*Mus musculus*) will not live past its 5th birthday, the oldest person on record—Jean Calment—died at age 122, but a bowhead whale (*Balaena mysticetus*) may live over 200 years (George *et al.*, 1999). Equally impressive, similar species tend to show great differences in longevity and aging rates. Among primates, for instance, while humans may live over 100 years, dwarf and mouse lemurs do not commonly live more than 20 years and, in their second decade of life, show age-related pathologies typical of elderly people.

Despite great differences in lifespan, the aging phenotype is remarkably similar across mammals (Finch, 1990; Miller, 1999). For example, aged (8–11 year-old) mouse lemurs (*Microcebus murinus*) show senile plaques comparable to those witnessed during human cerebral aging (Bons *et al.*, 1992). Consequently, the principle behind the comparative biology of aging is that studying why different species age at different rates may provide clues about the mechanistic basis of aging. Moreover, identifying which genetic factors determine the pace of aging in mammals could open the possibility of delaying aging and/or age-related diseases in people.

The focus of this work is on animal species and their selection for use in comparative studies of aging. Recently, we developed AnAge, an aging-oriented database featuring over 3,000 animals (de Magalhaes *et al.*, 2005a). All species mentioned in this chapter are featured in our database, and hence additional information and references are available in AnAge. My aims in this chapter are to (1) briefly discuss how to compare the aging process between different species; (2) provide a selection of species for comparative studies of aging; and (3) suggest species that may be models of antiaging strategies. Importantly, the purpose of biomedical research is to improve the human condition. The goal of gerontology is to preserve human health and well-being, and extend healthy life. Consequently, the choice of models employed by researchers must always have humans as the ultimate goal, and this is reflected in this work.

Although the focus of this chapter is not on how to perform comparative studies of aging, but rather on which species to employ, the selection process must take potential experiments into consideration. Numerous parameters may be studied between species with different rates of aging: DNA repair rates, cellular stress resistance, antioxidant concentrations, and many others (Finch, 1990). Some of these experiments require captive populations of the species under study, which may not be readily available and might even be impossible to obtain. Although in vivo studies may be highly informative, these may be difficult to conduct in many of the species mentioned herein—such as in bowhead whales. Modern high-throughput technologies like genomics, however, do not require captive populations or in vivo studies. Furthermore, cellular studies have been proposed as a means to study long-lived species (Austad, 2001; de Magalhaes, 2004), such as stem cells differentiating in culture. Therefore, intact organism studies may not be necessary in comparative biology, particularly since I predict that comparative genomics will become a major tool for comparative studies of aging (de Magalhaes and Toussaint, 2004). My choice of species hence does not take into account potential husbandry costs and difficulties.

Measures for Comparing Aging

In this work, lifespan is defined as the period of time in which the life events of a species typically occur. So far, I have been mostly referring to maximum lifespan (*tmax*) as a means to compare aging among different species. There are multiple problems, however, in using *tmax* as an estimate of aging. For example, feral animal populations may have their *tmax* limited by predation, accidents, or starvation. Even differences in *tmax* in captivity may reflect husbandry difficulties, and several species are impossible to maintain in captivity. Therefore, and since *tmax* is not the only way of comparing aging, it is worthwhile to consider how aging rates can be compared across species before selecting them. After all, since aging is one of the variables under study in comparative studies of aging, we must at least roughly quantify the rate of aging if we are to design appropriate experiments. As an example, I will examine the closest human relative, chimpanzees (*Pan troglodytes*). Chimpanzees live a maximum of 73 years while humans live 122 years, so *tmax* suggests that chimpanzees age about twice as fast as humans.

PHYSIOLOGICAL AGING

Aging can be defined as an age-related decline in physiological function (Austad, 2005). Studying aging in model organisms may include numerous anatomical, physiological, and biochemical age-related changes (Finch, 1990). Consequently, one way to determine rate of aging is to study the pace of age-related changes and/or the onset of age-related pathologies (Miller, 2001; de Magalhaes *et al.*, 2005b). This is arguably the most accurate and informative way of studying aging in a given species.

Briefly, the basic aim of physiological studies in aging animals is to investigate typical human age-related changes. These include the major human killers in old age: cancer, heart and neurodegenerative diseases. In fact, while it is not a measure of aging, it is informative to know what animals die of, particularly in captivity where the effects of accidents and predation are minimized. Determining common causes of death for model organisms is insightful regarding the onset of aging and regarding which age-related pathologies in a given animal model are similar to those seen in people. Equally relevant are reproductive changes with age, which include testis and ovary changes as well as the onset of reproductive senescence such as age of menopause. Many age-related changes and pathologies can also be studied and compared to human aging. A few parameters of interest include, but are not limited to, fat deposits, hormonal levels such as those of growth hormone, insulin and insulin-like hormones, and dehydroepiandrosterone (DHEA), atherosclerotic lesions, osteoporosis, arthritic changes, changes in reaction times with age, changes in senses, and the presence of cerebrovascular β-amyloid protein (Finch, 1990). There are also examples of comparative studies aimed at specific age-related pathologies, and readers should consult other chapters in this book.

In the case of chimpanzees, physiological deterioration appears to occur at earlier ages than in humans (Finch, 1990; Hill *et al.*, 2001; Erwin *et al.*, 2002). This is obvious in, for instance, bone aging: chimpanzees generally develop bone aging—such as fractures and loss of bone density—at earlier ages than people do (Morbeck *et al.*, 2002). Chimpanzees also show tooth erosion at earlier ages than humans (Hill *et al.*, 2001). While chimpanzees, in general, appear to show signs of aging at earlier ages than humans, little is known about the pace of aging in chimpanzees, some age-related changes typical of humans may not occur faster in chimpanzees. For example, cancer rates do not appear to be higher in chimpanzees, though little is known about age-related cancer rates in chimpanzees (Erwin *et al.*, 2002).

DEMOGRAPHIC AGING

Changes in physiological parameters are interesting for comparative studies of aging but they are potentially expensive and difficult to study. One alternative is to employ demographic measurements of aging. Aging can also be defined as an age-related increase in vulnerability and decrease in viability (Comfort, 1964). One of the features of aging in species with gradual senescence, like most mammals, is an exponential increase in mortality after maturity. For example, in humans, our chance of dying roughly doubles every 8 years after about age 30. This is remarkably similar among different human populations, independently of average lifespan (Finch 1990). Therefore, one way to compare rates of aging across different species is to calculate the rate at which mortality increases with age, which gives a measure of senescence (Pletcher *et al.*, 2000). As an example, Figure 2.1 shows the hazard function—which represents the probability of death—of chimpanzees according to age based on published mortality rates (Hill *et al.*, 2001).

In chimpanzees, hazard rates begin to increase near the end of the second decade of life, while human hazard rates generally begin to climb at the end of the third decade of life. This time it takes for mortality rates to climb has also been suggested as a measure of aging (Finch, 1990),

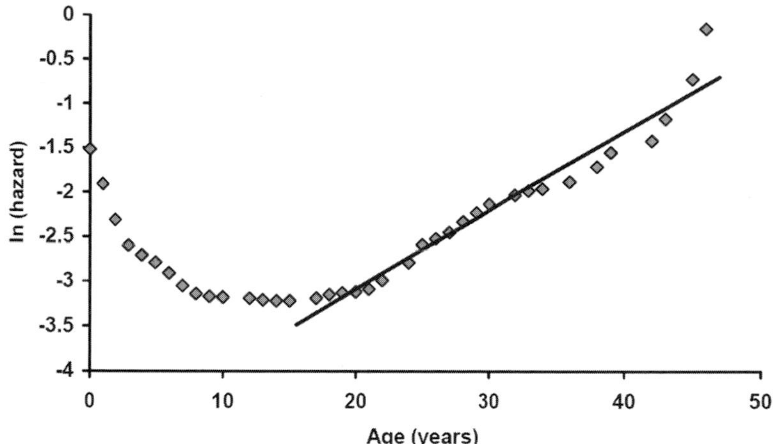

Figure 2.1. Natural logarithm of chimpanzee mortality rates as a function of age. The straight black line represents the estimated adult mortality trajectory based on Gompertz parameters calculated using a weighted linear regression. The data comes from five field studies of chimpanzees (Hill *et al.*, 2001) and was fitted using the T4253H smoothing algorithm from the SPSS package (SPSS Inc., Chicago, IL).

and in this case suggests aging commences earlier ages in chimpanzees than in humans. To calculate the age-related increase in mortality, the Gompertz function is typically used. Although other functions have been proposed (Wilson, 1994), the Gompertz function is generally the most adequate for these calculations, particularly when using small populations as is common in studies of higher vertebrates. It is also the most widely used function, making it a good term for comparisons. The Gompertz equation is $R_m = R_0 e^{\alpha t}$ where R_m is the chance of dying at age t—i.e., the hazard rate—R_0 is the nonexponential factor in mortality, and α is the exponential parameter. Based on the Gompertz equation it is possible to calculate the mortality rate doubling time (MRDT), which is an estimate of rate of aging given by MRDT $= 0.693/\alpha$ (Finch, 1990; Mueller *et al.*, 1995).

Depending on the quantity and quality of the data, there are different ways of calculating the Gompertz parameters (Mueller *et al.*, 1995), and a certain amount of subjectivity is unavoidable. In this case, and as previously described (de Magalhaes *et al.*, 2005b), the weighted linear regression was obtained from the ln-transformed Gompertz equation: ln (Rm) = ln (R0) + αt. The chimpanzee curve was estimated as: ln (Rm) = $-4.56 + 0.0798$t with r2 = 0.81. Hence, $\alpha = 0.0798$ with 95% confidence intervals of 0.0627 and 0.0969. This means that the MRDT for chimpanzees is around 8–9 years, similar to that of humans.

The great advantage of the Gompertz function and estimating α and the MRDT is that it allows us to quantify the rate of aging. As shown above, however, MRDT estimates indicate chimpanzees and humans age at similar paces, which may not be true from a physiological level. Our results from rodents also suggest that MRDT is a good but not perfect estimate of rate of aging (de Magalhaes *et al.*, 2005b). Therefore, even though the MRDT is a useful measurement of aging rates, it should be used in conjunction with physiological observations.

CONCLUDING REMARKS

While not being measurements of aging, lifehistory traits such as developmental schedules are relevant for comparative studies of aging. For instance, long development in mammals is typically associated with a long adult lifespan, independently of body size (Harvey and Zammuto, 1985). Age at sexual maturity, gestation or incubation time, and litter or clutch size are all important features of animals, particularly in the context of ecology and to understand the evolutionary forces that shape lifespan.

Other estimates of aging have been used such as adult mortality rates, average longevity, and adult lifespan. Adult mortality rates and average longevity did not correlate well with the MRDT or with physiological aging parameters in rodent cohorts (de Magalhaes *et al.*, 2005b). In the context of comparative studies of aging, there is no strong reason to use these estimates rather than maximum lifespan, though maximum adult lifespan may sometimes be more appropriate than *tmax*. In contrast, the large amounts of *tmax* data available make it a good term for comparisons.

In conclusion, the most adequate measure of aging is still *tmax*. Faster aging organisms will not be able to live as long as slower or nonaging species, which will be reflected in *tmax*. In fact, α has been shown to correlate with *tmax* (Finch and Pike 1996). We also recently showed that *tmax* correlates with MRDT in rodent cohorts (de Magalhaes *et al.*, 2005b). Certainly, there are inherited problems in quantifying aging using *tmax* and, at least for species with high mortality rates in the wild, *tmax* should be estimated from captive populations. Nonetheless, while the use of the methods described above is encouraged, particularly descriptions of physiological, biochemical, and anatomical changes with age, *tmax* will continue to be the most widely used estimate of rate of aging. In the remaining of this chapter, *tmax* is commonly used.

Species for the Comparative Biology of Aging

As mentioned above, the ultimate objective of aging research is to benefit people. Consequently, choosing species for the comparative biology of aging must be done having *Homo sapiens* in perspective. Whether model organisms are representative of the human aging process has been debated by many others (Gershon and Gershon, 2000). It is possible that mechanisms of aging are conserved across distant species, and it is possible that they are not (de Magalhaes, 2004). Since there is still no definitive answer to this debate, my position in this work is that species biologically and evolutionarily more distant from humans are less likely to share mechanisms of aging with people, and thus an effort was made to select species closer to humans.

Since among mammals there is a great diversity in the pace of aging, there is no scientific reason to employ nonmammalian species in the comparative biology of aging. On the contrary, incorporating nonmammalian species may lead to the use of species with different biology than humans and thus of more dubious use to understand human aging. In fact, mammals feature unique traits associated with aging such as diphyodont replacement—i.e., two sets of teeth—which is surprisingly common in mammals and is associated with tooth erosion, and a lack of oocyte regeneration, which makes reproductive senescence inevitable in all studied female mammals. These traits suggest that the evolution of aging in mammals may have had unique features (de Magalhaes and Toussaint, 2002). While there may be practical and economical reasons to employ nonmammalian species in aging research, these must be considered as secondary choices and more error-prone than mammalian models.

PRIMATES AND RODENTS

If the focus of gerontology is on the human species, then it makes sense for us to select our closest relatives as models of aging, provided these species indeed age differently than humans (Figure 2.2).

As mentioned above, our closest living relative is the chimpanzee, in which aging appears to occur earlier than in humans. Similarly, all the great apes show signs of aging at younger ages than humans, though it is unknown whether they age differently from each other (Erwin *et al.*, 2002). As we move further away from humans and great apes, species tend to be smaller, less intelligent, and shorter-lived. This is apparent among Old World monkeys (family: Cercopithecidae), which are generally shorter-lived than apes. Two species of Old World

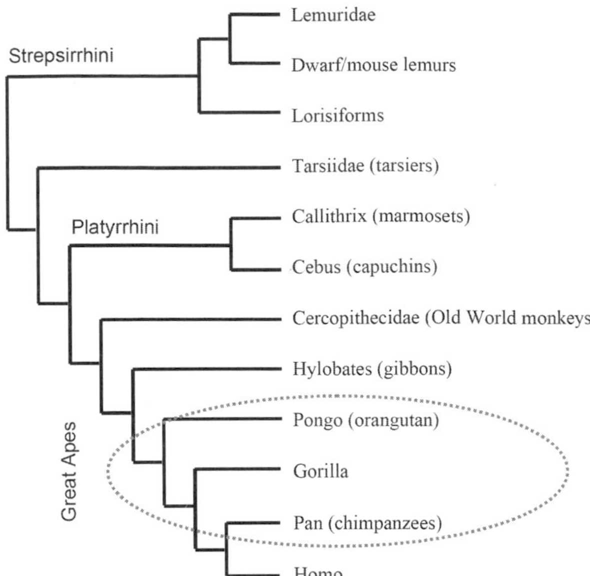

Figure 2.2. Primate phylogeny highlighting potential models for comparative studies of aging. The Platyrrhini infraorder represents New World monkeys. Phylogeny was drawn based on Goodman *et al.* (1998). Branch lengths are not to scale.

monkeys have already been studied in the context of aging: rhesus monkeys and baboons. Both appear to age considerably faster than humans and great apes, making them potentially useful models for comparative studies of aging. Interestingly, baboons have an MRDT of roughly 4 years (Bronikowsky *et al.*, 2002) while rhesus monkeys appear to have an MRDT not smaller than that of humans (Finch, 1990). Nonetheless, physiological studies suggest that rhesus monkeys age about twice as fast as humans (Finch, 1990; also see Chapter 38 by Roth and colleagues in this book and references in AnAge). Baboons and rhesus monkeys demonstrate how comparing aging rates among different species can be difficult and how the MRDT is not always an accurate estimate of rates of aging.

Among New World monkeys, also termed Platyrrhini, we find species much shorter lived than apes and humans. Marmosets are a good example, such as the common marmoset *Callithrix jacchus*. The record longevity for these animals is little over 16 years, and numerous age-related changes have been reported in their second decade of life (see AnAge for references). They also reach sexual maturity at about one year of age—which is much sooner than apes—suggesting shorter generation cycles, shorter lifespans, and hence in accordance with a faster aging process. Therefore, if our choice of species is aimed at discovering what determines rate of aging among primates, with humans as our ultimate goal, then these shorter lived primates are certainly a good choice. In contrast, some New World monkeys are longer lived, attaining sexual maturity at older ages. Examples include members of the genera Alouatta, Ateles, Cacajao, and Cebus. The white-faced capuchin (*Cebus capucinus*) is a good example with a record longevity of almost 55 years and attaining sexual maturity with at least 5 years of age. Therefore, New World monkeys offer a variety of aging phenotypes suitable for comparative studies of aging. The large variation in rates of aging among such closely related species argues, once again (Miller, 1999), that genetic factors determine rate of aging in primates and makes New World monkeys a valuable source of models of aging.

Moving further away from humans, tarsiers (family: Tarsiidae; genus: *Tarsius*) also appear to be short-lived with short generation cycles (Austad, 1997a). In contrast, a greater diversity is found among Strepsirrhini, one of the two primate suborders (Figure 2.2). Lemurs of the *Lemuridae* genus are relatively long-lived when compared to their closest relatives. The brown lemur can live 37 years, which is impressive considering it reaches sexual maturity at about age 2. It was also reported that a hybrid between a brown and a black lemur lived for 39 years (Jones, 1982). In contrast, dwarf and mouse lemurs (family: Cheirogaleidae) do not live more than 20 years, and age-related changes have been described in their second decade of life (see AnAge). For instance, the fat-tailed dwarf lemur (*Cheirogaleus medius*) has been argued as an example of a fast-aging primate (Austad, 1997a). Lorisiforms such as the slender loris (*Loris tardigradus*) also appear to be short-lived with a fast development (Austad, 1997a), although the slow loris (*Nycticebus coucang*) has been reported to live over 26 years. As in New World monkeys, the Strepsirrhini suborder appears to feature a variety of aging rates.

While there are reasons to focus only on primates in comparative studies of aging (Austad, 1997a), rodents may also serve as a potential models. First of all, mice and rats (*Rattus norvegicus*) are well-established models in biomedical and aging research. Secondly, rodents and primates diverged roughly 58 million years ago (mya), not long before the two primate suborders—Strepsirrhine and Haplorrhini—diverged 49 mya (Springer *et al.*, 2003). Lastly, the short life cycles and fast aging processes of mice and rats have not been observed in any primate. By incorporating rodents and primates, we thus obtain a range of aging rates close to that of the entire Mammalia class. In Table 2.1 I recap all of the species mentioned above.

If we aim to investigate the factors regulating aging in primates having the human species as our priority, then our choice of species need not go further than primates and rodents. As argued before (Austad, 2005), more is learned by the study of closely-related species that differ considerably in the trait of interest. Of course, diversity is always welcomed and other species can be incorporated into the comparative biology of aging. Nonetheless, solely using primates and rodents in the comparative biology of aging may be adequate to determine which genetic factors regulate the human aging rate. Certainly, there are major difficulties in studying primates, but that depends on which factor is being studied. In the modern age of genomics it may be necessary, not to keep animals in captivity, but rather to have their genome sequenced. It is with this prospect that I suggest these animals as choices for aging research. Hopefully, some of these animals, like short-lived primates, may also be incorporated as experimental models, as suggested before (Austad, 1997a).

THE INFLUENCE OF BODY SIZE

A number of factors correlate with *tmax*, and while this work is about species selection, not the methodology of comparative biology, there is one factor that must be mentioned: body size (Promislow, 1993). Clearly, bigger species, including mammals, live longer, on average, than shorter-lived species (Austad, 2005). Exceptions exist and, for example, gorillas (*Gorilla gorilla*) are typically bigger than humans and still do not live longer than us. Likewise, bats live longer than predicted from their body size. Nonetheless, when comparing parameters across species it is crucial to take body size into consideration. Otherwise we could make the mistake of correlating some physiological factor with body size, not with longevity or aging. For example, early studies indicated that DNA repair capacity was higher in longer-lived mammals, arguing that DNA repair was a factor in aging (Hart and Setlow, 1974). Yet it has been argued that the correlation between DNA repair and longevity is due to the fact that bigger animals live longer and, for reasons unrelated to aging, have better DNA repair mechanisms (Promislow, 1994). In other words, the evolution of aging rates and DNA repair may have been related to body size and thus independent from one another. Therefore, body size is a factor that comparative studies of aging must take into consideration. It is necessary that we devise appropriate methods to exclude or at least minimize the impact of body size in such studies, and a careful selection of species may also minimize these problems.

Among primates, longer-lived species tend to be bigger with bigger brains, and hence the problems cited above must also be taken into consideration. One way to minimize these problems is the inclusion of negative controls. For example, pairs of species that age similarly but that differ in body size may be employed: gorillas may age at the same pace as chimpanzees even though the former are considerably bigger. Choosing different species with similar aging processes may then be necessary. Likewise, choosing species that live longer than expected for their body size is important: the white-faced capuchin is a good example of a relatively small primate with a *tmax* comparable to that of apes (Table 2.1).

Assuming mechanisms of aging are conserved between rodents and humans, which is debatable in itself, it may be worthwhile to consider other rodents besides rats and mice. For instance, long-lived rodents like porcupines (Erethizontidae and Hystricidae families), which may live over 20 years, and the naked-mole rat (*Heterocephalus*

TABLE 2.1
Species with potential interest for comparative studies of aging, including comparative genomics

Taxon[a]	Name	Species	tmax[b]	tsex[c]	M[d]	Observations
Primates	Humans	*Homo sapiens*	122.5	13	60	
Apes	Chimpanzee	*Pan troglodytes*	73	9	45	
	Gorilla	*Gorilla gorilla*	54	9–15	140	
	Orangutan	*Pongo pygmaeus*	59	8	65	
	Gibbons	*Hylobates* genus	40–47	6–8	6–8	
Old World monkeys	Hamadryas baboon	*Papio hamadryas*	45	3–5	15–30	Examples of Old World monkeys
	Rhesus macaque	*Macaca mulatta*	40	4–6	8	
New World monkeys	Common marmoset	*Callithrix jacchus*	16.8	1–1.5	0.2–0.4	
	Golden lion marmoset	*Leontopithecus rosalia*	30	2–3	0.65	Longest-lived marmoset
	White-faced capuchin	*Cebus capucinus*	54.8	4–8	2	Example of a long-lived Platyrrhini
Tarsiidae	Tarsiers	*Tarsius* genus	15	1–2	0.1–0.2	Generally short-lived
Strepsirrhini	Brown lemur	*Eulemur fulvus*	37	2	2	Longest-lived lemur
	Fat-tailed dwarf lemur	*Cheirogaleus medius*	19.3	1	0.3	
	Lesser mouse lemur	*Microcebus murinus*	15.5	1	0.06	Fast aging for a primate
Lorisidae	Galago	*Galago senegalensis*	18.8	<1	0.2	
	Slender loris	*Loris tardigradus*	16.4	1	0.2–0.3	
	Slow loris	*Nycticebus coucang*	26.5	2	1	
Rodentia	House mouse	*Mus musculus*	5	0.1–0.2	0.02	One of the fastest aging mammals
	Norway rat	*Rattus norvegicus*	6	0.25	0.2	
	Slender-tailed cloud rat	*Phloeomys cumingi*	13.6	–	2	Long-lived murids
	Muskrat	*Ondatra zibethicus*	10	0.5–1	1	
Other rodents	Naked mole-rat	*Heterocephalus glaber*	28	<1	0.03	Longest-lived rodent
	Old World porcupine	*Hystrix brachyura*	27.3	1	8	
	European beaver	*Castor fiber*	25	2	25	

[a]Species are typically listed according to their evolutionary distance to humans.
[b]Maximum lifespan in years.
[c]Age at sexual maturity in years. Typical or range of values is displayed.
[d]Adult body mass (M), a standard measure of body size, in kilograms. Typical or range of values is displayed.

glaber), which may live up to 28 years, could be useful models. Likewise, while mice and rats are short-lived, some species of the Muridae family can live up to 10 years or more, namely, the slender-tailed cloud rat (*Phloeomys cumingi*) and the muskrat (*Ondatra zibethicus*). The phenotypic variation we witness across mammalian orders may bias comparative studies of aging, so again primates and rodents should be preferred (Table 2.1). Of course, we can consider other mammalian orders, and for practical reasons these may even be necessary. Still, I maintain my opinion that studies, such as comparative genomics studies, based on primates and rodents should suffice to study aging and are the most appropriate to identify genetic factors influencing human aging.

Putative Models of Antiaging Strategies

Due to obvious practical and economical reasons, the most widely employed models of aging are short-lived. It has been argued, however, that studying short-lived species may be irrelevant to humans because whatever mechanisms limit the lifespans of these species have been evolutionarily "solved" by long-lived species like us.

Studying long-lived species may then be potentially more beneficial to people (Strehler, 1986).

MAMMALIAN EXAMPLES OF LIFE-EXTENSION

It is well-established that longevity increased in the lineage leading to humans, yet the evolution of longevity occurred in other mammalian lineages as well (Figure 2.3).

Thus it is possible, and even likely, that life-extending strategies vary according to phylogeny. In other words, different mechanisms for long life may have evolved independently in different mammalian lineages. Identifying these mechanisms could potentially allow us to employ them in human medicine.

The best example is certainly the bowhead whale, which has been reported to live over 200 years (George *et al.*, 1999). There is little knowledge of diseases affecting these animals. Still, given that bowhead whales weigh over 75 tons, they must feature some sort of anticancer mechanism(s) to prevent cancer from developing among their huge mass of cells (Austad, 1997b). Other whales too appear to have long lifespans. Animals of the Balaenopteridae family are generally long-lived: examples include the blue whale (*Balaenoptera musculus*) and the fin whale (*Balaenoptera physalus*) which may live over a century. Understanding why these species live so long may yield clues about antiaging mechanisms that are absent from humans, such as anticancer mechanisms. Similar examples include elephants (*Elephas maximus* and *Loxodonta africana*), which can live up to 80 years, and the dugong (*Dugong dugon*), which can live up to 70 years. All these mammals feature a long lifespan, a rate of aging, from what we know, comparable to that of humans, and are considerably bigger than us. The hippopotamus (*Hippopotamus amphibius*), which has a maximum lifespan of 61 years and an MRDT of 7 years, rhinoceros (*Ceratotherium simum* or *Rhinoceros unicornis*), which can live up to 50 years, and maybe even horses (*Equus caballus*), which can live nearly 60 years, may also fit this category. Identifying anticancer mechanisms in these species is thus a promising prospect.

Other specific life-preserving mechanisms may exist in several mammals. For example, the nabarlek (*Petrogale concinna*), a wallaby from northern Australia, apparently features continuous tooth development, termed polyphyodonty (Department of the Environment and Heritage, 2000). Elephants also feature an unusual scheduling of tooth eruption and species of the Sirenia order—i.e., manatees (genus: *Trichechus*) and the dugong—may also feature some form of polyphyodonty (Finch, 1990). While progress in stem cells may allow teeth replacement in humans sooner than later (Ohazama *et al.*, 2004), animals like the nabarlek and manatees demonstrate how numerous species may feature unique mechanisms to cope with nearly universal age-related diseases among mammals that also afflict humans. Even among strains of a given species there may be potentially useful phenotypes, as exemplified in the regeneration capacity observed in the MRL mouse (Heber-Katz *et al.*, 2004).

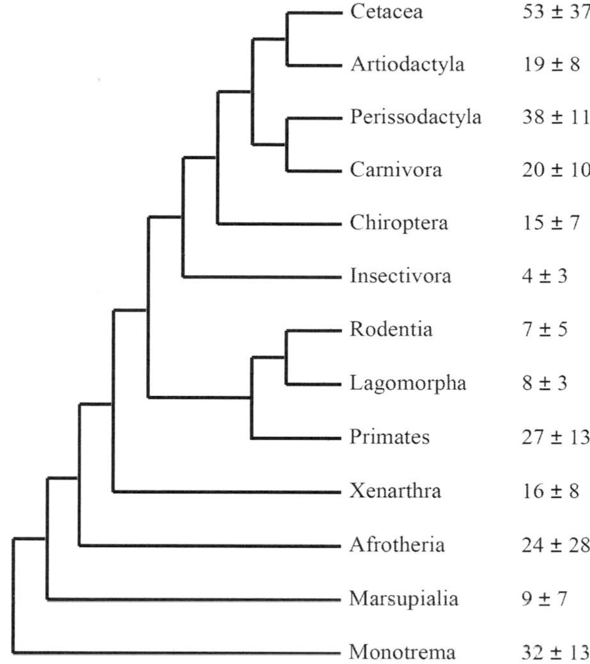

Figure 2.3. Maximum lifespan phylogentic tree for different mammalian orders. Obtained from AnAge, values represent the average *tmax* for species of each mammalian order and are expressed in years ± standard deviation. Afrotheria is not an order but rather a clade of mammals proposed, based on DNA analysis, to have a common origin. It includes the following families: Macroscelidea ($n = 4$), Tubulidentata ($n = 1$), Sirenia ($n = 3$), Hyracoidea ($n = 3$), Proboscidea ($n = 2$), and Tenrecidae ($n = 7$). Thus, it is normal for Afrotheria to feature a bigger standard deviation than other taxa. Phylogeny was drawn based on Springer *et al.* (2003). Branch lengths are not to scale.

Potential Nonmammalian Models of Antiaging Strategies

Long-lived nonmammalian species may also feature antiaging mechanisms of potential use in human medicine that obviate, at least, some human age-related pathologies. The best examples are species that appear not to age, such as many types of turtles (order: Testudines). Species like Blanding's turtle (*Emydoidea blandingii*) and the painted turtle (*Chrysemys picta*) have been reported not to show signs of aging in studies lasting decades (Congdon *et al.*, 2001, 2003). An increased reproductive output with age was also reported, in accordance with reports of *de novo* oogenesis in adult reptiles (Finch, 1990; Patnaik, 1994). Understanding the physiological basis of this phenomenon, also termed negligible senescence (Finch, 1990), has tremendous implications for gerontology but has so far been neglected. Further examples include the Aldabra tortoise (*Geochelone gigantea*) and the Galapagos tortoise (*Geochelone elephantopus*), which likely live over a century. Anecdotal evidence suggests the Galapagos tortoise reaches sexual maturity only after at least two decades, making it one of the vertebrates with the longest developmental period. Unfortunately, work on turtles is limited. There is some evidence that telomere biology is different in turtles (Girondot and Garcia, 1999), and some results suggest that the brains of turtles have enhanced mechanisms to protect against reactive oxygen species formation and damage (Lutz *et al.*, 2003). Likewise, neurogenesis may be predominant in reptiles (Font *et al.*, 2001). Since other turtles may feature negligible senescence and oocyte regeneration (Finch, 1990), turtles are promising models for antiaging medicine (de Magalhaes, 2004).

Apart from turtles, other species with negligible senescence include bullfrogs (*Rana catesbeiana*), certain fishes such as rockfishes (genus: *Sebastes*) and sturgeons (family: Acipenseridae), as well as many lower life forms (Finch, 1990). It is possible, of course, that many other species feature negligible senescence, or at least slower rates of aging than humans, of which we know nothing about. Since all studied mammals age, incorporating nonaging species in studies of the biology of aging is auspicious. Species with negligible senescence are also promising models for identifying mechanisms that can be used to fight specific human age-related pathologies. For example, it was shown that the rainbow trout (*Oncorhynchus mykiss*) features high levels of telomerase and a continuous molting which may be partly responsible for its continuous growth and negligible rate of aging (Klapper *et al.*, 1998). Moreover, species with negligible senescence are important in understanding how the genetic program, the genome, can be optimized for long-term survival. Certainly, there are great difficulties in studying, for instance, an animal that outlives humans and that is probably why most of these species have not been studied in detail. Modern high-throughput technologies, however, give researchers a host of new experimental opportunities (de Magalhaes and Toussaint, 2004). Sequencing the genome of these species should then be a priority.

Turtles are clearly the reptiles with the greatest potential as models of antiaging strategies. Nonetheless, while some short-lived reptiles show signs of aging, other long-lived reptilian species may be of interest. For example, *de novo* oogenesis has been reported in different reptiles, including alligators and lizards, plus the aforementioned turtles (Patnaik, 1994). The ability to regenerate oocytes in adulthood is crucial to avoid reproductive senescence and, according to evolutionary models, essential for the emergence of negligible senescence. Increased reproductive output with age has also been reported in other reptiles apart from turtles, such as in the northern fence lizard (*Sceloporus undulatus*) and in king snakes (*Lampropeltis getulus*), as well as other species (Finch, 1990; Patnaik, 1994). With the exception of turtles, the longest-lived reptile is the tuatara (*Sphenodon punctatus*), which lives at least 77 years, but possibly much longer (Patnaik, 1994). Tuataras are the only living descendants from the Rhynchocephalia order and thus have no closely related species. They are found only in New Zealand. Even though tuataras rarely exceed one kilogram in weight, they are long-lived, attaining sexual maturity after at least 10 years. Due to their unique evolutionary history and features, the tuatara is a potential model of antiaging strategies.

There are no confirmed birds with negligible senescence, though fulmars and the Andean condor age very slowly, if they age at all. The northern fulmar (*Fulmarus glacialis*), for example, likely ages more slowly than humans (Gosden, 1996). The longest-lived bird, however, is reported to be the Andean condor (*Vultur gryphus*), which can live up to 75 years. Senescence has not been described in these animals, though detailed studies are lacking (Finch, 1990). In the arctic tern (*Sterna paradisaea*) too no senescence has been demonstrated so far (Gosden, 1996). The record longevity for this species is only 34 years, but this particular 34-year-old individual appeared in excellent health and was actually released in the wild (Terres, 1980). Such cases again suggest that there may be many species aging more slowly than humans and about which we know little. The African grey parrot (*Psittacus erithacus*), the mute swan (*Cygnus olor*), the southern ground hornbill (*Bucorvus cafer*), and the Manchurian crane (*Grus japonensis*) have all been reported as living around 70 years. Interestingly, it has also been suggested that long-lived birds feature enhanced mechanisms of neurogenesis, protection against oxidative damage, and mechanisms against the formation of advanced glycosylation end products (Holmes *et al.*, 2001).

Another bird of potential interest to gerontologists is the raven (*Corvus corax*), a passerine. Typically, Passeriformes, corvids, and other species of the genus *Corvus* are short-lived, but ravens are clearly an exception. In the wild, ravens generally only live a few years, but in captivity their lifespan is likely above 70 years, with anecdotal reports of one raven living up to 80 years in captivity (Boarman and Heinrich, 1999). It would be interesting to know what physiological and genetic mechanisms make ravens live so much longer than their closest relatives. Likewise, more rigorous studies may reveal other long-lived species in the genus *Corvus*.

Although amphibians are not reported to be as long-lived as reptiles or mammals, they may prove useful for gerontology. The longest-lived amphibian is the Japanese giant salamander (*Andrias japonicus*), which reportedly can live up to 55 years. While this pales in comparison to whales and tortoises, amphibians do have some unique traits of potential use to medicine. One of them is how regenerative mechanisms in amphibians are more advanced than those of mammals. For example, amphibians can regenerate entire limbs while mammalian tissues, such as muscle, can regenerate only as isolated entities (Carlson, 2003). Limb regeneration has been particularly well-studied in newts, and it may have future applications in antiaging research. In one study, protein extracts derived from newts were able to dedifferentiate mouse muscle cells into stem cells. This process of dedifferentiation of adult cells appears then to be modulated by appropriate factors that can be potentially isolated in newts (McGann *et al.*, 2001). Future studies to implement the regenerative capacity of some amphibians to humans are of great medical interest. Furthermore, while short-lived amphibians show signs of aging, long-lived amphibians may feature negligible senescence, polyphyodonty, and oocyte regeneration (Kara, 1994).

Among the large diversity of animals in the world there are certainly multiple processes that can be useful to prevent age-related pathologies in humans. For example, loss of auditory hair cells (AHCs) is a major cause of deafness in people and hence regeneration of these cells has considerable medical interest (Hawkins and Lovett, 2004). It is interesting to note that most mammals, contrary to most birds and amphibians and maybe even some bats (Kirkegaard and Jorgensen, 2002), lose the capacity to regenerate AHCs early in life. Therefore, it has been suggested that genomic tools may be used to understand the basis of this regenerative capacity and eventually apply it to mammals (Hawkins and Lovett, 2004). Another example is heart regeneration. Mammals and amphibians typically have a limited regenerative capacity of the heart muscle. The zebrafish (*Danio rerio*) heart, however, appears to have a robust capacity for regeneration based on the proliferation of cardiomyocytes which can avoid scar formation and allow cardiac regeneration (Poss *et al.* 2002). Thus, zebrafish may also be a powerful system to study antiaging or life-prolonging strategies of specific human age-related diseases (see chapters 27 and 28 in this book about the zebrafish). With the emerging age of genomics, it may soon be possible to employ genomic tools to identify life-extending genes and pathways absent from humans. For example, mammals appear to have lost the CPD-photolyase DNA-repair enzyme (Thoma, 1999). Certainly, other such genes exist and some may turn out to have life-extending functions.

These examples are only the tip of the iceberg. Among the extraordinary diversity of life forms on earth, including the thousands of vertebrates, we are likely to find many novel antiaging strategies. In Table 2.2 I present the examples cited above plus the longest-lived species for a number of vertebrate classes and selected mammalian orders. These represent species in which longevity likely evolved and hence may feature antiaging mechanisms. In theory, the longest-lived animals in each mammalian family are capable of delaying aging in relation to similar species, and thus studying these animals may allow us to identify not only genetic factors regulating aging rates but even life-extending mechanisms.

Conclusion

Maximum lifespan will likely continue to be used as the measure of aging in animal species. Even though other measures exist and should be implemented, *tmax* does give an estimate of rate of aging; it is the easiest method presently at our disposal, and *tmax* data are widely available—including in AnAge—making comparisons straightforward. It is not a perfect measure for comparing aging across species, but it is arguably the best.

More animal diversity is necessary in comparative studies of aging. Implementing novel models of aging should be welcomed independently of the species used. In the context of comparative studies of aging, though, there is no need to drift away from primates and rodents and certainly not from mammals. With sequencing technology becoming cheaper, in a near future it will become possible to sequence the genome of multiple species, and I predict comparative genomics to become the predominant tool in comparative studies of aging (de Magalhaes and Toussaint, 2004). Choosing which species to investigate will then become crucial. My rationale is that the best way to perform comparative genomics studies of aging is by focusing on primates plus a few rodents (Table 2.2).

Mammalian species, with a major bias toward primates and rodents, may allow us to understand the genetic factors that determine the pace of aging. Yet numerous other species, including long-lived mammals, reptiles, amphibians, fishes, and birds, may hold secrets to delay human age-related pathologies and maybe even the aging process itself. From species that appear to have escaped senescence, to animals featuring extreme forms of regeneration, passing by animals possessing specific traits that may be used to delay human age-related pathologies, multiple species may feature applications to antiaging research.

Recommended Resources

Readers are encouraged to visit the Human Ageing Genomic Resources (http://genomics.senescence.info), which features the AnAge database (http://genomics.senescence.info/species/).

ACKNOWLEDGMENTS

Thanks to the many researchers who contributed their knowledge to AnAge, particularly Steven Austad. Further thanks to George Church and Joana Costa for comments on the manuscript. J. P. de Magalhães is supported by NIH-NHGRI CEGS grant to George Church.

TABLE 2.2
Species with potential interest as sources of antiaging strategies

Taxon[a]	Name (species)	tmax[b]	Observations
Mammalia: Cetacea	Bowhead whale (*Balaena mysticetus*)	211	Longest-lived vertebrate
	Fin whale (*Balaenoptera physalus*)	116	
	Blue whale (*Balaenoptera musculus*)	110	Biggest animal
Artiodactyla	Hippopotamus (*Hippopotamus amphibius*)	61	Long-lived artiodactyls
	Camel (genus: *Camelus*)	50	
Perissodactyla	Horse (*Equus caballus*)	60	Long-lived perissodactyls
	Rhinoceros (*Ceratotherium simum* or *Rhinoceros unicornis*)	50	
Afrotheria	Elephant (*Elephas maximus* or *Loxodonta africana*)	80	Biggest land animal
Sirenia	Manatees (genus: *Trichechus*) and the dugong (*Dugong dugon*)	>50	May feature polyphyodonty
Marsupialia	Nabarlek (*Petrogale concinna*)	>10	Appear to feature polyphyodonty
Reptilia: Testudines	Aldabra tortoise (*Geochelone gigantea*)	152	
	Mediterranean spur-thighed tortoise (*Testudo graeca*)	127	
	Galapagos tortoise (*Geochelone elephantopus*)	>100	Long developmental phase
	Blanding's turtle (*Emydoidea blandingii*)	75	Featuring negligible senescence
	Painted turtle (*Chrysemys picta*)	61	
Diapsida	Tuatara (*Sphenodon punctatus*)	90	Longest-lived reptile that is not a turtle
Aves	Andean condor (*Vultur gryphus*)	75	Longest-lived bird
	African grey parrot (*Psittacus erithacus*)	73	
	Northern fulmar (*Fulmarus glacialis*)	48	Likely age very slowly
	Artic tern (*Sterna paradisaea*)	34	
Passeriformes	Raven (*Corvus corax*)	69	Longest-lived passeriform
Amphibia	Japanese giant salamander (*Andrias japonicus*)	55	
	Common European toad (*Bufo bufo*)	40	
	Bullfrog (*Rana catesbeiana*)	16	Can increase reproductive output with age
	Red-spotted newt (*Notophthalmus viridescens*)	15	One of several species capable of limb regeneration
Osteichthyes	Lake sturgeon (*Acipenser fulvescens*)	152	
	Rockfish (*Sebastes aleutianus*)	>150	Featuring negligible senescence
	Orange roughy (*Hoplostethus atlanticus*)	149	Slow-growing, long-lived species
	Zebrafish (*Danio rerio*)	5.5	Capable of heart regeneration

[a]Species are typically listed according to their evolutionary distance to humans.
[b]Maximum lifespan in years.

REFERENCES

Austad, S.N. (1997a). Small nonhuman primates as potential models of human aging. *Ilar J 38*, 142–147.

Austad, S.N. (1997b). *Why We Age: What Science Is Discovering about the Body's Journey through Life*. New York: John Wiley.

Austad, S.N. (2001). An experimental paradigm for the study of slowly aging organisms. *Exp Gerontol 36*, 599–605.

Austad, S.N. (2005). Diverse aging rates in metazoans: targets for functional genomics. *Mech Ageing Dev 126*, 43–49.

Boarman, W.I., and Heinrich, B. (1999). Corvus corax: Common Raven. In Poole, A., and Gill, F., Eds. *The Birds of North America* (No. 476), pp. 1–32. Philadelphia: The Birds of North America, Inc.

Bons, N., Mestre, N., and Petter, A. (1992). Senile plaques and neurofibrillary changes in the brain of an aged lemurian primate, Microcebus murinus. *Neurobiol Aging 13*, 99–105.

Bronikowski, A.M., Alberts, S.C., Altmann, J., Packer, C., Carey, K.D., and Tatar, M. (2002). The aging baboon: Comparative demography in a non-human primate. *Proc Natl Acad Sci USA 99*, 9591–9595.

Carlson, B.M. (2003). Muscle regeneration in amphibians and mammals: passing the torch. *Dev Dyn 226*, 167–181.

Comfort, A. (1964). *Ageing: The Biology of Senescence*. London: Routledge & Kegan Paul.

Congdon, J.D., Nagle, R.D., Kinney, O.M., and van Loben Sels, R.C. (2001). Hypotheses of aging in a long-lived vertebrate, Blanding's turtle (*Emydoidea blandingii*). *Exp Gerontol 36*, 813–827.

Congdon, J.D., Nagle, R.D., Kinney, O.M., van Loben Sels, R.C., Quinter, T., and Tinkle, D.W. (2003). Testing hypotheses of aging in long-lived painted turtles (*Chrysemys picta*). *Exp Gerontol 38*, 765–772.

de Magalhaes, J.P. (2004). Modelling human ageing: Role of telomeres in stress-induced premature senescence and design of anti-ageing strategies. PhD thesis. University of Namur, Department of Biology, Namur, Belgium.

de Magalhaes, J.P., and Toussaint, O. (2002). The evolution of mammalian aging. *Exp Gerontol 37*, 769–775.

de Magalhaes, J.P., and Toussaint, O. (2004). How bioinformatics can help reverse engineer human aging. *Ageing Res Rev 3*, 125–141.

de Magalhaes, J.P., Costa, J., and Toussaint, O. (2005a). HAGR: the Human Ageing Genomic Resources. *Nucleic Acids Res 33* Database Issue, D537–D543.

de Magalhaes, J.P., Cabral, J.A., and Magalhaes, D. (2005b). The influence of genes on the aging process of mice: A statistical assessment of the genetics of aging. *Genetics 169*, 265–274.

Department of the Environment and Heritage (2000). Kangaroo Biology. http://www.deh.gov.au/biodiversity/trade-use/wild-harvest/kangaroo/biology.html.

Erwin, J.M., Hof, P.R., Ely, J.J., and Perl, D.P. (2002). One gerontology: Advancing understanding of aging through studies of great apes and other primates. In Erwin, J.M., and Hof, P.R., Eds., *Aging in Nonhuman Primates*, pp. 1–21. Basel: Karger.

Finch, C.E. (1990). *Longevity, Senescence, and the Genome*. Chicago and London: The University of Chicago Press.

Finch, C.E., and Pike, M.C. (1996). Maximum life span predictions from the Gompertz mortality model. *J Gerontol A Biol Sci Med Sci 51*, B183–B194.

Font, E., Desfilis, E., Perez-Canellas, M.M., and Garcia-Verdugo, J.M. (2001). Neurogenesis and neuronal regeneration in the adult reptilian brain. *Brain Behav Evol 58*, 276–295.

George, J.C., Bada, J., WZeh, J., Brown, S.E., O'Hara, T., and Suydam, R. (1999). Age and growth estimates of bowhead whales (*Balaena mysticetus*) via aspartic acid racemization. *Can J Zool 77*, 571–580.

Gershon, H., and Gershon, D. (2000). Paradigms in aging research: A critical review and assessment. *Mech Ageing Dev 117*, 21–28.

Girondot, M., and Garcia, J. (1999). Senescence and longevity in turtles: What telomeres tell us. In Miaud, C., and Guyétant, R., Eds., *9th Extraordinary Meeting of the Europea Societas Herpetologica*, Chambéry, France, 25–29 August 1998.

Goodman, M., Porter, C.A., Czelusniak, J., Page, S.L., Schneider, H., Shoshani, J., Gunnell, G., and Groves, C.P. (1998). Toward a phylogenetic classification of Primates based on DNA evidence complemented by fossil evidence. *Mol Phylogenet Evol 9*, 585–598.

Gosden, R. (1996). *Cheating Time*. New York: W.H. Freeman.

Hart, R.W., and Setlow, R.B. (1974). Correlation between deoxyribonucleic acid excision-repair and life-span in a number of mammalian species. *Proc Natl Acad Sci USA 71*, 2169–2173.

Harvey, P.H., and Zammuto, R.M. (1985). Patterns of mortality and age at first reproduction in natural populations of mammals. *Nature 315*, 319–320.

Hawkins, R.D., and Lovett, M. (2004). The developmental genetics of auditory hair cells. *Hum Mol Genet 13*, Spec No 2, R289–R296.

Hayflick, L. (1994). *How and Why We Age*. New York: Ballantine Books.

Heber-Katz, E., Leferovich, J.M., Bedelbaeva, K., and Gourevitch, D. (2004). Spallanzani's mouse: A model of restoration and regeneration. *Curr Top Microbiol Immunol 280*, 165–189.

Hill, K., Boesch, C., Goodall, J., Pusey, A., Williams, J., and Wrangham, R. (2001). Mortality rates among wild chimpanzees. *J Hum Evol 40*, 437–450.

Holmes, D.J., Fluckiger, R., and Austad, S.N. (2001). Comparative biology of aging in birds: An update. *Exp Gerontol 36*, 869–883.

Jones, M.L. (1982). Longevity of captive mammals. *Zool Garten 52*, 113–128.

Kara, T.C. (1994). Ageing in amphibians. *Gerontology 40*, 161–173.

Kirkegaard, M., and Jorgensen, J.M. (2001). The inner ear macular sensory epithelia of the Daubenton's bat. *J Comp Neurol 438*, 433–444.

Klapper, W., Heidorn, K., Kuhne, K., Parwaresch, R., and Krupp, G. (1998). Telomerase activity in 'immortal' fish. *FEBS Lett 434*, 409–412.

Lutz, P.L., Prentice, H.M., and Milton, S.L. (2003). Is turtle longevity linked to enhanced mechanisms for surviving brain anoxia and reoxygenation? *Exp Gerontol 38*, 797–800.

McGann, C.J., Odelberg, S.J., and Keating, M.T. (2001). Mammalian myotube dedifferentiation induced by newt regeneration extract. *Proc Natl Acad Sci USA 98*, 13699–13704.

Miller, R.A. (1999). Kleemeier award lecture: Are there genes for aging? *J Gerontol A Biol Sci Med Sci 54*, B297–B307.

Miller, R.A. (2001). Genetics of increased longevity and retarded aging in mice. In Masoro, E.J., and Austad, S.N., Eds. *Handbook of the Biology of Aging*, 5th ed., pp. 369–395. New York: Academic Press.

Morbeck, M.E., Galloway, A., and Sumner, D.R. (2002). Getting old at Gombe: Skeletal aging in wild-ranging chimpanzees. In Erwin, J.M., and Hof, P.R., Eds., *Aging in Nonhuman Primates*, pp. 48–62. Basel: Karger.

Mueller, L.D., Nusbaum, T.J., and Rose, M.R. (1995). The Gompertz equation as a predictive tool in demography. *Exp Gerontol 30*, 553–569.

Ohazama, A., Modino, S.A., Miletich, I., and Sharpe, P.T. (2004). Stem-cell-based tissue engineering of murine teeth. *J Dent Res 83*, 518–522.

Patnaik, B.K. (1994). Ageing in reptiles. *Gerontology*, *40*, 200–220.

Pletcher, S.D., Khazaeli, A.A., and Curtsinger, J.W. (2000). Why do life spans differ? Partitioning mean longevity differences in terms of age-specific mortality parameters. *J Gerontol A Biol Sci Med Sci 55*, B381–B389.

Poss, K.D., Wilson, L.G., and Keating, M.T. (2002). Heart regeneration in zebrafish. *Science 298*, 2188–2190.

Promislow, D.E. (1993). On size and survival: progress and pitfalls in the allometry of life span. *J Gerontol 48*, B115–B123.

Promislow, D.E. (1994). DNA repair and the evolution of longevity: A critical analysis. *J Theor Biol 170*, 291–300.

Springer, M.S., Murphy, W.J., Eizirik, E., and O'Brien, S. J. (2003). Placental mammal diversification and the Cretaceous-Tertiary boundary. *Proc Natl Acad Sci USA 100*, 1056–1061.

Strehler, B.L. (1986). Genetic instability as the primary cause of human aging. *Exp Gerontol 21*, 283–319.

Terres, J.K. (1980). *The Audubon Society Encyclopedia of North American Birds*. New York: Alfred A. Knopf.

Thoma, F. (1999). Light and dark in chromatin repair: Repair of UV-induced DNA lesions by photolyase and nucleotide excision repair. *Embo J 18*, 6585–6598.

Wilson, D.L. (1994). The analysis of survival (mortality) data: Fitting Gompertz, Weibull, and logistic functions. *Mech Ageing Dev 74*, 15–33.

3

Principles of Animal Use for Gerontological Research

Richard A. Miller

Animals, and in particular rats and mice, have long been a mainstay of experimental work in biological gerontology. This chapter presents ten key principles that should be considered in designing and interpreting reports that use laboratory rodents to learn about aging. In a nutshell, experimenters are implored (1) to use mice that are neither too old nor (2) too young; (3) to use more than two age groups; (4) to use rodents that are demonstrably specific pathogen-free; (5) to consider the use of genetically heterogeneous rodent populations; (6) to obtain necropsy data as a source of important covariates; (7) not to pool across individuals; (8) to reduce cost by judicious distribution of money across age classes; (9) to favor designs that use young mice destined to age at differing rates; and (10) to abandon—or at least subjugate—rodent-oriented research in favor of comparative biology.

Introduction

As of this writing, a PubMed search for "aging AND (mouse OR mice OR rat Or rats)" yields 46964 citations, of which 9256 appeared in the current millennium, and 1813 appeared in 2004, a rate of 5 papers per day. (For reference: substitute "fly OR flies OR Drosophila" and you obtain 117 papers in 2004; the analogous search produces 90 papers on aging worms.) Worms and flies, for all their obvious virtues, are organized along alien design principles, and seem sufficiently dissimilar to people, physiologically and developmentally, to make extrapolation of all but the most fundamental findings feel unsafe. Experimental studies of the aging process in humans are stymied by ethical constraints on most interventions of biological interest, inaccessibility of internal tissues, catch-as-catch-can genetics, and discouragingly long life spans. Mice and rats occupy the sweet spot: organized like humans in most ways that count, relatively short-lived, and willing to eat what we give them and to breed with whom we suggest. Rodent-oriented gerontologists are, in addition, blessed by a pre-existing and quickly expanding infrastructure that makes interesting mice and has developed powerful methods for assessing their genetic and physiological characteristics; "mice AND (transgenic or knockout)" gets you 9466 papers in 2004 alone.

This chapter aims to provide a broad overview, not of the nitty gritty of animal care and manipulation, but of the strategic planning that might help a researcher select a rodent model to answer questions of interest in the biology of aging. Emerging from the "Dear Abby" and Emily Post tradition of *ex cathedra* advice givers, it will employ the imperative voice more often than is typical for an academic review. It will also use the term "mice" to mean "mice and rats" except in those rare cases where the distinction is critical. The chapter will range over Ten Basic Principles for studies of aging rodents. Principles 1–4 and 6–8 are more-or-less conventional wisdom, or minor twists thereon. Principles #5, #9, and #10 are more radical proposals (though not entirely without adherents): these are the ones least likely to be taken seriously, but the ones most worthy of contemplation.

Principle #1: Do not Use Mice that are too Old

Newcomers to rodent gerontology show a strong preference for the oldest available mice or rats they can get their hands on, on the grounds that the older the animals are, the more they will differ from the young control group, the sooner the work will be finished, and the more striking the effects to be documented. There are three good reasons to avoid very old mice: they are expensive, sick, and unrepresentative.

Expensive: the Gompertz equation, though originally devised in another context, provides a good guide to the estimation of relative mouse costs, too; because the risk of mortality increases exponentially with age, so does the cost of producing a live mouse. Because the mortality rate doubling time for lab mice is about 4 months (Finch, 1990), the cost of producing a 30-month-old mouse is not 25% higher than the cost of a 24-month-old specimen, but roughly 400% higher, given reasonable estimates of the Gompertz parameters for laboratory mice. Table 3.1 presents a sample calculation illustrating the cost for producing mice at various ages, and provides a strong rationale for designs in which the "old" mice are as young

TABLE 3.1
Sample calculation of production costs for mice at various ages

Mice alive	Deaths/Month	Months of age	Cost/Month	Cumulative cost	Cost per mouse
1000	0	3	$7000	$7,000	$7
1000	0	5	$7000	$21,000	$21
1000	0	7	$7000	$35,000	$35
1000	0	9	$7000	$49,000	$49
1000	0	11	$7000	$63,000	$63
1000	12	13	$7000	$77,000	$77
973	17	15	$6814	$90,729	$93
935	24	17	$6548	$103,968	$111
882	34	19	$6174	$116,518	$132
808	46	21	$5659	$128,114	$158
710	59	23	$4973	$138,426	$195
586	72	25	$4101	$147,087	$251
438	79	27	$3067	$153,754	$351
281	74	29	$1969	$158,239	$563
141	55	31	$986	$160,674	$1,141
46	26	33	$320	$161,598	$3,534
6	5	35	$43	$161,779	$26,578

The values in Table 3.1 were calculated as follows: The cost of a 3-month-old mouse is estimated as $7. The cost per month thereafter is calculated as $7 times the number of mice alive at the start of the month. The colony size is 1000 mice initially. It is assumed that no mice die until age 12 months. Mortality rate doubling time is taken as 0.3 years. The risk of death in any given month (after age 12 months) is calculated as $m(t) = 0.01 * \exp(2.31 * t/12)$, where $t =$ (number of months of age $-$ 12). Cumulative cost is the sum of cost for all previous months. The cost per mouse is calculated as the cumulative cost divided by the number of live mice at the start of the interval. These calculations were performed for each month of a three-year period, but to save space Table 3.1 shows only the odd-numbered months. The table shows, for example, that the production cost of a 35-month-old mouse is approximately 100-fold higher than that of a 25-month-old mouse, which is itself about twice the cost of an 18-month-old mouse.

as possible consistent with the experimental question under consideration.

Even if one is fortunate enough to locate a supplier (see http://www.nia.nih.gov/ResearchInformation/ScientificResources/; and Chapter 33 by Dr. Nancy Nadon in this Handbook) willing to provide you with rodents whose cost is adjusted arithmetically rather than exponentially with age, the burden of illness provides a strong reason to avoid mice in the last third of their lifespan. Very old mice are far more likely than middle-aged mice to have one, or more than one, major form of illness. If the experimental goal is to learn more about a specific form of late life illness, then of course protocols will need to include animals old enough for the illness to have appeared. If the goal is instead to learn something about the aging process, which gradually converts healthy young adults into older ones progressively more vulnerable to multiple forms of debility and illness, then focusing attention on subjects not yet sick is more likely to be informative. A study of the ways in which thymic involution leads to immunodeficiency, for example, is likely to be spoiled by the presence of lymphoma, or indeed any systemic malignancy, in the experimental subjects, just as unsuspected metabolic adjustments secondary to glomerulonephritis would complicate studies of the effects of aging on fuel usage or hormone responsiveness.

Lastly, very old populations are likely to be unrepresentative, in that individuals subject to early and midlife illnesses, for whatever known or unknown reasons, have already been removed by death. Studies of centenarians (or other cohorts of very long-lived people) often show clearly, for instance, that they resemble much younger populations in many physiological parameters (Franceschi *et al.*, 1995; Perls *et al.*, 2002); cross-sectional tables of such traits would show a retardation, or reversal, of age-specific trends as those with typical patterns of aging are eliminated by death, leaving only atypical survivors. Among men who are healthy at age 60, for example, only about 30% are expected to be alive and healthy at age 80, but those destined for good health at age 80 are typically healthier than average at the age of 60 years (Metter *et al.*, 1992). Differences between 60- and 80-year-olds therefore confound effects of aging (and disease) with those of survivorship.

Thus studies that focus on very old rodents are not only far more expensive, they are on the whole less informative than those which use younger animals in the aged cohorts, because data on survivor animals, or sick ones, may give few insights into the life-long process of aging. In my own laboratory we prefer to evaluate animals at ages where 90% or more of the population is still alive, and we almost never make experimental use of mice older than the age of median survival.

Principle #2: Don't Use Mice that are too Young, Either

The goal of this precept is to avoid confusing developmental changes with the effects of aging. Although it takes a mere 8 weeks or so for mice to become reproductively competent, many physiological systems and body dimensions continue to change along developmental trajectories that can, in poorly designed studies, be confused with aging. Consider, for example, the trait shown in the top panel of Figure 3.1, which rises progressively until age 6 months and then remains stable thereafter.

A study which evaluated mice at ages 2 and 20 months would misleadingly conclude that the trait in question "goes up with aging," although a more judicious interpretation, based on a wider range of ages, would conclude instead that the trait shows increases only in juveniles and young adults, with no effects of aging per se. A human or dog that has completed 25% of its lifespan is likely to be 20 or 3 years old, respectively, well within the "mature young adult" stage of life; a corresponding stage for mice would recommend animals of 6–7 months as the "young" control group of a descriptive study of age trajectory in a variable of interest. Beginners tend to prefer designs that use the youngest available animals, again from a mistaken desire to see maximally-sized effects, and because these are the least expensive and are usually available on short notice. Certainly information on maturational process has its own merits and may even be useful in understanding ways in which early life changes modulate the pace of aging or risks of late-life illnesses, but the use of very young mice under the mistaken impression that they are typical of young adult animals may lead to misleading impressions of the ways in which aging alters the outcomes of interest.

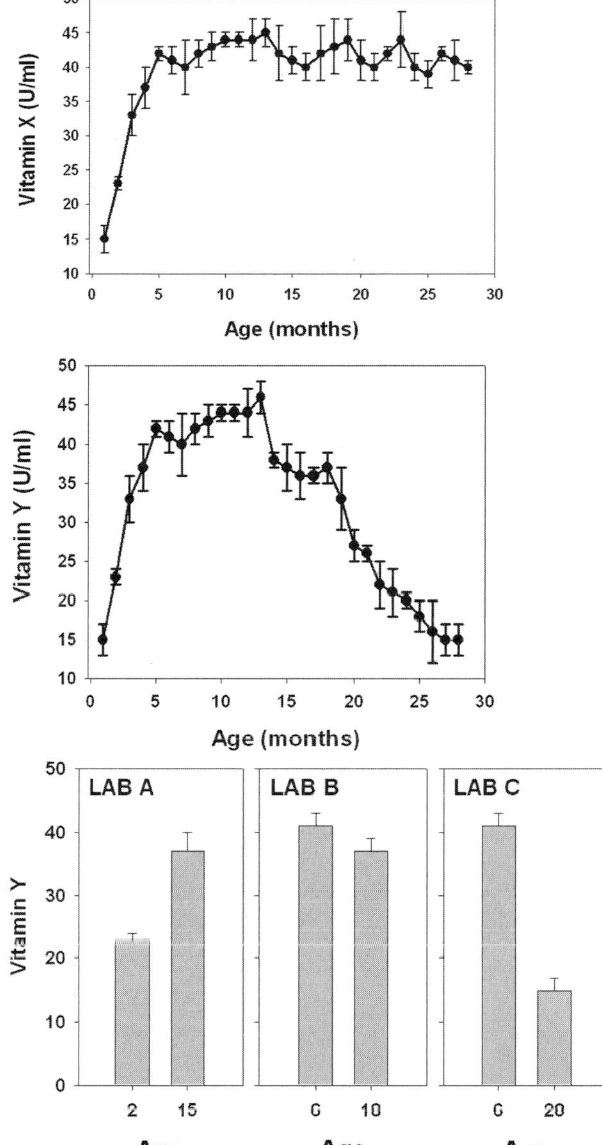

Figure 3.1. The top panel shows a hypothetical data set, as an illustration of errors that can occur when a survey of aging effects starts with mice that are too young to be considered fully mature; see text for interpretation. The middle panel shows a second hypothetical data set, as an illustration of the hazards of evaluating only two age groups. The bottom panels represent reports by three different laboratories of the data shown in the middle panel; each laboratory has selected different age groups. Laboratory A, for example, has reported data at 2 and 15 months of age, extracted from the complete data.

Principle #3: Don't Use too Few Age Groups

The common error here is to investigate whether a trait is age-sensitive by comparing its level in two groups, one allegedly young, the other supposedly old. The middle panel of Figure 3.1 shows another hypothetical data set, showing a trait that rises to a plateau in midlife and then declines thereafter. The bottom shows three possible misinterpretations of this data set, compiled by three laboratories, each of which has conducted assays at two arbitrary ages. Laboratory A concludes that the trait increases with age; Laboratory B finds no age effect; and Laboratory C infers that the trait declines with age. None of these conclusions agrees with the other two, and none is very helpful. Two ages may be sufficient for traits that show a simple, monotonic change over the entire age range, but this default assumption fails too often for comfort and cannot itself be tested without evaluation of a wider range of subject ages. A study of cytokine production in responses to schistosomal egg antigens (Chiu *et al.*, 2002), for example, found several examples of cytokines whose production increased between 6 and 18 months of age and then declined at later ages, helping to resolve conflicts among earlier papers that had disagreed on the extent, and even the direction, of age change in cytokine production based on less comprehensive data sets.

Principle #4: Use Mice that are Specific Pathogen Free and be able to Prove it

A specific pathogen-free (SPF) rodent colony contains mice or rats that are known not to be infected with any members of a specific, defined list of pathogenic micro-organisms and parasites. The animals are *not* free of all bacterial and viral species, i.e., they are not gnotobiotic. Vendors of SPF rodents, and managers of SPF colonies, are able to define the pathogens for which their mice or rats have been tested, and can produce documentation of the diagnostic testing. Our own mouse colonies, for example, are tested routinely for serological evidence of infection by mouse hepatitis virus, mouse parvovirus, minute virus of mice, ectromelia, Sendai, reovirus, lymphocytic choriomeningitis virus, and seven other viruses, and examined for pinworm by cecal inspection. Rat colonies are tested for exposure to each of 13 rat viruses. Testing for viral contamination typically involves looking for antibodies specific to viral antigens; such tests should be negative in rodents never exposed to the pathogen. Tests for pinworm involve direct examination of cecal samples for eggs. Most facilities use a sentinel system, in which the used bedding is pooled for a group of cages or racks, and then transferred to a fresh cage containing a group of mice from a strain known to be susceptible to the viruses of interest. After an interval of several weeks to allow the sentinels to become infected by the viruses or parasites—if these are present—and to form detectable antiviral antibodies, serum from the sentinels is checked for antiviral titers. This procedure is usually repeated 2–4 times per year for the most common viruses and at least annually for the others on the checklist.

Colonies that do not maintain mice under SPF conditions are referred to as "conventional" vivaria; these were in the clear majority until the 1980s, but are now fortunately becoming rare among top-level universities and medical centers. Conventional colonies may or may not have any particular virus or parasite present at any given time; the presence and prevalence of infection may fluctuate from year to year or month to month, and be reluctantly accepted as one source of undocumented "technical" variation in experimental outcomes.

Maintenance of an SPF colony depends upon strict adherence to well-known, but often violated, safety precautions. The rules seem simple: purchase mice only from a small, predefined list of vendors whose health reports document the SPF status of their colony; do not permit mice removed to a non-SPF colony or laboratory to be returned to the vivarium; be compulsive about use of head and shoe covers and protective gowns for each entry into the colony, and compulsive about the use of filter tops for each mouse cage; restrict access to the housing rooms to those whose duties require them to be there; never allow people or cages or equipment to go from a dirty (conventional) colony to an SPF colony. But the hazards are many. They include the peer review committee whose members wish to see the animal housing area (including one visitor whose own lab is a hotbed of pinworm contamination). They include the new faculty member whose laboratory work requires importation of several knock-out stocks whose construction was the key outcome of her postdoctoral work at her previous laboratory. They include the technician who keeps pet mice at home, or the student who stopped by the conventional colony to drop off some syringes on the way to the SPF part of the facility. Use of cage-washing facilities that service clean and unclean housing areas, or transport of water bottles or cage cards from one area to another are also common, but risky, practices. Hazards of this kind are compounded when animal rooms must be shared by multiple investigators; a slip by any one laboratory can lead to spread of infectious agents to rodents used by many colleagues. The introduction of pinworm eggs or a single virus-infected mouse can place an entire colony at risk, and in some cases eradication of the infection can require removal and elimination of all mice in the colony or a major section of it, a step that is always expensive and often impractical.

Why, then, go to all this fuss? The central basis for the emphasis on SPF rodent colonies, in aging research as in many other areas of science, is the need to be able to reproduce experimental findings at later times and in other places. Viral and parasitic infections have known effects on multiple biochemical and physiological outcomes, and are certain to have undocumented effects on many traits not formally studied in this context. Conventional colonies may well have infectious burdens that influence the outcome of a study of age effects or antiaging interventions, and the level and kind of infection may well fluctuate during the course of a single study with consequences that are unforeseen, unpredictable, irreproducible, and undocumented. The traits affected are not always those, like immune responses, most obviously linked to infectious status. Age-related changes in rat skeletal muscle fiber distribution, for example, have been shown to differ systematically between conventional and specific pathogen-free colonies (Florini, 1989).

A common scenario involves the importation of SPF rodents into a conventional colony, in the mistaken hopes that the experimental subjects can then be considered as "almost SPF." Such a situation can, unfortunately, lead to infection of the newcomers by whatever local agents are then current in the host colony, so that the experimental assessments are conducted on mice at varying stages of an acute infectious process.

Advocates, or apologists, for the use of conventional vivaria sometimes raise the issue that SPF colonies are artificial, and thus fail to mimic the constant exposure to infectious agents that accompanies, and may mold, the aging process in real life. It is fair to acknowledge the potential importance of infectious agents in aging outside the vivarium, and important to encourage analyses of how aging might alter, and be altered by, specific defined pathogens. The point of SPF protocols, however, is not to duplicate some "natural" condition, but to define a set of environmental conditions well enough to permit replication and extension of the study's results.

Principle #5: Consider the Use of Non-isogenic Stocks

The large majority of work done with aging mice and rats makes use of inbred stocks, such as the C57BL/6J line of inbred mice, and the F344 stock of inbred rats. These inbred stocks of rats and mice were originally developed by geneticists who wish to have available groups of animals whose genetic characteristics did not change over time and which were uniform from laboratory to laboratory. They were invaluable for working out the basic rules of transplantation biology and played a major role in the development of experimental tumor immunology. Nowadays, many studies of aging rodents start with the assumption that inbred mice or rats should be used, in part because these animals are easy to obtain, and because the published literature contains a great deal of background information about their characteristics. In part, the preference for the use of inbred mouse in rat stocks is based upon a mixture of tradition and inertia, the tendency to use the same animal types that were used for previous studies in one's own lab and in the laboratory of one's mentor, and one's mentor's mentor.

In many ways, this unthinking attachment to the same old stocks is unfortunate, because the use of inbred rodents has several disadvantages. The first disadvantage is that each inbred line contains only animals of a single genotype. For this reason, it is not possible to tell, without further experimentation, whether the observations about the effects of aging on any specific trait of interest in a given inbred stock will or will not prove to be reproducible when analogous experiments are carried out on any other given inbred stock. Many traits, of course, are strongly influenced by genetic alleles that are polymorphic among the wide range of inbred mouse and rat stocks, and it is for this reason that each stock will have its own particular idiosyncratic properties, including disease susceptibilities and rates of change in age-dependent traits. Experimental studies of aging are often sufficiently expensive and tedious that most researchers are reluctant to duplicate or triplicate their workload by conducting the same study several times, "merely" to see if they get similar results in a second or third kind of mouse. For this reason, it would seem advisable for the aging research community to develop and to make use of genetically heterogeneous mouse and rat stocks for routine investigation.

A second problem with the routine use of inbred lines is that these mice are not only genetically uniform, but they are also homozygous at every locus. The development of inbred lines from the starting population of genetically heterogeneous mice is, in a sense, an exercise in genetic compromise. Each person or mouse among us carries in our genomes a "genetic load," a set of genetic alleles each one of which, if homozygous, might lead to early life mortality or to sterility; we are spared these consequences because each of these alleles is rare enough to be heterozygous in most individuals who carry the allele at all. Developing an inbred population, however, requires forcing each locus to the homozygous state. Most homozygous genomes, therefore, produce individuals who die at an early age, are sterile, or show other traits that are rare within the genetically heterogeneous population from which the inbreeding was begun. Genetic combinations that lead to early death or sterility are eliminated during the development of inbred lines, and in fact producing a new inbred line often requires starting many such lines knowing that most will die out during the inbreeding process. Those lines of mice that emerge from this highly selective process contain animals that are able to survive to adulthood and produce live progeny, but may differ in many other ways from the starting population. In particular, inbred lines are almost invariably shorter-lived than mice produced by crosses between any two given inbred stocks (Smith *et al.*, 1967). This lack of robustness and vigor characteristic of inbred rodents, together with strain-specific idiosyncrasies, both well-known and hitherto undocumented, should render the stocks a questionable choice for routine work in biological gerontology.

There are a variety of other options, some attractive and others less so. A cross between two inbred stocks produces an F1 hybrid stock, which like its inbred parents is isogenic—all the mice are genetically identical—but unlike them is heterozygous at multiple loci, i.e., those loci where the two parents differ. F1 hybrid mice are more robust, i.e., longer-lived, than their inbred progenitors, but are vulnerable to the same objection of strain-specific idiosyncrasies that make it hazardous to generalize from data based on a single genotype.

The search for a source of genetic heterogeneity might prompt some researchers to purchase outbred rodents from commercial suppliers. Commercial vendors often sell mice and rats that are marketed as "outbred," but that in some cases could more justly be characterized as approximately inbred stocks. In at least two cases, detailed by Miller *et al.* (1999), the vendor's own catalogue copy states that the "outbred" stock originated in a single pair of inbred progenitors. Production of outbred stocks from a single homozygous genotype can only be recommended by someone unaware that the loss of genetic heterogeneity, like the loss of virginity, is not easily reversible by continued reproductive efforts. Leaving aside clear errors of this kind, genetic heterogeneity can be irretrievably lost, inadvertently, if the breeding nucleus is reduced to a single pair or a small number of pairs at any point in the long history of the stock. This seems to be a frequent occurrence: DNA fingerprint analyses of six allegedly outbred rat stocks (Festing, 1995) supports the idea that these stocks contain only limited genetic heterogeneity: within each stock 84–95% of the animals shared any one individual DNA marker, as contrasted to 34% sharing for rats chosen from different inbred strains.

To help mitigate the disadvantages of relying on isogenic stocks for research on aging, a committee chartered by the U.S. National Academy of Science recommended, in 1981, that researchers make greater use of populations that exhibit controlled genetic heterogeneity, and in particular recommended use of four-way cross populations in aging research (Committee on Animal Models for Research on Aging, 1981). Such a population is produced by a cross between males and females of two different F1 hybrid stocks, for example using (BALB/c × C57BL/6)F1 females bred to (C3H × DBA/2)F1 males. Because each of the F1 parents is heterozygous at many loci, each of their offspring will receive different alleles, at multiple loci, from each parent. From the perspective of the nuclear (i.e., nonmitochondrial) genome, each individual in the four-way cross population is a full sib of each other individual; each is genetically unique, but shares 50% of its alleles with any other mouse in the test population. Populations of this kind have genetic heterogeneity, but of a controlled sort, because additional populations with similar genetic structure can be produced at any time, at any place, and in any numbers, as long as the four grandparental inbred stocks are available. Production of such a colony requires no special expertise in genotyping or husbandry, and is rapid, because the F1 hybrids are commercially available and because breeding success and fecundity are typically high. Four-way cross stocks should be strongly considered for descriptive studies, in which the goal is to discover how a trait changes with age, for intervention studies, and for correlational studies, and they are particularly attractive when evaluation of the genetic control of the age-related phenomenon is potentially of interest. The virtues of these stocks have led to their selection by the National Institute on Aging for a multi-center mouse intervention project (Warner and Nadon, 2005), and one such stock has been selected for inclusion among stocks available, at multiple ages, from the NIA's aging rodent colonies (Nadon, 2005). There is now extensive information on late-life pathology of the population produced by the cross between (BALB/c × C57BL/6)F1 females bred to (C3H × DBA/2)F1 males (Lipman *et al.*, 2004).

Principle #6: Necropsy Data Provides Important Covariates

At a minimum, each researcher should conduct a careful gross inspection of each middle-aged or old mouse used in his/her study. This should include a notation of the presence or absence of masses in the skin, mammary glands, lungs, and abdominal organs, and a check for size of thymus, lymph nodes, and spleen suggestive of hematopoietic malignancy. Signs of bite wounds or scars on the skin should raise a suspicion of chronic or acute infection. Claims in the materials and methods section that the mice used were "apparently healthy" carry little conviction without a gross inspection of this kind, at a minimum. The best idea is to discard all data from mice with any lesions noted, although this advice becomes very expensive to follow, particularly if the mice are older than recommended by Principle #1 above. This recommendation is just as important for protocols in which animals are tested while alive—tests of antibody production or cognitive powers, for example; here, even though it is not necessary to euthanize the mouse to obtain the experimental data of interest, euthanasia as soon as possible after completion of the evaluation should be carried out to identify those mice in which a disease process may have influenced the outcome of the test.

Even better, of course, is to have the animal examined by a professional veterinary pathologist, or by a laboratory technician, with specialized training, working as part of the pathology team. This step will add a cost of approximately $10 for each mouse examined. Reports are usually returned from the pathology office within a few weeks, making it possible for researchers to go back and eliminate, retroactively, those animals found to have been diseased. A complete histopathological necropsy can cost between $25 and $100 per case, and should be strongly considered when the objectives of the study include characterization of a new mutant, drug, or experimental system.

Principle #7: Pooling Across Individuals is Hazardous

Because the proportion of individuals with an illness serious enough to affect the outcome of an experimental test increases dramatically with age, the use of pooled samples from multiple individuals should be avoided whenever possible. In a study of antibody production, for example, sensible experimental designs would exclude those with hematopoietic malignancy. If the proportion of mice with lymphoma is as low as 20%, the chance that a pool of five mice will consist only of lymphoma-free mice is only 33%, and pools of samples from 10 mice are 89% likely to contain at least one diseased mouse. In other circumstances, the investigator may be unaware of the ways in which her test outcome might be influenced by specific forms of illness.

For many traits variability may increase in older subjects, and the routine use of pooled samples obscures this variability, and may prevent an appreciation of its effects on the biological question of interest. If, for example, a measure of muscle fatigue differs in important ways in subjects that do or do not have compromised pulmonary function, a study of individuals might reveal a bimodal distribution, with a fatigable subgroup—consisting of those with pulmonary adenomas—at one mode. Even without necropsy information, analysis of unpooled subjects would reveal a bimodal or strongly skewed distribution on the muscle outcome, raising issues about population heterogeneity that require careful follow-up work. Combining subjects into pools, each of which has some compromised individuals, would obscure this relationship, and provide a misleading impression of age effects on muscle function.

In some cases pooling may be required, particularly when the assay method is too insensitive to provide a reliable measure using the amount of material available from an individual donor. In such cases it will be necessary to test multiple pools of individuals from each age or treatment group of interest in order to perform a statistical analysis of the hypothesis. The power of the statistical test, of course, depends on the number of individually tested subjects, or the number of different pools, for which results are available. Thus combining a group of 12 subjects into 4 pools (of 3 subjects each) is certain to diminish statistical power, and the individual protocol will need to balance the practicality, and cost, of testing individual subjects against the loss of power that results from pooling.

Principle #8: Cost-adjusted Power Analyses can Reduce Overall Expense

Most experimenters are familiar with the uses of statistical power analysis, in which the goal is typically to determine the number of subjects that will need to be examined in order to have a good chance of refuting a null hypothesis of interest. Such an analysis can tell us, for example, that if the mean value of some substance ("Vitamin X") in controls is 1200 ± 200 units, and we wish to see if the experimental group will differ from the control level by 200 units, we will need to use 17 control and 17 treated mice to have an 80% chance ("80% power") of documenting the difference at a level of $p < 0.05$. The number of mice needed will go up if the change induced by the experimental treatment is smaller; or if the standard deviation is larger; or if the significance criterion is made more stringent (e.g., $p < 0.01$); or if we wish to increase our chance of proving the matter from 80% to 90%; or if we plan to test more than two groups; or if we plan to test several hypotheses using the same set of mice. Power analyses are, appropriately, considered a critical element in designing experiments and seeking financial support for them; it may be hard to drum up support for a research protocol that has only a 10% chance of detecting an effect sufficiently large to be worth reporting. An experiment designed to see if mean lifespan is increased 10% by a specific diet, for example, may require 60 control and 60 treated mice to achieve 80% power; an experiment with only 20 mice per group might be judged not worth the effort.

This synopsis above has a hidden assumption, the assumption that the number of animals in the two comparison groups should be the same. The design is "balanced," in the sense that each group has the same size, and such balanced designs minimize the total number of animals tested. This makes good sense when the cost of each test is the same, but in a typical aging experiment the cost of obtaining and testing an elderly mouse may be a good deal higher than the cost for a young control. As shown in Table 3.1, for example, the production cost of a 25-month-old mouse, under plausible assumptions, may be 10-fold the cost of a 5-month-old mouse. Unbalanced designs, in which groups are permitted to have different numbers of subjects, can minimize the cost of the experimental protocol by using more mice of the less expensive variety. The procedure for conducting a "cost-adjusted" power analysis has two steps. First, you conduct a standard power analysis, along the lines shown above for "Vitamin X," to estimate the number needed to produce acceptable power using a balanced design. In the example, the balanced design would require $N_e = 17$ mice per group. Then one calculates N_Y and N_O, the numbers of young and old mice needed, using the following formula (developed by Dr. Andrzej Galecki of the University of Michigan's Geriatrics Center):

$$N_Y = 0.5 * N_e * (1 + \mathrm{SQRT}(C_O/C_Y))$$
$$N_O = 0.5 * N_e * (1 + \mathrm{SQRT}(C_Y/C_O))$$

where C_Y and C_O are respectively the cost of each experimental datum for young and old mice.

Consider a specific example, an experiment comparing 5-month-old to 25-month-old mice, for Vitamin X, with mean and standard deviation as given above, so that an experiment using 17 mice/group provides 80% power. In this example, a 5-month-old mouse costs $21 and a 25-month-old mouse costs $251 (from Table 3.1). Assuming the test kit and the technical labor add $10 per sample, the cost for each data point is $31 for young mice and $261 for old mice. The formula above suggests that the optimal distribution of resources would involve testing 33 young mice and 11 of the more expensive, old mice. The cost of this experimental series would be $4011, a savings of

$953 over the "balanced" design that uses 17 mice of each age. If half of the mice at age 25 months are found to have a tumor or some other illness that requires their exclusion from the test population, then the cost per tested, healthy aged mouse goes to $512, the optimal distribution changes to 43 young and 11 (tumor-free) old mice, and the savings to $2500 compared to the balanced design.

Principle #9: Prefer Protocols that Compare Young Adults Destined to Age at Different Rates

The large majority of experiments on rodent aging use an old-fashioned design, in which some trait is measured in rodents of two or more ages, to produce a description of what aging does. It is for this reason that the National Institute on Aging has committed itself to providing aged rodents of multiple ages, and for this reason that most of this chapter has implicitly focused on designs that involve comparisons among age groups. From a different perspective, though, the main goal of biological gerontology should not be to develop an exhaustive catalog of what aging does, at ever-deeper levels of molecular and cellular sophistication, but instead to develop a good idea of how aging works to produce aged individuals from young ones. Descriptions of how aged individuals differ from young ones are only a first, exploratory step in producing and testing hypotheses about aging mechanisms. An alternate design, already in fashion for studies of invertebrate aging, involves comparisons of young or middle-aged subjects that are known to be aging at different rates. There are now at least two diets that slow aging in both rats and mice, one based on caloric restriction (Weindruch and Sohal, 1997) and the other based on restriction of the amino acid methionine (Miller *et al.*, 2005; Orentreich *et al.*, 1993). There are at least eight published mutations that extend lifespan in mice (Bartke *et al.*, 2001; Bluher *et al.*, 2003; Holzenberger *et al.*, 2003; Miller, 2001; Miskin and Masos, 1997; Tatar *et al.*, 2003). Here the increases in maximal lifespan provide presumptive evidence that the aging process has been delayed or decelerated, and in some cases additional work has documented delays in aging effects on collagen cross-linking, immune changes, joint pathology, cataracts, kidney damage, cognitive decline, and tumor rates (Flurkey *et al.*, 2001; Ikeno *et al.*, 2003; Kinney *et al.*, 2001; Silberberg, 1972; Vergara *et al.*, 2004), thus building a strong case for broad effects on aging rate in these mutants. There is also good evidence that mouse stocks recently derived from wild-trapped progenitors retain genetic alleles, lost by inbred mouse stocks, that are responsible for increases in mean and maximal lifespan (Klebanov *et al.*, 2001; Miller *et al.*, 2002).

The availability of multiple varieties of slow-aging mice allows investigators to look at factors that act, throughout early adult life, to determine the rate at which age changes occur. It is misleading to assume that aging occurs mainly in old age, i.e., at ages at which the signs of aging first become apparent and inconvenient. Because causes precede effects, the processes that begin to induce clear signs of aging in 18-month-old mice (and 50-year-old people) must have been at work at earlier ages. Thus the mechanisms by which calorie-restricted diets or genetic variations and mutations retard the development of aging effects must also be in action during the months prior to the onset of geriatric symptoms. Research designs that compare pairs of strains, similar to one another except for an age-retarding mutation or exposure to an antiaging intervention, are thus powerful tools for seeking, and then testing, ideas about the ways in which the aging process is itself differentially timed. From this perspective, for example, a gene expression survey which focused on comparisons of control, food-restricted, and slow-aging dwarf mutants at early or middle adult ages is expected to be more fruitful than one which instead compiled lists of genes whose expression is age sensitive. Comparisons among differentially aging mice at relatively early ages also have the benefits of being faster, less expensive, and less confounded by disease and survivor effects than experiments which require data from aged organisms.

Principle #10: Avoid using Laboratory Rodents for Studies of Aging

Or, to be more diplomatic about it, avoid using *only* laboratory rodents for studies of aging. This principle has two subcomponents: (a) an argument that laboratory-adopted rodent stocks are a particularly poor choice on which to develop general ideas about aging, and (b) the more important point that important insights into mammalian aging are likely to require data on species that age at different rates.

Theoretical biologists have postulated, and experimentalists have confirmed, that genes whose natural selection depends on their beneficial effects on early life survival and fitness may have ill effects in old age. Studies have shown repeatedly that selection for genes that influence early-life maturation and reproductive performance (Luckinbill *et al.*, 1984; Rose and Charlesworth, 1980) or growth rate (Miller *et al.*, 2000) can have major effects on aging rate and longevity. Similar conclusions emerge from analysis of the actions of evolution in field studies (Austad, 1993) and in domesticated dogs (Li *et al.*, 1996; Miller and Austad, 2005; Patronek *et al.*, 1997). The evolutionary history of the inbred mouse and rat stocks typically used in experimental biology, including biogerontology, features over a hundred generations of selection for rapid early life growth, large body size (an indirect result of selection for large litter size), independence from reproductive linkage to day length, promiscuity in mate selection, tameness, slow speed, and a preference to go into cages rather than out of them. These selection pressures were not the result of deliberate experimental decisions, but represent adaptation of the genome to optimal fitness in the laboratory environment and to laboratory breeding schemes. On theoretical grounds, intensive selection for rapid early growth and early maturation might be expected to eliminate polymorphic alleles that delay aging. In confirmation, two analyses of populations of mice recently derived from wild-trapped progenitors have shown increases in mean and maximal longevity compared to inbred strains and to genetically heterogeneous mouse stocks produced by crosses among laboratory-adapted inbred stocks (Miller *et al.*, 2002). Unpublished data (Harper, Austad, and Miller *et al.*) have replicated these findings and shown further that hybrids produced by crosses between wild-derived and laboratory-adapted stocks have intermediate lifespans.

The laboratory mouse is a highly artificial construct, related to real mice in much the same way as a poodle is related to a wolf. Most pertinent for biogerontology, it is a short-lived construct, from which at least some significant antiaging genes have been stripped. Studies of the biology of aging in laboratory-adapted mice thus face some of the same critiques, detailed elsewhere (Miller, 2004a b), to which analyses of mouse models of so-called accelerated aging can be subjected.

More generally, the biogerontology community, by largely restricting its mammalian cadre to work on rodents, seems to have turned its back on the most obvious source of experimental leverage, i.e., availability in nature of species that age at radically different rates. The best that experimentalists can do within a homeothermic species is to tease out an increase in maximum lifespan of about 50%. Long- and short-lived breeds of dogs, single gene mutants in mice, diet-induced lifespan expansion—each produces changes of 50% or less in the pace of aging, functional decline, and change in mortality risks. Evolutionary selective pressures, working on a longer time scheme, can of course do much better. Maximum lifespan within rodents varies from about 4 years in mice to about 30 years in some porcupines and beavers (omitting the naked mole rat on the grounds of poikilothermy). Within the mammals, maximum lifespan seems likely to exceed 200 years in bowhead whales, and species with maximal longevity over 50 years are found within several orders and many genera. The theme of Principle #9—comparison among adults destined to age at different rates—goes double for comparative biology of aging. Gerontologists with an interest in discovering the fundamental basis for alterations in aging rate should be obsessed with exploiting this extremely rich but nearly untapped pool of natural experiments. Environmental niches suitable for evolution of long-lived species arise with regularity and become filled with birds, gliding mammals (Austad and Fischer, 1991), large predators, unpalatable porcupines, large-sized herbivores, whales and fish, and primates with complex social systems. Each of these many kinds of long-lived homeotherms has evolved separately from shorter-lived progenitors. Yet there is virtually nothing known as to the mechanisms exploited by evolution in pursuit of longevity, nor whether similar mechanisms are repeatedly employed in each circumstance. The challenges to evolutionary potency appear, from a naïve perspective, to be formidable: development of a human-sized animal with a 70-year lifespan from a mouse-size creature built for a maximum of 3–4 years requires the reduction of the rates of neoplastic transformation (per target cell, per day) by about five orders of magnitude (Miller, 1991), and evolution of whales calls for another 10,000-fold improvement. Studies that compare antineoplastic defenses, and more generally antiaging mechanisms, among sets of species that differ radically in aging rate deserve far more attention than they have hitherto received, although initial forays into this area look promising (Busuttil *et al.*, 2003; Kapahi *et al.*, 1999; Ku and Sohal, 1993; Ogburn *et al.*, 1998). Twenty years from now, biogerontologists may view mice and rats not as the main weapon for research on aging in mammals, but as one tool (the shortest-lived one) in a kit developed for disassembling and reconstructing the systems that regulate aging rate in mammals.

ACKNOWLEDGMENTS

This work has been supported by NIA grants AG08808 and AG13283. I thank Nancy Nadon for her collaboration on an earlier article on closely related topics, and Andrzej Galecki for advice and formulae related to cost-adjusted power analyses.

REFERENCES

Austad S.N. (1993). Retarded senescence in an insular population of Virginia opossums (*Didelphis virginiana*). *J Zoology 229*, 695–708.

Austad S.N., and Fischer K.E. (1991). Mammalian aging, metabolism, and ecology: evidence from the bats and marsupials. *J Gerontol Biol Sci 46*, B47–B53.

Bartke A., Coschigano K., Kopchick J., Chandrashekar V., Mattison J., Kinney B., and Hauck S. (2001). Genes that prolong life: Relationships of growth hormone and growth to aging and life span. *Journals of Gerontology Series A, Biological and Medical Sciences 56*, B340–B349.

Bluher M., Kahn B.B., and Kahn C.R. (2003). Extended longevity in mice lacking the insulin receptor in adipose tissue. *Science 299*, 572–574.

Busuttil R.A., Rubio M., Doll A.C., Campisi J., and Vijg J. (2003). Oxygen accelerates the accumulation of mutations during the senescence and immortalization of murine cells in culture. *Aging Cell 2*, 287–294.

Chiu B.C., Shang X., Frait K.A., Hu J.S., Komuniecki E., Miller R.A., and Chensue S.W. (2002). Differential effects of ageing on cytokine and chemokine responses during type-1 (mycobacterial) and type-2 (schistosomal) pulmonary granulomatous inflammation in mice. *Mech Ageing Dev 123*, 313–326.

Committee on Animal Models for Research on Aging (1981). *Mammalian Models for Research on Aging*. Washington, DC: National Academy Press.

Festing M.F. (1995). Use of a multistrain assay could improve the NTP carcinogenesis bioassay. *Environmental Health Perspectives 103*, 44–52.

Finch C.E. (1990) *Longevity, Senescence, and the Genome*. Chicago: University of Chicago Press.

Florini J.R. (1989). Limitations of interpretation of age-related changes in hormone levels: Illustration by effects of thyroid hormones on cardiac and skeletal muscle. *J Gerontol 44*, B107–B109.

Flurkey K., Papaconstantinou J., Miller R.A., and Harrison D. E. (2001). Lifespan extension and delayed immune and collagen aging in mutant mice with defects in growth hormone production. *Proceedings of the National Academy of Sciences USA 98*, 6736–6741.

Franceschi C., Monti D., Sansoni P., and Cossarizza A. (1995). The immunology of exceptional individuals: The lesson of centenarians. *Immunol Today 16*, 12–16.

Holzenberger M., Dupont J., Ducos B., Leneuve P., Geloen A., Even P.C., Cervera P., and Le Bouc Y. (2003). IGF-1 receptor regulates lifespan and resistance to oxidative stress in mice. *Nature 421*, 182–187.

Ikeno Y., Bronson R.T., Hubbard G.B., Lee S., and Bartke A. (2003). Delayed occurrence of fatal neoplastic diseases in Ames dwarf mice: Correlation to extended longevity. *Journals of Gerontology Series A-Biological Sciences & Medical Sciences 58*, 291–296.

Kapahi P., Boulton M.E., and Kirkwood T.B. (1999). Positive correlation between mammalian life span and cellular resistance to stress. *Free Radical Biology & Medicine 26*, 495–500.

Kinney B.A., Meliska C.J., Steger R.W., and Bartke A. (2001). Evidence that Ames dwarf mice age differently from their normal siblings in behavioral and learning and memory parameters. *Hormones & Behavior 39*, 277–284.

Klebanov S., Astle C.M., Roderick T.H., Flurkey K., Archer J. R., Chen J., and Harrison D.E. (2001). Maximum life spans in mice are extended by wild strain alleles. *Experimental Biology & Medicine* (Maywood, NJ), *226*, 854–859.

Ku H.H., and Sohal R.S. (1993). Comparison of mitochondrial pro-oxidant generation and anti-oxidant defenses between rat and pigeon: Possible basis of variation in longevity and metabolic potential. *Mech Ageing Dev 72*, 67–76.

Li Y., Deeb B., Pendergrass W., and Wolf N. (1996). Cellular proliferative capacity and life span in small and large dogs. *J Gerontol A Biol Sci Med Sci 51*, B403–B408.

Lipman R., Galecki A., Burke D.T., and Miller R. A. (2004). Genetic loci that influence cause of death in a heterogeneous mouse stock. *J Gerontol Biol Sci 59A*, 977–983.

Luckinbill L.S., Arking R., Clare M.J., Cirocco W.C., and Buck S.A. (1984). Selection for delayed senescence in *Drosophilia melanogaster*. *Evolution 38*, 996–1003.

Metter E.J., Walega D., Metter E.L., Pearson J., Brant L.J., Hiscock B.S., and Fozard J.L. (1992). How comparable are healthy 60- and 80-year-old men? *J Gerontol Med Sci 47*, M73–M78.

Miller R.A. (2004a). 'Accelerated aging': A primrose path to insight? *Aging Cell 3*, 47–51.

Miller R.A. (2004b). Rebuttal to Hasty and Vijg: 'Accelerating aging by mouse reverse genetics: A rational approach to understanding longevity'. *Aging Cell 3*, 53–54.

Miller R.A. (2001) Genetics of increased longevity and retarded aging in mice. In Masoro E.J., and Austad S.N., Eds., *Handbook of the Biology of Aging*, pp. 369–395. San Diego, CA: Academic Press.

Miller R.A. (1991). Gerontology as oncology: Research on aging as the key to the understanding of cancer. *Cancer 68*, 2486–2501.

Miller R.A., Austad S., Burke D., Chrisp C., Dysko R., Galecki A., and Monnier V. (1999). Exotic mice as models for aging research: polemic and prospectus. *Neurobiol Aging 20*, 217–231.

Miller R.A., and Austad S.N. (2005) Growth and aging: Why do big dogs die young? In Masoro E.J., and Austad S.N., Eds., *Handbook of the Biology of Aging*, pp. 369–395. San Diego, CA: Academic Press.

Miller R.A., Buehner G., Chang Y., Harper J.M., Sigler R., and Smith-Wheelock M. (2005). Methionine-deficient diet extends mouse life span, slows immune and lens aging, alters glucose, T4, IGF-I and insulin levels, and increases hepatocyte MIF levels and stress resistance. *Aging Cell 4*, 199–125.

Miller R.A., Chrisp C., and Atchley W.R. (2000). Differential longevity in mouse stocks selected for early life growth trajectory. *J Gerontol Biol Sci 55A*, B455–B461.

Miller R.A., Harper J.M., Dysko R.C., Durkee S.J., and Austad S.N. (2002). Longer life spans and delayed maturation in wild-derived mice. *Experimental Biology and Medicine 227*, 500–508.

Miskin R., and Masos T. (1997). Transgenic mice overexpressing urokinase-type plasminogen activator in the brain exhibit reduced food consumption, body weight and size, and increased longevity. *J Gerontol A Biol Sci Med Sci 52*, B118–B124.

Nadon N. 2005. Aged Rodent Colonies Handbook. http://www.nia.nih.gov/ResearchInformation/ScientificResources/AgedRodentColoniesHandbook/.

Ogburn C.E., Austad S.N., Holmes D.J., Kiklevich J.V., Gollahon K., Rabinovitch P.S., and Martin G.M. (1998). Cultured renal epithelial cells from birds and mice: Enhanced resistance of avian cells to oxidative stress and DNA damage. *J Gerontol [A] 53A*, B287–B292.

Orentreich N., Matias J.R., DeFelice A., and Zimmerman J. A. (1993). Low methionine ingestion by rats extends life span. *J Nutr 123*, 269–274.

Patronek G.J., Waters D.J., and Glickman L.T. (1997). Comparative longevity of pet dogs and humans: Implications for gerontology research. *J Gerontol A Biol Sci Med Sci 52*, B171–B178.

Perls T., Levenson R., Regan M., and Puca A. (2002). What does it take to live to 100? *Mech Ageing Dev 123*, 231–242.

Rose M., and Charlesworth B. (1980). A test of evolutionary theories of senescence. *Nature 287*, 141–142.

Silberberg R. (1972). Articular aging and osteoarthritis in dwarf mice. *Path Microbiol 38*, 417–430.

Smith G.S., Walford R.L., and Mickey M.R. (1967). Lifespan and incidence of cancer and other diseases in selected long-lived inbred mice and their F1 hybrids. *J Natl Cancer Inst 50*, 1195–1213.

Tatar M., Bartke A., and Antebi A. (2003). The endocrine regulation of aging by insulin-like signals. [Review] [74 refs]. *Science 299*, 1346–1351.

Vergara M., Smith-Wheelock M., Harper J.M., Sigler R., and Miller R.A. (2004). Hormone-treated Snell dwarf mice regain fertility but remain long-lived and disease resistant. *J Gerontol Biol Sci 59*, 1244–1250.

Warner H., and Nadon N., Eds. (2005). NIA Interventions Testing Program. http://www.nia.nih.gov/Research Information/ScientificResources/InterventionsTesting Program.htm.

Weindruch R. and Sohal R.S. (1997). Seminars in medicine of the Beth Israel Deaconess Medical Center. Caloric intake and aging. *New Engl J Med 337*, 986–994.

4

From Primary Cultures to the Aging Organism: Lessons from Human T Lymphocytes

Rita B. Effros

One of the prominent clinical features of human aging is the dramatic increase in morbidity and mortality due to infections. Aging is also the most significant risk factor for developing cancer. Both phenomena are related to the age-associated decline in immune function, particularly within the T cell compartment, the part of the immune system that patrols the body for cells that appear foreign, which would indicate they are infected or cancerous. Development of long-term cell culture protocols for analyzing the effect of chronic antigenic stimulation on primary T cells from young adult donors has led to the identification of multiple characteristics of the terminal stage of replicative senescence in this cell type. These include inability to divide, altered cytokine patterns, resistance to apoptosis, shortened telomeres, reduced antiviral cytolytic function, and loss of expression of a major signaling molecule, CD28. Many elderly persons have high proportions of T cells with similar characteristics, and the abundance of these cells has been correlated with such deleterious outcomes as poor response to vaccination, osteoporotic fractures, reduced immunity to infection, and even early mortality. Thus, cell culture studies have provided novel insights into the cellular basis for an important facet of immune system aging that has significant effects on a variety of human age-related pathologies.

Introduction

Among the most significant clinical problems associated with aging are infections and cancer. Indeed, influenza and pneumonia rank as the 5th leading cause of death in U.S. adults age 65 and older. In addition to actual mortality, morbidity and prolonged periods of illness due to infections are substantially increased with age. With respect to cancer, epidemiological studies show that old age—even more than known harmful lifestyle factors, such as smoking—is the greatest risk factor for the development of cancer. One of the major contributory factors to the age-related changes in infection and cancer is the waning protective function of the immune system.

The complex changes that occur within the immune system of aged humans are due both to intrinsic events, such as the decrease in thymic size and function, as well as to environmental factors, mainly the lifelong exposure to various pathogens. The combined effects of these intrinsic and extrinsic factors lead to major alterations in immune function with age, changes that have been implicated in the deleterious effects of pathogens and cancer in the elderly. Ironically, vaccination, which is aimed at manipulating the immune system in ways that would prevent infection or retard cancer progression, is far less effective in the elderly (McElhaney *et al.*, 1998). Even immune memory to certain pathogens that is generated early in life declines during aging.

In order to develop strategies for enhancing immune function of the elderly, a thorough understanding of the mechanisms responsible for age-associated immunological changes is clearly essential. In this chapter, we will focus on one particular component of the immune system, the T lymphocyte, and demonstrate how primary cell culture analysis of T cells has led to novel insights into an important and previously unrecognized facet of the immune system in elderly humans, namely, the accumulation of cells with characteristics of replicative senescence. Information from theses studies provides evidence suggesting that senescent T cells may affect not only immune function *per se*, but a variety of age-related pathologies. The high correlation between characteristics identified *in vitro* and T cells present *in vivo* suggests that the long-term T cell culture model will also be informative for evaluating therapeutic interventions to retard or prevent a variety of deleterious clinical problems associated with aging.

How Does the Immune System Work?

INNATE AND ADAPTIVE IMMUNITY

The fundamental purpose of the immune system is to distinguish between self and non-self. Foreign antigens are eliminated in a variety of ways by both the so-called innate and adaptive components of the immune system. The innate immune system deals with foreign invaders through rapid, albeit fairly nonspecific, responses. Moreover, there is no recall or memory within the innate immune system. By contrast, the adaptive immune system takes a bit longer to respond, but retains memory for the specific antigen, and is able to respond in an accelerated fashion in the event of re-encounter with the same antigen. Indeed, it is this ability to "learn" and remember specific antigens that is the basis for vaccination.

The two major types of lymphocytes that comprise the adaptive immune system are B cells and T cells. Both are derived from hematopoetic stem cells in the bone marrow, but they function in entirely different ways. B cells produce soluble proteins known as antibodies, which can neutralize or otherwise inhibit the activity of foreign pathogens. Thus, B cells are responsible for the so-called humoral immune response. T cells, on the other hand, cannot recognize anything foreign unless it has actually entered another cell. The infected cell, which expresses parts of the virus or bacterium on its surface, is recognized as non-self by the T cells, eliciting what is known as "cellular immunity."

How do B cells and T cells recognize foreign pathogens that enter the body? The recognition structures, known as antigen receptors, are generated through a unique and complex set of genetic events, which allows a limited number of genes to create an immune system with an enormous range of specificities. Briefly, during the development of lymphocytes, one member of a set of gene segments is randomly joined to other gene segments by an irreversible process of DNA recombination. The consequence of this mechanism is that just a few hundred different gene segments can combine in a variety of ways to create thousands of receptor chains. This diversity is further amplified by the pairing of two different chains, each encoded by distinct sets of gene segments, to form a functional antigen receptor. Each lymphocyte bears many copies of its antigen receptor, and once generated, the receptor specificity of a lymphocyte does not change. Thus, only one specificity can be expressed by a single lymphocyte and its progeny (Janeway Jr *et al.*, 2001).

CLONAL EXPANSION—WHAT ABOUT THE HAYFLICK LIMIT?

Because of the random nature of the genetic events that create lymphocyte receptors, a small amount of genetic material is utilized to generate at least 10^8 different specificities. The corollary to this is that since each lymphocyte bears a different antigen receptor, the number of lymphocytes that can recognize any single foreign antigen is exceedingly small. Therefore, when a mature lymphocyte interacts with a particular antigen that is recognized by its receptor, that lymphocyte becomes activated and must begin dividing, giving rise to a clone of identical progeny bearing identical receptors for antigen. Antigen specificity is thereby maintained as the dividing cells continue to proliferate and differentiate into effector cells. Once antigen is cleared, a small number of memory cells persist, all bearing the same antigen receptor. When the same antigen is encountered again, the process of activation and clonal expansion is repeated (Janeway Jr *et al.*, 2001).

From what has been described above, it becomes clear that cell proliferation is a central feature of adaptive immunity. One wonders, then, how the so-called Hayflick Limit might affect the behavior of cells within the immune system. This innate barrier to unlimited cell division, known as replicative senescence, has been documented for a variety of cell types, and would seem to be highly relevant to T cells, whose ability to fight infections is critically dependent on extensive cell division.

From the cell culture data on other cell types, a preliminary estimate would suggest that the degree of proliferation achievable by each T cell is so large that the finite replicative lifespan would not necessarily be biologically meaningful *in vivo*. For example, if a T cell has an average proliferative lifespan of 35 population doublings, and even if all daughter cells continue to grow unchecked, the resulting yield of more than 10^{10} cells would appear to be more than sufficient. However, because T-cell immune responses include both extensive proliferation and apoptotic removal of excess cells, the finite proliferative lifespan of T cells might allow only two or three rounds of antigen-driven expansion before the end stage of replicative senescence is reached. The above crude estimate suggests that the limited proliferative potential might indeed be detrimental *in vivo*, particularly by old age (Effros and Pawelec, 1997).

Based on the importance of cell proliferation in maintaining effective immune function, we sought to examine the changes that T cells undergo as they progressed through their proliferative lifespan. In order to ensure that we were studying the same population of T cells over time, the most suitable method to address this issue is in cell culture, where it is possible to conduct a virtual longitudinal study on a specific set of cells. Long-term cell culture analyses had been performed on other cell types, including fibroblasts, epithelial cells, endothelial cells and keratinocytes, to characterize the unique features of each cell type under conditions of enforced, extensive prolilferation (Campisi, 1997). Ironically, until fairly recently, T cells, whose function is critically dependent on clonal expansion, had never been examined with respect to the process of replicative senescence (Adibzadeh *et al.*, 1995; Effros, 1996). In the following section, we describe our adaptation of the long-term culture techniques to human T cells, and summarize the main features of replicative senescence in this cell type.

Primary Cultures of Human T Cells

SUMMARY OF THE CULTURE PROTOCOL

Our cell culture studies have focused on the analysis of the CD8$^+$ T cell subset, the cell type responsible for controlling viral infections, which are a major clinical problem in the elderly. In preliminary experiments, aimed at optimizing long-term growth and viability of human T cells, we verified that the most reproducible growth patterns of human T cells, whether from neonates or adults, were obtained in AIMV serum-free medium. In these early studies, we observed that some batches of fetal calf serum or even human serum inhibited the growth of T cells, particularly T cells derived from neonates (Perillo *et al.*, 1989).

Our initial cell culture protocol used in defining the proliferative lifespan for human T cells involved stimulation of peripheral blood mononuclear cells with an irradiated allogeneic lymphoblasoid cell line in the continued presence of the T cell growth factor, Interleukin-2 (IL-2). After an initial burst of proliferation over approximately 2–3 weeks, the cells reached quiescence, at which time the culture was restimulated with the same antigen and IL-2. This process was repeated until the point at which the culture showed no cell number increase in response to two rounds of antigen stimulation, at which time it was considered to have reached the end stage of replicative senescence.

Since T cells grow in suspension culture, accurate cell counts could be performed at each passage, allowing us to calculate the total number of population doublings achieved by that culture. Using this cell culture protocol, which favors the generation of CD8$^+$ T cell cultures, we followed over 100 T cell cultures, derived from peripheral blood samples from both adults and neonatal donors, and reported that the number of population doublings (PDs) ranged from 11 to 57, with a mean of 23 ± 7 (Perillo *et al.*, 1989). Similar ranges of proliferative potential of human T cells have been reported by other groups as well.

In our experiments, there was a significant difference in the PDs achieved by cells from adult versus neonatal donors ($p < 0.025$). However, among the adult donors, there was no correlation between *in vitro* lifespan and chronological age (Perillo *et al.*, 1989). In terms of function, our studies showed that for alloantigen-stimulated cultures, antigen-specific cytotoxic function was retained even at senescence, and the cells in senescent cultures were able to upregulate expression of the alpha chain of the IL-2 receptor in response to specific antigen, despite the inability to enter cell cycle when exposed to the same antigen (Perillo *et al.*, 1993).

CHARACTERISTICS OF SENESCENT T CELL CULTURES

Certain notable changes in critical cellular functions were observed in alloantigen-specific cultures that reached replicative senescence. Similar to senescent fibroblasts (Wang, Lee, and Pandey, 1994), CD8$^+$ T cell cultures that reach senescence became resistant to apoptosis and expressed increased levels of bcl2 (Spaulding *et al.*, 1999). Stimuli such as antibody to Fas, IL-2 withdrawal, mild heat shock, galectin-1 and staurosporine, all of which caused robust apoptosis in the early passage cells, caused only minimal cell death in the senescent cultures. A second major change involved the reduced ability of senescent cultures to respond to stress by upregulation of the major mammalian stress protein, hsp70 (Effros, Zhu, and Walford, 1994b). This defect is reminiscent of the overall reduction in responsiveness to physical and oxidative stress that is believed to play a major role in organismic aging (Golden *et al.*, 2002).

One of the main advantages of studying T cells in long-term culture is the ability to monitor changes in expression over time in the large spectrum of known T cell surface markers reflecting lineage, activation status, adhesion, and memory. Using flow cytometry, we demonstrated that for nearly all such markers, there was no change in expression between early passage and senescent cultures (Perillo *et al.*, 1993). The single exception was CD28, a key T cell-specific signaling molecule that plays diverse roles in T cell biology, including delivering the costimulatory second signal that is essential for activation/proliferation, stabilizing cytokine mRNAs, modulating cell trafficking, and regulating glucose metabolism. As T cells progress to senescence in culture, the proportion of cells that are CD28$^-$ increases, and senescent cultures are >99% CD28$^-$ (Effros *et al.*, 1994a). The loss of CD28 expression is associated with complete suppression of gene expression of this key T cell signaling molecule.

Whereas characterization of senescence-associated changes using long-term primary T cell cultures has the advantage of allowing longitudinal analysis of the same population of cells over time, the model admittedly suffers from the absence of the *in vivo* milieu, which undoubtedly plays a role in marker expression patterns changes that occur in the context of the whole organism. Indeed, although loss of CD28 expression has been presumed to be the ultimate senescence-associated change based on cell culture analysis, it is possible that other cell surface antigens identified on *ex vivo* samples may delineate a more precise phenotype for the true end-stage senescent CD8$^+$ T cell. One such marker change is the acquisition of CD57, which has been documented for virus-specific CD8$^+$ T cells from HIV-infected persons that have undergone multiple rounds of proliferation (Brenchley *et al.*, 2003). Interestingly, many features are shared by CD57$^+$ and CD28$^-$ T cells isolated *ex vivo*, reinforcing the notion that both the loss of CD28 expression and the acquisition of CD57 can be considered markers of senescent T cells (Demarest *et al.*, 2001; Mach *et al.*, 1997; Posnett *et al.*, 1999; Weekes *et al.*, 1999). Additional markers that have been identified on putatively senescent

CD28$^-$ T cells isolated *ex vivo* are the KLRG1 NK inhibitory lectin-like receptor and CD56, an NK marker bearing the HNK-1 epitope (Ouyang *et al.*, 2003a; Tarazona *et al.*, 2000), findings that may explain earlier reports of MHC-unrestricted NK function in senescent cultures (Pawelec *et al.*, 1986).

As CD8$^+$ T cells undergo increasing numbers of cell divisions in long-term culture, they show a variety of alterations that would be predicted to dramatically affect *in vivo* immune function. For example, alloantigen-specific cultures from healthy donors produce increasing amounts of two pro-inflammatory cytokines, IL-6 and TNFα, as they approach replicative senescence (Effros *et al.*, 2005), and virus-specific CD8$^+$ T cells show decreased antigen-specific production of IFNγ (Dagarag *et al.*, 2004). HIV-specific CD8$^+$ T cell cultures initiated from T cells of HIV-infected persons show a progressive decline in the ability to perform antigen-specific lysis of target cells pulsed with HIV peptides, a change that is accompanied by reduced expression of perforin (Dagarag *et al.*, 2004; Yang *et al.*, 2005). Moreover, one of the key antiviral activities believed to function protectively *in vivo*—inhibition of HIV replication—is markedly reduced in senescent HIV-specific CD8$^+$ T cells (Dagarag *et al.*, 2003). One can envision that such functional changes might exert pleiotropic influences on a variety of physiological processes *in vivo*, both in the context of aging and in chronic HIV infection.

TELOMERASE AND T CELLS

It is generally accepted that the "clock" that keeps track of cell divisions and signals cell cycle arrest in human cells is the telomere, a region at the end of each chromosome that consists of multiple repeats of a specific DNA sequence (Campisi *et al.*, 2001). Due to the end-replication problem in copying the full length of the lagging DNA strand, normal somatic cells undergo progressive telomere shortening with cell division. Once the telomere reaches a certain critical length, the DNA damage signaling pathway is activated, with the concomitant up-regulation of cell cycle inhibitors. The process of replicative senescence is a stringent characteristic of human somatic cells, whereas in germ cells, in certain stem cells, and in tumor cells, telomere shortening and replicative senescence are prevented by the activity of an enzyme called telomerase, which uses its RNA template to synthesize the telomere sequence.

Human and mouse cells show fundamental differences with respect to telomere size and telomerase activity. Because of the significantly longer telomeres in laboratory strains of inbred *Mus musculus*, and the high levels of telomerase present in most mouse tissues, it is unlikely that mouse cells undergo telomere-based senescence (Akbar *et al.*, 2000). Indeed, the barrier to unlimited proliferation may actually be less stringent in murine cells, since, unlike human cells, mouse cells undergo frequent spontaneous immortalization in cell culture. Thus, there is a major difference between mice and humans with respect to this important facet of cell biology. In terms of the aging immune system as well, the life-long exposure to pathogens also differentiates elderly humans from aged mice housed in barrier facilities, further underscoring the value of using a human cell culture model for analysis of the role of T cell replicative senescence in human aging.

Our cell culture analysis of human T cells has documented that telomere length undergoes progressive shortening with increasing rounds of antigen-driven proliferation, reaching 5–7 kb at senescence (Vaziri *et al.*, 1993) Although this telomere length was similar to that of other cell types that reach senescence in cell culture, we were somewhat perplexed by the observed telomere shortening in T cells, since lymphocytes are unique among human somatic cells in that they induce high levels of telomerase activity in concert with the activation process (Weng *et al.*, 1996). Indeed, the levels of telomerase activity in antigen or mitogen-stimulated T cells are comparable to those of tumor cells (Bodnar *et al.*, 1996).

To address this issue, we performed a detailed kinetic analysis in cell culture of CD8$^+$ T cell telomerase activity induced by activation. We showed that after mitogen or T cell receptor (TCR)-mediated activation, the telomerase activity peaks at 3–5 days, then undergoes a gradual decline, becoming undetectable at approximately 3 weeks. A second wave of telomerase activity can be induced by a subsequent exposure to the same antigen, and during the period of high telomerase activity, telomere length remains stable (Bodnar *et al.*, 1996). However, in CD8$^+$ T cells, the antigen-induced upegulation of telomerase in response to stimulation with antigen is markedly reduced by the third stimulation, and is totally absent in all subsequent encounters with antigen (Valenzuela and Effros, 2002).

One of the unexpected findings in our cell culture studies was the significant difference between helper (CD4$^+$) and cytotoxic (CD8$^+$) T cell subsets with respect to telomerase. This observation was made by culturing CD4$^+$ and CD8$^+$ T cell subsets that were isolated from the same individual, using the identical stimulatory schedule. The initial stimulation by alloantigen elicited a 45-fold and 53-fold increase in telomerase activity in the CD8$^+$ and CD4$^+$ cell cultures, respectively. However, by the 4th antigenic stimulation, telomerase activity was undetectable in the CD8$^+$ T cells, whereas CD4 T cells still showed robust telomerase activity even as late as the 10th round of antigenic stimulation.

The divergent patterns of telomerase activity between CD4$^+$ and CD8$^+$ T cells paralleled the pattern of CD28 expression changes. By the 7th antigenic stimulation, 90% of the cells in the CD8$^+$ culture no longer expressed CD28, whereas at that same stage, the CD4$^+$ cultures were still 75% CD28$^+$ (Valenzuela *et al.*, 2002). The intimate relationship between telomerase activation and CD28 signaling was further demonstrated in experiments using antibodies to block CD28 binding to its ligand on antigen-presenting cells, which resulted in a significant reduction in telomerase activity. Finally, the distinct contribution of CD28 to telomerase activation was evident in experiments using Cyclosporin, a TCR signaling inhibitor. Cyclosporin was not able to inhibit telomerase in T cells activated by a combination of antibodies to CD3 and CD28, whereas potent inhibition was observed when only anti-CD3 was used for stimulation (Valenzuela *et al.*, 2002).

REVERSAL/RETARDATION OF T CELL REPLICATIVE SENESCENCE IN CELL CULTURE

Given the central role of telomere shortening in the replicative senescence "program" in T cells, our main approach at modulating senescence has focused on strategies to enhance telomerase activity in $CD8^+$ T cells. An excellent model system for these studies is the virus-specific $CD8^+$ T cell response, which is known to decline with age as well as during chronic infections, such as HIV. Therefore, using the long-term culture system described above, we followed HIV-specific $CD8^+$ T cells that had been isolated from persons infected with HIV, and tested the effect of gene transduction with the catalytic component of telomerase (hTERT). Comparisons were made between the hTERT-transduced cultures and the empty-vector-transduced cultures.

Results of these experiments showed significant effects of hTERT on proliferative and functional aspects of the T cells. Briefly, we observed that hTERT transduction led to telomere length stabilization and reduced expression of the $p16^{INK4A}$ and $p21^{WAF1}$ cyclin-dependent kinase inhibitors, implicating both of these proteins in the senescence program (Dagarag *et al.*, 2004). Indeed, the transduced cultures showed indefinite proliferation, with no signs of change in growth characteristics or of karyotypic abnormalities. In terms of protective immune function, the "telomerized" HIV-specific $CD8^+$ T cells were able to maintain the production of IFNγ for extended periods, and showed significantly enhanced capacity to inhibit HIV replication. The loss of CD28 expression was delayed considerably, although ultimately not prevented, suggesting that additional genetic manipulation of the CD28 gene itself may be required for full correction of this important senescence-associated alteration. Similarly, virus-specific cytolytic function was not restored by hTERT transduction (except in selected clones). Thus, hTERT corrects most, but not all, the alterations associated with replicative senescence in $CD8^+$ T cells isolated from HIV-infected persons. Ongoing studies are addressing whether these same effects will be seen in hTERT transduced cells from healthy donors, and whether transduction at earlier timepoints along the trajectory to senescence will enhance the telomerase effects.

Telomerase enhancement may also be achieved using nongenetic strategies, which would offer more practical approaches to therapeutic interventions in the elderly. For example, it is known that estrogen is able to enhance telomerase activity in reproductive tissues. The complex formed when estrogen binds to its receptors migrates to the nucleus and functions as a transcription factor. In normal ovarian epithelial cells, this complex actually binds to the hTERT promoter region (Misiti *et al.*, 2000). It has been known for some time that T cells can bind to estrogen via specific estrogen receptors. Thus, we tested whether pre-incubation of T cells to 17β-estradiol prior to activation might augment telomerase activity. Our preliminary data suggest that estrogen does, in fact, enhance T cell telomerase activity. The enhancement is observed in both CD4 and CD8 subsets, and can also be seen when estrogen is conjugated to BSA, indicating that surface estrogen receptor interaction may be sufficient to mediate the telomerase effect (Effros, manuscript in preparation).

Our data on estrogen effects in T cells *in vitro* are reminiscent of an earlier study in which we documented the reversal of some of the age-related T cell changes in postmenopausal women treated with hormone replacement therapy (Porter *et al.*, 2001). In another set of preliminary experiments with small molecule activators of telomerase, we have shown a significant enhancement of telomerase activity in T cells from both healthy and HIV-infected persons (Fauce *et al.*, manuscript in preparation). Thus, therapeutic approaches that are based on telomerase modulation would seem to be promising candidates for clinical interventions in the elderly that are aimed at reversing or retarding the process of replicative senescence in T cells. The major question to be addressed is whether the process of replicative senescence, characterized so extensively in cell culture, has any relationship to events within the immune system during normal human aging. As will be described below, this certainly does seem to be the case.

Is T Cell Replicative Senescence Occurring *in vivo*?

SENESCENT $CD8^+$ T CELLS ACCUMULATE WITH AGE AND WITH CHRONIC INFECTION

The results of our cell culture studies were invaluable in transitioning to *in vivo* analysis of the possible occurrence of replicative senescence during normal aging. Based on the absence of CD28 expression as a marker of senescence, we compared 20 adults (age 25–69) and 21 healthy centenarians for the presence of cells with a similar phenotype, using flow cytometry. We showed that there was a significant increase ($p < 0.01$) in the proportion of T cells lacking CD28 expression in the elderly, with some aged individuals having $>60\%$ $CD28^-$ T cells within the $CD8^+$ T cell subset, compared to the mean young adult value of $<10\%$. Importantly, since the decrease in the percentage of $CD28^+$ T cells with age was not associated with an alteration in the intensity or standard deviation of mean fluorescence, our analysis indicated that the expression of CD28 was normal on those cells that were registered as being $CD28^+$ (Effros *et al.*, 1994a).

There was an intriguing correlation between the presence of high proportions of $CD28^-$ T cells and the reversal of the youthful ratio between $CD4^+$ and $CD8^+$ T cells. Our data showed that those elderly persons who had the highest proportion of $CD28^-$ T cells also had CD4/8 ratios that reflected an increased proportion of $CD8^+$ T cells (Effros *et al.*, 1994a). Interestingly, altered CD4/8 ratios have also been reported in elderly persons who have large expansions of clonal populations of $CD8^+$ T cells (Posnett *et al.*, 1994). These oligoclonally expanded populations actually resemble cells in senescent cultures in terms of their increased level of activation, the absence of CD28 expressions and their inability to proliferate.

Importantly, cells lacking CD28 expression do not suddenly appear in old age; there is a progressive increase over the lifespan in the proportion of T cells that lack CD28 expression (Boucher *et al.*, 1998). Moreover, chronological age is not unique in its association with T cell replicative senescence. Chronic infection with HIV is also associated with the progressive accumulation over time of $CD8^+$ T cells that are $CD28^-$ (Borthwick *et al.*, 1994). In early reports, this unusual subset was suggested to have arisen as a distinct lineage, possibly related to some unusual aspect of HIV disease pathogenesis. However, based on our cell culture studies, we suspected that these cells were the descendants of cells that previously did express CD28, but that had undergone extensive proliferation and reached the end stage of replicative senescence. To test this idea, we performed telomere analysis on purified cell populations from persons infected with HIV. We first isolated the $CD8^+$ T cells from peripheral blood, then sorted them further into $CD28^+$ and $CD28^-$ populations. Using Southern blot analysis, we showed that the telomere length of the $CD28^-$ population was significantly shorter than that of the $CD28^+$ population from the same donor. In fact, the mean telomere length of the $CD8^+CD28^-$ T cells from persons infected with HIV (mean age 43 years) was the same range as that of PBMC isolated from centenarians (Effros *et al.*, 1996).

As further evidence in support of the notion that replicative senescence was actually occurring *in vivo*, the sorted $CD8^+CD28^-$ T cells tested immediately *ex vivo* showed minimal proliferative ability, even when the stimulation bypassed cell surface-mediated activation signals. Although it is impossible to formally prove that the cells with characteristics of senescence arose by the same mechanism as those in senescent cell culture, the overwhelming similarity between the two cell populations is highly suggestive that replicative senescence is not a cell culture artifact. Indeed, the cell culture model is thus far highly predictive of the functional, genetic, and phenotypic traits of certain $CD8^+$ T cells present *in vivo*.

THE DRIVING FORCE

We have recently proposed that latent infection with herpes viruses may constitute a major antigenic stimulus leading to the accumulation of senescent $CD8^+$ T cells *in vivo* (Pawelec *et al.*, 2004). Elderly persons have large numbers of dysfunctional $CD8^+$ T cells bearing antigen receptors for a single dominant cytomegalovirus (CMV) epitope (Ouyang *et al.*, 2003b). Even in younger persons who are infected with HIV and whose immune systems are thought to age prematurely, there are substantial numbers of $CD8^+CD28^-$ T cells that are specific for CMV as well as for Epstein–Barr virus (EBV). These sorts of data suggest that the cost of maintaining control over these latent infections is the progressive generation of senescent $CD8^+$ T cells (Pawelec *et al.*, 2004). The apoptosis resistance of these cells leads to a situation where they occupy progressively more and more of the memory T cell pool in the elderly, restricting the repertoire of the remaining T cells.

Latent viruses associated with certain forms of cancer can also drive $CD8^+$ T cells to senescence, as illustrated by the accumulation of $CD8^+CD28^-$ T cells with reactivity to the human papilloma virus E7 antigen in cervical cancer patients (Pilch *et al.*, 2002). Other viruses associated with chronic infection, such as Hepatitis C, also seem to elicit expanded populations of $CD8^+$ T cells that lack CD28 expression (Kurokohchi *et al.*, 2003). The common thread in all of these situations is chronic antigenic stimulation, which seems to result in massive cell division of antigen-reactive $CD8^+$ T cells, ultimately causing them to reach what might be considered the end-stage of their differentiation pathway, namely replicative senescence. Clearly, most memory T cells encounter their nominal antigen only once or twice over an individual's lifespan, and it is only those $CD8^+$ T cells with reactivity to antigens that are never cleared from the body that have the potential to continue dividing extensively, eventually reaching senescence.

IN VIVO IMMUNE EFFECTS OF SENESCENT T CELLS

The $CD28^-$ T cells present *in vivo* are similar by a variety of criteria to $CD28^-$ cells in senescent cultures, suggesting that they arose by the same mechanism. Extensive research on replicative senescence in nonimmune cell types indicates that once senescent cells are generated, they not only suffer from an inability to enter the cell cycle, but can also affect a variety of physiological processes or organ system functions. For example, senescent human fibroblasts stimulate premalignant and malignant, but not normal, epithelial cells to proliferate in culture and also to form tumors in SCID mice, suggestive of a potential role in age-related cancers (Krtolica *et al.*, 2001). In addition, whereas *normal* fibroblasts function to create intracellular matrix, *senescent* fibroblasts secrete collagenase and other matrix-destroying enzymes, leading to altered tissue integrity (Campisi, 1998).

The significant correlation between high proportions of $CD8^+CD28^-$ T cells and poor antibody response to influenza vaccination documented in two independent clinical studies (Goronzy *et al.*, 2001; Saurwein-Teissl *et al.*, 2002) provides an example of putative suppressive effects of senescent $CD8^+$ T cells on the function of other immune cells. Senescent $CD8^+$ T cells have also been associated with suppressive effects in organ transplant patients. Donor-specific $CD8^+CD28^-$ T cells are detectable in the peripheral blood of those patients with stable function of heart, liver and kidney transplants, whereas no such cells were found in patients undergoing acute rejection (Cortesini *et al.*, 2001). Although in the context of organ transplantation, suppression may lead to a favorable outcome, in many other contexts, the $CD8^+CD28^-$ T cell populations are associated with deleterious effects. For example, expanded populations of $CD8^+CD28^-$ T cells are present in ankylosing spondylitis patients, and, in fact, correlate with a more severe course of this autoimmune disease (Schirmer *et al.*, 2002).

In addition to the role that putatively senescent $CD8^+$ T cells may play in regulating functions of other immune cell types, these cells also show alterations in the normal functional attributes of $CD8^+$ T cells. First, $CD8^+CD28^-$ T cells isolated *ex vivo* are unable to proliferate (like their cell culture counterparts), even in response to signals that bypass cell surface receptors, such as PMA and ionomycin (Effros *et al.*, 1996). This observation is consistent with extensive research on replicative senescence in a variety of cell types documenting the irreversible nature of the proliferative block, and its association with upregulation of cell cycle inhibitors and p53-linked checkpoints (Campisi, 2001). If the $CD8^+CD28^-$ T cells present in elderly persons are virus-specific, their inability to undergo the requisite clonal expansion in response to antigen re-encounter will compromise the immune control over that particular virus. Indeed, as noted above, senescent HIV-specific $CD8^+$ T cells are markedly reduced in lytic activity, IFNγ production, and antiviral suppressive function (Dagarag *et al.*, 2004). Thus, $CD8^+CD28^-$ T cells in elderly persons may contribute to emergence of latent infections, such as varicella zoster virus (shingles) and EBV (some lymphomas), as well to the reduced control over acute infection with a repeatedly encountered virus (influenza), well-documented in elderly persons (Effros, 2001). Second, since CD28 ligation enhances the binding affinity of T cells to endothelial cells, T cells lacking CD28 may be altered in their trafficking patterns between tissue and blood. Third, if the putatively senescent T cells present *in vivo* produce high levels of IL-6 and TNFα like their *in vitro* counterparts, their presence *in vivo* may be contributing to the well-documented pro-inflammatory milieu present in many elderly persons. Indeed, enhanced inflammation is now believed to play a role in many of the diseases of aging that had not been previously considered immune-mediated pathologies. Overiectomy-induced bone loss in mice, for example, has been specifically linked to TNFα-secreting T cells present within the bone marrow (Raggia *et al.*, 2001).

The apoptosis resistance of $CD8^+CD28^-$ T cells tested immediately *ex vivo* (Posnett *et al.*, 1999) leads to their persistence, which, in turn, affects the quality and composition of the total memory pool, as discussed above. Moreover, since the $CD28^-$ T cells are usually part of oligoclonal expansions (Posnett *et al.*, 1994), their accumulation would presumably also lead to a reduction in the overall spectrum of antigenic specificities within the T cell pool. Elderly persons with high proportions of $CD8^+$ T cell that are $CD28^-$ do, in fact, have reduced repertoires of antigenic specificities (Ouyang *et al.*, 2003b).

A final aspect of senescent T cells that could have broad physiological consequences relates to the role of stress in the aging process. T cells that undergo replicative senescence in culture show transcriptional down-regulation of the *hsp70* gene in response to heat shock (Effros *et al.*, 1994b), and T cells from elderly persons show attenuation in the molecular chaperone system hsp70, in the steroid binding hsp90, and the chaperonin hsp60. These immune cell changes may contribute to the well-documented reduction in ability to respond to stress that characterizes organismic aging.

Global Effects of Senescent T Cells on the Aging Organism

BONE HOMEOSTASIS

Senescent $CD8^+$ T cells may affect other organ systems as well. Indeed, there is accumulating evidence implicating chronic immune activation in bone loss (Arron and Choi, 2000). Although much of the research on "osteoimmunology" relates to $CD4^+$ T cell/bone interaction in the context of rheumatoid arthritis, there is increasing evidence suggesting a link between the $CD8^+$ T cell subset and bone resorption activity (John *et al.*, 1996) as well as with osteoporotic fractures in the elderly (Pietschmann *et al.*, 2001).

One of the central regulators of bone resorption is a molecule known as "RANKL" (receptor activator of NFkB ligand), which binds to RANK on osteoclasts, inducing these bone-resorbing cells to mature and become activated (Kong *et al.*, 2000). Importantly, RANKL is expressed on and secreted by activated T cells. Normally, the bone-resorbing activity induced by RANKL is kept in check by IFNγ, a cytokine also produced by the activated T cells. However, we have shown that $CD8^+$ T cell IFNγ production is markedly reduced when the cells reach replicative senescence (Dagarag *et al.*, 2004). A second facet of the T cell/bone connection relates to the fact that activated T cells can also modulate bone mass by producing cytokines that inhibit the bone-forming activity of osteoblasts. Specifically, the cytokine TNF-α whose production is increased in senescent cultures, inhibits osteoblast bones forming activity, and also affects bone mass by inducing formation of certain cytokines by osteoblasts that increase bone resorption (Lorenzo, 2000). Thus, senescent T cells have the potential to play a significant role in bone mass changes during aging.

ALZHEIMER'S DISEASE AND ATHEROSCLEROSIS

There is some evidence that chronic activation of T cells, leading to increased proliferation and telomere shortening, may be involved in other age-related diseases as well. The etiology of Alzheimer's disease (AD) is not known, but our recent studies suggest a possible involvement of T cells. We observed that the telomere length of T cells, but not of B cells or monocytes, correlates with mental function tests in AD patients (Panossian *et al.*, 2002). Those patients with lower Mini Mental Status Examination (MMSE) scores, which is a marker of disease status, had T cells with shorter telomeres than those persons with higher MMSE scores. These findings suggest that the immune system of AD patients is perturbed in some way and may not necessarily respond normally to therapeutic vaccines aimed at retarding AD disease progression. Interestingly, one such therapeutic vaccine trial was recently interrupted due to unanticipated brain inflammation in some participants (Nicoll *et al.*, 2003).

A second age-related pathology in which chronically-activated T cells may play a role is atherosclerosis. Immune involvement in cardiovascular disease (CVD) is suggested by both epidemiological data and experimental animal models. T cells are present in atherosclerotic lesions (Libby *et al.*, 1995), and interaction of CD40 on T cells with vascular endothelial cells, smooth muscle cells, and macrophages has been documented (Mach *et al.*, 1997).

Importantly, several types of infections have been hypothesized to increase the risk of CVD by causing systemic inflammation, or by triggering autoimmunity, for example, by cross-reactivity of heat shock proteins (hsp) with bacterial antigens (Mayr *et al.*, 1999). Indeed, clinically healthy volunteers with sonographically documented carotid artery atherosclerosis have significantly increased antibody titers to hsp 65 compared to controls with no lesions, and in follow-up studies, those with highest titers showed highest mortality. The blocking of the hsp65 effect by T cell immunosuppressive agents further implicates specific immunity in the pathogenesis of atherosclerosis. Most recently, there was a report showing expanded populations of senescent $CD8^+$ T cells in patients with coronary artery disease as compared to controls, further underscoring the potential involvement of chronic antigen-driven proliferation in atherosclerosis (Jonasson *et al.*, 2003).

SENESCENT T CELLS AND MORTALITY

The ultimate effect of T cells on aging is with respect to mortality itself. Early work suggested a connection, based on correlative data, between T cell proliferative responses in cell culture and mortality over the subsequent few years (Wikby *et al.*, 1998). More recently, telomere analysis of total lymphocytes in a group of 60 year olds was shown to be predictive of mortality many years later (Cawthon *et al.*, 2003). In these studies, it was shown that the individuals who had telomeres in the lowest quartile were 7–8 times more likely to die from infections compared with those with the longest telomeres. Longitudinal studies of elderly Swedes over several decades confirm the link between immune parameters and lifespan. These data show that early mortality is associated with a so-called immune risk phenotype, which includes a cluster of T cell parameters, including high proportions of senescent $CD8^+$ T cells (Nilsson *et al.*, 2003). Interestingly, the presence of these risk factors is strongly correlated with chronic CMV infection (Wikby *et al.*, 2002). Moreover, the predictive value of the immune profile is retained for a variety of causes of death. In sum, there is accumulating evidence that immune system function is intimately linked with a variety of age-related pathologies, some of which are actual causes of death.

Concluding Remarks

The phenomenon of replicative senescence has been documented and characterized in cell culture for a variety of cell types. The basic phenotype of a senescent cell is a dysfunctional, permanently growth-arrested cell with reduced ability to undergo apoptosis. It is now clear that cells with similar characteristics do increase in frequency during aging, particularly within the immune system. However, analysis of T cell replicative senescence has led to a paradigm shift regarding the role of replicative senescence in organismic aging.

Early data showing correlations between *in vitro* cell growth and species lifespan had reinforced the notion that analysis of cells in culture would yield mechanistic insights into the process of aging. In hindsight, it appears that this goal might not have been realistic. It has become evident that senescent cells do affect lifespan, but probably not in the sense originally proposed. In other words, rather than affecting the basic aging process, senescent cells exert their impact on the aging organism by contributing to or enhancing certain age-related pathologies. Thus, senescent cells may affect lifespan only indirectly, not by modulating the rate of aging, but rather by affecting the risk of mortality. This altered view of the relationship between aging in cell culture and *in vivo* aging does not diminish the value of using cell culture models in the study of aging. It merely changes the hypotheses and interpretations of the experiments.

ACKNOWLEDGMENTS

The research described in this chapter has been supported by various NIH grants, as well as by funding from the University of California Discovery Program, Geron Corporation, the Universitywide AIDS Research Program, and the Plott Endowment. The author holds the Elizabeth and Thomas Plott Endowed Chair in Gerontology.

REFERENCES

Adibzadeh, M., Pohla, H., Rehbein, A., and Pawelec, G. (1995). Long-term culture of monoclonal human T lymphocytes: Models for immunosenescence? *Mechanisms of Ageing and Development 83*, 171–183.

Akbar, A.N., Soares, M.V., Plunkett, F.J., and Salmon, M. (2000). Differential regulation of CD8+ T cell senescence in mice and men. *Mechanisms of Ageing and Development 121*, 69–76.

Arron, J.,R., and Choi, Y. (2000). Bone versus immune system. *Int Immunol 408*, 535–536.

Bodnar, A.G., Kim, N.W., Effros, R.B., and Chiu, C.P. (1996). Mechanism of telomerase induction during T cell activation. *Experimental Cell Research 228*, 58–64.

Borthwick, N.J., Bofill, M., and Gombert, W.M. (1994). Lymphocyte activation in HIV-1 infection II. Functional defects of CD28- T cells. *AIDS 8*, 431–441.

Boucher, N., Defeu-Duchesne, T., Vicaut, E., Farge, D., Effros, R.B., and Schachter, F. (1998). CD28 expression in T cell aging and human longevity. *Exp. Geronol. 33*, 267–282.

Brenchley, J.M., Karandikar, N.J., Betts, M.R., Ambrozak, D.R., Hill, B.J., Crotty, L.E. *et al.* (2003). Expression of CD57 defines replicative senescence and antigen induced apoptotic death of CD8+ T cells. *Blood 101*, 2711–2720.

Campisi, J. (1997). The biology of replicative senescence. *Eur. J. Cancer 33*, 703–709.

Campisi, J. (1998). The role of cellular senescence in skin aging. *Journal of Investigative Dermatology. Symposium Proceedings 3*, 1–5.

Campisi, J. (2001). From cells to organisms: Can we learn about aging from cells in culture? *Exp. Gerontol. 36*, 607–618.

Campisi, J., Kim, S.H., Lim, C.S., and Rubio, M. (2001). Cellular senescence, cancer and aging: the telomere connection. *Exp. Gerontol. 36*, 1619–1637.

Cawthon, R.M., Smith, K.R., O'Brien, E., Sivatchenko, A., and Kerber, R.A. (2003). Association between telomere length in blood and mortality in people aged 60 years or older. *Lancet 361*, 393–395.

Cortesini, R., LeMaoult, J., Ciubotariu, R., and Cortesini, N.S. (2001). CD8+CD28- T suppressor cells and the induction of antigen-specific, antigen-presenting cells-mediated suppression of Th reactivity. *Immunol. Rev. 182*, 201–206.

Dagarag, M.D., Evazyan, T., Rao, N., and Effros, R.B. (2004). Genetic manipulation of telomerase in HIV-specific CD8+ T cells:enhanced anti-viral functions accompany the increased proliferative potential and telomere length stabilization. *Journal of Immunology 173*, 6303–6311.

Dagarag, M.D., Ng, H., Lubong, R., Effros R.B., and Yang, O. O. (2003). Differential impairment of lytic and cytokine functions in senescent HIV-1-specific cytotoxic T lymphocytes. *Journal of Virology 77*, 3077–3083.

Demarest, J.F., Jack, N., Cleghorn, F.R., Greenberg, M.L., Hoffman, T.L., Ottinger, J.S. *et al.* (2001). Immunologic and virologic analyses of an acutely HIV type 1-infected patient with extremely rapid disease progression. *AIDS Res. Hum. Retroviruses 17*, 1333–1344.

Effros, R.B. (2001). Immune system activity. In Masoro, E., and Austad, S. (Eds.), *Handbook of the Biology of Aging*, 5th ed., pp. 324–350. San Diego: Academic Press.

Effros, R.B., Dagarag, M.D., Spaulding, C.C., and Man, J. (2005). The Role of CD8 T cell replicative senescence in human aging. *Immunological Reviews 205*, 147–157.

Effros, R.B. (1996). Insights on immunological aging derived from the T lymphocyte cellular senescence model. *Exp. Gerontol. 31*, 21–27.

Effros, R.B., Allsopp, R., Chiu, C.P., Wang, L., Hirji, K., Harley, C.B. *et al.* (1996). Shortened telomeres in the expanded CD28-CD8+ subset in HIV disease implicate replicative senescence in HIV pathogenesis. *AIDS/Fast Track 10*, F17–F22.

Effros, R.B., Boucher, N., Porter, V., Zhu, X., Spaulding, C., Walford, R.L. *et al.* (1994a). Decline in CD28+ T cells in centenarians and in long-term T cell cultures: A possible cause for both in vivo and in vitro immunosenescence. *Exp. Gerontol. 29*, 601–609.

Effros, R.B., and Pawelec, G. (1997). Replicative Senescence of T lymphocytes: Does the Hayflick Limit lead to immune exhaustion? *Immunology Today 18*, 450–454.

Effros, R.B., Zhu, X., and Walford, R.L. (1994b). Stress response of senescent T lymphocytes: Reduced hsp70 is independent of the proliferative block. *Journal of Gerontology 49*, B65–B70.

Golden, T.R., Hinerfeld, D.A., and Melov, S. (2002). Oxidative stress and aging: beyond correlation. *Aging Cell 1*, 117–123.

Goronzy, J.J., Fulbright, J.W., Crowson, C.S., Poland, G.A., O'Fallon, W.M., and Weyand, C.M. (2001). Value of immunological markers in predicting responsiveness to influenza vaccination in elderly individuals. *J. Virol. 75*, 12182–12187.

Janeway Jr, C.A., Travers, P., and Walpert, M.S. M. (2001). *The immune system in health and disease.* (5th ed.) Garland Publishing, Inc.

John, V., Hock, J.M., Short, L.L., Glasebrook, A.L., and Galvin, R.J. (1996). A role for CD8+ T lymphocytes in osteoclast differentiation in vitro. *Endocrinology 137*, 2457–2463.

Jonasson, L., Tompa, A., and Wikby, A. (2003). Expansion of peripheral CD8+ T cells in patients with coronary artery disease: relation to cytomegalovirus infection. *J. Intern. Med. 254*, 472–478.

Kong, Y.Y., Boyle, W.J., and Penninger, J.M. (2000). Osteoprotegerin ligand: A regulator of immune responses and bone physiology. *Immunology Today 21*, 445–502.

Krtolica, A., Parrinello, S., Lockett, S., Desprez, P.Y., and Campisi, J. (2001). Senescent fibroblasts promote epithelial cell growth and tumorigenesis: A link between cancer and aging. *Proc. Natl. Acad. Sci. USA 98*, 12072–12077.

Kurokohchi, K., Masaki, T., Arima, K., Miyauchi, Y., Funaki, T., Yoneyama, H. *et al.* (2003). CD28-negative CD8-positive cytotoxic T lymphocytes mediate hepatocellular damage in hepatitis C virus infection. *J. Clin. Immunol. 23*, 518–527.

Libby, P., Sukhova, G., Lee, R.T., and Galis, Z.S. (1995). Cytokines regulate vascular functions related to stability of the atherosclerotic plaque. *Journal of Cardiovascular Pharmacology 25 Suppl 2*, S9–S12.

Lorenzo, J. (2000). Interactions between immune and bone cells: New insights with many remaining questions. *Journal of Clinical Investigation 106*, 749–752.

Mach, F., Scheonbeck, U., Sukhova, G.K., Bourcier, T., Bonnefoy, J.Y., Pober, J.S. *et al.* (1997). Functional CD40 ligand is expressed on human vascular endothelial cells, smooth muscle cells, and macrophages: Implications for CD40-CD40 ligand signaling in atherosclerosis. *Proceedings of the National Academy of Sciences USA 94*, 1931–1936.

Mayr, M., Metzler, B., Kiechl, S., Willeit, J., Schett, G., Xu, Q. *et al.* (1999). Endothelial cytotoxicity mediated by serum antibodies to heat shock proteins of *Escherichia coli* and *Chlamydia pneumoniae*: Immune reactions to heat shock proteins as a possible link between infection and atherosclerosis. *Circulation 99*, 1560–1566.

McElhaney, J.E., Upshaw, C.M., Hooton, J.W., Lechelt, K.E., and Meneilly, G.S. (1998). Responses to influenza vaccination in different T-cell subsets: A comparison of healthy young and older adults. *Vaccine 16*, 1742–1747.

Misiti, S., Nanni, S., Fontemaggi, G., Cong, Y.S., Wen, J., Hirte, H.W. *et al.* (2000). Induction of hTERT expression and telomerase activity by estrogens in human ovary epithelium cells. *Molecular and Cellular Biology 20*, 3764–3771.

Nicoll, J.A., Wilkinson, D., Holmes, C., Steart, P., Markham, H., and Weller, R.O. (2003). Neuropathology of human Alzheimer disease after immunization with amyloid-beta peptide: A case report. *Nat. Med. 9*, 448–452.

Nilsson, B.O., Ernerudh, J., Johansson, B., Evrin, P.E., Lofgren, S., Ferguson, F.G. *et al.* (2003). Morbidity does not influence the T-cell immune risk phenotype in the elderly: Findings in the Swedish NONA Immune Study using sample selection protocols. *Mech. Ageing Dev. 124*, 469–476.

Ouyang, Q., Wagner, W.M., Voehringer, D., Wikby, A., Klatt, T., Walter, S. *et al.* (2003a). Age-associated accumulation of CMV-specific CD8+ T cells expressing the inhibitory killer cell lectin-like receptor G1 (KLRG1). *Exp. Gerontol. 38*, 911–920.

Ouyang, Q., Wagner, W.M., Wikby, A., Walter, S., Aubert, G., Dodi, A.I. *et al.* (2003b). Large numbers of dysfunctional CD8+ T lymphocytes bearing receptors for a single dominant CMV epitope in the very old. *J. Clin. Immunol. 23*, 247–257.

Panossian, L., Porter, V.R., Valenzuela, H.F., Masterman, D., Reback, E., Cummings, J. *et al.* (2002). Telomere shortening in T cells correlates with Alzheimer's disease status. *Neurobiology of Aging*.

Pawelec, G., Akbar, A., Caruso, C., Effros R.B., Grubeck-Loebenstein, B., and Wikby, A. (2004). Is immunosenescence infectious? *Trends Immunol. 25*, 406–410.

Pawelec, G., Schneider, E.M., and Wernet, P. (1986). Acquisition of suppressive activity and natural killer-like cytotoxicity by human alloproliferative "helper" T cell clones. *Journal of Immunology 136*, 402–411.

Perillo, N.L., Naeim, F., Walford, R.L., and Effros, R.B. (1993). The in vitro senescence of human lymphocytes: Failure to divide is not associated with a loss of cytolytic activity or memory T cell phenotype. *Mechanisms of Ageing and Development 67*, 173–185.

Perillo, N.L., Walford, R.L., Newman, M.A., and Effros, R.B. (1989). Human T lymphocytes possess a limited in vitro lifespan. *Exp. Gerontol. 24*, 177–187.

Pietschmann, P., Grisar, J., Thien, R., Willheim, M., Kerschan-Schindl, K., Preisinger, E. *et al.* (2001). Immune phenotype and intracellular cytokine production of peripheral blood mononuclear cells from postmenopausal patients with osteoporotic fractures. *Exp. Gerontol. 36*, 1749–1759.

Pilch, H., Hoehn, H., Schmidt, M., Steiner, E., Tanner, B., Seufert, R. *et al.* (2002). CD8+CD45RA+CD27-CD28-T-cell subset in PBL of cervical cancer patients representing CD8+T-cells being able to recognize cervical cancer associated antigens provided by HPV 16 E7. *Zentralbl. Gynakol. 124*, 406–412.

Porter, V., Greendale, G.A., Schocken, M., Zhu, X., and Effros, R.B. (2001). Immune effects of hormone replacement therapy in post-menopausal women. *Exp. Gerontol. 36*, 311–326.

Posnett, D.N., Edinger, J.W., Manavalan, J.S., Irwin, C., and Marodon, G. (1999). Differentiation of human CD8 T cells: Implications for in vivo persistence of CD8+ CD28-cytotoxic effector clones. *International Immunology 11*, 229–241.

Posnett, D.N., Sinha, R., Kabak, S., and Russo, C. (1994). Clonal populations of T cells in normal elderly humans: The T cell equivalent to "benign monoclonal gammopathy." *Journal of Experimental Medicine 179*, 609–618.

Roggia, C., Gao, Y., Cenci, S., Weitzmann, M.N., Toraldo, G., Isaia, G. *et al.* (2001). Up-regulation of TNF-producing T cells in the bone marrow: A key mechanism by which estrogen deficiency induces bone loss in vivo. *Proc. Natl. Acad. Sci. USA 98*, 13960–13965.

Saurwein-Teissl, M., Lung, T.L., Marx, F., Gschosser, C., Asch, E., Blasko, I. *et al.* (2002). Lack of antibody production following immunization in old age: Association with CD8(+)CD28(−) T cell clonal expansions and an imbalance in the production of Th1 and Th2 cytokines. *J. Immunol. 168*, 5893–5899.

Schirmer, M., Goldberger, C., Wurzner, R., Duftner, C., Pfeiffer, K.P., Clausen, J. *et al.* (2002). Circulating cytotoxic CD8(+) CD28(−) T cells in ankylosing spondylitis. *Arthritis Res. 4*, 71–76.

Spaulding, C.S., Guo, W., and Effros, R.B. (1999). Resistance to apoptosis in human CD8+ T cells that reach replicative senescence after multiple rounds of antigen-specific proliferation. *Exp. Gerontol. 34*, 633–644.

Tarazona, R., DelaRosa, O., Alonso, C., Ostos, B., Espejo, J., Pena, J. *et al.* (2000). Increased expression of NK cell markers on T lymphocytes in aging and chronic activation of the immune system reflects the accumulation of effector/senescent T cells. *Mech. Ageing Dev. 121*, 77–88.

Valenzuela, H.F., and Effros R.B. (2002). Divergent telomerase and CD28 expression patterns in human CD4 and CD8 T cells following repeated encounters with the same antigenic stimulus. *Clin. Immunol. 105*, 117–125.

Vaziri, H., Schachter, F., Uchida, I., Wei, L., Zhu, X., Effros, R. *et al.* (1993). Loss of telomeric DNA during aging of normal and trisomy 21 human lymphocytes. *American Journal of Human Genetics 52*, 661–667.

Wang, E., Lee, M.J., and Pandey, S. (1994). Control of fibroblast senescence and activation of programmed cell death. *Journal of Cellular Biochemistry 54*, 432–439.

Weekes, M.P., Wills, M.R., Mynard, K., Hicks, R., Sissons, J. G., and Carmichael, A.J. (1999). Large clonal expansions of human virus-specific memory cytotoxic T lymphocytes within the CD57+ CD28- CD8+ T-cell population. *Immunology 98*, 443–449.

Weng, N.P., Levine, B.L., June, C.H., and Hodes, R.J. (1996). Regulated expression of telomerase activity in human T lymphocyte development and activation. *Journal of Experimental Medicine 183*, 2471–2479.

Wikby, A., Johansson, B., Olsson, J., Lofgren, S., Nilsson, B. O., and Ferguson, F. (2002). Expansions of peripheral blood CD8 T-lymphocyte subpopulations and an association with cytomegalovirus seropositivity in the elderly: The Swedish NONA immune study. *Exp. Gerontol. 37*, 445–453.

Wikby, A., Maxson, P., Olsson, J., Johansson, B., and Ferguson, F.G. (1998). Changes in CD8 and CD4 lymphocyte subsets, T cell proliferation responses and non-survival in the very old: The Swedish longitudinal OCTO-immune study. *Mechanisms of Ageing and Development 102*, 187–198.

Yang, O.O., Lin, H.D., Ng, H., Effros R.B., and Uittenbogaart, C.H. (2005). Decreased Perforin and Granzyme B expression in senescent HIV-1-specific cytotoxic T lymphocytes. *Virol. 332*, 16–19.

5

Models of Systems Failure in Aging

Leonid A. Gavrilov and Natalia S. Gavrilova

Mathematical models of systems failure are critically important for understanding the mechanisms of aging because aging of organisms is associated with increased risk of failure of its physiological systems.

Theoretical analysis of systems failure in aging leads naturally to apply the existing general theory of systems failure, which is also known as the reliability theory. Reliability-theory approach to biological aging is useful for three reasons. (1) It provides a useful scientific language (definitions and cross-cutting principles) helping to create a general theoretical framework for organizing numerous and diverse observation on aging into a coherent picture. This is very important for researchers, because it helps them to understand each other despite a disruptive specialization of aging studies. (2) It allows researchers to develop a scientific intuition and understanding of the main principles of the aging process by considering simplified mathematical models of systems failure, having some general features of real aging organisms. (3) It helps to generate and test specific predictions on age-related dynamics of systems failure, and to get deeper insights in the mechanisms of aging by more creative analysis of already collected data.

This chapter reviews the existing theoretical reliability models and approaches, which help us to understand the mechanisms and age-dynamics of systems failure. Empirical observations on systems failure in aging are also reviewed (the Gompertz and Weibull failure laws, the compensation law of systems failure, and the late-life failure rate leveling-off), and are theoretically explained through the observed decline in system's redundancy with age. The causes of failure rate increase with age are discussed and explained using five simple mathematical models of systems failure in aging as an illustration.

Introduction

This introductory-overview chapter sets a stage for introducing theoretical models of systems failure in aging. Mathematical models of systems failure are important for the studying of human aging, because aging is associated with increased risk of failure in human physiological systems. Theoretical analysis of systems failure in aging invites us to consider the general theory of systems failure known as reliability theory (Barlow and Proshan, 1975; Barlow *et al.*, 1965; Gavrilov, 1978; Gavrilov and Gavrilova, 1991, 2001, 2003a, 2004a, 2005; Gavrilov *et al.*, 1978).

Reliability theory was historically developed to describe failure and aging of complex electronic (military) equipment, but the theory itself is a very general theory based on mathematics (probability theory) and systems approach (Barlow and Proschan, 1975; Barlow *et al.*, 1965). It may therefore be useful to describe and understand the aging and failure of biological systems too. Reliability theory may be useful in several ways: first, by providing a kind of scientific language (definitions and cross-cutting principles), which helps to create a logical framework for organizing numerous and diverse observations on aging into a coherent picture. Second, it helps researchers to develop an intuition and an understanding of the main principles of the aging process through consideration of simple mathematical models, having some features of a real world. Third, reliability theory is useful for generating and testing specific predictions, as well as deeper analyses of already collected data. The purpose of this chapter is to review the theoretical reliability models and approaches, which help to understand the mechanisms and dynamics of systems failure in aging.

Reliability Approach to System's Failure in Aging

Reliability theory is a body of ideas, mathematical models, and methods directed to predict, estimate, understand, and optimize the lifespan and failure distributions of systems and their components (adapted from Barlow and Proschan, 1975). Reliability theory allows researchers to predict the age-related failure kinetics for a system of given architecture (reliability structure) and given reliability of its components.

DEFINITIONS OF SYSTEM'S FAILURE AND AGING

The concept of failure is important to the analysis of system's reliability. In reliability theory failure is defined as the *event* when a required function is terminated (Rausand and Houland, 2003). In other words, failure is such an outcome when the system deviates from optimistically anticipated and desired behavior ("fails"). Failures are often classified into two groups:

1. degradation failures, where the system or component no longer functions properly, and
2. catastrophic or fatal failures—the end of system's or component's life.

Good examples of degradation failures in humans would be an onset of different types of health impairments, diseases, or disabilities, while catastrophic or fatal failures obviously correspond to death. The notions of aging and failure are related to each other in the following way: when the risk of failure outcomes increases with age ("old is not as good as new")—this is aging by definition. Note that according to reliability theory, aging is not just growing old; instead aging is a degradation leading to failure (adverse health outcomes)—becoming sick, disabled, frail and dead. Therefore, from a reliability-theory perspective the notion of "healthy aging" is an oxymoron like a healthy dying, or a healthy disease. More appropriate terms instead of "healthy aging" or "aging well" would be a delayed aging, postponed aging, slow aging, arrested aging, or negligible aging (senescence).

Because the reliability definition of biological aging is linked to health failures (adverse health outcomes, including death), aging without diseases is just as inconceivable as dying without death. Diseases and disabilities are an integral part (outcomes) of the aging process. Not every disease is related to aging, but every progression of disease with age has some relevance to aging: aging is a "maturation" of diseases with age.

Note that a system may have an aging behavior for one particular type of failure, but it may remain to be as good as new for some other type of failure. Thus the notion of aging is outcome-specific—it requires specifying for which particular type of failure (or group of failures) the system deteriorates. Consequently, the legitimate antiaging interventions may be outcome-specific too, and limited to postponing some specific adverse health outcomes. Aging is likely to be a summary term for many different processes leading to various types of degradation failures, and each of these processes deserves to be studied and prevented.

BASIC FAILURE MODELS

Reliability of the system (or its component) refers to its ability to operate properly according to a specified standard (Crowder *et al.*, 1991). Reliability is described by the *reliability function* $S(x)$, which is the probability that a system (or component) will carry out its mission through time x (Rigdon and Basu, 2000). The reliability function (also called the *survival function*) evaluated at time x is just the probability P, that the *failure time X*, is beyond time x. Thus, the reliability function is defined in the following way:

$$S(x) = P(X > x) = 1 - P(X \leq x) = 1 - F(x)$$

where $F(x)$ is a standard *cumulative distribution function* in the probability theory (Feller, 1968). The best illustration for the reliability function $S(x)$ is a survival curve describing the proportion of those still alive by time x (the l_x column in life tables).

Failure rate, $\mu(x)$, or instantaneous risk of failure, also called the *hazard rate*, $h(x)$, or mortality force is defined as the relative rate for reliability function decline:

$$\mu(x) = -\frac{dS_x}{S_x dx} = \frac{-dlnS_x}{dx}$$

In those cases when the failure rate is constant (does not increase with age), we have *nonaging system* (component) that does not deteriorate (does not fail more often) with age:

$$\mu(x) = \mu = \text{const}$$

The reliability function of nonaging systems (components) is described by the *exponential distribution*:

$$S(x) = S_0 e^{-\mu x}$$

This *failure law* describes "lifespan" distribution of atoms of radioactive elements, and, therefore, it is often called an exponential decay law. Interestingly, this failure law is observed in many wild populations with high extrinsic mortality (Finch, 1990; Gavrilov and Gavrilova, 1991). This kind of distribution is observed if failure (death) occurs entirely by chance, and it is also called a "one-hit model," or a "first order kinetics." The nonaging behavior of a system can be detected graphically when the logarithm of the survival function decreases with age in a linear fashion.

Recent studies found that at least some cells in the aging organism might demonstrate nonaging behavior. Specifically, the rate of neuronal death does not increase with age in a broad spectrum of aging-related neurodegenerative conditions (Heintz, 2000). These include 12 different models of photoreceptor degeneration, "excitotoxic" cell death *in vitro*, loss of cerebellar granule cells in a mouse model, and Parkinson's and Huntington's diseases (Clarke *et al.*, 2000). In this range of diseases, five different neuronal types are affected. In each of these cases, the rate of cell death is best fit by an exponential decay law with constant risk of death independent of age (death by chance only), arguing against models of progressive cell deterioration and aging (Clarke *et al.*, 2000, 2001a). An apparent lack of cell aging is also observed in the case of amyotrophic lateral sclerosis (Clarke *et al.*, 2001a), retinitis pigmentosa (Burns, 2002; Clarke *et al.*, 2000, 2001a; Massof, 1990) and idiopathic Parkinsonism (Calne, 1994; Clarke *et al.*, 2001b; Schulzer *et al.*, 1994). These observations correspond well with another observation that "an impressive range of cell functions in most organs remain unimpaired throughout the life span" (Finch, 1990, p. 425), and these unimpaired functions might reflect the "no-aging" property known as "old as good as new" property in survival analysis (Klein and Moeschberger, 1997, p. 38). Thus we come to the following fundamental question about the origin of aging: How can we explain the aging of a system built of nonaging elements? This question invites us to think about the possible systemic nature of aging and to wonder whether aging may be a property of the system as a whole. We would like to emphasize the importance of looking at the bigger picture of the aging phenomenon in addition to its tiny details, and we will suggest a possible answer to the posed question in this chapter.

If failure rate increases with age, we have an *aging system* (component) that deteriorates (fails more often) with age. There are many failure laws for aging systems, and the most famous one in biology is the *Gompertz law* with exponential increase of the failure rates with age (Finch, 1990; Gavrilov and Gavrilova, 1991; Gompertz, 1825; Makeham, 1860; Strehler, 1978):

$$\mu(x) = Re^{\alpha x}$$

An exponential (Gompertzian) increase in death rates with age is observed for many biological species including fruit flies *Drosophila melanogaster* (Gavrilov and Gavrilova, 1991), nematodes (Brooks *et al.*, 1994; Johnson, 1987, 1990), mosquitoes (Gavrilov, 1980), human lice, *Pediculus humanus* (Gavrilov and Gavrilova, 1991), flour beetles, *Tribolium confusum* (Gavrilov and Gavrilova, 1991), mice (Kunstyr and Leuenberger, 1975; Sacher, 1977), rats (Gavrilov and Gavrilova, 1991), dogs (Sacher, 1977), horses (Strehler, 1978), mountain sheep (Gavrilov, 1980), baboons (Bronikowski *et al.*, 2002) and, perhaps most important, humans (Finch, 1990; Gavrilov and Gavrilova, 1991; Gompertz, 1825; Makeham, 1860; Strehler, 1978). According to the Gompertz law, the logarithm of failure rates increases linearly with age. This is often used in order to illustrate graphically the validity of the Gompertz law—the data are plotted in the semilog scale (known as the Gompertz plot) to check whether the logarithm of the failure rate is indeed increasing with age in a linear fashion.

For technical systems one of the most popular models for failure rate of aging systems is the Weibull model, the power-function increase in failure rates with age (Weibull, 1939):

$$\mu(x) = \alpha x^{\beta} \text{ for } x \geq 0, \quad \text{where} \quad \alpha, \beta > 0$$

This law was suggested by Swedish engineer and mathematician W. Weibull in 1939 to describe the strength of materials (Weibull, 1939). It is widely used to describe aging and failure of technical devices (Barlow and Proschan, 1975; Rigdon and Basu, 2000; Weibull, 1951), and occasionally it was also applied to a limited number of biological species (Eakin *et al.*, 1995; Hirsch and Peretz, 1984; Hirsch *et al.*, 1994; Janse *et al.*, 1988; Ricklefs and Scheuerlein, 2002; Vanfleteren *et al.*, 1998). According to the Weibull law, the logarithm of failure rate increases linearly with the *logarithm* of age with a slope coefficient equal to parameter β. This is often used in order to illustrate graphically the validity of the Weibull law—the data are plotted in the log–log scale (known as the Weibull plot) to check whether the logarithm of the failure rate is indeed increasing with the *logarithm* of age in a linear fashion.

We will show later that both the Gompertz and the Weibull failure laws have a fundamental explanation rooted in reliability theory. Therefore it may be interesting and useful to compare these two failure laws and their behavior.

Figure 5.1a presents the dependence of the logarithm of the failure rate on age (Gompertz plot) for the Gompertz and the Weibull functions.

Note that in Figure 5.1a this dependence is strictly linear for the Gompertz function (as expected), and concave-down for the Weibull function. So the Weibull function looks like decelerating with age if compared to the Gompertz function.

Figure 5.1b presents the dependence of the logarithm of the failure rate on the *logarithm* of age (Weibull plot) for the Gompertz and the Weibull functions. Note that this dependence is strictly linear for the Weibull function (as expected), and concave-up for the Gompertz function. So the Gompertz function looks like the accelerating one with the *logarithm* of age if compared to the Weibull function.

There are two fundamental differences between the Weibull and the Gompertz functions.

First, the Weibull function states that the system is immortal at starting age—when the age X is equal to zero, the failure rate is equal to zero too, according to the Weibull formula. This means that the system should be initially ideal (immortal) in order for the Weibull law to be applicable to it. On the contrary, the Gompertz function states that the system is already vulnerable to failure at starting age—when the age X is equal to zero, the failure rate is already above zero, equal to parameter R in the Gompertz formula. This means that the partially damaged systems having some initial damage load are more likely to follow the Gompertz failure law, while the initially perfect systems are more likely to follow the Weibull law.

Second, there is a fundamental difference between the Gompertz and the Weibull functions regarding their response to misspecification of the starting age ("age zero"). This is an important issue, because in biology there is an ambiguity regarding the choice of a "true" age, when aging starts. Legally, it is the moment of birth, which serves as a starting moment for age calculation. However, from a biological perspective there are reasons to consider a starting age as a date either well before the birth date (the moment of conception in genetics, or a critical month of pregnancy in embryology), or long after the birth date (the moment of maturity, when the formation of a body is finally completed). This uncertainty in starting age has very different implications for data analysis with the Gompertz or the Weibull functions.

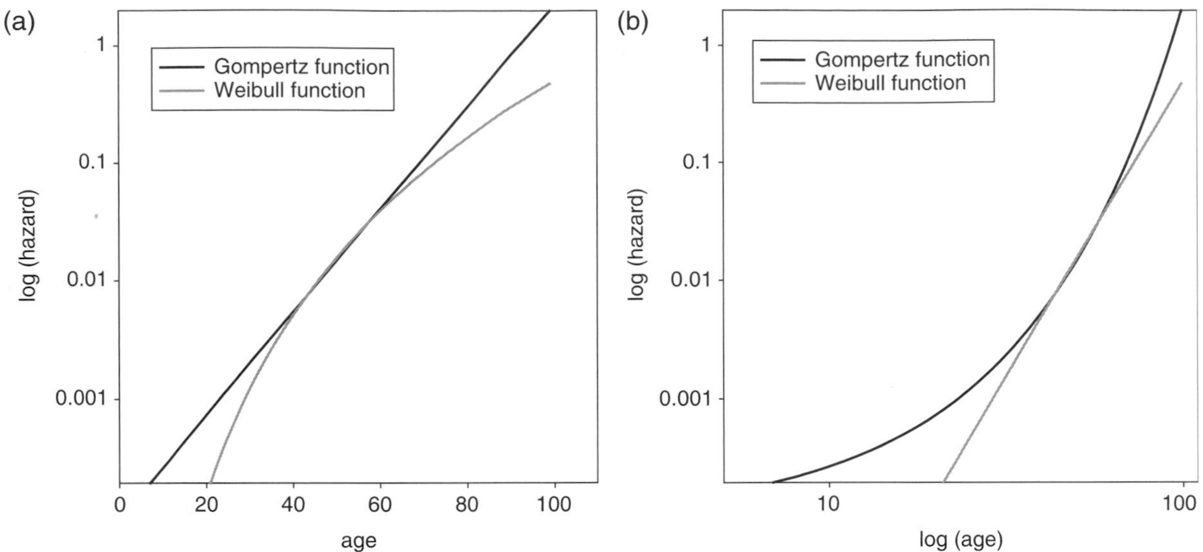

Figure 5.1. Plots of Gompertz and Weibull functions in different coordinates. (**a**) semilog (Gompertz) coordinates, (**b**) log-log (Weibull) coordinates. Source: Gavrilov and Gavrilova, 2005.

For the Gompertz function a misspecification of a starting age is not as important, because the shift in the age scale will still produce the same Gompertz function with the same slope parameter α. The data generated by the Gompertz function with different age shifts will all be linear and parallel to each other in the Gompertz plot. The situation is very different for the Weibull function—it is linear in the Weibull plot for only one particular starting age, and any shifts in a starting age produce a different function. Specifically, if a "true" starting age is larger than assumed, then the resulting function will be a nonlinear concave-up curve in the Weibull plot indicating model misspecification and leading to a bias in estimated parameters. Thus, researchers choosing the Weibull function for data analysis have first to resolve an uneasy biological problem—at what age does aging start?

An alternative graceful mathematical solution of this problem would be to move from a standard two-parameter Weibull function to a more general three-parameter Weibull function, which has an additional "location parameter" γ (Clark, 1975):

$$\mu(x) = \alpha(x - \gamma)^{\beta}, \quad x > \gamma, \quad \text{and equal to zero otherwise}$$

Parameters of this formula, including the location parameter γ, could be estimated from the data through standard fitting procedures, thus providing a computational answer to a question "when does aging start?" However, this computational answer might be shocking to researchers, unless they are familiar with the concept of initial damage load, which is discussed elsewhere (Gavrilov and Gavrilova, 1991; 2001; 2004b; 2005).

In addition to the Gompertz and the standard two-parameter Weibull laws, a more general failure law was also suggested and theoretically justified using the systems reliability theory. This law is known as the *binomial failure law* (Gavrilov and Gavrilova, 1991; 2001; 2005), and it represents a special case of the three-parameter Weibull function with a negative location parameter:

$$\mu(x) = \alpha(x_0 + x)^{\beta}$$

The parameter x_0 in this formula is called the *initial virtual age of the system, IVAS* (Gavrilov and Gavrilova, 1991; 2001; 2005). This parameter has the dimension of time and corresponds to the age by which an initially ideal system would have accumulated as many defects as a real system already has at the starting age (at $x = 0$). In particular, when the system is initially undamaged, the initial virtual age of the system is zero and the failure rate grows as a power function of age (the Weibull law). However, as the initial damage load is increasing, the failure kinetics starts to deviate from the Weibull law, and eventually it evolves to the Gompertz failure law at high levels of initial damage load. This is illustrated in Figure 5.2, which represents the Gompertz plot for the data generated by the binomial failure law with different levels of initial damage load (expressed in the units of initial virtual age).

Note that as the initial damage load increases the failure kinetics evolves from the concave-down curves typical to the Weibull function, to an almost linear dependence between the logarithm of failure rate and age (the Gompertz function). Thus, biological species dying according to the Gompertz law may have a high initial damage load, presumably because of developmental noise, and a clonal expansion of mutations occurred in the early development (Gavrilov and Gavrilova, 1991; 2001; 2003a; 2004b).

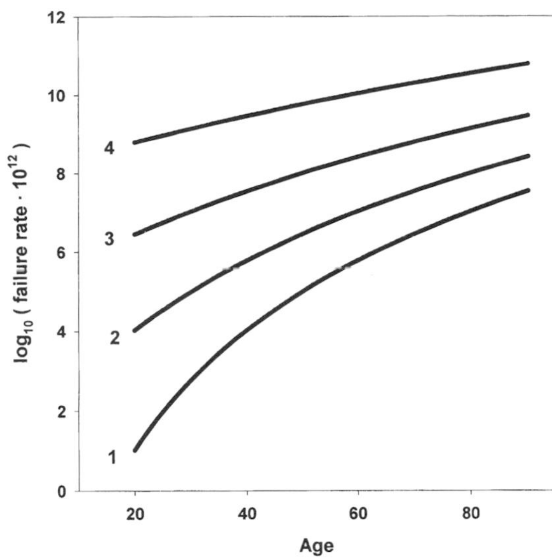

Figure 5.2. Failure kinetics of systems with different levels of initial damage. Dependence 1 is for initially ideal system (with no damage load). Dependence 2 is for system with initial damage load equivalent to damage accumulated by 20-year-old system. Dependencies 3 and 4 are for systems with initial damage load equivalent to damage accumulated respectively by 50-year-old and 100-year-old system. Source: Gavrilov and Gavrilova, 2005.

SYSTEM'S FAILURE AND RELIABILITY STRUCTURE

A branch of reliability theory, which studies reliability of an entire system given the reliability of its components and components' arrangement (reliability structure), is called system reliability theory (Rausand and Hoyland, 2003). System reliability involves the study of the overall performance of systems of interconnected components. The main objective of system reliability is the construction of a model that represents the times-to-failure of the entire system based on the life distributions of the components, from which it is composed. Consideration of some basic ideas and models of the system reliability theory is important because living organisms may be represented as structured systems comprised of organs, tissues and cells.

System reliability theory tells us that the component arrangement strongly affects the reliability of the whole system. The arrangement of components that are important for system reliability is also called reliability structure and is graphically represented by a schema of logical connectivity. It is important to understand that the model of logical connectivity is focused only on those components that are relevant for the functioning ability of the system. Components that do not play a direct role in the system's reliability usually are not included in the analyzed reliability structure (Rausand and Hoyland, 2003). For example, organs of vision are not included in the reliability structure of living organisms if death is the only type of failure to be analyzed (complete failure of vision does not cause an immediate death of the organism). On the other hand, if disability is the type of failure under consideration, then organs of vision should be included in the schema of reliability structure. Therefore, reliability structure does not necessarily reflect a physical structure of the object.

There are two major types of components arrangement (connection) in the system: components connected in series and components connected in parallel (Rausand and Hoyland, 2003). Here we consider a simple system of n statistically independent components, where failure of one component does not affect the failure rate of other components of the system.

Components connected in series

For a system of n independent components connected in series, the system fails if any one of the components fails, as in electrical circuits connected in series. Thus, failure of any one component results in failure of the whole system as in the Christmas tree lighting chains. Figure 5.3a shows a schema of the logical connectivity of the system in series.

This type of system is also called a weakest-link system (Ayyub and McCuen, 2003). In living organisms many organs and tissues (heart, lung, liver, brain) are vital for the organism's survival—a good example of series-connected components. Thus, the series connection means a logical connectivity, but not necessarily a physical or anatomical one.

The reliability of a system in series (with independent failure events of the components), P_s, is a product of reliabilities of its components:

$$P_s = p_1 p_2 \dots p_n$$

where $p_1 \dots p_n$ are reliabilities of the system's components. This formula explains why complex systems with many critical components are so sensitive to early failures of their components.

For example, for a system built of 458 critical components, the initial period of the components' life when their cumulative risk of failure is only 1% corresponds to the end of the system's life when 99% of systems have already failed. This difference between the lifetimes of systems and the potential lifetimes of their components is increasing further with system complexity (numbers of critical components). Therefore, the early failure kinetics of components is so important in determining the failure kinetics of a complex system for its entire life.

The failure rate of a system connected in series is the sum of failure rates of its components (Barlow *et al.*, 1965):

$$\mu_s = \mu_1 + \mu_2 + \mu_i \dots + \mu_n$$

If the failure rates of all components are equal, then the failure rate of the system with n components is $n\mu$. It follows from this formula that if the system's

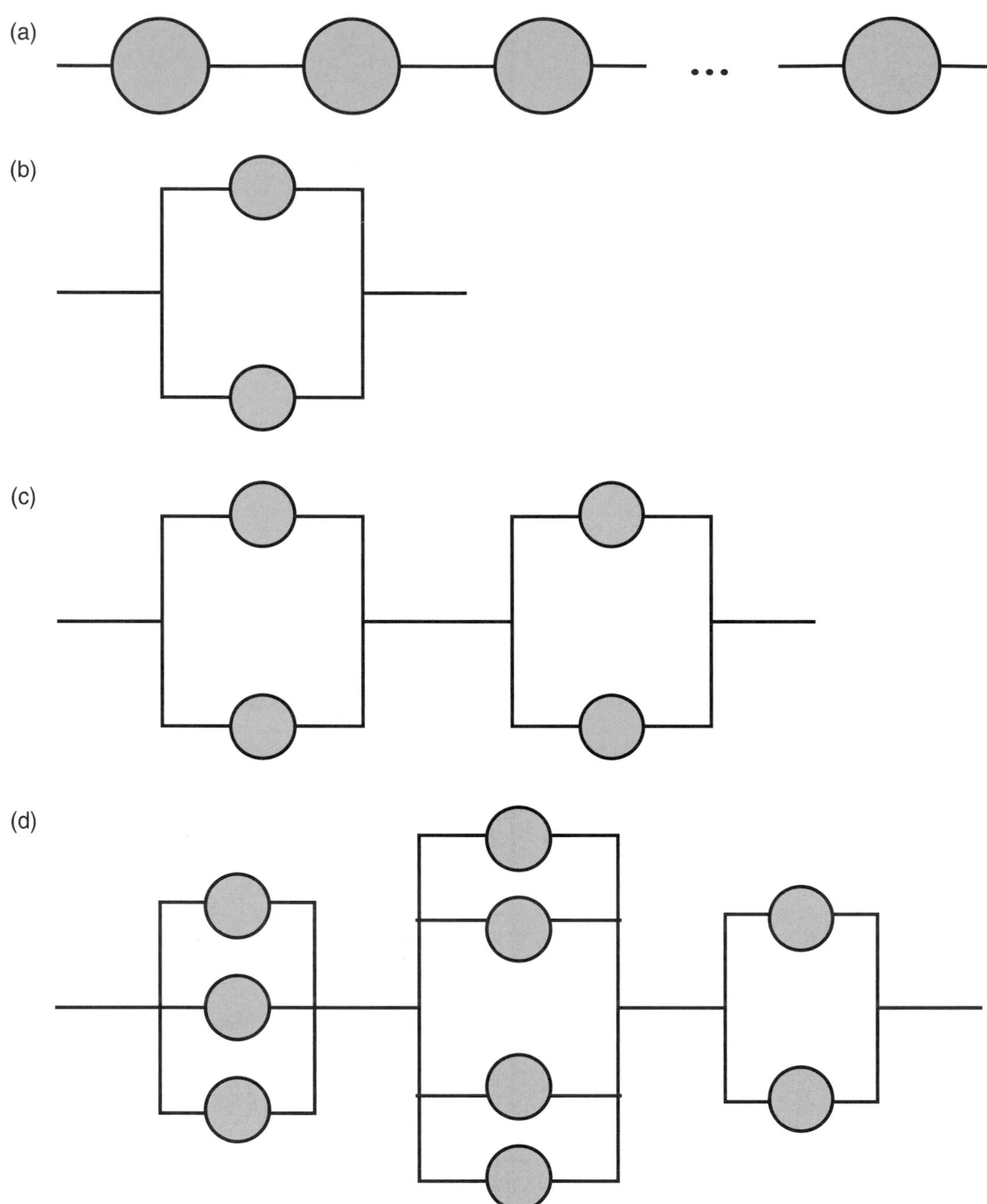

Figure 5.3. Logical schemas of systems with different types of elements connectivity: (**a**) system connected in series, (**b**) system connected in parallel, (**c**) series-parallel system, (**d**) series-parallel system with distributed redundancy, Source: Gavrilov and Gavrilova, 2005.

components do not age (μ_i = const), then the entire system connected in series does not age either.

Components connected in parallel

A parallel system of a n independent components fails only when all the components fail (as in electrical circuits connected in parallel). The logical structure of parallel system is presented in Figure 5.3b.

An example of a parallel system is a system with components all performing an identical function. This function will be destroyed only in the case when all the components fail. The number of additional components in parallel structure with one and the same function is called the redundancy or reserve of the system. In living organisms vital organs and tissues (such as liver, kidney, or pancreas) consist of many cells performing one and the same specialized function.

For a parallel system with n independent components the probability of the system's failure, Q_s, is the product of the probabilities of failure for its components, q_i:

$$Q_s = q_1 q_2 \ldots q_n$$

Hence the reliability of a parallel system, P_s, is related to the reliabilities of its components in the following way:

$$P_s = 1 - Q_s = 1 - (1 - p_1)(1 - p_2)\ldots(1 - p_n)$$

The reliability of a parallel system with components of equal reliability, p, is

$$P_s = 1 - (1 - p)^n$$

What is very important is the emergence of aging in parallel systems—a parallel system is aging even if it is built of nonaging components with a constant failure rate (see more details in the section on causes of failure rate increase with age).

In a real world most systems are more complex than simply series and parallel structures, but in many cases they can be represented as combinations of these structures.

More complex types of reliability structure

The simplest combination of the two reliability structures is a series–parallel system with equal redundancy shown in Figure 5.3c.

A general series–parallel system is a system of m subsystems (blocks) connected in series, where each block is a set of n components connected in parallel. It turns out that even if the components themselves are not aging, the system as a whole has an aging behavior—its failure rate grows with age according to the Weibull law and then levels off at advanced ages (Gavrilov and Gavrilova, 1991; 2001, 2003a). This type of system is important to consider, because a living organism can be presented as a system of critical organs and tissues connected in series, while each organ consists of specialized cells connected in parallel. A reliability model for this type of system is described in more detail in the section on causes of failure rate increase with age.

Another type of reliability structure, a series–parallel system with distributed redundancy, was introduced by Gavrilov and Gavrilova in 1991 (Gavrilov and Gavrilova, 1991; 2001). The series-connected blocks of this system have nonequal redundancy (different numbers of elements connected in parallel), and the elements are distributed between the system's blocks according to some particular distribution law (see schema in Figure 5.3d).

Gavrilov and Gavrilova (1991; 2001) studied the reliability and failure rate of series–parallel systems with distributed redundancy for two special cases: (1) the redundancy distributed within an organism according to the Poisson law or (2) according to the binomial law. They found that the failure rate of such systems initially grows according to the Gompertz law (in the case of the Poisson distributed redundancy) or binomial failure law in the case of the binomially distributed redundancy (Gavrilov and Gavrilova, 1991; 2001). At advanced ages the failure rate for both systems asymptotically approaches an upper limit (mortality plateau). Reliability models for this type of system are described in more detail in the section on theoretical models of systems failure in aging.

Now that the basic concepts of reliability theory have been discussed, we may proceed to linking them to empirical observations on aging and mortality.

Empirical Observations on Systems Failure in Aging

GENERAL OVERVIEW OF FAILURE KINETICS

There is a striking similarity between living organisms and technical devices in the general age pattern of their failures—in both cases the failure rate usually follows the so-called bathtub curve (Figure 5.4).

The bathtub curve of failure rate is a classic concept presented in all textbooks on reliability theory (Ayyub and McCuen, 2003; Barlow and Proshan, 1975; Rausand and Hoyland, 2003).

The bathtub curve consists of three periods. Initially the failure rates are high and decrease with age. This period is called the "working-in" period and the period of "burning-out" of defective components. For example, the

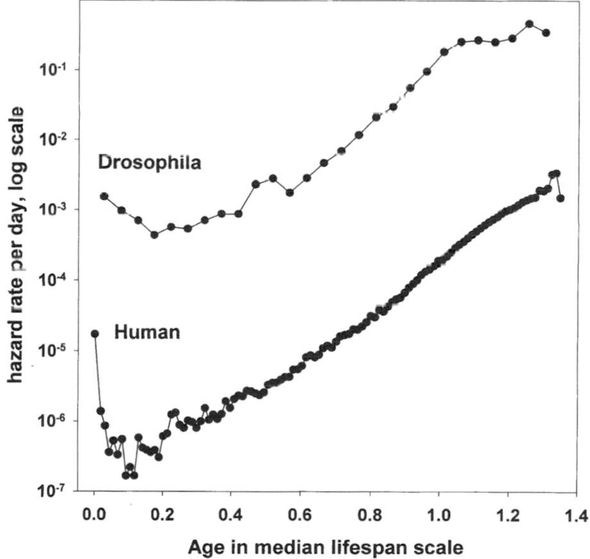

Figure 5.4. Bathtub mortality curves for humans and fruit flies. Mortality is estimated on a daily basis; age is expressed in a median lifespan scale (a similar approach was used by Pearl and Miner, 1935 and Carnes *et al.*, 1998). Mortality for *Drosophila melanogaster* was calculated using data published by Hall (1969). Mortality for humans was calculated using the official Swedish female life table for 1985 (ages 0-80 years), and the 1980-90 decennial life table for Swedish females available in the Kannisto-Thatcher Database on Old Age Mortality, http://www.demogr.mpg.de/databases/ktdb (ages over 80 years), Source: Gavrilov and Gavrilova, 2005.

risk for a new computer to fail is often higher at the very start, but then those computers that did not fail initially work normally afterwards. The same period exists early in life for most living organisms, including humans, and it is called the "infant mortality" period. Then follows the second period called "the normal working period," corresponding to an age of low and approximately constant failure rates. This period also exists in humans, but unfortunately it is rather short (10–15 years) and ends too soon. Then the third period, "the aging period," starts, which involves an inexorable rise in the failure rate with age. In most living organisms, including humans, this rise in failure rates follows an explosive exponential trajectory (the Gompertz curve). For humans, the aging period lies approximately within the interval 20–100 years. Thus there is a remarkable similarity in the failure patterns of technical and biological systems. This similarity is reinforced further by the fact that at extreme old ages there is one more, the fourth period common to both technical devices and living organisms (Economos, 1979). This period is known in biology as a period of late-life mortality leveling-off (Carey and Liedo, 1995; Clark and Guadalupe, 1995; Economos, 1979; Fukui *et al.*, 1993; 1996; Vaupel *et al.*, 1998), and also as the late-life mortality deceleration law (Fukui *et al.*, 1993; 1996; Khazaeli *et al.*, 1996; Partridge and Mangel, 1999).

FAILURE LAWS IN SURVIVAL STUDIES

Attempts to develop a fundamental quantitative theory of aging, mortality, and lifespan have deep historical roots. In 1825, the British actuary Benjamin Gompertz discovered a law of mortality (Gompertz, 1825), known today as the Gompertz law (Finch, 1990; Gavrilov and Gavrilova, 1991; Olshansky and Carnes, 1997; Strehler, 1978). Specifically, he found that the force of mortality increases in geometrical progression with the age of adult humans. According to the Gompertz law, human mortality rates double about every 8 years of adult age.

Gompertz also proposed the first mathematical model to explain the exponential increase in mortality rate with age (Gompertz, 1825). In reality, system failure rates may contain both nonaging and aging terms as, for example, in the case of the *Gompertz–Makeham law* of mortality (Finch, 1990; Gavrilov and Gavrilova, 1991; Makeham, 1860; Strehler, 1978):

$$\mu(x) = A + Re^{\alpha x}$$

In this formula the first, age-independent term (Makeham parameter, A) designates the constant, "nonaging" component of the failure rate (presumably due to external causes of death, such as accidents and acute infections), while the second, age-dependent term (the Gompertz function, $Re^{\alpha x}$) designates the "aging" component, presumably due to deaths from age-related degenerative diseases like cancer and heart disease.

The validity of the Gompertz–Makeham law of mortality can be illustrated graphically, when the logarithms of death rates without the Makeham parameter ($\mu_x - A$) are increasing with age in a linear fashion. The log–linear increase in death rates (adjusted for the Makeham term) with age is indeed a very common phenomenon for many human populations at ages 35–70 years (Gavrilov and Gavrilova, 1991).

Note that the slope coefficient α characterizes an "apparent aging rate" (how rapid is the age-deterioration in mortality)—if α is equal to zero, there is no apparent aging (death rates do not increase with age).

At advanced ages (after age 70), the "old-age mortality deceleration" takes place—death rates are increasing with age at a slower pace than expected from the Gompertz–Makeham law. This mortality deceleration eventually produces "late-life mortality leveling-off" and "late-life mortality plateaus" at extreme old ages (Curtsinger *et al.*, 1992; Economos, 1979; 1983; Gavrilov and Gavrilova, 1991; Greenwood and Irwin, 1939; Vaupel *et al.*, 1998). Actuaries (including Gompertz himself) first noted this phenomenon and proposed a logistic formula for mortality growth with age in order to account for mortality fall-off at advanced ages (Perks, 1932; Beard, 1959; 1971). Greenwood and Irwin (1939) provided a detailed description of this phenomenon in humans and even made the first estimates for the asymptotic value of human mortality (see also review by Olshansky, 1998). According to their estimates, the mortality kinetics of long-lived individuals is close to the law of radioactive decay with half-time approximately equal to 1 year.

The same phenomenon of "almost nonaging" survival dynamics at extreme old ages is detected in many other biological species. In some species the mortality plateau can occupy a sizable part of their life (see Figure 5.5).

Biologists have been well aware of mortality leveling-off since the 1960s. For example, Lindop (1961) and Sacher (1966) discussed mortality deceleration in mice. Strehler and Mildvan (1960) considered mortality deceleration at advanced ages as a prerequisite for all mathematical models of aging to explain. Later A. Economos published a series of articles claiming a priority in the discovery of a "non-Gompertzian paradigm of mortality" (Economos, 1979; 1980; 1983; 1985). He found that mortality leveling-off is observed in rodents (guinea pigs, rats, mice) and invertebrates (nematodes, shrimps, bdelloid rotifers, fruit flies, degenerate medusae *Campanularia Flexuosa*). In the 1990s the phenomenon of mortality deceleration and leveling-off became widely known after some publications demonstrated mortality leveling-off in large samples of *Drosophila melanogaster* (Curtsinger *et al.*, 1992) and medflies *Ceratitis capitata* (Carey *et al.*, 1992), including isogenic strains of *Drosophila* (Curtsinger *et al.*, 1992; Fukui *et al.*, 1993; 1996). Mortality plateaus at advanced ages are observed for some other insects: house fly *Musca vicina* and blowfly *Calliphora erythrocephala* (Gavrilov, 1980), bruchid

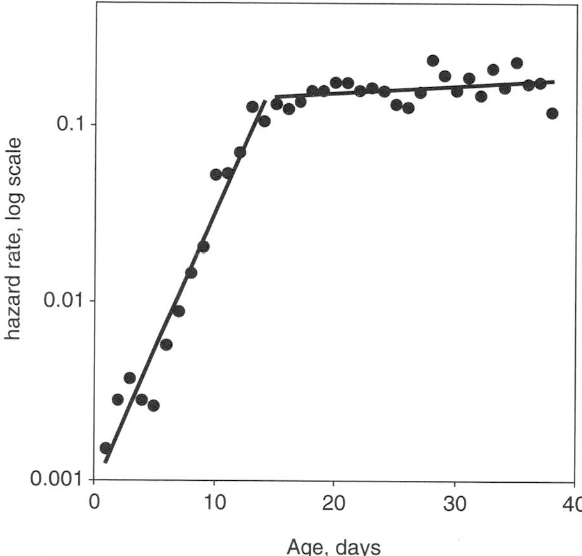

Figure 5.5. Mortality leveling-off in a population of 4,650 male house flies, Hazard rates were computed using life table of house fly, *Musca domestica*, published by Rockstein and Lieberman (1959). Source: Gavrilov and Gavrilova, 2005.

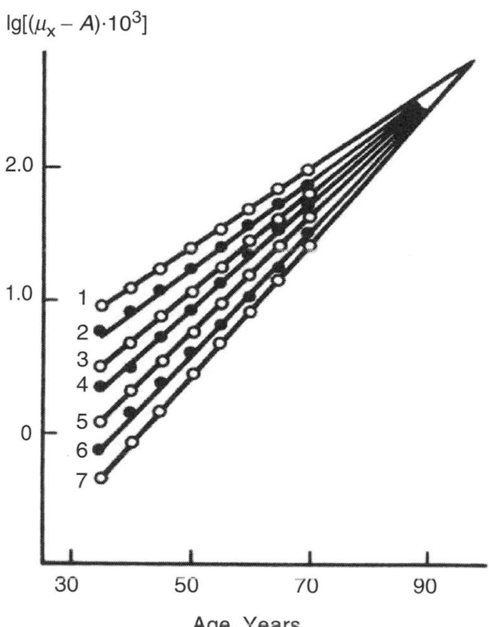

Figure 5.6. Compensation Law of Mortality. Convergence of mortality rates in different populations at advanced ages. Death rates (with removed age-independent external mortality component) are plotted in a log scale as a function of age in the following countries: 1 – India, 1941–1950, males. 2 – Turkey, 1950–1951, males. 3 – Kenya, 1969, males. 4 – Northern Ireland, 1950–1952, males. 5 – England and Wales, 1930–1932, females. 6 – Austria, 1959–1961, females. 7 – Norway, 1956–1960, females. Adapted from Gavrilov and Gavrilova, "The Biology of Life Span," 1991.

beetle *Callosobruchus maculates* (Tatar *et al.*, 1993), fruit flies *Anastrepha ludens*, *Anastrepha obliqua*, *Anastrepha serpentine* and a parasitoid wasp *Diachasmimorpha longiacaudtis* (Vaupel *et al.*, 1998).

Interestingly, the failure kinetics of manufactured products (steel samples, industrial relays, and motor heat insulators) also demonstrates the same "nonaging" pattern at the end of their "lifespan" (Economos, 1979). This phenomenon is presenting a theoretical challenge to many models and theories of aging. One interesting corollary from these intriguing observations is that there seems to be no fixed upper limit for individual lifespan (Gavrilov, 1984; Gavrilov and Gavrilova, 1991; Wilmoth, 1997).

This observation calls for a very general explanation of this apparently paradoxical "no aging at extreme ages" phenomenon, which will be discussed in this chapter.

Another empirical observation, the *compensation law of mortality*, in its strong form refers to *mortality convergence*, when higher values for the parameter α (in the Gompertz function) are compensated by lower values of the parameter R in different populations of a given species:

$$\ln(R) = \ln(M) - B\alpha$$

where B and M are universal species-specific invariants. Sometimes this relationship is also called the Strehler-Mildvan correlation (Strehler, 1978; Strehler and Mildvan, 1960), although that particular correlation was largely an artifact of the opposite biases in parameters estimation caused by not taking into account the age-independent mortality component, the Makeham term A (see Gavrilov and Gavrilova, 1991; Golubev, 2004). Parameter B is called the species-specific lifespan (95 years for humans), and parameter M is called the species-specific mortality rate (0.5 year^{-1} for humans). These parameters are the coordinates for convergence of all the mortality trajectories into one single point (within a given biological species), when extrapolated by the Gompertz function (Gavrilov and Gavrilova, 1979; 1991). This means that high mortality rates in disadvantaged populations (within a given species) are *compensated* for by a low apparent "aging rate" (longer mortality doubling period). As a result of this compensation, the relative differences in mortality rates tend to decrease with age within a given biological species (Figure 5.6).

In those cases when the compensation law of mortality is not observed in its strong form, it may still be valid in its weak form—i.e., the relative differences in mortality rates of compared populations tend to decrease with age in many species. Explanation of the compensation law of mortality is a great challenge for many theories of aging and longevity (Gavrilov and Gavrilova, 1991; Strehler, 1978).

There are some exceptions from both the Gompertz law of mortality and the compensation law of mortality that have to be understood and explained. There were reports that in some cases the organisms die according to the Weibull (power) law (see the section on basic failure models). The Weibull law is more commonly applicable to technical devices (Barlow and Proschan, 1975; Rigdon and Basu, 2000; Weibull, 1951), while the Gompertz law is more common in biological systems (Finch, 1990; Gavrilov and Gavrilova, 1991; Strehler, 1978). As was already noted, the exponential Gompertzian increase in age-specific mortality is observed for many biological species including fruit flies *Drosophila melanogaster*, nematodes, mosquitoes, human lice, flour beetles, mice, rats, dogs, horses, mountain sheep, baboons and humans. Comparative meta-analysis of 129 life tables for fruit flies as well as 285 life tables for humans demonstrates that the Gompertz law of mortality provides a much better data fit for each of these two biological species, compared to the Weibull law (Gavrilov and Gavrilova, 1991, pp. 55–56, 68–72). Possible explanations why organisms prefer to die according to the Gompertz law, while technical devices typically fail according to the Weibull law are provided elsewhere (Gavrilov and Gavrilova, 1991; 2001; 2005) and will be discussed later in this chapter (see the section on theoretical models of systems failure in aging).

Both the Gompertz and the Weibull failure laws have a fundamental explanation rooted in reliability theory (Barlow and Proschan, 1975) and are the only two theoretically possible *limiting extreme value distributions* for systems whose lifespans are determined by the first failed component (Gumbel, 1958; Galambos, 1978). In other words, as the system becomes more and more complex (contains more vital components, each being critical for survival), its lifespan distribution may asymptotically approach one of the only two theoretically possible limiting distributions—either Gompertz or Weibull (depending on the early kinetics of failure of system components). The two limit theorems in the statistics of extremes (Gumbel, 1958; Galambos, 1978) make the Gompertz and the Weibull failure laws as fundamental as are some other famous limiting distributions known in regular statistics, e.g., the normal distribution and the Poisson distribution. It is puzzling, however, why organisms prefer to die according to the Gompertz law, while technical devices typically fail according to the Weibull law. One possible explanation of this mystery is suggested later in this chapter.

Thus, a comprehensive theory of species aging and longevity should provide answers to the following questions:

1. Why do most biological species deteriorate with age (i.e., die more often as they grow older) while some primitive organisms do not demonstrate such a clear mortality growth with age (Austad, 2001; Finch, 1990; Haranghy and Balázs, 1980; Martinez, 1998)?
2. Specifically, why do mortality rates increase exponentially with age in many adult species (Gompertz law)? How should we handle cases when the Gompertzian mortality law is not applicable?
3. Why does the age-related increase in mortality rates vanish at older ages? Why do mortality rates eventually decelerate compared to predictions of the Gompertz law, occasionally demonstrate leveling-off (late-life mortality plateau), or even a paradoxical decrease at extreme ages?
4. How do we explain the so-called compensation law of mortality (Gavrilov and Gavrilova, 1991)?

Any theory of human aging has to explain these last three rules, known collectively as mortality, or failure, laws. And reliability theory, by way of a clutch of equations, covers all of them (see the section on theoretical models of systems failure in aging, and Gavrilov and Gavrilova, 1991, 2001, 2005).

DECLINE IN SYSTEMS' REDUNDANCY WITH AGE

Many age changes in living organisms can be explained by cumulative effects of cell loss over time. For example, the very common phenomenon of hair graying with age is caused by depletion of hair follicle melanocytes (Commo *et al.*, 2004). Melanocyte density in human epidermis declines gradually with age at a rate approximately 0.8% per year (Gilchrest *et al.*, 1979). Hair graying is a relatively benign phenomenon, but cell loss can also lead to more serious consequences.

Recent studies found that such conditions as atherosclerosis, atherosclerotic inflammation, and consequent thromboembolic complications could be linked to age-related exhaustion of progenitor cells responsible for arterial repair (Goldschmidt-Clermont, 2003; Libby, 2003; Rauscher *et al.*, 2003). Taking these progenitor cells from young mice and adding them to experimental animals prevents atherosclerosis progression and atherosclerotic inflammation (Goldschmidt-Clermont, 2003; Rauscher *et al.*, 2003).

Age-dependent decline in cardiac function is also linked to the failure of cardiac stem cells to replace dying myocytes with new functioning cells (Capogrossi, 2004). It was found that aging-impaired cardiac angiogenic function could be restored by adding endothelial precursor cells derived from the young bone marrow (Edelberg *et al.*, 2002).

Chronic renal failure is known to be associated with decreased number of endothelial progenitor cells (Choi *et al.*, 2004). People with diminished numbers of nephrons in their kidneys are more likely to suffer from hypertension (Keller *et al.*, 2003), and the number of glomeruli decreases with human age (Nyengaard and Bendtsen, 1992).

Humans generally lose 30–40% of their skeletal muscle fibers by age 80 (Leeuwenburgh, 2003), which contributes to such adverse health outcomes as sarcopenia and frailty. Loss of striated muscle cells in such places as rhabdosphincter from 87.6% in a 5-week-old child to only 34.2% in a 91-year-old has obvious implications for urological failure—incontinence (Strasser, 2000).

A progressive loss of dopaminergic neurons in substantia nigra results in Parkinson's disease, loss of GABAergic neurons in striatum produces Huntington's disease, loss of motor neurons is responsible for amyotrophic lateral sclerosis, and loss of neurons in cortex causes Alzheimer's disease over time (Baizabal *et al.*, 2003). A study of cerebella from normal males aged 19–84 years revealed that the global white matter was reduced by 26% with age, and a selective 40% loss of both Purkinje and granule cells was observed in the anterior lobe. Furthermore a 30% loss of volume, mostly due to a cortical volume loss, was found in the anterior lobe, which is predominantly involved in motor control (Andersen *et al.*, 2003).

The phenomenon of human aging of menopause also is caused by loss of ovarian cells. For example, the female human fetus at age 4–5 months possesses 6–7 million eggs (oocytes). By birth, this number drops to 1–2 million and declines even further. At the start of puberty in normal girls, there are only 0.3–0.5 million eggs—just only 4–8% of initial numbers (Gosden, 1985; Finch and Kirkwood, 2000; Wallace and Kelsey, 2004). It is now well established that the exhaustion of the ovarian follicle numbers over time is responsible for menopause (reproductive aging and failure), and women having higher ovarian reserve have longer reproductive lifespans (Wallace and Kelsey, 2004). When young ovaries were transplanted to old post-reproductive mice, their reproductive function was restored for a while (Cargill *et al.*, 2003). This example illustrates a general idea that aging largely occurs because of cell loss, which starts early in life.

Loss of cells with age is not limited to the human species and is observed in other animals as well. For example, a nematode *C. elegans* demonstrates a gradual, progressive deterioration of muscle, resembling human sarcopenia (Herndon *et al.*, 2002). The authors of this study also found that the behavioral ability of nematodes was a better predictor of life expectancy than chronological age.

Interestingly, caloric restriction can prevent cell loss (Cohen *et al.*, 2004; McKiernan *et al.*, 2004), which may explain why caloric restriction delays the onset of numerous age-associated diseases and can significantly increase lifespan in mammals (Masoro, 2003).

In terms of reliability theory the loss of cells with age is a loss of system redundancy, and therefore this chapter will focus further on the effects of redundancy loss on systems aging and failure.

Causes of Failure Rate Increase with Age

THE ORIGIN OF AGE-RELATED INCREASE IN FAILURE RATES

The aging period for most species occupies the greater part of their lifespan; therefore any model of mortality must explain the existence of this period. It turns out that the phenomena of mortality increase with age and the subsequent mortality leveling-off are theoretically predicted to be an inevitable feature of all reliability models that consider aging as a progressive accumulation of random damage (Gavrilov and Gavrilova, 1991). The detailed mathematical proof of this prediction for some particular models is provided elsewhere (Gavrilov and Gavrilova, 1991; 2001) and is briefly described in the next sections of this chapter.

The simplest schema, which demonstrates an emergence of aging in a redundant system, is presented in Figure 5.7.

If the destruction of an organism occurs not in one but in two or more sequential random stages, this is sufficient for the phenomenon of aging (mortality increase) to appear and then to vanish at older ages. Each stage of destruction corresponds to one of the organism's vitally important structures being damaged. In the simplest organisms with unique critical structures, this damage usually leads to death. Therefore, defects in such organisms do not accumulate, and the organisms themselves do not age—they just die when damaged. For example, the inactivation of microbial cells and spores exposed to a hostile environment (such as heat) follows approximately a nonaging mortality kinetics; their semilogarithmic survival curves are almost linear (Peleg *et al.*, 2003). This observation of nonaging survival

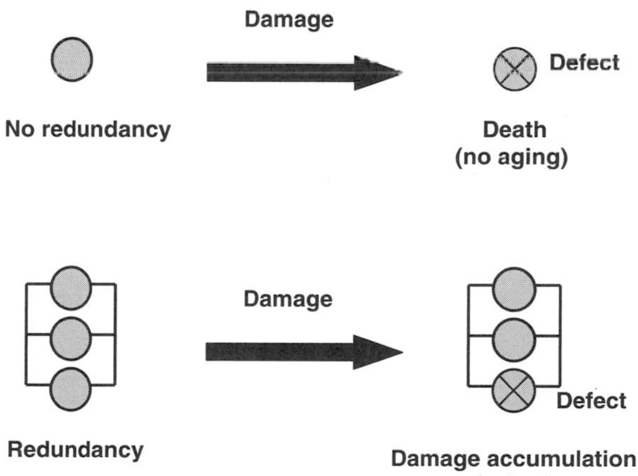

Figure 5.7. Redundancy creates both damage tolerance and damage accumulation (aging). Systems without redundancy (on the top) fail every time when they are damaged, and therefore damage is not accumulated among survivors (no aging). Redundant systems (on the bottom) can sustain damage because of their redundancy, but this damage tolerance leads to damage accumulation (aging).

dynamics is extensively used in the calculation of the efficacy of sterilization processes in medicine and food preservation (Brock *et al.*, 1994; Davis *et al.*, 1990; Jay, 1996). A similar nonaging pattern of inactivation kinetics is often observed for viruses (Andreadis and Palsson, 1997; Kundi, 1999) and enzymes (Kurganov, 2002; Gouda *et al.*, 2003).

In more complex systems with many vital structures and significant redundancy, every occurrence of damage does not lead to death (unless the environment is particularly hostile) because of their redundancy. Defects accumulate, therefore, giving rise to the phenomenon of aging (mortality increase). Thus, aging is a direct consequence (trade-off) of a system's redundancies, which ensure increased reliability and an increased lifespan of more complex organisms. As defects accumulate, the redundancy in the number of elements finally disappears. As a result of this *redundancy exhaustion*, the organism degenerates into a system with no redundancy (that is, a system with elements connected in series, in which any new defect leads to death). In such a state, no further accumulation of damage can be achieved, and the mortality rate levels off.

Reliability theory predicts that a system may deteriorate with age even if it is built from nonaging elements with a constant failure rate. The key issue here is the system's redundancy for irreplaceable elements, which is responsible for the aging phenomenon. In other words, each particular step of system destruction/deterioration may seem to be apparently random (no aging, just occasional failure by chance), but if a system failure requires a sequence of several such steps (not just a single step of destruction), then the system as a whole may have an aging behavior.

The positive effect of systems' redundancy is *damage tolerance*, which decreases the risk of failure (mortality) and increases lifespan. However damage tolerance makes it possible for damage to be tolerated and accumulated over time, thus producing the aging phenomenon.

The next section provides a mathematical illustration for these ideas.

THE SIMPLEST RELIABILITY MODEL OF AGING

In this section we show that a system built of nonaging components demonstrates an aging behavior (mortality growth with age) and subsequent mortality leveling-off.

Consider a parallel system built of n nonaging elements with a constant failure rate μ and reliability (survival) function $e^{-\mu x}$ (see also Figure 5.3b). We already showed (see the system's failure and reliability structure section) that in this case the reliability function of the entire parallel system is

$$S(x) = 1 - (1 - p)^n = 1 - (1 - e^{-\mu x})^n$$

This formula corresponds to the simplest case when the failure of elements is statistically independent. More complex models would require specific assumptions or prior knowledge on the exact type of interdependence in elements failure. One such model known as "the model of the avalanche-like destruction" is described elsewhere (see pp. 246–251 in Gavrilov, Gavrilova, 1991) and is briefly summarized in the theoretical models of systems failure in aging section.

Consequently, the failure rate of the entire system $\mu_s(x)$, can be written as follows:

$$\mu_s(x) = \frac{-dS(x)}{S(x)dx} = \frac{n\mu e^{-\mu x}(1 - e^{-\mu x})^{n-1}}{1 - (1 - e^{-\mu x})^n} \approx n\mu^n x^{n-1}$$

when $x \ll 1/\mu$ (early-life period approximation, when $1 - e^{-\mu x} \approx \mu x$);

$$\approx \mu$$

when $x \gg 1/\mu$ (late-life period approximation, when $1 - e^{-\mu x} \approx 1$).

Thus, the failure rate of a system initially grows as a power function n of age (the Weibull law). Then the tempo at which the failure rate grows declines, and the failure rate approaches asymptotically an upper limit equal to μ.

Here we should pay attention to three significant points. First, a system constructed of nonaging elements is now behaving like an aging object: aging is a direct consequence of the redundancy of the system (redundancy in the number of elements). Second, at very high ages the phenomenon of aging apparently disappears (failure rate levels off), as redundancy in the number of elements vanishes. The failure rate approaches an upper limit, which is totally independent of the initial number of elements, but coincides with the rate of their loss (parameter μ). Third, the systems with different initial levels of redundancy (parameter n) will have very different failure rates in early life, but these differences will eventually vanish as failure rates approach the upper limit determined by the rate of elements' loss (parameter μ). Thus, the compensation law of mortality (in its weak form) is an expected outcome of this illustrative model.

Note also that the identical parallel systems in this example do not die simultaneously when their elements fail by chance. A common view in biology is the idea that all the members of homogeneous population in a hypothetical constant environment should die simultaneously so that the survival curve of such a population would look like a rectangle. This idea stems from the basic principles of quantitative genetics, which assume implicitly that every animal of a given genotype has the same genetically determined lifespan so that all variation of survival time around a genotype mean results from the environmental variance. George Sacher (1977) pointed out that this concept is not applicable to longevity and used an analogy with radioactive decay in his arguments.

Even the simplest parallel system has a specific lifespan distribution determined entirely by a stochastic nature of the aging process. In order to account for this stochasticity it was proposed to use a stochastic variance component of lifespan in addition to genetic and environmental components of phenotypic lifespan variance (Gavrilov and Gavrilova, 1991). The stochastic nature of the system's destruction also produces heterogeneity in an initially homogeneous population. This kind of induced heterogeneity was observed in isogenic strains of nematodes, in which aging resulted in substantial heterogeneity in behavioral capacity among initially homogeneous worms kept in controlled environmental conditions (Herndon *et al.*, 2002).

The graph shown in Figure 5.8 depicts mortality trajectories for five systems with different degrees of redundancy.

System 1 has only one unique element (no redundancy), and it has the highest failure rate, which does not depend on age (no aging). System 2 has two elements connected in parallel (one extra element is redundant), and the failure rate initially increases with age (aging appears). The apparent rate of aging can be characterized by a slope coefficient that is equal to 1. Finally, the failure rate levels off at advanced ages. Systems 3, 4, and 5 have, respectively, three, four, and five elements connected in parallel (two, three, and four extra elements are redundant), and the failure rate initially increases with age at an apparent aging rate (slope coefficient) of 2, 3, and 4, respectively. Finally, the mortality trajectories of each system level off at advanced ages at exactly the same upper limit to the mortality rate.

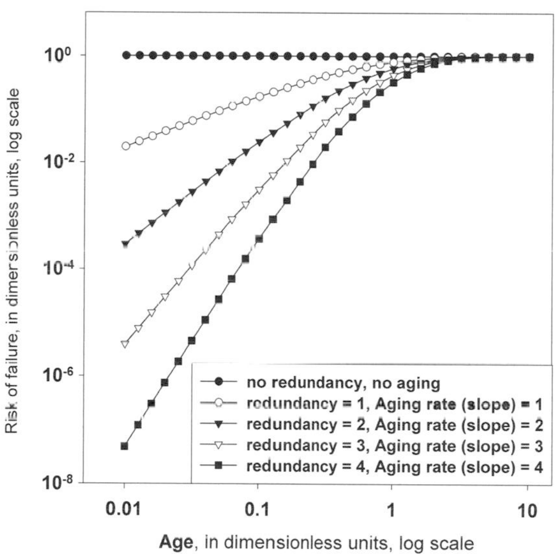

Figure 5.8. Failure kinetics of systems with different levels of redundancy. The dependence of the logarithm of mortality force (failure rate) on the logarithm of age in five systems with different levels of redundancy (computer simulation experiment). The scales for mortality rates (vertical axis) and for age (horizontal axis) are presented in dimensionless units (μ_s/μ) for mortality rates, and μx for age), to ensure the generalizability of the results (invariance of graphs on failure rate of the elements in the system, parameter μ). Also, the log scale is used to explore the system behavior in a wide range of ages (0.01–10 units) and failure rates (0.00000001–1.0 units). Dependence 1 is for the system containing only one unique element (no redundancy). Dependence 2 is for the system containing two elements connected in parallel (degree of redundancy = 1). Dependencies 3, 4 and 5 are for systems containing, respectively, 3, 4 and 5 elements connected in parallel (with increasing levels of redundancy). Source: Gavrilov and Gavrilova, 2005.

This computational example illustrates the following statements: (1) Aging is a direct consequence of a system's redundancy, and the expression of aging is directly related to the degree of a system's redundancy. Specifically, an apparent relative aging rate is equal to the degree of redundancy in parallel systems. (2) All mortality trajectories tend to converge with age, so that the compensation law of mortality is observed. (3) All mortality trajectories level off at advanced ages, and a mortality plateau is observed. Thus, the major aging phenomena (aging itself, the compensation law of mortality, late-life mortality deceleration, and late-life mortality plateaus) are already observed in the simplest redundant systems. However, to explain the Gompertz law of mortality, an additional idea of initial damage load should be taken into account (see next section).

Theoretical Models of Systems Failure in Aging

HIGHLY REDUNDANT SYSTEM REPLETE WITH DEFECTS

It was demonstrated in the previous section that the failure rate of a simple parallel system grows with age according to the Weibull law. This model analyzed initially ideal structures in which all the elements are functional from the outset. This standard assumption may be justified for technical devices manufactured from pretested components, but it is not justified for living organisms, replete with initial defects (see Gavrilov and Gavrilova, 1991; 2001; 2004b; 2005).

Following the tradition of the reliability theory, we start our analysis with reliability of an individual system (or homogeneous population). This model of series–parallel structure with distributed redundancy was suggested by Gavrilov and Gavrilova in 1991 and described in more detail in 2001.

Consider first a series–parallel model in which initially functional elements occur very rarely with low probability q, so that the distribution of the organism's subsystems (blocks) according to the initial functioning elements they contain is described by the Poisson law with parameter $\lambda = nq$. Parameter λ corresponds to the mean number of initially functional elements in a block.

As has already been noted, the failure rate of a system constructed out of m blocks connected in series is equal to the sum of the failure rates of these blocks, μ_b (Barlow *et al.*, 1965):

$$\mu_s = \sum \mu_b = \sum_{i=1}^{n} mP_i\mu_b(i) = mCe^{-\lambda}\sum_{i=1}^{n}\frac{\lambda^i\mu_b(i)}{i!}$$

where P_i is the probability of a block to have i initially functioning elements. Parameter C is a normalizing factor that ensures the sum of the probabilities of all possible outcomes being equal to unity (see Gavrilov, Gavrilova, 1991; 2001). For sufficiently high values of n and λ, the normalizing factor turns out to be hardly greater than unity.

Using the formula for failure rate of a block of elements connected in parallel (see the simplest reliability model of aging section), we obtain the final expression for the series–parallel system with distributed redundancy:

$$\mu_s = \mu\lambda mCe^{-\lambda}\sum_{i=1}^{n}\frac{(\lambda\mu x)^{i-1}}{(i-1)!} \approx R(e^{\alpha x} - \varepsilon(x)) \approx Re^{\alpha x}$$

where $R = Cm\lambda\mu e^{-\lambda}$, $\alpha = \lambda\mu$

$\varepsilon(x)$ is close to zero for large n and small x (initial period of life; see Gavrilov, Gavrilova, 1991, 2001 for more detail).

In the early-life period (when $x \ll 1/\mu$) the mortality kinetics of this system follows the exponential Gompertzian law.

In the late-life period (when $x \gg 1/\mu$), the failure rate levels off and the mortality plateau is observed:

$$\mu_s(x) \approx m\mu$$

If the age-independent mortality (A) also exists in addition to the Gompertz function, we obtain the well-known Gompertz–Makeham law described earlier. At advanced ages the rate of mortality decelerates and approaches asymptotically an upper limit equal to $m\mu$.

The model explains not only the exponential increase in mortality rate with age and the subsequent leveling-off, but also the compensation law of mortality:

$$\ln(R) = \ln(Cm\alpha) - \frac{\alpha}{\mu} = \ln(M) - B\alpha$$

where $M = Cm\alpha$, $B = 1/\mu$.

According to this model, the compensation law is inevitable whenever differences in mortality arise from differences in the parameter λ (the mean number of initially functional elements in the block), while the "true aging rate" (rate of elements' loss, μ) is similar in different populations of a given species (presumably because of homeostasis). In this case, the species-specific lifespan estimated from the compensation law as an expected age at mortality convergence (95 years for humans, see Gavrilov and Gavrilova, 1991) characterizes the mean lifetime of the elements ($1/\mu$).

The model also predicts certain deviations from the exact mortality convergence in a specific direction because the parameter M proved to be a function of the parameter α according to this model (see earlier). This prediction could be tested in future studies.

It also follows from this model that even small progress in optimizing the processes of ontogenesis and increasing the numbers of initially functional elements (λ) can potentially result in a remarkable fall in mortality and a significant improvement in lifespan.

The model assumes that most of the elements in the system are initially nonfunctional. *This interpretation of the assumption can be relaxed, however, because most nonfunctional elements (e.g., cells) may have already died and been eliminated by the time the adult organism is formed.* In fact, the model is based on the hypothesis that the number of *functional* elements in the blocks is described by the Poisson distribution, and the fate of defective elements and their death in no way affects the conclusions of the model. Therefore, the model may be reformulated in such a way that stochastic events in early development determine later-life aging and survival through variation in initial redundancy of organs and tissues (see, for example, Finch and Kirkwood, 2000). Note that this model does not require an assumption of initial population heterogeneity in failure risks. Instead the model is focused on distributed redundancy of physiological systems within a given organism, or a group of initially identical organisms.

PARTIALLY DAMAGED REDUNDANT SYSTEM

In the preceding section, we examined a reliability model for a system consisting of m series-connected blocks with numbers of elements distributed according to the Poisson law. In this section, we consider a more general case in which the probability of an element being initially functional can take any possible value: $0 < q \leq 1$ (see Gavrilov and Gavrilova, 1991; 2001 for more detail).

In the general case, the distribution of blocks in the organism according to the number of initially functional elements is described by the binomial rather than Poisson distribution.

If an organism can be presented as a system constructed of m series-connected blocks with binomially distributed elements, its failure rate is given by the following formula:

$$\mu_s \approx Cmn(q\mu)^n\left[\frac{1-q}{q\mu} + x\right]^{n-1} = Cmn(q\mu)^n(x_0 + x)^{n-1}$$

$$\text{where } x_0 = \frac{1-q}{q\mu}$$

It is proposed to call a parameter x_0 the *initial virtual age of the system, IVAS* (Gavrilov and Gavrilova, 1991; 2001). Indeed, this parameter has the dimension of time, and corresponds to the age by which an initially ideal system would have accumulated as many defects as a real system already has at the initial moment in time (at $x = 0$). In particular, when $q = 1$, i.e., when all the elements are functional at the beginning, the initial virtual age of the system is zero and the failure rate grows as a power function of age (the Weibull law), as described in the causes of failure rate increase with age section. However, when the system is not initially ideal ($q < 1$), we obtain the *binomial law of mortality* (see basic failure models).

In the case when $x_0 > 0$, there is always an initial period of time, such that $x \ll x_0$ and the following approximation to the binomial law is valid:

$$\mu_s \approx Cmn(q\mu)^n x_0^{n-1}\left[1+\frac{x}{x_0}\right]^{n-1}$$

$$\approx Cmn(q\mu)^n x_0^{n-1}\exp\left[\frac{n-1}{x_0}x\right]$$

Hence, for any value of $q < 1$ there always exists a period of time x when the number of newly formed defects is much less than the original number, and the failure rate grows exponentially with age.

So, if the system is not initially ideal ($q < 1$), the failure rate in the initial period of time grows exponentially with age according to the Gompertz law. A numerical example provided in Figure 5.2 (see the reliability approach to system's failure in aging section) shows that increase in the initial system's damage load (initial virtual age) converts the observed mortality trajectory from the Weibull to the Gompertz one.

The model discussed here not only provides an explanation for the exponential increase in the failure rate with age, but it also explains the compensation law of mortality (see Gavrilov and Gavrilova, 1991; 2001).

The compensation law of mortality is observed whenever differences in mortality are caused by differences in initial redundancy (the number of elements in a block, n), while the other parameters, including the "true aging rate" (rate of elements' loss μ), are similar in populations of a given species (presumably because of homeostasis—stable body temperature, glucose concentration, etc.). For lower organisms with poor homeostasis there may be deviations from this law. Our analysis of data published by Pletcher *et al.* (2000) revealed that in *Drosophila* this law holds true for male–female comparisons (keeping temperature the same), but not for experiments conducted at different temperatures, presumably because temperature may influence the rate of element loss.

The failure rate of the blocks asymptotically approaches an upper limit which is independent of the number of initially functional elements and is equal to μ. Therefore the failure rate of a system consisting of m blocks in series tends asymptotically with increased age to an upper limit $m\mu$, independently of the values of n and q.

Thus the reliability model described here provides an explanation for a general pattern of aging and mortality in biological species: the exponential growth of failure rate in the initial period, with the subsequent mortality deceleration and leveling-off, as well as the compensation law of mortality.

This model might also be called the model of series-connected blocks with varying degrees of redundancy or distributed redundancy. The basic conclusion of the model might be reformulated as follows: *if vital components of a system differ in their degree of redundancy, the mortality rate initially grows exponentially with age (according to the Gompertz law) with subsequent leveling-off in later life.*

HETEROGENEOUS POPULATION OF REDUNDANT ORGANISMS

In the previous sections, we examined a situation in which series-connected blocks have varying degrees of redundancy within each organism, while the organisms themselves were considered to be initially identical to each other and to have the same risk of death. This latter assumption can be justified in some special cases (see Gavrilov and Gavrilova, 1991) and also when the focus is on the analysis of the individual risks of failure. In a more general case the population heterogeneity needs to be taken into account, because there is a large variation in the numbers of cells for the organisms of the same species (Finch and Kirkwood, 2000).

In this section, we demonstrate that taking into account the heterogeneity of the population provides an explanation for all the basic laws of mortality. This model of heterogeneous redundant systems was proposed by Gavrilov and Gavrilova in 1991 (pp. 264–272).

The model considers the simplest case when the organism consists of a single vital block with n elements connected in parallel with q being the probability that an element is initially functional. Then the probability of encountering an organism with i initially functional elements out of a total number n of elements is given by the binomial distribution law.

The final formula for failure rate in heterogeneous population, $\mu_p(x)$, is (see Gavrilov and Gavrilova, 1991 for more details):

$$\mu_p(x) = \frac{F'(x)}{1-F(x)} = \frac{nq\mu e^{-\mu x}(1-qe^{-\mu x})^{n-1}}{1-(1-qe^{-\mu x})^n}$$

$$\approx Cnq\mu(1-q+q\mu x)^{n-1} \quad \text{for} \quad x \ll 1/\mu$$

$$\approx \mu \quad \text{for} \quad x \gg 1/\mu$$

where C is a normalizing factor.

Thus the hazard rate of a heterogeneous population at first grows with age according to the binomial law of mortality, then asymptotically approaches an upper limit μ:

$$\mu_p(x) \approx Cn(q\mu)^n\left[\frac{1-q}{q\mu}+x\right]^{n-1}$$

$$= Cn(q\mu)^n(x_0+x)^{n-1} \quad \text{for} \quad x \ll \frac{1}{\mu}$$

$$\mu_p(x) \approx \mu \quad \text{for} \quad x \gg \frac{1}{\mu}$$

where $x_0 = (1-q)/q\mu$, a parameter which we propose to call the initial virtual age of the population. This parameter has the dimension of time, and corresponds to the age by which an initially homogeneous population would have accumulated as many damaged organisms as a real population actually possesses at the initial moment in time (at $x = 0$). In particular, when $q = 1$, i.e., when all the elements in each organism are functional at the outset, the initial virtual age of the population is zero and the hazard rate of population grows as a power function of age (the Weibull law), this being the case described in causes of failure rate increase with age. However when the population is not initially homogeneous ($q < 1$), we arrive at the already mentioned binomial law of mortality. Thus, the heterogeneous population model proposed here can also provide a theoretical justification for the binomial law of mortality.

If a population is initially heterogeneous ($q < 1$), the hazard rate in the initial period of time grows exponentially with age (according to the Gompertz law).

The heterogeneous population model not only provides an explanation for the exponential growth in the failure rate with age, but also the compensation law of mortality (Gavrilov and Gavrilova, 1991). The compensation effect of mortality is observed whenever differences in mortality are brought about by inter-population differences in the number of elements in the organism (n), while the other parameters, including the rate of aging (the rate of irreversible elements failure μ), are similar for all compared populations of a particular species (presumably because of homeostasis in physiological parameters). It is not difficult to see the similarity between this explanation for the compensation effect of mortality and the explanations which emerge from the models of individual system described in preceding sections.

Figure 5.9 presents the age kinetics of failure rate in heterogeneous population where redundancy is distributed by the Poisson law (a special case of binomial distribution) with different mean number of functional elements ($\lambda = 1$, 5, 10, 15 and 20).

Note that the logarithm of the failure rate is increasing with age in almost a linear fashion, indicating a reasonable applicability of the Gompertz law in this case. Also note that the slope of the lines is increasing with higher mean redundancy levels (λ), and the lines have a tendency for convergence (compensation law of mortality).

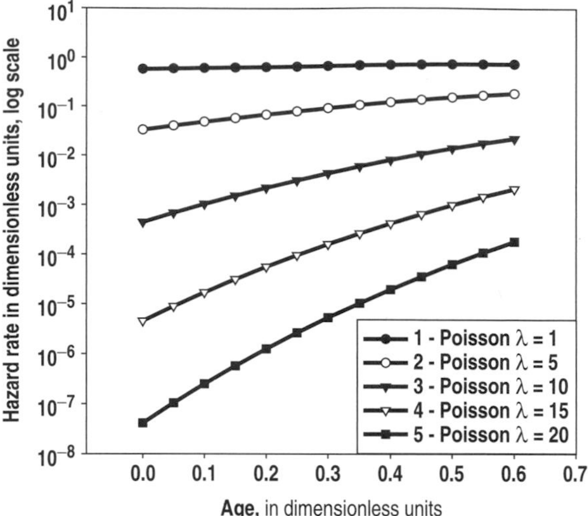

Figure 5.9. Failure kinetics in mixtures of systems with different redundancy levels. Initial period. The dependence of failure rate as a function of age in mixtures of parallel redundant systems having Poisson distribution by initial numbers of functional elements (mean number of elements, $\lambda = 1, 5, 10, 15, 20$). Source: Gavrilov and Gavrilova, 2005.

The heterogeneous population model leads in principle to the same conclusions as the previously discussed model of series-connected blocks with varying degrees of redundancy. However, we are dealing with two fundamentally different models: whereas in the first model the individual risk of death is the same for all organisms and grows exponentially with age, in the second model there initially exist n subpopulations of living organisms with different risks of death which grow as a power function rather than exponential function of age. However, these different models seem to lead to virtually coincident interpretations of certain mortality phenomena. For example, the compensation effect of mortality is only possible, according to any of the models, when the rate of irreversible age changes is approximately constant within a given species. This interpretation of the compensation effect of mortality is not only a feature of the three models examined in this chapter, but also of other models (Gavrilov, 1978; Gavrilov *et al.*, 1978; Strehler and Mildvan, 1960).

Thus, the heterogeneous population model provides an explanation for all the basic mortality phenomena (the exponential growth of the force of mortality in the initial period, with the subsequent mortality deceleration, as well as the compensation effect of mortality) even in the simplest case when the organism consists of a single vital block with n parallel elements. Generalizing the model to the case of m blocks connected in series in each organism does not present any problems if the blocks are independent of each other with respect to their reliability (Gavrilov and Gavrilova, 1991).

MODELS OF AVALANCHE-LIKE DESTRUCTION

> For want of a nail the shoe was lost,
> For want of a shoe the horse was lost,
> For want of a horse the rider was lost,
> For want of a rider the battle was lost,
> For want of a battle the kingdom was lost,
> And all for the want of a horseshoe nail.
> — English nursery rhyme (ca. 1390)

The models described in previous sections assumed that the failures of elements in the organism occur independently of each other. This assumption may be acceptable as the first approximation. In real biological systems many aging phenomena may be represented as a "cascade of dependent failures" which occurs when one of the organism's systems randomly fails (Gavrilov, 1978; Gavrilov *et al.*, 1978). The idea that an avalanche-like mechanism is involved in the destruction of an organism during natural aging is worth further consideration. In fact, it is well-known that defects in an organism have a tendency to multiply following an avalanche-like mechanism. For example, if there are n cancer cells in the organism, each of which is capable of division, the rate at which the organism is transformed into a state with $n+1$ cancer cells increases with the growth of the number of cancer cells (n) already accumulated. Infections of the organism follow similar regularities. The positive feedback between the degree and the rate of an organism's destruction also follows from the fact that when parts of the structure fail, the load on the remaining structures increases, accelerating the wearing-out. It seems that aging may be caused by similar cascades of dependent failures developing over long periods in a hidden, preclinical form. Therefore mathematical models of the avalanche-like destruction of the organism are of particular interest.

Consider the simplest model of the avalanche-like destruction of the organism (Gavrilov and Gavrilova, 1991). Let $S_0, S_1, \ldots, S_n$ denote the states of an organism with $0, 1, 2, \ldots, n$ defects. Let λ_0 be the background rate at which defects accumulate being independent on the stage of destruction, which the organism has reached. Correspondingly, let μ_0 be the age-independent mortality (the Makeham term). In the simplest case, both of these quantities arise from random harmful effects of the external environment. In tandem, there is also an induced rate of deterioration (parameter λ) and an induced failure rate (parameter μ) which grow as the number of defects increases. At a first approximation, it can be assumed that both the induced rate of deterioration and the induced failure rate are proportional to the number of defects, so that for an organism with n defects the induced rate of deterioration is equal to $n\lambda$, and the induced failure rate is $n\mu$.

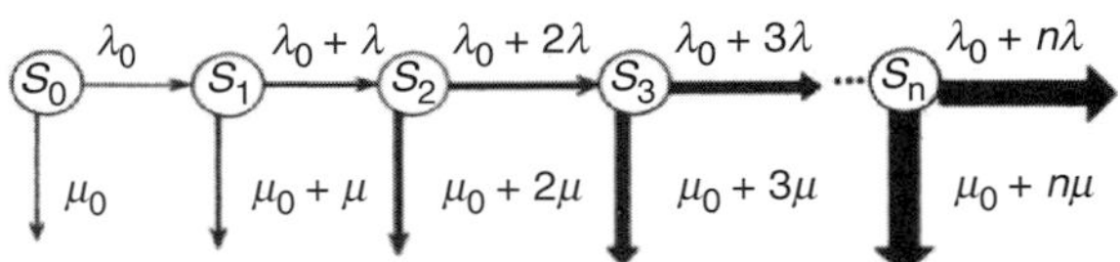

Figure 5.10. Avalanche-like mechanism of organism's destruction with age. In the initial state (S_0) organism has no defects. Then, as a result of random damage, it enters states $S_1, S_2, \ldots S_n$, where n corresponds to the number of defects. Rate of new defects emergence has avalanche-like growth with the number of already accumulated defects (horizontal arrows). Hazard rate (vertical arrows directed down) also has an avalanche-like growth with the number of defects.

With these assumptions, we can present the avalanche-like destruction of the organism by the schema presented in Figure 5.10.

This schema corresponds to the following system of differential equations:

$$dS_0/dx = -(\lambda_0 + \mu_0)S_0$$
$$dS_1/dx = \lambda_0 S_0 - (\lambda_0 + \mu_0 + \lambda + \mu)S_1$$
$$dS_n/dx = [\lambda_0 + (n-1)\lambda]S_{n-1} - [\lambda_0 + \mu_0 + n(\lambda + \mu)]S_n$$

A similar system of equations (not taking into account the age-independent mortality) was obtained and solved in a mathematical model linking the survival of organisms with chromosome damage (Le Bras, 1976). However, this "chromosomal" interpretation of the avalanche model could be applicable only to unicellular organisms, while for multicellular organisms including humans, where chromosomes are compartmentalized in separate cells, this model needs to be revised, or provided with a different "nonchromosomal" interpretation (as it is suggested in this section).

In the particular case when the rate at which defects multiply, the parameter λ is significantly greater than the induced failure rate, parameter μ,($\lambda \gg \mu$), the hazard rate of an organism in the initial stage (with low values of x) grows according to the Gompertz–Makeham law:

$$\mu(x) \approx \mu_0 + \frac{\mu\lambda_0(1 - e^{(\lambda+\mu)x})}{\lambda e^{(\lambda+\mu)x}} \approx A + Re^{\alpha x}$$
$$\text{where } A = \mu_0 - \frac{\mu\lambda_0}{\lambda}; \quad R = \frac{\mu\lambda_0}{\lambda}; \quad \alpha = \lambda + \mu$$

This model of the avalanche-like destruction of the organism not only provides a theoretical justification for the well-known Gompertz–Makeham law, but also explains why the values of the Makeham parameter A sometimes turn out to be negative (when age-independent mortality, μ_0, is small as for populations in the developed countries and the background rate of destruction, λ_0, is large).

Another advantage of the avalanche-like destruction model is that it correctly predicts mortality deceleration (deviations from the Gompertz–Makeham law) at very old ages. In this extreme age-range, the failure rate grows with age according to the formula

$$\mu(x) \approx \mu_0 + \lambda_0(1 - e^{-(\lambda+\mu)x})$$

Thus the model predicts an asymptotic growth of failure rate with age with an upper limit of $\mu_0 + \lambda_0$.

Alongside the strengths already listed, the avalanche-like destruction model has one significant limitation: it does not conform to the compensation law of mortality in its strong form (Gavrilov and Gavrilova, 1991). Nevertheless, the idea that organisms undergo cascade destruction is one of the promising ideas in further mathematical modeling of aging.

ACCUMULATION OF DEFECTS WITH CONSTANT RATE OF DAMAGE FLOW

A wide variety of concepts about the destruction of the organism can lead to the model where the rate of damage flow, numerically equal to the mean number of "hits" per unit of time, is practically independent of the state of the organism and is on average constant in time. In the simplest case, the model corresponds to a situation in which the organism is affected by a random flow of traumatic loads with an on average constant rate independent of the state of the organism (exogenous environmental damage like cosmic radiation, viruses, etc.)

However, there is also the possibility of other mechanisms of destruction leading to this particular model of the accumulation of defects. In particular, this model can be obtained after a critical reinterpretation of the assumptions underlying the previously described models. In fact, these models contain an assumption that the death of the organism occurs only when all the elements in a block fail. It is possible that this hypothesis may be justified for some of the organism's systems (stem cell populations, for example). However, in the majority of cases this hypothesis seems contentious. For example, it is hard to imagine that a single surviving liver cell (hepatocyte) can assume the functions of an entire destroyed liver. Significantly more realistic is the hypothesis that the system initially contains an enormous number of elements that greatly exceeds the critical number of defects leading to the death of the organism. In this case we arrive at a schema for the accumulation of damage in which the rate of damage flow (equal to the product of the number of elements and their failure rate) turns out to be practically constant in view of the incommensurability of the high initial numbers of elements, and the much smaller permitted number of defects (Gavrilov and Gavrilova, 1991).

Another advantage of this model is that it allows us to take into account the influence of living conditions on the value for the critical number of defects incompatible with the survival of the organism. The key to the solution of this problem is the replacement of the parallel connection hypothesis (assumed in previously described models) with the more realistic assumption that there exists a critical number of defects incompatible with the survival of the organism. In this case, it is natural to expect that under harsher conditions the critical number of defects leading to death might be less than under more comfortable living conditions. In particular, in the wild, when an animal is deprived of care and forced to acquire its own food, as well as to defend itself against predators, the first serious damage to the organism can lead to death. It is therefore not surprising that the mortality of many animals (in particular, birds) is practically independent of age in the wild. This follows directly from the single-stage destruction of the organism model. On the other hand, the greater the number of defects the organism can accumulate while remaining alive, the greater its lifespan will be.

If the rate of the damage flow equals k, and an organism dies after the accumulation of n defects, the density of the survival distribution is identical to the density of the gamma function (see Barlow and Proschan, 1965; 1975). At the initial moment in time, this distribution corresponds to a power (Weibull) law of mortality with an exponent equal to $(n-1)$.

A fundamentally different result is obtained when the initial damage of organisms is taken into account (Gavrilov and Gavrilova, 1991). If at the initial moment in time the average number of random defects in the population equals λ, the probability of encountering a living organism, P_i, with i defects may be approximated by the Poisson law (see Gavrilov and Gavrilova, 1991, pp. 272–276, for more detail).

Since the death of an organism with i defects occurs after $n-i$ additional hits, the density of the lifespan distribution for such organisms is given by

$$f_i(x) = \frac{k(kx)^{n-i-1}e^{-kx}}{(n-i-1)!}, \quad \text{where} \quad i < n$$

The density of the survival distribution for the whole population, which is a mixture of organisms with $i = 0, 1, 2, \ldots n-1$ initial defects, equals

$$f(x) = \sum_{i=0}^{n-1} P_i f_i(x) = Cke^{-(\lambda+kx)} \sum_{i=0}^{n-1} \frac{\lambda^i (kx)^{n-i-1}}{i!(n-1-i)!} = \frac{Ck(\lambda + kx)^{n-1} e^{-(\lambda+kx)}}{(n-1)!}$$

It is not difficult to see that at the initial moment in time this model leads to the binomial law of mortality, with an initial virtual age of the population equal to λ/k. A more detailed analysis of the model is formally similar to the analysis of the other models described in previous sections. We merely note that during the initial time period when $x \ll \lambda/k$, the model leads to an exponential growth of failure rate with age (the Gompertz law) with an exponent, α, of $k(n-1)/\lambda$ and a pre-exponential factor, R, of $Ck\lambda^{n-1}/(n-1)!$. It is easy to see that an inverse relationship between these Gompertz parameters (the compensation effect of mortality) can arise both as a result of variation in parameter λ (the degree to which the organisms are initially damaged) and of variation in parameter n (the critical number of defects, dependent on the harshness of living conditions).

Thus the basic mortality phenomena can equally be explained within the framework of the model of accumulation of defects with the constant rate of damage flow, as long as the organisms initially contain a significant number of defects.

Summarizing this brief review of reliability models, we note the striking similarity between the formulas and conclusions of the considered models. It must, however, be noted that we are dealing only with a superficial similarity in behavior between fundamentally different and competing models. The existence of a multitude of competing models is therefore compatible with the reliable and meaningful interpretation of a number of mortality phenomena, since pluralism of models does not preclude their agreement on a number of issues. All these models predict a mortality deceleration, no matter what assumptions are made regarding initial population heterogeneity, or its complete initial homogeneity. Moreover, these reliability models of aging produce mortality plateaus as the inevitable outcome for any values of considered parameters (Gavrilov and Gavrilova, 1991). The only constraint is that the elementary steps of the multistage destruction process of a system should occur only by chance, independent of age. The models also predict that an initially homogeneous population will become highly heterogeneous for risk of death over time (acquired heterogeneity).

Conclusions

Theoretical reliability models of system failure in aging considered in this book chapter lead to the following conclusions:

1. *Redundancy* is a key notion for understanding aging and the systemic nature of aging in particular. Systems, which are redundant in numbers of irreplaceable elements, do deteriorate over time (fail more often with age), even if they are built of nonaging elements. The positive effect of systems' redundancy is *damage tolerance*, which decreases mortality and increases lifespan. However damage tolerance makes it possible for damage to be tolerated and accumulated over time, thus producing the aging phenomenon.
2. An apparent aging rate or expression of aging (measured as age differences in failure rates, including death rates) is higher for systems with higher redundancy levels (all other things being equal). This is an important issue, because it helps to put a correct perspective on fascinating observations of negligible senescence (no apparent aging) observed in the wild and at extreme old ages. Reliability theory explains that some cases of negligible senescence may have a trivial mechanism (lack of redundancies in the system being exposed to challenging environment) and, therefore, will not help to uncover "the secrets of negligible senescence." The studies of negligible senescence make sense, however, when the death rates are also demonstrated to be negligible.
3. Reliability theory also persuades a re-evaluation of the old belief that aging is somehow related to limited economic or evolutionary investments in systems longevity. The theory provides a completely opposite perspective on this issue—aging is a direct consequence of investments into systems reliability and durability through enhanced redundancy. This is a significant statement, because it helps to understand why the expression of aging (differences in failure rates between the younger and the older age groups) may be actually more profound in more complicated redundant systems, designed for higher durability.
4. During the life course the organisms are exhausting the reserve numbers of their cells (Gosden, 1985; Herndon *et al.*, 2002), losing reserve capacity (Bortz, 2002; Sehl and Yates, 2001), and this *redundancy depletion* explains the observed "compensation law of mortality" (mortality convergence at older ages) as well as the observed late-life mortality deceleration, leveling-off, and mortality plateaus.
5. Living organisms seem to be formed with a high *load of initial damage*, and therefore their lifespan and aging patterns may be sensitive to *early-life conditions* that determine this initial damage load during early development. The idea of early-life programming of aging and longevity may have important practical implications for developing early-life interventions promoting health and longevity.

The theory also suggests that aging research should not be limited to the studies of qualitative changes (like age changes in gene expression), because changes in *quantity* (numbers of cells and other functional elements) could be an important driving force of aging process. In other words, aging may be largely driven by a process of redundancy loss.

The reliability theory predicts that a system may deteriorate with age even if it is built from nonaging elements with constant failure rate. The key issue here is the system's redundancy for irreplaceable elements, which is responsible for the aging phenomenon. In other words, each particular step of system destruction/deterioration may seem to be apparently random (no aging, just occasional failure by chance), but if a system failure requires a sequence of several such steps (not just a single step of destruction), then the system as a whole may have an aging behavior.

Why is this important? Because the significance of beneficial health-promoting interventions is often undermined by claims that these interventions are not proven to delay the process of aging itself, but instead simply delay or "cover-up" some particular manifestations of aging.

In contrast to these pessimistic views, reliability theory says that there may be no specific underlying elementary "aging process itself"—instead aging may be largely a property of a redundant system as a whole, because it has a network of destruction pathways, each being associated with particular manifestations of aging (types of failure). Therefore, we should not be discouraged by only partial success of each particular intervention, but instead we can appreciate an idea that we do have so many opportunities to oppose aging in numerous different ways.

Thus, the efforts to understand the routes and the early stages of age-related degenerative diseases should not be discarded as irrelevant to understanding the "true biological aging." On the contrary, the attempts to build an intellectual firewall between biogerontological research and clinical medicine are counterproductive. After all, the main reason why people are really concerned about aging is because it is related to health deterioration and increased morbidity. The most important pathways of age changes are those that make older people sick and frail (Bortz, 2002).

Reliability theory suggests general answers to both the "why" and the "how" questions about aging. It explains "why" aging occurs by identifying the key determinant of aging behavior—system redundancy in numbers of irreplaceable elements. Reliability theory also explains "how" aging occurs, by focusing on the process of redundancy loss over time as the major mechanism of aging.

Ageing is a complex phenomenon (Sehl and Yates, 2001), and a holistic approach using reliability theory may help to analyze, understand, and perhaps to control it. We suggest, therefore, adding theoretical reliability models of system failure in aging to the arsenal of methodological approaches for the studying of human aging.

ACKNOWLEDGMENTS

This work was supported in part by grants from the National Institute on Aging.

REFERENCES

Andersen, B.B., Gundersen, H.J., and Pakkenberg B. (2003). Aging of the human cerebellum: A stereological study. *J. Comp. Neurol. 466*, 356–365.

Andreadis, S., and Palsson, B.O. (1997). Coupled effects of polybrene and calf serum on the efficiency of retroviral transduction and the stability of retroviral vectors. *Hum. Gene Ther. 8*, 285–291.

Austad, S.N. (2001). Concepts and theories of aging. In Masoro, E.J., and Austad, S.N., *Handbook of the Biology of Aging*. San Diego, CA: Academic Press, pp. 3–22.

Aven, T., and Jensen, U. (1999). *Stochastic Models in Reliability*. New York: Springer-Verlag.

Ayyub, B.M., and McCuen, R.H. (2003). *Probability, Statistics, Reliability for Engineers and Scientists*. Boca Raton, FL: Chapman and Hall/CRC.

Baizabal, J.M., Furlan-Magaril, M., Santa-Olalla, J., and Covarrubias, L. (2003). Neural stem cells in development and regenerative medicine. *Arch. Med. Res. 34*, 572–588.

Barlow, R.E., and Proschan, F. (1975). *Statistical Theory of Reliability and Life Testing. Probability Models*. New York: Holt, Rinehart and Winston.

Barlow, R.E., Proschan, F., and Hunter, L.C. (1965). *Mathematical Theory of Reliability*. New York: John Wiley.

Beard, R.E. (1959). Note on some mathematical mortality models. In: Wolstenholme, G.E.W., and O'Connor, M. (Eds.). *The Lifespan of Animals* (pp. 302–311). Boston: Little, Brown.

Beard, R.E. (1971). Some aspects of theories of mortality, cause of death analysis, forecasting and stochastic processes. In: Brass, W. (Ed.), *Biological Aspects of Demography* (pp. 57–68). London: Taylor and Francis.

Bortz, W.M. (2002). A conceptual framework of frailty: A review. *J. Gerontol. Ser. A 57*, M283–M288.

Brock, T.D., Madigan, M.T., Martinko, J.M., and Parker, J. (1994). *Biology of Microorganisms* (7th ed.), Englewood Cliffs, NJ: Prentice-Hall.

Bronikowski, A.M., Alberts, S.C., Altmann, J., Packer, C., Carey, K.D., and Tatar, M. (2002). The aging baboon: Comparative demography in a non-human primate. *Proc. Natl. Acad. Sci. USA 99*, 9591–9595.

Brooks, A., Lithgow, G.J., and Johnson, T.E. (1994). Mortality rates in a genetically heterogeneous population of *Caenorhabditis elegans*. *Science 263*, 668–671.

Burns, J., Clarke, G., and Lumsden, C.J. (2002). Photoreceptor death: Spatiotemporal patterns arising from one-hit death kinetics and a diffusible cell death factor. *Bull. Math. Biol. 64*, 1117–1145.

Calne, D.B. (1994). Is idiopathic parkinsonism the consequence of an event or a process? *Neurology 44*, 5–10 (1994).

Capogrossi, M.C. (2004). Cardiac stem cells fail with aging: A new mechanism for the age-dependent decline in cardiac function. *Circ. Res. 94*, 411–413.

Carey, J.R., and Liedo, P. (1995). Sex-specific life table aging rates in large medfly cohorts. *Exp. Gerontol. 30*, 315–325.

Carey, J.R., Liedo, P., Orozco, D., and Vaupel, J.W. (1992). Slowing of mortality rates at older ages in large Medfly cohorts. *Science 258*, 457–461.

Cargill, Sh. L., Carey, J.R., Muller, H.-G., and Anderson, G. (2003). Age of ovary determines remaining life expectancy in old ovariectomized mice. *Aging Cell 2*, 185–190.

Carnes, B.A., Olshansky, S.J., and Grahn, D. (1998). An interspecies prediction of the risk of radiation-induced mortality. *Radiat. Res. 149*, 487–492.

Choi, J.H., Kim, K.L., Huh, W., Kim, B., Byun, J., Suh, *et al.* (2004). Decreased number and impaired angiogenic function of endothelial progenitor cells in patients with chronic renal failure. *Arterioscler. Thromb. Vas.c Biol. 24*, 1246–1252.

Clark, A.G., and Guadalupe, R.N. (1995). Probing the evolution of senescence in *Drosophila melanogaster* with P-element tagging. *Genetica 96*, 225–234.

Clark, V.A. (1975). Survival distribution. *Annual Review of Biophysics and Bioengineering 4*, 431–448.

Clarke, G., Collins, R.A., Leavitt, B.R., Andrews, D.F., Hayden, M.R., Lumsden, C.J., and McInnes, R.R. (2000). A one-hit model of cell death in inherited neuronal degenerations. *Nature 406*, 195–199.

Clarke, G., Collins, R.A., Leavitt, B.R., Andrews, D.F., Hayden, M.R., Lumsden, C.J., and McInnes, R.R. (2001a). Addendum: A one-hit model of cell death in inherited neuronal degenerations. *Nature 409*, 542.

Clarke, G., Lumsden, C.J., and McInnes, R.R. (2001b). Inherited neurodegenerative diseases: The one-hit model of neurodegeneration. *Hum. Mol. Genet. 10*, 2269–2275.

Cohen, H.Y., Miller, C., Bitterman, K.J., Wall, N.R., Hekking, B., Kessler, B., *et al.* (2004). Calorie restriction promotes mammalian cell survival by inducing the SIRT1 deacetylase. *Science 305*, 390–392.

Commo, S., Gaillard, O., and Bernard, B.A. (2004). Human hair greying is linked to a specific depletion of hair follicle melanocytes affecting both the bulb and the outer root sheath. *Br. J. Dermatol. 150*, 435–443.

Crowder, M .J., Kimber, A.C., Smith, R.L., and Sweeting, T.J. (1991). *Statistical Analysis of Reliability Data.* London: Chapman and Hall.

Curtsinger, J.W., Fukui, H., Townsend, D., and Vaupel, J.W. (1992). Demography of genotypes: Failure of the limited life-span paradigm in *Drosophila melanogaster. Science 258*, 461–463.

Davis, B.D., Dulbeco, R., Eisen, H.N., and Ginsberg, H.S. (1990). *Microbiology* (4th ed.), Philadelphia, PA: Lippincott.

Eakin, T., Shouman, R., Qi, Y.L., Liu, G.X. and Witten, M. (1995). Estimating parametric survival model parameters in gerontological aging studies. Methodological problems and insights. *J. Gerontol. Ser. A 50*, B166–B176.

Economos, A.C. (1979). A non-gompertzian paradigm for mortality kinetics of metazoan animals and failure kinetics of manufactured products. *AGE 2*, 74–76.

Economos, A.C. (1980). Kinetics of metazoan mortality. *J. Social Biol. Struct., 3*, 317–329.

Economos, A.C. (1983). Rate of aging, rate of dying and the mechanism of mortality. *Arch. Gerontol. and Geriatrics 1*, 3–27.

Economos, A. (1985). Rate of aging, rate of dying and non-Gompertzian mortality—Encore ... *Gerontology 31*, 106–111.

Edelberg, J.M., Tang, L., Hattori, K., Lyden, D., and Rafii, S. (2002). Young adult bone marrow-derived endothelial precursor cells restore aging-impaired cardiac angiogenic function. *Circ. Res. 90*, E89–E93.

Feller, W. (1968). *An Introduction to Probability Theory and Its Applications,* Vol. 1. New York: Wiley and Sons.

Finch, C.E., (1990). *Longevity, senescence and the genome.* Chicago: University of Chicago Press.

Finch, C.E., and Kirkwood, T.B. L. (2000). *Chance, Development, and Aging.* New York, Oxford: Oxford University Press.

Finger, S., Le Vere, T.E., Almli, C.R. and Stein, D.G. (Eds.) (1988). *Brain Injury and Recovery: Theoretical and Controversial Issues.* New York: Plenum Press.

Fukui, H.H., Ackert, L. and Curtsinger, J.W. (1996). Deceleration of age-specific mortality rates in chromosomal homozygotes and heterozygotes of *Drosophila melanogaster. Exp. Gerontol. 31*, 517–531.

Fukui, H.H., Xiu, L., and Curtsinger, J.W. (1993). Slowing of age-specific mortality rates in *Drosophila melanogaster. Exp. Gerontol. 28*, 585–599.

Galambos, J. (1978). *The Asymptotic Theory of Extreme Order Statistics.* New York: Wiley.

Gavrilov, L.A. (1978). Mathematical model of aging in animals. *Doklady Akademii Nauk SSSR Biological Sciences 238*, 53–55 (English translation).

Gavrilov, L.A. (1980). Study of Life Span Genetics Using the Kinetic Analysis. Thesis, Moscow, Russia: Moscow State University.

Gavrilov, L.A. (1984). Does a limit of the life span really exist? *Biofizika 29*, 908–911.

Gavrilov, L.A., and Gavrilova, N.S. (1979). Determination of species length of life. *Doklady Akademii Nauk SSSR Biological Sciences 246*, 905–908 (English translation).

Gavrilov, L.A., and Gavrilova, N.S. (1991). *The Biology of Life Span: A Quantitative Approach.* New York: Harwood Academic Publishers.

Gavrilov, L.A., and Gavrilova, N.S. (2001). Biodemographic study of familial determinants of human longevity. *Population: English Selection 13*, 197–222.

Gavrilov, L.A., and Gavrilova, N.S. (2003a). The quest for a general theory of aging and longevity. *Science's SAGE KE* (Science of Aging Knowledge Environment), 16 July 2003; *2003(28)*, 1–10. Available: http://sageke.sciencemag.org

Gavrilov, L.A., and Gavrilova, N.S. (2003b). Early-life factors modulating lifespan. In: Rattan, S.I.S. (Ed.). *Modulating Aging and Longevity* (pp. 27–50), Dordrecht, The Netherlands: Kluwer Academic Publishers.

Gavrilov, L.A., and Gavrilova, N.S. (2004a). The reliability-engineering approach to the problem of biological aging. *Ann. N.Y. Acad. Sci. 1019*, 509–512.

Gavrilov, L.A., and Gavrilova, N.S. (2004b). Early-life programming of aging and longevity: The idea of high initial damage load (the HIDL hypothesis). *Ann. N.Y. Acad. Sci. 1019*, 496–501.

Gavrilov, L.A., and Gavrilova, N.S. (2004c). Why we fall apart. Engineering's reliability theory explains human aging. *IEEE Spectrum 9*, 2–7.

Gavrilov, L.A., and Gavrilova, N.S. (2005). Reliability theory of aging and longevity. In: Masoro, E.J., and Austad, S.N., *Handbook of the Biology of Aging.* San Diego, CA: Academic Press 1–40.

Gavrilov, L.A., Gavrilova, N.S. and Iaguzhinskii, L.S. (1978). Basic patterns of aging and death in animals from the standpoint of reliability theory. *J. General Biology* (*Zhurnal Obshchej Biologii,* Moscow), *39*, 734–742 (In Russian).

Gilchrest, B.A., Blog, F.B., and Szabo, G. (1979). Effects of aging and chronic sun exposure on melanocytes in human skin. *J. Invest. Dermatol., 73*, 141–3.

Goldschmidt-Clermont, P.J. (2003). Loss of bone marrow-derived vascular progenitor cells leads to inflammation and atherosclerosis. *Am. Heart J. 146(4 Suppl)*, S5–S12.

Golubev, A. (2004). Does Makeham make sense? *Biogerontology* 5, 159–167.

Gompertz, B. (1825). On the nature of the function expressive of the law of human mortality and on a new mode of determining life contingencies. *Philos. Trans. Roy. Soc. London A 115*, 513–585.

Gosden, R.G. (1985). *The Biology of Menopause: The Cause and Consequence of Ovarian Aging*. San Diego, CA: Academic Press.

Gouda, M.D., Singh, S.A., Rao, A.G., Thakur, M.S., and Karanth, N.G. (2003). Thermal inactivation of glucose oxidase: Mechanism and stabilization using additives. *J. Biol. Chem. 278*, 24324–24333.

Greenwood, M., and Irwin, J.O. (1939). The biostatistics of senility. *Hum. Biol. 11*, 1–23.

Griffiths, A.J.F., Miller, J.H., Suzuki, D.T., Lewontin, R.C., and Gelbart, W.M. (1996). *An Introduction to Genetic Analysis* (6th ed.). New York: W.H. Freeman.

Gumbel, E.J. (1958). *Statistics of Extremes*. New York: Columbia University Press.

Hall, J.C. (1969). Age-dependent enzyme changes in *Drosophila melanogaster*. *Exp. Gerontol. 4*, 207–222.

Haranghy, L., and Balázs, A. (1980). Regeneration and rejuvenation of invertebrates. In: Shock, N.W. (Ed.), *Perspectives in Experimental Gerontology* (pp. 224–233). New York: Arno Press.

Heintz, N. (2000). One-hit neuronal death. *Nature*, *406*, 137–138.

Herndon, L.A., Schmeissner, P.J., Dudaronek, J.M., Brown, P.A., Listner, K.M., Sakano, Y., *et al.* (2002). Stochastic and genetic factors influence tissue-specific decline in ageing *C. elegans*. *Nature 419*, 808–814.

Hirsch, H.R., and Peretz, B. (1984). Survival and aging of a small laboratory population of a marine mollusc. *Aplysia californica*. *Mech. Ageing Dev. 27*, 43–62.

Hirsch, A.G., Williams, R.J., and Mehl, P. (1994). Kinetics of medfly mortality. *Exp. Gerontol. 29*, 197–204.

Janse, C., Slob, W., Popelier, C.M., and Vogelaar, J.W. (1988) Survival characteristics of the mollusc *Lymnaea stagnalis* under constant culture conditions: effects of aging and disease. *Mech. Ageing Dev. 42*, 263–174.

Jay, J.M. (1996). *Modern Food Microbiology*. New York: Chapman and Hall.

Johnson, T.E. (1987). Aging can be genetically dissected into component processes using long-lived lines of *Caenorhabditis elegans*. *Proc. Natl. Acad. Sci. USA 84*, 3777–3781.

Johnson, T.E. (1990). Increased life span of agc-1 mutants in *Caenorhabditis elegans* and lower Gompertz rate of aging. *Science 249*, 908–912.

Kaufmann, A., Grouchko, D. and Cruon, R. (1977). *Mathematical Models for the Study of the Reliability of Systems*. New York: Academic Press.

Keller, G., Zimmer, G., Mall, G., Ritz, E., and Amann, K. (2003). Nephron number in patients with primary hypertension. *N. Engl. J. Med. 348*, 101–108.

Khazaeli, A.A., Xiu, L., and Curtsinger, J.W. (1995). Stress experiments as a means of investigating age-specific mortality in *Drosophila melanogaster*. *Exp. Gerontol. 30*, 177–184.

Khazaeli, A.A., Xiu, L., and Curtsinger, J.W. (1996). Effect of density on age-specific mortality in *Drosophila:* A density supplementation experiment. *Genetica 98*, 21–31.

Klein, J.P., and Moeschberger, M.L. (1997). *Survival Analysis. Techniques for Censored and Truncated Data*. New York: Springer-Verlag.

Kundi, M. (1999). One-hit models for virus inactivation studies. *Antivir. Res. 41*, 145–152.

Kunstyr, I., and Leuenberger, H.-G.W. (1975). Gerontological data of C57BL/6J mice. I. Sex differences in survival curves. *J. Gerontol. 30*, 157–162.

Kurganov, B.I. (2002). Kinetics of protein aggregation. Quantitative estimation of the chaperone-like activity in test-systems based on suppression of protein aggregation. *Biochemistry* (Moscow), *67*, 409–422.

Le Bras, H. (1976). Lois de mortalité et age limité. *Population 31*, 655–692.

Leeuwenburgh, C. (2003). Role of apoptosis in sarcopenia. *J. Gerontol. A* 58, 999–1001.

Libby, P. (2003). Bone marrow: A fountain of vascular youth? *Circulation 108*, 378–379.

Lindop, P.J. (1961). Growth rate, lifespan and causes of death in SAS/4 mice. *Gerontologia 5*, 193–208.

Lloyd, D.K. and Lipow, M. (1962). *Reliability: Management, Methods, and Mathematics*. Englewood Cliffs, NJ: Prentice-Hall.

Makeham, W.M. (1860). On the law of mortality and the construction of annuity tables. *J. Inst. Actuaries 8*, 301–310.

Makeham, W.M. (1867). On the law of mortality. *J. Inst. Actuaries 13*, 325–358.

Martinez, D.E. (1998). Mortality patterns suggest lack of senescence in Hydra. *Exp. Gerontol. 33*, 217–225.

Masoro, E.J. (2003). Subfield history: caloric restriction, slowing aging, and extending life. *Sci. Aging Knowledge Environ. 2003(8)*, RE2.

Massof, R.W., Dagnelie, G., Benzschawel, T., Palmer, R.W., and Finkelstein, D. (1990). First order dynamics of visual field loss in retinitis pigmentosa. *Clin. Vision Sci. 5*, 1–26.

McKiernan, S.H., Bua, E., McGorray, J., and Aiken, J. (2004). Early-onset calorie restriction conserves fiber number in aging rat skeletal muscle. *FASEB J. 18*, 580–581.

Mildvan, A. and Strehler, B.L. (1960). A critique of theories of mortality. In: Strehler, B.L., Ebert, J.D., Glass, H.B., and Shock, N.W. (Eds.). *The Biology of Aging* (pp. 216–235). Washington, DC: American Institute of Biological Sciences.

Miller, A.R. (1989). The distribution of wearout over evolved reliability structures. *J. Theor. Biol. 136*, 27–46.

Mueller, L., and Rose, M.R. (1996). Evolutionary theory predicts late-life mortality plateaus. *Proc. Natl. Acad. Sci. USA 93*, 15249–15253.

Nyengaard, J.R., and Bendtsen, T.F. (1992). Glomerular number and size in relation to age, kidney weight, and body surface in normal man. *Anat. Rec. 232*, 194–201.

Olshansky, S.J. (1998). On the biodemography of aging: A review essay. *Population and Development Review 24*, 381–393.

Olshansky, S.J., and Carnes, B.A. (1997). Ever since Gompertz. *Demography 34*, 1–15.

Partridge, L., and Mangel, M. (1999). Messages from mortality: The evolution of death rates in the old. *Trends in Ecology and Evolution 14*, 438–442.

Pearl, R., and Miner, J.R. (1935). Experimental studies on the duration of life. XIY. The comparative mortality of certain lower organisms. *Quart. Rev. Biol. 10*, 60–79.

Peleg, M., Normand, M.D., and Campanella, O.H. (2003). Estimating microbial inactivation parameters from survival curves obtained under varying conditions—The linear case. *Bull. Math. Biol. 65*, 219–234.

Perks, W. (1932). On some experiments in the graduation of mortality statistics. *Journal of the Institute of Actuaries 63*, 12–57.

Pletcher, S.D., and Curtsinger, J.W. (1998). Mortality plateaus and the evolution of senescence: Why are old-age mortality rates so low? *Evolution 52*, 454–464.

Pletcher, S.D., Khazaeli, A.A., and Curtsinger, J.W. (2000). Why do life spans differ? Partitioning mean longevity differences in terms of age-specific mortality parameters. *J. Gerontol. 55A*, B381–B389.

Prescott, L.M., Harley, J.P., and Klein, D.A. (1996). *Microbiology* (3rd ed.), Dubuque, IA: WCB.

Rausand, M., and Hoyland, A. (2003). *System Reliability Theory: Models, Statistical Methods, and Applications* (2nd ed.), Hoboken, NJ: Wiley-Interscience.

Rauscher, F.M., Goldschmidt-Clermont, P.J., Davis, B.H., Wang, T., Gregg, D., *et al.* (2003). Aging, progenitor cell exhaustion, and atherosclerosis. *Circulation 108*, 457–63.

Ricklefs, R.E., and Scheuerlein, A. (2002). Biological implications of the Weibull and Gompertz models of aging. *J. Gerontol. Ser. A 57*, B69–B76.

Rigdon, S.E., and Basu, A.P. (2000). *Statistical Methods for the Reliability of Repairable Systems*. New York: John Wiley.

Rockstein, M., and Lieberman, H.M. (1959). A life table for the common house fly, *Musca domestica*. *Gerontologia 3*, 23–36.

Rose, M.R. (1991). *The Evolutionary Biology of Aging*. Oxford: Oxford University Press.

Sacher, G.A. (1966). The Gompertz transformation in the study of the injury-mortality relationship: Application to late radiation effects and ageing. In: Lindop, P.J., and Sacher, G.A. (Eds.). *Radiation and Ageing* (pp. 411–441). London: Taylor and Francis.

Sacher, G.A. (1977). Life table modification and life prolongation. In: Finch, C.E., and Hayflick, L., *Handbook of the Biology of Aging* (pp. 582–638). New York: Van Nostrand Reinhold.

Schulzer, M., Lee, C.S., Mak, E.K., Vingerhoets, F.J.G., and Calne, D.B. (1994). A mathematical model of pathogenesis in idiopathic parkinsonism. *Brain 117*, 509–516.

Sehl, M.E., and Yates, F.E. (2001). Kinetics of human aging: I. Rates of senescence between ages 30 and 70 years in healthy people. *J. Gerontol. Ser. A 56*, B198–B208.

Strasser, H., Tiefenthaler, M., Steinlechner, M., Eder, I., Bartsch, G., and Konwalinka, G. (2000). Age dependent apoptosis and loss of rhabdosphincter cells. *J. Urol. 164*, 1781–1785.

Strehler, B.L. (1960). Fluctuating energy demands as determinants of the death process (A parsimonious theory of the Gompertz function). In: Strehler, B.L., Ebert, J.D., Glass, H.B., and Shock, N.W. (Eds.). *The Biology of Aging* (pp. 309–314). Washington, DC: American Institute of Biological Sciences.

Strehler, B.L. (1978). *Time, Cells, and Aging* (2nd ed.). New York and London: Academic Press.

Strehler, B.L., and Mildvan, A.S. (1960). General theory of mortality and aging. *Science 132*, 14–21.

Strohman, R. (2002). Maneuvering in the complex path from genotype to phenotype. *Science 296*, 701–703.

Strohman, R. (2003). Thermodynamics-old laws in medicine and complex disease. *Nature, Biotechnol. 21*, 477–479.

Tatar, M., Carey, J.R., and Vaupel, J.W. (1993). Long-term cost of reproduction with and without accelerated senescence in *Callosobruchus maculatus*: Analysis of age-specific mortality. *Evolution 47*, 1302–1312.

Vanfleteren, J.R., De Vreese, A., and Braeckman, B.P. (1998). Two-parameter logistic and Weibull equations provide better fits to survival data from isogenic populations of *Caenorhabditis elegans* in axenic culture than does the Gompertz model. *J. Gerontol. Ser. A 53*, B393–B403.

Vaupel, J.W., Carey, J.R., Christensen, K., Johnson, T., Yashin, A.I., Holm, N.V., *et al.* (1998). Biodemographic trajectories of longevity. *Science 280*, 855–860.

Wallace, W.H., and Kelsey, T.W. (2004). Ovarian reserve and reproductive age may be determined from measurement of ovarian volume by transvaginal sonography. *Human Reproduction 19*, 1612–1617.

Weibull, W.A. (1939). A statistical theory of the strength of materials. *Ingeniorsvetenskapsakademiens Handlingar* Nr 151, 5–45.

Weibull, W.A. (1951). A statistical distribution function of wide applicability. *J. Appl. Mech. 18*, 293–297.

Wilmoth, J.R. (1997). In search of limits. In: Wachter, K.W., and Finch, C.E. (Eds.), *Between Zeus and the Salmon. The Biodemography of Longevity* (pp. 38–64). Washington, DC: National Academy Press.

6

Major Issues in Ethics of Aging Research

Michael D. Smith

This chapter discusses some of the significant issues that arise when principles for the ethical treatment of research subjects are applied to aging subjects. Some of the ways in which researchers have addressed those issues in the design and execution of their own research are identified. After a brief review of sources for ethical principles in research, several kinds of ethical issues are examined: the complexity of respecting the human autonomy of older research subjects in the consent process, how the nursing home environment creates new ethical issues for research, and a contemporary debate that questions the goodness and rightness of aging research itself.

Introduction

Ethics in human subject research has generated robust discussion and a growing body of literature for at least 50 years. During the same time period the scientific study of aging has emerged. There is now substantial agreement on the basic principles of human research ethics—principles that apply to all subjects regardless of age. Still, the process of normal aging, diseases associated with aging, and the environments in which we age all give rise to ethical issues and concerns not typically related to research with younger subjects. This chapter will discuss some of the significant issues that arise when principles for the ethical treatment of research subjects are applied to aging subjects. I shall also point to some of the ways in which researchers have addressed those issues in the design and execution of their own research.

After a brief review of sources for ethical principles in research, I will look at several kinds of ethical issues. First, we will look at the complexity of respecting the human autonomy of older research subjects. Then we will look at how the environment, in this case the nursing home environment, itself creates new ethical issues for the conduct of research. Finally, we will look at a contemporary debate that questions the goodness and rightness of aging research itself.

The Basic Principles of Research Ethics

Through the 1940s little explicit attention had yet been paid to issues of research ethics, but at the end of the decade the Nuremberg War Crime Trials changed that. Nazi physicians and soldiers were brought to trial before an international tribunal for atrocities committed in the Holocaust. The defendants justified their actions as scientific research. The Nuremberg Code was developed to serve as a set of 10 standards in judging that defense (Nuremberg Code, 1949). The code insisted that the free and informed consent of human subjects was essential to all ethical research. It also addressed the prevention of suffering by subjects and the necessity that researchers be qualified and their research well designed.

Several years later, the Helsinki Code described ethically important differences between clinical and nonclinical human research (World Medical Association, 1964). Research intended to be therapeutic for subjects is different from that in which the subjects are primarily a means to the welfare of others. That distinction moved the ethics of nontherapeutic research into the mainstream: misuse of research subjects did not have to be at the level of a Nazi atrocity to be unethical. The Helsinki Code proposed also that research consent by a proxy (a substitute decision-maker) might in some cases be ethical. The Helsinki Code has since then undergone several revisions, but consensus had begun to build about the fundamental ethical principles of human research ethics.

Soon after, the disclosure of several instances of research abuse in the United States made it clear that the recently articulated principles would have to become more specific and be embodied in policy and regulation. The Tuskegee Syphilis Study (Mitford, 1972), the Willowbrook Studies (Ramsey, 1970), and the Jewish Chronic Disease Hospital study (Langer, 1966) all used subjects whose free and informed consent to participate was at best questionable in studies in which potential harm to the subjects was disproportionate to the potential benefit. Federal committees and task forces worked throughout the 1970s to make clear and precise what is ethical in the use of human subjects in research. The most significant of their outputs was the *Belmont Report* (National Commission for the Protection of Human Subjects of Biomedical and Behavioral Research, 1979). That report is the basis for much informed dialogue about research ethics, the IRB process, and FDA and other government regulations.

The authors of the *Belmont Report* proposed three broad principles as fundamental to ethical human subjects research: respect for persons, beneficence, and justice.

These general principles would not by themselves solve particular ethical problems. Instead, they "provide an analytical framework that will guide the resolution of ethical problems."

RESPECT FOR PERSONS

The *Belmont Report* draws on a fundamental belief about what persons *are* in order to state how they *ought to be treated.* Human beings are autonomous, i.e., they are capable of self-determination by comprehending information and making considered judgments based on their own preferences. In ordinary life, this leads to the ethical principle that human beings should be respected by being given maximum freedom to make their own choices. In research, this same principle recognizes research participation as elective and that research subjects, with full information and comprehension, make a voluntary choice to participate. Voluntariness must be maintained; i.e., subjects are free to withdraw at any time. Informed consent includes all the processes leading up to and maintaining the voluntariness of the choice to participate in research, both before and during the research. It is not just the signed consent form or even the act of signing it.

Persons' abilities to receive and comprehend information, relate it to their own preferences, and then make a decision are sometimes limited. Their own immaturity or disability can limit free choice. So also can some feature of the environment in which the consent process takes place. Respect for persons requires that we protect from harm those whose self-determination is diminished. At the extreme, it may require overriding the individual's judgment in order to do what is in that person's best interests. Still, the first duty of respect is to honor the autonomy of persons. Research with older subjects can test the richness of this principle as an analytical framework. Some older adults are well able to make their own decisions; others may require accommodation or assistance in making decisions; and some cannot make their own decisions even with assistance. We will return to this topic. There are other implications to respect for autonomy. The duty to protect confidentiality has its roots not just in agreements made but in respect for persons; controlling disclosure of intimate knowledge concerning oneself is a way of preserving one's own autonomy.

BENEFICENCE

The Hippocratic maxim "First, do no harm" is important but not sufficient to guide the ethics of research. The risk of harm must be compared with the potential benefits, through a form of cost-benefit analysis which takes place on three levels: for the sake of the individual research subject, for all those affected by the protocol, and for society-at-large. Good research design and execution are ethical, insofar as they minimize harm and maximize benefit. The metaphor of "balancing" risks with benefits may, however, disguise some of the complexity and ambiguity involved in such a calculus (Weijer, 2000). Older adults have fewer remaining years than their younger counterparts to experience either the benefits or harm related to research participation. They may be more inclined to altruistic behavior than younger persons (Midlarsky *et al.*, 1994). While cost-benefit analysis provides an analytic technique, it does not itself resolve some of the underlying questions in ethics.

JUSTICE

The *Belmont Report* uses the term "justice" to refer to "fairness in distribution." This is different from the word's common association with enforceable rights and penalties within a legal system but consistent with general usage in the field of bioethics. Justice in this context involves the ethical allocation of a fair share of risks or possible harms incurred in research and the allocation of benefits expected to result from the research. Research risks can range from minor inconvenience, to discomfort, to actual harm. For an individual or group to carry a large share of risks of research without getting a proportionate share of the benefits seems unfair, even if it is difficult to say exactly what constitutes a fair and equitable distribution. The early history of human subject research is replete with examples of disadvantaged or vulnerable populations (prisoners, disabled elderly, developmentally disabled persons, etc.) serving as research subjects and risking harm in the quest for knowledge expected to benefit some other population. Study design and subject selection distribute potential harm among subjects. The knowledge acquired in research and the research activity itself (particularly in therapeutic clinical research) can be a source of tremendous benefits; the nature of the study itself and its subject recruitment and selection determine who will get those benefits.

Autonomy and Protection of Older Adults in Research: How Much Is Enough?

The aging process presents some unique challenges to respect for autonomy among older adults, particularly in relation to obtaining informed consent; and in the research environment those challenges are even more exquisitely complex. We will consider three possibilities that correspond roughly to the variations in decision-making capacities of older adults. The first two possibilities address recognizing and supporting the capacity of older adults to consent to research. The third addresses the possible and actual loss of that capacity.

Many older adults are as capable of informed consent for research as are other members of the population whose capacity to consent is not in question. The ethics of their participation as research subjects should not be presumed to be different from that of other adults. Some groups have been classified as vulnerable. Children, the developmentally disabled, the mentally ill, and prisoners and other institutionalized groups have all been at various times considered vulnerable groups, due to their inability to exercise fully independent and informed judgment, their lack of information or comprehension, their inability to decide, or some coercive influence. Identifying a group as vulnerable has important ethical implications for research: membership in the group confers protections that may limit or even prevent one from consenting to participate. Being identified with that group, rather than one's individual capacities, becomes the criterion for whether one is allowed to choose to participate or not to participate. Robert Butler, the first director of the National Institute on Aging, coined the term "ageism" to describe the process of systematic stereotyping and discrimination against people because they are old (Butler, 1969). In practice, it is most ethical to assume that older adults are as competent as others to make their own choices. If there is doubt in an individual case or the subject population for a specific study, the protocol should include ways of confirming the capacity to make a decision.

Some older adults, due to conditions commonly associated with aging, are capable of informed consent, but require additional accommodation to exercise it. Older adults typically undergo changes that may affect the informed consent process. Changes in vision and hearing are among them. More than 37% of noninstitutionalized persons 65 and over report trouble hearing and 17.5% report trouble seeing (National Center for Health Statistics, 2002). Visual acuity, color discrimination, and sensitivity all tend to decrease with age (Fozard *et al.*, 2001).

Cognitive changes include increased difficulty with selective and sustained attention (Rogers *et al.*, 2001) and slowing of information processing and retrieval (Madden, 2001). In making decisions, older adults typically use less information and have more difficulty accurately using comparative information (Park, 1999; Hibbard *et al.*, 2001).

These changes are sufficiently prevalent among the aging that they should be routinely considered in informed consent by older adults. The changes are typically moderate and their onset gradual, so that persons adapt (through eyeglasses and hearing aids, avoiding noisy restaurants, taking additional time for decision-making, etc.) and continue to lead autonomous lives. Accommodating these needs in the informed consent process is ethically important to ensure that older adults receive and comprehend the information they would use to make a considered and free judgment about participation. Such needs are not an indication that they should be protected by bypassing their own free choice.

Informed consent documents and recruiting materials should be high in visual contrast, with a simple large font. Discussions concerning participation should be held in an environment with a high light level, and minimal ambient noise and without visual and auditory distractions (Metlife, 1999). Completing the consent process in several stages on separate occasions can help some older adults to have sufficient time to comprehend the study and perhaps to consult with a trusted friend (Tymchuk *et al.*, 1990). These may be merely amenities or courtesies for younger subjects. With older adults they become ethically important as routine means of enabling them to exercise freely their autonomy.

Some older adults may not be able to provide informed consent. Various neurological, vascular, or psychiatric disorders, depression, or stroke can all affect an older person's capacity to consent. In the course of research a subject's lack of capacity may become evident. Concerns may develop during an initial interview or consent process, or in a run-in sometimes used prior to randomization (Ouslander *et al.*, 1993). Or they could arise in the course of neuropsychological testing integral to the protocol. In any case, study procedures for addressing such findings or concerns should be addressed explicitly, from the time of initial submission to an IRB for approval (Kapp, 1998). General guidelines are available for assessing the capacity of impaired individuals (National Bioethics Advisory Commission, 1998). Although tests are available to measure specific capacities, there is no consensus on which of these tests should be used for determining capacity to consent to research (Curry, 2002).

Testing for cognitive impairment in the research context may create additional ethical issues. The investigator may receive evidence of a previously undiagnosed condition in a potential research subject. Keeping that information confidential might prevent the subject from accessing needed therapeutic assistance. Disclosing it might violate an expectation of confidentiality. To manage such issues, some studies retain an appropriate health professional or ask subjects to consent to disclosure of relevant study information to an identified primary care physician.

Should those who have lost the capacity to consent be barred from being research subjects? While this might be consistent with an ethical principle that all research participation should be voluntary, it could work against the best interests of those same persons. Individually, it could prevent access to promising new therapies available only in clinical trials. On a broader level, it could stifle progress in the very diseases or conditions that render persons cognitively incapable of consenting. Nevertheless, it should always be determined whether a study *must* include subjects who have lost the capacity to consent. If the study could proceed as well without them, then it is best to use only subjects able to consent.

Federal regulations effectively defer to state law by insisting that consent in such cases involve the subject's legally authorized representative. States have laws to address decision-making for incapacitated persons, but those laws are for the most part designed to address the need for health care decision-making in urgent situations.

The fit of those rules to research consent is at best inexact, and at times irrelevant to the research environment (Hoffman *et al.*, 1998). As a result, there is active ethics discussion about how to act in the absence of laws and about what laws should be enacted. We will look specifically at two common features in state laws, proxy consent and advance directives, and discuss their application to the research environment.

In health care a proxy or surrogate makes decisions for the person who is incapable of consenting to treatment. While the specific method varies from state to state, there are generally two different ways. The person can, in advance of becoming incapable, name a proxy by granting power-of-attorney. In the absence of such a designation, the next of kin in an ordered list defined by state law becomes the decision-maker. The ethical expectation behind proxy consent is that the surrogate will have known the patient well enough and be sufficiently empathetic to the patient to make the decision the patient would have made. If what the patient would have decided is unknowable, the proxy must then make the decision that is in the best interests of the subject. Proxies in decision-making for nontherapeutic research are more problematic, because there is no expected benefit to the person beyond the altruistic satisfaction of contributing to the welfare of other humans in the future (Hoffman *et al.*, 1998; Kapp, 1994). In such situations proxy consent for research could result in abusively using demented persons to the benefit of others. For that reason, the American Geriatrics Society holds that proxy consent should not be used where the subject is incapacitated, is unlikely to directly benefit, and will undergo more than minimal risk (American Geriatrics Society, 1998). The Alzheimer's Association has taken a similar position (Alzheimer's Association, 1997).

Both of those organizations consider an advance directive for research as a tool that is useful in ways that a proxy consent is not. The health care advance directive, frequently embodied in a living will, is intended to direct end-of-life care. Just as in health care, an advance directive for research does not involve substituting one person's judgment for another's; it is a documented decision by a competent person which is to be honored if and when that person becomes incapacitated (Dresser, 2001). Advance directives differ from proxy consent in that they rely directly on a person's own previously expressed and documented choice. A common criticism of advance directives in health care is that persons are seldom able to envision the specific end-of-life circumstances in which others will be expected to apply the directive (Fagerlin *et al.*, 2004). It is at least as difficult to envision the kinds of research one might be a candidate for at some indefinite future date and how one's own needs and preferences might have changed by that time. For that reason, it is best not to assume an advance directive for research to be informed consent already given. It can serve as supportive documentation to guide a surrogate decision-maker (Sachs, 1994). Advance directives may also be helpful when a person is in the early stages of a progressive dementing illness, but still able to consent to participate in longitudinal research. Such an advance directive may guide the proxy when the subject is in later stages of the disease and no longer able to consent to continuing in or withdrawing from the study.

How great a risk may a surrogate consent to on behalf of an incapacitated research subject? What I shall call the "conservative approach" holds that nontherapeutic research that creates any risk of harm greater than minimal (i.e., greater than the risk of harm experienced in everyday living) should never be conducted on an incapacitated subject, even with proxy consent or an advance directive (Keyserlingk *et al.*, 1995). Positions more favorable to proxy consent for research have begun to emerge. The Alzheimer's Association has taken the position that, in research involving more than minimal risk, subjects who stand to benefit individually and have a proxy's consent should be allowed to participate. Scientific progress in understanding and fighting diseases that rob older adults of their ability to remain autonomous may require research on persons who are unable to consent to or benefit from that research.

Although respect for autonomy is ethically good, human beneficence (contributing to the common good) is also good; and respect for individual autonomy should not always take priority over beneficence. The American Geriatrics Society proposes developing a mechanism for future consideration of subjects who cannot consent and who have neither an advance directive nor reasonable expectation of benefit, but only in studies especially promising in the benefit they eventually provide to society. Similarly, Stephen Post has advocated recently that, recognizing that defeating Alzheimer disease (the most prevalent older adult dementia) is a high priority for our common good, we should think differently about risk in this category of research (Post, 2003). The issue should not be whether a study poses only "minimal risk," but where to set the upper threshold of allowable risk ("maximal potential risk"); and it should be set in a consensus conference of experts with due consideration of the social good.

The ethical waters do quickly become murky when we accept proxy consent or advance directives in research, or when we consider increasing the amount of risk an incapacitated subject may be asked to incur in support of some socially desirable outcome. When we do that, it becomes increasingly important to maintain other forms of respect for autonomy. A free consent can be withdrawn at any time. To maintain the freedom to withdraw, either the proxy or a "monitor" or "research intermediary" must be continuously involved on behalf of the incapacitated subject (Kapp, 1998). Monitors or proxies, along with the investigator, in such situations must watch for not only the best interests of the subject but also for the subject's continued assent to participate. Even a subject who is not cognitively able to consent to participate may at any point resist continued participation or express a strong preference for withdrawing, and such preferences should be noticed and honored.

In summary, there is ethical agreement that older adults should be able to consent or refuse to consent to participate in research, even if that requires some additional assistance. There is also agreement that incapacitated persons deserve special protection. The question is still open on whether the goal of controlling or eliminating diseases that affect older adults can be a societal good so important that it justifies increasing the maximum permissible risk to subjects who cannot consent.

Your Home/My Lab: The Ethics of Research in Nursing Homes

A VULNERABLE POPULATION

Long-term care includes not only nursing homes but other environments such as day health centers, day hospitals, assisted living facilities, and home health services. Long-term care services all deal with concentrations of older adults who have significant ongoing needs for health care and various forms of personal assistance, depend on professionals to meet those needs, and spend substantial time in environments controlled by those professionals. The nursing home will be the focus of this discussion, but much of what is said about it will be applicable to other sites of long-term care as well.

Data from the National Nursing Home Survey provide a fairly illustrative picture of nursing home residents in the United States (Jones, 2000). More than 1.6 million persons 65 years and over reside in nursing homes. More than 90% are age 65 or over, and 46% age 85 or over. The current population has an average length of stay of 892 days. Those discharged from nursing homes have an average stay of 272 days. Many nursing home residents require help with basic needs such as bathing (94%), dressing (87%), toileting (56%), and eating (47%); 47.7% have an active diagnosis of dementia (U.S. Department of Health and Human Services, 1998).

Together, these data show that nursing home populations are vulnerable in several important respects. They depend on others to meet the most basic of human needs as well as their specific health needs. A high percentage have limited or questionable capacity for decision-making. The facility is home for its residents; but they do not have the same control over their home environment that we ordinarily use to gain privacy. They are subject to schedules and routines imposed for the good of the whole. They can be solicited for research participation in their home.

The nursing home can be an attractive and efficient site for aging research. It has an unusually high concentration of older residents; human and environmental variables are monitored, measured, and controlled; health records are close by; and professional resources are available. These very features that make the nursing home attractive for research can also make its population vulnerable and make the ethical conduct of research more complex.

VULNERABILITY AND RESEARCH CONSENT IN THE NURSING HOME

Informed consent for research in the nursing home is ethically complex. The same health problems that result in nursing home admissions can also affect the capacity to consent. Ordinarily, we assume persons have the capacity to consent and then watch and check for exceptions *during* and after the recruitment and consent processes. In the nursing home, there is a higher probability that each individual is incapable of consent or requires some additional assistance. Consequently, potential subjects should be screened for capacity by a knowledgeable and disinterested party *before* recruitment or consent. Making this initial determination of capacity ensures that the appropriate approach is then taken to the consent process itself. Some advocate the use of an ethics or research committee for screening (Cassel, 1988). Others recommend using knowledgeable nursing home staff, such as nurses or social workers (Ouslander *et al.*, 1993). In either case, the researcher must still ensure that the consent process itself is monitored, that proxies are used as appropriate, and that the research is monitored for ongoing consent or assent.

Nursing home residents have significant health care needs and are accustomed to the continual presence of professionals charged with meeting those needs. They (and their families) do not typically regard the nursing home as a research site; teaching and research nursing homes are uncommon. When research is conducted in the same environment as the one in which persons typically receive health care, they may assume that the research is related to their care and that it is in their best interests to participate (Lidz *et al.*, 2002). This assumption, the therapeutic misconception, can result in a consent based on misunderstanding. Ethical researchers take steps to prevent such mistaken assumptions. To prevent such misconceptions, it may be important to have someone not identified as a regular caregiver to discuss consent with the subject and proxy and to conduct any interventions that are related to the study protocol.

Understanding the consent process for treatment can be helpful for those who seek research consent in the nursing home. That process can become complex. Staff may have an interest in providing correct health care and in an orderly routine to benefit the residents as a group. Family members of residents may vacillate between wanting the best health care and wanting them to be as free as possible to continue their preferred living patterns. Residents may experience the same ambivalence, complicated occasionally by confusion and forgetfulness.

Residents, family members and staff as a group must make decisions that direct health care, respect the autonomy of the resident, and maintain the orderly operation of the nursing home. This is frequently done in care planning meetings in which all groups and interests are represented. Afterwards, it may be difficult to identify a point in this process at which consent actually takes place. In some respects, it is more like a negotiation process (Moody, 1996). Still, it is highly adapted to the vulnerability and possible incapacity of the resident.

Researchers in nursing homes may find a similar process taking place with research consent. Multiple parties may participate, and they may bring various considerations to bear on the decision. It can be challenging to avoid deviating from the protocol during such a process. The researcher needs to view this unfamiliar and complex process as responsive to the unusual situation of a vulnerable population. To ignore it is to disregard the imperfect supports in place to protect persons in an ethically ambiguous situation.

VULNERABILITY AND DISTRIBUTIVE JUSTICE

To do research with a nursing home population solely for the convenience it presents for the researcher raises questions of distributive justice or fairness. Putting a vulnerable population at risk for the benefit of some other group can be unethical. Nontherapeutic research, not reasonably expected to provide medical benefit to vulnerable subjects, might appear unethical; but even the calculation of risks and benefits in the nursing home environment is complex. Rigorously insulating nursing home populations from risk can ignore other human needs and deprive them of stimulation, social involvement, and the opportunity to contribute to society, features already frequently lacking in the lives of nursing home residents. "Such participation in the human community should not be automatically withheld from a whole class of persons in the name of protecting them from exploitation" (Cassel, 1988). The opportunity for involvement should be considered in this cost-benefit analysis, and its value should be considered in relation to the nursing home resident's unique situation. It must, however, be used in good faith; as risk increases and the capacity to consent is diminished, that justification becomes less reasonable.

We should also consider studies that are especially promising in their potential to improve nursing home living. Such studies, by their nature, may have to involve members of the population they are intended to benefit. The vulnerability of the nursing home population should not by itself prevent that research. Research into the diseases that result in nursing home admission, into optimal nursing home practices or into conditions such as decubiti, incontinence, environmentally induced depression, and nosocomial infection will benefit the nursing home population as a whole, even if not all subjects will individually receive the benefits. The question of whether the nursing home population may ethically be recruited for such research is distinct from whether an individual resident may be recruited. Whether an individual resident should participate is still a function of the informed consent process, which still is especially complex in the nursing home.

MANAGING RESEARCH IN THE NURSING HOME

Nursing homes are neither designed nor staffed for research purposes. Their mission, and primary ethical obligation, is to provide the health care personal services needed while offering residents maximum autonomy in a homelike atmosphere. The researcher who is given access to a nursing home must design and conduct research that does not interfere with the nursing home's own obligations, which are also the rights of its residents.

The Institutional Review Board, or IRB, is a federally mandated committee whose role is to review research proposals and monitor research so as to protect human subjects. In reviewing proposals to conduct research in nursing homes, IRBs may require the investigator to submit documentation from the facility's administrator agreeing to the research, identifying an onsite person who will attest to the study's appropriateness with that facility's population, and ascertaining the facility's capabilities to perform the research. If nursing home staff are to be involved in data collection, the administrator may also need to provide assurance that they have appropriate expertise and will follow IRB-approved procedures. Such a requirement can elicit the kind of understanding, communication, and agreement between the investigator and the nursing home that is needed for nursing home research to be ethical and successful.

IRBs are typically university-based and are most familiar with research sites such as laboratories and acute and primary care facilities. They may lack the knowledge to oversee research in nursing homes and sometimes use a consultant to assist in reviewing and monitoring such research. The researcher will need to be prepared to explain to an IRB how the protocol meets its ethical standards in an environment unfamiliar to that committee.

The nursing home must make a considered decision about permitting a research project to take place within its walls. Nursing homes may find it difficult to review research opportunities due to the lack of familiarity with research. They need to address questions related to the rights and welfare of their residents during the research. They may need also to address facility-wide issues such as disruption of routine, resource consumption, and potential benefits to the facility. A nursing home's participation in research is elective; producing new and generalizable knowledge is usually not at the core of its mission and must be weighed against competing priorities. One author tells of a facility in which 17 different research proposals were received in one year (Daly *et al.*, 2000). It is unlikely that a facility would have the resources to accommodate that many requests; if it did, competition for enrollment could easily doom all studies. Research committees in nursing homes, as Daly describes, can analyze such issues. Such committees are still uncommon, but developing one is worth considering in a facility planning to be open to research. Nursing home ethics committees are somewhat more common and present another possible avenue for consideration of protocols (Cassel, 1988). Such committees function in ways analogous to hospital ethics committees, by consulting and sometimes educating on issues related to ethical decisions in the institution (Hoffman *et al.*, 1995).

In summary, research in the nursing home is complex ethically. The presence of a subject in the nursing home raises initial concerns for that person's ability to consent that must be addressed in study design and execution. The facility itself has an ethical mandate different from that of the researcher, and honoring it may require adaptation of the protocol and persistent communication. Research in nursing homes should be guided by an interest in the specific characteristics of its residents and structure, and not by the apparent convenient access to older subjects.

Is Aging Research Anti-Aging?

This is truly an odd question. It is a question about ethics, but one that operates at a level different from the "how-to" of ethical research practices discussed so far in this chapter. It has more to do with the fundamental values, direction, and purpose that underlie one's engagement in aging research. Such fundamental values influence one's choice of research areas and beliefs about the benefits of that research.

Much of aging research involves understanding and addressing the diseases and conditions that occur in an aging population. That sort of aging research is not ethically controversial and clearly not anti-aging; words like "disease" and "disability" already carry with them the implication that they should be controlled, avoided, or eradicated. Other research begins from the belief in an organism-wide process of aging, a unified process of senescence that is distinct from various specific processes of degeneration and must be dealt with as one would deal with disease. Discovering and controlling that process, just as one would research and address a disease, is "age retardation" (President's Council on Bioethics, 2003).

Age retardation seems to be a neutral or even a praiseworthy enterprise, but it has encountered significant objections with bases in ethics. Common to those objections is the belief that aging and mortality are so fundamental to human existence that, without them, we would lack something essential to human flourishing. "Old age is an inevitable human condition, one that should not be defined as a medical problem to be conquered. . . ." (Joint International Research Group, 1994). Let us consider several of those objections.

First, significant increases in lifespan could create significant societal problems (Capron, 2004). A longer lifespan could result in a larger aging population and a longer period of decline for humans. Significant gains in age retardation could upset delicate social institutions related to health care, employment, retirement, marriage, etc. In so doing they could be destructive of the common good and create issues of distributive justice and intergenerational equity.

Second, the enticement of eternal youth is a powerful tool for taking unfair advantage of those who most fear aging, disability, and mortality. Our culture places great value on staying young. A promise of a miracle treatment can waste money, actually cause harm, and dissuade the gullible from doing what is best known to support one's chances of aging well—a healthy lifestyle.

Third, the pursuit of a cure for biological aging seems to ignore or deny anything positive about psychosocial aging. Human life is shaped by our understanding of our own finitude and imperfection. It underlies our perception of youth and of maturity, and of unique wisdom that does not come without years of life and the recognition that it will end. In short the quest for age retardation is an expression of ageism, as described by Butler (1969).

It can be plausibly argued that a researcher in basic science is essentially neutral on the age retardation issue. The scientist does not choose how the knowledge developed in the laboratory might be used by others. Unlocking the secrets of cellular aging might just as well support the efforts to prevent or retard cancer as to retard aging. The legitimacy of that perspective begins to fade along a continuum that begins with basic science and culminates in clinical trials. Translational science moves one closer to exploring specific applications of the knowledge discovered. Clinical research and trials are farther along the same continuum.

It can also be argued that, with informed planning, the calamities that age retardation could rain upon us could just as well be blessings. Most importantly, the recurring debates about the uses of new knowledge in society would suffer dramatically without the involvement of the scientists who create that knowledge. The rate of scientific progress frequently outruns the adjustment of social policy that must occur with the new knowledge. So it was with nuclear energy, the Internet, and, more recently, stem cell therapies. We cannot afford to repeat the experience with the significant new knowledge emerging in biogerontology. Without scientific input, social policy would still change, but just in time and in ill-informed and counterproductive ways.

Conclusion

Applying principles of ethics to aging research is more than one project. It consists in part of artfully and ethically responding to the obvious, using accepted principles of ethics. We know, for example, that some persons are impaired, that impairment makes it difficult to get informed consent, and that we ought to take additional measures to protect those persons. We know some of the measures that can be effective in enhancing informed consent or in protecting those who cannot consent.

Some ethical problems are sufficiently identified and articulated, but still lack a satisfactory response around which consensus can be built. There are still open questions about whether the pursuit of the common good should be allowed to override the individual interests of a research subject with a surrogate decision-maker. Other problems are so new and the science supporting them so seminal that the best interests of society will be served only by a broad base of participation in establishing social policy sufficiently robust to accommodate new research findings in aging. "Doing ethics" becomes something more than learning and accepting rules and principles. It also involves active participation in developing that ethics.

Some Recommended Resources

Ethics in aging research is actually the intersection of three different studies, gerontology, ethics, and research methodology, each of which has its own literature. Among periodicals, consider the *Hastings Center Report*, *IRB: Ethics and Human Research*, the *Journal of the American Geriatric Society*, and the *American Journal of Bioethics*. Disease-specific periodicals can be helpful as well. The Alzheimer's research community has sustained a long and fruitful discussion related to capacity for consent, much of which is in *Alzheimer's Disease and Related Disorders*.

The literature of research ethics is in some respects different from publications that report research findings. Frequently authors, in trying to get to core issues, work with principles that were not recently discovered. It is not at all uncommon for a seminal book or article from several decades ago to continue to be valuable. See, for example, *The Patient as Person*, which appeared in the wake of the research scandals of the 1960s (Ramsey, 1970).

Consider also the work of associations with an interest in aging and research. Much of their contributions can be accessed through the respective websites of the Alzheimer's Association, the American Geriatric Society, and the Association for the Accreditation of Human Research Protection Programs. Websites for are listed in the References section.

REFERENCES

Alzheimer's Association (1997). Position Paper: Ethical Issues in Dementia Research. http://www.alz.org/AboutUs/Position Statements/overview.asp.

American Geriatrics Society (1998). Position Statement: Informed Consent for Research on Human Subjects with Dementia. http://www.americangeriatrics.org/products/positionpapers/infconsentPF.shtml.

Association for the Accreditation of Human Research Protection Programs. www.aahrpp.org.

Birren, J.E., and Schaie, K.W. (2001), Eds. *Handbook of the Psychology of Aging*. San Diego: Academic Press.

Butler, R.N. (1969). Age-ism: Another form of bigotry. *The Gerontologist 9*, 243–246.

Capron, A.M. (2004). Ethical aspects of major increases in life span and life expectancy. In Aaron, H.J., and Schwartz, W.B., Eds., *Coping with Methuselah: The Impact of Molecular Biology on Medicine and Society*, pp. 198–234. Washington, DC: Brookings Institution Press.

Cassel, C.K. (1988). Ethical issues in the conduct of research in long term care. *The Gerontologist 28*, 90–96.

Curry, L. (2002). Ethical and legal considerations in health services research. In Kapp, M.B. (Ed.), *Ethics, Law, and Aging Review*, 8. pp. 57–75. New York: Springer Publishing Company.

Daly, J.M., and Maas, M.L. (2000). Research review committees in long-term care settings. *Geriatric Nursing 21*, 13–15.

Dresser, R. (2001). Advance directives in dementia research: promoting autonomy and protecting subjects. *IRB: Ethics and Human Research, 23*, 1–6.

Fagerlin, A., and Schneider, C. (2004). Enough: The failure of the living will. *Hastings Cent Rep 34(2)*, 30–42.

Fozard, J.L., and Gordon-Salant, S. (2001). Changes in vision and hearing with aging. In Birren, J.E., and Schaie, K.W., Eds. *Handbook of the Psychology of Aging*, pp. 241–266. San Diego: Academic Press.

Hibbard, J.H., Slovic, P., Peters, E., Finucane, M.L., and Tusler, M. (2001). Is the informed-choice policy approach appropriate for medicare beneficiaries? *Health Aff*, May/June 2001, pp. 199–203.

High, D.M., and Doole, M.M. (1995). Ethical and legal issues in conducting research involving elderly subjects. *Behavioral Science and the Law 13(3)*, 319–335.

Hoffman, D.E., Boyle, P., and Levenson, S.A. (1995). *Handbook for Nursing Home Ethics Committees*. Washington, DC: American Association of Homes and Services for the Aging.

Hoffman, D., and Schwartz, J. (1998). Proxy consent to participation of the decisionally impaired in medical research—Maryland's policy initiative. *Journal of Health Care Law and Policy 1*, 123–153.

Joint International Research Group (1994). What do we owe the elderly? *Hastings Cent Rep 24(2)Suppl.*, 1–11.

Jones, A. (2000). National Nursing Home Survey, 1999 Summary. National Center for Health Statistics. Vital and Health Statistics 13 (152). http://www.cdc.gov/nchs/about/major/nnhsd/nnhsd.htm.

Juengst, E.T., Binstock, R.H., Mehlman, M., Post, S.G., and Whitehouse, P. (2003). Biogerontology, "anti-aging medicine," and the challenges of human enhancement. *Hastings Cent Rep 33*, 21–30.

Kapp, M.B. (1994). Proxy decision making in Alzheimer disease research: Durable powers of attorney, guardianship, and other alternatives. *Alzheimer Dis Assoc Disord 8 Suppl. 4*, 28–37.

Kapp, M. (1998). Decisional capacity, older human research subjects, and IRBs: Beyond forms and guidelines. *Stanford Law and Policy Review 9*, 359–371.

Keyserlingk, E., Glass, K., Kogan, S., and Gauthier, S. (1995) Proposed guidelines for the participation of persons with dementia as research subjects. *Perspect Biol Med 38*, 319–362.

Langer, E. (1966). Human experimentation: New York verdict affirms patient's rights. *Science 151*, 663–666.

Lidz, C.W., and Appelbaum, P.S. (2002). The therapeutic misconception: Problems and solutions. *Med Care 40(9 Suppl.)*, 55–63.

Madden, D. (2001). Speed and timing of behavioral processes. In Birren, J.E., and Schaie, K.W., Eds., *Handbook of the Psychology of Aging*, pp. 288–312. San Diego: Academic Press.

Metlife Mature Market Institute (1999). The Mature Market: Guidelines for Effective Communication http://www.metlife.com/Applications/Corporate/WPS/CDA/PageGenerator/0%2C1674%2CP2801%2C00.html.

Midlarsky, E., and Kahana, E. (1994). *Altruism in Later Life*. Thousand Oaks, CA: SAGE Publications.

Mitford, J. (1972). *Kind and Usual Punishment: The Prison Business*. New York: Alfred A. Knopf.

Moody, H.R. (1996). *Ethics in an Aging Society*. Baltimore: Johns Hopkins University Press.

National Bioethics Advisory Commission. (1998). Research involving persons with mental disorders that may affect decision-making capacity. Rockville, MD.

National Center for Health Statistics (2002). National Health Interview Survey, 2002. Centers for Disease Control and Prevention.

National Commission for the Protection of Human Subjects of Biomedical and Behavioral Research. (1979). The Belmont Report. Department of Health, Education and Welfare. http://www.hhs.gov/ohrp/humansubjects/guidance/belmont.htm.

Nuremburg Code. (1949). Trials of War Criminals Before the Nuremberg Military Tribunals Under Control Council Law No. 10, Vol. 2, Nuremberg, October 1946–April 1949. (Washington, DC: US Government Printing Office, 1949). pp. 181–182.

Ouslander, J.G., and Schnelle, J.F. (1993). Research in nursing homes: Practical aspects. *J Am Geriatr Soc 41*, 182–187.

Park, D.C. (1999). Aging and the controlled and automatic processing of medical information and medical intentions. In Park, D.C., Morrell, R.W., and Shifrenm, K. Eds. *Processing of Medical Information in Aging Patients: Cognitive and Human Factors Perspectives*, Mahwah, NJ: Erlbaum.

Post, S.G. (2003) Full-spectrum proxy consent for research participation when persons with Alzheimer disease lose decisional capacities: Research ethics and the common good. *Alzheimer Dis Assoc Disord 17(Suppl. 1)*, 3–11.

President's Council on Bioethics (2003). Age-retardation: Scientific possibilities and moral challenges. Working paper. http://bioethicsprint/bioethics.gov/background/age_retardation.html.

Ramsey, P. (1970). *The Patient as Person*. New Haven: Yale University Press.

Rogers, W., and Fisk, A. (2001). Understanding the role of attention in cognitive aging research. . In Birren, J.E., and Schaie, K.W., Eds., *Handbook of the Psychology of Aging*, pp. 267–287. San Diego: Academic Press.

Sachs, G. (1994) Advance consent for dementia research. *Alzheimer Dis Assoc Disord 8(Suppl. 4)*, 19–27.

Stocking, C., Hougham, G., Baron, A., and Sachs, G. (2004). Ethics reporting in publications about research with Alzheimer's disease patients. *J Am Geriatr Soc* 52, 305–310.

Tymchuk, A., and Ouslander, J. (1990). Optimizing the informed consent process with elderly people. *Educational Gerontology 16*, 245–257.

U.S. Department of Health and Human Services (1998). *Characteristics of Nursing Home Residents—1996*. Washington, DC: Agency for Health Care Policy and Research, Pub. No. 99-0006.

Weijer, C. (2000). The ethical analysis of risk. *Journal of Law, Medicine, and Ethics 28*, 344–361.

World Medical Association. (1964). "Declaration of Helsinki." Ethical Principles for Medical Research Involving Human Subjects. http://www.wma.net/e/policy/b3.htm.

7

Ethical Aspects of Research Involving Elderly Persons

Paul S. Mueller and C. Christopher Hook

The number of elders living in the U.S. is rapidly growing. Elders are uniquely burdened with illnesses and account for most deaths. In order to reduce morbidity and mortality experienced by elders, research involving elderly human subjects is needed. Contemporary codes of ethics and regulations governing research involving human subjects derive from the ethical principles of respect for persons, beneficence and justice. Investigators conducting research involving elders should be familiar with and adhere to these general ethical principles. In addition, investigators should acknowledge and address the potential ethical challenges of research involving elderly persons. These challenges include obtaining adequate informed consent by conveying sufficient information and ensuring subject voluntariness and decision-making capacity. Research involving elders with impaired decision-making capacity is especially challenging. In this chapter, the history of human subjects research, the general ethical principles of research, and ethical challenges specifically associated with conducting research involving elders are discussed. In addition, an approach to these challenges and a list of resources for investigators engaged in research involving elders are described.

Introduction

Because of advances in public health and medicine, Americans are living longer. By the year 2020, nearly 54 million elderly (older than 65 years) persons (also known as "elders") will be living in the United States (U.S. Census Bureau, 2000). However, compared to younger persons, elders are uniquely burdened with illnesses. On average, an elderly person has 3 to 4 illnesses and a 20% annual risk of hospitalization. Furthermore, elders are the largest consumers of prescription drugs and account for most deaths (Jahnigen, D., and Schrier, R., 1986; Swift, C., 1988; U.S. Census Bureau, 2000). As a result of these factors, clinicians will care for an increasing number of elderly persons with multiple medical problems, some of which are uniquely associated with aging itself (e.g., Alzheimer disease).

Medical care that improves the outcomes (e.g., mortality, morbidity, and quality of life) of elderly persons depends on research advances. This research, in turn, depends on the involvement of elderly patients in research studies. Research on health-related problems of elders is important not only because of demographic trends, but also because of a lack of previous research involving elders and poor understanding of the processes associated with aging itself and what constitutes normal aging (Zimmer *et al.*, 1985; Kaye, J. *et al.*, 1990; Sachs, G. and Cassel, C., 1990). Hence, research involving elders is needed. If one accepts the need for research involving elderly subjects, then the ethical aspects of human subjects research in general and research involving elders specifically should be considered (Denham, M., 1984). In this chapter, we discuss the history of human subjects research and the unique aspects and potential ethical challenges of conducting research involving elders. In addition, we provide suggestions for conducting research involving elders that yields ethically valid and fruitful results not only for the good of elders but also for society in general.

History of Human Subjects Research

THE NUREMBERG CODE

Before World War Two, no internationally acknowledged code of ethics for human subjects research existed. During the war, Nazi physicians conducted many experiments of dubious value on thousands of prisoners. The experiments were conducted without the prisoners' informed consent and many prisoners were mutilated and killed. The discovery of the atrocities committed by the Nazi physicians under the guise of experimentation led to the Nuremberg War Crimes Physicians Trial of Nazi physicians for "crimes against humanity" consisting of experments upon concentration camp prisoners and others without their voluntary consent resulting in "murders, brutalities, cruelties, tortures, atrocities and other inhuman acts" (The Nuremberg Code, 1947). The trial judges included in their 1947 verdict a list of rules for

TABLE 7.1.
The Nuremberg Code: "Permissible Medical Experiments" (Excerpted from The Nuremberg Code, 1947)

1. The voluntary consent of the human subject is absolutely essential.
2. The experiment should be such as to yield fruitful results for the good of society, unprocurable by other methods or means of study, and not random and unnecessary in nature.
3. The experiment should be so designed and based on the results of animal experimentation and a knowledge of the natural history of the disease or other problem under study that the anticipated results will justify the performance of the experiment.
4. The experiment should be so conducted as to avoid all unnecessary physical and mental suffering and injury.
5. No experiment should be conducted where there is an a priori reason to believe that death or disabling injury will occur, except, perhaps, in those experiments where the experimental physicians also serve as subjects.
6. The degree of risk to be taken should never exceed that determined by the humanitarian importance of the problem to be solved by the experiment.
7. Proper preparations should be made and adequate facilities provided to protect the experimental subject against even remote possibilities of injury, disability, or death.
8. The experiment should be conducted only by scientifically qualified persons. The highest degree of skill and care should be required through all stages of the experiment of those who conduct or engage in the experiment.
9. During the course of the experiment the human subject should be at liberty to bring the experiment to an end if he has reached the physical or mental state where continuation of the experiment seems to him to be impossible.
10. During the course of the experiment the scientist in charge must be prepared to terminate the experiment at any stage, if he has probably cause to believe, in the exercise of the good faith, superior skill and careful judgment required of him that a continuation of the experiment is likely to result in injury, disability, or death to the experimental subject.

"Permissible Medical Experiments" which later became known as the Nuremberg Code and was the first internationally recognized code of ethics for experimentation on human subjects. The rules included requirements that (a) subject voluntary consent be obtained; (b) the study benefits outweigh the risks; (c) the study should be conducted to avoid unnecessary harm, with no experiment to be conducted if there is *a priori* belief that death or injury will occur; and (d) the subject has the right to withdraw from the study at any time (Table 7.1).

WORLD MEDICAL ASSOCIATION DECLARATION OF HELSINKI

Notably, the Nuremberg Code only addresses research involving healthy subjects. In an effort to address the ethical aspects of research involving patients, the World Medical Association drafted the Declaration of Helsinki in 1964 (World Medical Association Declaration of Helsinki, 1964). As with the Nuremberg Code, informed consent, the need for favorable risk-to-benefit ratios, and subject voluntariness are central features of the Declaration. However, the Declaration also addresses proxy consent (e.g., when potential subjects have impaired decision-making capacity), the use of control groups and placebos, and nontherapeutic research.

Human Subjects Research in the United States after World War Two

Despite the Nuremberg Code and the Declaration of Helsinki, medical research after World War Two continued to be tainted by revelations of widespread abuse of human subjects. Henry K. Beecher described some of these revelations in an article published in the *New England Journal of Medicine* in 1966 (Beecher, H., 1966). In this article, Beecher described 22 studies conducted at prestigious institutions and published in leading medical journals in which human research subjects were subjected to excessive risks (i.e., risk to benefit ratio) often without their knowledge or consent. Beecher concluded that (a) it is "absolutely essential" to obtain informed consent from research subjects; (b) consent is not valid if the patient doesn't understand "what is to be undertaken" in the study; (c) "the gain anticipated from an experiment must be commensurate with the risk involved"; (d) research reports should explicitly state that ethical "proprieties have been observed"; and (e) data obtained unethically should not be published. Notably, Beecher hypothesized that these ethical breaches were due partly to the growth of public funding for research coupled with the need for investigators to publish to obtain such funding and advance professionally.

A number of studies cited by Beecher became notorious on their own. In a study of immunity to cancer at the Jewish Chronic Disease Hospital (New York), investigators injected live cancer cells into human subjects without obtaining informed consent. Another study involved the deliberate induction of infectious hepatitis (to understand better the natural history of the disease) in mentally impaired children who were residents at the Willowbrook State School for the Retarded (New York). The ethical concerns raised by this study were the deliberate exposure of the children to harm, and the deception and coercion that occurred during the parental informed consent process (Weyers, W., 2003).

Another study that achieved notoriety was the Tuskegee (Alabama) syphilis study. The purpose of this study, which was funded by the U.S. government and conducted by the U.S. Public Health Service from 1932 to 1972, was to determine the natural history of untreated late-stage syphilis in poor African–American men. The men were not told that they had syphilis, did not receive effective treatment for the disease, and were not informed that they were participating in an experiment. Instead, subjects were told they had "bad blood" and that the examinations they underwent were treatments. In fact, the study continued after effective treatment for syphilis became available. A widely publicized media report of the study resulted in public outrage, a class-action lawsuit, a congressional investigation, and the study's termination (Weyers, W., 2003).

The National Commission

Revelations of the aforementioned unethical studies led to public scrutiny and debate regarding human subjects research and ultimately regulatory attempts to prevent abuse. Particular concerns were respect for persons (i.e., research subjects) and the equitable distribution of the burdens and benefits of research. Congressional hearings led to the passage of the National Research Act in 1974. This act mandated the establishment of institutional review boards (IRBs) for the independent review of research at institutions receiving federal support for human subject research and created the National Commission for the Protection of Human Subjects of Biomedical and Behavioral Research. A major achievement of the National Commission was the influential Belmont Report (The Belmont Report, 1979).

THE BELMONT REPORT

The Belmont Report begins by recognizing that while research involving human subjects has produced important social benefits including reduced morbidity, greater longevity and improved quality of life, this research has also posed challenging and troubling ethical questions. The report also explicitly distinguishes clinical practice and medical research. The purpose of clinical practice is to enhance the well-being of the patient by using interventions for which there is an expectation for success. On the other hand, the purpose of medical research is to gain new knowledge; research involves testing hypotheses and drawing conclusions through experiments from which research subjects may or may not derive benefits. Notably, clinical practice and medical research often occur in the same setting. However, subjects in the clinical setting may not recall that they are participating in a research study (Riecken, H. and Ravich, R., 1982). It is important for research subjects to be informed of and understand these differences (American College of Physicians, 2005).

The Belmont Report also recognizes that the Nuremberg Code and later codes were drafted to assure the ethical conduct of human subjects research. However, these codes consist primarily of rules for conducting research that do not address every potential research scenario (e.g., a scenario that the rules do not cover or conflict with each other). To address these deficiencies of the codes, the authors of the Belmont Report describe three prima facie ethical principles for conducting human subjects research that provide a basis on which specific rules may be established, appraised and interpreted. These three principles are respect for persons, beneficence (nonmaleficence) and justice.

1. Respect for persons

The principle of respect for persons requires that investigators acknowledge that individual human research subjects are autonomous (the word *autonomy* derives from the Greek *autos* for "self" and *nomos* for "rule") agents with the right of self-determination (Beauchamp, T. and Childress J., 2001). The centrality of informed consent in research derives from this principle. Informed consent consists of three elements: (a) adequate information regarding the research study and its potential risks and benefits and subject understanding of the information; (b) subject decision-making capacity; and (c) subject voluntary involvement (i.e., without coercion). Respect for persons is maximized when the elements of informed consent are fully realized. Notably, not every person is capable of self-determination. Hence, this principle also requires that investigators protect subjects with diminished autonomy (e.g., due to impaired decision making capacity) from exploitation and harm.

2. Beneficence

The principle of beneficence requires that investigators act to secure the well-being of human research subjects, maximize benefits and minimize risks and harm. The Belmont Report, however, recognizes that the goal of avoiding harm may, in fact, require that research be done to determine what is harmful and what is beneficial and, hence, may involve exposing research subjects to risks. The dilemma for investigators is to determine when benefits should be forgone because of risks and when benefits should be sought despite the risks. Research protocols should be designed in ways that maximize benefit while at the same time minimizing harm. Proposed research questions must also be worth answering. Research studies involving human subjects, even those involving minimal risk, are not justifiable if the research does not generate scientifically valid and worthy new knowledge. Hence, proper study design and methods are not only scientific, but also ethical, obligations.

The Belmont Report also declares that: (a) inhumane treatment of human subjects is never morally justified;

(b) investigators should determine if human subjects are necessary and, if so, the risks should be reduced to those necessary or alternative means used to reach the research objective; (c) if the research involves risk of harm, the risk should be justified; (d) the appropriateness of involving vulnerable populations in research should be demonstrated; and (e) risks and benefits should be clearly stated in informed consent documents.

3. Justice

The principle of justice refers to the equitable distribution of the benefits and burdens of research. Injustice occurs when one receives (or is denied) benefits or when one bears (or does not bear) burdens without good reason. Applied to research involving human subjects, the benefits and burdens of participating in research should be distributed fairly. In fact, the Belmont Report explicitly notes the legacy of unjust prior research studies (and specifically mentions the Tuskegee study) in which the burdens of being research subjects fell primarily upon disadvantaged (e.g., poor) persons, while the benefits of improved healthcare was realized primarily by privileged patients.

Instead, the selection of research subjects should be based on the needs of the study. Furthermore, publicly-funded research should not unduly involve individuals who will not likely benefit from therapeutic innovations that derive from the research, and when such research results in therapeutic innovations, the innovations should not provide advantages only to those who can afford them.

General applications of the three prima facie ethical principles described in the Belmont Report are described in Table 7.2.

TABLE 7.2.
Ethical principles of the Belmont Report and their applications to human subjects research (data from The Belmant Report, 1979 and Cohen, J.)

Principles	Applications
Respect for Persons	• Informed consent
	• Protection of vulnerable research subjects (e.g., persons with impaired decision-making capacity and institutionalized persons)
	• Proxy consent and subject assent for persons with impaired decision-making capacity
	• Maintenance of subject confidentiality
Beneficence	• Scientifically valid study design
	• Research question worth answering
	• Study minimizes harms and maximizes benefits
Justice	• Equitable distribution of benefits and burdens of research (i.e., fair recruitment and selection of subjects)

UNITED STATES FEDERAL REGULATIONS (THE COMMON RULE)

While the principles described in the Belmont Report provide a basis for ethically conducting human subjects research, the report has been variably interpreted and used (High, D., 1992). Nevertheless, the Belmont Report became the basis for the Code of Federal Regulations Title 45 Part 46 ("Protection of Human Subjects") issued in 1981 by what is now known as the Department of Health and Human Services (DHHS). Since then, these regulations have undergone a number of modifications. Most, but not all, federal agencies that sponsor and fund research involving human subjects have formally adopted these regulations as the Federal Policy for the Protection of Human Subjects or "Common Rule" (45 CFR 46) (Department of Health and Human Services). The Common Rule articulates requirements for compliance by institutions involved in research, informed consent, and for IRB membership and responsibilities. The Common Rule also articulates measures for protecting especially vulnerable research subjects (e.g., children and prisoners).

Today, the Office for Human Research Protections (OHRP), which is part of the DHHS, oversees matters related to protecting human research subjects participating in studies conducted or supported by the DHHS. The OHRP (a) establishes criteria for and approves assurances of compliance for protecting human subjects with institutions engaged in research conducted or sponsored by the DHHS; (b) provides clarification and guidance on involving human subjects in research; (c) develops and implements educational programs and resource materials; and (d) promotes the development of approaches to enhance human subject protections. Under the direction of the OHRP, more than 10,000 research institutions have agreed to comply with the regulations for protecting human subjects found in the Common Rule (Office for Human Protections).

In addition to designing and conducting research studies that adhere to the ethical principles of the Belmont Report and comply with federal regulations, investigators engaged in human subjects research have a number of specific responsibilities regarding their local IRBs. These responsibilities are listed in Table 7.3.

Research Involving Elderly Persons

In general, the ethical principles for protecting elderly human subjects in research are the same as those for protecting younger subjects (Sachs, G. and Cassel C., 1990). However, elders who are potential research subjects are of two types; those who are vigorous, independent, and autonomous (the majority of elders), and those who

TABLE 7.3.
Responsibilities of investigators engaged in research involving human subjects (data from Cohen, J.)

1.	Design and conduct research in alignment with the ethical principles described in the Belmont Report
2.	Comply with all federal regulations related pertaining to the protection of human subjects
3.	Obtain approval for all research involving human subjects from the appropriate institutional IRB
4.	Comply with all IRB policies, procedures and decisions and other requirements
5.	Conduct research as approved by the IRB
6.	Obtain IRB approval for all changes to the study protocol
7.	Obtain and document informed consent and assent from subjects in compliance with federal regulations and as approved by the IRB
8.	Report progress of research to the IRB as prescribed by the IRB
9.	Report to the IRB any adverse events or unanticipated problems involving subjects or others
10.	Retain research documents (e.g., signed consent forms) for at least three years following completion of the study

are dependent, decisionally impaired, or dependent on others. Persons who comprise the former group do not differ from younger persons in any way except for chronological age, and the ethical principles governing research in general are sufficient to encompass research involving them. Research involving the latter group, however, is more complex; these elders are vulnerable, often institutionalized, and many lack decision-making capacity (Dubler, N., 1987). In fact, there are a number of unique aspects and potential ethical challenges of conducting research involving elderly subjects that merit special attention (Sachs, G. and Cohen, H., 2003). The remainder of this chapter will address these unique aspects and challenges.

Unique Aspects and Potential Ethical Challenges of Conducting Research Involving Elderly Persons

Compared to other research subjects, elders may be unique for a variety of reasons: (a) greater prevalence among elders of conditions [e.g., hearing and vision loss, diminished cognition, etc.] that may impair informed consent; (b) greater prevalence among elders of comorbid illnesses and other potential confounding variables that may make interpretation of study results difficult; (c) the captive nature of some populations of elders (e.g., residents of nursing homes) making them susceptible to coercion and breaches of confidentiality; and (d) evidence that elders have been unjustly excluded from research studies including those especially relevant to elders.

ELDERLY PERSONS' WILLINGNESS TO PARTICIPATE IN RESEARCH STUDIES

Elders are less willing to participate in research studies (Kaye *et al.*, 1990; Sachs, G. and Cassel, C., 1990). For elders who have sensory deficits, the informed consent process may be prolonged and frustrating, thereby reducing participation (Sugarman *et al.*, 1998). Furthermore, some elders refuse to sign, fear the implications of, or are otherwise inexperienced with consent forms, and some may insist that family members be involved in the informed consent process, thereby adding to the efforts of investigators. These factors may frustrate both potential research subjects and investigators and lead to reduced participation (Kaye, J., Lawton, P. and Kaye, D., 1990). Transportation, mobility issues and medical conditions that require frequent attention may reduce participation or cause some elders to drop out of studies (Sachs, G. and Cassel, C., 1990). When recruiting elders for research studies, investigators should consider and address these and other factors that may adversely affect participation.

OBTAINING INFORMED CONSENT FROM ELDERLY PERSONS

As articulated by the Nuremberg Code and the Belmont Report, and codified in federal regulations, research involving human subjects may be done only with the subjects' voluntary informed consent. However, any element of the informed consent process (relevant and sufficient information, decision-making capacity and subject voluntariness) may be compromised when conducting research involving elderly research subjects.

1. Information

Meaningful and ethically valid informed consent requires that research subjects be given relevant and sufficient information including the purpose of the study, potential risks and alternatives to participation, and the subject's right to withdraw from the study at any time. Furthermore, investigators should inform potential research subjects that the primary objective of research is to acquire new knowledge and that personal clinical benefit may or may not occur (American College of Physicians, 2005).

Subjects must also understand the disclosed information. Investigators should ensure that subjects understand the information conveyed during the informed consent process since harm may occur as a result of the subject making a misinformed choice (i.e., a choice they would not have made if they had understood the information) (Ratzan, R., 1980). However, many research subjects, especially those who are ill or poorly educated, do not understand the purposes and risks of the studies in which they are participating even after consent has been obtained (Sachs, G. and Cassel, C., 1990). Informed consent forms can be long, complex and difficult to understand (LoVerde *et al.*, 1989). Furthermore, research subjects participating in studies in a clinical setting may forget that they are, in fact, research subjects (Riecken, H. and Ravich, R., 1982).

Notably, systematic reviews of studies of the informed consent process have found that reduced understanding of conveyed information was associated with older age (Sugarman *et al.*, 1998; Flory, J. and Emanuel, E., 2004). In addition, compared to younger persons, elders may have more difficulty in recalling information conveyed (Sachs, G. and Cassel, C., 1990). Impaired understanding and recalling of information by elders may be due to sensory deficits (e.g., vision and hearing), comorbid illnesses, diminished cognition, and other factors (Sugarman *et al.*, 1998).

However, a number of strategies can improve the understanding of information. Simplified consent forms, multimedia approaches (e.g., video), quizzes, multiple disclosure sessions and especially generous one-on-one time with a study team member or educator are effective means of improving understanding (Sugarman *et al.*, 1998; Flory, J. and Emanuel, E., 2004). Another promising tool for maximizing informed consent among potential research subjects who are frail and elderly is "experienced consent." In a study of frail elders, a week-long trial of noninvasive testing to gain experience with a research study's methods resulted in significant increases in comprehension of the study methods and the number of subjects capable of weighing the risks associated with the study (Olde Rikkert, M., *et al.*, 1997).

2. *Voluntariness*

The first item of the Nuremberg Code is that "the voluntary consent of the human subject is absolutely essential" (Nuremberg Code, 1947) (Table 7.1). Subsequent codes, reports and regulations have reiterated this principle. Subjects, to the degree that they are capable, must be allowed to decide what shall and what shall not happen to them. Notably, despite the crucial role of voluntariness in the informed consent process, little empirical data regarding voluntariness has been published (Sugarman *et al.*, 1998).

Autonomy may be limited for residents of long-term care institutions (e.g., nursing homes), most of whom are elders. When to eat and go to bed, choosing a roommate and other activities are largely controlled by the institution. Hence, it is not surprising that concerns exist about the possibility of obtaining voluntary consent for research from residents of long-term care institutions. Residents depend on the institution for food, shelter, medications and care. In the context of consent for research, this dependency may foster coercion; i.e., residents may not feel free to refuse to participate in research out of fears that their care will suffer if they refuse, especially if their clinicians are also the investigators (Bell, J., *et al.*, 1987; Sachs, G. and Cassel, C., 1990; Sachs, G. and Cohen, H., 2003). Whereas independent research subjects can freely choose to continue or withdraw from a research study, institutionalized persons may perceive less freedom to choose because of needs for attention and care, and fear of rejection (Dubler, N., 1987).

3. *Decision-making Capacity*

Decision-making capacity refers to a potential research subject's ability to understand, make and express a reasoned and meaningful choice about whether to participate in a research study. Of the elements of the informed consent process, decision-making capacity is often the most problematic for elders, since elders represent an age group most susceptible to illnesses that affect mental functioning (Marson, D., et al., 1994). Nevertheless, society and law assume that all adults are competent. In fact, the term *competent* is a legal term, and only a court can declare a person incompetent. Clinicians and investigators, however, may care for and work with elders who cannot effectively comprehend or manipulate information in a way that allows for weighing of the risks and benefits of, and alternatives to, a proposed intervention or research protocol. These patients lack decision-making capacity. Unlike competency, clinicians and investigators determine if a person has decision-making capacity.

Having a mental illness or an illness that affects cognition does not necessarily mean an individual lacks decision-making capacity (AGS Ethics Committee, 1998; Alzheimer's Association, 2004). Indeed, many elders with diminished cognition are not only legally competent, but also have decision-making capacity and can consent to participate in research. Capacity to consent need not be based on an overall state of competence. A patient can have diminished cognition (e.g., due to dementia) and still understand the purpose of the study (e.g., that it is research and may not provide a therapeutic benefit), the risks of participating in the study, and that he or she may refuse to participate. Instead, consent for participating in research studies of varying complexity requires varying levels of capacity. For example, a person may be able to effectively consent to participate in a minimal risk study (i.e., a study in which the risk and magnitude of harm to the subject are no greater than what the subject would encounter in daily life or during the performance of routine physical or psychological examinations or tests), but not a trial of a new drug or procedure (Dubler, N., 1987; Sachs, G. and Cohen, H., 2003).

Assessing the decision-making capacity of potential research subjects is an important step in the informed consent process. Capacity to consent for participating in research should include the following abilities: (a) ability to evidence a choice (i.e., ability to reach a decision and effectively communicate the decision); (b) ability to understand the nature of the research study and other information relevant to participants disclosed by the investigator; (c) ability to understand and appreciate the risks and consequences of participating or not participating in the study, and the procedures to follow if adverse events occur and if withdrawal from participation is desired; and (d) ability to manipulate information rationally (Alzheimer's Association, 2004; American Psychiatric Association, 1998).

Unfortunately, clinicians and investigators are uncommonly trained to assess the decision-making capacity of potential subjects and thereby have difficulty assessing capacity. In fact, those who are experienced in assessing decision-making capacity may disagree with each other. Furthermore, no universally accepted standardized tool for assessing decision-making capacity for research consent exists. Because of these facts, investigators assessing capacity have relied on subjective impressions and brief mental status tests (Marson, D., *et al.*, 1994). One promising approach, however, is for investigators to incorporate details of a given study into open-ended questions that assess the aforementioned decision-making capacity abilities of a potential subject for the study (Karlawish, J., 2003).

Research protocols should describe how assessment of subject decision-making capacity will be done. The extent of the assessment should correlate with the risks of the research. For minimal risk studies, an informal assessment by a research team member should suffice. For higher risk studies, using an independent qualified professional skilled in assessing decision-making capacity should be considered (Alzheimer's Association, 2004).

Notably, some subjects may lose decision-making capacity during a study. If at the time of enrollment subjects have capacity to consent, but are at risk of losing capacity during the study, then investigators should describe in their protocols how periodic capacity reassessments will be done. Furthermore, investigators should offer subjects the opportunity the name a proxy decision-maker and ask the subject to provide guidance to the proxy on what to do should loss of capacity occur. In addition, some subjects with impaired capacity and enrolled in research studies via proxy consent may later regain capacity. In these situations, the investigator must obtain informed consent from the subject for continued participation (Alzheimer's Association, 2004).

RESEARCH INVOLVING ELDERLY PERSONS WITH IMPAIRED DECISION-MAKING CAPACITY

1. Background

Approximately 10 percent of elders older than 65 years and 22 percent older than 80 years have dementia. Furthermore, a majority of nursing home residents have some form of cognitive impairment (Cassel, C., 1988). In addition, many elders experience delirium during hospitalizations for acute illnesses (Rummans, T., *et al.*, 1995). Many of these patients are incapable of giving valid informed consent. Nevertheless, to better understand illnesses that uniquely afflict elders including those illnesses that impair decision-making capacity, research that involves decisionally impaired elders may be necessary. Restrictive approaches that bar subjects with impaired capacity from research may cause harm; these individuals would be deprived of research-derived medical advances on the very conditions that limit their capacity and be deprived of the benefits of participating in research. Nevertheless, informed voluntary consent to research requires decision-making capacity. Hence, is it ever legitimate to enroll in research studies individuals with impaired decision-making capacity?

The permissibility of enrolling decisionally impaired persons in research has evolved over time. The authors of the Nuremberg Code did not allow for the involvement of decisionally impaired persons in research even if such research was potentially therapeutic. The prevailing view was that studies involving subjects with impaired capacity that do not directly benefit or are potentially harmful to the subjects should not be done (Capron, A., 1999). The Declaration of Helsinki, however, allowed for legally recognized surrogates of decisionally impaired persons to provide consent for therapeutic research (Capron, A., 1999; Michels, R., 1999). Later the National Commission went beyond the Nuremberg Code and the Declaration of Helsinki by claiming that prohibiting such research might harm an entire class of decisionally-impaired persons by depriving them of potential benefits of research (Michels, R., 1999). Indeed, proxy consent for minimal risk studies and greater than minimal risk studies with potential direct benefits to subjects is now widely accepted (Capron, A., 1999).

The National Commission, however, noted that investigators may need to make special provisions for protecting subjects with impaired decision-making capacity. Later, in 1983, the President's Commission reiterated the National Commission's concern (Shamoo, A. and Khin-Maung-Gyi, F., 2002). Nevertheless, despite the reports of these two commissions, specific federal regulations aimed to protect research subjects with impaired decision-making capacity have not been adopted. Even so, the Common Rule (45 CFR 46) does state that "if an IRB regularly reviews research that involves a vulnerable category of subjects, such as ... mentally disabled persons, consideration shall be given to the inclusion of one or more individuals who are knowledgeable about and experienced in working with these subjects" (Department of Health and Human Services). Nevertheless, in the absence of federal regulations, IRBs must decide what constitutes impaired decision-making capacity, what constitutes greater than minimal risk, and when decisionally impaired subjects are not at excessive risk of harm (Shamoo, A. and Khin-Maung-Gyi, F., 2002).

In 1998, the National Bioethics Advisory Commission (NBAC) issued its report, "Research Involving Persons with Mental Disorders That May Affect Decisionmaking Capacity," in which it stated that a "case can be made for requiring additional special protections in research involving subjects persons with impaired decision making capacity" (National Bioethics Advisory Commission, 1998). Specific recommendations made by NBAC include: (a) IRBs involved in reviewing protocols involving populations with impaired decision-making capacity should contain at least two members who are familiar with the disorders causing the impaired capacity and with the concerns of the population being studied; (b) for greater than minimal risk protocols, IRBs should require independent and professionally qualified assessment of potential subjects' capacity to consent; (c) for greater than minimal risk protocols that offer no prospect of direct medical benefit to subjects, the protocol should be referred to a national Special Standing Panel for a decision. NBAC advised that its recommendations become part of the Common Rule and that, until the recommendations become federal regulations, IRBs adopt voluntarily the recommendations. To date, these recommendations have not become part of the Common Rule (Sachs, G. and Cohen, H., 2003).

2. Advance Directive for Research

Advance care planning consists of informal and formal healthcare planning by a decisionally capable person to guide healthcare decision-making for a future time in which they no longer have decision-making capacity. A discussion with family members, friends and healthcare providers is an example of informal advance care planning. A written advance directive for healthcare decisions is an example of formal planning (Sachs, G., 1994). For research involving persons with impaired decision-making capacity, NBAC recommended that these subjects could be enrolled in research studies if the subject gave prospective authorization via an advance directive for research completed at a time when the subject had decision-making capacity, and in the absence of an advance directive for research, consent from a legally authorized proxy is obtained and the subject assents to the research study (National Bioethics Advisory Commission, 1998).

Like the advance directive for healthcare decisions, the advance directive for research (also known as advance consent) is a legal document executed by a decisionally capable person that authorizes their enrollment in research studies for the time the person lacks decision-making capacity (Kapp, M., 1994; AGS Ethics Committee, 1998). In an advance directive for research, persons can designate their proxy decision-maker, the types of research and risks that would be acceptable, and other values (e.g., religious values) and goals (Sachs, G., 1994).

The advance directive for research, however, has important limitations. First, only 10–20% of Americans adults have advance directives for healthcare treatment decisions (Sachs, G., 1994; Hanson, L. and Rodgman, E., 1996), and it is likely that even fewer have advance directives for research. Many people who complete advance directives for healthcare decisions are motivated to avoid invasive procedures and burdensome life-sustaining treatments (e.g., respirators) at the end-of-life and to prevent prolongation of the dying process. There is no equivalent motivating factor for completing an advance directive for research. Second, by the time it is recognized that a person has lost decision-making capacity, it is unlikely that she or he can complete a detailed advance directive for research. Finally, requiring a written advance directive for research in order for persons with impaired decision-making capacity to participate in research would substantially limit the number of potential subjects and deprive them of the benefits of being research participants and deprive others with their condition of the benefits derived from the discovery of new knowledge (Sachs, G., 1994).

3. Proxy Consent for Research

In the absence of an advance directive for research, investigators must obtain consent for research from a legally authorized proxy (AGS Ethics Committee, 1998; Alzheimer's Association, 2004). Typically, the person at the top of the decision-making hierarchy is a court-appointed guardian followed by the person or persons named in an advance directive. If no advance directive exists, investigators should identify and seek consent from a legally authorized proxy. Notably, hierarchies of proxy decision-making vary from jurisdiction to jurisdiction (Karlawish, J., 2003).

Proxies should base their decisions to enroll the decisionally impaired subjects they represent in research studies on the subjects' previously expressed wishes, values and goals (i.e., substituted judgment). However, as with healthcare decision-making, proxies frequently do not know the previously expressed wishes, values and goals of subjects and, hence, do not consistently make substituted judgments for enrollment in research (Sachs, G., 1994; Karlawish, J.,2003). Indeed, in a study (Warren, J., *et al.*, 1986) of proxy consent, investigators examined the decisions by proxies for 168 nursing home residents about whether to permit the residents' participation in a minimal risk study. In all but one instance, the proxies were family members. Fifty-five proxies were of the opinion that the residents that they represented would refuse to participate (if capable) in the study. Of these proxies, however, 17 (31%) gave consent to participate. Another study (Sachs, G., *et al.*, 1994) involving patients with dementia, proxies and well elders found that some demented patients were capable of giving informed consent and most were capable of identifying a proxy decision-maker. The investigators commented that many patients regard designating a trusted proxy as more important than the decisions a proxy would make and that designating a proxy requires less decision-making capacity than the informed consent process for research. Finally, using research scenarios, the investigators found that proxies were more likely to take risks for themselves and protect patients from greater than minimal risk studies (e.g., trials involving drugs and procedures). On the other hand, proxies made decisions contrary to what the patient would want in scenarios in which the risk was perceived to be low and the benefit for others perceived to be present. The results of these studies and others suggest that while proxies do not always use substituted judgments for enrollment in research, they do make decisions that minimize harm to patients. In addition, evidence suggests that patients care more about who is making the decisions for them than the decisions being made (Sachs, G., 1994).

4. Subject Assent for Research

Despite impaired decision-making capacity and proxy consent, subject assent is essential and subjects should be allowed to refuse to participate. Assent can be judged based on subject behavior and cooperatives. Subject dissent should be respected, and when it occurs, subjects should be withdrawn from the study (Capron, A., 1999; Alzheimer's Association, 2004). Notably, in some situations, assent is not possible (e.g., coma and persistent vegetative state). In these situations, investigators must rely solely on the proxy decision-maker for consent.

5. Acceptable Risks of Research Involving Elders with Impaired Decision-Making Capacity

The American Geriatrics Society (AGS Ethics Committee, 1998), the Alzheimer's Association (Alzheimer's Association, 2004) and NBAC (National Bioethics Advisory Commission, 1998) have provided similar guidelines regarding acceptable risks of research involving individuals with impaired decision-making capacity. Provided that informed consent (via an advance directive for research or proxy consent) has been obtained and subject assent, subjects with impaired capacity may be enrolled in research if involvement in the study offers direct health-related benefit to the subject, and, if not, then the study should not expose the subject to more than a minor increment above minimal risk and should have the prospect of yielding generalizable new knowledge about the subject's illness or condition. Enrollment in studies of greater than a minor increment above minimal risk should be offered only to persons who have decision-making capacity or to persons with impaired capacity who have an advance directive for research that allows enrollment in such a study. However, the AGS and NBAC recommend a national panel for considering, on a case-by-case basis, approval of especially promising studies that pose risks greater than a minor increment above minimal risk involving subjects lacking decision-making capacity who have not executed an advance directive for research. To date, such a panel has not been established.

CONDUCTING RESEARCH FOR THE GOOD OF ELDERLY PERSONS

The principle of beneficence requires that investigators maximize benefit and minimize harm to human research subjects. This principle also demands that investigators protect subjects from exploitation. Indeed, the Belmont Report states that "the appropriateness of involving vulnerable populations in research should be demonstrated" (The Belmont Report, 1979).

Elders, especially those with diminished cognition and living in nursing homes or other institutions, are vulnerable to exploitation (e.g., they may be viewed as convenient subjects for research). Investigators and proxy decision-makers have a duty to protect potential research subjects, especially those who lack decision-making capacity, from harm. Persons who lack capacity should not be enrolled in research studies that provide no benefit to them or to persons with similar conditions, expose them to undue risks, or disrupt their normal routines (Bell *et al.*, 1987).

Beneficence requires that elders be included in research studies. Lack of research involving elderly human subjects leads to inadequate clinical care of elderly patients (Cassel, C., 1985). In fact, the results of clinical trials and other studies involving younger human subjects are often extrapolated to elders. However, changes associated with normal aging (e.g., altered drug metabolism, reduced glomerular filtration rate, etc.), comorbid illnesses, concurrent use of medications, and other factors make the extrapolation of the results of studies involving younger subjects to elders risky (Bell *et al.*, 1987).

Participating in research has a number of benefits aside from direct medical benefit to the individual elderly subject. These benefits include deriving meaning and purpose from the altruistic act of being a research subject, socialization, remuneration, and other benefits. Notably, in a study (Kaye *et al.*, 1990) of elders, those who consented to being research subjects had more positive feelings about being a research subject, helping others, and finding out about problems as a means of passing time compared to those who did not consent. Reasons for participating included interest in the project and benefiting others. This study and others (Leader, M. and Neuwirth, E., 1978; Lipsitz *et al.*, 1987) have also found that elders are more likely to participate in research that directly benefits them and less likely to participate in research that offers no direct benefit.

The principle of beneficence suggests that investigators avoid involving vulnerable elders in research. Yet, many elders suffer from conditions that not only leave them vulnerable, but also have a predilection for elders (e.g. dementia). Ideally, research of such conditions would involve subjects with those conditions. However, if vulnerable elders are excluded from research in order to avoid harm, then these elders would never benefit from research. Indeed, prohibiting research involving vulnerable elders may in fact cause significant harm by not allowing discovery of new knowledge that would help them (Ratzan, R., 1980).

Unfortunately, investigators who conduct studies involving elders infrequently or imprecisely describe ethical considerations (e.g., IRB processes, consent, decisional capacity, funding sources, and confidentiality) in their research reports even when the research involves vulnerable persons (Lane *et al.*, 1990). It is imperative that investigators describe these considerations in their protocols and research reports.

JUST INVOLVEMENT OF ELDERS IN RESEARCH

The burdens and benefits of research should be distributed equally, and elders should not bear burdens or receive benefits more than other age groups. Nevertheless, elders may be unjustly included or excluded from research studies. Investigators may find elderly residents of nursing homes and other institutions convenient subjects for research. In fact, before the 1970s, nursing homes were common sites for research primarily because of convenient access to captive subjects, most of whom were elders (Cassel, C., 1985). Furthermore, nursing home residents were commonly used for experiments that were not directly relevant to their own illnesses or elders in general (e.g., the Jewish Chronic Disease Hospital study). Instead, the selection of research subjects should be based on the needs of the study, not the convenience of the investigator or the accessibility of subjects.

The National Commission examined the issue of conducting research involving institutionalized human subjects. The Commission noted that investigators should preferentially involve subjects who are living freely in the community rather than those living in institutions. The Commission also stated that the convenience of subjects is not sufficient rationale to conduct research in an institution (Cassel, C., 1985).

On the other hand, elders, especially the oldest-old (age >85 years), have been unjustly excluded from research studies (Sachs, G. and Cohen, H., 2003). For example, a review of original research papers published in four journals during 1996 and 1997 found that one-third of the studies unjustifiably excluded elders (Bugeja *et al.*, 1997). Another study of research protocols on topics relevant to elders that were submitted to a hospital "ethics committee" (institutional review board) found that a majority of the protocols had unjustifiable upper age limits (Bayer, A. and Tadd, W., 2000). A study of human subjects consecutively enrolled in 164 study protocols of an oncology study group found substantial underrepresentation of elders (Hutchins, L., *et al.*, 1999). A recent review of 59 randomized controlled trials between 1985 and 1999 of interventions for congestive heart failure (a disease that afflicts elders more than any other age group) found that elders were underrepresented in the trials (Heiat *et al.*, 2002). Other studies have had similar results (Morse, A., *et al.*, 2004; Avorn, J., 1997). Elders bear more illnesses, use more medications, and experience more deaths than any other age group. Hence, investigators should not exclude elders from research studies and should include enough elders in order to generate valid results that can be generalized to elderly populations.

Investigators may be tempted to exclude elders from research for a number of reasons. For example, investigators may avoid elders with impaired decision-making capacity because involving proxy decision-makers is time-consuming and costly (Bugeja *et al.*, 1997). Investigators may be unwilling to enroll elders in research studies because elders are more likely to have sensory deficits, mobility issues, comorbid illnesses, and other confounding variables. Conducting long-term studies involving elders is difficult because of their relatively high mortality rates (Sachs, G. and Cassel, C., 1990). Finally, compared to other age groups, elders are less willing to participate in research studies (Kaye *et al.*, 1990; Sachs, G. and Cassel, C., 1990). Nevertheless, while these reasons for excluding elders from research are not trivial, investigators should make efforts to address them in order to conduct valid research, the results of which can be generalized to elderly populations for their benefit.

Injustice also occurs when elders are excluded from their fair share of the benefits of being involved in research. These benefits include altruistic feelings of meaning and purpose associated with being a research subject, attention and socialization that accompanies being a research subject, medical supervision and other benefits (Cassel, C., 1985; Sachs, G. and Cassel, C., 1990).

GENETIC RESEARCH INVOLVING ELDERS

Genetic research (i.e., the identification of genetic variants) has the potential for discovering important preventive and therapeutic interventions for diseases associated with aging. For example, the identification of genetic mutations in familial Alzheimer disease and other diseases has yielded information regarding the mechanisms of the sporadic, yet more prevalent, forms of these diseases (Banks, D. and Fossel, M., 1997; Blacker, D., *et al.*, 1997; Longo, V. and Finch, C., 2002). Hence, it is not surprising that the interest in and conducting of genetic research in elders are growing.

While the aforementioned principles of research also apply to genetic research, the implications of genetic information obtained through research can be complex for subjects, their blood relatives, clinicians, and investigators (American Society of Human Genetics, 1996).

Indeed, genetic research raises a number of important ethical concerns, particularly those related to informed consent and subject confidentiality that are applicable to all subjects regardless of age.

The American Society of Human Genetics (ASHG) has published a statement on informed consent that provides guidance to investigators who wish to conduct genetic research involving human subjects including elders (American Society of Human Genetics, 1996). Subjects should be informed not only about the physical discomforts associated with collecting specimens (e.g., blood), they should also be informed about the types of information that can result from genetic research including potentially unexpected findings (e.g., carrier status, paternity, children affected by genetic disease, etc.). Needless to say, these findings may be alarming to subjects and, hence, geneticists and/or genetic counselors should be directly involved or available in genetic studies in order to communicate accurately the results to subjects. Subjects should be informed if specimens will be stored for future studies and should be given options regarding the scope of future studies involving the specimens (including after the subject's death). Investigators should not seek "blanket consent" for unspecified future genetic

TABLE 7.4.
Checklist for addressing the unique aspects and potential ethical challenges of conducting research involving elderly persons

1. Adhere to responsibilities listed in Table 7.3
2. Employ beneficent research design and methods
   - Scientifically valid
   - Protocol clearly describes ethical considerations (e.g., IRB processes, informed consent, assessment of decisional capacity, etc.)
   - Requires the involvement of elders
   - Minimizes harms and maximizes benefits to elders
   - Protects vulnerable elderly subjects (e.g., due to impaired decision-making capacity)
3. Address barriers to enrollment of elders (e.g., sensory impairments, mobility issues, etc.)
4. Ensure elements of informed consent are realized
   - Adequate amount of information about the study is conveyed to and understood by subject
   - Subject voluntariness (i.e., free of coercion)
   - Subject decision-making capacity
5. Assess decision-making capacity
   - Ability to evidence a choice
   - Ability to understand the nature of the research study and other information relevant to participants disclosed by the investigator
   - Ability to understand and appreciate the risks and consequences of participating and the procedures to follow if adverse events occur or if withdrawal from participation is desired
   - Ability to manipulate information rationally
6. Adhere to requirements for enrolling subjects with impaired decision-making capacity
   - Consent articulated in an advance directive for research
   - Consent by a legally authorized proxy
   - Subject assent regardless of level of decision-making capacity
7. Adhere to acceptable standards of risk when conducting research involving subjects with impaired decision-making capacity
   - Study has direct therapeutic benefit to the subject
   - If no direct benefit to the subject, no more than a minimal increment greater than minimal risk and has the prospect of yielding generalizable new knowledge about the subject's illness or condition
   - For studies of greater than a minor increment above minimal risk, enrollment should be offered only to potential subjects who have an advance directive for research that allows enrollment in such a study
8. Ensure that research involving elders is just
   - Study does not unfairly include or exclude elders
   - Study includes sufficient numbers of elders to facilitate understanding of the physiologic processes, diseases and other factors that pertain to elders

research studies using the specimens. Investigators who use and maintain identified or identifiable specimens must scrupulously maintain subject confidentiality. Information derived from these specimens must not be divulged to anyone (e.g., family members, insurance companies, etc.) without the explicit written permission of the subject. Subjects should be given the opportunity to decide whether or not to receive the information discovered by the investigation (i.e., some subjects may not want to know the results of testing if nothing can be done constructively with the information).

Beyond the ASHG statement, investigators should consider additional ethical aspects of genetic research. First, because genetic research usually involves blood, buccal, and/or stool specimens, investigators may regard these studies as minimal risk. However, risk must be understood as something larger than the discomforts associated with collecting specimens. Indeed, the ASHG statement recognizes that the risks of genetic research include psychosocial risks such as disrupted family dynamics caused by the discovery of genetic information (e.g., carrier status) and employment and insurance discrimination (American Society of Human Genetics, 1996). Hence, these studies should be regarded as greater than minimal risk. Second, information derived from genetic research that is disclosed to the subject or the proxy decision-maker should be recorded in the subject's medical record, since such information may influence clinical practice. Care, however, must be taken to avoid inappropriate disclosure of this information. Third, investigators should inform subjects of situations in which disclosure of information to subjects may be ethically obligatory (e.g., information that, if not known and addressed by the subject, poses high risk of harm) and how such disclosure will be done. Fourth, genetic research may have implications for blood relatives of subjects. Investigators, for various reasons, may desire to contact relatives. Investigators should obtain consent from subjects to contact relatives where appropriate. Relatives should be contacted in a nonthreatening way (e.g., certified letter) that explains (a) how their name was obtained; (b) the nature of the research involving the subject (without divulging the research results pertaining to the subject); (c) the possible implications of the research for the relatives; and (d) how to contact the investigator for more information (e.g., counseling regarding the study).

Conclusions

The number of elders living in the United States is rapidly growing. Elders are uniquely burdened with illnesses (some of which are associated with aging) and account for most deaths. In order to reduce morbidity and mortality experienced by elders, research involving elderly human subjects is needed. Contemporary codes of ethics and regulations governing research involving human subjects derive from the ethical principles of respect for persons, beneficence, and justice. Investigators conducting research involving elders should be familiar with and adhere to these general ethical principles. In addition, investigators should acknowledge and address the unique aspects and potential ethical challenges of research involving elderly persons. A checklist for addressing these unique aspects and potential ethical challenges is found in Table 7.4. A list of useful Web-based resources for investigators engaged in research involving elderly persons is found in Table 7.5. Following this approach should yield ethically valid and fruitful results not only for the good of elders but also for society in general.

TABLE 7.5.
Useful Web-based resources for investigators engaged in research involving elderly persons

1. The World Medical Association Declaration of Helsinki: http://www.wma.net/e/policy/b3.htm
2. Belmont Report: http://www.hhs.gov/ohrp/humansubjects/guidance/belmont.htm
3. Common Rule: http://www.hhs.gov/ohrp/humansubjects/guidance/45cfr46.htm
4. American Geriatrics Society "The Responsible Conduct of Research": http://www.americangeriatrics.org/products/positionpapers/respcondresearch.shtml
5. American College of Physicians *Ethics Manual*, 5th edition: http://www.acponline.org/ethics/ethicman5th.htm
6. American Psychiatric Association "Guidelines for Assessing Decision-Making Capacities of Potential Research Subjects with Cognitive Impairment": http://www.psych.org/edu/other_res/lib_archives/archives/199811.pdf
7. National Bioethics Advisory Commission Report "Research Involving Persons with Mental Disorders That May Affect Decision-Making Capacity": http://www.georgetown.edu/research/nrcbl/nbac/capacity/TOC.htm
8. American Geriatrics Society "Informed Consent for Research on Human Subjects with Dementia": http://www.americangeriatrics.org/products/positionpapers/infconsent.shtml
9. American Society of Human Genetics "Statement on Informed Consent for Genetic Research": http://www.ashg.org/genetics/ashg/pubs/policy/pol-25.htm

REFERENCES

AGS Ethics Committee. Informed consent for research on human subjects with dementia. *J Am Geriatr Soc*. 1998;*46*:1308–1310.

Alzheimer's Association. Research consent for cognitively impaired adults: Recommendations for institutional review boards and investigators. *Alzheimer Dis Assoc Discord*. 2004;*18*:171–175.

American College of Physicians. Ethics manual, 5th ed. *Ann Intern Med*. 2005;*142*:560–582.

American Psychiatric Association. Guidelines for assessing the decision-making capacities of potential research subjects with cognitive impairment (1998). Available at: http://www.psych.org/edu/other_res/lib_archives/archives/199811.pdf

American Society of Human Genetics. Statement on informed consent for genetic research. *Am J Hum Genet*. 1996;*59*: 471–474.

Avorn J. Including elderly people in clinical trials. *BMJ*. 1997;*315*:1033–1034.

Banks DA and Fossel M. Telomeres, cancer, and aging: Altering the human life span. *JAMA*. 1997;*278*:1345–1348.

Bayer A and Tadd W. Unjustified exclusion of elderly people from studies submitted to research ethics committee for approval: Descriptive study. *BMJ*. 2000;*321*:992–993.

Beauchamp TL and Childress JF. *Principles of Biomedical Ethics*, 5th ed. (New York: Oxford University Press, 2001).

Beecher HK. Ethics and clinical research. *New Engl J Med*. 1966;*274*:1354–1360.

Bell JA, May FE, Stewart RB. Clinical research in the elderly: Ethical and methodological considerations. *Drug Intell Clin Pharm*. 1987;*21*:1002–1007.

The Belmont Report (1979). Ethical principles and guidelines for the protection of human subjects of research. Available at: http://www.hhs.gov/ohrp/humansubjects/guidance/belmont.htm

Blacker D, Haines JL, Rodes L, Terwedow H, Go RCP, Harrell LE, *et al. Neurology*. 1997;*48*:139–147.

Bugeja G, Kumar A, Banerjee AK. Exclusion of elderly people from clinical research: A descriptive study of published reports. *BMJ*. 1997;*315*:1059.

Capron AM. Ethical and human-rights issues in research on mental disorders that may affect decision-making capacity. *New Engl J Med*. 1999;*340*:1430–1434.

Cassel CK. Research in nursing homes. *J Am Geriatr Soc*. 1985;*33*:795–799.

Cassel CK. Ethical issues in the conduct of research in long term care. *Gerontologist*. 1988;*28*:90–96.

Cohen JM. Top ten investigator responsibilities when conducting human subjects research. http://irb.mc.duke.edu/ppt/investigator_top_ten–full–jeff_cohen–4-12-02.ppt

Denham MJ. The ethics of research in the elderly. *Age and Aging*. 1984;*13*:321–327.

Department of Health and Human Services. Protection of human subjects, 45 CFR 46. Available at: http://www.hhs.gov/ohrp/humansubjects/guidance/45cfr46.htm

Dubler NN. Legal judgments and informed consent in geriatric research. *J Am Geriatr Soc*. 1987;*35*:545–549.

Flory J and Emanuel E. Interventions to improve research participants' understanding in informed consent for research: A systematic review. *JAMA*. 2004;*292*:1593–1601.

Hanson LC and Rodgman E. The use of living wills at the end of life: A national study. *Arch Intern Med* 1996;*156*:1018–1022.

Heiat A, Gross CP, Krumholtz HM. Representation of the elderly, women, and minorities in heart failure clinical trials. *Arch Intern Med*. 2002;*162*:1682–1688.

High DM. Research with Alzheimer's disease subjects: Informed consent and proxy decision making. *J Am Geriatr Soc*. 1992;*40*:950–957.

Hutchins LF, Unger JM, Crowley JJ, Coltman CA, Albain KS. Underrepresentation of patients 65 years of age or older in cancer-treatment trials. *New Engl J Med*. 1999;*341*:2061–2067.

Jahnigen DW and Schrier RW. The doctor/patient relationship in geriatric care. *Clin Geriatr Med* 1986;*2*:457–464.

Kapp MB. Proxy decision making in Alzheimer disease research: Durable powers of attorney, guardianship, and other alternatives. *Alzheimer Disease Associated Disorders*. 1994; *8*(suppl):28–37.

Karlawish JHT. Research involving cognitively impaired adults. *New Engl J Med*. 2003;*348*:1389–1392.

Kaye JM, Lawton P, Kaye D. Attitudes of elderly people about clinical research on aging. *The Gerontologist*. 1990;*30*:100–106.

Lane LW, Cassel CK, Bennett W. Ethical aspects of research involving elderly subjects: Are we doing more than we say? *J Clinical Ethics*. 1990;*1*:278–285.

Leader MA and Neuwirth E. Clinical research and the noninstitutional elderly: A model for subject recruitment. *J Am Geriatr Soc*. 1978;*26*:27–31.

Lipsitz LA, Pluchino FC, Wright SM. Biomedical research in the nursing home: Methodological issues and subject recruitment results. *J Am Geriatr Soc*. 1987;*35*:629–634.

Longo VD and Finch CE. Genetics of aging and diseases: From rare mutations and model systems to disease prevention. *Arch Neurol*. 2002;*59*:1706–1708.

LoVerde ME, Prochazka AV, Byyny RL. Research consent forms. Continued unreadability and increasing length. *J Gen Intern Med*. 1989;*4*:410–412.

Marson DC, Schmitt FA, Ingram KK, Harrell LE. Determining the competency of Alzheimer patients to consent to treatment and research. *Alzheimer Disease Associated Disorders*. 1994;*8*(suppl):5–18.

Michels R. Are research ethics bad for our mental health? *New Engl J Med*. 1999;*340*:1427–1430.

Morse AN, Labin LC, Young SB, Aronson MP, Gurwitz JH. Exclusion of elderly women from published randomized trials of stress incontinence surgery. *Obstetrics and Gynecol*. 2004;*104*:498–503.

National Bioethics Advisory Commission. Research involving persons with mental disorders that may affect decisionmaking capacity. Volume I (1998). Available at: http://www.georgetown.edu/research/nrcbl/nbac/capacity/TOC.htm

The Nuremberg Code (1947). Available at: http://ohsr.od.nih.gov/guidelines/nuremberg.html

Office for Human Protections (OHRP). Available at: http://www.hhs.gov/ohrp/

Olde Rikkert MGM, van den Bercken JHL, ten Have HAMJ, Hoefnagels WHL. Experienced consent in geriatrics research: A new method to optimize the capacity to consent in frail elderly subjects. *J Med Ethics*. 1997;*23*:271–276.

Ratzan RM. 'Being old makes you different': The ethics of research with elderly subjects. *Hastings Center Report*. 1980;*10*:32–42.

Riecken HW and Ravich R. Informed consent to biomedical research in Veterans Administration hospitals. *JAMA*. 1982;*248*:344–348.

Rummans TA, Evans JM, Krahn LE, Fleming KC. Delirium in elderly patients: Evaluation and management. *Mayo Clin Proc*. 1995;*70*:989–98.

Sachs GA. Advance consent for dementia research. *Alzheimer Disease Associated Disorders*. 1994;*8*(suppl):19–27.

Sachs GA and Cassel CK. Biomedical research involving older human subjects. *Law, Medicine and Health Care*. 1990;*18*:234–243.

Sachs GA and Cohen HJ. Ethical challenges to research in geriatric medicine. In *Geriatric Medicine: An Evidence-Based Approach*, 4th ed. (Springer, 2003).

Sachs GA, Stocking CB, Stern R, Cox DM, Hougham G, Sachs RS. Ethical aspects of dementia research: informed consent and proxy consent. *Clin Res*. 1994;*42*:403–412.

Shamoo AE, Khin-Maung-Gyi FA. The use of decisionally impaired people in research. In *Ethics of the Use of Human Subjects in Research: A Practical Guide* (London: Garland Science, 2002).

Sugarman J, McCrory DC, Hubal RC. Getting meaningful informed consent from older adults: A structured literature review of empirical research. *J Am Geriatr Soc*. 1998;*46*: 517–524.

Swift CG. Ethical aspects of clinical research in the elderly. *Br J Hosp Med*. 1988;*40*:370–373.

U.S. Census Bureau. *Statistical Abstract of the United States: 2000*, 120th ed. (Washington, DC: U.S. Government Printing Office).

Warren JW, Sobal J, Tenney JH, Hoopes JM, Damron D, Levenson S, DeForge BR, Muncie HL. Informed consent by proxy: An issue in research with elderly patients. *New Engl J Med*. 1986;*315*:1124–8.

Weyers W. *The Abuse of Man: An Illustrated History of Dubious Medical Experimentation* (New York: Ardor Scribendi, 2003).

World Medical Association Declaration of Helsinki (1964). Ethical principles for medical research involving human subjects. Available at: http://www.wma.net/e/policy/b3.htm

Zimmer AW, Calkins E, Hadley E, Ostfeld AM, Kaye JM, Kaye D. Conducting clinical research in geriatric populations. *Ann Intern Med*. 1985;*103*:276–283.

8

SAGE KE and Other Online Sources Related to Aging

Evelyn Strauss and R. John Davenport

Researchers are making rapid headway in uncovering details about aging and its associated maladies. Yet the field faces a number of challenges. In particular, investigators from a wide range of disciplines who do not necessarily interact are generating daunting quantities of new data. A number of online resources can help researchers organize and manage the barrage of new results and can spark discussions. These Web sites publish summaries of the latest findings, offer tools with which to manipulate data, supply opportunities for direct communication with colleagues, and explore societal implications of the work. They are building bridges between different realms of the field and fostering creative thinking.

Introduction

Many of us wish for a 48-hour day—or that we could function on half as much sleep. Online resources in the field of aging can't alter planetary movements or physiology, but these Web sites can help researchers squeeze more out of their available time. They provide information, analysis, and tools that enhance efficiency and productivity—even in the wee hours before a grant deadline.

Online resources fulfill a variety of needs. Some offer up-to-date commentary on recent findings or high-level backgrounders on key topics in the field of aging; some supply tools such as databases of genes that have been implicated in aging or lists of animals and tissue sources that are of particular use for experiments in this arena; others post data and analysis in realms such as policy that influence progress in aging-related research. This chapter is not an exhaustive catalog of aging-related Web sites, nor does it completely explore the sites that it mentions; instead, it gives readers a taste of what's available on the Web.

Staying Informed; Digging Deep

Researchers from diverse subspecialties compose the field of aging, These human geneticists, molecular geneticists, evolutionary biologists, physiologists, neurobiologists, demographers, and cell, structural, and molecular biologists don't necessarily encounter one another while carrying out their professional activities: No single meeting brings everyone together, they don't all read one another's primary journals, nor does any journal publish papers from every discipline. Furthermore, research in the area is booming, posing a challenge to scientists struggling to keep up with relevant research even in their own corners of the field. In 2000, editors at the American Association for the Advancement of Science (AAAS) reasoned that a virtual community might catalyze interactions and creative thinking by bringing together researchers from many disciplines to exchange information and discuss ideas.

To that end, AAAS launched the Science of Aging Knowledge Environment in October 2001. The site aims to keep researchers in the field abreast of the latest scientific developments and to provide an online meeting place for the community. In particular, it strives to render information and commentary accessible to investigators with a broad range of backgrounds.

SAGE KE employs several strategies to inform scientists about research advances that have been published in other journals or presented at meetings. It posts critical summaries of the latest developments, written by both science journalists and investigators. The pieces by professional writers (News Focus) are based on interview material as well as literature research, and represent multiple viewpoints; their language and level of explanation assume scientific proficiency—but not that a reader is well informed about the particular matter at hand. Many of these stories attempt to entertain as well as educate (see Figure 8.1).

The articles by scientists (Perspectives) afford detailed commentary by experts. SAGE KE's editors attend meetings and maintain ongoing contact with researchers and journals, so news stories and Perspectives cover the latest findings as soon as they are publicly released. Editors also list additional articles of interest in each weekly issue. As a result, the site introduces newcomers to relevant topics in a timely fashion, and provides caveats and expert opinions to fully educate the reader as quickly as possible. Visitors can comment on the articles, a feature

Handbook of Models for Human Aging

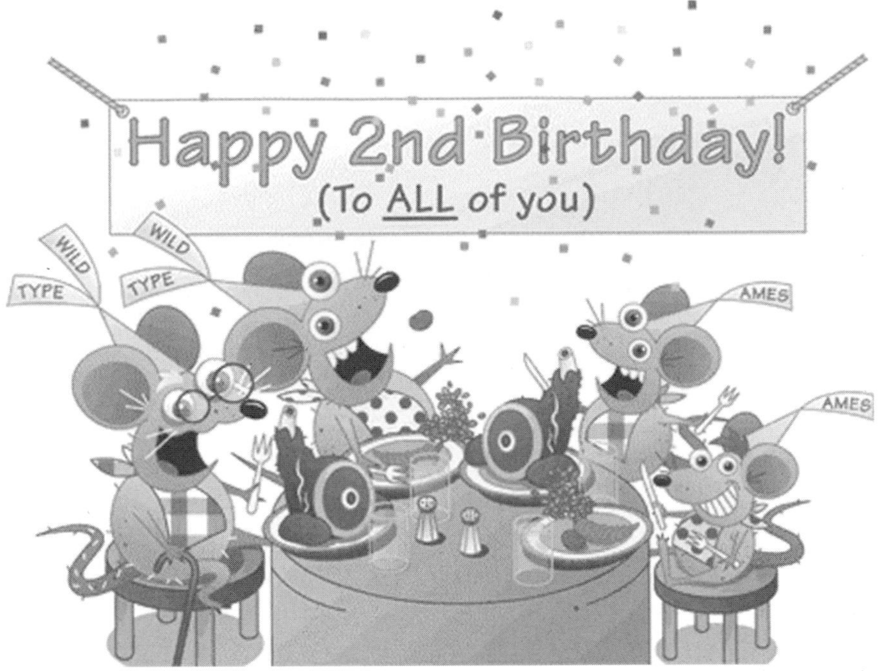
Happy 2nd Birthday!
(To ALL of you)
WILD TYPE
WILD TYPE
AMES
AMES

Figure 8.1. Party on. Calorie restriction and the *Prop-1* mutation collaborate to confer longer life than either one does alone [*Credit:* Terry E. Smith].

that provides an opportunity to extend the discussions further.

In addition to keeping readers informed about new discoveries in the field, some sites offer overview articles that provide in-depth information about key topics. The pieces differ in their styles and accessibility. SAGE KE's reviews are written by scientists and assume a fairly sophisticated audience. They cover diverse subjects, including oxidative mutagenesis and mismatch repair; a critical look at microarray analysis; senescence in plants; and ubiquitin, proteasomes, and brain aging. These articles provide a comprehensive look at research in particular areas. Other types of overviews present information in a less dense form. For example, SAGE KE's feature stories (News Synthesis) tie together multiple findings and place them in a broad context. Like the other journalist-written content, they rely on interview material and are informed by multiple opinions and viewpoints. Newcomers to the field should find SAGE KE's Hot Topic Orientations particularly worthwhile. In these pieces, writers introduce central and often controversial topics; the current collection includes subjects such as oxidative damage, the relation between cell and organismal aging, pain, the immune system, and Alzheimer's disease. Finally physicians have produced a series of case studies aimed at the basic researcher. These articles describe aspects of age-related diseases (mostly neurodegenerative ones so far) from the clinician's and pathologist's point of view. They put a human face on these illnesses for people whose professional home is the lab bench.

Other sites focus on single aspects of aging-related research. For example, Alzheimer Research Forum (Alzforum) targets Alzheimer's disease. It posts summaries of new findings, which include interview material, and houses a collection of seminars, online journal club discussions, recorded talks, and other presentations that describe a variety of hypotheses about the pathogenesis of Alzheimer's disease. Alzforum material assumes proficiency with the terminology of molecular biology.

Don't Know Much about History

SAGE KE's Classic Papers section offers PDFs of key papers published before 1990. This resource provides a way to gain historical perspective on aging-related research and sheds old light on unresolved problems. It includes, for example, Denham Harman's 1956 article on the free radical theory of aging and George C. Williams's 1957 article entitled Pleiotropy, Natural Selection, and the Evolution of Senescence as well as other seminal works.

The site also invites readers back in time through another route—with its historical reviews by luminaries in particular research areas. For instance, Edward Masoro's description of how the study of calorie restriction has unfolded reaches back to 1914 in its narrative. These articles include items of historical interest; Thomas Johnson's piece on *Caenorhabditis elegans* as a system for studying the genetics of aging contains the agenda for the 1979 Gordon Research Conference on the Biology of Aging.

Genes and Interventions That Influence Aging

These days, a significant proportion of research findings in the field relate to genes or environmental factors that adjust the rate of aging—usually in model organisms. A number of databases summarize key findings about such genes and interventions.

The U.S. National Library of Medicine's Online Mendelian Inheritance in Man (OMIM) catalogs human genes and disorders. Although it doesn't focus on aging-related conditions, it contains information about many diseases that disproportionately affect the elderly. For example, searching for "Parkinson's Disease" produces a list of several dozen genes. The summaries include information about the chromosomal location of the gene, activities of the protein it encodes and its purported or established role in disease, how the gene was cloned, a discussion of relevant animal models, and the history of its implication in disease. The write-ups are detailed and extensively referenced. NIH's Genetics Home Reference, too, supplies details about genes that have been associated with many aging-related disorders as well as other information on these illnesses. It includes entries for Alzheimer's disease, Parkinson's disease, and Hutchinson Gilford progeria syndrome, among many others.

For individuals who are interested in particular disorders with known or suspected genetic underpinnings, the Web serves up a number of focused resources. For example, Alzforum contains a database of genes and mutations that have been implicated in AD. The University of Washington's "Werner Syndrome" (WS) site hosts a repository for data on this premature aging disorder. The site's curators have compiled a list of mutations in the *WRN* gene that are associated with the condition, as well as diagnostic criteria, a historical overview of the topic, and a list of key papers. And the Diabetes Genome Anatomy Project homes in on the genetic underpinnings of this metabolic disease, whose risk increases with age.

Two databases focus specifically on genes that appear to alter the pace of aging: SAGE KE's Genes/Interventions Database and GenAge, directed by Pedro de Magalhães at Harvard University. SAGE KE's database catalogues published genes and interventions—such as calorie restriction—that affect longevity or selected age-related diseases in any organism. Each of the more than 200 entries for genes and 400 entries for interventions includes the organism, a description of the gene or treatment, a list of related genes in other organisms (for gene entries), pertinent references, and links to other databases such as WormBase and LocusLink. These write-ups function as crib sheets for the gene or intervention at hand and its association with aging. Visitors can search by organism, gene, key word, and other categories. Because few experiments have linked genes to mammalian aging, it contains only a few dozen mammalian longevity genes, a handful of which are from humans. GenAge takes a different tack, focusing on human genes that might influence the aging process. Its creators selected 20 genes that speed or slow mammalian decline, excluding some that might affect predisposition to disease rather than the aging process itself. Next, they picked other genes that work closely with those in the first set—for instance, those whose protein products operate in the same molecular pathway. This process yielded a list of more than 200 human genes that might alter aging, although solid data don't exist for every one. GenAge excludes genes in model organisms such as worms or yeast. Each entry includes a description of the rationale for inclusion, selected references, protein and DNA sequence information, and links to other databases such as Swiss-Prot and Ensembl. GenAge entries also supply a list of molecules that team up with the protein produced by each gene. For instance, the insulin receptor page specifies 11 molecules that grab the protein in cells, and one click reveals a diagram of those connections.

The sites mentioned thus far center on any genes that influence aging or its maladies, but another spotlights genetic changes in a specific cell structure that has been connected with aging. According to some theories, glitches in mitochondrial DNA accumulated over years might cause organisms to break down by hampering energy production and increasing the generation of pernicious free radicals. MitoMap can aid in probing that idea. The site, curated by researchers at the University of California, Irvine, contains the sequence of the human mitochondrial genome, and organizes mitochondrial mutations into different categories, such as mutations that cause disease, inversions, and deletions. The site also features illustrations such as a mitochondrial genome diagram, a map of world migrations by humans based on data from mitochondrial DNA sequencing, and a model of how metabolic changes in the mitochondria might contribute to diabetes. MitoMap also lists links to other Web sites related to mitochondria.

For a different way to manage the literature, check out Telemakus. Produced by researchers at the University of Washington, the resource aims to organize publications in particular research areas and illuminate connections between related studies. The first database created by the project covers calorie restriction, a treatment that extends lifespan in many organisms. Users can browse the database by author, research findings, or organism, or can search for keywords. The description of each piece of work offers a summary of the study design, including the organisms studied, and the number, sex, and age of animals used. Entries also include a list of tables and figures from the publication and, in many cases, the figures and tables themselves, enabling visitors to quickly review a study's findings without leaving Telemakus or having to track down the original paper.

Animals and Reagents

SAGE KE provides an experimental resources section that includes sources for tissues, cell lines, and animals of particular use in aging-related research, as well as a list of articles that consider issues of experimental design or data analysis. Of special interest are the write-ups on rodent strains and genetically-altered mice. The rodent-strain tables provide detailed information about commonly used inbred and hybrid laboratory strains, including their history and genetic background, caveats about using these animals, and the results of major studies on them. The entries aim to provide information so researchers can easily compare the strains and select an appropriate animal for a particular study. The genetically altered mice tables provide key references and information about the gene changed, the resulting phenotype, and the corresponding human phenotype for selected mutant, transgenic, and knock-out mice. These mice include strains that are exceptionally long lived, those that serve as models of neurodegenerative disease and other age-related conditions such as osteoarthritis, and animals that carry mutations in genes involved in processes related to aging, such as DNA repair.

The National Institute on Aging's (NIA's) "Scientific Resources" section offers information about the rhesus monkeys that are available for research on aging and the nonhuman primate tissue bank, which offers archived tissue to researchers in the field. The site also describes its rodent resources, human biospecimens, Aging Cell Repository, and microarrays, among other experimental tools available to scientists.

Population Studies

NIA's Scientific Resources section also highlights a different type of experimental tool: longitudinal studies. The site contains an extensive list of such studies and provides a searchable database that allows the user to identify those that relate to a keyword (or keywords) of interest.

Other sites also cover this topic. In SAGE KE, "Taking the Long View," the article discusses longitudinal studies in general and summarizes the goals of some on the NIA list as well as several others. Some population studies don't track people for many years; rather, they target—at least as their primary subjects—very old people with the hope of discovering keys to long life. The Okinawa Centenarian Study and the New England Centenarian Study, for instance, aim to uncover genetic and lifestyle characteristics that predispose people to outstanding health.

Demography, Mortality, and Health Statistics

The last century has seen a dramatic longevity rise in the industrialized world. Some Web sites aim to document this phenomenon and to provide information that might lead researchers to the factors that have caused this life-span gain. The Human Mortality Database, a joint effort between researchers at the University of California, Berkeley and the Max Planck Institute for Demographic Research in Rostock, Germany, currently provides detailed mortality and population data for 23 countries. Visitors can download and analyze these statistics to compare mortality trends in different regions over time. The site also provides links to other resources that contain useful information, such as cause of death, that is not included in the Human Mortality Database.

The National Center for Health Statistics at the United States Center for Disease Control and Prevention contains a Data Warehouse on Trends in Health and Aging on its aging activities page. Users can view, chart, and download data on life expectancy, disability, insurance utilization, socioeconomic status and other measures for United States citizens over the last century or so. Furthermore, the site provides downloadable software for manipulating the information and tailoring it to individual needs. Some sites document types of demographic data other than mortality trends. For instance, the Utah Population Database contains an extensive set of Utah family histories, including medical information for individual family members. This database contains a cancer registry and information about cause of death. Access is free, but requires advance approval for use of the data.

The United States Administration on Aging provides statistics on the elderly, and the U.S. Census Bureau compiles census numbers relevant to aging.

For researchers focused on species other than our own, the Web-accessible book, Longevity Records: Life Spans of Mammals, Birds, Amphibians, Reptiles, and Fish, contains data on the highest documented age for more than 3000 mammals, birds, amphibians, reptiles, and fish.

Policy Matters

As research in the field of aging is blossoming, so are questions about its implications for society. The importance of these issues is compounded by the fact that populations in industrialized nations are growing older. Several Web sites address policy-related topics that intersect the science of aging.

SAGE Crossroads, a collaboration between the Alliance for Aging Research and AAAS, wrestles with the policy implications of aging-related research. It has tackled numerous thorny questions with policymakers, journalists, and the public in mind. Some individuals worry, for example, that "artificially" extending human lives would cheapen our existence, whereas others point out that the modern medical enterprise has already drastically increased lifespans with no ill effects on society. Other subjects that the site has explored include the paucity of older people included in clinical trials; the wisdom of using human growth hormone to combat symptoms of aging despite data suggesting that the substance curtails lifespan; and how we might improve our flu-combating measures. It has discussed nanotechnology, hormone replacement therapy, guidelines for keeping bones strong, and chronic pain, as well as age-related voice changes and hearing loss. SAGE Crossroads ponders such topics in News and Views articles as well as through Webcasts in which experts debate and discuss such matters.

To gain insight into how lawmakers address these and other age-related policy issues, visit the U.S. Senate Special Committee on Aging Web site. Visitors can view video or read testimonies from hearings, which the committee uses to guide recommendations for new legislation to the United States Senate.

Talk amongst Yourselves

The Web fosters the opportunity to interact with peers in addition to providing an efficient conduit for collecting information. At SAGE KE's bulletin board, visitors can post questions and items for discussion with the goal of eliciting feedback. With the site's Listserv, individuals can communicate by Email with others who want to toss around ideas informally.

For stimulating, real-life contact with colleagues, attending scientific meetings is hard to beat. SAGE KE's Meetings and Events calendar can help with the planning.

Reaching beyond Researchers

A number of Web sites aim to inform the general public, but prove useful for researchers. They can help with teaching or setting scientific work in a broader context. The American Federation for Aging Research's Info-Aging, for example, offers explanations of a number of topics under several headings. Topics in the "Biology of Aging" section include oxidative damage, telomeres, stem cells, and biomarkers of aging. Each one summarizes crucial issues, addresses basic questions, provides links to related research, and points readers toward other resources; in addition, they are reviewed by experts in each field. The "Disease Center" similarly contains key information and questions on some age-related illnesses, such as Alzheimer's disease, macular degeneration, and osteoporosis, and the "Healthy Aging Center" discusses issues such as nutrition, stress, hearing, and immunization.

AgeLine, hosted by AARP, formerly known as the Association for the Advancement of Retired People, catalogs publications related to social gerontology as well as age-related topics in psychology, sociology, social work, economics, public policy, and the health sciences. The site features abstracts of journal articles, books and chapters, research reports, dissertations, and educational videos, and provides links to purchase or view the full text.

Other resources explain particular age-related diseases. The Centers for Disease Control Cardiovascular Health site contains information for lay people such as fact sheets on topics that include cholesterol, heart attacks, and high blood pressure. Of particular interest to researchers are the interactive maps that supply heart attack and stroke mortality rates for the state, gender, and racial/ethnic group of choice. The site includes a list of Morbidity and Mortality Reports that relate to cardiovascular disease as well as other statistical and public-health information. NIH's Osteoporosis and Related Bone Diseases National Resource Center offers background articles on topics of interest to researchers as well as lay people; these include "Vitamin A and Bone Health," "Phytoestrogens and Bone Health," and "Bone Mass Measurement: What the Numbers Mean."

The Merck Manual of Geriatrics provides detailed information and guidelines on the care of older people for health professionals. This online book is searchable and covers conditions from falls to dementia to urinary tract disorders. The Merck Manual of Health and Aging is a work in progress, offering demographic information and explanations about how the body ages in language that is intended for the general public.

The Web provides a wealth of tools to help researchers tackle the wide-ranging topics related to aging, tame the sea of data, and make contact with investigators in a variety of subspecialties. These resources can seem invaluable when burning the midnight oil, but they also hold up well in the light of day.

Recommended Resources

In addition to the Web sites mentioned in the text, see SAGE KE's Web links section.

Internet Resources

Science of Aging Knowledge Environment (SAGE KE) (http://sageke.sciencemag.org)
Alzheimer Research Forum (http://www.alzforum.org)
Online Mendelian Inheritance in Man (OMIM) (http://www.ncbi.nlm.nih.gov/entrez/query.fcgi?db=OMIM)
NIH's Genetics Home Reference (http://ghr.nlm.nih.gov/)
Alzforum's database of genes (http://www.alzforum.org/res/com/gen/default.asp)

Alzforum's database of mutations (http://www.alzforum.org/res/com/mut/default.asp)
University of Washington's Werner Syndrome site (http://www.pathology.washington.edu/werner/)
Diabetes Genome Anatomy Project (http://www.diabetesgenome.org/home/)
SAGE KE's Genes/Interventions Database (http://sageke.sciencemag.org/cgi/genesdb)
GenAge (http://genomics.senescence.info/genes/index.html)
MitoMap (http://www.mitomap.org/)
Telemakus (http://www.telemakus.net)
SAGE KE's Experimental Resources section (http://sageke.sciencemag.org/resources/experimental/)
NIA's Scientific Resources section (http://www.nia.nih.gov/ResearchInformation/ScientificResources/)
SAGE KE's "Taking the Long View" news article (http://sageke.sciencemag.org/cgi/content/full/2004/26/ns3)
Okinawa Centenarian Study (http://okinawaprogram.com/)
New England Centenarian Study (http://www.bumc.bu.edu/Dept/Home.aspx?DepartmentID=361)
The Human Mortality Database (http://www.mortality.org/)
National Center for Health Statistics at the United States Center for Disease Control and Prevention: Data Warehouse on Trends in Health and Aging (http://www.cdc.gov/nchs/agingact.htm)
Utah Population Database (http://www.hci.utah.edu/groups/ppr/)
United States Administration on Aging statistics on elderly Americans (http://www.aoa.gov/prof/Statistics/statistics.asp)
U.S. Census Bureau: census numbers relevant to aging (http://www.census.gov/population/www/socdemo/age.html)
Longevity Records: Life Spans of Mammals, Birds, Amphibians, Reptiles, and Fish, by James R. Carey and Debra S. Judge (http://www.demogr.mpg.de/longevityrecords/)
U.S. Senate Special Committee on Aging Web site (http://aging.senate.gov/public/)
SAGE KE's bulletin board (http://sageke.sciencemag.org/cgi/forum-display/sagekeForum;3)
SAGE KE's Listserv (http://mailman.aaas.org/mailman/listinfo/sagemail)
SAGE KE's Meetings and Events calendar (http://sageke.sciencemag.org/cgi/calendarcontent/)
InfoAging (http://www.infoaging.org/)
AgeLine (http://www.aarp.org/research/ageline/)
Centers for Disease Control Cardiovascular Health Information (http://www.cdc.gov/cvh/index.htm)
NIH's Osteoporosis and Related Bone Diseases—National Resource Center Fact Sheet on Osteoporosis (http://www.osteo.org/osteolinks.asp)
Merck Manual of Geriatrics (http://www.merck.com/mrkshared/mmg/home.jsp)
Merck Manual of Health and Aging (http://www.merck.com/pubs/mmanual_ha/contents.html)
SAGE KE's Web links (http://sageke.sciencemag.org/cgi/ul/sagekeUl;CAT_1)

9

Proteomics in Aging Research

Christian Schöneich

The process of biological aging is a complex phenomenon, depending on a manifold of different parameters, including nature of the organism, lifestyle, diet, and so forth. In order to compare different aging phenotypes, a global qualitative and quantitative proteomic analysis of different species is necessary. Proteomic data need to be interpreted relative to complementary genomic and functional analysis. The present article surveys several proteomic methods and their direct application and/or potential relevance for the characterization of the "aging proteome." Specific emphasis has been given to the analysis of post-translational protein modifications.

Introduction

Biological aging is controlled to various extents by several closely related parameters, which include metabolic rate, caloric intake, genetics, lifestyle, and environmental factors (Jazwinski, 1996; Sohal and Weindruch, 1996; Smith and Pereira-Smith, 1996; Finch and Tanzi, 1997; Morrison and Hof, 1997; Lamberts *et al.*, 1997). Over the years, a number of different theories for the aging process have been formulated (Masoro, 1993) such as the "rate-of-living theory," the "somatic mutation theory," the "error catastrophy theory," the "cross-linkage theory," and the "free radical theory of aging." Some of these theories are based on common phenomena. For example, the rate-of-living theory correlates higher metabolic rates with shorter lifespan. Higher metabolic rates lead to higher levels of reactive oxygen species, available for the transformation of biomolecules, linking the rate of living theory with the cross-linkage theory and the free radical theory of aging. Ultimately, each one of these theories seems to favor a rather unique mechanism as the predominant cause of aging, and this may be considered the general shortcoming of these theories.

Aging represents a complex developmental phenomenon, depending on the global interplay between genes and gene products. The rate of aging will certainly depend on gene identity, gene polymorphism, the rate of translation, developmental regulation of translation, the residence time of gene products in the organism, and post-translational modification of the gene products. A thorough understanding of the aging process requires the evaluation of all these processes, and this is where aging research will greatly benefit from genomics and proteomics studies. Various genomics studies have started to address the general quantification of age-dependent changes in gene expression (Kayo *et al.*, 2001) and the effects of nutrition and/or genetic modification (i.e., deletion or overexpression of genes affecting life span) on gene expression profiles. Currently, the role of proteomic studies is to provide quantitative information on the generation of gene products including the profiling of native proteins, protein isoforms, splice variants, mutants, and post-translationally modified species. In addition, proteomic studies need to define networks of protein–protein interactions. Bioinformatics studies are then necessary to combine both genomics and proteomics data into a multidimensional network of time-dependent, developmentally regulated interaction of genes. Such an effort is underway with the development of GenAge (available on the World Wide Web: http://genomics.senescence.info/genes/), a curated database of genes related to human aging (de Magalhaes and Toussaint, 2004). Ultimately, we hope that proteomic studies will not only further our basic understanding of the aging process but also yield reliable biomarkers for the early diagnosis of age-dependent diseases, preferentially in easily accessible biological fluids. The present article will review commonly used proteomic techniques and their application to the profiling of protein expression and post-translational modification.

Proteomic Techniques

TWO-DIMENSIONAL GEL ELECTROPHORESIS (2DE)

The last years have witnessed an immense improvement in the techniques available for the analysis of the proteome. This is largely due to advances in mass spectrometry (MS) analysis, where electrospray ionization (ESI) and matrix-assisted laser desorption ionization (MALDI) represent soft ionization techniques suitable for native and most post-translationally modified peptides (Aebersold and Goodlett, 2001). However, it has been realized that none of the individual methods will be sufficient to provide satisfactory answers to all questions of interest. Each of the proteomic techniques has certain strengths and shortcomings as outlined below. Two-dimensional gel electrophoresis (2DE) has been and continues to be a widely used technique due to its relatively low cost and maintenance requirements. Continuous improvements are made with regard to reproducibility, solubility (especially of membrane proteins), alternative protein stains, and the differential display of proteins during *d*ifferential *i*n-gel *e*lectrophoresis (DIGE). For DIGE, two separate pools of proteins from cells/tissue of different origin are labeled with two distinct fluorescent dyes, such as 1-(5-carboxypentyl)-1′-propylindocarbocyanine halide (Cy3) *N*-hydroxy-succinimidyl ester and 1-(5-carboxypentyl)-1′-methylindodi-carbocyanine halide (Cy5) *N*-hydroxy-succinimidyl ester, which can then be individually excited for exclusive monitoring of the labeled proteins from one specific pool (Zhou *et al.*, 2002a). Specific software allows for the three-dimensional representation of the individual protein spots on the gel. Importantly, the fluorescent dyes should be similar in molecular weight and charge so that identical proteins labeled with different dyes comigrate during 2DE. Two labeling strategies for DIGE have been developed, (i) minimal labeling and (ii) saturation labeling (Shaw *et al.*, 2003). During minimal labeling, fluorescent dyes are covalently attached to protein Lys residues. Based on the abundance of Lys residues in proteins, the labeling stoichiometry may exceed more than one molecule of dye per protein. Proteins with multiple dye molecules may migrate differently on 2DE compared to proteins with a single dye or precipitate due to the hydrophobicity of the dyes, enhancing the complexity of samples and rendering the relative quantitation of proteins from different tissues a difficult task. Hence, minimal labeling is run under conditions that ensure that not more than one dye molecule is attached to a single protein. Under these conditions, a significant fraction of proteins remains unlabeled, resulting in an overall loss of sensitivity. The latter may require larger sample volumes for the relative quantitation of low abundance proteins. A new generation of fluorescent dyes has been developed for saturation labeling (Shaw *et al.*, 2003). These dyes are covalently attached to protein Cys residues, which usually show a lower abundance in proteins relative to Lys residues. Saturation labeling is achieved under conditions where each protein Cys residue is labeled. This technique results in a greater sensitivity of the analysis but may still suffer from the precipitation of individual proteins. One drawback of the saturation labeling technique is the potential age-dependent oxidation of protein Cys residues, resulting in the age-dependent loss of labeling sites. In such a scenario the lower stoichiometric labeling of a protein from aged tissue could be misinterpreted as lower expression. The ICAT methodology, described below, suffers from the same problem.

MULTIDIMENSIONAL CHROMATOGRAPHY METHODS

Alternative to 2DE, proteins and peptides can be separated by multidimensional (micro) liquid chromatography methods and/or capillary electrophoresis on-line coupled to multidimensional mass spectrometry (MS^n) (Shen and Smith, 2002). Protein mixtures are proteolytically digested, and a large number of the resulting peptides are resolved and identified in a single run, a strategy termed "multidimensional protein identification technology" (MudPIT) (Washburn *et al.*, 2001; Wolters *et al.*, 2001). Orthogonal separation modes of any choice can be coupled, provided that the eluate composition of an earlier separation mode is compatible with the following separation mode. Prefractionation of protein families (e.g., through affinity purification, solution isoelectric focusing, etc.) (Righetti *et al.*, 2005), followed by one- or multidimensional separation, increases the dynamic range of the analytical method allowing for the monitoring of even low abundance proteins (Gygi *et al.*, 2002). This is necessitated by the MS detector, where large amounts of high-abundance peptides can suppress the ionization of lower abundant peptides.

To achieve relative quantitation of proteins during 2DE or chromatographic runs, Aebersold and coworkers have developed the isotope-coded affinity tag (ICAT) methodology (Gygi *et al.*, 1999): in the original approach proteins/peptides are derivatized with a bifunctional reagent (structure **1**, as shown in Figure 9.1) which contains an electrophile on one end and biotin on the other end.

The electrophile affords covalent derivatization of Cys, and the biotin moiety enables affinity purification of the labeled proteins/peptides. An organic linker between the functional groups of the reagent contains

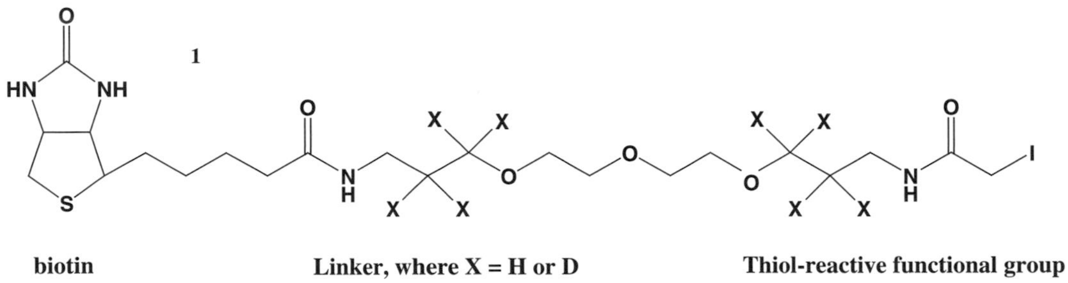

Figure 9.1. Structure **1**.

either normal (H) or heavy (D) hydrogen isotopes. When two pools of proteins are labeled with the normal or heavy isotope-containing ICAT reagent, their relative abundance can be determined by quantitative MS analysis of the ratio of normal to heavy ICAT-derivatized peptides of specific proteins. During 2DE, normal and heavy isotope ICAT-derivatized proteins comigrate, ensuring an accurate relative quantification of the proteins from different sources (Smolka *et al.*, 2002). However, slight differences in the elution profiles of normal and heavy isotope ICAT-labeled peptides have been noted during reverse-phase chromatography (Zhang *et al.*, 2001). Therefore, an accurate relative quantification of ICAT-labeled peptides requires MS analysis at the respective peak maxima of the individual chromatographic peaks of normal and heavy isotope ICAT-labeled peptides. Complications have also been noted with the recovery of ICAT-labeled peptides during biotin-avidin affinity purification (Gygi *et al.*, 2002), and with tandem MS sequencing of ICAT-labeled peptides.

Recent improvements of ICAT reagents include the design of a solid-phase isotope tagging method, avoiding biotin, and incorporation of a photocleavable linker (structure **2**, as shown in Figure 9.2); after solid-phase purification of ICAT-labeled peptides and photolysis, the remaining peptides essentially contain an additional normal or heavy isotope-containing Leu residue (Zhou *et al.*, 2002b).

Using the ICAT methodology, complex mixtures of peptides from digested proteins can be reduced to one or a few peptides per protein (essentially as many peptides as the protein contains reduced or reducible Cys residues). Such a reduction in sample size significantly enhances the dynamic range of the proteomic analysis. For example, using the codon bias value as a measure for protein expression, Gygi *et al.* (2000) showed that traditional 2D gel electrophoresis was not able to indicate low abundant proteins with codon bias values of <0.1, whereas many of these proteins were detected with a multidimensional separation strategy including ICAT-labeling and affinity purification (Gygi *et al.*, 2002). We note that irreversibly oxidized Cys residues (to cysteic acid) will not be amenable to ICAT labeling.

Surface-enhanced laser desorption/ionization (SELDI) represents a concept with great promise for sample size reduction and enrichment of specific classes of analytes (Merchant and Weinberger, 2000). Protein-chips with specifically modified surfaces allow the affinity purification of analytes prior to on-chip digestion and MALDI-TOF MS analysis. Various different chemical and biochemical surfaces have been designed containing immobilized hydrophobic, ionic, or mixed-mode phases or antibodies; IMAC supports; polynucleotides; or specific enzymes or receptors.

PROTEIN ARRAYS

The advent of high-throughput protein expression systems has enabled the construction of protein arrays for the rapid screening of protein–biomolecule interactions (Smith *et al.*, 2005). This includes the interaction of proteins with small molecules, other proteins, polynucleotides, phospholipids, and antibodies. For example, these platforms allow evaluation of the specificity (or cross-reactivity) of a given antibody toward a large matrix of different proteins. Another form of microarray is the tissue microarray (TMA). This can now be produced with good accuracy, permitting the rapid screening of a large number of human tissue sections for individual proteins (Uhlen and Ponten, 2005).

Protein Expression Profiling

The relative quantitation of protein expression profiles between young and normally aged or prematurely aged tissue as well as tissue suffering from age-dependent disease provides an important basis for the global proteomic analysis of aging. These analyses will be supplemented by the proteomic analysis of age-dependent

2

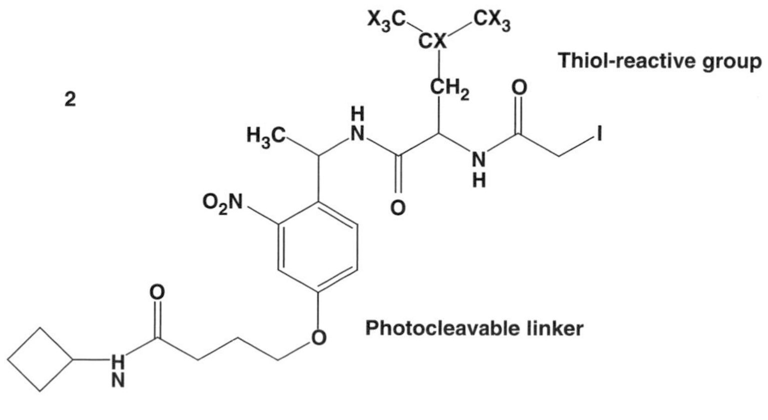

X_3C CX_3 CX CH_2 O Thiol-reactive group H_3C H N N H O O_2N I O O Photocleavable linker H N Beads

Figure 9.2. Structure **2**.

post-translational protein modification and functional proteomics, as described in more detail below. So far, 2DE has been the method of choice for profiling cell culture models of aging or aging tissue (Dierick *et al.*, 2002a; Gromov *et al.*, 2002; Benvenuti *et al.*, 2002a; 2002b) and the effect of environmental stresses (Dierick *et al.*, 2002b; 2002c). Chang *et al.* have characterized the reproducibility and sensitivity of proteomic analysis of mitochondrial proteins from aged mouse skeletal muscle, suggesting that a sample size of 10 animals will be sufficient to detect a 100% difference in 97% of the 505 mitochondrial proteins resolved in their 2D electrophoresis separation (Chang *et al.*, 2003). The senescent-accelerated mouse represents a convenient animal model for the proteomic characterization of aging and age-dependent pathologies. Cho *et al.* compared the liver proteome of the senescence-prone strain SAMP8 (senescence-accelerated mouse senescence prone) with that of the senescent-resistant SAMR1 (senescence-accelerated mouse senescence-resistant) and detected age-dependent changes of 64 proteins between both strains, whereas 18 proteins showed age-dependent changes in both SAMP8 and SAMR1 mice (Cho *et al.*, 2003). Surprisingly, Poon *et al.* quantified age-dependent changes between 12- and 4-month-old SAMP8 for only five brain proteins (Poon *et al.*, 2004). Proteomic analysis revealed a gender-specific alteration in the age-dependent relative expression of glycolytic and mitochondrial cardiac proteins in monkeys (Yan *et al.*, 2004). A limited proteomic analysis was also presented for the Hutchinson–Gilford Progeria Syndrome (Robinson *et al.*, 2003). This premature aging disease is associated with mutations in the gene for lamin; a comparison of lamin expression levels between 10 and 13 years old progeria patients with their age-matched controls showed significantly reduced lamin levels. Moreover, the lamin of the progeria patients displayed ca. 0.3 units more basic pI value, consistent with the loss of a C-terminal phosphorylation site. The proteome of human cerebrospinal fluid (CSF) was profiled as part of an ongoing search for biomarkers of age-dependent pathologies (Zhang *et al.*, 2005). Using shotgun proteomics in conjunction with the ICAT methodology, a series of proteins changing between 20 and 100% between the CSF of young and old donors was monitored, and, for specific proteins, these changes were confirmed by complementary Western blot analysis. An important aspect of these proteomic experiments is the elimination of highly abundant proteins such as albumin and immunoglobulin prior to the analysis, which was achieved with sequential precipitation of CSF proteins by an organic solvent, acetonitrile.

Proteomic Analysis of Post-translational Modifications

Post-translational protein modifications significantly expand the portfolio of proteins with specific properties encoded by the genetic code. They allow for the production of multiple variants of a single gene product through specific, potentially reversible, covalent alterations of amino acid side chains. To date, about 200 distinct post-translational protein modifications are known (Khidekel and Hsieh-Wilson, 2004). However, we are just at the beginning of a thorough qualitative and quantitative characterization of only a few of these post-translational modifications in the "aging proteome." Importantly, proteins will not necessarily only incorporate a single modification, but often multiple modifications accumulate specifically on long-lived proteins in tissues with low protein turnover (e.g., the crystallins in the lens). Considering the progressive age-dependent functional changes of most cell types and tissues, an accurate profile of age-dependent post-translational protein modifications is mandatory. The following paragraphs will focus on the proteomic characterization of selected post-translational protein modifications such as phosphorylation and oxidation.

PHOSPHORYLATION

Age-dependent changes in protein phosphorylation have been noted for individual proteins, e.g., the crystallins (Ueda *et al.*, 2002) and various sarcoplasmic reticulum proteins (Xu and Narayanan, 1998). The sensitive analysis of phosphopeptides and/or phosphoproteins requires a separation of phosphorylated peptides or proteins from excess nonphosphorylated species. While few proteomic studies have focused on the characterization of the "phosphoproteome" of aging tissue, much research effort has been placed on method development for the analysis of the phosphoproteome (Mann *et al.*, 2002; Conrads *et al.*, 2002). Importantly, antibodies against phosphoserine, phosphothreonine and phosphotyrosine allow for the enrichment of phosphoproteins prior to chromatographic separation and mass spectrometric analysis of phosphopeptides, resulting in a reduction of sample complexity (Grønborg *et al.*, 2002; Pandey *et al.*, 2002). During mass spectrometric analysis, phosphopeptides can be recognized through specific fragmentation processes, i.e., the loss of PO_3^- (79 Da) from all phosphoamino acids in the negative electrospray ionization (ESI) mode or the neutral losses of HPO_3 (80 Da) or H_3PO_4 (98 Da) from phosphoserine and phosphothreonine in the positive ESI mode (Schlosser *et al.*, 2001). Moreover phosphopeptides can be monitored through the appearance of characteristic immonium ions from phosphotyrosine (Steen *et al.*, 2002) or chemically modified (into dimethylamine-containing sulfenic acids) phosphoserine and phosphothreonine (Steen and Mann, 2002a). The resolution of such immonium ions from other small peptide fragments is possible because the reporter ions contain a higher incidence of mass-deficient atoms (O, P, S), creating an inherent *M*ass-*D*eficient *M*ass *T*ag (MaDMaT) (Steen and Mann, 2002b). The chemical modification of phosphoserine and phosphothreonine can be achieved after β-elimination at alkaline pH, generating dehydroalanine, which can be derivatized via Michael addition of appropriate nucleophiles. This chemistry enables biotinylation of original phosphoserine and phosphothreonine residues for affinity purification (Oda *et al.*, 2001), selective immobilization on solid phases (Zhou *et al.*, 2001), and introduction of a cleavage-site for a lysine-specific protease (Knight *et al.*, 2003).

A further reduction of sample complexity can be achieved by metal-affinity chromatography (IMAC) of phosphopeptides on chromatographic supports containing trivalent metal ions such as Fe^{3+} or Ga^{3+} (Zarling *et al.*, 2000; Riggs *et al.*, 2001; Ficarro *et al.*, 2002; Chen *et al.*, 2002). Optimal resolution of phosphorylated from nonphosphorylated peptides requires chemical esterification of peptide carboxylate groups (Ficarro *et al.*, 2002), and the selectivity of the method towards phosphopeptides can be improved when proteins are digested with endoproteinase Glu-C instead of trypsin, reducing the number of acidic residues per peptide (Seeley *et al.*, 2005). For relative quantitation of phosphopeptides, Ga(III) IMAC has been combined with stable isotope labeling of peptides at the *N*-terminal amino group (Riggs *et al.*, 2005).

OXIDATIVE MODIFICATIONS

Analysis of protein-associated carbonyls

Consistent with the "free radical theory" of aging, many tissues show an age-dependent increase of the steady-state concentrations of oxidized proteins. So far most reports on the accumulation of oxidized proteins have analyzed "protein-associated carbonyls." The term "protein-associated carbonyl" classifies a carbonyl-containing covalent protein modification, which results either from the direct chemical transformation of an amino acid residue into a carbonyl product or from the covalent attachment of a carbonyl-containing molecule (e.g., 4-hydroxynonenal, 4-HNE) (Berlett and Stadtman, 1997). The most frequently used analytical method for the detection of protein-associated carbonyls is derivatization with 2,4-dinitrophenylhydrazine (Scheme 1, as shown in Figure 9.3), followed by UV spectroscopy or Western blot detection with anti-2,4-dinitrophenyl antibodies (Shacter *et al.*, 1994).

The specificity of these antibodies was evaluated through specific reaction with DNP conjugated to proteins (Eshhar *et al.*, 1980; Shacter *et al.*, 1994), and 1 pmol was reported as a lower limit of detection of protein-associated carbonyls (Shacter *et al.*, 1994). A comparable detection limit (0.64 pmol) was recently achieved with a slight modification of the methodology, using biotin-hydrazide labeling of the carbonyls followed by staining with fluorescein isothiocyanate (FITC)-labeled avidin (Yoo and Regnier, 2004). A number of studies have used stationary phase bacterial cells as a model for aging somatic cells of higher eukaryotic organisms in order to delineate the routes leading to the accumulation of oxidized proteins (Dukan and Nyström, 1999; Nyström, 2002; Aguilaniu *et al.*, 2001; Ballesteros *et al.*, 2001). Experiments with growth-arrested *Escherichia coli* demonstrated that protein carbonylation is fairly selective to specific proteins. Misfolded proteins are especially susceptible to the formation of protein-associated carbonyls (Dukan *et al.*, 2000). Mechanistically, not the rate of respiration *per se* but the degree of coupling in the mitochondrial respiratory apparatus appears to be responsible for the increased accumulation of oxidized proteins (Aguilaniu *et al.*, 2001). A remarkable observation was that mother cells retain a large fraction of oxidized proteins during cell division, somehow protecting their daughter cells from the consequences of protein oxidation (Aguilaniu *et al.*, 2003). Such a result would suggest that old tissues would have a reduced ability to resist oxidative stress; however, recently experiments with *Arabidopsis thaliana* demonstrated a mechanism in plants, where old leaves can eliminate oxidized proteins prior to bolting and flowering of the plant (prior to reproduction) (Johansson *et al.*, 2004).

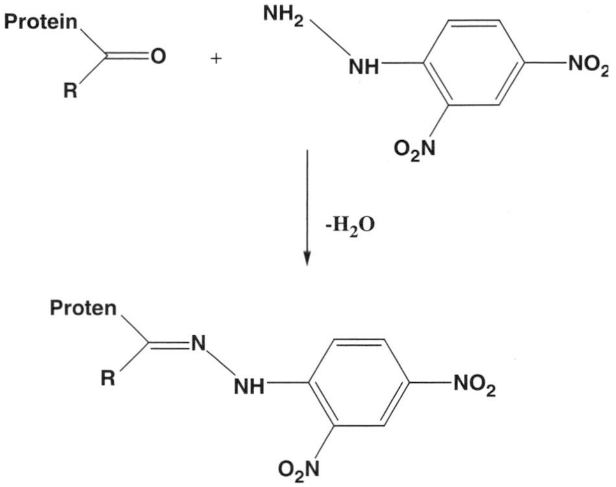

Protein, R, O, +, NH_2, NH, NO_2, O_2N, $-H_2O$, Proten, R, N, NH, NO_2, O_2N

Figure 9.3. Scheme 1.

Predominantly Western blot analysis demonstrated a quite selective age-dependent accumulation of carbonylated proteins in *Drosophila melanogaster* (Das *et al.*, 2001) and human Alzheimer's disease brain (Castegna *et al.*, 2002a; 2002b). Selective protein carbonyl-association was also detected in the brain of SAMP8 mice (Poon *et al.*, 2004) and model experiments where the Alzheimer's disease β-amyloid peptide was directly injected into rat brain (Boyd-Kimball *et al.*, 2005). However, all these Western blot-based experiments identified only a small subset of carbonylated proteins compared to the more than 100 carbonyl-containing proteins identified in brain via a complementary approach, where proteins were derivatized with a biotin-containing hydrazide, and the so biotinylated proteins immunoenriched with immobilized streptavidin (Soreghan *et al.*, 2003). An important caveat in the analysis of carbonylated proteins is their inherent instability towards further covalent modification such as Schiff base-formation (Mirzaei and Regnier, 2005). The latter would not be detected via any of the carbonyl-specific methods involving derivatization with hydrazines. Another problem with most of the proteomic data so far presented on protein carbonyl formation is the general lack of tandem mass spectrometry data which would (1) confirm the carbonyl content by a complementary technique, and (2) locate the modified amino acids. A potential source of error in the immunochemical identification of carbonyl-containing proteins only by Western blot could be the contamination of a nonmodified protein in a 2D gel spot by a trace amount of a second, carbonylated, protein. Mirzaei and Regnier (2005) demonstrated that tandem mass spectrometric information on the carbonyl-containing peptide sequences can be obtained after biotin hydrazide derivatization of protein carbonyls, followed by immunoenrichment on immobilized monomeric avidin columns.

Analysis of 3-Nitrotyrosine

Increasing evidence is accumulating that the formation of 3-nitrotyrosine *in vivo* is associated with changes in protein structure and function and represents a valid biomarker for conditions of oxidative stress (Ischiropoulos and Beckman, 2003). To date, most proteomic strategies for the detection of 3-nitrotyrosine utilized 2DE followed by Western blot detection of 3-nitrotyrosine (Aulak *et al.*, 2001; Miyagi *et al.*, 2002; Turko *et al.*, 2003; Casoni *et al.*, 2005). Analogous to the proteomic analysis of protein-associated carbonyls, the age-dependent accumulation of 3-nitrotyrosine is rather selective to a subset of proteins (Kanski *et al.*, 2003; 2005a; 2005b). Interestingly, predominantly cytosolic proteins displayed an age-dependent increase in 3-nitrotyrosine in skeletal muscle (Kanski *et al.*, 2003; 2005b) while cardiac aging caused 3-nitrotyrosine accumulation to a significant extent also on mitochondrial proteins (Kanski *et al.*, 2005a). It remains to be shown whether complementary analytical strategies can confirm this rather unexpected selectivity.

Most of the 2DE analysis of 3-nitrotyrosine-containing proteins *in vivo* suffer from the absence of tandem mass spectrometric sequence information, confirming the presence of 3-nitrotyrosine on the identified proteins. Exceptions are noted for the 2DE analysis of human pituitary (Zhan and Desiderio, 2004) and rat cardiac proteins (Kanski *et al.*, 2005a). This general lack of tandem mass spectrometric information is likely due to the actual yield and recovery of 3-nitrotyrosine-containing peptides/proteins from biological tissue. However, when skeletal muscle proteins were resolved by solution isoelectric focusing/SDS-PAGE instead of 2DE, permitting significantly higher sample loads, eleven 3-nitrotyrosine-containing proteins were identified and confirmed by tandem mass spectrometric data (Kanski *et al.*, 2005b). Information on the actual location of 3-nitrotyrosine in the identified proteins led to some interesting observations. In the cytosolic creatine kinase, age-dependent tyrosine nitration occurred predominantly on residues at positions Tyr^{14} and Tyr^{20}. Instead, the exposure of creatine kinase to peroxynitrite ($ONOO^-$) *in vitro* led to nitration of predominantly Tyr^{82}, a residue not affected *in vivo*. Peroxynitrite forms through the reaction of nitric oxide (NO) with superoxide ($O_2^{\bullet -}$) and represents one important tyrosine-nitrating species *in vivo*. However, additional nitrating systems are known such as the peroxidase-nitrite system, affording nitrogen dioxide ($^{\bullet}NO_2$). Moreover, while identifying nitrated proteins *in vivo* we must always be aware of the fact that any observed selectivity will be the result not only of the nitration chemistry, but also of protein turnover and repair. Nitrated proteins are subject to accelerated turnover, and Murad and coworkers have identified a potential repair enzyme for nitrated proteins, a putative "denitrase," which targets selected nitrated proteins such as histone H1.2 (Irie *et al.*, 2003). Proteomic studies in isolated mitochondria have indicated that nitrated proteins can be repaired quite rapidly when the oxygen tension decreases (Aulak *et al.*, 2004; Koeck *et al.*, 2004).

Analysis of Cys oxidation and S-glutathiolation

Cys oxidation is one of the most prevalent protein modifications under conditions of oxidative stress. Proteomic evidence for Cys oxidation has been obtained through tandem MS characterization of cysteic acid-containing peroxiredoxins in Jurkat T-cell lymphoma cells exposed to an organic peroxide or glucose oxidase (Rabilloud *et al.*, 2002). Lin *et al.* (2002) utilized a lipophilic cation, (4-iodobutyl)triphenylphosphonium (IBTP), which enriches inside the mitchondria, and an antibody directed against the triphenylphosphonium moiety, for the proteomic characterization of mitochondrial protein thiols, which are sensitive towards oxidation. Intracellular proteins encounter large concentrations of the endogenous antioxidant glutathione (GSH). Therefore, *S*-glutathiolation is a common endogenous process, and proteomic methods for the detection of *S*-glutathiolated proteins have been developed, using either biotinylated GSH ester for the selective immuno-affinity purification of glutathiolated proteins (Sullivan *et al.*, 2000), or [^{35}S]-labeled GSH for the specific detection of [^{35}S] incorporation into proteins resolved on 2D gels (Fratelli *et al.*, 2002). Obviously, these methods are applicable only to cell cultures or tissue homogenates but cannot be performed *in vivo*. *S*-glutathiolation *in vivo* would need to be characterized by direct tandem MS analysis of *S*-glutathiolated peptide sequences isolated from tissue. A subset of proteins, which are susceptible to *S*-glutathiolation by *S*-nitrosoglutathione, was identified utilizing *S*-nitrosoglutathione-sepharose (Klatt *et al.*, 2000).

Analysis of protein glycation

The accumulation of advanced glycation endproducts (AGEs) is a hallmark of age-dependent protein modification. AGEs represent a class of chemical structures generated via breakdown or cross-linking of initial sugar-protein adducts. Poggioli *et al.* (2002) could demonstrate that age-dependent glycation does not occur randomly but appears to selectively target a few proteins, though no mass spectrometric studies to characterize these proteins were presented. In contrast, Crabb *et al.* (2002) performed both HPLC-tandem MS and Western blot experiments to identify proteins, including AGE-modified proteins, present in debris-like material, referred to as "drusen," accumulating below the retinal pigment epithelium on Bruch's membrane during age-related macular degeneration (AMD).

Conclusion

To date, proteomics studies have just begun to unravel small details of the "aging proteome." Continuous improvements of proteomics methodology are necessary, specifically with regard to sample preparation and presentation, in order to cover as large parts of the entire proteome as possible and to extract biologically meaningful information. Experimental studies need to be accompanied by bioinformatics studies, which provide information about protein interaction networks. These studies are in progress and will yield important information on the "aging proteome" in, hopefully, not too distant time.

REFERENCES

Aebersold, R., and Goodlett, D.R. (2001). Mass spectrometry in proteomics. *Chem. Rev. 101*, 269–295.

Aguilaniu, H., Gustafsson, L., Rigoulet, M., and Nyström, T. (2001). Protein oxidation in G_0 cells of *Saccharomyces cervisiae* depends on the state rather than rate of respiration and is enhanced in *pos9* but not *yap1* mutants. *J. Biol. Chem. 276*, 35396–35404.

Aguilaniu, H., Gustafsson, L., Rigoulet, M., and Nyström, T. (2003). Asymmetric inheritance of oxidatively damaged proteins during cytokinesis. *Science 299*, 1751–1753.

Aulak, K.S., Koeck, T., Crabb, J.W., and Stuehr, D.J. (2004). Dynamics of protein nitration in cells and mitochondria. *Am. J. Physiol. Heart Circ. Physiol. 286*, H30–H38.

Aulak, K.S., Miyagi, M., Yan, L., West, K.A., Massillon, D., Crabb, J.W., and Stuehr, D.J. (2001). Proteomic method identifies proteins nitrated *in vivo* during inflammatory challenge. *Proc. Natl. Acad. Sci. USA 98*, 12056–12061.

Ballesteros, M., Fredrikson, A., Henriksson, J., and Nyström, T. (2001). Bacterial senescence: Protein oxidation in non-proliferating cells is dictated by the accuracy of the ribosomes. *EMBO J. 20*, 5280–5289.

Benvenuti, S., Cramer, R., Bruce, J., Waterfield, M.D., and Jat, P.S. (2002a). Identification of novel candidates for replicative senescence by functional proteomics. *Oncogene 21*, 4403–4413.

Benvenuti, S., Cramer, R., Quinn, C.C., Bruce, J., Zvelebil, M., Corless, S., *et al.* (2002b). Differential proteome analysis of replicative senescence in rat embryo fibroblasts. *Mol. Cell. Proteomics 1*, 280–292.

Berlett, B., and Stadtman, E.R. (1997). Protein oxidation in aging, disease, and oxidative stress. *J. Biol. Chem. 272*, 20313–20316.

Boyd-Kimball, D., Sultana, R., Poon, H.F., Lynn, B.C., Casamenti, F., Pepeu, G., *et al.* (2005). Proteomic identification of proteins specifically oxidized by intracerebral injection of amyloid *β*-peptide (1-42) into rat brain: implications for Alzheimer's disease. *Neuroscience 132*, 313–324.

Casoni, F., Basso, M., Massignan, T., Gianazza, E., Cheroni, C., Salmona, M., *et al.* (2005). Protein nitration in a mouse model of familial amyotrophic lateral sclerosis. *J. Biol. Chem. 280*, 16295–16304.

Castegna, A., Aksenov, M., Aksenova, M., Thongboonkerd, V., Klein, J.B., Pierce, W.M., *et al.* (2002a). Proteomic identification of oxidatively modified proteins in Alzheimer's disease brain. Part 1. Creatine kinase BB, glutatmine synthetase, and ubiquitin carboxy-terminal hydrolase L-1. *Free Radi. Biol. Med. 33*, 562–571.

Castegna, A., Aksenov, M., Thongboonkerd, V., Klein, J.B., Pierce, W.M., Booze, R., *et al.* (2002b). Proteomic identification of oxidatively modified proteins in Alzheimer's disease brain. Part 2. Dihydropyrimidinase-related protein 2, alpha-enolase and heat shock cognate 71. *J. Neurochem. 82*, 1524–1532.

Chang, J., van Remmen, H., Cornell, J., Richardson, A., and Ward, W.F. (2003). Comparative proteomics: Characterization of a two-dimensional gel electrophoresis system to study the effect of aging on mitochondrial proteins. *Mech. Ageing Dev. 124*, 33–41.

Chen, S.L., Huddleston, M.J., Shou, W., Deshaies, R.J., Annan, R.S., and Carr, S.A. (2002). Mass spectrometry-based methods for phosphorylation site mapping of hyperphosphorylated proteins applied to Net1, a regulator of exit from mitosis in yeast. *Mol. Cell. Proteomics 1*, 186–196.

Cho, Y.-M., Bae, S.-H., Choi, B.-K., Cho, S.Y., Song, C.-W., Yoo, J.-K., and Paik, Y.-K. (2003). Differential expression of the liver proteome in senescence-accelerated mice. *Proteomics 3*, 1883–1894.

Conrads, T.P., Issaq, H.J., and Veenstra, T.D. (2002). New tools for quantitative phosphoproteome analysis. *Biochem.Biophys. Res. Commun. 290*, 885–890.

Crabb, J.W., Miyagi, M., Gu, X., Shadrach, K., West, K.A., Sakaguchi, H., *et al.* (2002). Drusen proteome analysis: An approach to the etiology of age-related macular degeneration. *Proc. Natl. Acad. Sci. USA 99*, 14682–14687.

Das, N., Levine, R.L., Orr, W.C., and Sohal, R.S. (2001). Selectivity of protein oxidative damage during aging in *Drosophila melanogaster*. *Biochem. J. 360*, 209–216.

De Magalhães, J.P., and Toussaint, O. (2004). GenAge: A genomic and proteomic network map of human ageing. *FEBS Lett. 571*, 243–247.

Dierick, J.-F., Dieu, M., Remacle, J., Raes, M., Roepstorff, P., and Toussaint, O. (2002a). Proteomics in experimental gerontology. *Exp. Gerontol. 37*, 721–734.

Dierick, J.-F., Eliaers, F., Remacle, J., Raes, M., Fey, S.J., Larsen, P.M., and Toussaint, O. (2002b). Stress-induced premature senescence and replicative sensescence are different phenotypes. Proteomic evidence. *Biochem. Pharmacol. 64*, 1011–1017.

Dierick, J.-F., Kalume, D.E., Wenders, F., Salmon, M., Dieu, M., Raes, M., Roepstorff, P., and Toussaint, O. (2002c). Identification of 30 protein species involved in replicative senescence and stress-induced premature senescence. *FEBS Lett. 531*, 499–504.

Dukan, S., Farewell, A., Ballesteros, M., Taddei, F., Radman, M., and Nyström, T. (2000). Protein oxidation in response to increased transcriptional or translational errors. *Proc. Natl. Acad. Sci. USA 97*, 5746–5749.

Dukan, S., and Nyström, T. (1999). Oxidative stress defense and deterioration of growth-arrested *Escherichia coli* cells. *J. Biol. Chem. 274*, 26027–26032.

Eshhar, Z., Ofarim, M., and Waks, T. (1980). Generation of hybridomas secreting murine reaginic antibodies of anti-DNP specificity. *J. Immunol. 124*, 775–780.

Ficarro, S.B., McCleland, M.L., Stukenberg, P.T., Burke, D.J., Ross, M.M., Shabanowitz, J., *et al.* (2002). Phosphoproteome analysis by mass spectrometry and its application to *Saccharomyces cervisiae. Nat. Biotechnol. 20*, 301–305.

Finch, C.E., and Tanzi, R.E. (1997). Genetics of aging. *Science 278*, 407–411.

Fratelli, M., Demol, H., Puype, M., Casagrande, S., Eberini, I., Salmona, M., *et al.* (2002). Identification by redox proteomics of glutathionylated proteins in oxidatively stressed human T lymphocytes. *Proc. Natl. Acad. Sci. USA 99*, 3505–3510.

Gromov, P.S., Ostergaard, M., Gromova, I., and Celis, J.E. (2002). Human proteomic databases: A powerful reource for functional genomics in health and disease. *Prog Biophys. Mol. Biol. 80*, 3–22.

Grønborg, M., Kristiansen, T.K., Stensballe, A., Andersen, J.S., Ohara, O., Mann, M., Jensen, O.N., and Pandey, A. (2002). A mass spectrometry-based proteomic approach for identification of serine/threonine-phosphorylated proteins by enrichment with phospho-specific antibodies. *Mol. Cell. Proteomics 1*, 517–527.

Gygi, S.P., Corthals, G.L., Zhang, Y., Rochon, Y., and Aebersold, R. (2000). Evaluation of two-dimensional gel electrophoresis-based proteome analysis technology. *Proc. Natl. Acad. Sci. USA 97*, 9390–9395.

Gygi, S.P., Rist, B., Griffin, T.J., Eng, J., and Aebersold, R. (2002). Proteome analysis of low-abundance proteins using multidimensional chromatography and isotope-coded affinity tags. *J. Proteome Res. 1*, 47–54.

Irie, Y., Saeki, M., Kamisaki, Y., Martin, E., and Murad, F. (2003). Histone H1.2 is a substrate for denitrase, an activity that reduces nitrotyrosine immunoreactivity. *Proc. Natl. Acad. Sci. USA 100*, 5634–5639.

Ischiropoulos, H., and Beckman, J.S. (2003). Oxidative stress and nitration in neurodegeneration: Cause, effect, or association? *J. Clin. Invest. 111*, 163–169.

Jazwinski, S.M. (1996). Longevity, genes, and aging. *Science 273*, 54–59.

Johannson, E., Olsson, O., and Nyström, T. (2004). Progression and specificity of protein oxidation in the life cycle of *Arabidopsis thaliana. J. Biol. Chem. 279*, 22204–22208.

Kanski, J., Alterman, M., and Schöneich, Ch. (2003). Proteomic identification of age-dependent protein nitration in rat skeletal muscle. *Free Radic. Biol. Med. 35*, 1229–1239.

Kanski, J., Behring, A., Pelling, J., and Schöneich, Ch. (2005a). Proteomic identification of cardiac proteins in Fisher 344/BNF1 rats which undergo tyrosine nitration as a consequence of biological aging. *Am. J. Physiol. Heart Circ. Physiol. 288*, 371–381.

Kanski, J., Hong, S.J., and Schöneich, Ch. (2005b). Proteomic analysis of protein nitration in aging skeletal muscle and identification of nitrotyrosine-containing sequences in vivo by nanoelectrospray ionization tandem mass spectrometry. *J. Biol. Chem., 280*, 24261–24266.

Khidekel, N., and Hsieh-Wilson, L.C. (2004). A "molecular switchboard"-covalent modification to proteins and impact on transcription. *Org. Biomol. Chem. 2*, 1–7.

Klatt, P., Pineda Molina, E., Perez-Sala, D., and Lamas, S. (2000). Novel application of S-nitrosoglutathione-Sepharose to identify proteins that are potential targets for S-nitrosoglutathione-induced mixed-disulphide formation. *Biochem. J. 349*, 567–578.

Knight, Z.A., Schilling, B., Row, R.H., Kenski, D.M., Gibson, B.W., and Shokat, K.M. (2003). Phosphospecific proteolysis for mapping sites of protein phosphorylation. *Nat. Biotechnol. 21*, 1047–1054.

Koeck, T., Fu, X., Hazen, S.L., Crabb, J.W., Stuehr, D.J., and Aulak, K.S. (2004). Rapid and selective oxygen-regulated protein tyrosine denitration and nitration in mitochondria. *J. Biol. Chem. 279*, 27257–27262.

Lamberts, S.W.J., Van den Beld, A.W., and Van der Lely, A.-J. (1997). The endocrinology of aging. *Science 278*, 419–424.

Lin, T.-K, Hughes, G., Muratovska, A., Blaikie, F.H., Brookes, P.S., Darley-Usmar, V., Smith, R.A.J., and Murphy, M.P. (2002). Specific modification of mitochondrial protein thiols in response to oxidative stress. *J. Biol. Chem. 277*, 17048–17056.

Mann, M., Ong, S.E., Grønborg, M., Steen, H., Jensen, O.N., and Pandey, A. (2002). Analysis of protein phosphorylation using mass spectrometry: deciphering the phosphoproteome. *Trends Biotechnol. 20*, 261–268.

Masoro, E.J. (1993) Concepts and hypothesis of basic aging processes. In Yu, B.P. (Ed.). *Free Radicals in Aging*. Boca Raton: CRC Press, pp. 1–9.

Merchant, M., and Weinberger, S.R. (2000). Recent advancements in surface-enhanced laser desorption/ionization-time of flight-mass spectrometry. *Electrophoresis 21*, 1164–1167.

Mirzaei, H., and Regnier, F.E. (2005). Affinity chromatographic selection of carbonylated proteins followed by identification of oxidation sites using tandem mass spectrometry. *Anal. Chem. 77*, 2386–2392.

Miyagi, M., Sakaguchi, H., Darrow, R.M., Yan, L., West, K.A., Aulak, K.S., *et al.* (2002). Evidence that light modulates protein nitration in rat retina. *Mol. Cell. Proteomics 1*, 293–303.

Morrison, J.H., and Hof, P.R. (1997). Life and death of neurons in the aging brain. *Science 278*, 412–419.

Oda, Y., Nagasu, T., and Chait, B.T. (2001). Enrichment analysis of phosphorylated proteins as a tool for probing the phosphoproteome. *Nat. Biotechnol. 19*, 379–382.

Pandey, A., and Mann, M. 2000. Proteomics to study genes and genomes. *Nature 405*, 837–846.

Poggioli, S., Bakala, H., and Friguet, B. (2002). Age-related increase of protein glycation in peripheral blood lymphocytes is restricted to preferential target proteins. *Exp. Gerontol. 37*, 1207–1215.

Poon, H.F., Castegna, A., Farr, S.A., Thongboonkerd, V., Lynn, B.C., Banks, W.A., *et al.* (2004). Quantitative proteomics analysis of specific protein expression and oxidative modification in aged senescence-accelerated-prone 8 mice brain. *Neuroscience 126*, 915–926.

Rabilloud, T., Heller, M., Gasnier, F., Luche, S., Rey, C., Aebersold, R., *et al.* (2002). Proteomic analysis of cellular response to oxidative stress. *J. Biol. Chem. 277*, 19396–19401.

Riggs, L., Seeley, E.H., and Regnier, F.E. (2005). Quantification of phosphoproteins with global internal standard technology. *J. Chromatogr. B 817*, 89–96.

Riggs, L., Sioma, C., and Regnier, F.E. (2001). Automated signature peptide approach for proteomics. *J. Chromatogr. A 924*, 359–368.

Righetti, P.H., Castagna, A., Antonioli, P., and Boschetti, E. (2005). Prefractionation techniques in proteome analysis: The mining tools of the third millennium. *Electrophoresis 26*, 297–319.

Robinson, L.J., Karlsson, N.G., Weiss, A.S., and Packer, N.H. (2003). Proteomic analysis of the genetic premature aging disease Hutchinson Gilford Progeria Syndrome reveals differential protein expression and glycosylation. *J. Proteome Res. 2*, 556–557.

Schlosser, A., Pipkorn, R., Bossemeyer, D., and Lehmann, W.D. (2001). Analysis of protein phosphorylation by a combination of elastase digestion and neutral loss tandem mass spectrometry. *Anal. Chem. 73*, 170–176.

Seeley, E.H., Riggs, L.D., and Regnier, F.E. (2005). Reduction of non-specific binding in Ga(III) immobilized metal affinity chromatography for phosphopeptides by using endoproteinase glu-C as the digestive enzyme. *J. Chromatogr. B 817*, 81–88.

Shacter, E., Williams, J.A., Lim, M., and Levine, R.L. (1994). Differential susceptibility of plasma proteins to oxidative modification: examination by Western blot immunoassay. *Free Radic. Biol. Med. 17*, 429–437.

Shaw, J., Rowlinson, R., Nickson, J., Stone, T., Sweet, A., Williams, K., and Tonge, R. (2003). Evaluation of saturation labeling two-dimsnional difference gel electrophoresis fluorescent dyes. *Proteomics 3*, 1181–1195.

Shen, Y., and Smith, R.D. (2002). Proteomics based on high-efficiency capillary separations. *Electrophoresis 23*, 3106–3124.

Smith, J.R., and Pereira-Smith, O.M. (1996). Replicative senescence: Implications for in vivo aging and tumor suppression. *Science 273*, 63–67.

Smith, M.G., Jone, G., Ptacek, J., Devgan, G., Zhu, H., Zhu, X., and Snyder, M. (2005). Global analysis of protein function using protein microarrays. *Mech. Ageing Dev. 126*, 171–175.

Smolka, M., Zhou, H., and Aebersold, R. (2002). Quantitative protein profiling using two-dimensional gel electrophoresis, isotope-coded affinity tag labeling, and mass spectrometry. *Mol. Cell. Proteomics 1*, 19–29.

Sohal, R.S., and Weindruch, R. (1996). Oxidative stress, caloric restriction, and aging. *Science 273*, 59–63.

Soreghan, B.A., Yang, F., Thomas, S.N., Hsu, J., and Yang, A.J. (2003). High-throughput proteomic-based identification of oxidatively induced protein carbonylation in mouse brain. *Pharm. Res. 20*, 1713–1720.

Steen, H., Kuster, B., Fernandez, M., Pandey, A., and Mann, M. (2002). Tyrosine phosphorylation mapping of the epidermal growth factor receptor signaling pathway. *J. Biol. Chem. 277*, 1031–1039.

Steen, H., Mann, M. (2002a). A new derivatization strategy for the analysis of phosphopeptides by precursor ion scanning in positive ion mode. *J. Am. Chem. Mass Spectrom. 13*, 996–1003.

Steen, H., and Mann, M. (2002b). Analysis of bromotryptophan and hydroxyproline modifications by high-resolution, high-accuracy precursor ion scanning utilizing fragment ions with mass-deficient mass tags. *Anal. Chem. 74*, 6230–6236.

Sullivan, D.M., Wehr, N.B., Fergusson, M.M., Levine, R.L., and Finkel, T. (2000). Identification of oxidant-sensitive proteins: TNF-α induces protein glutathiolation. *Biochemistry 39*, 11121–11128.

Turku, I.V., Li, L., Aulak, K.S., Stuehr, D.J., Chang, J.-Y., and Murad, F. (2003). Protein tyrosine nitration in the mitochondria from diabetic mouse heart. *J. Biol. Chem. 278*, 33972–33977.

Ueda, Y., Duncan, M.K., and David, L.L. (2002). Lens proteomics: the accumulation of crystalline modifications in the mouse lens with age. *Invest. Ophtalmol. Vis. Sci. 43*, 205 215.

Uhlen, M., and Ponten, F. (2005). Antibody-based proteomics for human tissue profiling. *Mol. Cell. Proteomics* 4, 384–393.

Washburn, M.P., Wolters, D., and Yates III, J.R. (2001). Large-scale analysis of the yeast proteome by multidimensional protein identification technology. *Nat. Biotech. 19*, 242–247.

Wolters, D.A., Washburn, M.P., and Yates III, J.R. (2001). An automated multidimensional protein identification technology for shotgun proteomics. *Anal. Chem. 73*: 5683–5690.

Xu, A., and Narayanan, N. (1998). Effects of aging on sarcoplasmic reticulum Ca^{2+}-cycling proteins and their phosphorylation in rat myocardium. *Am. J. Physiol. 275*, H2087–H2094.

Yan, L., Ge, H., Li, H., Lieber, S.C., Natividad, F., Resuello, R.R.G., Kim, S.-J., Akeju, S., Sun, A., Loo, K., Peppas, A.P., Rossi, F., Lewandowski, E.D., Thomas, A.P., Vatner, S.F., and Vatner, D.E. (2004). Gender-specific proteomic alterations in glycolytic and mitochondrial pathways in aging monkey hearts. *J. Mol. Cell. Cardiol. 37*, 921–929.

Yoo, B.-S., and regnier, F. (2004). proteomic analysis of carbonylated proteins in two-dimensional gel electrophoresis using avidin-fluorescein affinity staining. *Electrophoresis 25*, 1334–1341.

Zarling, A.L, Ficarro, S.B., White, F.M., Shabanowitz, J., Hunt, D.F., and Engelhardt, V.H. (2000). Phosphorylated peptides are naturally processed by major histocompatibility complex I molecules in vivo. *J. Exp. Med. 192*, 1755–1762.

Zhan, X., and Desiderio, D.M. (2004) The human pituitary nitroproetome: detection of nitrotyrosyl-proteins with two–dimensional Western blotting, and amino acid sequence determination with mass spectrometry. *Biochem. Biophys. Res. Commun. 325*, 1180–1186.

Zhang, J., Goodlett, D.R., Peskind, E.R., Quinn, J.F., Zhou, Y., Wang, Q., Pan, C., Yi, E., Eng, J., Aebersold, R.H., and Montine, T.J. (2005). Quantitative proteomic analysis of age-related changes in human cerebrospinal fluid. *Neurobiol. Aging 26*, 207–227.

Zhang, R., Sioma, C.S., Wang, S., and Regnier, F.E. (2001). Fractionation of isotopically labeled peptides in quantitative proteomics. *Anal. Chem. 73*, 5142–5149.

Zhou, G., Li, H., DeCamps, D., Chen, S., Shu, H., Gong, Y., Flaig, M., Gillespie, J.W. Hu, N., Taylor, P.R., Emmert-Buck, M.R., Liotta, L.A., Petricoin III, E.F., and Zhao, Y. (2002a). 2D differential in-gel electrohoresis for the identification of esophageal scans cell cancer-specific protein markers. *Mol. Cell. Proteomics 1*, 117–124.

Zhou, H., Ranish, J.A., Watts, J.D., and Aebersold, R. (2002b). Quantitative proteome analysis by solid-phase isotope tagging and mass spectrometry. *Nat. Biotechnol. 19*, 512–515.

Zhou, H., Watts, J.D., and Aebersold, R. (2001). A systematic approach to the analysis of protein phosphorylation. *Nat. Biotechnol. 19*, 375–378.

10

Application of High-Throughput Technologies to Aging-Related Research

Matt Kaeberlein

The development and application of high-throughput methods to study aspects of aging-related biology are among the key forces driving the field. New hypotheses are being developed, and new questions are being asked on a genome-wide scale. High-throughput technologies offer many advantages over traditional methods, but they also present new pitfalls for the unwary. Rather than provide detailed protocols for different methods, this chapter attempts to give an overview of some of the ways that high-throughput methods are currently being applied to aging-related research, along with a discussion of both the successes and the difficulties associated with these new technologies.

Introduction

Many areas of biological research have benefited from the technological advances of the past several years. The human genome is sequenced, along with genomes from dozens of other organisms; genome-wide protein–protein interaction maps have been generated for most of the major model systems; simultaneous gene expression profiling for tens of thousands of genes has become routine; and an almost inconceivable amount of primary data are only a mouse-click away via the Internet.

One of the most important questions facing the field of biogerontology is how to integrate and optimize the use of new technologies for the study of aging and age-associated disease. Application of new technologies to aging-related biology has often lagged relative to other fields, such as cancer biology. In the past, aging-related research has been driven largely by gene-specific or model-driven studies based on prior assumptions or knowledge. More recently, however, that trend seems to be changing as researchers recognize the opportunities associated with genome-scale approaches. In many cases, new technologies are being developed with the specific goal of tackling a particular aspect of aging-related research.

Along with the advantages of high-throughput methodologies, however, there are also risks, such as higher false positive and false negative rates. This is particularly likely to be the case when a high-throughput method departs substantially from the standard method, and, in extreme cases, can result in artifacts that threaten the validity of entire lines of research (see the section on targeted screens for small molecules that slow aging). It is also often the case that statistical methods for dealing with new types of data generated from high-throughput methods are underdeveloped. This issue, which has plagued microarray studies for several years, is now better appreciated. Potential problems with large-scale methods can generally be avoided by independent replication of key data points using a more standard methodology, such as real-time quantitative polymerase chain reaction (PCR), to verify gene expression changes from microarray studies (see Applications of Microarrays to Aging-Related Research).

Gene Expression Microarrays in Aging-Related Research

Microarrays have provided researchers with the ability to monitor gene expression changes across tens of thousands of genes in a single experiment. The potential applications of this technology are profound, and there are many cases where global gene expression profiling has been particularly useful, for example, in identifying cell cycle and stress-dependent transcriptional networks and characterizing gene expression signatures associated with different types of human cancers. The application of microarrays to aging-related research was initially received with great enthusiasm. That enthusiasm has been tempered somewhat, as a realization of the technical difficulties and limitations, some of which are specific to aging-related features, has emerged.

When considering the application of microarray technology to an aging-related question, there are several important issues that determine appropriate experimental design, and there are numerous examples in the literature of poorly designed microarray experiments and over-interpretation of microarray data. Recent reviews discuss many of the most important considerations associated with microarrays and provide advice for appropriate ways to deal with them (Hudson *et al.*, 2005; Melov and Hubbard, 2004; Nair *et al.*, 2003). It is highly recommended that anyone considering the use of microarrays in their research program consult these resources and develop a detailed experimental plan prior to initiating experiments.

GENERAL CONSIDERATIONS WHEN USING MICROARRAYS

Choosing microarray technology

Microarrays afford the possibility of measuring gene expression levels for thousands of genes simultaneously. This is accomplished by obtaining RNA from a cell, tissue, or organism, and quantifying the amount of mRNA present for each gene being assayed. One of the most basic considerations when designing a microarray experiment is the type of microarray technology to use. There are two common types of gene expression microarrays: (1) "cDNA arrays," usually PCR amplified open reading frames (ORFs) spotted onto glass slides, and (2) oligonucleotide arrays. It is generally accepted that for most applications, oligonucleotide arrays, while more expensive than cDNA arrays, also tend to provide higher specificity (Hudson *et al.*, 2005). Several commercially available oligonucleotide array platforms exist, including Affymetrix GeneChip microarrays, Agilent Oligo microarrays, and Amersham Biosciences (GE Healthcare) CodeLink Bioarrays (Hudson *et al.*, 2005).

The most commonly utilized microarray platforms employ either a two-color or one-color design. Two-color experiments involve co-hybridization of cDNAs derived from two different RNA samples on the same slide. Each set of cDNAs is labeled with a different fluorescent dye (e.g., Cy3 and Cy5). For each gene being assayed the relative expression level in sample #1 versus sample #2 is obtained by the ratio of Cy3 fluorescence to Cy5 fluorescence. One-color platforms, such as Affymetrix ("Affy" chips), are simpler, in that only one labeled cDNA is hybridized per chip. For each experimental sample, a fluorescence value is associated with each gene present on the microarray. This value can then be compared against the fluorescence value for that gene obtained with a common reference sample, to generate a ratio value analogous to that of a 2-color design.

Replication, variation, and validation

A primary criticism against many aging-related microarray studies is a lack of sufficient replication (Melov and Hubbard, 2004). While the number of replicates required for interpretation of microarray data will vary based on many different factors, including the type of experimental design and the organism under study, there are standard approaches that can help determine the degree of replication needed to obtain statistically meaningful gene expression changes (Hudson *et al.*, 2005). Of particular import when considering replication is the difference between biological and technical replicates. Technical replicates are replicates derived from the same biological sample (e.g., the same pool of RNA), and can refer either to the same probe spotted at different places on a microarray slide or to parallel hybridization of the same sample to multiple slides. In either case, technical replication can provide information only about the error in the measurement and gives no indication of the variation within the population from which the samples originated. Biological replication refers to analysis of samples obtained from different individuals or pools of individuals. When considering the number of *independent* replicates necessary for statistical analysis, only biological replicates should be counted.

A higher number of replicates may be necessary for aging-related microarray studies relative to microarray studies that examine other aspects of biology. Unlike gene expression changes associated with cancer, for example, which can be several-fold in magnitude for the most up- or down-regulated transcripts, age-associated changes tend to be relatively small in magnitude and can easily be masked by variation between individuals (Hudson *et al.*, 2005). In addition, there is evidence that gene-specific variation increases with age, perhaps due to dysregulation of transcription in older individuals. Thus, the most relevant transcriptional changes in an age-related study may be smaller in magnitude and require a greater number of replicates to be statistically detectable.

The first look a researcher usually gets at the data from a microarray experiment is in the form of an image file, where each "spot" corresponds to the fluorescence intensity associated with the expression of a particular gene. The process of getting from the raw data to a list of genes that are up- or down-regulated involves several steps, each of which can have a substantial impact on the quality of the data set. The image must first be processed, which involves manual inspection of the image files for anomalies, followed by spot quantification, quality control, and normalization. Many software packages are available to assist with visual inspection and spot quantification, and the appropriate choice will depend of several factors, including platform and cost (Hudson *et al.*, 2005).

In the early days of microarray use, researchers would often carry out experiments with two or three replicates (sometimes only one), apply minimal normalization procedures, calculate the average fold-change in mRNA levels for each gene, select an arbitrary fold-change cutoff (usually 2-fold), and report a list of genes that are "significantly" up- or down-regulated (Melov and Hubbard, 2004). Fortunately, those days are (mostly) gone. Although there are no universally accepted standards for processing, analyzing, and presenting microarray data, it is now expected that rigorous statistical methods be applied to any microarray data prior to publication. Several detailed reviews are available on statistical methods for analyzing microarray data

(Churchill, 2002; Kerr and Churchill, 2001; Kerr *et al.*, 2000; Lee and Whitmore, 2002). In most cases a statistician should be consulted both during the design phase of the microarray experiment and during the data analysis phase.

A well-designed microarray experiment will result in a set of genes that, following appropriate statistical analysis, show statistically significant changes in mRNA level as a function of the experimental condition under study. Unfortunately, many studies go no further, in terms of validation, than to list the set of genes that meet this description. In any microarray experiment, independent validation of the observed changes in mRNA levels, or at least a subset of the most important observed mRNA changes, is essential. At a minimum, real-time quantitative PCR (RT-PCR) or some other method should be used to demonstrate the expected change in mRNA level. If biological relevance of a particular gene expression change is to be inferred, then a change in protein level, or even better protein activity, should be shown. Since translational or post-translational regulation can offset changes in mRNA level, there is no guarantee that the activity of the encoded protein has been altered even if mRNA levels are dramatically changed.

APPLICATIONS OF MICROARRAYS TO AGING-RELATED RESEARCH

Comparing young versus old

The most common application of microarrays to aging-related research is an experimental design that compares gene expression in young organisms to gene expression in old organisms. Studies of this type have been carried out in all of the major model systems, as well as in humans (Hudson *et al.*, 2005). Most often, the goal of this type of study is to identify genes for which transcription either increases or decreases as a function of age, in other words, biomarkers of age. It is important to recognize that the gene expression changes observed from this type of design don't confer any information about genes that determine longevity or rate of aging. Also, as is true of any microarray experimental design, the observed gene expression changes can be stated to correlate with the condition being studied (biological age, in this case), but no information is obtained regarding whether the gene products themselves play a causal role.

An important question when designing an experiment of this type is how to define the "young" and "old" populations. There is no single "correct" answer to this question; however, there are several considerations that should be taken into account. Without exception, two age-point designs (one young and one aged) are less favorable than multiple age-point designs where gene expression profiles are obtained at several different ages. As a rule of thumb, experiments of this type should examine the maximum number of different age-points possible while still maintaining sufficient replication at each age-point for meaningful statistical analysis.

The importance of appropriate timing and spacing of age-points in the interpretation of gene expression studies should not be underestimated. Data regarding the kinetics of age-associated gene expression changes can provide valuable information for developing hypotheses regarding the functional consequences of the observed changes. In addition, both the structure and interpretation of the data may differ substantially depending on the number and spacing of age-points and the type of gene expression changes that occur (Figure 10.1).

In most cases, it will be desirable that animals are reproductively and developmentally mature at the youngest age-point. In order to define the oldest age-point, statistical parameters of the population life span can be used as a guideline. For example, an old age-point could be defined as 50% or 75% of the median longevity. It must be kept in mind, however, that the older an animal is at the latest age-point, the more likely that age-associated degenerative changes will obscure the relevant age-associated gene expression changes.

A majority of the published microarray studies examining age-correlated gene expression suffer from an inadequate number of age-points (Melov and Hubbard, 2004), a fact that must be considered when analyzing and interpreting these data. Nonetheless, some interesting trends have been observed in multiple studies across a variety of species. For example, up-regulation of genes involved in the response to oxidative stress and other types of stress seems to be a common theme in aged invertebrates (Landis *et al.*, 2004; Pletcher *et al.*, 2002; Zou *et al.*, 2000) and mammals (Kayo *et al.*, 2001; Weindruch *et al.*, 2001). This is consistent with the idea that oxidative damage increases during aging, and is interesting in light of the observations that some long-lived mutants show increased expression of oxidative stress response genes as well as increased oxidative stress resistance as young animals (McElwee *et al.*, 2003; Murphy *et al.*, 2003).

Comparing short- and long-lived

There are currently no commonly accepted biomarkers of aging rate (biomarkers of longevity) (Butler *et al.*, 2004), and this lack is one of the key problems in aging-related research. Microarrays provide the opportunity to assay many thousands of potential gene expression biomarkers in order to detect a subset of genes whose expression predicts individual longevity. In order to identify gene expression biomarkers of aging rate, the gene expression profile of more slowly aging individuals must be compared to the gene expression profile of more quickly aging individuals. The most reliable method for accomplishing this is to carry out microarray analysis on long-lived individuals relative to individuals with a normal life span. In theory, short-lived "premature aging" mutants can also be used;

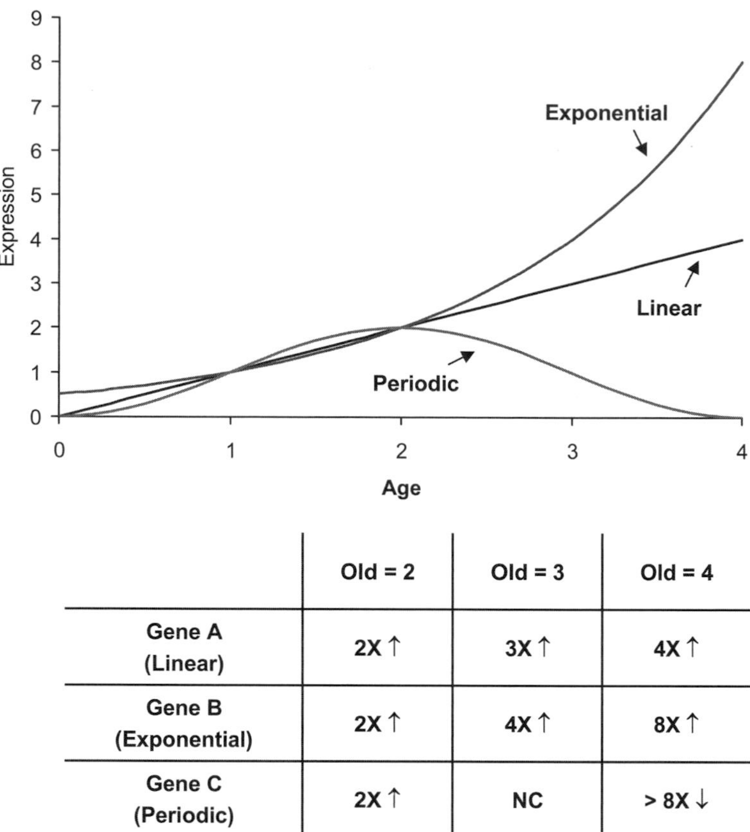

	Old = 2	Old = 3	Old = 4
Gene A (Linear)	2X ↑	3X ↑	4X ↑
Gene B (Exponential)	2X ↑	4X ↑	8X ↑
Gene C (Periodic)	2X ↑	NC	> 8X ↓

Figure 10.1 Importance of age-points in microarray analyses of aging. Age-related gene expression is shown for three hypothetical genes: expression of Gene A increases linearly with age; expression of Gene B increases exponentially with age; Gene C shows a periodic expression pattern, where expression increases at young age, then decreases during old age. For a two age-point design (one "young" and one "old") specifying age-point 1 as the young age-point, different conclusions are reached depending on which age-point is used as the old age-point. If age-point 2 is used, all three genes show the same 2-fold increase in expression. If age-point 3 is used, genes A and B both appear to be up-regulated, while gene C shows no age-associated change (NC) in expression. If age-point 4 is used, gene A appears to be up-regulated by 4-fold, gene B is dramatically up-regulated by 8-fold, and gene C is down-regulated by more than 8-fold with age. The only design that provides an accurate picture of the (relatively simple) age-associated gene expression kinetics for these genes employs at least 3 age-points.

however, there are no short-lived mutants that recapitulate all aspects of normal aging, and it is extremely difficult to differentiate premature aging from nonspecific deleterious effects.

Several studies have reported gene expression profiles corresponding to long-lived mammalian models, as a result of environmental changes such as calorie restriction (CR) (Park and Prolla, 2005b), as well as longevity-enhancing mutations, such as the Ames dwarf, the growth hormone receptor knock-out (GHR-KO) (Dozmorov *et al.*, 2001; Miller *et al.*, 2002; Tsuchiya *et al.*, 2004), and the fat-specific insulin receptor knock-out (FIRKO) (Bluher *et al.*, 2004). In *C. elegans*, the transcriptional changes associated with longevity-determining mutations in the insulin-like/IFG-1 pathway have been well characterized by microarray, resulting in the identification of several previously unknown aging genes (McElwee *et al.*, 2003; Murphy *et al.*, 2003).

One popular design for microarray studies of aging combines both a longevity component and an age component. This approach allows for the identification of several classes of gene expression biomarkers that would otherwise be obscured (Hudson *et al.*, 2005). A classic study of this type (Lee *et al.*, 1999) compared the gene expression profile in gastrocnemius muscle from young and old mice, either fed ad libetum or calorie restricted, and reported that many of the age-correlated gene expression changes are attenuated by CR. While the limitations of this study (small number of replicates and no statistical analysis) have been amply documented (Melov and Hubbard, 2004; Miller *et al.*, 2001), this represents the basic design strategy for all microarray studies of this type. Subsequent studies have validated the idea that CR retards age-associated gene expression changes in a variety of tissues (Park and Prolla, 2005a) and have begun to address the question of determining which CR-induced changes in mRNA might be relevant for increased life span (see Biomarkers of calorie restriction).

Biomarkers of calorie restriction

An important class of longevity biomarkers consists of biomarkers of CR. The discovery of CR mimetics—drugs that recapitulate the longevity benefits of CR without necessarily requiring a decrease in nutrient consumption—has obvious applications to human health. One approach that might be taken to identify CR mimetics is to use microarrays to define a pattern of gene expression changes that is characteristic of the calorie-restricted state. Animals can then be fed a putative CR mimetic and the corresponding effect on gene expression assayed. The higher the similarity between gene expression associated with CR and the observed gene expression profile, the greater the likelihood the compound will have a beneficial effect on longevity, at least in theory. Although yet to be proven, this approach is appealing because it does not require the time and expense of life-span assays—a limiting factor in mammalian aging studies—for each compound.

Gene expression biomarkers of CR have begun to be used to address important questions regarding the mechanism and temporal kinetics of CR. Dhahbi and colleagues used microarrays to compare the changes in hepatic gene expression of young and old mice in response to CR after 2, 4, and 8 weeks (Dhahbi *et al.*, 2004). The striking result of this study is that old mice switched to CR late in life showed a rapid shift toward the gene expression profile of animals subjected to long-term CR, while old mice switched from a long-term CR diet to a control diet showed a corresponding shift in gene expression profile toward animals maintained on a control diet for their entire life. These data are consistent with evidence from both mice (Dhahbi *et al.*, 2004) and flies (Mair *et al.*, 2003) that CR initiated late in life reduces mortality to a comparable extent as life-long CR, and suggests that at least some of the observed gene expression changes correlate well with the ability of CR to slow aging.

Gene expression meta-analyses

As the number of aging-related microarray studies increases, the opportunity presents itself to carry out bioinformatic comparisons between multiple organisms or multiple models of enhanced longevity. In the first such meta-analysis of aging, gene expression changes correlated with age were compared between worms and flies (McCarroll *et al.*, 2004). A phylogenetic analysis was used to first identify orthologous gene pairs for which the pattern of expression change with age has been reported from prior work. From this analysis, the authors define a "shared transcriptional profile of aging" involving genes involved in a variety of processes, including mitochondrial metabolism, DNA repair, catabolism, peptidolysis and cellular transport. As with many of the microarray studies already described, valid criticisms of the statistical methods employed in this meta-analysis have been raised (Melov and Hubbard, 2004), and it remains to be seen how much of the shared profile of aging is conserved in mammals. Nonetheless, this represents an important step forward in the application of bioinformatics to aging-related data sets.

At this writing, no large-scale meta-analysis of multiple models of enhanced longevity has been reported. An initial foray in this direction has been carried out by Miller and colleagues who have compared gene expression patterns in two long-lived mouse models, the GHR-KO and Snell dwarf, with CR (Miller *et al.*, 2002). More recently, a comparative analysis of longevity versus microarray and other data for 22 lines of inbred recombinant mice was reported (de Haan and Williams, 2005). As global gene expression profiles are generated for additional longevity models and bioinformatic approaches to analyzing microarray data improve, more opportunities to carry out meaningful comparative analyses of this sort will arise.

APPLICATIONS OF MICROARRAYS TO HUMAN AGING

The application of microarrays to study aging-related processes in humans is, for obvious reasons, more difficult than in model organisms. Availability of samples from healthy donors, genetic and environmental heterogeneity, and variation in sample quality and preparation are just a few of the possible confounding issues. Of particular concern in samples obtained from elderly people is the possibility that medications or other interventions prescribed for a variety of age-associated ailments might alter the normal gene expression profile.

Many studies have reported changes in gene expression as a function of age in humans, and age-correlated gene expression profiles have been described for several tissue types, including retina (Yoshida *et al.*, 2002), muscle (Welle *et al.*, 2004; Welle *et al.*, 2003), kidney (Rodwell *et al.*, 2004), and brain (Lu *et al.*, 2004). Microarrays have also been used to examine gene expression profiles of human cells cultured *in vitro*. This approach has the benefit of being more controlled and less resource limited than assaying expression in tissues directly from donors, but is subject to a host of caveats associated with the process of obtaining and maintaining stable cell lines *in vitro*. In addition, the relevance of *in vitro* replicative senescence to *in vivo* cellular aging has yet to be determined.

In vitro gene expression profiles have been generated for two progeroid syndromes, Werner syndrome (Kyng *et al.*, 2003) and Hutchinson–Guilford progeria syndrome (Csoka *et al.*, 2004). It has been suggested that most of the changes in gene expression associated with normal aging are recapitulated in cell lines derived from Werner syndrome patients (Kyng *et al.*, 2003), although methodological problems make this interpretation questionable (Prolla, 2005). Interestingly, the gene expression changes observed in fibroblasts from Hutchinson–Guilford progeria syndrome patients show almost no similarity to gene expression changes observed in fibroblasts from aged donors, nor do they correspond to age-related changes in tissues from mice (Prolla, 2005).

SAGE PROFILING OF GENE EXPRESSION IN AGING

Microarrays are not the only technology available for high-throughput analysis of gene expression. Serial analysis of gene expression (SAGE) is a technique that involves converting a mixture of cDNA into a linear concatemer of short sequence tags followed by DNA sequencing of the concatemer library (Velculescu *et al.*, 1995). The frequency at which each tag is present in the library represents the abundance of the mRNA transcript from which the tag was derived. SAGE is more technically difficult than microarray analysis and requires a large DNA sequencing capability, but has the advantage that it can detect an entire transcriptome (rather than only genes corresponding to the probes on a microarray chip) as well as changes in the frequency of different splice variants.

SAGE has been used only rarely in aging-related research. In *C. elegans*, gene expression of long-lived dauer animals relative to controls has been examined by SAGE (Jones *et al.*, 2001), and, more recently, a comparison of gene expression in *daf-2* mutants as a function of age has been reported (Halaschek-Wiener *et al.*, 2005). The latter study, in particular, is of interest because a comparison between the SAGE data and analogous microarray data (McElwee *et al.*, 2003; Murphy *et al.*, 2003) has identified a set of six genes, *hsp-12.6*, *vit-2*, *vit-5*, *fat-3*, *nid-1*, and *mtl-1*, that show reproducibly altered expression. SAGE has also been used along with microarray in a comparative analysis of age-correlated changes in muscle gene expression between humans and mice (Welle *et al.*, 2001) and to examine the age-correlated transcriptional changes in the mouse cerebellum (Popesco *et al.*, 2004).

High-Throughput Approaches to Measuring Life Span in Simple Eukaryotes

Simple eukaryotic models, such as yeast, worms, and flies, have had a significant impact on aging-related research, largely due to their short life span and genetic tractability (see Chapters 17–25). Nearly all model-based studies of aging have been driven either by candidate gene approaches, where a particular gene is studied based on its known or assumed function related to aging, or by genetic screens for secondary phenotypes correlated with longevity. These approaches, while often fruitful, are inherently biased. The development of true high-throughput life span assays, where longevity can be measured for thousands of individuals simultaneously, provides the opportunity to identify genetic and environmental regulators of aging in an unbiased, genome-wide manner.

ALTERNATIVES TO STANDARD LIFE-SPAN ASSAYS

Even in simple eukaryotes, such as yeast, worms, and flies, the length of time that it takes to measure life span can be a rate-limiting step in high-throughput longevity phenotyping. New approaches are being developed that decrease the time and effort necessary to predict whether a particular mutation or environmental intervention is likely to alter aging rate. For example, in *C. elegans* a high-throughput method has been developed that combines automated worm-handling technology with a fluorescent dye exclusion phenotype to screen for small molecules that impact oxidative stress resistance and aging (Gill *et al.*, 2003). While the utility of this method has yet to be proven, the approach appears promising.

A new method has been proposed that shortens the length of time required to carry out life-span analysis in flies by 80% (Bauer *et al.*, 2004). By coupling the expression of a lethal toxin to expression of a putative age-dependent biomarker, flies are prematurely killed. In theory, any intervention that alters the rate of aging should similarly alter the rate of toxin expression and, hence, life span of the toxin-expressing animals. The authors do a good job of validating their system by showing that several examples known to increase longevity in wild-type flies also increase life span in the toxin-expressing strain. Whether expression of the biomarker correlates with aging rate in every situation has yet to be determined, and it will be important to validate any putative longevity-altering intervention discovered with this system using a standard life span assay.

In yeast, where replicative life span is measured by the number of daughter cells produced by each mother cell (see Chapter 18: Longevity and Aging in the Budding Yeast), methods have also been developed to screen for increased replicative life span. In one case, a strain has been constructed such that an essential gene is produced in mother cells but fails to be expressed in daughter cells (Jarolim *et al.*, 2004). In theory, only mother cells should be able to divide under these conditions, greatly simplifying and accelerating measurement of replicative life span. Although this system, as described in the initial report, fails to recapitulate the standard life-span assay, this represents a first step toward a workable high-throughput replicative life-span assay.

Another variation on high-throughput screening for long-lived yeast strains has been developed in which the number of chitin bud scars, a surface marker of replicative age, is quantified fluorescently by FACS (Chen *et al.*, 2003). This study reported that expression of human ferritin light chain in yeast increases the number of cells with elevated bud scar counts. The authors failed to

failure to attain extreme longevity (Bellizzi *et al.*, 2005). SIRT3 was chosen as a candidate human aging gene based on reports that increased expression of SIRT3 homologs increases life span in yeast (Kaeberlein *et al.*, 1999), worms (Tissenbaum and Guarente, 2001), and flies (Rogina and Helfand, 2004). The insulin/IGF-1 signaling pathway is another highly conserved longevity-determining pathway that has been screened for longevity-associated polymorphisms in people (van Heemst *et al.*, 2005). As additional conserved aging genes are identified, further studies of this type will shed light on the role of specific genetic variation in human aging.

Other High-Throughput Approaches

New technologies continue to be developed for biomedical research, and application of these methods to aging-related problems will be an important force for advancing our understanding of the aging process. High-throughput proteomic (see Chapter 9 on proteomics) and metabolomic methods, in particular, offer the opportunity to dissect age-associated changes that go beyond mRNA. Protein microarrays, for example, may allow for genome-scale determination of protein levels (rather than mRNA) as a function of age and aging rate. Other high-throughput methods can detect macromolecular damage and modifications, such as glycation, that might play an important role in cellular aging (Schoneich, 2003). A particularly exciting prospect is the development of a noninvasive test for mammalian aging rate (perhaps serum based) that relies on protein or metabolite markers to determine whether a particular intervention alters aging in individual animals or people. The value of such a diagnostic method, both for disease treatment and aging research, would be immense.

Conclusion

The application and development of high-throughput technologies in aging-related research have the potential to dramatically enhance our understanding of human aging. Microarray studies are beginning to identify conserved age-associated transcriptional changes across model systems, and the identification of *bona fide* gene expression biomarkers will be essential for testing putative antiaging therapies in people.

Accelerated assays for measuring life span in simple eukaryotes will provide additional candidates for longevity studies in mammals. Genome-wide attempts to identify genetic polymorphisms associated with human longevity have already uncovered important age-associated disease alleles, and will perhaps result in candidate aging genes in people.

Indeed, there is reason to be optimistic that continued application of these new technologies will enhance our understanding of the molecular biology of aging and, ultimately, our ability to treat age-associated disease.

Recommended Resources

The institute for genomics research (TIGR) microarray resources: http://www.tigr.org/tdb/microarray/. A nice compilation of microarray-related information and links. TIGR also provides free software for processing, analyzing, and presenting array data. http://www.tigr.org/software/#m

Stanford microarray resources: http://genome-www5.stanford.edu/resources/. Another good collection of array resources and software.

Eisen lab software: http://rana.lbl.gov/EisenSoftware.htm. The classic Cluster and Treeview software along with additional software for array analysis and data presentation.

Significance analysis of microarrays (SAM): http://www-stat.stanford.edu/~tibs/SAM/. Statistical software for detecting significant changes in gene expression from microarray data. Can be used as a Microsoft Excel plug-in.

Bioconductor: http://www.bioconductor.org/. Open source software for bioinformatic analyses. More powerful than most of the other free software, but requires R, a software environment for statistical computing and graphics.

BASE BioArray Software Environment: http://base.thep.lu.se/index.phtml. An open-source database system for storage, retrieval, and analysis of microarray data.

GeneX-Lite: http://www.ncgr.org/genex/. Relational database system for managing, analyzing, and visualizing array data.

Gene Expression Omnibus: http://www.ncbi.nlm.nih.gov/geo/. NCBI database for depositing and retrieving microarray data.

ArrayExpress: http://www.ebi.ac.uk/arrayexpress/. European bioinformatics institute database for depositing and retrieving microarray data.

REFERENCES

Bauer, J.H., Goupil, S., Garber, G.B., and Helfand, S.L. (2004). An accelerated assay for the identification of lifespan-extending interventions in *Drosophila melanogaster*. *Proc Natl Acad Sci USA 101*, 12980–12985.

Bellizzi, D., Rose, G., Cavalcante, P., Covello, G., Dato, S., De Rango, F., *et al.* (2005). A novel VNTR enhancer within the SIRT3 gene, a human homologue of SIR2, is associated with survival at oldest ages. *Genomics 85*, 258–263.

Bluher, M., Patti, M.E., Gesta, S., Kahn, B.B., and Kahn, C.R. (2004). Intrinsic heterogeneity in adipose tissue of fat-specific insulin receptor knock-out mice is associated with differences in patterns of gene expression. *J Biol Chem 279*, 31891–31901.

Borra, M.T., Smith, B.C., and Denu, J.M. (2005). Mechanism of human SIRT1 activation by resveratrol. *J Biol Chem 280*, 17187–17195.

Butler, R.N., Sprott, R., Warner, H., Bland, J., Feuers, R., Forster, M., *et al.* (2004). Biomarkers of aging: From primitive organisms to humans. *J Gerontol A Biol Sci Med Sci 59*, B560–567.

Chen, C., Dewaele, S., Braeckman, B., Desmyter, L., Verstraelen, J., Borgonie, G., *et al.* (2003). A high-throughput screening system for genes extending life-span. *Exp Gerontol 38*, 1051–1063.

Churchill, G.A. (2002). Fundamentals of experimental design for cDNA microarrays. *Nat Genet 32 Suppl*, 490–495.

Csoka, A.B., English, S.B., Simkevich, C.P., Ginzinger, D.G., Butte, A.J., Schatten, G.P., *et al.* (2004). Genome-scale expression profiling of Hutchinson–Gilford progeria syndrome reveals widespread transcriptional misregulation leading to mesodermal/mesenchymal defects and accelerated atherosclerosis. *Aging Cell 3*, 235–243.

de Haan, G., and Williams, R.W. (2005). A genetic and genomic approach to identify longevity genes in mice. *Mech Ageing Dev 126*, 133–138.

Dhahbi, J.M., Kim, H.J., Mote, P.L., Beaver, R.J., and Spindler, S.R. (2004). Temporal linkage between the phenotypic and genomic responses to caloric restriction. *Proc Natl Acad Sci USA 101*, 5524–5529.

Dozmorov, I., Bartke, A., and Miller, R.A. (2001). Array-based expression analysis of mouse liver genes: Effect of age and of the longevity mutant Prop1df. *J Gerontol A Biol Sci Med Sci 56*, B72–80.

Fabrizio, P., and Longo, V.D. (2003). The chronological life span of *Saccharomyces cerevisiae*. *Aging Cell 2*, 73–81.

Fabrizio, P., Pozza, F., Pletcher, S.D., Gendron, C.M., and Longo, V.D. (2001). Regulation of longevity and stress resistance by Sch9 in yeast. *Science 292*, 288–290.

Geesaman, B.J., Benson, E., Brewster, S.J., Kunkel, L.M., Blanche, H., Thomas, G., *et al.* (2003). Haplotype-based identification of a microsomal transfer protein marker associated with the human lifespan. *Proc Natl Acad Sci USA 100*, 14115–14120.

Gill, M.S., Olsen, A., Sampayo, J.N., and Lithgow, G.J. (2003). An automated high-throughput assay for survival of the nematode *Caenorhabditis elegans*. *Free Radic Biol Med 35*, 558–565.

Halaschek-Wiener, J., Khattra, J.S., McKay, S., Pouzyrev, A., Stott, J.M., Yang, G.S., *et al.* (2005). Analysis of long-lived *C. elegans* daf-2 mutants using serial analysis of gene expression. *Genome Res. 15*, 603–615.

Howitz, K.T., Bitterman, K.J., Cohen, H.Y., Lamming, D.W., Lavu, S., Wood, J.G., *et al.* (2003). Small molecule activators of sirtuins extend *Saccharomyces cerevisiae* lifespan. *Nature 425*, 191–196.

Hudson, F.N., Kaeberlein, M., Linford, N., Pritchard, D., Beyer, R.P., and Rabinovitch, P.S., eds. (2005). *Microarray Analysis of Gene Expression Changes in Aging*, 6th ed. (Academic Press).

Imai, S., Armstrong, C.M., Kaeberlein, M., and Guarente, L. (2000). Transcriptional silencing and longevity protein Sir2 is an NAD-dependent histone deacetylase. *Nature 403*, 795–800.

Jarolim, S., Millen, J., Heeren, G., Laun, P., Goldfarb, D.S., and Breitenbach, M. (2004). A novel assay for replicative lifespan in *Saccharomyces cerevisiae*. *FEMS Yeast Res 5*, 169–177.

Jones, S.J., Riddle, D.L., Pouzyrev, A.T., Velculescu, V.E., Hillier, L., Eddy, S.R., *et al.* (2001). Changes in gene expression associated with developmental arrest and longevity in *Caenorhabditis elegans*. *Genome Res 11*, 1346–1352.

Kaeberlein, M. (2004). Aging-related research in the "-omics" age. *Sci Aging Knowledge Environ* 2004, pe39.

Kaeberlein, M., McDonagh, T., Heltweg, B., Hixon, J., Westman, E.A., Caldwell, S., *et al.* (2005a). Substrate specific activation of sirtuins by resveratrol. *J Biol Chem. 280*, 17038–17045.

Kaeberlein, M., McVey, M., and Guarente, L. (1999). The SIR2/3/4 complex and SIR2 alone promote longevity in *Saccharomyces cerevisiae* by two different mechanisms. *Genes Dev 13*, 2570–2580.

Kaeberlein, M., Powers, R.W., Steffen, K.K., Westman, E.A., Hu, D., Dang, N., *et al.* (2005b). Regulation of yeast replication life span by TOR and Sch9 in response to nutrients. *Science* in press.

Kammerer, S., Burns-Hamuro, L.L., Ma, Y., Hamon, S.C., Canaves, J.M., Shi, M.M., *et al.* (2003). Amino acid variant in the kinase binding domain of dual-specific A kinase-anchoring protein 2: A disease susceptibility polymorphism. *Proc Natl Acad Sci USA 100*, 4066–4071.

Kapahi, P., Zid, B.M., Harper, T., Koslover, D., Sapin, V., and Benzer, S. (2004). Regulation of lifespan in *Drosophila* by modulation of genes in the TOR signaling pathway. *Curr Biol 14*, 885–890.

Kayo, T., Allison, D.B., Weindruch, R., and Prolla, T.A. (2001). Influences of aging and caloric restriction on the transcriptional profile of skeletal muscle from rhesus monkeys. *Proc Natl Acad Sci USA 98*, 5093–5098.

Kerr, M.K., and Churchill, G.A. (2001). Statistical design and the analysis of gene expression microarray data. *Genet Res 77*, 123–128.

Kerr, M.K., Martin, M., and Churchill, G.A. (2000). Analysis of variance for gene expression microarray data. *J Comput Biol 7*, 819–837.

Kyng, K.J., May, A., Kolvraa, S., and Bohr, V.A. (2003). Gene expression profiling in Werner syndrome closely resembles that of normal aging. *Proc Natl Acad Sci USA 100*, 12259–12264.

Landis, G.N., Abdueva, D., Skvortsov, D., Yang, J., Rabin, B.E., Carrick, J., Tavare, S., and Tower, J. (2004). Similar gene expression patterns characterize aging and oxidative stress in *Drosophila melanogaster*. *Proc Natl Acad Sci USA 101*, 7663–7668.

Landry, J., Sutton, A., Tafrov, S.T., Heller, R.C., Stebbins, J., Pillus, L., and Sternglanz, R. (2000). The silencing protein SIR2 and its homologs are NAD-dependent protein deacetylases. *Proc Natl Acad Sci USA 97*, 5807–5811.

Lee, C.K., Klopp, R.G., Weindruch, R., and Prolla, T.A. (1999). Gene expression profile of aging and its retardation by caloric restriction. *Science 285*, 1390–1393.

Lee, M.L., and Whitmore, G.A. (2002). Power and sample size for DNA microarray studies. *Stat Med 21*, 3543–3570.

Lee, S.S., Lee, R.Y., Fraser, A.G., Kamath, R.S., Ahringer, J., and Ruvkun, G. (2003). A systematic RNAi screen identifies a critical role for mitochondria in *C. elegans* longevity. *Nat Genet 33*, 40–48.

Lu, T., Pan, Y., Kao, S.Y., Li, C., Kohane, I., Chan, J., and Yankner, B.A. (2004). Gene regulation and DNA damage in the ageing human brain. *Nature 429*, 883–891.

Mair, W., Goymer, P., Pletcher, S.D., and Partridge, L. (2003). Demography of dietary restriction and death in *Drosophila*. *Science 301*, 1731–1733.

McCarroll, S.A., Murphy, C.T., Zou, S., Pletcher, S.D., Chin, C.S., Jan, Y.N., *et al.* (2004). Comparing genomic expression patterns across species identifies shared transcriptional profile in aging. *Nat Genet 36*, 197–204.

McElwee, J., Bubb, K., and Thomas, J.H. (2003). Transcriptional outputs of the *Caenorhabditis elegans* forkhead protein DAF-16. *Aging Cell 2*, 111–121.

Melov, S., and Hubbard, A. (2004). Microarrays as a tool to investigate the biology of aging: A retrospective and a look to the future. *Sci Aging Knowledge Environ* 2004, re7.

Miller, R.A., Chang, Y., Galecki, A.T., Al-Regaiey, K., Kopchick, J.J., and Bartke, A. (2002). Gene expression patterns in calorically restricted mice: Partial overlap with long-lived mutant mice. *Mol Endocrinol 16*, 2657–2666.

Miller, R.A., Galecki, A., and Shmookler-Reis, R.J. (2001). Interpretation, design, and analysis of gene array expression experiments. *J Gerontol A Biol Sci Med Sci 56*, B52–57.

Murphy, C.T., McCarroll, S.A., Bargmann, C.I., Fraser, A., Kamath, R.S., Ahringer, J., *et al.* (2003). Genes that act downstream of DAF-16 to influence the lifespan of *Caenorhabditis elegans*. *Nature 424*, 277–283.

Nair, P.N., Golden, T., and Melov, S. (2003). Microarray workshop on aging. *Mech Ageing Dev 124*, 133–138.

Park, S.K., and Prolla, T.A. (2005a). Gene expression profiling studies of aging in cardiac and skeletal muscles. *Cardiovasc Res 66*, 205–212.

Park, S.K., and Prolla, T.A. (2005b). Lessons learned from gene expression profile studies of aging and caloric restriction. *Ageing Res Rev* 4, 55–65.

Pletcher, S.D., Macdonald, S.J., Marguerie, R., Certa, U., Stearns, S.C., Goldstein, D.B., and Partridge, L. (2002). Genome-wide transcript profiles in aging and calorically restricted *Drosophila melanogaster*. *Curr Biol 12*, 712–723.

Popesco, M.C., Frostholm, A., Rejniak, K., and Rotter, A. (2004). Digital transcriptome analysis in the aging cerebellum. *Ann N Y Acad Sci 1019*, 58–63.

Prolla, T.A. (2005). Multiple roads to the aging phenotype: Insights from the molecular dissection of progerias through DNA microarray analysis. *Mech Ageing Dev 126*, 461–465.

Puca, A.A., Daly, M.J., Brewster, S.J., Matise, T.C., Barrett, J., Shea-Drinkwater, M., *et al.* (2001). A genome-wide scan for linkage to human exceptional longevity identifies a locus on chromosome 4. *Proc Natl Acad Sci USA 98*, 10505–10508.

Rodwell, G.E., Sonu, R., Zahn, J.M., Lund, J., Wilhelmy, J., Wang, L., *et al.* (2004). A transcriptional profile of aging in the human kidney. *PLoS Biol 2*, e427.

Rogina, B., and Helfand, S.L. (2004). Sir2 mediates longevity in the fly through a pathway related to calorie restriction. *Proc Natl Acad Sci USA 101*, 15998–16003.

Rual, J.F., Ceron, J., Koreth, J., Hao, T., Nicot, A.S., Hirozane-Kishikawa, T., *et al.* (2004). Toward improving *Caenorhabditis elegans* phenome mapping with an ORFeome-based RNAi library. *Genome Res 14*, 2162–2168.

Schoneich, C. (2003). Proteomics in gerontological research. *Exp Gerontol 38*, 473–481.

Tanner, K.G., Landry, J., Sternglanz, R., and Denu, J.M. (2000). Silent information regulator 2 family of NAD-dependent histone/protein deacetylases generates a unique product, 1-O-acetyl-ADP-ribose. *Proc Natl Acad Sci USA 97*, 14178–14182.

Tissenbaum, H.A., and Guarente, L. (2001). Increased dosage of a sir-2 gene extends lifespan in *Caenorhabditis elegans*. *Nature 410*, 227–230.

Tsuchiya, T., Dhahbi, J.M., Cui, X., Mote, P.L., Bartke, A., and Spindler, S.R. (2004). Additive regulation of hepatic gene expression by dwarfism and caloric restriction. *Physiol Genomics 17*, 307–315.

van Heemst, D., Beekman, M., Mooijaart, S.P., Heijmans, B.T., Brandt, B.W., Zwaan, B.J., *et al.* (2005). Reduced insulin/IGF-1 signalling and human longevity. *Aging Cell 4*, 79–85.

Velculescu, V.E., Zhang, L., Vogelstein, B., and Kinzler, K.W. (1995). Serial analysis of gene expression. *Science 270*, 484–487.

Vellai, T., Takacs-Vellai, K., Zhang, Y., Kovacs, A.L., Orosz, L., and Muller, F. (2003). Genetics: Influence of TOR kinase on lifespan in C. elegans. *Nature 426*, 620.

Weindruch, R., Kayo, T., Lee, C.K., and Prolla, T.A. (2001). Microarray profiling of gene expression in aging and its alteration by caloric restriction in mice. *J Nutr 131*, 918S–923S.

Welle, S., Brooks, A., and Thornton, C.A. (2001). Senescence-related changes in gene expression in muscle: Similarities and differences between mice and men. *Physiol Genomics 5*, 67–73.

Welle, S., Brooks, A.I., Delehanty, J.M., Needler, N., Bhatt, K., Shah, B., and Thornton, C.A. (2004). Skeletal muscle gene expression profiles in 20–29 year old and 65–71 year old women. *Exp Gerontol 39*, 369–377.

Welle, S., Brooks, A.I., Delehanty, J.M., Needler, N., and Thornton, C.A. (2003). Gene expression profile of aging in human muscle. *Physiol Genomics 14*, 149–159.

Wood, J.G., Rogina, B., Lavu, S., Howitz, K., Helfand, S.L., Tatar, M., and Sinclair, D. (2004). Sirtuin activators mimic caloric restriction and delay ageing in metazoans. *Nature 430*, 686–689.

Yoshida, S., Yashar, B.M., Hiriyanna, S., and Swaroop, A. (2002). Microarray analysis of gene expression in the aging human retina. *Invest Ophthalmol Vis Sci 43*, 2554–2560.

Zou, S., Meadows, S., Sharp, L., Jan, L.Y., and Jan, Y.N. (2000). Genome-wide study of aging and oxidative stress response in *Drosophila melanogaster*. *Proc Natl Acad Sci USA 97*, 13726–13731.

11

Models of Alzheimer's Disease

Harry LeVine III and Lary C. Walker

The concepts that drive disease modeling are presented in the context of animal models for Alzheimer's disease (AD). A number of the best-characterized natural and transgenic animal models for AD are described along with the caveats that each presents for studying mechanisms of disease and for testing of potential therapeutic strategies.

Introduction

Animal models do not now exist that recapitulate all of the behavioral, physiological, and biochemical facets of Alzheimer's disease (AD). In the last dozen years, transgenic mouse models have been developed that display many of the hallmark neuropathological structures as well as some of the behavioral consequences predicted by the Amyloid Hypothesis. They have been useful for testing hypotheses for root causes, defining interactions, and in investigating therapeutic strategies for this most prevalent chronic neurodegenerative condition. A brief description of AD is provided that points out the key features of the disease and the evolution of the models that have been used to probe mechanisms and to search for therapeutics. Rationales for development of different kinds of disease models and the limits of their utility are explained. The bulk of the chapter summarizes models that have been the most thoroughly investigated or that have made seminal contributions to the understanding of AD. It is not intended to be a comprehensive review of AD animal models, and the authors apologize to those investigators whose work or animals were not included due to limits on scope.

Characteristics of AD

Alzheimer's disease (AD) is a progressive neurodegenerative disorder that is characterized by the relentless decline of cognitive function, judgment, perception and personality, and ultimately the loss of the distinctive and shared qualities that define an individual's existence (Cummings, 2004). For unknown reasons, the full behavioral and neurodegenerative phenotype of AD is unique to humans, a characteristic that has hindered the development of representative AD models. However, in recent years substantial progress has been made in the development of animal models of behavioral and pathological components of AD.

Histopathologically, AD is characterized primarily by the presence of senile plaques and neurofibrillary tangles (NFTs) in specific brain regions (Figure 11.1) (see Hauw and Duyckaerts, 2001; Hardy and Selkoe, 2002 for review). Senile plaques are intricate lesions centered about a core of aggregated, fibrillar amyloid-β (Aβ) peptide; neurofibrillary tangles are intracellular inclusions comprised of aberrant, microtubule-associated protein *tau*. A variety of additional pathologic changes accompany plaques and tangles in AD, including cerebral β-amyloid angiopathy (CAA; Figure 11.1B), granulovacuolar degeneration, inflammation, and loss of specific neurons and synapses (Hauw and Duyckaerts, 2001) (Cummings, 2004). NFTs occur in over 20 brain disorders besides AD, and mutations in the gene for tau on chromosome 17 have been linked to hereditary CNS tauopathies (FTDP-17) (Lee *et al.*, 2001, 2005). Despite some similarities, the genetic tauopathies differ in important ways from AD, one being the critical role that Aβ plays in Alzheimer pathogenesis.

Alzheimer's disease afflicts primarily the higher order processing regions of the cerebral cortex and associated subcortical nuclei. The pathogenic process begins stereotypically in the allocortex of the medial temporal lobe and progresses inexorably to other brain regions over the course of many years (Braak *et al.*, 1997). Structures that are heavily involved in the end-stages of the disease are the neocortex, hippocampus, and amygdala, whereas some regions (such as the cerebellum) remain relatively spared (Hauw and Duyckaerts, 2001). Within affected areas, certain neurons are selectively vulnerable, in particular long projection neurons and/or neurons that use glutamate, acetylcholine, gamma-amino butyric acid (GABA), dopamine, or norepinephrine as neurotransmitters.

Paradoxically, in spite of evidence that Aβ plays a primary role in the causation of AD (below), the atypical, intraneuronal accumulation of tau is the first lesion to appear in aging humans (Braak *et al.*, 1997). Tau protein, which normally stabilizes cellular microtubules, begins to polymerize separately in affected cells,

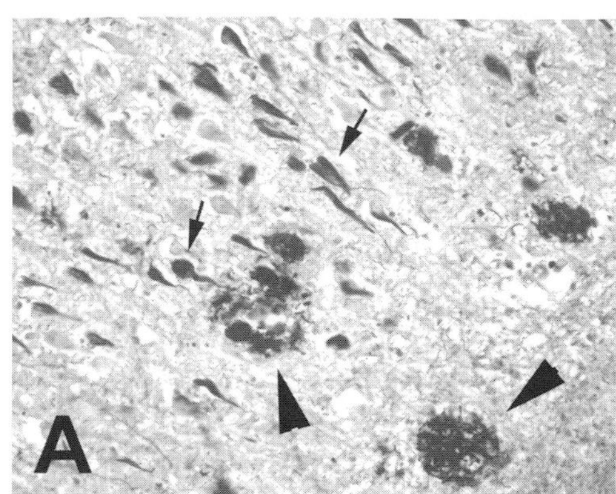

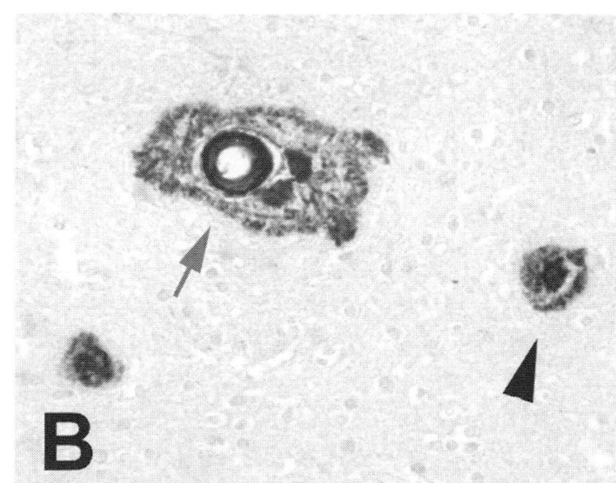

Figure 11.1 The Canonical Pathology of Alzheimer's Disease. (A) Gallyas silver-stained section showing neurofibrillary tangles (arrows) and senile plaques (arrowheads) in the hippocampal formation of an AD patient (10X objective). (B) Aβ-immunostained scction showing senile plaques (arrowhead) and CAA (grey arrow) in the neocortex (antibody 10D5; 20X objective).

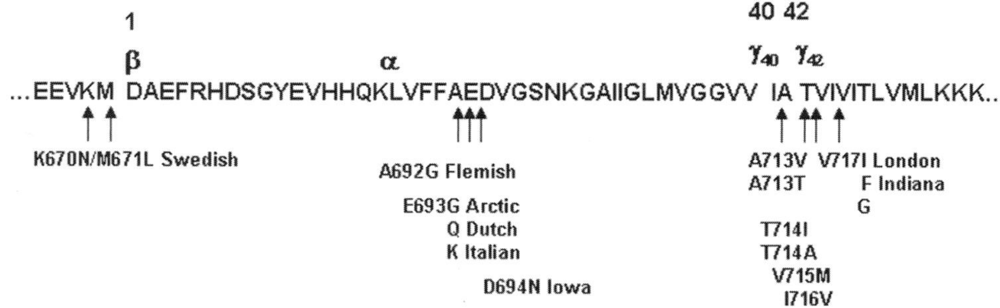

Figure 11.2 Familial AD Mutations in βAPP. The amino acid sequence of the region of the Amyloid Precursor Protein that contains the Aβ peptide is shown with the different secretase sites (α-, β-, γ-) marked. The sequence numbering for the Aβ peptide is above the sequence while the βAPP sequence numbering is below the sequence. Positions and amino acid changes of the various familial mutations in βAPP are indicated.

eventually forming neurofibrillary tangles, neuropil threads, and vacuolar granules (granulovacuolar degeneration). Tauopathy is first apparent in the entorhinal region, which receives heavy input from the sensory association areas of the neocortex, and then spreads progressively into other limbic structures, the neocortex, and specific subcortical neuronal groups. Senile plaques generally arise after the first tau lesions, and they do not consistently colocalize with neurofibrillary tangles, although there is evidence that they occur in terminal fields of tangle-bearing projection neurons (Schonheit *et al.*, 2004). The stereotypical localization of plaques and tangles suggests the importance of local biochemical conditions and neuronal interconnections in the instigation and spread of the lesions.

While neurofibrillary tangles become evident prior to senile plaques in aging humans, there is growing evidence that the anomalous aggregation of Aβ is a seminal event in AD pathogenesis (Hardy and Selkoe, 2002; Walker and LeVine, 2002) and that the corruption of tau occurs in response to initial abnormalities of Aβ (Walker and LeVine, 2002; Oddo *et al.*, 2004). Three compelling arguments support the primacy of Aβ in the Alzheimer's disease cascade: (1) The large quantity of Aβ deposits in the AD brain implicates the peptide in pathogenesis; (2) the most common autosomal dominant forms of AD all involve mutations either in the β-amyloid precursor protein (βAPP) (Figure 11.2) (Revesz *et al.*, 2003) or in the presenilins (PS1 and PS2, which form the probable catalytic subunit of the gamma-secretase complex that liberates Aβ at its C-terminus (Marjaux *et al.*, 2004); and (3) all known genetic and environmental risk factors for AD increase the production of Aβ and/or its tendency to aggregate (Hardy and Selkoe, 2002).

According to the Aβ-cascade hypothesis, the abnormal accumulation of multimeric Aβ triggers a progression of events leading to amyloid plaques, neurofibrillary tangles, inflammation, neuron- and synapse loss, and dementia. *In vitro* and *in vivo* studies are beginning to implicate a prefibrillar, oligomeric form of Aβ in this cascade (Kayed *et al.*, 2003). Indeed, the major genetic risk factor for AD (accounting for over 50% of the risk) is the inheritance of the $\varepsilon 4$ allele of apolipoprotein-E (ApoE); ApoE$\varepsilon 4$ is associated with increased Aβ(1–42) while decreasing the age of disease onset (Poirier, 1994).

NORMAL AGING OR DISEASE?

A key issue for AD model development is whether AD is a pathological process or whether it is part of the normal sequence of aging. It is not as easy to decide this as it might seem. Sporadic AD is a condition of advanced age; average onset in the general population is 80–85 years. In fact, advancing age is the single most important risk factor for AD. Some of the symptoms and many of the lesions of AD are observed in normal persons as they age, a significant number of whom never develop dementia. Would all of them develop dementia if they were to live long enough? This issue remains unresolved, although it is clear at least that the initiation and trajectory of AD pathogenesis vary widely among aging persons.

Advanced age is not a requirement for AD pathology. Familial (genetic) forms of AD clearly fit the criteria for a disease, as the pathology occurs decades earlier than for the sporadic form of AD. One mutation (presenilin-1, P117L) causes disease onset as early as the 20s (Wisniewski *et al.*, 1998). Early onset AD is not a progeric disorder, as other signs of advanced age are not observed. The difference between a disease and aging blurs when the processes involved overlap.

In terms of therapeutics, the prospects for blocking an aberrant process are significantly greater than for discovering a fountain-of-youth agent that halts aging. Disease models based on current hypotheses of what is driving AD pathology address the former condition while general aging models concentrate on the latter. The two approaches are not exclusive. Aging provides a substrate for the pathological processes in AD. Much can be learned from both types of models, and from considering how they interact and overlap.

Characteristics of an Animal Model: Modeling Pathology or Function?

Animal models of human disease are seldom comprehensive. Rarely does a single system recapitulate all aspects of the human pathological process. Defining the key characteristics of a disease to be reproduced requires some knowledge of the driving force for the pathology and the symptoms. Secondary co-morbid characteristics that may be observed in the disease, but that are not critical for disease progression, would clearly be poor choices for modeling. It is not always easy to tell the difference. Before the development of molecular targets and mechanism-based approaches, pharmaceutical research and drug discovery were heavily based on animal models that reproduced symptoms seen in humans. Animals with high blood pressure or hyperglycemia were treated to determine which compounds best normalized the condition. The success of such models in predicting efficacious agents in humans depended greatly on whether the mechanisms were similar.

This approach had been relatively successful for another chronic neurodegenerative disease, Parkinson's disease. Remarkable improvement was achieved with dopaminergic neurotransmitter replacement therapy (L-dopa). The first AD models and therapeutics were based on a similar principle of symptomatic relief, alleviating the functional deficits of cholinergic systems early in the disease. Cholinergic therapies for AD were significantly less effective than was L-dopa for Parkinson's disease, and clinical evidence indicates that supplementation of cholinergic function can slow, but fails to halt, the progression of AD. The lack of effect of L-dopa on disease progression also was recognized for Parkinson's disease, suggesting that the prime mover in both diseases remained to be addressed.

Symptom-based models gave way to pathology-based models as molecular knowledge of AD expanded, and the interplay of genetic factors and the metabolism of the precursor protein to the Aβ peptide found in the amyloid plaques were understood. The models based on this insight produced Aβ plaques or tau filaments in the brains of transgenic mice overexpressing βAPP or tau, respectively, but failed to develop robust neuronal cell death or atrophy that resemble these events in AD. Neurophysiological and behavioral deficits were observed in young βAPP-overexpressing animals; however, they were not linked to histologically demonstrable deposits of Aβ, which usually developed later.

PURPOSES OF MODELS

Since only humans develop AD, there are no "natural" models that display all of the pathological, physiological, and symptomatic features of the human disease. The same is true for genetically engineered models, as each model has both advantages and weaknesses in recapitulating the AD phenotype. It is thus important when choosing a model for study to consider how well it is suited to answering the specific questions being asked about AD.

Development of therapeutics

Testing of potential therapeutics was the motivation for developing a number of the early models of AD. A symptomatic approach was adopted similar to the one that produced effective therapy for Parkinson's disease, where the targeted deficit was in the nigrostriatal dopaminergic system and the control of movement was monitored. Cognitive deficits in AD were modeled by subjecting hippocampally deficient mice or aged monkeys to memory tests of different sorts. Reversal of pharmacologically or lesion-induced cholinergic dysfunction in behavioral tasks by test agents was another approach.

Cholinergic therapeutics—specifically inhibitors of acetylcholinesterase—have proven to provide some benefit to patients for a limited period of time. However, this first generation of cholinergic therapeutics failed to cure or halt AD, prompting the development of models based on other pathogenic mechanisms, such as the "Aβ-cascade" (Hardy and Selkoe, 2002). Such models could be used for monitoring the effects of therapeutics targeting such elements of the pathogenic cascade as plaque deposition, Aβ peptide levels, glial responses, and secondary pathology. These animal models lack the profound neurodegeneration of AD, and thus they are incomplete models of AD. Combining dominant transgenes for βAPP, PS1, and even tau had surprisingly little effect on neurodegeneration, the substrate for dementia. Nevertheless, these models, when judiciously chosen, are useful for developing possible therapeutic agents targeting key components of the pathogenic process, but the efficacy of such disease-modifying treatments in humans remains to be validated.

Probing mechanisms of AD neurodegeneration

The cell-selective neurodegeneration in AD and other chronic neurodegenerative diseases and the failure to produce models with comparable neuronal cell death are unexplained. The partial models of AD pathology have been useful for teasing out mechanistic details that may apply to AD. The human disease, or cohort of diseases as some believe, is a morass of overlapping pathologies where it is difficult to determine which one(s) drive(s) the disease process, and when, during the estimated forty years of (mostly silent) progression the key players act. Modeling individual components of the multifactorial process, assessing their impact, and then combining them in different ways provide information on how they might interact in a disease state. Incorporation into a single model with the correct temporal and spatial sequencing of events would be the Holy Grail of AD.

Optimizing clinical trials

A model that rapidly predicts the efficacy of an agent in producing the desired therapeutic effect, even if it is unknown whether that intervention will ultimately influence the disease, would invigorate clinical trials. The double unknown of pharmacologic efficacy and impact on the disease is discouraging. Another area in which models can contribute is in identifying potential side-effects or toxicities and to establish safe dosage ranges. Gamma secretase inhibitors have the potential to interfere with important signaling molecules, such as Notch in hematopoiesis, and this is assessed in the models.

The current models do not anticipate all possible side-effects. An Aβ immunization trial designed to lower Aβ levels (AN-1792, Elan) was halted by unexpected immune encephalopathy in 6% of the immunized patients. In addition, the patients who mounted an antibody response to Aβ-immunization, despite weak evidence for clinical improvement, paradoxically showed an augmented shrinkage of the brain substance. A search for models capable of detecting these serious side effects is underway.

MAMMALIAN VS NONMAMMALIAN SYSTEMS

A debate rages over the relevance of nonmammalian animal models to what is a uniquely human disease. Much has been learned about the basic biology of AD mechanisms from nonmammalian systems. Biochemical processes tend to follow general precepts that are comparable in simple and complex organisms. The yeast *Saccharomyces cerevisiae* allows the use of powerful classical and molecular genetic tools, although this organism lacks a nervous system. The roundworm *Caenorhabditis elegans* and the fruit fly *Drosophila melanogaster* are well-studied animals that are also genetically accessible. Both feature relatively simple, stereotyped nervous systems to analyze biochemical pathways and cell function. *C. elegans* (Rankin, 2004) and *Drosophila* (Rohrbough *et al.*, 2003) display certain aspects of learning behavior that have been dissected genetically. The genomes of all these organisms have been sequenced, so mammalian and human gene homologs can be readily identified. Short generation times shrink the timescale of experiments with these organisms, even for elderly individuals.

While possessing a number of advantages for studying specific instances of biochemical pathways, mechanisms, or physiological subsystems, there remain significant differences in complexity and organization between invertebrate and mammalian nervous systems that limit the simpler organisms as AD models. Although these organisms have been used as models of aging, and there are certain similarities, questions remain about the equivalence of two months of life in fruit flies to 80 years in humans.

Nonmammalian organism models

Drosophila and *C. elegans* provide both powerful genetic tools and a sufficiently complex behavioral repertoire to be able to detect alterations in brain function (Driscoll and Gerstbrein, 2003). They possess homologs to the human genes that are linked to familial AD. Unfortunately, neither the fly nor worm βAPP contains the amyloidogenic sequence, and thus natural AD β-amyloid models are not available. The fly, in particular, has been useful for studies in AD, in Huntington's disease (HD), and in Parkinson's disease (PD) when the human familial disease transgenes are expressed leading to neurodegeneration. By a judicious choice of promoters, the mutant gene is directed to an easily observed neural tissue, the compound eye, in which neurodegeneration can be easily monitored.

In *C. elegans* expression of human Aβ(1–42) in muscle leads to toxic effects (Fonte *et al.*, 2002). By searching for suppressor genes for the toxic phenotype in both flies and worms, potential pathways for countering the neurodegeneration have been identified. An example is the hsp70 chaperone protein, which reduces the accumulation of misfolded proteins. Mutation of negative regulators of hsp70 activity also suppresses the toxic phenotype. Toxicity of misfolded proteins linked to AD, PD, and HD in these organisms is ameliorated by increased hsp70 activity. However, implementing a therapeutic strategy of increased hsp70 levels is likely to be fraught with difficulties due to the multiple roles of hsp70 in cell biology and the consequences of a sustained stress response.

Ex-vivo models

In this category we include both isolated cell culture and tissue slice organotypic culture systems that approximate various aspects of AD. *Ex vivo* models are a step up in complexity—and hopefully disease relevance—from *in vitro* assays of biochemical components and biophysical processes. A variety of cell lines have been used via transfection of appropriate genes to study βAPP metabolism and to work out the consequences of the familial AD mutations in βAPP and the presenilins. Under the premise that many of the events are similar in all cells, even ones not thought to be altered in AD, these systems have been used to probe the cell biology of the amyloid cascade. Overall correspondence of results with those from neuronally derived cell lines is cited as evidence for the validity of these models. Indeed, the link between mutant presenilins and the increased production of Aβ in familial AD was accurately predicted from cell culture models.

Major caveats to blanket acceptance of the isolated cell systems as models of AD are that they are mostly transformed, relatively undifferentiated cells, often of nonneuronal origin or mixed neuronal–glial origin. Those cell lines of neuronal origin are frequently derived from the peripheral nervous system, which is spared in AD. Cultured cells also do not manifest the multiple connections or the extreme polarity and long-distance transport requirements of central neurons that are most affected in AD. Neurons cultured from embryonic or fetal brain regions are more representative of differentiated neurons, although they are mixtures of different kinds of neurons, in early stages of differentiation, that are removed from the surroundings in which they developed. There is much discussion about how similar these neurons are to *in situ* neurons because of the selection pressures *in vitro*. Fetal neurons from some brain regions survive to various degrees, while fully differentiated neurons from postnatal animals rarely are successfully cultured.

Organotypic brain-slice cultures are routinely used for neurotransmitter electrophysiology studies. The connectivity of various regions is more or less intact, depending on how the slices are made. Advantages are that the cells maintain their local contacts and are more highly differentiated than are embryonic cultures. Disadvantages are that they are labor- and resource-intensive, generally not long-term, and are difficult to prepare successfully from older animals. These systems have been useful for distinguishing neuronal toxicity of soluble monomeric, oligomeric and fibrillar β-amyloid species (Lacor *et al.*, 2004) and the effects of Aβ on electrophysiology, such as blocking LTP but not LTD (Walsh and Selkoe, 2004).

Cerebrovascular smooth muscle cells cultured from human, canine, and βAPP-transgenic mouse (Tg2576) leptomeninges actively produce Aβ peptides, secreting them into the medium and depositing them intracellularly and extracellularly (Frackowiak *et al.*, 2003; Frackowiak *et al.*, 2005). This is the only cell system that deposits Aβ in culture. The smooth muscle cells are susceptible to Aβ toxicity, particularly to a mutant peptide, Aβ E22Q, that produces a selective cerebrovascular smooth muscle amyloidosis with little parenchymal involvement in humans and in mouse models. This is a highly relevant system since these cells are involved in cerebral β-amyloid angiopathy (CAA), which is seen in virtually all AD patients and can lead to intracerebral hemorrhages.

BEHAVIORAL MODELS AND THE CHOLINERGIC HYPOTHESIS

The symptomatic approach to treating AD involves maintaining or restoring the neuronal pathways that become deficient during the course of the disease. In early AD, a prominent deficit occurs in cholinergic pathways, particularly in the basal forebrain cholinergic system, whose afferents project widely to the hippocampus, amygdala and neocortical areas. The Cholinergic Hypothesis for AD held that the deficiency of presynaptic neurotransmitter was a central etiologic factor. The drugs currently on the market for treatment of AD are designed to boost presynaptic levels of acetylcholine, usually by inhibition of the breakdown of acetylcholine by cholinesterases. These cholinesterase inhibitors were developed through the use of mice or rats whose cholinergic function had been impaired by genetics (hippocampally-deficient mice), reversal of acetylcholinergic antagonist drugs, or lesioning. The animals were then assessed for behavioral improvement in the presence of the test agent. The compounds developed had the expected pharmacological properties, but they do not alter the course of the disease in a major way.

MODELING OTHER BEHAVIORAL CONDITIONS

AD is characterized by a number of behavioral disturbances beyond cognitive function, particularly in the mid- to late stages of the disease. These include sleep disturbances, depression, wandering, and aggressiveness, which are frequently the cause of nursing home placement. These are conditions that also occur in the absence of AD symptoms. There is some question as to whether they are different in the presence and absence of dementia. This is an area in which better therapeutics could make a significant impact on quality of life for the patient and the caregivers. These behavioral problems are currently addressed by add-on medications, but the effects are somewhat different than in nondemented subjects. This topic is outside the scope of this review.

Pathology Models: Natural vs Engineered

AD symptoms are dominated by the progressive loss of cognitive function, although other modalities are affected, particularly in the later stages of the disease. Dementia, however, can result from multiple etiologies such as tumors, drugs, toxic agents, multiple cerebral infarcts, Lewy body disease, prionoses, and tauopathies, to name a few. Each disease generally presents a clinical picture that is distinct from the others, although areas of overlap are a persistent challenge for clinical diagnosis. The defining characteristic of AD is that the dementia develops in the context of the accumulation of β-amyloid peptide in plaque structures and the development of neurofibrillary tangles. In the absence of these lesions, in particular the amyloid deposition, the dementia is not considered to be of the Alzheimer's type.

"NATURAL" MODELS OF ALZHEIMER-LIKE PATHOLOGY

Several animal species naturally develop senile plaques, cerebral amyloid angiopathy (CAA), and (to a limited degree) tauopathy with age. The most comprehensively studied nonhuman animals have been primates and canines. These animals are well-suited for modeling AD neuropathology for the following reasons: (1) They have the human-like Aβ sequence and develop senile plaques and CAA with age; (2) tau abnormalities (but not fully developed tangles) occur naturally with age in some primates and dogs; (3) the behavioral complexity of monkeys and dogs enables in-depth analysis of cognitive, social and motoric components of neurodegeneration; (4) both groups manifest age-associated decline of certain behavioral capacities; and (5) their large brains allow detailed *in vivo* imaging (Walker and Cork, 1999; Bussiere *et al.*, 2002; Voytko and Tinkler, 2004).

Aging canine

Cerebral amyloid deposition was first noted in a nonhuman species in the 1950s by von Braunmuhl, who described senile plaques in elderly dogs. Since then, the characteristics of the deposits and the natural history of their emergence have been well established, as has their possible relationship to age-associated cognitive decline. In dogs, as in primates, the Aβ peptide is identical in sequence to human Aβ. Normal rats and mice differ in three amino acids from humans. The deposits that arise in the parenchyma of the aged canine brain are usually diffuse in nature; i.e., fully developed, dense-cored senile plaques are relatively rare. However, cerebral amyloid angiopathy (CAA) is common in older dogs (Wegiel *et al.*, 1995). CAA in canines, as in humans, primates, and transgenic mice, is associated with an increased incidence of intracerebral hemorrhage and possibly white matter lesions as well (Torp *et al.*, 2000).

Aβ accumulation correlates with behavioral impairments in aged dogs (Colle *et al.*, 2000), and with a regional loss of brain substance (particularly in the frontal lobes) beginning around 8 years of age (Tapp *et al.*, 2004). As in all affected species, there is substantial variation in age-associated changes among animals of comparable age; in addition, controlled comparative studies of the development and composition of lesions in different breeds of dogs are lacking. The age-related cognitive decline in aged dogs can be ameliorated by a diet rich in antioxidants and mitochondrial co-factors, as well as by behavioral enrichment (Milgram *et al.*, 2005; Siwak *et al.*, 2005), and there is evidence that drugs used to treat cognitive decline in humans can be usefully tested in aged canines (Studzinski *et al.*, 2005).

Aging primate

Information on the neurobiology of aging in nonhuman primates has grown steadily over the past four decades (Hof *et al.*, 2002). By far the most thoroughly investigated species are the rhesus monkey (*Macaca mulatta*) and the squirrel monkey (*Saimiri* spp), although there is a burgeoning literature on other nonhuman primate species, including great apes, marmosets (*Saguinus jacchus*), cynomolgus monkeys (*Macaca fascicularis*), green monkeys (*Chlorocebus aethiops*), baboons (*Papio hamadryas*), and mouse lemurs (*Microcebus murinus*). We will focus here primarily on rhesus monkeys and squirrel monkeys as natural primate models of Alzheimer-like pathology.

Rhesus monkeys. Rhesus monkeys are Old World monkeys with a maximum life span of approximately 40 years; they reach puberty at 3–4 years of age, and females go through menopause at approximately 25 years of age (Walker, 1995). Age-related cognitive decline is well-documented in rhesus monkeys, but a dementia-like state has not been reported. Rhesus monkeys develop senile plaques with age, usually in their early-mid 20's (Walker and Cork, 1999). These lesions are cytologically and biochemically similar to human plaques, except that the abnormal neurites that surround the core are devoid of tau filaments. Indeed, although primates can manifest tau abnormalities in brain, fully formed neurofibrillary tangles have not yet been detected in any nonhuman primate, including the apes.

Squirrel monkeys. In addition to widely varying phenotypes and lifespans, nonhuman primates show species-specific patterns of age-associated lesion development in brain. Squirrel monkeys are small, New World primates with a maximum lifespan of approximately 30 years (Walker and Cork, 1999). They begin to form Aβ deposits in the brain by the age of 13 years (around the age of menopause in females), and such lesions can be plentiful by 21 years. Unlike in rhesus monkeys, the Aβ-proteopathy in squirrel monkeys is predominantly in the walls of cerebral blood vessels. Senile plaques also are present in squirrel monkeys, but they are less common than is CAA. Infrequent neurons are immunoreactive for hyperphosphorylated tau, but as in all nonhuman primates studied to date there are no fully developed neurofibrillary tangles.

Apolipoprotein E (ApoE) is heterogeneous in humans, and one form (ApoE4) is linked to an increased risk of AD and CAA. Intriguingly, *all* nonhuman primates are homozygous for apoE4; that is, their apoE resembles human apoE4 with arginines at positions 112 and 158. However, in nonhuman primates, threonine replaces arginine at position 61 of the human apoE sequence, which causes simian apoE to interact with lipoproteins similarly to human apoE3. Thus, neither βAPP mutations nor apoE type account for the species-related variation in Aβ-pathology, at least in *non*human primates.

In summary, nonhuman primates and canines have been invaluable in illuminating the biochemistry, cytology and genetics of senile plaques, amyloid angiopathy and tau pathology in the aging brain, and they remain useful for testing emerging therapies for neurodegenerative diseases (Studzinski *et al.*, 2005; Walker *et al.*, 2005). However, for a variety of reasons, a major component of which is their longevity, research with these species is limited in scope. The emergence of genetically engineered rodent models has greatly accelerated the investigation of AD-like pathogenesis *in vivo*.

Engineered Pathology Models

Although aged dogs and primates provide some insight into spontaneous AD and can be invaluable in testing the safety and efficacy of diagnostic and therapeutic agents, they are long-lived and do not reproduce all of the pathological features of the human disease. Engineered models attempt to combine knowledge gained from the familial forms of AD with transgenic technology to individually reconstruct the major components of the pathology. In order for such an approach to completely succeed, either the prime mover in the disease process has to be addressed or the complex pathology has to be an approximately linear combination of two or more pathologies, such as plaques and tangles. In the case of overlapping pathologies, each transgene should be able to induce key characteristics of AD pathology. Finally, the organism must be capable of reflecting the impact of the pathology in a recognizable way, preferably with behavioral signs and symptoms similar to those in humans with AD.

AMYLOID HYPOTHESIS AND Aβ AMYLOIDOSIS

The characteristic pathological signature of AD noted by Alzheimer is the presence of deposits of Aβ peptide in extracellular plaques accompanied by tau deposits in intracellular tangles. The weight of the genetic evidence from familial forms of AD supports the Aβ peptide as a prime mover in the etiology of the disease (Hardy and Selkoe, 2002). While it is clear that mutations in βAPP *can* cause AD in the genetic cases, sporadic AD must involve other factors. If it is true that multimeric Aβ is either an initiating factor and/or a chronic stressor, strategies to alleviate these effects should alter the course of the disease.

SEEKING THE PRIME MOVER IN ANIMAL MODELS

The human sequence of the Aβ peptide is particularly prone to aggregation *in vitro* and is required for deposition *in vivo*. The murine sequence contains three amino acid substitutions, F4G, Y10F, H13R, all in the hydrophilic N-terminus of the peptide (Figure 11.2), resulting in greatly reduced fibril-forming activity, which may explain why rats and mice don't spontaneously develop plaques. Initial attempts at modeling amyloid deposition involved infusion of the human sequence peptide or plaque cores into the brains of recipient animals. In rat models, the infused peptide itself can form deposits in brain, but these lesions lack many features of bona fide plaques, and, unlike AD, the deposition is not sustained by endogenous processes. In a monkey model of synthetic Aβ fibril infusion (Geula *et al.*, 1998), some neurodegeneration at the site of injection was observed, but amyloid plaque pathology did not develop. Similar results were obtained in rodent brain (Frautschy *et al.*, 1996).

Aβ amyloid pathology has been successfully induced in animals by taking a lead from the prion field, where mouse models to study infectious prions were created in which the species barrier had been circumvented by overexpressing the cognate normal prion protein in mice. Seeding of new β-amyloid plaques in the parenchyma and the walls of the cerebrovasculature was engendered in Tg2576 animals with high interstitial fluid levels of Aβ by a single injection of dilute AD brain extract (Walker *et al.*, 2002). Aβ proteopathy was not inducible in age-matched, nontransgenic mice, and the injection of brain extracts from young subjects was ineffective. To date, injections of pure, synthetic Aβ(1–40) and Aβ(1–42) have failed to instigate β-amyloidogenesis in the same way as brain extracts, suggesting that there is something special about the Aβ in the extract that is not found in the synthetic material. Identifying the properties of the brain extracts that promote β-amyloidogenesis will yield important information about the events that initiate this process *in vivo*.

Transgenic expression models

Success in obtaining plaque deposition in transgenic mice initially required overexpression of the human βAPP relative to the endogenous mouse protein. Transgenic animals with human βAPP-overexpression under the control of neuron-selective or neuron–specific promoters deposit Aβ peptides in parenchymal plaques in many of the same areas as in the AD brain as well as around cerebral and leptomeningeal blood vessels. Deposition is age- and protein level–dependent, usually beginning at 6–10 months in the absence of accelerating mutations. Dystrophic neurites develop around condensed senile plaques, as do reactive microgliosis and astrogliosis. While phosphorylated tau epitopes become prominent in dystrophic neurites, true neurofibrillary tangles never develop, and large-scale neuronal cell death has not been documented. A number of βAPP transgenic models have been produced that employ a variety of promoters, expression levels, and βAPP splicing variants. The upshot is that human βAPP overexpression in mice reproduces CNS β-amyloidosis and (to a variable degree) amyloid angiopathy in specific brain regions, but the mice do not develop the full histopathology of AD. βAPP overexpression also produces deficits in synaptic physiology (particularly in long-term potentiation [LTP]) and in several behavioral paradigms thought to reflect memory function in humans well before Aβ deposits are histologically demonstrable. While potentially due to the overexpression of βAPP, which is believed to mediate cell–cell contact and signaling, these same effects can be induced by application of soluble oligomeric forms of Aβ, and the deficits are abolished by antibodies to Aβ peptide. Only some of the most widely used or most informative models are discussed here.

Caveats. In evaluating the histopathologic effects of murine transgene expression, it is important to recognize the presence of nonspecific lesions that develop with age in various strains of mice. Specifically, clusters of inclusions emerge most prominently in the hippocampus but to a lesser degree also in the cerebellum and other areas (Jucker *et al.*, 1992). These inclusions (sometimes referred to as *Jucker Bodies*) occur within astrocytes and do not closely resemble any known human lesions. The inclusions can react nonspecifically with many antibodies, particularly polyclonal antibodies, and their presence is governed by a variety of factors, including the age, strain, and possibly sex of the mice. It is imperative to distinguish these inclusions from transgene-related neuropathology.

It is also important to recognize that the gender of the mice can influence the degree of Aβ pathology. In Tg2576 βAPP-transgenic mice, amyloid deposition is significantly greater in females than in males (Callahan *et al.*, 2001).

PDAPP. The first compelling report of a transgenic mouse that deposited Aβ plaques used βAPP V717F familial AD mutation minigene construct containing some intronic sequences under the control of the platelet-derived growth factor-β (PDGF-β) promoter (Games *et al.*, 1995). The V717F mutation, which is near the gamma-secretase cleavage site, promotes the selective production of the highly amyloidogenic Aβ42 peptide. Plaque deposition is noticeable around 6 months of age. Between 6 and 12 months plaque deposition increases, and virtually all plaques up through this age are neuritic and Thioflavine S-positive. After 12 months, Aβ-deposition increases precipitously, much of which is diffuse and Thioflavine S-negative. The dentate gyrus and entorhinal cortex are heavily invested (Reilly *et al.*, 2003). There is no change in hippocampal volume from 3 to 22 months in the transgenic animals compared to nontransgenic littermates. Four to five months before plaque deposition there are significant differences in electrophysiology and behavior in the transgenic animals. This model has been a workhorse driving anti-Aβ-based therapeutic development for Elan (Athena) and Lilly, but PDAPP mice were not made generally available to the research community. At Elan, they were used for the studies that first demonstrated that immunization with the Aβ peptide would prevent or clear brain Aβ deposits, currently a promising therapeutic strategy for AD and an area of active research.

Tg2576 – Hsiao mouse. The human βAPP695 amino acid protein with a Swedish K670N/M671L mutation coupled to a mouse prion promoter was designed to express the human protein in neuronal cells (Hsiao *et al.*, 1996), although this promoter seems to be active in other cell types such as vascular smooth muscle cells. A five- to six-fold overexpression was achieved in this early model, which is sufficient to drive deposition by 9 months of age, increasing dramatically up to 30 months. The Swedish mutation increases only β-site cleavage; as a result, there is a higher ratio of Aβ40:Aβ42 produced, and the plaques are a mixture of diffuse Thioflavin S-negative and neuritic Thioflavin S-positive deposits. Neuritic plaques are associated with abnormal, tau-immunoreactive neurites and with a glial inflammatory response. An electrophysiological and behavioral phenotype that is typical of the βAPP overexpressing mouse models is present in these animals. These deficits are established before plaque deposition is apparent. Maintenance on a SJL/BL6 hybrid strain background and βAPP heterozygosity are required because of βAPP toxicity and of the site of insertion of the transgene array, respectively. These mice were made available both to industry and academia, and as a result, Tg2576 has become the most thoroughly studied of the murine βAPP models. They are now commercially available from Taconic.

Caveat. Several inbred mouse strains, including SJL, carry the *rd* (retinal degeneration) mutation, a recessive, null mutation in the β-subunit of rod-specific cyclic GMP phosphodiesterase. Homozygous *rd* animals lose their rod cells between postnatal days 8 and 20, followed by a more gradual disappearance of the cone cells, such that by 4 weeks of age, the retina is devoid of photoreceptors. Obviously, this condition can profoundly influence performance on vision-dependent behavioral tasks.

APP23 mice. These mice express βAPP751 with a Swedish K670N/M671L mutation under control of the neuron-specific Thy 1 promoter. The 751 isoform of βAPP is not normally expressed in neurons, which produce mostly βAPP695. Plaque deposition begins around 6 months of age (0.3% of the cortical area) rising to 9% area at 22 months. Electrophysiological and behavioral deficits are noted before the onset of deposition, and condensed plaques induce inflammatory responses in the surrounding glial elements. Phospho-tau epitope induction is documented in neurites, but as in other βAPP-transgenics, there are no neurofibrillary tangles. Some neurodegeneration is also reported, which is unusual in βAPP models, but neocortical synapses are not depleted even when amyloid load is high (Boncristiano *et al.*, 2005). APP23 mice have a particularly strong propensity to develop Aβ accumulation in the vascular wall, and thus are a useful model of cerebral amyloid angiopathy (CAA) (Vloeberghs *et al.*, 2004).

CRND8 mouse. The double βAPP695 Swedish K670N/M671L–Indiana V717F mutant under control of the hamster prion protein promoter produces a massive amount of Aβ and a particularly virulent β-amyloidosis. The Swedish mutation increases the total amount of peptide produced by altering the βAPP sequence immediately N-terminal to the β-secretase cleavage site, making it a much better substrate for BACE. The Indiana mutation alters the βAPP sequence immediately C-terminal to the γ-secretase cleavage site causing more Aβ(1–42) than Aβ(1–40) to be present after 8 weeks of age. The CRND8 mouse attains significant Thioflavine S-positive Aβ deposition at 3 months of age in 100% of the animals, and both diffuse and neuritic plaques are apparent by 6 months. Neurofibrillary tangles are not present, but studies of the phospho-tau epitopes in neurites, which are seen in all other βAPP models, have not been published. The lack of neuronal cell death with the high level of βAPP expression achieved in these animals is unusual. A possible explanation for this is the C3H genetic background, which is resistant to βAPP toxicity. Behavioral and electrophysiological effects are noted early and can be reversed by immunization with anti-Aβ antibodies.

Hereditary cerebral Aβ angiopathy. Several βAPP familial mutations are associated with pathologies other than pure AD. βAPP mutations that change specific amino acids within Aβ (at positions 21–23) cause rare, autosomal dominant Aβ-proteopathies characterized by profuse CAA (Revesz *et al.*, 2003). The Aβ(1–40) peptide is the main deposited species in these mutants; as deposition progresses, the smooth muscle cells of the tunica media are lost, and the vessel walls lose their elasticity and become susceptible to rupture. While hereditary CAA is rare, wild-type Aβ is deposited in the cerebrovasculature of nearly all AD subjects as well as Down Syndrome patients, increasing the probability of hemorrhage.

Until recently, CAA has been difficult to model in mice bearing the human familial mutations. Mice transgenic for βAPP770 Swedish K670N/M671L + Dutch E22Q and Iowa D23N under control of the Thy 1.2 promoter express very low levels of βAPP770, less than the endogenous mouse βAPP (Davis *et al.*, 2004). Nevertheless, the mice develop significant accumulations of mostly fibrillar vascular and perivascular Aβ by 3 months of age. After 6 months, about 50% of vessels have deposits, and diffuse plaques appear in brain forebrain parenchyma. By one year of age there is robust deposition of Aβ in microvessels and within the brain parenchyma. Part of the reason for the accumulation of the (Dutch, Iowa) Aβ(1–40) is that, at physiologic concentration, the mutant peptides are 10-fold less readily cleared than the wild-type peptide.

In another model of CAA, neuronal overexpression of Dutch mutant E693Q hβAPP driven by the Thy-1 promoter produced a phenotype characterized predominantly by CAA, whereas overexpression of wild-type βAPP caused mainly parenchymal (plaque) amyloidosis (Herzig *et al.*, 2004). Interestingly, when the Dutch mutant mice are made doubly transgenic by crossing with mutant presenilin-1-transgenic mice, the most abundant form of brain Aβ is changed from Aβ40 to Aβ42, and the amyloid pathology is shifted from the vasculature to the brain parenchyma.

Double transgenics

In an effort to produce animals that more rapidly develop plaque pathology and a more severe phenotype, presenilin (PS) mutants were crossed with hβAPP-expressing animals. Aβ deposition requires the presence of the human Aβ peptide, as transgenic mice expressing only mutant PS fail to develop plaque pathology or CAA. A number of different PS1 mutant double transgenics reproduce the pattern of elevated Aβ42/40 ratios seen in the human familial AD cases (Borchelt *et al.*, 1996; Duff *et al.*, 1996; Citron *et al.*, 1997). Plaque formation in the transgenic animals mimics the aggressiveness of the familial disease as judged by the age of onset and rate of progression of the human cognitive symptoms. Plaques are detected as early as three months of age in the double mutants. There are some differences depending on which PS1 mutant is used.

βAPPSWE × PS1(M146L) (Duff mouse). This mouse was constructed by crossing the human βAPPSWE Tg2576 (Hsiao mouse section) with human PS1 (A246E) mutant mice (Holcomb *et al.*, 1998). Since the transgenes are both under the control of the mouse prion protein promoter, they are expressed in the same cells.

βAPPSWE × PS1(A246E) (Borchelt Mouse). These mice overexpress murine βAPP695 in which the mouse βAPP Aβ region is replaced with the human Aβ sequence with the Swedish K670N/M671L mutation (Borchelt *et al.*, 1997). The mice were crossed with human PS1 (A246E) mutant mice, and both transgenes are under control of the mouse prion promotor. A 50% increase in the ratio of Aβ42/Aβ40 is observed in the brains of these animals. Aβ accumulation is accelerated by several months, although the eventual degree of deposition is similar in the APPSWE and the APPSWE/PS1 animals.

Caveat. While useful in screening for agents that will prevent amyloid deposition, transgenic mice expressing mutant PS1 come with complications for studying mechanisms of neurodegeneration. The sporadic form of AD does not involve PS1 mutations or βAPP mutations. PS1 is thought to be the catalytic component of the intramembrane γ-secretase complex, which includes a number of proteins of unknown function. Mutations in PS1 alter the processing of other γ-secretase substrates besides βAPP, such as Notch as well as unknown substrates. There is one PS1 mutant (out of over 150 different mutations) that demonstrates frontotemporal dementia-like neurodegeneration in the absence of changes in βAPP metabolism (Dermaut *et al.*, 2004). Thus, mutations in PS1 could have effects on cellular physiology beyond βAPP.

Even with both transgenes present, the amount of neurodegeneration observed in βAPP/PS1 animals is disappointingly meager compared to that occurring in AD brain. The reason for the lack of extensive neuronal death is unknown. Possible explanations include an incomplete inflammatory response resulting from a deficiency in complement components in many mouse strains, augmented metabolism or sequestration of intracellular Aβ, or a missing linkage between PKR and JNK/p38 stress kinase systems in mice (Peel and Bredesen, 2003).

Non-overexpressing transgenic models

Early experiences in trying to create mice that would produce Aβ plaques appeared to dictate that levels of βAPP 5–6 times the endogenous mouse βAPP were required for deposition. Several laboratories produced models that were expected to be more like the sporadic AD situation, making do with less expression and leaving the βAPP gene in its normal chromosomal context.

βAPP Knock-in mice. Murine βAPP was modified by inserting the Swedish mutation immediately N-terminal to the β-secretase cleavage site and humanizing the three residues in the mouse Aβ sequence that differ from those in humans (H:M = R5G, Y10F, H13R) (Siman *et al.*, 2000). The hybrid full-length βAPP was under the control of the endogenous mouse promoter and retained the native mouse introns and splicing signals. In these animals humanized βAPP is produced in the absence of the mouse peptide in homozygotes at a normal level. The Swedish mutation causes a 9-fold increase in the amount of Aβ present as a result of its enhancement of β-secretase cleavage. These mice produce human sequence Aβ in the absence of the mouse sequence protein and develop plaques around 20 months of age. Other characteristics of the pathology are the same as in the overexpressors.

YAC mice. Another approach designed to maintain appropriate promoter control and splice variant production employed inserting the genomic sequence for the entire human βAPP gene, including introns and exons for the 770 residue protein (~400 kb) plus flanking sequences (~250 kb) in a yeast artificial chromosome construct (Lamb *et al.*, 1999). Expression levels are modest, 2–3 times the endogenous mouse protein, and the tissue-specific ratios of splice variants are retained. The Swedish mutation (K670N, M671L) increases the amount of Aβ peptides produced while (V717I) increases the proportion of Aβ(x-42). The Swedish mutation animals produce plaques at 14 months but with a different anatomical distribution than the Tg2576 cDNA-equivalent overexpressing mice. Most transgenic βAPP models employ neuron-specific/selective promoters. The results with the native βAPP promoter and introns suggest that βAPP splicing to produce isoforms and/or promoter activity in different brain regions or cell types such as glia can influence the development of pathology. This is a particularly important concept to consider when employing transgenic models to study mechanisms.

THE TAU HYPOTHESIS AND TAU PATHOLOGY

Since neurofibrillary pathology is the first lesion observed in most AD cases (see Characteristics of AD), often preceding amyloid plaques, and deranged tau function can be mechanistically related to impaired microtubular function, a logical hypothesis was that altered tau was the primary etiologic agent in AD, with Aβ as a secondary factor. The two competing dogmas attracted supporters and detractors, the "Tauists" and the "βAP-tists." Although the sequence of histopathological changes supported the preeminence of tau, the genetics of the familial, early-onset forms of AD highlighted the importance of Aβ.

Tau transgenics

The discovery of mutations in the tau gene in frontotemporal dementia-17 (FTDP-17) familial tauopathy opened up the possibility that similar advantage could be taken of tau mutants to model pathology as had been so useful with βAPP. There was also the chance to settle the long-standing debate over the primary insult in AD. Although familial forms of various tauopathies were mapped to the tau gene, no tau mutations have been linked to AD, despite ample tau deposition in neurofibrillary tangles in AD. Tau is expressed as multiple splice variants in humans such that up to six forms are produced in developmental-, tissue-, and cell-specific patterns. Abnormal polymerization of tau is caused by mutations in coding or intronic regions of the tau gene, each somehow resulting in a characteristic tangle morphology causing a recognizable clinical phenotype resulting in different diseases such as Pick's disease, progressive supranuclear palsy, and multiple system tauopathy. Both the fibril morphology and dementia profile differ from those found in AD. Aβ usually is not deposited in these diseases.

Unlike the case for mouse models of β-amyloidosis, generating murine neurofibrillary tangles that mimic those in humans has been more challenging. Unlike humans, which express 3- and 4-repeat tau, mice produce only the four-repeat form. Overexpression of a number of proteins such as tau kinases increases the phosphorylation and accumulation of tau in axons, but the phenotype seldom resembles that seen in AD (Tesseur *et al.*, 2000; Bian *et al.*, 2002). Transgenic mice expressing human tau protein produce tangle-like structures in the CNS (Lewis *et al.*, 2000; Gotz *et al.*, 2004). When co-expressed with mutant human βAPP transgenes (Lewis *et al.*, 2001; Oddo *et al.*, 2003a; Oddo *et al.*, 2003b), tangle-like pathology is exacerbated in these mice.

The fibril morphologies in tau-transgenic mice resemble human tauopathy in the disease from which the mutant tau was derived, not the twisted organization of true NFTs that are common in AD. In most instances, tau in transgenic mice is expressed and deposited in areas where it is not seen in AD and yet is missing from areas in which it is found in AD (Lewis *et al.*, 2001). Major pathology in these models occurs in the spinal cord and brain stem, with much less in cortical areas where the pathology is prominent in humans. Relative amounts of expression of the different splice variants seem to be part of the explanation. No Aβ deposits have been detected in tau-only transgenic models. The current state of tauopathy models is summarized by Lee *et al.* (2005).

Combined Aβ and tau pathology

Critical evidence consistent with a role for Aβ as a driving force in AD was obtained with mice doubly transgenic for βAPP and for P301L tau (Lewis *et al.*, 2001). Tg 2576 mice were crossed with JNPL3 mice carrying a four-repeat form of tau without the N-terminal repeats under control of the mouse prion promoter. Tau expression does not significantly alter regional Aβ deposition patterns, while βAPP expression results in tau deposition in AD-relevant areas where the tau is not deposited in the single tau transgenic animals. The morphology of the tau fibrils is not PHF-like, resembling, instead, the tauopathy from which the mutant tau had been derived. These observations and microinjection studies of Aβ(1–42) fibrils into P301L tau–expressing mice (Gotz *et al.*, 2001) indicate that Aβ, and not tauopathy, is the primary insult in AD. Tissue culture models are being used to tease apart the complex biochemical network that connects the two pathologies (Gotz *et al.*, 2004).

Triple transgenics (APP, PS1, P301L tau). Human βAPP Swedish mutant K670N/M671L and human tau 4R P301L cloned separately behind neuron-specific Thy1.2 promoters were co-injected into the pronucleus of oocytes of homozygous PS1 M146V knock-in mice in which the human sequence I145V and human mutation M146V had been engineered into the mouse gene behind its natural promoter (Oddo *et al.*, 2003a; Oddo *et al.*, 2003b). The βAPP and tau genes both incorporate at the same locus, greatly simplifying the breeding by ensuring that they are co-inherited. These animals develop synaptic dysfunction before plaques or tangles appear, and the deficits in LTP correlate with the accumulation of intraneuronal Aβ. The patterns and relative timing of Aβ and tau deposition, which are distinct, closely resemble those in AD brain. While closer to AD-like tangle morphology, the tau deposits have not been definitively characterized as NFTs. Interestingly, Aβ immunotherapy in these animals results in the clearance of amyloid plaques and of early, but not established, tau pathology (Oddo *et al.*, 2004).

Models Omitted

It is not possible in the space of this chapter to consider models of other important aspects of AD. These include recapitulation of brain inflammation, oxidative stress, and apolipoprotein E isotype effects, along with the role of cholesterol. Reviews on mouse models of these subjects in relation to AD are available (Eikelenboom *et al.*, 2002; Mattson, 2002; DeMattos, 2004).

Conclusions

The modeling of AD, much like the modeling of many other human diseases, has been partially successful, but is in need of further refinement. Many, but not all, of the aspects of the AD phenotype have been reproduced in animal models. It is too early to know whether the models will be predictive of therapeutic efficacy in humans of the different agents currently being tested. That is a hurdle that all models for testing interventions must clear. The models have already proven extremely valuable for hypothesis testing and exploration of molecular mechanisms of disease.

PROGRESS IN RECAPITULATING ALZHEIMER'S DISEASE

The original models for AD attempted to mimic the neurochemical deficits, mainly in the cholinergic pathways. With a better understanding of the neuropathological lesions at a molecular level, transgenic models were devised that recapitulated a surprising degree of AD pathology. These include reasonably faithful age dependence, brain region specificity, and appropriate behavioral effects. There is evidence of neuroinflammation in microglial activation, even though many of the mouse strains are deficient in the inflammatory response (Schwab *et al.*, 2004). There is also evidence of oxidative stress, and some of the neurochemical changes are similar to those in AD. Some of the behavioral changes in the βAPP overexpressing mice also resemble facets of early AD dementia.

DEFICIENCIES OF AD MODELS

The missing link in current animal models for AD is the lack of the profound neurodegeneration of AD. In the context of animal models of other diseases, as mentioned earlier, this is common. Often, different species model particular aspects of the human disease, but not others, so multiple models are used for each disease. A compounding factor for AD is that it is a disease of aging, and extreme age at that. Mice may simply not live long enough to produce the decrements in neuronal structure and function. Longer lived models, on the order of the human lifespan, that recapitulated the disease would be of academic and mechanistic interest, but not practical for testing therapeutic interventions. It is possible that critical pathways that couple insults such as Aβ aggregation to toxicity and neurodegeneration are deficient in mice, or that there is a compensating pathway. Processes that magnify the toxic effects of Aβ, such as inflammation, may be attenuated in mice. Compounding this could be an intrinsic difference in the plaque structure (Klunk *et al.*, 2004) or composition compared to the AD brain.

FUTURE OUTLOOK

Mouse models are likely to remain the workhorses for the *in vivo* modeling of AD pathogenesis. The advantages of speed, economy, and reasonably compelling lesion development are likely to improve as new models are developed and refined. There remains a disconnect between current models and the profound neurodegeneration that is prominent in AD. Filling this gap is the most important mechanistic need. Present models are sufficient for testing many of the current therapeutic avenues being explored. However, if time is an essential and immutable element in the ultimate manifestation of AD, and many years are required for the full phenotype to emerge, then the expression of AD-related transgenes in longer-lived species, such as nonhuman primates, could provide an important bridge between mouse models and the human disease. To this end, the expression of disease-related transgenes in adult animals via viral vectors, which has produced a remarkably Parkinsonian phenotype in nonhuman primates (Kirik *et al.*, 2003), has potential for more faithfully recapitulating the full neuropathological phenotype of AD. At the other end of the taxonomic spectrum, advances in modeling AD pathology in lower organisms such as fruit flies and worms will be a boon to testing mechanistic hypotheses at the cellular and molecular levels.

Since AD is a uniquely human disorder, the thoughtful integration of experimental information from cellular, nonmammalian and mammalian models will be needed to achieve a comprehensive view of the natural history of the Alzheimer's disease process.

REFERENCES

Bian, F., Nath, R., Sobocinski, G., Booher, R.N., Lipinski, W.J., Callahan, M.J., *et al.* (2002). Axonopathy, tau abnormalities, and dyskinesia, but no neurofibrillary tangles in p25-transgenic mice. *J Comp Neurol 446*, 257–266.

Boncristiano, S., Calhoun, M.E., Howard, V., Bondolfi, L., Kaeser, S.A., Wiederhold, K.H., *et al.* (2005). Neocortical synaptic bouton number is maintained despite robust amyloid deposition in APP23 transgenic mice. *Neurobiol Aging 26*, 607–613.

Borchelt, D.R., Ratovitski, T., van Lare, J., Lee, M.K., Gonzales, V., Jenkins, N.A., *et al.* (1997). Accelerated amyloid deposition in the brains of transgenic mice coexpressing mutant presenilin 1 and amyloid precursor proteins. *Neuron 19*, 939–945.

Borchelt, D.R., Thinakaran, G., Eckman, C.B., Lee, M.K., Davenport, F., Ratovitsky, T., *et al.* (1996). Familial Alzheimer's disease-linked presenilin 1 variants elevate Abeta1-42/1-40 ratio in vitro and in vivo. *Neuron 17*, 1005–1013.

Bussiere, T., Friend, P.D., Sadeghi, N., Wicinski, B., Lin, G.I., Bouras, C., *et al.* (2002). Stereologic assessment of the total cortical volume occupied by amyloid deposits and its relationship with cognitive status in aging and Alzheimer's disease. *Neuroscience 112*, 75–91.

Callahan, M.J., Lipinski, W.J., Bian, F., Durham, R.A., Pack, A., and Walker, L.C. (2001). Augmented senile plaque load in aged female beta-amyloid precursor protein-transgenic mice. *Am J Pathol 158*, 1173–1177.

Citron, M., Westaway, D., Xia, W., Carlson, G., Diehl, T., Levesque, G., *et al.* (1997). Mutant presenilins of Alzheimer's disease increase production of 42-residue amyloid beta-protein in both transfected cells and transgenic mice. *Nat Med 3*, 67–72.

Colle, M.A., Hauw, J.-J., Crespau, F., Uchihara, T., Akiyama, T., Checler, F., *et al.* (2000). Vascular and parenchymal Abeta deposition in the aging dog: Correlation with behavior. *Neurobiol Aging 21*, 695–704.

Cummings, J.L. (2004). Alzheimer's disease. *N Engl J Med 351*, 56–67.

Davis, J., Xu, F., Deane, R., Romanov, G., Previti, M., Zeigler, K., *et al.* (2004). Early-onset and robust cerebral microvascular accumulation of amyloid beta-protein in transgenic mice expressing low levels of a vasculotropic Dutch/Iowa mutant form of amyloid beta-protein precursor. *J Biol Chem 279*, 20296–20306.

DeMattos, R.B. (2004). Apolipoprotein E Dose-dependent modulation of beta-amyloid deposition in a transgenic mouse model of Alzheimer's disease. *J Mol Neurosci 23*, 255–262.

Dermaut, B., Kumar-Singh, S., Engelborghs, S., Theuns, J., Rademakers, R., Saerens, J., *et al.* (2004). A novel presenilin 1 mutation associated with Pick's disease but not beta-amyloid plaques. *Ann Neurol 55*, 617–626.

Driscoll, M., and Gerstbrein, B. (2003). Dying for a cause: Invertebrate genetics takes on human neurodegeneration. *Nat Rev Genet 4*, 181–194.

Duff, K., Eckman, C., Zehr, C., Yu, X., Prada, C.M., Perez-tur, J., *et al.* (1996). Increased amyloid-beta42(43) in brains of mice expressing mutant presenilin 1. *Nature 383*, 710–713.

Eikelenboom, P., Bate, C., Van Gool, W.A., Hoozemans, J.J., Rozemuller, J.M., Veerhuis, R., and Williams, A. (2002). Neuroinflammation in Alzheimer's disease and prion disease. *Glia 40*, 232–239.

Fonte, V., Kapulkin, V., Taft, A., Fluet, A., Friedman, D., and Link, C.D. (2002). Interaction of intracellular beta amyloid peptide with chaperone proteins. *Proc Natl Acad Sci USA 99*, 9439–9444.

Frackowiak, J., Miller, D.L., Potempska, A., Sukontasup, T., and Mazur-Kolecka, B. (2003). Secretion and accumulation of Abeta by brain vascular smooth muscle cells from AbetaPP-Swedish transgenic mice. *J Neuropathol Exp Neurol 62*, 685–696.

Frackowiak, J., Potempska, A., LeVine, H., Haske, T., Dickson, D., and Mazur-Kolecka, B. (2005). Extracellular deposits of Abeta produced in cultures of Alzheimer disease brain vascular smooth muscle cells. *J Neuropathol Exp Neurol 64*, 82–90.

Frautschy, S.A., Yang, F., Calderon, L., and Cole, G.M. (1996). Rodent models of Alzheimer's disease: Rat Abeta infusion approaches to amyloid deposits. *Neurobiol Aging 17*, 311–321.

Games, D., Adams, D., Alessandrini, R., Barbour, R., Berthelette, P., Blackwell, C., *et al.* (1995). Alzheimer-type neuropathology in transgenic mice overexpressing V717F beta-amyloid precursor protein. *Nature 373*, 523–527.

Geula, C., Wu, C.K., Saroff, D., Lorenzo, A., Yuan, M., and Yankner, B.A. (1998). Aging renders the brain vulnerable to amyloid beta-protein neurotoxicity. *Nat Med 4*, 827–831.

Gotz, J., Chen, F., van Dorpe, J., and Nitsch, R.M. (2001). Formation of neurofibrillary tangles in P301l tau transgenic mice induced by Abeta 42 fibrils. *Science 293*, 1491–1495.

Gotz, J., Schild, A., Hoerndli, F., and Pennanen, L. (2004). Amyloid-induced neurofibrillary tangle formation in Alzheimer's disease: Insight from transgenic mouse and tissue-culture models. *Int J Dev Neurosci 22*, 453–465.

Hardy, J., and Selkoe, D.J. (2002). The amyloid hypothesis of Alzheimer's disease: Progress and problems on the road to therapeutics. *Science 297*, 353–356.

Hauw, J.-J., and Duyckaerts, C. (2001). Alzheimer's Disease. In Duckett, S., and De La Torre, J.C. (Eds.), *Pathology of the Aging Human Nervous System*, pp. 207–263. New York: Oxford University Press.

Herzig, M.C., Winkler, D.T., Burgermeister, P., Pfeifer, M., Kohler, E., Schmidt, S.D., *et al.* (2004). Abeta is targeted to the vasculature in a mouse model of hereditary cerebral hemorrhage with amyloidosis. *Nat Neurosci 7*, 954–960.

Hof, P.R., Gilissen, E.P., Sherwood, C.C., Duan, H., Lee, P.W.H., Delman, B.N., *et al.* (2002). Comparative neuropathology of brain aging in primates. In Erwin, J.M., and Hof, P.R. (Eds.), *Aging in Nonhuman Primates*, pp. 130–154. Basel: Karger.

Holcomb, L., Gordon, M.N., McGowan, E., Yu, X., Benkovic, S., Jantzen, P., *et al.* (1998). Accelerated Alzheimer-type phenotype in transgenic mice carrying both mutant amyloid precursor protein and presenilin 1 transgenes. *Nat Med 4*, 97–100.

Hsiao, K., Chapman, P., Nilsen, S., Eckman, C., Harigaya, Y., Younkin, S., *et al.* (1996). Correlative memory deficits, Abeta elevation, and amyloid plaques in transgenic mice. *Science 274*, 99–102.

Jucker, M., Walker, L.C., Martin, L.J., Kitt, C.A., Kleinman, H.K., *et al.* (1992). Age-associated inclusions in normal and transgenic mouse brain. *Science 255*, 1443–1445.

Kayed, R., Head, E., Thompson, J.L., McIntire, T.M., Milton, S.C., Cotman, C.W., and Glabe, C.G. (2003). Common structure of soluble amyloid oligomers implies common mechanism of pathogenesis. *Science 300*, 486–489.

Kirik, D., Annett, L., Burger, C., Muzyczka, N., Mandel, R.J., and Bjorklund, A. (2003). Nigrostriatal alpha-synucleinopathy induced by viral vector-mediated overexpression of human alpha-synuclein: A new primate model of Parkinson's disease. *PNAS 100*, 2884–2889.

Klunk, W.E., Lopresti, B.J., Debnath, M.L., Holt, D.P., Wang, Y., Huang, G.-F., *et al.* (2004). Amyloid deposits in transgenic PS1/APP mice do not bind the amyloid PET tracer, PIB, in the same manner as human brain amyloid. *Neurobiology of Aging 25*, 232.

Lacor, P.N., Buniel, M.C., Chang, L., Fernandez, S.J., Gong, Y., Viola, K.L., *et al.* (2004). Synaptic targeting by Alzheimer's-related amyloid beta oligomers. *J Neurosci 24*, 10191–10200.

Lamb, B.A., Bardel, K.A., Kulnane, L.S., Anderson, J.J., Holtz, G., Wagner, S.L., *et al.* (1999). Amyloid production and deposition in mutant amyloid precursor protein and presenilin-1 yeast artificial chromosome transgenic mice. *Nat Neurosci 2*, 695–697.

Lee, V.M., Goedert, M., and Trojanowski, J.Q. (2001). Neurodegenerative tauopathies. *Annu Rev Neurosci 24*, 1121–1159.

Lee, V.M., Kenyon, T.K., and Trojanowski, J.Q. (2005). Transgenic animal models of tauopathies. *Biochim Biophys Acta 1739*, 251–259.

Lewis, J., Dickson, D.W., Lin, W.L., Chisholm, L., Corral, A., Jones, G., *et al.* (2001). Enhanced neurofibrillary degeneration in transgenic mice expressing mutant tau and APP. *Science 293*, 1487–1491.

Lewis, J., McGowan, E., Rockwood, J., Melrose, H., Nacharaju, P., Van Slegtenhorst, M., *et al.* (2000). Neurofibrillary tangles, amyotrophy and progressive motor disturbance in mice expressing mutant (P301L) tau protein. *Nat Genet 25*, 402–405.

Marjaux, E., Hartmann, D., and De Strooper, B. (2004). Presenilins in memory, Alzheimer's disease, and therapy. *Neuron 42*, 189–192.

Mattson, M.P. (2002). Oxidative stress, perturbed calcium homeostasis, and immune dysfunction in Alzheimer's disease. *J Neurovirol 8*, 539–550.

Milgram, N.W., Head, E., Zicker, S.C., Ikeda-Douglas, C.J., Murphey, H.L., Muggenburg, B., *et al.* (2005). Learning ability in aged beagle dogs is preserved by behavioral enrichment and dietary fortification: A two-year longitudinal study. *Neurobiol Aging 26*, 77–90.

Oddo, S., Billings, L., Kesslak, J.P., Cribbs, D.H., and LaFerla, F.M. (2004). Abeta immunotherapy leads to clearance of early, but not late, hyperphosphorylated tau aggregates via the proteasome. *Neuron 43*, 321–332.

Oddo, S., Caccamo, A., Kitazawa, M., Tseng, B.P., and LaFerla, F.M. (2003a). Amyloid deposition precedes tangle formation in a triple transgenic model of Alzheimer's disease. *Neurobiol Aging 24*, 1063–1070.

Oddo, S., Caccamo, A., Shepherd, J.D., Murphy, M.P., Golde, T.E., Kayed, R., *et al.* (2003b). Triple-transgenic model of Alzheimer's disease with plaques and tangles: intracellular Abeta and synaptic dysfunction. *Neuron 39*, 409–421.

Peel, A.L., and Bredesen, D.E. (2003). Activation of the cell stress kinase PKR in Alzheimer's disease and human amyloid precursor protein transgenic mice. *Neurobiol Dis 14*, 52–62.

Poirier, J. (1994). Apolipoprotein E in animal models of CNS injury and in Alzheimer's disease. *Trends Neurosci 17*, 525–530.

Rankin, C.H. (2004). Invertebrate learning: What can't a worm learn? *Curr Biol 14*, R617–618.

Reilly, J.F., Games, D., Rydel, R.E., Freedman, S., Schenk, D., Young, W.G., *et al.* (2003). Amyloid deposition in the hippocampus and entorhinal cortex: Quantitative analysis of a transgenic mouse model. *Proc Natl Acad Sci USA 100*, 4837–4842.

Revesz, T., Ghiso, J., Lashley, T., Plant, G., Rostagno, A., Frangione, B., and Holton, J.L. (2003). Cerebral amyloid angiopathies: A pathologic, biochemical, and genetic view. *J Neuropathol Exp Neurol 62*, 885–898.

Rohrbough, J., O'Dowd, D.K., Baines, R.A., and Broadie, K. (2003). Cellular bases of behavioral plasticity: Establishing and modifying synaptic circuits in the *Drosophila* genetic system. *J Neurobiol 54*, 254–271.

Schonheit, B., Zarski, R., and Ohm, T.G. (2004). Spatial and temporal relationships between plaques and tangles in Alzheimer-pathology. *Neurobiol Aging 25*, 697–711.

Schwab, C., Hosokawa, M., and McGeer, P.L. (2004). Transgenic mice overexpressing amyloid beta protein are an incomplete model of Alzheimer disease. *Exp Neurol 188*, 52–64.

Siman, R., Reaume, A.G., Savage, M.J., Trusko, S., Lin, Y.G., Scott, R.W., and Flood, D.G. (2000). Presenilin-1 P264L knock-in mutation: Differential effects on abeta production, amyloid deposition, and neuronal vulnerability. *J Neurosci 20*, 8717–8726.

Siwak, C.T., Tapp, P.D., Head, E., Zicker, S.C., Murphey, H.L., Muggenburg, B.A., *et al.* (2005). Chronic antioxidant and mitochondrial cofactor administration improves discrimination learning in aged but not young dogs. *Prog Neuropsychopharmacol Biol Psychiatry 29*, 461–469.

Studzinski, C.M., Araujo, J.A., and Milgram, N.W. (2005). The canine model of human cognitive aging and dementia: Pharmacological validity of the model for assessment of human cognitive-enhancing drugs. *Prog Neuropsychopharmacol Biol Psychiatry 29*, 489–498.

Tapp, P.D., Siwak, C.T., Gao, F.Q., Chiou, J.Y., Black, S.E., Head, E., *et al.* (2004). Frontal lobe volume, function, and beta-amyloid pathology in a canine model of aging. *J Neurosci 24*, 8205–8213.

Tesseur, I., Van Dorpe, J., Spittaels, K., Van den Haute, C., Moechars, D., and Van Leuven, F. (2000). Expression of human apolipoprotein E4 in neurons causes hyperphosphorylation of protein tau in the brains of transgenic mice. *Am J Pathol 156*, 951–964.

Torp, R., Head, E., Milgram, N.W., Hahn, F., Ottersen, O.P., and Cotman, C.W. (2000). Ultrastructural evidence of fibrillar beta-amyloid associated with neuronal membranes in behaviorally characterized aged dog brains. *Neuroscience 96*, 495–506.

Vloeberghs, E., Van Dam, D., Engelborghs, S., Nagels, G., Staufenbiel, M., and De Deyn, P.P. (2004). Altered circadian locomotor activity in APP23 mice: A model for BPSD disturbances. *Eur J Neurosci 20*, 2757–2766.

Voytko, M.L., and Tinkler, G.P. (2004). Cognitive function and its neural mechanisms in nonhuman primate models of aging, Alzheimer disease, and menopause. *Front Biosci 9*, 1899–1914.

Walker, L.C., Callahan, M.J., Bian, F., Durham, R.A., Roher, A.E., and Lipinski, W.J. (2002). Exogenous induction of cerebral beta-amyloidosis in betaAPP-transgenic mice. *Peptides 23*, 1241–1247.

Walker, L.C., and Cork, L.C. (1999). The neurobiology of aging in nonhuman primates. In Terry, R.D., Katzman, R., Bick, K.L., and Sisodia, S.S. (Eds.), *Alzheimer Disease*, pp. 233–243. Philadelphia: Lippincott Williams and Wilkins.

Walker, L.C., Ibegbu, C.C., Todd, C.W., Robinson, H.L., Jucker, M., LeVine, H.R., and Gandy, S. (2005). Emerging prospects for the disease-modifying treatment of Alzheimer's disease. *Biochem Pharmacol 69*, 1001–1008.

Walker, M.L. (1995). Menopause in female rhesus monkeys. *Am J Primatology 35*, 59–71.

Walsh, D.M., and Selkoe, D.J. (2004). Oligomers on the brain: The emerging role of soluble protein aggregates in neurodegeneration. *Protein Pept Lett 11*, 213–228.

Wegiel, J., Wisniewski, H.M., Dziewiatkowski, J., Tarnawski, M., Nowakowski, J., Dziewiatkowska, A., and Soltysiak, Z. (1995). The origin of amyloid in cerebral vessels of aged dogs. *Brain Res 705*, 225–234.

Wisniewski, T., Dowjat, W.K., Buxbaum, J.D., Khorkova, O., Efthimiopoulos, S., Kulczycki, J., *et al.* (1998). A novel Polish presenilin-1 mutation (P117L) is associated with familial Alzheimer's disease and leads to death as early as the age of 28 years. *Neuroreport 9*, 217–221.

12

Age-Related Hippocampal Dysfunction: Early Alzheimer's Disease vs. Normal Aging

Scott A. Small

As we age, all of us will experience an inexorable slide into forgetfulness. Age-related memory decline localizes, in part, to the hippocampal formation, a brain circuit made up of separate but interconnected hippocampal subregions. Human studies have established that Alzheimer's disease targets the hippocampal circuit early in its course, and since Alzheimer's disease affects older individuals it is one cause of age-related hippocampal dysfunction. Animal studies, however, have established that the aging process itself targets the hippocampal circuit, contributing to age-related hippocampal dysfunction observed in all mammalian species. These independent observations have led to a continued debate among investigators of the aging human brain, summarized by the following questions: Is age-related hippocampal dysfunction in humans etiologically homogeneous, or is age-related hippocampal dysfunction caused by both AD and by normal aging? If age-related hippocampal dysfunction is caused by both AD and normal aging how can they be distinguished from each other? If age-related hippocampal dysfunction is caused by both AD and normal aging what are the molecular underpinnings of each? This chapter will review a series of recent studies that rely on in vivo imaging, the results of which have begun addressing these important questions.

Introduction

As commonly experienced, and as neuropsychologically documented, our cognitive abilities decline with advancing aging (Zelinski and Burnight, 1997). Luckily for us, age-related cognitive decline is not diffuse, but rather aging targets select cognitive domains. The ability to consciously memorize new and complex experiences—for example, learning the name of a new acquaintance—is one cognitive domain particularly sensitive to the aging process (Small, Stern *et al.*, 1999). This cognitive ability requires the hippocampal formation (Amaral and Witter, 1989), a brain structure nestled deep in the temporal lobes (Figure 12.1).

As clinicians, we are interested in the etiology of age-related hippocampal dysfunction. One cause is undoubtedly Alzheimer's disease (AD), a gradually progressive disorder that typically manifests in later life. Anatomically, AD begins by targeting the hippocampal formation, presenting as mild forgetfulness, but ultimately sweeps throughout the neocortical mantle, devastating most cognitive abilities in its wake (Masur, Sliwinski *et al.*, 1994; Jacobs, Sano *et al.*, 1995) and leading to dementia. Within each affected area, AD progressed through different pathophysiological stages. Early on, AD causes neurons to malfunction (Selkoe, 2002), manifesting as metabolic and synaptic failure, before causing neurons to die. Accordingly, a distinction is sometimes made between the early "cell sickness" stage versus the later "cell death" stage of AD (Small, 2005).

Not every aging individual with age-related hippocampal dysfunction progresses to AD dementia, raising the possibility that the aging process itself might affect hippocampal function. A wide range of nonhuman studies support this possibility (Barnes, 1994; Gallagher and Rapp, 1997; Erickson and Barnes, 2003). All aging nonhuman mammals manifest hippocampal dysfunction, yet no species besides our own develops AD. Thus, all species develop non-AD age-related memory decline, and it would seem unlikely that humans would be spared this species-wide process. Nevertheless, the possibility still exists that in humans age-related hippocampal dysfunction uniformly reflects the early stages of AD, and that if humans live long enough all will develop full-fledged AD.

This chapter will review a combination of human and animal studies that have set out to address two interrelated questions: First, is age-related hippocampal dysfunction etiologically homogeneous—uniformly reflecting the early stages of AD—or is age-related hippocampal caused by both AD and by normal aging? Second, if age-related hippocampal dysfunction is caused by both AD and normal aging, how can they be distinguished from each other?

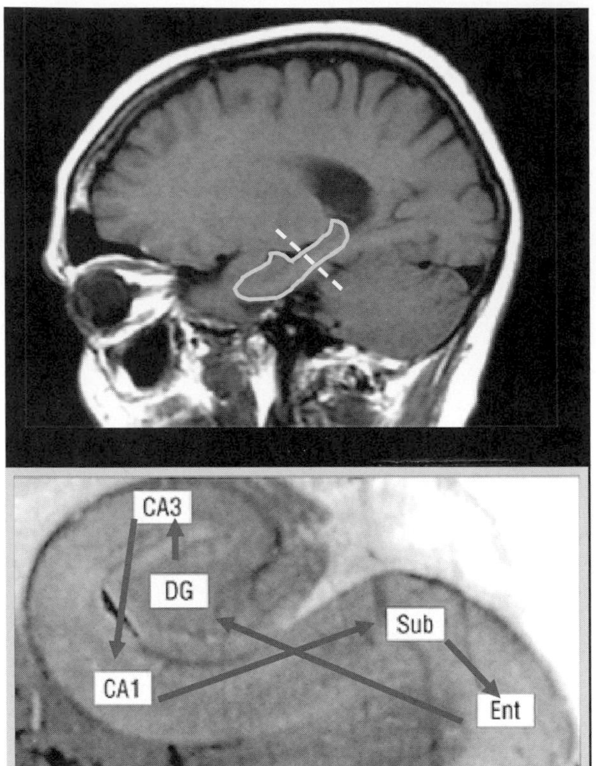

Figure 12.1. The functional organization of the hippocampal formation. The hippocampal formation is a cylindrical structure located in the medial temporal lobes (demarcated in the upper panel). The microanatomy of the hippocampal formation (bottom panel) is best appreciated by viewing a transverse slice through the body of the hippocampal formation (stippled line in the upper panel). The hippocampal formation is made up of the anatomically and molecularly distinct subregions—the entorhinal cortex (EC), the dentate gyrus (DG) and the CA1 and CA3 subfields (bottom panel). The hippocampal subregions are interconnected, giving rise to the hippocampal circuit. The circuit organization of the hippocampal formation accounts for why dysfunction in any individual hippocampal subregion will equivalently interrupt the circuit, causing overlapping memory deficits. The molecular organization of the hippocampal formation accounts for why each hippocampal subregion is differentially vulnerable to mechanisms of dysfunction.

The Functional and Molecular Organization of the Hippocampal Formation

In theory, the microanatomy of the hippocampal formation may provide an answer to both questions. The hippocampal formation is a complex structure made up of separate but interconnected subregions (Amaral and Witter, 1989): the entorhinal cortex, the dentate gyrus, the CA1 and CA3 subfields, and the subiculum (Figure 12.1). Because the subregions are connected in a unidirectional manner, the hippocampal formation functions as a circuit. Thus, a lesion in any individual hippocampal subregion will equivalently interrupt the circuit, leading to overlapping memory deficits.

Importantly, each hippocampal subregion houses a distinct population of neurons, unique in their molecular expression profiles (Zhao, Lein *et al.*, 2001). It is this molecular uniqueness that accounts for why each hippocampal subregion is differentially vulnerable to mechanisms of dysfunction (Small, 2001). So, for example, transient hypoxemia causes memory deficits by targeting the CA1 subfield because of high expression of glutamate receptors in CA1 neurons, while, in contrast, an adrenalectomy causes overlapping memory deficits by targeting the dentate gyrus because neurons in this subregion express relatively high concentrations of corticosteroid receptors.

Based on this anatomical and molecular organization, the following hypothesis can be made: If AD and normal aging are indeed pathologically separate processes, then the odds are that they should targets different hippocampal subregions (Small, 2001). Establishing whether this anatomical dissociation exists, therefore, is an effective approach for answering the first question (Is age-related hippocampal dysfunction etiologically homogeneous?); and if it does exist, then this anatomical dissociation can potentially be used in dissociating one cause from the other.

A Classification of Brain Imaging

In order to test this hypothesis, an imaging technique is needed that fulfills two requirements. First, a technique needs to be sensitive to neuronal function—not just structure. As already mentioned, the early stages of AD are characterized by cell sickness, not cell death. Animal studies have established that insofar as aging causes memory decline, it does so by interrupting neuronal physiology—again, a form of cell sickness—with a notable absence of cell loss (Rapp and Gallagher, 1996). Second, the technique needs to have sufficient spatial resolution to interrogate the hippocampus as a circuit. Because of its circuit organization, a lesion in one hippocampal subregion will secondarily affect the function of other subregions, and will affect the circuit as a whole. Thus, in order to pinpoint the primary subregion targeted by a particular mechanism of dysfunction, a technique needs to assess each hippocampal subregion individually but also simultaneously to account for circuitwide effects.

With these goals in mind, a number of imaging approaches have been developed that have fulfilled both requirements—sensitivity to neuronal function and resolution sufficient to visualize individual hippocampal subregions (Small, 2003). As in any field, a shorthanded terminology is typically used to describe different imaging approaches, and terms are often confusing or even misleading. In this regard, a brief review of the field of functional imaging is worthwhile, pinning down which aspects of the brain are actually being imaged (Figure 12.2).

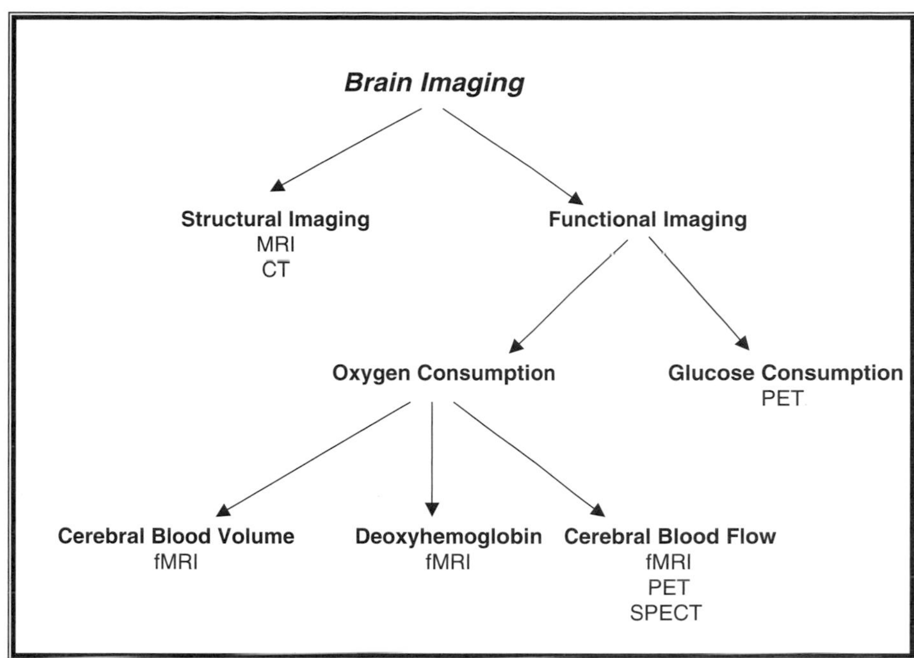

Figure 12.2. Classification of brain imaging. Brain imaging is dichotomized into structural versus functional imaging. Brain structure is imaged using either magnetic resonance imaging (MRI) or computerized tomography (CT). Functional imaging indirectly assesses regional energy metabolism by relying on the neuronal consumption of two ingredients of ATP production—glucose and oxygen. Glucose consumption is imaged with positron emission tomography (PET). Oxygen consumption is measured by imaging its three correlates—cerebral blood volume (CBV), deoxyhemoglobin content, or cerebral blood flow (CBF). CBV and deoxyhemoglobin content can be imaged with functional magnetic resonance imaging (fMRI), and CBF can imaged with fMRI, PET, or single photon emission tomography (SPECT). Among these, CBV and deoxyhemoglobin content imaged with fMRI are best suited for pinpointing functional defects in individual hippocampal subregions.

Historically, *in vivo* imaging has been subdivided into *structural imaging*, such as magnetic resonance imaging (MRI) or computerized axial tomography (CT) imaging, versus *functional imaging*—single photon emission tomography (SPECT), positron emission tomography (PET) or functional magnetic resonance imaging (fMRI). Of course, in principle, functional imaging techniques are more likely to be sensitive to cell sickness. What exactly is meant by the "function" in functional imaging? Since the early studies performed by Kety and Schmidt (Small, 2004), functional brain imaging has come to imply a method that detects changes in regional energy metabolism. Energy metabolism is best defined as the rate with which cells produce ATP, which in neurons requires the consumption of oxygen and glucose from the blood stream. Visualizing ATP directly is challenging, but imaging techniques have been developed that can visualize correlates of oxygen and glucose consumption. With the use of radiolabeled glucose, PET can quantify the regional rates of glucose uptake. In contrast, MRI-based techniques have typically relied on the second ingredient of ATP production, oxygen consumption, to visualize correlates of energy metabolism. Because of hemodynamic coupling, oxygen consumption is correlated with cerebral blood flow, cerebral blood volume, and deoxyhemoglobin content, and all these correlates can be estimated with MRI.

The cell-sickness stage of any disease typically affects the basal metabolic rate of oxygen consumption, and relying on the basal state to map anatomical sites of dysfunction enhances parametric quantification and spatial resolution. Indeed, the basal changes of energy metabolism associated with disease have been detected relying on all metabolic correlates—glucose uptake, CBF, CBV, and deoxyhemoglobin content. Among these variables, however, only MRI measures of CBV and deoxyhemoglobin content can achieve the spatial resolution required to visualize individual hippocampal subregions. Indeed, studies have used MRI measures of basal CBV or deoxyhemoglobin content to investigate the hippocampal circuit in aging and AD, and these will be reviewed in the next sections.

Human Studies Interrogating the Hippocampal Circuit in AD and Aging

By quantifying cell loss in postmortem tissue of AD patients, studies have suggested that either the entorhinal cortex or the CA1 subfield is the hippocampal subregion most vulnerable to AD (Braak and Braak, 1996; Fukutani, Cairns *et al.*, 2000; Price, Ko *et al.*, 2001; Shoghi-Jadid, Small *et al.*, 2002; Giannakopoulos, Herrmann *et al.*, 2003; Schonheit, Zarski *et al.*, 2004). In many of these studies, the entorhinal cortex and the CA1 subfield were not assessed simultaneously, accounting in part for the reported inconsistencies. More generally, however, isolating the hippocampal subregion most vulnerable to AD is difficult relying on postmortem studies alone. Not only are postmortem series biased against the earliest and most discriminatory stages of disease, but these studies cannot assess the cell-sickness stage of AD (Selkoe, 2002).

As discussed above, variants of fMRI sensitive to basal correlates of neuronal function are well suited to aid in resolving this debate. In one study, an MRI measure sensitive to basal levels of deoxyhemoglobin was used to assess the hippocampal subregions in patients with AD dementia compared to age-matched controls (Small, Nava *et al.*, 2000). This MRI measure has proven capable to detect cell sickness in individual hippocampal subregions. Univariate analysis revealed that normalized signal intensity was reduced in all hippocampal subregions in patients compared to controls. Nevertheless, when the hippocampus was analyzed as a circuit—namely, using a multivariate model to analyze signals from all hippocampal subregions simultaneously—the entorhinal cortex was found to be the primary site of dysfunction in AD (Small, Nava *et al.*, 2000).

This study suggests that the entorhinal cortex, not the CA1 subfield, is the hippocampal subregion most vulnerable to AD—agreeing with some, though not all, postmortem studies. Nevertheless, the patients assessed in this study already had full-blown dementia, indicating that they had already progressed from the cell-sickness to the cell-death stage of AD. Furthermore, this study does not inform us about the hippocampal subregions most vulnerable to normal aging.

Both of these issues were addressed in a second study, in which 70 subjects across the age span—from 20 to 88 years of age—were imaged with the same MRI measure (Small, Tsai *et al.*, 2002). Importantly, all subjects were healthy. The older age groups in particular were carefully screened against any evidence of dementia. The starting assumption made in this study was that some of the older subjects were in the earliest stage of AD and some subjects were aging normally. The question was how to make this distinction. Remember, there is no independent indicator to determine who had early AD or not. This is true even if the hippocampal formation of all subjects could be examined postmortem, because, as mentioned, the earliest stages of AD may be invisible to the microscope. Instead, formal parametric criteria were used to distinguish a "pathological pattern" of decline (i.e., related to Alzheimer's disease) versus a "normal pattern" of decline. Specifically, since the effect of normal aging on the brain is, by definition, a stochastic process, the variance of signal intensity among an older age group should be equal to the variance among a younger age group, although a shift in the mean is expected. In contrast, since it is a disease, AD should affect a subgroup within an older age group, which should significantly broaden the variance of signal intensity compared to a younger age group.

Applying this and other criteria, the results of this study showed that age-related changes in the entorhinal cortex fulfilled criteria for pathological decline; in contrast, age-related changes in the dentate gyrus, and to a lesser extent in the subiculum, fulfilled criteria for normal aging (Small, Tsai *et al.*, 2002). These findings not only confirm but also extend the results of the previous study. First, the entorhinal cortex indeed appears to be the hippocampal subregion most vulnerable to AD, even during the early cell-sickness stage. Second, these findings provided the first evidence that the dentate gyrus might be the hippocampal subregion most vulnerable to normal aging.

This study had a number of limitations. First, despite the strict criteria, independent verification of which older subjects did or did not have early AD was not possible. Second, although the MRI measure used is sensitive to basal deoxyhemoglobin levels, these images are also sensitive to other, nonmetabolic, tissue constituents that are potential confounds (Small, Wu *et al.*, 2000; Small, 2003).

These potential limitations were addressed in a third study. First, a cohort of aging individuals was needed that indisputably were free of AD. Because this cohort is difficult, or even impossible, to identify in human subjects, we turned to aging nonhuman primates instead. Like all mammals, monkeys develop age-related hippocampal dysfunction, yet they do not develop the known molecular or histological hallmarks of AD. Second, because of the stated limitations of imaging techniques sensitive to deoxyhemoglobin content, we relied on MRI to generate regional measures of cerebral blood volume (CBV). Previous studies have established that CBV is a hemodynamic variable tightly correlated with brain metabolism, capable of detecting brain dysfunction in the hippocampus and other brain regions (Gonzalez, Fischman *et al.*, 1995; Harris, Lewis *et al.*, 1998; Wu, Bruening *et al.*, 1999; Bozzao, Floris *et al.*, 2001).

In the third study, the hippocampal subregions of 14 rhesus monkeys were imaged across the age span from 7 to 31 years of age (Small, Chawla *et al.*, 2004). In a remarkable parallel to the previous human study, age-related decline in CBV was observed only in the dentate gyrus, and to a lesser extent the subiculum. Notably, CBV measured from the entorhinal cortex and the CA1 subregion remained stable across the life span. Indeed, when all subregions were analyzed simultaneously—in accordance with the circuit organization of the hippocampus—the dentate gyrus was the primary subregion that declined with age. Furthermore, since all monkeys were assessed cognitively, we found that a decline in dentate gyrus CBV was the only subregion that correlated with a decline in memory performance (Small, Chawla *et al.*, 2004).

Despite the reliance on CBV to investigate aging monkeys, this third study also had a number of limitations. The first limitation applies to all functional imaging: As derived from Fick's principle (Small, 2004), all hemodynamic variables—deoxyhemoglobin, CBV, or cerebral blood flow (CBF)—are correlates of oxygen metabolism; nevertheless, they are only *indirect* correlates. The possibility always exists that these measures are confounded by changes in vascular physiology, and not underlying neuronal physiology. Thus, we cannot exclude the possibility that there is something unique to the vascular system within the dentate gyrus that caused shrinkage of CBV, independent of dentate gyrus physiologic dysfunction. The second limitation of the monkey MRI study has to do with the cellular complexity of any brain subregion, including the dentate gyrus. Although the granule cells are the primary neurons of the dentate gyrus, the dentate gyrus contains other types of neurons as well as glial cells. Even if the CBV measure does reflect underlying cellular function, MRI cannot be relied on to isolate the cells that govern this observed effect.

A fourth study was designed to address these concerns. Here, *in vitro* imaging was used, directly visualizing correlates of neuronal physiology. Aging rats were investigated, who like humans and monkeys develop age-related hippocampal dysfunction. Immunocytochemisty was used to visualize the behaviorally-induced expression of *Arc* in the hippocampal subregions of aging rats. *Arc* is an immediate early gene whose expression has been shown to correlate with spike activity and with long-term plasticity in hippocampal neurons (Guzowski, McNaughton *et al.*, 1999; Guzowski, Lyford *et al.*, 2000; Guzowski, Setlow *et al.*, 2001). Rats of different ages were allowed to explore a novel place and sacrificed and processed for *Arc* staining. *Arc* expression was quantified in the granule cells of the dentate gyrus and in the pyramidal neurons of the CA1 and CA3 subregions. The dentate gyrus was the only hippocampal subregion whose neurons were found to have a significant age-related decline in *Arc* expression (Small, Chawla *et al.*, 2004). Thus, this study confirms and extends the prior studies, showing that it is in fact neuronal, not vascular, physiology that underlies the aging effect. Moreover, this study established that aging primarily targets the granule cells of the dentate gyrus.

To summarize, by using different imaging techniques across three different mammalian species (Small, Tsai *et al.*, 2002; Small, Pierce *et al.*, 2003), a consensus has emerged from these complementary studies: That the dentate gyrus is the hippocampal subregion differentially vulnerable to the aging process, and that it is the primary subregion underlying age-related hippocampal dysfunction and memory decline.

Conclusions

By interrogating the functional integrity of the hippocampal circuit in humans and animals, a double anatomical dissociation has emerged distinguishing early AD from normal aging. During its earliest stages, AD targets the entorhinal cortex and spares the dentate gyrus, while, in contrast, normal aging spares the entorhinal cortex but targets the dentate gyrus (Figure 12.3).

This anatomical profiling has three important implications. First, the anatomical dissociation establishes that AD and normal aging are pathogenically separate processes, forevermore putting an end to the possibility that age-related memory decline might solely represent AD. Second, the anatomical dissociation, and the ability to visualize this dissociation in living subjects, can be exploited as a diagnostic tool. Although we currently do not have effective treatments for AD, on theoretical

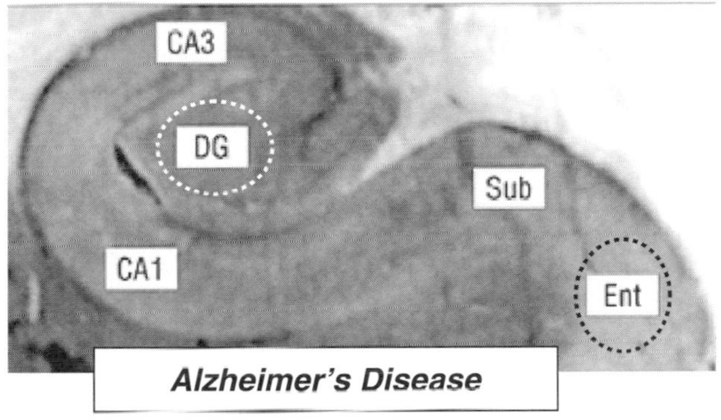

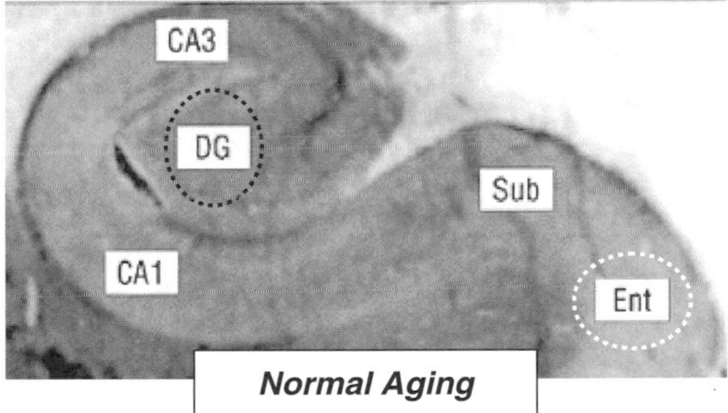

Figure 12.3. A double-anatomical dissociation distinguishes early Alzheimer's disease from normal aging. Alzheimer's disease targets the neurons of the entorhinal cortex with relative sparing of the neurons of the dentate gyrus. In contrast, normal aging targets the neurons of the dentate gyrus with relative sparing of the neurons of the entorhinal cortex. This dissociation establishes that Alzheimer's disease and normal aging are separate processes, and that both contribute to age-related hippocampal dysfunction. Furthermore, this dissociation, and the ability to visualize dysfunction in individual hippocampal subregions in living subjects, provide a method for distinguishing the early stages of Alzheimer's disease from normal age-related hippocampal dysfunction. Finally, this dissociation sets the stage for uncovering the molecular underpinnings of both Alzheimer's disease and normal age-related memory decline.

grounds arresting or even reversing the cell-sickness stage of AD is more likely than treating the cell-death stage of AD. Currently, relying on cognitive measures alone, we cannot accurately diagnose AD during its early cell-sickness stage because it cognitively overlaps with normal aging. Imaging techniques that can assess the functional integrity of the hippocampal subregions—in particular, the entorhinal cortex and the dentate gyrus—are well suited to achieve this diagnostic goal. Testing the diagnostic capabilities of any technique requires large-scale, epidemiologically rigorous, prospective studies. One such study is currently underway, testing whether the imaging approaches discussed in this chapter can be used to diagnose AD during its earliest stages.

Finally, pinpointing the hippocampal neurons most vulnerable to AD and to aging is a required first step for uncovering the molecular causes of each process. By isolating the molecular defects that underlie the rare autosomal-dominant form of AD, and by expressing these molecules in cell culture and in transgenic mice, tremendous strides have been made uncovering the molecular biology of AD. Nevertheless, the primary molecules whose defects underlie autosomal-dominant AD are normal in sporadic AD, the common form that accounts for over 95% of all cases. Thus, the primary molecular defects of the vast majority of AD remain unknown. Pinpointing the entorhinal cortex as the site of greatest vulnerability provides an anatomical handle with which to tackle this problem. Specifically, comparing the molecular profiles of the entorhinal cortex of affected and unaffected brains, at the mRNA or protein level, holds great promise for uncovering heretofore unidentified pathogenic molecules underlying sporadic AD. In a similar fashion, mapping age-related changes in the molecular profiles of the dentate gyrus, among healthy brains, may lead to insights into the molecular causes of memory decline associated with normal aging.

Age-related hippocampal dysfunction has emerged as a serious societal problem. As life expectancy is expanding, most of us do not simply want to live longer, but rather we would like to age with cognitive grace, remaining intellectually engaged in our information-rich environments. As discussed in this chapter, and in accordance with fundamental principles of clinical neuroscience, pinpointing the population of neurons differentially vulnerable to aging and to AD is an important first step towards developing effective diagnostics and, one day, even ameliorating the age-related slide into forgetfulness.

Recommended Resources

1. Erickson, C.A., and Barnes, C.A.: The neurobiology of memory changes in normal aging. *Exp Gerontol* 2003, *38*:61–9.
2. Small, S.A.: Age-related memory decline; current concepts and future directions. *Archives of Neurology* 2001, *58*:360–364.
3. Gallagher, M., and Rapp, P.R.: The use of animal models to study the effects of aging on cognition. *Annu Rev Psychol* 1997, *48*:339–370.

ACKNOWLEDGMENTS

Dr. Small's work is supported in part by federal grants AG07232 and AG08702, the Beeson Faculty Scholar Award from the American Federation of Aging, the McKnight Neuroscience of Brain Disorders Award, and the McDonnell Foundation.

REFERENCES

Amaral, D.G., and M.P. Witter (1989). "The three-dimensional organization of the hippocampal formation: A review of anatomical data." *Neuroscience 31(3)*: 571–591.

Barnes, C.A. (1994). "Normal aging: Regionally specific changes in hippocampal synaptic transmission." *Trends Neurosci 17(1)*: 13–18.

Bozzao, A., R. Floris, *et al.* (2001). "Diffusion and perfusion MR imaging in cases of Alzheimer's disease: Correlations with cortical atrophy and lesion load." *AJNR Am J Neuroradiol 22(6)*: 1030–1036.

Braak, H., and E. Braak (1996). "Evolution of the neuropathology of Alzheimer's disease." *Acta Neurol Scand Suppl 165*: 3–12.

Erickson, C.A., and C.A. Barnes (2003). "The neurobiology of memory changes in normal aging." *Exp Gerontol 38(1–2)*: 61–69.

Fukutani, Y., N.J. Cairns, *et al.* (2000). "Neuronal loss and neurofibrillary degeneration in the hippocampal cortex in late-onset sporadic Alzheimer's disease." *Psychiatry Clin Neurosci 54(5)*: 523–529.

Gallagher, M., and P.R. Rapp (1997). "The use of animal models to study the effects of aging on cognition." *Annu Rev Psychol 48*: 339–370.

Giannakopoulos, P., F.R. Herrmann, *et al.* (2003). "Tangle and neuron numbers, but not amyloid load, predict cognitive status in Alzheimer's disease." *Neurology 60(9)*: 1495–1500.

Gonzalez, R.G., A.J. Fischman, *et al.* (1995). "Functional MR in the evaluation of dementia: Correlation of abnormal dynamic cerebral blood volume measurements with changes in cerebral metabolism on positron emission tomography with fludeoxyglucose F 18." *AJNR Am J Neuroradiol 16(9)*: 1763–1770.

Guzowski, J.F., G.L. Lyford, *et al.* (2000). "Inhibition of activity-dependent arc protein expression in the rat hippocampus impairs the maintenance of long-term potentiation and the consolidation of long-term memory." *J Neurosci 20(11)*: 3993–4001.

Guzowski, J.F., B.L. McNaughton, *et al.* (1999). "Environment-specific expression of the immediate-early gene Arc in hippocampal neuronal ensembles." *Nat Neurosci 2(12)*: 1120–1124.

Guzowski, J.F., B. Setlow, *et al.* (2001). "Experience-dependent gene expression in the rat hippocampus after spatial learning: A comparison of the immediate-early genes Arc, c-fos, and zif268." *J Neurosci 21(14)*: 5089–5098.

Harris, G.J., R.F. Lewis, *et al.* (1998). "Dynamic susceptibility contrast MR imaging of regional cerebral blood volume in Alzheimer disease: A promising alternative to nuclear medicine." *AJNR Am J Neuroradiol 19(9)*: 1727–1732.

Jacobs, D.M., M. Sano, *et al.* (1995). "Neuropsychological detection and characterization of preclinical Alzheimer's disease [comment] [see comments]." *Neurology 45(5)*: 957–962.

Masur, D.M., M. Sliwinski, *et al.* (1994). "Neuropsychological prediction of dementia and the absence of dementia in healthy elderly persons [see comments]." *Neurology 44(8)*: 1427–1432.

Price, J.L., A.I. Ko, *et al.* (2001). "Neuron number in the entorhinal cortex and CA1 in preclinical Alzheimer disease." *Arch Neurol 58(9)*: 1395–1402.

Rapp, P.R., and M. Gallagher (1996). "Preserved neuron number in the hippocampus of aged rats with spatial learning deficits." *Proc Natl Acad Sci USA 93(18)*: 9926–9930.

Schonheit, B., R. Zarski, *et al.* (2004). "Spatial and temporal relationships between plaques and tangles in Alzheimer-pathology." UI *25(6)*: 697–711.

Selkoe, D.J. (2002). "Alzheimer's disease is a synaptic failure." *Science 298(5594)*: 789–791.

Shoghi-Jadid, K., G.W. Small, *et al.* (2002). "Localization of neurofibrillary tangles and beta-amyloid plaques in the brains of living patients with Alzheimer disease." *Am J Geriatr Psychiatry 10(1)*: 24–35.

Small, S., E. Wu, *et al.* (2000). "Imaging physiologic dysfunction of individual hippocampal subregions in humans and genetically modified mice." *Neuron (28)*: 653–664.

Small, S.A. (2001). "Age-related memory decline; Current concepts and future directions." *Archives of Neurology 58*: 360–364.

Small, S.A. (2003). "Measuring correlates of brain metabolism with high-resolution MRI: A promising approach for diagnosing Alzheimer disease and mapping its course." *Alzheimer Dis Assoc Disord 17(3)*: 154–161.

Small, S.A. (2004). "Quantifying cerebral blood flow: Regional regulation with global implications." *J Clin Invest 114(8)*: 1046–1048.

Small, S.A. (2005). "Alzheimer disease, in living color." *Nat Neurosci 8(4)*: 404–405.

Small, S.A., M.K. Chawla, *et al.* (2004). "From the Cover: Imaging correlates of brain function in monkeys and rats isolates a hippocampal subregion differentially vulnerable to aging." *Proc Natl Acad Sci USA 101(18)*: 7181–7186.

Small, S.A., A.S. Nava, *et al.* (2000). "Evaluating the function of hippocampal subregions with high-resolution MRI in Alzheimer's disease and aging [In Process Citation]." *Microsc Res Tech 51(1)*: 101–108.

Small, S.A., A. Pierce, *et al.* (2003). *Combining functional imaging with microarray; identifying an unexplored cellular pathway implicated in sporadic Alzheimer's disease*. Society for Neuroscience, New Orleans.

Small, S.A., Y. Stern, *et al.* (1999). "Selective decline in memory function among healthy elderly." *Neurology 52(7)*: 1392–1396.

Small, S.A., W.Y. Tsai, *et al.* (2002). "Imaging hippocampal function across the human life span: Is memory decline normal or not?" *Ann Neurol 51(3)*: 290–295.

Wu, R.H., R. Bruening, *et al.* (1999). "MR measurement of regional relative cerebral blood volume in epilepsy." *J Magn Reson Imaging 9(3)*: 435–440.

Zelinski, E.M., and K.P. Burnight (1997). "Sixteen-year longitudinal and time lag changes in memory and cognition in older adults." *Psychol Aging 12(3)*: 503–513.

Zhao, X., E.S. Lein, *et al.* (2001). "Transcriptional profiling reveals strict boundaries between hippocampal subregions." *J Comp Neurol 441(3)*: 187–196.

13

Epidemiology in Aging Research

Hermann Brenner and Volker Arndt

In this chapter, we outline the definition of epidemiology and its historical development as a scientific discipline. Various conceptual approaches to epidemiology in aging research are introduced and discussed. We present the major epidemiological study designs and epidemiological measures, with a particular emphasis on peculiarities of their application in aging research. We review major fields of application of epidemiology in aging research, and we give examples of past and current contributions of epidemiology to those fields. We outline the specific challenges, difficulties and opportunities encountered by epidemiologists in aging research. We end up with an outlook on major challenges and opportunities for further development of epidemiology in aging research.

Introduction

It has long been known that the complex and intertwined causes and consequences of aging of populations demand an interdisciplinary approach including the application of epidemiological skills. Nevertheless, epidemiology has only recently emerged as a substantial contributor and as an integrating activity within aging research, drawing upon the clinical sciences, biology and genetics, social science, demography, economics and policy/planning methods and using numeric and biostatistical and experimental techniques. Epidemiologic research provides answers to questions on how much age-related burden of disease and functional impairment there is within various populations, who is affected, and what specific factors put individuals at risk.

The term *epidemiology* was originally used almost exclusively to mean the study of epidemics of infectious diseases, but the definition has broadened during the past 80 years due to the marked change of patterns of morbidity and mortality in developed countries. It is now generally understood as comparing all phenomena related to health in populations and is defined as "the study of the distribution and determinants of health-related states in specific populations, and the application of this study to control of health problems" (Last, 2001).

Key Concepts of Epidemiology

In the most basic classification of epidemiological study designs, two major fields are to be distinguished: descriptive epidemiology and analytical epidemiology. Occasionally, a third category—experimental or interventional epidemiology—is added to this list. A common feature of all these studies is that they focus on populations rather than on individuals, cells or molecules. Figure 13.1 illustrates how descriptive, analytical and experimental epidemiology are interrelated and how observational studies contribute to the development of public health interventions.

DESCRIPTIVE EPIDEMIOLOGY

Data sources

As expressed in the title, descriptive epidemiology deals with the description of the occurrence of diseases or functional impairments in the population without regard to causal or other hypotheses. Depending on the legal regulations, various sources may provide data for descriptive morbidity statistics (a more detailed description can be found in Lilienfeld and Stolley, 1994):

- Disease control programs such as disease reporting systems in case of communicable disease or case registries for cancer, cardiovascular, and other diseases
- Tax-financed public-assistance programs (public aid to the disabled, department of veterans affairs, . . .)
- Records of industrial absenteeism and periodic physical examination in industry
- Data from medical care plans, public or private health insurance plans, state disability insurance plans, data from retirement boards, hospital discharge data
- Morbidity surveys on population samples

However, one has to have in mind that most sources of morbidity statistics provide information only on special population groups, such as the group covered by a particular health insurance plan. Also, the underlying population served by a facility, such as a hospital, is not well defined. Permanent population-based registries may provide valuable epidemiologic data for some specific disease, but completeness is crucial and makes it necessary to collect information from many sources. Mortality data are also of direct interest to the epidemiologist, as they may serve as proxies for morbidity information about a population. Nationwide or statewide death registration

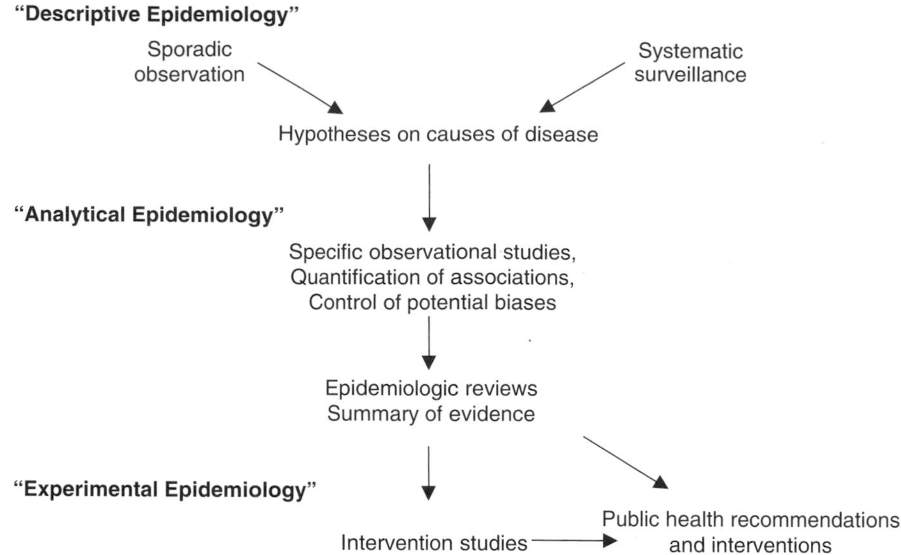

Figure 13.1. Cascade from observational studies to public health intervention.

based on standardized death certificates has been legally mandated in many developed countries. The cause of death, in fact the underlying cause, is classified according to the International Classification of Disease (ICD). Revisions of the ICD, which are implemented about every 8 to 10 years, have to be considered in analysis of mortality trends. Further specific methodological issues, such as the accuracy of the cause of death statements on the certificate and problems with the use of a single cause of death have to be considered and are further discussed in standard textbooks (e.g., Lilienfeld and Stolley, 1994). In countries where a National Death Index has been established, computerized mortality data may be linked to other databases through some common identifier such as the Social Security Number. Mortality data for descriptive statistics also may be obtained in some countries from other sources such as autopsy, hospital, occupational, and financial records (e.g., insurance, pension funds), but these data sources may not represent the general population.

Measures

Basic measures of descriptive epidemiology include the incidence (which quantifies the occurrence of new diseases or functional impairments among persons at risk), the mortality (the occurrence of deaths), and the prevalence (the proportion of people with a certain disease or a certain functional impairment at a given point or at some point during a given period of time). The terms "risk" and "rate" are sometimes used synonymously, but strictly speaking they represent two different measures. Risk describes the probability that a person will develop a disease or die within a given time frame, and is usually derived from the proportion of those who develop the disease among a large group of people. Although the concept of risk is easily understood, it is almost impossible to measure risk over any appreciable time interval as some people inevitably either will be withdrawn from the study population due to competing risks such as dying from causes other than the outcome under study, or will be lost to follow-up. To overcome the problem of competing risks, a different measure of disease occurrence—the incidence (or mortality) *rate*—has been introduced and is widely used in epidemiology. A rate is calculated as the number of cases that occur in a study population, over the person time experienced by the population followed. Unlike risk, the rate measures not the proportion of the population that is affected, but rather the ratio of the number of cases to the time at risk for disease.

In addition, there are a large number of more complex measures derived from these basic measures, such as the (healthy) life expectancy, defined as the average length of (healthy) life from birth or from a given age, the years of life lost (with or without "quality adjustment"), the maximum lifespan, defined as the average maximum length of time people can be expected to survive, and so on.

For many chronic diseases and functional impairments, incidence, mortality and prevalence strongly increase with age, and they often vary by sex even within the same age groups. Therefore, it is often crucial that these measures are reported by age and sex, as so-called age and sex specific measures. However, in analyses of time trends or comparisons between populations, it is often desirable to come up with a single summary measure of disease (or functional impairment) frequency rather than a whole bunch of age- and sex-specific measures. On the other hand, it is essential that such comparisons are not biased by possible changes in the age structure of the population over time or between various populations to be compared. In such instances, calculation of age-standardized measures of incidence, mortality and prevalence may often be reasonable. With this procedure, the respective measures for the populations to be compared are recalculated assuming a common fixed age structure of some "standard population." Depending on the kind of study, the world population, or some regional or national population, may be used as standard.

ANALYTICAL EPIDEMIOLOGY

The aim of analytical epidemiology is to identify risk factors or protective factors for diseases and functional impairments, and to quantify their impact on disease (or functional impairment) occurrence by measures such as the relative risk, the risk difference or more recently developed measures which may be particularly relevant for aging research, such as risk advancement periods (Brenner *et al.*, 1993).

In the simplest case of a binary exposure and a binary outcome (disease), the data collected in an epidemiologic study can be tabulated in the form of a fourfold table (see Table 13.1). Basically, two prototypes of study designs, case-control studies and cohort (longitudinal) studies, can be distinguished. The choice of study design primarily depends on the frequency of the risk factors and the diseases (or impairments) under study.

Case-control studies

For rare health outcomes, such as certain rare cancers, a case-control approach is often used, in which the cases (people with newly acquired disease or functional impairment) are compared with the controls (people without this outcome) with respect to the frequency of certain potential risk factors or preventive factors. In such studies, utmost care has to be taken that the controls are selected in such a way that they can be assumed to be representative of the population base from which the cases are recruited. This is often best done in a population-based study. For example, one might decide to recruit all cases diagnosed with a certain disease within some time window in a state, and to select a control group of comparable age and sex by some stratified random sampling from the general population of the same state. Case-control studies usually comprise more cases with age-related diseases than the current cohort studies. Several hundreds of cases and a similar (or an up to four times larger) number of controls are typically included, but even much larger studies are needed for the assessment of specific questions, such as the interaction of certain environmental and genetic factors in the development of chronic diseases.

TABLE 13.1
The distinction between cohort and case-control study

		Case-control study ↓	
	Exposure (Risk factor)	Diseased group (cases)	Nondiseased group (controls)
Cohort Study →	Present (exposed)	a	b
	Absent (not exposed)	c	d

Relative risk (cohort studies only): $(a/(a+b))/(c/(c+d))$
Risk difference (cohort studies only): $(a/(a+b)) - (c/(c+d))$
Odds ratio (cohort and case-control studies): ad/bc

Cohort studies

In cohort studies, participants are classified with respect to potential risk factors or protective factors in the first place, and they are then followed over time with respect to the occurrence of certain health outcomes. Unlike case-control studies, this study design allows for the assessment of etiologic factors of multiple health outcomes (all of which may be ascertained during follow-up), but it may be inefficient for rare health outcomes. Given that the frequency of multimorbidity strongly increases with age, the former argument strongly favors the use of cohort studies in epidemiologic aging research in many instances. Also, the quality of data on risk factors or protective factors is often superior in cohort studies, where this information is prospectively collected, compared to case-control studies, where such information has to be collected retrospectively, often over many decades. The cohort approach also provides more unequivocal evidence regarding the temporal relation between the occurrence of putative risk or preventive factors and the health outcome, and is therefore more suitable for establishing causal effects. Cohort studies do have their drawbacks, though, as conduction of large-scale cohort studies poses major challenges in terms of costs and logistics. Typical cohort studies include thousands (sometimes even tens of thousands and occasionally even hundreds of thousands) of participants who are followed over many years.

Prominent examples of cohort studies in aging research include the Baltimore Longitudinal Study on Aging, the Longitudinal Aging Study Amsterdam, the Rotterdam Study, the Health and Retirement Study (USA), and many others. A comprehensive overview of longitudinal studies on aging has been prepared by Health Canada and can be accessed online (Health Canada, 2002).

Cross-sectional studies

Somewhere in-between cohort studies and case-control studies are cross-sectional studies, in which the prevalence of certain health outcomes is assessed in relation with the prevalence of certain putative risk factors or protective factors at a given point of time. This approach is often less challenging in terms of costs and logistics, particularly in comparison with cohort studies, but is more prone to certain biases, which may be particularly relevant at old age. For example, the association between physical inactivity and presence of a certain disease, such as cardiovascular disease, may be difficult to interpret in a cross-sectional study, as temporality and causality of the association may be ambiguous.

INTERVENTIONAL STUDIES, EXPERIMENTAL STUDY DESIGNS

Once risk factors have been identified by observational studies, the impact of their reduction or elimination on health outcomes may be assessed in randomized trials, and positive results of such studies are commonly regarded as the definitive (and sometimes necessary) proof of causality of epidemiological associations. Well-known examples include reduction of cardiovascular disease endpoints by lipid lowering or antihypertensive medication in randomized trials after hyperlipidemia and hypertension had been identified as major risk factors in observational epidemiologic studies (e.g., Hebert *et al.*, 1997; Psaty *et al.*, 1997) or randomized clinical trials to prevent falls in elderly patients as summarized by Tinetti (2003).

Such intervention studies, which may address measures of primary, secondary or tertiary prevention, are sometimes summarized under the heading of "experimental epidemiology."

DERIVING CAUSAL INFERENCES FROM EPIDEMIOLOGICAL STUDIES

Much of epidemiologic research is aimed at uncovering the causes of disease and identifying potential risk or protective factors. The demonstration of a statistical association between a disease and a potential risk factor does not necessarily imply a causal relationship; chance, confounding or other forms of bias have to be carefully discussed as further explanations for any observed statistical association.

Even if chance and bias can be ruled out, further careful evaluation is warranted. A well-known and widely used framework for deriving causal inference has been proposed by Hill (1965) and provides a helpful orientation for causal inference (see Table 13.2). However, it should not be considered as a checklist as it does not allow clearly distinguishing causal from noncausal relations. For a more in-depth discussion of the Hill criteria and some encountered problems, we refer to some standard textbooks (e.g., Rothman and Greenland, 1998; Rothman, 2002).

TABLE 13.2
Causal criteria proposed by Hill (1965)

- Strength of the association
- Consistency of the association
- Specificity of the association
- Temporal sequence of events
- Dose-response relationship, biologic gradient
- Plausibility
- Coherence with existent theories and knowledge
- Experimental evidence
- Analogy

GENERAL METHODOLOGICAL CONSIDERATIONS OF OBSERVATIONAL STUDIES

With the exception of experimental studies, epidemiologic research is based on observational studies, and as such, in theory prone to bias by "confounding." Confounders are "extraneous factors" that may lead to an apparent (or conceal a true) association between putative risk factors (or protective factors) and disease, due to their own association with both the former and the latter. For example, various lifestyle factors, such as dietary habits, physical activity, smoking and alcohol consumption, which are clearly related to a variety of health outcomes at old age, are often also interrelated. Therefore, when the impact of one of these factors on some health outcome is assessed, it is crucial that the other factors, as well as additional relevant factors, such as age or gender, are carefully measured and controlled for in the analysis. Control for confounding is typically done by means of multivariable analysis, such as multiple logistic regression or the Cox proportional hazards model (Hosmer and Lemeshow, 1999 and 2000). But even if this caveat is taken into account, one can rarely rule out confounding from still other, unmeasured factors. The only design to guarantee absence of this possibility is large-scale randomized trials. Obviously, for ethical reasons, such trials cannot be conducted to experimentally assess the impact of putative risk factors on health outcomes in humans. Therefore, carefully conducted observational studies will always be in the center of etiologic epidemiologic research.

Besides confounding, selection bias and information bias represent other sources of systematic errors and have to be carefully addressed in planning, conducting and interpreting epidemiologic research. In addition, random variability and the role of chance due to a finite number of observations have to be considered. Whereas random variability has an effect on the precision of the study result, systematic errors compromise the validity of a study.

Selection bias occurs when the association between exposure and disease differs for those who participate and those who do not participate in the study and it is mainly due to systematic differences in characteristics between participants and nonparticipants. For example, a hospital-based study on cases with myocardial infarction will exclude those cases who die before admission to hospital, and such a selection may invalidate conclusions and generalizations.

Information bias arises if the information collected about or from the study participants is less than perfect. It can apply to either exposure or disease status or both. Imperfect measurement is often referred to as misclassification if the variable is measured on a categorical scale.

Misclassification of subjects can be either differential or nondifferential. The distinction between these two terms refers to the question of whether misclassification of exposure (disease) relates to disease (exposure) status. A more thorough discussion about sources and consequences of information bias and misclassification can be found in standard textbooks (e.g., Rothman and Greenland, 1998).

Specific Challenges of Epidemiology in Aging Research

When looking at the epidemiologic literature, it is surprising to see how limited evidence from epidemiologic studies is available on health outcomes for the elderly. Similar to the situation in clinical studies, older people have often been excluded from epidemiologic studies, and evidence from studies conducted among younger age groups have often been generalized without adequate attention to the limited age range studied. There may be multiple reasons why epidemiologic findings for the elderly are so limited.

DIFFICULTIES OF INCLUDING ELDERLY STUDY PARTICIPANTS IN EPIDEMIOLOGIC STUDIES

A primary prerequisite for any epidemiological study is informed consent of study participants. Among the elderly, this may often be a difficult matter given the higher prevalence of cognitive and functional impairment compared to younger populations. Often, extensive data collections needed in many epidemiological studies may also be too exhausting for potential study participants with reduced general health status. In case of major cognitive impairment or dependence on nursing care, additional persons (relatives, professional care providers) have to be involved, which poses additional challenges with regard to legal issues, cooperation and validity of data.

DIFFICULTIES OF CONSIDERING LONG TIME SPANS

There is increasing evidence that many chronic diseases at old age have their roots quite early in life, which requires a life course approach in analytical epidemiologic research. While prospective longitudinal studies from the prenatal period to the oldest age, which is a reasonable option in laboratory research with short-living animals, will probably never play a relevant role in epidemiological studies among humans for obvious reasons, obtaining high-quality data on early life exposures retrospectively collected in epidemiologic studies is a major challenge, given that imperfect or incomplete memory, lack of pertinent records and so on are the rule rather than the exception. Another difficulty related to aging studies lies in "cohort" or "generation" effects in which variation in health status arises from different causal factors to which each birth cohort in the population is exposed as the environment and society change.

SELECTIVE SURVIVAL

Due to their lower costs and shorter duration, cross-sectional studies have remained a common epidemiologic study design even among the elderly. In these studies, the role of risk factors potentially associated with lower odds of surviving up to old age needs to be interpreted with particular caution, however. For example, the decrease in prevalence of major cardiovascular risk factors at higher ages, such as hypertension, hyperlipidemia or smoking, or even of certain chronic diseases, may reflect selective survival in addition to rather than changes of risk factors over time which have to be studied longitudinally (Corti *et al.*, 1996).

MULTIMORBIDITY

In the past, most epidemiologic studies have focused on single health outcomes, depending on the clinical specialty of the principal investigator. Also, many epidemiological measures and methods have been primarily developed for single health endpoints. An obvious example is studies on cause-specific mortality which typically relied on single causes of death. Such approaches may be inadequate for studies among the elderly who often suffer from multiple diseases and functional impairments which may share etiologic factors and influence each other. For example, depressive illness may lead to reduced activity and consequent muscle weakness, which then may lead to increased joint pain and a diagnosis of osteoarthritis (Ebrahim, 1996). Comorbidity may also lead to treatment or changes in behavior (e.g., eating habits) that modify risk factors or the natural history of the disease (or functional impairment) under study. Also comorbidity itself may alter risk factors under study and bias the results of epidemiologic studies unless such patterns are carefully taken into account in the analysis (e.g., a previous myocardial infarction may lower the blood pressure and attenuate the association between blood pressure and risk of stroke).

Epidemiology of Common Major Diseases Among Older Adults

CARDIOVASCULAR DISEASE

Despite some reduction in recent decades, cardiovascular disease continues to be the most common cause of death, accounting for up to 50% of deaths in developed countries. Incidence and mortality strongly increase with age. In the following, the epidemiology of three major clinical manifestations of cardiovascular disease, coronary heart disease, stroke and heart failure (which to a large extent have common etiologies), will be addressed.

Despite a major decline in mortality by more than 50% in the second half of the 20th century, coronary heart disease (CHD) remains the single largest killer, accounting for 20% of all deaths in developed countries such as the United States, where mean age of manifestation of a first heart attack is 65–70 years (American Heart Association, 2005). The major risk factors for CHD, which include hypertension, hyperlipidemia, smoking and diabetes, are well established, and 80–90% of all CHD patients have prior exposure to at least one of these risk factors (Khot *et al*., 2003). In the United States, about 700,000 patients have a new heart attack each year. In recent years, the proportion of affected people surviving the acute stage of a heart attack has substantially increased, but the survivors have a risk of another heart attack, stroke and heart failure that is substantially higher than that of the general population (Hurst, 2002). Although there is evidence that much of the subsequent disease burden could be prevented by cardiac rehabilitation, this opportunity appears to be largely underused. For example, only a minority (32%) of patients aged 70 or older participate in cardiac rehabilitation in the United States (Witt *et al*., 2004).

Although stroke also accounts for a large share of mortality in developed countries (e.g., about 160,000 deaths annually in the United States [American Heart Association, 2005]), it has an even larger impact as a disabling disease, accounting for a large share of disability among the elderly. For example, in Germany, stroke is responsible for about 15 percent of cases of dependency on permanent nursing care (Ramroth *et al*., 2005). Mortality has been declining worldwide in the last decades (American Heart Association, 2005), mainly due to improved clinical management, whereas trends for incidence have been less consistent. International comparative studies have found major variation of incidence between countries. For example, within Europe, incidence was found to be threefold higher in some populations from Northern Europe than in populations from middle and Southern Europe (Thorvaldsen *et al*., 1995). Incidence rates are higher for men than for women, but women generally have a higher stroke prevalence, because they have a longer life expectancy and are more likely to survive a stroke (Sacco, 1997).

Regarding etiology and risk factors, three major types of stroke have to be distinguished: ischemic stroke (IS), intracerebral hemorrhage (ICH), and subarachnoid hemorrhage (SAH), accounting for about 88%, 9%, and 3% of all strokes, respectively (American Heart Association, 2005). Major modifiable risk factors for IS identified in large-scale epidemiologic case-control and cohort studies include hypertension, diabetes, lack of physical activity, smoking and coronary artery disease (Boden-Albala and Sacco, 2004). Hypertension is clearly the most important modifiable risk factor for IS, but other factors, including heavy alcohol consumption, anticoagulant therapy and potentially low cholesterol levels may also play a role. For SAH, smoking appears to be a particularly strong risk factor (Longstreth *et al*., 1992).

Whereas age-adjusted death rates of coronary heart disease and stroke decreased within the past decades, there have been significant increases in the prevalence of chronic heart failure (HF) as well as in associated morbidity and mortality. The lifetime risk of developing HF is now 1 in 5 for both men and women, and it is considerably higher among victims of a myocardial infarction. The prevalence of HF strongly increases with age, and 50% of patients are older than 65 years. Mortality is as high as 50% in 24 months in symptomatic men. In the United States, HF has become the most common hospital discharge diagnosis in patients >65 years of age and the primary cause of readmission within 60 days of discharge (Young, 2004; American Heart Association, 2005). Major risk factors include hypertension, coronary heart disease, diabetes and overweight. With the rise of the diabetes and overweight epidemic in many countries, the burden of disease is expected to rise further in the years to come in many countries.

CANCER

Cancer is a major health problem in developing countries, in many of which it is the second most common cause of death behind cardiovascular disease for all ages combined, and it will become of increasing importance in developing countries in the future as well. All of the major malignancies primarily affect the elderly, and the incidence of most common cancer types as well as of all tumors combined sharply increases with age.

The incidence of cancer at different sites shows extreme variations between populations and also strongly varies over time within populations. Furthermore, migrant studies have shown that migrants adopt cancer rates of the countries they are going to. Taken together, these patterns strongly support a major role of environmental, cultural and behavioral factors for the occurrence of different types of cancer. Although genetic factors undoubtedly also play a role, hereditary forms of cancer often account for small fractions of cancers only.

Prognosis of cancer patients strongly varies by cancer site, with 5-year survival rates ranging from almost 0% for patients with pancreatic cancer to almost 100%, for example, for patients with thyroid and prostate cancer, in some developed countries (Brenner, 2002; Brenner and Arndt, 2005). However, even for cancers of the same site, there is often strong variation of prognosis according to stage at diagnosis. For example, 5-year survival for patients with colorectal cancer nowadays exceeds 80% for patients with localized cancer, whereas it remains as low as 10% for patients with distant tumor spread. For that reason, there is much hope that the cancer burden can be strongly reduced by effective early detection programs. For some forms of cancer, such as cancer of the uterine cervix, early detection programs have been shown to be very effective indeed in lowering mortality. For other forms of cancer, such as colorectal cancer and breast cancer, the effectiveness of early detection measures has been demonstrated or is currently being assessed in large-scale clinical trials, and their implementation is likely to contribute to major reductions in mortality.

At the same time, progress in therapy will also continue to reduce cancer mortality. It certainly has contributed to major increases in survival of patients with a variety of cancers, including cancers of the breast, colon and rectum, testis and thyroid. Unfortunately, however, improvements have often been less pronounced for older adults, so that the age gradient in survival, which exists for many forms of cancer, has further increased in recent years (Brenner and Arndt, 2004). This is not too surprising, though, since older age groups, despite accounting for the majority of cancer patients, have often been and continue to be excluded from clinical trials evaluating new therapies (Hutchins *et al.*, 1999), and older patients less often receive effective therapy (Bouchardy *et al.*, 2003). With increasing expectations of survival, quality of life will become more and more important as an outcome measure for patients with cancer (Arndt *et al.*, 2004 and 2005).

Probably the most powerful tool for reducing the cancer burden in the elderly would be primary prevention. For example, it is well established by large-scale epidemiologic studies that at least 20% of all cancers and more than 90% of lung cancers are attributable to smoking and could be prevented by reducing or eliminating this most harmful habit in the population. There also seems to be a large potential to reduce the cancer burden by a diet that is rich in vegetables and fruits. Although these facts have been well known for a long time, progress in primary prevention is slow and even absent in many countries of the world. Given the long latency period between tumor initiation and clinical cancer manifestation, primary prevention measures need to start early in life; many cancers in the elderly could be best prevented by primary prevention in childhood, adolescence and early and middle adulthood.

NEUROLOGIC DISORDERS

Neurologic disorders are much less common as causes of death than cardiovascular disease and cancer, but account for a tremendous share of morbidity, disability, and dependence on nursing care in the elderly. This particularly applies to cognitive decline and dementia, the epidemiology of which we will focus on in this section.

The prevalence of dementia has been found to increase exponentially with age, with prevalence doubling every five years. Overall prevalence has been estimated to be about 2% between ages 65 and 74 and reaching 30% for ages 85 and over (Borenstein Graves, 2004). Age-specific overall prevalences of dementia appear to be quite similar in different countries.

Two major forms of dementia are commonly distinguished: Alzheimer's disease (AD) and vascular dementia. In most studies, the majority of cases of dementia have been classified as AD, but there have been substantial variation in estimates of the relative frequency of both disorders between studies from different populations. Furthermore, there is considerable overlap between both disorders: Between 18% and 46% of dementia cases share both Alzheimer and vascular lesions, and this overlap increases with age. Recent epidemiologic studies have consistently found cardiovascular risk factors to be related to both forms of dementia, suggesting they may share a common etiology (Launer, 2002).

Although analytical epidemiologic studies on dementia are facing particular logistic challenges (e.g., the need to rely on proxy respondents in case-control studies), a number of risk factors have now been quite consistently established in more recent large-scale prospective cohort studies. Genetic factors undoubtedly play some role, particularly among early onset cases, with the ApoE-ε4 alleles being the best established single markers. The ApoE-ε4 allele is also an established risk factor for cardiovascular disease (CVD). Other risk factors of CVD linked to the occurrence of dementia include diabetes, hypertension, hyperlipedemia, and high levels of plasma homocysteine. As is the case for CVD, moderate alcohol consumption as well as intake of nonsteroidal anti-inflammatory drugs seem to be protective (Borenstein Graves, 2004).

MUSCULOSKELETAL DISORDERS

Musculoskeletal disorders represent another group of diseases whose incidence steeply increases with age and which are rarely fatal by themselves, but which account for a major share of detriments in quality of life, disability and costs for medical and nursing care among older adults. Up to 10% of cases of severe disability are mainly caused by these disorders (Ramroth *et al.*, 2005). The most important disabling musculoskeletal disorders include osteoporosis and osteoarthrits. The former is the main reason for the strong increase in the incidence of fractures with age, particularly among women. Osteoarthrits (OA) affects a variety of joints, with OA of the hip and knee accounting for the largest share in morbidity, disability and costs. Causes and risk factors are still rather incompletely understood. Apart from congenital malformations and injury, "systemic" factors, such as overweight and related metabolic disorders, may play a major role, and their reduction may provide possibilities of primary prevention (Stürmer *et al.*, 1998, 2000).

Conclusion and Outlook

Epidemiology has been well established as an indispensable component of the disciplinary spectrum for aging research in recent years. Its contributions to aging research will continue to grow in the decades to come, mainly due to the contributions from recently and newly setup large-scale longitudinal studies. The largest benefits are to be expected from interdisciplinary approaches which keep determinants of health throughout the life span in mind. The unique contributions of this discipline to aging research may become even more fruitful, however, by taking the following aspects into account:

1. Strengthening interdisciplinarity
   Given the high prevalence of multimorbidity at old age, the horizon of single clinical specialties, which are mostly focused on a single (group of) diagnosis, may often be much too narrow for epidemiological studies among the elderly. Simply addressing multiple different health outcomes separately does not overcome the problem. What is needed are integrative approaches with a particular emphasis on functional impairments. Also, development of new methods is required to adequately deal with multiple, complexly interrelated health outcomes. The rapidly emerging fields of molecular aging research and molecular genetics provide new opportunities for interdisciplinary cooperation in epidemiologic studies in which biological materials (such as blood samples) are collected and stored.
2. From epidemiology among the elderly to epidemiology in aging research
   The etiology of chronic diseases and impairments among the elderly cannot be studied by restricting the focus to health outcomes and their determinants at old age. Major efforts are needed to incorporate measures of relevant determinants throughout the life span, starting from the genetic predisposition and intrauterine growth, and including factors that may act in childhood, adolescence or various parts of adulthood. Achievements to this end may again best be made by integrating expertise from such diverse fields as human genetics, prenatal and neonatal care, pediatrics, internal and family medicine, and developmental psychology (Kuh *et al.*, 2003).
3. Large-scale longitudinal studies
   Most of the study questions in epidemiologic aging research can best be answered by large-scale longitudinal (cohort) studies, on either a regional, national or international level. Although investments in such studies in terms of time and funds are comparably large in the beginning, this investment is often more than paid off after a few years of follow-up. International studies are confronted with more difficult logistics (e.g., for standardization and validation of instruments), but may often benefit from a wider range of possible health determinants and outcomes. A number of well-planned large-scale cohort studies have meanwhile been set up among older adults in different parts of the world. While they steadily provide a wealth of data, their contribution to aging research will further increase with each additional year of follow-up.
4. Epidemiology of medical and nursing care
   Apart from studying health outcomes, epidemiologic methods can also be used and should be more widely used to study patterns of medical and nursing care and their determinants (e.g., Kliebsch *et al.*, 1998; Ramroth *et al.*, 2005). The epidemiology of medical and nursing care might prove particularly useful in the process of modernization of health and nursing care systems that is required to meet the challenges imposed by demographic aging and that is now ongoing in many countries around the world.
5. Translating epidemiologic study results into the practice of prevention
   In the last 50 years, epidemiologic research has identified a large number of risk factors and preventive factors of multiple chronic diseases, yet the transfer of these findings into applied disease prevention has often remained unsatisfactory. For example, half a century after the deleterious health effects of smoking have been disclosed by carefully conducted epidemiologic studies, the global number of smokers and prevalence of smoking keep rising. A similar development appears to be seen for physical inactivity, which is likewise related to a large number of severe chronic diseases. Therefore, further development of epidemiology in aging research has to go along with research on how to more effectively translate epidemiologic study results into the practice of prevention. Preventive efforts again have to keep the entire life span in mind.

Recommended Resources

SELECTION OF REVIEWS AND BOOKS ON EPIDEMIOLOGY AND AGING RESEARCH

Brenner, H., and Arndt, V. (2004). Epidemiology in aging research. *Exp. Gerontol.* 39: 679–686.

Brody, J.A., and Maddox, G.L. (1991). *Epidemiology and Aging—An International Perspective*. Springer Publishing Company, New York.

Davies, A.M. (1993). Aging and epidemiology. *Public Health Rev.* 21: 225–242.

Ebrahim, S., and Kalache, A. (1996). *Epidemiology in Old Age*. BMJ Publishing Group. London.

Fried, L.P. (2000). Epidemiology of aging. *Epidemiol. Rev.* 22: 95–106.

Health Canada. (2002). Review on longitudinal studies on aging. Division of Aging and Seniors, for the Institute of Aging of the Canadian Institutes of Health Research. http://www.fhs.mcmaster.ca/clsa/en/links.htm.

Kalache, A., and Gatti A. (2003). Active ageing: A policy framework. *Adv. Gerontol.* 11: 7–18.

Miettenen, O.S. (1991). Epidemiological research on ageing: An orientation. *Int J Epidemiol* 20 Suppl. 1: 2–7.

Satariano, W. (2005). *Epidemiology of Aging: An Ecological Approach*. Jones and Bartlett Publishers, Boston.

Wallace, R.B. (1992). "Epidemiology and aging: How gerontology has changed noncommunicable disease epidemiology in the United States of America." *World Health Stat. Q.* 45: 75–79.

Wallace, R.B., and Woolson, R.F. (1992). *The Epidemiologic Study of the Elderly*. Oxford University Press, New York, Oxford.

Weinstein, M., Hermalin, A.I., and Stoto, M.A. (2001). "Population health and aging. Strengthening the dialogue between epidemiology and demography." *Ann NY Acad Sci* 954: 1–321.

World Health Organization Scientific Group on the Epidemiology of Aging. (1984). The uses of epidemiology in the study of the elderly. *World Health Organ. Tech. Rep. Ser.* 706, 1–84.

SELECTION OF MODERN AND CLASSIC TEXTBOOKS IN EPIDEMIOLOGY

Gordis, L. (2004). *Epidemiology*. (4th ed.). Saunders, Philadelphia.

Kleinbaum, D.G., Kupper, L.L., and Morgenstern, H. (1982). *Epidemiologic Research*. John Wiley and Sons, New York.

Last, J.M. (2001). *A Dictionary of Epidemiology*. (4th ed.). Oxford University Press, New York, Oxford.

Lilienfeld, D.E., and Stolley, P.D. (1994). *Foundations of Epidemiology*. (3rd ed.) Oxford University Press, New York, Oxford.

Rothman, K.J., and Greenland, S. (1998). *Modern Epidemiology*. (2nd ed.) Lippincott-Raven Publishers, Philadelphia.

Rothman, K.J. (2002). *Epidemiology—An Introduction*. Oxford University Press, New York.

Woodward, M. (2005). *Epidemiology—Study Design and Data Analysis*. (2nd ed.). Chapman and Hall. Boca Raton.

REFERENCES

American Heart Association (2005). Heart disease and stroke statistics—2005 update. http://www.americanheart.org/downloadable/heart/1105390918119HDSStats2005Update.pdf.

Arndt, V., Merx, H., Stegmaier, C., Ziegler, H., and Brenner, H. (2004). Quality of life in patients with colorectal cancer 1 year after diagnosis compared with the general population: A population-based study. *J. Clin. Oncol. 22*, 4829–4836.

Arndt, V., Merx, H., Stegmaier, C., Ziegler, H., and Brenner, H. (2005). Persistence of restrictions in quality of life from the first to the third year after diagnosis in women with breast cancer. *J. Clin. Oncol. 23*, 4945–4953.

Boden-Albala, B., and Sacco, R.L. (2004). Stroke. In L.M. Nelson, C.M. Tanner, S.K. Van Den Eden, and V.M. McGuire, eds., *Neuroepidemiology. From Principles to Practice*, pp. 223–253. New York: Oxford University Press.

Borenstein Graves, A. (2004). Alzheimer's disease and vascular dementia. In L.M. Nelson, C.M. Tanner, S.K. Van Den Eden, and V.M. McGuire, eds., *Neuroepidemiology. From Principles to Practice*, pp. 102–130. New York: Oxford University Press.

Bouchardy, C., Rapiti, E., Fioretta, G., Laissue, P., Neyroud-Caspar, I., Schafer, P., *et al.*. (2003). Undertreatment strongly decreases prognosis of breast cancer in elderly women. *J. Clin. Oncol. 21*, 3580–3587.

Brenner, H. (2002). Long-term survival rates of cancer patients achieved by the end of the 20th century: A period analysis. *Lancet. 360*, 1131–1135.

Brenner, H., and Arndt, V. (2004). Recent increase in cancer survival according to age: Increase in all age groups, but widening age gradient. *Cancer Causes Control. 15*, 903–910.

Brenner, H., and Arndt, V. (2005). Long-term survival rates of patients with prostate cancer in the PSA screening era: population-based estimates for the year 2000 by period analysis. *J. Clin. Oncol. 23*, 441–447.

Brenner, H., Gefeller, O., and Greenland, S. (1993). Risk and rate advancement periods as measures of exposure impact on the occurrence of chronic diseases. *Epidemiology. 4*, 229–236.

Corti, M.-C., Guralnik, J.M., and Bilato, C. (1996). Coronary heart disease risk factors in older persons. *Aging Clin. Exp. Res. 8*, 75–89.

Ebrahim, S. (1996). Principles of epidemiology in old age. In S. Ebrahim and A. Kalache, eds., *Epidemiology in Old Age*, pp. 12–21. London: BMJ Publishing Group.

Health Canada (2002). Review on longitudinal studies on aging. Division of Aging and Seniors, for the Institute of Aging of the Canadian Institutes of Health Research. http://www.fhs.mcmaster.ca/clsa/en/links.htm.

Hebert, P.R., Gaziano, J.M., Chan K.S., and Hennekens, C.H. (1997). Cholesterol lowering with statin drugs, risk of stroke, and total mortality. *JAMA. 278*, 313–321.

Hill, A.B. (1965). The environment and disease: Association or causation? *Proc. R. Soc. Med. 58*, 295–300.

Hosmer, D.W., and Lemeshow, S. (1999). *Applied Survival Analysis: Regression Modelling of Time to Event Data.* New York: Wiley.

Hosmer, D.W., and Lemeshow, S. (2000). *Applied Logistic Regression.* 2nd ed. New York: Wiley.

Hurst, W. (2002). *The Heart, Arteries and Veins.* (10th ed.) New York: McGraw-Hill.

Hutchins, L.F., Unger, J.M., Crowley, J.J., Coltman, C.A. Jr., and Albain, K.S. (1999) Underrepresentation of patients 65 years of age or older in cancer-treatment trials. *N. Engl. J. Med. 341*, 2061–2067.

Khot, U.N., Khot, M.B., Bajzer, C.T., Sapp, S.K., Ohman, E.M., Brener, S.J., *et al.* (2003). Prevalence of conventional risk factors in patients with coronary heart disease. *JAMA. 290*, 898–904.

Kliebsch, U., Stürmer, T., Siebert, H., and Brenner, H. (1998). Risk factors for institutionalization in an elderly disabled population. *Eur. J. Public Health 8*, 106–112.

Kuh, D., Ben-Shlomo Y., Lynch, J., Hallqvist, J., and Power, C. (2003). Life course epidemiology. *J. Epidemiol. Comm. Health 57*, 778–783.

Last, J.M. (2001). *A Dictionary of Epidemiology.* New York: Oxford University Press.

Launer, L.J. (2002). Demonstrating the case that AD is a vascular disease: Epidemiologic evidence. *Ageing Res. Rev. 1*, 61–77.

Lilienfeld, D.E., and Stolley, P.D. (1994). *Foundations of Epidemiology.* (3rd ed.). New York: Oxford University Press.

Longstreth, W.T. Jr., Nelson, L.M., Koepsell, T.D., and van Belle, G. (1992). Cigarette smoking, alcohol use, and subarachnoid hemorrhage. *Stroke 23*, 1242–1249.

Psaty, B.M., Smith, N.L., Siscovick, D.S., Koepsell, T.D., Weiss, N.S., Heckbert, S.R., *et al.* (1997). Health outcomes associated with antihypertensive therapies used as first-line agents. A systematic review and meta-analysis. *JAMA. 277*, 739–745.

Ramroth, H., Specht-Leible, N., and Brenner, H. (2005). Hospitalisations before and after nursing home admission: a retrospective cohort study from Germany. *Age Ageing 34*, 291–294.

Rothman, K.J., and Greenland, S. (1998). *Modern epidemiology.* (2nd ed.) Philadelphia: Lippincott-Raven Publishers.

Rothman, K.J. (2002). *Epidemiology—An Introduction.* New York: Oxford University Press.

Sacco, R.L. (1997). Risk factors, outcomes, and stroke subtypes for ischemic stroke. *Neurology. 49 Suppl. 4*, 39–44.

Stürmer, T., Günther, K.-P., and Brenner, H. (2000). Obesity, overweight and patterns of osteoarthritis: The Ulm Osteoarthritis Study. *J. Clin. Epidemiol. 53*, 75–81.

Stürmer, T., Sun, Y., Sauerland, S., Zeißig, I., Günther, K.-P., Puhl, W., and Brenner H. (1998). Serum cholesterol and osteoarthritis. The baseline examination of the Ulm Osteoartritis Study. *J. Rheumatol. 25*, 1827–1832.

Thorvaldsen, P., Asplund, K., Kuulasmaa, K., Rajakangas, A.M., and Schroll, M. (1995). Stroke incidence, case fatality, and mortality in the WHO MONICA project. World Health Organization Monitoring trends and Determinants in Cardiovascular Disease. *Stroke 26*, 361–367.

Tinetti, M.E. (2003). Clinical practice. Preventing falls in elderly persons. *N. Engl. J. Med. 348*, 42–49.

Witt, B.J., Jacobsen, S.J., Weston, S.A., Killian, J.M., Meverden, R.A., Allison, T.G., *et al.* (2004). Cardiac rehabilitation after myocardial infarction in the community. *J. Am. Coll. Cardiol. 44*, 988–996.

Young, J.B. (2004). The global epidemiology of heart failure. *Med. Clin. North. Am. 88*, 1135–1143.

14

Statistical Issues for Longevity Studies in Animal Models

Chenxi Wang, Scott W. Keith, Kevin R. Fontaine, and David B. Allison

In this chapter we provide an overview of basic statistical concepts and procedures that are germane to researchers interested in aging. We include discussions of hypothesis testing, research design, statistical power, data collection, statistical significance, parametric and nonparametric statistical methods, and choosing an appropriate statistical test. We also provide brief introductions to the different types of data (categorical versus continuous), summary statistics, and a selection of parametric and nonparametric statistical tests including t-tests, analysis of variance, ordinary least squares regression, logistic regression, and survival analysis. We place special emphasis on statistics for maximum lifespan using the example of animal research on caloric restriction. We also include discussions of the major methods of significance testing for statistics of maximum lifespan. We conclude the chapter by offering a series of recommendations that will greatly increase the chances of conducting a valid statistical analysis.

Introduction

Although findings from animal experiments cannot be directly applied to humans, well-designed animal studies remain powerful tools for advancing scientific knowledge, especially in biomedical fields including aging research. Most applied researchers share the idea with statisticians that statistics is an essential component for successful scientific research. This appreciation is not always clearly reflected in appropriate analysis and interpretation of results in published studies (Olsen, 2003; Williams *et al.*, 1997; Murphy, 2004). Therefore, a brief review of basic statistical concepts and considerations is important not only for the completeness of this comprehensive book but also for quality of research practice. In this chapter, we review some basic statistical concepts, summary statistics, hypothesis testing, and study design considerations. We then discuss statistical methods to test differences in maximum lifespan. Finally, using a maximum lifespan example, we illustrate how to choose an appropriate design and statistical methods.

Our goal is to provide applied researchers on aging with a better understanding of basic statistical concepts to help them communicate more effectively with the statistical support staff who actually conduct the analyses. Therefore, the primary task of this chapter is to provide a general overview of statistical concepts and issues, not to provide a detailed and exhaustive discussion. We will focus on statistical hypothesis testing and statistical methods useful for animal experiments in which, typically, the researcher can control factors that affect the outcomes, but not have to face issues that are common in human clinical trials such as loss to follow-up, missing data, and noncompliance to treatment. Motivated readers looking for more extensive discussions are referred to some excellent texts (Daniel, 1998; Alterman, 1999; Fisher and van Belle, 1993).

Brief Review of Statistical Concepts

Biomedical researchers try to find answers for questions pertaining to populations of interest. A hypothesis is a formal statement of or prediction for the scientific question of interest. In other words, most research activities are designed to test a given hypothesis in one or more populations. Hypothesis testing involves a number of steps (Daniel, 1998): (A) developing a formal hypothesis; (B) designing a study that tests the hypothesis; (C) collecting data from a sample of the target population; and (D) calculating the test statistics from the data and drawing conclusions as to whether the hypothesis is supported.

Each of these steps is summarized below.

A. DEVELOPING A FORMAL HYPOTHESIS

In the planning stage of research, the researcher should generate a formal hypothesis or set of hypotheses based on previous research and/or theories that have yet to be formally tested. The hypothesis is usually a statement or prediction that the researcher seeks to evaluate with a study. For example, suppose a researcher wants to test the hypothesis that the average lifespan of mouse line A is longer than the average lifespan of mouse line B. Implicit in this hypothesis are two distinct possibilities represented individually by the null hypothesis, denoted H_0, and the alternative hypothesis, denoted H_a. The null and alternative hypotheses can be expressed as follows:

H_0: there is no difference in average lifespan between mouse line A and mouse line B ($\mu_A = \mu_B$);
H_a: the average lifespan of mouse line A is longer than mouse line B ($\mu_A > \mu_B$).

This is an example of a one-sided hypothesis (i.e., the researcher expects mouse line B to live longer, on average.)

If the researcher has no particular reason to believe that the average lifespan of mouse line A will be longer than the average lifespan of mouse line B, or vice versa, he or she will need to test a two-sided hypothesis. The null and alternative hypotheses would then be as follows:

H_0: there is no difference in average lifespan between line A and line B ($\mu_A = \mu_B$);
H_a: there is a difference in average lifespan between line A and line B ($\mu_A \neq \mu_B$).

Depending on the form of the hypotheses, the researcher uses either a two-sided or one-sided statistical test to determine the statistical significance of any observed difference in average lifespan before either accepting H_0 or rejecting H_0 in favor of H_a. Most statistical analysis software will calculate both one-sided and two-sided tests at the same time, and the researcher simply needs to pick the proper one based on the nature of their hypothesis.

B. DESIGNING A STUDY

In the design stage, one needs to select a test statistic, significance level, desired power, and the sample size required to adequately test the hypothesis.

1. Statistical test

A simple approach is to choose a statistical test according to the type of data to be collected. We will discuss this in greater detail in the next section. In short, to compare the lifespans of two mouse lines from our example an independent *t*-test is appropriate if the lifespans of both mouse lines are approximately normally distributed or can be transformed to produce a normal distribution and the sample variances for the two lines are approximately equal.

2. Significance level

An investigator always runs the risk of observing significant-looking results by chance alone. The significance level reflects the investigator's tolerance for committing a type I error, which occurs when a true null hypothesis is rejected by chance resulting in a false positive test. That chance is expressed in terms of probability and is conventionally preset at 0.05 or 0.01. In other words, the researcher has sufficient control over other aspects of the study in order to set the significance level (sometimes called alpha (α) level) to 0.05 or 0.01.

It is also possible to accept the null hypothesis when the alternative is true. This is known as a type II error or false negative. The probability of committing a type II error is called the beta (β) level. One minus β is the power of a statistical test, which represents the probability of finding a true difference when the alternative hypothesis is true (i.e., finding a true difference when there actually is one). In general, with all other factors held constant, the smaller α is, the higher the power is; and the larger α is, the lower the power is.

Sometimes the true type I error rate of certain statistical tests may not be equal to the preset α level. When it is smaller than the preset α level, we say that the statistical test is conservative, and, as a result, the type II error rate increases and the power of the test decreases. When the type I error rate is larger than the α level, which may be due to a violation of the test assumptions, we may consider the statistical test to be invalid. Readers can find further discussion of these issues in Statistics for Maximum Lifespan.

3. Sample size calculation and power analysis

Sample size calculation is a procedure for calculating the sample size required to achieve a desirable degree of statistical power. The calculation is based upon a selected statistical test, an estimate of the variation in the population, an established significance level, and an expected effect size. Power analysis estimates the power of a study given the sample size used, the selected statistical test, the significance level, the variance of the outcome variables, and the effect size. If the researcher has limited resources or has any other reason to conduct research with a fixed number of subjects, the researcher will need to conduct a power analysis to determine whether the study would be adequately powered. If it is determined that the study would have low power (typically $\beta < 0.80$) the researcher may decide to alter the significance level and/or the expected effect size to increase the power.

In practice, we usually calculate sample size instead. When we calculate the sample size, the statistical power is chosen arbitrarily anywhere between 0.8 and 0.95 and the type I error rate is set at 0.05 (or 0.01). Sometimes, deciding on the effect size to be detected is challenging. For example, holding all other factors constant, a test with very good power to detect a 20% difference in mean lifespan between mouse lines A and B may have very low power to detect a 10% difference using the same sample size. A practical guideline is to choose the effect size according to biological or clinical importance. If the researcher thinks a 10% difference in average lifespan is not important or does not care if the study cannot detect the 10% difference, a smaller sample size can be used to detect a larger difference. If a 10% difference is biologically or clinically meaningful, the sample size has to be recalculated according to the 10% effect size.

As previously stated, in order to calculate sample size, a researcher will need to have reasonable variance estimates for the outcome variables of interest. While they may be based on pilot studies or other sources, such estimates can be highly inaccurate and can thus result in underpowered studies. Suppose, for example, that a group of researchers have underestimated the population variance at the outset of their study. Consequently, they would then be apt to underestimate the sample size required to detect the difference for which they are looking. Suppose further that there truly was a difference, yet the results of their underpowered study yielded p-values close to, but still greater than, the significance level. As a result of their insufficient sample, the researchers were not successful in detecting the true difference. Therefore, it may be necessary, in general, to adjust the sample size during and/or at the proposed end of a study using information from the observed sample.

Researchers can recalculate the sample size based on conditional power. This method uses the power of the proposed statistical tests, calculated conditionally on the data from the current sample, to suggest the extension of the study to collect a larger and/or more comprehensive sample. The original data can then be combined with the new data to retest the hypothesis.

Under certain circumstances, more advanced sampling methods can be useful and cost-effective. Some studies require the use of expensive animals, such as nonhuman primates, and investigators may not have the resources to recruit the entire sample at one time. Other studies are longitudinal, and data will be collected two or more times on each subject followed over time. In cases such as these, it is a common practice to do interim data analysis or group sequential power analysis to determine if the study may be terminated early due to obtaining enough evidence either to accept or reject the null hypothesis.

It is important to note that both conditional power analysis and group sequential analysis are complicated methods in which one must control for the inflated type I error rate resulting from the multiple comparisons. Motivated readers are referred to texts by Proschan and Hunsberger (1995); Brannath and Bauer (2004); DeMets and Lan (1994); and Jennison and Turnbull (1999).

Bootstrapping—a resampling with replacement procedure—can be a useful approach to studying the properties (e.g., variance) of estimates and test statistics. In the bootstrap approach, a sample of size m is drawn with replacement from the observed sample of size n drawn originally from the population of interest. This sample may then be combined with the original sample, and the $m+n$ observations may be analyzed together. If this resampling procedure is reiterated a sufficient number of times, one can obtain empirical estimates of the power of proposed tests based on samples of size $m+n$ from the population while controlling for type I errors. For more information and instruction on bootstrapping, the interested reader is referred to Mooney and Duval (1993).

Many formulas, tables, nomograms (for example, Machin *et al.*, 1987; Schoenfeld and Richter, 1982) and software packages are available for power and sample size calculations. For example, when the type I error rate is α and expected power is $1-\beta$, the sample size needed for each group in order to detect a difference in average lifespan of size, δ, between two groups with equal sample size, n, and equal standard deviation, s, can be calculated as

$$n = 2s^2\left(\frac{t_{\alpha/2} + t_\beta}{\delta}\right)^2$$

where $t_{\alpha/2}$ and t_β are critical values from the t-distribution. Some of these equations are self-explanatory, while some of them are not so straightforward. Applied researchers are encouraged to consult with statisticians when necessary.

C. COLLECTING DATA

The third step in hypothesis testing is to collect the study data. A population is defined as the entire set of individuals of interest. In our example, all the mice of line A and all the mice of line B are the populations of interest. Most of the time, it is impossible and unnecessary to collect data from the entire population in order to test a hypothesis. In practice, researchers usually collect data from a subset of the population and generalize the finding from this subset to the original population. This subset is called a sample. Ideally, the sample used for a study is a random sample, which implies that every individual in the population has an equal probability of being selected. This ensures that the sample represents the population well with respect to the variation within the population. Sampling is a complex issue that is beyond the scope of this chapter. The interested reader is referred to Thompson (2002).

D. CALCULATING STATISTICS AND DRAWING CONCLUSIONS

Finally, one needs to use the data to calculate test statistics and the associated p-values which provide the basis for testing hypotheses and drawing conclusions. Statistical testing is analogous to finding the signal-to-noise ratio (Carlin and Doyle, 2001). In our mice example, when sample means are compared, the signal is the difference between the means of the two mice lines and the noise is the standard error, a measurement of variability. The test statistic would be a ratio of these two quantities, and the general formula for a test statistic can be expressed as (Carlin and Doyle, 2001)

$$\text{Test statistic} \propto \frac{\text{signal}}{\text{variation}/\sqrt{n}} \tag{1}$$

where n is the sample size.

A p-value is the probability of obtaining a test statistic as extreme as or more extreme than the test statistic observed from the sample given that the null hypothesis is true. In other words, large negative or large positive values for the ratio in Equation (1) will result in small p-values. When the p-value for a test is equal to or smaller than the significance level (often set at 0.05 or 0.01), one rejects the null hypothesis in favor of the alternative hypothesis. Note that, as shown in Equation (1), the test statistic and therefore the p-value, are functions of the sample size, n. This implies that even a small difference between means can become statistically significant given a sufficiently large sample size.

Choosing the Proper Statistical Test

TYPE OF DATA

Loosely speaking, there are two types of data: categorical data and continuous data. The categorical data can be further divided into nominal data and ordinal data.

The possible values for continuous data typically will form a whole interval or range. For example, data collected from measuring the body weight of adult mice in line A could range from very low, say 150 grams, to very high, say 450 grams. The body weight of a randomly selected member of this population could assume any value in this range. For instance, a random sample of $n = 5$ subjects from this population could have the following set of weight measurements: {177, 283, 222, 155, 399}.

Categorical data are a collection of observations that can be categorized by classification or on an ordered scale. Nominal data are based on classifications. Suppose that, as a researcher, you are interested in collecting information on the distribution of body weight throughout a given mouse line according to the breeders from which they were bred. Each subject would be measured for body weight and then classified by the breeder. The body weights of mice could also be categorized according to relative size. For instance, mice with body weight less than the 25th percentile may be categorized as "lean"; mice with body weight between the 25th and 75th percentile may be categorized as "normal weight"; and those over the 75th percentile may be categorized as "overweight." These categories have a natural order or scale to them, and this type of data is called ordinal. The information on the scale of ordinal data can be used to the advantage of the researcher by way of testing for trends that would not be possible were the data treated as nominal.

The distinctions between these data types are not always clear. One must look beyond the measurements themselves and examine the quantities or qualities being measured before giving meaning to the numbers in a dataset. Continuous data may be divided into categories that can be treated as being either ordinal or nominal. Although there may also be many justifiable reasons for doing this, such as nonlinear relationships between factors under study, continuous data may be categorized simply to ease the interpretation of the results of an experiment. In our previous example, we showed how the mice could be categorized according to preset cut points into either lean, normal weight, or overweight classifications by their body weights. In this case, researchers may prefer the ordinal categorization in order to make statements about the relationship between some factor(s) and being normal weight or overweight rather than trying to relate the continuous measure of body weight with the factor(s). Another example is that we can categorize animals into those with hypertension and those with normal blood pressures based on their systolic blood pressure. In this case, we transform a continuous variable into a nominal one. The ease in interpretation from such analyses does come at a cost. Categorizing continuous data will strip it of some portion, perhaps a very significant portion, of the information on the relationship the researcher is investigating.

SUMMARY STATISTICS

Every experiment will produce a set of data. We denote the original data without any statistical process as raw data. Summary statistical analysis is always the first step of statistical treatment that will give a systemic overview of the features of the data and can guide further presentation and analysis of the data. Moreover, it is often the case that producing both graphical and numerical summaries of a set of data can provide the investigator with important insights that could inform subsequent hypothesis testing (Altman, 1999). An initial summary of the data determines whether parametric or nonparametric statistical methods are most appropriate when one seeks to address issues of inference (see Section "Statistical Inference Methods," below).

In general, investigators will want to summarize the data as simply as possible so that they can acquire a general sense of what the data look like. For example, nominal variables such as sex and years of education can be summarized by tabulating the frequency of responses in a given category (i.e., the number of males and the number of respondents with a high school education) or by converting these frequencies into percentages (i.e., the number of males divided by the total number of respondents). These summary data can be presented in a table or bar diagram.

For ordinal or continuous data, it is important to derive point estimates of the center of the distribution, as well as the spread or dispersion of the distribution. The former numerical summary is often called a measure of central tendency, while the latter is called a measure of variability. The most common measures of central tendency are the arithmetic mean (i.e., the sum of all of the observations divided by the number of observations), the median (i.e., the value that comes half way when the data are ranked in order) and the mode (i.e., the most common value observed).

The mean is by far the most common measure of central tendency because it ties in well with most approaches to inferential statistical analysis (Fisher and van Belle, 1993). However, because the mean is sensitive to extreme values in the distribution (sometimes called outliers), it is often the case that the median provides the "best" estimate of the center of a distribution.

With regard to summarizing the variability of data, the most common measures are the range (i.e., the smallest value subtracted from the largest), quartiles (i.e., an estimate of the four quarters of the distribution), the interquartile range (i.e., the difference between the third and first quartile), and percentiles (i.e., the value below which a given percentage of values occur). In general these measures of dispersion are useful in getting a general sense of the data, but their mathematical properties do not lend themselves to inferential statistical techniques.

Another way to quantify variability is to calculate and standardize the average distance of each value for the mean of the distribution. This summary measure, the standard deviation, is a point estimate of the variability of values in a given distribution.

Both the mean and standard deviation of a given set of ordinal or continuous data provide the cornerstone for parametric methods of statistical inference. Once an investigator derives a general sense of the data and calculates the appropriate summary measures, he or she is well placed to begin to use these data to test a given hypothesis.

STATISTICAL INFERENCE METHODS

We will now discuss the differences between parametric and nonparametric methods, then describe some of the most common and effective statistical methods being used in the field. For a comprehensive listing of tests based on these methods see Table 14.1, and for a listing of the underlying assumptions for each test see Table 14.2.

1. Parametric vs. nonparametric methods

Before applying a particular statistical test of a hypothesis, the analyst must verify that the data being tested meets the requirements (assumptions) for that test (see Table 14.1). In particular, when the hypothesis compares the measures of central tendency of two groups, the researcher has the option of using either parametric or nonparametric methods (see Table 14.2). A parametric method is used for testing hypotheses about parameters in a population described by a specified distributional form such as the normal distribution. Alternatively, a nonparametric method is useful for testing hypotheses using information based on a function of the sample observations (often the ranks) whose probability distribution does not depend on a complete specification of the probability distribution of the population from which the sample was drawn, as is generally the case with parametric methods. Hence, a nonparametric method will be valid under relatively general assumptions about the underlying population.

Parametric methods, on the other hand, are valid only under certain distributional conditions. Most parametric methods, such as the *t*-test described in more detail below, require that observations be approximately normally distributed, and both groups should have equal sample variances. Implicit in these requirements is that the data should be continuous, although ordinal data may be suitable as well, especially when the sample size is large.

Nonparametric methods ignore many of the distributional aspects of the data in favor of having the flexibility to handle nominal data as well as continuous and ordinal data for which we either (a) have insufficient information about the distribution or (b) know that the distributional requirements for parametric methods have not been adequately satisfied. The nonparametric methods offer a suitable alternative under these conditions, but they are not as powerful and efficient as the analogous parametric methods when the data do not violate the distributional assumptions.

With either method, the data must be from a random sample of the population of interest. In addition to generating samples that adequately represent the population as we have already mentioned, random sampling also gives a sample the desirable property of having independent observations. Independence between observations is a critical assumption for virtually every common statistical test. For more information and in-depth discussion of nonparametric methods we suggest that the reader refer to Conover (1999).

2. Analysis of continuous data

The *t*-test is a parametric statistical method used for testing the difference in a mean from a hypothesized value or the difference in means between two normally distributed populations with equal variances

Analysis of Variance (ANOVA) is another parametric statistical method. One-way ANOVA is a popular tool for comparing the means from several samples. For example, Weindruch *et al.* (1986) collected data from mice on the relationship between caloric intake and life expectancy. They randomly assigned female mice to feeding regimen groups where scientists regulated the caloric intake as well as the composition and quality of the nutrition in the diets of the mice. In this situation, comparisons of mean life expectancy between feeding groups can be made by using ANOVA. Keep in mind, however, that ANOVA is a parametric method and the validity of the assumptions underlying this method must be verified prior to performing this analysis.

Ordinary least squares regression (OLS) is a parametric method that is used to test for a linear relationship between a continuous dependent response variable and a set of independent predictor variables that can be either continuous or categorical. The parameters

TABLE 14.1.
Statistical methods and their assumptions

Assumption[b] Test[a]	Independent observations[c]	Equal standard deviations[d]	Normal distriibution[e]	Adequate model fit[f]	Typical Hypothesis Tested
T-test	X	X	X	–	$\mu_1 = \mu_2$
ANOVA	X	X	X	–	$\mu_1 = \mu_2 = \cdots = \mu_k$
Wilcoxon Rank Sum test	X			–	$m_1 = m_2$ (equal medians)
Kruskal-Wallis test	X			–	$m_1 = m_2 = \cdots = m_k$
Linear Regression	X	X	X	X	$\beta_1 = \beta_2 = \cdots = \beta_k = 0;\ \beta_i = 0$
Correlation coefficient[g] (r)	X			X	Y and X linearly related
Kernel Regression	X				Y linear combination of X's
LOESS[h]	X				Y linear combination of X's
ANCOVA	X	X	X	X	$\mu_1 = \mu_2 = \cdots = \mu_k$ controlling for continuous covariate
Likelihood ratio	X		X[i]	–	$\beta_i = 0$; Y independent of X; goodness of fit
Cochran-Armitage trend test	X			X	Linear trend between ordinal variables
Logistic Regression	X		X[i]	X	$\beta_1 = \beta_2 = \cdots = \beta_k = 0;\ \beta_i = 0$
Poisson Regression	X		X[i]	X	$\beta_1 = \beta_2 = \cdots = \beta_k = 0;\ \beta_i = 0$
χ^2 test	X			–	Y independent of X; goodness of fit
Fisher's Exact Test	X			–	Y independent of X
Score Test	X			–	Y independent of X; goodness of fit
CMH test	X			–	Y independent of X; Y independent of X controlling for covariates
Parametric regression	X[i]		X[i]	X	$\beta_1 = \beta_2 = \cdots = \beta_k = 0;\ \beta_i = 0$ (handles censoring)
Cox-Mantel test	X[i]			–	$\mu_1 = \mu_2$ (handles censoring)
Log rank test	X[i]			–	$\mu_1 = \mu_2$ (handles censoring)
Cox proportional hazards regression	X[i]			X[k]	$\beta_1 = \beta_2 = \cdots = \beta_k = 0;\ \beta_i = 0$ (handles censoring)

[a] Textbook references we suggest for these statistical tests include the following: for basic statistical methods try Ramsey and Schafer (2002) or Ott (1993); for regression try Montgomery *et al.* (2001); for categorical methods try Agresti (1996); for nonparametric methods try Conover (1999); for time-to-event (survival) analysis try Lee and Wang (2003).

[b] The statistical and graphical methods used to verify these assumptions are beyond the scope of this chapter. Most of these methods are detailed in the text by Ramsey and Schafer (2002). A reference for categorical data methods is the text by Agresti (1996).

[c] Observations must be free of cluster and serial effects. Random sampling from the population of interest implies that the observations will be independent of one another.

[d] Standard deviation must be the same between groups being compared, and the variance of a dependent variable should be homogeneous over the range of the independent variable(s) being considered.

[e] This assumption may be ignored if the sample sizes involved are large enough. How large depends on how far from normality the data seem to stray.

[f] Adequate model fit typically requires that the dependent response varies as a linear function of the independent predictors and no insignificant (nuisance) parameters are allowed to remain in the model.

[g] Both variables must be from random samples.

[h] Loess local regression is a nonparametric technique for describing bivariate relationships where the functional form is not known in advance.

[i] This method has underlying distributional requirements but not necessarily that of normality.

[i] Censored observations are typically assumed to be censored at random.

[k] Assumes that the hazard functions of different individuals are proportional and independent of time.

TABLE 14.2.
Appropriate statistical method according to the type of data

Dependent variable		Independent variables: Continuous	Categorical	Combined
Continuous	Parametric	Linear regression	t-test	Linear regression
		Correlation coefficient (r)	ANOVA	ANCOVA
	Nonparametric	Kernel regression	Wilcoxon rank sum test	Kernel regression
		Loess	Kruskal–Wallis test	LOESS
Categorical	Parametric	Logistic regression	Likelihood ratio	Logistic regression
		Poisson regression		Poisson regression
	Nonparametric		CMH test or trend test	
			Chi–squared test	
Time to event	Parametric	Parametric regression	Likelihood ratio	Parametric regression
	Nonparametric	Cox proportional hazards regression	Cox–Mantel test	Cox proportional hazards regression
			Log rank test	

estimated by this method describe the expected change in response per unit increase in each continuous predictor, independently. When the predictor variable is categorical, the associated parameters represent the expected change in response for each particular category relative to a chosen reference category. For more information and in-depth discussion, the interested reader is referred to Ramsey and Schafer (2002); Ott (1993) and Montgomery *et al.* (2001).

3. Analysis of categorical data

The chi-squared (χ^2) test is typically applied when an investigator needs to tell if the categories of one variable occur independently of the categories of another variable. The χ^2 test also may be utilized for the purpose of testing the goodness of fit of a more complicated statistical model.

Logistic regression is a parametric method used for examining the relationship between a binary response variable (one that is categorical having only two categories) and a set of independent predictor variables that can be either continuous or categorical. Unlike OLS, the natural exponent of an estimated parameter represents the contribution to the odds of response occurring, where we can think of the response as being the more interesting event of the two possible outcomes. For continuous predictor variables, the natural exponent of the estimated parameter represents the contribution to the odds of response per unit increase in the predictor variable. In cases where a predictor is a categorical variable, the natural exponent of the parameter represents the contribution to the odds of the response occurring for that category relative to a reference category chosen by the investigator. For more information and in-depth discussion of these categorical statistical methods see Agresti (1996).

4. Analysis of time-to-event data

In aging studies, researchers may be interested in not only the occurrence of a certain event but also in the timing of the event. This type of data is called time-to-event data. Statistical methods applicable to this type of data are generally known as survival analysis. Time-to-event data have two distinguishing features: censoring and time-dependent covariates (Allison, 1995). For example, suppose that a young investigator gets a one-year pilot grant to follow the effect of a new anti-hypertension agent on the occurrence of heart attack in a certain rodent model. By the end of the one-year period, both the treatment group and the control group have some subjects that had the event (the heart attack) and some had not. The status of animals without events is censored. In this context, censored means that we cannot know whether, much less when, they would have a heart attack after the follow-up period. As another example of censoring data, we may wish to study lifespan and mortality rate by conducting an aging study. For some animal models with a relatively long lifespan, such as nonhuman primates, it is difficult or impractical to follow the animals until death. By the end of the study, one can expect that there will be some subjects with unknown life expectancy (i.e., censored). Moreover, during the follow-up period, the values of some covariates, such as blood pressure and heart function, may also change over time. Conventional statistical methods such as logistic regression and linear regression cannot model the event and the timing of event simultaneously, nor can they incorporate changes in covariates over time. Modern survival analysis methods are capable of handling these complexities inherent in longitudinal time-to-event data analysis (Singer and Willett, 2003).

Survival analysis techniques model the event and timing of the event simultaneously by estimating the hazard function or the survivor function. The hazard function, $h(t)$ is the rate, not the probability, of an event (failure) in a very short time interval. The survivor function, $S(t)$, is the probability that the time to event is greater than t. The hazard function, survivor function, and probability density function of the event time, T, are equivalent. That is, we can derive all of these three functions if we know any one of them (Allison, 1995). Some widely used nonparametric, semiparametric, and parametric survival analysis methods, their assumptions, and the survivor and hazard functions to be estimated are listed in Table 14.3. In summary, the proportional hazards model (Cox, 1972) is the most popular model because, as a semiparametric method, it is the most robust. The nonparametric methods such as Kaplan–Meier and life-table methods are useful for comparing survival curves and evaluating model fit for regression methods (Allison, 1995).

Given the unique features of survival analysis, there are some specific considerations for sample size calculation for studies using time-to-event data. For example, in addition to the information needed for sample size calculation using conventional methods, the researcher may also need to know the follow-up time, an estimate of the overall follow-up event rate, the underlying assumption of event time, and/or the ratio of median/mean survival time of different groups depending on the study design. The most popular approach for sample size calculation of survival analysis is based on the assumption that the survival times are random draws from an exponential distribution (Schoenfeld and Richer, 1982). Several software packages have implemented either this approach or similar approaches (Iwane *et al.*, 1997). One property of the exponential distribution is that the hazard rate is constant over time, but this is not always true in reality. Some other distributions, such as the Weibull distribution, may be more appropriate to characterize the distribution of survival time especially when the follow-up period is long and the hazard rate is accelerated with time. Heo *et al.* (1997) developed an approximate sample calculation method for the Weibull regression

TABLE 14.3.
Comparison of widely used survival analysis methods

Method		Assumption	Survivor/hazard function to be estimated
Nonparametric	Kaplan–Meier method	N/A	$\hat{S}(t) = \prod_{j:t_j \leq i} \left[1 - \frac{d_i}{n_i}\right]$ 1
	Life-table method	N/A	$\hat{S}(t_i) = \prod_{j=1}^{i-1} (1 - q_i)$ 2
Parametric (Accelerated failure time model)	Exponential model	Event time is a random draw from the exponential distribution	$\log h(t) = \mu + \beta_1 X_1 + \beta_2 X_2 + \cdots + \beta_k X_k$ 3
	Weibull model	Event time is a random draw from the Weibull distribution	$\log h(t) = \mu + \alpha \log(t) + \beta_1 X_1 + \beta_2 X_2 + \cdots + \beta_k X_k$ 3
	Gompertz model	Event time is a random draw from the Gompertz distribution	$\log h(t) = \mu + \alpha t + \beta_1 X_1 + \beta_2 X_2 + \cdots + \beta_k X_k$ 3
Semiparametric	Propotional hazard model	Hazard ratio is constant over time	$h_i(t) = \lambda_0(t) \exp(\beta_1 x_{i1} + \beta_2 X_{i2} + \cdots + \beta_k x_{ik})$ 4

1. $\hat{S}(t)$ is the survival function; d_i is the number of events at time t_i; n_i is the number of individual at risk at time t_i.
2. $\hat{S}(t)$ is the survival function of the ith time interval with start time t_i; q_i is the probability of event conditional on no event at time t_i.
3. $h(t)$ is the hazard function at time t and α, μ, and $\beta_1, \beta_2, \ldots, \beta_k$ are parameters to be estimated. $X_{i1}, \ldots, X_{ik}$ are covariates.

method that extended the method developed by Schoenfeld and Richer (1982). Investigators can implement Heo *et al.*'s method by using existing software (Heo *et al.*, 1997). There are also other recently developed methods to calculate sample size for Weibull and proportional hazard models (Vaeth and Skovlund, 2004; Halabi and Singh, 2004).

Statistics for Maximum Lifespan

Interesting research topics unique to aging research include comparing the "maximum lifespan" for different populations or the examination of the effects of different treatments on lifespan. As mentioned previously, it is generally impractical or impossible to collect data from all of the individuals in the population of interest. As such, we collect data on samples taken from the population and attempt to generalize our sample-specific findings to the larger population. As a result, one can only observe the maximum lifespan of a sample which is sensitive to sample size (David and Nagaraja, 2003). Therefore, in practice, the phrase "maximum lifespan" is used to refer to upper percentiles, for example, the 90th percentile (Speakman *et al.*, 2002). Seeking and evaluating interventions that can extend maximum lifespan is an exciting and active field in aging research. For instance, evidence that caloric restriction (CR) increases both the maximum and mean lifespan of many species has been accumulating (Weindruch and Walford, 1988). In this context, the null hypothesis is that there is no difference in maximum lifespan between two independent groups, say one experiencing CR and one not. What is a little surprising is that many studies, including some recent, well-known studies (Hochschild, 1973; Flurkey *et al.*, 2001; and Anisimov *et al.*, 1998) did not conduct any formal statistical hypothesis testing to compare maximum lifespan between treatment groups. Moreover, there is no statistical test accepted as being the "best" for testing the difference in lifespan.

COMPARE MEANS

Because lifespan is a continuous variable, it is straightforward to apply a *t*-test to compare the maximum lifespan between two groups, or to apply ANOVA to compare maximum lifespan among multiple groups. We call this the conditional *t*-test (CTT) approach. It can be easily generalized to compare means across multiple groups by conditional ANOVA (Goodrick *et al.*, 1990). If the lifespan of the sample is normally distributed, it is apparent that the distribution of the lifespan in the upper percentile has a truncated normal distribution, not a symmetric distribution. We already know that the *t*-test is a parametric method and that one of its assumptions is that the data are derived randomly from a normally distributed population. Therefore, in this instance, the application of the CTT is questionable. In fact, in a simulation study, Wang *et al.* (2004) showed that the CTT does have an inflated type I error rate and is invalid for comparing maximum lifespan.

COMPARE PERCENTILES

An alternative approach is to compare percentiles or quantiles across groups. Quantile regression is such an approach (Koenker and Bassett, 1978). It is used to estimate conditional quantile functions by minimizing the weighted sum function. Redden *et al.* (2004) recently developed a simplified quantile regression method using logistic regression which has an appropriate type I error rate and good power. For comparing maximum lifespan, one needs to first find the 90th percentile for all animals combined. Then the animals are categorized into two categories (i.e., constituting a binary variable): lifespan longer than the 90th percentile versus lifespan shorter than the 90th percentile. This binary variable can then be regressed on the predictors including the group assignment by logistic regression to test for differences in maximum lifespan. Although Redden *et al.*'s method performs very well when the sample size is reasonably large, this approach is not informative when there is a cell count of zero or near zero in the two-by-two contingency table, which is often likely given the sample sizes in animal experiments.

It should be noted that Redden *et al.*'s approach represents a form of categorical data analysis. The methods suitable for contingency tables with small sample sizes, such as Fisher's exact test, may be a better choice in this context. As shown by Wang *et al.* (2004), apart from Fisher's exact test, an ordinary chi-squared test, Boschloo's test, or a score test could also be used to test for significance. Mehrotra *et al.* (2003) thoroughly studied the properties of these four methods and found that when the sample size is small, the ordinary chi-squared test inflates the type I error rate; the Fisher's exact test is conservative but has good power; and the Boschloo's test and score test have relatively appropriate type I error rate and good power even when the sample sizes are as small as 50 per group (i.e., only 10 subjects in two groups having a lifespan equal to or longer than the 90th percentile). In summary, Fisher's exact test, Boschloo's test, and the score test are valid and suitable when testing for significant differences in maximum lifespan and they each possess reasonably good power. Wang *et al.*'s (2004) simulation study also provides practical guidelines for choosing the appropriate sample size for the given effect size and type I error rate.

FUTURE STUDY

In addition to the methods discussed, some other nonparametric methods may also be applicable to test for differences in maximum lifespan. These include the Wilcoxon rank-sum test (or the Mann–Whitney U-test) for two independent samples and the Kruskal–Wallis one-way ANOVA for multiple groups. Indeed, the Wilcoxon rank-sum test and Mann–Whitney U-test are analogous to the t-test and can be appropriately used to test for the difference in median between two independent groups by using the ranks of the raw data. In general, nonparametric methods are more robust when the assumptions of parametric methods are not satisfied and/or when the sample size is small. Of course, there is a trade-off in that nonparametric methods are less powerful than parametric methods when the distributional requirements have been met. Further statistical evaluations are required to confirm the validity of these approaches when applied to maximum life span studies.

Practical Recommendations

Many excellent statistical software packages available commercially (e.g. SAS®, SPSS®, S-Plus®) can perform the statistical procedures outlined in this chapter. Some of these software packages, such as SPSS, are very user friendly. In addition to procedures for data analysis, some software, such as SAS, can be used to assist in developing a study design. With the help of such software, we can perform statistical tasks much more efficiently and with greater power than ever before. Indeed, statistical procedures that once took months to calculate can now be performed in less than 5 seconds. Although this is a blessing, it can also become problematic. That is, in the wrong hands these powerful statistical software packages can produce misleading if not downright false results.

One must exercise great care and use caution when conducting complex statistical analyses. As such, to increase the chances of producing a valid analysis, we offer the following recommendations: (1) Whenever possible, and ideally at the study design stage, consult with a statistician regarding the best statistical approach to addressing a given research question. (2) Begin with graphical and/or tabular displays of the data to develop a sense of what the data look like and to assess possible errors in data input and processing. (3) Carefully examine your data to assess whether the assumptions required for the use of parametric methods are adequately met (sometimes a simple data transformation can transform skewed data into a normal distribution, thereby meeting a parametric assumption). (4) Always opt for the simplest statistical analysis possible to test a given hypothesis.

Conclusions

Statistics are important and powerful tools for conducting sound scientific research. Statistical methods can affect the validation of such research at almost every stage beginning with the design of the study through to the interpretation of the results and statements of the conclusions. To be valid, a study must have a testable hypothesis, a properly chosen statistical method to test that hypothesis with a suitable type I error rate, and a sufficient number of study subjects in order to achieve the degree of statistical power necessary for detecting a meaningful difference or effect. Descriptive statistics can help to summarize the data, check assumptions, and guide further analysis. While many statistical software packages are powerful tools for data analysis, applied researchers should understand the statistical basis of the procedures they use and avoid careless operation of such software.

Many topics are not included in this chapter, and aging researchers are collecting data with increasing levels of complexity, such as microarray and other high-dimension biological data. We strongly suggest that the applied researchers seek assistance from statisticians when necessary. The basic concepts and considerations discussed in this chapter will be helpful for communication between applied researchers and statisticians.

REFERENCES

Agresti, A. (1996). *Introduction to Categorical Data Analysis*. John Wiley, New York.

Allison, P. (1995). *Survival Analysis Using the SAS System: A Practical Guide*. SAS Institute, Inc. Cary.

Altman, D. (1999). *Practical Statistics for Medical Research*. Chapman & Hall/CRC, New York.

Anisimov, V., Mylnikov, S., and Khavinson, V. (1998) Pineal peptide preparation epithalamin increases the lifespan of fruit flies, mice and rats. *Mech Ageing Dev. 103*, 123–132.

Brannath, W., and Bauer, P. (2004). Optimal conditional error functions for the control of conditional power. *Biometrics. 60*, 715–723.

Carlin, J., and Doyle, L. (2001). Statistics for clinicians: 4: Basic concepts of statistical reasoning: hypothesis tests and the t-test. *J Paediatr Child Health. 37*, 72–77.

Conover, W. (1999). *Practical Nonparametric Statistics*. John Wiley, New York.

Cox, D. (1972). Regression model and life-tables (with discussion). *J. Roy. Statist. Soc. Ser. B. 34*, 187–220.

Daniel, W. (1998). *Biostatistics: A Foundation for Analysis in the Health Sciences*. John Wiley, New York.

David, H., and Nagaraja, H. (2003). *Order Statistics* (3rd ed.). Wiley-Interscience, New York.

DeMets, D., and Lan, K. (1994). Interim analysis: The alpha spending function approach. *Stat Med. 13*, 1341–1352; discussion 1353–1356.

Fisher, L., and van Belle, G. (1993). *Biostatistics: A Methodology for the Health Sciences*. John Wiley, New York.

Flurkey, K., Papaconstantinou, J., Miller, R., and Harrison, D. (2001). Lifespan extension and delayed immune and collagen aging in mutant mice with defects in growth hormone production. *Proc Natl Acad Sci USA 98*, 6736–6741.

Goodrick, C., Ingram, D., Reynolds, M., Freeman, J., and Cider, N. (1990). Effects of intermittent feeding upon body weight and lifespan in inbred mice: Interaction of genotype and age. *Mech. Ageing. Dev. 55*, 69–87.

Halabi, S., and Singh, B. (2004). Sample size determination for comparing several survival curves with unequal allocations. *Stat Med. 23*, 1793–1815.

Heo, M., Faith, M., and Allison, D. (1998). Power and sample size for survival analysis under the Weibull distribution when the whole lifespan is of interest. *Mech Ageing Dev. 102*, 45–53.

Hochschild, R. (1973). Effect of dimethylaminoethanol on the life span of senile male A-J mice. *Exp Gerontol. 8*, 185–191.

Iwane, M., Palensky, J., and Plante, K. (1997). A user's review of commercial sample size software for design of biomedical studies using survival data. *Control Clin Trials. 18*, 65–83.

Jennison, C., and Turnbull, B. (1999). *Group Sequential Methods with Applications to Clinical Trials.* Chapman & Hall/CRC, New York.

Koenker, R., and Bassett, G. (1978). Regression quantiles. *Econometrica. 46*, 33–50.

Lee, E., and Wang, J. (2003). *Statistical Methods for Survival Data Analysis.* John Wiley, New York.

Machin, D., Campbell, M. (1987). *Statistical Tables for the Design of Clinical Trials.* Oxford, Blackwell.

Mehotra, D., Chan, I., and Berger, R. (2003). A cautionary note on exact unconditional inference for a difference between two independent binomial proportions. *Biometrics. 59*, 441–450.

Montgomery, D., Peck, E., and Vining, G. (2001). *Introduction to Linear Regression Analysis.* John Wiley, New York.

Mooney, C., and Duval, R. (1993). *Bootstrapping A Nonparametric Approach to Statistical Inference.* Sage Publications, Newbury Park.

Murphy, J. (2004). Statistical errors in immunologic research. *J Allergy Clin Immunol. 114*, 1259–1263.

Olsen, C. (2003). Review of the use of statistics in infection and immunity. *Infect Immun. 71*, 6689–6692.

Ott, R. (1993). *An Introduction to Statistical Methods and Data Analysis.* Duxbury Press, Belmont.

Proschan, M., and Hunsberger, S. (1995). Designed extension of studies based on conditional power. *Biometrics. 51*, 1315–1324.

Schoenfeld, D., and Richter, J. (1982). Nomograms for calculating the number of patients needed for a clinical trial with survival as an endpoint. *Biometrics. 38*, 163–170.

Speakman, J., Selman, C., McLaren, J., and Harper, E. (2002). Living fast, dying when? The link between aging and energetics, *J. Nutr. 6 Suppl. 2*, 1583S–1597S.

Ramsey, F., and Schafer, D. (2002). *The Statistical Sleuth: A Course in Methods of Data Analysis.* Duxbury, Pacific Grove.

Redden, D., Fernandez, J., and Allison, D. (2004). A simple significance test for quantile regression. *Stat Med. 23*, 2587–2597.

Singer, J., and Willett, J. (2003). *Applied Longitudinal Data Analysis: Modeling Change and Event Occurrence.* Oxford University Press, New York.

Thompson, S. *Sampling.* John Wiley, New York.

Wang, C., Li, Q., Redden, D., Weindruch, R., and Allison, D. (2004). Statistical methods for testing effects on "maximum lifespan." *Mech Ageing Dev. 125*, 629–632.

Weindruch, R., Walfor, R., Fligiel, S., and Guthrie, D. (1986). The retardation of aging mice by dietary restriction: Longevity, cancer, immunity and lifetime energy intake. *Journal of Nutrition 116*, 641–654.

Weindruch, R., and Walford, R. (1998). *The Retardation of Aging and Disease by Dietary Restriction.* C.C. Thomas Publisher, Springfield, IL.

Williams, J., Hathaway, C., Kloster, K., and Layne, B. (1997). Low power, type II errors, and other statistical problems in recent cardiovascular research. *Am J Physiol. 273*, H487–H493.

Vaeth, M., and Skovlund, E. (2004). A simple approach to power and sample size calculations in logistic regression and Cox regression models. *Stat Med. 23*, 1781–1792.

15

Models for the Study of Infection in Populations

John R. Williams

This chapter provides an overview of the modeling of transmission dynamics of infectious diseases, with particular focus on the use of compartmental differential equation models, the most commonly used for such work. An introduction including a brief description of historical antecedents is followed by a section putting such modeling in its ecological context. The next section discusses some of the characteristics of infection in populations that are determinants of the observed population dynamics of infection. This is followed by a brief section considering the scope and limitations of dynamic models, followed by a section summarizing some of the key concepts relevant to this type of modeling work. Simple ordinary differential equation models are introduced in the next section. Demography and the relevance of population age structure to infection transmission dynamics, and partial differential equation models incorporating age structure and age-related processes of infection and disease, are explored in the following two sections. The section after this considers three examples of infections in which age-related processes are important. Next there is a brief look at alternative approaches to modeling, and the penultimate section introduces further uses for dynamic models in health economic analysis, immune system dynamics, and exploring the impact of strain variation in infections. The concluding section is followed by a short appendix on the solution of differential equation system models.

Introduction

Infectious agents are no respecters of age. The population as a whole is their natural habitat, so a focus on the population therefore does not preclude, but rather facilitates, investigation of how aging and life span influence and are influenced by the public health impact of infections. Thus the population in any given epidemiological setting is the sensible unit to consider when using mathematical models to address issues relating to aging and infectious diseases.

The first attempts to model infections in populations appear to have been undertaken by Bernouilli in 1760 in relation to smallpox. A few instances occur also in the 19th century, but the true origins of today's mathematical modeling of infection transmission in populations can be found in the work of Hamer and of Ross in the early years of the 20th century on malaria. Further developed in the 1920s by Soper, and Kermack and McKendrick, this has led to a rapidly expanding literature on the dynamics of infection transmission in populations (see Anderson and May (1991) for an overview and a comprehensive introduction to the field). In essence, infectious disease transmission dynamics consists of the ebb and flow of infection within populations, as mediated by the distribution of immunity in the population and patterns of contacts leading to exposure. While a substantial proportion of the relevant literature is largely theoretical and to be found in mathematical journals, increasingly work involving transmission dynamics modeling is concerned with questions involving real data, future trends, and what may be expected from specific control interventions. Such work may be found with increasing frequency in journals with an orientation towards public health.

This chapter largely focuses on the use of a particular class of mathematical models to investigate the transmission dynamics of infectious diseases. Mathematical modeling, in general, is a very wide field from which many new approaches to the modeling of infection transmission have arisen, but the class of model considered here is one of the most generally useful. These models are known as deterministic compartmental differential equation models. In simple terms, differential equations describe the relationship between the value of a variable (e.g., number of infected individuals at a particular point in time) and the way in which that variable changes (e.g., how the rate of change increases or decreases as the number of infected individuals changes); if they are deterministic, their results are completely determined by the initial model parameters and initial conditions (i.e., there are no stochastic or random processes included in these models), and the models are described as compartmental because the population

Handbook of Models for Human Aging

under consideration is divided between compartments representing different states of susceptibility, infection and disease. This chapter will describe how this initially simple approach can usefully be expanded to take into account, among other things, demographics, age-related processes of infection and immunity, patterns of contact and risk behaviors, and public health interventions. First, however, it may be helpful to say something about the ecological context in which such models operate, as many useful developments and insights from the field of modeling population ecology have found their way into that of modeling infections in human populations. Infectious agents are, after all, simply organisms which operate in a particular and specialized environment.

The Ecological Context of Infection

As with other biological organisms, infectious agents have evolved through natural selection to fill a particular niche in the global ecosystem, but in this case the organism is a parasite (Begon *et al.*, 1996) having the "body" of another organism as the environment in which to grow or reproduce and from which to disseminate in order to colonize other suitable environments. Here we are, of course, interested in infections of humans, but it is useful to bear in mind that infection is a widespread phenomenon across the biosphere, including bacteriophages infecting bacteria, viral infections of plants, bacterial infections of insects and nematodes, and so forth.

Numerous strategies have evolved allowing infections to continue to reproduce and disseminate (Mims *et al.*, 2001; Davies *et al.*, 1999). Rapid reproduction facilitates dissemination before the host's immune system can suppress it; alternatively a very slow rate of reproduction may allow the infection to establish and persist "below the radar" of the immune system. A highly virulent infection may kill the host before it has had the opportunity to disseminate (although in some cases consumption of the dead host by another potential host may be a potential route for further dissemination, as in hydatid disease); in some cases an infection may be highly virulent only when infecting a species not its usual host (e.g., arenaviruses causing hemorrhagic fevers or meningitis in humans, but little apparent disease in rodent reservoirs). Alternatively the infection may evolve with reduced virulence, providing a longer time window within which to spread to a new host. The duration of immunity evoked by infection is a significant determinant of observed infection behavior; for example, if immunity from measles infection were of only short duration, it would no longer simply be classifiable as an infection of childhood, whereas the long duration of immunity that it does produce necessitates a continual supply of newly susceptible infants.

The size of the infectious organism is also a factor in its reproductive strategy; the fact that single-cell organisms invest fewer resources in development than multicellular ones means that rapid reproduction and dissemination are easier to accomplish, whereas for multicellular organisms a longer lifespan is desirable to allow an adequate return on investment in development, which in turn implies more resources being invested also in defenses against the host's immune response. Broadly speaking, human infectious agents (and those of other animals) can usefully be divided into microparasites and macroparasites (Anderson and May, 1991; Thomas and Weber, 2001), although the distinction between the two is pragmatic rather than absolute. Microparasites are those organisms which reproduce directly in the host with relatively short generation times. They do so in such large numbers that it is impracticable to make a count of the numbers of the organism; in general upon recovery from infection there tends to be a period of immunity against reinfection. Viruses and bacteria are typical microparasites. Macroparasites, on the other hand, are generally larger organisms, as the name implies, which do not in general complete their reproductive cycle in a single host; their life cycles can be quite complex, with perhaps another animal species forming an intermediate host, or a free-living stage in the environment before maturity is reached in the definitive host. Infections with macroparasites result in many fewer organisms than with microparasites, and numbers of individuals in each individual stage in the life cycle can often be measured to provide a quantitative indicator of intensity of infection, typically correlating with the severity of disease experienced (but see page 178). Macroparasite infections tend to be of relatively long duration—a significant proportion of the host life time—and a degree of immune tolerance is usually evoked; if infection should be eliminated, for example as a result of treatment, immunity against further infection tends to be short-lived, so that repeated infections tend to be the norm. For reasons of space, the remainder of this chapter will concentrate on modeling microparasitic infections, with the modeling of macroparasite infections (a topic in itself) only briefly being discussed.

Infections in Human Populations

There are many clinical characteristics of human infections that are relevant to modeling of infection transmission dynamics in populations (Thomas and Weber, 2001) and that determine whether they are endemic (i.e., sustained at similar levels over a long period) or epidemic (i.e., with a substantial excess of cases over and above the norm). The time spent in each stage of infection is particularly important, bearing in mind that the "goal" of an infectious agent is to reproduce and disseminate itself through the population. Thus the length of the period of infectivity and its intensity (generally related to the probability of infecting a contact) are clearly important to establish. However the latent period, the period between being infected and becoming infectious, is also a factor to be considered as this also affects how rapidly an infection may spread in the population. One more factor which may or may not be significant is the length of the prepatient period, the time between infection and symptoms becoming apparent, as the onset of symptoms may result in relative isolation from the rest of the population. Some infections, such as herpes simplex or hepatitis B (HBV), may be symptomatic in some individuals but to a greater or lesser degree asymptomatic in others with corresponding differences shown in infectivity, and the tendency to symptomatic vs. asymptomatic infection may vary according to age, as is shown very strongly in the case of hepatitis B (Medley *et al.*, 2001). HBV is also a good example of an infection that may manifest itself as an initial asymptomatic infection or an acute primary infection (in this case lasting a few weeks) leading to recovery or to a persistent chronic infection which for HBV may last several decades or be effectively lifelong. The existence and duration of immunity following infection, ranging for different infections from several months to more or less lifelong immunity, is a further strong determinant of an infection's transmission dynamics in the population. The case fatality rate may or may not be another important determinant. For example, the extremely rapid virulence of the Ebola virus is probably the reason why it has so far failed to propagate itself beyond its local environment; on the other hand, the substantial mortality arising from HBV infection over the long term does not significantly impede its transmission. All these factors may also vary according to the age of infected individuals, so that the age distribution of infection is one further determinant of transmission dynamics (Anderson and May, 1991).

The route or routes of transmission characteristic of an infection also determine the population dynamics of an infection. The means by which the infection leaves its host, the means by which it is transported from one host to another, and the means by which it enters the new host are topics in themselves, but for the purposes of transmission dynamics modeling routes can be classified as horizontal transmission through direct or very close contact between hosts (e.g., measles, rubella), vertical transmission from mother to child at or around birth (e.g., HBV, toxoplasmosis), sexual transmission between sexual partners (often considered to be in a separate category from horizontal transmission) (e.g., gonorrhea, syphilis), environmental transmission in which the infective agent is disseminated in the air, water, food or soil (e.g., Legionnaire's disease, hepatitis A, hookworm), and vector transmission in which the agent is transported, usually by an arthropod, from one host to another (e.g., malaria, river blindness, dengue fever). Additionally some infections make use of more than one host species to complete their transmission cycle (e.g., snail–human for schistosome flukes). As well as the transmission dynamics themselves, these transmission routes determine the structure of the models to be used to investigate the dynamics; the intensity of these different modes of transmission is also often age-dependent, with such age-dependencies forming another determinant of the epidemiological dynamics (Anderson and May, 1991).

Philosophy Underlying Modeling of Infection

Before proceeding further, it is perhaps useful to emphasize what transmission dynamics models can do and what they cannot. In order for a model to be useful, many assumptions and generalizations need to be made if its behavior is not to become so complex that it is impossible to interpret the results or to understand how the various processes interact in the model. Unless we understand why a model produces the results it does we cannot sensibly interpret the results, nor answer the questions we wish to ask (and nor can we identify when an error has crept into the design or implementation of the model!). The value of the results is directly related to the skill with which the complexity of the real-world system is simplified while still retaining the essential features of the epidemiology. When undertaking modeling work, and when reviewing the results of other peoples' models, it should always be borne closely in mind that the results of such work can never be predictions of the future course of an epidemic with the precision that the term "prediction" implies. What such models can do is to make qualitative projections of possible future trends under specific scenarios allowing such questions to be addressed as follows: How should we interpret the epidemiological trends in infection that are being observed, and what might be the underlying processes involved? What data do we need to gather to gain a better understanding of these trends and processes? If a specific infection is introduced into a population, is there the potential for an epidemic, and how many people might be infected? How best might we optimize the design of control programs? What might be the relative advantages and disadvantages of one health intervention versus another?

Key Concepts in Mathematical Modeling of Infection

Before proceeding to look at some simple models, we should first consider some of the key concepts which underpin this approach to modeling the transmission dynamics of infectious disease.

SUSTAINABILITY OF INFECTION IN A POPULATION

The ability of an infection to transmit from an infectious individual to another who is susceptible to that infection depends on many factors, but an essential component is that there should be a point of contact between the two which is either direct—such as through droplets, skin to skin contacts, or sexual transmission, and so on—or indirect, such as via insect vectors or through ingestion or other contact with infective particles which have been disseminated into the environment, for example, through food or water, or contaminated objects. No matter how the infective contact is made, if on average each infection in an individual is only able to newly infect, directly or indirectly, less than one other individual, the infection itself will inevitably die out in this population; the operation of chance effects may result in shorter or longer chains of infection, but in the longer term the infection will be unable to sustain itself. Thus, in order to persist in a population, each infection must, on average, result in the infection of at least one further individual, that is, the infection must reproduce itself at least once.

THE EFFECTIVE REPRODUCTIVE NUMBER

The effective reproductive number, R, is a measure of how many new infections on average result from each existing infection (Anderson and May, 1991); R is also known as the effective reproductive ratio or, incorrectly, as it is not strictly a rate, the effective reproductive rate. When $R=1$, on average each infection produces only one further infected individual. If there are sufficient numbers of infections in the population to ensure that it does not die out simply through chance effects, the infection will be at equilibrium in the population and if this equilibrium is self-sustaining the infection will be endemic; where on the other hand R is significantly greater than one, a growing number of infections, i.e., an epidemic, will result. Although R is a useful measure of the speed with which an infection in a population is spreading, it changes over time as infection spreads through the population and does not give an indication of the potential rate of increase of infection in other populations because the value of R is governed not only by the characteristics of the infection itself but also by the proportion of the population which is immune through past infection or otherwise.

THE BASIC REPRODUCTIVE NUMBER

The basic reproductive number, R_0 (also known as the basic reproductive ratio or, again incorrectly, rate), is the measure used to characterize the potential for an infectious organism to spread through a population in which there is no prior immunity and thus gives a measure of the maximum potential rate of spread in a given population (though differing social, economic, demographic and health characteristics of populations may provide widely differing opportunities for an infectious organism to disseminate) (Anderson and May, 1991). Clearly when everyone in a population is susceptible to infection R and R_0 will have the same value, but assuming some degree of immunity is produced, however short term, R will decrease as the infection spreads whereas R_0 by definition remains constant.

When an infection is at equilibrium, $R=1.0$, as noted above. If R_0 is greater than R ($R_0 > R$), a proportion of the potential transmission events implied by R_0 will fail because a proportion of potential contacts are already immune to infection in these circumstances, and only effective contacts with susceptible individuals will result in transmission. The symbol X is often used to represent the number of susceptible individuals in a population of N individuals, and x ($=X/N$) to represent the proportion of susceptible individuals in the population. In a theoretically uniformly homogeneous population, if x^* represents the proportion of susceptible individuals when the infection is at equilibrium, x^* can be used to estimate R_0 as $R_0x^* = R = 1.0$. Anderson and May (1991) quote from their earlier work a range of values for R_0 for different infections and different epidemiological settings; that for measles, for example, varying from 5 to 6 in post–World War I Kansas, USA to 16 to 18 in post–World War II England and Wales. Although in theory when $R_0=1$ an infection has the capacity to spread in a wholly susceptible population, in practice it needs to exceed this value by a sufficient amount to ensure that the chain of infection is not terminated purely through chance events.

FORCE OF INFECTION

The incidence (total yearly number of new cases or yearly proportion of the population newly infected) and prevalence of an infection (proportion of the population with current infection) in a population are basic and essential epidemiological measures, and are in principle directly observable or deducible, given an adequate surveillance system, clear case definition, and either unambiguous clinical symptoms or suitable laboratory techniques for confirmation. However, incidence and prevalence cannot be used directly as inputs to a model because these measures are a reflection, among other things, of both the capacity of the infectious agent to spread and also the distribution of prior immunity in the population. What is needed is a measure of the intrinsic ability of the infectious agent to spread from an infected individual to a susceptible individual in the population. The *force of infection* (FOI, often assigned the Greek letter lambda, λ) is the measure that is needed and plays an integral role in the operation of transmission dynamic models. This measure corresponds to the yearly incidence of infection per capita among those individuals who are susceptible to infection, that is, those who are not immune as a result of past infection, the presence of maternal antibody, or effective immunization, or those who are currently infected with the same infectious agent (it will be seen that there are parallels here with R_0, the basic reproductive number; see Anderson and May (1991) for a detailed exposition of the relationship between the two). In fact the FOI is a composite of (a) the rate of contacts with other individuals in the population, whether infectious or not; (b) the risk of infection actually being transmitted to another individual given a suitable contact; and (c) the proportion of contacts who are in fact infectious. Depending on the complexity of the model, many simplifying assumptions need to be made if these components of the FOI are to be measured. However, it is also possible for the FOI to be inferred from serological data (prior to introduction of any vaccination) if infection results in long-lasting immunity to further infection and case mortality is relatively small (Farrington, 1990). An additional requirement for this approach is that the infection, to a rough approximation, can be considered to be more or less at equilibrium in the population over the longer term so that the distribution of immunity by age does not change significantly over time. Such stability in the age profile of immunity over time means that measurement at a given time (i.e., cross-sectional measurement) of the age distribution of exposure to infection in a population (i.e., the proportion at each age with the appropriate antibody) may be taken to correspond to a longitudinal measurement over time of exposure to infection of any birth cohort of the population. This cumulative risk can be analyzed in the same way as other cumulative risks by using survival analysis (Farrington, 1990) and making the assumption that everyone entering the population at birth is either susceptible to infection or becomes so following the loss of maternal antibody. The "failure rate" resulting from this analysis is the FOI which may be either independent of age or, if the data is sufficiently detailed to warrant it, age-dependent. An alternative to estimation of the FOI in such a population is to make use of case notifications, but the potential weakness of this latter approach lies in the common problem of failures and biases intrinsic to reporting systems; the use of sentinel surveys is likely to prove the more reliable approach. If an infection is newly introduced into a previously unexposed population, which therefore has no immunity, a useful estimate of the FOI can also be derived from R_0, which in turn can be estimated from the time taken for the number of cases of the newly introduced infection to double (Anderson *et al.*, 1986; Anderson and May, 1991). When there are no long-lasting markers of infection, mortality is high, infection is not at equilibrium, or there are substantial heterogeneities in patterns of infection in different subgroups of the population, this last method is particularly useful for estimating the FOI. The case of HIV/AIDS is a notable example where this latter technique has been used in the initial stages of an epidemic (Anderson *et al.*, 1986).

HERD IMMUNITY

Herd immunity is essentially a simple concept describing the totality of naturally acquired and vaccine-based immunity to a given infectious agent as a proportion of the whole population. While the individual objective of vaccination is clearly to prevent or reduce the risk of infection for the individual concerned, the public health objective of vaccination is to increase the level of herd immunity to that required for control or elimination of the infection from the population, and in the longer term on a regional or global scale to eradicate the infection altogether. (Note the distinction between *elimination* where an infectious agent is no longer present in a particular population and *eradication* in which the agent is eliminated world- or region-wide; the smallpox virus remains, at the time of writing, the only infection for which global eradication has been achieved.) The term *herd immunity* is occasionally used to describe the level of population immunity that will result in elimination of a specific infection from a population, but here *herd immunity for elimination* would be more appropriate. This level of herd immunity for elimination is that at which an infection cannot propagate effectively in the population; at this level of immunity there may be some secondary cases or even short chains of infection, but these chains are sooner or later broken and prove insufficient to prevent the infection from dying out. In other words, the effective reproduction number, R, in these circumstances is less than 1.0. Herd immunity is obviously dynamic, as natural or vaccine-based immunity is lost over time through waning of immunological memory or deaths of immune individuals, and newly susceptible individuals arrive through births or migration. Thus to maintain the effectiveness of vaccination programs, vaccine coverage and herd immunity need to be monitored at regular intervals and if necessary a strategy planned, informed by dynamic modeling, of supplementary vaccination programs introduced to boost herd immunity to the necessary level (Nokes and Anderson, 1988).

CONTACT MATRICES

The various patterns of contacts between individuals, which are necessary for transmission of infection to occur, clearly are not dependent on the presence of a particular infection (although it is true that the presence of infection may lead to changes in patterns of behavior that might result in contacts being made). As prevalence and perhaps intensity or duration of an infection will vary between age groups and between the various subgroups that make up a population, the patterns of contact between these may be important determinants of the dynamics of the infection in the population and the age distribution of infection and hence of the burden of disease. It is therefore advantageous to be able to include a representation of such contact patterns when modeling the transmission dynamics of infection. Although such a representation cannot hope to reproduce the full richness of patterns of contact found in everyday life, nevertheless there are greatly simplified ways of representing such patterns, which nonetheless allow some of the essence of these patterns to be usefully captured. In the compartmental models described in this chapter, this is typically achieved by the use of a matrix specifying the proportion of contacts made by each group with every other group represented in the model (i.e., contacts which would result in transmission of infection if made with an infectious individual). Typically, for infections such as measles which may be acquired simply through close proximity to a infective case, the contact matrix is presented in the form of a "Who Acquires Infection from Whom" (WAIFW) matrix (Anderson and May, 1985; Anderson and Grenfell, 1986; Anderson and May, 1991) in which the individual elements of the matrix represent the probability per unit of time that a susceptible individual in one subgroup (often an age group) may be infected by an infective individual from the same or one of the other subgroups. There is not normally sufficient data to be able to specify the elements of the WAIFW matrix directly, so estimates of the force of infection for each group may be used in combination with estimates of the proportion of the precontrol population in the infective state to estimate the matrix indirectly (there are also strong constraints on the form which the WAIFW matrix may take using this procedure) (Anderson and May, 1991). In the case of sexually transmitted infections (STIs) the contact matrix might simply describe the proportion of its sexual partnerships (or sexual acts) that each subgroup has with each of the other subgroups; then the numbers of partners and/or acts per unit time for individuals in each subgroup together with the probability of transmission per partnership (or per act) are specified as separate parameters (Anderson and May, 1991; Williams and Anderson, 1994).

AVERAGE AGE AT INFECTION (A)

Average age at infection (A) is a useful summary measure indicating the arithmetic mean age at infection of all cases over some (often unspecified) period of time. For a childhood infection such as measles, it also provides an approximate indication of how narrow is the age window for vaccination which public health programs should aim for between the loss of passive immunity from maternal antibodies and the age at which the majority of children will already have been infected. The average age at infection will also provide some indication of the likely disease burden from an infection in which processes of morbidity or mortality are age-related. For infections provoking long-lasting immunity the average age at infection will change according to the evolution of the age profile of herd immunity in the population, so that it is likely to be higher when an infection is introduced into the population for the first time and lower as the infection becomes endemic in the population and many older individuals are immune following recovery from infection; the infectious agent is then primarily reliant on births to supply new susceptible individuals to the population. If an infection is characterized by epidemics repeated at longer intervals of time, the average age at infection will rise and fall accordingly. Note that the introduction of a vaccination program, through its impact on the age distribution of immunity, will itself change the average age at infection, and as infection becomes more rare as a result of a successful vaccination program, those who have not been vaccinated will themselves be less at risk of infection (herd immunity effect). If these individuals do eventually become infected it is likely to be at an older age than would otherwise have been the case in the absence of vaccination. Should morbidity increase with age it is therefore theoretically possible, dependent on circumstances, for vaccination to result in an increased burden of disease (Williams and Manfredi, 2004). Rubella infection constitutes a prime example of such a risk, being a mild infection in childhood, but should the average age at infection be delayed there is likely to be an increase in risk of infection for women in their fertile years, with a resulting risk of congenital rubella if infection occurs in the first trimester of pregnancy (Edmunds *et al.*, 2000). Processes of demographic change whether a result of increase or reduction in the population growth rate or the onset of population decline, by changing the population age structure (and indirectly therefore the age profile of susceptibility), may also change the average age at infection (Williams and Manfredi, 2004). The arithmetic mean, of course, tells us little about the variance in ages at infection which may itself be important—if there is substantial variance in ages at infection, a substantial proportion of cases may occur in younger or older (perhaps much older) ages, so that when considering how changes in the age distribution of infection may affect age-dependent morbidity or mortality, median and percentile measures also become important.

MODEL VALIDATION AND SENSITIVITY AND UNCERTAINTY ANALYSIS

An essential aspect of the use of mathematical models in infectious disease epidemiology is validation of model results against real data, validation here referring simply to the ability to satisfy oneself that the model results are consistent with the available data relating to the population which is being modeled (or in its absence, data from a population sharing similar characteristics). It is not necessary for this process to be one of fitting, in the statistical sense, as we are dealing with model results which are qualitative rather than quantitative, and it is usually therefore more important that the model can reproduce the change in shape over time of the data being used for validation rather than absolute values. Thus the process is more one of inspection and fitting by eye rather than statistical fitting. Given that we can establish the validity of the model results in this way, it is important to know how sensitive these results are to the values of the model parameters. Depending upon the structure of the model and the role played by each parameter in the model, very small changes in the values of some parameters can lead to large variations in model results; for other parameters the situation may be reversed and relatively large changes in values may have little impact on the results. It is the role of sensitivity analysis to establish how variation in parameter values might impact on model outputs; if the model should prove to be too sensitive, the results will be useless. This can either be done simply by varying the values of each parameter in turn and observing what effect each has, or more systematically by the use of "Latin hypercube" sampling (cf. Latin square), which involves specifying a distribution for the values of each parameter (which could simply be a uniform distribution if the true distribution is not known) and sampling at random and without replacement parameter values from the combined set of distributions (Seaholm *et al.*, 1988). Once the sensitivity of the model to its parameters has been established, it is necessary to consider how much uncertainty there is in our knowledge about the true values of each parameter in relation to the population being considered. In uncertainty analysis we are considering what the plausible range of values for each parameter might be, and exploring the variation in model results which arises when parameter values are varied within this set of ranges; the variation in model outputs then provides an indication of uncertainty about the likely way in which, for example, prevalence or incidence of an infection may change over time in the population being studied.

Simple Compartmental Models

FLOW DIAGRAMS

A key stage in the design and definition of a transmission dynamics model is preparation of a flow diagram. This comprises (1) a set of compartments representing that part of the population found in each of the various states of susceptibility, infection or disease to be included in the model and (2) the transitions or flows of population from one state to another upon initial infection, progression of disease, recovery etc. Such diagrams may often appear simple in the extreme (Figure 15.1), but they provide an invaluable aid to thinking about the epidemiological system being modeled by ensuring that the modeler specifies very precisely which stages of infection will be incorporated in the model (and what, precisely, is the meaning of each stage), and also how each stage is entered and how it is left; this should be done bearing in mind that simplicity will facilitate understanding and that unnecessary complexity will have the opposite result.

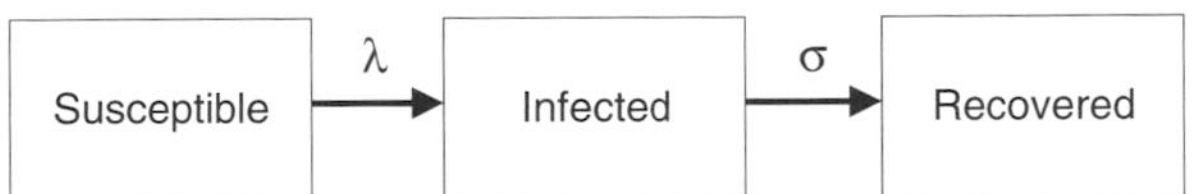

Figure 15.1. A simple flow diagram. The diagram shows the compartments representing the susceptible (S), infected (I) and recovered (R) proportions of the population and arrows representing the flows or transitions between compartments upon infection, at rate λ (the force of infection) per capita, and recovery from infection at the per capita rate σ; arrows representing births into the population and deaths leaving the population may also be included if desired or useful. This is often referred to as an S-I-R model, although the letters X, Y and Z are commonly used in place, respectively, of S, I and R.

MODEL EQUATIONS

The design of the flow diagram also specifies the structure of the system of differential equations that constitutes the compartmental model. There is a direct correspondence between the flow diagram compartments and the model's state variables (representing the proportion or numbers in the population in each stage), and between the flows in the diagram and how the rates of change in the equations are specified. (The model equations may also incorporate subsidiary population structure such as different age groups or different behavioral groups which might not be included in the flow diagram.) The simplest example of a differential equation is the exponential growth curve in which the rate of increase over time of, say, a population N depends only on a constant per capita growth rate parameter r, and on the size of N (known as the equation's state variable).

$$\frac{dN}{dt} = rN$$

Here dN/dt is the rate at which the value of N changes with time and is equivalent to the slope of the curve of N at any point in time. This example, of course, assumes no deaths. A more realistic simple example incorporating also infection and recovery to permanent immunity would be the equation system corresponding to the flow diagram of Figure 15.1.

$$\frac{dX}{dt} = \mu N - (\lambda + \mu)X$$
$$\frac{dY}{dt} = \lambda X - (\sigma + \mu)Y$$
$$\frac{dZ}{dt} = \sigma Y - \mu Z$$
$$N = X + Y + Z$$

(NB: Addition of the equations will give the rate of change of the whole population (dN/dt) so that, if population size is constant, the sum of the equations will be zero, a useful check for errors in specifying the equations.)

In this set of equations, X (the susceptible population), Y (the infected population), and Z (the recovered population) are the "state variables" corresponding to the compartments in the flow diagram, and the various terms in the equations represent the different flows into and out of the compartments in the form of the product of the values of the state variables at that moment in time and the values of the parameters determining the rates of flow. (Here λ represents the force of infection, σ the rate of recovery from infection and μ the per capita death rate and also, for convenience in order to ensure constant population size, the per capita birth rate.) Note that the model is expressed as rates of change of each of the state variables. In simple cases, the values of the state variables at any point in time (an analytic solution) can be found through a mathematical solution of the equation system (see Appendix). In many cases, however, it is necessary to rely on a numerical solution of the equations using either computer modeling tools, or in the more complex cases involving partial differential equations (see below) computer programs written *ad hoc*. Various types of intervention can also be incorporated into such models, perhaps by explicitly adding further compartments/variables (e.g., for individuals who are vaccinated and thus at reduced risk of infection, or for those receiving some therapeutic intervention speeding recovery or reducing infectiousness) together with a corresponding further flow from the appropriate compartment (e.g., from the susceptible compartment in the case of prophylactic intervention or from an infection compartment for a therapeutic intervention). In the case of vaccination at or shortly after birth, the entry flow into the population could be divided into those entering as susceptible and those entering as immune through vaccination (in other cases intervention might be included implicitly by assuming that only a proportion of the population might be susceptible to infection) (Figures 15.2, 15.3, and 15.4) (Anderson and May, 1991).

The model population can also be stratified into different behavioral or other relevant subgroups (it may not be necessary to represent this stratification in the flow diagram), and contact matrices specifying contacts between the subgroups can then become a component of the force of infection. A simple example of the latter is for sexually transmitted infections in which the force of infection term experienced by individuals in subgroup i (λ_i) is composed of a term describing probability of infection, β, as a result of a sexual contact with an infected individual, the contact matrix itself, ρ_{ij}, specifying the proportion of sexual contacts that an individual in group i might have with an individual in group j, and the number of sexual contacts per year, c_i, by individuals in group i:

$$\lambda_i = c_i \beta \rho_{ij}$$

PARAMETER VALUES

Values for some model parameter values, such as birth or death rates, may be easily available from data; in other cases, such as vaccination rates, it may be appropriate to investigate a range of plausible values to see how they affect the model results. Often the most important and at the same time most difficult to estimate will be the value of the force of infection (see above).

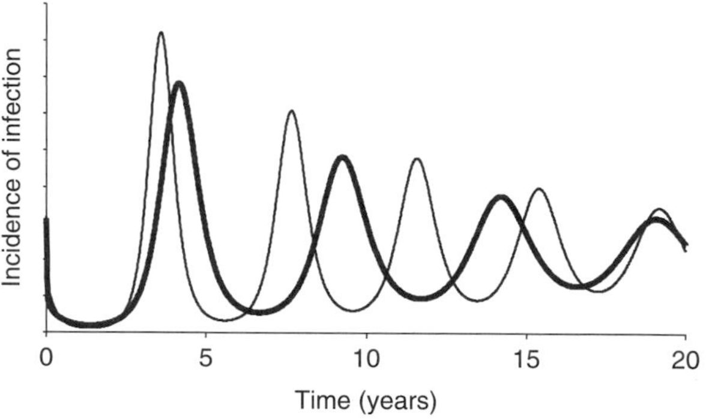

Figure 15.3. Influence of latent period of infection on dynamics. Outputs from simple model shown in Figure 15.2 showing epidemic peaks in prevalence of infection (compartment Y) in absence of vaccination but with different durations for the period of latent infection prior to becoming infectious. It can be seen that increasing the latent period (here from 0.5 month (thin line) to 1 month (thick line)) increases the time interval between epidemic peaks.

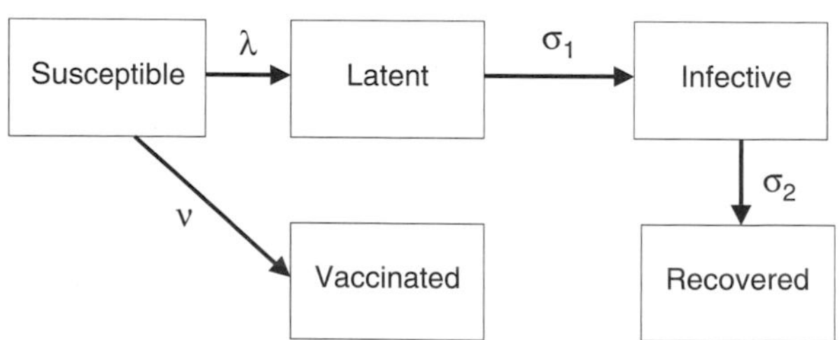

Figure 15.2. A flow diagram with vaccination. As Figure 15.1 but with the addition of a latent stage following infection prior to becoming infective at the per capita rate σ_1, with recovery at rate σ_2, and a compartment representing vaccination with permanent immunity of susceptible individuals at a per capita rate ν. Note that, with the possible exception of lambda, λ, representing the force of infection, there are no rules about which symbol should be used to label transitions in the model (equivalent to parameters in the equations).

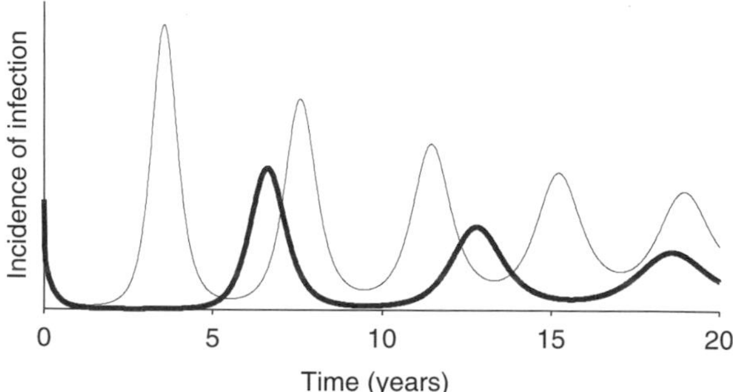

Figure 15.4. Influence of vaccination on dynamics. More outputs from the simple model of Figure 15.2 showing the impact of vaccination in this model. Though the model is over simplistic, the results do show the increase in period between epidemics when a moderate level of vaccination is introduced (thick line) compared with a scenario with no vaccination (thin line) (doubling the rate of vaccination leads to immediate elimination of the infection).

The Role of Demography

AGE DISTRIBUTIONS AND FERTILITY

The three basic processes of fertility, mortality and migration determine observed population age profiles. Grossly simplified age profiles that are stable over time are often used as convenient caricatures of real-world populations (Figure 15.5): (1) an exponentially declining age distribution curve for exponentially growing populations in the Less Developed Countries (LDC) in the developing world, and (2) a uniform age distribution for the Industrialized Developed Countries (IDC); for a number of older industrialized economies, however (3) a more appropriate age distribution is one in which the proportion of older individuals exceeds that of the younger as fertility is below the level necessary for replacing deaths.

Clearly the first of these is unsustainable over the longer term as it would lead to infinite population size and (3), with fertility below replacement level, would lead to population extinction unless supplemented by immigration. More realistically fertility, mortality, and migration evolve over time in response to influences such as better health care, socio-economic factors, and people's expectations about the future (e.g., basic fertility may increase as a result of better health care, but individuals, for a wide range of reasons, may also have, or choose to have, fewer children, the latter trend, in general, appearing to dominate over the long term). Also important is the time lag between birth and reproduction; an increase or decrease in births will lead to an increase or decrease in individuals of reproductive age some two decades later so that the changes observed now in numbers of births will, as those born now reach their reproductive years, be echoed by increases or decreases in birth numbers two or three decades hence. Thus to reverse the decline of an aging population (i.e., one with an age distribution increasingly skewed towards older ages) simply by means of an increasing per capita birth rate becomes increasingly difficult over the short term (i.e., less than several decades). In these circumstances inward migration becomes the major defense against a declining workforce, which, as migrants may well have had different previous experiences of infection to that of the host population, in turn may bring changes to the age distributions of susceptibility and immunity in the combined population and have implications for epidemiology and the design of control programs.

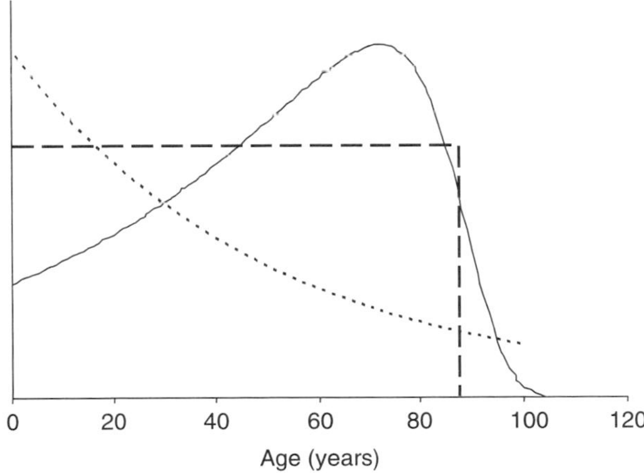

Figure 15.5. Stylized population age profiles. Two simple population age profiles often employed in modeling: (1) an exponentially declining age profile corresponding to an exponentially growing population (dotted line); (2) a uniform age distribution for a population of constant size (dashed line); and (3) a less simple, theoretical stable age distribution corresponding to a declining population size (solid line).

CHANGING DEMOGRAPHY AND ITS IMPACT

The age distribution of infection is governed by the intrinsic transmissibility of the infection, by contact patterns between age groups, and by the age distribution of immunity from past infection. Thus, changes in age distribution of the population itself will impact upon the transmission dynamics of infection, perhaps in complex ways, and these in turn will impact upon the future age distribution of infection and disease and of susceptibility and immunity; the "echoes" of such perturbations in the dynamics of infection have the potential therefore to persist for a number of years (Williams and Manfredi, 2004). The processes of infection and disease are often strongly age related, so that changes in age at infection may have important consequences for the number of deaths or cases of serious disease. Well-known examples are rubella, mumps, and poliomyelitis in which infection of young children is likely to have few long-term consequences, but infection of young adults may have severe consequences, such as congenital rubella when infection occurs in the first trimester of pregnancy; meningitis or encephalitis, and orchitis in males, in the case of mumps; paralysis in the case of poliomyelitis (Mims *et al.*, 2001). Age-related phenomena are found in many infections, affecting how the infection manifests itself in terms of symptoms, course, duration or outcome, and patterns of contact which vary by age also determine the likelihood of infection. In particular a number of infections manifest increasing severity with increasing age, so that in aging populations in which individuals may have not had the "opportunity" to be exposed to infection as a result of partial control (e.g., vaccination without elimination) they may run a greater risk of experiencing significant morbidity (Williams and Manfredi, 2004). Another zexample of age-related phenomena is responsiveness to immunization; for example, older individuals are less likely to generate a satisfactory immune response to hepatitis B vaccine. Such age-related processes can have substantial implications for the epidemiology of infectious disease, but often ones which are difficult to intuit (Medley *et al.*, 2001). Modeling can help to elucidate the ways in which these processes may interact. Although simple compartmental models can be used to model in a simple way the population size effects of basic demographic processes of fertility, mortality and migration, to consider impacts of age-related processes of infection, models explicitly incorporating age structure and age-related processes are desirable. These are considered in the next section.

Age-Structured Models

Simple compartmental models (i.e., ODE models), as described above, in effect represent populations in which the risk of mortality and infection processes does not change with age, which as a result would have an age distribution that is exponentially declining with increasing age. The mean age at death for such a population is $1/\mu$, where μ is the per capita death rate. However, with a mean age at death of 75, this distribution would imply a substantial proportion of the population would be over 100 years old and some would be very much older—several hundreds of years with the oldest tending to infinite age. Nevertheless, despite this lack of realism in terms of age distribution, such models are extremely useful for preliminary investigations of transmission dynamics.

Simple representations of age can be introduced into ODE models by the straightforward means of adding further series of compartments, such as for children, young adults and older adults (Figure 15.6), with flows representing aging between, for example, compartments for children and young adults and between young adults and older adults; by this means some age-related infection processes can be incorporated, so that risk of infection, rate of recovery, mortality etc. can vary according to the subset of compartments representing a particular age grouping; also contact patterns between the different age groupings can be specified using a contact or mixing matrix.

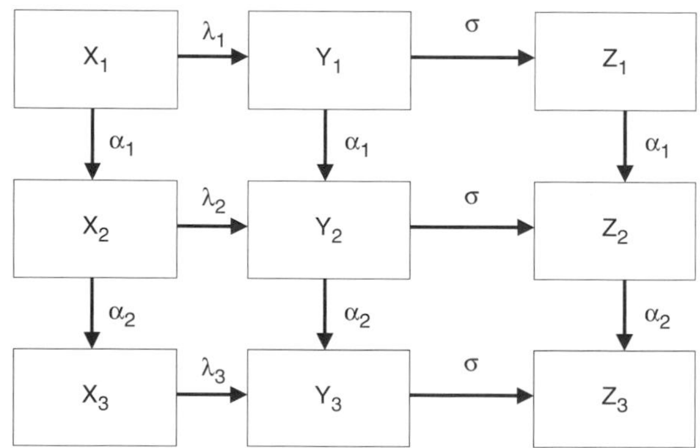

Figure 15.6. Simple model with different ages. A development of the simple model in Figure 15.1 representing three successive age groups, e.g., children (X_1, Y_1, Z_1), young adults (X_2, Y_2, Z_2) and older adults (X_3, Y_3, Z_3) and the rate of aging α_1 and α_2 from each age group to the next. In this instance the value of the force of infection is shown to differ from age group to age group (λ_1, λ_2, λ_3) although the rate of recovery from infection, σ, does not change.

There is no restriction on the number of compartments that can be added in this way, but the model will become increasingly cumbersome, and it needs to be borne in mind that in each "age grouping" so created there will effectively be an exponential distribution of ages, so that, for example, although the average time spent in a compartment representing the first 5 years of life may be 5 years (corresponding to a rate of 0.2 per year = 1/5 years), as with a single compartment representing all age groups, a proportion of this exponentially distributed population will be far older with no limit on maximum age. (A further drawback of this scheme is that the rate of flow from one compartment to another in the same age group, say, upon infection or upon recovery from infection, corresponds to an exponentially distributed waiting time in the first compartment. For a flow, for example, from the susceptible children compartment via infected and recovered children's compartments to that of recovered adolescents, the overall mean time to reach adolescence is greater than that for a flow from susceptible children to susceptible adolescent—the mean time to reach the oldest age group represented is not the same for all routes through the system.)

A great improvement on this strategy is achieved by the use of a more complex class of models using partial differential equations (PDE). In essence, while ODE models describe how the state variables change over time, PDE models describe how they change both with time and with age; that is, whereas ODE models can be visualized as epidemiology evolving in one dimension along the arrow of time, PDE models incorporating age structure can be thought of as epidemiology evolving two-dimensionally through both time and by age. (NB: Such PDE models are a special case of PDE because population age and time advance in step at the same rate as in Figure 15.7; this greatly facilitates approaches to solution of the equations.)

When using PDE models, in addition to specifying how entries into the population at birth (i.e., at age = 0) are distributed between the various states of susceptibility, infection and immunity, the initial age distribution (i.e., at time = 0) must also be specified (these are known as the boundary conditions) as inputs to the model. Using PDE models allows achievement of much more realistic age distributions through the use of age-related mortality and fertility rates. An age-structured version of the simple ODE model of Figure 15.1 might be

$$\frac{\partial X}{\partial t}+\frac{\partial X}{\partial a}=-[\lambda(a)+\mu(a)]X(a)$$

$$\frac{\partial Y}{\partial t}+\frac{\partial Y}{\partial a}=\lambda(a)X(a)-[\sigma(a)+\mu(a)]Y(a)$$

$$\frac{\partial Z}{\partial t}+\frac{\partial Z}{\partial a}=\sigma(a)Y(a)-\mu(a)Z(a)$$

Here the differential on the left-hand side of the equation represents the rate of change of the state

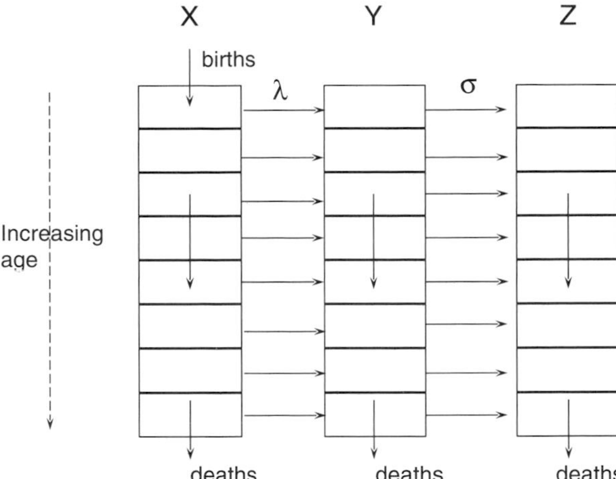

Figure 15.7. Schematic diagram of an age-structured model. A schematic diagram of a partial differential equation (PDE) model with full age structure. As before, X, Y and Z represent susceptibles, infecteds and recovereds, with horizontal arrows representing infection and recovery; however, with each time step individuals also increase in age by one age step (typically time steps and age steps are of equal duration), thus gradually progressing vertically downwards until reaching maximum age, when death occurs.

variable with age, a, and time, t, and the parameters all vary with age. Typically, however, when modeling growing populations in developing countries, mortality rates may be kept constant over age and time (commonly referred as Type II mortality, a usage adopted by epidemiological modelers from demography and ecology). This results in an exponentially decreasing age distribution, but, to avoid unrealistically high ages, it is truncated at a predetermined maximum age (e.g., 75 years) so that when reaching this age all die. For populations in the so-called developed world an alternative scheme is often adopted in which it is assumed that no one dies until the limiting maximum age is reached so that the age distribution, in the absence of disease induced mortality, is completely uniform (referred to as Type I mortality). Use of these distributions providing a stable age distribution makes it easier to understand the transmission dynamics of a system than it is with one in which the age distribution is changing over time at the same time as processes of infection and disease and behaviors may also be changing with age. However, in the real world, of course, age distributions do indeed change with time, and once a good understanding of the nature of the dynamics has been achieved through the use of theoretical rates, it is relatively simple to incorporate age-specific mortality rates derived from data. In a similar way, age-specific fertility rates can be incorporated into the model so that a much better representation of demography may be obtained. It should be borne in mind, however, that it is necessary also to specify the initial age distribution of the population. Clearly, if the majority of the population is in the fertile age range, the shape of the age distribution of the population will, over the short and medium term, evolve in a different way to that observed if the majority of the adult population have passed their fertile years. Provided that the per capita age-related fertility and mortality rates are constant over time, the final equilibrium age distribution is determined simply by the rates specified. This will, however, be attained only over a generational time scale. It should also be borne in mind that even though a stable age distribution may be achieved, this does not necessarily mean that population size itself is at equilibrium. A declining population may have attained a stable age distribution skewed towards upper ages (Figure 15.5) but, in the absence of migration, population numbers will continue to decline as fewer individuals are entering the population through births than are leaving it through deaths. Age-specific migration also may be incorporated into the model through additional terms in the state variable equations, but this does increase the challenge of interpreting model results and of maintaining a suitable age distribution. In theoretical terms, also, this adds a further layer of difficulty in terms of gaining theoretical insight into the PDE equation system, although in practice PDE models are solved numerically using a computer so that migrational flows into and out of the model population can be dealt with in a relatively straightforward way. For practical considerations, much epidemiological modeling has been and remains concerned with populations at demographic equilibrium. With the prospect of substantial demographic change occurring in many parts of the world, however, often leading to a significantly older population age distribution, it becomes desirable to consider possible epidemiological scenarios under such conditions of change, as there may be the potential for these demographic changes to drive epidemiological dynamics in unexpected ways (Figures 15.8 and 15.9) (Williams and Manfredi, 2004).

Often the population in PDE (and ODE) models is not divided between the two sexes—although in many instances this is not of great significance particularly if we are concerned solely with population levels of infection and disease, as control or treatment issues that relate to males or females can be simply considered by assuming a 50:50 split. Even in the case, for example, of congenital rubella in which the concern is the proportion of females reaching fertile age ranges without prior exposure or immunization, the impact of a given universal vaccination strategy can usefully be assessed without specific representation of males and females, as the age at infection remains the same for both. In some circumstances, however, it will be useful to explicitly divide the population into male and female. Examples are health provisions specifically directed at males or females, and cases of significant differences in epidemiology between males and females. One instance might be the modeling of sexually transmitted infections (STI) in heterosexual populations in which transmission risks or proportions

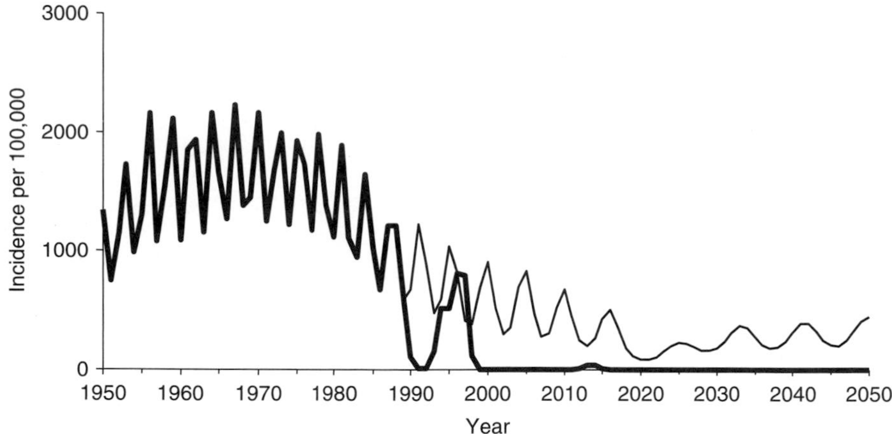

Figure 15.8. Examples of age-structured model outputs for measles incidence under two regimes of measles vaccination in an aging population. Outputs from fully age-structured (PDE) model with realistic demography. For a population with declining birth rate leading to an increasingly aging population the incidence of measles infection over time is shown under two scenarios: (i) from 1976 onwards moderate continuous infant vaccination coverage insufficient to achieve elimination (thin line) and (ii) the same level of vaccination but with additional vaccination campaigns every 4 years from 1989 onwards, which achieves elimination (thick line), albeit after a significant epidemic in 1995 and a miniscule one in 2015. (Williams and Manfredi, 2004)

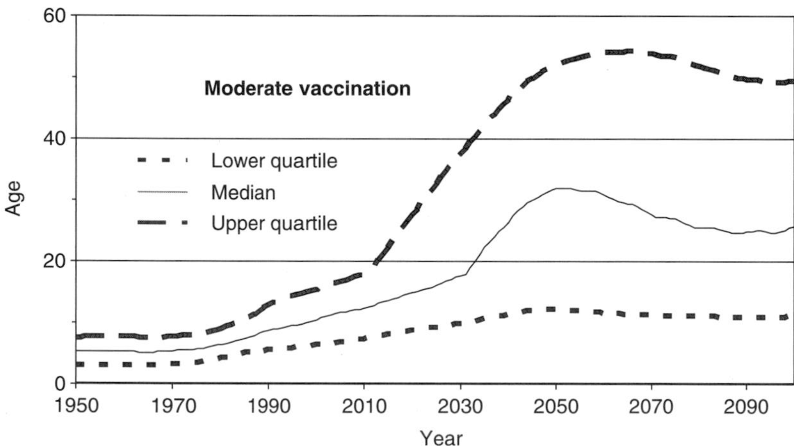

Figure 15.9. Examples of age-structured model outputs showing the influence of suboptimal measles vaccination on age at infection in an aging population. Further outputs from the same PDE model as shown in Figure 15.8. These show for a population with declining birth rate leading to an increasingly aging population how the median and upper and lower quartiles of the distribution of the age at infection change through time under a scenario of moderate vaccination coverage insufficient to achieve elimination. This scenario highlights the potential for a substantial proportion of cases of ostensibly childhood infection to occur among older individuals. (Williams and Manfredi, 2004)

of asymptomatic (and hence probably untreated) infection may differ between males and females. In the case of heterosexual transmission of HIV/AIDS in sub-Saharan Africa while the risk of transmission from an infectious partner for women may be significantly higher, males in general may tend to have more partners and so may be more likely to have sex with an infectious partner. The interaction between the two effects is difficult to tease out without incorporating both sexes in the model. Note that when a model population is explicitly divided into males and females for modeling STI epidemiology, it is necessary to ensure that the numbers of partnerships experienced by females with males corresponds to the number of partnerships that females have with males; where numbers in male or female populations change at different rates, a mechanism must be included in the model to allow the balance in the numbers of partnerships to be maintained over time.

AGE-RELATED PROCESSES

The age structure of PDE models facilitates the inclusion of parameters representing age-related processes of infection and disease (Anderson and May, 1991). These can be processes related to exposure, such as patterns of behavior and of contacts (including sexual contacts), or to the initial establishment and subsequent course of infection or to the transmission of infection from an infected individual as some function of processes of maturation or aging. Patterns of exposure will be determined by the changing intensity and patterns of social and familial contacts (and whether families are nuclear or extended) that an individual has through his or her lifetime, or by more specific patterns such as sexual partner choice and sexual lifestyles. Nursery and primary schools are prime points of contact for exchange of viruses for young children, though in different regions children may enter these institutions at different ages. Young adults may be more likely to have many sexual partners, or to have, for the first time, significant contacts with those from other parts of the country or the world during higher education, military service or travel (illustrative examples are, in Italy, a peak in measles cases in males at military age or, in the UK, recent outbreaks of mumps among university students). Older people are more likely to spend significant time in hospitals or nursing homes and be exposed to the particular range of infections which may have found a niche there among the frail and the sick. Examples of age-determined factors relating to establishment of disease are, for the very young, the degree of protection remaining from passive (i.e., maternal) antibody, or, for older individuals, the possibly decreasing degree of protection from acquired active immunity arising from past infection or from vaccination many years previously, or diminished lung function or reduced effectiveness of the mucous membranes leading to easier establishment of infections. Disease processes in many infections are age-determined; for example, for hepatitis B the age at infection is a very strong determinant of the risk of persistent infection—neonates and the very young being at very much greater risk than older children and adults even less so, although older individuals are significantly less responsive to HBV vaccine. In the case of varicella zoster (chicken pox virus), its secondary manifestation as shingles or zoster is essentially a disease of older ages (probably a result of reactivation following a diminution of immune function perhaps following ill health or simply as a result of loss of immune function with age) (Brisson *et al.*, 2003).

Control measures also may be distributed according to age. For example often vaccination may be targeted at people of a specific age (e.g., young children for measles or the elderly for influenza) or a specific group (e.g., those with many sexual partners for hepatitis B). In such cases vaccination in the model can be effected by specifying a transition at a particular age to a vaccinated compartment for age cohort vaccination, or by specifying that those in a particular compartment are continuously vaccinated at a specified rate. Vaccination campaigns may also be simply effected in the computer program, providing the numerical solution to a model through the device of switching vaccination on and off at specified time points (Figure 15.8) (Manfredi *et al.*, 2005).

Examples of Infections in Which Population Dynamics Is Governed by Age-Related Processes

MEASLES

A great deal of modeling work has focused upon the population dynamics of measles infection (see Anderson and May, 1991). In part this is because there are good data sets resulting from a long history of case notifications against which model performance may be judged; in some cases, there are data also from serological surveys carried out prior to the introduction of vaccination. However, it is also in part because measles provides the classic example of an infection with strong epidemic cycles: in the case of England and Wales, for example, with numbers of cases oscillating over a 2-year period, whereas in others the period of oscillation is greater (Anderson *et al.*, 1984; Manfredi *et al.*, 2005). From a global public health perspective, however, the prime interest is the fact that until recently up to 1 million children each year are believed to have died as a result of measles infection. Even now, with safe and effective vaccination widely available, substantial numbers of deaths and serious disease occur in the developing world. Measles case mortality rates decline sharply with age in the first few months and early years of life, but then increase again towards adult years so that by early adulthood the risk is of a similar order to that seen in infants only a few months old, and case mortality rates appear to continue to increase towards old age. Thus although the majority of older individuals will have experienced measles infection in childhood and, because of the particular patterns of contact between age groups, may in any event be at reduced risk of infection, those who do become infected in later life may be at greatly enhanced risk of death or disease. As noted above, interventions in the form of vaccination and demographic change can result in increases in the average age at infection with a resulting skewing of the distribution of infection towards older age groups, so that there is the potential for these processes to bring about an increase in disease burden at older ages (Figure 15.9) (Williams and Manfredi, 2004). In such circumstances, the modeling of plausible scenarios of vaccination and demographic change can help (1) to indicate which age groups are more at risk, (2) to quantify the broad range of the increase in disease burden, (3) to identify to what extent this is a function of a transient change in demography or a side effect of gradual elimination of the infection from the population and to what extent it is a more long lasting phenomenon, and (4) to inform design of vaccination strategies. An approach of this type can be applied to any infection where case fatality rates or case morbidity rates change with age.

HEPATITIS B

Age-related processes play a very important role in the population dynamics of hepatitis B virus (HBV) (Medley *et al.*, 2001). This infection has similarly been estimated to result in 1 million deaths each year, but mainly in adulthood as a result of liver cancer and cirrhosis; as with measles, however, there is a safe and effective vaccine. In contrast to measles, infection with HBV can result in persistent infection over a period of decades, and additionally the probability of persistent infection is much greater if infection occurs in early childhood. The modes of transmission of HBV are similar to those of HIV (though HBV is very much more infectious), such as through sexual contacts, health interventions, intravenous drug use (IVU) or at birth from mother to child (Edmunds *et al.*, 1996; Williams *et al.*, 1996). These processes all have a strongly age-related or age-determined component. Also, in general, the endpoint of many persistent HBV infections, such as liver cancer or cirrhosis, is not reached for several decades, so that persistent HBV infection arising in childhood (e.g., through maternal transmission) or in young adulthood (perhaps through sexual contacts or IVU) often becomes a cause of severe disease or death in middle-aged or older adults. This long time span of infection means that the population dynamics of HBV is quite different from that of measles, showing no regular oscillations and, in the absence of sharp changes in behavioral trends, prevalence of infection will change only over a period of decades. In these circumstances even a program vaccinating all susceptibles in every age with 100% efficacy will take decades before persistent infection can be eliminated, and over this extended period the reservoir of persistent infection and associated disease would be found increasingly in older age groups.

MACROPARASITE INFECTIONS

For macroparasite infections, disease tends to be associated with past or present intensity of infection, that is, the numbers of parasites infecting the human host. Intensity of exposure and host genetics are components contributing to intensity of infection. However, as macroparasites may live for many years in the human host, the duration of exposure to infection is also a determinant of infection intensity and, in general, duration of exposure correlates with age and with behaviors associated with particular age and sex factors (e.g., being exposed while working in fields, fishing or watering cattle), so that older individuals may be expected to have higher burdens of disease from macroparasite infections and perhaps also higher mortality. An additional factor to consider is the degree to which immune tolerance develops towards the macroparasite infection, so that a high parasite worm burden may be acquired with little accompanying disease, although when such immunotolerance breaks down the host's immune reaction may exacerbate pathology—disease is a result of the immune response to macroparasite infection rather than due to the infection itself. (In some circumstances there may be a reduction in level of disease with increasing age, although some changes may be irreversible such as the corneal opacities giving rise to river blindness which are generated by the immune response to certain parasite stages dying in the eye (Maizels and Lawrence, 1991).) Because intensity of infection is the main determinant of disease rather than infection itself (low-intensity infections causing little if any disease), the modeling of these infections concentrates on the distribution of intensity of infection in the exposed population rather than simply prevalence of infection, and age-structured models are necessary to capture observed age profiles of infection and disease. Often a vector or other secondary host may play an essential role in the transmission of such infections, such as simulium flies as vectors of onchocerciasis, or snails as intermediate hosts in schistosomasis and these, in addition to direct treatment of the human host, may also be subjected to measures aimed at controlling infection spread; in these circumstances it becomes most important to consider how to incorporate these stages into the modeling framework. There is insufficient space here to do more than mention the importance of such considerations in relation to modeling, but there are good examples in the literature devoted to this topic. Useful and instructive examples of modeling macroparasite infections and the associated complexities may be found in Anderson and May (1991), Anderson and Medley (1985), Basanez and Ricardez-Esquinca (2001), Brown and Grenfell (2001), Chan *et al.* (1995), and Medley and Bundy (1996).

Alternative Approaches

The type of model described here, compartmental and deterministic, is one of the most widely adopted for investigating the transmission dynamics of infections in populations. As noted earlier, the results from these models are completely determined by their structure, the values specified for the parameters, and the initial values of the state variables. One drawback of this is that when an infection is first introduced into a population, when it is fading out, when it is very rare, or when the population is very small, the effects of chance can be an important determinant of whether the infection is able to continue to propagate itself through the population. In such cases a model incorporating random or stochastic elements into the transmission dynamics process can help to determine the distribution of possible outcomes (Bailey (1975) provides a useful introduction to this approach); in a sense, a deterministic model provides information about the mean of such a possible distribution of outcomes (they are sometimes called "mean field" models). In the limited space available it would not be possible to discuss adequately the full range of types of models used in infectious disease epidemiology including, among others, individual-based models and network models; for this purpose the reader is referred to the references quoted in the Resources section.

Going Further

OTHER APPLICATIONS FOR TRANSMISSION DYNAMICS MODELS

There are several other areas in which dynamic compartmental models can provide useful insights into aspects of the understanding, treatment and control of human infections. Some examples are as follows:

ECONOMIC ANALYSES

The outputs of models which incorporate some kind of intervention, say, treatment or vaccination, can provide useful inputs to economic analyses. In many cases health economics analyses ignore the importance of herd immunity effects in the control of infections. Dynamics models allow these nonlinear effects to be taken into account in the analysis (Brisson and Edmunds, 2003). By running a model both with and without intervention, the numbers of prevented cases of infection or disease can be calculated. Likewise the number of treatments or vaccinations can be output so that an indication of the number of cases prevented by the program per individual intervention may be calculated, and similarly comparisons between levels of intervention or between different interventions may be undertaken.

WITHIN HOST/IMMUNE SYSTEM MODELS

The compartmental differential equation models described earlier are also adaptable to the study of the dynamics of the immune system in response to infection. Such models can provide novel and useful insights into the observed time course of quantitative clinical measures of infection within the human host and how these might relate to the probable course which may be taken by the infection; by providing explanations for observed dynamical changes in such measures they also offer the prospect of illuminating some of the reasons why response to infection appears to differ between hosts. Useful examples of such work may be found in work on HIV by Nowak and Bangham (1996) and Nowak *et al.* (1997), and on viral hepatitis by Bocharov *et al.* (2004).

STRAIN VARIATION

For a number of infections, previous exposure to different strains of the infection can be an important determinant of eventual outcome of infection, whether as a result of a degree cross-immunity between closely related strains which might therefore mitigate the seriousness of disease (e.g., influenza) or, as appears to be the case for dengue virus, a degree of "antigenic enhancement" resulting in increased morbidity (e.g., dengue hemorrhagic shock syndrome). Transmission dynamics models are eminently suitable for the investigation of the epidemiology arising from such phenomena, and there are a number of examples in the literature (e.g., Koella and Antia, 2003; Turner and Garnett, 2002), although as the possible number of co-circulating strains of an infection increases, the complexity of such models increases greatly and the difficulty in providing satisfactory estimates for the increasing number of parameters greatly increases. Another aspect of strain variation which can usefully be tackled using these types of models relates to the evolution of resistance to control measures in some strains but not in others. Here modeling can provide insights in a number of ways, such as how long it might take for the less controlled or uncontrolled strain to predominate or how best control measures might be designed to counter the danger of emergence of new strains (Wilson *et al.*, 2000).

ISSUES RELATING TO AGE

Age-related processes can be introduced into the types of models described in this section in a number of ways. Examples of this might be, for economic analyses, the targeting of interventions at those in a particular age group or efficacy that varies with age; for immune system dynamics, factors relating to the effectiveness of the immune response; or for strain variation, levels of past exposure to the different strains of infection that are a function of age.

Conclusion

Transmission dynamics models are capable of providing a valuable tool with which to investigate the epidemiology of infectious diseases. The process of simplification of the real world inherent in the design and implementation of such a model is of itself an important step in achieving epidemiological understanding; indeed, in contrast to so-called black box models in which the relative importance of interactions giving rise to results remains obscure, it has often been said that mathematical models are tools for thinking about epidemiology in a precise way and are, in a sense, thought experiments.

The ability of the modeling framework to include population age structure and age-specific parameters allows exploration of many facets of infection in the context of age and aging. An appreciation of the theoretical abilities of such models, however, should not distract from the fundamental importance of having sufficient good data with which to parameterize the models and against which to measure model performance. The modeling process itself can help to highlight what data are needed to further epidemiological understanding and to assess prospects for control, but a lack of reliable data inevitably limits in turn the reliability of further modeling work, although sensitivity and uncertainty analysis are useful tools for assessing how much faith may be placed in the results being produced.

Among the areas where good data are often lacking are the quantification of risk of infection per contact, the nature of contact patterns, and how these change over time. A further challenge lies in establishing and understanding the importance of heterogeneity in behaviors and contact patterns. In the field of sexually transmitted infections, behavioral data are vital but particularly difficult to acquire and validate. Insights from the field of genetics have the potential to greatly increase our understanding of variation in responses to infection and differing patterns of disease, but also to increase the complexity and to bring new challenges for modelers. Infections with multiple strains, reassortment of genetic material between strains, and significant cross-immunity between strains pose yet another challenge. Changing demography, including migrational trends, has the potential to profoundly influence the epidemiology of many infections but also to substantially increase the difficulty of the task of specifying and acquiring the necessary data for modeling.

As far as the techniques and approaches used in infectious disease modeling are concerned, historically these have been adapted from uses in other fields, primarily the physical sciences, and the introduction of new techniques often occurs when those entering infectious disease modeling from another field bring with them new insights and approaches to modeling from that field. With continually increasing computing power and no lack of potentially useful modeling techniques, given sufficient suitable and reliable data, the major challenge remains that of achieving a satisfactory balance between simplicity and explanatory power and that of understanding and interpreting model results.

Appendix: Solution of Ordinary and Partial Differential Equation Systems

SOLUTION OF ODE MODELS

The solution at epidemic equilibrium of the simple set of equations on page 171 be arrived at analytically by noting that under equilibrium the values of the state variables remain constant so that therefore the rates of change of these variables (the differentials) become zero. From this fact we have

$$\frac{dX}{dt} = \mu N - (\lambda + \mu)X = 0$$

$$\frac{dY}{dt} = \lambda X - (\sigma + \mu)Y = 0$$

$$\frac{dZ}{dt} = \sigma Y - \mu Z = 0$$

$$N = X + Y + Z$$

Thus at equilibrium

$$\mu N = (\lambda + \mu)X$$
$$\lambda X = (\sigma + \mu)Y$$
$$\sigma Y = \mu Z$$

and from this set of equations expressions can be derived for the values for the state variables at equilibrium in terms of the parameters:

$$X = \frac{\mu}{(\lambda + \mu)}N$$

$$Y = \frac{\lambda\mu}{(\sigma + \mu)(\lambda + \mu)}N$$

$$Z = \frac{\lambda\sigma}{(\sigma + \mu)(\lambda + \mu)}N$$

Further examples of the analytic solutions of transmission dynamics models, both at equilibrium and during the dynamic stages prior to equilibrium, are provided by Anderson and May (1991), to which reference should be made if more detailed exposition is sought.

A number of easy-to-use computer-based tools are available to facilitate the task of solving ODE models, including Berkeley Madonna, ModelMaker, and Stella (see Recommended Resources).

SOLUTION OF PDE MODELS

While some aspects of PDE models may be amenable to an analytic approach, or, in very straightforward cases, solution, in general it is necessary to resort to numerical approaches to solution. Although good computer modeling tools are available for the solution of ODE models, the picture is different for PDE models for which the usual approach is for computer programs to be written ad hoc in a high-level programming language such as C, C++ or Fortran; although often tedious, this approach is usually relatively straightforward. Suitable algorithms for numerical solutions can be found in reference works such as Numerical Recipes series (see Recommended Resources). Essentially the procedure is for a set of arrays, or one multidimensional array to be used to represent the proportion of the population in each compartment of the model with consecutive locations in the arrays representing consecutive age steps. As before, at each time step the appropriate transitions occur between the different epidemiological compartments; but also at each time step, starting from the oldest age step, the contents of adjacent age steps are moved to the next (i.e., older) age step (the contents of oldest age step being discarded on the assumption that for this age step death is the next step). As a rule of thumb the time step used should, for convenience, be of the same duration as the age step and, to avoid numerical errors, preferably be about an order of magnitude less than the mean duration corresponding to the fastest transition rate in the equation system; that is, if the time from infection to the development of symptoms is 10 days and is the shortest period represented in the model, the time and age steps should be around 1 day.

Recommended Resources

BOOKS

1. *Infectious Diseases of Humans. Dynamics and Control* by Roy M. Anderson and Robert M. May. Oxford University Press (1991) Oxford. A unique and comprehensive reference giving an in-depth exposition of transmission dynamics modeling considering both deterministic and stochastic models but largely focusing on the former. The book provides much mathematical detail for those who would like it, but for those who do not wish to immerse themselves in the mathematics, a great deal can be gained from simply reading the text and skimming over the mathematical details.
2. *Parasitic and Infectious Diseases: Epidemiology and Ecology* by Marilyn E. Scott and Gary Smith. Academic Press; 1st ed. (1994). An easily accessible introduction to modeling infectious disease transmission, which introduces the mathematics in a clear and easily understandable fashion.
3. *Modern Infectious Disease Epidemiology* by Johan Giesecke. Arnold Publication; 2nd ed. (2001). An excellent and easily accessible initial introduction to current ideas in infectious disease epidemiology including dynamic modeling.
4. *Epidemiologic Methods for the Study of Infectious Diseases* by J.C. Thomas and D.J. Weber (eds). Oxford University Press (2001): New York. Not a modeling book but an excellent introduction to many of the concepts used in infectious disease modeling as well as to infectious disease epidemiology in general.
5. *Mathematical Epidemiology of Infectious Diseases: Model Building, Analysis and Interpretation* (Wiley Series in Mathematical and Computational Biology) by O. Diekmann and J.A.P. Heesterbeek. John Wiley Sons; New Ed edition (2000). A thorough, more mathematical treatment aimed at theoretical biologists, epidemiologists and applied mathematicians, which covers both deterministic and stochastic approaches to epidemiological modeling and includes exercises for the reader throughout.
6. *The Mathematical Theory of Infectious Diseases* by Norman T.J. B. Griffin; 2nd ed London. A very comprehensive coverage of stochastic infectious disease modeling, currently out of print but it is very much worth trying to locate a copy in specialist bookstores or libraries.
7. *Models for Infectious Human Diseases: Their Structure and Relation to Data* by Valerie Isham and Graham Medley (Editors) and H.K. Moffatt (Series Editor). Cambridge University Press (1996). *Epidemic Models: Their Structure and Relation to Data* by Denis Mollison (Editor) and H.K. Moffatt (Series Editor). Cambridge University Press (1995). Two books arising from a workshop held at the Newton Institute, University of Cambridge, whose relatively short chapters cover a wide and interesting but, above all, relevant series of topics related to all aspects of infectious disease modeling by leaders in the field.
8. *Population Ecology: A Unified Study of Animals and Plants* by Michael Begon, Martin Mortimer and David J. Thompson. Blackwell Science, Oxford. 3rd ed. (1996). A useful introduction to the fundamental principles of population ecology covering animals and plants, including an introduction to parasitism.
9. *A Dictionary of Epidemiology* by the International Epidemiological Association (Corporate Author), John M. Last, Robert A. Spasoff, Susan S. Harris, and Michel C. Thuriaux (editors). Oxford University Press; 4th ed. (2000) New York. An excellent and wide-ranging epidemiological reference tool.
10. *Numerical Recipes in C++: The Art of Scientific Computing* by William H. Press *et al.* (eds.). Cambridge University Press (2002). *Numerical Recipes in C: The Art of Scientific Computing* by William H. Press *et al.* Cambridge University Press; 2nd ed. (1992). *Numerical Recipes in Fortran: The Art of Scientific Computing* by William H. Press *et al.* Cambridge University Press. 2nd ed. (1992). A very useful series of source books of methods for tackling numerical tasks arising when creating *ad hoc* computer programs to solve ODE or PDE models; included in each section are algorithms set out in computer code which implement these methods.

MODELING SOFTWARE

Among the software packages available for constructing and solving ordinary differential equation models, good examples are the following which are also straightforward to use:

Berkeley Madonna, Robert I. Macey and George F. Oster	http://www.berkeleymadonna.com/
ModelMaker, FamilyGenetix Ltd	http://www.modelkinetix.com/
Stella, ISEE Systems, Inc	http://www.iseesystems.com/

Flow diagrams can also be designed with these packages and then automatically transformed into systems of ODEs.

REFERENCES

Anderson, R.M., and Grenfell, B.T. (1986) Quantitative investigations of different vaccination policies for the control of congenital rubella syndrome (CRS) in the United Kingdom. *J. Hyg. (Lond). 96*, 305–333.

Anderson, R.M., Grenfell, B.T., and May, R.M. (1984) Oscillatory fluctuations in the incidence of infectious disease and the impact of vaccination: Time series analysis. *J. Hyg. (Lond.). 93*, 587–608.

Anderson, R.M., and May, R.M. (1985) Age-related changes in the rate of disease transmission: Implications for the design of vaccination programmes. *J. Hyg. (Lond). 94*, 365–436.

Anderson, R.M., and May, R.M. (1991) *Infectious Diseases of Humans. Dynamics and Control*. Oxford University Press, Oxford.

Anderson, R.M., and Medley, G.F. (1985) Parasitology. Community control of helminth infections of man by mass and selective chemotherapy. *Parasitology 90*, 629–660.

Anderson, R.M., Medley, G.F., May, R.M., and Johnson, A.M. (1986) A preliminary study of the transmission dynamics of the human immunodeficiency virus (HIV), the causative agent of AIDS. *IMA J. Math. Appl. Med. Biol. 3*, 229–263.

Bailey, N.T.J. (1975) *The Mathematical Theory of Infectious Diseases* (2nd ed.) Griffin, London.

Basanez, M.G., and Ricardez-Esquinca, J. (2001) Models for the population biology and control of human onchocerciasis. *Trends Parasitol. 17*, 430–438.

Begon, M., Harper, J.L., and Townsend, C.R. (1996) *Ecology: Individuals, Populations and Communities*. 3rd ed. Blackwell Science, Malden.

Bocharov, G., Ludewig, B., Bertoletti, A., Klenerman, P., Junt, T., Krebs, P., *et al.* (2004) Underwhelming the immune response: Effect of slow virus growth on CD8+-T-lymphocyte responses. *J. Virol. 78*, 2247–2254.

Brisson, M., and Edmunds, W.J. (2003) Varicella vaccination in England and Wales: Cost–utility analysis. *Arch. Dis. Child. 88*, 862–869.

Brisson, M., Edmunds, W.J., and Gay, N.J. (2003) Varicella vaccination: Impact of vaccine efficacy on the epidemiology of VZV. *J. Med. Virol. 70 Suppl 1*, S31–S37.

Brown, S.P., and Grenfell, B.T. (2001) An unlikely partnership: Parasites, concomitant immunity and host defence. *Proc. Biol. Sci. 268*, 2543–2549.

Chan, M.S., Guyatt, H.L., Bundy, D.A., Booth, M., Fulford, A.J., and Medley, G.F. (1995) The development of an age structured model for schistosomiasis transmission dynamics and control and its validation for *Schistosoma mansoni*. *Epidemiol. Infect. 115*, 325–344.

Davies, D.H., Halablab, M.A., Clarke, J., Cox, F.E.G., and Young, T.W.K. (1999) *Infection and Immunity*. Taylor and Francis, London.

Edmunds, W.J., Medley, G.F., Nokes, D.J., O'Callaghan, C.J., Whittle, H.C., and Hall, A.J. (1996) Epidemiological patterns of hepatitis B virus (HBV) in highly endemic areas. *Epidemiol Infect. 117*, 313–325.

Edmunds, W.J., van de Heijden, O.G., Eerola, M., and Gay, N.J. (2000) Modelling rubella in Europe. *Epidemiol. Infect. 125*, 617–634.

Farrington, C.P. (1990) Modelling forces of infection for measles, mumps and rubella. *Stat. Med. 9*, 953–967.

Koella, J.C., and Antia, R. (2003) Epidemiological models for the spread of anti-malarial resistance. *Malar. J. 2*, 3.

Maizels, R.M., and Lawrence, R.A. (1991) Immunological tolerance: The key feature in human filariasis? *Parasitol Today 7*, 271–276.

Manfredi, P., Cleur, E.M., Williams, J.R., Salmaso, S., and Atti, M.C. (2005) The pre-vaccination regional epidemiological landscape of measles in Italy: Contact patterns, effort needed for eradication, and comparison with other regions of Europe. *Popul. Health Metr. 3*, 1.

Manfredi, P., Williams, J.R., Ciofi Degli Atti, M.L., and Salmaso, S. (2005) Measles elimination in Italy: Projected impact of the National Elimination Plan. *Epidemiol Infect. 133*, 87–97.

Medley, G.F., and Bundy, D.A. (1996) Dynamic modeling of epidemiologic patterns of schistosomiasis morbidity. *Am. J. Trop. Med. Hyg. 55(5 Suppl)*, 149–158.

Medley, G.F., Lindop, N.A., Edmunds, W.J., and Nokes, D.J. (2001) Hepatitis-B virus endemicity: Heterogeneity, catastrophic dynamics and control. *Nat. Med. 7*, 619–624.

Mims, C.A., Nash, A., and Stephen, J. (2001) *Mims' Pathogenesis of Infectious Disease*. 5th ed. Academic Press, London.

Nokes, D.J., and Anderson, R.M. (1988) The use of mathematical models in the epidemiological study of infectious diseases and in the design of mass immunization programmes. *Epidemiol Infect. 101*, 1–20.

Nowak, M.A., and Bangham, C.R. (1996) Population dynamics of immune responses to persistent viruses. *Science 272*, 74–79.

Nowak, M.A., Bonhoeffer, S., Shaw, G.M., and May, R.M. (1997) Anti-viral drug treatment: Dynamics of resistance in free virus and infected cell populations. *J. Theor. Biol. 184*, 203–217.

Seaholm, S.K., Ackerman, E., and Wu, S.C. (1988) Latin hypercube sampling and the sensitivity analysis of a Monte Carlo epidemic model. *Int. J. Biomed. Comput. 23*, 97–112.

Thomas, J.C., and Weber, D.J. (eds.). (2001) *Epidemiologic Methods for the Study of Infectious Diseases*. Oxford University Press: New York.

Turner, K.M., and Garnett, G.P. (2002) The impact of the phase of an epidemic of sexually transmitted infection on the evolution of the organism. *Sex. Transm. Infect. 78 Suppl 1*, i20–i30.

Williams, J.R. and Anderson, R.M. (1994) Mathematical models of the transmission dynamics of human immunodeficiency virus in England and Wales: Mixing between different risk groups. *J. R. Stat. Soc. [Ser A]. 157*, 69–87

Williams, J.R., and Manfredi, P. (2004) Ageing populations and childhood infections: The potential impact on epidemic patterns and morbidity. *Int. J. Epidemiol. 33*, 566–572.

Williams, J.R., Nokes, D.J., Medley, G.F., and Anderson, R.M. (1996) The transmission dynamics of hepatitis B in the UK: A mathematical model for evaluating costs and effectiveness of immunization programmes. *Epidemiol. Infect. 116*, 71–89.

Wilson, J.N., Nokes, D.J., and Carman, W.F. (2000) Predictions of the emergence of vaccine-resistant hepatitis B in The Gambia using a mathematical model. *Epidemiol. Infect. 124*, 295–307.

16

Estimation of the Rate of Production of Oxygen Radicals by Mitochondria

Alberto Sanz and Gustavo Barja

Oxygen radical production by mitochondria seems to be implicated in various degenerative diseases and aging. In order to estimate the rate of generation of reactive oxygen species, it is necessary to use adequate methods. In this article we describe a fluorometric method appropriate to measure the rate of generation of H_2O_2 in isolated functional mitochondria. The method is specific for H_2O_2 and is sensitive enough to assay mitochondrial H_2O_2 generation in the presence of respiratory substrates without the presence of inhibitors of the respiratory chain. Just after isolating functional mitochondria from fresh tissues, rates of generation of H_2O_2 are measured by fluorometry in the presence of homovanillic acid and horseradish peroxidase. Simultaneous measurement of mitochondrial oxygen consumption allows calculation of the percent of electrons out of sequence, which reduce oxygen to oxygen radicals along the mitochondrial respiratory chain instead of reducing oxygen to water at the terminal cytochrome oxidase. This is known as the free radical leak. This method is also appropriate to study the effect of different inhibitors and modulators on the rate of mitochondrial oxygen radical production, allowing the localization of the sites of generation in the respiratory chain where reactive oxygen species are specifically formed.

Abbreviations

ETC Electron transport chain
ESR Electron spin resonance
H_2O_2 Hydrogen peroxide
HRP Horseradish peroxidase
$O_2^{\bullet-}$ Superoxide
ROS Reactive oxygen species
SOD Superoxide dismutase

Introduction

Since Denham Harman published his Free Radical Theory of Aging in 1956, there has been growing evidence that reactive oxygen species (ROS) of biological origin are implicated in pathological processes. Free radicals damage cellular macromolecules including carbohydrates, lipids, proteins, and most importantly, the nucleic acids of nuclear and mitochondrial DNA. In addition, ROS are continuously generated by aerobic tissues. These two properties make ROS potentially responsible in part for degenerative processes like diabetes, cancer, Parkinson's or Alzheimer's diseases, as well as aging (Barja, 2004; Sohal *et al.*, 2002).

Mitochondria are the main generator of ROS in healthy cells. The mitochondrial electron transport chain (ETC) is responsible for more than 90% of cellular oxygen consumption. During the flow of electrons in the ETC, a small percent of them incompletely reduce oxygen to superoxide and hydrogen peroxide. The first reactive species produced in the ETC is superoxide radical ($O_2^{\bullet-}$), resulting from the univalent reduction of oxygen. $O_2^{\bullet-}$ dismutates to hydrogen peroxide (H_2O_2), which can diffuse out of mitochondria to their surrounding medium. In submitochondrial particles $O_2^{\bullet-}$ is directly secreted outside. For this reason ROS generation is measured as $O_2^{\bullet-}$ in submitochondrial particles and as H_2O_2 in intact mitochondria. Although submitochondrial particles are adequate for various particular reasons including the possibility of using NADH directly as a substrate, assays in intact functional mitochondria are closer to the real physiological situation. The ideal situation would be to measure mitochondria ROS production *in vivo* in the whole animal, but techniques allowing this are still not available.

In the present paper we describe a reliable method for measuring H_2O_2 production in isolated functional mitochondria. This method was originally designed to measure H_2O_2 in macrophages and neutrophils (Ruch *et al.*, 1983), and it was afterwards adapted to isolated mitochondria (Barja, 1999; Barja, 2002). We described the method in detail, including the latest improvements.

Characteristics of Different Mitochondrial ROS Production Assays

ROS production can be measured with different techniques including chemiluminescence, electron spin resonance (ESR), spectrophotometry, and fluorometry. These techniques have been used to estimate ROS levels in submitochondrial particles, mitochondria and whole cells. Any appropriate method for estimating ROS production must be highly sensitive since the amount of ROS produced by intact mitochondria in the absence of inhibitors is small. In many physiological comparisons (e.g., related to aging) it is essential to be able to measure basal ROS production without inhibitors. Chemilumiescent methods are highly sensitive (Chance and Gao, 1994), but unfortunately have low chemical specificity. This is why they are seldom used to assay mitochondrial ROS production. On the other hand, spin-trap ESR techniques can have enough sensitivity and specificity, and their main advantage is their capacity to detect free radicals directly. These methods have been employed to measure ROS levels in brain mitochondria (Dykens, 1994), heart submitochondrial particles (Giulivi *et al.*, 1995), cultured vascular cells (Inoguchi *et al.*, 2000), or liver mitoplasts (Han *et al.*, 2001). However, ESR techniques require expensive equipment not frequently present in biochemistry laboratories, and in many occasions need the use of spin trap intermediates.

The two more classical methods of estimating free radical production in mitochondria use spectrophotometry and fluorometry. The measurement of $O_2^{\bullet-}$ production by spectrophotometry in mitochondrial preparations has been commonly performed by kinetic assays of superoxide dismutase-sensitive epinephrine reduction to adrenochrome or reduction of acetylated or succinylated cytochrome *c* (Boveris *et al.*, 1976; Takeshige and Minakami, 1979; Lass and Sohal, 2000). They have been also applied to submitochondrial particles or to isolated complexes (Takeshige and Minakami, 1979; Cadenas *et al.*, 1977). However, the detection of ROS production in functional mitochondria needs methods which measure H_2O_2 rather than $O_2^{\bullet-}$. Chance and co-workers developed a method for measuring the rate of mitochondrial H_2O_2 production (Boveris and Chance, 1973). They used double wavelength spectrophotometry to follow the enzyme-substrate complex between H_2O_2 and cytochrome *c* peroxidase. However cytochrome *c* peroxidase is not commercially available, and it must be prepared from yeast or other sources, which complicates routine assays (Prat *et al.*, 1991). Although substitution of cytochrome *c* peroxidase by horseradish is possible (Turrens *et al.*, 1985), it further decreases the intrinsically low sensitivity of spectrophotometric techniques.

Fluorometric techniques have the advantage that they are more sensitive. One of the earliest fluorometric methods developed for evaluating H_2O_2 production (Loschen *et al.*, 1971) was scopoletin (6-methyl-7-hydroxy-1,2-benzopyrone), and sometimes it is still employed (Mattiasson, 2004). During the assay, fluorescent scopoletin is oxidized by H_2O_2 to a nonfluorescent substance in the presence of horseradish peroxidase. This assay is specific, but it has the inconvenience that it is a negative method because it is based on the disappearance of fluorescence. It requires the use of graded quantities of scopoletin in order to get the best range for measurements (Loschen *et al.*, 1971).

There are other fluorescent probes available for the measurement of ROS production in mitochondria: diacetyldichlorfluorescin, *p*-hydroxyphenylacetate, homovanillic acid (4-hydroxy-3-methoxy-phenylacetic acid) and Amplex Red (10-acetyl-3,7-dihydroxyphenoxazine), all of them specific for H_2O_2 due to the presence of horseradish peroxidase. Nowadays, the last two probes are the ones most frequently used. The general principle is similar for all these substances (Tarpey *et al.*, 2004): in the presence of H_2O_2, hydrogen donors (AH2) are oxidized by horseradish-peroxidase (HRP) generating a fluorescent compound:

$$HRP + H_2O_2 \rightarrow HRP - H_2O_2 \text{ (Compound I)}$$

$$HRP - H_2O_2 + AH_2 \rightarrow HRP + 2H_2O + A$$

In the assay described here, homovanillic acid is used since it is less expensive than Amplex Red and does not spontaneously generate fluorescence in the absence of H_2O_2. Amplex Red can have interferences with NADH or reduced glutathione (Votyakova and Reynolds, 2004; Towne *et al.*, 2004). However, Amplex Red is being frequently used (Zhou *et al.*, 1997) and can produce interesting results (Muller *et al.*, 2004) when properly handled. Homovanillic has been used to specifically detect H_2O_2 production in isolated mitochondria from a wide variety of tissues and animal species (Drew *et al.*, 2003; Gredilla *et al.*, 2001, Hagopian *et al.*, 2005). The method, which is described in detail below, is useful to (1) quantify basal ROS production, (2) localize the main sites of oxygen radical generation in the respiratory chain, (3) determine the free radical leak (see below), and (4) study the effect of different compounds on mitochondrial ROS production.

Isolation of Mitochondria and Measurement of Oxygen Consumption

H_2O_2 production must be measured always in functional mitochondria obtained from fresh tissue, and never from frozen tissue samples. The measurement of H_2O_2 in functional intact mitochondria requires the use of appropriate protocols of isolation. There are methods specifically designed to obtain functional mitochondria from different tissues. Possible choices are those of Mela and Seitz (1979) for heart mitochondria, the method of Lai and Clark (1979) for brain mitochondria (which uses Ficoll gradients specially useful in this tissue), and the protocol described by López-Torres *et al.* (2002) for liver mitochondria. Using these methods, well-coupled mitochondria can be isolated in a few hours. During all the steps, including homogenization, centrifugation and resuspensions, the mitochondrial preparations must be maintained at 4°C. Between isolation and measurements the tube containing the mitochondria must be kept over ice, and the concentration of mitochondria must be high. This helps avoid loss of mitochondrial functional properties during a few hours.

Just after this isolation, the mitochondrial protein concentration must be measured. Immediately after isolation is finished, oxygen consumption and H_2O_2 production are assayed at the same temperature (37°C), using the same buffer and with the same concentrations of substrates and inhibitors. This allows calculating the percent free radical leak (see below).

Oxygen consumption is measured with a Clark-type electrode calculating the respiratory control index (RCI), which is the ratio state 3/state 4 respiration. State 3 is the mitochondrial oxygen consumption in the presence of saturating ADP (phosphorylating state), and state 4 is the mitochondrial oxygen consumption without ADP (nonphosphorylating state). The RCI indicates the degree of coupling and metabolic activity of the mitochondrial preparations. A RCI of 1 or less indicates damaged nonfunctional mitochondria. The appropriate RCI must be substantially higher than 1, with values varying depending on the tissue and the substrate used.

Fluorescent Assay of Mitochondrial H_2O_2

PRACTICAL PROCEDURE

H_2O_2 produced by mitochondria is measured by reacting it with homovanillic acid in the presence of horseradish peroxidase (see above). This reaction produces a fluorescent dimer at 312 nm excitation and 420 nm emission.

The incubation medium contains 145 mM KCl, 30 mM Hepes, 5 mM KH_2PO_4, 3 mM $MgCl_2$, 0.1 mM EGTA, and 0.1% fatty-acid free albumin at pH 7.4. The pH of the medium must be adjusted at the same temperature used during the assay (37°C). Solutions of substrates, ADP and enzymes are prepared in this medium without albumin at the following (initial) concentrations: 70 Units/ml of high purity horseradish peroxidase, 4 mM homovanillic acid, pyruvate/malate (125 mM or 250 mM depending on the tissue) and succinate neutralized to pH 7.4 (250 mM in heart and liver; 500 mM in brain).

The different components of the assay are added to tubes in the following order after adding a large volume of incubation medium: (1) mitochondria, (2) horseradish peroxidase, (3) homovanillic acid, (4) superoxide dismutase, and (5) the substrates (pyruvate/malate, glutamate/malate or succinate+rotenone) to start the reaction. The volume of incubation medium added should be around 85% of the total reaction volume (e.g., 1.5 ml of total reaction volume). The volumes added of the rest of the reactants are those needed to reach the following final concentrations: 0.25 mg of mitochondrial protein per ml in heart and liver, 0.4 mg of mitochondrial protein per ml in brain, 6 U/ml of horseradish peroxidase, 0.1 mM homovanillic acid, 50 U/ml of SOD, 5 mM succinate + 2 μM rotenone, 2.5 mM pyruvate/2.5 mM malate or 2.5 mM glutamate/2.5 mM malate in heart and liver. However, in brain, it is advisable to increase the concentration of substrate to 10 mM for succinate (+ 2 μM rotenone) and to 5 mM for pyruvate. At those concentrations H_2O_2 production is not substrate-dependent. To localize the place where ROS are produced inside the electron transport, chain inhibitors must be employed. Rotenone (2 μM final concentration) is used to inhibit at complex I, thenoyltrifluoroacetone (TTFA, 11 μM final concentration) for complex II, and antimycin A (10 μM final concentration) for complex III. Solutions of inhibitors are prepared in pure high-grade ethanol. The reaction is performed during 15 minutes with constant agitation in a temperature-controlled water bath at 37°C. After 15 minutes of incubation, the reaction is stopped, the samples are transferred to an ice-cold bath, 0.5 ml of the stop buffer (2 M glycine, 2.2 M NaOH, 50 mM EDTA) is added (per each 1.5 ml of reaction volume), and the fluorescence (312 nm excitation, 420 nm emission) is measured. With the addition of the glycine-NaOH-EDTA the final pH is around 12.4, which increases the sensitivity and makes the final fluorescence essentially pH-independent. This procedure highly decreases the variability of results compared to measuring the fluorescence at neutral pH at which it is strongly pH dependent.

In the absence of SOD, the rates represent H_2O_2 production. SOD added in excess converts $O_2^{\bullet-}$ produced (if any) to H_2O_2. Thus, in the presence of SOD, the assay estimates the mitochondrial production of $O_2^{\bullet-}$ plus H_2O_2. Since the respiratory chain univalently reduces oxygen to $O_2^{\bullet-}$ which then dismutates to H_2O_2, the measurement of mitochondrial H_2O_2 production represents the rate of oxygen radical generation. Moreover, the addition of SOD can prevent the underestimation of the rate of H_2O_2 production due to reaction of $O_2^{\bullet-}$ with HRP or HRP-Compound I (Muller *et al.*, 2004).

BLANKS

Appropriate blanks are also run during the assay to correct for the positive fluorescence of the mitochondria themselves. These blanks have mitochondria and all the reaction components but do not contain substrate. Values are obtained by subtracting the fluorescence of the blanks from the fluorescence of the samples and dividing the results by the 15 minutes of incubation. Special blanks (also without substrate) must be included to correct for the fluorescence of antimycin A when this mitochondrial respiratory inhibitor is included in the reaction.

STANDARDS

The arbitrary fluorescence units must be converted to amounts of H_2O_2. There are different possibilities to do this. One of them is to use H_2O_2 standards. However, μM H_2O_2 solutions are unstable, and they should be prepared just before use from stable mM H_2O_2 solutions.

An alternative is to use a glucose–glucose oxidase system as standard. In the presence of excess glucose, this couple generates H_2O_2 at a rate that depends on the amount of glucose oxidase added. For this purpose the following is added to standard tubes: incubation medium, 6 Units/ml of horseradish peroxidase, 0.1 mM homovanillic acid, glucose oxidase, and 14 mM glucose (total volume 1.5 ml). Another advantage of this procedure is that the standards are incubated in parallel in the same conditions as the samples (15 min at 37°C, transfer to the ice-cold bath, and addition of 0.5 ml of 2 M glycine, 2,2 M NaOH, 50 mM EDTA). Glucose oxidase is added in amounts generating 1 nanomol of H_2O_2/min, and the fluorescence of samples and standards is compared. This is used to calculate the final mitochondrial production of oxygen radicals, which is expressed in nanomoles of H_2O_2/min. mg of protein. When using this kind of standard, care should be taken that no limiting losses of activity have occurred during transport to or storage of glucose oxidase and horseradish peroxidase at the laboratory.

SPECIFICITY

The horseradish peroxidase enzyme gives the assay specificity for H_2O_2. Furthermore, H_2O_2 secreted to the outside of mitochondria reacts only with the H_2O_2 detection system, since there are no antioxidants in the incubation medium. On the other hand, addition of catalase to the incubation buffer prevents the increase in fluorescence elicited by H_2O_2, whereas addition of external pulses of H_2O_2 during a kinetic assay shows that the response of the detection system to the peroxide is instantaneous.

VALIDITY

Any useful assay of ROS production should not interfere with mitochondrial function. This can be checked by measuring mitochondrial respiration in the presence of the molecular probes constituting the chemical detection system. Addition of horseradish peroxidase and homovanillic acid, at the same final concentration used in the fluorometric H_2O_2 assay, does not change the rates of mitochondrial state 4 or state 3 respiration or the RCI. High purity horseradish peroxidase and superoxide dismutase should be used. Commercial solution of these two enzymes stabilized with agents capable of altering mitochondria should be avoided. The appropriateness of the particular commercial reactants used can be easily checked in pilot experiments measuring mitochondrial respiration in their absence and in their presence.

STABILITY AND REPRODUCIBILITY

The final fluorescence of the samples does not vary significantly during at least 2 hours. Variations between duplicated samples of the same preparation of mitochondria assayed on the same day are less than 4%.

RECOMMENDATIONS

The following recommendations can help to obtain better measurements:

1. The use of highly purified ion-free water is recommended for preparation of all solutions.
2. The pH of the incubation buffer (7.4) should be carefully checked, and it should be readjusted if needed, since ROS production can be affected by this parameter.
3. Excessive mitochondrial concentration during the incubation at 37°C can cause decreases in fluorescence and should be avoided.
4. A chemical (in the absence of mitochondria) H_2O_2 pulse experiment can be easily performed each day before starting the measurements with mitochondria, or even before sacrificing the animal to isolate them. This reaction can be very useful to check the quality of the horseradish peroxidase and homovanillic acid reactants, in order to avoid erroneously attributing an absence or very low rate of ROS production to the mitochondrial preparations if a recently received or stored reactant is not in good condition or has lost enzymatic activity. For this purpose H_2O_2 is added from a standard H_2O_2 solution to the homovanillic-HRP detection system, and the occurrence of the corresponding increase in fluorescence is checked.
5. The use of soap to clean the materials (glassware, etc.) that will be in direct contact with the mitochondria should be avoided.
6. Tubes with isolated mitochondria must be kept on ice and at high mitochondrial concentrations. The mitochondria must be used between 2 and 3 hours after isolation. If longer time periods are needed, it is necessary to check again the functionality of the mitochondria (RCI) after the assays.

Mitochondrial Free Radical Leak

It is frequently assumed that mitochondrial ROS production is a direct function of mitochondrial O_2 consumption. While this is sometimes true (Ku *et al.*, 1993), in other situations, including comparisons between birds and mammals or caloric restriction (Barja, 2004), this is not the case. A well-known example is the transition from state 4 to state 3, during which mitochondrial O_2 consumption increases strongly but ROS production decreases or is even totally abolished. In this last case ROS production per unit oxygen consumption decreases acutely during the energy transition. In other words, during state 3 mitochondria are more efficient than in state 4, avoiding ROS generation per unit electron flow in the respiratory chain, which is clearly adaptive. This can be quantified by measuring the "free radical leak": the fraction (%) of electrons out of sequence which reduce oxygen to ROS in the mitochondrial respiratory chain

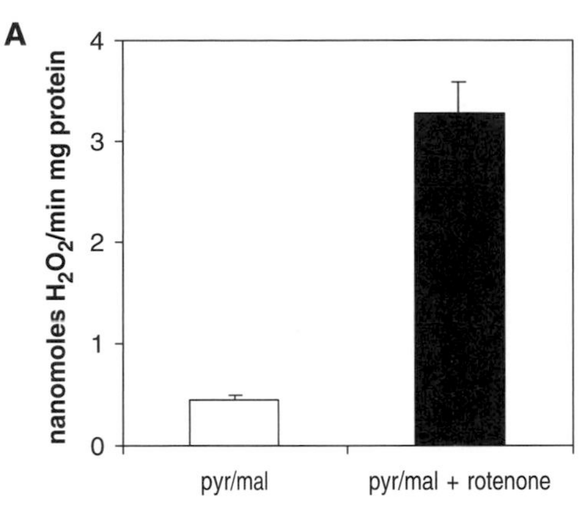

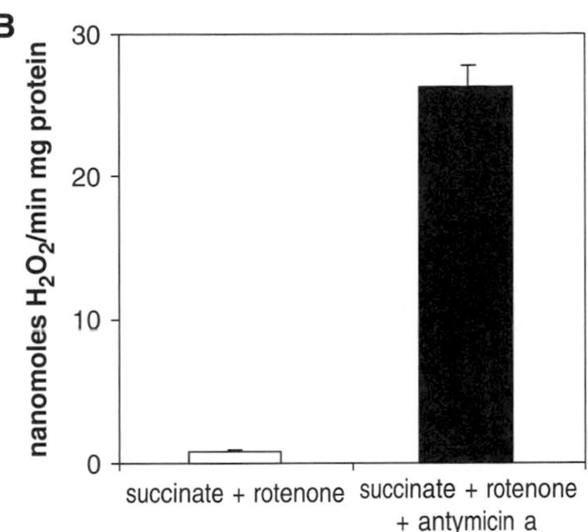

Figure 16.1. Effects of inhibitors of the respiratory chain on the rate of H_2O_2 generation of rat heart mitochondria. (A) Addition of rotenone (complex I inhibitor) to pyruvate/malate-supplemented rat heart mitochondria increases H_2O_2 production. (B) Addition of antimycin A (complex III inhibitor) to succinate (+rotenone)-supplemented rat heart mitochondria increases H_2O_2 production.

instead of reducing oxygen to water at cytochrome oxidase. If mitochondrial H_2O_2 production and oxygen consumption are measured in parallel using the same incubation medium, temperature and concentrations of substrates and modulators in each mitochondria preparation, the free radical leak can be calculated. Since two electrons are needed to reduce one molecule of oxygen to H_2O_2, whereas four electrons are needed to reduce one molecule of oxygen to water, the free radical leak is easily calculated by dividing the rate of ROS production by two times the rate of oxygen consumption, the result being multiplied by 100.

Localization of Mitochondrial Sites of H_2O_2 Production

The method allows localizing the sites responsible for ROS production inside the electron transport chain. The sites of ROS production are identified by measuring the rate of H_2O_2 production with different combinations of substrates and inhibitors specific for different segments of the respiratory chain. For example, pyruvate/malate and glutamate/malate are complex I-linked substrates, and succinate is a complex II-linked substrate. Rotenone inhibits specifically at complex I, TTFA at complex II and antimycin A at complex III.

It is well known that the rate of oxygen radical production increases as a function of the degree of reduction of the autoxidazable electron carrier responsible for ROS generation (Boveris and Chance, 1973). Blocking the respiratory chain with an inhibitor increases the reduction state of electron carriers on the substrate side of the inhibitor, whereas those in the oxygen (opposite) side change to a more oxidized state. Thus, an increase in oxygen radical production following the addition of an inhibitor means that the oxygen radical generator is located on the substrate side of the block. Conversely, if oxygen radical production decreases after addition of the inhibitor, the generator must be situated on the oxygen side. Thus, the higher H_2O_2 production observed in the presence than in the absence of rotenone in pyruvate/malate-supplemented rat mitochondria (Figure 16.1A) indicates that they produce ROS at complex I since this is the only complex situated on the substrate side of the inhibitor in this experiment.

Similarly, the classically described increase in H_2O_2 production after addition of antimycin A to succinate(+rotenone)-supplemented rat heart mitochondria (Figure 16.1B) is due to ROS production at complex III. On the other hand, in contrast with the experiment with pyruvate/malate, addition of rotenone to mitochondria respiring with succinate decreases H_2O_2 production, indicating that part of the ROS generated with this substrate comes from complex I (Herrero and Barja, 1997; Lambert and Brand, 2004). In this experiment rotenone blocks the reverse flow of electrons from succinate to complex I and thus its capacity for ROS production. Similar experiments can be used to localize the sites involved in changes in ROS generation induced by experimental manipulations in animals.

Conclusions

An efficient and reliable method for measuring ROS production in intact functional mitochondria is described. The method is specific for H_2O_2 and is sensitive enough to assay basal H_2O_2 production in the respiratory chain. It shows high reproducibility, generates stable final fluorescence, and does not interfere with mitochondrial function. The assay system shows instantaneous response to H_2O_2, and is thus useful for studying the effect of inhibitors or modulators on the rate of ROS production. It also allows the calculation of the free radical leak (the percentage of electrons out of sequence which reduce O_2 to ROS instead of to water at the respiratory chain). While other fluorescent methods are available to measure

ROS production in isolated mitochondria, the one presented here has various advantages: it is based on increases (instead of decreases) in fluorescence, reactants are not expensive, and homovanillic acid does not spontaneously generate fluorescence. The method, similarly to the available alternatives, can be applied only to isolated mitochondria. The measurement of ROS production (independent of ROS scavenging) in intact cells or animals must wait for future technical developments.

Recommended Resources

RESOURCES IN THE INTERNET

Pages about different complexes of mitochondrial electron transport chain:

1. Complex I: www.scripps.edu/biochem/CI
2. Complex II: www.mpibp-frankfurt.mpg.de/lancaster/complexII/
3. Complex III: www.life.uiuc.edu/crofts/bc-complex_site/

In these pages structures, genes and proteins, and main researchers working on the topic and recent references are included.

PAGE ABOUT HUMAN MITOCHONDRIAL DNA

DNA: http://www.mitomap.org/. Organization of mitochondrial DNA, mitochondrial diseases, code of translation and more frequent mutations are included.

BOOKS

1. Tyler, D. (1992). *The Mitochondrion in Health and Disease*. VCH Publisher, New York. A classical book about mitochondria. An essential book for anyone working in the mitochondrial area.
2. Nicholls, D.G., and Ferguson, S.J. (2002). *Bioenergetics 3*. Academic Press, San Diego. Essential book exclusively dedicated to cellular bioenergetics. The information included concerning mitochondria is extensive.

ACKNOWLEDGMENTS

Supported in part by a grant from Spanish Education and Science Ministry (SAF2002-01635). Alberto Sanz received a PhD fellowship from Complutense University of Madrid.

REFERENCES

Barja, G. (1999). Measurements of mitochondrial oxygen radical production. In Yu, B.P., Ed., *Methods in Aging Research*, pp. 533–549, CRC, Boca Raton.

Barja, G. (2002). The quantitative measurement of H_2O_2 generation in isolated mitochondria. *J. Bioenerg. Biomembr. 34*, 227–233.

Barja, G. (2004). Aging in vertebrates, and the effect of caloric restriction: A mitochondrial free radical production-DNA damage mechanism? *Biol. Rev. Camb. Philos. Soc. 79*, 235–251.

Boveris, A., and Chance, B. (1973). The mitochondrial generation of hydrogen peroxide. General properties and effect of hyperbaric oxygen. *Biochem. J. 134*, 707–716.

Boveris, A., Cadenas, E., and Stoppani, O.M. (1976). Role of ubiquinone in the mitochondrial generation of hydrogen peroxide. *Biochem. J. 156*, 435–444.

Cadenas, E., Boveris, A., Ragan, I., and Stoppani, A.O.M. (1977). Production of superoxide radical and hydrogen peroxide by NADH-ubiquinone reductase and ubiquinol-cytochrome c reductase from beef-heart mitochondria. *Arch. Biochem. Biophys. 180*, 248–257.

Chance, B., and Gao, G. (1994). In vivo detection of radicals in biological reactions. *Environm. Health Persp. 102*, 29–32.

Drew, B., Phaneuf, S., Dirks, A., Selman, C., Gredilla, R., Lezza, A., Barja, G., and Leeuwenburgh, C. (2003). Effects of aging and caloric restriction on mitochondrial energy production in gastrocnemius muscle and heart. *Amer. J. Physiol. 284*, R474–R480.

Dykens, J.A. (1994). Isolated cerebral and cerebellar mitochondria produced free radicals when exposed to elevated Ca^{2+} and Na^{+}: Implications for neurodegeneration. *J. Neurochem. 63*, 584–591.

Giulivi, C., Boveris, A., and Cadenas, E. (1995). Hydroxyl radical generation during mitochondrial electron transfer and the formation of hydroxydesoxyguanosine in mitochondrial DNA. *Arch. Biochem. Biophys. 316*, 909–916.

Gredilla, R., Sanz, A., López-Torres, M., and Barja, G. (2001). Caloric restriction decreases mitochondrial free radical generation at Complex I and lowers oxidative damage to mitochondrial DNA in the rat heart. *FASEB J. 15*, 1589–1591.

Hagopian, K., Harper, M.E., Ram, J.J., Humble, S.J., Weindruch, R., and Ramsey, J.J. (2005). Long-term calorie restriction reduces proton leak and hydrogen peroxide production in liver mitochondria. *Am. J. Physiol. 288*, E674–678.

Han, D., Williams, E., and Cadenas, E. (2001). Mitochondrial respiratory chain-dependent generation of superoxide anion and its release into the intermembrane space. *Biochem. J. 353*, 411–416.

Harman, D. (1956). A theory based on free radical and radical chemistry. *J. Gerontol. 11*, 298–300.

Herrero, A., and Barja, G. (1997). Sites and mechanisms responsible for the low rate of free radical production of heart mitochondria in the long lived pigeon. *Mech. Ageing Dev. 98*, 95–111.

Inoguchi, T., Li, P., Umeda, F., Yu, H.Y., Kakimoto, M., Imamura, M., *et al.* (2000). High glucose level and free fatty acid stimulate reactive oxygen species production through protein kinase C-dependent activation of NAD(P)H oxidase in cultured vascular cells. *Diabetes 49*, 1939–1945.

Ku, H.H., Brunk, U.T., and Sohal, R.S. (1993). Relationship between mitochondrial superoxide and hydrogen peroxide production and longevity of mammalian species. *Free Rad. Biol. Med. 15*, 621–627.

Lai, J.C.K., and Clark, J.B. (1979). Preparation of synaptic and nonsynaptic mitochondria from mammalian brain. *Methods Enzymol. 55*, 51–60.

Lambert, A.J., and Brand, M.D. (2004). Superoxide production by NADH: ubiquinone oxidoreductase (complex I) depends on the pH gradient across the mitochondrial inner membrane. *Biochem. J. 382*, 511–517.

Lass, A., and Sohal, R.S. (2000). Effect of coenzyme Q(10) and alpha-tocopherol content of mitochondria on the production of superoxide anion radicals. *FASEB J. 14*, 87–94.

López-Torres, M., Gredilla, R., Sanz, A., and Barja, G. (2002). Influence of aging and long-term caloric restriction on oxygen radical generation and oxidative DNA damage in rat liver mitochondria. *Free Rad. Biol. Med. 32*, 882–889.

Loschen, G., Flohé, L., and Chance, B. (1971). Respiratory chain linked H_2O_2 production in pigeon heart mitochondria. *FEBS Lett. 18*, 261–274.

Matiasson, G. (2004). Analysis of mitochodrial generation and release of reactive oxygen species. *Cytometry Part A. 62*, 89–96.

Mela, L., and Seitz, S. (1979). Isolation of mitochondria with emphasis on heart mitochondria from small amounts of tissue. *Methods Enzymol. 55*, 39–46.

Muller, F.L., Liu, Y., and Van Remmen, H. (2004). Complex III releases superoxide to both sides of the inner mitochondrial membrane. *J. Biol. Chem. 279*, 49064–49073.

Prat, A.G., Bolter, C., Chavez, U., Taylor, C., Chefurka, W., and Turrens, J. (1991). Purification of cytochrome c peroxidase for monitoring H_2O_2 production. *Free Rad. Biol. Med. 11*, 537–544.

Ruch, W., Cooper, P.H., and Baggiolini, M. (1983) Assay of H_2O_2 production by macrophages and neutrophils with homovanillic acid and horse-radish peroxidase. *J. Immunol. Meth. 63*, 347–357.

Sohal, R.S., Mockett, R.J., and Orr, W.C. (2002). Mechanisms of aging: An appraisal of the oxidative stress hypothesis. *Free Rad. Biol. Med. 33*, 575–586.

Takeshige, K., and Minakami, S. (1979). NADH- and NADPH-dependent formation of superoxide anions by bovine heart submitochondrial particles and NAD-ubiquinone-reductase preparation. *Biochem. J. 180*, 129–135.

Tarpey, M.M., Wink, D.A., and Grisham, M.B. (2004). Methods for detection of reactive metabolites of oxygen and nitrogen: in vitro and in vivo considerations. *Am. J. Physiol. Regul. Integr. Comp. Physiol. 286*, R431–R444.

Towne, V., Will, M., Oswald, B., and Zhao, Q. (2004). Complexities in horseradish peroxidase-catalyzed oxidation of dihdryoxyphenoxazine derivatives: Appropriate ranges for pH values and hydrogen peroxide concentrations in quantitative analysis. *Anal. Bioch. 334*, 290–296.

Turrens, J.F., Alexandre, A., and Lehninger, A.L. (1985). Ubisemiquinone is the electron donor for superoxide formation by complex III of heart mitochondria. *Arch. Biochem. Biophys. 237*, 408–414.

Votyakova, T.V., and Reynolds, I.J. (2004). Detection of hydrogen peroxide with Amplex Red: intereference by NADH and reduced glutathione auto-oxidation. *Arch. Bioch. Biophys. 431*, 138–144.

Zhou, M., Diwu, Z., Panchuk-Voloshine, N., and Haugland, R.P. (1997). A stable nonfluorescent derivative of resorufin for the fluorometric determination of trace hydrogen peroxide: Applications in detecting the activity of phagocyte NADPH oxidase and other oxidases. *Anal. Bioch. 253*, 162–168.

17

Telomeres and Aging in the Yeast Model System

Kurt W. Runge

Telomeres are the physical ends of linear eukaryotic chromosomes. In many organisms, including humans and yeasts, telomeres are composed of short repeated DNA sequences and their associated proteins. These repeats are lost gradually due to incomplete DNA synthesis of the chromosome end, or by degradation from nucleases, and can be resynthesized by the enzyme telomerase. Many human somatic cells do not express sufficient telomerase activity to prevent telomere repeat loss, resulting in cell senescence or death when telomeres shorten to a critical length. This telomere length checkpoint for aging and cell growth is also seen in yeast whose genes for telomerase components have been deleted, allowing yeast to serve as a model for telomere-linked senescence and aging in human cells. Telomeres also serve as a reservoir of bound proteins that are released as the telomere DNA shortens, and work in yeast has shown that these telomere-associated proteins play important roles in yeast replicative aging. The advantages of yeast as an aging model include rapid growth and aging, a small well-defined and well-annotated genome, powerful molecular genetics for modifying this genome, simple but robust assays for the activity and location of telomeric proteins, publicly available collections of mutants in every gene, and multiple assays for replicative and chronological aging. This chapter will describe how the budding yeast Saccharomyces cerevisiae has contributed to our knowledge of telomeres and aging, and the emerging role of the evolutionarily divergent fission yeast Schizosaccharomyces pombe as another important model system. The powerful genetics of these two different yeast systems should identify central evolutionarily conserved processes that control cellular aging.

Telomere Replication, the Telomere Length Checkpoint and Growth without Telomerase

TELOMERE STRUCTURE

Telomeres in the majority of model systems have the general DNA structure of a simple sequence repeat at the end of the chromosome that is adjacent to a middle-repetitive family of repeats. Experiments with chromosome truncations in yeast and the discovery of viable chromosome truncations in humans indicate that the simple sequence repeats are all that are required to maintain a stable chromosomal telomere in mitosis and meiosis (Gottschling *et al.*, 1990; Wilkie *et al.*, 1990). In contrast, broken DNA ends lacking these repeats are highly recombinagenic, as are yeast telomeres that have lost their simple sequence repeats (Hackett *et al.*, 2001). In humans, the 3′ end of the chromosome bears the repeat sequence TTAGGG while *S. cerevisiae* has the more divergent repeat $(TG_{2-3})(TG)_{1-6}$, abbreviated as TG_{1-3}, and *S. pombe* has a more divergent sequence with a core repeat of G_nTTACA that can be interrupted by additional bases (Hiraoka and Chikashige, 2004; Smogorzewska and De Lange, 2004). The current model for telomere end structure in humans and yeast is that the 3′ end extends past the 5′ end by several telomere repeats (Makarov *et al.*, 1997; McElligott and Wellinger, 1997; Wellinger *et al.*, 1993).

TELOMERASE AND TELOMERE REPLICATION

The structure of the telomere end reflects its unique mode of replication. Normally, replication of a linear DNA molecule from internal origins of replication would generate to daughter molecules, each of which has one blunt end and one end with a 3′ overhang after removal of the terminal RNA primer. The current model from work in budding yeast is that at the end of S-phase, telomeres undergo a processing event in which the 5′ strand (sometimes called the CA strand to reflect the predominant bases in the telomere repeats) is degraded to produce a long 3′ overhang (possibly 50–100 bases in yeast) which is then partially filled-in to leave a shorter 3′ overhang of ~12 bases (Figure 17.1).

The removal of the RNA primer, or the action of nucleases on the repeats, causes telomeres to shorten each time the cell divides. In the absence of a mechanism to replicate the telomere repeats, the telomeres continuously shorten. In this "mitotic clock" hypothesis (Harley and Villeponteau, 1995), the size of the telomere repeat tract is related to the number of divisions the cell has undergone. In old cells where the telomere tract becomes too short, the cell senses this state and induces a "short telomere checkpoint" that causes cell cycle arrest (discussed below).

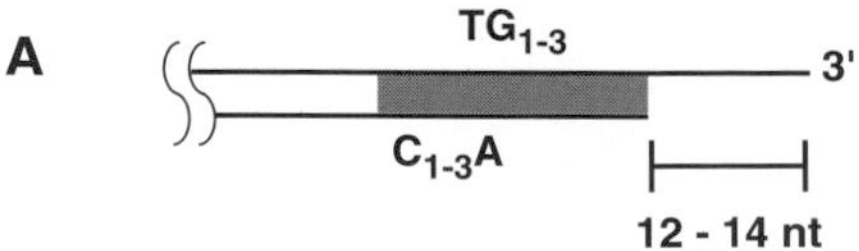

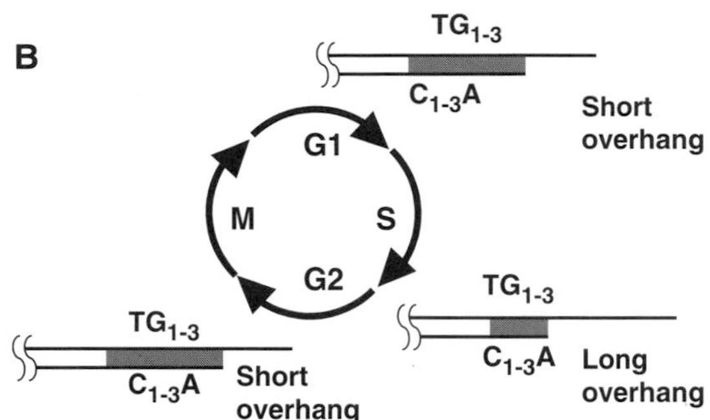

Figure 17.1. Yeast telomere end structure. (A) Yeast telomere repeat tracts have 250–400 bp of the irregular sequence TG_{1-3} at their very ends. The terminus of the chromosome has a 3′ overhang in the G1 phase of the cell cycle which is 12–14 nt long (Larrivee *et al.*, 2004). The telomeres of human cells also possess 3′ overhangs (McElligott and Wellinger 1997). (B) The 3′ overhang is elongated in S phase in a telomerase-independent manner. At the end of S-phase after telomere replication, the overhang is expanded to greater than 50 nt and then returns to a shorter overhang which is presumed to have the G1 structure. Because this long overhang is detected in cells lacking *in vivo* telomerase activity, it is thought that the overhang is produced by a nuclease acting on replicated telomeres (Wellinger *et al.*, 1996).

In yeast and human germ cells, this arrest is prevented by the synthesis of new telomere repeats by the activity of the enzyme telomerase.

Telomerase is the name given to the core enzyme consisting of a protein (the TERT subunit for TElomerase Reverse Transcriptase) and RNA (the TER subunit for TElomerase RNA, also called TERC and TR). The RNA serves as an internal template for the synthesis of new telomere repeats (reviewed by Smogorzewska and De Lange (2004)). A number of other protein subunits that make up the telomerase holoenzyme are known in several organisms, but most conserved components are TERT and TER. While growing cultures of human and yeast cells that lack telomerase eventually senesce and/or die from loss of telomere function, cultures of cells that express telomerase activity form cultures that continuously double (Bodnar *et al.*, 1998). Consequently, the presence of telomerase can prevent the short telomere-mediated cell senescence or death of all cells in the culture.

When human and yeast cells express telomerase, the size of their telomere repeat tracts is usually kept within a certain range (as opposed to elongating continuously). A great deal of work on telomerase and the genetics of telomere length control has yielded a model in which much of the control of telomere length is due to telomeric chromatin regulating the access of telomerase to the 3′ end of the chromosome (reviewed by Smogorzewska and De Lange (2004)). The proteins that bind directly to the telomere repeats, or the co-factors that they recruit, are thought to form a structure that sequesters the chromosome end from telomerase and other cellular activities. Short telomeres are preferentially elongated over longer telomeres (Hemann *et al.*, 2001; Ouellette *et al.*, 2000; Teixeira *et al.*, 2004), and it is thought that shorter telomeres bind fewer of these proteins, which makes them more likely to be lengthened. This interplay between telomerase and the many telomere chromatin components is an area of intensive research, and a greater understanding of the intricacies of these processes is likely in the coming years.

TELOMERE REPLICATION WITHOUT TELOMERASE

Failure to elongate very short telomeres, as occurs in cells lacking telomerase, induces a short telomere checkpoint. As this growth arrest can be bypassed in human cells by the expression of transforming genes without the re-expression of telomerase, this arrest represents a true cell cycle checkpoint (Harley and Villeponteau, 1995). In cultures of human and yeast cells, the majority of cells arrest. In yeast, this arrest appears as a prolonged delay at the G2/M boundary of the cell cycle (Enomoto *et al.*, 2002; IJpma and Greider, 2003). However, rare cells can undergo mutagenic events that allow them to grow out of these cultures. For transformed human cells, these rare cells go on to form cell lines. In yeast, these mutant cells that can grow without telomerase are often referred to as "survivors."

At this point it is worth asking: is the senescence observed in yeast due to short telomeres a true senescence, or is it cell death? Senescence is defined as a quiescent but metabolically active state. In yeast, short telomere-induced senescence has been demonstrated by the ability to return these nongrowing cells to growth by reintroducing active telomerase. While defining the minimal portions of yeast telomerase RNA required for function, Livengood *et al.* (2002) grew cells lacking the telomerase RNA gene to the point of senescence and prepared these cells for transformation. Transforming cells with an empty vector yielded very few transformants, while transforming cells with a vector bearing a functional telomerase RNA gene gave many transformants. These data suggest that these arrested cells can be returned to the cell cycle and normal growth by taking up a new gene, transcribing and processing the RNA and assembling an active telomerase enzyme. These activities suggest that many of the senescent cells are metabolically active. A more defined set of experiments where telomere lengthening is re-established in senescent cells would provide the opportunity to analyze the reversible cellular changes associated with this growth arrest.

Yeasts lacking telomerase are constructed by deletion of the gene for a telomerase component such as yeast TERT (yTERT) or yeast TER (yTER or the *TLC1* gene). Since the haploid yeast have no copy of the telomerase component in its genome, the only way to escape senescence and death due to loss of telomere repeats is to find an alternative mechanism to maintain these repeats that does not involve telomerase. In the budding yeast *S. cerevisiae*, there are two types of survivors that can replicate telomeres, called Type I and Type II. Type I survivors are yeast that have rearranged their genomes such that each telomere contains copies of the subtelomeric repeat called Y′ followed by a short stretch of TG_{1-3}. These telomeres are thought to use nonreciprocal recombination to replicate their TG_{1-3} repeats. The generation of Type I survivors requires a number of recombination genes including *RAD52*, *RAD51*, *RAD54* and *RAD57*. In contrast, Type II survivors contain long stretches of TG_{1-3} at the chromosome end and require the recombination genes *RAD52*, *RAD50* and *SGS1* (Chen *et al.*, 2001; Huang *et al.*, 2001; Teng *et al.*, 2000; Teng and Zakian, 1999).

Postsenescent survivors have also been isolated in the fission yeast, *S. pombe*. Cells lacking the TERT subunit can give rise to two types of survivors: a recombination-driven mode of growth with amplification of subtelomeric sequences to give telomeres of heterogeneous lengths, and a chromosome circularization mode in which the 3 linear *S. pombe* chromosomes are converted to circular versions (Nakamura *et al.*, 1997). The *S. pombe* genome is similar in size to that of *S. cerevisiae*, but organized into 3 chromosomes instead of the 16 in budding yeast. This reduced chromosome number apparently allows shortening telomeres on the same chromosome to undergo head-to-head fusions and generate circular chromosomes that allow stable growth at a detectable frequency. In contrast, the 16 chromosomes of *S. cerevisiae* provide 32 telomeres that may compete with each other for telomere–telomere fusion events and reduce the chance of forming a cell where all of the cell's chromosomes are circularized. However, circularized chromosomes can be detected in some survivor strains of budding yeast, indicating that telomere–telomere fusions of this type are a general phenomenon (Liti and Louis, 2003).

In contrast to yeast deletion mutants, human cells that lack telomerase activity have often repressed the expression of the gene for the hTERT subunit. Cells that grow out of cultures that have bypassed senescence to form cell lines have often reactivated this gene and now express telomerase activity. Increased telomerase activity is also found in many, but not all, human tumors (Kim *et al.*, 1994). However, telomere replication in the absence of telomerase activity has also been found in human cells and some human tumors (reviewed by Henson *et al.* (2002)). This Alternative Lengthening of Telomeres, or ALT, pathway also appears to involve recombination pathways that involve copying sequences from one telomere to another, as well as more complex recombination events (Fasching *et al.*, 2005; Londono-Vallejo *et al.*, 2004). Thus, both telomerase-mediated and telomerase-independent modes of telomere replication are conserved in yeasts and humans, strengthening the use of yeast as a model system for telomere function.

YEAST TELOMERE PROTEIN COMPONENTS

Telomerase

The core of the telomerase enzyme is the TERT and TER subunits. In budding yeast, the *EST2* gene encodes the protein subunit while the *TLC1* gene encodes the telomerase RNA (Lingner *et al.*, 1997; Singer and Gottschling, 1994). The *EST2* gene name stands for Ever Shorter Telomeres 2, because the telomere repeat tracts in these mutants that have inactivated the *EST2* gene continuously shorten until the most of the cells in the culture senesce. Four *EST* genes were isolated in the screen that identified *EST2*, yielding the additional protein-encoding genes *EST1*, *EST3* and *EST4* (*EST4* was found to be the previously characterized *CDC13* gene, and the *EST4* mutant is commonly referred to as *cdc13–2* or $cdc13^{est}$) (Lendvay *et al.*, 1996). The mutants isolated in these genes all show the same phenotype, indicating a loss of telomerase activity *in vivo*. However, cell extracts from *est1*, *est3* or $cdc13^{est}$ mutants all yield telomerase activity *in vitro* (Lingner *et al.*, 1997). Elegant work has since demonstrated that the *EST1*, *EST3* and *CDC13* gene, products serve as adaptor proteins to help recruit the telomerase enzyme to the telomere, and the molecular dynamics of this process is under intensive study by many groups (Evans and Lundblad, 1999; Smith *et al.*, 2003; Taggart *et al.*, 2002). One *EST1* paralog has been identified in budding yeast. Two orthologs in fission yeast and three *EST1* orthologs in human cells have been identified, and some of these proteins associate with telomerase and telomerase RNA (Lundblad, 2003; Sanger_Institute 2005; Zhou *et al.*, 2000). While *CDC13* has no ortholog beyond budding yeasts, it has a similar structure compared to the telomere end-binding factor POT1 in *S. pombe* and mammals.

Telomere structural proteins

Double-stranded yeast telomere repeats are bound predominantly by Repressor Activator Protein 1 or *RAP1* protein. This protein represses transcription when bound to the yeast silent mating type cassettes (described below) and telomeres, activates the transcription of many housekeeping genes, and serves as a crucial telomere length regulator and chromatin component. *RAP1* protein contains an ~230 amino acid DNA binding domain and an ~170 amino acid C-terminal domain which serves as an interaction site for many telomere-associated proteins (Hardy *et al.*, 1992; Henry *et al.*, 1990; Konig *et al.*, 1996; Moretti *et al.*, 1994; Wotton and Shore, 1997). Thus, *RAP1* encodes a multifunctional protein whose activities are dependent upon its DNA binding context. At the telomere, *RAP1* protein is known for its association with the gene-silencing proteins *SIR2*, *SIR3* and *SIR4* and the telomere length regulatory proteins encoded by *RIF1* and *RIF2*.

Gene silencing in budding yeast, a chromatin-mediated effect that prevents the transcription of genes, was first discovered in the late 1970s (Rine *et al.*, 1979). When reporter genes are placed adjacent to telomere repeats in the chromosome, their expression is repressed or silenced. Similar types of telomere-associated silencing have been reported in *S. pombe*, *Drosophila melanogaster* and humans (Baur *et al.*, 2001; Levis *et al.*, 1985; Nimmo *et al.*, 1994) in addition to other organisms. In budding yeast, silencing has been found to be effected by a number of chromatin proteins and chromatin modifying and remodeling complexes. The "classic" proteins involved are encoded by *SIR2*, *SIR3* and *SIR4*. These proteins also act with the *SIR1* protein to silence two specialized loci, the silent mating type cassettes, and *SIR2* protein also acts with other proteins to repress RNA polymerase II transcription and recombination in the array of ribosomal RNA genes called the rDNA array (Figure 17.2).

Of *SIR2*, *SIR3* and *SIR4*, only *SIR2* has orthologs in a large number of other organisms. *SIR2* encodes an NAD^+-dependent deacetylase that is important in maintaining gene silencing and prolonging yeast lifespan (reviewed by Blander and Guarente (2004)). Many organisms encode multiple *SIR2* family members, or sirtuins, and the suggestion has been made that sirtuins may alter protein posttranslational modification to regulate responses to stress that also affect lifespan (Blander and Guarente, 2004).

In budding yeast, the *SIR* proteins are one of the first examples of telomeres serving as a reservoir of proteins that can be mobilized to move to other genetic loci.

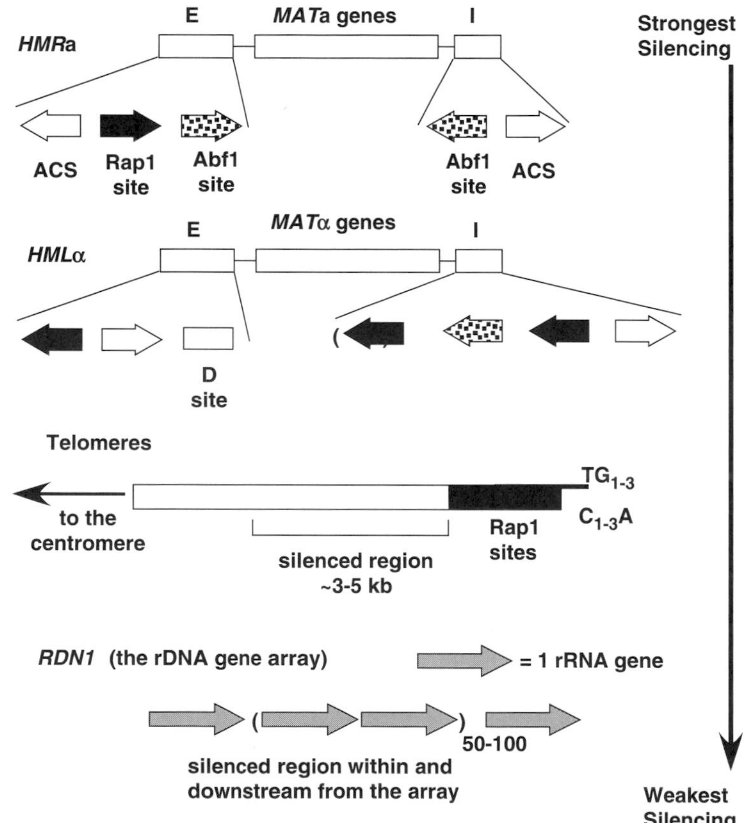

Figure 17.2. Silenced loci in yeast. The 4 major silent loci are shown, which fall into 3 classes: The silent mating type cassettes *HMRa* and *HMLα*, telomeres and the tandem array of ribosomal RNA genes called the rDNA array or *RDN1* (the genetic designation of this locus). In yeast, mating type is determined by the sets of genes expressed at the *MAT* locus, either a and α. Yeast has 3 copies of this locus, one which is expressed (*MAT*) and two which are strongly silenced (*HMR* and *HML*). These silent mating type cassettes contain flanking DNA elements, called E and I, which silence the *MAT* genes between them. The E and I sites in turn contain unidirectional binding sites for known DNA binding factors, *RAP1* protein (which binds to the Rap1 site), *ABF1* protein (which binds to the Abf1 site), and Origin Recognition Complex (which binds to the ACS element) (Laurenson and Rine 1992). The proteins encoded by *SIR1*, *SIR2*, *SIR3* and *SIR4* are required for silencing at the silent mating type cassettes. The TG_{1-3} repeats in telomeres contain arrays of *RAP1* protein sites, which tether *SIR2*, *SIR3* and *SIR4* proteins to telomeres and silence nearby genes (Gottschling *et al.*, 1990). The rDNA array binds a different set of proteins that include *SIR2* protein and silence RNA polymerase II transcribed genes placed within these repeats (Straight *et al.*, 1999).

Under a variety of mutant conditions that alter telomere chromatin structure, *SIR* proteins appeared to be released from the telomere and to relocalize at the silent mating type cassettes (Buck and Shore, 1995). Subsequently, *SIR3* protein was shown to move from telomeres to newly made double-strand breaks (Martin *et al.*, 1999; Mills *et al.*, 1999). Finally, this relocalization of *SIR* proteins from telomeres plays an important role in the replicative aging of yeast, illustrating how release of proteins from telomeres can have an impact on lifespan (see Telomeres and Yeast Replicative Aging, below).

In addition to *SIR* proteins, *RIF1* and *RIF2* proteins also interact with the C-terminus of *RAP1* protein bound at telomeres (Hardy *et al.*, 1992; Wotton and Shore, 1997). One clear function of the *RIF* proteins is in telomere length control: cells that lack the C-terminal 160 amino acids of *RAP1* protein have telomeres that grow from ~330 bp of TG_{1-3} to 2–4 kb of TG_{1-3}, and cells deleted for both *RIF1* and *RIF2* also have 2–4 kb TG_{1-3} telomere tracts (Kyrion *et al.*, 1992; Wotton and Shore, 1997). Recent evidence also suggests that *RIF* proteins may interact with proteins or DNA independent of *RAP1* protein while regulating telomere length (Levy and Blackburn, 2004).

Orthologs for *RAP1* and *RIF1* proteins have been identified in *S. pombe* and in humans, and show differences from budding yeasts. While *RAP1* protein binds directly to DNA in *S. cerevisiae*, *S. pombe* and human cells have different Myb-related double-stranded telomere DNA binding proteins called $taz1^{+}$ (in fission yeast) and TRF1 and TRF2 (in human cells). The *RAP1* of fission yeast and humans lacks the DNA binding domain, and instead is tethered to telomeres by interactions with *taz1* protein or TRF2, respectively. As in *S. cerevisiae*, the *RIF1* protein ortholog also interacts with the C-terminus of the Rap1 ortholog in *S. pombe* and humans. While fission yeast *rap1* and *rif1* proteins and human Rap1 protein behave as negative regulators of telomere length (reviewed in detail by Smogorzewska and De Lange (2004)), human Rif1 protein apparently leaves telomeres to play a role in the ATM-dependent DNA damage response (Silverman *et al.*, 2004). Recruitment of the human telomere binding protein TRF2 to DSBs has also been recently reported (Bradshaw *et al.*, 2005). These properties of human Rif1 and TRF2 suggest that human telomeres may also serve as a reservoir of factors for other cellular processes such as the response to DSBs. The release of such factors could potentially be regulated by stochastic processes, e.g., a DSB activating a protein kinase cascade, or could be gradual as telomeres shorten over repeated cell divisions. A DNA damage function for the yeast Rif1 proteins has not been tested yet.

Telomere proteins that act at double-strand breaks

Telomeres can be viewed as specialized double-strand breaks (DSBs). While telomeres have specific sequences and associated proteins, many of the proteins that interact with and process telomeres also play important roles in the recognition and processing of DSBs at internal chromosomal loci. These proteins include the *S. cerevisiae* DNA damage checkpoint kinases Tel1p and Mec1p (ATM and ATR in humans), the multifunctional MRX complex (MRN in humans), and the Yku70p-Yku80p DNA-end binding heterodimer (Ku70-Ku86 in humans) (Maser and DePinho, 2004). Yeast cells lacking these proteins maintain telomeres with fewer simple sequence repeats, indicating their role in telomere replication, and have defects in responding to and processing DSBs (Lustig and Petes, 1986; Morrow *et al.*, 1995; Porter *et al.*, 1996; Ritchie *et al.*, 1999; Ritchie and Petes, 2000). The simple sequence repeats that make up telomere DNA and the combination of proteins that associate with these sequences prevent them from being processed as DSBs by the cellular machinery.

The first DSB-associated protein found to directly associate with telomeres was the Yku70/Yku80 heterodimer. This DNA end-binding protein, first found in mammalian cells, binds to DNA breaks and activates DNA-activated protein kinase catalytic subunit (DNA-PK_{cs}), a member of the ATM family (Anderson and Lees 1992). The yeast Ku proteins were found to associate with the telomere and play a role in telomere replication by recruiting telomerase (Fisher *et al.*, 2004; Gravel *et al.*, 1998; Peterson *et al.*, 2001). Since then, Ku heterodimer association with the telomere in fission yeast and humans has also been demonstrated (Bailey *et al.*, 1999; Baumann and Cech, 2000).

Upon induction of a DSB, several proteins recognize and process this DNA lesion and signal the cell cycle machinery to pause. An elegant study investigating the choreography of these events in yeast found that the first proteins to bind are the MRX complex (composed of proteins encoded by *MRE11*, *RAD50* and *XRS2*) and *TEL1* protein, followed by recruitment of the RPA complex (Lisby *et al.*, 2004). RPA then recruits *MEC1* protein and MRX and *TEL1* protein leave the DSB. Importantly, phenotypes for mutants in each of these genes include changes in the length of the TG_{1-3} repeats in budding yeast (Ritchie *et al.*, 1999; Schramke *et al.*, 2004; Smith *et al.*, 2000; Tsukamoto *et al.*, 2001). So what are these proteins? *TEL1* and *MEC1* are DNA damage protein kinases of the ATM family, whose orthologs are, respectively, $tel1^{+}$ and $rad3^{+}$ in *S. pombe* and ATM and ATR in humans. MRX is a multifunctional complex *in vivo* that has helicase and nuclease activity *in vitro*, whose orthologs in fission yeast and humans are called MRN complex (for Mre11-Rad50-Nbs1) (reviewed by Smogorzewska and De Lange (2004)). RPA is a conserved complex that functions in DNA synthesis and repair (reviewed by Schramke *et al.*, (2004) and Smith *et al.*, (2000)). Interestingly, cells lacking *TEL1* and *MEC1* in budding yeast, or $tel1^{+}$ and $rad3^{+}$ in fission yeast, have telomeres that gradually shorten as telomerase cannot access the telomere (Chan *et al.*, 2001; Naito *et al.*, 1998;

Ritchie *et al.*, 1999). Experiments in budding yeast have shown that *TEL1* protein associates with telomeres when they reach ~1/3 their normal length, and *TEL1* association is a step in the pathway that allows telomere elongation by telomerase. In contrast, *MEC1* protein telomere association is observed when survivor/ALT cells arise in the culture, suggesting a role for *MEC1* protein when the telomere repeats become short enough for the telomere to lose its characteristic protection of the chromosome end (Hector *et al.*, submitted). These data indicate different roles for these checkpoint kinases in maintaining and monitoring telomere length. As all of these proteins have a role in DNA damage signaling, they most likely play some yet-to-be defined role in how the cell senses a short telomere to pause the cell cycle. This function appears to be conserved in humans, as senescing cells show increased association of ATM with telomeres.

TEL2 protein may be another yeast telomere protein that plays a role in the cellular response to DSBs. The original *TEL2* mutation, *tel2-1*, has telomeres one-half the length of wild-type cells and appears to control telomere length through the *TEL1* pathway (Lustig and Petes, 1986). *TEL2* protein binds to double and single-stranded telomere repeats *in vitro*, suggesting a direct role at the telomere similar to *TEL1* protein (Kota and Runge 1998; Kota and Runge, 1999), and preliminary data indicate that *TEL2* protein associates with telomeres *in vivo* (R. Kota and K.W. Runge, in preparation). However, deletion of the *TEL2* gene is lethal, while deletion of the *TEL1* gene is not, suggesting that *TEL2* protein may act in another pathway as well (Runge and Zakian, 1996). Work in *Caenorhabditis elegans* suggests a role for *TEL2* protein in aging and the response to DSBs. The *C. elegans TEL2* ortholog was identified twice by mutation: once as *clk-2*, a mutation that slows the rate of aging, and once as *rad-5*, a DNA damage checkpoint mutation (Ahmed *et al.*, 2001; Benard *et al.*, 2001). The human ortholog of *TEL2* has also been cloned and overexpressed in tissue culture cells, where it localizes in the cytoplasm (Jiang *et al.*, 2003), but it is unclear if this overexpression reveals all of the normal locations for human Tel2 protein activity. Thus, while the *in vivo* functions of *TEL2* are currently obscure, the efforts in many model organisms should soon reveal its mode of action at telomeres and in aging.

Chromatin remodeling complexes and telomere length

While yeast telomeres form a nonnucleosomal complex based on micrococcal nuclease mapping (Wright *et al.*, 1992), mutations in proteins known to modify nucleosomes can alter telomere length. Every open reading frame in yeast has been deleted in a systematic fashion, and this library of strains is publicly available. A screen of each of these strains for changes in telomere length has revealed a number of unexpected gene deletions that alter telomere length. The genes identified include *RSC2* (a member of the RSC remodeling complex), *FMP26* (which interacts with the SAGA complex) and nine members of various histone deacetylase, histone methylase and histone ubiquitination complexes (Askree *et al.*, 2004). Their effect on telomere length raises the possibility that many of these complexes may also modify telomere proteins to alter their functions or control the expression of telomere proteins. A third possibility was recently shown in *Tetrahymena*, where the placement of ordered nucleosome arrays adjacent to telomere repeats altered the length of the telomeric tract (Jacob *et al.*, 2004), raising the possibility that chromatin-modifying proteins may alter telomere length in a similar way.

Unknown players in telomere metabolism

The more telomeres are investigated, the more new processes are uncovered that require explanation. As mentioned previously, yeast telomeres have a 3′ overhang of 12–14 bp during most of the cell cycle, but in late S-phase this end is resected to an overhang of >50 nt in a manner that does not require telomerase activity (Wellinger *et al.*, 1996; Wellinger *et al.*, 1993) (Figure 17.1). These data suggest that a nuclease degrades the 5′ strand as part of normal telomere processing each cell cycle. The identity of this nuclease (or nucleases) and how it links telomeres to DNA replication will be of great interest. The process by which the 5′ strand is resected also has important implications for cell senescence and aging. When telomeres are short, degradation of the 5′ strand would further reduce the number of double-stranded telomere repeats, and could convert short telomeres into structures that activate the short telomere checkpoint. Identification of the 5′ telomere strand degrading nuclease may allow a direct test of this hypothesis.

Monitoring Yeast Senescence and Identifying Important Genes

A major advantage of yeast is that one can easily generate a cell that has normal-length telomeres and completely lacks a protein essential for telomere elongation. This cell gives rise to a population of cells that lack active telomerase and whose telomeres gradually shorten until the majority of cells arrest. This shortening time course typically requires 50–70 population doublings, which provides the opportunity to generate sufficient quantities of cells for different analyses during the course of the experiment. Yeast genetics also allows one to remove telomerase from a variety of mutant backgrounds to judge the role of a gene product in the pathway to short telomere-induced senescence.

INDUCED TELOMERASE LOSS AND BEHAVIOR OF THE RESULTING CULTURE

Two ways to lose telomerase

Telomerase loss is typically induced by deleting a gene for an essential telomerase component (usually the catalytic

TERT subunit or the TER template RNA) and then maintaining that strain by providing this gene in *trans*. One common method is to construct a diploid yeast strain and then delete one copy of the gene using standard techniques. The diploid is phenotypically wild type because one active copy of the gene remains in the diploid cell. The diploid yeast can then be sporulated to produce two haploid wild-type spores and two haploid spores bearing the gene deletion (e.g., Lendvay *et al.*, 1996). Because the gene deletion is accomplished by replacing the gene with a selectable marker, the deletion spores can be identified on medium requiring the selectable marker for growth. These haploid spores are born with wild-type length telomeres that gradually shorten over repeated mitotic divisions.

A second method is to delete the gene for the telomerase component in a haploid cell, identify the correct transformant, and introduce a normal copy of the gene on a plasmid that replicates as an episome in the cell. Episomal yeast plasmids are lost at rates that vary from 1 to 50% per cell division even when grown under selection (Murray and Szostak, 1983). Since most yeast selectable markers complement auxotrophic markers, cells that have lost the plasmid continue to divide until the gene product is diluted away or degraded and then arrested due to starvation for the auxotrophy. The fraction of plasmid-free cells in a selectively grown culture can vary from 10 to 70%, depending on the type of plasmid used. These cells can grow again if plated on medium that supplements the auxotrophic requirement (Newlon, 1988). Thus, plating cells from a selectively grown culture onto complete medium and testing portions of the resulting colonies for the presence of the plasmid's selectable marker allows one to identify the colony that lacks the gene for the telomerase component. The original colony can then be grown and tested in the same way as the haploid spore generated in the method described earlier. The disadvantage of this method is that the initial transformant lacks telomerase activity, and some mutant combinations with lack of telomerase cause rapid death (e.g., haploid spores bearing deletions of a telomerase component gene and the *YKU70* gene die very rapidly (Nugent *et al.*, 1998)). While this disadvantage can be overcome using more complex yeast methods to disrupt the chromosomal copy of the gene in a cell that already bears a plasmid-borne copy of the same gene, it is probably easier for the beginner to use the diploid method described earlier.

Observing senescence in yeast

Two common methods are used for different purposes in yeast. Serial streaking of individual colonies is a method used to demonstrate that senescence occurs, while serial dilution and regrowth of small cultures are used to show that the culture senesces and to isolate survivor/ALT cells whose rapid growth allows these cells to quickly overtake the slow growing cells with very short telomere tracts.

Serial streaking is streaking a colony of yeast on a plate to isolate single cells and to allow them to grow into colonies. A freshly grown colony is then restreaked on a fresh plate. A yeast colony ~2 mm in diameter contains 3×10^5 to 10^6 cells. If one approximates yeast cell growth as cell number $= 2^N$ where N is the number of cell doublings, then each yeast colony is 18–20 population doublings. Cells that have just lost a gene for a telomerase component lose 3–5 bp per cell doubling, and so give colonies for the first 3 streaks, and then show slower growth on the fourth streak (Lundblad and Szostak, 1989; Singer and Gottschling 1994). Not all cells senesce at the same time, which explains why some cells continue to grow on the fourth streak. This difference may reflect the fact that telomere tract length is not clonal and telomeres do not shorten at the same rate (e.g., Li and Lustig, 1996), and some small amount of lengthening may occur in these cells by nonreciprocal gene conversion mechanisms (Pluta and Zakian, 1989). Some cells in the colony may therefore have different telomere lengths than other cells, and so senesce after different numbers of cell divisions. Because each colony is a single cell that has grown into ~10^6 cells, there has only been ~10^6 cell divisions in which mutation(s) can occur to give rise to a survivor/ALT cell that can elongate its telomeres in the absence of active telomerase. Survivors can be readily identified on the fourth restreak because they grow much faster than the cells that are senescing, and form larger colonies (Teng and Zakian, 1999).

Serial dilutions of liquid cultures involve growing cells in a liquid culture, often 10 ml or so, for 24 hours. Usually, yeast grow to densities of ~10^8 cells/ml in the first growth phase without telomerase, in the same way wild-type cells do. Cells are then diluted to a constant number (from 10^4 cells/ml to 5×10^5 cells/ml, depending on the lab) in fresh medium and grown for another 24 hours for the second cycle (Le *et al.*, 1999; Teng and Zakian, 1999). Each subsequent 24-hr cycle involves diluting cells down to 5×10^5 cells/ml and allowing regrowth; however, cells do not grow to saturation by the 4th or 5th day. Instead, they begin to show slower rates of growth as the cells in the population begin to senesce, and the number of cells/ml that grow up in 24 hours steadily decreases on days 4 to 6. By the 7th day, cells begin to grow rapidly again as survivor/ALT cells take over the culture. It should be noted that this serial dilution method selects for faster growing mutants compared to the serial restreaking method because while serial restreaking restarts from a single cell each time, serial dilution restarts from 5×10^6 cells in a culture. Thus, any mutants that arose in an earlier dilution culture can be transferred to the new culture and undergo further selection for rapid growth. If the goal of the experiment is to isolate fast-growing survivors, the serial dilution method is superior. If the goal is to determine if the cells senesce, it is probably faster to use the serial restreaking method because more individual strains can be easily and rapidly assayed in parallel. The serial restreaking method may also allow one to isolate suppressors that grow at different rates (Teng and Zakian, 1999).

The serial dilution method has been frequently used to monitor the requirements for cell senescence and the two types of survivor/ALT cells that form in yeast cells lacking active telomerase. By starting with cells that lack active telomerase and one DNA damage checkpoint gene, it has been shown that a subset of checkpoint genes are required for the yeast G2/M cell cycle arrest caused by short telomeres, namely, *MEC1*, *DDC2*, *MEC3* and *RAD24* (Enomoto *et al.*, 2002; IJpma and Greider, 2003). Similar experiments have used cells lacking active telomerase and one or more recombination proteins to determine the requirements for forming Type I survivors and Type II survivors (Chen *et al.*, 2001).

Monitoring telomere structure during cell senescence

The slow loss of telomere repeats in yeast cells lacking active telomerase, about 3–5 bp per generation (Lundblad and Szostak, 1989), allows the experimenter to isolate large numbers of cells at different population doublings for analysis. Examining the length of the terminal TG_{1-3} repeat tracts is necessary to ensure that the cells are behaving as predicted. Two methods are routinely used: Southern blotting and Telomere PCR. Once telomere shortening has been verified, the chromatin components of telomeres can by monitored by chromatin immunoprecipitation at different time points during the telomere shortening.

Standard Southern blotting of Xho I cut yeast DNA using TG_{1-3} or TG sequences as probes has long been used to monitor telomere length. Most lab yeast strains have two types of subtelomeric middle repetitive elements, X and Y′ (reviewed by Louis 1995) (Figure 17.3).

Y′ is a highly conserved family of elements that contain an Xho I site 0.83–0.86 kb from the beginning of the TG_{1-3} repeats. As more than half of the telomeres in the common lab yeast strains have Y′ elements adjacent to the TG_{1-3} repeats, the 1.1–1.3 Y′ telomere restriction fragment provides an indicator of the behavior of many telomeres at once. In contrast, the X family of elements is less well conserved, and the Xho I restriction site is present at varying distances from the beginning of the TG_{1-3} repeat tract. Thus, the Xho I digest provides information on individual telomeres, which run as bands in the 2–4 kb range in many strains. When telomerase activity is absent, all of these bands shorten. When Type I survivors containing many tandem Y′ elements take over the culture, all of the X telomere bands disappear. When Type II survivors with heterogeneous lengths of TG_{1-3} arise, the telomere band pattern becomes highly variable (see Lundblad and Blackburn (1993); Teng and Zakian (1999)).

Telomere PCR is a more recent technique that allows one to monitor the length and sequence of the TG_{1-3} tract at the end of an individual telomere (Förstemann

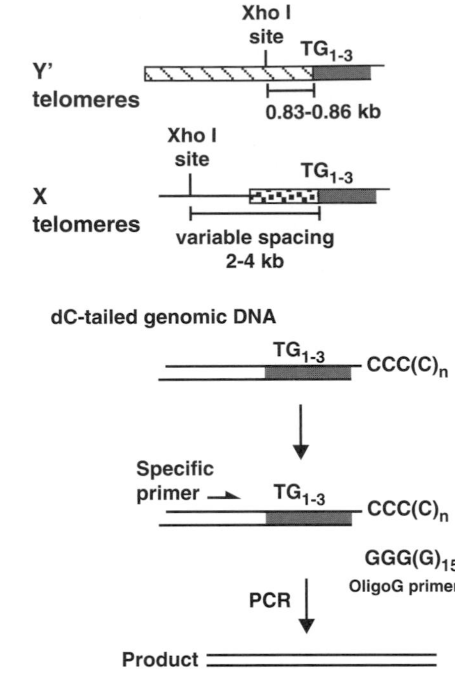

Figure 17.3. Monitoring telomere length in budding yeast. A. The telomeres in *S. cerevisiae* end with two types of middle repetitive elements, Y′ and X. The conserved Y′ repeat has an Xho I site a defined distance from the TG_{1-3} repeat tract, while the less conserved X element contains upstream Xho I sites whose distance from the TG_{1-3} repeat tract is more variable. Thus, a Southern blot of Xho I digested DNA probed with TG_{1-3} or TG probe shows several telomeres at once in the Y′ 1.1–1.3 kb band and individual X telomeres in the 2–4 kb size range (reviewed by Louis, 1995). B. Telomere PCR method to measure TG_{1-3} length of a unique telomere. Genomic DNA is tailed with terminal transferase, which tails telomeres and fragmented DNA. A specific primer is then used with an oligo dG primer to amplify the TG_{1-3} repeats of an individual telomere. Because the sequence of the DNA flanking the TG_{1-3} repeats is known, the size of the TG_{1-3} repeats can be easily determined by agarose gel electrophoresis.

et al., 2000) (Figure 17.3). Briefly, genomic DNA is treated with terminal transferase and dCTP to add an oligo-dC tail to all free DNA ends. This mix is then PCR amplified using an oligo-dG primer and a unique primer internal to the TG_{1-3} repeats. The resulting product has TG_{1-3} repeats flanked by DNA of known sequence, so the range of TG_{1-3} lengths can be easily determined on agarose gels. In the first demonstration of this technique, a synthetic telomere constructed *in vitro* was used to replace a chromosomal telomere and thereby place unique sequences adjacent to the TG_{1-3} repeats (Förstemann *et al.*, 2000). In subsequent uses, primers that hybridize to X and Y′ elements have been used to monitor telomere–telomere fusions (Mieczkowski *et al.*, 2003), and a primer that hybridizes to the unique sequences on the right telomere of chromosome VI has been used to monitor the length of that telomere (Hector *et al.*, submitted).

The use of Chromatin Immunoprecipitation (ChIP) and the serial dilution method for observing cell senescence allows one to monitor the components of telomeric chromatin as the telomere shortens. If the original cell lacking a gene for a telomerase component is grown for 31 divisions, one can obtain $\sim 2 \times 10^9$ cells, or one liter of cells at 2×10^6 cells/ml. This number of cells is sufficient to provide DNA for multiple Southern blots and cells for a standard ChIP experiment and to seed a second one-liter culture for 5 generations of growth. In most ChIP protocols, cells are cross-linked with formaldehyde, the chromatin is isolated and fragmented, chromatin fragments are immunoprecipitated with Abs to the protein of interest, purified, de-crosslinked and amplified by PCR using primers to the region of interest (Strahl-Bolsinger *et al.*, 1997). Because of its unique sequence, the right telomere of chromosome VI has been studied by ChIP to monitor the assembly of silenced chromatin (Luo *et al.*, 2002) and the association of *TEL1* and *MEC1* proteins with shortening telomeres (Hector *et al.*, submitted).

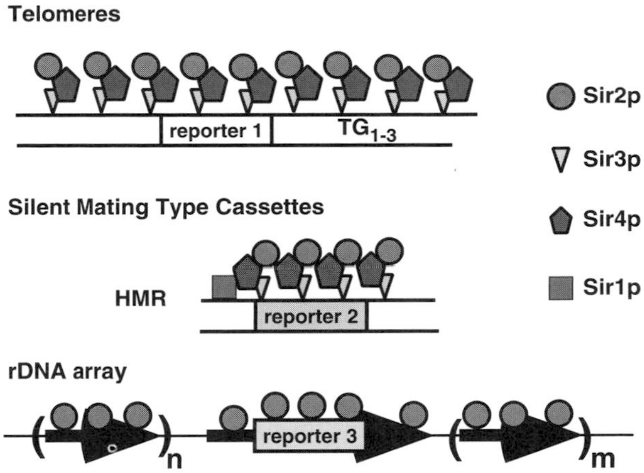

Figure 17.4. Triple silencer yeast strains. To monitor silencing at the 3 types of silenced yeast loci in a single population of yeast cells, 3 different reporter genes are inserted into the silenced loci in the same strain. In order to monitor both increases and decreases in silencing, a mutant version of *HMR* can be used where the *RAP1* protein binding site in the E box (Figure 17.2 top) is deleted. Because the amount of *SIR* silencing protein in the cell appears to be limited, such strains can monitor the redistribution of silencing function. Shortening telomeres would bind less *SIR2, SIR3* and *SIR4* protein, and so would free up some of these proteins that could then bind to the rDNA array or mutant silent mating type cassette.

Telomeres and Budding Yeast Replicative Aging

As described in the discussion of Sir proteins in the Yeast Telomere Protein Components section, yeast telomeres can serve as a reservoir of proteins that can act at other chromosomal loci. One of the clearest demonstrations of this phenomenon is the role of silencing proteins in yeast replicative aging. As described in other chapters of this volume, yeast replicative aging is a measure of the number of times a cell can divide or bud before it dies. Work by Guarente, Sinclair and colleagues has illustrated how one cause of yeast aging, the production of extrachromosomal rDNA circles, is related to telomeres acting as a reservoir of silencing proteins for use in other cellular functions. Understanding this example requires understanding the basics of silencing in yeast.

SILENCED LOCI AND METHODS FOR MONITORING SILENCING

Yeast have 3 types of silenced loci: silent mating type cassettes, telomeres and the rDNA array (Figure 17.2). Silencing at these loci is usually monitored by examining the expression of reporter genes inserted into these loci. Strains with reporters at one of each of these silenced loci have been constructed so the effect of silencing can be monitored at each locus (e.g., Ray *et al.*, 2003) (Figure 17.4).

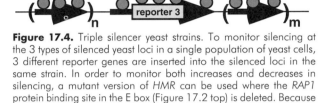

To be useful, the reporter constructs must be able to show both increases and decreases in silencing. Since silencing at some telomeres and in the rDNA locus occurs in only 1–10% of the cells, both increases and decreases in silencing can be readily detected. This property is not shared by the silent mating type cassettes *HMR***a** and *HML*α as only about 1 in 10^6 cells expresses information from these cassettes and an increase in silencing is very difficult to detect. Mutated cassettes show weaker silencing such that reporter genes placed within the cassettes are expressed in 10% of the cells. Strains bearing these three types of reporters allow one to examine silencing at these three types of loci and determine the relative level of silencing using a simple technique called a spot test.

Spot tests are performed by diluting a freshly grown culture of cells, typically a single yeast colony, into sterile water and by making serial dilutions of this suspension, usually 10-fold dilutions. Aliquots of 3 to 5 microliters of each suspension are spotted onto different media to monitor the total number of cells that can grow and reporter gene expression (Gottschling *et al.*, 1990). Markers with both positive and negative selections are used as reporters. In one triple silencer strain (Ray *et al.*, 2003), the *hmr* locus was marked by the *TRP1* gene. The expression of *TRP1* is monitored by growth on medium lacking tryptophan, which requires the *TRP1* gene product. This assay is a *positive* selection for *TRP1* expression, so more expression leads to more growth which equals less silencing. In contrast, the telomere and rDNA array were marked, respectively, with *URA3* and *CAN1*. Expression of these two genes can be monitored on medium containing drugs (5-fluoro orotic acid and canavanine, respectively) that kill cells which express these genes. These assays are *negative* selections for gene expression, so less expression leads to more growth which equals more silencing. Understanding these two different types of yeast reporters is essential for evaluating the silencing data, but once they are understood the assay becomes simple and extremely rapid. Six colonies can be assayed on one set of plates, allowing the screening of many different strains.

An important aspect of silencing is that the factors that accomplish it are limited. An excess of Sir proteins is toxic to the cells, and their levels are controlled (reviewed by Kahana and Gottschling (1999)). Consequently, concentrating more Sir proteins at one silenced locus can result in a decrease in silencing at another. The significance of this observation is that old yeast cells and some long-lived mutant yeast have a "silencing configuration" in which the relative level of silencing function is shifted to increase silencing at the rDNA array and decrease it at telomeres and the silent mating type cassettes.

REPLICATIVE AGING, SILENCING AND THE ERC MODEL

A series of papers from the Guarente lab demonstrated that Sir proteins in old yeast cells (i.e., cells that had budded many times) leave silencers and telomeres and move to the nucleolus, the site of rDNA transcription (Kennedy *et al.*, 1997; Smeal *et al.*, 1996). This lab also isolated a *SIR4* mutation that truncated the C-terminus and allowed the release of other Sir proteins from telomeres and silencers in young cells (Kennedy *et al.*, 1995). These observations established the aforementioned "silencing configuration" for long-lived cells and suggested that events in the nucleolus might play some role in aging. The only known function of Sir proteins in the nucleolus at the time was suppression of rDNA recombination: direct repeats such as the rDNA array are prone to intrachromosomal and interchromosomal recombination that can lengthen and shorten the repeats, and this recombination is repressed in yeast in part by the action of the *SIR2* gene product (Gottlieb and Esposito, 1989).

Work by Sinclair and Guarente later established that extrachromosomal rDNA circles (ERCs) can cause one form of yeast aging (Sinclair and Guarente, 1997) (Figure 17.5).

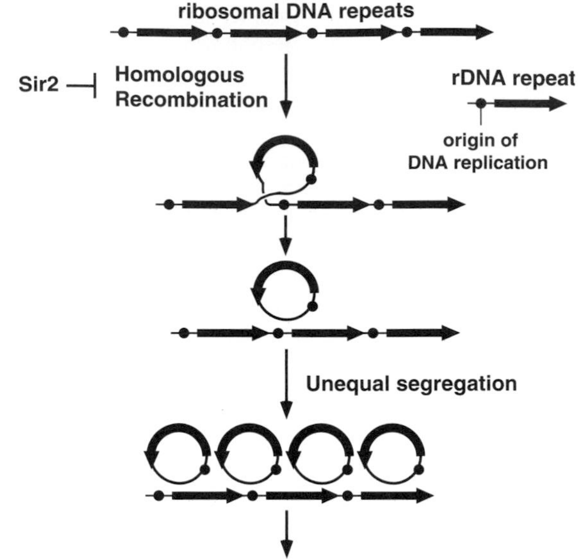

Figure 17.5. The ERC model for one cause of replicative aging in yeast. As described in the text, one cause of yeast aging is the production of **e**xtrachromosomal **r**DNA **c**ircles (ERCs) (Sinclair and Guarente 1997). Each rDNA repeat in the head-to-tail tandem array contains an origin of DNA replication sequence. Intrachromosomal crossing over by homologous recombination can loop out one or more repeats as an extrachromosomal circle. These circles can then replicate as episomal plasmids by virtue of the origin of DNA replication. These types of plasmids do not segregate equally at mitosis, but instead stay with the larger of the two cells at division (the Mother cell in the Mother–Daughter pair). Plasmids thus build up in the Mother cell over subsequent divisions. When plasmids reach large numbers (hundreds per cell), they are thought to compete for essential proteins involved in normal transcription and DNA metabolism, resulting in gene misregulation and cell death. *SIR2* protein (Sir2) can repress homologous recombination within the rDNA repeats (Gottlieb and Esposito, 1989), so the relocation of *SIR* proteins from telomeres to the rDNA can slow this cause of yeast aging. Other causes of yeast cell aging most certainly exist, but the mechanisms by which they cause cells to age are less defined.

ERCs are episomal plasmids that arise within yeast by means of recombination within the rDNA repeats to loop out a circular form of the repeat. Each repeat contains an origin of DNA replication, and so each circular form can replicate as an extrachromosomal plasmid. Budding yeast divides asymmetrically to produce a large mother cell and a smaller daughter cell, and extrachromosomal plasmids containing just an origin of DNA replication tend to stay with the mother cell at mitosis for unknown reasons (Murray and Szostak, 1983). Thus, once a plasmid is formed, its progeny accumulate in the mother cell quickly. Sinclair and Guarente showed that introduction of these plasmids early in life caused rapid replicative aging. Given the role of *SIR2* protein in repressing rDNA recombination, one explanation for the migration of silencing proteins from telomeres to the nucleolus prolonging replicative lifespan is that the *SIR2* protein released from telomeres can suppress the formation of ERCs. Subsequent work did show that increasing *SIR2* protein dosage could increase lifespan, but also indicated that suppression of rDNA recombination was not the only effect of *SIR2* protein on lifespan (Kaeberlein *et al.*, 1999). Thus, release of *SIR* proteins from telomeres may affect yeast lifespan in multiple ways.

The "silencing configuration" of long-lived cells established above provided a mechanism to search for other long-lived mutants. A mutation in the MAP kinase encoded by *SLT2* was isolated in a screen looking for mutants that have low telomere silencing and higher rDNA silencing. The *SLT2* kinase was found to phosphorylate *SIR3* protein (Ai *et al.*, 2002; Ray *et al.*, 2003). Mutation of one of the consensus *SIR3* protein phosphorylation sites to an unphosphorylatable residue

(*SIR3-S275A*) caused changes in silencing and an increase in lifespan, which did not appear to occur through an ERC-related mechanism (Ray *et al.*, 2003). Because the *SLT2* kinase is activated by continuous cell growth, these results suggested a feedback loop in which rapid growth stimulates *SIR3* phosphorylation which shortens lifespan while slower growth (which usually occurs in yeast when nutrients are limiting, i.e., a state resembling caloric restriction) results in extended lifespan. However, the actual mechanism by which lifespan is changed by *SIR3* protein phosphorylation is unknown.

The *SIR3* phosphorylation story illustrates a second important point in yeast research: the genetic variation between different lab strains. While the ERC model and the *SIR3* work were done in the same strain background, subsequent work in another strain that has a longer average lifespan (S288C) found that the *SIR3-275A* mutation did not cause a significant change in lifespan (Kaeberlein *et al.*, 2005). The genetic differences between these strains are unknown, but must include modifiers of lifespan that can be corrected by mutation of *SIR3*. As individual humans are genetically diverse, the yeast case illustrates how some changes may increase the lifespan of some individuals but not others. The utility of the yeast model system might be significantly enhanced if the genomic sequences of several common lab yeast strains were known and the genetic differences, and thus potential modifier genes of aging, were identified.

THE FISSION YEAST *S. POMBE* AS AN EMERGING MODEL SYSTEM IN AGING

As mentioned previously in the Yeast Telomere Protein Components section, fission yeast utilizes the same telomere maintenance machinery as budding yeast and humans, and in some cases contain orthologs that show more sequence similarity to the human sequences than do those of budding yeast (e.g., $pot1^+$ of *S. pombe* and Pot1 of humans are more similar than either protein is to *S. cerevisiae CDC13*). Fission yeast also exhibits gene silencing at telomeres, silent mating type cassettes, the rDNA, and centromeres. Thus, many of the characteristics that make budding yeast a useful model system for both short telomere-induced senescence and release of factors from telomeres are also present in fission yeast. Because these two yeasts are evolutionarily quite distant and show many physiological and genomic differences (e.g., fission yeast has fewer genes than budding yeast, and only 3/4 of the fission yeast genes have clear budding yeast orthologs (Sanger_Institute, 2005)), analysis of fission yeast aging could reveal evolutionarily conserved mechanisms that control lifespan and guide the work in more difficult mammalian systems.

One provocative report has been published that claims that fission yeast shows replicative aging. While fission yeasts divide to produce two equally sized sister progeny, after several cell divisions an asymmetry develops such that the "older" cell becomes more round and visually distinguishable from the "younger" sister (Barker and Walmsley, 1999). Chronological aging, the length of time cells in culture can survive in stationary phase and form colonies when transferred to fresh medium, has also been tested in *S. pombe* and provides similar results to work in budding yeast (Fabrizio and Longo, 2003) (B.-R. Chen and K.W. Runge, in preparation). Following up these results and development of high-throughput replicative and chronological aging assays will greatly enhance the utility of fission yeast as a model system for aging.

The Universality of Yeast Aging Mechanisms and Future Outlook

The short telomere senescence phenotypes of yeast have clear parallels with human cells. Both systems utilize telomerase and ATM family members in telomere metabolism and short telomere signaling. Both systems have telomere-associated proteins that can be released to function at other sites (the *SIR* proteins in yeast and the Rif1 and TRF2 proteins in human cells). Thus, telomere shortening in both systems has the potential to release associated proteins that may play roles in lifespan regulation. While the orthologs affected in these processes may not always show an exact one-to-one correspondence, the conservation of general biological mechanisms from one system can guide the model building in the other.

The yeast strains that can replicate telomeres without telomerase have telomeres similar to those of human ALT cell lines and tumors. It therefore seems likely that some of the mechanisms that give rise to these cell types are conserved. The advantage of the yeast system is that one can test a variety of candidate genes for changes in how cells survive shortening telomeres and if this mode of survival in the absence of telomerase is susceptible to different anti-cancer drugs. One can then identify a class of protein targets and families of chemical compounds to study in human cells.

Another major advantage of yeast is the rapid phenotypic testing of candidate longevity genes. For example, the ease of gene deletion in yeast means that one can find a gene whose expression is up-regulated in a microarray experiment under one growth condition, and then delete this gene to determine if this up-regulation is actually required for this growth condition. When this experiment was done with all budding yeast genes, it was found that only 7% of yeast genes that were up-regulated were actually required for optimal growth under the test condition (Giaever *et al.*, 2002). This sobering result means that many of the genes identified by microarray approaches in organisms such as humans are probably not the most important genes affecting the aging process, and some sort of validation is required. Since such gene deletion studies and aging experiments are difficult and long in mammalian systems, budding and fission yeast will be good first steps for identifying evolutionarily conserved processes that alter lifespan to augment the discoveries made in microarray experiments. Research in the yeast aging field is expanding rapidly, and the biggest challenge to the researcher may be sorting the future flow of information to define the biological processes that are universally conserved.

ACKNOWLEDGMENTS

I apologize to any of my colleagues whose work was not mentioned here due to space limitations. This work was supported by NIH grants GM 50752 and AG19960.

REFERENCES

Ahmed, S., A. Alpi, M.O. Hengartner, and A. Gartner (2001). *C. elegans RAD-5/CLK-2* defines a new DNA damage checkpoint protein. *Curr. Biol. 11(24)*, 1934–1944.

Ai, W., P.G. Bertram, C.K. Tsang, T.F. Chan, and X.F. Zheng (2002). Regulation of subtelomeric silencing during stress response. *Mol. Cell 10(6)*, 1295–1305.

Anderson, C.W., and M.S. Lees (1992). The nuclear serine/threonine protein kinase DNA-PK. *Critical Reviews in Eukaryotic Gene Expression 2(4)*, 283–314.

Askree, S.H., T. Yehuda, S. Smolikov, R. Gurevich, J. Hawk, *et al.*, (2004). A genome-wide screen for *Saccharomyces cerevisiae* deletion mutants that affect telomere length. *Proc. Natl. Acad. Sci. U. S. A. 101(23)*, 8658–8663.

Bailey, S.M., J. Meyne, D.J. Chen, A. Kurimasa, G.C. Li, B.E. Lehnert, and E.H. Goodwin (1999). DNA double-strand break repair proteins are required to cap the ends of mammalian chromosomes. *Proc. Natl. Acad. Sci. U. S. A. 96(26)*, 14899–14904.

Barker, M.G., and R.M. Walmsley (1999). Replicative ageing in the fission yeast *Schizosaccharomyces pombe. Yeast 15(14)*, 1511–1518.

Baumann, P., and T.R. Cech (2000). Protection of telomeres by the Ku protein in fission yeast. *Mol. Biol. Cell 11(10)*, 3265–3275.

Baur, J.A., Y. Zou, J.W. Shay, and W.E. Wright (2001). Telomere position effect in human cells. *Science 292(5524)*, 2075–7.

Benard, C., B. McCright, Y. Zhang, S. Felkai, B. Lakowski, and S. Hekimi (2001). The C. elegans maternal-effect gene clk-2 is essential for embryonic development, encodes a protein homologous to yeast Tel2p and affects telomere length. *Development 128(20)*, 4045–4055.

Blander, G., and L. Guarente (2004). The Sir2 family of protein deacetylases. *Annu. Rev. Biochem. 73*, 417–435.

Bodnar, A.G., M. Ouellette, M. Frolkis, S.E. Holt, C.-P. Chiu, *et al.*, (1998). Extension of life-span by introduction of telomerase into normal human cells. *Science 279(5349)*, 349–352.

Bradshaw, P.S., D.J. Stavropoulos, and M.S. Meyn (2005). Human telomeric protein TRF2 associates with genomic double-strand breaks as an early response to DNA damage. *Nat. Genet. 37(2)*, 193–197.

Buck, S.W., and D. Shore (1995). Action of a RAP1 carboxy-terminal silencing domain reveals an underlying competition between HMR and telomeres in yeast. *Genes Dev. 9(3)*, 370–384.

Chan, S.W., J. Chang, J. Prescott, and E.H. Blackburn (2001). Altering telomere structure allows telomerase to act in yeast lacking ATM kinases. *Curr. Biol. 11(16)*, 1240–1250.

Chen, Q., A. Ijpma, and C.W. Greider (2001). Two survivor pathways that allow growth in the absence of telomerase are generated by distinct telomere recombination events. *Mol. Cell. Biol. 21(5)*, 1819–1827.

Enomoto, S., L. Glowczewski, and J. Berman (2002). MEC3, MEC1, and DDC2 are essential components of a telomere checkpoint pathway required for cell cycle arrest during senescence in *Saccharomyces cerevisiae. Mol. Biol. Cell 13(8)*, 2626–2638.

Evans, S.K., and V. Lundblad (1999). Est1 and Cdc13 as comediators of telomerase access. *Science 286(5437)*, 117–120.

Fabrizio, P., and V.D. Longo (2003). The chronological life span of *Saccharomyces cerevisiae. Aging Cell 2(2)*, 73–81.

Fasching, C.L., K. Bower, and R.R. Reddel (2005). Telomerase-independent telomere length maintenance in the absence of alternative lengthening of telomeres-associated promyelocytic leukemia bodies. *Cancer Res. 65(7)*, 2722–2729.

Fisher, T.S., A.K. Taggart, and V.A. Zakian (2004). Cell cycle-dependent regulation of yeast telomerase by Ku. *Nat. Struct. Mol. Biol. 11(12)*, 1198–1205.

Förstemann, K., M. Hoss, and J. Lingner (2000). Telomerase-dependent repeat divergence at the 3′ ends of yeast telomeres. *Nucleic Acids Res. 28(14)*, 2690–2694.

Giaever, G., A.M. Chu, L. Ni, C. Connelly, L. Riles, *et al.*, (2002). Functional profiling of the *Saccharomyces cerevisiae* genome. *Nature 418(6896)*, 387–391.

Gottlieb, S., and R.E. Esposito (1989). A new role for a yeast transcriptional silencer gene, *SIR2*, in regulation of recombination in ribosomal DNA. *Cell 56(5)*, 771–776.

Gottschling, D.E., O.M. Aparicio, B.L. Billington, and V.A. Zakian (1990). Position effect at yeast telomeres: Reversible repression of polII transcription. *Cell 63*, 751–762.

Gravel, S., M. Larrivee, P. Labrecque, and R.J. Wellinger (1998). Yeast Ku as a regulator of chromosomal DNA end structure. *Science 280(5364)*, 741–744.

Hackett, J.A., D.M. Feldser, and C.W. Greider (2001). Telomere dysfunction increases mutation rate and genomic instability. *Cell 106(3)*, 275–286.

Hardy, C.F.J., D. Balderes, and D. Shore (1992). Dissection of a carboxy-terminal region of the yeast regulatory protein *RAP1* with effects on both transcriptional activation and silencing. *Mol. Cell. Biol. 12*, 1209–1217.

Hardy, C.F.J., L. Sussel, and D. Shore (1992). A *RAP1*-interacting protein involved in transcriptional silencing and telomere length regulation. *Genes Dev. 6*, 801–814.

Harley, C.B., and B. Villeponteau (1995). Telomeres and telomerase in aging and cancer. *Curr. Opin. Genetics Devel. 5(2)*, 249–255.

Hector, R.E., A. Ray, T. Nyun, K.L. Berkner, and K.W. Runge (submitted). Tel1p preferentially associates with short telomeres as part of the process for telomere elongation.

Hemann, M.T., M.A. Strong, L.Y. Hao, and C.W. Greider (2001). The shortest telomere, not average telomere length, is critical for cell viability and chromosome stability. *Cell 107(1)*, 67–77.

Henry, Y.A.L., A. Chambers, J.S.H. Tsang, A.J. Kingsman, and S.M. Kingsman (1990). Characterisation of the DNA binding domain of the yeast *RAP1* protein. *Nucleic Acids Res. 18*, 2617–2623.

Henson, J.D., A.A. Neumann, T.R. Yeager, and R.R. Reddel (2002). Alternative lengthening of telomeres in mammalian cells. *Oncogene 21(4)*, 598–610.

Hiraoka, Y., and Y. Chikashige (2004). Telomere Organization and Nuclear Movements. In Egel, R., *The Molecular Biology of Schizosaccharomyces pombe. Genetics, Genomics and Beyond*, pp. 191–205. Berlin, Heidelberg, New York: Springer-Verlag.

Huang, P., F.E. Pryde, D. Lester, R.L. Maddison, R.H. Borts, I.D. Hickson, and E.J. Louis (2001). SGS1 is required for telomere elongation in the absence of telomerase. *Curr. Biol. 11(2)*, 125–129.

IJpma, A.S., and C.W. Greider (2003). Short telomeres induce a DNA damage response in *Saccharomyces cerevisiae. Mol. Biol. Cell 14(3)*, 987–1001.

Jacob, N.K., A.R. Stout, and C.M. Price (2004). Modulation of telomere length dynamics by the subtelomeric region of tetrahymena telomeres. *Mol. Biol. Cell 15(8)*, 3719–3728.

Jiang, N., C.Y. Benard, H. Kebir, E.A. Shoubridge, and S. Hekimi (2003). Human CLK2 links cell cycle progression, apoptosis, and telomere length regulation. *J. Biol. Chem. 278(24)*, 21678–21684.

Kaeberlein, M., K.T. Kirkland, S. Fields, and B.K. Kennedy (2005). Genes determining yeast replicative life span in a long-lived genetic background. *Mech. Ageing Dev. 126(4)*, 491–504.

Kaeberlein, M., M. McVey, and L. Guarente (1999). The SIR2/3/4 complex and SIR2 alone promote longevity in *Saccharomyces cerevisiae* by two different mechanisms. *Genes Dev 13(19)*, 2570–2580.

Kahana, A., and D.E. Gottschling (1999). DOT4 links silencing and cell growth in *Saccharomyces cerevisiae. Mol. Cell. Biol. 19(10)*, 6608–6620.

Kennedy, B.K., N.J. Austriaco, J. Zhang, and L. Guarente (1995). Mutation in the silencing gene *SIR4* can delay aging in *S. cerevisiae. Cell 80(3)*, 485–496.

Kennedy, B.K., M. Gotta, D.A. Sinclair, K. Mills, D.S. McNabb, *et al.*, (1997). Redistribution of silencing proteins from telomeres to the nucleolus is associated with extension of life span in *S. cerevisiae. Cell 89(3)*, 381–391.

Kim, N.W., M.A. Piatyszek, K.R. Prowse, C.B. Harley, M.D. West, *et al.* (1994). Specific association of human telomerase activity with immortal cells and cancer. *Science 266(5193)*, 2011–2015.

Konig, P., R. Giraldo, L. Chapman and D. Rhodes (1996). The crystal structure of the DNA-binding domain of yeast RAP1 in complex with telomere DNA. *Cell 85*, 125–136.

Kota, R.S., and K.W. Runge (1998). The yeast telomere length regulator *TEL2* encodes a protein that binds to telomeric DNA. *Nucleic Acids Res. 26*, 1528–1535.

Kota, R.S., and K.W. Runge (1999). Tel2p, a regulator of yeast telomere length *in vivo*, binds to single-stranded telomeric DNA *in vitro. Chromosoma 108(5)*, 278–290.

Kyrion, G., K.A. Boakye, and A.J. Lustig (1992). C-terminal truncation of *RAP1* results in the deregulation of telomere size, stability and function in *Saccharomyces cerevisiae. Mol. Cell. Biol. 12*, 5159–5173.

Le, S., J.K. Moore, J.E. Haber, and C.W. Greider (1999). RAD50 and RAD51 define two pathways that collaborate to maintain telomeres in the absence of telomerase. *Genetics 152(1)*, 143–152.

Lendvay, T.S., D.K. Morris, J. Sah, B. Balasubramanian, and V. Lundblad (1996). Senescence mutants of *Saccharomyces cerevisiae* with a defect in telomere replication identify three additional *EST* genes. *Genetics 144*, 1399–1412.

Levis, R., T. Hazelrigg, and G.M. Rubin (1985). Effects of genomic position on the expression of transduced copies of the white gene of *Drosophila. Science 229*, 558–561.

Levy, D.L., and E.H. Blackburn (2004). Counting of Rif1p and Rif2p on *Saccharomyces cerevisiae* telomeres regulates telomere length. *Mol. Cell. Biol. 24(24)*, 10857–10867.

Li, B., and A.J. Lustig (1996). A novel mechanism for telomere size control in *Saccharomyces cerevisiae. Genes Dev. 10*, 1310–1326.

Lingner, J., T.R. Cech, T.R. Hughes, and V. Lundblad (1997). Three ever shorter telomere (EST) genes are dispensable for in vitro yeast telomerase activity. *Proc. Natl. Acad. Sci. U S A 94(21)*, 11190–11195.

Lingner, J., T.R. Hughes, A. Shevchenko, M. Mann, V. Lundblad, and T.R. Cech (1997). Reverse transcriptase motifs in the catalytic subunit of telomerase. *Science 276(5312)*, 561–567.

Lisby, M., J.H. Barlow, R.C. Burgess and R. Rothstein (2004). Choreography of the DNA damage response: Spatiotemporal relationships among checkpoint and repair proteins. *Cell 118(6)*, 699–713.

Liti, G., and E.J. Louis (2003). NEJ1 prevents NHEJ-dependent telomere fusions in yeast without telomerase. *Mol. Cell 11(5)*, 1373–1378.

Livengood, A.J., A.J. Zaug, and T.R. Cech (2002). Essential regions of *Saccharomyces cerevisiae* telomerase RNA: Separate elements for Est1p and Est2p interaction. *Mol. Cell. Biol. 22(7)*, 2366–2374.

Londono-Vallejo, J.A., H. Der-Sarkissian, L. Cazes, S. Bacchetti, and R.R. Reddel (2004). Alternative lengthening of telomeres is characterized by high rates of telomeric exchange. *Cancer Res. 64(7)*, 2324–2327.

Louis, E.J. (1995). The chromosome ends of *Saccharomyces cerevisiae. Yeast 11*, 1553–1573.

Lundblad, V. (2003). Telomere replication: An Est fest. *Curr. Biol. 13(11)*, R439–R441.

Lundblad, V., and E.H. Blackburn (1993). An alternative pathway for yeast telomere maintenance rescues *est1*⁻ senescence. *Cell 73*, 347–360.

Lundblad, V., and J.W. Szostak (1989). A mutant with a defect in telomere elongation leads to senescence in yeast. *Cell 57(4)*, 633–643.

Luo, K., M.A. Vega-Palas, and M. Grunstein (2002). Rap1-Sir4 binding independent of other Sir, yKu, or histone interactions initiates the assembly of telomeric heterochromatin in yeast. *Genes Dev. 16(12)*, 1528–1539.

Lustig, A.J., and T.D. Petes (1986). Identification of yeast mutants with altered telomere structure. *Proc. Natl. Acad. Sci. USA 83*, 1398–1402.

Makarov, V.L., Y. Hirose, and J.P. Langmore (1997). Long G tails at both ends of human chromosomes suggest a C strand degradation mechanism for telomere shortening. *Cell 88(5)*, 657–666.

Martin, S.G., T. Laroche, N. Suka, M. Grunstein, and S.M. Gasser (1999). Relocalization of telomeric Ku and SIR proteins in response to DNA strand breaks in yeast. *Cell 97(5)*, 621–633.

Maser, R.S., and R.A. DePinho (2004). Telomeres and the DNA damage response: Why the fox is guarding the henhouse. *DNA Repair (Amst) 3(8–9)*, 979–88.

McElligott, R., and R.J. Wellinger (1997). The terminal DNA structure of mammalian chromosomes. *EMBO J. 16(12)*, 3705–3714.

Mieczkowski, P.A., J.O. Mieczkowska, M. Dominska, and T.D. Petes (2003). Genetic regulation of telomere-telomere fusions in the yeast *Saccharomyces cerevisae. Proc. Natl. Acad. Sci. USA 100(19)*, 10854–10859.

Mills, K.D., D.A. Sinclair, and L. Guarente (1999). MEC1-dependent redistribution of the Sir3 silencing protein from telomeres to DNA double-strand breaks. *Cell 97(5)*, 609–620.

Moretti, P., K. Freeman, L. Coodly, and D. Shore (1994). Evidence that a complex of SIR proteins interacts with the silencer and telomere-binding protein RAP1. *Genes Dev. 8(19)*, 2257–2269.

Morrow, D.M., D.A. Tagle, Y. Shiloh, F.S. Collins, and P. Hieter (1995). *TEL1*, an *S. cerevisiae* homolog of the human gene mutated in *ataxia telangiectasia*, is functionally related to the yeast checkpoint gene *MEC1. Cell 82*, 831–840.

Murray, A.W., and J.W. Szostak (1983). Pedigree analysis of plasmid segregation in yeast. *Cell 34(3)*, 961–970.

Naito, T., A. Matsuura, and F. Ishikawa (1998). Circular chromosome formation in a fission yeast mutant defective in two ATM homologues. *Nat. Genet. 20(2)*, 203–206.

Nakamura, T.M., G.B. Morin, K.B. Chapman, S.L. Weinrich, W.H. Andrews, *et al.* (1997). Telomerase catalytic subunit homologs from fission yeast and human. *Science 277(5328)*, 955–959.

Newlon, C.S. (1988). Yeast chromosome replication and segregation. *Microbiol. Rev. 52*, 568–601.

Nimmo, E.R., G. Cranston, and R.C. Allshire (1994). Telomere-associated chromosome breakage in fission yeast results in variegated expression of adjacent genes. *EMBO J 13(16)*, 3801–3811.

Nugent, C.I., G. Bosco, L.O. Ross, S.K. Evans, A.P. Salinger, *et al.*, (1998). Telomere maintenance is dependent on activities required for end repair of double-strand breaks. *Curr. Biol. 8(11)*, 657–660.

Ouellette, M.M., M. Liao, B.S. Herbert, M. Johnson, S.E. Holt, *et al.*, (2000). Subsenescent telomere lengths in fibroblasts immortalized by limiting amounts of telomerase. *J. Biol. Chem. 275(14)*, 10072–10076.

Peterson, S.E., A.E. Stellwagen, S.J. Diede, M.S. Singer, Z.W. Haimberger, *et al.* (2001). The function of a stem-loop in telomerase RNA is linked to the DNA repair protein Ku. *Nat. Genet. 27(1)*, 64–67.

Pluta, A.F., and V.A. Zakian (1989). Recombination occurs during telomere formation in yeast. *Nature 337(6206)*, 429–433.

Porter, S.E., P.W. Greenwell, K.B. Ritchie, and T.D. Petes (1996). The DNA-binding protein Hdf1p (a putative Ku homologue) is required for maintaining normal telomere length in *Saccharomyces cerevisiae. Nucleic Acids Res. 24*, 582–585.

Ray, A., R.E. Hector, N. Roy, J.H. Song, K.L. Berkner, and K.W. Runge (2003). Sir3p phosphorylation by the Slt2p pathway effects redistribution of silencing function and shortened lifespan. *Nat. Genet. 33(4)*, 522–526.

Rine, J., J.N. Strathern, J.B. Hicks, and I. Herskowitz (1979). A suppressor of mating-type locus mutations in *Saccharomyces cerevisiae*: Evidence for and identification of cryptic mating-type loci. *Genetics 93(4)*, 877–901.

Ritchie, K., J. Mallory, and T.D. Petes (1999). Interactions of *TLC1, TEL1* and *MEC1* in regulating telomere length in the yeast *Saccharomyces cerevisiae. Mol. Cell. Biol. 19(9)*, 6065–6075.

Ritchie, K.B., and T.D. Petes (2000). The Mre11p/Rad50p/Xrs2p complex and the Tel1p function in a single pathway for telomere maintenance in yeast. *Genetics 155(1)*, 475–479.

Runge, K.W., and V.A. Zakian (1996). *TEL2*, an essential gene required for telomere length regulation and telomere position effect in *Saccharomyces cerevisiae. Mol. Cell. Biol. 16*, 3094–3105.

Sanger_Institute 2005 The S. pombe genome project http://www.sanger.ac.uk/Projects/S_pombe/

Schramke, V., P. Luciano, V. Brevet, S. Guillot, Y. Corda, *et al.*, (2004). RPA regulates telomerase action by providing Est1p access to chromosome ends. *Nat. Genet. 36(1)*, 46–54.

Silverman, J., H. Takai, S.B. Buonomo, F. Eisenhaber, and T. de Lange (2004). Human Rif1, ortholog of a yeast telomeric protein, is regulated by ATM and 53BP1 and functions in the S-phase checkpoint. *Genes Dev. 18(17)*, 2108–2119.

Sinclair, D.A., and L. Guarente (1997). Extrachromosomal rDNA circles—A cause of aging in yeast. *Cell 91(7)*, 1033–1042.

Singer, M.S., and D.E. Gottschling (1994). TLC1: Template RNA component of *Saccharomyces cerevisiae* telomerase. *Science 266(5184)*, 404–409.

Smeal, T., J. Claus, B. Kennedy, F. Cole, and L. Guarente (1996). Loss of transcriptional silencing causes sterility in old mother cells of *S. cerevisiae. Cell 84(4)*, 633–642.

Smith, C.D., D.L. Smith, J.L. DeRisi, and E.H. Blackburn (2003). Telomeric protein distributions and remodeling through the cell cycle in *Saccharomyces cerevisiae. Mol. Biol. Cell 14(2)*, 556–570.

Smith, J., H. Zou, and R. Rothstein (2000). Characterization of genetic interactions with RFA1: The role of RPA in DNA replication and telomere maintenance. *Biochimie 82(1)*, 71–78.

Smogorzewska, A., and T. De Lange (2004). Regulation of telomerase by telomeric proteins. *Annu. Rev. Biochem. 73*, 177–208.

Strahl-Bolsinger, S., A. Hecht, K. Luo, and M. Grunstein (1997). SIR2 and SIR4 interactions differ in core and extended telomeric heterochromatin in yeast. *Genes Dev. 11*, 83–93.

Taggart, A.K., S.C. Teng, and V.A. Zakian (2002). Est1p as a cell cycle-regulated activator of telomere-bound telomerase. *Science 297(5583)*, 1023–1026.

Teixeira, M.T., M. Arneric, P. Sperisen, and J. Lingner (2004). Telomere length homeostasis is achieved via a switch between telomerase- extendible and -nonextendible states. *Cell 117(3)*, 323–335.

Teng, S.C., J. Chang, B. McCowan, and V.A. Zakian (2000). Telomerase-independent lengthening of yeast telomeres occurs by an abrupt Rad50p-dependent, Rif-inhibited recombinational process. *Mol. Cell 6(4)*, 947–952.

Teng, S.C., and V.A. Zakian (1999). Telomere-telomere recombination is an efficient bypass pathway for telomere maintenance in *Saccharomyces cerevisiae*. *Mol. Cell. Biol. 19(12)*, 8083–8093.

Tsukamoto, Y., A.K. Taggart, and V.A. Zakian (2001). The role of the Mre11-Rad50-Xrs2 complex in telomerase-mediated lengthening of *Saccharomyces cerevisiae* telomeres. *Curr. Biol. 11(17)*, 1328–1335.

Wellinger, R.J., K. Ethier, P. Labrecque, and V.A. Zakian (1996). Evidence for a new step in telomere maintenance. *Cell 85*, 423–433.

Wellinger, R.J., A.J. Wolf, and V.A. Zakian (1993). Origin activation and formation of single-strand TG1-3 tails occur sequentially in late S phase on a yeast linear plasmid. *Mol. Cell. Biol. 13(7)*, 4057–4065.

Wellinger, R.W., A.J. Wolf, and V.A. Zakian (1993). *Saccharomyces* telomeres acquire single-strand TG_{1-3} tails late in S phase. *Cell 72*, 51–60.

Wilkie, A.O.M., J. Lamb, P.C. Harris, R.D. Finney, and D.R. Higgs (1990). A truncated human chromosome 16 associated with a thalassaemia is stabilized by addition of telomeric repeat $(TTAGGG)_n$. *Nature 346*, 868–871.

Wotton, D., and D. Shore (1997). A novel Rap1p-interacting factor, Rif2p, cooperates with Rif1p to regulate telomere length in *Saccharomyces cerevisiae*. *Genes Dev. 11*, 748–760.

Wright, J., D. Gottschling, and V.A. Zakian (1992). *Saccharomyces* telomeres assume a non-nucleosomal structure. *Genes Dev. 6*, 197–210.

Zhou, J., K. Hidaka, and B. Futcher (2000). The Est1 subunit of yeast telomerase binds the Tlc1 telomerase RNA. *Mol. Cell. Biol. 20(6)*, 1947–1955.

18

Longevity and Aging in Budding Yeast

Matt Kaeberlein

This chapter presents an overview of the current understanding of how yeast ages and the genes and pathways that play a role in determining yeast chronological and replicative life span. Several genes, as well as calorie restriction, have been found to regulate aging similarly in yeast and multicellular eukaryotes, and these potentially conserved determinants of longevity are emphasized. Descriptions of the chronological and replicative life span assay are provided in enough detail to allow a researcher with common knowledge of yeast methods to carry out his or her own aging studies.

Introduction

The budding yeast *Saccharomyces cerevisiae* has served as an exemplary model of cellular aging for more than 50 years (Kaeberlein *et al.*, 2001). Yeast provides several advantages over other model systems, including short life span, well-characterized genetic and molecular methods, low relative cost, cell-type homogeneity, and a vast organismal information base. Two distinct types of aging have been studied in yeast: replicative and chronological (Figure 18.1).

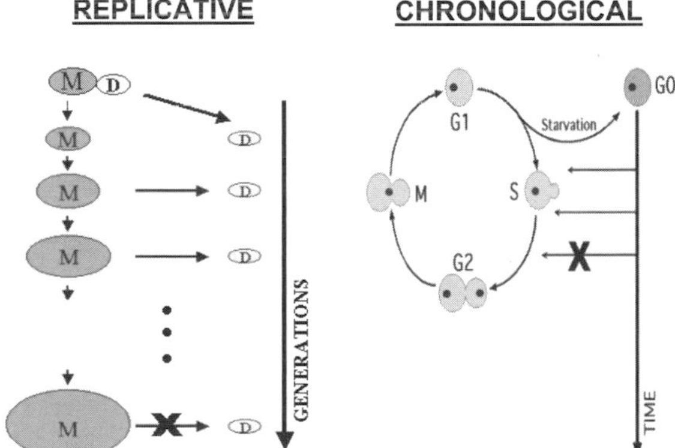

Figure 18.1. Two types of yeast aging. Replicative life span is defined as the number of daughter cells produced by a given mother cell prior to senescence. Chronological life span is defined as the length of time that a yeast cell can survive during quiescence. Chronological life span is typically measured by growing cells into stationary phase, which induces a starvation response and exit from the cell cycle.

The replicative life span of a yeast cell refers to the number of daughter cells produced by a mother cell prior to senescence (Mortimer and Johnston, 1959); while chronological life span measures the time a yeast cell can survive under nonproliferative conditions (Fabrizio and Longo, 2003).

The ability to monitor both the replicative and chronological aging of a yeast cell is fortuitous, as it allows for independent analysis of the aging process in both dividing and nondividing cell types. Yeast replicative aging may serve as a suitable model for the aging of mitotically active cell types in multicellular eukaryotes, such as human stem cell populations. Chronological aging, on the other hand, models the aging process of postmitotic cell types like muscle and brain. The surprising degree of conservation, at least at the level of individual genes, between aging in yeast and aging in multicellular eukaryotes has made *S. cerevisiae* one of the premier model organisms in aging-related research.

Replicative Aging in Yeast

The replicative life span of a yeast cell is determined by the number of daughter cells produced. Like other eukaryotic species, yeast replicative mortality follows Gompertz–Makeham kinetics, consistent with the hypothesis that similar processes underlie aging in yeast and aging in higher eukaryotes (Kaeberlein *et al.*, 2001). Several studies have demonstrated that replicative aging is under both genetic and environmental regulation, and the SAGE KE Aging Genes and Interventions Database (Kaeberlein *et al.*, 2002b) (see Chapter 8 on SAGE KE) has catalogued more than fifty genes reported to alter replicative life span in various strain backgrounds. This section describes the current understanding of the most important genetic pathways and molecular mechanisms underlying yeast replicative aging.

EXTRACHROMOSOMAL rDNA CIRCLES: A YEAST-SPECIFIC AGING MECHANISM

Several important cellular processes have been implicated in the regulation of yeast replicative aging, including glucose sensing, DNA damage response, stress response, mitochondrial function, and transcriptional silencing (Bitterman *et al.*, 2003; Jazwinski, 2002; Sinclair *et al.*, 1998). The roles that some of these processes play in life-span determination are beginning to be elucidated at a molecular level; however, only one molecular cause of replicative senescence has been demonstrated: the mother cell specific accumulation of extrachromosomal rDNA circles (ERCs).

ERCs are self-replicating circular DNA molecules formed through homologous recombination events at the rDNA (Sinclair and Guarente, 1997). The yeast rDNA is a tandem array of 100–200 copies of a 9.1-kb repeat unit, with each repeat unit containing all of the information needed to code for rRNA precursors. Due to the tandem nature of the rDNA array, homologous pairing and recombination can occur between adjacent repeats, resulting in the formation of ERCs containing one or more repeat units. ERCs can be observed by either 1-D or 2-D gel electrophoresis and Southern blotting with a probe for rDNA sequence, and mutations that block homologous recombination, such as deletion of *RAD52*, prevent ERC formation (Park *et al.*, 1999).

Once formed, a single ERC has the potential to undergo exponential amplification as a function of mother cell age. The age-associated accumulation of ERCs in yeast is likely due to two features: self-replication and asymmetric segregation. Each rDNA repeat unit contains an origin or replication (ARS element), but lacks a centromere-like sequence (CEN element), resulting in preferential segregation of ERCs to the mother cell during cell division (Sinclair and Guarente, 1997). Quantitation of ERCs in aged cells shows a dramatic increase in ERC levels with age, and artificial induction of a single ERC in a virgin daughter cell, through the use of a CRE recombinase system, shortens life span by about 50% (Sinclair and Guarente, 1997). Thus, ERCs accumulate in normally aging mother cells and can lead to senescence.

An important prediction of the ERC model of yeast aging is that a mutation resulting in decreased ERC formation (or accumulation) should increase life span, assuming said mutation does not also have a detrimental effect on fitness. This prediction was validated with the finding that deletion of *FOB1* both dramatically reduces ERC levels and increases mean and maximum life span by approximately 35% (Defossez *et al.*, 1999). The Fob1 protein promotes ERC formation by binding to the rDNA and causing a recombinogenic unidirectional replication fork block (Kobayashi and Horiuchi, 1996). In the absence of Fob1, rDNA recombination is reduced approximately 10-fold (Defossez *et al.*, 1999).

A second protein that regulates yeast replicative life span by altering ERC levels is Sir2 (Kaeberlein *et al.*, 1999). Sir2 is an NAD+-dependent histone deacetylase (Imai *et al.*, 2000; Landry *et al.*, 2000; Smith *et al.*, 2000; Tanner *et al.*, 2000), conserved from bacteria to man (Blander and Guarente, 2004). In yeast, Sir2, along with Sir3 and Sir4, promotes transcriptional silencing near telomeres (Aparicio *et al.*, 1991) and silent mating (*HM*) loci (Ivy *et al.*, 1986; Rine and Herskowitz, 1987). Sir2, acting independently of Sir3 and Sir4, localizes to the nucleolus where it transcriptionally represses polII transcribed genes (Bryk *et al.*, 1997; Smith and Boeke, 1997) and inhibits rDNA recombination (Gottlieb and Esposito, 1989). Deletion of *SIR2* causes an approximately 10-fold increase in rDNA recombination and shortens life span by about 50% (Kaeberlein *et al.*, 1999). Overexpression of *SIR2* in wild-type cells has the opposite effect, resulting in a 30–40% increase in life span, comparable to that observed upon deletion of *FOB1* (Kaeberlein *et al.*, 1999); however, overexpression of *SIR2* fails to further increase the life span of long-lived *fob1Δ* cells, consistent with the model that Sir2 and Fob1 both impact aging by altering ERC levels.

	Yeast	Worms	Flies	Mice
CR	✓	✓	✓	✓
Hsf1	✓	✓	?	?
Rpd3	✓	?	✓	?
Sch9	✓	✓	?	?
Sir2	✓	✓	✓	?
Sod1/Sod2	✓	✓	✓	?
Tor1/Tor2	✓	✓	✓	?

Figure 18.2. Evolutionarily conserved determinants of longevity in yeast. CR increases life span from yeast to mammals. In addition, orthologs to the yeast-aging genes Hsf1, Rpd3, Sch9, Sir2, Sod1/Sod2, and Tor1/Tor2 similarly modify aging in at least one multicellular eukaryote.

Sir2 represents the first example of a conserved determinant of longevity that was initially discovered in yeast (Figure 18.2).

Following on the finding that overexpression of Sir2 increases yeast replicative life span, two groups have independently reported that overexpression of the Sir2-orthologs, Sir-2.1 and dSir2, increases life span in the nematode, *Caenorhabditis elegans*, and the fly, *Drosophila melanogaster*, respectively (Rogina and Helfand, 2004; Tissenbaum and Guarente, 2001). While it remains unclear what role, if any, Sir2-like proteins play in mammalian aging, several proteins involved in important cellular processes, including Foxo3a (Motta *et al.*, 2004), p53 (Luo *et al.*, 2001; Vaziri *et al.*, 2001), and PGC1-α (Nemoto *et al.*, 2005), have been suggested as targets for deacetylation by the mammalian Sir2 ortholog, SirT1.

SIR2 AND CALORIE RESTRICTION

Calorie restriction (CR) is the only intervention demonstrated to increase life span in yeast, worms, flies, and mammals (Kaeberlein and Kennedy, 2005). CR can be accomplished in yeast by reducing the glucose concentration of the growth media, or by a number of genetic models of CR (Table 18.1) thought to mimic the physiological state of the cell under growth on low

TABLE 18.1.
Proposed genetic models of CR in yeast. Growth on low glucose media is the commonly accepted mechanism for CR in yeast. Several mutations (CR alleles) have been described that increase life span and are thought to mimic the physiological response of yeast cells to CR.

Gene(s)	Function	CR Allele(s)
CDC25	RAS GTP/GDP exchange factor	cdc25–10, a temperature-sensitive hypomorphic allele
CYR1 (CDC35)	Adenylate cyclase	cdc35–10, a temperature-sensitive hypomorphic allele
GPA2	GTPase upstream of PKA	gpa2Δ
GPR1	G protein-coupled receptor coupled to GPA2	gpr1Δ
HXK2	Hexokinase	hxk2Δ
SCH9	Akt-like kinase	sch9Δ
TOR1	PI3-like kinase	tor1Δ
TPK1/TPK2/TPK3	Protein kinase A catalytic subunits	tpk1Δ tpk2–63 tpk3Δ

glucose (Kaeberlein *et al.*, 2005a; Lin *et al.*, 2000). CR is reported to increase replicative life span in multiple yeast strain backgrounds from 30 to 50% (e.g., see Anderson *et al.*, 2003a; Anderson *et al.*, 2003b; Kaeberlein *et al.*, 2002a; Kaeberlein *et al.*, 2004a; Kaeberlein *et al.*, 2004b; Lin *et al.*, 2000; Lin *et al.*, 2002), comparable in magnitude to the effect of CR in other organisms (Houthoofd *et al.*, 2003; Lakowski and Hekimi, 1998; Weindruch and Walford, 1988).

The mechanism(s) by which CR increases life span in yeast and other organisms remains a mystery. It was initially proposed that CR slows aging in yeast by activating Sir2 (Lin *et al.*, 2000). This idea was supported by the fact that deletion of *SIR2* prevents life span extension by growth on low glucose (Kaeberlein *et al.*, 2004a) or by genetic models of CR (Lin *et al.*, 2000). Several models have described possible molecular mechanisms by which CR might enhance Sir2 activity, including elevated NAD^+ (a substrate of Sir2), resulting from a metabolic shift toward respiratory growth (Lin *et al.*, 2002); decreased nicotinamide (an inhibitor of Sir2), due to transcriptional up-regulation of the gene coding for nicotinamidase, *PNC1* (Anderson *et al.*, 2003a); and decreased NADH (an inhibitor of Sir2) (Lin *et al.*, 2004).

The link between Sir2 and CR has been called into question, however, with the observation that CR slows aging even in the absence of Sir2, as long as ERC levels are kept low (Kaeberlein *et al.*, 2004b). Deletion of *FOB1* suppresses the short life span of cells lacking Sir2 and dramatically reduces ERC levels, even below that observed in wild-type cells (Kaeberlein *et al.*, 1999). In cells deleted for both *SIR2* and *FOB1*, CR increases life span to a greater extent than in wild-type cells (Kaeberlein *et al.*, 2004b), demonstrating the existence of a Sir2-independent pathway by which CR slows aging. Further support for Sir2 and CR acting in parallel pathways is provided by the observation that growth of cells overexpressing *SIR2* on reduced glucose media results in an additive increase in life span (Kaeberlein *et al.*, 2004b). It remains to be determined whether CR acts in both a Sir2-dependent and Sir2-independent fashion, or if the longevity effects of CR are completely independent of Sir2.

CONSERVED NUTRIENT SENSING PATHWAYS AS A MEDIATOR OF CR IN YEAST

The dissociation of Sir2 from CR in yeast has profound implications for the likelihood that downstream molecular events associated with CR are conserved across evolutionarily divergent organisms. It seems certain that ERCs are a mechanism of aging private to yeast, as there is no evidence that ERCs accumulate with age or cause senescence in the cells of multicellular eukaryotes. CR, on the other hand, slows aging in nearly every organism studied. If CR is not regulating yeast longevity by altering ERC levels through up-regulation of Sir2, this raises the possibility that the downstream effectors of CR might also be conserved (Kaeberlein and Kennedy, 2005).

Many of the pathways responsible for mediating the response of yeast cells to limited nutrients are well characterized. Among these pathways, the glucose-activated kinases protein kinase A (PKA) and Sch9 play an important role in replicative aging. Deletion of Sch9 (Fabrizio *et al.*, 2004b; Kaeberlein *et al.*, 2005a) or one of several mutations resulting in decreased PKA activity, including *gpa2Δ*, *gpr1Δ*, *cdc25–10*, and *cyr1-1* (Lin *et al.*, 2000), result in a 30–40% increase in replicative life span. CR by growth on low glucose is known to decrease both PKA and Sch9 activity (Kaeberlein *et al.*, 2005a), suggesting that mutations in these pathways are genetic mimetics of CR.

From an ongoing genome-wide study of yeast replicative aging (Kaeberlein and Kennedy, 2005), we have uncovered evidence that a third nutrient sensing pathway, defined by the nitrogen responsive kinases Tor1 and Tor2, also plays a profound role in determining replicative life span (Kaeberlein *et al.*, 2005b). Tor1 and Tor2 regulate many of the same downstream targets as Sch9 and PKA, including genes involved in ribosome biogenesis, genes involved in autophagy, regulators of cell size and cell cycle progression, and the stress responsive transcription factors Msn2 and Msn4 (Beck and Hall, 1999). Interestingly, mutations that decrease the activity of Sch9 (Fabrizio *et al.*, 2001) or PKA (Fabrizio *et al.*, 2001) are also reported to increase chronological life span (see Nutrient Sensing and Chronological Aging). The fact that decreased activity of proteins orthologous to Sch9 or Tor1/Tor2 increases life span in worms (Vellai *et al.*, 2003) and flies (Kapahi *et al.*, 2004) indicates the evolutionary conservation of these nutrient responsive kinases as regulators of eukaryotic aging. The potential relevance of these observations is discussed further in Relationship between Replicative and Chronological Aging.

At this point it remains unclear which of the downstream targets shared by these nutrient sensing pathways are ultimately responsible for enhanced longevity in response to CR. The Msn2/Msn4-mediated stress response can be ruled out as necessary for increased replicative life span, since deletion of both *MSN2* and *MSN4* fails to prevent replicative life-span extension in response to either CR (Lin *et al.*, 2000) or deletion of Sch9 (Fabrizio *et al.*, 2004b). Decreased ribosome production or protein translation may be important for the effect of CR on replicative aging, as evidenced by the fact that deletion of individual genes coding for redundant ribosomal subunits is sufficient to confer replicative life-span extension comparable to that of CR (Kaeberlein *et al.*, 2005b). Although the molecular mechanism accounting for this effect remains poorly understood, an intriguing parallel can be drawn between yeast and flies, with the observation that mutation of S6 kinase, which functions downstream of TOR to promote ribosomal function and translation, increases life span in *D. melanogaster* (Kapahi *et al.*, 2004).

ADDITIONAL PATHWAYS THAT IMPACT REPLICATIVE AGING

Several additional genes have been suggested to play a role in replicative life-span determination that cannot be easily ascribed to the relatively well-characterized pathways discussed thus far. Many of these genes affect aging in a strain-specific manner, and their relevance is uncertain. This class includes *RTG1*, *RTG3*, *LAG1*, *LAG2*, and *RPD3* (Kaeberlein and Kennedy, 2005). Others, such as *SGS1*, *DNA2*, and *ATP2*, shorten life span when mutated, which could be due to accelerated aging, but this effect is most likely the result of a nonspecific reduction in fitness. Several reviews present a more comprehensive analysis of the aging phenotypes associated with these strain-specific modifiers of life span (Bitterman *et al.*, 2003; Jazwinski, 2002; Sinclair *et al.*, 1998).

Chronological Aging in Yeast

The chronological life span of a yeast cell is defined as the length of time that a cell can maintain viability in a nondividing state. Chronological aging in yeast has been studied using a variety of different methods involving culturing cells into stationary phase, a quiescent state in which cells are metabolically active but nonreplicative. Compared to replicative aging, relatively few genes have been studied with respect to their effect on chronological life span; yet, some of the important pathways regulating this process have already emerged. Unlike laboratory growth conditions, the natural environment of a yeast cell is likely to consist of relatively rare periods of exponential growth followed by prolonged periods of starvation-induced quiescence. Chronological aging may, therefore, play an important part in the ecology of wild yeast populations, as well as provide insight into the aging process of nondividing cells in higher eukaryotes.

WHAT DO CHRONOLOGICALLY AGED CELLS DIE FROM?

The chronological life span of a yeast cell begins under conditions highly favorable for growth: low cell density, optimal temperature, high nutrient availability, and the presence of a preferred carbon source (glucose). These conditions allow cells to enter an exponential growth phase, during which cells generate ATP primarily through glycolysis and fermentation of pyruvate to ethanol. As glucose becomes depleted, yeast cells progress through the diauxic shift, a growth phase characterized by large transcriptional changes resulting in enhanced expression of many enzymes involved in the TCA cycle, mitochondrial function, and respiration. Associated with this transition to a less favorable environment is an up-regulation of many stress responsive and antioxidant genes. Eventually, as nutrients are depleted and cell density increases, a postdiauxic stationary phase is achieved in which cells exit from the cell cycle and enter into a G0-like quiescent state.

Entry of yeast cells into stationary phase is accompanied by a starvation response in which storage carbohydrates, such as glycogen and trehalose, are synthesized and maintained at high levels in the cytoplasm (Gray *et al.*, 2004). Storage carbohydrates serve as the main source of energy production during stationary phase (Fabrizio and Longo, 2003) and adequate production of storage carbohydrates is essential for long-term survival. Interestingly, some chronologically long-lived mutants show dramatically increased glycogen stores, even under logarithmic growth conditions, suggesting that depletion of reserve carbohydrates might be one factor resulting in cell death. This idea is supported by one study in which intracellular glycogen and trehalose levels were reported to decrease dramatically between the second and third week of chronological aging (Samokhvalov *et al.*, 2004). In contrast to this, however, Fabrizio and Longo (Fabrizio and Longo, 2003) have reported that glycogen stores are not significantly depleted even after 70% of cells have senesced during a typical chronological aging experiment. A more comprehensive analysis of reserve carbohydrate levels during chronological aging, particularly in long-lived mutants, will be necessary to definitively address this important question.

A second mechanism by which yeast cells might senesce during chronological aging is apoptosis. Mammalian cells undergo apoptosis in response to specific environmental stimuli, and it has been demonstrated that yeast cells can undergo a similar process (Madeo *et al.*, 2004). Indeed, chronologically aged cells show markers consistent with apoptotic death (Herker *et al.*, 2004). Blocking apoptosis through deletion of the gene coding for yeast caspase, *YCA1*, failed to substantially increase chronological life span, however, indicating that the apoptosis-like event may be a secondary response to the primary lethal event.

Yeast cells maintained in stationary phase generally do not reenter the cell cycle unless diluted into fresh media. On rare occasions, a yeast cell will escape from the stationary phase–induced cell cycle arrest and begin vegetative growth in the aged culture. It has recently been speculated that this "gasping" effect is an altruistic phenomenon, whereby the majority of cells in an aging population die through a process resembling apoptosis in order to facilitate the outgrowth of a few remaining viable cells (Fabrizio *et al.*, 2004a). The probability that a cell will undergo a "gasping" event was observed to be inversely correlated with resistance to superoxide and chronological life span, but positively correlated with mutation frequency. These findings suggest a plausible mechanism by which an apoptotic pathway might evolve in a single-celled eukaryote.

A third mechanism by which quiescent yeast cells might senesce is due to damage generated by oxidative stress. The free radical theory of aging posits that one cause of aging is the accumulation of macromolecular damage due to oxidative free radicals (Harman, 1956). There are several lines of evidence suggesting that oxidative damage plays a causal role in the chronological aging process of yeast cells. For example, loss of respiratory capacity increases with time spent in stationary phase, suggesting that mitochondrial damage accumulates during chronological aging (Fabrizio and Longo, 2003). Also consistent with the idea that oxidative damage is correlated with chronological longevity, mutation of either mitochondrial superoxide dismutase (Sod2) or cytosolic superoxide dismutase (Sod1) results in a substantial decrease in stationary phase survival (Longo *et al.*, 1996). Finally, overexpression of both Sod2 and Sod1 increases chronological life span by about 30%, suggesting that oxidative stress is one factor limiting the survival of quiescent yeast cells (Fabrizio *et al.*, 2003).

NUTRIENT SENSING AND CHRONOLOGICAL AGING

Based on the hypothesis that oxidative damage is one cause of chronological aging, Fabrizio and Longo carried out a screen for mutants with increased chronological life span by selecting for mutations that confer a survival advantage in the presence of paraquat, a superoxide generating agent (Fabrizio *et al.*, 2001). From this screen two genes were identified that play a central role in regulating chronological aging, *SCH9* and *CYR1*. Sch9 is a nutrient responsive kinase with homology to mammalian Akt proteins, and *CYR1* codes for adenylate cyclase, an activator of PKA. Deletion of Sch9 increases yeast chronological life span by up to 300%, while a partial loss of function allele in *CYR1*, *cyr1::mTn*, increases life span by approximately 70% (Fabrizio *et al.*, 2001). Both of these genes have also been shown to similarly regulate yeast replicative aging (discussed in Conserved nutrient sensing pathways as a mediator of CR in yeast), and RNAi knock-down of the Sch9 ortholog, Sgk-1, increases life span in worms (Hertweck *et al.*, 2004).

CHRONOLOGICAL AGING AND RESPONSE TO STRESS

It has been proposed that aging in nondividing yeast cells is largely under the control of the transcription factors Msn2 and Msn4 (Fabrizio *et al.*, 2001). Msn2 and Msn4 bind to stress response elements (STRE) contained in the promoters of many genes coding for proteins involved in adaptation to starvation and stress, such as heat shock proteins, catalase, superoxide dismutase, and glycogen and trehalose biosynthetic enzymes (Smith et al., 1998). Msn2 and Msn4 are repressed by the nutrient responsive kinases TOR, PKA, and Sch9, which promote phosphorylation and exclusion of Msn2/4 from the nucleus. Mutation of *CYR1* or deletion of *SCH9* fails to increase chronological life span in an *msn2Δ msn4Δ* double mutant, consistent with the idea the enhanced longevity seen in these mutants is due to activation of Msn2/4-dependent targets (Fabrizio *et al.*, 2001).

In many ways the function of Msn2 and Msn4 as transcriptional regulators of the yeast chronological aging program parallels the role of Daf-16 in the *C. elegans* aging process. Msn2/4 and Daf-16 are downstream targets of pathways that regulate the rate of aging in response to nutrients or growth factors, and both sets of proteins are transcriptional activators of genes involved in stress response and starvation response.

The similarity between yeast chronological aging and adult aging in the nematode is perhaps not surprising, as adult *C. elegans* are thought to be completely postmitotic (with the exception of the germ line). This similarity extends beyond transcriptional regulation in response to nutrients, as evidenced by the fact that at least some of the downstream effectors impacting longevity are also conserved. As is the case for yeast chronological life span, Daf-16-dependent up-regulation of superoxide dismutase accounts for a portion of the life span extension seen in long-lived insulin/IGF-1 pathway mutants in *C. elegans* (Honda and Honda, 1999), and activation of the heat shock responsive transcription factor Hsf1 increases both chronological life span in yeast (Harris *et al.*, 2001) and adult life span in the nematode (Morley and Morimoto, 2004). Further studies will likely uncover additional shared longevity determinants, and it will be particularly interesting to see how highly conserved the aging process is for nondividing cells in evolutionarily divergent eukaryotes.

NUTRIENTS
GLUCOSE/NITROGEN
PKA
Sch9
TOR
TARGET GENES
↑CELL SIZE | ↑ RIBOSOME BIOGENESIS | ↓ STRESS RESPONSE | METABOLIC EFFECTS
REPLICATIVE AGING
CHRONOLOGICAL AGING

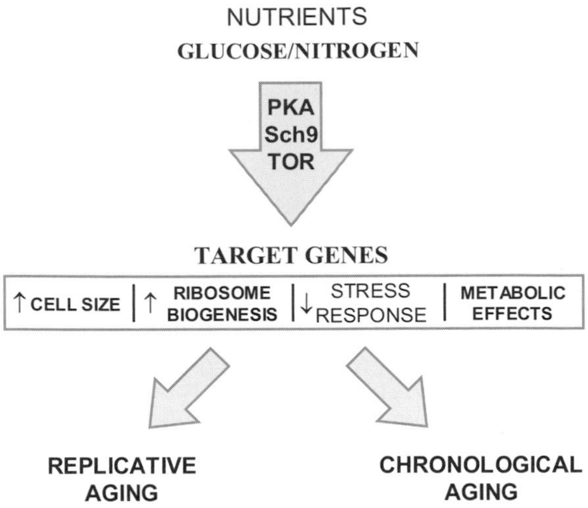

Figure 18.3. Nutrient responsive pathways that promote aging in yeast. PKA, SCH9, and TOR activate overlapping downstream targets in response to environmental nutrients and limit both replicative and chronological life span. The downstream effectors, although unidentified at present, appear to be different for replicative and chronological aging.

Relationship between Replicative and Chronological Aging

Cells that have been maintained in stationary phase for a sufficient length of time (chronologically aged) demonstrate reduced replicative capacity (Ashrafi *et al.*, 1999), suggesting that chronological and replicative aging are linked in some way. This link appears to be unrelated to ERCs, as chronologically aged cells do not have a detectable increase in ERC levels relative to young cells (Ashrafi *et al.*, 1999). One attractive hypothesis is that accumulation of oxidatively damaged proteins during chronological aging might contribute to premature replicative senescence. It has been reported that oxidatively damaged proteins accumulate with replicative age (Reverter-Branchat *et al.*, 2004); however, thus far, no direct link between oxidative damage and replicative capacity in yeast has been demonstrated. In fact, deletion of *SOD2*, which results in sensitivity to oxidative stress and dramatically shortens chronological life span, has no effect on replicative life span (Kaeberlein *et al.*, 2005a). Thus, it seems unlikely that oxidative damage limits replicative capacity, at least under normal conditions. It may be the case, however, that in chronologically aged cells, an abnormally high level of oxidative damage is sufficient to detrimentally affect replicative capacity.

Another link between replicative and chronological aging is seen in the response of cells to CR. The same nutrient sensing pathways play an important role in determining the rate at which cells age both chronologically and replicatively, as evidenced by the fact that decreased activity of PKA or Sch9 increases both chronological and replicative life span (see Conserved Nutrient Sensing Pathways as a Mediator of CR in Yeast and Nutrient Sensing and Chronological Aging). Intriguingly, the molecular mechanisms by which nutrient depletion slows aging appear to be quite different in dividing and nondividing yeast cells.

The mechanistic divergence for replicative versus chronological life-span extension by CR is of particular interest in light of the fact that CR slows aging in both mitotic and postmitotic cells of multicellular organisms. The yeast model provides a molecular explanation for how such a system might have evolved from a unicellular progenitor. TOR, Sch9, and PKA are known to converge on a shared set of downstream targets that impact a variety of cellular processes, including regulation of cell size, metabolic flux through many of the major biosynthetic and degradative pathways, ribosome biosynthesis and translation, and stress response (Figure 18.3).

Through modulation of specific subsets of these downstream targets, it is possible to imagine how aging can be regulated in both dividing and nondividing cells in response to similar environmental parameters, such as nutrient availability.

Goals and Challenges for the Future

EMBRACING DIVERSITY: UNDERSTANDING STRAIN-SPECIFIC DIFFERENCES

As with other model systems used for aging-related research, strain-specific effects due to genetic diversity can have a large impact on longevity and other age-associated phenotypes in yeast. The importance of strain diversity for studies of aging consists of two distinct components. The first component of strain diversity is the large genetic variation between different laboratory strains commonly used in scientific research. Laboratory strains can have dramatically different life spans, ranging from an average of less than 10 generations to nearly 30 generations, for replicative life span (Kaeberlein *et al.*, 2005a). This type of diversity is analogous to that seen between different inbred strains of mice, which also can have substantially different longevity and aging disease phenotypes. There have been no attempts to systematically characterize strain-specific effects on chronological life span, and only one attempt has been made to determine which genes are strain-specific and which are strain-independent with respect to replicative life span (Kaeberlein *et al.*, 2005a).

The second type of diversity relevant to aging-related research is the genetic divergence between "domesticated" laboratory yeast and wild isolates of *S. cerevisiae*. This type of diversity and its impact on yeast aging is almost completely unstudied. Preliminary analysis of the aging properties of a polyploid lager yeast has been reported (Maskell *et al.*, 2003; Powell *et al.*, 2000), but it is currently unknown whether the same genes and pathways that influence longevity of lab yeast will be shared among yeast obtained from other environments. The aging properties of "wild" yeast obtained from natural populations have not been examined at all. In order to begin to address this question, it will be important to determine whether ERCs accumulate and cause replicative senescence in wild yeast as well as whether CR slows aging in natural isolates.

AGING IN OTHER YEAST SPECIES

Given the relative ease of studying aging in *S. cerevisiae*, it is surprising that few aging-related studies have been carried out in other yeast species. The chronological aging assay, in particular, would be easily adapted to a wide variety of budding, filamentous, and fission yeast species. One study examined replicative senescence in the fission yeast *Schizosaccharomyces pombe* (Barker and Walmsley, 1999). Unlike *S. cerevisiae*, cell division in *S. pombe* is morphologically symmetric, making differentiation of mother and daughter cells problematic. By the second division, however, the progenitor mother cell (now two generations old) is both longer and thinner than the daughter cells and can be separated by microdissection from progeny cells in a manner identical to the *S. cerevisiae* replicative life-span assay (see The Replicative Life-Span Assay). Using this method, it was demonstrated that fission yeast undergoes a senescence process with mortality kinetics similar to budding yeast. Unfortunately, no additional studies of this process have been published. A system for studying aging in a yeast species that is evolutionarily divergent from *S. cerevisiae*, such as *S. pombe*, would be of great value, both for verifying the generality of findings and for potentially identifying new determinants of cellular aging.

DEVELOPING HIGH-THROUGHPUT METHODOLOGIES FOR LIFE-SPAN ANALYSIS

Until recently, discovery of genetic and environmental determinants of longevity in any organism has been driven largely by gene-specific studies based on prior knowledge or hypotheses. The development of new methods and technologies for moderate to high-throughput longevity phenotyping in yeast offers the promise of analyzing the replicative and chronological aging properties of thousands of strains simultaneously (see Chapter 10: Application of High-Throughput Technologies to Aging-Related Research). Recently, a method for high-throughput chronological life-span determination carried out in a 96-well format has been developed (T. Powers, M. Kaeberlein, B. Kennedy, S. Fields, unpublished data). This approach should provide the ability to carry out both large-scale genetic screens for mutations that alter chronological life span and screens for small molecules that alter the rate of aging in nondividing cells.

The ability to measure replicative life span in a high-throughput manner has been difficult to develop due to the nature of the replicative life-span assay, which requires the separation of daughter cells from mother cells (see The Replicative Life-Span Assay). Automated microdissection of daughter cells away from mother cells has proven difficult to implement for several reasons, and other methods of enriching for aged cells (for example, see Park *et al.*, (2002)) are not sufficiently stringent to permit quantitative life-span determination. We have recently developed an iterative method that allows for moderate-throughput analysis of replicative life span for ~100 strains at one time (Kaeberlein and Kennedy, 2005). This is an improvement over past efforts; however, development of a true high-throughput method would be of immense value to the field.

The most obvious method by which high-throughput replicative life-span analysis might be accomplished is through the development of a system in which daughter cells are selectively killed. In theory, such a system could be engineered by the expression of a toxic product under the control of a daughter-specific promoter or by the expression of an essential product only in mother cells. In either case, the system would need to be inducible so that the strain can be propagated. The first system of this type to be developed uses the latter approach by expressing an essential gene, *CDC6*, under the control of the mother cell specific *HO* promoter (Jarolim *et al.*, 2004). Unfortunately, this system appears to have serious flaws, as all three mutations observed to increase mother cell survival with this method fail to increase replicative life span as measured by the standard life-span assay (Jarolim *et al.*, 2004). This may be due to a large amount of premature mother cell death, as evidenced by the fact that mother cell life span is shorted by about 70% when *CDC6* is expressed from the *HO* promoter (Jarolim *et al.*, 2004). Although not useful in its current form, this system represents a first step toward the development of a true high-throughput replicative life-span assay.

Methods for Measuring Life Span in Yeast

Of all the model systems used in aging-related research, yeast is perhaps the most accessible to a wide variety of scientists. Assays have been developed that allow the measurement of yeast chronological and replicative life span which require little more than a microscope and an incubator. This section described the most common yeast life-span assays and important considerations when designing an experiment to study yeast aging.

THE REPLICATIVE LIFE-SPAN ASSAY

The goal of the replicative life-span assay is to determine how many times each mother cell buds before senescence. Cell division in yeast is an asymmetric budding process resulting in the production of a larger mother cell and a smaller daughter cell. The mother and daughter cells can be easily differentiated by an experienced researcher using a standard light microscope (total magnification 160×) such as the Zeiss Axioscope 40 or another comparable model. Physical separation of daughter cells from mother cells is achieved using a manual micromanipulator equipped with a fiber-optic needle (see Recommended Resources for information on obtaining needles). Currently, there is no automated method for determining replicative life span (see Developing High-Throughput Methodologies for Life-Span Analysis).

Prior to initiating the replicative life-span experiment, it is important that all strains to be analyzed are freshly removed from frozen stock and allowed to enter a logarithmic growth phase for several divisions, as growth into stationary phase is known to depress replicative life span (see The Replicative Life-Span Assay). The standard growth conditions for replicative life-span experiments are growth on solid YPD (2% bacto peptone, 1% yeast extract, 2% glucose, 1.7% agar) plates at 30°C. Replicative life-span analysis can also be carried out on synthetically defined medium; however, this is generally not recommended as growth on synthetic media shortens life span dramatically (Jiang *et al.*, 2000), complicating phenotypic analysis (Kaeberlein *et al.*, 2004b). Cells can be placed at 4–10°C overnight, or the experiment can be carried out continuously by maintaining optimal growth temperature. It has been observed in multiple wild-type backgrounds that overnight incubation at a reduced temperature has no significant effect on longevity (Kennedy *et al.*, 1994); although, it is possible that certain mutant backgrounds could be differentially affected by growth at reduced temperature.

There are a variety of similar methods that can be used to prepare cells for a replicative life-span experiment. One preferred method is to remove the strains from frozen stock and allow the formation of small colonies on YPD plates. Cells from a single colony are then patched lightly onto fresh YPD and cultured overnight. The following evening, cells are again patched lightly onto fresh YPD and allowed to grow for approximately 8–12 hours. The patches should be placed near one edge of the plate, and, depending on the number of cells to be analyzed per strain, up to 5 patches can be arranged on the same plate (Figure 18.4).

From this point on, it is essential to keep the plates wrapped in parafilm at all times, except during micromanipulation, in order to prevent moisture loss and excessive drying of the agar.

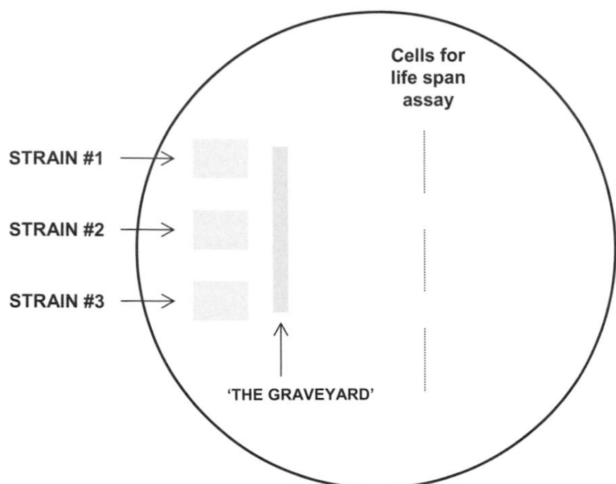

Figure 18.4. Yeast replicative life-span assay. Strains are lightly patched onto a 100-mm diameter YPD plate and allowed to grow overnight. 40–50 cells from each strain are arrayed for life-span analysis away from the patches. Daughter cells are discarded in "the graveyard" throughout the experiment.

Following the overnight incubation, the cells should be growing under near optimal conditions. The next step is to position the cells away from the patches for life-span analysis. For each strain, transfer approximately 100 cells to a position on the plate distal to the patched cells using the dissecting needle. Then arrange the appropriate number of cells (generally 40–50 per strain) in a line with 1–3 needle diameters (~100 μm) between each cell. The cells should be allowed to go through at least one division (~2 hours at 30°C), at which time *daughter cells* should be selected and the mother cells discarded. This guarantees that every cell for which replicative life span is determined started as a virgin cell. From this point on, the life-span assay is an iterative process of allowing the cells to divide 1–2 generations in the incubator; dissecting daughter cells away from mother cells and counting the number of daughters produced by each mother; and discarding daughter cells by moving them to a distal portion of the plate ("the graveyard"). Once all of the mother cells have failed to divide after incubation for greater than 8 hours at 30°C, the experiment is complete. Statistical analysis of replicative life-span data is generally carried out using a Wilcoxon Rank-Sum test to determine whether a significant change in median life span has been observed.

THE CHRONOLOGICAL AGING ASSAY

In its most general form, the chronological aging assay requires maintaining cells in a nondividing state for a prolonged period of time, while intermittently challenging a subset of the cell population for the ability to reenter the cell cycle and successfully begin vegetative growth. Several variations of this assay have been described (Fabrizio and

Longo, 2003; MacLean *et al.*, 2001), and many others can be imagined. The most commonly utilized variation involves growing cells into stationary phase in chemically defined media with glucose as the carbon source and maintaining the cells in culture for a period of several weeks (Fabrizio and Longo, 2003). An alternative method, in which cells are grown to stationary phase in rich media and then transferred to water, has also been described. A major difference between these two methods is the metabolic state of the cells in the quiescent state; cells aged in synthetic media maintain a high metabolic rate, whereas cells transferred to water from rich media enter a so-called hypometabolic state (Fabrizio and Longo, 2003). Survival time is greatly enhanced for cells maintained in water relative to cells maintained in synthetic medial. In general, it has been observed that mutations altering chronological life span in one of these assays have the same effect on life span as measured by the other assay variant; however, this has not been examined in a systematic manner.

In addition to the composition of the culture media, another important variant in the chronological aging assay is the condition under which cells are maintained during aging. Temperature and oxygenation are two of the most important environmental parameters that can alter the rate at which cells age chronologically. The importance of temperature is demonstrated by the observation that chronological longevity of cells maintained in water is substantially reduced as temperature is increased (MacLean *et al.*, 2001). Survival is also reduced as oxygenation is increased. For example, cells cultured in flasks on a rotating shaker have a chronological life span that is up to 50% shorter than cells cultured in a tube on a rotating drum, while cells maintained under low aeration (no agitation) in 96-well plates have a median life span that is extended.

In the chronological aging assay, viability is determined by the fraction of cells reintroduced to favorable growth conditions that successfully reenter the cell cycle (Figure 18.1). The most common method for assaying viability involves removing an aliquot of cells from the aging culture and determining the density of colony forming units (CFUs) by plating onto YPD media. Cells aged in SC media typically reach a saturation density of $\sim 5 \times 10^7$ CFUs/mL by the third day in culture, which can be considered the initial viability (100%). Over time, the density of CFUs will decrease, with a rate dependent on environmental and genetic parameters, but with median survival on the order of 1–3 weeks.

In most cases, viability for each strain should be determined with time points spaced every 1–2 days. When designing a chronological aging experiment, it is important to determine whether any of the strains being examined exhibits an abnormal growth rate or stationary phase density. Extreme slow growth, in particular, should be taken into consideration when defining time points for viability measurements. Each strain should be analyzed in triplicate, at least, with replicates grown as independent cultures, rather than measuring viability from the same culture in triplicate at each time point. Stochastic variability in culture conditions and the possibility of "gasping," a phenomenon where a small fraction of aged cells escapes the G0-like state and takes over the culture population (see What Do Chronologically Aged Cells Die From?), make independent replication essential.

Conclusion

As with other model organisms, the ultimate utility of yeast as a model for human aging has yet to be determined. Thus far, at least six genes and one environmental intervention (calorie restriction) have been found to increase life span in yeast and similarly impact longevity in one or more multicellular models of aging (Figure 18.2). Although it remains to be seen whether these potential conserved determinants of longevity are affecting aging through a similar mechanism in different organisms, there is reason for optimism that this is, indeed, the case. In particular, the recent findings that highly conserved nutrient responsive kinase pathways regulate aging in both dividing and nondividing yeast cells through divergent downstream components suggest a plausible mechanism by which CR might slow aging in both mitotic and postmitotic cell types of multicellular eukaryotes. Dissecting the genetic and molecular components of these nutrient responsive, longevity-determining pathways in yeast will provide direction for further study in complex systems.

Recommended Resources

Cora Styles Needles and Blocks—http://www.corastyles.com/. The place to purchase your yeast dissection paraphernalia if you want to perform replicative life-span assays.

SAGE KE Genes/Interventions Database—http://sageke.sciencemag.org/cgi/genesdb. A comprehensive catalog of longevity experiments from yeast and other organisms.

Saccharomyces Genome Database—
http://www.yeastgenome.org.

REFERENCES

Anderson, R.M., Bitterman, K.J., Wood, J.G., Medvedik, O., and Sinclair, D.A. (2003a). Nicotinamide and PNC1 govern lifespan extension by calorie restriction in *Saccharomyces cerevisiae*. *Nature 423*, 181–185.

Anderson, R.M., Latorre-Esteves, M., Neves, A.R., Lavu, S., Medvedik, O., Taylor, C., Howitz, K.T., Santos, H., and Sinclair, D.A. (2003b). Yeast life-span extension by calorie restriction is independent of NAD fluctuation. *Science 302*, 2124–2126.

Aparicio, O.M., Billington, B.L., and Gottschling, D.E. (1991). Modifiers of position effect are shared between telomeric and silent mating-type loci in *S. cerevisiae*. *Cell 66*, 1279–1287.

Ashrafi, K., Sinclair, D., Gordon, J.I., and Guarente, L. (1999). Passage through stationary phase advances replicative aging in *Saccharomyces cerevisiae*. *Proc Natl Acad Sci USA 96*, 9100–9105.

Barker, M.G., and Walmsley, R.M. (1999). Replicative ageing in the fission yeast *Schizosaccharomyces pombe*. *Yeast 15*, 1511–1518.

Beck, T., and Hall, M.N. (1999). The TOR signalling pathway controls nuclear localization of nutrient-regulated transcription factors. *Nature 402*, 689–692.

Bitterman, K.J., Medvedik, O., and Sinclair, D.A. (2003). Longevity regulation in *Saccharomyces cerevisiae*: Linking metabolism, genome stability, and heterochromatin. *Microbiol Mol Biol Rev 67*, 376–399, table of contents.

Blander, G., and Guarente, L. (2004). The Sir2 family of protein deacetylases. *Annu Rev Biochem 73*, 417–435.

Bryk, M., Banerjee, M., Murphy, M., Knudsen, K.E., Garfinkel, D.J., and Curcio, M.J. (1997). Transcriptional silencing of Ty1 elements in the RDN1 locus of yeast. *Genes Dev 11*, 255–269.

Defossez, P.A., Prusty, R., Kaeberlein, M., Lin, S.J., Ferrigno, P., Silver, P.A., *et al.* (1999). Elimination of replication block protein Fob1 extends the life span of yeast mother cells. *Mol Cell 3*, 447–455.

Fabrizio, P., Battistella, L., Vardavas, R., Gattazzo, C., Liou, L.L., Diaspro, A., *et al.* (2004a). Superoxide is a mediator of an altruistic aging program in *Saccharomyces cerevisiae*. *J Cell Biol 166*, 1055–1067.

Fabrizio, P., Liou, L.L., Moy, V.N., Diaspro, A., Selverstone-Valentine, J., Gralla, E.B., and Longo, V.D. (2003). SOD2 functions downstream of Sch9 to extend longevity in yeast. *Genetics 163*, 35–46.

Fabrizio, P., and Longo, V.D. (2003). The chronological life span of *Saccharomyces cerevisiae*. *Aging Cell 2*, 73–81.

Fabrizio, P., Pletcher, S.D., Minois, N., Vaupel, J.W., and Longo, V.D. (2004b). Chronological aging-independent replicative life span regulation by Msn2/Msn4 and Sod2 in *Saccharomyces cerevisiae*. *FEBS Lett 557*, 136–142.

Fabrizio, P., Pozza, F., Pletcher, S.D., Gendron, C.M., and Longo, V.D. (2001). Regulation of longevity and stress resistance by Sch9 in yeast. *Science 292*, 288–290.

Gottlieb, S., and Esposito, R.E. (1989). A new role for a yeast transcriptional silencer gene, SIR2, in regulation of recombination in ribosomal DNA. *Cell 56*, 771–776.

Gray, J.V., Petsko, G.A., Johnston, G.C., Ringe, D., Singer, R.A., and Werner-Washburne, M. (2004). "Sleeping beauty": Quiescence in *Saccharomyces cerevisiae*. *Microbiol Mol Biol Rev 68*, 187–206.

Harman, D. (1956). Aging: A theory based on free radical and radiation chemistry. *J Gerontol 11*, 298–300.

Harris, N., MacLean, M., Hatzianthis, K., Panaretou, B., and Piper, P.W. (2001). Increasing *Saccharomyces cerevisiae* stress resistance, through the overactivation of the heat shock response resulting from defects in the Hsp90 chaperone, does not extend replicative life span but can be associated with slower chronological ageing of nondividing cells. *Mol Genet Genomics 265*, 258–263.

Herker, E., Jungwirth, H., Lehmann, K.A., Maldener, C., Frohlich, K.U., Wissing, S., *et al.* (2004). Chronological aging leads to apoptosis in yeast. *J Cell Biol 164*, 501–507.

Hertweck, M., Gobel, C., and Baumeister, R. (2004). C. elegans SGK-1 is the critical component in the Akt/PKB kinase complex to control stress response and life span. *Dev Cell 6*, 577–588.

Honda, Y., and Honda, S. (1999). The daf-2 gene network for longevity regulates oxidative stress resistance and Mn-superoxide dismutase gene expression in *Caenorhabditis elegans*. *Faseb J 13*, 1385–1393.

Houthoofd, K., Braeckman, B.P., Johnson, T.E., and Vanfleteren, J.R. (2003). Life extension via dietary restriction is independent of the Ins/IGF-1 signalling pathway in *Caenorhabditis elegans*. *Exp Gerontol 38*, 947–954.

Imai, S., Armstrong, C.M., Kaeberlein, M., and Guarente, L. (2000). Transcriptional silencing and longevity protein Sir2 is an NAD-dependent histone deacetylase. *Nature 403*, 795–800.

Ivy, J.M., Klar, A.J., and Hicks, J.B. (1986). Cloning and characterization of four SIR genes of *Saccharomyces cerevisiae*. *Mol Cell Biol 6*, 688–702.

Jarolim, S., Millen, J., Heeren, G., Laun, P., Goldfarb, D.S., and Breitenbach, M. (2004). A novel assay for replicative lifespan in *Saccharomyces cerevisiae*. *FEMS Yeast Res 5*, 169–177.

Jazwinski, S.M. (2002). Growing old: Metabolic control and yeast aging. *Annu Rev Microbiol 56*, 769–792.

Jiang, J.C., Jaruga, E., Repnevskaya, M.V., and Jazwinski, S.M. (2000). An intervention resembling caloric restriction prolongs life span and retards aging in yeast. *Faseb J 14*, 2135–2137.

Kaeberlein, M., Andalis, A.A., Fink, G.R., and Guarente, L. (2002a). High osmolarity extends life span in *Saccharomyces cerevisiae* by a mechanism related to calorie restriction. *Mol Cell Biol 22*, 8056–8066.

Kaeberlein, M., Andalis, A.A., Liszt, G., Fink, G.R., and Guarente, L. (2004a). *Saccharomyces cerevisiae* SSD1-V confers longevity by a Sir2p-independent mechanism. *Genetics 166*, 1661–1672.

Kaeberlein, M., Jegalian, B., and McVey, M. (2002b). AGEID: A database of aging genes and interventions. *Mech Ageing Dev 123*, 1115–1119.

Kaeberlein, M., and Kennedy, B.K. (2005). Large-scale identification in yeast of conserved ageing genes. *Mech Ageing Dev 126*, 17–21.

Kaeberlein, M., Kirkland, K.T., Fields, S., and Kennedy, B.K. (2004b). Sir2-independent life span extension by calorie restriction in yeast. *PLoS Biol 2*, E296.

Kaeberlein, M., Kirkland, K.T., Fields, S., and Kennedy, B.K. (2005a). Genes determining replicative life span in a long-lived genetic background. *Mech Ageing Dev 126*, 491–504.

Kaeberlein, M., McVey, M., and Guarente, L. (1999). The SIR2/3/4 complex and SIR2 alone promote longevity in *Saccharomyces cerevisiae* by two different mechanisms. *Genes Dev 13*, 2570–2580.

Kaeberlein, M., McVey, M., and Guarente, L. (2001). Using yeast to discover the fountain of youth. *Sci. Aging Knowledge Environ. Oct 3*; 2001 (1): pe1.

Kaeberlein, M., Powers, R.W., Steffen, K.K., Westman, E.A., Hu, D., Dang, N., *et al.* (2005b). Regulation of yeast replicative life span by TOR and Sch9 in response to nutrients. *Science* in press.

Kapahi, P., Zid, B.M., Harper, T., Koslover, D., Sapin, V., and Benzer, S. (2004). Regulation of lifespan in *Drosophila* by modulation of genes in the TOR signaling pathway. *Curr Biol 14*, 885–890.

Kennedy, B.K., Austriaco, N.R., Jr., and Guarente, L. (1994). Daughter cells of *Saccharomyces cerevisiae* from old mothers display a reduced life span. *J Cell Biol 127*, 1985–1993.

Kobayashi, T., and Horiuchi, T. (1996). A yeast gene product, Fob1 protein, required for both replication fork blocking and recombinational hotspot activities. *Genes Cells 1*, 465–474.

Lakowski, B., and Hekimi, S. (1998). The genetics of caloric restriction in *Caenorhabditis elegans*. *Proc Natl Acad Sci USA 95*, 13091–13096.

Landry, J., Sutton, A., Tafrov, S.T., Heller, R.C., Stebbins, J., Pillus, L., and Sternglanz, R. (2000). The silencing protein SIR2 and its homologs are NAD-dependent protein deacetylases. *Proc Natl Acad Sci USA 97*, 5807–5811.

Lin, S.J., Defossez, P.A., and Guarente, L. (2000). Requirement of NAD and SIR2 for life-span extension by calorie restriction in *Saccharomyces cerevisiae*. *Science 289*, 2126–2128.

Lin, S.J., Ford, E., Haigis, M., Liszt, G., and Guarente, L. (2004). Calorie restriction extends yeast life span by lowering the level of NADH. *Genes Dev 18*, 12–16.

Lin, S.J., Kaeberlein, M., Andalis, A.A., Sturtz, L.A., Defossez, P., Culotta, V.C., *et al.* (2002). Calorie restriction extends *Saccharomyces cerevisiae* life span by increasing respiration. *Nature 418*, 344–348.

Longo, V.D., Gralla, E.B., and Valentine, J.S. (1996). Superoxide dismutase activity is essential for stationary phase survival in *Saccharomyces cerevisiae*. Mitochondrial production of toxic oxygen species in vivo. *J Biol Chem 271*, 12275–12280.

Luo, J., Nikolaev, A.Y., Imai, S., Chen, D., Su, F., Shiloh, A., Guarente, L., and Gu, W. (2001). Negative control of p53 by Sir2alpha promotes cell survival under stress. *Cell 107*, 137–148.

MacLean, M., Harris, N., and Piper, P.W. (2001). Chronological lifespan of stationary phase yeast cells: A model for investigating the factors that might influence the ageing of postmitotic tissues in higher organisms. *Yeast 18*, 499–509.

Madeo, F., Herker, E., Wissing, S., Jungwirth, H., Eisenberg, T., and Frohlich, K.U. (2004). Apoptosis in yeast. *Curr Opin Microbiol 7*, 655–660.

Maskell, D.L., Kennedy, A.I., Hodgson, J.A., and Smart, K.A. (2003). Chronological and replicative lifespan of polyploid *Saccharomyces cerevisiae* (syn. *S. pastorianus*). *FEMS Yeast Res. 3*, 201–209.

Morley, J.F., and Morimoto, R.I. (2004). Regulation of longevity in *Caenorhabditis elegans* by heat shock factor and molecular chaperones. *Mol Biol Cell 15*, 657–664.

Mortimer, R.K., and Johnston, J.R. (1959). Life span of individual yeast cells. *Nature 183*, 1751–1752.

Motta, M.C., Divecha, N., Lemieux, M., Kamel, C., Chen, D., Gu, W., *et al.* (2004). Mammalian SIRT1 represses forkhead transcription factors. *Cell 116*, 551–563.

Nemoto, S., Fergusson, M.M., and Finkel, T. (2005). SIRT1 functionally interacts with the metabolic regulator and transcriptional coactivator PGC-1alpha. *J Biol Chem.*

Park, P.U., Defossez, P.A., and Guarente, L. (1999). Effects of mutations in DNA repair genes on formation of ribosomal DNA circles and life span in *Saccharomyces cerevisiae*. *Mol Cell Biol 19*, 3848–3856.

Park, P.U., McVey, M., and Guarente, L. (2002). Separation of mother and daughter cells. *Methods Enzymol 351*, 468–477.

Powell, C.D., Quain, D.E., and Smart, K.A. (2000). The impact of media composition and petite mutation on the longevity of a polyploid brewing yeast strain. *Lett Appl Microbiol 31*, 46–51.

Reverter-Branchat, G., Cabiscol, E., Tamarit, J., and Ros, J. (2004). Oxidative damage to specific proteins in replicative and chronological-aged *Saccharomyces cerevisiae*: Common targets and prevention by calorie restriction. *J Biol Chem 279*, 31983–31989.

Rine, J., and Herskowitz, I. (1987). Four genes responsible for a position effect on expression from HML and HMR in *Saccharomyces cerevisiae*. *Genetics 116*, 9–22.

Rogina, B., and Helfand, S.L. (2004). Sir2 mediates longevity in the fly through a pathway related to calorie restriction. *Proc Natl Acad Sci USA 101*, 15998–16003.

Samokhvalov, V., Ignatov, V., and Kondrashova, M. (2004). Reserve carbohydrates maintain the viability of *Saccharomyces cerevisiae* cells during chronological aging. *Mech Ageing Dev 125*, 229–235.

Sinclair, D., Mills, K., and Guarente, L. (1998). Aging in *Saccharomyces cerevisiae*. *Annu Rev Microbiol 52*, 533–560.

Sinclair, D.A., and Guarente, L. (1997). Extrachromosomal rDNA circles—a cause of aging in yeast. *Cell 91*, 1033–1042.

Smith, A., Ward, M.P., and Garrett, S. (1998). Yeast PKA represses Msn2p/Msn4p-dependent gene expression to regulate growth, stress response and glycogen accumulation. *Embo J 17*, 3556–3564.

Smith, J.S., and Boeke, J.D. (1997). An unusual form of transcriptional silencing in yeast ribosomal DNA. *Genes Dev 11*, 241–254.

Smith, J.S., Brachmann, C.B., Celic, I., Kenna, M.A., Muhammad, S., Starai, V., *et al.* (2000). A phylogenetically conserved NAD^{+}-dependent protein deacetylase activity in the Sir2 protein family. *Proc Natl Acad Sci USA 97*, 6658–6663.

Tanner, K.G., Landry, J., Sternglanz, R., and Denu, J.M. (2000). Silent information regulator 2 family of NAD-dependent histone/protein deacetylases generates a unique product, 1-*O*-acetyl-ADP-ribose. *Proc Natl Acad Sci USA 97*, 14178–14182.

Tissenbaum, H.A., and Guarente, L. (2001). Increased dosage of a sir-2 gene extends lifespan in *Caenorhabditis elegans*. *Nature 410*, 227–230.

Vaziri, H., Dessain, S.K., Ng Eaton, E., Imai, S.I., Frye, R.A., Pandita, T.K., *et al.* (2001). hSIR2(SIRT1) functions as an NAD-dependent p53 deacetylase. *Cell 107*, 149–159.

Vellai, T., Takacs-Vellai, K., Zhang, Y., Kovacs, A.L., Orosz, L., and Muller, F. (2003). Genetics: Influence of TOR kinase on lifespan in *C. elegans*. *Nature 426*, 620.

Weindruch, R.H., and Walford, R.L. (1988). *The Retardation of Aging and Disease by Dietary Restriction.* (Springfield, IL., Thomas).

19

From Yeast Methuselah Genes to Evolutionary Medicine

Paola Fabrizio and Valter D. Longo

The recent identification of many genes that regulate the life span of yeast, worms, flies, and mice has greatly enhanced our understanding of the mechanisms of aging. Saccharomyces cerevisiae *has emerged as the simplest of the major model systems to study aging, thanks in part to the development of a chronological aging paradigm that has allowed a more direct comparison with higher eukaryotes. Remarkably, similar pathways regulate the chronological life span of yeast and of the other major model systems, suggesting that the "test-tube" approach to study aging and death can provide a simple but valuable contribution to the process of identification of the genes and pathways that regulate aging in humans. Furthermore, comparative studies in unicellular and higher eukaryotes can shed light on the best strategies to delay human aging and prevent age-related diseases without causing significant side-effects.*

Introduction

Our current knowledge of the genetics of aging has relied greatly on studies in simple model systems such as *S. cerevisiae*, *Caenorhabditis elegans*, and *Drosophila melanogaster*. The recent discovery that aging, similarly to other fundamental biological processes, is regulated by a conserved set of genes has attracted many researchers interested in the basic mechanisms of human aging and diseases to the "model system" field. Yeast are particularly amenable to aging studies because of their relatively short life span, the straightforward genetic manipulation techniques available, and the high-throughput technologies recently developed specifically for this unicellular eukaryote. Yeast life span can be measured as replicative potential (replicative or budding life span) by counting the number of buds produced by individual mother cells (Mortimer, 1959) or chronologically by monitoring mean and maximum survival of populations of nondividing yeast (chronological life span). *C. elegans* represents the second simplest and perhaps the more widely studied model system for aging research. Being made up of only about 1000 somatic cells, it provides the advantages of both a multicellular organism and those of a relatively simple genetic system. Together with *D. melanogaster*, *C. elegans* is playing a key role in elucidating both the cell autonomous and non-autonomous regulation of aging. The fourth major model system, *Mus musculis*, has the disadvantage of being much more complex and difficult to study but it is obviously an essential system because of its much closer phylogenetic relationship to humans. Thus, yeast, worms, and flies are simple systems—amenable to rapid genetic manipulation, highly characterized—and have a short life span (6 to 60 days). By contrast, the mouse has a much longer life span (30 months and more) and is much more difficult to manipulate genetically, but it is a key model system to begin to face the complexity of human aging and diseases. Given the existence of evolutionary conserved aging pathways (Kenyon, 2001; Longo and Finch, 2003), a possibility offered to the geneticists is to study simple organisms such as yeast, worms, or flies to perform genome-wide screens/selections for long-lived mutants and then test whether analogous mutations can cause similar effects in mice. In fact, some of the proteins whose modified activity was shown to extend the life span of the three simple model systems have been shown to play a similar role in mice. For example, insulin/IGF-1-like pathways have been implicated in the regulation of aging in worms, flies and mice. Notably, homologs of two of the major proteins in the insulin/IGF-1-like pathway in mice were shown to regulate the life span of *S. cerevisiae* (Figure 19.2) (Longo and Finch, 2003). Furthermore, increased antioxidant activity has been shown to cause small but significant extension of the life span of all the genetics model systems of aging (Fabrizio *et al.*, 2003; Harris *et al.*, 2003; Melov *et al.*, 2000; Orr and Sohal, 1994; Parkes *et al.*, 1998; Schriner *et al.*, 2005; Sun and Tower, 1999).

In this chapter we will provide methods to perform yeast chronological survival measurements and comprehensive genome-wide selections to isolate novel long-lived mutants. We will review the genetics of aging in yeast with particular emphasis on the genes that affect the chronological life span. We will also review the genetics of aging in worms, flies, and mice, focusing mainly on the insulin-IGF-1 signaling and on the conserved characteristics shared by the long-lived mutants of different species.

The Life Span of Yeast

The chronological life span is determined by measuring the survival time of populations of nondividing yeast. Alternatively, yeast life span is measured by monitoring the replicative potential of single mother cells. Each system has led to the identification of genes involved in either chronological or replicative aging (Bitterman *et al.*, 2003). The activity of the products of some of these genes (*SCH9*, *CYR1*; see The Genetics of Chronological Aging: Yeast Methuselah Genes) consistently affects both replicative and chronological life span (Fabrizio *et al.*, 2004b). Conversely, some genes encoding for stress resistance proteins (*MSN2*, *SOD1/2*) promote chronological longevity but negatively affect replicative life span, suggesting that there is only a partial overlap between the mechanisms that regulate replicative potential and survival of postmitotic yeast (Fabrizio *et al.*, 2004b). In the following section we review both paradigms with emphasis on the chronological life span.

CHRONOLOGICAL LIFE SPAN: SURVIVAL IN THE POSTDIAUXIC AND STATIONARY PHASES

Microorganisms have evolved to survive under adverse conditions, such as starvation, that are commonly encountered in the wild. In fact, most microorganisms are estimated to survive in a low-metabolism stationary phase under nutrient-depleted conditions (Werner-Washburne *et al.*, 1996). In the wild, yeast organisms are likely to exit stationary phase only during the rare periods when all the nutrients required for growth become available. For this reason we perform most of our experiments in either a medium containing a limited amount of nutrients [synthetic dextrose complete (SDC)] or in water. Wild-type DBY746 or SP1 yeast grown in SDC medium survive 5 to 6 days while maintaining high metabolic rates for the majority of the life span (Figure 19.1).

When yeast grown in SDC are switched to water between days 1 and 5, metabolic rates decrease and survival is extended (Fabrizio *et al.*, 2004a). However, since long-lived mutants isolated by incubation in SDC also live longer when incubated in water, we believe that analogous pathways and mechanisms regulate survival in both paradigms. Yeast grown and incubated in the nutrient-rich YPD medium also survive for months in a low metabolism stationary phase. However, it is not clear whether YPD medium allows some growth to occur during the supposedly "stationary" phase (see Survival in Water/YPD).

To understand how yeast age and to identify conserved pathways that regulate longevity in many eukaryotes,

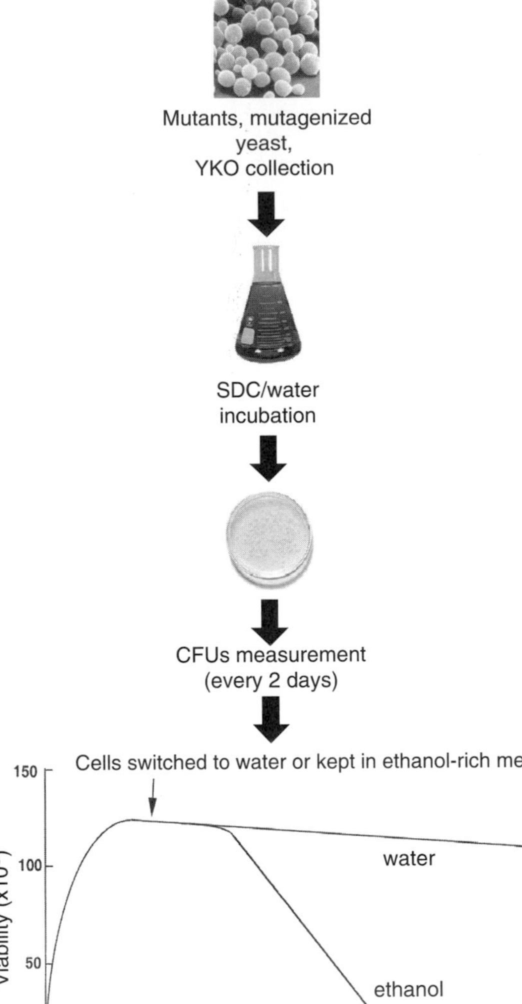

Figure 19.1. Chronological life-span measurement and its use for the isolation of long-lived mutants. Populations of mutagenized yeast or a pool of deletion mutants obtained from the Yeast Knock-out (YKO) collection are grown in minimal medium containing glucose (SDC). After 2–3 days, cell growth stops and ethanol accumulates in the medium. At day 3 yeast are either kept in this ethanol-rich medium or switched to water. Cell viability is measured every two days by diluting the yeast cultures and plating an appropriate number of cells onto rich medium (YPD) plates to monitor the colony forming units (CFUs). When yeast are switched to water, the cultures are washed every two days to avoid the cell division that might be caused by the accumulation of nutrients released from the dead yeast. Mutants that are still alive when the majority of the population is dead are isolated and then retested individually to monitor their mean and maximum life span.

it is of key importance to reproduce conditions similar to those under which these pathways have evolved. Although the chronological life-span paradigm may appear to be a starvation phase that does not resemble the life span of higher eukaryotes, nondividing yeast are not starving but are slowly utilizing the nutrients stored intracellularly at the end of the growth phase. An environment that lacks nutrients may not be common for certain mammals, but it is very common for microorganisms. In some circumstances even mammals have learned how to respond to long periods of starvation. For example, black bears and turkish hamsters alternate between a high and a low metabolism hibernation phase, in which stored nutrients are utilized to survive. The longer the period turkish hamsters spend under hibernation, the longer the life span (Lyman, 1981). Similarly, yeast forced to enter the low metabolism stationary phase by incubation in water survive longer than yeast grown and incubated in SDC medium, which maintain high metabolic rates (Fabrizio *et al.*, 2004a).

In addition to the high metabolism postdiauxic life span (SDC), and the low metabolism stationary phase, under particularly severe starvation conditions, diploid *S. cerevisiae* can form haploid spores that may survive for years in a dormant state. However, most yeast diploid organisms enter and remain in stationary phase, and only a minority of diploid organisms form spores (Codon *et al.*, 1995). All of our life-span studies are performed using haploid strains that behave similarly to diploid cell under most conditions but do not sporulate. Yeast spores may be the equivalent of the worm dauer larva, which also live much longer than adult worms (Guarente, 2001; Riddle, 1988). The food supply determines whether worms grow and become metabolically active adults or exit development at the L2 larva stage to enter the low-respiration dauer larva stage. In the following sections we will describe how the ability to survive of long-lived *S. cerevisiae* and *C. elegans* mutants appears to be linked to the entry into phases with similarities to starvation-response phases such as the spore or dauer.

Survival in SDC: Postdiauxic phase

Most of our chronological life-span studies are performed by monitoring survival in the high metabolism postdiauxic phase (SDC medium). The SDC studies are started by diluting overnight cultures to an initial density of 1–2 10^6 cells/ml (OD_{600} of 0.1–0.2) in 10–50 ml of synthetic complete medium containing 2% glucose (SDC) as well as a 4-fold excess of the supplements Trp, Leu, Ura, and His (for DBY746-derived strains). The SDC medium contains glucose, yeast nitrogen base, agar, ammonium sulfate (nitrogen source), sodium phosphate, vitamins, metals, and salts. Yeast cultures are incubated at 30°C in flasks with a volume/medium ratio of 5:1, shaking at 220 rpm. After approximately 10 hours of growth, the glucose concentration in the medium reaches very low levels, and yeast switch from a fermentation- to a respiration-based metabolism. During fermentative growth, ethanol is accumulated and released from the cells. In wild-type DBY746 and SP1 cultures the level of ethanol undergoes an age-dependent decline, suggesting that it is used as a carbon source (VL, unpublished results). When yeast organisms are incubated in SDC, the diauxic shift is followed by a postdiauxic phase, in which growth continues slowly until approximately 48 hours, and then stops (Figure 19.1). In the postdiauxic phase metabolic rates remain high until days 4–6 (day 0 = dilution day). The final density reached at day 3 varies from strain to strain and is usually between 7 and 15 (OD_{600}). The mean survival of wild-type strains depends on their genetic background and ranges from 6 to 7 days (DBY746 or SP1) to 15–20 days (S288C or BY4700). A diauxic-shift-like switch from fermentation to respiration may also occur after reducing the glucose concentration in the medium from 2 to 0.5%. This form of calorie restriction increases respiration rates and causes an extension of the yeast replicative life span (Lin *et al.*, 2002).

In a standard postdiauxic experiment we monitor survival by measuring the ability of an individual yeast cell/organism to form a colony (colony forming units or CFUs) within three days of plating onto YPD plates. CFUs are normally monitored until at least 99.9% of the population dies. The number of CFUs at day 3 is considered to be the initial survival (100% survival) and is used to determine the age-dependent mortality. Day 3 was selected considering that in our wild-type strains DBY746 and SP1 the population density does not normally increase after day 3, suggesting that the great majority of the cells have stopped dividing. To confirm that the loss of CFUs correlates with death, we have used a live/dead fluorescence assay to monitor the percentage of live cells over time. After staining a sample of cells with the FUN-1 dye, which confers red fluorescence to live cells and green/yellow fluorescence to dead cells, we have estimated the live/dead ratio and found a very significant correlation with the CFUs-based viability data (Fabrizio *et al.*, 2003).

The "postdiauxic phase" differs for organisms incubated in SDC and those incubated in rich YPD medium (Werner-Washburne *et al.*, 1996). In fact, incubation in YPD promotes a 6–7 day postdiauxic phase characterized by slow growth and low respiration followed by entry into a nondividing hypometabolic stationary phase in which organisms are highly resistant to multiple stresses and survive for up to 3 months. By contrast, incubation in SDC triggers the entry into an alternative postdiauxic phase in which only minimal growth occurs after 48 hours and metabolic rates remain high until the population begins to die.

Survival in water/YPD: Stationary phase

Yeast incubated in YPD or water survive much longer than yeast grown and maintained in SDC/ethanol medium (Figure 19.1). In fact, the mean life span of strains DBY746 and SP1 in water is approximately 3 times longer than in SDC (15–20 days). Our experiments are usually repeated in water to simulate an alternate environment that may be commonly encountered by yeast in the wild and also to confirm that the extended life span of a particular mutant is not an artifact caused by regrowth. In fact, we do not monitor survival in YPD, since this rich medium may promote growth after the culture reaches the maximum density. After more than 99% of wild-type DBY746 and SP1 yeast incubated in SDC dies, in about 50% of the studies a better-adapted subpopulation is able to grow back by utilizing the nutrients released by dead cells (Fabrizio *et al.*, 2004a). A similar phenomenon called "gasping" is observed for populations of bacteria (Zambrano and Kolter, 1996). By contrast, incubation of yeast in YPD appears to promote major increases in viability before the majority of the population has died, suggesting that some growth may occur when viability is high. Growth would create a mixed population containing both young and old organisms and possibly only young organisms, which would invalidate the survival studies.

For life-span studies in water, yeast are grown in and incubated for 3 days in SDC and are then washed with sterile distilled water and resuspended in sterile water (Figure 19.1). Viability is monitored by measuring CFUs every 2 days. The cells are washed 3 times with water every 2 days to remove all the nutrients released by dead yeast. Incubation in water and the removal of nutrients released by dead organisms minimize the chance of growth during long-term survival in stationary phase. Incubation in water decreases metabolic rates and may increase life span simply by promoting a slower rate of senescence.

REPLICATIVE LIFE SPAN

The asymmetrical division characteristic of *S. cerevisiae* is an essential for replicative life-span measurements. Daughter cells are normally smaller than mother cells and can be easily distinguished and removed from their progenitors by micromanipulation (Mortimer, 1959). The average replicative life span is 20 divisions. "Replicative aged" cells divide more slowly, become sterile, and when cell division stops, they are considered dead, although their postreproductive survival time has never been estimated (Bitterman *et al.*, 2003). Whereas few genes are known to regulate both life spans, the relationship between replicative and chronological aging has yet to be established. Notably, yeast replicative life span is analogous to the replicative life span of mammalian fibroblasts and lymphocytes, which undergo a limited number of population doublings in culture. Thus, the "budding life span" is a model for studying aging of mitotic cells but can also provide insights on fundamental mechanisms of organismal aging.

Replicative aging can be caused by a form of genomic instability that leads to the accumulation of extrachromosomal ribosomal DNA circles (ERCs) (Sinclair and Guarente, 1997) and is delayed by increasing the activity of the silencing regulator Sir2 (Kaeberlein *et al.*, 1999). Sir2 is a NAD-dependent histone-deacetylase whose activity is required to promote chromatin silencing at the telomeres, mating type loci, and rDNA (Braunstein *et al.*, 1993; Tanny *et al.*, 1999). Increased dosage of *SIR2* delays replicative aging by inhibiting rDNA recombination and consequently the formation of ERCs (Kaeberlein *et al.*, 1999). Although this aging mechanism has not been observed in any other species, Sir2 was shown to play a conserved antiaging role in higher eukaryotes. In fact, increased dosage of the Sir2 homologs extends the life span of both *C. elegans* and *Drosophila* by up to 50%, and Sir2 activity has been associated with the longevity extension caused by calorie restriction—an intervention known to extend the life span of all model organisms (Rogina and Helfand, 2004; Tissenbaum and Guarente, 2001; Wood *et al.*, 2004). However, despite the extensive experimental effort to link the Sir2 family of proteins (sirtuins) to mammalian longevity, a conclusive role for the sirtuins in mediating life-span regulation has not been established.

Other genes implicated in the regulation of replicative aging have been identified. Among these are *RAS1/RAS2* and *LAG1/LAG2*. *RAS1* and *RAS2*, which encode for highly conserved pro-growth signaling G-protein, play opposite roles in replicative aging. The deletion of *RAS1* extends replicative life span. By contrast, lack of *RAS2* shortens replicative longevity (Sun *et al.*, 1994). Intriguingly, lack of Ras2 promotes chronological survival (see The Genetics of Chronological Aging: Yeast Methuselah Genes). Deletion of Lag1, a protein implicated in ceramides synthesis, extends replicative life span, and so does the overexpression of Lag2, a protein of unknown function (D'Mello N *et al.*, 1994).

The activation of the retrograde response also triggers replicative life-span extension. This response is activated by an intracellular signaling pathway from the mitochondrion to the nucleus and leads to the transcription of several genes encoding for metabolic enzymes (Kirchman *et al.*, 1999).

The Genetics of Chronological Aging: Yeast Methuselah Genes

Using this aging paradigm, we have identified several mutations that promote life-span extension and resistance to both heat and oxidative stress. Among these is the deletion of the gene coding for the serine–threonine kinase Sch9. Lack of Sch9 promotes high-stress resistance and extends the life span up to 3-fold (Fabrizio *et al.*, 2001). Sch9 is part of a glucose-sensing pathway, which regulates cell division, cell size, ribosomal synthesis, and the expression of stress resistance proteins including mitochondrial superoxide dismutase (Sod2) (Fabrizio *et al.*, 2003; Jorgensen *et al.*, 2002; Jorgensen *et al.*,

2004; Toda *et al.*, 1988). Importantly, Sch9 appears to be a homolog of Akt/PKB, a component of the conserved pro-aging pathways of worms, flies and mice (see Evolutionary Conserved Pro-Aging Pathways) (Geyskens *et al.*, 2000) (Figure 19.2–19.3).

Another glucose-sensing pathway known to regulate chronological aging is the Cyr1/Ras/PKA pathway. A reduced activity of adenylate cycalse (Cyr1) promotes stress resistance and longevity, and so does the deletion of *RAS2*, (Fabrizio *et al.*, 2003; Fabrizio *et al.*, 2001). The down-regulation of the Ras/PKA pathway promotes chronological survival via the activation of stress resistance transcription factors Msn2/Msn4 (Fabrizio *et al.*, 2001), which in turn activate the expression of the detoxifying enzymes catalase and superoxide dismutase and of several heat shock proteins and promote the accumulation of reserve carbohydrate glycogen (Boy-Marcotte *et al.*, 1998; Schmitt, 1996; Smith *et al.*, 1998) (Figure 19.2). The Sch9 and Ras/PKA pathways share several gene targets although in some cases their regulation of gene expression is opposite (Roosen *et al.*, 2005). The exact relationship between these two pathways is still unclear mainly because the Sch9 pathway components upstream and downstream of Sch9 have been elusive. A recent *in vitro* study showed that the protein kinase Pkh1 can phosphorylate and activate Sch9 and that this activation is stimulated by phytosphingosine (Liu *et al.*, 2005). This is important because Pkh1 is a yeast homolog of PDK1, a protein also found in the pro-aging insulin/IGF-1 pathways of worms, flies, and mice and supports the hypothesis that the Sch9 and the insulin/IGF-1 pathways originated from a common ancestral pathway (Evolutionary Conserved Pro-Aging Pathways; Figure 19.2).

The ability to withstand oxidative stress is one of the conserved features of long-lived mutants (see Evolutionary Conserved Pro-Aging Pathways). We have shown that Sod2 functions as a mediator of longevity extension in both the Ras and Sch9 pathway and is required for chronological longevity extension (Fabrizio *et al.*, 2003). In fact, the TCA cycle enzyme aconitase is a key target of mitochondrial superoxide toxicity, and loss of aconitase activity precedes death in yeast aging chronologically (Fabrizio *et al.*, 2003; Fabrizio *et al.*, 2001).

The activity of the Hsp90 chaperone also affects chronological survival. Reducing the activity of Hsp82, one of the yeast Hsp90 proteins, extends chronological life span by overactivating the heat-shock transcription factor HSF1 and consequently the heat shock response (Harris *et al.*, 2001). Further genes involved in the regulation of chronological aging are *YAP1*, *YCA1*, and *AIF1*. Overexpression of *YAP1*, which encodes for an oxygen stress response transcription factor, reduces the accumulation of reactive oxygen species during chronological aging and promotes life-span extension (Herker *et al.*, 2004). Deletion of either *YCA1*, coding for a yeast caspase, or *AIF1*, coding for a homolog of the mammalian apoptosis-inducing factor (AIF), extends chronological survival (Madeo *et al.*, 2002; Wissing *et al.*, 2004).

Novel Methods for the Identification of Genes that Regulate Chronological Aging

Chronological life-span experiments are conducted using yeast cultures of billions of organisms and are very well suited for the screening of long-lived mutants. In the past we used a transposon mutagenesis technique to generate a pool of yeast carrying mutations that decrease or abolish the expression of the corresponding genes. The mutagenized population was subject to either heat shock or a treatment with the superoxide generator paraquat to select for stress resistance mutants, which were subsequently tested for chronological survival in SDC. Yeast that were viable after 9–15 days were isolated and retested individually to monitor their survival (Fabrizio *et al.*, 2001). The identification of the insertions associated with life-span extension was obtained by sequencing the region adjacent to the transposon, a rather straightforward technique. The approach of preselecting the stress resistant mutants was based on the association between ability to withstand stress and life-span extension, which applies to all model organisms, and allowed us to reduce the representation of non-long lived mutants (false positives) among the day 9–15 survivors.

Recently a more sophisticated genetic tool to study how each individual gene can affect the life span of yeast has become available: the yeast knock-out (YKO) collection. Currently, the collection covers 96% of the yeast open reading frames (ORFs) and is constructed in a way that each deletion represents a complete loss of function of the gene and is uniquely tagged with two 20-nucleotide sequences (UPTAG and DNTAG) (Wach *et al.*, 1994). The abundance of specific deletion mutants in a pool can be measured quantitatively by amplifying the tag sequences and hybridizing them to a high-density oligonucleotide arrays (Affymetrix Tag3) (Giaever *et al.*, 2002). Once completed, the yeast gene-deletion collection will overcome the main limitation of the standard mutagenesis methods used for mutant screening—under-representing the yeast genome. However, with only 4% of the ORFs missing, the YKO collection already represents a remarkable genetic tool for a comprehensive genomic analysis of chronological aging. In a typical experiment, a pool generated using approximately the same number of cells for each deletion strain is (~600) grown in SDC, and viability is measured every 48 hours as described in Survival in SDC: Postdiauxic Phase. Every 48 hours samples of yeast (OD = 0.2–2) are collected and genomic DNA is extracted. 0.2 μg of DNA is used to amplify the UPTAG and DNTAG molecular bar codes in two

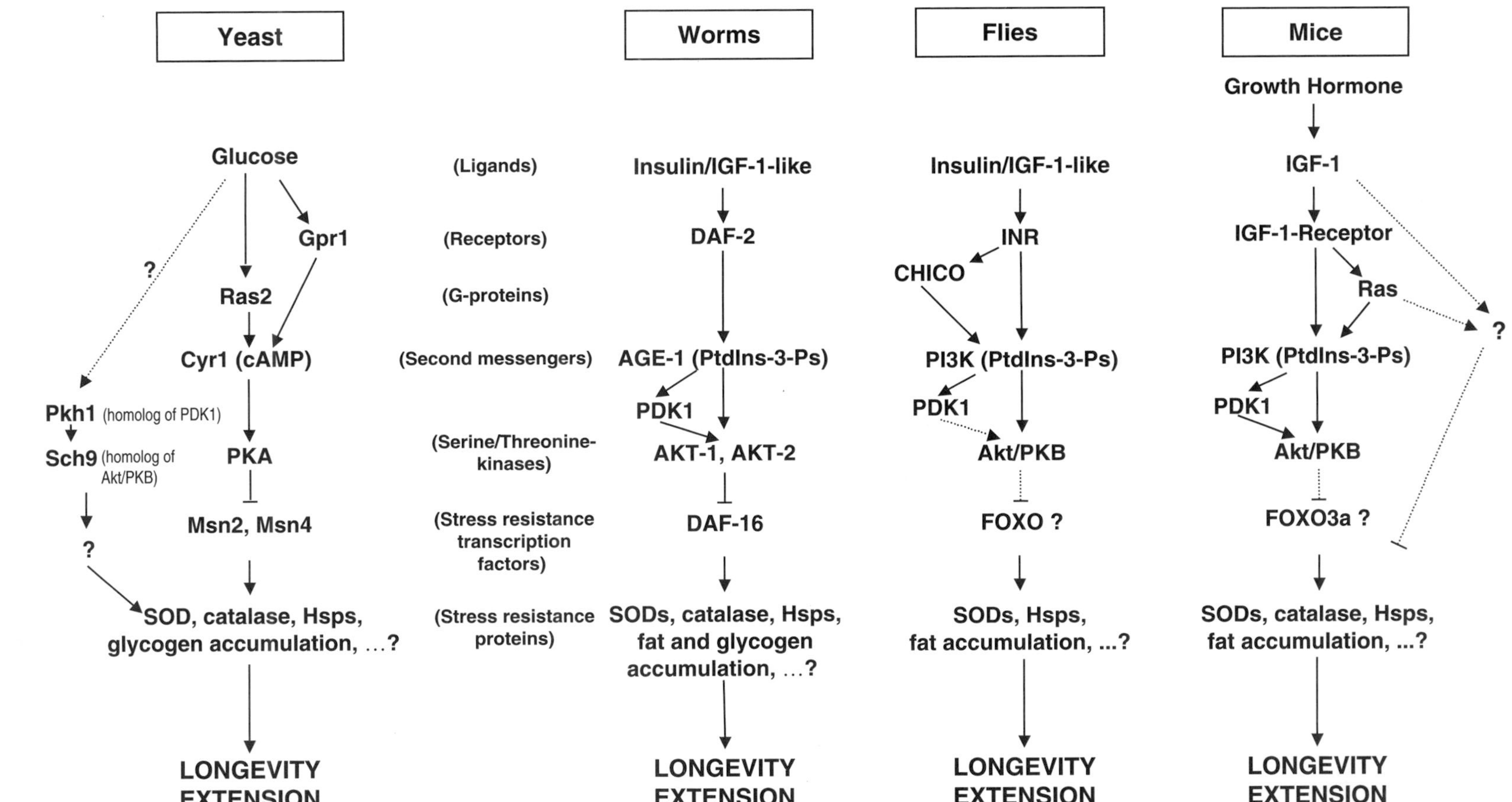

Figure 19.2. Conserved regulation of longevity. In yeast, worms, flies, and mice the down-regulation of partially conserved glucose or insulin/ insulin-like growth factor 1 (IGF-1) pathways promotes the expression of antioxidant enzymes and heat-shock proteins, induces the accumulation of glycogen or fat, and extends life span. In yeast and worms the induction of stress resistance is required for longevity extension. In flies and mice a conclusive role for stress resistance induction in promoting life span has not been established yet. Sch9 and Pkh1 are functional homologs of Akt1 and PDK1, respectively.

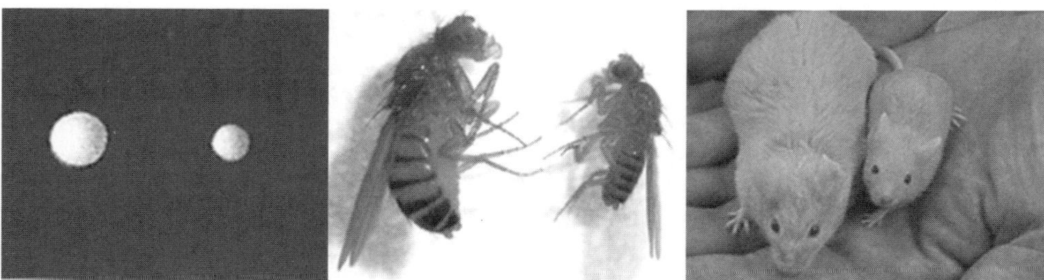

Figure 19.3. Wild-type (left) and long-lived "dwarf" (right) yeast, flies and mice with mutations that decrease glucose or insulin/IGF-I-like signaling. Yeast *sch9* null mutants form smaller colonies (left panel). *sch9* mutants are also smaller in size, grow at a slower rate, and survive three times longer than wild-type yeast. *Chico* homozygous mutant female flies are dwarfs and exhibit an increase in life span of up to 50% (center panel) (figure provided by D. Gems). Chico functions in the fly insulin/IGF-I-like signaling pathway. The GHR/BP mice are dwarfs deficient in IGF-I and exhibit a 50% increase in life span (right panel) (figure provided by A. Bartke). Other yeast and worm mutants exhibit life-span extension of more than 100% but do not have detectable growth defects. (Figure reproduced from *Science*, Vol. 299, pp. 1342–1346, 2003.)

separate PCR reactions. The UPTAG amplification uses primers B-U1 (5′biotin-GATGTCCACGAGGTCTCT) and B-U2- comp (5′biotin-GTCGACCTGCAGCG TACG); the DNTAG amplification uses B-D1 (5′biotin-CGGTGTCGGTCTCGTAG) and B-D2-comp (5′biotin-CGAGCTCGAATTCATCG). Biotinylated amplicons are combined and used to probe high-density oligonucleotide arrays. The arrays are stained with phycoerythrin–streptavidin and scanned at an emission wavelength of 560 nm. The enrichment or depletion of any specific deletion over time is determined by monitoring the changes in TAG intensities after normalizing using day 3 arrays. Based on the relative abundance of each strain on a time course, it is possible to identify genes whose expression is required for long-term survival (the corresponding deletion mutants disappear early in the experiment), and genes whose activity reduces the life span (the corresponding deletion mutants are found in the pool after the death of the majority of the population). We expect that most deletions will have either no effect or a negative effect on life span and that only a few deletions will cause major increases in life span. However, this method should allow an accurate classification of each deletion based on its negative, positive or neutral effect on survival. After identifying the potential long-lived deletion mutants, we will test each of them individually to confirm their life-span extension phenotype. We predict that this system will allow us to identify novel long-lived deletion mutants we previously missed because of the limitations of the mutagenesis method used.

Evolutionary Conserved Pro-Aging Pathways

Research conducted in the last decade has shown that aging is genetically regulated. More importantly, similar pro-aging pathways have been identified in all model organisms, suggesting that a strategy to regulate life span may have appeared early during evolution (Kenyon, 2001; Longo and Finch, 2003) (Figures 19.2–19.3).

As described in The Genetics of Chronological Aging: Yeast Methuselah Genes, two glucose-sensing pathways are responsible for the regulation of chronological aging in yeast: the Sch9 and the Ras/PKA pathways (Figure 19.2). Down-regulating the activity of these pathways promotes life-span extension by increasing thermotolerance and oxidative stress resistance and possibly by reducing cell metabolism (Fabrizio *et al.*, 2003; Fabrizio *et al.*, 2001).

Research conducted in *C. elegans* has identified the insulin/IGF-1-like pathway as a major pro-aging pathway (Figure 19.2). The similarities between yeast and worm aging pathways are remarkable. Analogously to the yeast Ras/PKA pathway, the insulin/IGF-1-like pathway senses the presence of nutrients and regulates entry into a hypometabolic stage (dauer larva) (Kimura *et al.*, 1997). Worm life span can be extended up to three times by reducing the activity of some of the components of the insulin/IGF-1-like pathway such as the cellular receptor DAF-2 and PI-3 kinase AGE-1 (Kimura *et al.*, 1997; Morris, 1996). Importantly, AGE-1 activates kinase Akt/PKB, which was shown to be homolog of yeast Sch9 and can also be activated by PDK-1, homolog of yeast Pkh1 (Figure 19.2) (Paradis *et al.*, 1999). Life-span extension in both daf-2 and age-1 mutants requires the activity of stress resistance transcription factor DAF-16, which belongs to the FOXO family transcription factors, and of the heat-shock transcription factor HSF-1, a highly conserved heat-shock protein (Hsu *et al.*, 2003; Ogg *et al.*, 1997). The mediators of longevity extension downstream of DAF-16 are also partially conserved between yeast and worms and include mitochondrial superoxide dismutase, catalase, and several heat-shock proteins (Figure 19.2). Long-lived mutants of both species store carbon in the form of glycogen (yeast and worm) or fat (worm).

The insulin-IGF-1 pathway has also been linked to the regulation of aging in *Drosophila* (Figures 19.2–19.3).

Reducing the activity of this pathway by mutating the insulin receptor (*InR*) or the insulin receptor substrate (*chico*) extends the life span of fruit fly by up to 85%. This life-span extension is associated with increased levels of superoxide dismutase activity and fat accumulation (Figure 19.2) (Clancy *et al.*, 2001; Tatar *et al.*, 2001). Notably, as shown in yeast, the mitochondrial enzyme aconitase is oxidatively modified and inactivated in old flies (see The Genetics of Chronological Aging: Yeast Methuselah Genes) (Yan *et al.*, 1997). Thus, impairing mitochondrial respiration by inactivating aconitase appears to be an age-dependent phenomenon shared between species, increasing superoxide dismutase activity—a common mechanism that contributes to longevity extension. Consistently, the overexpression of *SOD1/SOD2* in yeast and flies causes a modest but significant extension of life span (Fabrizio *et al.*, 2003; Orr and Sohal, 1994; Parkes *et al.*, 1998; Sun and Tower, 1999). The life span of *Drosophila* is also extended by overexpressing dFOXO, homolog of the worm DAF-16, in the peripheral fat body (Giannakou *et al.*, 2004; Hwangbo *et al.*, 2004).

Mammals have separate receptors for IGF-1 and insulin. Research in mice has connected both receptors to life-span regulation. Dwarf mice with defective pituitary gland, consequently deficient in growth hormone (GH), IGF-1, and insulin, live up to 65% longer than the wild type and are stress resistant (Brown-Borg *et al.*, 1996; Flurkey *et al.*, 2002) (Figures 19.2–19.3). The effect of dwarf mutations on life span appears to be caused by reduction in GH and IGF-I signaling. In fact, mice lacking the GH receptor are long-lived (Coschigano *et al.*, 2000), and IGF-1 receptor heterozygous knock-out mice live 30% longer than the wild type (Holzenberger *et al.*, 2003). Furthermore, mice lacking the insulin receptor in the adipose tissue live 18% longer than the wild type (Bluher *et al.*, 2003). Stress resistance also appears to be regulated by GH and IGF-I. In fact, the activities of superoxide dismutases and catalase are decreased after exposure of murine hepatocytes to GH or IGF-1 and in transgenic mice overexpressing GH (Brown-Borg and Rakoczy, 2000; Brown-Borg *et al.*, 2002). Like the worm daf-2 and the fly *InR* mutants, dwarf mice accumulate fat, suggesting that the accumulation of reserve carbon sources is an important and conserved portion of a maintenance mode aimed at slowing down aging and surviving through periods of starvation. Analogously, long-lived yeast mutants accumulate glycogen, their main reserve carbon source during starvation. Mammalian FOXOs transcription factors, homologs of the life-span extending DAF-16 and dFOXO transcription factors, have not been conclusively linked with life-span regulation in mammals. However, FOXO activity is associated with increased stress resistance and elevated mitochondrial superoxide dismutase activity in quiescent cells (Figure 19.2) (Kops *et al.*, 2002).

Taken together, the remarkable similarities between the life-span regulatory pathways of organisms ranging from yeast to mice suggest that they may have originated from a common ancestral pathway that regulated mechanisms of cell maintenance, protection against stress, and carbon storage in order to minimize aging during periods of starvation.

Conclusions

Ten years ago the genes and pathways that regulate the chronological life span of eukaryotes were unknown. Since then, studies mostly performed in *S. cerevisiae*, *C. elegans*, *Drosophila*, and mice have resulted in the identification of many genes and a few conserved pathways that can be activated or inactivated to extend the life span of the organism. These pathways also regulate stress resistance, the storage of reserve carbon sources, and entry into hypometabolic starvation response phases.

Worms, flies and mice are excellent model systems to study aging because of their progressively closer relationship to humans. By contrast, the unicellular *S. cerevisiae* is a valuable model system because it is very simple and amenable to powerful techniques and technologies such as transposon mutagenesis and high-density oligonucleotide genome-wide arrays of tagged deletion mutations. The information on the function or putative function of the majority of *S. cerevisiae* proteins contributes further to making this unicellular eukaryote one of the simplest and most valuable model systems to study the fundamental mechanisms of aging. Whereas aging in *S. cerevisiae* has been studied for 50 years by measuring the number of buds generated by an individual mother cell, studies of the chronological life span of yeast populations have been mostly published in the past 10 years. These studies have indicated that yeast and higher eukaryotes use similar "molecular strategies" to regulate entry into maintenance phases that extend life span. These strategies, which include down-regulation of glucose- or IGF-I-like receptor activated signal transduction proteins, up-regulation of antioxidant enzymes and heat shock proteins, and increased storage of reserve nutrients, are likely to also extend to many additional biological processes including repair and replacement systems. We predict that we will continue to observe many similarities and some differences between the genes and pathways that regulate aging and life span in yeast and higher eukaryotes. An important aim should be to determine whether the knowledge of these conserved "antiaging" pathways can be applied to the development of drugs that cause a switch to an antidisease mode in humans. Whereas modern medicine is focused on the treatment of diseases, the identification of Methuselah genes could ignite a novel "evolutionary medicine" approach in which multiple diseases of aging including cancer, Alzheimer's, and cardiovascular diseases are prevented pharmacologically.

REFERENCES

Bitterman, K.J., Medvedik, O., and Sinclair, D.A. (2003). Longevity regulation in *Saccharomyces cerevisiae*: Linking metabolism, genome stability, and heterochromatin. *Microbiol Mol Biol Rev 67*, 376–399, table of contents.

Bluher, M., Kahn, B.B., and Kahn, C.R. (2003). Extended longevity in mice lacking the insulin receptor in adipose tissue. *Science 299*, 572–574.

Boy-Marcotte, E., Perrot, M., Bussereau, F., Boucherie, H., and Jacquet, M. (1998). Msn2p and Msn4p control a large number of genes induced at the diauxic transition which are repressed by cyclic AMP in *Saccharomyces cerevisiae*. *J Bacteriol 180*, 1044–1052.

Braunstein, M., Rose, A.B., Holmes, S.G., Allis, C.D., and Broach, J.R. (1993). Transcriptional silencing in yeast is associated with reduced nucleosome acetylation. *Genes Dev 7*, 592–604.

Brown-Borg, H.M., Borg, K.E., Meliska, C.J., and Bartke, A. (1996). Dwarf mice and the ageing process. *Nature 384*, 33.

Brown-Borg, H.M., and Rakoczy, S.G. (2000). Catalase expression in delayed and premature aging mouse models. *Exp Gerontol 35*, 199–212.

Brown-Borg, H.M., Rakoczy, S.G., Romanick, M.A., and Kennedy, M.A. (2002). Effects of growth hormone and insulin-like growth factor-1 on hepatocyte antioxidative enzymes. *Exp Biol Med 227*, 94–104.

Clancy, D.J., Gems, D., Harshman, L.G., Oldham, S., Stocker, H., Hafen, E., Leevers, S.J., and Partridge, L. (2001). Extension of life-span by loss of CHICO, a *Drosophila* insulin receptor substrate protein. *Science 292*, 104–106.

Codon, A.C., Gasent-Ramirez, J.M., and Benitez, T. (1995). Factors which affect the frequency of sporulation and tetrad formation in *Saccharomyces cerevisiae* baker's yeasts [published erratum appears in Appl Environ Microbiol 1995 Apr; 61(4):1677]. *Appl Environ Microbiol 61*, 630–638.

Coschigano, K.T., Clemmons, D., Bellush, L.L., and Kopchick, J.J. (2000). Assessment of growth parameters and life span of GHR/BP gene-disrupted mice. *Endocrinology 141*, 2608–2613.

D'Mello, N.P., Childress, A.M., Franklin, D.S., Kale, S.P., Pinswasdi, C., and Jazwinski, S.M. (1994). Cloning and characterization of LAG1, a longevity-assurance gene in yeast. *J Biol Chem 269*, 15451–15459.

Fabrizio, P., Battistella, L., Vardavas, R., Gattazzo, C., Liou, L.L., Diaspro, A., *et al.* (2004a). Superoxide is a mediator of an altruistic aging program in *Saccharomyces cerevisiae*. *J Cell Biol 166*, 1055–1067.

Fabrizio, P., Liou, L.L., Moy, V.N., Diaspro, A., Selverstone-Valentine, J., Gralla, E.B., and Longo, V.D. (2003). SOD2 functions downstream of Sch9 to extend longevity in yeast. *Genetics 163*, 35–46.

Fabrizio, P., Pletcher, S.D., Minois, N., Vaupel, J.W., and Longo, V.D. (2004b). Chronological aging-independent replicative life span regulation by Msn2/Msn4 and Sod2 in *Saccharomyces cerevisiae*. *FEBS Lett 557*, 136–142.

Fabrizio, P., Pozza, F., Pletcher, S.D., Gendron, C.M., and Longo, V.D. (2001). Regulation of longevity and stress resistance by Sch9 in yeast. *Science 292*, 288–290.

Flurkey, K., Papaconstantinou, J., and Harrison, D.E. (2002). The Snell dwarf mutation Pit1(dw) can increase life span in mice. *Mech Ageing Dev 123*, 121–130.

Geyskens, I., Kumara, S., Donaton, M., Bergsma, J., Thevelein, J., and Wera, S. (2000). Expression of mammalian PKB complements deletion of the yeast protein kinase Sch9. *Nato Science Series A316*, 117–126.

Giaever, G., Chu, A.M., Ni, L., Connelly, C., Riles, L., Veronneau, S., *et al.* (2002). Functional profiling of the *Saccharomyces cerevisiae* genome. *Nature 418*, 387–391.

Giannakou, M.E., Goss, M., Junger, M.A., Hafen, E., Leevers, S.J., and Partridge, L. (2004). Long-lived *Drosophila* with overexpressed dFOXO in adult fat body. *Science 305*, 361.

Guarente, L. (2001). SIR2 and aging—The exception that proves the rule. *Trends Genet 17*, 391–392.

Harris, N., Costa, V., MacLean, M., Mollapour, M., Moradas-Ferreira, P., and Piper, P.W. (2003). MnSOD overexpression extends the yeast chronological (G(0)) life span but acts independently of Sir2p histone deacetylase to shorten the replicative life span of dividing cells. *Free Radic Biol Med 34*, 1599–1606.

Harris, N., MacLean, M., Hatzianthis, K., Panaretou, B., and Piper, P.W. (2001). Increasing *Saccharomyces cerevisiae* stress resistance, through the overactivation of the heat shock response resulting from defects in the Hsp90 chaperone, does not extend replicative life span but can be associated with slower chronological ageing of nondividing cells. *Mol Genet Genomics 265*, 258–263.

Herker, E., Jungwirth, H., Lehmann, K.A., Maldener, C., Frohlich, K.U., Wissing, S., *et al.* (2004). Chronological aging leads to apoptosis in yeast. *J Cell Biol 164*, 501–507.

Holzenberger, M., Dupont, J., Ducos, B., Leneuve, P., Geloen, A., Even, P.C., *et al.* (2003). IGF-1 receptor regulates lifespan and resistance to oxidative stress in mice. *Nature 421*, 182–187.

Hsu, A.L., Murphy, C.T., and Kenyon, C. (2003). Regulation of aging and age-related disease by DAF-16 and heat shock factor. *Science 300*, 1142–1145.

Hwangbo, D.S., Gersham, B., Tu, M.P., Palmer, M., and Tatar, M. (2004). *Drosophila* dFOXO controls lifespan and regulates insulin signalling in brain and fat body. *Nature 429*, 562–566.

Jorgensen, P., Nishikawa, J.L., Breitkreutz, B.J., and Tyers, M. (2002). Systematic identification of pathways that couple cell growth and division in yeast. *Science 297*, 395–400.

Jorgensen, P., Rupes, I., Sharom, J.R., Schneper, L., Broach, J.R., and Tyers, M. (2004). A dynamic transcriptional network communicates growth potential to ribosome synthesis and critical cell size. *Genes Dev 18*, 2491–2505.

Kaeberlein, M., McVey, M., and Guarente, L. (1999). The SIR2/3/4 complex and SIR2 alone promote longevity in *Saccharomyces cerevisiae* by two different mechanisms. *Genes Dev 13*, 2570–2580.

Kenyon, C. (2001). A conserved regulatory system for aging. *Cell 105*, 165–168.

Kimura, K.D., Tissenbaum, H.A., Liu, Y., and Ruvkun, G. (1997). *daf-2*, an insulin receptor-like gene that regulates longevity and diapause in *Caenorhabditis elegans*. *Science 277*, 942–946.

Kirchman, P.A., Kim, S., Lai, C.Y., and Jazwinski, S.M. (1999). Interorganelle signaling is a determinant of longevity in *Saccharomyces cerevisiae*. *Genetics 152*, 179–190.

Kops, G.J., Dansen, T.B., Polderman, P.E., Saarloos, I., Wirtz, K.W., Coffer, P.J., *et al.* (2002). Forkhead transcription factor FOXO3a protects quiescent cells from oxidative stress. *Nature 419*, 316–321.

Liu, K., Zhang, X., Lester, R.L., and Dickson, R.C. (2005). The sphingolipid long chain base phytosphingosine activates AGC kinases in *Saccharomyces cerevisiae* including Ypk1, Ypk2 and Sch9. *J Biol Chem. 280*, 22679–22687.

Longo, V.D., and Finch, C.E. (2003). Evolutionary medicine: From dwarf model systems to healthy centenarians. *Science 299*, 1342–1346.

Lyman, C.P., O'Brien, R.C., Greene, G.C., and Papagrangos, E.D. (1981). Hybernational longevity in the Turkish hamster *Mesocricetus brandti. Science 212*, 668–670.

Madeo, F., Herker, E., Maldener, C., Wissing, S., Lachelt, S., Herlan, M., *et al.* (2002). A caspase-related protease regulates apoptosis in yeast. *Mol Cell 9*, 911–917.

Melov, S., Ravenscroft, J., Malik, S., Gill, M.S., Walker, D.W., Clayton, P.E., *et al.* (2000). Extension of life-span with superoxide dismutase/catalase mimetics. *Science 289*, 1567–1569.

Morris, J.Z., Tissenbaum, H.A., and Ruvkun G. (1996). A phospatidylinositol-3-OH kinase family member regulating longevity and diapause in *Caenorhbditis elegans. Nature 382*, 536–539.

Mortimer, R.K. (1959). Life span of individual yeast cells. *Nature 183*, 1751–1752.

Ogg, S., Paradis, S., Gottlieb, S., Patterson, G.I., Lee, L., Tissenbaum, H.A., and Ruvkun, G. (1997). The Fork head transcription factor DAF-16 transduces insulin-like metabolic and longevity signals in *C. elegans. Nature 389*, 994–999.

Orr, W.C., and Sohal, R.S. (1994). Extension of life-span by overexpression of superoxide dismutase and catalase in *Drosophila melanogaster. Science 263*, 1128–1130.

Paradis, S., Ailion, M., Toker, A., Thomas, J.H., and Ruvkun, G. (1999). A PDK1 homolog is necessary and sufficient to transduce AGE-1 PI3 kinase signals that regulate diapause in *Caenorhabditis elegans. Genes Dev 13*, 1438–1452.

Parkes, T.L., Elia, A.J., Dickinson, D., Hilliker, A.J., Phillips, J.P., and Boulianne, G.L. (1998). Extension of *Drosophila* lifespan by overexpression of human SOD1 in motorneurons. *Nat Genet 19*, 171–174.

Riddle, D.L. (1988). *The Nematode C. elegans* (Cold Spring Harbor, NY, Cold Spring Harbor Laboratory Press).

Rogina, B., and Helfand, S.L. (2004). Sir2 mediates longevity in the fly through a pathway related to calorie restriction. *Proc Natl Acad Sci USA 101*, 15998–16003.

Roosen, J., Engelen, K., Marchal, K., Mathys, J., Griffioen, G., Cameroni, E., *et al.* (2005). PKA and Sch9 control a molecular switch important for the proper adaptation to nutrient availability. *Mol Microbiol 55*, 862–880.

Schmitt, A.P., and McEntee K. (1996). Msn2p, a zinc finger DNA-binding protein, is the transcriptional activator of the multistress response in *Saccharomyces cerevisiae. PNAS 93*, 5777–5782.

Schriner, S.E., Linford, N.J., Martin, G.M., Treuting, P., Ogburn, C.E., Emond, M., *et al.* (2005). Extension of murine lifespan by overexpression of catalase targeted to Mitochondria. *Science 808*, 1909–1911.

Sinclair, D.A., and Guarente, L. (1997). Extrachromosomal rDNA circles—A cause of aging in yeast. *Cell 91*, 1033–1042.

Smith, A., Ward, M.P., and Garrett, S. (1998). Yeast PKA represses Msn2p/Msn4p-dependent gene expression to regulate growth, stress response and glycogen accumulation. *Embo J 17*, 3556–3564.

Sun, J., Kale, S.P., Childress, A.M., Pinswasdi, C., and Jazwinski, S.M. (1994). Divergent roles of RAS1 and RAS2 in yeast longevity. *J Biol Chem 269*, 18638–18645.

Sun, J., and Tower, J. (1999). FLP recombinase-mediated induction of Cu/Zn-superoxide dismutase transgene expression can extend the life span of adult *Drosophila melanogaster* flies. *Mol Cell Biol 19*, 216–228.

Tanny, J.C., Dowd, G.J., Huang, J., Hilz, H., and Moazed, D. (1999). An enzymatic activity in the yeast Sir2 protein that is essential for gene silencing. *Cell 99*, 735–745.

Tatar, M., Kopelman, A., Epstein, D., Tu, M.P., Yin, C.M., and Garofalo, R.S. (2001). A mutant *Drosophila* insulin receptor homolog that extends life-span and impairs neuroendocrine function. *Science 292*, 107–110.

Tissenbaum, H.A., and Guarente, L. (2001). Increased dosage of a sir-2 gene extends lifespan in *Caenorhabditis elegans. Nature 410*, 227–230.

Toda, T., Cameron, S., Sass, P., and Wigler, M. (1988). *SCH9*, a gene of *Saccharomyces cerevisiae* that encodes a protein distinct from, but functionally and structurally related to, cAMP-dependent protein kinase catalytic subunits. *Genes Dev 2*, 517–527.

Wach, A., Brachat, A., Pohlmann, R., and Philippsen, P. (1994). New heterologous modules for classical or PCR-based gene disruptions in *Saccharomyces cerevisiae. Yeast 10*, 1793–1808.

Werner-Washburne, M., Braun, E.L., Crawford, M.E., and Peck, V.M. (1996). Stationary phase in *Saccharomyces cerevisiae. Mol Microbiol 19*, 1159–1166.

Wissing, S., Ludovico, P., Herker, E., Buttner, S., Engelhardt, S.M., Decker, T., *et al.* (2004). An AIF orthologue regulates apoptosis in yeast. *J Cell Biol 166*, 969–974.

Wood, J.G., Rogina, B., Lavu, S., Howitz, K., Helfand, S.L., Tatar, M., and Sinclair, D. (2004). Sirtuin activators mimic caloric restriction and delay ageing in metazoans. *Nature 430*, 686–689.

Yan, L.J., Levine, R.L., and Sohal, R.S. (1997). Oxidative damage during aging targets mitochondrial aconitase [published erratum appears in Proc Natl Acad Sci USA 1998 Feb 17;95(4):1968]. *Proc Natl Acad Sci USA 94*, 11168–11172.

Zambrano, M.M., and Kolter, R. (1996). GASPing for life in stationary phase. *Cell 86*, 181–184.

20

Strongyloides ratti: A Nematode with Extraordinary Plasticity in Aging

Michael P. Gardner, Mark E. Viney and David Gems

Aging has been characterized in detail in relatively few animal species. Here we describe the aging process of a nematode with an unusual life cycle, Strongyloides ratti. *This organism has distinct parasitic and free-living reproductive adult forms, which are genetically identical.* S. ratti *exhibits a remarkably high degree of phenotypic plasticity of aging: the maximum lifespan of parasitic adults is 80 times greater than that of free-living adults (403 and 5 days, respectively). Free-living* S. ratti *adults are short-lived even by terrestrial nematode standards; their lifespan is approximately only 30% of that of the short-lived free-living nematode model species* C. elegans. *Phenomenologically, aging appears similar in* S. ratti *free-living adults and* C. elegans, *except that it unfolds much more rapidly in* S. ratti. *Demographic senescence (a hallmark of aging) occurs in free-living* S. ratti, *with a mortality rate doubling time (MRDT) of 0.8 ± 0.1 days (females), compared with 2.0 ± 0.3 in* C. elegans. *Likewise, parasitic* S. ratti *undergo senescence, but have an MRDT approximately 30 times greater than that of free-living adults of* S. ratti. *Among nematodes, parasitic species are generally longer-lived than free-living species. This presumably reflects the evolutionary consequences of differences in levels extrinsic mortality experienced in their respective niches. Here, we describe in detail the aging process in the two adult forms of* S. ratti *and explore how these different lifespans might have evolved, despite sharing the same genome. In this species, an evolved and vast difference in the rate of aging appears to be determined by gene expression alone. This implies that, at least in this one species, "late-acting deleterious mutations" correspond to regulated differences in gene expression that generate a shorter lifespan. Potentially, differences in lifespan between species might evolve via similar mechanisms, involving mutationally driven alterations in gene expression.*

Introduction

Our understanding of aging in certain model species such as the nematode *Caenorhabditis elegans*, the fruitfly *Drosophila melanogaster*, and the mouse is well advanced (Longo and Finch, 2003). However, there are still relatively few animal species for which there are even basic descriptions of how they age. Among nematodes, patterns of aging are highly diverse, and lifespans can vary over more than a 1,000 fold range (Gems, 2001). *Strongyloides ratti*, the subject of this chapter, is a nematode that has previously been used as a model organism in parasitological studies (Grove, 1989). As a biogerontological model, it is attractive because of its unique level of phenotypic plasticity in aging and the genetics of its life cycle.

Much has been learned about the genetics of lifespan by the use of mutational studies in model organisms. In *C. elegans*, increases in lifespan of up to 7-fold have been observed in long-lived mutants (Houthoofd *et al.*, 2004). While substantial, such differences are relatively small, compared with evolved differences in lifespan between different animal species. The genetic basis of such evolved differences remains unknown. It is also unclear whether similar genes and mechanisms underlie both the altered aging in model organisms as uncovered by the analysis of mutants and the evolved differences in aging between different species. These issues may be explored via a comparative approach and through insights gained into the biology of aging from the existing diversity in evolved patterns of aging in the animal kingdom. Thus, it is worthwhile to study the basic phenomenology of aging in species with interesting life histories, such as *S. ratti*.

Many animal species show phenotypic plasticity in aging, of which there are two major types. The first is the relatively limited response to a changing environment by a given stage in the life cycle. For example, dietary restriction extends lifespan in many species, including rodents (McCay *et al.*, 1935), *Drosophila* (Nusbaum and Rose, 1999), and *C. elegans* (Lakowski and Hekimi, 1998). A more dramatic form of phenotypic plasticity in aging is associated with the development of different morphs within a given life cycle. For example, in *C. elegans* there is a facultative diapausal form of the third-stage larva, known as the dauer larva. This long-lived stress-resistant dispersal form develops when food is scarce and population density high (Golden and Riddle, 1984) and can survive for up to 3 months (Klass and Hirsh, 1976). This compares to a two- or three-week lifespan in *C. elegans* adults (Klass, 1977). Striking differences in lifespan between adult morphs also occur in social insects (Finch, 1990), where honey bee queens survive for up to 40-times longer than genetically identical summer worker bees. Understanding the evolutionary and physiological determinants of such plasticity of aging and lifespan can provide insight into the biology of aging.

In this chapter we review what is known about *S. ratti* aging. We describe optimization of culture conditions for aging studies, environmental factors that affect lifespan, and age changes in behavior, pathology and mortality that accompany aging in this unusual nematode. In the concluding section, we consider the question of how the phenotypic plasticity in *S. ratti* may have evolved.

Aging in *S. ratti*

WHAT IS *S. RATTI*?

Strongyloides is a genus of parasitic nematodes that infect a wide variety of vertebrates (mammals, birds, amphibians, reptiles); two species (*S. stercoralis* and *S. fuelleborni*) infect humans (Speare, 1989). Some 50 million individuals are infected with *Strongyloides* spp. worldwide (Grove, 1989). For most individuals there are often no overt signs of infection. However, in individuals that are immunocompromised the infection can disseminate throughout the body and is fatal in the absence of anti-*Strongyloides* therapy. *S. ratti* has been used for some years as a model organism for investigating the biology of nematode parasitic infections (Viney, 1999).

Strongyloides spp. have an unusual and complex life cycle involving both free-living and parasitic phases (Figure 20.1).

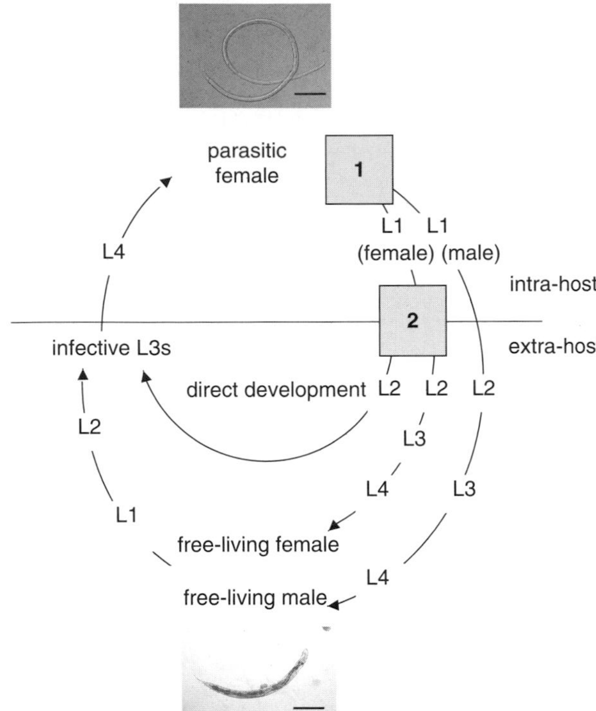

Figure 20.1. Life cycle of *Strongyloides ratti* with two discrete developmental switches, shown as grey boxes: (1) a sex determination event; (2) a female-only developmental switch. Adapted from Harvey *et al.*, (2000). Also included are larval stages L1–L4. The life cycle contains both parasitic and free-living generations; an adult parasitic female (left) and free-living adult female (right). Bars = 200 μm.

Parasitic adult females dwell in the gut of the host (which in the case of *S. ratti*, as its name implies, is the rat). Here they burrow into the intestinal mucosa and reproduce by mitotic parthenogenesis (Viney, 1994), passing eggs via the feces into the external environment. These eggs can either moult through two larval stages into infective third-stage larvae (iL3s) or through four larval stages into free-living adult females and males (Figure 20.1). These adults mate by conventional sexual reproduction and produce progeny which (as above) can develop into iL3s (Viney *et al.*, 1993; Harvey *et al.*, 2000). Infective L3s infect new hosts by skin penetration. Experimental genetic studies found that reproduction of the parasitic females of *S. ratti* is functionally mitotic (Viney, 1994), and so the progeny of the parasitic female are genetically identical to each other and to their mother. Anecdotal observations had noted a large difference in the lifespan potential of the adult free-living and parasitic female morphs: approximately one week and one year, respectively (Viney, 1994; Gemill *et al.*, 1997). However, the role of aging in this apparent difference was unknown.

CULTURE CONDITIONS FOR *S. RATTI*

Parasitic S. ratti

The parasitic stages of *S. ratti* are maintained in the laboratory by infecting rats. Immunologically normal animals mount an immune response against these infections, such that the infections are lost after four to six weeks (Wilkes *et al.*, 2004). However, long-term infections can be established in immunologically deficient (nude) rats (Gemill *et al.*, 1997). Feces collected from infected rats contain the eggs or first-stage larvae. These feces can be collected and used to make fecal cultures, from which all the free-living stages of the life cycle can be grown. Infective L3s obtained from such cultures are used to initiate new infections, which is done by the subcutaneous administration of iL3s to naïve rats (Gemill *et al.*, 1997; Wilkes *et al.*, 2004).

Free-living S. ratti

For the analysis of aging and lifespan, the culture conditions used for the free-living adult *S. ratti* are based on those used for *C. elegans*. The latter are typically maintained on NGM agar seeded with *Escherichia coli* strain OP50 (a uracil auxotroph) as a food source (Sulston and Hodgkin, 1988). For *S. ratti*, L4 female and male worms are taken from 2-day old rat fecal cultures (19°C), cleaned by repeated washing in sterile distilled water to remove associated bacteria, and then introduced onto NGM plates under optimized culture conditions (see below). To measure lifespan, survival of the free-living stages of *S. ratti* is measured at least daily, with scoring for death as described for *C. elegans* (Klass, 1977).

Cultures of *C. elegans* are monoxenic; that is, only the *E. coli* food source is present. In contrast, *S. ratti* larval stages derived from fecal cultures are inevitably contaminated with fecal bacteria, which may reduce their lifespan. To minimize this problem, the agar plates on which these *S. ratti* free-living stages are cultured contain 400 μg/ml streptomycin and are seeded with a streptomycin-resistant (SR) *E. coli* OP50 food source. Under these conditions, visible contamination by other microbes is reduced but not prevented. With these conditions the maximum mean lifespan ($\pm$ SE) of *S. ratti* females was 4.2 $\pm$ 0.2 days. This lifespan is significantly greater than that of *S. ratti* maintained without the presence of streptomycin (Gardner *et al.*, 2004; Figure 20.2A).

MEASURING AGING IN *S. RATTI*

Analysis of age-specific mortality

One feature of aging that has been observed throughout the animal kingdom is the exponential acceleration of

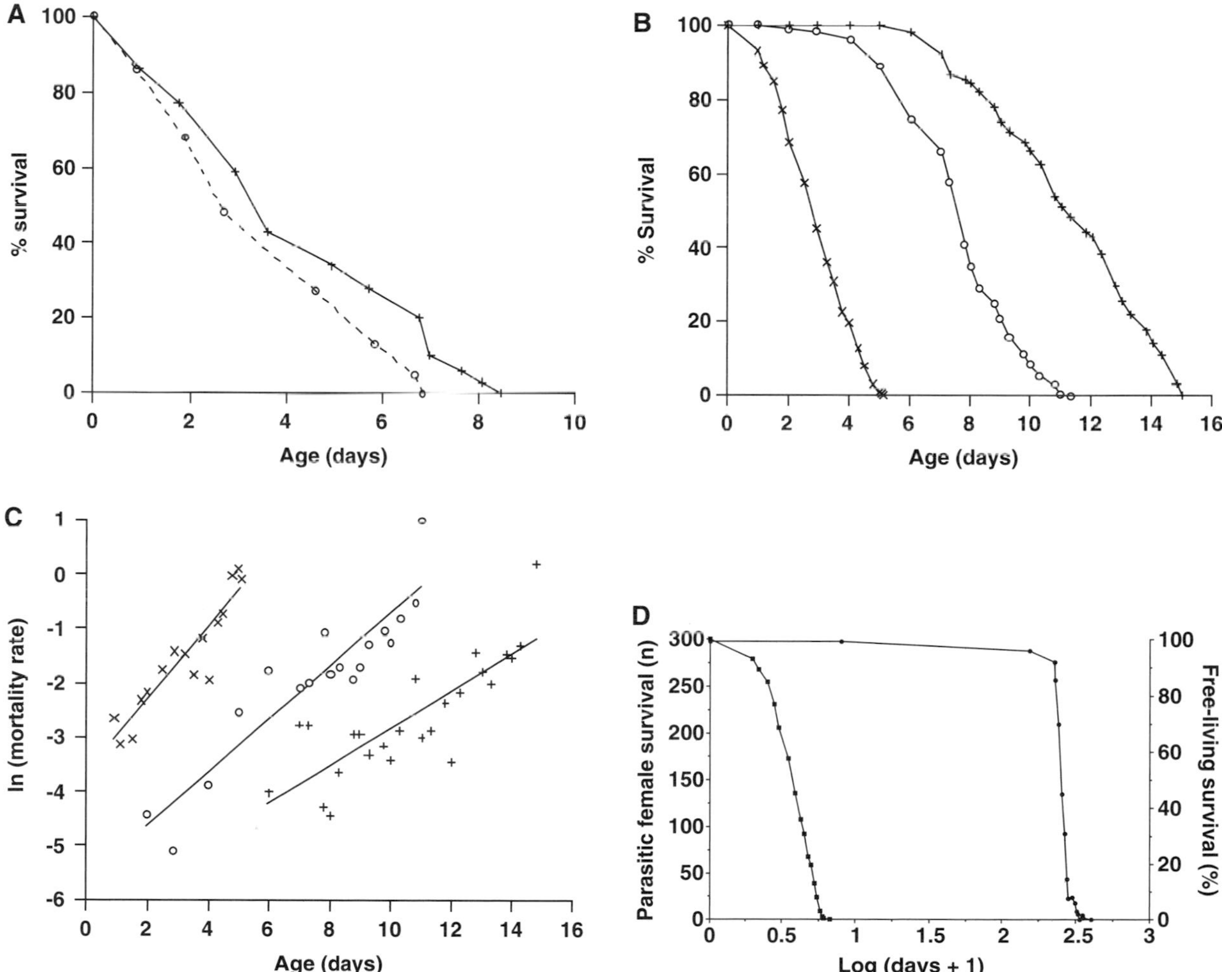

Figure 20.2. Factors affecting *S. ratti* lifespan. (A) Survivorship of virgin free-living females under optimized culture conditions (400mg/μl streptomycin and *E. coli* SR) (x, ——) and on *E. coli* OP50 (o, - - - -). (B) Survival and (C) Plots of ln($m(t)$) against age for *S. ratti* (x, ——) and *C. elegans* (o, ——) both in the *S, ratti*-optimized culture conditions (400mg/μl streptomycin and *E. coli* SR) and *C. elegans* (+, ——) in monoxenic culture conditions *E. coli* OP50. (D) The estimated number of parasitic females (•) and the percent survival of free-living females (■) over time, which is shown on a log scale. Figures 20.2D, 20.3C, and 20.4C are from Gardner, Gems and Viney, submitted. Figures 20.1, 20.2A–C, 20.3A–B and 20.4A–B are reprinted from Gardner, Gems and Viney, Aging in a very short-lived nematode, *Experimental Gerontology* Volume 39, 1267–1276 (2004) with permission from Elsevier.

the mortality rate with increasing age (Finch, 1990). The pattern of age-specific mortality in many species (including humans) can be described by the Gompertz equation, $m(t) = Ae^{\alpha t}$, where $m(t)$ is the mortality rate at time t, A is the initial mortality rate (IMR) and α is the Gompertz exponential function (Finch, 1990). Population cohorts may be extinguished as the result of mortality that is related or unrelated to aging; therefore, differences in lifespan *per se* do not necessarily reflect differences in the rate of aging. Limitations of lifespan by aging, as opposed to some other extrinsic cause of mortality (e.g., predation or disease), may be established by testing for the occurrence of an exponential increase in mortality rate with increasing age (Wachter and Finch, 1997). From plots of ln(mortality rate) against age, the IMR and the Gompertz exponential function can be calculated. The latter may be expressed in a form that is easier to grasp: the mortality rate doubling time (MRDT). These mortality parameters for free-living *S. ratti* females and parasitic *S. ratti* females are described below.

Age-specific mortality in S. ratti *free-living adult females*

The survival of free-living *S. ratti* females under optimized *S. ratti* culture conditions are shown in Figure 20.2B. This shows that its maximum lifespan is 4.5 ± 0.8 days. In our studies of free-living *S. ratti* we were at pains to distinguish whether the very short lifespan resulted from rapid aging, or from some form of pathology distinct from aging. To this end, we compared age changes in *S. ratti* with those in *C. elegans*. The latter was cultured either monoxenically (i.e., with *E. coli* OP50 alone), or under the same conditions as *S. ratti* (i.e. with SR OP50 and low-level contamination with other microbes). (Figure 20.2B).

The mean lifespan of *C. elegans* hermaphrodites under either culture condition (*S. ratti* conditions: 7.7 ± 0.1 days; monoxenic: 11.2 ± 0.1 days) was substantially and significantly longer than that of *S. ratti* (3.0 ± 0.1 days) (Gardner *et al.*, 2004; Figure 20.2B). Unsurprisingly, *C. elegans* lifespan was greater in monoxenic culture conditions than in *S. ratti* optimized culture conditions, presumably due to the presence of contaminating microbes in the *S. ratti* culture conditions (Figure 20.2B).

In all cases, an age-specific mortality rate acceleration was observed (Figure 20.2C), consistent with the occurence of senescence (i.e., intrinsic aging). For *S. ratti* the MRDT (±SE) was lower and the IMR (±SE) higher (0.8 ± 0.1 days; 0.025 ± 0.002 days^{-1}, respectively) than in *C. elegans* (in either culture condition). For *C. elegans* under the two culture conditions, there was no difference in the MRDT (*S. ratti*-conditions: 1.4±0.2 days; monoxenic conditions: 2.0±0.3 days), but the IMR for *C. elegans* kept under *S. ratti* culture conditions was almost twice that of monoxenically cultured populations (*S. ratti* conditions: 0.0036 ± 0.0003 days^{-1}; monoxenic: 0.0018 ± 0.0002 days^{-1}). Overall, these findings imply that *S. ratti* is shorter lived than *C. elegans* because (a) it is more frail, as reflected by higher IMR, and (b) it ages more quickly, as reflected by a lower MRDT.

Age-specific mortality in S. ratti *parasitic females*

In *S. ratti* parasitic females, maximum lifespan is 403 days (Gardner, Gems and Viney, submitted; Figure 20.2D), which compares to 5 days in the free-living morph (Figure 20.2D).

The maximum lifespan of *S. ratti* parasitic females is 403 days, which is some 80 times greater than the 5-day lifespan of the free-living females. The parasitic females underwent an exponential increase in mortality rate with age, thereby showing that senescence was occuring. The IMR of the parasitic females was 0.0056 days^{-1}, which is approximately 25% of that of the free-living females. The MRDT of the parasitic females was 22.7 days, which is some 30 times longer than that of the free-living females. Overall, this comparison of the parasitic and free-living females implies that free-living morphs are shorter-lived due to their increased frailty (as reflected by the greater IMR) and a faster rate of aging (as reflected by lower MRDT). *S. ratti* is the first parasitic nematode in which the occurrence of demographic senescence has been demonstrated in the laboratory.

FACTORS AFFECTING LIFESPAN IN FREE-LIVING *S. RATTI* AND *C. ELEGANS*

The lifespan of the free-living adult female *S. ratti* is really very short; in fact it is the shortest-lived nematode reported. One possibility is that this very short lifespan is not the result of aging in the usual sense. For example, mortality might result from failure to feed, or a gross anatomical defect not seen in other nematodes. To address these issues, we compared aging in free-living *S. ratti* with that in *C. elegans* in two ways. First, we tested the effect of factors known to affect aging in *C. elegans* and in *S. ratti* free-living adults. Second, we asked whether the age-associated changes in *C. elegans* behavior, morphology and appearance are also seen in *S. ratti*. Overall, our findings strongly support the view that the short lifespan in *S. ratti* free-living adults is the result of typical nematode aging, but which is happening at an unusually swift pace.

In *C. elegans*, lifespan is reduced by various factors, including the *E. coli* food source (Gems and Riddle, 2000; Garigan *et al.*, 2002), higher temperature (Klass, 1977), mating between the sexes (Gems and Riddle, 1996) and attempted mating between males (Gems and Riddle, 2000). In *S. ratti*, lifespan (Figure 20.3A) and lifetime fecundity (Figure 20.3B) were reduced by higher temperatures, as in *C. elegans* (Klass, 1977).

However, mating did not affect lifespan in *S. ratti* in the same way as it does in *C. elegans*. Thus, mating (manipulated by adjusting the male:female ratio from 0 to 4.0) had no effect on *S. ratti* free-living female lifespan,

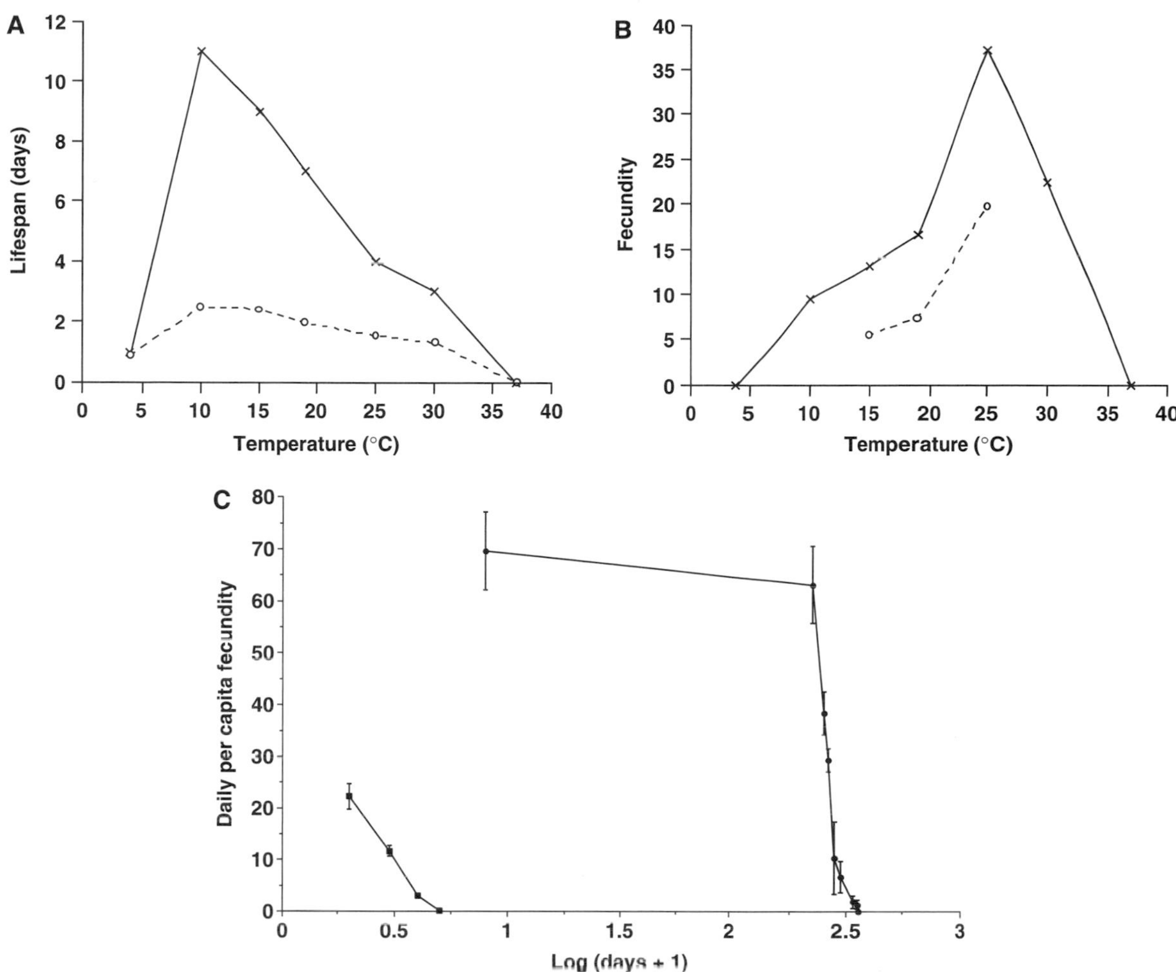

Figure 20.3. (A) Effects of temperature on mean (○, - - - -) and maximum (x, ——) lifespan of virgin free-living females. *S. ratti* adults die within 24 hours at 37°C. (B) Effect of temperature on mean *per capita* lifetime fecundity of *S. ratti* females, mated on day one only (○, - - - -) or mated throughout life (x, ——). (C) The mean (±1 SE) daily *per capita* fecundity of the parasitic females (●) and of the free-living females (■) (mean ±1 SE; adapted from Gardner *et al.*, 2004) over time, which is shown on a log scale.

whereas in males it actually increased lifespan. Thus lifespan in *S. ratti* and *C. elegans* is affected in the same way by some factors (temperature, food source in data not shown, proliferating bacteria) but in different ways by others (mating).

BEHAVIORAL CHANGES ACCOMPANYING AGING IN *S. RATTI*

Fecundity

The daily *per capita* fecundity of free-living *S. ratti* females fell rapidly with age, as in *C. elegans*, but more rapidly, halving between the first and second days of adult life (Figure 20.3C). The resultant maximum lifetime fecundity was less than 40 progeny per female, compared to over 1,400 in *C. elegans* (Hodgkin and Barnes, 1991). By contrast, the daily *per capita* fecundity of the parasitic adult morph was >50 for *c.* 250 days before it declined, giving a lifetime fecundity of ~16,000 (Gardner, Gems and Viney, submitted; Figure 20.3C).

Pharyngeal pumping rate and movement

In *C. elegans*, the rate of pharyngeal pumping (reflecting the rate of ingestion of food) declines gradually with age (Kenyon *et al.*, 1993). We observed a similar age-related decline in pharyngeal pumping rate in *S. ratti*. We also saw a similar age-related decline in movement in *S. ratti*, as in *C. elegans* (Herndon *et al.*, 2002). In each case the pattern of age-related change in *S. ratti* was similar, but more rapid than that in *C. elegans*.

MORPHOLOGICAL CHANGES ACCOMPANYING AGING IN *S. RATTI*

Autofluorescence

In *C. elegans*, there is an increase in intestinal autofluorescence with age (Garigan *et al.*, 2002), similar to accumulation of age-pigment (lipofuscin) seen during mammalian aging. There is a similar increase in autofluorescence with age in free-living *S. ratti* morphs (Gardner *et al.*, 2004). By contrast, little such autofluorescence was seen in parasitic females, even in 11-month-old individuals (Gardner, Gems and Viney, submitted). Lipofuscin accumulation reflects organismal failure to detoxify and excrete molecular waste products. The paucity of autofluorescence in *S. ratti* parasitic females suggests reduced generation, and/or increased excretion, of damaged molecular constituents. This is consistent with aging occurring in the two *S. ratti* female morphs, but at very different rates.

Microscopic examination of aging nematodes

The integrity of major anatomical features was compared in young and old *S. ratti* adults using differential interference contrast (DIC) and transmission electron microscopy (TEM) (Gardner *et al.*, 2004; Gardner, Gems and Viney, submitted). Overall, the appearance of aging *S. ratti* free-living females was similar to that of aging *C. elegans* (Herndon *et al.*, 2002). The pharynxes of older free-living *S. ratti* were frequently distended and blocked with bacteria. Such pharyngeal blockage has also been observed in older *C. elegans* (Garigan *et al.*, 2002). The most striking morphological age changes in free-living *S. ratti* occurred in the intestine (Gardner *et al.*, 2004). Whilst in one-day-old animals there were large, healthy looking refractile intestinal cells (Figure 20.4A), in the majority of four-day-old animals these cells were severely atrophied and the cytoplasm had a ragged appearance (Figure 20.4B).

By contrast, older parasitic females showed no marked degenerate changes.

TEM observations of free-living females showed numerous inclusions in the intestinal cytoplasm whose

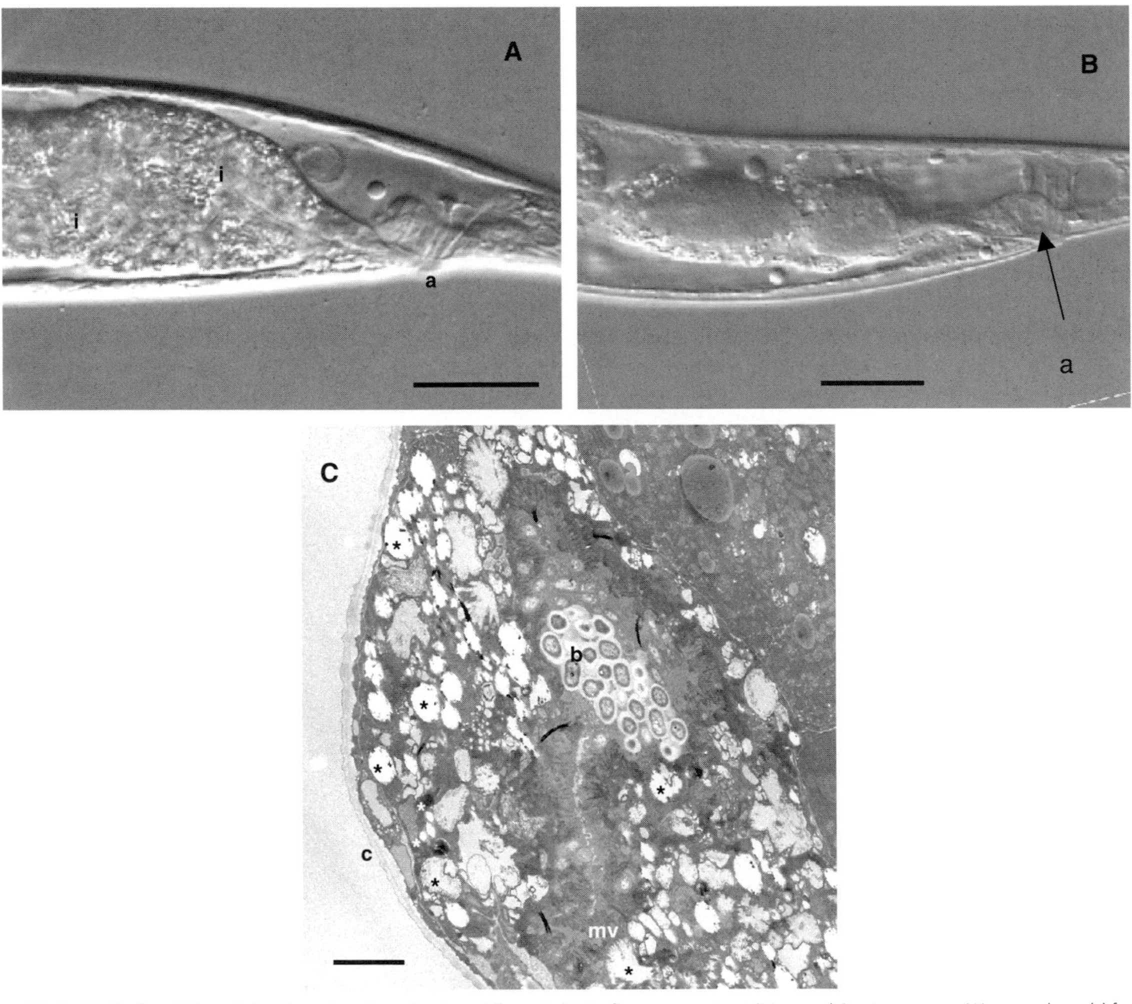

Figure 20.4. (A–B) *S. ratti* free-living females viewed using differential interference contrast (Nomarski) microscopy. (A): one-day-old female; (B), four-day-old adults. (A) and (B): posterior intestine. In (A), note the large, healthy refractile intestinal cells (i). In (B), the intestine is strikingly atrophied. Anus (a). Bars = 20 μm. (C) TEM of four-day-old free-living females with electron-dense inclusions of intestinal cells indicated by * (Bar = 2 μm); c, cuticle; mv, microvilli; b, clump of bacteria in lumen.

number increased with age (Figure 20.4C). Most of these resembled lipid droplets (or possibly secondary lysosomes) within which have accumulated electron-opaque particles with a sooty appearance. By contrast, there were very few such inclusions in the intestines of parasitic females and their number did not change with age. These observations suggest that degeneration of the intestine, possibly associated with accumulation of fluorescent/electron opaque waste material, represents a pathology of aging that contributes to nematode pathology. This idea was previously put forward based on TEM studies of aging in *Caenorhabditis briggsae* (Epstein *et al.*, 1972). The fact that this pathology was not detected in the intestine of the parasitic *S. ratti* adult is consistent with the idea that the absence of this pathology contributes to parasitic longevity.

The parasitic and free-living females morphs of *S. ratti* are genetically identical. Therefore differences between these morphs must be due to differences in gene expression. This being so, these differences in intestinal pathology might reflect differences in regulated biochemical processes which determine longevity and aging. One intriguing and attractive possibility is that in parasitic females there is an increase in biochemical processes promoting detoxification. Recent microarray studies of long-lived insulin/IGF-1 signalling mutants of *C. elegans* have implicated a broad range of detoxification processes in longevity assurance (Murphy *et al.*, 2003; McElwee *et al.*, 2004; Gems and McElwee, 2005). These include phase 1 and phase 2 drug detoxification, as well as antioxidant enzyme and chaperonin activities. Most of these processes require energy input, and excretion of solubilized toxic metabolites by the drug detoxification system occurs via the smooth endoplasmic reticulum. Interestingly, intestinal cells of parasitic *S. ratti* adults are rich with mitochondria and smooth endoplasmic reticulum.

Conclusion

LEARNING ABOUT LIFESPAN EVOLUTION FROM *S. RATTI*

In this chapter we have described the uniquely high level of phenotypic plasticity in aging in *Strongyloides ratti*, corresponding to an 80-fold difference in lifespan, accompanied by a 400-fold difference in maximum fecundity. While these represent something of a comparative gerontological party trick, does it provide any real insight into the biology of aging? Arguably, the existence of plasticity of this sort has implications for the genetic mechanisms underlying lifespan evolution.

Evolutionary theory predicts that organisms in environments with a low rate of extrinsic mortality will evolve slower rates of aging than those in environments with a high rate of extrinsic mortality (Medawar, 1952; Williams, 1957). This is because high levels of extrinsic mortality reduce selection against alleles which produce deleterious effects later in life. As a consequence, populations experiencing higher extrinsic mortality will accumulate such late-acting deleterious alleles, which cause aging. If alleles are pleiotropic, and capable of producing phenotypic effects at different time in an animal's life, there may be selection for alleles which enhance fitness due to early effects, despite later deleterious effects (antagonistic pleiotropy).

The relationship between extrinsic mortality rate and aging has been supported by numerous comparative studies. For example, bats generally live longer than rodents of a similar size, presumably since flight aids predator evasion, reducing extrinsic mortality (Wilkinson and South, 2002). Evolution results in intraspecific as well as interspecific differences in lifespan. For example, in social insect species there are intercaste differences in lifespan which may reflect the evolutionary effects of different levels of extrinsic mortality on rates of aging (Page and Peng, 2001; Chapuisat and Keller, 2002). However, the extent to which these lifespan differences are the result of differences in the rate of aging remains unclear. For example, Chapuisat and Keller (2002) compared survival in large and small worker ants, and found that the smaller workers lived significantly longer, which they hypothesized was because the larger morphs were fighting and getting killed more quickly.

Thus, here lifespan differences are not due to differences in aging but rather, just differences in extrinsic mortality rates.

Although the evolutionary theory of aging provides an explanation for how different aging rates evolve, in terms of molecular or developmental genetics, the concept of "late-acting deleterious mutations" remains frustratingly abstract. Potentially, the pattern of aging in *S. ratti* provides a clue as to the molecular genetic basis of lifespan evolution, as follows. Free-living nematodes are typically much shorter lived than parasitic nematodes, some of which have lifespans of over a decade (Gems, 2001). These evolved differences are likely to reflect differences in extrinsic mortality experienced by free-living versus parasitic species. Hence the difference in lifespan of free-living and parasitic *S. ratti* seems consistent with the evolutionary theory of aging. What is interesting about *S. ratti* is that the two adult forms have evolved such a vast difference in aging rate, despite the fact that they are the same species, sharing a common genome.

That this is possible sheds some light on the nature of "late-acting deleterious mutations." According to an evolutionary interpretation, free-living *S. ratti* have evolved a short lifespan due to high extrinsic mortality rate and accumulation of alleles with deleterious late-acting effects. However, one might expect that these alleles would be purged from the population by selection against them in the parasitic adult. The nature of *S. ratti* clearly demonstrates that this has not happened, and in this sense its evolution represents a useful experiment of nature. What is also clear from *S. ratti* is that the evolved difference in lifespan between the two adult forms is the product of differential gene expression. This tells us that, at least in this one species, "late-acting deleterious mutations" actually reflect regulated differences in gene expression leading to shorter lifespan.

Aging is a trait which shows remarkable evolutionary plasticity and is able to evolve rapidly. For example, humans and chimpanzees have evolved a difference in maximum lifespan of some 50 years since divergence from a common ancestor only 6–7 million years ago. It has been suggested that there are "lifespan regulatory modules," which are regulated sets of genes which control the rate of aging (Kenyon, 2005). The existence of these makes possible the observed rapid rates of evolutionary change in aging rates. Some clues to the possible nature of the genes involved in lifespan are emerging from new genetic studies of aging in model organisms.

BETWEEN THE GENETICS AND EVOLUTION OF LIFESPAN

Major advances have recently been made in terms of the genetics of lifespan, particularly using *C. elegans* and *D. melanogaster*. For example, the insulin/insulin-like growth factor (IGF-1) signalling pathway has been shown to be a powerful regulator of lifespan in nematodes, flies and probably rodents (Kenyon, 2005). The relationship between the lifespan-determining genes and pathways identified, and those involved in lifespan evolution, remain unclear. One possibility is that at least some of the genes and processes identified by model organism lifespan genetics are the same as those involved in lifespan evolution. In the case of *S. ratti*, insulin/IGF-1 signalling is a good candidate for a regulator of phenotypic plasticity of aging. In *C. elegans*, this pathway controls the differences in lifespan between the long-lived dauer larva and the shorter lived adult (Riddle and Albert, 1997).

In *C. elegans*, DAF-16, a FOXO-family transcription factor, controls the rate of aging in response to insulin/IGF-1 signalling. Recently, microarray studies have begun to identify the transcriptional targets of DAF-16, which are predicted to include the ultimate genetic determinants of longevity and aging in *C. elegans* (Murphy *et al.*, 2003; McElwee *et al.*, 2004). DAF-16 alters the expression of a wide range of genes, involved in many life processes, including defenses against stress, toxins and microbial invasion. To date, these analyses of the role of IIS and DAF-16 have been based on the analysis of mutants, where lifespan differences of up to 2.5 fold can be achieved (Kenyon *et al.*, 1993). While substantial, such differences are much less than evolved, interspecific differences in lifespan, or the 80-fold differences in lifespan between the different adult morphs of *S. ratti*. Therefore, a plausible hypothesis is that *S. ratti* lifespan plasticity is determined by differential expression of the same sorts of genes and processes regulated by DAF-16 in *C. elegans*. Further, one may speculate that this is also the case for lifespan differences between species, such as that between human and chimpanzee. A graphic representation of this hypothesis is presented in Figure 20.5.

Overall, this discussion of the implications of *S. ratti* aging suggests a view of lifespan as a highly plastic, regulated trait that is consistent with the rapid evolution of interspecific differences in lifespan.

WHY ARE FREE-LIVING *S. RATTI* SO VERY SHORT LIVED?

One remaining oddity of *S. ratti* is that the free-living adults are really very short-lived, even by the standards of short-lived free-living nematode species. There are several possible explanations for this. First, the free-living adult phase of the life cycle is facultative (Viney, 1996). Hence when it does not occur, this may weaken selection on lifespan in the same manner as high extrinsic mortality. Second, it might result from antagonistic pleiotropy between the effects of genes on fitness in the free-living and parasitic forms. Aging may reflect action of alleles that increase early-life fitness (e.g., by increasing reproductive output) but have deleterious late-life effects (Williams, 1957). Such antagonistic pleiotropy is supported by experimental investigation (Kirkwood and Austad, 2000; Partridge and Gems, 2002). Hence, in the case of *S. ratti*, the short life of the free-living adults may result from the greater fecundity of the parasitic female, which may favor pleiotropic alleles that increase parasitic fecundity but reduce lifespan of free-living adults.

LEARNING ABOUT AGING FROM COMPARATIVE STUDIES

Studies concentrating on a small number of model organisms have figured strongly in recent biogerontological

Figure 20.5. A hypothetical scheme for the mechanism of lifespan regulation and evolution. (A) Evolved intraspecific differences in lifespan between parasitic and free-living adults are generated by differences in gene expression, regulated by endocrine and cellular signalling systems via regulated transcription factors. We propose that, as in *C. elegans* (Murphy *et al.*, 2003), parasitic adult longevity in *S. ratti* results from up-regulation of longevity assurance genes and down-regulation of genes which promote aging. A arrows = stimulation, and T bars = inhibition. (B) Potentially, differences in aging rate between species may evolve via similar mechanisms. Here, the environment of an ancestral species changes, such that the extrinsic mortality rate is lowered, and selection against deleterious late-life effects is increased. This leads to the evolution of slower aging and increased longevity, which might occur via alterations in regulation of longevity assurance and aging genes. This predicts that several types of gene are likely to be altered during lifespan evolution: those encoding endocrine, signalling proteins and transcription factors. In (B), asterisks represent alterations in the trait resulting from random mutation, and selection.

A

Free-living development

S. ratti genome

Parasitic development

Endocrine/ signalling

Endocrine/ signalling

Transcription factors

Transcription factors

Longevity assurance genes

Aging genes

Longevity assurance genes

Aging genes

Short-lived free-living adult

Long-lived parasitic adult

B

Shorter-lived ancestral species

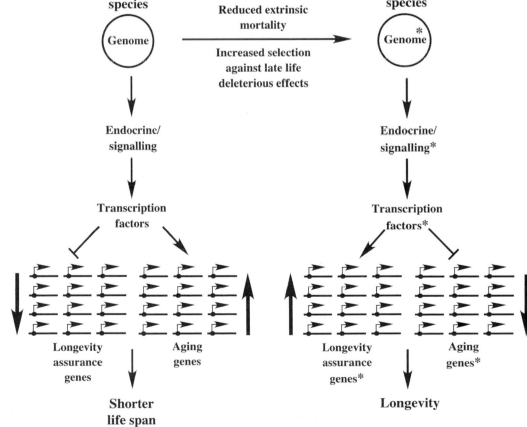

Genome

Reduced extrinsic mortality

Increased selection against late life deleterious effects

Longer-lived descendant species

Genome*

Endocrine/ signalling

Endocrine/ signalling*

Transcription factors

Transcription factors*

Longevity assurance genes

Aging genes

Longevity assurance genes*

Aging genes*

Shorter life span

Longevity

research. While this approach has been very fruitful indeed, studies of *S. ratti* aging illustrate the value of limited investigations of the biology of aging in selected animal species. Such studies in the comparative biology of aging can yield fundamental facts about the biology of aging. A good example of this is the study of *Hydra vulgaris* which revealed an apparent absence of senescence in this species (Martinez, 1998). This demonstrates that aging is not a necessary feature of adult metazoan biology. It seems likely that there are many unusual and informative patterns of aging to be discovered, particularly among lower invertebrates, which may include the absence of senescence, facultative nonsenescence and examples of phenotypic plasticity of aging even more extreme than in *S. ratti*. The possible value of organisms with exotic patterns of aging is likely to increase as the ease of genome sequencing increases and its expense falls. Comparative functional genomic approaches, using whole genome microarray analysis, applied to such organisms, have the potential to yield insights into both the biology of lifespan determination and the evolution of aging and longevity.

Recommended Resources

Below are listed useful Web sites and suggested further reading (books and review articles).

S. RATTI REVIEWS/PAPERS

Aging has been characterized in detail in relatively few animal species. In his review article and book chapter below, David Gems underlines the potential importance of comparative studies of aging in nematodes.

Gems, D., 2001. Longevity and aging in parasitic and free-living nematodes. Biogerontology 1, 289–307.

Gems, D., 2002. Ageing. In: Lee, L.D. (Ed.). *The Biology of Nematodes*. Taylor and Francis, London and New York, pp. 413–455.

In the study below, we described the aging process in free-living adults of the parasitic nematode *Strongyloides ratti*.

Gardner, M.P., Gems, D., and Viney, M.E., 2004. Aging in a very short-lived nematode. Exp. Gerontol. 39, 1267–1276.

Gardner, M.P., Gems, D., and Viney, M.E. 2005. Extraordinary plasticity of ageing in a nematode. Submitted.

S. RATTI/PARASITIC NEMATODE WEBSITES

ESTs of S. ratti http://www.nematode.net/Species.Summaries/Strongyloides.ratti/index.php

Genome sequence of parasitic nematode *B. malayi* http://www.tigr.org/tdb/e2k1/bma1/

GENERAL AGING BOOKS

Finch, C.E., 1990. *Longevity, Senescence and the Genome*, University of Chicago Press, Chicago.

ACKNOWLEDGMENTS

MPG was supported by a grant to MEV and DG from the Experimental Research on Ageing Programme of the BBSRC and we thank them for their support. MEV is supported by the MRC, NERC and the Wellcome Trust. DG is also supported by funds from the EU (Framework V), the Wellcome Trust, and the Royal Society.

REFERENCES

Chapuisat, M., and Keller, L., 2002. Division of labour influences the rate of ageing in weaver ant workers. *Proc. R. Soc. London Ser. B 269*, 909–913.

Epstein, J., Himmelhoch, S., and Gershon, D., 1972. Studies on aging in nematodes III. Electronmicroscopical studies on age-associated cellular damage. *Mech. Ageing Dev. 1*, 245–255.

Finch, C.E., 1990. *Longevity, Senescence and the Genome*, University of Chicago Press, Chicago.

Gardner, M.P., Gems, D., and Viney, M.E., 2004. Aging in a very short-lived nematode. *Exp. Gerontol. 39*, 1267–1276 (2004).

Garigan, D., Hsu, A -L., Fraser, A.G., Kamath, R.S., Ahringer, J., and Kenyon, C., 2002. Genetic analysis of tissue aging in *Caenorhabditis elegans*: A role for heat-shock factor and bacterial proliferation. *Genetics 161*, 1101–1112.

Gemmill, A.W., Viney, M.E., and Read, A.F., 1997. Host immune status determines sexuality in a parasitic nematode. *Evolution 51*, 393–401.

Gems, D., 2001. Longevity and ageing in parasitic and free-living nematodes. *Biogerontology 1*, 289–307.

Gems, D., and McElwee, J.J., 2005. Broad spectrum detoxification: The major longevity assurance process regulated by insulin/IGF-1 signalling? *Mech. Ageing Dev. 126*, 381–387.

Gems, D., and Riddle, D.L., 1996. Longevity in *Caenorhabditis elegans* reduced by mating but not gamete production. *Nature 379*, 723–725.

Gems, D., and Riddle, D.L., 2000. Genetic, behavioural and environmental determinants of male longevity in *Caenorhabditis elegans*. *Genetics 154*, 1597–1610.

Golden, J.W., and Riddle, D.L., 1984. The *Caenorhabditis elegans* dauer larva: Developmental effects of pheromone, food and temperature. *Dev. Biol. 102*, 368–378.

Grove, D.I., 1989. Historical introduction. In Grove, D.I. (Ed.). *Strongyloidiasis: A Major Roundworm Infection of Man*. Taylor and Francis, London and New York, pp. 1–9.

Harvey, S.C., Gemill, A.W., Read, A.F., and Viney, M.E., 2000. The control of morph development in the parasitic nematode *Strongyloides ratti*. *Proc. R. Soc. London Ser. B 267*, 2057–2063.

Herndon, L.A., Schmeissner, P.J., Dudaronek, J.M., Brown, P.A., Listner, K.M., Sakano, Y., *et al.*, 2002. Stochastic and genetic factors influence tissue-specific decline in ageing *C. elegans*. *Nature 419*, 808–814.

Hodgkin, J., and Barnes, T.M., 1991. More is not better: brood size and population growth in a self-fertilizing nematode. *Proc. R. Soc. London Ser. B 246*, 19–24.

Houthoofd, K., Braeckman, B.P., Johnson, T.E., and Vanfleteren, J.R., 2004. Extending life-span in *C. elegans*. *Science 305*, 1238–1239.

Kenyon, C., 2005. The plasticity of aging: Insights from long-lived mutants. *Cell 120*, 449–460.

Kenyon, C., Chang, J., Gensch, E., Rudener, A., and Tabtiang, R.A., 1993. A *C. elegans* mutant that lives twice as long as wild type. *Nature 366*, 461–464.

Kirkwood, T.B.L., and Austad, S.N., 2000. Why do we age? *Nature 408*, 233–238.

Klass, M.R., 1977. Aging in the nematode *Caenorhabditis elegans*: Major biological and environmental factors influencing life span. *Mech. Ageing Dev. 6*, 413–429.

Klass, M.R., and Hirsh, D.I., 1976. Non-ageing development variant of *Caenorhabditis elegans*. *Nature 260*, 523–525.

Lakowski, B., and Hekimi, S., 1998. The genetics of caloric restriction in *Caenorhabditis elegans*. *Proc. Natl. Acad. Sci. USA 95*, 13091–13096.

Longo, V.D., and Finch, C.E., 2003. Evolutionary medicine: From dwarf model systems to healthy centenarians? *Science 299*, 1342–1346.

Martínez, D.E., 1998. Mortality patterns suggest lack of senescence in hydra. *Exp. Gerontol. 33*, 217–225.

McCay, C., Crowell, and M., Maynard, L., 1935. The effect of retarded growth upon the length of the life span and upon the ultimate body size. *J. Nutr. 10*, 63–79.

McElwee, J.J., Schuster, E., Blanc, E., Thomas, J.H, and Gems, D., 2004. Shared transcriptional signature in *C. elegans* dauer larvae and long-lived *daf-2* mutants implicates detoxification system in longevity assurance. *J. Biol. Chem. 279*, 44533–44543.

Medawar, P.B., 1952. *An Unsolved Problem of Biology*. H.K. Lewis, London.

Murphy, C.T., McCarroll, S.A., Bargmann, C.I., *et al.*, 2003. Genes that act downstream of DAF-16 to influence the lifespan of *Caenorhabditis elegans*. *Nature 424*, 277–284.

Nusbaum, T., and Rose, M., 1999. The effects of nutritional manipulation and laboratory selection on lifespan in *Drosophila melanogaster*. *J. Gerontol. A Biol. Sci. Med. Sci. 54*, B192–B198.

Page, R.E., and Peng, C.Y.-S., 2001. Aging and development in social insects with emphasis on the honey bee, *Apis mellifera* L. *Exp. Gerontol. 36*, 695–711.

Partridge, L., and Gems, D., 2002. Mechanisms of ageing: Public or private? *Nat. Rev. Genet. 3*, 165–175.

Riddle, D.L., and Albert, P.S., 1997. Genetic and environmental regulation of dauer larva development. In *C. elegans II* (eds. D.L. Riddle, T. Blumenthal, B.J. Meyer, J.R. Priess), pp. 739–768. Cold Spring Harbor Laboratory Press, New York.

Speare, R., 1989. Identification of species of Strongyloides. In: Grove, D.I. (Ed.). *Strongyloidiasis: A Major Roundworm Infection of Man*. Taylor and Francis, London and New York, pp. 11–83.

Sulston, J., and Hodgkin, J., 1988. Methods. In: Wood, W.B. (Ed.). *The Nematode Caenorhabditis elegans*. Cold Spring Harbor Press, New York, pp. 587–606.

Viney, M.E., 1994. A genetic analysis of reproduction in *Strongyloides ratti*. *Parasitology 109*, 511–515.

Viney, M.E., 1996. Developmental switching in the parasitic nematode *Strongyloides ratti*. *Proc. R. Soc. London Ser. B 263*, 201–208.

Viney, M.E., 1999. Exploiting the life-cycle of *Strongyloides ratti*. *Parasitology Today 15*, 231–235.

Viney, M.E., Matthews, B.E., and Walliker, D., 1993. Mating in the nematode parasite *Strongyloides ratti*: Proof of genetic exchange. *Proc. R. Soc. London Ser. B 254*, 213–219.

Wachter, K.W., and Finch, C.E., 1997. *Between Zeus and the Salmon*, National Academy Press, Washington DC.

Wilkes, C.P., Thompson, F.J., Gardner, M.P., Paterson, S., Viney, M.E., 2004. The effect of the host immune response on the parasitic nematode *Strongyloides ratti*. *Parasitology 128*, 661–669.

Wilkinson, G., and South, J., 2002. Life history, ecology and longevity in bats. *Aging Cell 1*, 124–131.

Williams, G.C., 1957. Pleiotropy, natural selection and the evolution of senescence. *Evolution 11*, 398–411.

21

Insect Models for the Study of Aging

Klaus-Günter Collatz

*The aim of the following chapter is to show that different insect species can be used to answer many questions relevant in mammalian or human aging studies. Insects share with vertebrates, including man, many basic similarities in structural components, energy metabolism, and signal transduction mechanisms. Many insects are easy and cheap to rear in mass cultures. With few exceptions they have short life and generation times. After a short survey of the principles of insect anatomy and function, biotic and abiotic factors are considered which are responsible for modifying an insect's life span. I then describe insects that we use in our own laboratory (*Phormia terraenovae, Gastrophysa viridula *and* Panorpa vulgaris*) and their rearing conditions, as well as those of two other flies frequently used (*Musca domestica and Drosophila *species). I further present various studies relevant for aging investigations, including biodemographic statistics, examples of age-dependent ultrastructural tissue changes, and different metabolic measurements. The metabolic section raises issues of caloric restriction, studies of redox systems, trade-offs between physical activities, reproduction, and longevity and chronobiological effects.*

Introduction

Insects are a huge group of arthropods in the animal kingdom, comprising about two million described but up to 30 million estimated species. They are distributed over extremely different habitats ranging from the sea cost to high mountains. One can find them in deserts as well as in aquatic regions. Only the open sea lacks this extremely prosperous animal group.

WHY INSECTS AS MODELS

At first sight, insects seem to be very different from vertebrates and therefore poorly qualified to act as models in our context. A closer look, however, reveals many similarities on tissue and basic metabolic levels. Aging insect tissues, for instance, are characterized by structural changes that also occur in mammalian tissues. The deposition of the age pigment lipofuscin and the more or less abundant "whorllike" structures of mitochondrial origin are examples of common signs of aging or otherwise degenerating tissues (see below). A further peculiarity is that adult insects are composed of post-mitotic cells—except for their hemocytes and germ cells. Therefore all lifelong changes on the tissue level can easily be detected.

Most insect species are short-lived organisms. Therefore many generations can be studied in a short time. Insects can be raised in large quantities and with low costs.

The use of insects as model systems in gerontological studies has a long tradition. Loeb and Northrop (1917) were the first to use *Drosophila* in this way. They conducted experiments on metabolic rates and life span, and these early attempts can be acknowledged as the beginning of a comparative biology of aging. These *Drosophila* studies were based on results of Rubner (1908). Working with mammals, he showed that the amount of lifelong metabolic energy per gram body weight is more or less constant. These results stimulated further studies on the rate of living theory (Pearl, 1928). This old problem was then elucidated in greater detail by Sohal and coworkers using modern methods and the house fly—*Musca domestica*. The rate of living theory was then consequently redefined as follows: "The rate of ageing is directly related to the rate of unrepaired molecular damage inflicted by the by-products of oxygen metabolism and it is inversely related to the efficiency of antioxidant and repair mechanisms" (Sohal, 1986). Since that time many investigations have addressed the influence of oxidative stress, free radical damage, and repair on aging and longevity in insects. Regardless of the acceptance of the rate of living theory, these factors are generally accepted as being of central importance for the understanding of aging mechanisms.

Extensive studies on aging mechanisms are mostly restricted to dipterans. The fruit fly *Drosophila*, of course, is the most intensively studied insect even in this sense. Other dipterans more often studied are the house fly *Musca domestica* and blowflies, including our own model organism *Phormia terraenovae* (Collatz, 1997). The scorpion fly *Panorpa vulgaris* and the chrysomelid beetle *Gastrophysa viridula* attracted particular attention in our laboratory due to special questions, which are outlined in more detail below.

For the biologist interested in comparative aging studies, large differences in life-history strategies of insects of the same genus could offer the opportunity to test phylogenetic causes of aging. In the last years special attention was given to social hymenoptera like bees, wasps, and ants with their remarkable long living queens (see below).

GENERAL FEATURES OF THE INSECT BODY PLAN

In contrast to the various life habits and life histories, the insect body plan is quite uniform with its basic body plan (see Figure 21.1).

The body is composed of three parts—head, thorax, and abdomen—and covered with a chitinous cuticle of varying thickness. Three pairs of legs and, in winged insects, two pairs of wings, are attached to the thorax.

The central nervous system consists of a supraesophageal and a subesophageal ganglion in the head and a rope ladder-like ventral nerve cord. The supraesophageal ganglion or brain is the most complex part of the nervous system. It includes the optic center, areas of behavioral regulation and centers of integrative learning. The alimentary canal consists of three parts. It begins, behind the mouth, with an ectodermic foregut or stomodeum with pharynx and stomach, followed by the entodermic midgut or mesodeum, which is the main region of digestion. An ectodermic hind gut or

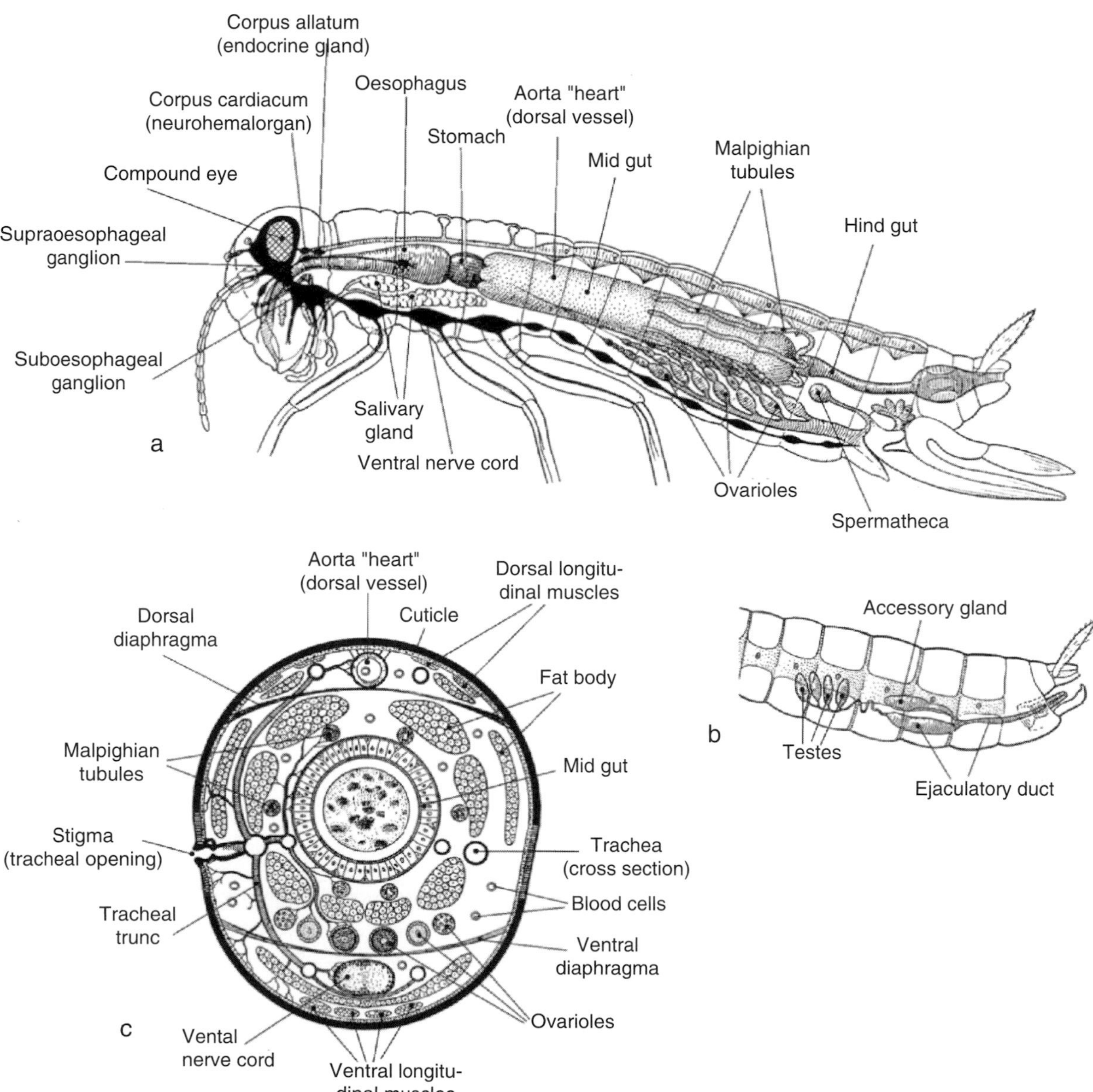

Figure 21.1. Basic body plan of an insect: (a) lateral view of the female insect body (fat body omitted); (b) lateral view of the male insect abdomen; (c) cross section of the female insect abdomen. (All charts modified after Weber, 1966)

proctodeum opens into the anus. The excretory system consisting of the malpighian tubules is connected to the proctodeum.

The blood circulation system of insects is an open system; their body fluid—hemolymph—is therefore comparable to a mix of extracellular fluid ("lymph") and blood in animals with closed circulatory systems. The respiratory system is separated from the circulatory system. Tracheae that start with spiracles transport the respiratory gases. There are no respiratory proteins, and the distribution of oxygen and carbon dioxide is achieved by diffusion.

The body cavity is filled with the prominent fat body. This is not simply a storage organ like the white fat of vertebrates. It is very active metabolically, most comparable to the liver of vertebrates.

The male sex organs consist of the paired testes accompanied with glands for accessory fluids. The female ovaries are composed of a varying number of ovarioles and adjacent parts (e.g., spermatheca).

Life-Span Characteristics and Factors Which Are Responsible for Modifying an Insect's Life Span

Although the aging pattern of insects, like that of other organisms, is doubtless under genetic control, it is extremely flexible, depending on several biotic and abiotic factors. Life span includes the longevity of all developmental stages an individual passes through during its life cycle. Individuals of insect species (as well as those of other species) experience a number of critical points in time during their life cycles, which influence the life span from eggs over larvae up to pupae and adult stages. Without knowledge of such modifying factors the life span of an insect species is unpredictable.

Insects are ectothermic organisms. The ambient temperature is therefore a key life-span modifying factor. It is easy to manipulate the metabolic rate simply by changing ambient temperature. The mentioned work of Loeb and Northrop used this regimen as an experimental tool. The light regime also acts as a prominent abiotic stimulus together with the temperature. Both factors are essential in habitats with distinctive seasons; they determine in many species whether phases of dormancy occur or not. A phase of low metabolism can be induced experimentally by changing the photoperiod from long day (16:8) to short day (8:16). This treatment evidently interrupts the aging process (see below).

All insects dealt with in the present contribution are holometabolic. Their development from egg to adult is interrupted by a metamorphosis. Preimaginal conditions are important for the adult life course. A controlled underfeeding of larvae does not terminate the development but results in dwarf adult forms. They can be used to study the interrelationship of body size, fecundity, and longevity.

Fecundity and reproductive success are also essential for the determination of the following course of life. As we will see in the case of the blowfly *Phormia*, reproductive success depends not only on the availability of mates but equally on the presence of proteins as specific food for the development of eggs. This in turn is of great influence for longevity.

Physiological trade-offs between physical performance, reproduction, and longevity are also important and gave rise to numerous studies. We will refer to this in a later section.

As mentioned above, a particular situation is given in eusocial insects as wasps, bees, ants and termites. They live in colonies with cooperating members of different castes, sharing a high level of genetic similarity with the queen. Aging process and life span of the colony members are widely determined by extrinsic factors such as nutrition and kind of work. The remarkable longevity of the queen ranging from 4 to 8 years in wasps and up to 30 years in termites is of great interest (Page and Peng, 2001). This topic is further dealt with in Chapter 23, "Models of Aging in Honeybee Workers," and Chapter 24, "Ants as Naturally Long-Lived Insect Models for Aging." For a more detailed description of aging and environmental conditions in insects see Collatz (2003).

Finally, caloric restriction in general can act as a life-prolonging strategy not only in vertebrates, but also in insects. It is proposed that the basic mechanisms and effects are almost the same in such different organisms.

Biology and Rearing Conditions of Insects Used in Our Own Laboratory (Figure 21.2)

PHORMIA TERRAENOVAE

The blowfly *Phormia terraenovae* (= *Protophormia terraenovae*) is a holarctic distributed calliphorid fly. It is abundant in the cooler regions and was found in Spitsbergen as well as within 550 miles of the North Pole. This synanthropic fly plays an important role as indicator in forensic biology since especially calliphorids are recognized as the first wave of the faunal succession on human cadavers.

Under free-living conditions both sexes can be found on umbels of Apiaceae. The compact body of these flies is shiny metallic blue. Their eyes and wings are well developed. The mouth parts operate as licking proboscis. Males and females are easily distinguished by the different positions of their eyes; there is a broad interspace in females and a negligible one in males. The natural food of both sexes is nectar.

Phormia belongs to the group of anautogenous insects in contrast to autogenous insects. The term *autogenous*, particularly used for dipterans, means that during metamorphosis larval protein is transferred into the

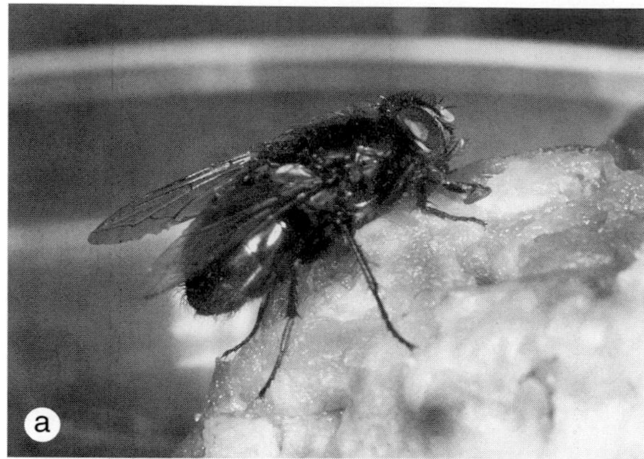

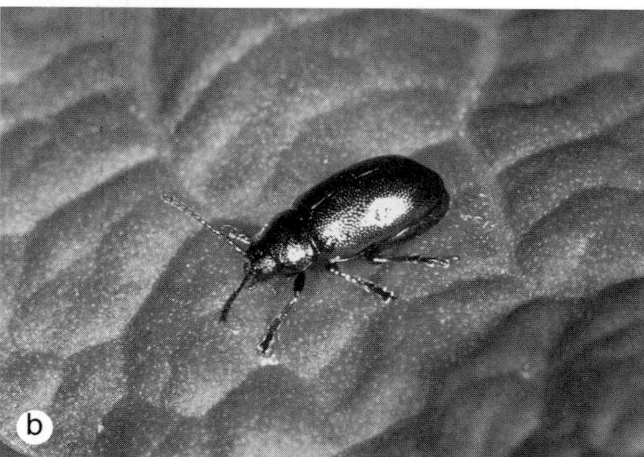

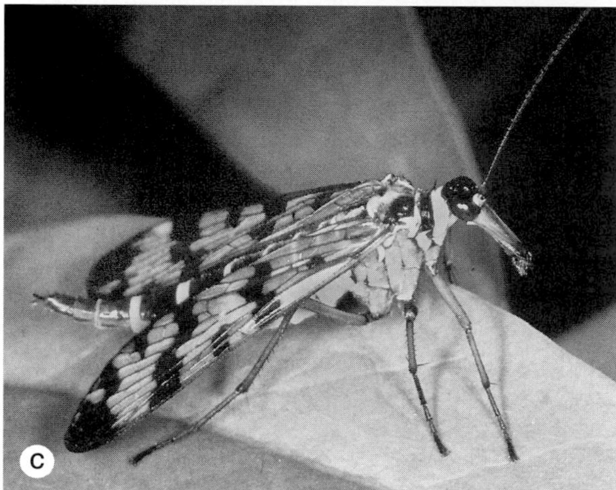

Figure 21.2. Insects used in our laboratory: (a) *Phormia*, (b) *Gastrophysa*, (c) *Panorpa*

adult. In female adults this protein is an indispensable requisite for the development of eggs. In male adults it often serves as source for the synthesis of the accessory genital gland fluids: a prerequisite for the insemination of females. Anautogenic insects such as *Phormia* rely on exogenic protein sources. Under natural conditions protein is a rare and ephemeric substrate. Time and the opportunity of acquisition influence the aging process.

Rearing conditions

We perform the stock culture of flies under a 16:8 (l:d) light regime with a temperature of 25°C and a relative humidity of 60 to 75%. The raising room is illuminated with "Lumilux-Eco Daylight" lamps (Osram). The cages are cubic with an edge length of 50 cm. This is sufficient for a population of 400 flies. The cages are covered on top and on two sides with gauze. The third side is attached with black cloth containing a sleeve. The front site is covered with a removable Plexiglas pane.

Three plastic Petri dishes with lump sugar, minced meat and water (on filter paper to avoid drowning of the flies) are placed inside the cage. If provided with meat, newly emerged flies start to lay eggs after about three days. Half a teaspoon of eggs will provide about 2500 individuals for a new generation. The eggs are placed together with meat in plastic containers (25 × 20 × 15 cm l/w/h) filled up to one-third with sawdust. The sawdust must always be moist to avoid drying of the meat and to fix the ammonia, which is produced by the maggots. The larvae hatch after about 24 hours: they need an increasing amount of meat. During the last days of larval development this amount can reach up to 500 g per day. After 7 to 10 days after hatching, the larvae stop feeding and start to pupate. The pupae are now transferred to fresh sawdust and placed into a new cage. Here the new generation of adult flies emerge after 5 to 8 days. To obtain a cohort with definite age structure, the emergence can be better synchronized by placing the cage for several hours in a cooling chamber at about 4°C.

GASTROPHYSA VIRIDULA

The chrysomelid beetle *Gastrophysa viridula* was formerly restricted to alpine regions, but now it has expanded its distribution to northern, middle, and eastern Europe. In North America this species is replaced by *G. formosa*. The oligophagous beetles are found on Polygonaceae, mostly *Rumex* plants but also on *Rheum*, and were reported to be a pest on vine in Arizona. The 4 to 6 mm long beetles are metallic green with a black ventral side. Females with eggs are easy to distinguish from males by their swollen abdomen. The eggs are deposited in batches of 20 to 45 on the underside of leaves. The emerging larvae moult two times. The developing time from egg to the adult beetle takes about 50 days (eggs: 7–10, larvae: 21–30, pupae: 6–9 days). Normally, *Gastrophysa* produces three generations per year. Adults of the autumn generation enter diapause up to the next spring.

Rearing conditions

We rear the stock culture of beetles under a 16:8 (l:d) light regime with a temperature of 20°C and a relative humidity of 50% in a climate chamber (Rubarth Apparatus 3201). Twenty to 30 beetles are placed in Petri dishes of 12 cm diameter. The dishes are covered with paper pulp, and the beetles are fed daily with fresh *Rumex* leaves. The newly emerged animals start to copulate after 3 days and deposit the first eggs after 5–7 days. Larvae get *Rumex* leaves up to the end of the third stage. Thereafter they stop feeding and seek deeper places in the paper sheets. The pupae are extremely sensible against touching and they should not be disturbed.

PANORPA VULGARIS

The over 100 species of scorpion fly *Panorpa* (Mecoptera) have a world-wide distribution. Both sexes are characterized by a snout-shaped elongated head, and the males have a tail-like grasping apparatus resembling a scorpion's tail, which is used to hold the female during copulation. During mating, the male presents a "nuptial gift" to the female, a proteinaceous bowl produced by the salivary gland. The adults are common on shrubs in shady areas. They feed on dead organisms, mostly insects. Under mid-European environmental conditions two generations per year—a spring and an autumn generation—can be produced. The last larval stage of the second generation enters an overwintering diapause.

Panorpa is remarkable in that it shows senescence like histological degenerations even under free-living conditions.

Rearing conditions

Adults can be maintained in the laboratory on long day (18:6 h) conditions at 23°C and 60–75% relative humidity. Cages (40 × 20 × 35 cm) for 50 individuals are covered on top and on the four sides with gauze and can be placed on paper sheets. These insects are such lazy fliers that the cages can easily be handled without special opening devices. Mealworm larvae are suited as food. Under this treatment, males and females reach a maximum life span of about 110 days, which is in accordance with free-living populations. Life expectancy at the day of emergence is 61–63 days for both males and females. After sampling egg-clusters from moist peat-soil used as egg-laying substrate, they are transferred to Petri dishes containing the same substrate. The emerging larvae are fed on pieces of mealworm larvae. Under the same conditions, the larvae hatch after 6 days, pass through 4 larval stages in 3 weeks and emerge after an additional 3 weeks. Adult males emerge 3 days after the females.

Rearing Conditions of Other Frequently Used Insects

MUSCA DOMESTICA

The common house fly was often used besides *Drosophila* in early studies on aging in insects. As in *Phormia* (and other diptera), males and females can easily be distinguished by the different positions of their eyes.

The flies are easy to raise in gauze-covered boxes as used for *Phormia*.

Rearing conditions

The rearing temperature should be 27 to 28°C and the relative humidity about 60%.

The cages contain a Petri dish with humidified blotting paper. Another dish contains the larval food composed of a mixture of alfalfa flour, wheat bran, yeast and water (1:1:0, 2:5). This mixture is fermented for 3 days at 26°C. For adults, this mixture should be covered with powdered milk. Another larval food mix contains equal parts dry yeast and milk powder (10%) dissolved in 2% boiling agar solution.

After egg deposition, the food dishes are taken away and covered with gauze. After two days, the larvae are about 3 mm in length. Depending on population density, the food mixture has to be divided among additional food dishes. (About 1 kg food mixture is sufficient for breeding of 1000 maggots.) After about 6 days the larvae stop feeding and move to the dry surface of the food. They pupate after another 4 to 8 days. The dark brown pupae can be washed out with water from the food and stored in slightly wet sawdust. The adult flies emerge after 4 to 5 days. They can be fed on powdered milk, sugar and/or larval food.

DROSOPHILA

Rearing conditions of *Drosophila* can be found in different handbooks and internet pages (see the link at the end of the References). It should therefore suffice to give only a short comment.

Breeding temperature is recommended between 18 and 25°C. Relative humidity in the breeding chamber should not be lower than 60%.

A recipe for standard medium used in our institute is given as follows:

Add together: 2.4 l water, 19.2 g agar, 192 g corn powder, 24 g soy flour (low fat), 43.2 g yeast, 180 g treacle, 90 g barley malt extract, 18 ml propionic acid and 2.5 g nipagin.

All ingredients are boiled up under constant stirring and filled in portions of about 50 ml into plastic ("*Drosophila*") vials (10 cm height and 5 cm diameter). The indicated amount is sufficient for about 50 vials. After cooling the medium congeals. Before transferring flies on to the medium it is recommended to add some yeast on the surface. This stimulates the egg deposition and development of larvae.

Kinds of Aging Studies

BIODEMOGRAPHIC STUDIES

It has been proven to be advantageous—and we recommend it—to accompany all forms of biodemographic studies with a control population. This has a simple reason. Carey (2000) emphasized how difficult it is to speak on life span in general and, in particular, in insects. In contrast to life expectancy and age specific

TABLE 21.1.
Diagram of a mortality table

Days	l_x	d_x	q_x	e_x	$\log q_x$
1					
2					
n					

x: age interval (days); l_x: survivors at the beginning of age interval; d_x: deads during the age interval (absolute death rate); q_x: age-specific death rate; e_x: life expectancy and a = number of days in the age interval

$$d_x = l_x - l_{(x+1)}$$

$$q_x = \frac{d_x}{l_x}$$

$$e_x = \frac{T_{x.a}}{L_x}$$

$$L_x = \frac{l_x + l_{(x+1)}}{2}$$

$$T_x = L_x + L_{(x+1)} \dots\dots\dots + L_w = \sum_x^w L_x$$

mortality, which are measurable values, "life span" is weakly defined as time after which no member of a given species can survive even under the most favorable conditions. "Maximum life-span potential" is another description. It is evident therefore that maximum life span depends on the number of individuals under observation; it is higher when large numbers of individuals are observed. On the other hand, data on longevity obtained under laboratory conditions may have nothing to do with data recorded under free-living conditions. The determination of maximum life spans of ectothermic organisms as insects is even more problematical. Insects are extremely sensible to abiotic factors like temperature, humidity or light regime. It is therefore meaningless—as Carey pointed out—"to consider life-span for any species without considering environmental, ecological and evolutionary contexts."

Preparing mortality data

To get survival and mortality data of *Phormia* in a longitudinal study, we start with a population of 400 individuals. Dead flies are counted daily, and mortality statistics are calculated after scaling the data to 1000. (Table 21.1; see Lamb, 1977).

Plotting the logarithm of q_x against age in days results in the Gompertz curve of mortality.

It is easy to put the single calculation steps into an Excel table, so that you only have to count the dead flies per day.

Age-Dependent Ultrastructural Changes in Insect Tissues

As mentioned above, adult insects are composed of nondividing (postmitotic) cells. Tissue degeneration with advancing age resembles that of brain and other postmitotic tissues in mammals. The observed changes in dipterans like *Drosophila* or *Musca*, however, are not uniform, ranging from "total degeneration" to "poorly developed changes." We use *Panorpa* as a model organism not only for comparative reasons but also because, as said above, this insect shows senescent tissue degeneration even under free-living conditions (Collatz and Collatz, 1981). Figure 21.3 shows an example of tissue degeneration in senescent *Panorpa*. It should be possible in such an organism to demonstrate protective effects of various drugs (e.g., antioxidants) on tissue degeneration.

The Possibility of Continuously Measuring Energy Metabolism

The small body size of insects offers the opportunity of continuously monitoring the total energy metabolism of a whole population over their total life span. This results in a "metabolic picture." One can then test the influence of different treatments (e.g., temperature, light program, drugs, mating, virginity) on the energy consumption. We performed such measurements with *Phormia* using an infrared CO_2 monitoring system (URAS). Due to the restriction on carbohydrates as energy-providing substrate, the CO_2 output equals the O_2 input and therefore gives a true picture of energy metabolism. Thirty-five flies were placed in a respiration chamber and fed in the usual manner with sugar and water. The relatively big volume of the chamber allows unrestricted flying and walking activity. Figure 21.4 shows an example of such a measurement.

The CO_2 production per 30 min was calculated from the continuous monitoring. Males and females exhibit a very different energy profile. In both sexes, however, a well-developed day–night rhythm of activity could be found. With increasing age, a decline of maximum (flight) and minimum (walking) activity can be observed. The basal metabolic rate (night values) in contrast is independent from age and is constant over the life span in males.

Different light regimes influence the adult life span. At least in *Drosophila*, constant light has a life-shortening effect (Sheeba *et al.*, 2000). Under such conditions, a very high egg production rate can be observed, which might be responsible for the early death. After results from Pittendrigh (1972), the light–dark cycle under which larvae of *Drosophila* were reared had strong influence on the longevity of the adults. It is generally known that a desynchronization of endogenous rhythms affects many physiological parameters and is therefore of major

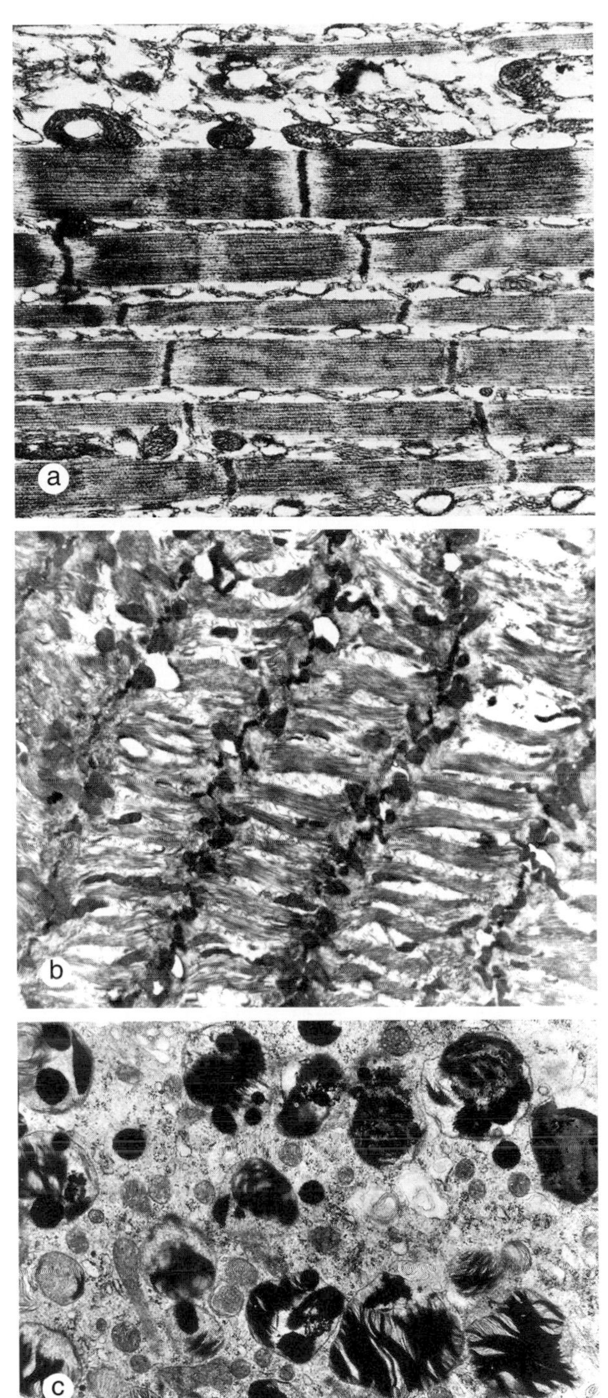

Figure 21.3. Example for senescent tissue degeneration in *Panorpa* ultrastructure of (a) young flight muscle, (b) flight muscle deterioration, (c) malpighian tubule with lipofuscine like inclusions and degenerated mitochondria.

influence on aging and disease. *Phormia* has proven to be a suited experimental animal to study such chronobiological aspects. After keeping the flies in non–24-h light-dark cycles or subjecting them to a jet lag, a life-shortening effect could be detected (Saint Paul, 1978). Only few attempts have been made up to now to gain more insight into the mechanisms of circadian dyschronism and aging. Aging changes in glycolytic oscillations—a basic biochemical rhythm—were described for *Phormia* by Collatz and Horning (1990) and Horning and Collatz (1990).

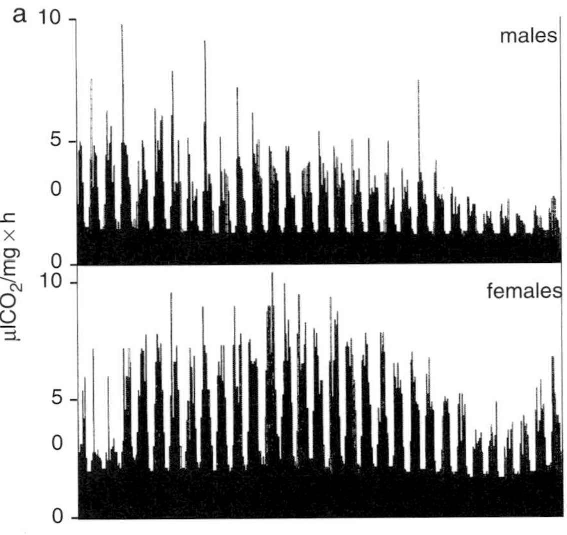

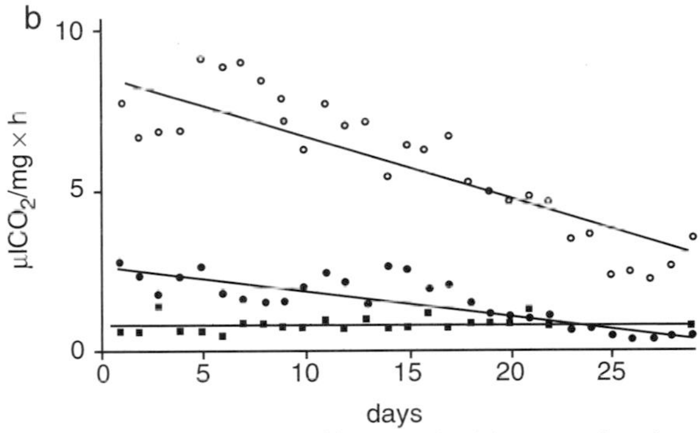

Figure 21.4. (a) Energy profile over the life span of male and female *Phormia* flies measured as CO_2 production with an infrared analyzer. (b) Decline of maximum (flight) and minimum (walking) activity and constant basal metabolic rate (night values) over the life span of males. Data taken from (a).

Interrupting the Aging Process by Induction of a Phase of Low Metabolic Rate

Insect diapause is a particular form of prospective dormancy, comparable to adaptations like hibernation in small mammals or dauer forms in nematods. It seems reasonable to assume that the underlying mechanisms, including the signal transduction mechanisms which trigger the intrinsic metabolic rearrangements during this phase of reduced energy metabolism, are similar in different animals. The blowfly *Phormia* and *Drosophila* could be promising models to study aging in diapause—see Tatar and Yin (2001), Stoffolano (1974), and Yin and Stoffolano (1994, 1997).

We used *Gastrophysa viridula* to show that reproductive diapause is characterized as a life period with negligible senescence (Albonetti and Becker in our laboratory).

Under experimental conditions, 75% of adult *Gastrophysa* beetles enter diapause after changing the photoperiod from long-day conditions (16:8) to short-day conditions (8:16) without lowering the normal rearing temperature of 20°C. The survival curves of diapausing and nondiapausing beetles are very different. The survival curve of beetles in diapause resembles an exponential function, which is characteristic for nonaging systems. In accordance with this, the age-specific mortality is constant over a long period. The survival curve and age-specific mortality of nondiapausing beetles follow the usual type of aging under senescence conditions. The average life span of beetles in diapause surpasses that of nondiapausing animals about fourfold (Figure 21.5).

Despite the high ambient temperature, which should enable a high activity spectrum of the beetles, the metabolic rate of diapausing animals slows down to only 20% of that of nondiapausing beetles (Figure 21.6).

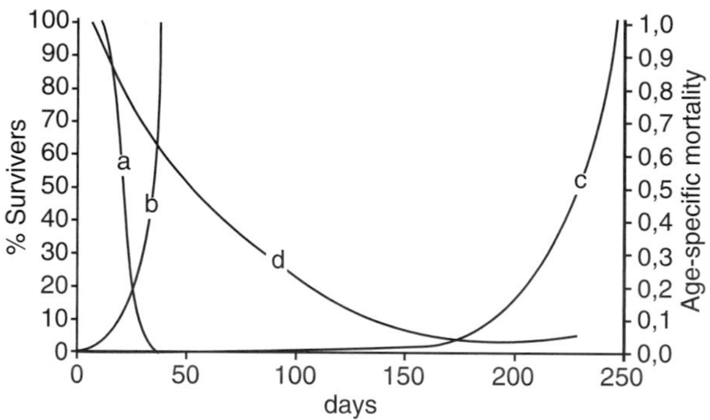

Figure 21.5. Survival curve (d) and age-specific mortality rate (c) of *Gastrophysa* females in diapause compared to survival (a) and mortality (b) under long-day (nondiapause) conditions.

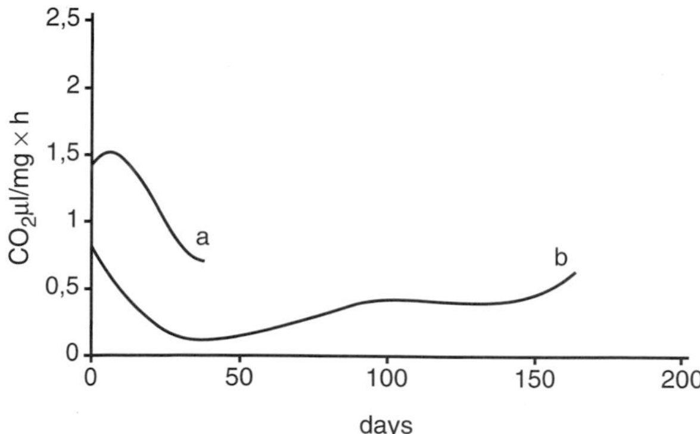

Figure 21.6. Metabolic rate of *Gastrophysa* females under diapause (b) and long day (nondiapause) conditions (a).

The feeding activity persists almost completely, and males and females accumulate high lipid values.

It would be interesting to study if the suppression of reproduction favors an allocation of metabolic reserves for maintenance of body integrity in the sense of the "disposable soma theory" (see Study of Trade-offs Between Physical Activities, Reproduction, and Longevity; Kirkwood and Holliday, 1979). However, the metabolic consequences that are responsible for this drastic variation in life cycle are nearly unknown.

Caloric Restriction

Beginning with the early work of McCay and Maynard (1935) who reported a life-prolonging effect of caloric restriction in rats, numerous attempts have been made to study the underlying causes of this obviously general mechanism. It could be shown that a reduction of caloric intake of 30 to 50% prolonged the life of rodents up to 60%. The same results were obtained in young animals and in older adults which received the reduced diet later in life. The results of the studies on rodents could be confirmed in numerous studies on other vertebrates, nematodes and even protozoa (see Masoro, 2000). Evidence for enhanced survival under dietary restriction in insects was provided by studies on waterstriders (Kaitala, 1991), carabid beetles (Ernsting and Isaaks, 1991), and *Drosophila* (see chapters in this book). Long-time studies using primates started in the eighties and continue up to now, revealing exciting results (Mattison *et al.*, 2003).

The influence of dietary restriction on the organism is manifold. Obviously, the reduction of oxidative stress by reducing the accumulation of reactive oxygen molecules and the protection of the antioxidant system plays a central role.

It is often reported that a dietary restriction leads to a reduction of fertility. It was argued that the energy resources are used for the maintenance of body function instead for reproduction with the result of prolonging the life span. The evolutionary implications of such a life-history strategy were discussed by Shanley and Kirkwood (2000).

Recently the influence of dietary restriction on gene expression has attracted more and more attention. It could be shown that the expression of gluconeogenetic genes was stimulated in rodents after caloric restriction (Spindler, 2001).

Regarding the change in intermediary metabolism, a gene family came into consideration which is called SIR2 (Brachman *et al.*, 1995). Studies with yeast show that the gene product of SIR2 is a NAD-dependent histone deacetylase which inactivates chromosomal regions (Guarente and Kenyon, 2000). With increasing age, a partial loss of inactivation results in errors in gene expression. This process can be delayed by high bioavailability of NAD. A reduced glycolytic flow as shown after caloric restriction is therefore sufficient to provide the SIR2 system with more NAD.

The ultimate reasons for the evolution of the beneficial effects of caloric restriction are more speculative. Holliday (1989) considered the life prolongation as an adaptation to temporary periods with insufficient food. Animals which survive these periods due to a reduced energy metabolism and interrupted reproduction are able to reproduce when the situation becomes more favorable.

This short summary shows that a major effect of caloric restriction is visible in the glycolytic pathway and its regulation. Since *Phormia*—as pointed out—is exclusively dependent on carbohydrates as energy fuel, the fly could be a very promising subject for corresponding studies. This will be further illustrated below.

Braun in our laboratory used copulated *Phormia* flies to study the effect of caloric restriction induced by intermittent sugar feeding on mortality characteristics, fertility, and metabolic rate. Two experimental groups with starvation periods of 24 or 48 hours against a control group with ad libitum feeding were taken for the experiments. The fertility was calculated over the average number of laid eggs per day. The metabolic rate was determined by measurement of CO_2 production.

The specific activity of arginine phosphokinase (APK) in the thorax was measured as biomarker of muscle (flight) activity. APK represents the phosphagen cleaving enzyme in insects and other invertebrates and is comparable to creatine phosphokinase in vertebrates.

The most remarkable result was that under these experimental conditions the life expectancy and the maximum life span of males were reduced against the control group whereas that of females was increased.

Females with a starvation period of 24 hours produced significantly more eggs than the control group. After 48 hours intermittent starvation, the egg production was reduced and shifted to the last period of life. Males fed ad libitum exhibited a significantly higher metabolic rate than females. Under dietary restriction we found a reduction of metabolic rate up to 90% in the males (Figure 21.7).

In contrast, dietary restriction had no effect on metabolic rate in females. The specific activity of APK is generally higher in fully fed flies.

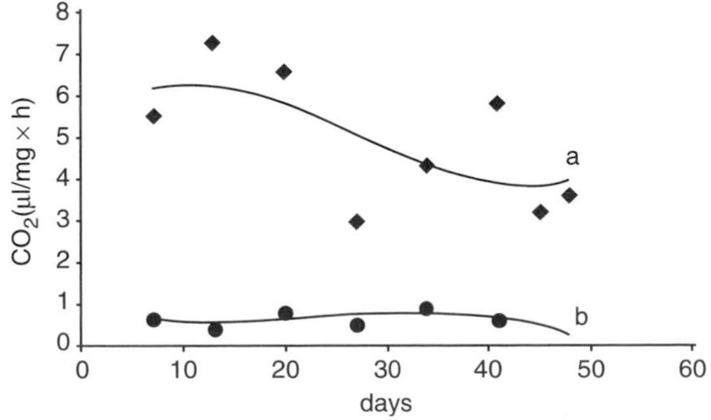

Figure 21.7. Metabolic rate of male *Phormia* flies under ad libitum feeding (a) and two days intermittent starvation (b).

In summary, caloric restriction has a sex-specific effect and does not necessarily result in a reduction of metabolic rate and fertility. In our example, the higher fertility and life span of females with caloric restriction is obviously reached at the expense of reduced activity.

Study of Trade-offs Between Physical Activities, Reproduction, and Longevity

The comparative gerontologist often uses a theory which is assumed to explain the different longevities of organisms. This theory known as "disposable soma theory" was introduced into the studies of aging by Kirkwood (1977). The central thought is that the life history of a species in general is characterized by limited resources (constraints) of variable nature. That means that trade-offs exist between key life history variables and such trade-offs favor the allocation of energy between reproduction and maintenance of body constituents. Kirkwood argued that this universal theory should also be adaptable to humans. Together with Westendorp he had the opportunity to study the birth and death rates of about 35,000 males and females of the British aristocracy living between 740 and 1875. The main result was a negative correlation between longevity of females and the number of progeny (Westendorp and Kirkwood, 1998). Recent studies do not agree with these data (Lycett *et al.*, 2000). Accepted or not, the theory is testable with insects as models. Trade-offs between flight capability, reproduction, and longevity were indeed found in two cricket species (Tanaka and Suzuki, 1998, Zera *et al.*, 1998). In fruit flies deprived of protein as a source for egg development, the time of reproduction can be delayed with the result of a remarkable elongation of life span (Carey *et al.*, 1998). The same life-prolonging effect can be induced in *Phormia* (Wilker in our laboratory), which is an anautogenic insect as mentioned above. Feeding protein at the first time after 17 days of adult life decreases the age-specific mortality rate. This effect was particularly obvious when virgin females were used (Figure 21.8).

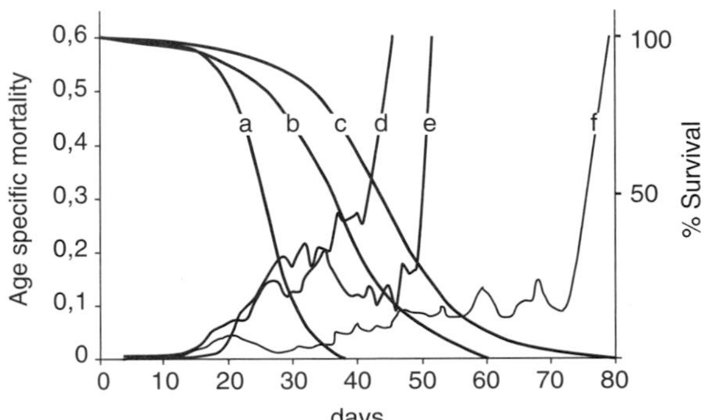

Figure 21.8. Survival curves (a,b,c) and age-specific mortality rates d,e,f) of virgin female *Phormia* under conditions of "no protein," "protein ad libitum," and first protein access after 17 days (after Collatz, 2003), with permission).

Metabolic Aging Studies

All metabolic aging studies on substrate and enzymatic level can profit by the basic similarity of the insect metabolism with that of other organisms, including man. It is therefore not surprising that many studies deal with enzyme activity or substrate changes in aging insects. Their antioxidative system garnered more attention with increasing knowledge of the role of free radicals and oxidative stress in aging and disease. Before showing some examples of such measurements, it seems advantageous to give some technical comments for the work with insects like *Phormia*.

RECOMMENDED PREPARATION OF *PHORMIA* FOR ENZYME AND SUBSTRATE DETERMINATION

Enzyme determination. Take 5 to 10 flies total or separate thorax and abdomen after decapitation.

Homogenize in 5-fold volume of ice cold TRA-buffer, 100 mM with 10 mM EDTA at pH 7.5 with a glass homogenizer. Centrifuge 20 minutes at 4°C with 5000 g. Take the supernatant and precipitate the dissolved proteins with 80% ammonium sulphate. Dissolve the precipitant with 1 ml homogenizing buffer after centrifugation as above.

Substrate determination. Place 10 flies into liquid nitrogen. This separates head, thorax, abdomen and extremities. Take the desired parts and grind them in liquid nitrogen after addition of 1 ml of 0.6 N $HClO_4$. Transfer the mixture into centrifuge tubes and centrifuge after thawing 30 min at 4°C and 5000 g. Neutralize the supernatant with solid $KHCO_3$ and store at −20°C until substrate determination.

Isolation of mitochondria. Put 10 thoraces (or abdomina) in 10 ml ice cold buffer (100 mM Tris/HCl, 10 mM EDTA, 320 mM sucrose, pH 7.5) and crush the material in a glass homogenizer with a Teflon pestle by raising and lowering it 20 times. Put the crude homogenate onto a nylon filter to remove chitin, myofibrills and tracheae fragments and wash it with buffer up to an end volume of 50 ml. Centrifuge 20 min at 100 g in the cold. Take the supernatant and centrifuge once more for 10 min at 3000 g and 4°C. The mitochondria are now in the precipitate and can be redissolved in 4-ml buffer.

EXAMPLES OF METABOLIC DETERMINATIONS

Redox state and influence of cell milieu on enzymatic activities

The thiole glutathione (GSH) is the most important nonenzymatic antioxidant in organisms and exists in considerably high concentrations in all cell types. GSH can react with electrophilic compounds or free radicals. The content of GSH in aging tissues generally declines, and it is assumed that this decline reduces the capacity to defend toxic effects of free radicals. Buthionin sulfoximine (BSO) is an irreversible inhibitor of the γ-glutamylcystein synthetase, which is a key enzyme for the synthesis of GSH. BSO can be used to empty the intracellular stores of GSH. This allows conclusions about the protective role of GSH.

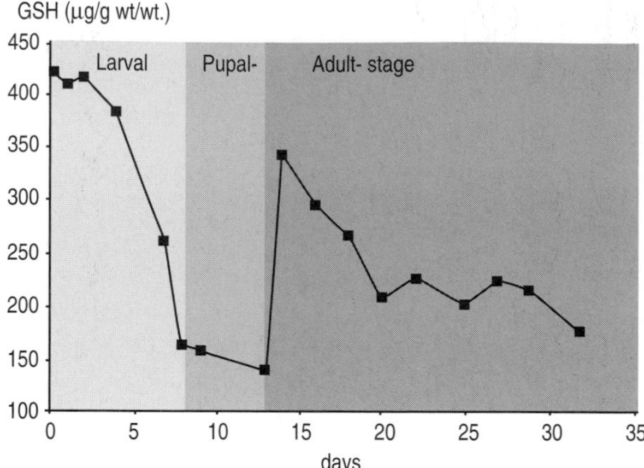

Figure 21.9. Glutathione content of *Phormia* flies in different life stages.

In *Phormia* there is a strong correlation between life stage and the GSH content (Figure 21.9).

Treatment with BSO for 11 days reduces the GSH content to 10% compared with the control. After this treatment, a resynthesis of GSH is observed only in younger flies.

Similarly, *Phormia* can be used to study the age-dependent capability of xenobiotics via the GSH-S-transferase (GST) system for detoxification (Collatz and Flury, 1992). Using the analgetic drug Paracetamol, we were able to show that both a reduced GSH level and a diminished activity of GST lead to an increasing mortality of old flies after drug injection.

It is a common phenomenon that the redox state of an old organism is shifted towards the oxidized site. *Phormia* is no exception. Together with the reduced GSH content, the quotient of the NAD/NADH and NADP/NADPH redox system is responsible for the redox state of the cell (Figure 21.10).

It is important to note that a change of the redox state, and with this the cell milieu, can alter enzyme activities. Jaekel in our laboratory showed this for purified glyceraldehyde-3-phosphate dehydrogenase (GAPDH) from young and old flies (Figure 21.11).

The kinetic properties of "young" and "old" enzymes are determined by the age-appropriate *in vivo* concentrations of NAD and NADH. "Old" enzyme reacts under "young" physiological conditions with an increase of V_{max} and K_m. In contrast "young" enzyme reacts under "old" physiological conditions with a reduction of V_{max} and K_m.

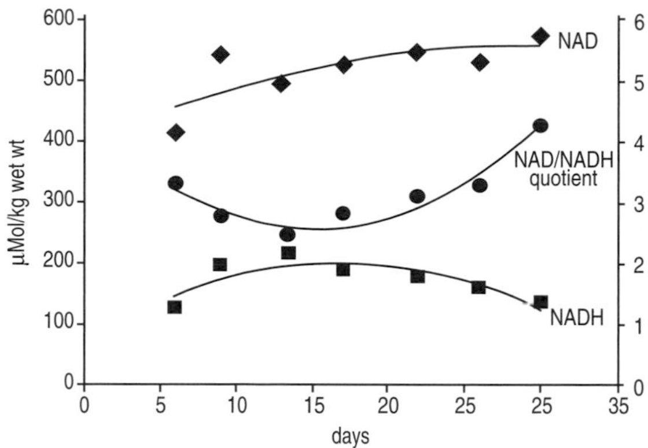

Figure 21.10. NAD and NADH content and NAD/NADH-quotient over the life span of *Phormia* flies to show the shift of the redox system to more oxidized state with increasing age.

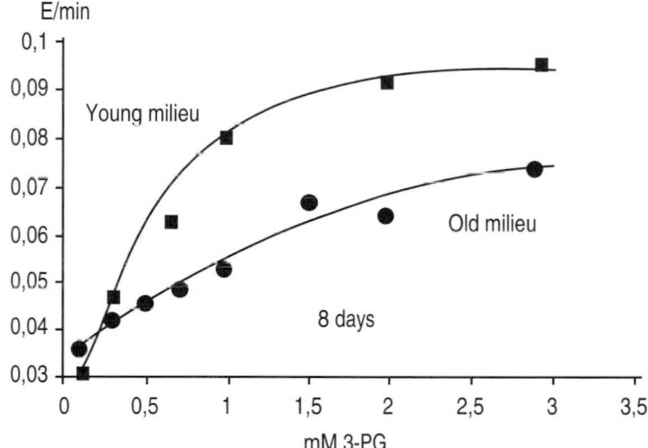

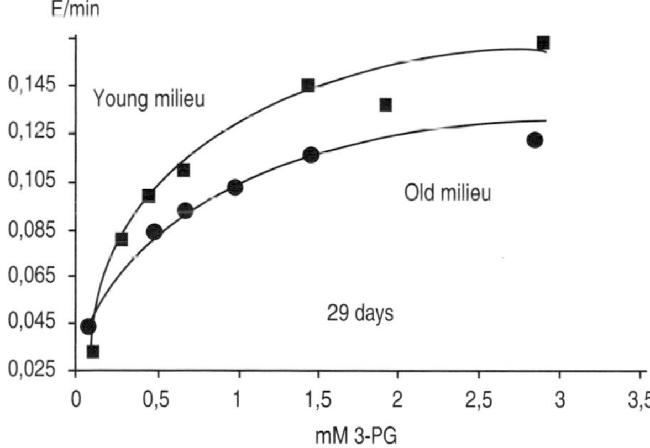

Figure 21.11. Influence of the cell milieu in aged *Phormia* flies on enzyme activity. Kinetics of purified GAPDH from young (8 days) and old (29 days) flies in mixture of NAD 0.4 mM/NADH 0.2 mM ("young milieu") and NAD 0.8 mM/NADH 0.1 mM ("old milieu"), after Collatz *et al.* (1993), with permission.

Conclusion

When comparative aging studies began in the eighties of the last century, it was a frequently quoted question whether insects are appropriate as model systems for aging studies. In the meantime insects cannot be dismissed as experimental animals for gaining insight in aging mechanisms in general. It was already addressed that the underlying chemical and cytological processes through which aging becomes visible are shared throughout the animal kingdom and, in part, even by plants.

In the last decade, several attempts have been made to unravel the similarities and differences from yeast to man that exist in signal transduction mechanisms, in particular those of the insulin/IGF signalling pathway. According to Rincon *et al.* (2004), the disruption of the insulin/IGF-1 receptor in nematodes and flies increases life span significantly. Mammals with genetic defects in the insulin signalling pathway, however, are at risk for increased mortality. Indeed, even these contradictory results and the paradox of the insulin/IGF-1 signalling pathway in longevity were recognized only after careful examinations of invertebrate models, including flies.

REFERENCES

Brachman, C.B., Sherman, S.E., Devine, E.E., Cameron, E.E., Pillus, L., and Boeke, J.D. (1995) The SIR2 gene family, conserved from bacteria to humans, functions in silencing, cell cycle progression, and chromosome stability. *Genes & Dev. 9*, 2888–2902.

Carey, R. (2000) Insect biodemography. *Ann. Rev. Entomol. 46*, 79–110.

Carey, J.R., Liedo, P., Müller, H.G., Wang, J.L., and Vaupel W. (1998) Dual modes of ageing in Mediterranean fruit fly females. *Science 281*, 996-998.

Collatz, K.-G. (1997) Fifteen years of *Phormia*—On the value of an insect for the study of aging. *Arch. Gerontol. Geriatr. 25*, 83–90.

Collatz, K.-G. (2003) Ageing and environmental conditions in insects. In *Aging of Organisms* (H.D. Osiewacz, ed.), pp. 99–123. Kluwer Academic Publishers, Dordrecht, Boston, London.

Collatz, K.-G., and Collatz, S. (1981) Age dependent ultrastructural changes in different organs of the mecopteran fly *Panorpa vulgaris. Exp. Gerontol. 16*, 183–193.

Collatz, K.-G., and Flury, T. (1992) Glutathione S-transferase and paracetamol detoxication in young and aged *Phormia* blowflies. *Verh. Dtsch. Zool. Ges. 85*, 135.

Collatz, K.-G., and Horning, M. (1990) Age dependent changes of a biochemical rhythm—The glycolytic oscillator of the blowfly *Phormia terraenovae. Comp. Biochem. Physiol. 96B*, 771–774.

Collatz, K.-G, Jaekel, K., Haebe, M., and Flury, T. (1993) Insects as models for aging mechanism studies. In *Recent Advances in Aging Science* (E. Beregi, I.A. Gergely and K. Rajczi, eds.), pp. 75-83. Monduzzi Editore S.p.A., Bologna.

Ernsting, G., and Isaaks, J.A. (1991) Accelerated ageing: A cost of reproduction in the carrabid beetle *Notiophilius biguttatus* F. *Funct. Ecol. 5*, 299–203.

Guarente, L., and Kenyon, C. (2000) Genetic pathways that regulate ageing in model organisms. *Nature 408*, 255–262.

Holliday, R. (1989) Food, reproduction and longevity: Is the extended lifespan of calorie-restricted animals an evolutionary adaptation? *BioEssays 10*, 125–127.

Horning, M., and Collatz, K.-G. (1990) First description of the glycolytic oscillator of an insect, the blowfly *Phormia terraenovae*. *Comp. Biochem. Physiol. 95B*, 613–618.

Kaitala, A. (1991) Phenotypic plasticity in reproductive behavior of waterstriders: Trade-offs between reproduction and longevity during food stress. *Funct. Ecol. 5*, 12–18.

Kirkwood, T.B. (1977) Evolution of ageing. *Nature 270*, 301–304.

Kirkwood, T.B.L., and Holliday, R. (1979) The evolution of ageing and longevity. *Proc. R. Soc. Lond. Ser. B 205*, 531–546.

Lamb, M.J. (1977) *Biology of Ageing*. Blackie & Son, Glasgow.

Loeb, J., and Northrop, J.H. (1917) On the influence of food and temperature on the duration of life. *J. Biol. Chem. 32*, 103–121.

Lycett, J.E., Dunbar, R.I.M., and Voland, E. (2000) Longevity and the costs of reproduction in a historical human population. *Proc. R. Soc. Lond. Ser. B 267*, 31–35.

Masoro, E.J. (2000) Caloric restriction and aging: An update. *Exp. Geront. 35*, 299–305.

Mattison, J.A., Lane, M.A., Roth, G.S., and Ingram, D.K. (2003) Calorie restriction in rhesus monkey. *Exp. Gerontol. 38*, 35–46.

McCay, C.M., and Maynard, L. (1935) The effect of retarded growth upon length of life and upon ultimate size. *J. Nutr. 10*, 63–79.

Page Jr., R.E., and Peng, C.Y.S. (2001) Ageing and development in social insects with emphasis on the honey bee, *Apis mellifera*. L. *Exp. Gerontol. 36*, 695–711.

Pearl, R. (1928) *The Rate of Living*. Knopf, New York.

Pittendrigh, C.S., and Minis, D.H. (1972) Circadian systems: Longevity as a function of circadian resonance in *Drosophila melanogaster*. *Proc. Natl. Acad. Sci. USA 69*, 1537–1539.

Rincon, M., Muzumdar, R., Atzmon, G., and Barzilai, N. (2004) The paradox of the insulin/IGF-1 signaling pathway in longevity. *Mech. Ageing Dev. 125*, 397–403.

Rubner, M. (1908) *Das Problem der Lebensdauer*. Berlin.

Saint Paul, U. (1978) Longevity among blowflies *Phormia terraenovae* R.D. kept in non-24-h light-dark cycle. *J. Comp. Physiol. A. 127*, 191–195.

Shanley, D.K., and Kirkwood, T.B.L. (2000) Caloric restriction and ageing: A life-history analysis. *Evolution 54*, 740–750.

Sheeba, V., Sharma, V.K., Shubha, K., Chandrashekaran, M.K., and Joshi, A. (2000) The effect of different light regimes on adult life span in *Drosophila melanogaster* is partly mediated through reproductive output. *J. Biol. Rhythm. 15*, 380–392.

Sohal, R.S. (1986) The rate of living theory: A contemporary interpretation. In *Insect Ageing* (K.-G. Collatz and R. Sohal, eds.), pp. 9–22. Springer, Berlin, Heidelberg, New York, Tokyo.

Spindler, S.R. (2001) Calorie restriction enhances the expression of key metabolic enzymes associated with protein renewal during aging. *Ann. N.Y. Acad. Sci. 928*, 296–304.

Stoffolano, J.G. (1974) Influence of diapause and diet on the development of the gonads and accessory reproductive glands of the black blowfly, *Phormia regins* (Meigen). *Can. J. Zool. 52*, 981–988.

Tanaka, S., and Suzuki, Y. (1998) Physiological trade-offs between reproduction, flight capability and longevity in a wing-dimorphic cricket, *Modicogryllus confirmatus*. *J. Insect Physiol. 44*, 121–129.

Tatar, M., and Yin, C.M. (2001) Slow ageing during insect reproductive diapause: Why butterflies, grasshoppers and flies are like worms. *Exp. Gerontol. 36*, 723–738.

Weber, H. (1966) *Grundriss der Insektenkunde*. VEB Gustav Fischer Verlag, Jena.

Westendorp, R., and Kirkwood, T.B. (1998) Human longevity at the cost of reproductive success. *Nature 396*, 743–746.

Yin, C.M., and Stoffolano Jr., J.G. (1994) Endocrinology of vitellogenesis in blowflies. In *Perspectives in Comparative Endocrinology* (K.G. Davey, R.E. Peter and S.S. Tobe, eds.), pp. 291–298. National Research Council of Canada, Ottawa.

Yin, C.M., and Stoffolano Jr., J.G. (1997) Juvenile hormone regulation of reproduction in the *Cyclorrhapuos Diptera* with emphasis on oogenesis. *Arch. Insect. Biochem. Physiol. 35*, 513–537.

Zera, A., Potts, J. and Kobus, K. (1998) The physiology of life-history trade-offs: Experimental analysis of a hormonally induced life-history trade-off in *Gryllus assimilis*. *Am. Nat. 152*, 7–23. http://fly.bio.indiana.edu/

22

Drosophila Models of Aging

Satomi Miwa and Alan Cohen

The fruit fly, Drosophila melanogaster, *is one of the most studied organisms in a variety of biological research fields, including studies on aging. The* Drosophila *model has approached aging from a range of angles and contributed significantly to our understanding of aging. It has been a valuable model organism in the field and is expected to remain so. This chapter aims to introduce* Drosophila *as a model organism for the study of aging. First, the basic biology of* Drosophila *is described within the context of aging, including its life history, characteristics of aging and physiology, and factors that affect lifespan. Next, various types of experimental approaches that can be used with* Drosophila *are presented, such as demographic, genetic, and physiological approaches. Lastly, a review of* Drosophila *studies on aging is presented, with emphasis on major achievements that* Drosophila *studies have accomplished. They illustrate types of studies particularly suited for flies, and how to combine different experimental approaches into one integrated study. We also raise limitations and technical problems, as well as unsolved problems; such issues are discussed with possible future directions.*

Introduction

The common fruit fly, *Drosophila melanogaster*, is one of the most studied organisms in biological research, with a history of use going back to the early 1900s. The first person known to have cultured *Drosophila* in quantity is Charles W. Woodworth, who suggested to colleagues that this organism be used for genetic work. Shortly after, *Drosophila* was introduced to Thomas Hunt Morgan, who made significant advances in genetics using this organism, leading him to win a Nobel Prize in Physiology or Medicine in 1933.

Drosophila is a convenient model organism in laboratories because it is easy to culture, inexpensive, available with a highly homogeneous genetic background, and has high reproductive capacity and a short lifespan. The system has traditionally been used in genetics, but more recently has become a staple in developmental biology. Furthermore, it has proven a useful model on which to study basic physiology such as circadian rhythms, learning, and memory. It even provides a genetic model for human neurodegenerative diseases including Huntington's disease, Alzheimer's disease, and Parkinson's disease. A potential new field may be the use in nociception research (Manev and Dimitrijevic, 2005), since there are no serious ethical considerations for insects like there are for higher model organisms.

The sequencing and annotation of the entire eukaryotic component of the *Drosophila* genome (about 13,600 genes) was completed in March 2000. Humans have about twice as many genes as flies, but the extra genes rarely represent novel functions; they simply allow for more complex regulation of fundamental molecular pathways. This is one of the main reasons the *Drosophila* model has implications for biological understandings of higher organisms.

Drosophila has also been one of the major model organisms on which to study fundamental mechanisms of aging. Although aging has been studied in various model organisms, a unique feature the *Drosophila* model has relative to other organisms is the wealth of resources already available. Its embryonic development, physiology, and behavior have all been studied by experts in these areas, and experimental techniques including advanced genetic tools are readily accessible. Furthermore, different stocks are available from stock centers around the world, and related information is publicly available on the Internet. Thus, although there are merits to working on novel animals, working with well-characterized organisms like *Drosophila* can facilitate research immensely. In addition, there are some biological characteristics that may be useful in aging studies. First, the period of growth and development (egg, larva and pupa) is clearly distinguishable from adult phase, where aging manifests. The transition to adult phase is not always so discrete in some animals. Next, the adult fly consists of mostly postmitotic cells, except for a few cells in the gonads and gut. Thus, the changes that occur during aging in cells and tissues are readily measurable.

The purpose of this chapter is to introduce *Drosophila* as a model organism for the study of aging. It includes a description of *Drosophila* life history, *Drosophila* as an aging organism, types of studies that can be done, and a brief review of aging research on *Drosophila*. Basic fly culturing techniques are also outlined. From this, one might consider whether *Drosophila* is a suitable model for a particular question to be investigated and whether it is feasible to culture flies in a given laboratory. Although *Drosophila* is often associated with genetic approaches, a detailed explanation of genetic techniques is beyond the scope of this chapter. More detailed laboratory protocols and experimental procedures as well as genetic technologies available are described elsewhere. See the Recommended Resources section at the end of this chapter for many excellent review articles, books and Internet resources on *Drosophila*.

Basic Biology of *Drosophila* as It Relates to Aging Studies

LIFE HISTORY OF *DROSOPHILA*

Development and maturation

There are three distinct morphological stages during development of *Drosophila*: egg, larva, and pupa. Approximate durations of each stage (at 25°C) are shown in Table 22.1. At 25°C, it takes around 10 days for a fertilized egg to become adult. Eggs are laid on the surface of the food medium. The egg is very small, shiny white, and ovoid (about 0.5 mm). The larva is a worm-like creature that feeds extensively. The larva molts twice, and the periods between the molts are called instars; thus the larva undergoes three stages as the first, second and third instars. It rapidly expands during molting before the new cuticle hardens (2–3 mm long at the third instar). The third instar larva eventually stops feeding and crawls out of the food medium and becomes still. After several hours a white prepupa (about 2 mm) is formed. It becomes brown within an hour, and air bubbles come out from the abdomen making it buoyant. Most pupae are stuck to the wall of the container or on the stopper. During pupation, imaginal discs develop in the tissues of the adult fly (about 3 mm).

Flies tend to eclose just before dawn. Newly eclosed adult flies have a soft cuticle and folded wings. It takes several hours for the wings to become unfolded, dry out and harden. Very young flies are light colored and have dark meconium in the gut, visible through the ventral abdominal wall. Flies do not mate for 8 hours after eclosion; this is a critical period in which virgin females can be collected. The lifespan of adult flies is dependent on strain and environment. Under standard conditions, wild-type flies live up to 2–3 months.

TABLE 22.1
Developmental stages and durations of *Drosophila*

Stages		Times after egg laying	Duration
Egg		–	≈1 day
Larva	1st instar	22 hours	≈1 day
	2nd instar	46 hours	≈1 day
	3rd instar	70 hours	≈2 days
Pupa		120 hours	≈5 days

Characteristics of aging

Finch (1990) has identified three major patterns of aging in animals: rapid, which is typified by semelparous organisms such as Atlantic salmon and mayflies (Ephemeroptera); negligible, which is typified by colonial invertebrates and some turtles and fish; and gradual, which is found in most birds and mammals, including humans (Finch, 1990). Unlike many insects, *Drosophila* aging is gradual, an important feature for an organism serving as a model for human aging. However, unlike humans, *Drosophila* does not have a very long post-reproductive lifespan. Some examples of manifestations of senescence are shown in Table 22.2 (Rockstein and Miquel, 1973).

In general, marked degenerative changes occur in *Drosophila* tissues with advancing age. It is perhaps

TABLE 22.2
Manifestation of aging in *Drosophila*

Flight muscles

- Formation of giant mitochondria by fusing, "swirls" in matrix
- Decrease in glycogen content, almost absent in very old individuals
- Decrease in oxidative phosphorylation enzyme activity
- Myofibrillar degeneration
- Inability to fly in very old individuals

Reproductive system

- In male testis, decreases in the number of spermatogonia and spermatocytes
- Decrease in numbers of egg production in females

Digestive system

- Accumulation of numerous large lamellated cytoplasmic inclusions in the midgut
- Increases in lipid droplets and vacuoles

Fat body

- Decrease in fat content
- Decrease in cell size and shrunken appearance
- Uneven distribution of glycogen within a cell

Nervous system

- Nerve-cell degeneration in brain
- Decrease in the amount of cytoplasm and ribosomes in neurosecretory cells
- Decrease in negative geotaxis ability

Others

- Decrease in heart rate
- Structural and functional alterations in Malpighian tubules in excretory system

due to the fact that cells in *Drosophila* are mostly postmitotic and are not replaced except for a small part of the reproductive tissues. Causes of death in *Drosophila* are not well established. Suggestions include starvation, fat body degeneration, failure of the digestive system, failure of the excretory organs, and failure of the nervous system, among others (Rockstein and Miquel, 1973).

COMMENTS ON PHYSIOLOGY

The appearance of male and female flies is described elsewhere; see the Recommended Resources section. Like the mammals for which it often serves as a proxy, *Drosophila* has a nervous system, hormonal system, and circulatory system. However it lacks several systems present in mammals, and many shared systems function somewhat differently. First, as a poikilotherm, temperature has a direct effect on metabolic rate, and lifespan of the flies can be significantly extended when they are kept at lower temperatures (see below). Because the adult fly consists mostly of postmitotic cells, issues such as replicative senescence, cell proliferation in aging, and cancer development have not been considered in flies; however, these factors may be important in higher organisms that have many mitotic cells.

In the mammalian insulin signaling pathway, functions of growth and metabolism in mammals are regulated by different receptors, the IGF-1 and insulin receptors. In contrast, in *Drosophila*, diverse physiological functions (including growth, metabolism, and reproduction) are regulated by a single hormonal receptor in the insulin signaling pathway (Tatar, 2004). The insulin-signaling pathway influences the levels of other insect hormones including juvenile hormone and the sterol ecdysone, which themselves may affect aging (Garofalo, 2002).

The respiration of *Drosophila* is mediated by simple diffusion; oxygen uptake is achieved by diffusion through the trachea (Weis-Fogh, 1964). In flight muscles, mitochondria are located almost adjacent to tracheole. Flight muscle mitochondria in insects have an exceptionally high oxidative metabolism capacity capable of supporting around 100-fold increases in oxygen consumption on initiation of flight (Sacktor, 1974). Recently, mitochondria have been at the center of attention in aging research. First, mitochondria are implicated as a major endogenous source of reactive oxygen species that can damage surrounding molecules; second, many experimental manipulations that extend lifespan are also known to alter glucose and lipid metabolism, and logically mitochondria are thought to play an important role. Finally, mitochondria are thought to be responsible for apoptosis, at least in part. Thus, together with the fact that mitochondria undergo significant morphological alterations with age (Sohal, 1976), highly active insect flight muscle mitochondria could be an interesting research subject.

The fat body, the organ that has been implicated as playing a role in regulating lifespan (Hwangbo *et al.*, 2004; Giannakou *et al.*, 2004), is equivalent to liver and white adipose tissue in mammals. It stores fat and glycogen, and is also responsible for immune function by producing antimicrobial peptides upon infection. In contrast to mammals and many other vertebrates, insects have only an innate immune system.

FACTORS THAT AFFECT LIFESPAN

When conducting aging studies, it is most important to control genetic and environmental factors that affect lifespan. Uncontrolled variables can lead to erroneous interpretation of the results. The information below should be used both as a guide for variables that are particularly important to control, and as a primer on lifespan-related variables for further exploration.

Intrinsic/genetic factors

Genetic background plays a major role in lifespan. It is important that the effects of mutant gene actions or any experimental manipulations be studied on a standard genetic background with an appropriate control group. However, because genetic influences on longevity are described in detail in Chapter 25 of this volume, no more will be said here.

Adult survival and fecundity show significant inbreeding depression, presumably because deleterious recessive mutations present are more likely to become homozygous and have deleterious phenotypic effects on the offspring of matings between relatives. Adult survival and fecundity evolve rapidly in laboratory culture. In a typical fly lab, the newly emerged adult flies are collected into new culture bottles, allowed to lay eggs, and then discarded. When this regime is applied to flies collected from nature, there is a rapid increase in early fecundity (which is selectively favored under this culture regime) and also a large decrease in adult survivorship as a correlated response to the early fecundity (Partridge and Pletcher, 2003).

There is no evidence to suggest sex differences in lifespan; however, males and females respond differently to interventions known to extend lifespan (e.g., dietary restriction (Magwere *et al.*, 2004)). Physiological differences, for example, differences in nutrient demand, differences in resource allocation (females for egg production; males for activity and courtship), and differences in sensitivity to hormonal signaling pathways that are known to determine lifespan (such as insulin/insulin-like growth factor signaling (IIS) pathway) may be responsible.

Extrinsic factors

The lifespan of *Drosophila* is also affected by factors unrelated to genetics (Table 22.3), many of which have

TABLE 22.3
Extrinsic factors that affect lifespan in *Drosophila*

Factors	Condition	Effects
Pre-adult development	Higher larval density	Prolongs the duration of development time and extends adult lifespan; results in smaller adult size
	Lower ambient temperature	Prolongs the duration of development time and extends adult lifespan; results in larger adult size
Parental age	Older parents	Fewer viable eggs and offspring have shorter lifespan
Fecundity	Higher reproductive activity	Shortens lifespan; Virgins live longer than mated flies in both sexes, but the magnitude of increase in lifespan is greater in females
Ambient temperature	Lower ambient temperature	Extends lifespan; Flies cultured at 18°C live more than twice as long as those at 25°C
Mild stress	Heat shock, cold stress, hypergravity, low levels of radiation	Extends lifespan
Diet	Dietary restriction	Extends lifespan
Physical activity	Reduced flight activity	Extends lifespan

been used as experimental manipulations to extend lifespan in order to elucidate factors that affect longevity. However, a mechanistic explanation of these factors is still unclear (see below).

Probably the strongest environmental stimulus that affects lifespan is environmental temperature. Adult flies cultured at 18°C live more than twice as long as those cultured at 25°C. Various mild stressors, including heat shock (37°C for less than 1 hour), cold stress, hypergravity, and low levels of irradiation, have been shown to extend lifespan. It has been proposed that mild stressors may induce protective systems that will be beneficial for forthcoming events. However, the effects could be secondary in some cases, as some stressors such as irradiation have negative effects on reproduction, which alone can extend lifespan.

Dietary yeast is important in survival and reproduction in adult *Drosophila*. In the absence of yeast, *Drosophila* arrest reproduction and increase mortality in both males and females (Good and Tatar, 2001). Dietary restriction extends lifespan in a variety of organisms including *Drosophila*. The females have greater responses to dietary restriction, even in sterile or *ovaryless* females (Mair *et al.*, 2004). The maximum extension of lifespan in females is achieved at a less severe level of dietary restriction than in males (Magwere *et al.*, 2004).

Prevention of flight activity has been shown to extend lifespan in blowflies (Yan and Sohal, 2000) as well as in *Drosophila* (Tapi Magwere, personal communications). In accord with this, mutant flies that move more than normal (*shaker* mutants) have shorter lifespan (Trout and Kaplan, 1970). Thus levels of physical activity in flies appear to negatively correlate with lifespan (see the "*Drosophila* in Aging Studies" section for further discussion).

Types of Experimental Approaches in Aging Studies

DEMOGRAPHIC STUDIES

In aging studies it is of course important to measure the rate of aging. However, the rate at which an individual ages is difficult to measure. There is no consensus on biomarkers of aging. Furthermore, if one were to follow the changes in a biomarker, the assay would need to be noninvasive to avoid biasing the measure, and certainly could not kill the organisms. In contrast, the measurement of the rate of aging in a population can be achieved easily by analyzing patterns of age-at-death. Age-at-death is an unambiguous and easily measurable end point. Age-specific mortality is a measure of the instantaneous hazard of death for an individual at a given age. It allows independent comparisons of vulnerability to death at different ages. The main drawback of such demographic studies is that they require very large population sizes, especially for estimates of age-specific mortality and maximum lifespan. *Drosophila* is ideally suited for demographic analyses because it is easier to culture and monitor large numbers of individuals than with other short-lived model organisms such as yeast (*Saccharomyces cerevisiae*) and nematode worms (*Caenorhabditis elegans*). One assumption of such demographic measures of aging is that physiological and functional declines correlate with increases in death rate, which might not be the case. Therefore, ideally studies should be supplemented with some physiological measures such as the number of eggs laid and locomotive function.

The mortality rate (μ_x) at age x can be expressed mathematically as

$$\mu_x = -\ln(P(x)) \tag{1}$$

where $P(x)$ is the probability of an individual alive at age x surviving to age $x+1$ (Carey, 1993). The data are often gathered so as to fit explicit models in order to (a) reduce complexity and day-to-day variations of mortality data, and (b) allow parametric statistical tests. The most popular model is the Gompertz model:

$$\mu_x = ae^{bx} \tag{2}$$

where the constant a is the intrinsic baseline mortality rate and b is the rate at which mortality rates accelerate with age (Promislow and Haselkorn, 2002). The natural logarithm of the Gompertz equation gives a linear function:

$$\ln(\mu_x) = a + bx \tag{3}$$

which is analogous to a straight line with slope b and intercept a on the vertical axis. The slope b represents the rate of aging (Magwere *et al.*, 2004; Mair *et al.*, 2003). In the Gompertz model, the baseline mortality rate is not independent of aging rate. It should be noted that the Gompertz model assumes a constant, exponential increase in mortality rate throughout adulthood.

However, the early and very late mortality rates do not appear to fit the model completely: the increase in mortality rates slows down at the end of the lifespan.

Using this approach, experimental manipulations to extend lifespan can be classified into two types depending on the pattern of changes in mortality trajectory: treatments that change the slope (i.e., the rate of aging) and treatments that change the intercept (i.e., the underlying baseline mortality rate is changed) (Finch, 1990). A good illustration is a study by Mair *et al.* (2003) which performed a demographic analysis of effects of dietary restriction in flies (see "*Drosophila* in aging studies" Figure 22.1).

GENETIC APPROACHES

Genetic tools in *Drosophila* have been well developed and can be used for a variety of purposes. There are ways to explore genes that control lifespan (e.g., quantitative trait loci (QTLs), longevity screens, candidate genes), and to identify genes that change their expression patterns in response to a particular treatment and/or with age (e.g., enhancer traps, microarray analysis). There are ways in which to manipulate the cellular environment by altering gene expressions in a time-dependent and tissue-specific manner (e.g., candidate gene approach). Below is an overview of such methods; comprehensive review articles on genetic approaches in aging studies in *Drosophila* can be found elsewhere (Partridge and Pletcher, 2003; Helfand and Rogina, 2003; Poirier and Seroude, 2005).

Quantitative Trait Locus (QTL) approaches

QTL is a method for associating variation in quantitative genetic traits with specific regions of the genome. Backcrosses and intercrosses can be used to find markers on a genomic map that correlate with variation in the quantitative trait. The amount of variation in the trait that is explained by each locus can be quantified, and this information can then be used to target specific areas of the genome for further investigation. Ultimately, the utility of the QTL approach depends on a detailed genomic map and the ability to characterize the functions of genes in the regions identified, making *Drosophila* an excellent organism for this technique. Moreover, the cross-breeding and inbreeding process is facilitated in *Drosophila* by the wide variety of lineages available.

In particular, the combination of candidate gene approaches (see below) and QTL can be a powerful tool for identifying genes responsible for quantitative variation in traits such as lifespan. However, it must be cautioned that QTL results may be specific to the environment and/or genetic background under which the experiment is conducted, and care should be used in generalizing the results.

Phenotype (longevity) screening

This is a method for identifying genes affecting lifespan by observing phenotypes (i.e., longevity) of flies that are generated through random gene mutations. Identification of mutated genes can be simplified by using transposition for mutagenesis: the *P*-element transposon is a commonly used mutagen. *P*-elements are transposable elements that are widely used to make mutations and manipulate the genome. Often random insertion of transposons into genes or their regulatory elements decreases gene activity (Cooley *et al.*, 1988). For example, the *methuselah* gene, which encodes G-protein-coupled receptor, was identified by this method; loss of function in this by a *P*-element transposon resulted in 40% increases in average lifespan (Lin *et al.*, 1998).

Enhancer Traps

With enhancer traps, detailed gene expression patterns in specific tissues or cells can be characterized. In enhancer traps, a promoter, usually a *P*-transposable element, is inserted into the genome together with a reporter gene such as lacZ and GAL4. Enhancer regulation is expected to affect the reporter gene as well as its usual targets, so expression patterns of the reporter gene can be characterized and taken as a proxy for expression patterns of genes nearby the insertion locus. Then the region around the insertion can be identified and studied further in order to pinpoint what nearby gene(s) may be involved in the expression pattern and may thus be relevant to the phenomenon of interest (see O'Kane, 1998 for details). The gene *Indy* (*I'm Not Dead Yet*), which is associated with extended lifespan, was originally identified with an enhancer trap (Rogina *et al.*, 2000).

Microarray Analysis

Microarray analysis is a method that makes use of gene chips to which thousands of different mRNAs can bind and be quantified. By using such chips to quantify mRNA levels in different tissues or in individuals under different treatments, tens or hundreds of specific genes which vary in relation to the tissue or treatment can be identified, aiding in a mechanistic understanding of the differences. Further work can then be conducted using candidate locus approaches (see below). In contrast to QTL, which looks at allelic variation, microarray analysis looks at gene regulation: potentially, but not necessarily, a result of allelic variation.

As with QTLs, care must be exercised not only to control for genetic background and environment, but also to limit interpretation of results to the genetic background and environment studied. Also, it must be remembered that microarray analysis is by its nature correlative, and that further study of patterns is generally necessary for clear interpretation. That said, microarray analysis remains one of the most powerful techniques for examining genetic processes underlying physiological variation.

Drosophila in particular are well suited to microarray analysis (a) because the genome is relatively small, meaning that most of it can be analyzed with a single microarray and that potentially important patterns are less likely to be missed, and (b) because the functions of many genes have already been studied, facilitating interpretation of results. Microarray analysis has been used in *Drosophila* to characterize gene expression changes during dietary restriction and with aging (Pletcher *et al.*, 2002).

Candidate gene approaches

The major use of candidate gene approaches is to test specific genes selected based on educated guesses as to which genes affect the process in question. The genes of interest can be deleted, overexpressed, or induced, and phenotypes of the mutant flies are observed accordingly. Mutation methods usually involve *P*-element mediated transgenes. They can be used to introduce foreign DNA into the *Drosophila* genome. However, depending on its position in the genome, the expression of an inserted transgene may vary and the insertion can have considerable effects on lifespan. Therefore, methods that allow the experimental and the control groups to have a transgenic insert in the same genomic location are desirable (Partridge and Pletcher, 2003; Helfand and Rogina, 2003; Venken and Bellen, 2005; Poirier and Seroude, 2005).

There are techniques for "inducible" mutation that allow conditional expression of genes in a time- and tissue-specific manner. In principle, gene expression is initiated upon application of the inducer. The "flip-out" system uses a heat pulse as the inducer. However, the heat pulse can itself affect lifespan, potentially complicating the results. Two other systems, the "gene-switch" and the "tet-on" systems, use antiprogestin, RU486, and tetracycline or its analogue deoxycycline respectively, to feed flies to initiate gene expression.

PHYSIOLOGICAL AND BIOCHEMICAL APPROACHES

In order to elucidate mechanisms of aging, downstream effects of experimental manipulations that extend lifespan need to be fully characterized. For example, identification of a gene for a mutation that extends lifespan does not by itself explain how the gene achieves this. Here, physiological, biochemical, and cell biological studies become essential.

Biochemical and cell biological approaches in *Drosophila* are well developed and easy to utilize. A large number of protocols for procedures such as DNA and RNA extractions and purification of mitochondrial DNA can be found in the literature (see Recommended Resources section).

Usually most types of measurements that have been performed in other model species such as rodents can also be applied to *Drosophila*. Preparation of tissue homogenate is easy, and potential aging biomarkers such as protein, lipid and DNA oxidative damage can be measured, as well as various metabolites and enzyme activities. Mitochondria are easily prepared from the homogenates (Miwa *et al.*, 2003), and respiration rate, reactive oxygen species production, membrane potentials and mitochondrial enzyme activities can be measured.

Physiological measures are important because they can provide insight into the nature of aging processes, which may not be apparent from the "age-at-death" measure that is used in demographic studies. A number of different types of behavioral assays such as learning and memory have been established (Connolly and Tully, 1998). Also there are other measures that are relevant to aging; number of eggs laid, negative geotaxis, immune function (DeVeale *et al.*, 2004), heart function (Wessells *et al.*, 2004), and circadian rhythm (Driver, 2000). Metabolic rate can be assayed by respirometry/calorimetry (Hulbert *et al.*, 2004), and stress resistance can be tested in various forms, including hydrogen peroxide, paraquat feeding, cold, starvation, and desiccation.

Drosophila in Aging Studies

Drosophila studies have been involved in many aging-related topics and have been instrumental in shaping our current view of aging. The success of the *Drosophila* model is no doubt helped by the availability of the variety of experimental approaches indicated above, which have been successfully used in combination on one topic, namely, demographic and genetic approaches in combination. Contributions of *Drosophila* studies can be roughly divided into four main areas: selection experiments on the evolution of aging; tests of metabolic and oxidative damage hypotheses of aging; dietary restriction; and searches for evolutionarily conserved genetic mechanisms of lifespan regulation. Though not necessarily mutually exclusive, each of these is presented below. They illustrate practical uses of various experimental approaches and how they can be combined to perform integrative studies; in addition, problems and future directions are also discussed.

SELECTION AND DEMOGRAPHIC EXPERIMENTS

In 1957, G.C. Williams proposed antagonistic pleiotropy as an explanation for the evolution of aging (Williams, 1957). According to the theory, the declining force of selection with age results in selection for pleiotropic genes that enhance fitness early in life but reduce it later. The accumulation of many such genes could result in a deterioration of condition with age. This hypothesis became a driving force for most evolutionary studies of aging. Current research on the topic is less explicitly genetic, referring more to "trade-offs" than "pleiotropy": a recognition that constraints may come from physiological, developmental, or even behavioral conflicts.

Because of its short generation time, *Drosophila* is ideally suited to selection experiments testing trade-off hypotheses. In a series of seminal experiments, Rose (1984) confirmed antagonistic pleiotropy for aging in *Drosophila*, demonstrating a tight correlation between early fecundity and lifespan. Selection for early fecundity produced short lifespans; selection for late fecundity produced long lifespans. Moreover, the results were highly reproducible. Further experiments in a number of labs have examined other trade-offs with lifespan. Development time was found to not be directly associated with lifespan, disproving the developmental theory of aging (Lints, 1978), at least for *Drosophila* (Chippindale *et al.*, 1994). Stress resistance was found to correlate positively with lifespan, though this response could eventually be broken down with strong selection over many generations (Phelan *et al.*, 2003). Mating itself was found to be toxic to females, mediating the lifespan–fecundity trade-off (Chapman *et al.*, 1993).

Large population sizes in *Drosophila* have also facilitated demographic studies examining fine details of mortality rate changes with age. Late-life mortality plateaus, a common phenomenon in a number of species, has been examined in depth in *Drosophila*. Also, studies have been conducted with large populations testing antagonistic pleiotropy in contrast to simple mutation accumulation, though the interpretation of the results is still debated (Hughes *et al.*, 2002). Both mutation accumulation and antagonistic pleiotropy predict age-specific effects of mutations on mortality; this also has been tested and found (Yampolsky *et al.*, 2000).

It is a testament to the strength of the *Drosophila* model that most of the above studies, especially the detailed demographic explorations of mortality, have been done only in *Drosophila*. However, this also produces the caveat that the results may apply only to *Drosophila*, or at least may apply less broadly than some of the genetic mechanisms of aging described below. For example, while there do appear to be trade-offs between reproduction and longevity in mammals, the correlation is much less tight than in *Drosophila* and the mechanisms may be indirect (Cohen, 2004).

RATE OF LIVING, METABOLISM, AND OXIDATIVE DAMAGE

The first substantive biological theory of aging, the rate of living theory, was developed from studies on *Drosophila*. The early work of Loeb and Northorp (1917) demonstrated that temperature was negatively associated with lifespan in *Drosophila*. Raymond Pearl, a biostatistician who worked on population genetics, put forward this phenomenon as the "rate of living theory." He found that the coefficient relating lifespan to ambient temperature in flies had a magnitude between two and three, which was similar to that of chemical reactions; he interpreted this as signifying that all the biochemical reactions for living processes occurred faster at higher temperatures in flies.

Thus, increased lifespan in flies at lower temperatures was originally thought to be due to slowing down of *all* biochemical processes. However, the interpretation of effects of temperature may not be so simple because not all enzyme activities are affected by temperature to the same degree. Concentration of a molecule "X" depends on its production and consumption, and if the activities of the producer and the consumer have different Q10 values (thus differently affected by temperature) the concentration of molecule "X" could go up or down, depending on the balance. Furthermore, there are certain physiological responses to cold (temperature compensation) that are independent of metabolic rate, such as changes in membrane fatty acid composition, that can affect susceptibility to oxidative damage (unpublished observation). It is not known how circadian rhythms, which are known to control various physiological functions, are affected by temperature, although a constant 12:12 hour light:dark cycle in laboratory culture conditions can force them to follow this circadian cycle. Nevertheless, the demographic study of mortality trajectories has shown that lowering temperature changes the slope, suggesting the rate of aging was slowed down (Mair *et al.*, 2003).

The rate of living theory stated that the metabolic rate of an organism is directly and causally linked to its longevity; that is, "live fast, die young." A mechanistic explanation of the rate of living theory was provided by the oxidative damage theory. Originally proposed by Harman (1956), its modified and refined version states that reactive oxygen species produced as byproducts by mitochondria during normal aerobic respiration can attack and damage surrounding molecules, and accumulation of such damage causes aging (Harman, 1972; Sohal and Weindruch, 1996; Beckman and Ames, 1998). It is thought that the phenomenon of increased physical activity in flies shortening lifespan is due to a higher metabolic cost in these flies, which in turn increases mitochondrial reactive oxygen species production. However, this concept is confusing because mitochondrial reactive oxygen species production will be lower, rather than higher, under state 3 respiration (active respiration state, such as during exercise, producing ATP in the presence of ADP) compared with state 4 respiration (resting state, no production of ATP). This is because mitochondrial reactive oxygen species production correlates with membrane potential, and membrane potential is lower in state 3 than state 4. Furthermore, in mammals, elevated metabolic rate by wheel running exercise (Holloszy, 1997) or cold exposure (Holloszy and Smith, 1986) in rats does not shorten lifespan, and mice with higher metabolic rates (with lower membrane potential due to more mitochondrial uncoupling) were reported to live longer than those with lower metabolic rates (Speakman *et al.*, 2004), demonstrating a dissociation of increased metabolic rate and longevity. Similarly, it has been shown that extended lifespan in *Drosophila* was not accompanied by lowered metabolic rate (van Voorhies *et al.*, 2003; Hulbert *et al.*, 2004; Khazaeli *et al.*, 2005).

Nonetheless, the elevation of respiration rates between rest and flight in *Drosophila* is much larger (~100 fold) than that seen in mammalian models, so intense oxygen uptake in flies might indeed have detrimental effects. Further investigations exploring effects of flight activity on longevity in flies are of great interest.

In addition, many *Drosophila*-based studies have tested the oxidative damage hypothesis; a popular approach has been to reduce the level of oxidative stress and see if lifespan can be extended. For example, using the candidate gene approach, attempts have been made to lower levels of oxidative stress either by overexpressing antioxidant enzymes or by lowering mitochondrial reactive oxygen species production through elevating proton conductance (Miwa *et al.*, 2004; Fridell *et al.*, 2005). Dietary antioxidant supplementation has also been performed (reviewed in Le Bourg, 2001).

However, not all studies support the hypothesis. Initial studies genetically inducing increased antioxidant defenses had technical problems: use of short-lived flies, different sized inserts between control and experimental groups, and uncontrolled position effects in transgene constructs (Tower, 2000; Partridge and Pletcher, 2003). Later work found that overexpression of Cu,Zn-SOD, Mn-SOD, or both with the FLP/FRT system increased lifespan (Sun *et al.*, 2002; Sun *et al.*, 2004; Sun and Tower, 1999), Cu,Zn-SOD overexpression in motorneurons extended lifespan (Parkes *et al.*, 1998), but overexpression of various combinations of Cu,Zn-SOD, Mn-SOD, catalase and thioredoxin reductase did not extend lifespan (Orr *et al.*, 2003). In addition, most studies involving altering antioxidant status did not check whether damage was actually reduced.

The effects of lowered mitochondrial reactive oxygen species on lifespan have been examined using transgenic flies that have higher proton conductance. Expression of human uncoupling protein 2 (hUCP2) in nervous tissue lowered reactive oxygen species production and extended lifespan but not when it was expressed in muscles (Fridell *et al.*, 2005). Overexpression of adenine nucleotide translocase in whole fly also lowered mitochondrial membrane potential and reactive oxygen species production, but lifespan was shortened (Miwa *et al.*, 2004). Although such negative results are difficult to interpret due to potential unknown side effects, there could be tissue-specific effects of this type of manipulation on lifespan. Alternatively, it is possible that hUCP2 induction in neurons in flies extended lifespan through mechanisms which are not related to oxidative stress, for example, by impairing insulin signaling. Further examination of this issue will be enlightening.

Other studies—some of them on houseflies—have aimed to establish correlational evidence of the oxidative damage theory, as has been done in mammalian systems. Oxidative damage was found to increase with age (Sohal *et al.*, 1993; Yan *et al.*, 1997; Yan and Sohal, 1998). Mitochondrial reactive oxygen species production was found to increase with age (Sohal and Sohal, 1991; Sohal, 1993; Ross, 2000), and it was lower in long-lived lines of flies than controls (Farmer and Sohal, 1989). However, no such correlation was found when lifespan was extended by dietary restriction (Miwa *et al.*, 2004).

Although there is much correlative evidence to support it, confirmation of the oxidative damage theory still requires establishment of (a) which specific forms of damage (DNA, proteins or lipids) are important; (b) how the balance between ROS formation, ROS removal, and damage repair is regulated; and (c) which tissues or cell types are most critically affected. Then the appropriate direct tests should be performed accordingly. The *Drosophila* model will be a major player in this ongoing research area.

DIETARY RESTRICTION

Dietary restriction is the only environmental manipulation that can bring robust extension of lifespan in a variety of model organisms, and is one of the most important themes in aging studies. Despite a great deal of effort, the precise mechanisms by which it works are not clear. Exploration of its mechanism has also been attempted in *Drosophila*, and though the picture is incomplete, progress is being made.

Using demographic analyses, it has been shown that dietary restriction extends lifespan in flies by altering baseline mortality rate without altering the rate of aging (Mair *et al.*, 2003). (Figure 22.1).

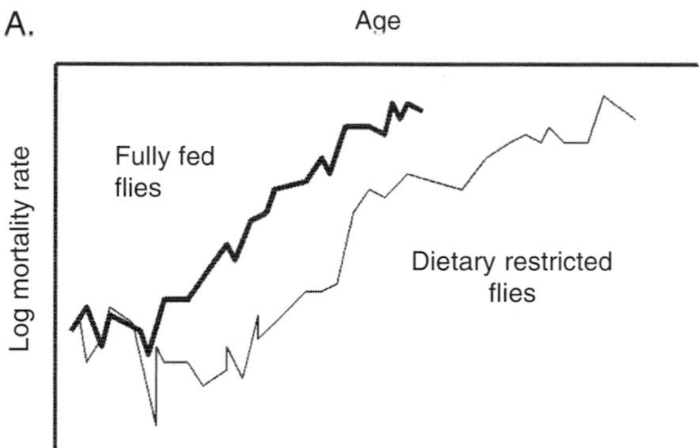

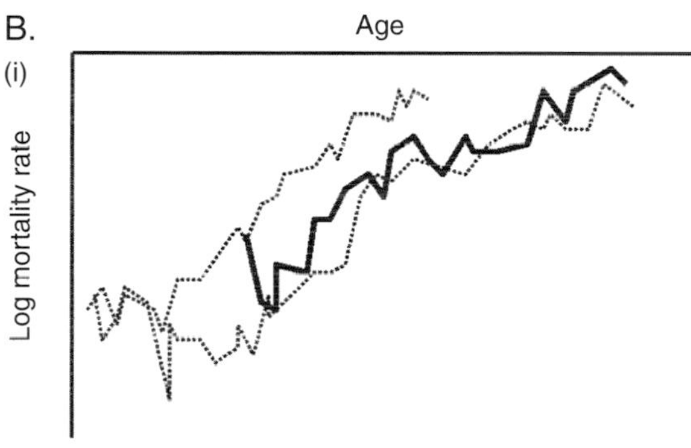

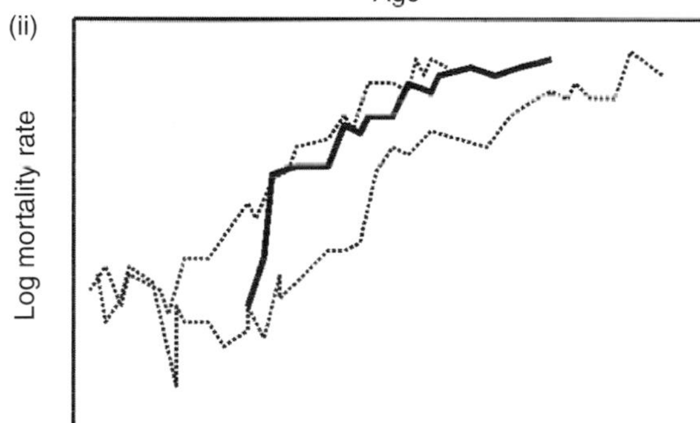

Figure 22.1. (A) Age-specific mortality trajectories in *Drosophila* subjected to different dietary regimes. Dietary restriction lowers initial mortality rate (intercept) but does not affect the rate of increase (slope).c (B) Rapid adjustment in mortality trajectories after changes in diet regime (post-switching trajectories are shown in solid lines; the trajectories in Figure 22.1-A are shown in dashed lines). (i) Switching from fully fed to dietary restriction diet; (ii) switching from dietary restriction to fully fed diet. Subsequent mortality trajectories after the diet switch are not affected by the previous dietary experiences, and only reflect the current dietary status. (Mair *et al.*, 2003). Figures re-drawn from (Mair *et al.*, 2003), with permission.

This study also suggests that dietary restriction does not affect irreversible, time-dependent accumulation of damage because the mortality was rapidly and completely reversed when the dietary restriction was removed (and vice versa). Thus, the effect of diet on mortality rate is only real-time, and not affected by past history (Mair *et al.*, 2003). Examining the reversibility of a treatment is therefore particularly informative, and it will be enlightening to conduct this type of treatment-switching experiment in other experimental models that extend lifespan. However, it is debatable whether this response is unique to flies (Partridge *et al.*, 2005). Similar demographic studies in mammals have not been performed to clarify this issue, perhaps due to a difficulty in conducting the study involving a large number of animals.

Next, microarray analysis of gene expression in response to dietary restriction showed that genes regulating cell growth, metabolism and reproduction were down regulated (Pletcher *et al.*, 2002). However, there are many other molecular, biochemical and physiological studies that can be performed on the *Drosophila* dietary restriction model, as in the case of rodent models.

SEARCH FOR EVOLUTIONARILY CONSERVED GENETIC MECHANISMS AFFECTING LIFESPAN

Drosophila has been used to identify evolutionarily conserved aging mechanisms by assessment of whether particular genes/genetic pathways that extend lifespan in other organisms such as yeast and nematodes also work in flies. Any mechanisms that are conserved across distant species are likely to have implications for humans.

Genes in the insulin/insulin-like growth factor signaling pathway have been examined based on the knowl edge that homologues such as *daf-2* extend lifespan in *C. elegans*. The *Drosophila* equivalent of *daf-2 (Inr)*, *chico*, a *Drosophila* insulin receptor substrate, were also found to extend lifespan in flies when mutated, suggesting conserved mechanisms of the IIS pathway in the control of lifespan.

Another example is the role of the sirtuin family of genes. SIR2 is a NAD-dependent histone deacetylase that is involved in silencing at mating type loci in yeast. In yeast, a single extra copy of SIR2 increases lifespan, whereas its deletion shortens lifespan, and SIR2 also mediates the effect of dietary restriction. In *C. elegans*, the closest homologue is *sir-2.1*, and increased dosage extended lifespan in a *daf-2*-dependent manner. Following these findings, effects of increasing *Drosophila* Sir2 (dSir2) were examined; dSir2 was also reported to regulate lifespan in flies, and the effect was linked with that of dietary restriction (Rogina and Helfand, 2004). Again, it suggests that there is a conserved mechanism of Sir2 in the regulation of lifespan.

Phenotype screening, candidate locus approaches, and QTL mapping have resulted in discovery of a number of genes in *Drosophila* that extend lifespan. The first example of such a gene was *methuselah* (*mth*), which codes for a G-coupled membrane receptor-like protein, reported in 1998 (Lin *et al.*, 1998) by longevity screens. Since then almost 50 additional genes have been identified. Whether these genes also affect lifespan in other species is yet to be determined, but just as *Drosophila* has served as a test species for genes identified in other organisms, others may serve to explore patterns initially found in *Drosophila*.

Drosophila in Practice

BASIC FLY HANDLING

In general, *Drosophila* are cultured at 25°C on a 12-hour light:dark cycle with 60–70% humidity. Flies may be kept in bottles or vials that have food on the bottom. Appropriately sized foam stoppers may be convenient to seal the top; however, a chunk of cotton wool may also be used. As has been mentioned, temperature has a significant effect on lifespan in flies. The minimum permissive temperature is 18°C, and the upper restrictive temperature is 29°C. If there are only a few hundred flies of a few stocks, one or two 25°C incubators are sufficient. However, if there are going to be large numbers of flies, a 25°C room will be a preferred choice.

Fly stocks can be successfully cultured by regular mass transfer to fresh food. The frequency of the transfer needs to be established depending on the fly strains, the temperature and the density of the cultures. Stocks kept at 25°C (200–300 adults per half-pint bottle) should be transferred to fresh food at least once every 2 weeks. In older stocks, mites and mold may appear and cause problems, so the stocks should be monitored from time to time regardless of the intervals. This period can be extended by keeping the stocks at a lower temperature (e.g., 18°C); however, not all strains survive well at 18°C, and mold can be a serious problem for certain strains.

To obtain healthy adults, optimum numbers of parental flies need to be established. In most cases, 300–600 flies are obtained from a bottle, in which around 100 females (and a few tens of males) are left for a day and allowed to lay eggs. All the parental flies need to be emptied afterwards. If larvae become overcrowded, baker's yeast should be added to provide additional nutrition.

There are many types of fly food used by different laboratories. Food is commercially available, but can also be cooked in laboratories (for recipes, see the "Recommended Resources" section: Roberts and Standen (1998), website for Bloomington stock center). The food may be kept at 4°C for about a month. Nipagin M (*p*-hydroxy benzoic acid methyl ester) is an antioxidant that is often included in food. *In vitro*, it is able to scavenge hydrogen peroxide production by mitochondria effectively at relatively high concentrations, although there is no report of the effects of Nipagin on lifespan.

Dietary restriction in flies has been applied by food dilution, and this method can extend lifespan in flies. However, there have been concerns about how much flies eat, since flies are cultured on food in a bottle and have access to food all the time; the flies on diluted food may eat more to make up the calories. Indeed, a recent study measuring food intake using isotope labeling reported that this is the case (Carvalho *et al.*, 2005). Further work will be needed to verify the dietary restriction effect of the dilution method if any, as well as to develop alternative methods for dietary restriction in flies.

ANESTHETICS

Anesthetization of flies is required when sorting out by sex or by genotype, and also when preparing tissue homogenate. Common methods are ether and carbon dioxide, but cooling can also be used in some cases.

Although the carbon dioxide method requires setting up of some devices (see Roberts and Standen, 1998), it has a number of advantages over the ether (ethyl ether or triethylamine) method; it is much less likely to kill or sterilize *Drosophila*. Additionally it is odorless and neither flammable nor reactive. With carbon dioxide, use of the diffusion pad enables application of continuous anesthetization. Flies can be kept unconscious for up to 20 minutes under the carbon dioxide air and still recover quickly once the carbon dioxide is removed, although too strong or too long exposure to carbon dioxide can kill flies. On the other hand, the effects of ether will wear off in less than 10 minutes. Thus, carbon dioxide is a preferred choice.

While they are anesthetized, flies can be placed on a glass plate or carbon dioxide plate to be examined under the microscope. The flies are moved around using a small paintbrush on the plate, and care must be taken not to damage the wings and so forth.

COLLECTING VIRGIN FEMALES

Female *Drosophila* store sperm after mating and are capable of laying fertile eggs for many days. Therefore in order to set up a cross between males and females of known genotypes, it is essential to collect virgin females. To do this, in the morning, empty all the flies from bottles that have adult flies just emerging from pupae. Then collect flies that eclose over the next 8 hours and separate into sexes. Virgins have dark meconium in the gut, visible through the ventral abdominal wall. Virgin females do lay some eggs; however, these are unfertilized and will not hatch.

Conclusions

Drosophila is a versatile model for investigating a variety of questions. The *Drosophila* model enables researchers to perform synergetic, integrated studies in a relatively short period of time. Powerful genetic tools are available, and it has advantages for demographic analysis and is suitable for molecular and biochemical studies. One can identify a gene of interest by phenotype screening or candidate locus approaches. The gene can be expressed, overexpressed, or deleted by genetic tools, and this can be done in a tissue- and time-specific manner. Its effect on lifespan can be monitored, and patterns of aging can be characterized by demographic analysis; downstream effects at the molecular level, as well as physiological and behavioral effects, can all be studied. Studies through gene homology will have great implications for higher organisms including humans.

However, there are some downsides to use of *Drosophila* as a model. Because *Drosophila* is small relative to mammals and birds, it is difficult to perform physiological and biochemical studies which require manual tissue isolation or dissection. *Drosophila* strains can rapidly evolve in laboratory culture; it is possible that deleterious mutations can accumulate and thus make closely related stocks genetically differentiated. This can give rise to serious confounding results, particularly when crosses are generated from these stocks.

In addition, there are theoretical considerations that should be taken into account. Aging may involve different processes in different species, and its underlying mechanisms may be different. Flies are short-lived, so they may not have evolved good longevity-promoting systems such as efficient damage-repair/defense systems. Furthermore, there are distinct biological differences between flies and mammals as indicated above. For these reasons, one cannot always translate results on *Drosophila* directly into mammals.

Nonetheless, there is no doubt that the *Drosophila* model has contributed significantly to our understanding of aging. Bearing in mind its limitations and knowing its advantages, in balance, *Drosophila* will still long continue to be an extremely useful model organism to understand basic mechanisms of aging and to give important clues for aging in the more complex mammalian systems.

Recommended Resources

BOOKS AND ARTICLES

Drosophila: A Laboratory Handbook and Manual. Ashburner, M. (1989, Cold Spring Harbor Laboratory Press, New York). Covers a wide range of molecular biology protocols.

Drosophila, a Practical Approach. D.B. Roberts, Ed. (2nd ed., 1998, Oxford University Press, Oxford). Covers laboratory culturing, biology, genetics, mutagenesis, protocols for preparation of nucleic acid, enhancer traps, and behavioral studies.

Fly Pushing: The Theory and Practice of Drosophila Genetics. Greenspan, R.J. (2nd ed., 2004, Cold Spring Harbor Laboratory Press, New York). An easy-to-read book describing fly genetics.

Emerging Technologies for Gene Manipulation in Drosophila melanogaster, Venken, K.J. and Bellen, H.J. (2005). *Nat. Rev. Genet.* 6, 167–178. Explains major genetic techniques used for *Drosophila*.

Research resources for Drosophila: The expanding universe. Matthews, K.A., Kaufman, T.C. and Gelbart, W.M. (2005). *Nat. Rev. Genet.* 6, 179–193. An excellent guide and information on *Drosophila* resources.

INTERNET RESOURCES

Fly base: The major internet resource for *Drosophila* researchers, providing information on stocks, genes, mutants, other researchers, publications and much more. The U.S. (Indiana) site is the original, with mirrors around the world.

http://flybase.net/

Drosophila images are also available: http://flybase.net/images/

Bloomington stock center: An excellent website of the largest of stock center in the world, including available stocks, information on culturing flies, practical suggestions and media recipes.

http://flystocks.bio.indiana.edu/

Other stock centers can be found via the link:

http://flystocks.bio.indiana.edu/other-centers.htm

Virtual library: The directory that points to internet resources for research on *Drosophila*.

http://www.ceolas.org/VL/fly/

Various protocols can be found: http://ceolas.org/VL/fly/protocols.html

Drosophila Information Service: A journal that aims to share out information useful to researchers, teachers and students, containing new techniques, research reports and so on.

http://www.ou.edu/journals/dis/index.html

REFERENCES

Beckman, K.B., and Ames, B.N. (1998). The free radical theory of ageing matures. *Physiol. Rev. 78*, 547–581.

Carey, J.R. (1993). *Applied Demography for Biologists*. Oxford University Press, Oxford.

Carvalho, G.B., Kapahi, P., and Benzer, S. (2005). Compensatory ingestion upon dietary restriction in *Drosophila melanogaster*. *Nature Methods 2*, 813–815.

Chapman, T., Hutchings, J., and Partridge, L. (1993). No reduction in the cost of mating for *Drosophila melanogaster* females mating with spermless males. *Proc. Royal Soc. Lon. 253*, 211–217.

Chippindale, A.K., Hoang, D.T., Service, P.M., and Rose, M.R. (1994). The evolution of development in *Drosophila melanogaster* selected for postponed senescence. *Evolution 48*, 1880–1899.

Cohen, A.A. (2004). Female post-reproductive lifespan: A general mammalian trait. *Biol. Rev. 79*, 733–750.

Connolly, J.B., and Tully, T. (1998). Behaviour, learning, and memory. In *Drosophila—A Practical Approach* (D.B. Roberts, ed.), pp. 265–318. Oxford University Press, Oxford.

Cooley, L., Kelley, R., and Spradling, A. (1988). Insertional mutagenesis of the *Drosophila* genome with single *P* elements. *Science 239*, 1121–1128.

DeVeale, B., Brummel, T., and Seroude, L. (2004). Immunity and aging: the enemy within? *Aging Cell 3*, 195–208.

Driver, C. (2000). The circadian clock in old *Drosophila melanogaster*. *Biogerontology 1*, 157–162.

Farmer, K.J., and Sohal, R.S. (1989). Relationship between superoxide anion radical generation and aging in the housefly, *Musca domestica*. *Free Radic. Biol. Med. 7*, 23–29.

Finch, C.E. (1990). *Longevity, Senescence, and the Genome*. University of Chicago Press, Chicago.

Fridell, Y.W.C., Sánchez-Blanco, A., Silvia, B.A., and Helfand, S.L. (2005). Targeted expression of the human uncoupling protein 2 (hUCP2) to adult neurons extends life span in the fly. *Cell Metab. 1*, 145–152.

Garofalo, R.S. (2002). Genetic analysis of insulin signaling in *Drosophila*. *Trends Endocrinol. Metab. 13*, 156–162.

Giannakou, M.E., Goss, M., Junger, M.A., Hafen, E., Leevers, S.J. and Partridge, L. (2004). Long-lived *Drosophila* with overexpressed dFOXO in adult fat body. *Science 305*, 361.

Good, T.P., and Tatar, M. (2001). Age-specific mortality and reproduction respond to adult dietary restriction in *Drosophila melanogaster*. *J. Insect Physiol. 47*, 1467–1473.

Harman, D. (1956). Aging: A theory based on free radical and radiation chemistry. *J. Gerontol. 11*, 298–300.

Harman, D. (1972). The biologic clock: The mitochondria? *J. Am. Geriatr. Soc. 20*, 145–147.

Helfand, S.L., and Rogina, B. (2003). Genetics of aging in the fruit fly, *Drosophila melanogaster*. *Annu. Rev. Genet. 37*, 329–348.

Holloszy, J.O. (1997). Mortality rate and longevity of food-restricted exercising male rats: A reevaluation. *J. Appl. Physiol. 82*, 399–403.

Holloszy, J.O., and Smith, E.K. (1986). Longevity of cold-exposed rats: A reevaluation of the "rate-of-living theory." *J. Appl. Physiol. 61*, 1656–1660.

Hughes, K.A., Alipaz, J.A., Drnevich, J.M., and Reynolds, R.M. (2002). A test of evolutionary theories of aging. *Proc. Nat. Acad. Sci. USA 99*, 14286–14291.

Hulbert, A.J., Clancy, D.J., Mair, W., Braeckman, B.P., Gems, D., and Partridge, L. (2004). Metabolic rate is not reduced by dietary restriction or by lowered insulin/IGF-1 signalling and is not correlated with individual lifespan in *Drosophila melanogaster*. *Exp. Gerontol. 39*, 1137–1143.

Hwangbo, D.S., Gershman, B., Tu, M.P., Palmer, M., and Tatar, M. (2004). *Drosophila* dFOXO controls lifespan and regulates insulin signalling in brain and fat body. *Nature 429*, 562–566.

Khazaeli, A.A., Van Voorhies, W., and Curtsinger, J.W. (2005). Longevity and metabolism in *Drosophila melanogaster*: Genetic correlations between life span and age-specific metabolic rate in populations artificially selected for long life. *Genetics 169*, 231–242.

Le Bourg, E. (2001). Oxidative stress, aging and longevity in *Drosophila melanogaster*. *FEBS Lett. 498*, 183–186.

Lin, Y.J., Seroude, L., and Benzer, S. (1998). Extended life-span and stress resistance in the *Drosophila* mutant *methuselah*. *Science 282*, 943–946.

Lints, K.A. (1978). *Genetics and Ageing*. Karger, Basel.

Loeb, J., and Northrop, J.H. (1917). On the influence of food and temperature on the duration of life. *J. Biol. Chem. 32*, 103–121.

Magwere, T., Chapman, T., and Partridge, L. (2004). Sex differences in the effect of dietary restriction on life span and mortality rates in female and male *Drosophila melanogaster*. *J. Gerontol. Appl. Biol. Sci. Med. Sci. 59*, 3–9.

Mair, W., Goymer, P., Pletcher, S.D., and Partridge, L. (2003). Demography of dietary restriction and death in *Drosophila*. *Science 301*, 1731–1733.

Mair, W., Sgro, C.M., Johnson, A.P., Chapman, T., and Partridge, L. (2004). Lifespan extension by dietary restriction in female *Drosophila melanogaster* is not caused by a reduction in vitellogenesis or ovarian activity. *Exp. Gerontol. 39*, 1011–1019.

Manev, H., and Dimitrijevic, N. (2005). Fruit flies for anti-pain drug discovery. *Life Sci. 76*, 2403–2407.

Matthews, K.A., Kaufman, T.C., and Gelbart, W.M. (2005). Research resources for *Drosophila*: The expanding universe. *Nat. Rev. Genet. 6*, 179–193.

Miwa, S., Riyahi, K., Partridge, L., and Brand, M.D. (2004). Lack of correlation between mitochondrial reactive oxygen species production and life span in *Drosophila*. *Ann. N. Y. Acad. Sci. 1019*, 388–391.

Miwa, S., St-Pierre, J., Partridge, L., and Brand, M.D. (2003). Superoxide and hydrogen peroxide production by *Drosophila* mitochondria. *Free Radic. Biol. Med. 35*, 938–948.

O'Kane C.J. (1998). Enhancer traps. In *Drosophila—Practical Approach* (D.B. Roberts, ed.), pp. 131–178. Oxford University Press, Oxford.

Orr, W.C., Mockett, R.J., Benes, J.J., and Sohal, R.S. (2003). Effects of overexpression of copper-zinc and manganese superoxide dismutases, catalase, and thioredoxin reductase genes on longevity in *Drosophila melanogaster*. *J. Biol. Chem. 278*, 26418–26422.

Parkes, T.L., Elia, A.J., Dickinson, D., Hilliker, A.J., Phillips, J.P., and Boulianne, G.L. (1998). Extension of *Drosophila* lifespan by overexpression of human SOD1 in motorneurons. *Nat. Genet. 19*, 171–174.

Partridge, L., and Pletcher, S.D. (2003). Genetics of aging in *Drosophila*. In *Aging of Organisms* (H.D. Osiewacz, ed.), pp. 125–161. Kluwer Academic Publishers, Dordrecht, The Netherlands.

Partridge, L., Pletcher, S.D., and Mair, W. (2005). Dietary restriction, mortality trajectories, risk and damage. *Mech. Ageing Dev. 126*, 35–41.

Phelan, J.P., Archer, M.A., Beckman, K.A., Chippindale, A.K., Nusbaum, T.J., and Rose, M.R. (2003). Breakdown in correlations during laboratory evolution. I. Comparative analyses of *Drosophila* populations. *Evolution 57*, 527–535.

Pletcher, S.D., Macdonald, S.J., Marguerie, R., Certa, U., Stearns, S.C., Goldstein, D.B., and Partridge, L. (2002). Genome-wide transcript profiles in aging and calorically restricted *Drosophila melanogaster*. *Curr. Biol. 12*, 712–723.

Poirier, L., and Seroude, L. (2005). Genetic approaches to study aging in *Drosophila melenogaster*. *Age 27*, in press.

Promislow, D.E., and Haselkorn, T.S. (2002). Age-specific metabolic rates and mortality rates in the genus *Drosophila*. *Aging Cell 1*, 66–74.

Roberts, D.B., and Standen, G.N. (1998). The elements of *Drosophila* biology and genetics. In *Drosophila—A Practical*

Approach. (D.B. Roberts, ed.), pp. 1–54. Oxford University Press, Oxford.

Rockstein, M., and Miquel, J. (1973). Aging in insects. In *The Physiology of Insecta* (M. Rockstein, ed.), pp. 371–478. Academic Press Inc., New York.

Rogina, B., and Helfand, S.L. (2004). Sir2 mediates longevity in the fly through a pathway related to calorie restriction. *Proc. Natl. Acad. Sci. USA 101*, 15998–16003.

Rogina, B., Reenan, R.A., Nilsen, S.P., and Helfand, S.L. (2000). Extended life-span conferred by cotransporter gene mutations in *Drosophila. Science 290*, 2137–2140.

Rose, M.R. (1984). Laboratory evolution of postponed senescene in *Drosophila. Evolution 38*, 1004–1010.

Ross, R.E. (2000). Age-specific decrease in aerobic efficiency associated with increase in oxygen free radical production in *Drosophila melanogaster. J. Insect Physiol. 46*, 1477–1480.

Sacktor, B. (1974). Biological oxidations and energetics in insect mitochondria. In *The Physiology of Insecta* Vol. IV (M. Rockstein, ed.), pp. 271–353. Academic Press, New York.

Sohal, R.S. (1976). Aging changes in insect flight muscle. *Gerontology 22*, 317–333.

Sohal, R.S. (1993). Aging, cytochrome oxidase activity, and hydrogen peroxide release by mitochondria. *Free Radic. Biol. Med. 14*, 583–588.

Sohal, R.S., Agarwal, S., Dubey, A., and Orr, W.C. (1993). Protein oxidative damage is associated with life expectancy of houseflies. *Proc. Natl. Acad. Sci. USA 90*, 7255–7259.

Sohal, R.S., and Sohal, B.H. (1991). Hydrogen peroxide release by mitochondria increases during aging. *Mech. Ageing Dev. 57*, 187–202.

Sohal, R.S., and Weindruch, R. (1996). Oxidative stress, caloric restriction, and aging. *Science 273*, 59–63.

Speakman, J.R., Talbot, D.A., Selman, C., Snart, S., McLaren, J.S., Redman, P., *et al.* (2004). Uncoupled and surviving: Individual mice with high metabolism have greater mitochondrial uncoupling and live longer. *Aging Cell 3*, 87–95.

Sun, J., Folk, D., Bradley, T.J., and Tower, J. (2002). Induced overexpression of mitochondrial Mn-superoxide dismutase extends the life span of adult *Drosophila melanogaster. Genetics 161*, 661–672.

Sun, J., Molitor, J., and Tower, J. (2004). Effects of simultaneous over-expression of Cu/ZnSOD and MnSOD on *Drosophila melanogaster* life span. *Mech. Ageing Dev. 125*, 341–349.

Sun, J., and Tower, J. (1999). FLP recombinase-mediated induction of Cu/Zn-superoxide dismutase transgene expression can extend the life span of adult *Drosophila melanogaster* flies. *Mol. Cell Biol. 19*, 216–228.

Tatar, M. (2004). The neuroendocrine regulation of *Drosophila* aging. *Exp. Gerontol. 39*, 1745–1750.

Tower, J. (2000). Transgenic methods for increasing *Drosophila* life span. *Mech. Ageing Dev. 118* , 1–14.

Trout, W.E., and Kaplan, W.D. (1970). A relation between longevity, metabolic rate, and activity in *shaker* mutants of *Drosophila melanogaster. Exp. Gerontol. 5*, 83–92.

van Voorhies, W.A., Khazaeli, A.A., and Curtsinger, J.W. (2003). Selected contribution: Long-lived *Drosophila melanogaster* lines exhibit normal metabolic rates. *J. Appl. Physiol. 95*, 2605–2613.

Venken, K.J., and Bellen, H.J. (2005). Emerging technologies for gene manipulation in *Drosophila melanogaster. Nat. Rev. Genet. 6*, 167–178.

Weis-Fogh, T. (1964). Diffusion in insect wing muscle, the most active tissue known. *J. Exp. Biol. 41*, 229–256.

Wessells, R.J., Fitzgerald, E., Cypser, J.R., Tatar, M., and Bodmer, R. (2004). Insulin regulation of heart function in aging fruit flies. *Nat. Genet. 36*, 1275–1281.

Williams, G.C. (1957). Pleiotropy, natural selection and the evolution of senescence. *Evolution 11*, 398–411.

Yampolsky, L.Y., Pearse, L.E., and Promislow, D.E.L. (2000). Age-specific effects of novel mutations in *Drosophila melanogaster*: I. Mortality. *Genetica (Dordrecht) 110*, 11–29.

Yan, L.J., Levine, R.L., and Sohal, R.S. (1997). Oxidative damage during aging targets mitochondrial aconitase. *Proc. Natl. Acad. Sci. USA 94*, 11168–11172.

Yan, L.J., and Sohal, R.S. (1998). Mitochondrial adenine nucleotide translocase is modified oxidatively during aging. *Proc. Natl. Acad. Sci. USA 95*, 12896–12901.

Yan, L.J., and Sohal, R.S. (2000). Prevention of flight activity prolongs the life span of the housefly, *Musca domestica*, and attenuates the age-associated oxidative damage to specific mitochondrial proteins. *Free Radic. Biol. Med. 29*, 1143–1150.

23

Models of Aging in Honeybee Workers

Gro V. Amdam and Olav Rueppell

*Understanding the control of senescence and lifespan constitutes one of the most intriguing but difficult goals in modern biology. Fully exploring the regulatory architectures of aging will likely require the use of a broad range of animal systems—many of which are not currently regarded as mainstream models in aging research. One such species is the honeybee (*Apis mellifera*) that is characterized by a facultative aging machinery under social control. Epigenetic regulation is responsible for the differentiation of females into workers and queens—two castes with strongly diverging lifespan potential—and a plastic pattern of worker longevity that appears to be determined by the social colony setting rather than chronological age. Compared to solitary model species, the honeybee is in a prime position to contribute to a deeper understanding of the aging phenomenology in organisms that live in complex social environments.*

Introduction

The honeybee is a eusocial insect, which means that it is characterized by reproductive division of labor and by the presence of a facultatively sterile worker caste that engages in alloparental care behaviors such as brood care and foraging. Eusocial insect societies are found in the orders *Hymenoptera* (ants, wasps, and bees) and *Isoptera* (termites). Within these genera, the honeybee is among the most socially advanced. It is also the species with the best developed tool kit for husbandry, and constitutes, by far, the best studied social insect (reviewed by Winston, 1987).

The honeybee receives considerable attention in studies that aim to understand how complex collective patterns emerge from interactions between individuals. It is, consequently, a key research model in behavioral ecology (e.g., Calderone and Page, 1992; Huang and Robinson, 1996; Trumbo *et al.*, 1997; Pankiw and Page, 2001), neurobiology (Scheiner *et al.*, 2001; Humphries *et al.*, 2003), and systems theory (e.g., Omholt, 1987; Bonabeau, 1998; Page and Erber, 2002; Amdam and Omholt, 2003). In addition, eusocial insects can make important contributions to our understanding of aging across levels of biological complexity (Rueppell *et al.*, 2004). This is in part because of caste-specific gene expression programs, which have emerged through social insect evolution (Evans and Wheeler, 2001). These programs may underlie trajectories of senescence and longevity regulation that show considerable variation between castes, both within and between species of the social *Hymenoptera* and *Isoptera* (for further information see Finch, 1990; Rueppell *et al.*, 2004). In this context, the honeybee worker caste also provides an additional regulatory layer of interest (Omholt and Amdam, 2004): within this caste the rate of senescence does not appear to be a function of chronological age (Amdam and Page, 2005). Rather, aging in honeybee workers is state-dependent (reviewed by Amdam, 2005), and longevity is—as a result—a function of a plastic progression through life-cycle stages with distinct behavioral and physiological profiles. This succession generates a facultative age-determination pattern of particular interest to research on aging and longevity (Omholt and Amdam, 2004; Amdam, 2005). It has therefore, been predicted that, in parallel with the development of new functional genomic tools (Beye *et al.*, 2002; Amdam *et al.*, 2003b) and the availability of the honeybee genome sequence (www.hgsc.bcm.tmc.edu), the bee will grow to become the most noteworthy social invertebrate model for senescence (for discussions see Rueppell *et al.*, 2004; Amdam and Page, 2005).

Rooted in these perspectives, we here provide an introductory overview aimed at researchers who are interested in using the honeybee as a gerontological model. We present a summary of the general biology of the bee, and outline the behavioral and physiological life trajectories that are specific to the different honeybee castes. The link between the plasticity of these trajectories and the dynamics of the honeybee society as a whole is emphasized. Subsequently, we present a preparative review of key handling procedures and sources of methods for studies of the bee, in which we elucidate how social integrity can be maintained under the experimental management of free-flying colonies as well as for individuals kept in a laboratory setting. We next provide examples of the use of honeybees in aging research—a section that also serves to outline the current status of the field in mechanistic and biodemographic terms. Finally, we discuss how social insects, in a wider taxonomic perspective, can contribute to the understanding of aging, and we outline future prospects for use of the honeybee as a gerontological model.

The Honeybee Society

In contrast to the classic models of biological aging research, honeybees represent a species in an advanced state of social evolution. They live their entire lives as part of a complex society, the colony, and cannot survive or reproduce as solitary individuals. The honeybee society rivals traditional human societies in many societal parameters, such as group size, cohesiveness, information exchange, integration, and differentiation of roles (Wilson, 1980), including reproductive division of labor. Honeybees are characterized by a strong colony-level selection component, which has led to functional differentiation of colony members into separate castes and to the concept of regarding the colony as a superorganism (Moritz and Fuchs, 1998): workers fulfill the various roles of the soma (food acquisition, processing, and distribution, homeostasis, and protection), while the mature queen represents the unique germ line and stem cell (meristem), and males and young queens can be regarded as the gametes.

Typically, a honeybee colony contains one reproductive queen and tens of thousands of female workers that are functionally sterile in the presence of a reproductive queen (de Groot and Voogd, 1954). During the reproductive season, several thousand males (drones) are also found in the nest. Additionally, all stages of the developing juveniles (brood, i.e., eggs, larvae and pupae) and extensive food resources (honey and pollen) are found in the colony. The brood, honey and pollen are stored in the main nest structure, the wax combs. These combs are typically arranged in sheets. The center of the nest is filled with brood, surrounded by a sphere of pollen storage, and the outer areas of the nest are used to store honey (Winston, 1987). All demographic variables have a strong seasonal component, at least in the temperate regions where the majority of studies have been conducted (Winston, 1987). Workers are produced throughout most of the year except for the first part of winter. However, the peak in the production of new workers precedes the production of drones and new queens in the early summer when resources are abundant.

In contrast to individual honeybees, colonies are perennial and potentially immortal through the continuous replacement of their members. The queen, as the only reproducing individual, can live several years (see below), but is regularly replaced by her own daughters (reviewed by Page and Peng, 2001). As part of the regular reproductive cycle, replacement queens are raised and the old queen leaves the nest in a swarm with the majority (50–90%) of the workers present to establish a new colony. One of the new queens takes over the remaining colony, killing all other young queens and engaging in mating flights (Severson, 1984). In contrast, the male reproductive role of honeybee colonies is exerted throughout the mating season by the continuous production of drones. These seek out matings from unrelated virgin queens during mating flights (Winston, 1987). After having been successfully mated, the young queen assumes the reproductive role in the colony, using her stored sperm (over five million) for several years of reproduction, producing up to 2000 eggs per day (Winston, 1987). During this time, the queen does not fulfill any other colony tasks and is attended by a retinue of young workers that clean and feed her.

Honeybees are haplo-diploid (drones are haploid), and their sex is determined by a single gene (Beye *et al.*, 2003). Female caste determination is nutritional: more abundant and higher quality food causes the female larva to develop into a queen, whereas less and lower quality food leads to worker development. It has been shown in cross-fostering experiments that the developmental trajectories start diverging in the bipotent third larval stage. Queens will continue to be fed royal jelly, a highly nutritional food that triggers a juvenile hormone (JH) peak that shifts global gene expression patterns compared to workers (Evans and Wheeler, 1999) and ultimately accelerates their development rate. Worker-destined larvae are reared on an inferior diet which causes them to emerge as adults with half of the body weight of queens (reviewed by Page and Peng, 2001).

The Lifespan of Worker Bees

The lifespan of honeybee workers is extremely plastic (e.g., Sakagami and Fukuda, 1968). This plasticity emerges because the behavioral trajectories of worker bees are sensitive to changes in the intra- and extra-colonial environment (e.g., Huang and Robinson, 1996), and the phasing and layout of these trajectories translates into specific physiological signatures and patterns of lifespan (for a review see Amdam and Page, 2005).

BEHAVIORAL SENSITIVITY IN A DYNAMIC SOCIAL CONTEXT

The worker population of a honeybee colony normally segregates into a temporal hive bee caste that performs a series of tasks inside the nest (cell cleaning, brood rearing and cell building), and a temporal forager caste that specializes in collecting nectar, pollen, water and propolis (reviewed by Winston, 1987). A worker starts out as a hive bee and subsequently switches to foraging—typically after 18–28 days. The timing of this shift, however, is elastic (7–135 days: Haydak, 1963; Free, 1965), and this plasticity is, in part, controlled by colony demography. Specifically, bees in the foraging population produce a pheromonal cue that inhibits hive bees from initiating foraging (Pankiw, 2004; Toth and Robinson, 2005). Consequently, as foragers progressively are lost from colonies they are replaced by hive bees that are not efficiently inhibited (Huang and Robinson, 1996) (but see Regulation of Aging through Social Control of Behavioral Plasticity as well for an expansion of the concept of inhibition of foraging behavior). The regulatory mechanisms responsible for the hive bee to go on to the forager transition deserve attention in a gerontological context because the timing of the switch largely determines the overall lifespan of the worker. This is because the age at onset of foraging is normally much more variable than the length of the foraging period (for a review see Omholt and Amdam, 2004), which suggests that the duration of the hive bee phase is a dynamic entity mainly determined by the intracolonial conditions, while the duration of the forager phase is more dependent on the extracolonial conditions.

Reversion of Task-Associated Trajectories

Worker bees can, moreover, revert from foraging duties to hive activities (Robinson *et al.*, 1992). This phenomenon constitutes an inversion of the above-mentioned behavioral progression and appears to require a substantial perturbation of colony demography: behavioral reversion can be triggered experimentally through removal of the entire hive bee population. Under this condition, a proportion of the remaining foragers initiate hive tasks such as brood rearing (Huang and Robinson, 1996). It is likely that this reversion, which withdraws bees from risky foraging tasks and causes them to engage in labor within the sheltered nest, is associated with an extension of lifespan.

Temporal Cessation of Behavioral Development

As foraging opportunities decline at the onset of the unfavorable season (the winter or drought period), a third and exceedingly long-lived temporal caste emerges. This group constitutes the *diutinus* stage (formerly referred to as the "winter bee" phenotype; Omholt and Amdam, 2004), and the appearance of these workers is intimately linked to the reduction of brood rearing that precedes the onset of the unfavorable season in honeybee colonies (Maurizio, 1950). The *diutinus* workers, like hive bees, reside within the protected nest. They thermoregulate the colony and take care of the queen, and do not initiate brood rearing or foraging until the next favorable period. Shorter intervals of reduced brood rearing can, nonetheless, arise for various reasons throughout the season (e.g., when swarming, replacement, or loss of the reproductive queen results in a reduction of the number of eggs, larvae and pupae in a colony). Therefore, *diutinus* bees can emerge during the favorable period also, when workers—as a rule—segregate into the hive- and forager populations, exclusively.

PHYSIOLOGICAL SIGNATURES AND PATTERNS OF LIFESPAN

Foragers have a high extrinsic mortality risk compared to hive bees, and the life of a forager is therefore short (typically 1–2 weeks: Neukirch, 1982) relative to the typical duration of the hive bees phase (normally 3–8 weeks: Free and Spencer-Booth, 1959) and the *diutinus* stage (up to 280 days: reviewed by Omholt and Amdam, 2004). Consequently, the transitions among those three distinct life history states are key determinants of the lifespan of any individual worker (reviewed by Amdam and Page, 2005). Within each temporal caste, however, longevity is further conditional on physiological factors (Maurizio, 1950) (see below).

Metabolic Rate (MR)

MR is one physiological factor that may underlie the temporal, caste-associated mortality rates of honeybee workers. Forager MR is significantly higher than the MR of hive bees (for a discussion see Suarez *et al.*, 1996), and the MR of a foraging bee constitutes one of the highest known mass-specific aerobe MRs among animals (approximately 3-fold higher than hummingbird flight muscle). Such intense activity is a major source of mechanical senescence in insects and causes mortality to increase as a function of age (reviewed by Finch, 1990). In accordance with their longevity, *diutinus* bees periodically exhibit low MRs compared to hive bees—and thus also relative to foragers (Crailsheim, 1986; Nerum and Buelens, 1997). The MR of *diutinus* workers can fall to half the MR of hive bees. Elevated MR causes an increase in the release of free radicals that can induce oxidative impairment (reviewed by Jazwinski, 1996), which has led to the suggestion that oxidative stress is a mediator of stage-dependent physiological frailty in honeybee workers (Amdam and Omholt, 2002).

Endocrine Status

Juvenile hormone (JH) and ecdysteroids are systemic hormones that are implicated in the regulation of invertebrate lifespan by orchestrating several suites of physiological processes (Tatar *et al.*, 2003).

The JHs form a family of related sesquiterpenoid compounds secreted by the corpora allata (CA) complex, and although insects (e.g., *Lepidoptera*) may secrete a blend of JHs, JH III is the only naturally occurring JH in the honeybee (Tobe, 1985). The JH titer of worker bees increases at the onset of foraging, and a comparable rise in the JH level is associated with accelerated rates of senescence in invertebrate models like *Drosophila* spp. (Tatar and Yin, 2001). *Diutinus* workers and hive bees, however, have very low JH titres (Fluri *et al.*, 1982). In many insect species, this hormonal signature is associated with diapause, and removal of the CA complex often results in diapause-associated characteristics, e.g., low MR, reduced activity levels, regression of ovary development, and enlargement of the fat body—a storage organ analogous to the mammalian liver and white adipose tissue. Yet, removal of the CA does not trigger a diapause-like state in worker bees: workers without the CA progress through a period of hive tasks and initiate foraging (Sullivan *et al.*, 2000). Moreover, MR increases in allatectomized foragers that do not have detectable JH titers (Sullivan *et al.*, 2003). Therefore, the role of JH in the regulation of honeybee longevity may not be directly comparable with its role in solitary insect species (see Regulation of Aging through Social Control of Behavioral Plasticity for further information).

The dominant ecdysteroid in the honeybee is Makisterone A (Robinson *et al.*, 1991). Steroids generally have multiple and complex regulatory effects that may affect longevity (Tatar *et al.*, 2003). Robinson *et al.* (1991), however, demonstrated that the ecdysteroid titer of adult worker bees is low (independent of age), and it is therefore unlikely that Makisterone A plays an important role in the regulation of adult honeybee physiology and lifespan. Yet, it has not been fully determined if ecdysteroids are involved in the control of worker reproductive maturation and oogenesis, a state that can be triggered if the queen is lost from a colony (Robinson *et al.*, 1991; Hartfelder *et al.*, 2002).

Nutritional State

The protein content of worker bees is low at emergence, but it increases sharply during the first 10–12 days of adult life through pollen feeding. In the broodless *diutinus* workers, protein may subsequently accumulate to extreme concentrations because nutritional resources are retained in the adult bees rather than being transferred to young larvae (Fluri *et al.*, 1977; Fluri *et al.*, 1982). This state is associated with an overall increase in longevity (Maurizio, 1950). Buildup of stored protein reserves (storage protein) is commonly linked to reduced mortality in insects. A comparable pattern to that observed in the bee is found in the ant *Camponotus festinatus*, where the presence of brood also has an inhibitory effect on the accumulation of storage proteins in workers (Martinez and Wheeler, 1994).

At the onset of foraging, protein levels in the hemolymph (blood), fat body and hypopharyngeal glands (brood food producing head glands) are significantly reduced in the bee, and a similar pattern is seen for stored lipids (Toth and Robinson, 2005). This loss of stored nutrients from individuals that perform risky exterior hive activities has parallel examples from other social *Hymenopterans* (Porter and Jorgensen, 1981; O'Donnell and Jeanne, 1995) and has led to the proposition that foragers are stripped of nutritional resources as part of a colony-level resource-saving strategy (O'Donnell and Jeanne, 1995; Amdam and Omholt, 2002). Accordingly, foraging bees have fewer resources that can be allocated to individual somatic maintenance—a state that appears to translate into a higher level of physiological frailty.

Immunity

The insect immune cells, or hemocytes, are involved in defense mechanisms such as phagocytosis, encapsulation and nodule formation (reviewed by Rolff and Siva-Jothy, 2002). The immune cells also produce antibacterial peptides and contain most of the recruitable enzyme prophenoloxidase, which catalyses crucial steps in the melanization immune response. The number of functional circulating hemocytes at any give time, therefore, reflects the organism's capacity to cope with immunogenic challenges.

Hive bees and *diutinus* workers have high numbers of functional hemocytes (5,000–12,000 immune cells per μl hemolymph: Fluri *et al.*, 1977; Amdam *et al.*, 2004a). JH, however, affects the number of normal hemocytes in honeybee worker hemolymph, and causes the cellular immune system of foragers to become suppressed (Rutz *et al.*, 1976). Specifically, under the influence of high JH titers, hemocytes change into inactive pycnotic forms. One effect of this loss of immunity is a complete deterioration of the nodulation response (Bedick *et al.*, 2001).

The Lifespan of Queens and Drones

In comparison to workers, little is known about the life history of drones and queens, including the determinants of their lifespan. This is particularly true with regard to mechanistic, causative studies. The lack of research effort can be explained in part by practical considerations (only workers are abundantly available all year), but it is particularly challenging because much of the appeal of the honeybee model in aging research hinges on intraspecific comparisons.

Drone life history dramatically differs from the patterns described above for workers. These males lead a quasi-solitary life (in a social environment), as they do not actively integrate in any colony-level activities. No social influences on their life history have been demonstrated, even though some of the underlying hormonal controls (e.g., JH) may be identical to workers (Giray and Robinson, 1996). The overall mortality pattern of drones is similar to that of workers in midreproductive season (Rueppell *et al.*, 2005), and their lifespan does not significantly exceed that of workers (reviewed by Page and Peng, 2001). Due to their flight activity, the external mortality risks of drones are similar to workers: predation, misorientation, exhaustion, and other environmental hazards (e.g., rain). Mortality risk increases during their flight tenure, as in workers, probably due to wear and tear, but drones also seem to age without fulfilling any significant task before their onset of flight (Rueppell *et al.*, 2005).

No significant demographic data exist on queens for three reasons. Large data sets require a disproportionate experimental effort since only one queen exists in each colony. Moreover, queens are long-lived. Finally, the lifespan of queens may be socially controlled (reviewed by Page and Peng, 2001), and it is difficult to distinguish a swarming event from replacement of the old queen by a daughter (supersedure). Longevity records demonstrate a much higher potential lifespan for queens than for either workers or drones. Their lifespan regularly exceeds one year, and maximal reported queen longevity is above eight years (reviewed by Page and Peng, 2001). This pronounced lifespan extension in social insect queens relative to solitary insects is general and associated with low external mortality and thus favors the evolutionary theory of aging over purely mechanistic explanations (Keller and Genoud, 1997).

Practical Aspects of Honeybee Research

There are several excellent sources for information on how to establish and maintain an apiary or a honeybee breeding program (e.g., Atkins *et al.*, 1975). Moreover, there are special resources available that describe experimental handling procedures and protocols for behavioral (Frisch, 1967; Seeley, 1995) and physiological (Snodgrass, 1956) data collection. Yet, we will provide a brief overview of tools, protocols and experimental considerations that are of specific relevance for research on aging and longevity.

HONEYBEE HUSBANDRY

Honeybee colonies are normally accommodated in standard commercial hive bodies, and a host of literature for laypersons and experts exists on the practical aspects of keeping honeybees (for more information see Atkins *et al.*, 1975; Laidlaw and Page, 1997). They can also easily be kept in hives or in sheltered milieus designed for specific research purposes, allowing for experimental manipulations or efficient censusing under seminatural conditions. Bees can be kept in indoor observation hives with access to the outside to facilitate behavioral observations and accurate censuses (for a discussion see Frisch, 1967). These hives can be designed to various sizes, but they require intense management. Egg-collection hives (Aase *et al.*, 2005) consist of a single-frame hive body with two aluminum frames that hold 6 Jenter frame modules (Karl Jenter, Nurtingen, Germany). This design allows the collection and introduction of eggs and larvae by simple extraction and insertion of individual cell bases. Egg collection hives are used for *in vivo* rearing of genetically manipulated bees (Amdam *et al.*, 2003b), and is an alternative to laborious *in vitro* rearing procedures (for a discussion see Aase *et al.*, 2005). An alternative to letting the bees fly into the wild is flight cages and flight rooms. They provide a controlled environment for studies of behavioral development and mortality (Jay, 1964; van Praagh and Velthuis, 1971) but need to be designed carefully (Omholt *et al.*, 1995). Most external mortality risk factors can be excluded, and flight activity can be controlled and measured accurately (Neukirch, 1982).

EXPERIMENTAL PROCEDURES AND MANIPULATIONS

The transition between field and laboratory procedures is gradual in honeybee research, and often a combination of both is desirable. Honeybees prove unproblematic in both contexts, but a few points have to be kept in mind. As members of a social group, honeybees are greatly affected by their social environment, and individuals readily adjust their life history to environmental conditions (Schulz *et al.*, 1998; Pankiw, 2003). For this reason, experimental handling and stress (including social isolation) ought to be minimized or at least carefully controlled.

Through demographic hive manipulations, introduction of comb, or brood grafting, colonies can be controlled to produce large cohorts of workers, drones, or queens (Atkins *et al.*, 1975). Artificial rearing of brood is also possible in the laboratory, but the described procedures to date are laborious and often produce individuals that do not span a normal phenotypic range. Upon emergence in a temperature- and humidity-controlled incubator, cohorts can be reliably marked for life with enamel paint, numbered color discs, or radio frequency identification tags (Streit *et al.*, 2003). Subsequently, marked bees can be introduced into a natural colony for studying their aging. Bees of older ages can also be transferred (grafted) between colonies, but special precautions have to be taken to avoid allo-recognition and rejection.

Physiological parameters such as hormone or protein titers can be investigated by taking hemolymph samples through the intersegmental membranes in the abdomen at different ages—also during larval and pupal development. Similarly, honeybees can be injected with various substances into the abdomen (e.g., JH: Muller and Hepburn, 1994) or brain (e.g., double-stranded RNA: Farooqui *et al.*, 2004) to study the physiological regulation of aging. These and other handling procedures are greatly facilitated by chilling bees to 8–12°C, keeping in mind that low temperature is a serious stressor (Jones *et al.*, 2004). Different protocols exist for investigating honeybee behavior and cognitive abilities in the laboratory (Scheiner *et al.*, 2004), and large samples, even at advanced ages, can be readily drawn from a single hive. Even though the honeybee does not compare with classic aging models for their genetic resources and versatility, some progress has been made (Robinson *et al.*, 2000; Beye *et al.*, 2002; Amdam *et al.*, 2003b; Kunieda and Kubo, 2004), and selective breeding using artificial insemination is well established (Laidlaw and Page, 1997).

Research on Aging in Honeybee Workers

The honeybee offers a point of entry to experimental research on aging that cannot easily be addressed in any of the classic—solitary—model organisms (Rueppell *et al.*, 2004). In the following, we present a set of recent studies that exemplify how the bee is starting to contribute to our understanding of longevity.

REGULATION OF AGING THROUGH SOCIAL CONTROL OF BEHAVIORAL PLASTICITY

It was recently suggested (Amdam and Omholt, 2003) that the hive bee and *diutinus* worker states are governed by an age-neutral regulatory structure that incorporates the glycolipoprotein vitellogenin. Vitellogenin is a yolk precursor that is produced by oviparous animals (for a review see Omholt and Amdam, 2004). In the honeybee worker caste, though, vitellogenin has evolved a novel function—it is utilized in the production of brood food (Amdam *et al.*, 2003a). The hypothesized regulatory link among vitellogenin, behavioral plasticity and longevity (Amdam and Omholt, 2003) has been explored in several studies with fundamental implications for our understanding of the evolvability of circuits that control the rate of aging (reviewed by Amdam, 2005). Specifically, *vitellogenin* genes are normally downstream of a female-specific regulatory cascade that has negative effects on lifespan (Murphy *et al.*, 2003). In the honeybee, however, the effect is inverted so that *vitellogenin* gene expression extends life (Seehuus *et al.*, 2005). This counterintuitive association may be caused by the novel, negative feedback regulation between vitellogenin and JH (Guidugli *et al.*, 2005).

Studies of the genetic control machinery responsible for the link among vitellogenin, behavioral plasticity and longevity in the honeybee are currently utilizing selected strains bred by Page and Fondrk (1995) that differ in JH- and vitellogenin titers in concert with dissimilar trajectories of longevity (reviewed by Amdam *et al.*, 2004b).

IMMUNOSENESCENCE

Another study has explored the putative role of vitellogenin in the regulatory control of the decline in immunity that characterizes honeybee foragers (Amdam *et al.*, 2004c). The data from this work demonstrate that vitellogenin is the main zinc carrier in honeybee workers, and that lack of zinc induces pycnosis of honeybee hemocytes *in vitro*. The authors therefore suggested that depletion of vitellogenin, a protein that normally constitutes 30–50 % of the plasma protein pool in hive bees and *diutinus* workers but is down-regulated to undetectable levels in foragers (see Nutritional State), causes the plasma level of zinc to become so low that it triggers a loss of immunity. This phenomenon may further elucidate how natural selection works on circuits that control aging in social insect societies (reviewed by Omholt and Amdam, 2004): turning off vitellogenin synthesis in foragers can serve to economize the colony's protein household, as it prevents build-up of a storage protein that will be lost when the forager perishes in the field. Furthermore, as immune system maintenance is costly in solitary as well as social insects, the down-regulation of the honeybee forager immune system fits well into an explanatory framework where foragers constitute a disposable caste (O'Donnell and Jeanne, 1995) with an accelerated aging rate and level of physiological frailty (reviewed by Amdam, 2005).

BIODEMOGRAPHIC RESEARCH

Honeybees provide multiple, practical advantages over other models in biodemographic research: worker cohorts are readily obtainable and maintainable in large numbers from either genetically homogeneous or heterogeneous sources (Laidlaw and Page, 1997). Honeybee workers return to their hive daily as long as they live. Thus, their activity and lifespan can be directly monitored in observation hives without disturbance and under seminatural conditions.

Due to its commercial importance and widespread public interest, the honeybee was also one of the earliest insects with a recorded lifespan (Langstroth, 1866). Early studies were based on small sample sizes or indirect estimations, but they provided the first data on the intraspecific variability and plasticity in aging that remain today one of the major reasons to study honeybee aging (Omholt and Amdam, 2004). Larger, demographic studies showed that honeybee workers have a type I (convex) survivorship curve, which is rare in insects (Sakagami and Fukuda, 1968) but common in social organisms with extended brood care, such as humans. The pattern of age-specific mortality in honeybee workers is largely due to the hive bee to forager transition, which is accompanied not only by major physiological changes, but also by a dramatic increase in external mortality risk (see above). More than 90% of all worker deaths are reported to occur outside of the colony under natural conditions (Lundie, 1925). Thus, it is difficult to identify the exact cause of death for the majority of workers (reviewed by Page and Peng, 2001), and biodemographic studies of the mortality dynamics are important for our understanding of aging and mortality in the honeybee.

The seasonality of worker lifespan is one of the most striking features of the honeybee aging model system (see Temporal Cessation of Behavioral Development). The few studies addressing seasonality from a comparative demographic perspective reveal that not only the average life expectancy, but also the variation in life expectancy (Sakagami and Fukuda, 1968) and life history trade-offs that determine life expectancy vary seasonally (Neukirch, 1982). In general, the *diutinus* phase over the winter period seems to slow aging effectively without any adverse, compensatory effects before or after this stage (Omholt and Amdam, 2004), but more work on the mechanistic and demographic aspects of this retardation of aging remains to be done.

The age at the onset of foraging activity is a major determinant of lifespan for honeybee workers, although some aging may also occur pre-foraging (honeybees that initiate flight later in life have a shorter foraging lifespan: Guzmán-Novoa *et al.*, 1994). Sharply increasing mortality dynamics indicates that foragers senesce (Sakagami and Fukuda, 1968) either as a consequence of regulatory processes (see Endocrine Status), or wear-and-tear, or expenditure of internal resources (Neukirch, 1982).

However, there is also a report of a constant mortality rate, relative to the intensity of foraging (Visscher and Dukas, 1997). Comprehensive data on larger samples are needed to resolve this issue, as well as their late-life mortality dynamics, and the quantification of genetic versus environmental influences on lifespan.

One further interesting aspect, which is unique to the honeybee model, is the connection between social structure and individual life history and aging. Isolated studies have indicated that the caregiver-to-dependent (worker-to-brood) ratio is of crucial importance to the individual longevity of the progeny (Eischen *et al.*, 1982), and possibly all other workers (Winston and Fergusson, 1985). The amount of brood and resources in a colony, and the age structure of the worker force, influence the age of foraging initiation of individual workers, and thus their lifespan (Winston, 1987). Furthermore, larger colony size confers a longevity advantage to the individuals presumably because individual workers in smaller colonies work harder, raising more offspring per adult bee (Harbo, 1986). These plastic reactions to social conditions are ultimately the result of dynamic colony-level resource allocation and optimization (Oster and Wilson, 1978). However, comprehensive quantitative models and experiments are rare because the combination of colony demography, resource flows, and individual physiology and behavior proves complex (Amdam and Omholt, 2002).

Comparative Aspects

While we argue here that the honeybee is an emerging model organism in aging research, it has already attained the status of a model organism in several other biological disciplines and it serves as the model social insect. Social evolution has generated a wide variety of social systems with unique selection pressures and adaptations that provide many opportunities for testing ultimate theories of aging, as well as study the proximate causes of naturally evolved aging differentials. Sociality with overlapping generations, cooperative brood care, and (reproductive) division of labor, as in the honeybee, has evolved multiple times in insects, with termites, ants, wasps, and bees as prominent representatives (for other groups see Choe and Crespi, 1997).

The multiple, independent evolution of sociality offers the prospects of analyzing phylogenetic trends in a comparative context, such as the analysis of the evolution of lifespan itself (Keller and Genoud, 1997). We can study in detail the phylogenetic correlation between the degree of social evolution (such as societal complexity, colony size, or morphological queen–worker dimorphism) and the lifespan extension in reproductives. Furthermore, any lifespan-extending mechanism identified in honeybee queens can be tested for its generality and its natural evolutionary history reconstructed by studying it in related, less socially advanced species (Parker *et al.*, 2004). The broad taxonomic array of social insects with widely differing social systems and biology provides many opportunities for comparative research. Particularly valuable "wide-scale" comparisons would seem to be between flying and nonflying, predatory and herbivorous, or monogynous (groups with a single reproductive queen) and polygynous (multiple reproductive queens) groups as these life history variables seem to have some impact on longevity (Finch, 1990; Keller and Genoud, 1997). If we are to understand how social evolution has affected lifespan, it is not sufficient to compare solitary and highly social species but to study intermediates and follow plausible trends in social evolution. This can lead to insights into the ultimate factors that lead to long-lived reproductives and social evolution, as well as the reinforcement between the two (Carey, 2001; Carey and Judge, 2001). All four species of honeybees are highly social, but in their family (the Apidae) solitary species and numerous intermediates exist (Michener, 2000). One such intermediate are bumblebees whose colonies are annual and all individuals except for the newly produced (and mated) queens die at the end of the season. This life history should select for very different longevity patterns at the individual level, with an even more pronounced seasonal plasticity than in the honeybee. Another interesting feature of bumblebees is the large size variation among workers that leads to a division of labor that is not age-dependent. Therefore, we have life-long behavioral specialists with differences in external mortality and consequently predicted differences in endogenous aging rates.

Like bumblebees, some ant species also exhibit division of labor that is related to functional size divergence (Hölldobler and Wilson, 1990) and cannot be regarded as an adaptation to aging (Tofilski, 2002). However, this has been used to confirm that a higher extrinsic mortality of outside workers has led to the evolution of a shorter intrinsic lifespan, relative to workers that work inside the protected colony (Chapuisat and Keller, 2002). Other ant species follow the honeybee model of age-dependent division of labor, probably with similar mortality patterns. In general, lifespans in ants are much longer than in honeybees. This makes the evolution of their lifespan extension more extreme, and significant research efforts are geared towards elucidating mechanisms of their great queen longevity (Hartmann and Heinze, 2003; Parker *et al.*, 2004; Schrempf *et al.*, 2005), which will provide interesting comparisons to the results from honeybees. However, the much longer lifespan also makes the practical aspects of aging studies in ants more difficult than studies in the honeybee.

Conclusion

It is now widely realized that the study of biological models can considerably advance our understanding of the processes that lead to aging and determine lifespan.

However, it is also realized that the classic models are all short-lived laboratory organisms. This may limit their value as models for human aging, and a broader comparative basis is currently sought in the scientific community. Aging research directed towards social insects, and the honeybee in particular, is still in its infancy. Nevertheless, some interesting patterns start to emerge with mutually corroborating proximate and ultimate explanations of lifespan. The large, experimentally accessible plasticity in aging rate in the honeybee provides a prime opportunity to study a strong case of epigenetic regulation of lifespan (Omholt and Amdam, 2004). We are beginning to understand how resource optimization at the colony level is driving multiple, physiological changes in the individual with drastic consequences for aging. In this context, it seems possible that the honeybee can become a key invertebrate model for understanding the molecular regulatory control of facultative longevity extension, a research area that is currently dominated by the nematode *Caenorhabditis elegans*. The honeybee model may also prove ideal to integrate these mechanistic studies with biodemographic concepts: we can apply the essence of biodemographic research—actuarial analysis of biological patterns in large-scale experiments—to more phenomena than just organismal death. In sum, the temporal dynamics of honeybee behavior, physiology, and gene expression can be explored in relation to social lifespan, implying that the aging process can be studied at ascending levels of biological organization from molecules to colonies (Rueppell *et al.*, 2004).

ACKNOWLEDGMENT

We would like to thank John Tomkiel and Jennifer Tsuruda for improving the manuscript with helpful suggestions. G.V.A. was supported by the Norwegian Research Council, project # 157851/432, and funding was provided to G.V.A. and O.R. by the National Institute on Aging, PO1 AG 22500.

REFERENCES

Aase, A.L.T.O., Amdam, G.V., Hagen, A., and Omholt, S.W. (2005). A new method for rearing genetically manipulated honey bee workers. *Apidologie 36*, 293–299.

Amdam, G.V., and Omholt, S.W. (2002). The regulatory anatomy of honeybee lifespan. *J. Theor. Biol. 216*, 209–228.

Amdam, G.V., Norberg, K., Hagen, A., and Omholt, S.W. (2003a). Social exploitation of vitellogenin. *Proc. Natl. Acad. Sci. USA* 100, 1799–1802.

Amdam, G.V., and Omholt, S.W. (2003). The hive bee to forager transition in honeybee colonies: The double repressor hypothesis. *J. Theor. Biol. 223*, 451–464.

Amdam, G.V., Simões, Z.L.P., Guidugli, K.R., Norberg, K., and Omholt, S.W. (2003b). Disruption of vitellogenin gene function in adult honeybees by intraabdominal injection of double-stranded RNA. *BMC Biotechnology 3*, 1–8.

Amdam, G.V., Hartfelder, K., Norberg, K., Hagen, A., and Omholt, S.W. (2004a). Altered physiology in worker honey bees (Hymenoptera: Apidae) infested by the mite *Varroa destructor* (Acari: Varroidae): A factor in colony loss during over-wintering? *J. Econ. Entomol. 97*, 741–747.

Amdam, G.V., Norberg, K., Fondrk, M.K., and Page, R.E. (2004b). Reproductive ground plan may mediate colony-level selection effects on individual foraging behavior in honey bees. *Proc. Natl. Acad. Sci. USA 101*, 11350–11355.

Amdam, G.V., Simões, Z.L.P., Hagen, A., Norberg, K., Schroder, K., Mikkelsen, O., *et al.* (2004c). Hormonal control of the yolk precursor vitellogenin regulates immune function and longevity in honeybees. *Exp. Gerontol. 39*, 767–773.

Amdam, G.V. (2005). In *Longevity and Frailty* (J.R. Carey, J.-M. Robine, J.-P. Michel, and Y. Christen, eds.), pp. 17–26, Springer-Verlag, Berlin.

Amdam, G.V., and Page, R.E. (2005). Intergenerational transfers may have decoupled physiological and chronological age in a eusocial insect. *Aging Res. Rev.* in press.

Atkins, E.L., Banker, R.B., Butler, C.G., Cale, Jr., G.H.J., Cale, G.H.J., Crane, E., and Dadant, C.C. (1975). *The Hive and the Honey Bee*, Datant & Sons, Hamilton.

Bedick, J.C., Tunaz, H., Aliza, A.R.N., Putnam, S.M., Ellis, M.D., and Stanley, D.W. (2001). Eicosanoids act in nodulation reactions to bacterial infections in newly emerged adult honey bees, *Apis mellifera*, but not in older foragers. *Comp. Biochem. Physiol. 130*, 107–117.

Beye, M., Hartel, S., Hagen, A., Hasselmann, M., and Omholt, S.W. (2002). Specific developmental gene silencing in the honey bee using a homeobox motif. *Insect Mol. Biol. 11*, 527–532.

Beye, M., Hasselmann, M., Fondrk, M.K., Page, R.E., and Omholt, S.W. (2003). The gene csd is the primary signal for sexual development in the honeybee and encodes an SR-type protein. *Cell 114*, 419–429.

Bonabeau, E. (1998). Social insect colonies as complex adaptive systems. *Ecosystems 1*, 437–443.

Calderone, N.W., and Page, R.E. (1992). Effects of interactions among genotypically diverse nestmates on task specialization by foraging honey bees (*Apis mellifera*). *Behav. Ecol. Sociobiol. 30*, 219–226.

Carey, J.R. (2001). Demographic mechanisms for the evolution of long life in social insects. *Exp. Gerontol. 36*, 713–722.

Carey, J.R., and Judge, D.S. (2001). Life span extension in humans is self-reinforcing: A general theory of longevity. *Popul. Dev. Rev.* 27.

Chapuisat, M., and Keller, L. (2002). Division of labour influences the rate of ageing in weaver ant workers. *Proc. R. Soc. Lond. B. 269*, 909–913.

Choe, J.C., and Crespi, B.J. (1997). *The Evolution of Social Behavior in Insects and Arachnids.* Cambridge University Press, Cambridge.

Crailsheim, K. (1986). Dependence of protein metabolism on age and season in the honeybee (*Apis mellifica carnica* pollm). *J. Insect Physiol. 32*, 629–634.

de Groot, A.P., and Voogd, S. (1954). On the ovary development in queenless worker bees (*Apis mellifica* L.). *Experientia 10*, 384–385.

Eischen, F.A., Rothenbuhler, W.C., and Kulincevic, J.M. (1982). Length of life and dry weight of worker honeybees reared in colonies with different worker-larva ratios. *J. Apic. Res. 21*, 19–25.

Evans, J.D., and Wheeler, D.E. (1999). Differential gene expression between developing queens and workers in the honey bee, *Apis mellifera*. *Proc. Natl. Acad. Sci. USA 96*, 5575–5580.

Evans, J.D., and Wheeler, D.E. (2001). Gene expression and the evolution of insect polyphenisms. *Bioessays 23*, 62–68.

Farooqui, T., Vaessin, H., and Smith, B.H. (2004). Octopamine receptors in the honeybee (*Apis mellifera*) brain and their disruption by RNA-mediated interference. *J. Insect Physiol. 50*, 701–713.

Finch, C.E. (1990). *Longevity, Senescence and the Genome*, University of Chicago Press, Chicago.

Fluri, P., Wille, H., Gerig, L., and Lüscher, M. (1977). Juvenile hormone, vitellogenin and haemocyte composition in winter worker honeybees (*Apis mellifera*). *Experientia 33*, 1240–1241.

Fluri, P., Lüscher, M., Wille, H., and Gerig, L. (1982). Changes in weight of the pharyngeal gland and haemolymph titres of juvenile hormone, protein and vitellogenin in worker honey bees. *J. Insect Physiol. 28*, 61–68.

Free, J.B., and Spencer-Booth, Y. (1959). The longevity of worker honey bees (*Apis mellifera*). *Proc. R. Ent. Soc. Lond. 34*, 141–150.

Free, J.B. (1965). The allocation of duties among worker honeybees. *Zool. Soc. Lond. 14*, 39–59.

Frisch, K.V. (1967). *The Dance Language and Orientation of Bees*, Harvard University Press, Cambridge.

Giray, T., and Robinson, G.E. (1996). Common endocrine and genetic mechanisms of behavioral development in male and worker honey bees and the evolution of division of labor. *Proc. Natl. Acad. Sci. USA 93*, 11718–11722.

Guidugli, K.R., Nascimento, A.M., Amdam, G.V., Barchuk, A.R., Angel, R., Omholt, S.W., *et al.* (2005). Vitellogenin regulates hormonal dynamics in the worker caste of a eusocial insect. *FEBS Letters 579*, 4961–4965.

Guzmán-Novoa, E., Page, R.E., and Gary, N.E. (1994). Behavioral and life-history components of division of labor in honey bees (*Apis mellifera* L.). *Behav. Ecol. Sociobiol. 34*, 409–417.

Harbo, J.R. (1986). Effect of population size on brood production, worker survival and honey gain in colonies of honeybees. *J. Apic. Res. 25*, 22–29.

Hartfelder, K., Bitondi, M.M.G., Santana, W.C., and Simões, Z.L.P. (2002). Ecdysteroid titer and reproduction in queens and workers of the honey bee and of a stingless bee: Loss of ecdysteroid function at increasing levels of sociality? *Insect Biochem. Mol. Biol. 32*, 211–216.

Hartmann, A., and Heinze, J. (2003). Lay eggs, live longer: Division of labor and life span in a clonal ant species. *Evolution 57*, 2424–2429.

Haydak, M.H. (1963). Age of nurse bees and brood rearing. *Minnesota Agric. Exp. Station, Scientific J. Series No. 5122*, 101–103.

Hölldobler, B., and Wilson, E.O. (1990). *The Ants*, Belknap Press of Harvard University Press, Cambridge.

Huang, Z.-Y., and Robinson, G.E. (1996). Regulation of honey bee division of labor by colony age demography. *Behav. Ecol. Sociobiol. 39*, 147–158.

Humphries, M.A., Muller, U., Fondrk, M.K., and Page, R.E. (2003). PKA and PKC content in the honey bee central brain differs in genotypic strains with distinct foraging behavior. *J. Comp. Physiol. A 189*, 555–562.

Jay, S.C. (1964). A bee flight and rearing room. *J. Apic. Res. 3*, 41–44.

Jazwinski, S.M. (1996). Longevity, genes, and aging. *Science 273*, 54–59.

Jones, J.C., Myerscough, M.R., Graham, S., and Oldroyd, B.P. (2004). Honey bee nest thermoregulation: Diversity promotes stability. *Science 305*, 402–404.

Keller, L., and Genoud, M. (1997). Extraordinary lifespans in ants: A test of evolutionary theories of ageing. *Nature 389*, 958–960.

Kunieda, T., and Kubo, T. (2004). In vivo gene transfer into the adult honeybee brain by using electroporation. *Biochem. Biophys. Res. Comm. 318*, 25–31.

Laidlaw, H.H., and Page, R.E. (1997). *Queen Rearing and Bee Breeding*, Wicwas Press, Cheshire.

Langstroth, L.L. (1866). *A Practical Treatise on the Hive and the Honey-Bee*, J. B. Lippincott & Co, Philadelphia.

Lundie, A.E. (1925). The flight activity of the honeybee. *Department Bulletin USDA 1328*, 1–37.

Martinez, T., and Wheeler, D.E. (1994). Storage proteins in adult ants (*Camponotus festinatus*): Roles in colony founding by queens and in larval rearing by workers. *J. Insect Physiol. 40*, 723–729.

Maurizio, A. (1950). The influence of pollen feeding and brood rearing on the length of life and physiological condition of the honeybee preliminary report. *Bee World 31*, 9–12.

Michener, C.D. (2000). *The Bees of the World*, Johns Hopkins University Press, Baltimore.

Moritz, R.F.A., and Fuchs, S. (1998). Organization of honeybee colonies: Characteristics and consequences of a superorganism concept. *Apidologie 29*, 7–21.

Muller, W.J., and Hepburn, H.R. (1994). Juvenile hormone III and wax secretion in honeybees (*Apis mellifera capensis*). *J. Insect Physiol. 40*, 873–881.

Murphy, C.T., McCarroll, S.A., Bargmann, C.I., Fraser, A., Kamath, R.S., Ahringer, J., *et al.* (2003). Genes that act downstream of DAF-16 to influence the lifespan of *Caenorhabditis elegans*. *Nature 424*, 277–284.

Nerum, K.V., and Buelens, H. (1997). Hypoxia-controlled winter metabolism in honeybees (*Apis mellifera*). *Comp. Biochem. Physiol. 117A*, 445–455.

Neukirch, A. (1982). Dependence of the life span of the honeybee (*Apis mellifera*) upon flight performance and energy consumption. *J. Comp. Physiol. 146*, 35–40.

O'Donnell, S., and Jeanne, R.L. (1995). Worker lipid stores decrease with outside-nest task performance in wasps: Implication for the evolution of age polytheism. *Experientia 51*, 749–752.

Omholt, S.W. (1987). Thermoregulation in the winter cluster of the honeybee, *Apis mellifera*. *J. Theor. Biol. 128*, 219–231.

Omholt, S.W., Hagen, A., Elmholdt, O., and Rishovd, S. (1995). A laboratory hive for frequent collection of honeybee eggs. *Apidologie 26*, 297–304.

Omholt, S.W., and Amdam, G.V. (2004). Epigenic regulation of aging in honeybee workers. *Sci. Aging Knowl. Environ. 26*, pe28.

Oster, G.F., and Wilson, E.O. (1978). *Caste and Ecology in the Social Insects*, Princeton University Press, Princeton.

Page, R.E., and Fondrk, M.K. (1995). The effects of colony-level selection on the social organization of honey bee (*Apis mellifera* L.) colonies: Colony-level components of pollen hoarding. *Behav. Ecol. Sociobiol. 36*, 135–144.

Page, R.E., and Peng, Y.-S.C. (2001). Aging and development in social insects with emphasis on the honey bee, *Apis mellifera* L. *Exp. Gerontol. 36*, 695–711.

Page, R.E., and Erber, J. (2002). Levels of behavioral organization and the evolution of division of labor. *Naturwissenschaften 89*, 91–106.

Pankiw, T., and Page, R.E. (2001). Genotype and colony environment affect honeybee (*Apis mellifera* L.) development and foraging behavior. *Behav. Ecol. Sociobiol. 51*, 87–94.

Pankiw, T. (2003). Directional change in a suite of foraging behaviors in tropical and temperate honey bees (*Apis mellifera* L.). *Behav. Ecol. Sociobiol. 54*, 458–464.

Pankiw, T. (2004). Worker honey bee pheromone regulation of foraging ontogeny. *Naturwissenschaften 91*, 178–181.

Parker, J.D., Parker, K.M., and Keller, L. (2004). Molecular phylogenetic evidence for an extracellular CuZn superoxide dismutase gene in insects. *Insect Mol. Biol. 13*, 587–594.

Porter, S.D., and Jorgensen, C.D. (1981). Foragers of the harvester ant, *Pogonomyrmex-owyheei*—A disposable caste. *Behav. Ecol. Sociobiol. 9*, 247–256.

Robinson, G.E., Strambi, C., Strambi, A., and Feldlaufer, M.F. (1991). Comparison of juvenile hormone and ecdysteroid haemolymph titres in adult worker and queen honey bees (*Apis mellifera*). *J. Insect Physiol. 37*, 929–935.

Robinson, G.E., Page, R.E., Strambi, C., and Strambi, A. (1992). Colony integration in honey bees: Mechanisms of behavioral reversion. *Ethology 90*, 336–348.

Robinson, K.O., Fergusson, H.J., Cobey, S., Vaessin, H., and Smith, B.H. (2000). Sperm-mediated transformation of the honey bee, *Apis mellifera*. *Insect Mol. Biol. 9*, 625–634.

Rolff, J., and Siva-Jothy, M.T. (2002). Copulation corrupts immunity: A mechanism for a cost of mating in insects. *Proc. Natl. Acad. Sci. USA 99*, 9916–9918.

Rueppell, O., Amdam, G.V., Page, R.E., and Carey, J.R. (2004). From genes to societies. *Sci. Aging Knowl. Environ. 5*, pe5.

Rueppell, O., Fondrk, M.K., and Page, R.E. (2005). Biodemographic analysis of male honey bee mortality. *Aging Cell 4*, 13–19.

Rutz, W., Gerig, L., Wille, H., and Lüscher, M. (1976). The function of juvenile hormone in adult worker honeybees, *Apis mellifera*. *J. Insect Physiol. 22*, 1485–1491.

Sakagami, S.F., and Fukuda, H. (1968). Life tables for worker honeybees. *Res. Popul. Ecol. 10*, 127–139.

Scheiner, R., Page, R.E., and Erber, J. (2001). Responsiveness to sucrose affects tactile and olfactory learning in pre-foraging honey bees of two genetic strains. *Behav. Brain Res. 120*, 67–73.

Scheiner, R., Page, R.E., and Erber, J. (2004). Sucrose responsiveness and behavioral plasticity in honey bees (*Apis mellifera*). *Apidologie 35*, 133–142.

Schrempf, A., Heinze, J., and Cremer, S. (2005). Sexual cooperation: Mating increases longevity in ant queens. *Current Biol. 15*, 267–270.

Schulz, D.J., Huang, Z.Y., and Robinson, G.E. (1998). Effects of colony food shortage on behavioral development in honey bees. *Behav. Ecol. Sociobiol. 42*, 295–303.

Seehuus, S.C., Norberg, K., Gimsa, U., Krekling, T., and Amdam, G.V. (2005). Reproductive protein protects sterile honey bee workers from oxidative stress. *Proc. Natl. Acad. Sci. USA, in revision.*

Seeley, T.D. (1995). *The Wisdom of the Hive*, Harvard University Press, Cambridge.

Severson, D.W. (1984). Swarming behavior of the honey bee. *Am. Bee J. 124*, 204–210.

Snodgrass, R.E. (1956). *Anatomy of the Honey Bee*, Comstock Publishing Associates, New York.

Streit, S., Bock, F., Pirk, C.W.W., and Tautz, J. (2003). Automatic life-long monitoring of individual insect behaviour now possible. *Zoology 106*, 169–171.

Suarez, R.K., Lighton, J.R.B., Joos, B., Roberts, S.P., and Harrison, J.F. (1996). Energy metabolism, enzymatic flux capacities, and metabolic flux rates in flying honeybees. *Proc. Natl. Acad. Sci. USA 93*, 12616–12620.

Sullivan, J.P., Jassim, O., Fahrbach, S.E., and Robinson, G.E. (2000). Juvenile hormone paces behavioral development in the adult worker honey bee. *Hormon. Behav. 37*, 1–14.

Sullivan, J.P., Fahrbach, S.E., Harrison, J.F., Capaldi, E.A., Fewell, J.H., and Robinson, G.E. (2003). Juvenile hormone and division of labor in honey bee colonies: Effects of allatectomy on flight behavior and metabolism. *J. Exp. Biol. 206*, 2287–2296.

Tatar, M., and Yin, C.M. (2001). Slow aging during insect reproductive diapause: Why butterflies, grasshoppers and flies are like worms. *Exp. Gerontol. 36*, 723–738.

Tatar, M., Bartke, A., and Antebi, A. (2003). The endocrine regulation of aging by insulin-like signals. *Science 299*, 1346–1350.

Tobe, S.S. (1985). Structure and regulation of the corpus allatum. *Adv. Insect Physiol. 18*, 305–432.

Tofilski, A. (2002). Influence of age polyethism on longevity of workers in social insects. *Behav. Ecol. Sociobiol. 51*, 234–237.

Toth, A.L., and Robinson, G.E. (2005). Worker nutrition and division of labour in honeybees. *Anim. Behav. 69*, 427–435.

Trumbo, S.T., Huang, Z.-Y., and Robinson, G.E. (1997). Division of labor between undertaker specialists and other middle-aged workers in honey bee colonies. *Behav. Ecol. Sociobiol. 41*, 151–163.

van Praagh, J.P., and Velthuis, H.H.W. (1971). Is the lux an appropriate measure for brightness in a bee flight room? *Bee World 52*, 25–26.

Visscher, P.K., and Dukas, R. (1997). Survivorship of foraging honey bees. *Insectes Soc. 44*, 1–5.

Wilson, E.O. (1980). *Sociobiology*, Harvard University Press, Cambridge.

Winston, M.L., and Fergusson, L.A. (1985). The effect of worker loss on temporal caste structure in colonies of the honeybee (*Apis mellifera* L.). *Can. J. Zool. 63*, 777–780.

Winston, M.L. (1987). *The Biology of the Honey Bee*, Harvard University Press, Cambridge.

24

Ants as Naturally Long-lived Insect Models for Aging

Joel D. Parker and Karen M. Parker

This chapter explains in what respects ants can be useful models in understanding the mechanisms of aging. It includes an introduction highlighting how ants fulfill a need for long-lived model systems in aging research. Three ant model systems are then described including their relevant natural history characteristics, collection and laboratory maintenance. Practical considerations are given for molecular studies and techniques. Finally, an overview is given of the available genomic resources and types of comparative studies that are possible.

Why Ants?

Humans owe their relatively long life span to living in societies that reduce the risk of extrinsic mortality. Other organisms in organized societies are also expected to exhibit a similar lengthening of life span over evolutionary time. One hundred million years before the first human stood up and walked, social insects existed in societies with cities, roads, division of labor, farming, slave making, and organized group defenses (Hölldobler and Wilson, 1990). Sociality has resulted in a 10- to 100-fold increase in the life span of queens in ants, bees, and termites, a trend that was rigorously demonstrated using phylogenetic methods to compare life span and social structure across the insects (Figure 24.1; Keller and Genoud, 1997). The evolution of sociality and its associated increase in life span show a general trend that has independently evolved several times.

Ants represent an ideal system for studying how evolution effects the changes necessary for long life. In addition to the differences in life span among species, there are also order-of-magnitude differences in life span between different castes in a single species. For example, queens of the ant *Lasius niger* have been known to live nearly 29 years in a lab, while workers live for only a few years and males a few weeks (Kutter and Stumper, 1969; Hölldobler and Wilson, 1990). Given that the same egg can become either a queen or a worker, differential gene expression seems to be the key difference between those two castes.

The traditional model systems used to study aging (*Drosophila melanogaster, Caenborabditis elegans, Mus musculus and Saccharomycies cerivisiae*) all share a short generation time, making them ideal experimental systems in terms of laboratory rearing and experimental manipulations. Unfortunately, this has introduced a bias in the types of life histories that have been sampled in modern aging research as almost all the mechanisms proposed for aging have been limited to these systems. Some of these mechanisms are not thoroughly understood in an evolutionary context and may not truly represent adaptations necessary for long life. Hence, these mechanisms need verification in long-lived species like humans. In addition, studies of long-lived species such as ants may also reveal new and novel life span extending processes and mechanisms that have withstood the test of evolutionary time.

The Ant Model Systems

Ants as a group share certain important life history characteristics, such as living in family groups with overlapping generations. Ants are haploid–diploid; the queens and workers are diploid and female, whereas males are haploid and develop from unfertilized eggs. In monogynous colonies, there is one reproductive queen per colony, with sterile workers who do not contribute directly to the reproduction of the colony. Sexual winged queens and males are produced by the colony at specific times of the year. Queens of monogynous colonies remove their wings after mating and found a new colony independently (claustral founding). For polygynous species, where there is more than one reproductive queen per nest, newly mated queens are accepted back into their colonies. In these cases, new colonies are typically formed by budding.

For aging research, there are two ant species and one genus that are particularly well suited for development into model systems. The species *Lasius niger* and the genus *Pogonomyrmex* have considerable life spans and are easy to rear in laboratory settings. The third species, *Solenopsis invicta*, has a variety of modern genomic tools available such as a large microarray and a large cDNA

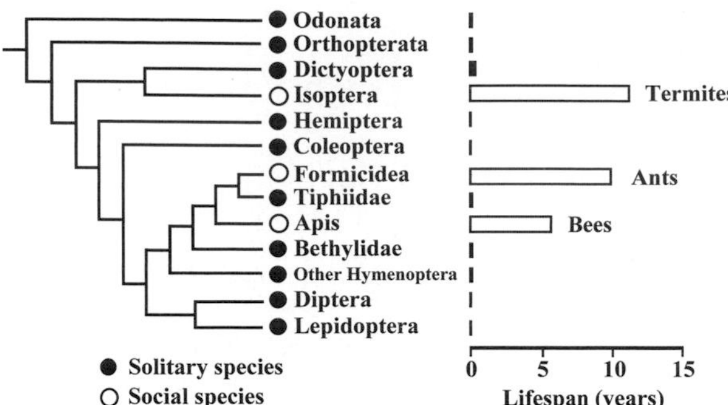

Figure 24.1. Sociality causes an increase in longevity. Redrawing of Figure 2 from Keller and Genoud 1997 showing how extreme life spans evolved multiple times in association with the evolution of sociality.

sequence database. These species are all very common in the Holartic, western North America, and the southern United States, respectively.

LASIUS NIGER

Queens of the common black ant, *Lasius niger*, have the longest recorded life span in the laboratory of 28 and 3/4 years (Kutter and Stumper, 1969). This monogynous species occurs in the Holartic region in forests and farm land. In central and northern European meadows, they occur in densities up to 1 mature colony per square meter. Colonies can be marked by placing a concrete paving slab over the colony entrance. The colony places brood underneath the slab for warming during the nonwinter months, which simplifies collection. The colonies do not seem to migrate, facilitating long-term monitoring and collection. Colonies can be huge with 10,000 or more workers, although smaller young colonies are easily maintained under laboratory conditions. *Lasius niger* has been extensively used in ecological studies as well as in genetic studies assessing colony relatedness, mating number, and sex ratio evolution (Fjerdingstad *et al.*, 2002; Fjerdingstad et al., 2003; Jemielity and Keller, 2003; Fjerdingstad and Keller, 2004). A recent search of the Web of Science Internet database yielded 141 publications on *L. niger*.

This species has large mating flights in mid- to late summer when hundreds of newly mated deallate queens can be collected. New laboratory colonies can be started in glass test tubes filled halfway with water with a tight wad of cotton holding the water back. The founding queen is placed in the tube which is closed with a cotton plug (Figure 24.2).

The tubes are placed in the dark for approximately six weeks, until the first minims emerge. The cotton plugs are removed from the tubes, which are placed inside plastic boxes with additional water tubes. The inside walls of the plastic boxes are painted with Fluon®, a fluoropolymer that most insects have difficulty climbing (available from Whitford Worldwide). Colonies will produce full-sized workers after approximately one year and can be transferred to progressively larger boxes as the colony grows. Best results are obtained when colonies are kept at 22°C with 60% constant humidity. *Lasius niger* prefers liquid food, and our current food mix is 1:1:2 ground meal worms:eggs:honey plus 1% volume of liquid baby vitamins. To facilitate pipetting, the meal worms are flash frozen with liquid nitrogen and ground into a fine powder with a mortar and pestle. Aliquots of the mixture are stored frozen at −20°C and diluted 1:1 with water just before use. Colonies are fed three times a week and are given one or several drops of food, depending on their size.

TABLE 24.1
Internet resources

Description
Codehop program and degenerate PCR recommendations:
http://bioinformatics.weizmann.ac.il/blocks/codehop.html
Fire ant BAC library:
https://www.genome.clemson.edu/cgi-bin/orders?page=productGroupandservice=bacrcandproductGroup=133
Fluon® manufacturer:
http://www.whitfordww.com
Formis ant literature database:
http://cmave.usda.ufl.edu/~formis/
Robert Johnson's *Pogonomyrmex* display nests:
http://lsweb.la.asu.edu/sirg/pogonomyrmex/culturingPogonomymrexqueens.htm
Robert Johnson's North American Pogonomyrmex distribution maps and pictures:
http://lsweb.la.asu.edu/sirg/pogonomyrmex/NORTHAMERICANPOGOS.htm
Texas A & M fire ant collection and maintenance:
http://fireant.tamu.edu/materials/factsheets/FAPFS008.2002rev.pdf
Texas A & M fireant research and management project:
http://fireant.tamu.edu
General ant information and images:
http://www.antweb.org/index.jsp http://myrmecology.info/portal/news.php

POGONOMYRMEX

The approximately 20 North American species of the seed harvester ant genus *Pogonomyrmex* are possibly the most studied genera of ants in the world with two books and a large body of primary literature is dedicated to them (Cole, 1968; Taber, 1998; Johnson, 2000; 2001).

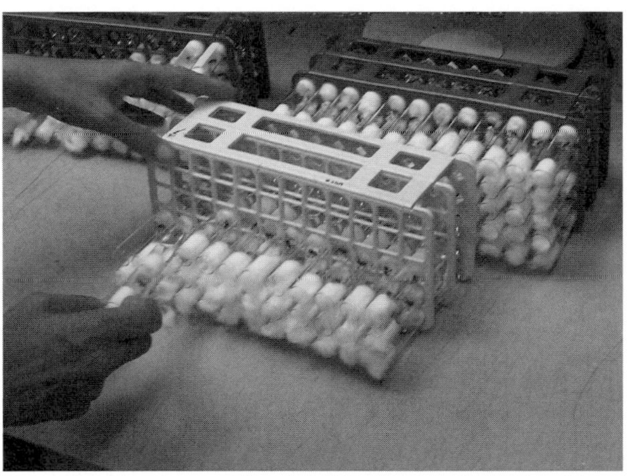

Figure 24.2. Founding *Lasius niger* queens. Queens being placed into water tubes after collection and stored in the dark until the first minims emerge.

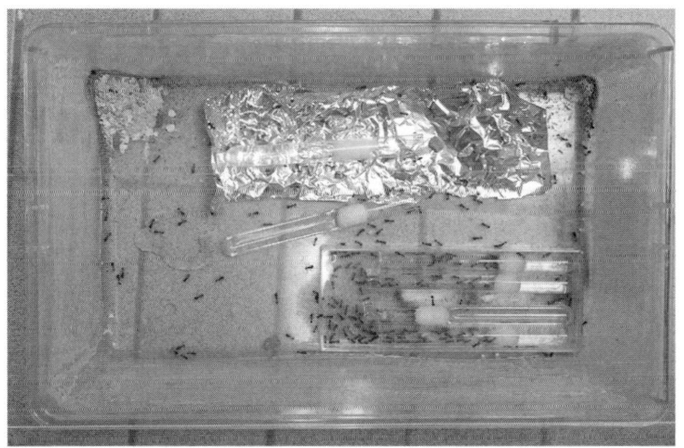

Figure 24.3. *Pogonomyrmex rugosus* laboratory colony. The colonies are kept in plastic boxes normally used for rodent housing. There is an additional small box with water tubes for the area where the queen and brood live.

Pogonomyrmex contains the longest lived ant species recorded in the field, 30 years for *P. salinus* (Porter and Jorgensen, 1988). The best candidate model species within the genus *Pogonomyrmex* are *P. rugous*, *P. barbatus* and *P. occidentalis*.

These monogynous, multiple mating species are extremely common in the western deserts of North America, forming large conspicuous disc- or mound-shaped colonies. The colonies rarely move, facilitating permanent marking and long-term demographic studies. All of these species sting and can be very aggressive. The mating flights are usually rain triggered in the mid- to late summer months. Queens can be collected after mating flights and colonies started in water tubes as for *L. niger*, transferring them to larger boxes with additional water tubes as needed (Figure 24.3).

Being desert ants, they should be kept at 30 to 35°C. Seed harvesters are poor climbers, but Fluon® is recommended to help contain them within their plastic boxes. A more elegant design is a sandwich style nest with either soil or plaster (see Johnson website for pictures and details). *Pogonomyrmex* should be fed pesticide-free grass seed or small bird seed, dead insects such as frozen crickets or meal worms, and a 1:1 mixture of honey and water. Colonies can be raised to large numbers and, in many cases, can produce sexuals in 2 to 3 years.

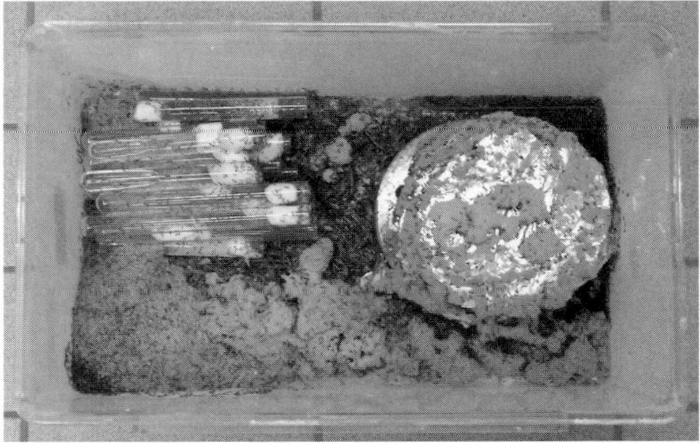

Figure 24.4. *Solenopsis invicta* laboratory colony. The colonies are kept in plastic boxes used for small rodent housing.

SOLENOPSIS INVICTA

From a molecular biology viewpoint, the most attractive model ant species is the red imported fire ant, *Solenopsis invicta*. Although queens live only 2 to 5 years, they have the advantage of existing in polygynous and monogynous colonies. This ant has the most extensively developed genomic tools available with a large cDNA EST database and a microarray chip nearing completion (J. Wang and L. Keller, pers. comm.) A BAC library is also available for purchase (see website list). Primary tissue culture and gene expression studies have been successfully employed using *S. invicta* (Chen, 2004). In addition, the first gene directly affecting social structure (i.e., queen number) was discovered and cloned from *S. invicta* (Krieger and Ross, 2002).

Solenopsis invicta are common where introduced and easily cultured in the laboratory. Their transient, shallow nests make it easy, if not sometimes painful, to collect mature colonies with queens. An entire nest can be shoveled into a Fluon® -coated bucket and water added slowly. *Solenopsis invicta* form living rafts in response to flooding, and the floating colony raft can be scooped from the water and placed into plastic boxes treated with Fluon® (Figure 24.4).

Newly mated queens can also be collected after mating flights in the early summer and colonies started in water tubes as for *L. niger* and *Pogonomyrmex* . Their optimal laboratory temperature is 25 to 30°C. Their dietary requirements are more demanding, requiring freshly killed insects and a constant source of water. Specific method descriptions and food recipes can be found online (see Internet section of the appendices).

There are two problems that must be considered when working with *S. invicta*. First, it is impossible to avoid being stung on a regular basis when working with these small, aggressive ants. Some people develop sensitivity to the stings and can experience life-threatening anaphylactic shock (Solley *et al.*, 2002). Second, this is a highly destructive and invasive species that should never be transported to, or kept in, warm moist regions of the world where they have not already been established.

Sampling at the Colony Level

Mature queens of single-queen colonies such as *Pogonomyrmex* and *L. niger* are almost impossible to collect due to the depth and size of the colonies. Fortunately, the genotype of a queen can be determined by genotyping male allates from the colony. As males are the product of unfertilized eggs, a sample size of 6 will cover 99% of the queen's genome. The genotype of the father(s) of the colony, as well as the queen's, can also be reconstructed by sampling workers. In both cases, such sampling will not negatively impact large colonies and represents a benign way to monitor the genetic structure of extant, wild long-lived populations.

Social insects should be sampled at the level of colony or group of colonies for molecular studies. When the queen has been fertilized by only one male, all of her daughters are full sisters and share the same haploid father and diploid mother. Thus, workers from a monogynous colony headed by a singly mated queen are identical for 75% of their genome. This can lead to pseudo-replication, as colonies represent closely related families with related genetic backgrounds. Measurements of a group of 25 workers consisting of 5 workers from 5 different colonies cannot be considered 25 independent samples because of within-colony relatedness. Instead, this example contains measurements of 5 independent colonies, each consisting of the average from 5 workers. Thus, in most cases, worker colony samples should be averaged and one value taken per colony for statistical tests.

Molecular Methods

There are some practical considerations one should keep in mind when isolating DNA, RNA and protein from ants. Queens tend to be very high in fat content before their mating flight as well as in their physogastric form. Supplementary extractions with ether to remove this fat can be helpful for DNA and RNA isolation. Ants also tend to have much harder exoskeleton and higher surface-to-mass ratio than *Drosophila*, and complete homogenization of tissue can be difficult without a bead-type shaker homogenizer.

Some experiments are better conducted on dissected tissues or body sections. Physogastric queens lay large quantities of eggs and the mRNA profiles of the queens can become dominated by that of the eggs. Males contain a large amount of sperm and subsequently large amounts of DNA for their body weight. Beginning a DNA extraction with dissected vas deferens containing sperm represents an immediate 10-fold purification. The formic acid in Formicine ants can also be problematic as was found in protein preparations from *L. niger* workers (Parker *et al.*, 2004a). The acidity can effect isolation and gel loading buffers as well as interfere with enzyme activity assays. The efficiency of phenol extractions in DNA isolations can also be adversely affected by the acid.

Genetics

Recently, the standard of proof in molecular biology has required demonstration of gene function by knocking out or overexpressing a gene in an experimental system. This comparison is not yet possible at the organismal level in ants either through selective breeding or gene transfer, but has been successfully achieved for primary tissue culture in *S. invicta* (Cônsoli, 2002; Chen, 2004). To date, no one has developed an immortal cell line for any social insect. Eventually, one may find a way to breed the ant model systems above, either by simulating the natural mating conditions or by artificial insemination as is done for honey bees, but neither has yet been accomplished.

The lack of a genome sequence for ants does not pose as much of a practical problem as one might think. Although *S. invicta* is the only ant species with a very large cDNA sequence database, differential gene expression studies with specifically targeted genes or suppressive subtractive hybridization are still possible using genomes already sequenced. Specific genes can be cloned by aligning sequences from the honeybee, fruit fly, mosquito, silk worm and fire ant sequence databases using the program CODEHOP (Rose *et al.*, 1998) with the *Lasius niger* codon usage table selected. This technique has been successfully employed to clone numerous *L. niger* genes, including an extracellular SOD, which was not thought to exist in insects (Parker *et al.*, 2004b).

Comparative Studies

Ants as a group are extremely diverse, and this diversity lends itself to many types of comparative studies across species and across populations. There are also exploitable differences across caste and sex within a single species. Some of these represent reversals of typical life span correlations with size and longevity as observed in humans and birds. For example, there are two sizes of workers in the weaver ant, *Oecophylla smaragdina*. The major (large) workers perform the dangerous tasks outside the colony and have shorter life spans than the minor (small) workers who remain within the highly protected nest. But this difference in life span remains intact even in a protected laboratory environment (Chapuisat and Keller, 2002). It would be interesting to investigate if there are metabolic differences between these two sizes of worker ants.

The phenomena of monogynous/polygynous colonies have evolved independently many times across a wide range of ants and other social insect taxa. There is evidence that, within the same species, queens of monogynous populations live longer than queens of polygynous populations as predicted by evolutionary theory (Keller and Genoud, 1997). *Solenopsis invicta* is an excellent system to investigate life-span variation within a single species but across populations with different social structure as it has both polygynous and monogynous populations. In addition, the genetic basis for this difference in queen number is already known (Krieger and Ross, 2002).

One possibility for cross-species comparisons is the many cases of social parasites. Socially parasitic ants lack a worker caste and invade a host colony where their reproductive brood are raised by the host colony workers. In the genus *Pogonomyrex,* there are socially parasitic ants who live only 1–3 years and have recently evolved from a shared common ancestor of their longer lived hosts (*P. barbatus* and *P. rugous* (Johnson *et al.*, 1996; Parker and Rissing, 2002). They represent an opportunity to investigate the evolution to a shorter life span once the relevant processes are discovered.

Reproductive rate correlates with life span such that highly fertile individuals have shorter life spans than less fertile members of the same species (Williams, 1957; Charlesworth, 1980; Partridge and Gems, 2002). Yet this fecundity/longevity tradeoff is reversed for queens and workers. The queen of a large social insect nest must lay eggs at a rapid rate to maintain the number of sterile workers in the colony, and yet she has an extremely long life span (Rueppell *et al.*, 2004). This reversal of the fecundity/longevity tradeoff has been shown true even without the morphological and physiological differences which are present between queen and worker ants. In the Ponerine ant *Platytyrea punctata*, all workers are capable of producing diploid workers, yet the reproductive workers live significantly longer than their non-reproductive counterparts (Hartmann and Heinze, 2003).

Given that castes share the same genome, the differences in life span must be based on differential gene expression at some point(s) in their life history. This provides the foundation for testing gene expression differences already associated with aging in model systems. If the mechanisms hypothesized for life span extension in model systems are truly general, then there should be evidence of these same mechanisms being used in queen ants. One such mechanism, the resistance to oxidative stress conferred by superoxide dismutase (SOD), was recently tested in a comparison of cytoplasmic SOD activity and expression levels across all castes (Parker *et al.*, 2004a). The study found that a high level of cytoplasmic SOD does not correlate with life span as for previous work in *Drosophila* (Orr and Sohal, 1994; Sohal *et al.*, 1995; Hari *et al.*, 1998; Sun and Tower, 1999; Arking *et al.*, 2002; Spencer *et al.*, 2003) and is in agreement with previous comparative studies (Perez-Campo et. al, 1998; Barja, 2002).

These small, highly fecund and extraordinarily long-lived queens must overcome all of the physiological problems of maintaining mitochondria, proteins which are degraded, damaged and/or incorrectly folded, as well as accumulative damage to DNA and membranes that are associated with long life. Queens in particular must do all of these things an order of magnitude longer than workers, and while reproducing at a high enough rate to sustain a colony. All of these individual molecular processes represent potentially fruitful lines of inquiry that could reveal novel aging resistance mechanisms.

Conclusions

It should not be overlooked that only those processes verified by both unnatural life-span manipulations in the laboratory and naturally occurring evolved differences can be considered as true proven causes of life-span variation. Without verification, one will never know whether the mechanisms uncovered in the traditional model systems are artifacts of laboratory stress or specific to short-lived organisms. Testing in the laboratory will guard against making up "just-so" stories based solely on observed natural correlations. The challenge is to combine studies across both types of systems to discover what processes truly underlie the human aging process. Ants offer one of the best insect models to build this bridge.

ACKNOWLEDGMENTS

We thank Michel Chapuisat and Stephanie Jemielity for providing helpful comments and suggestions. The authors are supported by grants to Laurent Keller from the AETAS, Foundation for Research into Ageing (Geneva), The Fondation A.R. and J. Leenards (Lausanne) and the Swiss National Science Foundation.

REFERENCES

Arking, R., Buck, S., Novoseltev, V.N., Hwangbo, D., and Lane, M. (2002). Genomic plasticity, energy allocations, and the extended longevity phenotypes of *Drosophila. Ageing Res. Rev. 1*, 209–228.

Barja, G. (2002). Rate of generation of oxidative stress-related damage and animal longevity. *Free Radical Biol. Med. 33*, 1167–1172.

Chapuisat, M., and Keller, L. (2002). Division of labour influences the rate of ageing in weaver ant workers. *Prod. R. Soc. Lond. B. 269*, 909–913.

Charlesworth, B. (1980). *Evolution in Age-Structured Populations.* Cambridge University Press, Cambridge.

Chen, M.-E., Lewis, D.K., Keeley, L.L., and Pietrantonio, P.V. (2004). cDNA cloning and transcriptional regulation of the vitellogenin receptor from the imported fire ant, *Solenopsis invicta* Buren (Hymenoptera: Formicidae). *Insect Mol. Biol. 13*, 195–204.

Cole, A.C., Jr. (1968). *Pogonomyrmex Harvester Ants. A Study of the Genus in North America.* University of Tennessee Press, Knoxville.

Cônsoli, F.L., and Vinson, S. B. (2002). Hemolymph of reproductives of *Solenopsis invicta* (Hymenoptera: Formicidae) amino acids, proteins and sugars. *Comp. Biochem. Physiol. 132*, 711–719.

Fjerdingstad, E.J., Gertsch, P.J., and Keller, L. (2002). Why do some social insect queens mate with several males? Testing the sex-ratio manipulation hypothesis in *Lasius niger. Evolution. 56*, 553–562.

Fjerdingstad, E.J., Gertsch, P.J., and Keller, L. (2003). The relationship between multiple mating by queens, within-colony genetic variability and fitness in the ant *Lasius niger. J. Evol. Biol. 16*, 844–853.

Fjerdingstad, E.J., and Keller, L. (2004). Relationships between phenotype, mating behavior, and fitness of queens in the ant *Lasius niger. Evolution. 58*, 1056–1063.

Hari, R., Burde, V., and Arking, R. (1998). Immunological confirmation of elevated levels of CuZn superoxide dismutase protein in an artificially selected long-lived strain of *Drosophila melanogaster. Exp. Gerontol. 33*, 227–237.

Hölldobler, B., and Wilson, E.O. (1990). *The Ants.* Springer-Verlag, Berlin.

Jemielity, S., and Keller, L. (2003). Queen control over reproductive decisions: No sexual deception in the ant *Lasius niger. Mol. Ecol. 12*, 1589–1597.

Johnson, R.A., Parker, J.D., and Rissing, S.W. (1996). Rediscovery of the workerless inquiline ant *Pogonomyrmex colei* and additional notes on natural history (Hymenoptera, Formicidae). *Insectes Sociaux. 43*, 69–76.

Johnson, R.A. (2000). Seed harvester ants (Hymenoptera: Formicidae) of North America: An overview of ecology and biogeography. *Sociobiology 36*, 89–122. [Erratum: 2000. v. 36,597].

Johnson, R.A. (2001). Biogeography and community structure of North American seed-harvester ants. *Annu. Rev. Entomol., 46*, 1–29.

Keller, L. and Genoud, M. (1997). Extraordinary lifespans in ants—A test of evolutionary theories of ageing. *Nature 389*, 958–960.

Krieger, M.J.B., and Ross, K.G. (2002). Identification of a major gene regulating complex social behavior. *Science 295*, 328–332.

Kutter, H., and Stumper, R. (1969). Hermann Appel, ein leidegeadelter Entomologe (1892–1966). *Proceedings of the Sixth International Congress of the IUSSI (Bern)*, pp. 275–279.

Orr, W.C., and Sohal, R.S. (1994). Extension of life-span by overexpression of superoxide dismutase and catalase in *Drosophila melanogaster. Science 263*, 1128–1130.

Parker, J.D., Parker, K.M., Sohal, B.H., Sohal, R.S., and Keller, L. (2004). Decreased expression of Cu-Zn Superoxide Dismutase 1 in ants with extreme lifespan. *Proc. Nat. Acad. Sci. USA 101*, 3486–3489.

Parker, J.D., Parker, K.M., and Keller, L. (2004). Molecular phylogenetic evidence for an extracellular Cu Zn superoxide dismutase gene in insects. *Insect Mol. Biol. 13*, 587–594.

Parker, J.D., and Rissing, S.W. (2002). Molecular evidence for the origin of workerless social parasites in the ant genus *Pogonomyrmex. Evolution 56*, 2017–2028.

Partridge, L., and Gems, D. (2002). Mechanisms of ageing: Public or private? *Nat. Rev. Genet. 3*, 165–175.

Perez-Campo, R., Lopez-Torres, M., Cadenas, E., Rojas, C., and Barja, G. (1998). The rate of free radical production as a determinant of the rate of aging: Evidence from the comparative approach. *J. Comp. Physiol. B. 168*, 149–158.

Porter, S.D., and Jorgensen, C.D. (1988). Longevity of harvester ant colonies in southern Idaho. *Journal of Range Management 41*, 104–107.

Rose, T.M., Schultz, E.R., Henikoff, J.G., Pietrokovski, S., McCallum, C.M., and Henikoff, S. (1998). Consensus-degenerate hybrid oligonucleotide primers for amplification of distantly related sequences. *Nucleic Acids Res. 26*, 1628–1635.

Rueppell, O., Amdam, G.V., Page, R.E., and Carey, J.R. (2004). From genes to societies. *Sci. Aging Knowl. Environ. 5*, pe5.

Sohal, R.S., Agarwal, A., Agarwal, S., and Orr, W.C. (1995). Simultaneous overexpression of copper- and zinc-containing superoxide dismutase and catalase retards age related oxidative damage and increases metabolic potential in *Drosophila melanogaster. J. Biol. Chem. 270*, 15671–15674.

Solley, G.O., Vanderwoude, C., and Knight, G.K. (2002). Fire ants in Australia: A new medical and ecological hazard. *Med. J. Aust. 176*, 521–523.

Spencer, C.C., Howell, C.E., Wright, A.R., and Promislow, D.E.L. (2003). Testing an 'aging gene' in long-lived *Drosophila* strains: Increased longevity depends on sex and genetic background. *Aging Cell 2*, 123–130.

Sun, J., and Tower, J. (1999). FLP recombinase-mediated induction of Cu/Zn-superoxide dismutase transgene expression can extend the life span of adult *Drosophila melanogaster* flies. *Mol.Cell. Biol. 19*, 216–228.

Taber, S.W. (1998), *The world of the harvester ants.* Texas A and M University Press, College Station.

Williams, G.C. (1957). Pleiotropy, natural selection, and the evolution of senescence. *Evolution 11*, 398–411.

25

Gene Expression and the Extended Longevity Phenotypes of *Drosophila melanogaster*[1]

Robert Arking

Flies show three different types of longevity phenotypes, only one of which is characterized by significant increases in both the mean and maximum life span. This arises as a result of an experimentally induced delay in the onset of senescence. The net result of this phenotype is a significant increase in the length of the "health span," coupled with no significant change in the "senescent span." It is the purpose of this chapter to summarize what we know about the gene expression patterns and pathways that appear to be critically involved in allowing the expression of the one longevity phenotype which extends longevity by delaying the onset of senescence.

Introduction

There was once a time when the view that model organisms would actually lead us to informative views regarding human aging was but a pious hope. That time has passed. Much of what we now know or suspect about human aging is based on studies originally done in model organisms. It turns out that the major gene systems regulating aging are highly conserved public mechanisms; the characterization of the genetic and metabolic *pathways* involved in longevity regulation, and the environmental conditions necessary for their expression, required the integration of data from the four most commonly used species: yeast, worm, fly, and mouse. A good review of the various genetic attributes and tools that make *Drosophila melanogaster* such an excellent experimental tool for investigation of the aging phenomenon is found in chapter 22 by Miwa and Cohen. This chapter will be concerned with the three different longevity phenotypes known in this organism and the nature of the gene expression patterns characteristic of each, with special emphasis on the extended longevity phenotype brought about by a delayed onset of senescence.

The laboratory experiments done over the past few decades have allowed the robust identification of four different—but intertwined—genetic and physiological pathways which seem to regulate longevity in all four of our model systems. These four major public longevity processes may be summarily listed as follows: (1) *Metabolic Control*, (2) *Stress Resistance*, (3) *Genetic Stability*, and (4) *Reproductive Effects*. Information regarding different patterns of senescence is still sketchy but we will deal with it under the fifth heading of *Patterns of Senescence*. [A more extensive discussion of these topics in all four model systems is given by Arking (2005a)]. Each of these categories should be regarded, not as an autonomous set of metabolic reactions, but rather as sets of regulatory reactions that are more closely linked to one another than to any of the other categories. Such a view obviously permits the existence of crosstalk between these several network hubs. Much of the variation inherent in aging may stem from such cross-reactions. Table 25.1 contains an outline summary of these major processes which play an important role in bringing about differential longevity and senescence *in Drosophila melanogaster*. These processes may be induced or repressed by a variety of stimuli, including pharmaceutical interventions.

The Three Longevity Phenotypes of *Drosophila*

One fact that has emerged from the past several decades of aging research is that aging is not simple. The work that my colleagues and I have done on *Drosophila* longevity bears this out. We reported that aging in our *Ra* strain of wild-type flies is rather complex, being characterized by at least three different extended longevity phenotypes, each of which was induced by specific stimuli and had different demographic mortality and survival profiles (Arking *et al.*, 2002). As shown in Figure 25.1A, the first longevity phenotype (Type 1) is a delayed onset of senescence that leads to a significant increase in both mean and maximum life span of the experimental strain.

[1]Adapted from Chapter 7 of book by Arking (2005a).

TABLE 25.1
Summary comparison of main longevity pathways in *Drosophila melanogaster*

Process	Major genes or pathway	Effect
Metabolic control		
via CR	*indy, rpd3, Sir2*	CR slows rate of gene expression change relative to WT. Downregulates synthesis, turnover, & reproduction. No consistent up-regulation pattern. CR effect is relatively rapid.
via ISP	*InR, chico, forkhead*	ISP affects hormones which indirectly affect longevity by altering stress resistance levels. See "Repro Effects" below. Forkhead is key transcription factor which increases stress resistances.
via Nuclear-mito interactions	–	Cybrids show longevity intermediate between nuclear & mitochondrial donors.
Stress resistance	*CuZnSOD, MnSOD, catalase, Gpx, hsp*, others	Up-regulation of different ADS genes by various techniques usually leads to increased oxidative/other stress resistance. Likely basis of extended longevity; QTL confirmation of ADS basis in one strain. Tissue-specific protective effects.
Genetic stability	–	Genome appears to be highly stable in normal flies. No evidence for regional or overall genomic dysregulation.
Reproductive effects	ISP, JH, Ecdysone, *EcR, DTS-3*	ISP induces JH synthesis which induces egg production and 20HE synthesis. At high levels, 20HE represses resistance to various stressors, & reduces life span. At moderate levels, longevity & stress resistance significantly increase.
Patterns of senescence	–	Various sensory & locomotor abilities do not age in unison. Long-lived mutants do not delay the senescence of all their functions but retain some & lose others as do normal-lived animals.

The second longevity phenotype (Type 2), shown in Figure 25.1B, is an increased early survival that leads to a significant increase in mean but not in maximum life span. The third longevity phenotype (Type 3), shown in Figure 25.1C, is an increased later survival, which leads to a change in the maximum (LT_{90}) but not in the mean life spans.

Analysis of the mortality data supports these statements. The Type 1 phenotype yields a Gompertz curve which is significantly different from that of the control strain (Figure 25.2A).

Analysis of the data suggests that the Type 1 phenotype involves a ~50% reduction in the mortality rate doubling time (MRDT) of the long-lived strain (8.8 days) relative to the normal-lived strain (5.8 days). Although not a direct measure, the MRDT is a commonly used proxy indicator of comparative aging rates. However neither the Type 2 long-lived populations (Figure 25.2B) nor the Type 3 long-lived populations (Figure 25.2C) show any sustained alteration in aging rates relative to their controls, but rather show only a transient decrease in either early or late life but not both.

Moreover, it should be pointed out that the same phenotype may be induced by multiple different stimuli. For example, the Type 1 delayed onset of senescence phenotype may be induced in flies by (a) caloric restriction (Pletcher *et al.*, 2002), (b) by the down-regulation of the insulin-like signaling pathway (Tatar, Partridge refs), (c) by up-regulation of the antioxidant defense system (ADS) plus altered mitochondrial properties (Arking *et al.*, 2002), (d) by drugs which inhibit histone deacetylases (Kang *et al.*, 1999), and by other mechanisms as discussed below. What is it that unites all these varied stimuli and mechanisms into bringing about a Type 1 phenotype? What is it that distinguishes them from the stimuli which yield only the Type 2 or 3 phenotypes? The remainder of this chapter will attempt to answer these questions.

Gene Expression Pathways Yielding an Extended Longevity

METABOLIC CONTROL OF LONGEVITY

Metabolic control of longevity via caloric restriction

Although the effect of dietary restriction (CR) was first demonstrated in rodents in 1934, and although there have been a number of investigations of nutritional effects on longevity of *Drosphila*, it was not until 1996 that the first repeatable report appeared showing that CR was effective in altering the fly's life span (Chapman and Partridge,

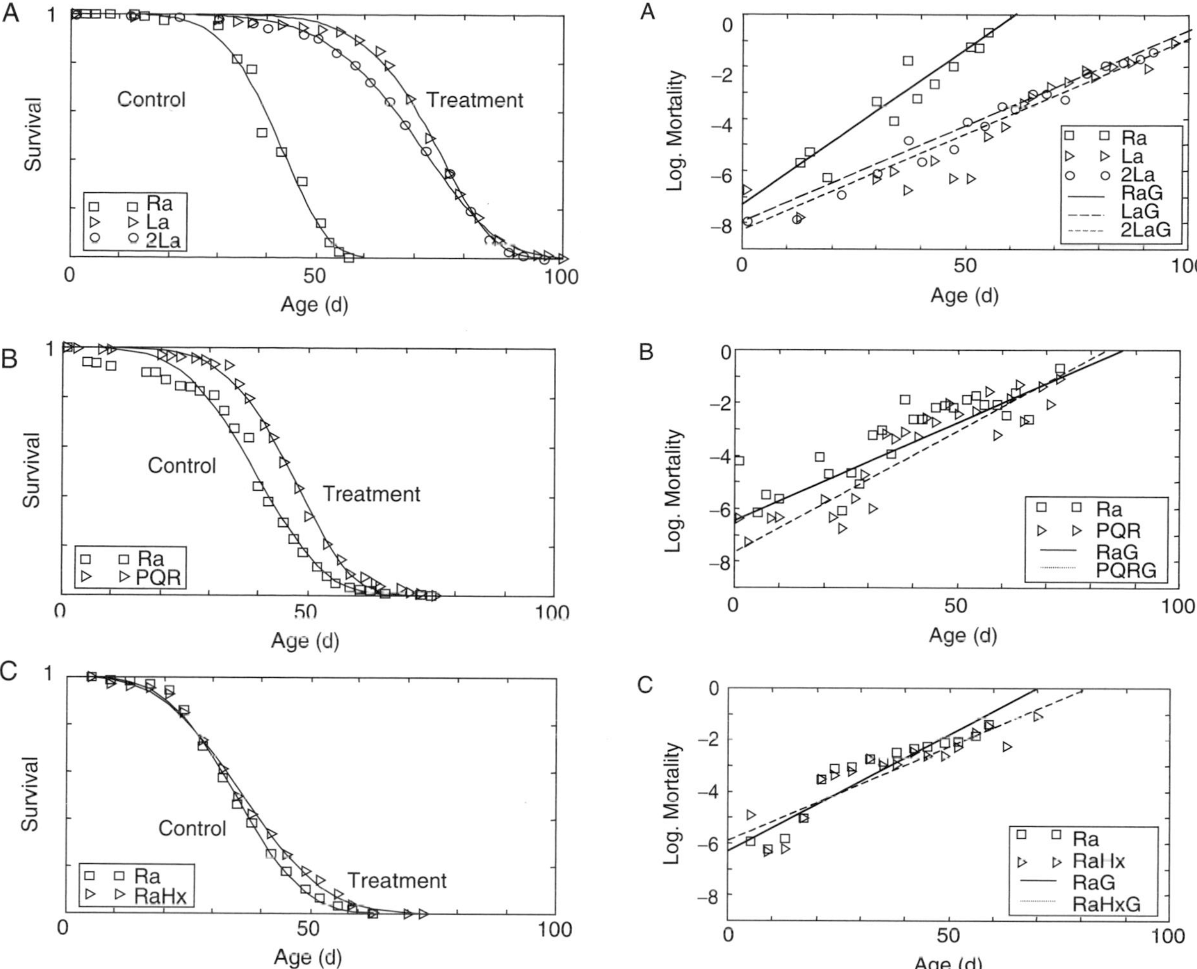

Figure 25.1. (A) Survival curves of the normal-lived Ra strain and of two long-lived strains (La and 2La) sequentially derived from it by a direct selection for delayed female fecundity. Each survival curve is based on the age-specific values obtained from two or three replicate cohorts consisting of at least 250 mixed sex individuals each. The Ra, La and 2La curves are significantly different (log-rank test = 530.16, df = 2, $P < 0.0001$). See Arking *et al.* (2000a) for experimental details. (B) Survival curves of the normal-lived Ra strain and the PQR strain selected from it by direct selection for paraquat resistance. Each survival curve is based on the age-specific values obtained from mixed sex cohorts of 250–450 animals each. The two curves are significantly different (log-rank test = 24.76, df = 1, $P < 0.00005$). See Vettraino *et al.* (2001) for experimental details. (C) Survival curves of the normal-lived Ra control strain and the longer-lived Ra heat-treated strain. The animals were subjected to a nonlethal heat shock (37°C for 90 minutes) early in life at days 5–7 after eclosion. They were then maintained under controlled optimal conditions, and their survival was monitored. The two curves are significantly different (log rank test = 17.84, df = 1, $P < 0.00005$). See Keuther and Arking (1999) for experimental details. (After Arking *et al.*, 2002)

Figure 25.2. (A) The hazard or force of mortality curves of the normal-lived Ra strain and of two long-lived strains (La and 2La) sequentially derived from it by a direct selection for delayed female fecundity. Each mortality curve is based on the age-specific values obtained from two or three replicate cohorts consisting of at least 250 mixed sex individuals each and was calculated using the Kaplan–Meier survival procedure in SPSS v.7. See Figure 25.1A for statistical significance. (B) The hazard or force of mortality curves of the normal-lived Ra strain and the PQR strain selected from it by direct selection for paraquat resistance. Each mortality curve is based on the age-specific values obtained from mixed sex cohorts of 250–450 animals each and was calculated using the Kaplan–Meier survival procedure in SPSS v.7. See Figure 25.1B for statistical significance. (C) The hazard or force of mortality curves of the normal-lived Ra control strain and the longer-lived Ra heat-treated strain. The animals were subjected to a nonlethal heat shock (37°C for 90 minutes) early in life at days 5–7 after eclosion. They were then maintained under controlled optimal conditions, and their survival was monitored. The mortality curve was calculated using the Kaplan–Meier survival procedure in SPSS v.7. See Figure 25.1C for statistical significance. (After Arking *et al.*, 2002)

1996). Raising the adults on food which contained only 33% of the nutrients found in the standard food allowed a ~34-day increase in the median life span and a ~31-day increase in the maximum life span (Pletcher *et al.*, 2002). Analysis of the age-specific mortality rates for this experiment showed that they did not begin to increase from the minimal values observed in the young until ~15 days in the control animals and about ~45 days in the CR animals. If this increase in the age-specific mortality is taken as indicating the age of onset of senescence, then the ~30-day delay in the age of onset of senescence in the CR animal essentially accounts for all the extra longevity noted in the survival curves. From a demographic point of view, the population enters what appears to be a period of stasis in which the age-specific mortality rate does not increase, and so this results in an extension of the young and healthy portion of the life span, as suggested in Figure 25.1A.

Gene expression analysis of the ad libitum (AL) and CR animals showed that >1% of the assayed genes showed a significant change in their expression. The genome is normally quite stable, and so our interest is focused on those few genes that do change. As a general rule, these changes occur more slowly in the CR set than in the control set. Those genes that increase with age in both sets comprise mostly genes involved with innate immunity and detoxification, enzyme inhibitors, and all sorts of genes involved in the response to various stresses. These data suggest that aging animals—regardless of their diet or chronological age—are under increasing stress from pathogens. It appears as if the proximate cause of death in old flies is infection (Tower *et al.*, 2004). An upstream cause of these proximate stresses may well be a loss of mitochondrial function, and the 458 gene probes down-regulated with age are consistent with this idea. The loss of energy production associated with decreased mitochondrial function is a major factor in the loss of function characteristic of aging. Most interesting is the CR-induced down-regulation of at least one gene (*methuselah* (*mth*), see below) known to significantly extend longevity when mutated. Its down-regulation under CR conditions suggests that the wild-type *mth* might act as a negative regulator of extended longevity. There is no obvious reduction in reproductive activities in the CR animals, and so it cannot be attributed only to a shift of energy from reproduction to somatic maintenance (Mair *et al.*, 2004). CR appears to extend longevity in the fly by ameliorating many of the normal transcriptional changes that occur with age. A model for the mechanisms involved in the onset of senescence is presented below and by Arking (2005b).

As was noted with CR in the mouse, different strains or mutants may have different sensitivity spectrums to CR. The *chico* mutant expresses its maximum life span at a higher food concentration than does the wild-type control (Clancy *et al.*, 2002). Other mutants show similar changes in their optimal food concentration. Thus the amount of food needed to trigger the CR response is not fixed in a species but is itself the outcome of the organism's genotype and nutritional environment. It is known that the organism actually has several pathways that sense its nutritional state. The TOR signaling pathway (see Figure 25.3) senses the amino acid levels so as to modulate growth or longevity.

There may well be other specific nutrient-sensing pathways. Their variable interactions with the nutritional environment and with each other may well account for the existence of different sensitivity spectrums to CR noted above.

The preceding discussion describes what CR does to a fly. But how does it do it? What gene pathways are involved? The evidence here is less detailed but still informative. Two different histone deacetylases are involved in mediating the CR response. Flies carrying a mutant *rpd3* deacetylase gene and raised on normal media have a mean and median life span about 40% longer than that of their wild-type controls (Rogina *et al.*, 2002). But *rpd3* mutants raised on low caloric food have a life span identical to that obtained if they are raised on normal food. The fact that the CR treatment has no effect on these mutants implies that the wild-type allele of the *rpd3* gene plays a role in the CR response. Even more interesting is the response of the *Drosophila Sir2* gene to CR and to *rpd3*. Wild-type animals subjected to CR show an approximate doubling in the level of *Sir2* gene expression, while *rpd3* mutants raised on normal food also show an approximate doubling in the level of *Sir2* gene expression. Thus the normal allele of *rpd3* seems to inhibit the *Sir2* gene expression that is necessary for the CR effect. In another series of experiments, it was shown that if the *Sir-2* histone deacetylase gene of Drosophila is up-regulated by feeding the animal a known sirtuin activator such as resveratrol (the longevity extending component of red wine), then life span is significantly extended even though the animals are fed AL (Wood *et al.*, 2004). Conversely, flies lacking a functional *Sir-2* gene failed to extend their longevity when fed resveratrol. Thus activation of *Sir-2* seems to be essential for the expression of CR-dependent extended longevity. It is reasonable to conclude that both these genes are components of the genetic pathway mediating CR expression, related perhaps in the manner suggested in Figure 25.3. It should be noted that there is much disagreement over the details of this interaction, and this is now an active area of investigation.

Another gene possibly involved in CR is the *indy* gene which encodes a metabolite transporter protein responsible for the uptake and transport of Krebs and citric acid cycle intermediates through the gut epithelium and into the appropriate organs (Knauf *et al.*, 2002). Homologous genes exist in nematodes and mammals. Flies carrying a mutation in this gene display a 90% increase in their mean life span and a 50% increase in their maximum life span (Rogina *et al.*, 2000). In flies, the *indy* gene is normally expressed primarily in the midgut, fat body (liver equivalent) and oenocytes, which are the main sites of intermediary metabolism. It is not unreasonable to assume that the mutant-induced down-regulation in the activity of this metabolite co-transporter protein brings about a lower effective concentration of essential metabolites in the cell, thus creating a metabolic state similar to that induced by CR. One possible interpretation of its role in the CR pathway is shown in Figure 25.3.

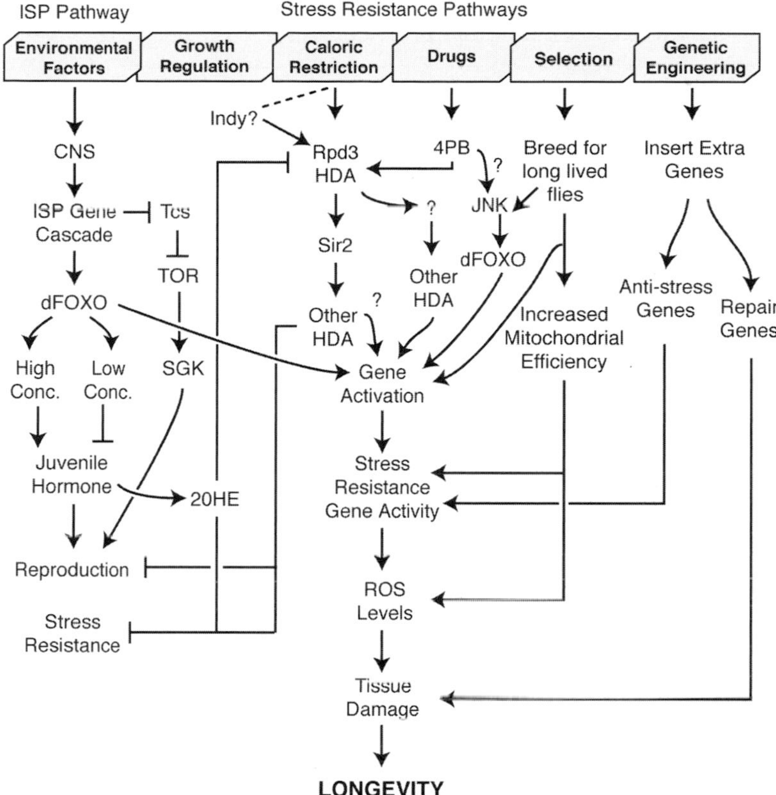

Figure 25.3. A schematic diagram integrating all the pathways empirically known to yield a Type 1 (delayed onset of senescence) longevity phenotype in *Drosophila melanogaster* (after Arking, 2005a).

A very important insight into the nature of the CR response was provided by an experiment in which flies were initially raised on either a CR or AL dietary regime and were then switched at various ages to the alternative diet (Mair *et al.*, 2003). AL-raised flies normally have a higher age specific mortality rate than do CR-raised animals. But after a AL → CR shift, the animals rapidly adopt the age-specific mortality rate characteristic of animals who have been raised on a CR regime for their entire life. A corresponding rapid upward shift in mortality rate is observed following a CR → AL shift. What this means is that the *age-specific mortality rates have no cellular memory;* change the physiological state of the cell and you change the resulting mortality rate. An AL → CR shift, for example, induces the animal to alter its regulatory pathways and shift its gene expression pattern from a pro-growth pattern to a pro-stress resistance pattern. The consequent change in damage patterns affects the mortality rate. The mortality rate is due only to the current levels of damage occurring in the organism. The animal's prior history does not directly play a determining role in its current mortality rate, although certainly the existence of prior unrepaired damage must have some effect. This finding implies that CR/ISP-dependent aging is an environmentally dependent cell level function, and the presence of the systemic regulatory mechanisms in multicellular eucaryotes does not invalidate this statement.

A cautionary note is in order here: not all flies react to CR in the same manner as described above. Our selected La and Ra strains have a different response pattern (Arking, unpublished data). Mediterranean fruit flies (*Ceratitis capitata*) are distantly related to *Drosophila* and might reasonably be expected to react to CR in the same manner if one assumes that the CR mechanism is highly conserved and public. However, a recent study reported that the Mediterranean fruit fly shows a more or less constant longevity at various levels of diet restriction with a sharp decrease in mortality once the diet falls below 50% of the ad libitum level (Carey *et al.*, 2002). There is no evidence for an increase in longevity at some consistent level of dietary restriction. Reproduction occurred across the range of diets tested. The mortality increase occurred in both sexes even though males have no obvious counterpart to the energetic demands of egg production in females. On the other hand, these same flies lived longer when subjected to a "feast or famine" dietary regime (Carey *et al.*, 2004). This latter regime likely resembles the normal situation in the wild, and so perhaps that environment selects for animals that can go into a survival mode when food becomes transiently scarce. These data suggest that there are intra- and interspecific differences in the CR response, which is thus a highly conserved but not universal mechanism.

Metabolic control of longevity via insulin-like signaling pathway

The insulin-like signaling pathway (ISP) was initially investigated for its effects on growth and size of the fly, and it was demonstrated that mutants affecting the activity of ISP did affect these parameters (Weinkove and Leevers, 2000). The ISP also affects blood sugar levels. The fly possesses five insulin-like proteins with significant homology to the mouse and human insulin proteins. These proteins are expressed in several tissues but most particularly in small clusters of insulin-producing cells (IPCs) in the brain (Rulifson *et al.*, 2002). These workers showed that ablation of these IPCs caused retarded growth and elevated carbohydrate levels, and that a normal phenotype could be restored by expressing one of the *Drosophila* insulin-like proteins. Thus there is a remarkable conservation of the insulin-based glucoregulatory mechanisms in flies and mammals with respect to its effects on growth and blood sugar. Once the experimental data allowed the concept of a conserved longevity regulation mechanism to become clear from the work done with yeast and nematode, then the fly's ISP was investigated to see if it also regulated the fly's longevity. There are some obvious phenotypic differences between homozygous and heterozygous mutants in genes comprising the ISP, but the important point made clear by these investigations is that certain of these mutants can significantly increase longevity.

As you might expect, flies with no ISP activity at all are lethal. But in rare cases, one can construct homozygous flies which contain two different mutations, each with a defect in a different part of the gene. Such unusual animals have a low but detectable level of ISP activity (~25% or less) and can survive through adulthood. These "heteroallelic" homozygotes contain two different mutations in their insulin receptor gene (*InR*; homologous to the *C. elegans daf-2* gene) and gave rise to dwarf adults with different longevity effects on the two sexes (Tatar *et al.*, 2001). Females expressed a delayed onset of senescence, with an 87% increase in their mean life span and a ~45% increase in their maximum life span. These homozygous mutant females are small because the ISP controls cell size, and the low activity levels result in small cells and slow growth. They are sterile because the low ISP activity results in a significant decrease in the juvenile hormone levels which are known to be essential for reproduction (see Reproductive Effects). Male homozygotes are also small and semisterile, for the same reasons. On the other hand, the males show no statistical change in their mean life span even though they have an increased mortality during early to mid-adult life followed by a lower mortality rate thereafter. Incidentally, the smaller effect of the ISP on males seems to be a general phenomenon, and we will touch on it in Reproductive Effects.

Both heterozygous and homozygous *InR* mutants have an impaired synthesis of the steroid hormone, ecdysone (Tu *et al.*, 2002). This suggests that the increased longevity associated with the heterozygous InR mutants is likely dependent on a decreased level of juvenile hormone synthesis and the consequent reduction of ecdysone synthesis to levels that do not repress the animal's level of stress resistance (see Reproductive Effects for a description of the mechanisms which tie these several observations together).

Flies which are either heterozygous or homozygous for a certain mutation in their IRS proteins (associated with the cytoplasmic side of the InR) also yield long-lived females but not males (Clancy *et al.*, 2001). These flies were also observed to be more resistant to oxidative stress than their controls. Thus disabling the *InR* and/or *IRS* genes is sufficient to down-regulate the entire ISP.

Finally, the *dFOXO* gene of *Drosophila* was shown to have sequence homology with the *daf-16* gene of *C. elegans*, and to function in the regulation of growth (Kramer *et al.*, 2003). Flies heterozygous for the *dFOXO* gene are incapable of expressing the extended longevity otherwise resulting from a mutational down-regulation of the *InR* gene (Hwangbo *et al.*, 2004). This functional test demonstrates that the *dFOXO* gene is downstream of *InR*. Thus the structure of the ISP is the same in yeast and nematode and fly, for effects on the upstream genes such as *InR* must be mediated through the downstream *dFOXO* transcription factor. If the latter is mutationally inactivated, then the upstream signals are ignored. This factor is believed to activate various stress-resistance genes and repress various pro-growth genes in a manner similar to that demonstrated in the nematode. Both of these actions will result in a slower accumulation of age-related oxidative damage and in a delayed onset of senescence, as described in Stress Resistance and External Longevity.

The simplest conclusion of these several experiments is that the modulation of longevity via the ISP is highly conserved from yeast to mammals. The fact that longevity regulation in the fly is intertwined in the same system with the regulation of growth, cell size, and fertility suggests that the fly ISP has multiple specific regulatory functions compared to a nematode. This is consistent with the fact that the fly has at least four independent isoloci of the PI3K gene, each of which apparently controls different sets of processes, while humans have at least 16 PI3K genes (Samuels *et al.*, 2004). This increased signaling complexity, which might have arisen as a consequence of the increased size and morphological complexity of the fly, might well account for its apparent greater genetic complexity.

Important though it is, the ISP is not the only signaling pathway involved in assaying nutrient availability.

The TOR signaling pathway is an important regulator of growth and size and is found in organisms from yeast to humans. Experiments with *Drosophila* show that the TOR pathway senses amino acid availability and uses this information to modulate activity of the S6 kinase regulatory gene so as to enhance growth and repress extended longevity (Kapahl *et al.*, 2004). It also plays an important role in regulating autophagy, or the digestion of the cell's own components for energy (Klionsky, 2004). It was found that either over-expression of the upstream *Tsc1* and *Tsc2* genes, or dominant–negative mutations in in the *TOR* or *S6K* genes, gave rise to extended longevity. As briefly summarized in Figure 25.3, these data suggest that the two upstream genes act as negative regulators of the TOR or S6K genes, which themselves act as a negative regulator of longevity and a positive regulator of growth. It seems likely that the TOR pathway acts in parallel with, and perhaps even overlaps, the ISP.

Metabolic control of longevity via nuclear–mitochondrial interaction

There exists a large body of information regarding the role of mitochondria in aging. But there is almost no definitive data regarding the role of nuclear–mitochondrial interaction in the *Drosophila* aging process. This, however, does not mean that nuclear–mitochondrial interaction does not occur in flies, for there are at least three lines of suggestive evidence to the contrary. Taken together, they suggest but do not prove that the observed changes stem from some alteration in nuclear–mitochondrial communication.

First, Ballard and James (2003) found that mitochondria and nuclei taken from animals indigenous to different parts of the species' geographic range yielded low fitness flies when combined. This might come about if the mitochondria had evolved so as to be most effective in certain environments. Combining a (genetically different?) mitochondria from one area with a nucleus which evolved in a different region might result in organelle incompatibilities and hence a decreased life span.

Second, the same laboratory collected strains of *Drosophila simulans* (a close relative of *D. melanogaster*) from comparable environments and assayed their longevity as well as aspects of their mitochondrial function. They found that a particular long-lived strain was characterized by a high mitochondrial efficiency. Complex IV of their mitochondria's electron transport chain is more efficient than is the case in normal-lived control strains, as evidenced by their lower than normal oxygen consumption but normal levels of ATP production (Melvin *et al.*, 2005). The nuclear encoded protein subunits of the complex responsible for the increased efficiency turned out to contain several point mutations which resulted in amino acid changes, the presence of which are highly correlated with the altered mitochondrial function. It is reasonable to suspect that the selection of chance mutations in nuclear encoded mitochondrial proteins bespeaks the likely existence of metabolic signals that coordinate nuclear and mitochondrial activities and provide the feedback signals necessary to the selection process.

Third, as a result of the selection experiment summarized in Figure 25.1A, we wound up with a long-lived La strain and a normal-lived Ra control strain. But their extended longevity arises in part from the fact that the La mitochondria produce from ~20 to ~40% less H_2O_2 than do the normal Ra mitochondria (Ross, 2001). Using the Ra and La strains, Driver and Tawadros (2000) set up various crosses that allowed them to combine mitochondria from different selected strains with the same normal-lived Ra nucleus. They then examined the resulting "cybrid" strains to see if any of the combined genomes had an effect on longevity. They showed that combining mitochondria from either normal-lived strain (Ra or Rb) with the Ra nucleus led to no change in longevity; but combining either of the long-lived mitochondria (La or Lb) with the Ra nucleus led to a significant change. Thus, the Lamt strain achieves about 40% of the extended longevity seen in the La strain solely because it has La type mitochondria. It would seem that mitochondria can make a significant contribution to longevity. Possible mechanisms for this phenomenon have been put forth elsewhere (Arking *et al.*, 2002). The important point here is that different mitochondrial genomes appear to set up different stable metabolic equilibrium settings with the Ra nucleus, and each of these permits different longevities to be expressed.

Whether any of these three cases constitutes nuclear–mitochondrial interaction is still to be determined. The fact that two different labs using different strains and different approaches have observed similar sorts of data

TABLE 25.2
Effect of nonlethal stressors on longevity*

Stressor	% Response of experimental	Molecules involved**
Animals over controls		
Cold	5%	hsp
Heat	10%	hsp & ADS
Hypergravity	12%	hsp
Physical activity	20%	ADS
Irradiation	20%	ADS & hsp
Caloric restriction	50%	ADS & others
Oxidative Stress Resistance	33–60%***	ADS & others

*data adapted from Figure 1 of Minois (2000).

**hsp = heat shock proteins; ADS = antioxidant defense system proteins.

***response noted after selection or transgenic modification of genome.

suggests that nuclear–mitochondrial interactions might also take place in *Drosophila*.

STRESS RESISTANCE AND EXTENDED LONGEVITY

It has long been observed that mild or nonlethal stress often has the apparently paradoxical effect of benefiting the organism by increasing its longevity (Minois, 2000). Conversely, it has also been suggested that all long-lived strains and mutants exhibit some form of stress resistance (Parsons, 1995; Johnson *et al.*, 1996). This relationship is thought to reflect the fact that their natural environment usually exerts substantial, albeit variable, stresses on organisms. Evolutionary considerations of Darwinian fitness will thus impose a premium on genotypes conferring metabolic efficiency and stress resistance (Parsons, 1997, 2003). The magnitude of the effects of stress resistance on longevity are summarized in Table 25.3.

We will examine four complementary lines of evidence bearing on the relationship of stress resistance and extended longevity in *Drosophila*. The first involves the use of strains selected for extended longevity, followed by an analysis of the mechanisms responsible for the altered phenotype. The second involves standard mutational techniques in which candidate genes thought to play an important role in longevity are inactivated, and the life span of the experimental animals is assayed to see if the original hypothesis was correct or not. The third approach involves "genetic engineering" or transgenic work in which extra copies of candidate genes are inserted into experimental animals and their longevity is then assayed to determine if the added gene has a significant effect on the life span. The fourth approach involves the environmental induction of stress response genes and the analysis of their effect on the longevity of the tested animals.

As a result of our studies on the biochemistry and stress resistance properties of the long-lived La strains, we knew that the only predictive factor clearly and significantly associated with extended longevity in our strains was an enhanced resistance to oxidative stress (Arking *et al.*, 1991; Force *et al.*, 1995). Thus it seemed logical to conclude that the long-lived La animals probably live long because of higher-than-normal activity of the antioxidant defense system genes early in life. Quantitative trait loci (QTL) mapping is a genetic method of identifying small chromosome regions which have a significant statistical effect on longevity, and may be viewed as a genome-wide scan that allows one to identify interesting genes for further investigation. Curtsinger and Khazaeli (2002) did such a procedure on recombinant inbred strains derived from the La and Ra strains discussed above. They found four QTLs located on chromosomes 2 and 3 of the (La × Ra) recombinant inbred strains that accounted for almost all of the selection response. The major QTLs for both paraquat resistance and longevity are coincident with each other and are centered over a small region of chromosome 3L which contains the loci of the CuZnSOD

TABLE 25.3
Summary of genetic interventions testing the relationship between resistance to oxidative stress and altered longevity

Manipulation	Genes involved	Effect on life span	Effect on stress resistance	Reference
Selection for long life	CuZnSOD, MnSOD	Increased	Increased	Arking *et al.* (2000a)
	Catalase	Increased	Increased	Arking *et al.* (2000b)
	CuZnSOD?	Increased	Increased ox stress, also increased starvation & dessication resistance	Rose (1984)
Catalase reduced	Cat	Decreased	No data	Mackay & Bewley (1989)
Catalase increased	Cat	No effect	Increased	Orr & Sohal (1992)
SOD1 reduced	CuZnSOD	Decreased	Decreased	Phillips *et al.* (1989)
SOD1 increased	CuZnSOD	Increased	Increased	Parkes *et al.* (1998)
				Sun & Tower (1999)
		Increased (some strains)	Increased (some strains)	Orr & Sohal (1993)
SOD1 & cat increased	CuZnSOD, cat	Increased	Increased	Orr & Sohal (1994)
		.........No increase over SOD alone.........		Sun & Tower (1999)
SOD2 reduced	MnSOD	Decreased	Decreased	Kirby *et al.* (2002)
SOD2 increased	MnSOD	Increased	No data	Sun *et al.* (2002)
		No effect	No effect	Mockett et *al.* (1999)

gene, and of several heat shock protein (hsp) genes. Both of these gene sets are involved in stress resistance. The other QTLs seem to be involved in maintaining female fertility. (One of these other QTLs appears to involve the ecdysone receptor (EcR) gene, which is involved in reproductive processes; see the section on Reproductive Effects.) The several genes involved exert their effects over the first six weeks of life but not thereafter. There are other minor contributors to the extended longevity phenotype (Curtsinger *et al.*, 1998), but the available data strongly indicates that the La strains live long primarily because of a specific up-regulation of antioxidant defense genes.

This finding supported our candidate gene approach in which we assayed the quantitative changes in the mRNA levels and the antioxidant enzyme activity levels of several loci during the development and early adult life of the normal-lived Ra and long-lived La strains (Dudas and Arking, 1995). In addition, we used antibodies to measure the actual amount of CuZnSOD protein present in these strains (Hari *et al.*, 1997). The mRNA data demonstrate that, at day 5 in the L strain, there appears to be a coordinately regulated significant increase in the mRNA levels of CuZnSOD, CAT, and xanthine dehydrogenase (XDH). There is a nonsignificant increase in glutathione-*S*-transferase (GST) mRNA during the same time period. These increases in mRNA levels are accompanied by significant increases in the enzyme activity of CuZnSOD, CAT, and GST. Other experiments showed that the amount of SOD-specific protein is proportionately increased in the La strain during the same time period (Hari *et al.*, 1998). Thus it seems reasonable to conclude that these alterations in gene expression in the long-lived strain are the result of a transcription-level change that alters the enzymatic arsenal available to the organisms. But these changes in gene expression have biological meaning only if they reduce the amount of oxidative damage in the long-lived animals.

The higher level of antioxidant gene expression and enzyme activities do in fact bring about a life-long and significant reduction in the levels of the most common oxidative damages in proteins or lipids in the long-lived L strain. There exists an inverse correlation between the levels of antioxidant enzyme activity (Dudas and Arking, 19956) and the levels of oxidative damage (Arking *et al.*, 2000a). It seems reasonable to conclude that these animals developed the ability, as a consequence of artificial selection, to turn on a regulatory process that coordinately activates the antioxidant defense genes early in life, thereby protecting the animals against the oxidative damage to vital molecules and thus delaying the onset of senescence until their antioxidant defenses fall to normal levels. Reverse-selecting these long-lived strains for shortened longevity (Arking *et al.*, 2000a,b) reverts their antioxidant gene expression patterns to control levels. Only the antioxidant genes (and certain other enzymes operationally connected to them) show these correlated and coordinate changes in gene expression. Other metabolically important enzymes which do not affect the antioxidant proteins do not show any significant changes as a result of selection (Arking *et al.*, 2000a). The reversal in life span was accompanied by a specific reversal in the expression of only the antioxidant genes and genes necessary to their function. Incidentally, an independent replicate strain (Lb) has the same longevity patterns as does the La line but uses different specific patterns of antioxidant gene expression (Arking *et al.*, 2002b). One interpretation of these data is that the overall oxidative stress level of the organism may be more important than which particular antioxidant gene is over-expressed. Another is that different signaling pathways may be involved.

Taken all together, this series of experiments reveals the existence of a causal relationship between antioxidant gene expression, oxidative stress resistance, levels of oxidative damage, and longevity in these selected strains of *Drosophila*.

In a parallel, simultaneous, and independent experiment, Michael Rose (1984) used a different wild-type progenitor stock but the same indirect selection protocols as used for the Wayne State University (WSU) lines to create a set of long-lived strains termed the University of California-Irvine (UCI) long-lived lines. Interestingly enough, the physiological traits associated with the UCI selected lines overlap those associated with the WSU lines, for both sets of strains of strains are significantly more resistant to environmental stresses than their respective controls. The two are resistant to a different spectrum of stressors, which may well be the result of the different genetic backgrounds used in their different progenitor stocks. The UCI lines are resistant to starvation, dessication, and oxidative stress; and selection for increased starvation or dessication resistance was later shown to lead to increased longevity (Rose *et al.*, 1992; Harshman *et al.*, 1999). The WSU lines are mildly resistant to dessication but mostly resistant to oxidative stress (Force *et al.*, 1995). Although several kinds of stress resistance are associated with extended longevity, it may not be a coincidence that the only common stress resistance in all these strains is that of oxidative stress.

Genetic data generally support these selection experiments. Phillips *et al.* (1989) created a CuZnSOD-null mutant of *Drosophila* and showed that the absence of this enzyme activity significantly decreased viability and longevity. Subsequent analysis by the same group (Parkes *et al.*, 1998) showed that the absence of the CuZnSOD gene has a number of important pleiotropic effects such as (1) adult sensitivity to paraquat, (2) male sterility, (3) female semisterility, (4) adult hyperoxia sensitivity, (5) larval radiation sensitivity, (6) developmental sensitivity to glutathione depletion (an important antioxidant molecule), and (7) adult life-span reduction. Before one could confidently interpret these results, it was necessary to determine whether these alterations stemmed from an increase in the rate of aging or from some abnormal pathology. An experiment was done showing that these CuZnSOD-null mutants showed an acceleration, relative to the wild-type control, of the normal age-related temporal changes in the expression of certain other genes (Rogina *et al.* 2000). Since the acceleration in the temporal expression of these other genes was proportional to the shortened life span, then this was interpreted as showing that the shortened life span of the CuZnSOD-null mutants is due, not to an abnormal pathological process, but to an increase in the rate of aging. This interpretation suggests that the aging rate is directly proportional to the animals' level of antioxidant capacity and resistance to oxidative stress, a finding in keeping with the selection results discussed above.

In contrast to the SOD data, acatalesemic mutants of *Drosophila* are essentially normal when reared under standard conditions as long as they have at least 3% of the normal catalase expression level (Mackay and Bewley, 1989), a finding consistent with the transgene work done on this gene (Orr and Sohal, 1992), which suggests that catalase is not normally a rate-limiting factor in longevity.

Transgenic technology, which allowed the insertion of an extra gene(s) into an otherwise normal organism, was early used to test the effects of increasing the level of CuZnSOD gene expression on the longevity and aging of the altered animals. The early experiments inserted single copies of either CuZnSOD or catalase into the test organisms, but their results were inconclusive for a variety of reasons. However, the tandem over-expression of both CuZnSOD and catalase in the same animal did extend median and maximum longevity by up to 34% in some lines while simultaneously retarding oxidative damage and increasing oxidative resistance (Orr and Sohal, 1994; Sohal *et al.*, 1995). Sun and Tower (1999) used a controllable transgenic system that allowed them to control when CuZnSOD over-expression would take place in adult flies. This system allowed increases in mean life span of up to 48%. These two transgenic alterations of gene expression ostensibly affected all tissues of the organism at all stages. But there is much information showing that most genes have characteristic tissue and stage-specific expression patterns. Thus it was important when Parkes *et al.* (1998, 1999) showed that a GAL4-UAS transgene expression system which selectively targeted CuZnSOD expression to the adult motor neuron was capable both of (a) restoring the normal adult life span of CuZnSOD-null mutants and (b) extending by 40% the adult life span of an otherwise wild-type fly. Over-expression of CuZnSOD in the adult central nervous system, adult muscle or larval body has no effect on adult longevity. It turns out that adult *Drosophila* have a surprising lack of CuZnSOD activity in their central nervous system relative to the rest of the body (Klichko *et al.*, 1999). It may be that the flies' motor neurons may have the lowest age-related failure threshold of the whole body and would normally be the first critical tissue to fail. Thus using transgenes to increase their resistance to oxidative stress may have the effect of postponing the age at failure of this critical tissue and thus result in lengthening the life span.

Scientific progress does not occur in a straight line. The validity of the three transgene experiments described above have been challenged by two of the researchers involved on the basis that an increased longevity was observed only in those cases where the control flies had a comparatively short life span (Orr and Sohal, 2003). In their rethinking of the matter, shorter lived control lines are helped by CuZnSOD over-expression, but genetically robust controls showed little or no effect. This reassessment casts doubt only on the efficacy of increasing life span by increasing only CuZnSOD expression; it does not affect experiments showing that suites of antioxidant genes are over-expressed in long-lived strains (e.g., Table 25.3) or that different antioxidant genes act together in a cooperative manner in the fly (Missirlis *et al.*, 2001) or experiments involving robust control flies. It is a likely possibility that the reason for the failure of some transgenes to significantly affect the life span of some flies is that an organism with an inefficient metabolism and low levels of available ATP is simply not in a position to effectively reallocate the energy saved due to lowered oxidative damage levels to increased somatic maintenance. In the La strain, the effective use of the increased antioxidative defense enzymes requires the simultaneous alterations of metabolism (e.g., shifting from glycolysis to the pentose shunt) so as to support the enzyme functions, as well as mitochondrial changes that yield an increased efficiency and thus increase the levels of available ATP (Arking *et al.*, 2002). Pathways—both genetic and metabolic—need to be changed if an animal is to live long. Altering the expression of one gene without altering the necessary pathways may bring about only a weak effect.

MnSOD is the mitochondrial version of superoxide dismutase. Given the crucial role of mitochondria in energy metabolism and ROS generation, it seemed logical that this gene product would likely play an important role in modulating the life span. This assumption is borne out by our selection data (Arking *et al.*, 2000a) and by the transgenic data of Sun *et al.* (2000). These researchers used their controllable transgene system to induce the over-expression of MnSOD only in adult flies but not in the developmental stages, thus avoiding complications in the analysis. They reported that MnSOD showed increases in expression of up to 75%. This yielded a 33% increase in mean life span and a 37% increase in maximum life span. The simultaneous over-expression of both CuZnSOD and MnSOD led to a complicated situation wherein each transgene partially inhibited the over-expression of the other, but nonetheless still resulted in the two genes having partially additive effects on life span (Sun *et al.*, 2004). Phillips and his colleagues (2000) have also used transgenes to over-express the MnSOD gene in wild-type animals and find that they obtain life span extensions of about 30%. They also note that the over-expressed MnSOD gives an incomplete rescue of the CuZnSOD-null mutant, thus establishing that the two enzymes operate in functionally different compartments. Conversely, destroying the MnSOD mRNA and thus silencing this one gene in a normal animal results in a disruption of mitochondrial function, an increased sensitivity to oxidative stress, and a striking ~80% reduction in mean and maximum life span (Kirby *et al.*, 2002). In contrast, Mockett *et al.* (1999) reported that their transgenic MnSOD lines did over-express MnSOD mRNA, protein and enzyme activity but did not show an increased life span relative to the controls. This finding may well have to do with the genetic background of their control strain; if so, it represents a limitation, but not a refutation, of the ability of any one specific antioxidant gene to increase life span for the reasons presented above.

Given the complexity of the stress resistance process, it is inevitable that other genes are involved. Glutathione is perhaps the most abundant low molecular weight antioxidant present in the animal and represents a potential clue to other candidate genes. Mockett *et al.* (1999) over-expressed the glutathione reductase gene in transgenic *Drosophila* and obtained up to 100% over-expression of the enzyme. Longevity was significantly enhanced under hyperoxic conditions but not under normoxic condtions, suggesting that glutathione reductase may not be a rate-limiting factor in antiaging defenses under normal conditions but may well be one when the level of oxidative stress is elevated. This is very similar to the effects of glutathione-*S*-transferase on nematode longevity (Leiers *et al.*, 2003).

Another set of candidate genes are those which regulate the expression of the antioxidant structural genes. Four different mutant searches have identified such genes. In the first, Lin *et al.* (1998) did P-element mutagenesis of the 3rd chromosome and screened for long life (relative to the *white* control strain) at 29°C. One homozygous mutant, named *methuselah* (*mth*), lived up to 35% longer and was more resistant to paraquat, starvation and high temperature. The *mth* gene appears to code for a transmembrane G protein-coupled receptor presumably involved in the regulation of stress response genes. Other data suggest it may be a negative regulator of these genes. Recent data suggest that the ligand for this *mth* receptor is the stunted (sun) protein, but the functional pathways involved are not yet known. The second search also used P-element mutagenesis but focused on the second chromosome and identified two groups of trans-acting mutants, one of which acted as if they were normally positive regulators of CuZnSOD and catalase in wild-type animals and the other of which acted as if they were normally negative regulators. The third approach showed that up-regulation of the JNK signaling pathway made the animals much more resistant to oxidative stress while increasing both their mean and maximun life spans (Wang *et al.*, 2003). Finally, the fourth approach used microarrays to conduct a genome-wide search for genes which responded to chronic exposure to oxidative and other stresses (Giradot *et al.*, 2004). The data show the existence of both general and specific responses to these different stressors, and indicate the existence of a complex interlocking network of stress response genes. The point is that four independent experiments have demonstrated that single genes seem to extend longevity by up-regulating the animal's ability to withstand various types of stress, and that these individual genes may well be components of a larger network of stress response genes.

The heat-shock protein (HSP) genes were initially found in *Drosophila*. Much work has demonstrated that these proteins have significant effects on stress resistance and longevity in all organisms. There are two complementary findings: first, the expression of the HSP genes is affected by aging; and second, the up-regulation of some (but not all) of these genes can significantly affect longevity. Aging animals usually express abnormal patterns of HSP expression relative to young animals (Niedzwiecki and Fleming, 1990). Two reports (Wheeler *et al.*, 1995; King and Tower, 2000) show that hsp22 mRNA is up-regulated during aging, particularly in the head. In addition, an earlier onset of hsp22 and hsp23 mRNA accumulation in *Drosophila* flies selected for increased longevity was also reported (Kurapati *et al.*, 2000), suggesting a possible correlation between hsp22 levels and longevity. Using genetic techniques to over-express hsp22 in motorneurons led to a 30% increase in longevity and stress resistance (Morrow *et al.*, 2004a). Conversely, knocking out the hsp22 gene so that flies could not express the HSP22 protein led to a 40% decrease in their longevity, coupled with an increased sensitivity to stress (Morrow *et al.*, 2004b). Finally, a ubiquitous over-expression of hsp22 throughout the entire body also led to a reduction in life span as well as an increased sensitivity to heat and oxidative stress (Bhole *et al.*, 2004). Looking at the data as a whole, we can see that increased longevity and stress resistance depend not just on the over-expression of the hsp22 gene, but on its being expressed in the appropriate tissues at the appropriate time and in a balanced manner relative to the expression of stress resistance genes in other tissues. Failure to achieve this balanced expression harms, rather than helps, the organism. This may come about because an unbalanced expression of one stress response gene may inappropriately down-regulate other stress response genes. This hypothesis assumes that there exists a stress response gene network of some sort, as has been noted in the nematode (Morley and Miramoto, 2004). Empirical evidence to support this assumption is provided by a DNA hybridization screen which identified at least 13 genes which were activated by exposure to heat, oxidants, and starvation (Wang *et al.*, 2004). The involvement of the HSP in extended longevity is shown by the fact that a beneficial effect of HSPs on aging and stress resistance is observed when organisms are preconditioned by exposure to a mild stress before being exposed to a subsequent damaging stress (hormesis: see LeBourg *et al.*, 2001; Hercus *et al.*, 2003).

Taken all together, the different types of experiments discussed above show that (1) there are a variety of different but interacting stress resistance pathways and (2) almost all tested long-lived animals are also stress-resistant. Both Parsons (2003) and Rattan (2004) have long argued the existence of a tight relationship between stress resistance and longevity. The reciprocal experiments in which one directly up-regulates a known stress response gene, such as *hsp26* or *hsp27*, have been done and results in flies having a significant increase in both stress resistance and longevity (Wang *et al.*, 2004). This experiment shows that at least some stress resistant animals are also long-lived. Taken together, the several sets of experiments verify the fundamentals of Parsons's (2003) argument.

GENETIC STABILITY

There are two aspects to genetic stability in *Drosophila*. One aspect has to do with the structural integrity of the DNA and the genome. The other has to do with the nonstructural epigenetic modification of the genome. We shall discuss them in sequence.

It was once hypothesized that aging might be the result of genomic instability and/or gene dysregulation, but recent data indicates instead that the genome is actually very stable during the adult period. For example, even though 86% of the genes assayed significantly changed their expression during the entire life cycle (i.e., embryo to young adult; Arbeitman *et al.*, 2002), only 9% of the genes in the *Drosophila* genome showed significant age-dependent changes in their levels of expression during adult aging. Furthermore, plotting the genomic distribution of this small set of changeable genes reveals no obvious clustering of the genes at particular chromosomal regions, such as telomeres or centromeres, once thought to be particularly unstable (Pletcher *et al.*, 2002). In addition, there is also no evidence for a genome-wide gene dysregulation. There is, however, extensive evidence supporting the idea that gene expression during adult aging is a precisely regulated process and probably represents a continuation or alteration of that experienced early in life. Independent studies using enhancer-trap techniques show that the expression of many genes changes in their own stereotypical patterns with age (Helfand and Rogina, 2000). If these aging changes were the result of some stochastic loss of function, then one would not expect such a random process to yield different but predictable signature patterns. A different enhancer-trap study found that the rate of change of expression in some cases was correlated with changes in longevity under various conditions (i.e., temperature), suggesting that the changes are indicators of physiological function and not of some stochastic loss of genome stability (Seroude *et al.*, 2002). Genes encoding functionally related proteins, such as cell-cycle proteins or metabolic enzymes, tend to be expressed at similar times during the life cycle, again suggesting a functional basis for the observed changes (Arbeitman *et al.*, 2002). Finally, a spatial analysis of individual gene patterns of expression throughout the entire adult body revealed that each gene had its own characteristic signature tissue localization; a finding not compatible with stochastic genomic instability (Seroude *et al.*, 2002). Each of these phenomena can be best understood as reflecting the operation of signal transduction mechanisms over the life course.

Of course, genetic stability is affected by the relative levels of mutation and repair processes. As was documented for the other model organisms, decreased DNA repair activity leads to widespread somatic mutations and a consequent loss of function. For example, Leffelaar and Grigliatti (1984) isolated several temperature-sensitive DNA repair mutants which acted so as to significantly decrease adult longevity relative to controls when raised under restrictive conditions. Another DNA repair protein (Rrp1) was shown, when over-expressed, to be capable of reducing the level of somatic mutations in animals exposed to oxidative stress (Szakmary *et al.*, 1996). The normal functioning of these and other repair genes likely plays an important role in maintaining genetic stability.

Woodruff and Nitikin have reinvestigated the somatic mutation theory of aging using the technique of P-element insertional mutagenesis (Nitikin and Woodruff, 1995; Woodruff and Nitikin, 1995). This technique has the advantage over radiation in that it allows the experimenter to induce defined and controllable numbers of random single mutations. They find convincing evidence that the induction of somatic genetic damage can reduce life span in *Drosophila* but that the effect is dependent on the particular species of fly involved and the type of transposable element used. The literature suggests that even in the heterozygous condition, recessive mutations can reduce life span by ~1–2%, and synergistic interactions between different deleterious mutations have the potential to further increase this effect to a statistically significant level. This possibility was tested by Woodruff and Thompson (2003), and their data indicate that the accumulation of undetected somatic mutations could, under special circumstances, reduce longevity by as much as ~22% over a period of 16 generations in a *Drosophila* system. These data suggest that a direct relationship between increased somatic genetic damage and the age of onset of senescence does actually exist.

Taken all together, the data suggest that the genome is remarkably stable during the aging process, that most of the genes do not show significant alterations in gene expression during this process, and that the observed changes in gene expression represent the dynamic regulation of specific genes in response to the changing physiological status of the organism. Note that none of the foregoing implies that these regulated gene expression patterns constitute an aging program.

If the genome of an organism is so stable, then how can environmental influences affect its operation? Epigenetic regulation of gene expression occurs when somatic cells use either DNA methylation to modify the genetic material itself, or histone acetylation/methylation to modify those proteins that intimately interact with the genetic material (Jaenisch and Bird, 2003; Czermin and Imhof, 2003). These epigenetic modifications arise in an orderly fashion during development, or stochastically during aging, or as the result of long-term external influences such as diet. This phenomenon was first detected in *Drosophila* in 1930 as the occurrence of variable phenotypes in neighboring somatic cells of an individual fly. Neighboring cells in the same tissue had different patterns of gene expression, suggesting a particular instability of their genomes. A gene later shown to be important in that process, *Su(var)3-9*, is now known to be a histone methyltransferase and has conserved orthologs in yeast and humans (Schotta *et al.*, 2003). The importance of these phenomena for the topic of aging is that the repression of various stress-resistant genes in normal-lived *Drosophila* is brought about in part by the epigenetic effects of histone deacetylation in those nucleosomes about which the chromatin is coiled. The absence of acetyl groups on the histone causes a tight winding of the chromatin about the nucleosome, making it difficult for various transcription factors to gain access to the gene promoters. Acetylation of the histone causes a loosening or partial unwinding of the chromation about the nucleosome, allowing the genes to be activated by the various factors. It turns out that a drug approved by the FDA for use with various diseases, 4-phenylbutyrate (4PB), inhibits the action of histone deacetylases and thereby induces hyperacetylation of the histones. Kang *et al.* (2002) fed this drug to normal-lived *Drosophila* and found that the optimal concentrations yielded a Type 1 phenotype, increasing the mean and maximum survival in both sexes by ~30 to 52% , depending on the sex and genetic background. The drug had no effect on the fly's fecundity or body weight. Furthermore, the treated flies are resistant to starvation, oxidative stress, and loss of locomotor ability. All of these observations are consistent with a heightened stress resistance. Assays of gene expression showed that a number of stress-resistant genes (including CuZnSOD) were induced by the drug, and that their induction was accompanied by altered levels of histone acetylation. These findings are intriguing for several reasons. First, they show that manipulation of the epigenetic code to specifically affect genetic stability is sufficient to significantly alter gene expression. Second, they demonstrate that pharmaceutical intervention is capable of significantly altering longevity. Third, they show that treatment of middle-aged adults yields significant delays in the onset of senescence.

REPRODUCTIVE EFFECTS

The antagonistic interaction between the soma and germ line cells first observed in the nematode also is found in the fly. In fact, there is much more information available in *Drosophila* on the several hormones involved and their various inhibitory and stimulatory effects on longevity (Tatar *et al.*, 2002, 2003; Hwangbo *et al.*, 2004)).

Cells of the CNS, the par intercerebralis, secrete insulin-like peptides (ILPs), which are directed to certain target cells as well as being released systemically. These insulin-like peptides (particularly dILP2) directly or indirectly stimulate certain neuroendocrine cells such as the corpora allata to produce one of the two key hormones in the insect, juvenile hormone (JH). dILP2 acts so as to activate the ISP and thus inactivate dFOXO and the stress resistance/somatic maintenance pathways. The ISP likely operates in the cells of the CNS as well as in the peripheral tissues. In the fly, the fat body cells in the head play a particularly important role, since these cells appear to regulate dFOXO, and thus control the aging of the organism, when activated (Hwangbo *et al.*, 2004). The ISP operating in the gonad–somatic cell axis can activate or inhibit the synthesis of juvenile hormone (JH). Thus the longevity-extending effects of mutants affecting the ISP presumably arise out of interference with the operation of the ISP portion of the process. Longevity arises from the interaction of control centers in the gonads, central nervous system, and head fat body cells with the various peripheral somatic tissues.

JH is essential for reproduction. It is known to promote vitellogenesis and reproduction in insects, and to inhibit adult diapause (a nonreproductive long-lived somatic state characteristic of, for example, overwintering adults). In the gonad, JH stimulates egg development and also stimulates the synthesis of the active form of the second key insect hormone involved in our story, 20-hydroxy-ecdysone (20HE). This steroid hormone is well known for its effects on development, and the molecular details of its action within the cell have been worked out—particularly the fact that the 20HE must bind with a bipartite receptor protein in the nucleus if it is to specifically activate its target genes (Riddiford *et al.*, 2000; Tatar, 2003). What is particularly interesting in the current context is that the known inhibitory effect of JH on the stress resistance of the adult may well be mediated through 20HE. The relationships of these two hormones are quite complex, and the interested reader should refer to Pu *et al.* (2005) for details.

Simon *et al.* (2003) have shown that animals bearing heterozygous mutations in the ecdysone receptor (EcR) protein, one component of the nuclear receptor protein complex, exhibit increased longevity relative to control animals. This locus is the probable site of a QTL known to be involved in longevity (Curtsinger *et al.*, 1998). The animals have a higher metabolic rate coupled with a lower rate of spontaneous activity. More interestingly, they are also significantly more resistant to oxidative stress, heat, and starvation than are normal animals. This implies that the increased life span and the increased stress resistance both are the result of a decrease in the effective concentration of the 20HE in the cells. Interestingly enough, female age-specific fecundity was increased in these heterozygous mutants relative to normal animals, suggesting that moderate levels of 20HE are compatible with both an extended longevity and an enhanced fecundity. A comparable increase (~42%) in life span was obtained in a separate experiment by use of a temperature-sensitive mutant (*DTS-3*) that affects ecdysone synthesis in females. Because this gene product is inactivated at high temperatures, then one can effectively turn it on or off simply by transferring the fly from a permissive temperature (20°C) to a restrictive temperature (29°C). Doing such shifts at different times indicates that the greatest effect of the decreased hormone levels on longevity takes place within the first two or three weeks of adult life. Finally, feeding 20HE to these mutant female flies abolished that extended longevity in a dose-sensitive manner and also reversed their resistance to the stress of starvation. As little as 10^{-3} M 20HE added to the food allowed the females to have a normal life span.

Absence of ecdysone is lethal. But these three experiments taken together clearly show that high levels of 20HE have a negative effect on longevity and on stress resistance. Thus the JH stimulation of the gonads to synthesize and secrete the high levels of 20HE leads to a shorter (i.e., normal) life span. This decreased life span may well arise from the concomitant repression of stress resistance observed in these experiments. Using mutants to reduce the level of 20HE to a moderate (~50%) level brings about an extended longevity and an enhanced fecundity, as do experiments in which the effective level of the receptor protein is manipulated. Note that the Type 1 phenotype obtained with either manipulation yields a ~45% increase in mean life span in both sexes and is about equal to the increase in life span obtained with selection, caloric restriction, or ISP mutants.

There is another aspect to the topic of reproductive effects on longevity. Reproduction requires the female fly to expend a considerable amount of energy. Individuals in which the energy demands of the reproductive system are not synchronized with the energy production ability of the somatic cells are likely to die when the demands exceed the supply. A formal analysis of the interplay between the age-related energy demand and supply led to a hypothesis about a mechanism which predicts two critical periods in the life history of an individual fly (Novoseltsev *et al.*, 2003). The first crisis occurs at early ages when the increased energy demand becomes greater than the available energy supply. This would often result in a "premature" or nonsenescent death and would presumably involve females in which their intrinsic rate of egg production is greater than can be supported by their intrinsic mitochondrial energy production. In other words, the weaker flies would preferentially die at this first stressful period in their lives. The stronger and surviving flies lay eggs at some more or less constant rate while their available energy supply is gradually decreased by various senescent processes. Eventually, they do not produce enough energy to simultaneously maintain their reproductive activities and to resist the various environmental stresses associated with living. The initially strong flies perferentially die late in life from a senescent-caused death precipitated by their inability to meet the cumulative energy demands placed upon them.

The reader will observe that these two mechanisms of reproductive effects on longevity—the hormonal mechanisms and the energy demands—are not contradictory but are really the same process as described on the one hand from the cell and tissue level of the geneticist, and on the other hand from the organismic level of life history theory.

Patterns of Senescence

Do all tissues of the fly age together and at the same rate? Our early work suggested that both normal- and long-lived animals undergo the same sort of senescent process, losing different traits in the same sequence and at the same stage (Arking and Wells, 1992). Since the animals do not lose all functions at the same time, it also implies that different tissues age at different rates. Is there any data to support this implication? The fact that there is a defined spatio–temporal pattern of gene expression during the aging process (Seyroude *et al.*, 2002), coupled with the fact that at least 9% of the genes are known to undergo transcriptional changes during aging (Pletcher *et al.*, 2002), suggests that it is unlikely that all tissues of the fly age together and at the same rate. Some data to support this supposition were presented by Cook-Wiens and Grotewiel (2002). They showed that different behaviors of the fly, utilizing different sensory systems, age at different rates. For example, locomotor and olfactory performance decreases with age even while the aging animal maintains its ability to respond to electric shock and light. Different sensory–motor behaviors decline at different rates within the same animal. What is most interesting is the fact that these olfactory and locomotor declines occurred at the same rate and at the same times in normal-lived control animals as they did in long-lived stress-resistant (*mth*) mutants. Thus genetic manipulations that enhance resistance to oxidative stress and extend life span do not necessarily protect against functional senescence in all pathways. We not only age in an individual manner, but each individual ages in a heterogeneous manner.

How Do Different Pathways Yield a Common Type I Phenotype?

Figure 25.3 summarizes the known activation and/or inhibition signals generated by each of the several longevity-extending mechanisms known to be operative in flies, which we have discussed above. The schematic is somewhat speculative in detail, but its tying together of the several known methods of inducing stress resistance with the expression of extended longevity as described in the foregoing text is most likely correct in concept. The important point to note is that all the interventions listed are known to induce the Type 1 longevity phenotype (i.e., delayed onset of senescence) (see Figure 25.1A). The ISS pathway, certainly, and the JNK pathway, probably, are involved in producing this phenotype. The details of the CR pathway are still being worked out. Even given our incomplete knowledge, it seems as if all inducers of the Type 1 phenotype work by effecting some common regulatory nexus, probably the dFOXO3 transcription factor that is known to activate or repress various stress resistance genes.

The interesting thing about the Type 1 phenotype is that delaying the onset of senescence means that the inflection point characteristic of such survival and mortality curves is shifted to some later time (see Figures 25.1A, 25.2A). What happens at that inflection point, regardless of its chronological value, that shifts the population from a state of health into a state of senescence? Senescence is the stochastic and nonprogrammed loss of function which becomes obvious as the reproductive period ends. This is a time-independent process, occurring at about two years in a mouse but at about fifty-five years in a human. What triggers its onset? In the fly, it has been shown that the repression of the ISP results in the activation of the dFOXO gene, and in the activation or repression of a whole suite of downstream genes under its singular or joint control (Murphy *et al.*, 2003). These downstream genes include a variety of stress resistance genes, including a number of molecular chaperones (hsp genes). Mutational inactivation of these downstream hsp genes reverses the extended longevity brought about by ISP repression. This leads to the emerging view that the beneficial effects of the ISP are mediated in part via these downstream hsps, which protect the cells in various ways against the accumulation of unrepaired damage to the cell's proteome (Marsh and Thompson, 2004) as well as the deleterious effects of ROS on the mitochondria and other cell structures. Up-regulation of the ISP, possibly via the increased production of the ILPs or growth factors such as IGF-1 under the control of the fly's glucoregulatory system, represses the expression of these downstream hsps and presumably of various antioxidant defense genes as well. This results in the down-regulation of damage control systems, the accumulation of unrepaired damage, and the gradual onset of senescence as various critical thresholds within the cell are exceeded. The individual nature of aging may be explained by individual and environmental variations in gene product levels, damage rates, repair levels, and so forth; all of which may be the outcome of various gene epistatic effects. A more extensive description of this model may be found in Chapter 9 of Arking (2005a).

REFERENCES

Arbeitman, M.N., E.E.M. Furlong, F. Imam, E. Johnson, B.H. Hull, B.S. Baker, *et al.* 2002. Gene expression during the life cyle of *Drosophila melanogaster*. *Science 297*:2270 2275.

Arking, R., J. Novoseltsev, D.-S. Hwangbo, V. Novoseltsev and M. Lane. 2002. Different age-specific demographic profiles are generated in the same normal-lived *Drosophila* strain by different longevity stimuli. *J. Gerontol.: Biol. Sci. 57A*:B390–B3999.

Arking, R., Buck, S. Berrios, A., Dwyer, S., and Baker, G.T., III. (1991). Elevated paraquat activity can be used as a biomarker for longevity in a selected strain of *Drosophila. Devel. Genetics 12*:362–370.

Arking, R.S. Buck, V.N. Novoseltsev, D.-S. Hwangbo, and M. Lane. 2002. Genomic plasticity, energy allocations, and the extended longevity phenotypes of *Drosophila. Aging Research Reviews 1*:209–228.

Arking R., V. Burde, K. Graves, R. Hari, E. Feldman, A. Zeevi, *et al.* 2000. Forward and reverse selection for longevity in *Drosophila* is characterized by alteration of antioxidant gene expression and oxidative damage patterns. *Exp Gerontol. 35*:167–85.

Arking, R., S. Buck, V.N. Novoseltsev, S.-D. Hwangbo, and M. Lane. 2002b. Genomic plasticity, energy allocations, and the extended longevity phenotypes of *Drosophila. Aging Research Reviews 1*:209–228.

Arking, R. 2005a. *Biology of Aging: Observations and Principles*, 3rd ed. Oxford Univ. Press. In press.

Arking, R. 2005b. *A Mechanistic View of the Transition from the Health Span to the Senescent Span*. Annals NY Acad Science: in press.

Bhole, D., M.J. Akkikian, and J. Tower. 2004. Doxcycline-regulated over-expression of hsp22 has negative effects on stress resistance and life span in adult *Drosophila melanogaster*. Mech. *Ageing Develop. 125*:651–663.

Carey J.R., Liedo, P., Harshman, L., Zhang, Y., Muller, H.G., Partridge, L., and Wang, J.L. 2002. Life history response of Mediterranean fruit flies to dietary restriction. *Aging Cell 1*:140–148.

Carey, J.R., P. Liedo, H.-G. Muller, J.-L. Wang, Y. Zhang, and L. Harshmann. 2005. Stochastic dietary restriction using a Markov-chain feeding protocol elicits complex, life history response in medflies. *Aging Cell 4*:31–40.

Chapman, T., and L. Partridge. 1996. Female fitness in *Drosophila melanogaster*: An interaction between the effect of nutrition and of encounter rate with males. *Proc. R. Soc. London, Series B 263*:755–759.

Clancy, D.J., D. Gems, E. Hafen, S.J. Leevers, and L. Partridge. 2002. Dietary restriction in long-lived dwarf flies. *Science 296*:319.

Clancy, D.J., D. Gems, L.G. Harshman, S. Oldham, H. Stocker, E. Hafen, S.J. Leevers, and L. Partridge. 2001. Extension of life-span by loss of CHICO, a *Drosophila* insulin receptor substrate protein. *Science 292*:104–107.

Cook-Wiens, E., and M.S. Grotewiel. 2002. Dissociation between functional senescence and oxidative stress resistance in *Drosophila. Exp Gerontol. 37*:1347–1357.

Curtsinger, J.W., and A.A. Khazaeli. 2002. Lifespan, QTLs, age-specificity, and pleiotropy in *Drosophila. Mech Ageing Dev. 123*:81–93.

Curtsinger, J.W., H.H. Fukui, A.S. Resler, K. Kelly and A.A. Khazaeli. 1998. Genetic analysis of extended life span in *Drosophila melanogaster*. I. RAPD screen for genetic divergence between selected and control lines. *Genetica 104*:21–32.

Czermin, B., and A. Imhof. 2003. The sounds of silence—Histone deacetylation meets histone methylation. *Genetica 117*: 159–164.

Driver, C., and N. Tawadros. 2000. Cytoplasmic genomes that confer additional longevity in *Drosophila melanogaster*. *Biogerontology 1*:255–260.

Dudas, S.P., and Arking, R. (1995) A coordinate up-regulation of antioxidant gene activities is required prior to the delayed onset of senescence characteristic of a long-lived strain of *Drosophila. J. Gerontology: Biological Sciences 50A*: B117–B127.

Force, A., Staples, T., Sherif, S., and Arking, R. (1995). Comparative biochemical and stress analysis of genetically selected *Drosophila* strains with different longevities. *Devel. Genetics 17*:340–351.

Giradot, F., V. Monnier, and H. Tricoire. 2004. Genome wide analysis of common and specific stress responses in adult *Drosophila melanogaster. BMC Genomics 2004, 5*:74 doi:10.1186/1471-2164-5-74.

Hari, R., V. Burde, and R. Arking. 1998. Immunological confirmation of elevated levels of CuZn superoxide dismutase protein in an artificially selected long-lived strain of *Drosophila melanogaster. Exp. Gerontol. 33*:227–238.

Harshman, L.G., K.M. Moore, M.A. Sty, and M.M. Magwire. 1999. Stress resistance and longevity in selected lines of *Drosophila melanogaster. Neurobiol Aging. 1999 Sep–Oct; 20(5)*:521–529.

Helfand, S.L., and B. Rogina. 2000. Regulation of gene expression during aging. *Results Probl. Cell Differ. 29*:67–80.

Helfand, S.L., and B. Rogina. 2003. Molecular genetics of aging in the fly: Is this the end of the beginning? *BioEssays 25*:134–141.

Hercus, M.J., V. Loeschcke, and S.I.S. Rattan. 2003. Lifespan extension of *Drosophila melanogaster* through hormesis by repeated mild heat stress. *Biogerontology 4*:149–156.

Hwangbo, D.-S., B. Gersham, M.-P. Tu, M. Palmer, and M. Tatar. 2004. *Drosophila* dFOXO controls lifespan and regulates insulin signalling in brain and fat body. Nature. Published online as [doi:10.1038/nature02549]www.nature.com/nature

Jaenisch, R., and A. Bird. 2003. Epigenetic regulation of gene expression: How the genome integrates intri signals. *Nature Genetics 33 (supplement)*:245–254. nsic and environmental.

James, A.C., and J.W.O. Ballard. 2003. Mitochondrial genotype affects fitness in *Drosophila* simulans. *Genetics 164*:173–186.

Johnson, T.E., G.I. Lithgow, and S. Murakami. 1996. Hypothesis: Interventions that increase the response to stress offer the potential for effective life prolongation and increased health. *J Gerontol A Biol Sci Med Sci. 51*:B392–B395.

Kang, H.-L., S. Benzer, and K.-T. Min. 2002. Life extension in *Drosophila* by feeding a drug. *PNAS 99*:838–843.

Kapahl, P., B.M. Zid, T. Harper, D. Koslover, V. Sapin, and S. Benzer. 2004. Regulation of lifespan in *Drosophila* by modulation of genes in the TOR signaling pathway. *Curr. Biol. 14*:885–890.

King, V., and J. Tower. 1999. Aging-specific expression of *Drosophila* hsp22. *Dev Biol. 207*:107–18.

Kirby, K., J. Hu, A.J. Hilliker, and J.P. Phillips. 2002. RNA interference-mediated silencing of Sod2 in *Drosophila* leads to early adult-onset mortality and elevated endogenous oxidative stress. *PNAS 99*:16162–16167.

Klichko, V.I., S.V. Radyuk, and W.C. Orr. 1999. CuZnSOD promoter-driven expression in the *Drosophila* central nervous system. *Neurobiol. of Aging 20*:557–543.

Klionsky, D.J. 2004. Regulated self-cannibalism. *Nature 431*: 31–32. (News & views.)

Knauf, F., B. Rogina, Z. Jiang, P.S. Aronson, and S.L. Helfand. 2002. Functional characterization and immunolocalization of the transporter encoded by the life extending gene Indy. *PNAS 99*:14312–14319.

Kramer, J.M., Davidge, J.T., Lockyer, J.M., and Staveley, B.E. 2003. Expression of *Drosophila* FOXO regulates growth and can phenocopy starvation. *BMC Dev Biol. 3*:5.

Kurapati, R., Passananti, H.B., Rose, M.R., and Tower, J. 2000. Increased hsp22 RNA levels in *Drosophila* lines genetically selected for increased longevity. *J Gerontol A Biol Sci Med Sci. 55*:B552–B559.

Landis, G.N., A.D. Skvortsov, J. Yang, B.E. Rabin, J. Carrick, S. Tavare, and J. Tower. 2004. Similar gene expression patterns characterize aging and oxidative stress in *Drosophila melanogaster. PNAS U S A. 101*:7663–7668.

Le Bourg, E., Valenti, P., Lucchetta, P., and Payre, F. (2001) Effects of mild heat shocks at young age on aging and longevity in *Drosophila melanogaster. Biogerontology 2*, 155–164.

Leffelaar, D., and T.A. Grigliatti. 1984. A mutation in *Drosophila* that appears to accelerate aging. *Devel. Genet. 4*: 199–210.

Leiers, B., A. Kampkotter, C.G. Grevelding, C.D. Link, T.E. Johnson, and K. Henkle-Duhrsen. 2003 A stress responsive glutathione-S-transferase confers resistance to oxidative stress in *Caenorhabiditis elegans. Free Rad. Biol. Med. 34*:1405–1415.

Lin, Y.-J, L. Seroude, and S. Benzer. 1998. Extended life-span and stress resistance in the *Drosophila* mutant methuselah. *Science 282*:943–946.

Mackay, W.J., and G.C. Bewley. 1989. The genetics of catalase in *Drosophila melanogaster*: Isolation and characterization of acatalesemic mutants. *Genetics 122*: 643–652.

Mair, W., P. Gomeyer, S.D. Pletcher, and L. Partridge. 2003. Demography of dietary restriction and death in *Drosophila. Science 301*:1731–1733.

Marsh, J.L., and L.M. Thompson. 2004. Can flies help humans treat neurodegenerative diseases? *BioEssays 26*:485–496.

Melvin, R.G., J.T. Miller, D.R. Spitz, and J.W.O. Ballard. 2005. Interspecific variation in mitochondrial oxidative phosphorylation, oxygen consumption, and survival in *Drosophila* simulans. Submitted.

Missirlis, F., J.P. Phillips, and H. Jackle. 2001. Cooperative action of antioxidant defense systems in *Drosophila. Current Biology 11*:1272–1277.

Mockett, R.J., W.C. Orr, J.J. Rahmandar, J.J. Benes, S.V. Radyuk, V.I. Klichko, and R.S. Sohal. 1999. Overexpression of Mn-containing superoxide dismutase in transgenic *Drosophila melanogaster*. *Arch. Biochem. Biophys. 371*:260–269.

Morley, J.E., and R.I. Morimoto. 2004. Regulation of longevity in *Caenorhabditis elegans* by heat shock factor and molecular chaperones. *Mol. Biol. Cell 15*:657–664.

Morrow G., Samson, M., Michaud, S., and Tanguay, R.M. 2004a. Overexpression of the small mitochondrial Hsp22 extends *Drosophila* life span and increases resistance to oxidative stress. *FASEB J. Mar;18(3)*:598–599.

Morrow, G., S. Battistini, P. Zhang, and R.M. Tanguay. 2004b. Decreased lifespan in the absence of expression of the mitochondrial small heat shock protein hsp22 in *Drosophila*. *J. Biol. Chem. 279*:43382–43385.

Murphy, C.T., McCarroll, S.A., Bargmann, C.I., Fraser, A., Kamath, R.S., Ahringer, J., Li, H., and Kenyon, C. 2003. Genes that act downstream of DAF-16 to influence the lifespan of *Caenorhabditis elegans*. *Nature 424*:277–283.

Niedzwiecki, A., and J.E. Fleming. 1990. Changes in protein turnover after heat shock are related to accumulation of abnormal proteins in aging *Drosophila melanogaster*. *Mech Ageing Dev. 52*:295–304.

Novoseltsev, V.N., J.A. Novoseltseva, and A.I. Yashin. 2003. What does a fly's individual fecundity pattern look like? The dynamics of resource allocation in reproduction and ageing. *Mech. Ageing Develop. 124*:605–617.

Orr, W.C., and R.S. Sohal. 2003. Does overexpression of CuZnSOD extend life span in *Drosophila melanogaster*? *Exp. Gerontol. 38*:227–230.

Orr, W.C., and R.S. Sohal, 1994. Extension of life-span by overexpression of superoxide dismutase and catalase in *Drosophila melanogaster*. *Science 263*:1128–1130.

Orr, W.C., and R.C. Sohal. 1992. The effects of catalase gene overexpression on life span and resistance to oxidative stress in transgenic *Drosophila melanogaster*. *Arch. Biochem. Biophys. 297*:35–41.

Parkes, T.L., A.J. Hilliker, and J.P. Phillips. 1999. Motorneur ons, reactive oxygen and life span in *Drosophila*. *Neurobiol. of Aging 20*:531–535.

Parkes, T.L., A.J. Elia, D. Dickinson, A.J. Hilliker, J.P. Phillips, and G.L. Boulianne. 1998. Extension of *Drosophila* lifespan by overexpression of human SOD1 in motorneurons. *Nature Genetics 19*:171–174.

Parsons, P.A. 1995. Inherited stress resistance and longevity: A stress theory of aging. *Heredity 75*:216–221.

Parsons, P.A. 2003. From the stress theory of aging to energetic and evolutionary expectations for longevity. *Biogerontology. 4(2)*:63–73.

Parsons, P.A. 1997. Success in mating: A coordinated approach to fitness through genotypes incorporating genes for stress resistance and heterozygous advantage under stress. *Behav. Genet. 27*:75–81.

Phillips, J.P., T.L. Parkes, and A.J. Hilliker. 2000. Targeted neuronal gene expression and longevity in *Drosophila*. *Exp. Gerontol. 35*:1157–1164.

Pletcher, S.D., S.J. Macdonald, R. Marguerie, U. Certa, S.C. Stearns, D.B. Goldstein, and L Partridge. 2002. Genome-wide transcript profiles in aging and calorically restricted *Drosophila melanogaster*. *Current Biology 12*:712–723.

Pu, M.-P., T. Flatt, and M. Tatar. 2005. Juvenile and steroid hormones in *Drosophila melanogaster* longevity. In E.J. Masoro and S.N. Austad (eds.), *Handbook of the Biology of Aging*, 6th ed., Chap. 16. In press.

Rattan, S.I. 2004. Aging intervention, prevention, and therapy through hormesis. *J Gerontol:Biol Sci. 59*:705–709.

Riddiford, L.M., P. Cherbas, and J.W. Truman. 2000. Ecdysone receptors and their biological actions. *Vitamins and Hormones 60*:1–73.

Rogina, B., R.A. Reenan, S.P. Nilsen, and S.L. Helfand. 2000. Extended life span conferred by cotransporter gene mutations in *Drosophila*. *Science 290*:2137–2140.

Rogina, B., S.L. Helfand, and S. Frankel. 2002. Longevity regulation by *Drosophila* Rpd3 deacetylase and caloric restriction. *Science 298*:1745–1747.

Rose, M.R., L.N. Vu, S.U. Park, and J.L. Graves, Jr. 1992. Selection on stress resistance increases longevity in *Drosophila* melanogaster. *Exp. Gerontol. 27*: 241–250.

Rose, M.R. 1984. Laboratory evolution of postponed senescence in *Drosophila melanogaster*. *Evolution 38*: 1004–1010.

Ross, R.E. 2000. Age specific decreases in aerobic efficiency associated with increase in oxygen free radical production in *Drosophila melanogaster*. *J. Insect Physiol. 46*:1477–1480.

Rulifson, E.J., S.K. Kim, and R. Nusse. 2002. Ablation of insulin-producing neurons in flies: growth and diabetic phenotypes. *Science 296*:1118–1120.

Samuels, Y., Wang, Z., Bardelli, A., Silliman, N., Ptak, J., Szabo S., *et al.* 2004. High frequency of mutations of the PIK3CA gene in human cancers. *Science 304*:554.

Schotta, G., A. Ebert, and G. Reuter. 2003. SU(VAR)3-9 is a conserved key function in heterochromatic gene silencing. *Genetics 117*:149–158.

Seroude, L., T. Brummel, P. Kapahi, and S. Benzer. 2002. Spatiotemporal analysis of gene expression during aging in *Drosophila*. *Aging Cell 1*:47–56.

Simon, A.F., C. Shih, A. Mack, and S. Benzer. 2003. Steroid control of longevity in *Drosophila melanogaster*. *Science 299*:1407–1410.

Sohal, R.S., A. Agarwal, and W.C. Orr. 1995. Simultaneous overexpression of copper- and zinc-containing superoxide dismutase and catalase retards age-related oxidative damage and increases metabolic potential in *Drosophila melanogaster*. *J Biol Chem. 270*:15671–15674.

Sun, J., and J. Tower. 1999. FLP recombinase-mediated induction of CuZn-superoxide dismutase transgene expression can extend the life span of adult *Drosophila melanogaster* flies. *Mol. Cell. Biol. 19*:216–228.

Sun, J., D. Folk, T.J. Bradley, and J. Tower. 2002. Induced over-expression of the mitochondrial Mn-superoxide dismutase extends the life span of adult *Drosophila melanogaster*. *Genetics 161*:661–672.

Szakmary, A., S.-M. Huang, D.T. Chang, P.A. Beachy, and M. Sander. 1996. Overexpression of a Rrp1 transgene reduces the somatic mutation and recombination frequency induced by oxidative DNA damage in *Drosophila melanogaster*. *Proc. Natl. Acad. Sci. USA 93*:1607–1612.

Tatar, M., A. Bartke, and A. Antebi. 2003. The endocrine regulation of aging by insulin-like signals. *Science 299*:1346–1351.

Tatar, M., A. Bartke, and A. Antebi. 2003. The endocrine regulation of aging by insulin-like signals. *Science 299*:1346–1351.

Tatar, M., A. Kopelman, D. Epstein, M.P. Tu, C.M. Yin, and R.S. Garofalo. 2001. A mutant *Drosophila* insulin receptor homolog that extends life-span and impairs neuroendocrine function. *Science 292*:107–110.

Tu, M.-P., C.-M. Yeng, and M. Tatar. 2002. Impaired ovarian ecdysone synthesis of *Drosophila melanogaster* insulin receptor mutants. *Aging Cell 1*:158–160.

Wang, H.D., P. Kazemi-Esfarjani, and S. Benzer. 2004. Multiple stress analysis for isolation of *Drosophila* longevity genes. *PNAS 101*:12610–12615.

Wang, M.C., D. Bohmann, and H. Jasper. 2003. JNK signaling confers tolerance to oxidative stress and extends lifespan in *Drosophila. Develop. Cell 5*:811–816.

Weinkove, D., and S.J. Leevers. 2000. The genetic control of organ growth: Insights from *Drosophila. Curr. Opin. Genet. Develop 10*:75–80.

Wheeler, J.C., Bieschke, E.T., and Tower, J. 1995. Muscle-specific expression of *Drosophila* hsp70 in response to aging and oxidative stress. *Proc. Natl. Acad. Sci. USA 92*:10408–10412.

Wiens, E., and M.S. Grotewiel, 2002. Dissociation between functional senescence and oxidative stress resistance in *Drosophila. Exp. Gerontology 37*:1347–1357.

Wood, J.G., B. Rogina, S. Lavu, K. Howitz, S.G. Helfand, M. Tatar, and D. Sinclair. 2004. Sirtuin activators mimic caloric restriction and delay ageing in metazoans. www.nature.com/nature/doc.10.1038/nature02789.

Woodruff, R.C., and J.N. Thompson, Jr. 2003. The role of somatic and germline mutations in aging and a mutation interaction model of aging. *J. Anti. Aging. Med. 6*:29–39.

Woodruff, R.C., and A.G. Nikitin. 1995. P DNA element movement in somatic cells reduces lifespan in *Drosophila melanogaster*: Evidence in support of the somatic mutation theory of aging. *Mutation Res. 338*: 35–42.

26

Annual Fish as a Genetic Model for Aging

Pudur Jagadeeswaran

Nothobranchius fish have a lifespan of approximately one year whereas zebrafish live up to 4–5 years. This finding suggested that if classical genetic approaches could be adapted to Nothobranchius, these annual fish would become an ideal vertebrate genetic model for studying longevity genes. In this chapter, we provide arguments and approaches for utilizing Nothobranchius to study the genetics of aging. Because Nothobranchius has a relatively short lifespan, has multiple strains, is a diploid organism, has high fecundity and most importantly is able to lay eggs until the end of their lives, this fish is an excellent animal model for studying genetics of vertebrate longevity. Various approaches to isolate long-lived mutants are described along with their utility for discovering antiaging drugs.

Introduction

Aging is a universal process conserved in evolution, which cripples the organism at the end stages of life, ultimately resulting in death (Hamet and Tremblay, 2003). Since the dawn of time, man wanted to be eternal and always wished to conquer aging and death. While ecologically conquering aging may not be compatible for normal evolution, improving the quality of life and extending the lifespan remain the major goals of aging research. For example, in classical studies on dietary restriction, it has been shown that a caloric restriction extends the lifespan (Masoro, 2005). In addition, reduction of oxidative stress by antioxidants has been shown to extend the lifespan in several organisms (Droge, 2003). Since all biological pathways are controlled by genes and their products, one would anticipate that there will be genes whose function, if they are modulated, may result in the extension of lifespan, including those involved in the processes mentioned above such as dietary restriction and oxidative stress (Johnson and Wood, 1982). In fact, recently such information on genes conferring longevity has been gathered using different model organisms and using both classical genetic methods as well as surrogate genetic approaches (Kenyon, 2005). In model organisms such as *Drosophila* and *C. elegans*, long-lived mutants have been selected by genetic approaches (Helfand and Rogina, 2003; Luo, 2004). In mice, the extension of the lifespan has been noted by modulating the gene dosage, utilizing transgenic methods and by using knockout methods (Liang *et al.*, 2003). In these two approaches, the identification of mutant phenotypes by classical genetic methods is a powerful genetic approach that allows the identification of genes in an "unbiased" manner in a given pathway, as opposed to the gene-by-gene approach employed by knockout studies as well as by transgenic methods. Furthermore, even if one has to overexpress genes or knock out the genes to identify the players involved in aging, large-scale mutagenesis methods by retroviral insertion and expression methods would be suitable in a global search for genes conferring longevity. At present, neither classical genetic approaches nor large-scale insertion mutagenesis methods and overexpression studies have been applied to study aging in vertebrates, largely because of the difficulties of applying these approaches in the classical vertebrate model organism, the mouse.

Recently, fish have become genetic models for studying vertebrate development and disease (Kimmel, 1989; Patton and Zon, 2001). We and others have conceived the utility of fish as a model organism for studying genetics of aging (Gerhard *et al.*, 2002, Herrera and Jagadeeswaran, 2002). In this chapter, arguments are put forth that fish are excellent genetic models for studying aging, and opinions are provided for why annual fish are better models for studying the genetics of aging as compared to other species of fish (Herrera and Jagadeeswaran, 2004). Furthermore, the applications of annual fish to study aging and the detailed approaches and their advantages are described.

Aging Genetic Models

The gene mutations extending the lifespan are more important in understanding molecular basis for aging than the mutations in genes resulting in shorter lifespans. This is because studies on shorter lifespans are debatable due to the fact that the observed effect could be due to pathological consequences of the mutations rather than a result of true aging. Over the past decade, information on the longevity genes has accumulated and now we have an impressive list of longevity genes provided by SAGE KE from yeast through mice. In *C. elegans*, *daf* and *age-1* genes control the dauer state, an alternative larval state where these larvae are able to thrive despite the fact that food is scarcely available (Dorman *et al.*, 1995; Kimura *et al.*, 1997; Van Voorhies and Ward, 1999). These larvae could live up to two months in contrast to well-fed worms which live for about three weeks. Daf-2 is homologous to the insulin receptor. In this organism, an insulin-like hormone initiates a signaling cascade via daf-2 which ultimately activates AKT kinases to phosphorylate the forkhead transcription factor Daf-16 so that it is retained in the cytoplasm to favor the reproductive growth of the organism (Paradis and Ruvkun, 1998). When daf-2 is mutated, the forkhead transcription factor translocates to the nucleus and induces a group of stress resistance genes required for the dauer state, including super oxide dismutase gene. However, such a pathway may not be significant for vertebrates, because a mutation in an insulin receptor would develop insulin resistance and even diabetes—not a longer lifespan.

One of the best studies with known experimental evidence for extending life is dietary restriction, which extends life in every organism tested (Hursting *et al.*, 2003). Studies to understand the basis of dietary restriction resulted in identification of altered expression of several genes using microarray analysis (Weindruch *et al.*, 2001). However, deciphering the details of the molecular basis for extending the lifespan through restricting the diet is difficult and requires other approaches such as the use of genetics. Recently, Guarente and his colleagues have identified the sir-2 locus coding for NAD-dependent histone acetylase, which silences large regions of DNA and slows down aging in yeast (Guarente and Picard, 2005). Interestingly, caloric restriction, which produces more NAD, also slows down aging in other organisms, including humans. When an extra copy of the sir-2 homologue is placed in *C. elegans* and a similar homologue was placed in yeast, these organisms lived substantially longer (Tissenbaum and Guarente, 2001). Presently, this pathway seems to be common to organisms tested and also fits with dietary restriction, but it still remains to be tested in higher organisms.

In *Drosophila*, mutations like *methuselah*, and overexpression of Cu/Zn super oxide dismutase, can extend the maximum lifespan (Lin *et al.*, 1998; Parkes *et al.*, 1998). In mice, SHC gene product has been shown to respond to reactive oxygen species, and a mutation in this gene has been shown to increase the lifespan (Migliaccio *et al.*, 1999). Several such examples support the theory of oxidative damage and appear to display a common theme, although exceptions exist.

Comparison of gene expression between phylogenetically related organisms with different lifespans may reveal the critical differences between these organisms. Although this approach may produce the comprehensive differences between two organisms, it is difficult to pinpoint the genes which are responsible for lifespan differences since there may be tremendous variations in gene expression. Furthermore, a given pathway in an organism is more or less efficient depending upon the threshold levels of the factors involved in that pathway. The threshold levels of the factors may be different for different organisms, even though they are normal to the organism. Sifting for the true gene expression related to the lifespan differences over the background of normal threshold value differences will be difficult. Centenarian studies using SNPs to detect the longevity genes have yielded certain markers; however, this may not yield other possible genes affecting the lifespan (Perls *et al.*, 2002). The above impressive list of genes and multiple theories imply that there are several mechanisms that may operate to prolong the lifespan. However, given the multifactorial nature of aging, the current list of genes may not be complete. Since vertebrate genes are more numerous, more novel genes that are not conserved in the lower model organisms that are specific to vertebrates may be identified. Therefore, a vertebrate genetic model that is amenable for large-scale genetic screens for aging is needed.

Fish as Vertebrate Models of Aging

Earlier studies have suggested that fish age in a way that is similar to other vertebrates (Woodhead, 1998). Several factors that are thought to be important in the aging process have been studied in fish. For example, oxidative stress as a causative agent of senescence and the protective role of antioxidant enzymes were tested in the teleostei, taking peroxidase as the representative enzyme (Nayak *et al.*, 1999). O6-Methylguanine-DNA methyltransferase, an enzyme considered to play an important role in the repair of DNA lesions induced by alkylating carcinogens, showed a significant decrease in its activity in the liver with advancing age (Aoki *et al.*, 1993). Antagonistic pleiotropy between attractiveness and survival, or linkage disequilibrium between attractive and deleterious alleles, has been observed in fish (Brooks, 2000). Dietary restriction and lower environmental temperature retard the aging processes in a few fish species, showing gradual senescence (Patnaik *et al.*, 1994). Furthermore, given the large number of fish species (approximately 25,000), there is a larger selection from which to study the aging process. These observations strongly suggest that fish in general are a good model for studying aging. However, fish genetics has not yet been expanded as a model for aging.

Consideration of Zebrafish as Models for Aging

Since its introduction by Streisinger, the zebrafish has become a popular genetic model for studying development and disease because of its many advantages (Jagadeeswaran *et al.*, 2005; Streisinger *et al.*, 1981). One advantage is that zebrafish embryos are transparent, so a developing embryo and its morphology could be easily observed. Breeding zebrafish under laboratory conditions is extremely easy; the embryos grow for 72 hours until they hatch. Other advantages include high fecundity (the female fish can lay up to 200 eggs), short generation times, ease of *in vitro* fertilization, and amenability for large-scale mutagenesis. In addition, features such as transparency of embryos and generation of diploids from haploid eggs make the model even more attractive for identifying recessive mutations. Described below are the principles of genetics in zebrafish and how mutants are isolated and mapped to identify the genes that are affected. Mutagenesis is performed by dipping zebrafish males in ethylnitrosourea (ENU) to cause multiple, random point mutations throughout the genome of the germ cells (spermatogonia). Mating of an ENU-treated male with a wild-type female zebrafish will yield the F1 progeny that will carry as many as 1000 random mutations. Thus, saturating the genome with mutations is possible because theoretically, in 100 fish, 10^5 mutations can be generated. The fish from the F1 generation is then bred to a wild-type fish to generate the heterozygous F2 progeny. Homozygous fish are generated by performing brother–sister matings of the F2 generation. A screen on this F3 progeny for mutant phenotypes constitutes a classical three-generation screen. More than 1000 developmental mutants have been isolated using this strategy. Recently, several imaginative screens have been performed to isolate mutants related to thrombosis, lipid absorption, bone defects, and so forth. Adult screens are more difficult when compared to embryonic and larval screens, because rearing the F3 generation fish to adulthood requires more time and space. In identifying embryonic mutant phenotypes, many laboratories have also used two-generation screens as an alternative method. In this method, haploid or homozygous mutant progeny can be generated directly from the F1 females. Haploid embryos are generated by the *in vitro* fertilization of eggs obtained from a heterozygous F1 female with male sperm whose DNA was destroyed by treatment with ultraviolet light. Although these sperm do not contribute DNA, they can still initiate fertilization and allow the development of haploid embryos, which are viable for up to 3 days postfertilization. If these eggs are subjected to early high-pressure treatment (EP) immediately after fertilization, these haploids will become diploid embryos, which are fully viable. In the EP treatment, hydrostatic pressure causes disruption of spindle formation, which is required for the separation of sister chromatids and polar body extrusion following fertilization. The resulting gynogenetic diploid larvae possess only maternally derived genes that are homozygous for most loci (heterozygosity may arise from recombination events in meiosis I). Thus, this EP treatment allows for a two-generation mutagenesis screen that will identify mutant-carrier females one generation ahead of classical approaches. Once a mutant of interest is identified, the mutant loci can be identified by a positional cloning strategy as described below.

An F1 female mutant carrier is crossed with a male zebrafish that is polymorphic for many loci when compared with the strain used to generate mutations. From this progeny, homozygous mutants are generated by brother–sister mating. To map the mutant locus, two pools of genomic DNA are created from normal and mutant zebrafish (20 zebrafish per genomic DNA preparation) in the above progeny of brother–sister mating. Multiple sets of primers are then used to amplify known microsatellite markers that span the zebrafish genome at an average resolution of 10 cM. Due to the fact that recombination will shuffle both genes and markers in meiosis, markers not linked to the mutant loci, or distal to the loci, will be present in both normal and mutant pools, while linked markers will be present in only one of the two pools. Once a marker is identified showing linkage to a mutant gene, further analysis using additional flanking markers and a larger number of genomes will establish close linkage. Bacterial artificial chromosomes that contain the linked markers could then be sequenced to identify the mutant gene. However, with the availability of genome information, the painstaking efforts of positional cloning will be replaced by the candidate gene approach once a closer linkage is identified. By rescuing the mutant through introducing the functional cDNA or by inhibiting the gene function by antisense approaches, the mutant gene could be confirmed.

In addition to the above approach, there has recently been a major success in the retroviral insertion mutagenesis approach, which identified several hundred genes involved in development (Amsterdam *et al.*, 2004). It has been shown that mouse retroviral vectors pseudotyped with a VSV-G envelope infect the fish germ line after injecting the virus into blastula-stage embryos at the 1000–2000-cell stage. Retroviruses are attractive candidates for insertional mutagenesis, because they had been shown to integrate into many different sites in mammalian and avian chromosomes. Importantly, they integrate without rearrangement of their own sequences or significant alterations to host DNA sequences at the site of insertion—essential features for easily cloning genes disrupted by insertions. Once the infectious retrovirus is injected into the zebrafish embryos and the founder lines are generated, they are mated pairwise and the resulting F1 fish are tested for multiple insertions of the retroviral genome. Those with multiple insertions are then pair-mated and F2 families are raised. Again mating six pairs of siblings will generate homozygous insertional mutants, and one could score for the phenotypes similar to the screening done in ENU mutagenesis. However, the relatively low efficiency of insertional mutagenesis in contrast to the ENU mutagenesis limits the utility of this method for small laboratories. Also, this method will result in the inactivation of the gene rather than producing hyperactive and hypoactive alleles that are possible by the ENU mutagenesis.

Because of the above advantages of the zebrafish model, we tested its utility as a genetic model for studying aging by initially establishing the zebrafish lifespan (Gerhard *et al.*, 2002; Herrera and Jagadeeswaran, 2002; Herrera and Jagadeeswaran, 2004). Another group independently performed such studies (Gerhard *et al.*, 2002). Both of these studies revealed that zebrafish have a lifespan of approximately 4 years. Furthermore, Kishi and his colleagues have identified several potential aging biomarkers such as senescent associated β-galactosidase activity in skin and oxidized protein accumulation in muscle (Kishi, 2004). In contrast, markers such as accumulation of lipofuschin granules (which accumulate in muscle cells with advancing age) were not found. Another study revealed the decline of muscle function with advancing age by studying the bone curvature (Gerhard *et al.*, 2002). Even though some differences exist in the expression of biomarkers when compared to mammals, zebrafish nevertheless showed gradual senescence as observed in other fish species. In spite of this information on biomarkers, classical genetic studies will take long periods of study since zebrafish have long lifespans. Therefore, we suggested that zebrafish do not qualify as an ideal model because of their long lifespan. However, Gerhard and Cheng have recently argued that studying more than one fish may be useful for comparative aging (Gerhard *et al.*, 2004). While it is a good argument, the utility of such comparative studies in identifying longevity genes is questionable.

Genetics of Aging

Unlike performing genetic studies for development and disease, aging genetics is more complicated because of certain features that are unique to this phenotype. For example, the organism becomes old in the process of selecting for longevity and, thus, even if we find a long-lived organism, its reproductive ability would have declined, making it difficult to recover the organism. Thus, the parental population must be continuously bred until we are able to identify the progeny that has a long span. This could also be achieved by preserving parental sperm. In some organisms like *C. elegans*, they can be maintained in a cryogenically frozen state, facilitating the easy maintenance of large numbers of strains (Johnson, 2003). Thus, it is possible to identify the progeny of those that have long-lived survivors and recover them from a frozen state. While such advantages exist in lower organisms, the logistics of large-scale screens in vertebrates, like mice, to recover the organism from frozen sperm samples is not particularly practical. A similar situation exists in zebrafish as well because even if we preserve sperm, by the time we identify the long-lived survivors and then recover the mutation, it becomes an arduous task. Thus, a vertebrate model organism that circumvents these problems is needed.

Annual Fish as Models for Aging

We believe that *Nothobranchius rachovvi*, a killifish, is a better vertebrate model for longevity genetics because their maximum lifespan is about ten months (Herrera and Jagadeeswaran, 2004). *Nothobranchius rachovvi* are teleostei like zebrafish and have already been used in aging studies. They have been shown to begin senescent changes at approximately four months of age. They are relatively easy to breed and are approximately 2 inches in size. The females lay approximately 20 eggs per day. *Nothobranchius rachovvi* can breed even at an old age until the very end of their lives. This occurs because the natural habitat of these fish dries out seasonally. In order to preserve their species, these annual fish developed schemes to lay eggs up to the time of death. In the laboratory, eggs are collected in peat moss and then stored in a dry container for four months. The eggs hatch when placed in water, and they grow at 28–30°C. The larvae mature by the age of 3–4 weeks when males develop colors and are easy to distinguish from females. Since they belong to the cyprinodontiformes form of fish, the information on the zebrafish and fugu fish gene sequences should be useful in obtaining polymorphic EST markers for *Nothobranchius*. There are about 40 species of *Nothobranchius*, and most *Nothobranchius* species have a diploid number of chromosomes ranging from 2N = 16 to 28. Recently, another group claimed that *Nothobranchius furzeri* has the shortest lifespan of 2 months under circulating water conditions, which is similar to what we observed for *Nothobranchius rachovvi* under these same conditions. We do not know the normal lifespan of *Nothobranchius furzeri* under stagnant water conditions. Furthermore, different strains of *Nothobranchius rachovvi* are available, whereas for *furzeri* we do not know whether multiple strains are available. A prerequisite for genetic mapping is the availability of strains. Thus, *Nothobranchius rachovvi* is an ideal vertebrate organism that has a short lifespan if we could adapt the mutagenesis methods that are well established in zebrafish and medaka. These protocols for mutagenesis are standard and should be easily adaptable for the annual fish. In addition, several genetic markers for *Nothobranchius* have already been isolated.

From our published work, *Nothobranchius* would be a good vertebrate model for studying the genetics of longevity due to its shorter lifespan. However, the survivorship curves as presented appear to be less rectangular than the one we obtained for zebrafish (Austad, 2004). Furthermore, in the work of Walford on *Cynolebias*, the curves are rectangular (Liu and Walford, 1969). The difference between their work and our work is the difference in temperature at which the fish were maintained. Thus, optimization of survivorship curves is required using different temperatures. In addition, another possible cause for a nonrectangular curve is the existence of pathogens. We believe the alternation of one or two degrees in temperature maintenance of *Nothobranchius* as well as a clean water system will make a significant impact on the survivorship curves. Before using this fish, conditions for optimal growth and maintenance should be established. Since these fish have been used in commercial sales and the conditions for growth and maintenance are available from vendors, they should be helpful. For example, water quality, temperature, presence of good amounts of denitrifying bacteria, elimination of bacterial contamination, and appropriate monitoring of pH and ammonia are some of the conditions which might provide us with the desired rectangular shape of the survivorship curves. Since bubbles generated in the water circulation system may be causing the early deaths, the efficiency could be improved by using tanks that are connected at the bottom, whose water is recirculated slowly.

It is well established that heterosis or hybrid vigor exists in organisms. Thus, the effects of heterosis on longevity using progeny derived from the crossing of two strains should be determined. Studies on several parameters such as the body weight, growth, their physical activity measurable by analyzing images of locomotion captured by a video monitor system, the gill movements per minute, and lateral line responses observable by movements in response to a pendulum should help in determining any differences among the strains and their progeny. Additional important information on differences between survivorship curves among the parental strains and their hybrid progeny is also needed. A compilation of these curves will assist us in forming an appropriate baseline for the survivorship curves. Any noticeable increase in longevity among these hybrids would help determine an accurate time point for the selection of longevity mutants. In *Nothobranchius*, embryos must be kept dormant for four to twelve months before they can be hatched. The effect of dormancy over the lifespan needs to be investigated by keeping the eggs under dry conditions for different periods of time. We still do not know whether there is a decline in reproductive activity with age, so measurement of the egg-laying activity of *Nothobranchius* as a function of age is important. Due to the fact that fish embryos can be diploidized from haploid eggs, we can increase the speed of generating homozygous mutant fish (one generation is needed rather than two) for recessive mutations. The principle of generating the gynogenetic diploids is described above. This should be easily adaptable for this annual fish. The haploid eggs of females of the F1 progeny are fertilized *in vitro* with UV irradiated sperm and subjected to high pressure to rapidly generate diploid F2 progeny. The embryos can then be kept under dry conditions as described above. The lifespan of the F2 progeny can be analyzed for their similarities to normal survivorship curves. This information would provide us with two facts: first, the diploidization is feasible; and second, the gynogenetic diploids behave as wild-type normal fish as far as their survivorship curves are concerned. Important information that is also needed is the histology to look for any observable pathology. Since zebrafish histology and other fish histology and pathology are available, again it should be relatively easy to extend this information for the annual fish.

Mutagenesis of Annual Fish

CHEMICAL MUTAGENESIS

The ENU mutagenesis has been applied to many organisms and should be applicable to *Nothobranchius*. However, this requires the demonstration of efficiency of ENU mutagenesis in this species. Such results would form the basis for pursuing large-scale saturation mutagenesis in *Nothobranchius* to identify mutant fish with extended lifespan. To identify longevity mutants of *Nothobranchius*, the male *Nothobranchius* should be mutagenized with ENU and mated with normal females generating progeny with many heterozygous mutations representing either a gain of function or a loss of function. The specific mutation rate could be estimated by using phenotypic pigmentation patterns. To estimate a specific locus mutation rate, mutagenized males from a blue strain are mated with a red strain partner. The number of fish expressing these traits when they are homozygous in the progeny will predict the efficiency of ENU mutagenesis and the mutation rate. In ENU mutagenesis of zebrafish, the specific locus mutation frequency is as high as $0.9–1.3 \times 10^{-3}$ (Solnica-Krezel *et al.*, 1994). With the mutation rate of 1.27×10^{-3} if the distribution of mutations in the genome could be approximated by Poisson distribution, about 87% of the genes would be detected with an average of two mutations per locus, and for this approximately 1600 genomes must be screened to obtain one mutation for a given locus. Given the established methods in zebrafish, one would expect that high mutation rates will be achieved in *Nothobranchius*. The following scheme as a screen for selection of long-lived mutant fish is proposed: first, females from ENU mutagenized F1 progeny are used that generate gynogenetic diploids from each of these females. From this progeny, males and females are separated and kept in large tanks. This will prevent further breeding, although the density of the fish should be taken into consideration. Since the longest survivor in *Nothobranchius* is about 10 months, fish are selected for 12 months as lifespan. This gives approximately 20% longer life. The long-lived F2 diploid survivors are used to generate F3 homozygous. The survivorship curves of wild-type progeny of the two strains are compared to the survivorship curves of the above homozygous mutant progeny. The shift of the mutant progeny lifespan curve to the right compared to controls will confirm the longevity mutant. This homozygous progeny is then bred to a different strain of *Nothobranchius*, which would be polymorphic for many loci for mapping the mutant locus. Once the long-lived mutants are isolated for identification of the gene responsible for the phenotype, it should be possible to map the longevity mutant locus by using linkage methods. Since large chunks of DNA are syntenic in the *Nothobranchius* genome when compared to the zebrafish genome, the maps and the synteny of genes in zebrafish as well as those from mammals should be useful to predict candidate genes once a marker linked to the longevity phenotype is identified. For this, approximately 250 markers that are spaced approximately 10 cM and spanning the entire genome are needed for mapping longevity mutants. Since a large number of zebrafish EST sequences and a significant amount of genomic sequence from fugu fish as well as zebrafish are already available, it should be possible to choose a number of conserved EST marker primers in order to identify polymorphism that span the entire *Nothobranchius* genome. Based upon the existing linkage maps of zebrafish, the marker (EST) primers located approximately 10 cM can be selected. It should then be possible to amplify the total RNA using the above primers to find polymorphisms between two strains of *Nothobranchius* by SSCP or by DNA sequencing.

INSERTIONAL MUTAGENESIS

The insertional inactivation of genes by retroviral mutagenesis has been successfully employed in zebrafish as described above. How will this be useful in longevity selection? The underlying rationale for insertional mutagenesis in aging studies is that the inactivation of genes that have negative influence on the lifespan might increase the lifespan. Since it is easy to detect dominant genes, first dominant screens should be conducted by simply injecting the retroviruses into the *Nothobranchius* embryos and then the fish should be selected that are long lived and should be used further to identify the genes that are affected. This concept could also be extended further for recessive screens either by diploidization or by three-generation screens to identify the long-lived *Nothobranchius*. The methods that are used in zebrafish for insertional mutagenesis should be applicable for the annual fish.

Transgenesis and Overexpression of Genes in Annual Fish

Transgenic technology has been recently introduced in zebrafish, and many promoters have been expressed in a tissue-specific manner. Conditional misexpression of genes in certain tissue has been achieved by using GAL4-UAS system (Scheer and Camnos-Ortega, 1999). In this system two different kinds of transgenic strains, called activator and effector lines, are developed. In the activator line, the GAL4 (yeast transcriptional activator) gene is placed under the control of a tissue/cell specific promoter, while in the effector line the gene of interest is fused UAS (Upstream Activating Sequences, the DNA-binding motif of GAL4). Once the effector line is crossed to the activator line, the effector gene is expressed in a specific tissue because the GAL4 is supplied by the tissue specific promoter and will bind to the UAS and drive the effector gene transcription. Recently, the utility of the Cre/lox system has been demonstrated in the zebrafish model by developing a conditional myc-induced T cell acute lymphoblastic leukemia (Langenau *et al.*, 2005). Thus, in addition to GAL4-UAS system, this technology is available for fish. Depending upon the strength of the promoter and taking into account the positional effects, the gene expression could be modulated and the effects on longevity could be studied. Thus, it is conceivable that one could express genes that affect metabolism or oxidative stress pathways or insulin receptor mediated pathways to overexpress these genes. The information gained from studying invertebrate genes could also be used to verify whether mechanisms that are operative in invertebrates are conserved in vertebrates. However, this is a biased approach and would require prior knowledge of the genes that may be involved in lifespan extension. Furthermore, due to the fact that such studies could be performed in mice, one may question the utility of the fish model in such studies. However, since the *Nothobranchius* is amenable for large-scale unbiased overexpression of genes by using the above vectors that could specifically express genes in certain tissues, with the knowledge of information gained from large scale microarrays depicting the tissue-specific genes, one could construct libraries of such genes and generate transgenic lines on a large scale to verify which ones will have prolonged lifespan. These approaches require further testing.

Dietary Restriction and Oxidative Stress in Annual Fish Mutants

Once the mutagenesis is achieved, dietary resistant mutants and oxidative stress resistant mutants could be selected which might suggest genes involved in such a mechanism. For example a paraquat resistance mutant could be selected and then tested for lifespan extension. Similarly, mutants could be fed with a high fat and high nutrient diet which, in contrast to dietary restriction, should shorten the lifespan and the mutants that live under these conditions could be selected. However, these require careful feeding experiments. Likewise, by feeding ω-3 fatty acids, the mutants that do not prolong the lifespan in the presence of ω-3 fatty acids could be selected. All these imaginative screens will be feasible once the *Nothobranchius* model is available as a genetic model.

Annual Fish as a Tool for Screening for Antiaging Drugs

In 1999, we suggested that zebrafish could be used as a model for drug discovery (Jagadeeswaran *et al.*, 1999). Due to the availability of a large number of chemical compounds and the ease of screening the larvae, a number of mutants are being investigated to reverse the phenotype with these chemicals. Such reversal of phenotypes has been applied to aortic coarctation (Peterson *et al.*, 2004). This phenotypic reversal is feasible because the larvae are small and it is possible to accommodate screening in a 96-well format in tiny volumes such that only small amounts of chemical are used. However, in longevity studies such screening depends on the availability of compounds on a large scale and continuous replacement of the chemicals to accommodate for their half-lives. Interestingly, there are several naturally occurring compounds that are either antioxidants or participate in metabolic pathways that affect aging. Thus, in the future, it is anticipated that large-scale screens could be undertaken using *Nothobranchius* as a model to discover more new natural products that may have an effect on the extension of lifespans. For example, individual leaf extracts could be placed in tanks of *Nothobranchius* fish to see which of these extracts would prolong the lifespan. Once the extract is identified, the active compounds could be characterized and be synthesized by pharmaceutical companies. Thus, *Nothobranchius* could be useful in rapidly discovering drugs that will extend vertebrate lifespan.

Conclusions

The above suggestion that *Nothobranchius* would be a useful model for studying longevity genes is novel, and it is the first time that the genetic approach utilizing the annual fish is suggested, although Walford first noted the utility of annual fish in aging research (Liu and Walford, 1969). Such a utility will depend upon establishing conditions for chemical mutagenesis, isolating markers for linkage analysis, and identifying long-lived *Nothobranchius* mutants. Since these are straightforward, this is a feasible goal. This model will also be used in overexpression of genes by transgenesis and identification of antiaging drugs. Future identification of longevity genes may ultimately allow the identification of human homologues involved in aging. Only time will tell whether this beautiful aquarium fish will be useful in furthering the knowledge on aging. May the genome sequencers embrace this annual fish for eventually sequencing its genome!

Recommended Resources

1. http://zfin.org This site has much to offer regarding the zebrafish genetics and methodology.
2. www.aka.org This site has a collection of many annual fish species and information on resources.
3. http://sageke.sciencemag.org/cgi/genesdb This site has a collection of genes that affect the lifespan.

ACKNOWLEDGMENTS

This work was supported by National Institutes of Health grants HL63792, HL77910 and AG20863. I thank Jo Gail Stark for editorial help.

REFERENCES

Amsterdam, A., Nissen, R.M., Sun, Z., Swindell, E.C., Farrington, S., and Hopkins, N. (2004). Identification of 315 genes essential for early zebrafish development. *Proc Natl Acad Sci USA 101*, 12792–12797.

Aoki, K., Nakatsuru, Y., Sakurai, J., Sato, A., Masahito, P., and Ishikawa, T. (1993). Age dependence of O6-methylguanine-DNA methyltransferase activity and its depletion after carcinogen treatment in the teleost medaka (*Oryzias latipes*). *Mutat Res 293*, 225–231.

Austad, S.N. (2004). On Herrera and Jagadeeswaran's "Annual fish as a genetic model for aging". *J Gerontol A Biol Sci Med Sci 59*, 99–100.

Brooks, R. (2000). Negative genetic correlation between male sexual attractiveness and survival. *Nature 406*, 67–70.

Dorman, J.B., Albinder, B., Shroyer, T., and Kenyon, C. (1995). The age-1 and daf-2 genes function in a common pathway to control the lifespan of *Caenorhabditis elegans*. *Genetics 141*, 1399–1406.

Droge, W. (2003). Oxidative stress and aging. *Adv Exp Med Biol 543*, 191–200.

Gerhard, G.S., Kauffman, E.J., Wang, X., Stewart, R., Moore, J.L., Kasales, C.J., *et al.* (2002). Life spans and senescent phenotypes in two strains of Zebrafish (*Danio rerio*). *Exp Gerontol 37*, 1055–1068.

Gerhard, G.S., Malek, R.L., Keller, E., Murtha, J., and Cheng, K.C. (2004). Zebrafish, killifish, neither fish, both fish? *J Gerontol A Biol Sci Med Sci 59*, B873–B875.

Guarente, L., and Picard, F. (2005). Calorie restriction—the SIR2 connection. *Cell 120*, 473–482.

Hamet, P., and Tremblay, J. (2003). Genes of aging. *Metabolism 52*, 5–9.

Helfand, S.L., and Rogina, B. (2003). From genes to aging in *Drosophila*. *Adv Genet 49*, 67–109.

Herrera, M., and Jagadeeswaran, P. (2002). Killifish: A vertebrate model for aging. *International Meeting on Zebrafish Development and Genetics: Abstracts 5*, 244.

Herrera, M., and Jagadeeswaran, P. (2004). Annual fish as a genetic model for aging. *J Gerontol A Biol Sci Med Sci 59*, 101–107.

Hursting, S.D., Lavigne, J.A., Berrigan, D., Perkins, S.N., and Barrett, J.C. (2003). Calorie restriction, aging, and cancer prevention: Mechanisms of action and applicability to humans. *Annu Rev Med 54*, 131–152.

Jagadeeswaran, P., Gregory, M., Day, K., Cykowski, M., and Thattaliyath, B. (2005). Zebrafish: A genetic model for hemostasis and thrombosis. *J Thromb Haemost 3*, 46–53.

Jagadeeswaran, P., Sheehan, J.P., Craig, F.E., and Troyer, D. (1999). Identification and characterization of zebrafish thrombocytes. *Br J Haematol 107*, 731–738.

Johnson, T.E. (2003). Advantages and disadvantages of *Caenorhabditis elegans* for aging research. *Exp Gerontol 38*, 1329–1332.

Johnson, T.E., and Wood, W.B. (1982). Genetic analysis of life-span in *Caenorhabditis elegans. Proc Natl Acad Sci USA 79*, 6603–6607.

Kenyon, C. (2005). The plasticity of aging: Insights from long-lived mutants. *Cell 120*, 449–460.

Kimmel, C.B. (1989). Genetics and early development of zebrafish. *Trends Genet* **5**, 283–288.

Kimura, K.D., Tissenbaum, H.A., Liu, Y., and Ruvkun, G. (1997). daf-2, an insulin receptor-like gene that regulates longevity and diapause in *Caenorhabditis elegans. Science 277*, 942–946.

Kishi, S. (2004). Functional aging and gradual senescence in zebrafish. *Ann N Y Acad Sci 1019*, 521–526.

Langenau, D.M., Feng, H., Berghmans, S., Kanki, J.P., Kutok, J.L., and Look, A.T. (2005). Cre/lox-regulated transgenic zebrafish model with conditional myc-induced T cell acute lymphoblastic leukemia. *Proc Natl Acad Sci USA 102*, 6068–6073.

Liang, H., Masoro, E.J., Nelson, J.F., Strong, R., McMahan, C.A., and Richardson, A. (2003). Genetic mouse models of extended lifespan. *Exp Gerontol 38*, 1353–1364.

Lin, Y.J., Seroude, L., and Benzer, S. (1998). Extended life-span and stress resistance in the *Drosophila* mutant methuselah. *Science 282*, 943–946.

Liu, R.K., and Walford, R.L. (1969). Laboratory studies on life span, growth, aging, and pathology of the annual fish, *Cynolebias bellotti* Steindachner. *Zoologica 54*, 1–16.

Luo, Y. (2004). Long-lived worms and aging. *Redox Rep. 9*, 65–69.

Masoro, E.J. (2005). Overview of caloric restriction and ageing. *Mech Ageing Dev.*

Migliaccio, E., Giorgio, M., Mele, S., Pelicci, G., Reboldi, P., Pandolfi, P.P., *et al.* (1999). The p66shc adaptor protein controls oxidative stress response and life span in mammals. *Nature 402*, 309–313.

Nayak, S.B., Jena, B.S., and Patnaik, B.K. (1999). Effects of age and manganese (II) chloride on peroxidase activity of brain and liver of the teleost, *Channa punctatus. Exp Gerontol 34*, 365–374.

Paradis, S., and Ruvkun, G. (1998). *Caenorhabditis elegans* Akt/PKB transduces insulin receptor-like signals from AGE-1 PI3 kinase to the DAF-16 transcription factor. *Genes Dev 12*, 2488–2498.

Parkes, T.L., Elia, A.J., Dickinson, D., Hilliker, A.J., Phillips, J.P., and Boulianne, G.L. (1998). Extension of *Drosophila* lifespan by overexpression of human SOD1 in motorneurons. *Nat Genet 19*, 171–174.

Patnaik, B.K., Mahapatro, N., and Jena, B.S. (1994). Ageing in fishes. *Gerontology 40*, 113–132.

Patton, E.E., and Zon, L.I. (2001). The art and design of genetic screens: Zebrafish. *Nat Rev Genet 2*, 956–966.

Perls, T., Kunkel, L.M., and Puca, A.A. (2002). The genetics of exceptional human longevity. *J Am Geriatr Soc 50*, 359–368.

Peterson, R.T., Shaw, S.Y., Peterson, T.A., Milan, D.J., Zhong, T.P., Schreiber, S.L., *et al.* (2004). Chemical suppression of a genetic mutation in a zebrafish model of aortic coarctation. *Nat Biotechnol 22*, 595–599.

Scheer, N., and Camnos-Ortega, J.A. (1999). Use of the Gal4-UAS technique for targeted gene expression in the zebrafish. *Mech Dev 80*, 153–158.

Solnica-Krezel, L., Schier, A.F., and Driever, W. (1994). Efficient recovery of ENU-induced mutations from the zebrafish germline. *Genetics 136*, 1401–1420.

Streisinger, G., Walker, C., Dower, N., Knauber, D., and Singer, F. (1981). Production of clones of homozygous diploid zebra fish (*Brachydanio rerio*). *Nature 291*, 293–296.

Tissenbaum, H.A., and Guarente, L. (2001). Increased dosage of a sir-2 gene extends lifespan in *Caenorhabditis elegans. Nature 410*, 227–230.

Van Voorhies, W.A., and Ward, S. (1999). Genetic and environmental conditions that increase longevity in *Caenorhabditis elegans* decrease metabolic rate. *Proc Natl Acad Sci USA 96*, 11399–11403.

Weindruch, R., Kayo, T., Lee, C.K., and Prolla, T.A. (2001). Microarray profiling of gene expression in aging and its alteration by caloric restriction in mice. *J Nutr 131*, 918S–923S.

Woodhead, A.D. (1998). Aging, the fishy side: An appreciation of Alex Comfort's studies. *Exp Gerontol 33*, 39–51.

27

The Use of Mature Zebrafish (*Danio rerio*) as a Model for Human Aging and Disease

Evan T. Keller, Jill M. Keller, and Gavin Gillespie

Zebrafish (Danio rerio) have been extensively utilized for understanding mechanisms of development. These studies have led to a wealth of resources including genetic tools, informational databases, and husbandry methods. In spite of all these resources, zebrafish have been underutilized for exploring the pathophysiology of disease and the aging process. Zebrafish offer several advantages over mammalian models for these studies, including the ability to perform saturation mutagenesis and the capability to contain thousands of animals in a small space. In this review, we will discuss the use of mature zebrafish as an animal model. The challenges of developing and maintaining a colony of aging zebrafish will be addressed. Specific examples to support the use of mature zebrafish as an animal model will be provided, including the demonstration of clinical pathology and that age-associated changes in various phenotypes can be observed in aging zebrafish.

Introduction

Zebrafish (*Danio rerio*) have proven to be an outstanding animal model for exploring vertebrate development and genetics (Detrich *et al.*, 1999). Zebrafish have several advantages for study of developmental biology, including conservation of developmental genes across vertebrates, small size (which allows for large numbers of animals to be kept in a relatively small area), their external fertilization and transparent embryos (allowing direct visualization of development), the ease with which water soluble drugs and chemicals can be administered, and their amenability to large-scale saturation mutagenesis studies. These are unique aspects of zebrafish among currently used vertebrate animal models. Ongoing activities in the zebrafish community have resulted in a multitude of resources available to researchers using this animal model. For example, the formation of a National Zebrafish Stock Center (University of Oregon) has provided a central resource for wild-type stocks, mutant and transgenic lines, and extensive information on genetics of zebrafish. In addition, a variety of antibodies and cDNA libraries are available, and an extensive informatic web-based network has been created (Sprague *et al.*, 2003). Furthermore, the extensive genetic characterizations that zebrafish have undergone, including a detailed microsatellite genetic linkage map (Knapik *et al.*, 1998) and the ability to select for mutagenized genes (Wienholds *et al.*, 2003), provides a cutting edge ability to rapidly take advantage of this animal model.

The widespread resources and genetic characterization of these animals have led to many exciting discoveries related to developmental biology. However, this wealth of resources has been underexploited for evaluation of biology or pathophysiology of mature zebrafish. Most scientists evaluate zebrafish at the embryonic/neonate stages after mutagenesis or toxin exposure. Thus, it is plausible that many mutation- or toxic-mediated effects that occur in late life will not be identified. It follows that a wealth of information with great relevance to human biology and disease is being overlooked (Dooley *et al.*, 2000).

Husbandry of an Aging Zebrafish Colony

There are several excellent manuals regarding zebrafish husbandry (Westerfield 1995). However, development and maintenance of aging zebrafish poses some unique challenges which we will describe.

DISEASE PREVENTION

In any zebrafish colony, the appearance of disease could impact the whole colony, resulting even in death of the entire colony. Thus, disease prevention in a colony is critical. In an aging colony, this takes on a great urgency as one cannot readily replace the old fish that die and several years of work can be destroyed through introduction of a lethal pathogen or water impurity. Several filtration and detoxification methods are used in zebrafish facilities (Figure 27.1). These include methods such as ultraviolet filtration, to kill pathogenic bacteria from reaching the tank, and biological filters, to harvest bacteria that can denitrify the water. Accordingly, it is best to maintain an aging colony as an isolated colony in a barrier facility.

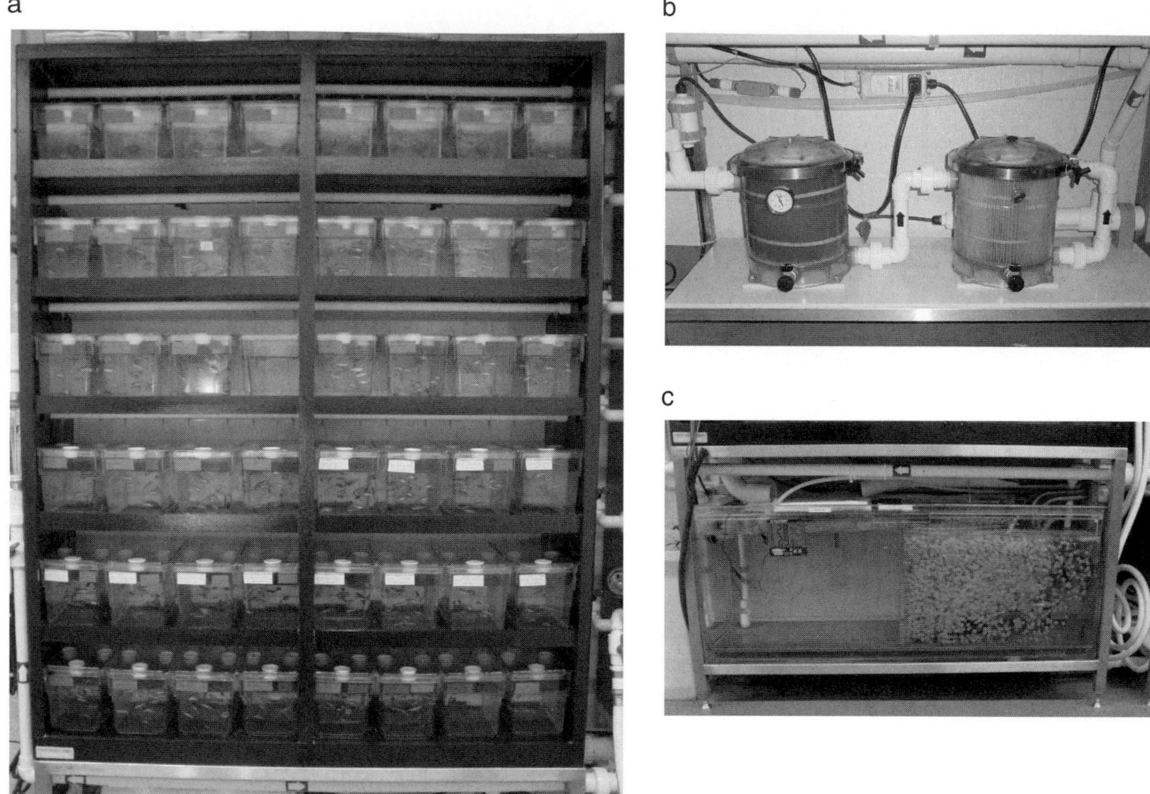

Figure 27.1. Zebrafish facility. (A) ZMod setup showing individual tanks that each hold between 20 and 30 fish. (B) Physical filtration system that uses filters to clear water. (C) Biological filtration system that uses beads with large surface area to allow for growth of bacteria that diminish nitrates in the water.

Stocking of a zebrafish colony should be performed using internal breeding.

POPULATION DENSITY

Population density can clearly affect the environment that the fish live in. In an aging colony, as individual fish die and are removed from a tank, the overall population density in that tank will be altered. This may confound studies when comparisons are made among different tanks. Thus, one should consider their experimental goals if this is an important issue. One method to minimize the impact of population density changes is to replace a dead fish with another fish. We typically use another zebrafish strain that we can clearly identify as different from the experimental strain (e.g., longfin versus shortfins).

ANIMAL AGE IDENTIFICATION

Clearly, in an aging colony, accurate identification of individuals' ages must be provided. Thus, attention must be given to establishing a record-keeping system and housing method that allow fish ages to be identified. We typically maintain approximately 20–30 fish from any one birthdate in a tank that is clearly labeled with the birthdate of the fish. When using animals, consideration should be given to the fish's ages in order to minimize time of the experiment. For example, if one needs fish at 6 months and 2 years of age, it would be more efficient to start the 2 year fish aging, and then approximately 1.5 years later, start the 6 month fish aging. This will result in both groups reaching their target ages at the same time and thus allow for consistency during animal collection and test procedures. Additionally, it will serve to minimize overall experimental time (in this example, to approximately 2 years) as opposed to aging the 6-month-old animals and then starting the 2-year-old animals.

Zebrafish as Model for Human Disease

Zebrafish have been used extensively in a variety of medical and scientific disciplines including cardiology, neurology, ophthalmology, and environmental toxicology. However, the majority of these studies have explored developmental aspects. Studies in mature zebrafish, and even their normal anatomy, have been largely unexplored, though they have tremendous potential as animal models for diseases that occur later in life. Their small size makes

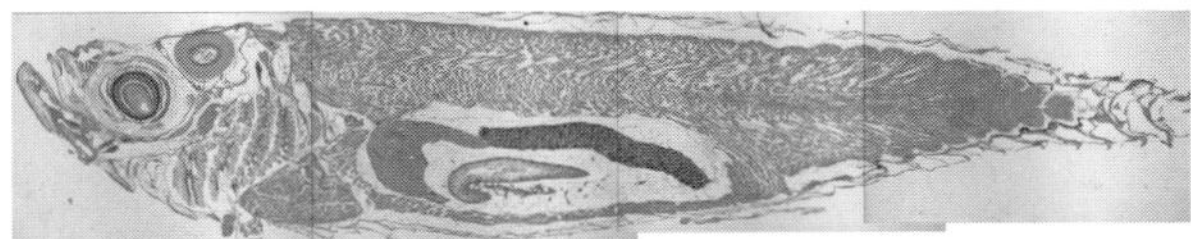

Figure 27.2. Sagittal section of zebrafish. This demonstrates a reconstruction of several individual sections of a zebrafish to create a high-resolution sagittal section. Stained with hematoxylin and eosin.

zebrafish amenable to rapid histological analysis (Figure 27.2).

We must understand their normal anatomy in order to detect pathology. In terms of serving as animal models for human disease, there are several examples. For instance, the recent cloning of the Huntington's disease gene homologue in zebrafish (Karlovich *et al.*, 1998) has broad implications for the importance that a mature zebrafish model may provide towards understanding this disease's pathophysiology. A mutation in *vHnf1* has also been recently cloned in zebrafish, which is orthologous to a gene mutated in human polycystic kidney disease (PKD) (Sun *et al.*, 2001). As in human disease, this zebrafish mutant forms cysts in its kidneys, representing a potential model of human glomerulocystic kidney disease. Zebrafish have also been found to express amyloid precursor protein (APP), presenilin (PS)-1, and apolipoprotein E (apoE), which have all been implicated in familial Alzheimer's disease (FAD) (Leimer *et al.*, 1999; Monnot *et al.*, 1999). Zebrafish PS-1 has been found to promote aberrant secretion of Abeta42 similar to FAD-associated PS1 mutations (Leimer *et al.*, 1999). Zebrafish have been proposed as an ideal vertebrate system in which to model cancer as well (Amatruda *et al.*, 2002; Stern *et al.*, 2003). Thus, the mature zebrafish has tremendous potential as a model of adult and late-life human diseases.

Zebrafish Models of Blood Disorders

In order to capitalize on zebrafish for exploring pathophysiology, a thorough understanding of its normal physiology is required. For example, the zebrafish is especially suitable for studies involving hematopoiesis (reviewed by Ward *et al.*, 2002). The anatomical and morphological features of hematopoiesis are comparable to those in mammals (Amatruda *et al.*, 1999). Zebrafish possess both erythroid and myeloid compartments, and there is strong conservation of hematopoietic gene expression, including transcription factors and signaling pathways (Conway *et al.*, 1997; Liao *et al.*, 1998; Oates *et al.*, 1999). Large-scale genetic screens have resulted in the identification of hundreds of mutant phenotypes, including many with hematopoietic disorders (Weinstein *et al.*, 1996). Several of these mutants present almost identical phenotypes to those of human hematopoietic diseases. For example, the *sauternes* mutant has anemia due to a defect in the erythroid δ-animolevulinate synthase (ALAS2) gene, an enzyme involved in heme biosynthesis (Brownlie *et al.*, 1998). Mutations in ALAS2 in humans cause congenital sideroblastic anemia, with many characteristics that resemble the *sau* phenotype. The *sau* mutant is the first animal model of this human disease. These mutants being recovered have tremendous potential for increasing our knowledge of normal hematopoietic processes as well as the pathophysiology of hematopoietic disorders. However, there is a serious lack of data describing the normal hematological characteristics of zebrafish. Normal hematological reference values for zebrafish are critical for interpreting results seen in mutant fish due to mutagenesis studies, transgenic applications, environmental stresses, or xenobiotic exposure.

Towards this goal, normal hematological and clinical chemistry parameters in adult zebrafish have been reported (Murtha *et al.*, 2003b). Hematological values for zebrafish, including leukocyte differential counts and total erythrocyte counts, were within the ranges reported for mammalian species and fish. The predominant leukocyte seen in zebrafish was the lymphocyte, with smaller numbers of monocytes, neutrophils, eosinophils, and basophils. With the exception of increases in alanine transaminase (ALT), amylase, and phosphorus values, results of serum biochemical analysis were also within the normal ranges reported for mammalian species and fish. Serum biochemical studies of healthy fish are scarce, and results vary widely. Phosphorus values were only slightly higher than the upper range reported in some publications. ALT and amylase activities were most likely falsely increased due to some hemolysis in the samples. In summary, we believe these values will be useful in future studies that examine various disease models in zebrafish, normal aging of zebrafish, and screens of mutagenic zebrafish lines.

Zebrafish as a Model for Aging

Many species of fish have been used as an experimental model for aging (Woodhead 1978; Patnaik *et al.*, 1994; Woodhead 1998); thus in addition to defining mechanisms of disease, zebrafish may be useful for exploring the process of aging. Recent studies have provided initial evidence that zebrafish have a median lifespan of approximately 36 to 42 months with a maximum lifespan of up to 66 months (Gerhard *et al.*, 2002b), indicating that zebrafish undergo an age-related increase in mortality rate. More recently, a shorter median and maximum lifespan was reported for zebrafish, with 31 and 45 months, respectively (Herrera *et al.*, 2004). The different results in these two studies may be a reflection of strain variation and differences in housing and environmental parameters. These findings, however, set the groundwork for identification of genes that control longevity. Aging zebrafish have been demonstrated to develop several phenotypes similar to aging mammals (Table 27.1), including the

TABLE 27.1
Aging phenotypes recognized in zebrafish

Phenotype	Finding	Reference
Median lifespan	36–42 months	(Gerhard *et al.*, 2002b)
Maximum lifespan	66 months	(Gerhard *et al.*, 2002b)
Heat shock protein 70	Decreased with age	(Murtha *et al.*, 2003a)
Heat shock factor 1	Increased with age	(Murtha *et al.*, 2003a)
Senescence-associated β-galactosidase staining	Observed in skin with aging	(Kishi *et al.*, 2003)
Protein oxidation	Increased with age in muscle	(Kishi *et al.*, 2003)
Spinal curvature	Observed with aging	(Gerhard *et al.*, 2002b)

appearance of senescence-associated β-galactosidase staining and oxidized protein (Kishi *et al.*, 2003). Additionally, spinal curvature occurs with age in zebrafish (Gerhard *et al.*, 2002b).

Fish have been said to show three types of senescence: rapid, gradual, and negligible. Teleost fish, of which zebrafish are members, generally undergo gradual senescence, as observed in most vertebrates (Kishi *et al.*, 2003). Whether or not zebrafish undergo gradual senescence as well is not yet fully understood, though they are reported to show increasing senescent morphology with aging, including spinal curvature and muscle degeneration (Gerhard *et al.*, 2002b). It has also been suggested that zebrafish may undergo "very gradual senescence" based on molecular changes, including senescence-associated β-galactosidase activity and accumulation of oxidized protein with age in the face of continuously proliferating myocytes and constitutive telomerase activity in adult zebrafish (Kishi *et al.*, 2003). While Kishi *et al.* (2003) did not find age-related changes in BrdU incorporation, telomerase activity, and lipofuscin accumulation in zebrafish, it is important to note that the oldest fish examined in that study were 24–31 months old, which is less than the median lifespan reported for zebrafish, and may not reflect what occurs in truly "old" fish. In many teleost fish, age-related increases in mortality rate, accumulation of lipofuscin, lipid peroxidation, collagen cross-linking and decreases in growth rate, reproductive capacity and protein utilization are clearly observed (Patnaik *et al.*, 1994). Zebrafish demonstrate an age-related increase in mortality rate (Gerhard *et al.*, 2002b; Herrera *et al.*, 2004) though accumulation of lipofuscin (Kishi *et al.*, 2003), and decreases in growth rate (Gerhard *et al.*, 2002b) have not been observed in zebrafish thus far. Other parameters, including lipid peroxidation, collagen cross-linking, reproductive capacity, and protein utilization, have not yet been examined specifically in zebrafish with respect to aging.

Populations of guppies kept under various conditions of culture have shown survival curves similar to those seen in populations of small mammals (Comfort 1960; Comfort 1961; Comfort 1963; Woodhead 1998). In these studies, guppies showed a median and maximum lifespan of approximately 36–44 and 55–60 months, respectively, which is quite similar to what has been reported in survival curves for zebrafish (Gerhard *et al.*, 2002b). In addition, the tissues of these guppies showed marked aging changes comparable to those seen in the tissues of aging mammals, including senile changes in the gonads, liver, kidneys, and brain (Woodhead *et al.*, 1983; Woodhead 1984; Woodhead *et al.*, 1984). These anatomical changes in various organs during aging have also been noted in other teleost species, confirming an increase in degenerative changes and pathological symptoms with age (Patnaik *et al.*, 1994). One method of manipulating longevity, caloric restriction, has been documented to extend the lifespan of some mammals (Weindruch 1996). Similarly, dietary restriction has been shown to retard the aging processes in several teleost species showing gradual senescence (Patnaik *et al.*, 1994), underscoring the similarities between the biology of aging in fish and mammals. While caloric restriction studies utilizing zebrafish have not yet been reported, preliminary studies are underway to determine its effects in zebrafish (Gerhard *et al.*, 2002a). Taken together, these results support a commonality in mechanism of aging processes in vertebrates.

Fish have several advantages for use as a model for the study of aging (reviewed by Woodhead 1978; Patnaik *et al.*, 1994), including the availability of large cohorts of offspring from single matings, their ectothermic nature which facilitates modulation by external environmental changes, and lower costs for breeding and maintenance. Zebrafish may serve as an excellent model of the biology of aging, particularly allowing for the identification of longevity assurance genes (genes that promote longevity). The zebrafish is readily amenable to large-scale mutagenesis studies which may detect and discover genes involved in pathways of the aging process. Generation of mutations and screening for mutant phenotypes can be achieved faster, on a larger scale, and more cost effectively than in mammalian systems (reviewed in

Gerhard *et al.*, 2002b). Thus, the zebrafish is an experimentally expedient organism similar to invertebrate models such as *C. elegans* and *Drosophila*, but with the anatomic and physiological complexities of a vertebrate.

While there are many advantages to the zebrafish as a model of aging, there are also some disadvantages which must be taken into consideration. Much like the mouse, zebrafish have a substantially longer lifespan than invertebrate models of aging such as *C. elegans* and *Drosophila*. Thus, while as a vertebrate they are phylogenetically much closer to humans than are these invertebrate models, their generation time is much longer, so aging studies utilizing zebrafish are likely to be more time consuming than with invertebrate models. Physiologically, the respiratory system of the zebrafish is very different from that of mammals, making them a poor model for studies involving respiratory physiology or respiratory diseases. In addition, zebrafish have considerable ability to regenerate tissues such as the heart (Poss *et al.*, 2002), which shows only minimal regeneration in mammals following injury, making the zebrafish a useful model for dissecting the molecular mechanisms of cardiac regeneration and comparative studies of regeneration, but perhaps limiting its usefulness for direct comparisons of regeneration in aging studies. Finally, fish are greatly influenced by their environment (Beverton 1987), and many environment variables, including temperature (Liu *et al.*, 1975), lighting (Raymond *et al.*, 1988), population density (Lorenzen *et al.*, 2002), water quality (Klontz 1995), and nutrition (Comfort 1960; Comfort 1963), must be tightly controlled in order to accurately interpret data obtained from aging studies. Despite these disadvantages, zebrafish still have many advantages and the potential for contributing to our knowledge of aging and complementing what has been learned in other organisms. Information regarding age-related changes specifically in zebrafish is very scarce. It is critical to characterize normal age-related changes in order to understand the effects of mutagenesis and transgenes in mature zebrafish.

Heat Shock Proteins

AGING AND HEAT SHOCK PROTEINS

A characteristic feature of aging is a progressive impairment in the ability to maintain homeostasis in the face of environmental challenges. Heat shock proteins (Hsps) consist of a family of proteins that modulate stresses to the body. Hsps are ubiquitous, highly conserved proteins that have been found in the cells of all organisms studied thus far, including plants, bacteria, yeast, flies, and vertebrates. They are part of a multigene family that has been divided into 6 subfamilies based on molecular size, ranging from 8 to 150 kD (Jaattela 1999). Some are expressed constitutively, whereas others are induced by various types of metabolic or environmental stresses such as heat, ischemia, heavy metal ions, ethanol, nicotine, viral agents, surgical stress, and reactive oxygen species. Hsps are expressed in response to a mild stress which allows the cells to adapt to gradual changes in their environment and survive otherwise lethal conditions (Welch 1992; Whitley *et al.*, 1999). Transcription of Hsp genes requires the activation and translocation to the nucleus of heat shock transcription factors (Hsfs), which recognize sequence elements (heat shock elements — HSEs) located within the Hsp gene promoters. The HSE consists of a series of pentameric units (5′-nGAAn-3′) (Santoro 2000). Inactive Hsfs exist as monomers bound to Hsp70 and other chaperones. Once activated, they trimerize into an active form that is capable of binding to the promoter site of the stress protein gene and initiating transcription and translation (Whitley *et al.*, 1999).

The expression of various types of Hsp protein and mRNA levels in response to heat stress has been shown to decrease with age in a variety of species from flies to rats. Old fruit flies were found to have a loss of resistance to oxidative stress induced by heat shock. This loss correlated with an increase in protein damage and a decrease in protection from the heat shock proteins (Fleming *et al.*, 1992). The expression of protein and mRNA levels in members of the Hsp70 family in response to heat shock was found to be decreased with age in rat neurons (Pardue *et al.*, 1992), hepatocytes (Rogue *et al.*, 1993; Wu *et al.*, 1993), and myocardium (Locke *et al.*, 1996). Based on measurements of Hsp70 mRNA stability and transcription in rat hepatocytes, it was demonstrated that the age-related decline in Hsp70 expression was a result of a decline in Hsp70 transcription. Interestingly, this age-related decrease in Hsp70 expression was reversible with caloric restriction. Caloric restriction is the only experimental manipulation known to retard aging and increase survival in mammals (Heydari *et al.*, 1993). In addition, this decline in Hsp70 transcription correlated with a decrease in the binding of Hsf1 to the heat shock element. This decreased binding activity was not due to reduced levels of Hsf1. In fact, Hsf1 levels were actually higher in hepatocytes from old rats, apparently due to a decrease in the degradation of Hsf1 since Hsf1 mRNA levels do not change and the synthesis of Hsf1 decreases with age (Heydari *et al.*, 2000). Similarly, hearts from aged rats exposed to heat stress demonstrated a reduction in Hsf1 activation, Hsp72 mRNA, and Hsp72 protein content, though myocardial Hsf1 protein content was similar between age groups (Locke *et al.*, 1996). Thus, it appears that during aging, the levels of Hsf1 remain constant, but the ability of this transcription factor to bind DNA is decreased in aged animals.

An age-related decline in Hsp72 expression was also seen in organ-cultured samples of normal human skin. Although the time course of Hsp72 expression was similar in both young and aged groups, a lower level of induction was achieved in the aged group (Muramatsu *et al.*, 1996). A similar decline in Hsp47 expression is seen in aged mouse and human fibroblasts exposed to heat stress.

Hsp47 is a collagen-specific chaperone which participates in the processing and secretion of procollagen in the ER. This decline was regulated by transcriptional mechanisms and was characterized by a greater retention of procollagen molecules in the ER lumen of cells from old subjects (Miyaishi *et al.*, 1995). Similarly, cultures of primary human peripheral lymphocytes exposed to heat stress revealed an age-related attenuation in the expression of many heat shock proteins, including Hsp70, Hsp90, Hsp60 (Rao *et al.*, 1999). Murine and human fibroblasts also showed a decline in heat shock protein expression with age upon heat treatment (Miyaishi *et al.*, 1995).

Given the central role of Hsps in cellular homeostasis, it seems likely that an impaired ability to produce Hsps in aging cells in response to stress could contribute to the increased incidence of infections and general morbidity and mortality that is seen in the elderly when exposed to stress.

ZEBRAFISH AND HSPS

A variety of heat shock proteins and the heat shock transcription factor Hsf1 have been identified and cloned from zebrafish (Krone *et al.*, 1994; Graser *et al.*, 1996; Lele *et al.*, 1997b; Santacruz *et al.*, 1997; Rabergh *et al.*, 2000). Many of these heat shock genes exhibit complex patterns of constitutive and inducible expression during embryonic development (Krone *et al.*, 1997). For example, the Hsp90alpha gene is expressed at low levels constitutively but is strongly upregulated during heat shock, whereas Hsp90beta is expressed at much higher levels constitutively but is only weakly induced following heat shock in all stages of development examined in zebrafish embryos (Krone *et al.*, 1994). Hsp70 and Hsp47 mRNA levels have also been shown to increase dramatically in response to heat stress, whereas the constitutively expressed heat shock cognate hsc70 exhibits only a slight increase. In contrast, exposure of zebrafish embryos to ethanol strongly induced Hsp47 but not Hsp70, demonstrating a differential response of the Hsps in zebrafish embryos (Lele *et al.*, 1997a). Two isoforms of Hsf1, termed zHsf1a and zHsf1b, have been identified and cloned in zebrafish and are expressed in a tissue-specific fashion upon exposure to heat stress. Specifically, both forms are expressed in the gonads under all conditions, but in the liver zHsf1a is increased with heat shock whereas zHsf1b is decreased, indicating a unique, tissue-specific regulation of Hsf1 upon exposure to increased temperatures (Rabergh *et al.*, 2000).

We have shown that mature zebrafish respond to heat shock with both nuclear translocation of Hsf1 and production of several Hsps in a variety of tissues (Murtha *et al.*, 2003a), similar to what has been reported in other species. More specifically, we found that Hsp70 and Hsp47 were induced in response to heat stress in a tissue-specific manner, while Hsp90α, Hsp90β, and Hsf1 were expressed constitutively and not induced by heat stress. Though Hsf1 RNA levels did not change with heat stress, Hsf1 protein translocated to the nucleus following heat stress, indicating activation of this transcription factor. Mammalian species show a similar pattern of Hsp and Hsf expression and Hsf activation in response to heat stress (Santoro, 2000). Furthermore, we found that aging modulates heat shock responsiveness and Hsp70 expression in zebrafish. Specifically, both basal and induced levels of Hsp70 were less in mature versus young zebrafish, which is consistent with previous reports in a variety of other species (Heydari *et al.*, 1994; Kregel *et al.*, 1995; Lee *et al.*, 1996; Liu *et al.*, 1996; Pahlavani *et al.*, 1996). We also observed that Hsf1 mRNA levels were elevated in mature compared to young zebrafish and that heat shock did not induce Hsf1 mRNA expression in either age group but did induce nuclear translocation. This is also consistent with previous reports on Hsf1 expression and induction in other species (Locke *et al.*, 1996; Heydari *et al.*, 2000; Locke, 2000), in which Hsp70 levels are diminished with age in the face of increased Hsf1 levels, which is thought to be due to a decreased ability of Hsf1 to bind DNA in aged animals. This provides evidence that zebrafish can serve as a novel vertebrate model to study the mechanisms of aging and response to environmental stress. In addition, these results also have the potential to elucidate the mechanisms underlying many disease processes which show abnormal Hsp expression, including atherosclerosis, congestive heart failure, fever, infection, Alzheimer's disease, cancer, and autoimmune disease (Whitley *et al.*, 1999).

Summary

The zebrafish has tremendous potential as a model of human disease and aging. It is already proving to be an excellent model for several human diseases, and there is an increasing wealth of resources available to the zebrafish community. In addition, aging phenotypes and age-associated molecular changes in pathways such as the heat shock response have been demonstrated in zebrafish, and zebrafish have been shown to have many similarities to aging mammals including gross, cellular, and molecular characteristics. Despite the many advantages to using mature zebrafish as an animal model, it has been underutilized in studies of aging and adult-onset or age-related diseases. Studies regarding normal physiology and age-related changes in zebrafish are very scarce, and it is critical to more fully characterize mature zebrafish in order to understand the effects of mutagenesis and transgenes in mature zebrafish. Characterization of normal zebrafish biology and physiology, as well as defining molecular mechanisms of stress response and aging, should help provide a foundation for future studies utilizing adult zebrafish.

ACKNOWLEDGMENTS

This work was supported by National Institute of Aging grant #R01-AG-21866.

REFERENCES

Amatruda, J.F., Shepard, J.L., Stern, H.M., Zon, L.I., 2002. Zebrafish as a cancer model system. Cancer Cell 1, 229–231.

Amatruda, J.F., Zon, L.I., 1999. Dissecting hematopoiesis and disease using the zebrafish. *Dev Biol 216*, 1–15.

Beverton, R.J., 1987. Longevity in fish: Some ecological and evolutionary considerations. *Basic Life Sci 42*, 161–185.

Brownlie, A., Donovan, A., Pratt, S.J., Paw, B.H., Oates, A.C., Brugnara, C., *et al.*, 1998. Positional cloning of the zebrafish sauternes gene: A model for congenital sideroblastic anaemia. *Nat Genet 20*, 244–250.

Comfort, A., 1960. The effect of age on growth-resumption in fish (Lebistes) checked by food restriction. *Gerontologia 4*, 177–186.

Comfort, A., 1961. Age and reproduction in female Lebistes. *Gerontologia 5*, 146–149.

Comfort, A., 1963. Effect of delayed and resumed growth on the longevity of a fish (*Lebistes reticulatus*, Peters) in captivity. *Gerontologia 49*, 150–155.

Conway, G., Margoliath, A., Wong-Madden, S., Roberts, R.J., Gilbert, W., 1997. Jak1 kinase is required for cell migrations and anterior specification in zebrafish embryos. *Proc Natl Acad Sci USA 94*, 3082–3087.

Detrich, H.W., 3rd, Westerfield, M., Zon, L.I., 1999. Overview of the Zebrafish system. *Methods Cell Biol 59*, 3–10.

Dooley, K., Zon, L.I., 2000. Zebrafish: A model system for the study of human disease. *Curr Opin Genet Dev 10*, 252–256.

Fleming, J.E., Reveillaud, I., Niedzwiecki, A., 1992. Role of oxidative stress in *Drosophila* aging. *Mutat Res 275*, 267–279.

Gerhard, G.S., Cheng, K.C., 2002a. A call to fins! Zebrafish as a gerontological model. *Aging Cell 1*, 104–111.

Gerhard, G.S., Kauffman, E.J., Wang, X., Stewart, R., Moore, J.L., Kasales, C.J., *et al.*, 2002b. Life spans and senescent phenotypes in two strains of Zebrafish (*Danio rerio*). *Exp Gerontol 37*, 1055–1068.

Graser, R.T., Malnar-Dragojevic, D., Vincek, V., 1996. Cloning and characterization of a 70 kd heat shock cognate (hsc70) gene from the zebrafish (*Danio rerio*). *Genetica 98*, 273–276.

Herrera, M., Jagadeeswaran, P., 2004. Annual fish as a genetic model for aging. *J Gerontol A Biol Sci Med Sci 59*, B101–107.

Heydari, A.R., Takahashi, R., Gutsmann, A., You, S., Richardson, A., 1994. Hsp70 and aging. *Experientia 50*, 1092–1098.

Heydari, A.R., Wu, B., Takahashi, R., Strong, R., Richardson, A., 1993. Expression of heat shock protein 70 is altered by age and diet at the level of transcription. *Mol Cell Biol 13*, 2909–2918.

Heydari, A.R., You, S., Takahashi, R., Gutsmann-Conrad, A., Sarge, K.D., Richardson, A., 2000. Age-related alterations in the activation of heat shock transcription factor 1 in rat hepatocytes. *Exp Cell Res 256*, 83–93.

Jaattela, M., 1999. Heat shock proteins as cellular lifeguards. *Ann Med 31*, 261–271.

Karlovich, C.A., John, R.M., Ramirez, L., Stainier, D.Y., Myers, R.M., 1998. Characterization of the Huntington's disease (HD) gene homologue in the zebrafish *Danio rerio*. *Gene 217*, 117–125.

Kishi, S., Uchiyama, J., Baughman, A.M., Goto, T., Lin, M.C., Tsai, S.B., 2003. The zebrafish as a vertebrate model of functional aging and very gradual senescence. *Exp Gerontol 38*, 777–786.

Klontz, G.W., 1995. Care of fish in biological research. *J Anim Sci 73*, 3485–3492.

Knapik, E.W., Goodman, A., Ekker, M., Chevrette, M., Delgado, J., Neuhauss, S., *et al.*, 1998. A microsatellite genetic linkage map for zebrafish (*Danio rerio*) [see comments]. *Nat Genet 18*, 338–343.

Kregel, K.C., Moseley, P.L., Skidmore, R., Gutierrez, J.A., Guerriero, V., Jr., 1995. HSP70 accumulation in tissues of heat-stressed rats is blunted with advancing age. *J Appl Physiol 79*, 1673–1678.

Krone, P.H., Lele, Z., Sass, J.B., 1997. Heat shock genes and the heat shock response in zebrafish embryos. *Biochem Cell Biol 75*, 487–497.

Krone, P.H., Sass, J.B., 1994. HSP 90 alpha and HSP 90 beta genes are present in the zebrafish and are differentially regulated in developing embryos. *Biochem Biophys Res Commun 204*, 746–752.

Lee, Y.K., Manalo, D., Liu, A.Y., 1996. Heat shock response, heat shock transcription factor and cell aging. *Biol Signals 5*, 180–191.

Leimer, U., Lun, K., Romig, H., Walter, J., Grunberg, J., Brand, M., Haass, C., 1999. Zebrafish (*Danio rerio*) presenilin promotes aberrant amyloid beta-peptide production and requires a critical aspartate residue for its function in amyloidogenesis. *Biochemistry 38*, 13602–13609.

Lele, Z., Engel, S., Krone, P.H., 1997a. hsp47 and hsp70 gene expression is differentially regulated in a stress- and tissue-specific manner in zebrafish embryos. *Dev Genet 21*, 123–133.

Lele, Z., Krone, P.H., 1997b. Expression of genes encoding the collagen-binding heat shock protein (Hsp47) and type II collagen in developing zebrafish embryos. *Mech Dev 61*, 89–98.

Liao, E.C., Paw, B.H., Oates, A.C., Pratt, S.J., Postlethwait, J.H., Zon, L.I., 1998. SCL/Tal-1 transcription factor acts downstream of cloche to specify hematopoietic and vascular progenitors in zebrafish. *Genes Dev 12*, 621–626.

Liu, A.Y., Lee, Y.K., Manalo, D., Huang, L.E., 1996. Attenuated heat shock transcriptional response in aging: Molecular mechanism and implication in the biology of aging. *Exs 77*, 393–408.

Liu, R.K., Walford, R.L., 1975. Mid-life temperature-transfer effects on life-span of annual fish. *J Gerontol 30*, 129–131.

Locke, M., 2000. Heat shock transcription factor activation and hsp72 accumulation in aged skeletal muscle. *Cell Stress Chaperones 5*, 45–51.

Locke, M., Tanguay, R.M., 1996. Diminished heat shock response in the aged myocardium. *Cell Stress Chaperones 1*, 251–260.

Lorenzen, K., Enberg, K., 2002. Density-dependent growth as a key mechanism in the regulation of fish populations: Evidence from among-population comparisons. *Proc R Soc Lond B Biol Sci 269*, 49–54.

Miyaishi, O., Ito, Y., Kozaki, K., Sato, T., Takechi, H., Nagata, K., Saga, S., 1995. Age-related attenuation of HSP47 heat response in fibroblasts. *Mech Ageing Dev 77*, 213–226.

Monnot, M.J., Babin, P.J., Poleo, G., Andre, M., Laforest, L., Ballagny, C., Akimenko, M.A., 1999. Epidermal expression of apolipoprotein E gene during fin and scale development and fin regeneration in zebrafish. *Dev Dyn 214*, 207–215.

Muramatsu, T., Hatoko, M., Tada, H., Shirai, T., Ohnishi, T., 1996. Age-related decrease in the inductability of heat shock protein 72 in normal human skin. *Br J Dermatol 134*, 1035–1038.

Murtha, J.M., Keller, E.T., 2003a. Characterization of the heat shock response in mature zebrafish (*Danio rerio*). *Exp Gerontol 38*, 683–691.

Murtha, J.M., Qi, W., Keller, E.T., 2003b. Hematologic and serum biochemical values for zebrafish (*Danio rerio*). *Comparative Medicine 53*, 37–41.

Oates, A.C., Brownlie, A., Pratt, S.J., Irvine, D.V., Liao, E.C., Paw, B.H., *et al.*, 1999. Gene duplication of zebrafish JAK2 homologs is accompanied by divergent embryonic expression patterns: Only jak2a is expressed during erythropoiesis. *Blood 94*, 2622–2636.

Pahlavani, M.A., Harris, M.D., Moore, S.A., Richardson, A., 1996. Expression of heat shock protein 70 in rat spleen lymphocytes is affected by age but not by food restriction. *J Nutr 126*, 2069–2075.

Pardue, S., Groshan, K., Raese, J.D., Morrison-Bogorad, M., 1992. Hsp70 mRNA induction is reduced in neurons of aged rat hippocampus after thermal stress. *Neurobiol Aging 13*, 661–672.

Patnaik, B.K., Mahapatro, N., Jena, B.S., 1994. Ageing in fishes. *Gerontology 40*, 113–132.

Poss, K.D., Wilson, L.G., Keating, M.T., 2002. Heart regeneration in zebrafish. *Science 298*, 2188–2190.

Rabergh, C.M., Airaksinen, S., Soitamo, A., Bjorklund, H.V., Johansson, T., Nikinmaa, M., Sistonen, L., 2000. Tissue-specific expression of zebrafish (*Danio rerio*) heat shock factor 1 mRNAs in response to heat stress [In Process Citation]. *J Exp Biol 203 Pt 12*, 1817–1824.

Rao, D.V., Watson, K., Jones, G.L., 1999. Age-related attenuation in the expression of the major heat shock proteins in human peripheral lymphocytes. *Mech Ageing Dev 107*, 105–118.

Raymond, P.A., Bassi, C.J., Powers, M.K., 1988. Lighting conditions and retinal development in goldfish: Photoreceptor number and structure. *Invest Ophthalmol Vis Sci 29*, 27–36.

Rogue, P.J., Ritz, M.F., Malviya, A.N., 1993. Impaired gene transcription and nuclear protein kinase C activation in the brain and liver of aged rats. *FEBS Lett 334*, 351–354.

Santacruz, H., Vriz, S., Angelier, N., 1997. Molecular characterization of a heat shock cognate cDNA of zebrafish, hsc70, and developmental expression of the corresponding transcripts. *Dev Genet 21*, 223–233.

Santoro, M.G., 2000. Heat shock factors and the control of the stress response. *Biochem Pharmacol 59*, 55–63.

Sprague, J., Clements, D., Conlin, T., Edwards, P., Frazer, K., Schaper, K., *et al.*, 2003. The Zebrafish Information Network (ZFIN): The zebrafish model organism database. *Nucleic Acids Res 31*, 241–243.

Stern, H.M., Zon, L.I., 2003. Cancer genetics and drug discovery in the zebrafish. *Nat Rev Cancer 3*, 533–539.

Sun, Z., Hopkins, N., 2001. vhnf1, the MODY5 and familial GCKD-associated gene, regulates regional specification of the zebrafish gut, pronephros, and hindbrain. *Genes Dev 15*, 3217–3229.

Ward, A.C., Lieschke, G.J., 2002. The zebrafish as a model system for human disease. *Front Biosci 7*, d827–833.

Weindruch, R., 1996. The retardation of aging by caloric restriction: Studies in rodents and primates. *Toxicol Pathol 24*, 742–745.

Weinstein, B.M., Schier, A.F., Abdelilah, S., Malicki, J., Solnica-Krezel, L., Stemple, D.L., *et al.*, 1996. Hematopoietic mutations in the zebrafish. *Development 123*, 303–309.

Welch, W.J., 1992. Mammalian stress response: Cell physiology, structure/function of stress proteins, and implications for medicine and disease. *Physiol Rev 72*, 1063–1081.

Westerfield, M., 1995. *The Zebrafish Book. Guide for the Laboratory Use of Zebrafish (Danio rerio)*. Univ. of Oregon Press, Eugene, OR.

Whitley, D., Goldberg, S.P., Jordan, W.D., 1999. Heat shock proteins: A review of the molecular chaperones. *J Vasc Surg 29*, 748–751.

Wienholds, E., van Eeden, F., Kosters, M., Mudde, J., Plasterk, R.H., Cuppen, E., 2003. Efficient target-selected mutagenesis in zebrafish. *Genome Res 13*, 2700–2707.

Woodhead, A.D., 1978. Fish in studies of aging. *Exp Gerontol 13*, 125–140.

Woodhead, A.D., 1984. Aging changes in the heart of a poeciliid fish, the guppy *Poecilia reticulatus*. *Exp Gerontol 19*, 383–391.

Woodhead, A.D., 1998. Aging, the fishy side: An appreciation of Alex Comfort's studies. *Exp Gerontol 33*, 39–51.

Woodhead, A.D., Pond, V., 1984. Aging changes in the optic tectum of the guppy *Poecilia* (Lebistes) *reticulatus*. *Exp Gerontol 19*, 305–311.

Woodhead, A.D., Pond, V., Dailey, K., 1983. Aging changes in the kidneys of two poeciliid fishes, the guppy *Poecilia reticulatus* and the Amazon molly *P. formosa*. *Exp Gerontol 18*, 211–221.

Wu, B., Gu, M.J., Heydari, A.R., Richardson, A., 1993. The effect of age on the synthesis of two heat shock proteins in the hsp70 family. *J Gerontol 48*, B50–56.

28

Zebrafish as Aging Models

Shuji Kishi

Zebrafish (Danio rerio) are well recognized as a powerful model for genetic studies in developmental biology. The zebrafish system has also given insights into several human diseases such as neurodegenerative, hematopoietic and cardiovascular diseases and cancer. The aging process affects these and various other human disorders, and it is important to compare age-related disfunctions at the organismal levels among vertebrates. From the point of view in comparative and evolutionary biology of aging, the aging process of zebrafish remains largely unexplored, and little is known about functional aging and senescence, compared with higher vertebrates including mammals. In our recent studies to assess aging phenotypes in zebrafish, we identified several potential biomarkers of zebrafish aging. In aging zebrafish, we have detected senescence-associated β-galactosidase activity in skin and oxidized protein accumulation in muscle. In contrast, our initial study showed that lipofuscin granules, which accumulate in postmitotic cells, were not obvious in muscle of zebrafish at fairly advanced age. In agreement with this observation, there were continuously proliferating myocytes in muscle tissues of aged fish. More intriguingly, we found that zebrafish have constitutively abundant telomerase activity in adult somatic tissues, implicating the unlimited replicative ability of cells throughout their lives. Taken together, some stress-associated markers are up-regulated, and minor histological alterations and lesions are occasionally observed during the aging process of zebrafish. However, our current studies and other evidence of remarkable reproductive and regenerative abilities suggest that zebrafish show very gradual senescence. By using those biological and biochemical aging markers already characterized in normal zebrafish, analyses of transgenic and mutant fish be readily performed for development of zebrafish aging models for age-dependent human diseases and progeroid syndromes. These efforts will help to elucidate the role and molecular mechanisms of common or different pathways of aging among vertebrates from fish to humans and also will contribute to the discovery of possible therapeutic interventions and potential drugs applicable to many age-associated diseases in the future.

Introduction

The bony fishes (Osteichthyes) represent the largest class of vertebrates, with some 24,000 extant species. However, only limited data are available on aging and senescence of just a few of these species (Patnaik *et al.*, 1994). Several small tropical species, such as the guppy (*Lebistes reticularis*) (Reznick *et al.*, 2001; Reznick, 1997), and a species of annual fish (*Cynelobias bellottii*) (Valdesalici and Cellerino, 2003), manifest increased mortality with age typical of gradual senescence and definite lifespan (Belinsky *et al.*, 1997; Finch and Austad, 2001; Finch and Ruvkun, 2001). In addition, age-related degenerative changes characteristic of gradual senescence, such as loss of muscle fibers, endocrine abnormalities, decline in reproductive capacity, increased cancer incidence, and increases in various pathological lesions, have been documented in other fish species (Patnaik *et al.*, 1994). In comparison to these fish, the aging process of zebrafish has not yet been addressed adequately.

A number of aging theories have been proposed, including oxidative or genotoxic stress and damage, telomere metabolism, regulation of caloric restriction (CR), and control of metabolic energy rate. A growing body of evidence suggests that reactive oxygen species (ROS) may regulate the aging process and may participate in cellular replicative senescence. Consistent with a role for ROS in senescence, examination in cell-culture systems showed that older cells have higher levels of ROS than younger ones (Finkel and Holbrook, 2000). Moreover, treatment with sublethal concentrations of hydrogen peroxide induces a senescence-like phenotype in primary human and rodent fibroblast (Chen and Ames, 1994; Sohal and Weindruch, 1996; Wolf *et al.*, 2002), termed "stress-induced premature senescence" (Toussaint *et al.*, 2000). On the other hand, antioxidant treatment or low-oxygen condition prolongs the lifespan of cells (Finkel and Holbrook, 2000). The free radical theory of aging, which proposes that oxidative stress increases with age, may provide some clues to this phenomenon. Specifically, reactive oxygen intermediates (ROI) act as second messengers culminating in activation of signal transduction pathways and subsequently changes in the activity of various transcription factors. Another theory holds that cellular replicative senescence is regulated by factors that govern the shortening of telomeres in dividing cells of the adult tissues and organs.

Telomeric TTAGGG repeats in vertebrates, which protect chromosome ends, are shortened with each division of most cells in the adult due to lack of telomerase activity (Blackburn, 2001). However, compelling evidence indicates that the ability of telomerase to elongate telomeres is regulated by several other telomere-binding factors with multiple interacting proteins, which construct a huge "telosome" complex (Blackburn, 2001; Liu *et al.*, 2004; Rodier *et al.*, 2005).

The CR paradigm provides additional support for this hypothesis. CR, which decreases oxidative stress, delays the appearance of expression of several age-associated genes (Sohal and Weindruch, 1996). Use of high-density oligonucleotide arrays and genome-wide transcript profiles in mice and flies revealed that aging was accompanied by a differential gene expression pattern with indications of a marked stress response and lower expression of metabolic and biosynthetic genes (Lee *et al.*, 1999; Pletcher *et al.*, 2002; Zou *et al.*, 2000). Most alterations were either completely or partially prevented by caloric restriction, the only intervention known to retard aging in mammals. Transcriptional patterns of calorie-restricted animals suggest that caloric restriction retards the aging process by causing a metabolic shift toward increased protein turnover and decreased macromolecular damage. On the other hand, oxidative damage is repaired less well in telomeric DNA than elsewhere in the chromosome, and oxidative stress accelerates telomere loss, whereas antioxidants decelerate it. Therefore, oxidative stress is also an important modulator of telomere loss, and telomere-driven replicative senescence is primarily a stress response. Among oxidative stress, regulation of CR, and telomere metabolism, there also seems to be a significant cross-talk mechanism with each other in the course of the aging process. However, genetic evidence of this mechanism in higher vertebrates has not been elucidated yet.

The propagation of a species could depend in principle either on the unlimited maintenance of its individuals or on the ability to renew the population with young members. Nature most commonly has chosen the latter option. Renewal is typically achieved by the setting aside of a pristine lineage of genetic information in the germ line, which is passed on by sexual reproduction. In contrast, the somatic lineage of all animals declines and degenerates with age, giving rise to phenotypic changes recognized as aging. Studies in model organisms have begun to map out important genes and pathways that seem to regulate the pace of aging and that are remarkably conserved from yeast to worm and insect. These studies have the great advantage that one can use genetic approaches to search directly for mutations that change lifespan. This makes it possible to identify mechanisms in a way that is independent of any preconceived model of aging. Recently, the analysis of such mutations that affect lifespan has revealed several different pathways that influence the aging process. These include, notably, signaling molecules from the Insulin-like growth factor-1 (IGF-1)-FoxOs (the FoxO subfamily of forkhead transcription factors) pathway which are highly conserved in evolution and have been identified in yeast, flies, and worms as regulating aging (Guarente and Picard, 2005; Kenyon, 2005; Murphy *et al.*, 2003). Thus once a gene has been identified as regulating aging in lower organisms it can be tested in mice by knockout or transgenic technologies. However, our inability to do forward genetics in vertebrates places serious restrictions on the types of genes we might find. Moreover, it seems quite likely that genetic screening in invertebrates will miss genes affecting cellular proliferation in adults, which confers on mammals with their relatively longer lifespan. Additionally, those unique genes and their functions related to longevity in vertebrates are not likely to be found in unicellular organisms and other invertebrate model systems. To address these questions in a more tractable and high-throughput setting, alternative vertebrate model systems are needed. Since zebrafish offer a number of advantages for the study of diseases and for tissue and organ development, we begun utilizin zebrafish as a new vertebrate model to explore the aging and senescence process with pathophysiological phenotypes. As part of this ongoing effort, mutagenesis and transgenesis approaches are expected to be extremely useful.

Zebrafish have proven to be an outstanding animal model system for studying vertebrate development using both genetic and genomic approaches. For instance, large-scale chemical mutagenesis strategies have been used to identify numerous zebrafish mutants with developmental abnormalities or defects. However, current approaches lack the ability to demonstrate developmental imprinting and identify adult or late-age onset mutants that can perturb the aging process. Although *C. elegans* and *Drosophila* are well-established aging models which have been used to identify a number of single gene mutations resulting in extended or shortened lifespan, these relatively shorter-lived invertebrates are unlikely to provide information on essential genes and molecular mechanisms that are unique to longer-lived vertebrates as described above. For instance, it is difficult to address the organo-specific aging process in nervous, cardiovascular, immune, and musculoskeletal system of invertebrates. Moreover, invertebrates cannot be utilized to explore developmental and aging functions of vertebrate-specific features such as the kidney, a multichambered heart, multilineage hematopoiesis, a notochord, and neural crest cells.

Mutagenesis is one of the best approaches for identifying a gene function. Of vertebrates studied to date, mutations can be generated and recovered most readily in zebrafish. Furthermore, as a result of recent advances in technology, zebrafish can be utilized for both forward genetics and, importantly, reverse genetics. For example, transgenesis coupled with chemical mutagenesis can be employed for the analysis of promoter activity and specificity utilizing an effective *in vivo* reporter system such as GFP (Dodd *et al.*, 2000). It is also possible to use high-throughput transgenic approaches such as GFP-positive embryos to study the function of gene products by taking advantage of the transparency of fish during its developmental stages. More recently, the Targeting Induced Local Lesions in Genomes (TILLING) approach coupled with a direct resequencing strategy of a target gene in mutagenized genomic DNA has been developed in the zebrafish system (Henikoff *et al.*, 2004; Wienholds *et al.*, 2002; Wienholds *et al.*, 2003). This approach, along with other related methods, brings zebrafish reverse genetics to a level equivalent with that of mice. Therefore, functional genetic and genomic analysis of signaling pathways involved in aging of zebrafish will be readily possible, once we identify effective and robust aging markers.

The zebrafish system is already well established in developmental biology, and recently zebrafish models have been used in disease-based biomedical studies. In marked contrast, the aging process of zebrafish has not been significantly addressed, so that there is little known with respect to the aging process and cellular senescence in zebrafish. Susceptibility to most human chronic diseases is affected by the aging process. Therefore, it is crucial to know how zebrafish aging is compared with aging in mammals, particularly since we also view zebrafish as a useful surrogate model for multiple human diseases. Moreover, through comparative studies of aging among vertebrates, we may be able to learn how we can take advantage of the certain unique properties in lower vertebrates, such as multiple organs' regeneration and indeterminate growth, which have been lost during mammalian evolution.

Identification of Biomarkers of Zebrafish Aging and Senescence

As has already been mentioned, compared with other model organisms, the aging process of zebrafish is in a very early stage of investigation, and we are currently unable to tell precisely how the fish age physiologically, and what the pathophysiological symptoms and lesions are, in zebrafish aging and in their age-associated diseases, respectively. Therefore, first and foremost, it is important to set forth some principles for evaluating the functional aging process in zebrafish.

To determine effective biomarkers of aging in zebrafish, we have analyzed the following potential markers in zebrafish aging: (a) age-dependent accumulation of oxidative damage in proteins and lipofuscin accumulation (oxidation aging marker); (b) senescence-associated β-galactosidase (SA-β-gal) activity (enzymatic aging marker); (c) age-dependent telomere length and metabolism, and telomerase activity (telomeric aging marker); (d) age-dependent competence for caudal (tail) fin regeneration (regeneration aging marker); (e) age-associated growth rate and size in a restricted space and time period (growth size aging marker); (f) age-related changes in locomotor activity (behavioral aging marker) and age-dependent changes of activity in circadian rhythm and decline of melatonin secretion (circadian aging marker).

AGING MARKERS BASED ON OXIDATION OF MACROMOLECULES

Aerobic metabolism and the corresponding generation of ROS is the most widely recognized cause of aging, although many questions remain regarding the detailed mechanism of action of ROS in organismal aging (Chien and Karsenty, 2005; Hadley *et al.*, 2005). Several lines of evidence argue that macromolecular oxidation by ROS is responsible for functional declines or inappropriate roles of proteins, lipids, and DNA (Balaban *et al.*, 2005). It seems likely that the accumulation of these oxidized dysfunctional macromolecules becomes a hallmark of progression of aging in zebrafish, as commonly recognized in other aging animals.

Protein oxidation has been detected by estimating its carbonyl content by Western blotting analysis (Dalle-Donne *et al.*, 2003). In current studies, we have identified increasing accumulation of oxidized proteins with age in skin, muscle, and brain of zebrafish, when we examined the samples from 6 30-month-old fish. However, we have not detected difference in ovary where we observed a constant amount of oxidized proteins. We have also measured the accumulation of the oxidized lipid by-product, lipofuscin, as the "age pigment," one of the most prominent age-related cellular alterations reported in many organisms (Brunk and Terman, 2002; Terman and Brunk, 2004). Although in our initial studies, we did not detect lipofuscin accumulation in 24-month old fish, our currently updated results indicate that gradually increased accumulation of lipofuscin occurs at 30 months and even more significantly at 42-months. In addition to muscle tissues, lipofuscin accumulation was observed in brain, liver, kidney, but not intestine, with advancing age. For each experiment, we examined 10–15 fish samples, and quantified the results by image intensities of Western blotting for oxidized proteins and by capturing images to count fluorescent spots for lipofuscin. Statistical analysis of these oxidative-stress-associated markers is currently in progress, but the relevance of the markers is already evident.

SENESCENCE-ASSOCIATED (SA)-β-GALACTOSIDASE AS AN ENZYMATIC AGING MARKER

Acidic senescence-associated-β-galactosidase (SA-β-gal) is histochemically detectable at pH 6 upon senescence in cultured cells *in vitro* and aged skin *in vivo* (Dimri *et al.*, 1995). This SA-β-gal marker can differentiate between the replicatively senescent state and the simply quiescent state during growth-arrest. This marker has been used to identify senescent cells in selected tissues from several aging animal models *in vivo* (Cao *et al.*, 2003;

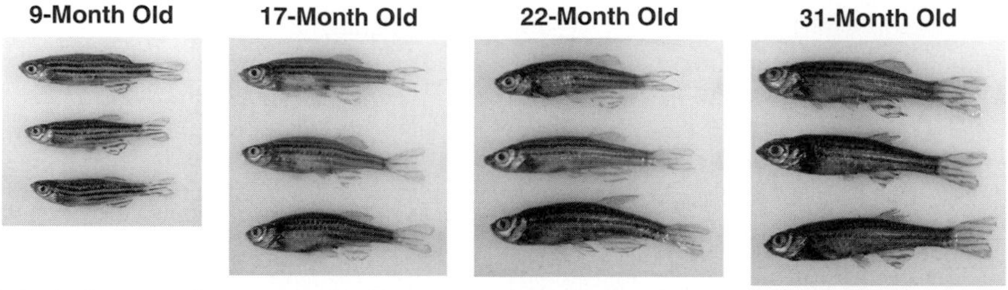

9-Month Old 17-Month Old 22-Month Old 31-Month Old

Figure 28.1. Whole-body detection of SA-β-gal activity in adult zebrafish of different ages (Kishi *et al.*, 2003). After whole-mount fixation of adult zebrafish with whole body, SA-β-gal staining was performed at pH 6 in 9, 17, 22, and 31-month-old zebrafish samples. As shown in this figure, younger 9-month-old fish exhibited very faint background staining in some abdominal regions, whereas several different levels of staining in individual fish were observed in 17- and 22-month-old fish. The staining patterns of each fish varied in these age groups. Some individuals showed fairly strong staining, while others were relatively variable. On the other hand, all examined 31-month-old fish exhibited notably intense staining over their entire bodies.

Keyes *et al.*, 2005; Varela *et al.*, 2005). We previously reported on SA-β-gal induction during the aging process in zebrafish *in vivo* (Kishi, 2004; Kishi *et al.*, 2003). We demonstrated significant increases of SA-β-gal activity in skin from aged (more than 31 months) versus young (less than 17 months) zebrafish (Kishi *et al.*, 2003) (Figure 28.1).

The presence of SA-β-gal has been determined further in 6, 18, 30, and 42-month-old fish for more than 10 fish in each age group. We have newly developed a quantitative approach through conversions of captured actual images into pixel images scored in zebrafish embryos and adults. Based on scanning of the fixed parts of the trunk region in adult fish, the images were converted into pixels, and a prominent increase of SA-β-gal intensity was found with age. In our studies, SA-β-gal activity of zebrafish appeared to correlate well with their chronological ages.

On the other hand, in zebrafish embryos under genotoxic or oxidative stress, induction of SA-β-gal was successfully measured qualitatively and quantitatively (Figure 28.2).

This will open up a new avenue for screening of potential aging mutants by the embryonic senescence phenotype in zebrafish without spending lengthy time-of-lifespan analyses.

TELOMERIC AGING MARKERS

All vertebrate telomeres contain a characteristic 6-base repeated sequence, TTAGGG (Meyne *et al.*, 1989). According to the telomere hypothesis, DNA replication in somatic cells leads to telomere shortening, which forms the basis of a cellular mitotic clock (Sherr and DePinho, 2000). Moreover, several premature aging syndromes lead to accelerated loss of telomeric DNA, which eventually results in accelerated replicative senescence of the cells (Kipling *et al.*, 2004; Metcalfe *et al.*, 1996; Pandita, 2002; von Zglinicki *et al.*, 2005). Cumulatively, these results suggest that it is also possible to ascertain aging and senescence phenotypes in zebrafish by qualitative and quantitative measurements of telomere metabolism and maintenance.

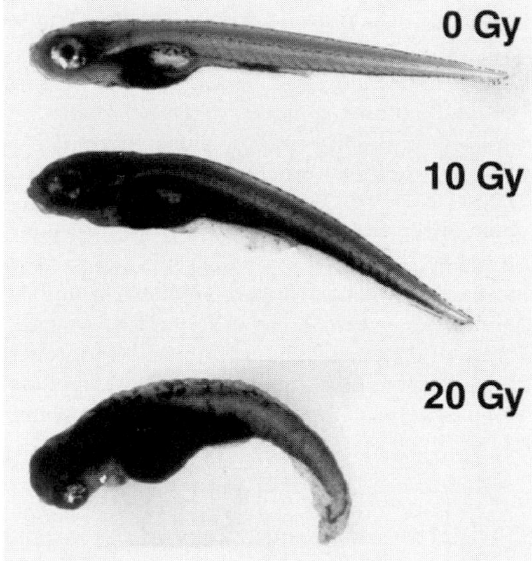

Figure 28.2. Whole-mount SA-β-gal detection of genotoxic stress-induced embryonic senescence. Wild-type zebrafish embryos were treated with IR (0, 10, and 20 Gy) at 6 hpf. Subjected embryos were raised by 6 dpf. The 6-day larval fish were fixed and stained for SA-β-gal. Both 10 and 20 Gy of IR obviously induced SA-β-gal in larval zebrafish. While 10 Gy-treated larval fish did not exhibit a particularly abnormal phenotype with more than 90% survival rate, 20 Gy-treated larval fish showed severe malformation and did not subsequently survive at all.

To detect and measure telomeric DNA in zebrafish, we have adopted a previously established procedure utilizing quantitative measurement of *in situ* hybridization (Q-FISH) with a fluorescence-labeled telomere-specific probe (Miller *et al.*, 1992). Importantly, telomeric repeat sequences of TTAGGG are conserved in all vertebrates, from fish to humans. Thus, zebrafish telomeric sequences can be detected by the same procedure used for human telomeres, utilizing a fluorescein- or Cy3-conjugated peptide nucleic acid (PNA) probe as confirmed previously (Baerlocher and Lansdorp, 2004; Sola and Gornung, 2001). Since zebrafish embryos are transparent, we can easily detect the telomere signals through fluorescence microscopy by staining with the PNA probe. We could quantify the fluorescence intensity of zebrafish telomeres by the telomere analysis program, TEL-TELO V1.0a, developed and provided by Peter Lansdorp at the Terry Fox Laboratory, as previously performed for human and mouse telomeres (Baerlocher and Lansdorp, 2004).

We have also performed Southern blot analysis to confirm telomere lengths in muscle from 6, 18, 30, and 42-month-old fish for 10 fish in each age group. Southern analysis can demonstrate length of terminal restriction fragments (TRF), containing DNA with uniform telomeric TTAGGG repeats, obtained by digestion of genomic DNA using *Hinf* I and *Rsa* I restriction enzymes in zebrafish, as well as in humans and mice. Through Southern analysis in adult fish muscle samples, we found that the telomere lengths were stochastically shortened late in the life of the fish (e.g., at more than 30 months), irrespective of their constitutive telomerase activity throughout their lives.

Telomerase is a ribonucleoprotein complex that consists of two main subunits: TR, the telomerase RNA template for addition of TTAGGG repeat sequence (telomerase RNA complex, TERC); and TERT, telomerase reverse transcriptase catalytic subunit of telomerase and other associated proteins. While TR is expressed ubiquitously and constitutively in various types of cells, TERT is not expressed in most normal somatic cells. However, stem cells and germ cells as well as approximately 80–85% of cancer cells express TERT in humans.

Zebrafish telomerase activity has been examined by Telomeric Repeat Amplification Protocol (TRAP) assay, which is a sensitive and efficient PCR-based telomerase detection method (Wright *et al.*, 1995). There is a causal relationship between telomerase expression, telomere maintenance and extension of cellular lifespan in mammalian cells. Due to tightly regulated expression of TERT as described above among normal tissues of adult humans, telomerase activity is almost undetectable except in germ-line cells, although very small amounts of activity are detectable in bone marrow, peripheral blood lymphocytes, and skin epidermis. In addition, mice normally exhibit telomerase activity in colon, liver, ovary, and testis but not in brain, heart, stomach, and muscle. However, strikingly in zebrafish, the results showed the constitutive activation of telomerase in nearly all the tissues, including muscle, heart, and brain, throughout their lives (Kishi *et al.*, 2003) (Figure 28.3).

Once the unlimited growth potential and remarkable regeneration ability of zebrafish is appreciated, the above results may not seem surprising. On the other hand, strong link between cell proliferation and telomerase activity is biologically and evolutionarily very intriguing.

REGENERATIVE CAPACITY AS AN AGING MARKER

Several vertebrates display the ability to regenerate parts of their body after amputation. Teleost fish,

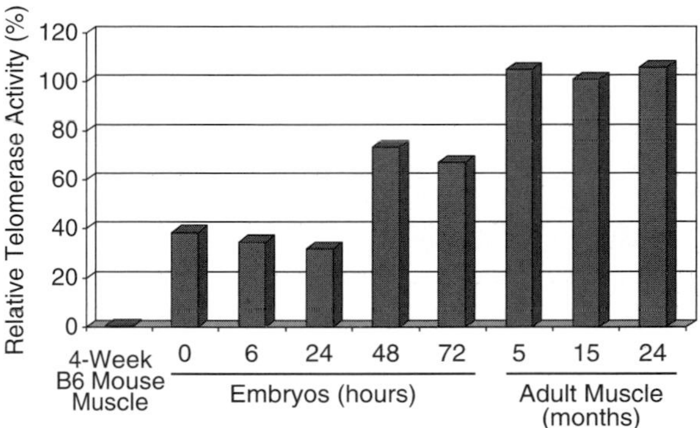

Figure 28.3. Relative telomerase activity in whole zebrafish embryos at various developmental stages (0, 6, 24, 48, and 72 hpf), and in skeletal muscle from adult fish of various ages (5, 15, and 24 months old) (Kishi *et al.*, 2003). Telomerase activity was examined by TRAP assay in extracted protein samples ($n = 3$ in each bar). Samples of B6 mouse skeletal muscle (4 weeks old) were almost undetectable levels in telomerase activity.

including zebrafish, can regenerate multiple tissues and organs, including spinal cord, retina, heart, and fins even at mature adult stages (Keating, 2004; Poss *et al.*, 2003). We have analyzed the age-dependent alterations in the ability of zebrafish to regenerate its caudal (tail) fin. Zebrafish fins normally regenerate rapidly following amputation. Regeneration occurs within a few weeks via processes resembling amphibian limb regeneration. Following amputation, differentiated bone cells apparently dedifferentiate and enter the cell cycle, rapidly divide, and migrate from the stump to form a regenerated blastema. Formation of the blastema is followed by a period of rapid growth with continued proliferation of some blastema cells matched by withdrawal of other cells to form new bone. There was clear difference in regeneration ability of caudal fin between young fish and old fish. This ability to regenerate declines with age in zebrafish as in most other fish reported. Thus, statistical analysis of data from the 18-month and 30-month-old fish provided baseline information for age-dependent decline of wound-healing and regenerative ability.

At the molecular levels in regeneration, previous experiments with regenerating fins in zebrafish have shown that members of the Msx family of homeodomain-containing transcription factors play key roles during blastema formation and patterning. Importantly, adult zebrafish have a remarkable capacity to regenerate the heart in a process that involves up-regulation of *msxB* and *msxC* genes. In addition, the hearts of zebrafish with mutations in the Mps1 mitotic checkpoint kinase, a critical cell cycle regulator, failed to regenerate and formed scars (Poss *et al.*, 2003; Poss *et al.*, 2002a; Poss *et al.*, 2002b). Preceding Msx activation (Akimenko *et al.*, 1995), there is a marked increase in the expression of Notch1b and DeltaC, which have been shown to be up-regulated during fin and heart regeneration (Raya *et al.*, 2003), suggesting a role for the Notch signaling pathway in the activation of the regenerative response. In this regard, Notch activation is at the base of the decisive event for proliferation and/or differentiation in a number of resident stem cells (Conboy *et al.*, 2005; Raya *et al.*, 2003), including those of hematopoietic, neural, gastrointestinal, and skeletal muscle lineages. Whether such stem or progenitor cells exist in zebrafish regenerative tissues and organs, whether they play a role in the regenerative response, and whether they are the origin of constitutive telomerase activity remain to be elucidated. The involvement of the Notch signaling pathway during regeneration is of biological and biomedical importance and warrants further investigation in connection with by telomerase and telomere regulation. Thus, in the next stage of regeneration studies on zebrafish aging, it will be required to investigate the molecular network in detail, taking into consideration aging stem cells. Advances in regeneration studies in zebrafish aging will undoubtedly aid in the implementation of strategies for regenerative medicine in human aging.

GROWTH RATE AND OVERALL SIZE AS AGING MARKERS

Most organisms exhibit determinate growth—up to the point at which growth no longer occurs. However, indeterminate growth may occur when it offers advantages in fitness or reproductive prowess. It was already hypothesized that zebrafish exhibit a capacity for unlimited growth (Gerhard *et al.*, 2002), and our study supported this notion. This is clearly different from humans and other mammals that cease growing after reaching sexual maturation (Figure 28.4).

This indefinite growth regulation may indicate an evolutional attempt to compensate for senescence with age. Similarly, age did not seem to simply deter continued growth, as small aged fish retained comparable ability to grow as small young fish. Instead, growth merely slowed as body size increased regardless of age.

On a different note, other factors such as environmental conditions can play a pivotal role in modulating growth regulation. Indeed, we have demonstrated that given adequate nourishment, living space available or density conditions directly governed the mean final size reached by fish in each tank. It may be postulated that density could act as a trigger to stop growth and to affect other processes by stimulating some sort of "space" sensors in zebrafish that allow them monitor their own surroundings, analogous to normal cells that stop division in response to contact inhibition. Alternatively, high density conditions may stimulate some form of communication with other members within close proximity, simulating the function of pheromones in insects. While this remains to be elucidated in future studies, it was important for us to establish

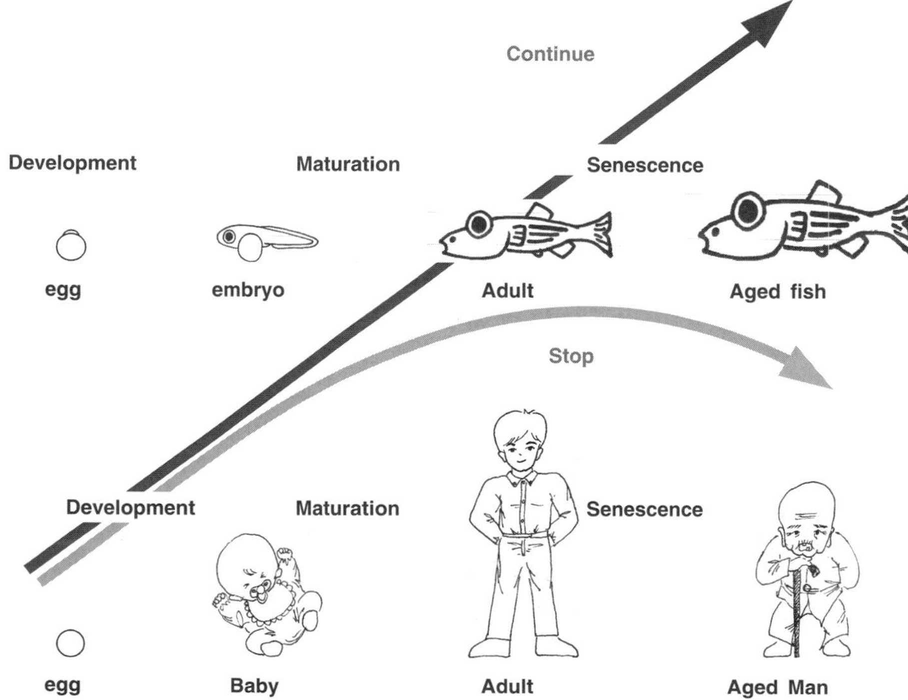

Figure 28.4. Potential differences in growth and aging between zebrafish and humans. Zebrafish continue growth past sexual maturation throughout life, with remarkable regenerative capability given adequate food, space, and good husbandry. On the other hand, human and other mammals cease growing after reaching sexual maturation as their function of age. The illustration provided here is modified from the original Japanese literature, having the translated title "Learning Biology through Medaka Fish," which was written by Nobuo Egami in 1989.

density-dependence of growth before undertaking further experiments on zebrafish growth and aging.

Our current data suggest that the propensity to grow can decrease with increased size, but not simply chronological age. Both older (18–30 months) and younger (6–18 months) fish exhibited similar patterns of growth throughout their lives as long as their sizes are almost same, indicating that they are similar in "biological age" albeit different in chronological ages. Subsequently, growth never clearly plateaued or stopped altogether up to the end of the final measurement, supporting the indefinite growth in zebrafish.

IGF-1 is known to play crucial roles in growth and development in all vertebrates. Several lines of evidence from studies in a variety of vertebrate species suggest that the ligands (IGFs), receptors (IGF receptors), and ligand-binding proteins (IGF-binding proteins) evolved early during vertebrate evolution (Barbieri *et al.*, 2003; Katic and Kahn, 2005). While central action sites of IGF-1 in invertebrates and higher vertebrates are currently well understood, little is known in the teleost models where their tissues and organs sometimes undergo continual and indeterminate growth, except for some fish of commercial importance. However, the IGF-1 signal that involves downstream signaling molecules, such as members in the protein deacetylase Sir2 family or the forkhead transcription factors FoxO subgroup, is believed to be one of the most prominent aging-associated pathways. Actually, CR definitely links up with the IGF-1 signaling pathway. In this respect, there is an exception to the common notion that CR extends lifespan in some fish, because "ferox trout" achieve long life by eating more, not less (Mangel and Abrahams, 2001). Most recently, the life span of guppies with CR (low food) was not extended, compared with the high-food population, and total fecundity are higher in high-food population with reproduction throughout their lives and with subsequent reproductive senescence (Reznick *et al.*, 2004). Thus apparent patterns of senescence in guppies derived from natural populations, with respect to either mortality or reproduction, were not simply controlled by levels of food availability in the laboratory, according to the common notion. Therefore, fish may have alternative or different control mechanisms of the IGF-1/Sir2/FoxO pathways in their fitness. Further investigations of this pathway in the zebrafish model may reveal a novel control mechanism between CR and aging in lower vertebrates.

AGING MARKERS BASED ON BEHAVIOR AND CIRCADIAN RHYTHMS

We are also attempting to document age-related changes in behavior and circadian rhythms of adult zebrafish. These studies on zebrafish aging markers have been pursued in collaboration with Irina Zhdanova at the Boston University School of Medicine.

It has been reported that zebrafish is a diurnal vertebrate with a clear circadian pattern of daytime activity and nighttime rest (Cahill, 1996; Cahill, 2002; Dekens *et al.*, 2003; Delaunay *et al.*, 2000; Hurd *et al.*, 1998; Kazimi and Cahill, 1999). Zhdanova has been studying the sleep-like state in zebrafish, using a high-throughput image-analysis system (Zhdanova *et al.*, 2001). Previous studies have shown that the sleep-like state in zebrafish has fundamental similarities with sleep in mammals, including characteristic postures, elevated arousal threshold to sensory stimulation and a compensatory rest rebound following rest deprivation (Zhdanova *et al.*, 2001). "Sleep" in zebrafish can be induced by conventional hypnotics, diazepam and sodium pentobarbital, and the circadian hormone melatonin (Zhdanova *et al.*, 2001). While the age-related decline in human sleep is a well-known phenomenon, it is not yet established whether this is true in lower vertebrates.

In order to determine whether sleep alteration could be a sensitive behavioral marker of aging, we have assessed the effects of zebrafish age on the sleep-like state. Using image analysis of locomotor activity, we documented the overall duration and continuity of sleep-like behavior (defined as period of immobility of 3 min or more, with increased arousal threshold) and changes in arousal threshold during this behavioral state in young and aged zebrafish adults. Our results on the intrinsic circadian rhythm of activity in larval and adult zebrafish maintained under constant conditions have also shown that the endogenous circadian period becomes more variable in adults, compared with larval fish. This might result from the weakening of the circadian oscillator with age or reduction in nighttime melatonin secretion.

By conducting a continuous 10-day analysis of zebrafish locomotor activity under constant conditions, we have compared the amplitude and period of the circadian rhythm in fish of 12 and 36 months of age and determined whether these circadian parameters might serve as a useful marker of aging. Preliminary results comparing locomotor activity in young (12-month-old) and old (36-month-old) zebrafish suggest that aging may be associated with an increased stochastic variability in locomotion. If these results are confirmed in a larger sample, extreme changes in locomotor activity might potentially represent an interesting biological marker of aging in zebrafish.

We have also assessed the circadian rhythm of melatonin production (levels in the pineal gland) and excretion (levels in the surrounding water). There are two major reasons to use melatonin levels as a prospective biological marker in zebrafish aging studies. In humans, melatonin secretion is known to be highest in children of 3–5 years of age, and to decline with age. Similar age dependency of melatonin levels was documented in other species as well. In our preliminary results, adult zebrafish also have significantly lower melatonin production, compared to zebrafish larvae. We are assessing whether melatonin levels further decline in aged fish, by comparing melatonin production in young and old zebrafish. In addition, the assessment of the circadian rhythm of melatonin production is widely considered to be the most sensitive way to document individual phases of the circadian rhythm and its changes. In zebrafish, a temporal pattern of melatonin secretion can be determined by measuring melatonin levels in different tissues, including the pineal gland or brain. Importantly, the relatively high amounts of melatonin excreted into the medium (surrounding water) allow the melatonin rhythm to be repetitively sampled without disturbing the animal. We have successfully used both methods in our studies of zebrafish circadian physiology. Thus, we can longitudinally measure melatonin excretion in individual fish from young to old age (6-months to 42-months old), in order to establish whether the decline in the circadian amplitude and/or the degree of entrainment to environmental cues can serve as useful biomarkers of aging in zebrafish.

Effects of Oxidative Stress and Genotoxic Stress on Zebrafish Aging and Senescence

Several lines of evidence suggest that genotoxic or oxidative stress promote the aging process (Campisi, 2005; Finkel and Holbrook, 2000; Lombard *et al.*, 2005). It is well known that the aging process diminishes the capability to adapt to environmental stresses. We hypothesized that genotoxic and oxidative stress leads to mutations and general declines in reproductive ability, ultimately producing the spectrum of age-related characteristics in zebrafish. Support for this idea comes from the fact that radiation increases genetic mutations and leads to premature aging in animals, such as mice and Medaka fish (*Oryzias latipes*) (Curtis, 1963; Egami and Eto, 1973; Ferbeyre and Lowe, 2002; Trifunovic *et al.*, 2004; Tyner *et al.*, 2002; Celeste *et al.*, 2002). Therefore, we have subjected embryos and adult zebrafish to genotoxic or oxidative stress and measured aging markers over the lifespan of the fish. To determine the effects of genotoxic and oxidative stresses on zebrafish aging, we have analyzed the effects of ionizing radiation (IR) and hydrogen peroxide (HP)/t-butyl hydroperoxide (tBH) on both embryos and adults using the markers already described. For quantitative aging markers we expect to see changes in activity that correlate with age; the rate of change should also correlate with the stress applied. In this manner, we can detect changes in aging in fish in a much shorter time intervals than would be required to measure mortality rates.

Typical features of cells derived from humans with premature aging syndromes include hypersensitivity to genotoxic stress and DNA damage such as IR (Cheng *et al.*, 2004; Naka *et al.*, 2004; Nove *et al.*, 1986; Smith and Paterson, 1980; Thacker, 1994). It has been reported that IR during embryogenesis shortens the lifespan in Medaka fish (Egami and Eto, 1973). Although shortened lifespan was demonstrated, no other phenotypic markers of aging were reported at that time. An aging phenotype induced by IR was also observed in mice (Curtis, 1963). IR has been used to perform mutagenesis in zebrafish, whereas the biological effects of IR on the fish themselves have not been examined in detail. To address this question, we initially exposed zebrafish adults and embryos to several doses of IR and observed the short-term as well as long-term biological effects. We have already examined radiation doses of 5 to 40 Gy for embryos (6–24 hours post fertilization, hpf) and adult fish (3 to 30 months old). Overall cell-cycle profiles and the level of apoptotic cells were studied in whole embryos by flow cytometry at 48 hpf. When embryos were irradiated at 6 hpf with 20 Gy, we observed an aberrant increase in apoptotic cells at 48 hpf, followed by subsequently causing malformation of the entire embryos later on, with decreased survival by 5 days post fertilization (dpf). In contrast, the survival rate is greater than 90% at 5 dpf in 10 Gy–irradiated animals, without obvious malformation as well as abnormal apoptosis induction in early development. Moreover, no embryos survived for more than 10 days following 20 Gy of irradiation, which may be due to an inability to start eating. Intriguingly, these embryos exposed to IR induced SA-β-gal activity by 6 dpf, indicating genotoxic stress-induced premature senescence, can be observed during the early development of zebrafish (Figure 28.2). We have raised group of embryos irradiated with 10 Gy at 6 hpf in groups at 6, 18, 30, and 42 months of ages. Each age group of embryos need to be raised to adulthood to examine the radiation effects late in life, as compared with irradiated control animals. These experiments are currently in progress.

It is noteworthy that 25–40 Gy of irradiation killed a large number of adult fish in a dose-dependent manner within 3 months after IR exposure, with possible acute lesions, as recently reported in the literature (Traver *et al.*, 2004). On the other hand, 20 Gy did not significantly affect survival rates even after 6 months postirradiation. Therefore, based on these pilot studies, we intend to examine the chronic effects of 20 Gy on adult fish during aging.

There are several lines of evidence that suggest that oxygen free radicals can contribute in an undetermined way to the aging process (Balaban *et al.*, 2005). Physiologically, superoxide is generated by the mitochondrial respiratory chain. The transformation of superoxide into HP and then, under certain conditions, into hydroxyl radicals appears to play an important role in various respiratory chain diseases (Taylor *et al.*, 2003). These may influence the aging process through mutagenesis of mitochondrial DNA (mtDNA) and an increased rate of shortening of telomeric DNA. Therefore, we are interested in the relationship between ROS production and telomere metabolism resulting from genotoxic and oxidative stress in zebrafish by measuring protein oxidation, lipid peroxidation, and the extent of oxidized DNA. The effects of ROS on telomeres seem to be mediated through the susceptibility of the telomeric GGG sites to DNA damage. ROS actively attack these telomeric regions, predisposing to DNA strand breaks and damage leading to increased telomere shortening. Importantly, fibroblasts from donors of several premature aging syndromes, such as ataxia–telengiectasia (A–T) with mutations in the *ataxia telangiectasia mutated* (*ATM*) gene and Hutchinson–Gilford progeria syndrome (HGPS) with mutations in the *lamin AC* gene (*lmna*), have short telomeres (Allsopp *et al.*, 1992; Metcalfe *et al.*, 1996; Smilenov *et al.*, 1997), consistent with reduced cell division potential *in vitro*. Recently, it has been suggested that ATM functions in the cellular response to oxidative damage (Ito *et al.*, 2004; Reliene *et al.*, 2004; Rotman and Shiloh, 1997; Watters, 2003). Support for this hypothesis comes from observations that ATM-deficient cells are very sensitive to the toxic effects of hydrogen peroxide, nitric oxide and superoxide treatment, as well as to exposure of IR (Green *et al.*, 1997; Takao *et al.*, 2000; Ziv *et al.*, 2005). Moreover, ATM-deficient mice have elevated markers of oxidative stress, particularly in organs such as the cerebellum, which are consistently affected in individuals with A–T (Barlow *et al.*, 1999a). In addition, elevated levels of Cu/Zn superoxide dismutase exacerbate specific features of the murine ATM-deficient phenotype, including abnormalities in hematopoiesis and radiosensitivity (Peter *et al.*, 2001). Accordingly, we have employed both hydrogen peroxide (HP) and t-butyl hydroperoxide (tBH) as sources of oxidative stress to zebrafish to establish baseline information. Because tBH is poorly hydrolyzed by catalase, we can examine the effect of oxidative damage irrespective of variation and difference in catalase activities in organisms. We hace exposed embryos to HP (100 μM) or tBH (300 μM) from 6 hpf for 3 days, and then raised them for 6, 18, 30, and 42 months, to observe late-onset aging phenotypes by oxidative stress early in life. These stress exposure studies examining multiple aging biomarkers already described above are currently underway.

Significance of Telomere and Telomerase in Zebrafish Aging and Senescence

As mentioned above with respect to the telomeric aging markers, the end of chromosomes termed telomeres consists of repeat sequences of TTAGGG, which are conserved in all vertebrates, from fish to humans. Telomerase is essential for maintaining telomere length and chromosome stability in stem cells, germline cells, and cancer cells. The telomerase ribonucleoprotein complex consists of two essential components, a catalytic protein component and an RNA molecule, that provide the template for telomeric repeat synthesis. Telomere shortening and telomerase activation in human somatic cells have been implicated in cell immortalization and cellular senescence. We previously reported that zebrafish have constitutive telomerase activity throughout life (Kishi, 2004; Kishi *et al.*, 2003). To study the role of telomerase and telomere in cellular immortalization and organismal mortality, we assayed telomerase activity and telomere length in primary zebrafish fibroblasts, in spontaneously immortalized cell clones, and in zebrafish embryos and adult tissues. In both primary fibroblasts and spontaneously immortalized clones, telomeres were maintained at stable lengths with telomerase activity during a certain number of passages. During early development *in vivo*, telomere length was also stably maintained and telomerase activity was prominently detectable at all stages, indicating that there is maternal carryover of telomerase before the embryonic gene expression. To determine if telomere shortening occurs with concomitant maintainance of telomerase activity throughout life *in vivo*, we monitored both telomerase and telomere in muscle tissues from zebrafish of many different ages. Telomere length was similar among different ages up to 24-months, whereas stochastic variation of telomere length appeared with more advancing age, as describe already. Differences in telomere lengths among several different tissues from organs in adult zebrafish have not been determined but need to be elucidated, while we know that zebrafish have constitutive telomerase activity in all of the examined tissues throughout their lives. These findings suggest that there is a unique regulation of zebrafish telomerase during development and aging *in vivo*. In contrast to human tissues, since all zebrafish tissues examined had constitutively active telomerase, there must be some differences in tissue homeostasis via the species-specific telomerase and telomere regulation *in situ* among vertebrates during evolution. In any case, the presence of telomerase in these tissues may reflect the ease of immortalization of primary fish cells relative to human cells in culture, indeterminate growth, and remarkable regenerative ability throughout life.

It should be noted that telomere shortening may limit the regenerative capacity of cells *in vivo* by inducing cellular senescence characterized by a permanent growth arrest of cells with critically short telomeres. To examine whether organ regeneration is impaired by telomerase inhibition and telomere shortening in zebrafish *in vivo*, we monitored caudal fin regeneration after amputation in telomerase-knockdown adult zebrafish. Our study has shown that telomere shortening is caused in regenerated fins and inhibits a subpopulation of cells with critically short telomeres from entering the cell cycle. This subpopulation of regenerated cells with impaired proliferative capacity exhibited induction of SA-β-gal activity. These studies provide experimental evidence for the existence of an *in vivo* process of premature senescence induced by telomerase knockdown and critical telomere shortening that has functional impact on tissue regeneration in zebrafish.

Potential Model Systems for Premature Aging Syndromes in Zebrafish

There are no perfect models for human aging, but zebrafish are vertebrates, and therefore are more closely related to human than commonly used invertebrate models. They are more likely to be similar to humans in many biological and biomedical traits such as genes, developmental processes, anatomy, physiology, behaviors, and diseases. This is an obvious advantage because invertebrate animals do not share these traits with humans. The invertebrates are more extensively used in identifications and comparisons of fundamental aging mechanisms, likely conserved in entire organisms rather than biologically complex traits in pathophysiology at the cellular and biochemical levels of organization where zebrafish share many features with humans.

Most premature aging models in vertebrates are derived from mutant and genetically manipulated mice. Zebrafish will probably become an alternative model for study of premature aging to recapitulate some of the human progeroid syndromes, such as ataxia telengiectasia (A–T), Fanconi anemia (FA), dyskeratosis congenita (DC), and Hutchinson–Gilford progeria syndrome (HGPS), because we have known that the molecular structures and functions of the genes and proteins responsible for these diseases are highly conserved between zebrafish and humans.

Functional aberrations of ATM protein cause a genetic disease A–T. We have recently demonstrated that zebrafish ATM (zATM) is functionally conserved at least in part because zebrafish embryos with disrupted ATM showed radiation hypersensitivity as observed in A–T patients and ATM-knockout mice (Imamura and Kishi, 2005). Since multiple aging/senescence-associated markers are readily monitored, it is worthwhile trying to identify premature senescence phenotypes in ATM-deficient zebrafish embryos as a representative model. Moreover, once a stable model system of zebrafish for human progeroid syndromes including A–T is established, it will become a powerful tool for characterizing molecular functions in the signal transduction pathway and using chemical genetic approaches for drug screening.

ZEBRAFISH MODEL OF ATAXIA TELANGIECTASIA

A–T is an autosomal recessive disorder characterized by progressive cerebellar degeneration, immunodeficiency, cancer predisposition, gonadal atrophy, growth retardation, premature aging, and hypersensitivity to IR (Lavin and Shiloh, 1997; McKinnon, 2004). Cells from A–T patients generally have short telomeres and are also highly sensitive to IR (Kishi and Lu, 2002; Metcalfe, *et al.*, 1996; Meyn, 1995; Pandita *et al.*, 1995; Shiloh, 1995; Smilenov *et al.*, 1997). The molecular cloning of the gene responsible for A–T, *ATM*, has allowed a better understanding of both ATM function and the A–T pleiotropic phenotypes (Savitsky *et al.*, 1995a; Savitsky *et al.*, 1995b; Taylor, 1998). The ATM gene encodes a nuclear phosphoprotein (Chen and Lee, 1996; Scott *et al.*, 1998), with serine/threonine protein kinase activity for which many downstream molecules, such as p53, Chk2, Mdm2, NBS1, BRCA1, 53BP1 SMC1, FANC2, H2AX, Pin2/TRF1, and TRF2, which control cell cycle check points, DNA double-strand break or repair pathway, and telomere metabolism, have been identified as substrates (Kastan and Lim, 2000; Kishi and Lu, 2002; Kishi *et al.*, 2001; Pandita, 2002; Shiloh, 2003; Tanaka *et al.*, 2005). ATM functions as a potent protein kinase that is activated by DNA damage, such as IR, to phosphorylate target substrates. The identification of these potential substrates places ATM in a signal transduction pathway, through which it functions to regulate cell-cycle checkpoints that mediate the DNA damage response and telomere homeostasis (Verdun *et al.*, 2005).

As a model system, ATM-knockout mice have been created in several laboratories by specific germline inactivation of the ATM gene (Barlow *et al.*, 1996; Elson *et al.*, 1996; Herzog *et al.*, 1998; Xu *et al.*, 1996). Fibroblasts isolated from ATM-knockout mice display similar cellular phenotypes to those observed in cells from A–T patients (Elson *et al.*, 1996). Also, phenotypically, ATM-deficient mice display a variety of growth defects, meiotic defects, immunological abnormalities, radiation hypersensitivity and cancer predisposition, similar to those seen in A–T patients, confirming the most common pleiotropic roles of ATM. Early resistance to apoptosis in the developing central nervous system (CNS) of ATM-knockout mice has been observed after IR, especially in diverse regions of the CNS including the cerebellum (Herzog *et al.*, 1998), which is markedly affected in A–T. Interestingly, the neurological defects in A–T become apparent early in life, suggesting that they likewise originate during development (Herzog *et al.*, 1998). However, little is known about ATM expression and function during early development in lower vertebrates, such as zebrafish.

To develop a zebrafish A–T model, we first isolated zebrafish ATM (zATM) cDNA. We recently provided the zATM cDNA sequence as a predicted primary structure (Imamura and Kishi, 2005). At the amino acid level, the overall identity was 58% between zATM and hATM. The high degree of conservation between zATM and hATM especially within the kinase domains (81% identity) strongly suggests that the catalytic activity of these proteins is conserved. The decreasing levels of identity outside the catalytic domains may reflect potential differences in regulation of these proteins between species, though this remains to be elucidated. Importantly, a number of amino acids corresponding to sites that are found to be mutated in A–T patients are highly conserved between hATM and zATM (Gilad *et al.*, 1996). In actuality, Garg *et al.* recently reported that a kinase-inactive form of the zATM catalytic domain exhibited dominant-negative activity in human and zebrafish cell lines (Garg *et al.*, 2004). The presence of these conserved amino acid sites further attests that corresponding zATM mutants from chemically point-mutated zebrafish genomes can probably be identified.

We also outlined zATM expression patterns during early development of zebrafish embryos. We observed that zATM mRNA was ubiquitously expressed during gastrulation and early neurulation. Differential tissue expression was evidenced by increased mRNA levels at later developmental stages in the eye, brain, and somites, with relatively weak expression in the trunk and tail. The profile of zATM expression is consistent with previous observations in *Xenopus* (Hensey *et al.*, 2000) and mice (Chen and Lee, 1996; Soares *et al.*, 1998), which also show increased expression of ATM in CNS, suggesting a common importance in early development of the nervous system among vertebrates.

By using antisense-morpholino oligonucleotides (MOs) to achieve *in vivo* elimination of zATM expression, we observed that loss of zATM leads to abnormal development and increased lethality in the early stages of development upon IR-induced DNA damage. Our results strongly support a model for structural and functional conservation of ATM's role in the DNA damage response among vertebrates from fish to human.

Our reported results also support the notion that ATM heterozygous phenotypes resemble those caused by protein dosage reduction, in genomic chromosomal instability and cancer susceptibility, which may all be due to diminished cell-cycle checkpoint function. We suspect that this hypothesis would be relevant not only to human A–T carriers, but also to heterozygous A–T zebrafish. However, there are conflicting data on the role of *ATM* heterozygosity in cancer risk (Concannon, 2002; FitzGerald *et al.*, 1997; Laposa *et al.*, 2004; Spring *et al.*, 2002). On the one hand, Barlow *et al.* argued that *ATM* heterozygous mice showed no evidence of increased acute radiation toxicity, although the mice intriguingly displayed premature greying and decreased survival at higher sublethal doses of irradiation (Barlow *et al.*, 1999b), suggesting progressive senescence with DNA damage.

ATM function is essential for telomere metabolism as well as DNA damage response. ATM is required for telomere maintenance and chromosome stability because inactivation of ATM causes telomere shortening (Metcalfe *et al.*, 1996; Pandita, 2002). Importantly, terminal deletions of *Drosophila* chromosomes can be stably protected from end-to-end fusion despite the absence of all telomere-associated sequences. The sequence-independent protection of these telomeres suggests that recognition of chromosome ends might contribute to the epigenetic protection of telomeres. In zebrafish as well as in mammals, ATM can be activated by DNA damage and could act through a telomerase-independent mechanism to regulate telomere length, protection, and homeostasis. It has been demonstrated that the *Drosophila* homolog of ATM is encoded by the telomere fusion (*tefu*) gene (Bi *et al.*, 2004; Oikemus *et al.*, 2004; Queiroz-Machado *et al.*, 2001; Silva *et al.*, 2004; Song *et al.*, 2004). In the absence of ATM, telomere fusions occur even though telomere-specific Het-A sequences are still present in *Drosophila*. Highly spontaneous apoptosis is observed in ATM-deficient tissues, indicating that telomere dysfunction induces apoptosis in *Drosophila*. Suppression of this apoptosis by p53 mutations suggests that loss of ATM activates ATM-independent but p53-dependent apoptosis through an alternative DNA damage-response mechanism. Furthermore, loss of ATM reduces the levels of heterochromatin protein 1 (HP1) at telomeres and suppresses telomere position effect, suggesting that recognition of chromosome ends by ATM prevents telomere fusion and apoptosis by recruiting chromatin-modifying complexes to telomeres (Oikemus *et al.*, 2004).

Epigenetic control apparently provides a mechanism not only for the position effect at telomeres on the transcription of nearby genes but also for the reversible silencing of telomerase expression that occurs as a natural consequence of cellular proliferation and differentiation. There exists significant overlap between indirect telomeric regulation pathways and cell-cycle checkpoint pathways, suggesting that these discrete genetic elements—namely, ATM, p53, p21, and TERT—synergistically cooperate to inhibit tumorigenesis and to govern aging. Mutations in these pathways have been known to contribute to cancer formation and senescence occurence in mammals. Besides genetic control, the incorporation of epigenetic regulatory mechanisms provides another line of defense against these negative occurrences. Although the debate still continues, there is significant evidence to view the process of cellular senescence as an *in vitro* model for human aging. In addition to A–T, other disorders such as Werner's syndrome, dyskeratosis congenita, ulcerative colitis, and atherosclerosis have been linked to aberration of telomere homeostasis, and other aging-related lesions could be related to changes in cellular microenvironment resulting from the presence of senescent cells. Therefore, simply restoring direct telomerase activity as a putative therapeutic strategy rather than fine-tuning telomere homeostasis necessitates further study to elucidate the link between genetic and epigenetic modulations of telomerase in humans (Lai *et al.*, 2005). This is a relevant argument considering our observation of zebrafish telomerase and telomere regulation *in vivo* because as mentioned above, their telomere metabolism is not simply regulated by detectable telomerase activity, particularly very late in life with stochastic telomere shortening in the presence of constitutive telomerase activity.

In any case, once a stable line of zebrafish with ATM disruption or inactivation has been obtained, it will be possible to use the zebrafish A–T model to identify candidate therapeutic interventions. On a broad scope, zebrafish additionally couple the power of genetics and functional genomics for efficient mutant screening. As such, a zebrafish model system for A–T will be amenable to studies directed towards identifying functional modifier genes that affect the ATM signaling pathway, as well as ultimately identifying small molecules that can ameliorate functional disorders caused by ATM mutations.

With respect to a future direction of this study, pilot screens of genetic mutants have been conducted using F2 heterozygous embryos under genotoxic or oxidative stress. Developmental defects and premature senescence phenotype have been confirmed in F3 homozygous recessive embryos. These results imply that a large-scale screen using a chemical mutagen will allow us to identify physiologically relevant players in the stress-associated signaling pathway as targets for the interventions in aging and age-associated diseases. However, positional cloning of the point mutations of a target gene will still be time consuming for identifying whether *ATM* or the other related gene is critical for readout of the zebrafish mutants.

Further studies of DNA damage response and ATM function in zebrafish may serve to unravel the regulation of genomic integrity and pleiotropic features, including progeroid manifestation, as the functional roles of ATM seem to have been commonly conserved or have commonly evolved among vertebrates from fish to humans.

ZEBRAFISH MODEL OF FANCONI ANEMIA

Regarding Fanconi anemia (FA), researchers have recently turned to zebrafish to help them unravel conserved signaling pathways (Liu *et al.*, 2003). Although FA is a relatively rare genetic disease, the genes involved in FA function as part of a large network of DNA damage response/repair, and the phenotypic features of FA consist of a combination of developmental and somatic abnormalities, including alterations reminiscent of premature aging (Giannelli, 1986; Tischkowitz and Hodgson, 2003; Willingale-Theune *et al.*, 1989). Liu and colleagues have recapitulated some of the clinical manifestations of human FA by knocking down the zebrafish *FANC-D2* gene, thereby providing a new model for probing the underlying causes of these phenotypes (Liu *et al.*, 2003). They have identified the zebrafish homolog of human FANCD2, which encodes a nuclear effecter protein that is monoubiquitinated in response to DNA damage, targeting it to nuclear foci where it preserves chromosomal integrity. Fancd2-knockdown zebrafish embryos developed defects similar to those found in children with FA, including shortened body length, microcephaly, and microophthalmia, which are due to extensive cellular apoptosis. Intriguingly, developmental defects and increased apoptosis in Fancd2-knockdown zebrafish are corrected by injection of human Fancd2 or zebrafish bcl-2 mRNA, or by knockdown of p53, indicating that in the absence of Fancd2, developing tissues spontaneously undergo p53-dependent apoptosis. Thus, Fancd2 is essential during embryogenesis to prevent inappropriate apoptosis in neural cells and other tissues undergoing high levels of proliferative expansion, implicating this mechanism in the congenital abnormalities observed in human infants with FA.

Although characterizations of premature senescence phenotypes in the zebrafish FA model are still needed, taking into account molecular interaction and signaling crosstalk between Fancd2 and ATM (Taniguchi *et al.*, 2002), FA and A–T will be one of the most prominent genetic diseases for the zebrafish models of human "premature aging syndromes."

TARGETED KNOCKDOWN OF ZEBRAFISH TELOMERASE TO RECAPITULATE DYSKERATOSIS CONGENITA

Dyskeratosis congenita (DC) is a severe, inherited, bone marrow failure syndrome, with associated cutaneous and noncutaneous abnormalities. DC patients also show signs of premature aging and have an increased occurrence of cancer. Accelerated telomeric erosion is a molecular hallmark of DC (Mitchell *et al.*, 1999; Ruggero *et al.*, 2003). DC can originate through (i) mutations in *DKC1*, which result in X-linked recessive DC; (ii) mutations in the RNA component of telomerase (TERC), which result in autosomal dominant DC; and (iii) mutations in other, currently uncharacterized, genes, which result in autosomal recessive DC. As *DKC1* encodes dyskerin, a protein component of small nucleolar ribonucleoprotein (snoRNP) particles, which are important in ribosomal RNA processing, DC was initially described as a disorder of defective ribosomal biogenesis. Subsequently, dyskerin and TERC were shown to closely associate with each other in the telomerase complex, and DC has since come to be regarded as a telomerase deficiency disorder characterized by shorter telomeres. These findings demonstrate the importance of telomerase in humans and highlight how its deficiency (through *DKC1* and *TERC* mutations) results in multiple abnormalities including premature aging, bone marrow failure and cancer. Identification of the gene(s) involved in autosomal recessive DC will help to define the pathophysiology of DC further, as well as expand our insights into telomere function, aging and cancer. Through the challenge with targeted knockdown of zebrafish telomerase, it is likely that a novel vertebrate model system can be developed for studies of DC. In this respect, studies of evolutionary and comparative biology in telomerase and telomere metabolism are important because zebrafish have a constitutive telomerase activity that is apparently different from the human telomerase regulation. There is first and foremost a need to compare the importance of telomerase in zebrafish and in humans, by trying to recapitulate DC phenotypes in a zebrafish model.

Prospective Basic Studies of Aging and Senescence in Zebrafish

The potential maximum lifespan of zebrafish is more than five years (Gerhard *et al.*, 2002), though the differences among strains as well as betwen genders need to be clarified. Thus, while searching for late age-onset disease models and long-lived mutants is extremely important and worthwhile trying, it will be tough and tedious work because of current paucity of baseline information on zebrafish aging. On the other hand, we have been planning to isolate zebrafish mutants like progeroid syndromes in humans as described above. Genetic manipulations of several genes related to pathophysiological aging symptoms into zebrafish embryos have the potential to unveil some important aspects of the molecular mechanisms of senescence through the use of easier traceable developmental stages. Without performing lengthy lifespan analyses and long-term studies of age-associated alterations and lesions in the animal, it may be possible to pick up predictable late-age onset phenotypes in early developmental stages. Although an "antagonistic pleiotropy" theory of aging is needed concerning phenomena early- versus late-in-life, antagonistically pleiotropic genes and processes that benefit organisms turn out to be detrimental immediately after stress rather than later in life. Based on the fact that senescence induced by stress exposure is recognized as "stress-induced premature senescence" at cellular levels in the cell culture system (Toussaint *et al.*, 2000), probably it is amenable at organismal levels in animal model systems. During mouse embryogenesis, the absence of the BRCA1 full-length isoform causes embryonic senescence that is carried out by p53 (Cao *et al.*, 2003). Usually, p53, the clearest example of an antagonistically pleiotropic gene product, has early-life benefit suppressing cancer development, but has late-life detrimental cost compromising tissue functions with age. However, once BRCA1 is disrupted, p53 turns out to be harmful to embryonic survival by inducing senescence during development. Thus, DNA-damaging stress as well as BRCA1 deficiency triggers p53-dependent stress-induced premature senescence in cells and in organisms. Moreover, embryonic senescence in p63-deficient mice as well as accelerated aging phenotypes in conditional p63-disrupted adult mice have been most recently reported in the literature (Keyes *et al.*, 2005). These lines of recent evidence strongly support the notion that it is possible to assess biological aging phenomena in model organisms without having to perform more time-consuming chronological aging studies.

Importantly, nematodes and fruitflies have no cancer or other abnormal growth during aging, in contrast to their common occurrence in vertebrates from fish to humans with advancing age. Having relevance to these phenomena with regard to cell growth characteristics, nematodes with a constant number of cells lack somatic cell replacement, whereas insects such as the fruitfly have limited but detectable cell proliferation in some adult tissues. On the other hand, mammalian tissues contain different proportions of the cells that are continuously replaced in adults but are of great importance to outcomes of organismal aging through replicative senescence of critical cells. However, humans possess only a limited capacity to restore their missing or injured body parts. Therefore, stimulating regenerative capability may circumvent some tissue deterioration in aging humans. Adult zebrafish have been shown to possess a remarkable capacity for regeneration. Zebrafish regenerate almost all tissues and organs such as fins, spinal cord, retina, and heart. By dissecting molecular mechanisms of zebrafish regeneration, it may be possible to illuminate novel factors that can stimulate a regenerative response in higher vertebrates. Thus, research of regeneration in zebrafish during the aging process will contribute to aging medicine as well as to regenerative medicine in humans.

With respect to amenability of genetic manipulations through forward genetic and reverse genetic approaches, robust zebrafish genetics will obviously hold the key to success. However, zebrafish have a relatively long generation time and fairly long lifespan compared with those of nematodes and flies, which slows down experiments that require breeding and analyzing offspring as well as longitudinal aging studies. Nevertheless, zebrafish are one of the most genetically pliable/tractable (visually traceable) and biologically attractive animal models. Presumably, specific gene expression and its function and a role of tissue-specific stem and progenitor cells in aging will be actively and progressively investigated in zebrafish, closely connected with regeneration studies.

POSSIBLE INVOLVEMENT OF TUMOR SUPPRESSOR GENE PRODUCTS, P53 AND PRB, IN ZEBRAFISH AGING

The tumor suppressor proteins p53 and pRB regulate cellular replicative senescence and organismal aging. Tumor suppressor mechanisms may represent evolutionary antagonistic pleiotropy because tumor suppressor genes benefit organisms early in life due to suppression of cancer. However, these genes may become harmful later during the aging process, compromising tissue functions. Importantly, telomere attrition in cells induces replicative senescence accompanied by activation of the p53 and pRB pathways. In zebrafish, the p53 pathway is known to exist with relevant functional conservation (Cheng *et al.*, 1997; Langheinrich *et al.*, 2002), but zebrafish pRB pathway has not been reported. Recent studies demonstrated that zebrafish p53 is involved in the tumor suppressor mechanism *in vivo* (Berghmans *et al.*, 2005; Patton *et al.*, 2005).

There are diverse stimuli for inducing cellular senescence. Both extrinsic and intrinsic factors are involved in these stimuli. Particularly, within intrinsic factors, tumor suppressors play an important role in the initiation, establishment, and maintenance of the cellular senescence phenotype. For example, the fundamental signaling pathways are governed by p53 and pRB in relation to telomeric homeostasis (Jacobs and de Lange, 2004; Zhang *et al.*, 2005). The downstream targets of these two tumor suppressors are the cyclin-dependent kinase inhibitors

(CDKIs) p21 and p16^{INK4a}, respectively. p21 and p16^{INK4a} as well as other CDKIs inhibit the cell-cycle progression, and in some cases these CDKIs also induce a cellular senescence phenotype. Moreover, ARF, another upstream tumor suppressor which regulates p53, is a crucial mediator of senescence in mammalian cells, whereas it is likely that zebrafish may have an alternative or different upstream pathway, given the insight that teleost fish apparently lack an *ARF* gene (Gilley and Fried, 2001; Langenau *et al.*, 2005), as discussed later.

p53 is a key player in DNA damage response and cell-cycle checkpoints as well as in mammalian cancer development. Activation of the transcriptional functions of p53 through DNA damage or other stresses can result in cell-cycle arrest, apoptosis, or senescence depending on the cellular environment and the upstream signal. It is well established that loss of p53 function abrogates replicative senescence in mammalian cells. Importantly, critically short and/or dysfunctional telomeres, resembling damaged DNA, trigger the p53-mediated DNA damage response (Campisi, 2005).

To characterize p53 signaling in zebrafish, Langheinrich *et al.* (2002) have studied the roles of p53 and its main negative regulator, Mdm2, in zebrafish by generating early embryonic knockdowns and examining the involvement of p53 in DNA damage-induced apoptosis. p53-deficient embryos, induced by injection of MOs, were morphologically indistinguishable from control embryos, when unperturbed, whereas Mdm2 knockdown embryos were severely apoptotic and arrested very early in development. Double knockdowns showed that p53 deficiency rescued Mdm2-deficient embryos completely, was seen earlier in mice (Jones *et al.*, 1995; Montes de Oca Luna *et al.*, 1995). p53 deficiency also markedly decreased DNA damage-induced apoptosis in zebrafish embryos, elicited by ultraviolet irradiation or the anticancer drug compound camptothecin. Zebrafish p21 appeared to be a downstream target of p53, as revealed by relative p21 mRNA levels determined by real-time RT-PCR analysis. As far as can be predicted on the basis of results with zebrafish p53 knockdown by MOs, zebrafish embryos are presumably amenable for studying p53-mediadted DNA damage response and cell-cycle regulation at the downstream pathways.

Most recently, stable p53-deficient zebrafish mutant lines were isolated by using target-selected mutagenesis strategy, from 2,679 individual *N*-ethyl-*N*-nitrosourea (ENU)-mutagenized F1 male fish (Berghmans *et al.*, 2005). Homozygote p53^{M214K} mutant fish were characterized for DNA damage (IR) response, and the mutants appeared resistant to apoptosis induction in response to irradiation. Unlike wild-type control fish embryos, irradiated p53 mutants were resistant to apoptosis induction and failed to up-regulate p21 with aberrant cell-cycle checkpoint. More importantly, within 1 year of age, more than one quarter of the mutant fish developed malignant peripheral nerve sheath tumors. With the use of mutant fish as a unique platform, further functional modifier gene screens and small molecule screens will be readily available in the future. Although aging and senescence phenotypes in p53 mutant fish have not been addressed in the literature, our ongoing studies of aging in these fish may be able to elucidate functional roles of zebrafish p53 in DNA damage- and telomere-associated senescence response.

In addition to p53, zebrafish p53 family members, p63 and p73, have been identified and their cDNAs cloned (Bakkers *et al.*, 2002; Lee and Kimelman, 2002; Rentzsch *et al.*, 2003; Satoh *et al.*, 2004). Furthermore, they appear to be more highly conserved than p53 among vertebrates. Functional analysis of zebrafish p63 in embryonic senescence might be interesting because a recent report showed that p63-deficient mouse embryos express high levels of SA-β-gal activity (Keyes *et al.*, 2005).

In terms of the upstream pathways that signal through p53, the functional links involving phosphorylation of p53 by kinases such as ATM/ATR/DNA-PK have not been fully elucidated in zebrafish. Nevertheless, zebrafish represent a promising model organism for future compound-based and genetic screens. Zebrafish-based efforts will also help to identify and characterize new drugs and new targets to ameliorate human genome instability diseases including cancer. However, to realize this goal, the comparative genetic pathways in vertebrates from fish to humans need to be elaborated.

A wide variety of genotoxic stresses, including IR and ultraviolet (UV) radiation, lead to p53 activation (Sancar *et al.*, 2004). As part of this activation, posttranslational modifications of p53, phosphorylation and ubiquitination have paramount impacts on protein stability and functional regulation (Wahl and Carr, 2001). While several pathways can lead to p53 stabilization, one of the most prominent key regulators is Mdm2, which functions as a ring-finger ubiquitin ligase, although Mdm2 may have other additional mechanisms of p53 inactivation than degradation through ubiquitination. Importantly, Mdm2-mediated ubiquitination of p53 is controlled by ATM-dependent mechanisms that regulate the ability of Mdm2 to bind p53 (Maya *et al.*, 2001). ATM-dependent phosphorylation of human Mdm2 on Ser395 is one of the most rapid responses to IR, which presumably compromises p53 degradation. However, in zebrafish Mdm2, the serine residue corresponding to Ser395 in human is not present (Thisse *et al.*, 2000), suggesting that relatively stable zebrafish p53 may not be necessary to be compromised by phosphorylated Mdm2 for degradation, or that it may be constitutively degraded by unphosphorylated Mdm2 more rapidly than in mammals.

ATM is a main Ser/Thr protein kinase for phosphorylation of p53, especially in response to IR in mammals (Figure 28.5).

In humans, ATM, as well as ATR and DNA-PK, directly phosphorylate p53 on Ser15, which is within the N-terminal transactivation domain (Kim *et al.*, 1999;

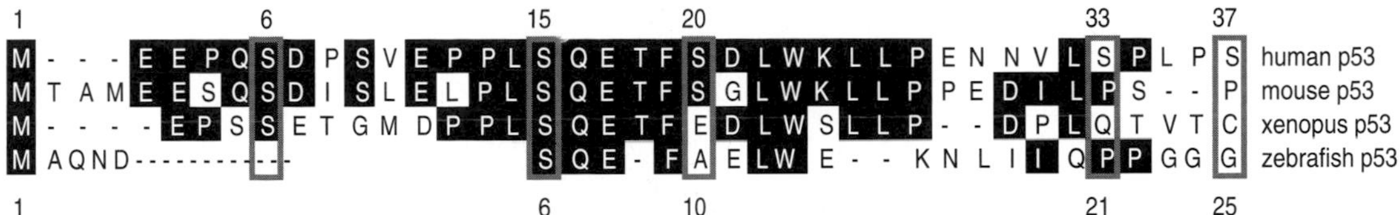

Figure 28.5. Sequence comparison of the N-terminal amino acids corresponding to 1–37 in human p53 between human, mouse, *Xenopus*, and zebrafish. The N-terminal phosphorylation sites, S6, S15, S20, S33, and S37, of p53 are compared among the species. Only S15 in human p53, which corresponds to S6 in zebrafish, is a well-conserved site.

Lavin and Khanna, 1999; Shiloh, 2001; Shiloh, 2003). This site is putatively conserved, but in zebrafish p53 the position is Ser6 followed by S(6)QE (Cheng *et al.*, 1997). In humans, Ser15 phosphorylation interferes with Mdm2 binding to p53 (Shieh *et al.*, 1997). Moreover, DNA damage induced by IR also results in ATM-dependent activation of Chk2 (Chehab *et al.*, 2000; Hirao *et al.*, 2000; Matsuoka *et al.*, 2000; Shieh *et al.*, 2000). Activated Chk2 phosphorylates Ser20 of human p53, which is also within the Mdm2-binding region and the phosphorylation of Ser 20, reduces the binding of Mdm2 (Chehab *et al.*, 1999; Unger *et al.*, 1999). However, zebrafish p53 does not contain a phosphorylation site equivalent to Ser20. Phosphorylation sites equivalent to Ser33 and Ser37 of human p53 are likewise lacking in zebrafish p53. Intriguingly, it has been shown that a Ser20 to Ala mutation generates a less stable form of human p53 (Chehab *et al.*, 1999; Unger *et al.*, 1999), whereas wild-type zebrafish p53 contains Ala10 followed by FA(10)E at the site equivalent to FS(20)D in human (Cheng *et al.*, 1997) (Figure 28.5), suggesting permanent instability or basic lack of function through the Mdm2 pathway. More importantly, the zebrafish genome contains homologues of those checkpoint regulators and kinases, but thus far, to our knowledge, apparently lacks an ARF homologue. ARF is a small protein generated from the CDKN4 locus, and the same region also encodes the CDK4 inhibitor p16. ARF is a tumor suppressor and an important inhibitor of the ubiquitin ligase Mdm2, thus antagonizing p53 degradation. In addition, nucleolar relocalization of Mdm2 by ARF connotes a novel mechanism for preventing p53 turnover and provides a framework for understanding how stress signals cooperate to regulate p53 function. In mammals, ARF also connects pathways regulated by the pRB and p53. ARF inactivation reduces p53-dependent apoptosis induced by oncogenic signals. If is also in zebrafish, the consequences may reveal that zebrafish don't utilize the protein turnover machinery to regulate p53 activity through the ARF-Mdm2-p53 pathway. Furthermore, since zebrafish p53 lacks the potentially targeted Chk1 and Chk2 phosphorylation sites Ser33 and Ser37, the Chk1/Chk2-p53 pathway might differentially function through an alternative mechanism in zebrafish. This is worthwhile investigating from the comparatively biological and evolutionary point of view among vertebrates because p53, as a critical tumor suppressor, is among the most commonly mutated genes in human cancers (Vogelstein, 1990; Vogelstein and Kinzler, 1992; Vogelstein and Kinzler, 2004; Vogelstein *et al.*, 2000). In humans, the Chk2 kinase is also a known tumor suppressor, and a wide variety of cancer-associated mutations and defects have been identified (Bartek and Lukas, 2003; Motoyama and Naka, 2004). Importantly, consistent with the tumor suppressor function of Chk2, recent studies demonstrated that Chk2 activation, caused by telomere attrition, triggers replicative senescence in human cells (Gire, 2004; Gire *et al.*, 2004; Oh *et al.*, 2003). In contrast, cancer-related defects in Chk1 are rare, and so far seem limited to some gastrointestinal carcinomas (Bartek and Lukas, 2003). Therefore, the zebrafish Chk1/Chk2 pathways need required to be characterized in terms of their role in cancer biology as well as for DNA damage and senescence response in zebrafish.

Collectively, p53 is a crucial molecule for regulation of the responses to DNA damage, cell-cycle arrest, apoptosis, and senescence. Critically short or dysfunctional telomeres trigger a p53-dependent DNA damage response possibly through ATM activation (Bakkenist *et al.*, 2004; d'Adda di Fagagna *et al.*, 2003; Herbig *et al.*, 2004). Moreover, telomere dysfunction enhances sensitivity to IR in mice. Loss of p53 function delays or abrogates the replicative senescence of human cells irrespective of the ATM states. However, both p53-independent ATM pathways and ATM-independent p53 pathways must be involved in the diversified regulations of senescence response (Figure 28.6).

Importantly, p53-dependent senescent growth arrest is reversible at least in some human cells, whereas the other senescent arrest, which is induced by the p16/pRB pathway, is irreversible even with subsequent inactivation of p53, p16, or pRB (Beausejour *et al.*, 2003; Dirac and Bernards, 2003). So far, the involvement of the p53/p21 pathway in cell-cycle regulation and apoptosis has been demonstrated in several experiments using zebrafish, and we have already confirmed p53-dependent premature senescence induction during development and adult fin regeneration of zebrafish. The importance of the pRB pathway in zebrafish aging and senescence response remains to be characterized, and further elucidation of the signaling pathways and their network may reveal evolutionary conservation of mechanisms among vertebrates.

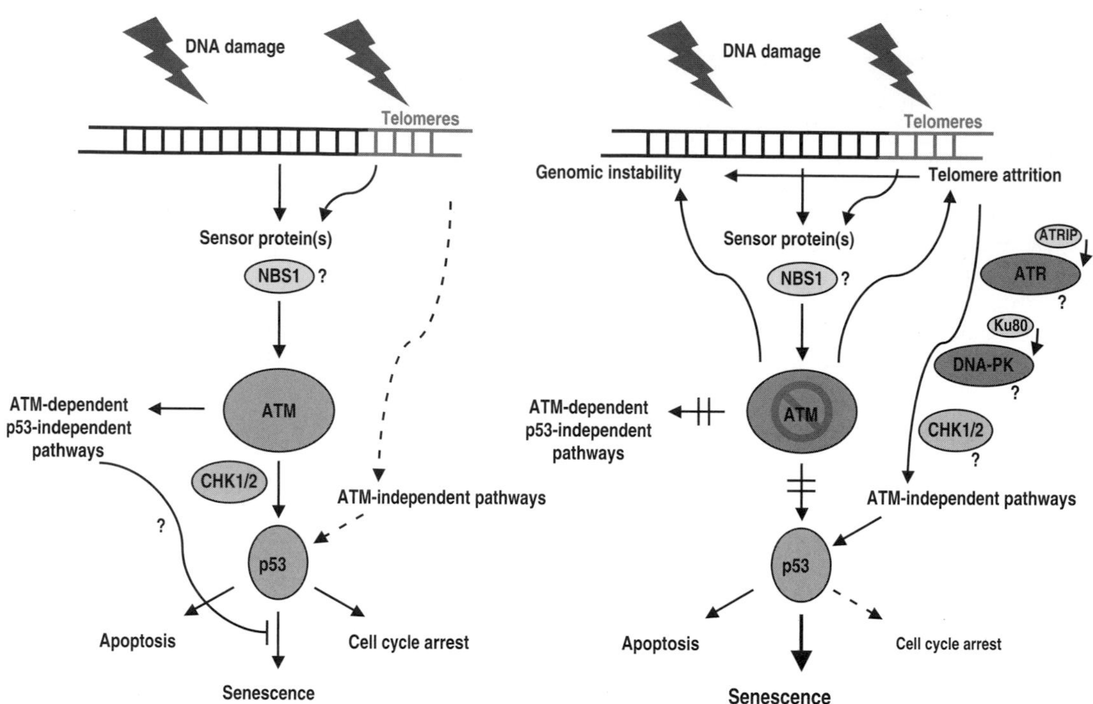

Figure 28.6. Possible schematic presentation of a model for DNA damage-mediated senescence response in the ATM-p53 axis. In the presence or absence of ATM, a different balance of ATM-dependent and ATM-independent senescence response probably occurs through p53. ATM can maintain genome and telomere integrity. In the absence of ATM, genomic instability and telomere attrition are aberrantly induced by DNA damage and p53 is still activated through an ATM-independent pathway. This ATM-independent p53 activation leads to much more prominent induction of senescence, in other words accelerated premature senescence, in an A–T patient. The ATM-independent p53-dependent pathway may involve ATR, DNA-PK, and Chk1/2. ATRIP and Ku80 seem to function as sensor proteins of DNA damage to ATR and DNA-PK, respectively (Falck *et al.*, 2005). NBS1 could be another sensor protein responsible for ATM (Falck *et al.*, 2005).

ZEBRAFISH FOR A MODEL OF NUTRITION-RELATED AND AGE-DEPENDENT CHRONIC DISEASES WITH OXIDATIVE STRESS

Oxidants are generated under various physiological conditions that include mitochondrial electron transport, peroxisomal fatty acid metabolism, phagocytosis by macrophages, and bone resorption by osteoclasts. However, increased oxidative stress has been correlated to a varying extents with common age-related diseases, such as adult-onset diabetes mellitus, atherosclerosis, some types of cancer, and some forms of neurodegeneration including cerebellar ischemia.

The increasing prevalence of obesity and other nutrition-related chronic diseases, which usually accompany aging, has prompted considerable efforts to understand their pathogenesis and treatment. One experimental approach is to overexpress, inactivate, or manipulate specific genes that regulate energy metabolism and fat storage. Many such techniques are fully amenable and have been established as routine tools in zebrafish, as well as in *Drosophila* and *C. elegans*. In the future, these elegant models will be complementarily helpful in dissecting endocrine problems and metabolic pathways, associated with aging and senescence. Particularly, once zebrafish counterparts of essential signaling molecules, such as Sir2 and FoxOs, involved in regulation of energy metabolism are available, development of model systems appear to be within of our current technologies and fat storage, are obtained, development of new vertebrate aging models appears to be within the scope of our current technologies.

AGING IMMUNITY IMPORTANCE OF INNATE IMMUNITY IN ZEBRAFISH

Finch and Crimmins proposed that the reduction in lifetime exposure to infectious diseases and other sources of inflammation has made an important contribution to the historical decline in old-age mortality (Finch and Crimmins, 2004). This will likely also be true in zebrafish, because one of the most critical problems in their husbandry late in life derives from multiple microbial infections. Resistance to microbial infectious diseases obviously declines with age in adult zebrafish. The cellular components involved in defense against pathogens/microbial agents are beyond the scope of this article. However, it should be noted that zebrafish have an almost complete set of the Toll-like receptors (TLRs) (Jault *et al.*, 2004; Meijer *et al.*, 2004). The TLR family is an evolutionarily conserved component of the innate immune system that responds to specific pathogen-associated molecular patterns (Takeda *et al.*, 2003), and important lines of evidence indicate that the innate immune system in zebrafish can be the primary layer of defense against microbial pathogens. Rag-1-deficient zebrafish that lack adaptive immunity have normal life expectancy in regular fish water, which notoriously contains multiple pathogens (Wienholds *et al.*, 2002). Importantly, adult zebrafish have a strikingly high expression of TLRs in the skin (Jault *et al.*, 2004), which may be highly relevant to their primary mechanism of defense against pathogens by the innate immune system. Aged adult zebrafish are naturally more susceptible to tuberculosis caused by *Mycobacterium marinum*, where TLRs and innate immunity play prominent roles of defense. This implies that age-dependent functional declines of the innate immune system including the TLRs expression levels are crucial for infectious diseases followed by inflammations late in life of zebrafish. However, zebrafish aging-associated immunity has not been investigated so far in detail. Due to declines of both innate and adaptive immune functions with age, leading to increased susceptibility to infectious diseases and cancer in vertebrate animals, importance of the immune system in aging zebrafish needs to be recognized and immunological senescence should adequately be studied with respect to various age-dependent diseases.

Zebrafish Aging and Senescence Research for Drug Discovery and Geriatric Medicine

Zebrafish have become a widely used model organism because of their fecundity, their morphological and physiological similarity to mammals, the existence of many genomic tools, and the ease with which large-scale and phenotype-based screens can be performed. Because of these attributes, zebrafish may provide opportunities to accelerate the process of drug discovery (Goldsmith, 2004; Yeh and Crews, 2003; Zon and Peterson, 2005). By combining the scale and throughput of *in vitro* screens with the physiological complexity of animal studies, the zebrafish system promises to contribute to several aspects of the drug development process, including identification of the molecular target, recapitulation of the disease, lead compound discovery and toxicology testing (Hill *et al.*, 2005; Parng, 2005). At present, assessment of toxicity often occurs independently from efforts to discover lead compounds and improve their potency. High-throughput zebrafish toxicity assays combine many of the advantages of *in vitro* and *in vivo* toxicity models, making it possible to assess toxicity much earlier in the drug development process.

Moreover, large-scale genetic and MO-based screens allow unbiased discovery of genes that cause a desired phenotype (Dodd *et al.*, 2004; Rubinstein, 2003). Zebrafish screens for genetic or epigenetic perturbations that suppress a disease phenotype can be used to discover novel therapeutic targets. These attributes might also enhance the efficiency of several steps in the drug development process for aging and age-associated diseases.

Historically, numerous drugs have been discovered by observing phenotypic changes in whole animals exposed to small molecules, but these discoveries have often been serendipitous and are usually arduous. However, if we can utilize zebrafish through the power of functional genomics and phenomics, the genome-wide study of gene dispensability by quantitative analysis of phenotypes can be performed as a large-scale and systematic screen in zebrafish to identify small molecules that can suppress multiple disease phenotypes (Love *et al.*, 2004; MacRae and Peterson, 2003; Pichler *et al.*, 2003). This apparently has the potential to contribute so enormously in the search for drugs against complex diseases that zebrafish aging can truly become a paradigm in gerontology diseases and geriatric medicine when we adopt zebrafish aging as a paradigm of gerontology.

Many genetic or environmental manipulations that alter lifespan in model organisms also alter survival following acute stresses such as oxidative damage, genotoxic stress, and thermal stress. Thus, in flies and worms, mutations that enhance lifespan also increase resistance to oxidative stress. This is also true for most of the small number of mutations that increase lifespan in mice. In lower organisms, this coupling of stress responses and aging mechanisms has proved a useful tool in identifying new genes that affect the aging process without the need for performing lengthy lifespan analyses. Therefore, it is quite possible that this approach may also be applied to the identification of zebrafish aging mutants and pharmacological agents that slow the aging process or extend lifespan through enhanced resistance to oxygen radicals or other stresses. To facilitate high-throughput mutant and drug screens in zebrafish aging, we have developed SA-β-gal-based colormetric and fluorometric quantitation assays to monitor a marker of premature senescence in zebrafish embryos. We have first verified that the signal intensity of SA-β-gal is dramatically increased both in aging fish and in embryos exposed to stress. We are further validating the assay by demonstrating that known signaling molecules and genetic mutations, which would be expected to modulate oxidative stress response or telomere metabolism, are linked to SA-β-gal induction in embryos. Screening for potential aging mutants in zebrafish is also in progress. In these screens, chemical/radiation-induced oxidative/genotoxic stress is used to identify mutant fish, which either enhance or suppress activity of the SA-β-gal depending on the sensitizing regimen. We have already isolated several candidate mutants that show enhanced response to stress. Our novel approach of mutant analysis in zebrafish has the potential to accelerate the identification of new aging mutants and to contribute to future drug discovery for pharmaceutical interventions in geriatric medicine.

Finally, although this chapter has not dealt with aging histopathology in zebrafish, traditional histopathological analysis is important for assessing aging phenotypes in animals versus humans. We previously reported some age-dependent histological and/or pathologic alterations in a few selected organs of zebrafish at fairly advanced age (Kishi *et al.*, 2003). However, we still need to extensively examine aging tissues and organs. We also need to investigate the possible relationship of age-related functional impairments of organs as a cause of exponentially increasing mortality in aging zebrafish.

Conclusions

The genetics-based study of zebrafish aging will be an invaluable approach in determining many common aspects of age-associated diseases among vertebrates. While the progressive discoveries of fundamentally common mechanisms of aging in *C. elegans* and *Drosophila*, as well as in mice, are of great importance in the field, more extensive groundwork will be required for in-depth studies of complex issues in aging, using a powerful vertebrate model organism. Zebrafish have been extensively exploited for developmental studies, and currently a number of research scientists are aiming to utilize this animal as an alternative model for multiple human diseases. However, only minimal data are available regarding late adult-onset and age-related alterations or aging lesions in any of the commonly used wild-type and mutant lines of zebrafish. Therefore, to fully utilize the potential of zebrafish as an animal model for understanding human aging and diseases, we need to advance our knowledge of zebrafish diseases and pathology with age. The future use of this model organism in biomedical science will contribute to own ability to intervene in human aging and will be relevant to the discovery of small molecules as drugs to ameliorate human disease states.

ACKNOWLEDGMENTS

I greatly acknowledge the contributions of Junzo Uchiyama, Irina Zhdanova, and Shintaro Imamura to this work. I am grateful to Peter Bayliss and Eriko Koshimizu for their contributions in our laboratory. I am also very grateful to Thomas Roberts for his support and continued encouragement. I really thank Andre Rosowsky for his critical reading of this manuscript. Finally, I thank Junko Kishi, Shunsuke Kishi, and Shota Kishi for their helpful preparation of this manuscript. This work is funded by research grants from A–T Children's Project, the Ellison Medical Foundation, and NIA/NIH to S.K.

REFERENCES

Akimenko, M.A., Johnson, S.L., Westerfield, M., and Ekker, M. (1995). Differential induction of four msx homeobox genes during fin development and regeneration in zebrafish. *Development 121*, 347–357.

Allsopp, R.C., Vaziri, H., Patterson, C., Goldstein, S., Younglai, E.V., Futcher, A.B., *et al.* (1992). Telomere length predicts replicative capacity of human fibroblasts. *Proc Natl Acad Sci USA 89*, 10114–10118.

Baerlocher, G.M., and Lansdorp, P.M. (2004). Telomere length measurements using fluorescence in situ hybridization and flow cytometry. *Methods Cell Biol 75*, 719–750.

Bakkenist, C.J., Drissi, R., Wu, J., Kastan, M.B., and Dome, J.S. (2004). Disappearance of the telomere dysfunction-induced stress response in fully senescent cells. *Cancer Res 64*, 3748–3752.

Bakkers, J., Hild, M., Kramer, C., Furutani-Seiki, M., and Hammerschmidt, M. (2002). Zebrafish DeltaNp63 is a direct target of Bmp signaling and encodes a transcriptional repressor blocking neural specification in the ventral ectoderm. *Dev Cell 2*, 617–627.

Balaban, R.S., Nemoto, S., and Finkel, T. (2005). Mitochondria, oxidants, and aging. *Cell 120*, 483–495.

Barbieri, M., Bonafe, M., Franceschi, C., and Paolisso, G. (2003). Insulin/IGF-I-signaling pathway: an evolutionarily conserved mechanism of longevity from yeast to humans. *Am J Physiol Endocrinol Metab 285*, E1064–E1071.

Barlow, C., Dennery, P.A., Shigenaga, M.K., Smith, M.A., Morrow, J.D., Roberts, L.J., 2nd, *et al.* (1999a). Loss of the ataxiA–Telangiectasia gene product causes oxidative damage in target organs. *Proc Natl Acad Sci USA 96*, 9915–9919.

Barlow, C., Eckhaus, M.A., Schaffer, A.A., and Wynshaw-Boris, A. (1999b). Atm haploinsufficiency results in increased sensitivity to sublethal doses of ionizing radiation in mice. *Nat Genet 21*, 359–360.

Barlow, C., Hirotsune, S., Paylor, R., Liyanage, M., Eckhaus, M., Collins, F., *et al.* (1996). Atm-deficient mice: a paradigm of ataxia telangiectasia. *Cell 86*, 159–171.

Bartek, J., and Lukas, J. (2003). Chk1 and Chk2 kinases in checkpoint control and cancer. *Cancer Cell 3*, 421–429.

Beausejour, C.M., Krtolica, A., Galimi, F., Narita, M., Lowe, S.W., Yaswen, P., and Campist, J. (2003). Reversal of human cellular senescence roles of the p53 and p16 pathways. *Embo J 22*, 4212–4222.

Belinsky, S.A., Swafford, D.S., Finch, G.L., Mitchell, C.E., Kelly, G., Hahn, F.F., Anderson, M.W., and Nikula, K.J. (1997). Alterations in the K-ras and p53 genes in rat lung tumors. *Environ Health Perspect 105 Suppl 4*, 901–906.

Berghmans, S., Murphey, R.D., Wienholds, E., Neuberg, D., Kutok, J.L., Fletcher, C.D., Morris, J.P., Liu, T.X., Schulte-Merker, S., Kanki, J.P., *et al.* (2005). tp53 mutant zebrafish develop malignant peripheral nerve sheath tumors. *Proc Natl Acad Sci USA 102*, 407–412.

Bi, X., Wei, S.C., and Rong, Y.S. (2004). Telomere protection without a telomerase; The role of ATM and Mre11 in *Drosophila* telomere maintenance. *Curr Biol 14*, 1348–1353.

Blackburn, E.H. (2001). Switching and signaling at the telomere. *Cell 106*, 661–673.

Brunk, U.T., and Terman, A. (2002). Lipofuscin: Mechanisms of age-related accumulation and influence on cell function. *Free Radic Biol Med 33*, 611–619.

Campisi, J. (2005). Senescent cells, tumor suppression, and organismal aging: good citizens, bad neighbors. *Cell 120*, 513–522.

Cahill, G.M. (1996). Circadian regulation of melatonin production in cultured zebrafish pineal and retina. *Brain Res 708*, 177–181.

Cahill, G.M. (2002). Clock mechanisms in zebrafish. *Cell Tissue Res 309*, 27–34.

Cao, L., Li, W., Kim, S., Brodie, S.G., and Deng, C.X. (2003). Senescence, aging, and malignant transformation mediated by p53 in mice lacking the Brca1 full-length isoform. *Genes Dev 17*, 201–213.

Celeste, A., Petersen, S., Romanienko, P.J., Fernandez-Capetillo, O., Chen, H.T., Sedelnikova, O.A., *et al.* (2002). Genomic instability in mice lacking histone H2AX. *Science 296*, 922–927.

Chehab, N.H., Malikzay, A., Appel, M., and Halazonetis, T.D. (2000). Chk2/hCds1 functions as a DNA damage checkpoint in G(1) by stabilizing p53. *Genes Dev 14*, 278–288.

Chehab, N.H., Malikzay, A., Stavridi, E.S., and Halazonetis, T.D. (1999). Phosphorylation of Ser-20 mediates stabilization of human p53 in response to DNA damage. *Proc Natl Acad Sci USA 96*, 13777–13782.

Chen, G., and Lee, E. (1996). The product of the ATM gene is a 370-kDa nuclear phosphoprotein. *J Biol Chem 271*, 33693–33697.

Chen, Q., and Ames, B.N. (1994). Senescence-like growth arrest induced by hydrogen peroxide in human diploid fibroblast F65 cells. *Proc Natl Acad Sci USA 91*, 4130–4134.

Cheng, R., Ford, B.L., O'Neal, P.E., Mathews, C.Z., Bradford, C.S., Thongtan, T., *et al.* (1997). Zebrafish (Danio rerio) p53 tumor suppressor gene: cDNA sequence and expression during embryogenesis. *Mol Mar Biol Biotechnol 6*, 88–97.

Cheng, W.H., von Kobbe, C., Opresko, P.L., Arthur, L.M., Komatsu, K., Seidman, M.M., *et al.* (2004). Linkage between Werner syndrome protein and the Mre11 complex via Nbs1. *J Biol Chem 279*, 21169–21176.

Chien, K.R., and Karsenty, G. (2005). Longevity and lineages: Toward the integrative biology of degenerative diseases in heart, muscle, and bone. *Cell 120*, 533 544.

Conboy, I.M., Conboy, M.J., Wagers, A.J., Girma, E.R., Weissman, I.L., and Rando, T.A. (2005). Rejuvenation of aged progenitor cells by exposure to a young systemic environment. *Nature 433*, 760–764.

Concannon, P. (2002). ATM heterozygosity and cancer risk. *Nat Genet 32*, 89–90.

Curtis, H.J. (1963). Biological mechanisms underlying the aging process. *Science 141*, 686–694.

D'Adda di Fagagna, F., Reaper, P.M., Clay-Farrace, L., Fiegler, H., Carr, P., Von Zglinicki, T., Saretzki, G., Carter, N.P., and Jackson, S.P. (2003). A DNA damage checkpoint response in telomere-initiated senescence. *Nature 426*, 194–198.

Dalle-Donne, I., Rossi, R., Giustarini, D., Milzani, A., and Colombo, R. (2003). Protein carbonyl groups as biomarkers of oxidative stress. *Clin Chim Acta 329*, 23–38.

Dekens, M.P., Santoriello, C., Vallone, D., Grassi, G., Whitmore, D., and Foulkes, N.S. (2003). Light regulates the cell cycle in zebrafish. *Curr Biol 13*, 2051–2057.

Delaunay, F., Thisse, C., Marchand, O., Laudet, V., and Thisse, B. (2000). An inherited functional circadian clock in zebrafish embryos. *Science 289*, 297–300.

Dimri, G.P., Lee, X., Basile, G., Acosta, M., Scott, G., Roskelley, C., *et al.* (1995). A biomarker that identifies senescent human cells in culture and in aging skin in vivo. *Proc Natl Acad Sci USA 92*, 9363–9367.

Dirac, A.M., and Bernards, R. (2003). Reversal of senescence in mouse fibroblasts through lentiviral suppression of p53. *J Biol Chem 278*, 11731–11734.

Dodd, A., Chambers, S.P., Nielsen, P.E., and Love, D.R. (2004). Modeling human disease by gene targeting. *Methods Cell Biol 76*, 593–612.

Dodd, A., Curtis, P.M., Williams, L.C., and Love, D.R. (2000). Zebrafish: Bridging the gap between development and disease. *Hum Mol Genet 9*, 2443–2449.

Egami, N., and Eto, H. (1973). Effect of x-irradiation during embryonic stage on life span in the fish, *Oryzias latipes*. *Exp Gerontol 8*, 219–222.

Elson, A., Wang, Y., Daugherty, C.J., Morton, C.C., Zhou, F., Campos-Torres, J., and Leder, P. (1996). Pleiotropic defects in ataxiA–Telangiectasia protein-deficient mice. *Proc Natl Acad Sci USA 93*, 13084–13089.

Falck, J., Coates, J., and Jackson, S.P. (2005). Conserved modes of recruitment of ATM, ATR and DNA-PKcs to sites of DNA damage. *Nature 434*, 605–611.

Ferbeyre, G., and Lowe, S.W. (2002). The price of tumour suppression? *Nature 415*, 26–27.

Finch, C.E., and Austad, S.N. (2001). History and prospects: Symposium on organisms with slow aging. *Exp Gerontol 36*, 593–597.

Finch, C.E., and Crimmins, E.M. (2004). Inflammatory exposure and historical changes in human life-spans. *Science 305*, 1736–1739.

Finch, C.E., and Ruvkun, G. (2001). The genetics of aging. *Annu Rev Genomics Hum Genet 2*, 435–462.

Finkel, T., and Holbrook, N.J. (2000). Oxidants, oxidative stress and the biology of ageing. *Nature 408*, 239–247.

FitzGerald, M.G., Bean, J.M., Hegde, S.R., Unsal, H., MacDonald, D.J., Harkin, D.P., *et al.* (1997). Heterozygous ATM mutations do not contribute to early onset of breast cancer. *Nat Genet 15*, 307–310.

Garg, R., Geng, C.D., Miller, J.L., Callens, S., Tang, X., Appel, B., and Xu, B. (2004). Molecular cloning and characterization of the catalytic domain of zebrafish homologue of the ataxiA–Telangiectasia mutated gene. *Mol Cancer Res 2*, 348–353.

Gerhard, G.S., Kauffman, E.J., Wang, X., Stewart, R., Moore, J.L., Kasales, C.J., Demidenko, E., and Cheng, K.C. (2002). Life spans and senescent phenotypes in two strains of Zebrafish (*Danio rerio*). *Exp Gerontol 37*, 1055–1068.

Giannelli, F. (1986). DNA maintenance and its relation to human pathology. *J Cell Sci Suppl 4*, 383–416.

Gilad, S., Khosravi, R., Shkedy, D., Uziel, T., Ziv, Y., Savitsky, K., *et al.* (1996). Predominance of null mutations in ataxiA Telangiectasia. *Hum Mol Genet 5*, 433 439.

Gilley, J., and Fried, M. (2001). One INK4 gene and no ARF at the Fugu equivalent of the human INK4A/ARF/INK4B tumour suppressor locus. *Oncogene 20*, 7447–7452.

Gire, V. (2004). Dysfunctional telomeres at senescence signal cell cycle arrest via Chk2. *Cell Cycle 3*, 1217–1220.

Gire, V., Roux, P., Wynford-Thomas, D., Brondello, J.M., and Dulic, V. (2004). DNA damage checkpoint kinase Chk2 triggers replicative senescence. *Embo J 23*, 2554 2563.

Goldsmith, P. (2004). Zebrafish as a pharmacological tool: The how, why and when. *Curr Opin Pharmacol 4*, 504–512.

Green, M.H., Marcovitch, A.J., Harcourt, S.A., Lowe, J.E., Green, I.C., and Arlett, C.F. (1997). Hypersensitivity of ataxiA–Telangiectasia fibroblasts to a nitric oxide donor. *Free Radic Biol Med 22*, 343–347.

Guarente, L., and Picard, F. (2005). Calorie restriction—the SIR2 connection. *Cell 120*, 473–482.

Hadley, E.C., Lakatta, E.G., Morrison-Bogorad, M., Warner, H.R., and Hodes, R.J. (2005). The future of aging therapies. *Cell 120*, 557–567.

Henikoff, S., Till, B.J., and Comai, L. (2004). TILLING. Traditional mutagenesis meets functional genomics. *Plant Physiol 135*, 630–636.

Hensey, C., Robertson, K., and Gautier, J. (2000). Expression and subcellular localization of X-ATM during early Xenopus development. *Dev Genes Evol 210*, 467–469.

Herbig, U., Jobling, W.A., Chen, B.P., Chen, D.J., and Sedivy, J.M., (2004). Telomere shortening triggers senescence of human cells through a pathway involving ATM, p53, and p21 (CIP1), but not p16 (INK4a). *Mol Cell 14*, 501–513.

Herzog, K.H., Chong, M.J., Kapsetaki, M., Morgan, J.I., and McKinnon, P.J. (1998). Requirement for Atm in ionizing radiation-induced cell death in the developing central nervous system. *Science 280*, 1089–1091.

Hill, A.J., Teraoka, H., Heideman, W., and Peterson, R.E. (2005). Zebrafish as a model vertebrate for investigating chemical toxicity. *Toxicol Sci 86*, 6–19.

Hirao, A., Kong, Y.Y., Matsuoka, S., Wakeham, A., Ruland, J., Yoshida, H., *et al.* (2000). DNA damage-induced activation of p53 by the checkpoint kinase Chk2. *Science 287*, 1824–1827.

Hurd, M.W., Debruyne, J., Straume, M., and Cahill, G.M. (1998). Circadian rhythms of locomotor activity in zebrafish. *Physiol Behav 65*, 465–472.

Imamura, S., and Kishi, S. (2005). Molecular cloning and functional characterization of zebrafish ATM. *Int J Biochem Cell Biol 37*, 1105–1116.

Ito, K., Hirao, A., Arai, F., Matsuoka, S., Takubo, K., Hamaguchi, I., Nomiyama, K., Hosokawa, K., Sakurada, K., Nakagata, N., *et al.* (2004). Regulation of oxidative stress by ATM is required for self-renewal of haematopoietic stem cells. *Nature 431*, 997–1002.

Jacobs, J.J., and de Lange, T. (2004). Significant role for p16INK4a in p53-independent telomere-directed senescence. *Curr Biol 14*, 2302–2308.

Jault, C., Pichon, L., and Chluba, J. (2004). Toll-like receptor gene family and TIR-domain adapters in *Danio rerio*. *Mol Immunol 40*, 759–771.

Jones, S.N., Roe, A.E., Donehower, L.A., and Bradley, A. (1995). Rescue of embryonic lethality in Mdm2-deficient mice by absence of p53. *Nature 378*, 206–208.

Kastan, M.B., and Lim, D.S. (2000). The many substrates and functions of ATM. *Nat Rev Mol Cell Biol 1*, 179–186.

Katic, M., and Kahn, C.R. (2005). The role of insulin and IGF-1 signaling in longevity. *Cell Mol Life Sci 62*, 320–343.

Kazimi, N., and Cahill, G.M. (1999). Development of a circadian melatonin rhythm in embryonic zebrafish. *Brain Res Dev Brain Res 117*, 47–52.

Keating, M.T. (2004). Genetic approaches to disease and regeneration. *Philos Trans R Soc Lond B Biol Sci 359*, 795–798.

Kenyon, C. (2005). The plasticity of aging: Insights from long-lived mutants. *Cell 120*, 449–460.

Keyes, W.M., Wu, Y., Vogel, H., Guo, X., Lowe, S.W., and Mills, A.A. (2005). p63 deficiency activates a program of cellular senescence and leads to accelerated aging. *Genes Dev 19*, 1986–1999.

Kim, S.T., Lim, D.S., Canman, C.E., and Kastan, M.B. (1999). Substrate specificities and identification of putative substrates of ATM kinase family members. *J Biol Chem 274*, 37538–37543.

Kipling, D., Davis, T., Ostler, E.L., and Faragher, R.G. (2004). What can progeroid syndromes tell us about human aging? *Science 305*, 1426–1431.

Kishi, S. (2004). Functional aging and gradual senescence in zebrafish. *Ann N Y Acad Sci 1019*, 521–526.

Kishi, S., and Lu, K.P. (2002). A critical role for Pin2/TRF1 in ATM-dependent regulation. Inhibition of Pin2/TRF1 function complements telomere shortening, radiosensitivity, and the G(2)/M checkpoint defect of ataxiA–Telangiectasia cells. *J Biol Chem 277*, 7420–7429.

Kishi, S., Uchiyama, J., Baughman, A.M., Goto, T., Lin, M.C., and Tsai, S.B. (2003). The zebrafish as a vertebrate model of functional aging and very gradual senescence. *Exp Gerontol 38*, 777–786.

Kishi, S., Zhou, X.Z., Ziv, Y., Khoo, C., Hill, D.E., Shiloh, Y., and Lu, K.P. (2001). Telomeric protein Pin2/TRF1 as an important ATM target in response to double strand DNA breaks. *J Biol Chem 276*, 29282–29291.

Lai, S.R., Phipps, S.M., Liu, L., Andrews, L.G., and Tollefsbol, T.O. (2005). Epigenic control of telomerase and modes of telomere maintenance in aging and abnormal systems. *Front Biosci 10*, 1779–1796.

Langenau, D.M., Feng, H., Berghmans, S., Kanki, J.P., Kutok, J.L., and Look, A.T. (2005). Cre/lox-regulated transgenic zebrafish model with conditional myc-induced T cell acute lymphoblastic leukemia. *Proc Natl Acad Sci USA 102*, 6068–6073.

Langheinrich, U., Hennen, E., Stott, G., and Vacun, G. (2002). Zebrafish as a model organism for the identification and characterization of drugs and genes affecting p53 signaling. *Curr Biol 12*, 2023–2028.

Laposa, R.R., Henderson, J.T., Xu, E., and Wells, P.G. (2004). Atm-null mice exhibit enhanced radiation-induced birth defects and a hybrid form of embryonic programmed cell death indicating a teratological suppressor function for ATM. *Faseb J 18*, 896–898.

Lavin, M.F., and Khanna, K.K. (1999). ATM: The protein encoded by the gene mutated in the radiosensitive syndrome ataxiA–Telangiectasia. *Int J Radiat Biol 75*, 1201–1214.

Lavin, M.F., and Shiloh, Y. (1997). The genetic defect in ataxiA–Telangiectasia. *Annu Rev Immunol 15*, 177–202.

Lee, C.K., Klopp, R.G., Weindruch, R., and Prolla, T.A. (1999). Gene expression profile of aging and its retardation by caloric restriction. *Science 285*, 1390–1393.

Lee, H., and Kimelman, D. (2002). A dominant-negative form of p63 is required for epidermal proliferation in zebrafish. *Dev Cell 2*, 607–616.

Liu, D., O'Connor, M.S., Qin, J., and Songyang, Z. (2004). Telosome, a mammalian telomere-associated complex formed by multiple telomeric proteins. *J Biol Chem 279*, 51338–51342.

Liu, T.X., Howlett, N.G., Deng, M., Langenau, D.M., Hsu, K., Rhodes, J., *et al.* (2003). Knockdown of zebrafish Fancd2 causes developmental abnormalities via p53-dependent apoptosis. *Dev Cell 5*, 903–914.

Lombard, D.B., Chua, K.F., Mostoslavsky, R., Franco, S., Gostissa, M., and Alt, F.W. (2005). DNA repair, genome stability, and aging. *Cell 120*, 497–512.

Love, D.R., Pichler, F.B., Dodd, A., Copp, B.R., and Greenwood, D.R. (2004). Technology for high-throughput screens: The present and future using zebrafish. *Curr Opin Biotechnol 15*, 564–571.

MacRae, C.A., and Peterson, R.T. (2003). Zebrafish-based small molecule discovery. *Chem Biol 10*, 901–908.

Mangel, M., and Abrahams, M.V. (2001). Age and longevity in fish, with consideration of the ferox trout. *Exp Gerontol 36*, 765–790.

Matsuoka, S., Rotman, G., Ogawa, A., Shiloh, Y., Tamai, K., and Elledge, S.J. (2000). Ataxia telangiectasia-mutated phosphorylates Chk2 in vivo and in vitro. *Proc Natl Acad Sci USA 97*, 10389–10394.

Maya, R., Balass, M., Kim, S.T., Shkedy, D., Leal, J.F., Shifman, O., *et al.* (2001). ATM-dependent phosphorylation of Mdm2 on serine 395: Role in p53 activation by DNA damage. *Genes Dev 15*, 1067–1077.

McKinnon, P.J. (2004). ATM and ataxia telangiectasia. *EMBO Rep 5*, 772–776.

Meijer, A.H., Gabby Krens, S.F., Medina Rodriguez, I.A., He, S., Bitter, W., Ewa Snaar-Jagalska, B., and Spaink, H.P. (2004). Expression analysis of the Toll-like receptor and TIR domain adaptor families of zebrafish. *Mol Immunol 40*, 773–783.

Metcalfe, J.A., Parkhill, J., Campbell, L., Stacey, M., Biggs, P., Byrd, P.J., and Taylor, A.M. (1996). Accelerated telomere shortening in ataxia telangiectasia. *Nat Genet 13*, 350–353.

Meyn, M.S. (1995). AtaxiA–Telangiectasia and cellular responses to DNA damage. *Cancer Res 55*, 5991–6001.

Meyne, J., Ratliff, R.L., and Moyzis, R.K. (1989). Conservation of the human telomere sequence (TTAGGG)n among vertebrates. *Proc Natl Acad Sci USA 86*, 7049–7053.

Miller, B.M., Werner, T., Weier, H.U., and Nusse, M. (1992). Analysis of radiation-induced micronuclei by fluorescence in situ hybridization (FISH) simultaneously using telomeric and centromeric DNA probes. *Radiat Res 131*, 177–185.

Mitchell, J.R., Wood, E., and Collins, K. (1999). A telomerase component is defective in the human disease dyskeratosis congenita. *Nature 402*, 551–555.

Montes de Oca Luna, R., Wagner, D.S., and Lozano, G. (1995). Rescue of early embryonic lethality in mdm2-deficient mice by deletion of p53. *Nature 378*, 203–206.

Motoyama, N., and Naka, K. (2004). DNA damage tumor suppressor genes and genomic instability. *Curr Opin Genet Dev 14*, 11–16.

Murphy, C.T., McCarroll, S.A., Bargmann, C.I., Fraser, A., Kamath, R.S., Ahringer, J., Li, H., and Kenyon, C. (2003). Genes that act downstream of DAF-16 to influence the lifespan of *Caenorhabditis elegans*. *Nature 424*, 277–283.

Naka, K., Tachibana, A., Ikeda, K., and Motoyama, N. (2004). Stress-induced premature senescence in hTERT-expressing ataxia telangiectasia fibroblasts. *J Biol Chem 279*, 2030–2037.

Nove, J., Little, J.B., Mayer, P.J., Troilo, P., and Nichols, W.W. (1986). Hypersensitivity of cells from a new chromosomal-breakage syndrome to DNA-damaging agents. *Mutat Res 163*, 255–262.

Oh, H., Wang, S.C., Prahash, A., Sano, M., Moravec, C.S., Taffet, G.E., *et al.* (2003). Telomere attrition and Chk2 activation in human heart failure. *Proc Natl Acad Sci USA 100*, 5378–5383.

Oikemus, S.R., McGinnis, N., Queiroz-Machado, J., Tukachinsky, H., Takada, S., Sunkel, C.E., and Brodsky, M.H. (2004). *Drosophila* atm/telomere fusion is required for telomeric localization of HP1 and telomere position effect. *Genes Dev 18*, 1850–1861.

Pandita, T.K. (2002). ATM function and telomere stability. *Oncogene 21*, 611–618.

Pandita, T.K., Pathak, S., and Geard, C.R. (1995). Chromosome end associations, telomeres and telomerase activity in ataxia telangiectasia cells. *Cytogenet Cell Genet 71*, 86–93.

Parng, C. (2005). In vivo zebrafish assays for toxicity testing. *Curr Opin Drug Discov Devel 8*, 100–106.

Patnaik, B.K., Mahapatro, N., and Jena, B.S. (1994). Ageing in fishes. *Gerontology 40*, 113–132.

Patton, E.E., Widlund, H.R., Kutok, J.L., Kopani, K.R., Amatruda, J.F., Murphey, R.D., *et al.* (2005). BRAF mutations are sufficient to promote nevi formation and cooperate with p53 in the genesis of melanoma. *Curr Biol 15*, 249–254.

Peter, Y., Rotman, G., Lotem, J., Elson, A., Shiloh, Y., and Groner, Y. (2001). Elevated Cu/Zn-SOD exacerbates radiation sensitivity and hematopoietic abnormalities of Atm-deficient mice. *Embo J 20*, 1538–1546.

Pichler, F.B., Laurenson, S., Williams, L.C., Dodd, A., Copp, B.R., and Love, D.R. (2003). Chemical discovery and global gene expression analysis in zebrafish. *Nat Biotechnol 21*, 879–883.

Pletcher, S.D., Macdonald, S.J., Marguerie, R., Certa, U., Stearns, S.C., Goldstein, D.B., and Partridge, L. (2002). Genome-wide transcript profiles in aging and calorically restricted *Drosophila melanogaster*. *Curr Biol 12*, 712–723.

Poss, K.D., Keating, M.T., and Nechiporuk, A. (2003). Tales of regeneration in zebrafish. *Dev Dyn 226*, 202–210.

Poss, K.D., Nechiporuk, A., Hillam, A.M., Johnson, S.L., and Keating, M.T. (2002a). Mps1 defines a proximal blastemal proliferative compartment essential for zebrafish fin regeneration. *Development 129*, 5141–5149.

Poss, K.D., Wilson, L.G., and Keating, M.T. (2002b). Heart regeneration in zebrafish. *Science 298*, 2188–2190.

Queiroz-Machado, J., Perdigao, J., Simoes-Carvalho, P., Herrmann, S., and Sunkel, C.E. (2001). tef: A mutation that causes telomere fusion and severe genome rearrangements in *Drosophila melanogaster*. *Chromosoma110*, 10–23.

Raya, A., Koth, C.M., Buscher, D., Kawakami, Y., Itoh, T., Raya, R.M., *et al.* (2003). Activation of Notch signaling pathway precedes heart regeneration in zebrafish. *Proc Natl Acad Sci USA 100 Suppl 1*, 11889–11895.

Reliene, R., Fischer, E., and Schiestl, R.H. (2004). Effect of N-acetyl cysteine on oxidative DNA damage and the frequency of DNA deletions in atm-deficient mice. *Cancer Res 64*, 5148–5153.

Rentzsch, F., Kramer, C., and Hammerschmidt, M. (2003). Specific and conserved roles of TAp73 during zebrafish development. *Gene 323*, 19–30.

Reznick, D., Buckwalter, G., Groff, J., and Elder, D. (2001). The evolution of senescence in natural populations of guppies (*Poecilia reticulata*): A comparative approach. *Exp Gerontol 36*, 791–812.

Reznick, D.N. (1997). Life history evolution in guppies (*Poecilia reticulata*): Guppies as a model for studying the evolutionary biology of aging. *Exp Gerontol 32*, 245–258.

Reznick, D.N., Bryant, M.J., Roff, D., Ghalambor, C.K., and Ghalambor, D.E. (2004). Effect of extrinsic mortality on the evolution of senescence in guppies. *Nature 431*, 1095–1099.

Rodier, F., Kim, S.H., Nijjar, T., Yaswen, P., and Campisi, J. (2005). Cancer and aging: The importance of telomeres in genome maintenance. *Int J Biochem Cell Biol 37*, 977–990.

Rotman, G., and Shiloh, Y. (1997). AtaxiA–Telangiectasia: Is ATM a sensor of oxidative damage and stress? *Bioessays 19*, 911–917.

Rubinstein, A.L. (2003). Zebrafish: From disease modeling to drug discovery. *Curr Opin Drug Discov Devel 6*, 218–223.

Ruggero, D., Grisendi, S., Piazza, F., Rego, E., Mari, F., Rao, P.H., *et al.* (2003). Dyskeratosis congenita and cancer in mice deficient in ribosomal RNA modification. *Science 299*, 259–262.

Sancar, A., Lindsey-Boltz, L.A., Unsal-Kacmaz, K., and Linn, S. (2004). Molecular mechanisms of mammalian DNA repair and the DNA damage checkpoints. *Annu Rev Biochem 73*, 39–85.

Satoh, S., Arai, K., and Watanabe, S. (2004). Identification of a novel splicing form of zebrafish p73 having a strong transcriptional activity. *Biochem Biophys Res Commun 325*, 835–842.

Savitsky, K., Bar-Shira, A., Gilad, S., Rotman, G., Ziv, Y., Vanagaite, L., *et al.* (1995a). A single ataxia telangiectasia gene with a product similar to PI-3 kinase. *Science 268*, 1749–1753.

Savitsky, K., Sfez, S., Tagle, D.A., Ziv, Y., Sartiel, A., Collins, F.S., Shiloh, Y., and Rotman, G. (1995b). The complete sequence of the coding region of the ATM gene reveals similarity to cell cycle regulators in different species. *Hum Mol Genet 4*, 2025–2032.

Scott, S.P., Zhang, N., Khanna, K.K., Khromykh, A., Hobson, K., Watters, D., and Lavin, M.F. (1998). Cloning and expression of the ataxiA–Telangiectasia gene in baculovirus. *Biochem Biophys Res Commun 245*, 144–148.

Sherr, C.J., and DePinho, R.A. (2000). Cellular senescence: Mitotic clock or culture shock? *Cell 102*, 407–410.

Shieh, S.Y., Ahn, J., Tamai, K., Taya, Y., and Prives, C. (2000). The human homologs of checkpoint kinases Chk1 and Cds1 (Chk2) phosphorylate p53 at multiple DNA damage-inducible sites. *Genes Dev 14*, 289–300.

Shieh, S.Y., Ikeda, M., Taya, Y., and Prives, C. (1997). DNA damage-induced phosphorylation of p53 alleviates inhibition by MDM2. *Cell 91*, 325–334.

Shiloh, Y. (1995). AtaxiA–Telangiectasia: Closer to unraveling the mystery. *Eur J Hum Genet 3*, 116–138.

Shiloh, Y. (2001). ATM and ATR: Networking cellular responses to DNA damage. *Curr Opin Genet Dev 11*, 71–77.

Shiloh, Y. (2003). ATM and related protein kinases: Safeguarding genome integrity. *Nat Rev Cancer 3*, 155–168.

Silva, E., Tiong, S., Pedersen, M., Homola, E., Royou, A., Fasulo, B., *et al.* (2004). ATM is required for telomere maintenance and chromosome stability during *Drosophila* development. *Curr Biol 14*, 1341–1347.

Smilenov, L.B., Morgan, S.E., Mellado, W., Sawant, S.G., Kastan, M.B., and Pandita, T.K. (1997). Influence of ATM function on telomere metabolism. *Oncogene 15*, 2659–2665.

Smith, P.J., and Paterson, M.C. (1980). Defective DNA repair and increased lethality in ataxia telangiectasia cells exposed to 4-nitroquinoline-1-oxide. *Nature 287*, 747–749.

Soares, H.D., Morgan, J.I., and McKinnon, P.J. (1998). Atm expression patterns suggest a contribution from the peripheral nervous system to the phenotype of ataxiA–Telangiectasia. *Neuroscience 86*, 1045–1054.

Sohal, R.S., and Weindruch, R. (1996). Oxidative stress, caloric restriction, and aging. *Science 273*, 59–63.

Sola, L., and Gornung, E. (2001). Classical and molecular cytogenetics of the zebrafish, *Danio rerio* (Cyprinidae, Cypriniformes): an overview. *Genetica 111*, 397–412.

Song, Y.H., Mirey, G., Betson, M., Haber, D.A., and Settleman, J. (2004). The *Drosophila* ATM ortholog, dATM, mediates the response to ionizing radiation and to spontaneous DNA damage during development. *Curr Biol 14*, 1354–1359.

Spring, K., Ahangari, F., Scott, S.P., Waring, P., Purdie, D.M., Chen, P.C., *et al.* (2002). Mice heterozygous for mutation in Atm, the gene involved in ataxiA–Telangiectasia, have heightened susceptibility to cancer. *Nat Genet 32*, 185–190.

Takao, N., Li, Y., and Yamamoto, K. (2000). Protective roles for ATM in cellular response to oxidative stress. *FEBS Lett 472*, 133–136.

Takeda, K., Kaisho, T., and Akira, S. (2003). Toll-like receptors. *Annu Rev Immunol 21*, 335–376.

Tanaka, H., Mendonca, M.S., Bradshaw, P.S., Hoelz, D.J., Malkas, L.H., Meyn, M.S., and Gilley, D. (2005). DNA damage-induced phosphorylation of the human telomere-associated protein TRF2. *Proc Natl Acad Sci USA 102*, 15539–15544.

Taniguchi, T., Garcia-Higuera, I., Xu, B., Andreassen, P.R., Gregory, R.C., Kim, S.T., *et al.* (2002). Convergence of the fanconi anemia and ataxia telangiectasia signaling pathways. *Cell 109*, 459–472.

Taylor, A.M. (1998). What has the cloning of the ATM gene told us about ataxia telangiectasia? *Int J Radiat Biol 73*, 365–371.

Taylor, R.W., Barron, M.J., Borthwick, G.M., Gospel, A., Chinnery, P.F., Samuels, D.C., *et al.* (2003). Mitochondrial DNA mutations in human colonic crypt stem cells. *J Clin Invest 112*, 1351–1360.

Terman, A., and Brunk, U.T. (2004). Lipofuscin. *Int J Biochem Cell Biol 36*, 1400–1404.

Thacker, J. (1994). Cellular radiosensitivity in ataxiA–Telangiectasia. *Int J Radiat Biol 66*, S87–96.

Thisse, C., Neel, H., Thisse, B., Daujat, S., and Piette, J. (2000). The Mdm2 gene of zebrafish (*Danio rerio*): Preferential expression during development of neural and muscular tissues, and absence of tumor formation after overexpression of its cDNA during early embryogenesis. *Differentiation 66*, 61–70.

Tischkowitz, M.D., and Hodgson, S.V. (2003). Fanconi anaemia. *J Med Genet 40*, 1–10.

Toussaint, O., Medrano, E.E., and von Zglinicki, T. (2000). Cellular and molecular mechanisms of stress-induced premature senescence (SIPS) of human diploid fibroblasts and melanocytes. *Exp Gerontol 35*, 927–945.

Traver, D., Winzeler, A., Stern, H.M., Mayhall, E.A., Langenau, D.M., Kutok, J.L., *et al.* (2004). Effects of lethal irradiation in zebrafish and rescue by hematopoietic cell transplantation. *Blood 104*, 1298–1305.

Trifunovic, A., Wredenberg, A., Falkenberg, M., Spelbrink, J.N., Rovio, A.T., Bruder, C.E., *et al.* (2004). Premature ageing in mice expressing defective mitochondrial DNA polymerase. *Nature 429*, 417–423.

Tyner, S.D., Venkatachalam, S., Choi, J., Jones, S., Ghebranious, N., Igelmann, H., *et al.* (2002). p53 mutant mice that display early ageing-associated phenotypes. *Nature 415*, 45–53.

Unger, T., Juven-Gershon, T., Moallem, E., Berger, M., Vogt Sionov, R., Lozano, G., *et al.* (1999). Critical role for Ser20 of human p53 in the negative regulation of p53 by Mdm2. *Embo J 18*, 1805–1814.

Valdesalici, S., and Cellerino, A. (2003). Extremely short lifespan in the annual fish *Nothobranchius furzeri*. *Proc Biol Sci 270 Suppl 2*, S189–191.

Varela, I., Cadinanos, J., Pendas, A.M., Gutierrez-Fernandez, A., Folgueras, A.R., Sanchez, L.M., Zhou, Z., Rodriguez, F.J., Stewart, C.L., Vega, J.A., *et al.* (2005). Accelerated ageing in mice deficient in Zmpste24 protease is linked to p53 signalling activation. *Nature 437*, 564–568.

Verdun, R.E., Crabbe, L., Haggblom, C., and Karlseder, J. (2005). Functional human telomeres are recognized as DNA damage in g2 of the cell cycle. *Mol Cell 20*, 551–561.

Vogelstein, B. (1990). Cancer. A deadly inheritance. *Nature 348*, 681–682.

Vogelstein, B., and Kinzler, K.W. (1992). p53 function and dysfunction. *Cell 70*, 523–526.

Vogelstein, B., and Kinzler, K.W. (2004). Cancer genes and the pathways they control. *Nat Med 10*, 789–799.

Vogelstein, B., Lane, D., and Levine, A.J. (2000). Surfing the p53 network. *Nature 408*, 307–310.

von Zglinicki, T., Saretzki, G., Ladhoff, J., d'Adda di Fagagna, F., and Jackson, S.P. (2005). Human cell senescence as a DNA damage response. *Mech Ageing Dev 126*, 111–117.

Wahl, G.M., and Carr, A.M. (2001). The evolution of diverse biological responses to DNA damage: Insights from yeast and p53. *Nat Cell Biol 3*, E277–286.

Watters, D.J. (2003). Oxidative stress in ataxia telangiectasia. *Redox Rep 8*, 23–29.

Wienholds, E., Schulte-Merker, S., Walderich, B., and Plasterk, R.H. (2002). Target-selected inactivation of the zebrafish rag1 gene. *Science 297*, 99–102.

Wienholds, E., van Eeden, F., Kosters, M., Mudde, J., Plasterk, R.H., and Cuppen, E. (2003). Efficient target-selected mutagenesis in zebrafish. *Genome Res 13*, 2700–2707.

Willingale-Theune, J., Schweiger, M., Hirsch-Kauffmann, M., Meek, A.E., Paulin-Levasseur, M., and Traub, P. (1989). Ultrastructure of Fanconi anemia fibroblasts. *J Cell Sci 93 (Pt 4)*, 651–665.

Wolf, F.I., Torsello, A., Covacci, V., Fasanella, S., Montanari, M., Boninsegna, A., and Cittadini, A. (2002). Oxidative DNA damage as a marker of aging in WI-38 human fibroblasts. *Exp Gerontol 37*, 647–656.

Wright, W.E., Shay, J.W., and Piatyszek, M.A. (1995). Modifications of a telomeric repeat amplification protocol (TRAP) result in increased reliability, linearity and sensitivity. *Nucleic Acids Res 23*, 3794–3795.

Xu, Y., Ashley, T., Brainerd, E.E., Bronson, R.T., Meyn, M.S., and Baltimore, D. (1996). Targeted disruption of ATM leads to growth retardation, chromosomal fragmentation during meiosis, immune defects, and thymic lymphoma. *Genes Dev 10*, 2411–2422.

Yeh, J.R., and Crews, C.M. (2003). Chemical genetics: Adding to the developmental biology toolbox. *Dev Cell 5*, 11–19.

Zhang, X., Li, J., Sejas, D.P., and Pang, Q. (2005). The ATM/p53/p21 pathway influences cell fate decision between apoptosis and senescence in reoxygenated hematopoietic progenitor cells. *J Biol Chem 280*, 19635–19640.

Zhdanova, I.V., Wang, S.Y., Leclair, O.U., and Danilova, N.P. (2001). Melatonin promotes sleep-like state in zebrafish. *Brain Res 903*, 263–268.

Ziv, S., Brenner, O., Amariglio, N., Smorodinsky, N.I., Galron, R., Carrion, D.V., Zhang, W., Sharma, G.G., Pandita, R.K., Agarwal, M., *et al.* (2005). Impaired genomic stability and increased oxidative stress exacerbate different features of Ataxia-telagiectasia. *Hum Mol Genet 14*, 2929–2943.

Zon, L.I., and Peterson, R.T. (2005). In vivo drug discovery in the zebrafish. *Nat Rev Drug Discov 4*, 35–44.

Zou, S., Meadows, S., Sharp, L., Jan, L.Y., and Jan, Y.N. (2000). Genome-wide study of aging and oxidative stress response in *Drosophila melanogaster*. *Proc Natl Acad Sci USA 97*, 13726–13731.

29

Telomeres in Aging: Birds

Susan E. Swanberg and Mary E. Delany

This chapter describes the use of avian species (the domestic chicken Gallus domesticus in particular) as model organisms for research in telomere biology and aging. Presented here are key concepts of avian telomere biology including characteristics of the model: the karyotype, telomere arrays, telomere shortening as a measure of the senescence phenotype or organismal aging, and telomerase activity in avian systems, including chicken embryonic stem cells, chicken embryo fibroblasts, the gastrula embryo and DT40 cells. Key methods used to measure telomere shortening and telomerase activity, and to conduct expression profiling of selected genes involved in telomere length maintenance are noted, as are methods for conducting gain- and loss-of-function studies in the chicken embryo. Tables containing references on general topics related to avian telomere biology and poultry husbandry as well as specific information regarding chicken orthologs of genes implicated in telomere maintenance pathways are provided. Internet resources for investigators of avian telomere biology are listed.

Introduction: The Chicken as a Model Organism

The versatility and utility of the domestic chicken as a developmental model was recently celebrated in a special issue of the journal *Developmental Dynamics* [(2004) 229, 413–712]. The chicken is one of the primary models for vertebrate developmental biology and a model organism for the study of virology, immunology, cancer and gene regulation (Tickle, 2004; Antin and Konieczka, 2005). With a 6.6X draft sequence of its genome completed, the chicken is poised to become even more valuable in traditional fields of study and also in aging research.

The earliest recorded descriptions of the chicken as a model for biological processes are attributed to Hippocrates and Aristotle, who wrote about embryonic development in fertilized chicken eggs. Twentieth-century embryologists authored numerous treatises describing, diagramming, and providing detailed photographs of the chicken during development (Hamburger and Hamilton, 1951; Romanoff, 1960; Eyal-Giladi and Kochev, 1976), which promoted use of the chicken embryo as a model for study of mechanisms including morphogenesis; neurogenesis; somatogenesis; limb, limb-digit and craniofacial development; left–right symmetry; axis development and others. The extensive use of the chicken as a model for early vertebrate development and its role in biomedical research has of necessity produced a detailed and comprehensive body of knowledge about basic chicken biology (Scanes *et al.*, 2004; Stern, 2005). Add to all of this the accessibility of the chicken embryo, the relative economy of breeding and maintaining chickens and the ease of manipulation of embryonic and adult tissues and the chicken becomes an obvious choice as a model for the study of organismal and cellular senescence.

Aging and Replicative Senescence

Cellular or replicative senescence (*in vitro*) is often utilized as a model for the aging process (*in vivo*) due to the hypothesis that cellular aging recapitulates organismal aging (Wadhwa *et al.*, 2005). The central dogma of replicative senescence holds that cultures of vertebrate fibroblasts have a limited capacity for proliferation. After a finite number of cell divisions, proliferation slows and culture arrest ensues. The barrier represented by culture arrest, termed the Hayflick Limit, is accompanied by a number of morphological changes including increased cell size, increased nuclear and nucleolar sizes, increased vacuolation of the cytoplasm and endoplasmic reticulum, expression of senescence-associated markers such as beta-galactosidase, and other changes in morphology and gene expression (Cristafalo *et al.*, 2004 and references therein).

A genomic alteration associated with cellular or replicative senescence in a variety of organisms, including the chicken, is the shortening of telomeres (Prowse and Greider, 1995; Taylor and Delany, 2000; Swanberg and Delany, 2003). Shortened telomeres induce a DNA damage response, signaling cell cycle arrest. If the damage cannot be repaired, a checkpoint response results in further arrest or apoptosis. An alternative or complementary model for telomere-induced replicative senescence is loss of the protective effect of accessory proteins, such as TRF2, at the telomeres (Karlseder *et al.*, 2002). Reactivation of telomerase or induction of the ALT (alternate lengthening of telomeres) pathway may provide protection against apoptosis or senescence and facilitate transformation and immortalization by stabilizing telomeres (Swanberg and Delany, 2003 and references therein).

The prevailing explanation for telomere shortening, the end-replication problem, is based on the inability of DNA polymerase to replicate the ends of a linear chromosome, resulting in the incomplete replication of the 5′ end of the daughter strand. Telomerase is able to offset telomere shortening by adding telomere repeats to the parent strand which generates a longer telomere in the daughter strand. The telomerase holoenzyme is composed of two elements, telomerase rNA, TR, which contains the template for addition of telomeric repeats (Greider and Blackburn, 1989) and telomerase reverse transcriptase, TERT, the component which catalyzes the addition of repeats to the parent-strand chromosome end (Lingner *et al.*, 1997). Most normal, adult vertebrate somatic cells, with the exception of cells from the lab mouse (*Mus musculus*), do not exhibit telomerase activity (Levy *et al.*, 1992; Kim *et al.*, 1994; Wright and Shay 2002; Levy *et al.*, 1992). Not only does telomerase maintain telomeres of proliferating cells, it is also implicated in oncogenesis (Greider and Blackburn, 1989).

In addition to the end-replication problem and the compensating function of telomerase, telomere length is impacted by proteins that bind to and contribute to the architecture of the telomere. The thousands of duplex DNA telomere repeats are, for the most part, packaged in closely-spaced nucleosomes (Blackburn, 2001). However, the G-rich 3′ overhang assumes a terminal loop (t-loop), which displaces one of the duplex strands forming a related structure (D-loop). The D-loop t-loop is stabilized by telomere-binding proteins and their interaction partners (Greider 1999; Griffith *et al.*, 1999; Wei and Price, 2003). Closed chromatin loops resembling t-loops have been observed in chicken using electron microscopy (Nikitina and Woodcock, 2004).

Telomere-repeat-binding factors 1 and 2 (TRF1 and 2) bind to double-stranded telomeric DNA (Wei and Price, 2003). TRF1, which induces telomeric DNA strands to bend, loop and pair (Bianchi *et al.*, 1997; Smogorzewska *et al.*, 2000), may produce shortening of telomeres by sequestering the 3′ overhang from telomerase (van Steensel and de Lange, 1997). TRF2 is described as protective of telomeres in some studies (Karlseder, 2003) and as a negative regulator of telomere length in other studies (Smogorzewska *et al.*, 2000; Stansel *et al.*, 2001). Overexpression of TRF1 or TRF2 produces a progressive shortening of telomeres (Ohki and Ishikawa, 2004 and references therein). Tankyrase 1 and 2 have the ability to bind TRF1, resulting in the ADP-ribosylation of TRF1 and the release of TRF1 from telomeric DNA. Overexpression of tankyrase 1 results in the removal of TRF1 from the telomeres followed by telomere elongation (Smith and de Lange, 2000).

In addition to the tankyrases, TRF1 and TRF2, Rap 1 and Pot 1 are involved in telomere maintenance. Rap1 interacts with TRF2, and Pot 1 may coat and protect both G-strand overhangs and the displaced G strand of a t loop (Bauman and Cech, 2001; Tan *et al.*, 2003). Other proteins known to be relevant to telomere length regulation include c-myc, an oncogenic transcription factor which regulates cell proliferation, differentiation and apoptosis (Piedra *et al.*, 2002). Down-regulation of c-myc is believe to be a prerequisite to differentiation (Skerka *et al.*, 1993; Baker *et al.*, 1994) and c-myc reactivates telomerase in transformed cells by inducing expression of its catalytic subunit TERT (Wu *et al.*, 1999).

Chicken orthologs of TRF1 and 2, tankyrase 1 and 2, TR, TERT, c-myc, Rap 1 and Pot 1 have been characterized. In addition, chicken orthologs of the helicases that are missing or mutated in the progeroid disorders, Werner and Bloom Syndrome, have been identified but not studied. The Werner (WNR) and Bloom (BLM) proteins, both Req-Q helicases, have been implicated in telomere maintenance pathways (Du *et al.*, 2004). Table 29.1 lists chicken genes related to telomere length regulation, their human orthologs and relevant references.

The Chicken as a Paradigm for Aging Research

Organisms frequently used in aging studies include yeast, *Drosophila*, *C. elegans*, and *M. musculus*, the laboratory mouse. With all of these well-characterized models available, particularly a mammalian vertebrate as well-studied as the lab mouse, why use an avian model? The advantages of using a vertebrate are obvious, and the mouse would at first glance appear to be a better choice than the chicken except for shortcomings of the mouse vis-à-vis the study of aging and oncogenesis. For example, mice have a very short lifespan. In contrast, maximum life expectancies of many species of birds approach the human life expectancy (Forsyth *et al.*, 2002; Austad, 1997). Lifespan is significant, as cellular and genetic mechanisms governing cell proliferation are likely conserved in longer-lived species.

In addition to the issue of lifespan, laboratory mouse somatic cells retain telomerase activity and do not appear to display division-dependent telomere shortening (Prowse and Greider, 1995; Forsyth *et al.*, 2002; Kim *et al.*, 2002). Mouse models of telomere shortening have been developed, but it takes several generations in the telomerase knockout mouse (TR-/TR-) to achieve a phenotype that demonstrates division-dependent telomere shortening (Cheong *et al.*, 2003). In contrast, human and chicken somatic cells lack telomerase, with down-regulation of telomerase occurring early in development. Division-dependent telomere shortening is established in chicken chromosomes (*in vivo* and *in vitro*) and human chromosomes. In human, mouse and chicken, highly proliferative tissues such as embryonic cells and intestine as well as transformed cells exhibit telomerase activity

TABLE 29.1
Chicken and human orthologs of genes involved in telomere maintenance pathways

Gene	Description	Accession	Chromosome or locus	References
hTERT	H. sapiens telomerase reverse transcriptase	AF015950	5p15.33	Nakamura *et al.*, 1007
cTERT	G. gallus telomerase reverse transcriptase	AY502592	2q21	Delany and Dainels, 2004
hTR	H. sapiens telomerase RNA	NR_001566	3q26	Feng *et al.*, 1995
cTR	G. gallus telomerase RNA	AY312571	9q-terminal	Delany and Daniels, 2003
tankyrase 1	H. sapiens tankyrase 1	NM_003747	8p23.1	Broccoli *et al.*, 1997
tankyrase 1	G. gallus tankyrase 1	AY142108	4	DeRyker *et al.*, 2003
tankyrase 2	H. sapiens tankyrase 2	AF438201	10q23.3	Kaminker *et al.*, 2001
tankyrase 2	G. gallus tankyrase 2	AY142107	unknown	DeRyker *et al.*, 2003
TERF1/TRF1	H. sapiens telomeric repeat binding factor 1	NM_003218	8q13	Zhong *et al.*, 1992
TERF1/TRF1	G. gallus telomeric repeat binding factor 1	AY237359	2	DeRyker *et al.*, 2003
TERF2/TRF2	H. sapiens telomeric repeat binding factor 2	BC024890	16q22.1	Broccoli *et al.*, 1997
TERF2/TRF2	G. gallus telomeric repeat binding factor 2	AJ133783	11	Konrad *et al.*, 1999
Rap 1	H. sapiens TRF2-interacting telomeric RAP1 protein	NM_204468	4	Tan *et al.*, 2003
Rap 1	G. gallus TRF2-interacting telomeric RAP1 protein (RAP1) mRNA	AY083908	11	Tan *et al.*, 2003
Pot 1	H. sapiens protection of telomeres 1	NM_015450	7q31.33	Bauman and Cech, 2001
Pot 1	G. gallus POT1 single-strand telomeric DNA-binding protein	AY555718	1	Wei and Price, 2004
WRN	H. sapiens Werner Syndrome (WRN) protein	NM_000553	8p12-p11.2	Gray *et al.*, 1997
WRN	G. gallus Werner Syndrome protein (WRN)	NM_001012888	4	Caldwell *et al.*, 2005
BLM	H. sapiens Bloom Syndrome (BLM) protein	NM_000057	15q26.1	Ellis *et al.*, 1995
BLM	G. gallus Bloom Syndrome (BLM) protein	NM_001007087	10	Caldwell *et al.*, 2005
c-myc	H. sapiens c-myc oncogene	V00568	8q24	Watt *et al.*, 1983
c-myc	G. gallus c-myc oncogene	X68073	2	Harris *et al.*, 1992

(Taylor and Delany, 2000; Forsyth *et al.*, 2002; Swanberg and Delany 2003; Delany *et al.*, 2003).

Unlike mouse fibroblasts, both chicken and human primary fibroblast cells are generally refractory to spontaneous immortalization (Lima and Macieira-Coelho, 1972; Lima *et al.*, 1972; Macieira-Coelho and Azzarone, 1988; Prowse and Greider, 1995). In addition, critically short human telomeres induce senescence either by activating p53 or by inducing the p16/RB pathway, and suppression of both pathways is required to suppress senescence of aged human cells. In mouse, the p16/RB response to telomere dysfunction is not active (Smogorzewska and de Lange, 2002). In contrast, the senescence pathways of chicken and human fibroblast systems thus far seem to share more similarities than differences (Kim *et al.*, 2002); see Table 29.2. For an

TABLE 29.2
Telomerase activity, telomere shortening and ease of immortalization in vertebrate model systems

Mouse	Human	Chicken
Telomerase activity in somatic cells	No telomerase activity in most somatic cells	No telomerase activity in most somatic cells
No division-dependent telomere shortening	Division-dependent telomere shortening	Division-dependent telomere shortening
Fibroblasts spontaneously immortalize	Fibroblasts refractory to spontaneous immortalization	Fibroblasts refractory to spontaneous immortalization

excellent review of the developmental regulation of telomerase activity in human, mouse, chicken and flowering plants, see Forsyth *et al.* (2002).

Features of the Chicken Genome Relevant to the Study of Aging

The chicken karyotype consists of 39 pairs of chromosomes, which is typical of most avian species. The genome is organized as eight pairs of cytologically distinct macrochromosomes, the Z and W sex chromosomes and thirty pairs of small cytologically indistinguishable microchromosomes (ICSGS, 2004). As in other vertebrates, chicken telomeres consist of a highly conserved hexanucleotide repeat, 5′ $TTAGGG_{(n)}$ 3′. The cytogenetic features of the telomere repeat were first described in chicken by Nanda and Schmid (1994). Molecular features of telomeric DNA in the chicken genome were described in 2000 (Delany *et al.*). Although the avian genome is one-third the size of the human genome (1.25 pg versus 3 pg/haploid cell), the amount of telomeric DNA sequence is five to ten times more abundant in birds than in humans (Delany *et al.*, 2000; Nanda *et al.*, 2002). Higher telomere repeat content in the chicken is likely due to the high number of chromosome ends ($2n = 78$ or 156 chromosome termini), the load of interstitial telomeric DNA and the presence of an unusual category of ultra-long telomeric arrays (see Figure 29.1).

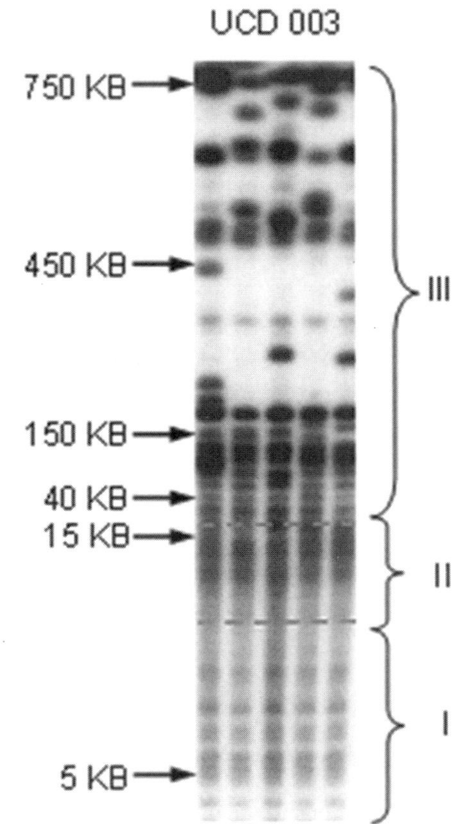

Figure 29.1. Image of pulse-field gel showing chicken Class I, II and III telomere arrays. Class II arrays are analyzed for telomere shortening.

Telomeric DNA in the chicken can be categorized into three main array size classes. Class I telomere repeats are 0.5–10 kb in length and exhibit discrete and genotype-specific banding patterns. Class I repeats are interstitially located and show no evidence of telomere shortening. Class II repeats are 10–40 kb and appear on Southern blots as the typical overlapping smear of TRFs; Class II arrays show evidence of terminal location based on digestion by *Bal* 31 and exhibit division-dependent shortening in somatic tissues. Class III telomeres are hundreds of kilobases in size and range to 3 megabases. Shortening of these arrays has not been established because of the inability to resolve changes of 100s of nucleotides (typical telomere erosion) in the context of 100s to 1000s of kilobases of the Class III arrays (Delany *et al.*, 2000). In order to resolve Class III arrays on a gel, special pulse field gel electrophoresis parameters are required (Delany *et al.*, 2000).

Not all avian species exhibit the Class III arrays (Delany *et al.*, 2000; Nanda *et al.*, 2002). Current models suggest that the Class III arrays of the chicken map to a subset of microchromosomes, perhaps serving to protect these small genetic elements from erosion and/or contributing to high microchromosome recombination rates (Delany *et al.*, 2000; Delany *et al.*, 2003). It is important to note that the existence of megabase telomere arrays in chicken does not diminish the power of the chicken as a model for division-dependent telomere shortening as it appears to be the shortest telomere or the unprotected telomere which triggers genome instability (Hemann *et al.*, 2001; Karlseder *et al.*, 2002).

Telomerase activity and telomere-shortening profiles in avian cells *in vivo* and *in vitro* mirror what is observed in human cells. Telomerase activity is developmentally regulated *in vivo* with high levels of telomerase in early-stage chicken embryos (preblastula through neurula) and during organogenesis all organs surveyed up to 10 days of embryonation (E10) followed by down-regulation for most somatic tissues. Constitutive telomerase activity continues for "renewable" tissues, including intestine, spleen, and organs or cells of the reproductive system. An average decrease of 3.2 kb in telomere length was observed from the early embryo to the adult (Taylor and Delany, 2000). *In vitro* observations include absence of telomerase from nontransformed primary cells (CEFs) contrasted with telomerase activity in cultured blastodermal cells, cES cells and in every transformed avian cell type surveyed to date (Table 29.3).

As measured by mean TRF, the *in vitro* rate of telomere shortening observed in Class II arrays in CEFs is approximately 50 bp of telomeric DNA per population doubling. Yet calculation of percent telomeric DNA at representative passages revealed that an average of 63% of the telomeric DNA was eroded in CEFs by senescence. The greatest loss of telomeric DNA occurred precipitously in later passages. These data suggest two mechanisms of telomere shortening: (1) telomere attrition due to the end-replication problem and (2) catastrophic erosion preceding culture arrest (Swanberg and Delany, 2003).

TABLE 29.3
Telomerase Positive Transformed Avian Cell Lines (Adapted from Swanberg and Delany, 2003)

Cell name	Description
RP-19	Turkey B cell
DT40	Chicken B cell (bursal lymphoma)
RP-9	Chicken B cell (bursal lymphoma)
MSB-1	Chicken T cell (spleen tumor cells in vitro)
MQ-NCSU	Chicken macrophage (peripheral blood)
QT6	Quail fibroblast (fibrosarcoma)
QT35	Quail fibroblast (fibrosarcoma)
LMH & LMH/2A	Chicken hepatocyte (hepatocellular carcinoma)

Tools for Utilizing the Chicken in Aging Studies

A variety of techniques for the study of telomere biology are available, including telomere terminal restriction fragment (TRF) analysis, fluorescence *in situ* hybridization (FISH), variations of polymerase chain reaction (PCR), and the telomere repeat amplification protocol (TRAP). For an excellent summary of selected methods utilized to measure telomere length, see Nakagawa *et al.*, (2004). A list of references pertaining to techniques used in the study of telomere biology is contained in Table 29.4.

TABLE 29.4
References for the study of Avian Telomere Biology

Telomere cytogenetics
Nanda and Schmid, 1994
Nanda *et al.*, 2002
Delany *et al.*, 2000
Replicative senescence in chicken cell culture
Lima *et al.*, 1972
Lima and Macieira-Coelho, 1972
Measuring telomeres
Harley *et al.*, 1990
Nakagawa *et al.*, 2004
Telomere shortening in birds
Talyor and Delany, 2000
Delany *et al.*, 2003
Swanberg and Delany, 2003
Telomeres as tool for age determination
Vleck *et al.*, 2003
Haussmann *et al.*, 2003
Hall *et al.*, 2004
TRAP assay
Kim *et al.*, 1994
Saldanha *et al.*, 2003
Telomerase in birds
Talyor and Delany, 2000
Delany *et al.*, 2000
Swanberg and Delany, 2003
Venkatesan and Price, 1998
Haussman *et al.*, 2004
Gene expression patterns: telomere maintenance pathways
Swanberg *et al.*, 2004
Swanberg and Delany, 2005

(Continued)

TABLE 29.4
Continued

Quantitative PCR
Bustin, 2004
Gain- and loss-of-function techniques in chick embryo
Krull, 2004 (electroporation)
Bourikas and Stoeckli, 2003 (RNAi)
Pekarik *et al.*, 2003 (RNAi)
Sato *et al.*, 2004 (RNAi)
Kos *et al.*, 2003 (morpholinos)
Chicken genome sequence and genomic resources
ICGSC, 2004
Antin and Konieczka, 2005
Dequeant and Pourquie, 2005

TELOMERE TERMINAL RESTRICTION FRAGMENT ANALYSIS

First described in Harley *et al.*, 1990, telomere terminal restriction fragment analysis establishes mean telomere length in a tissue or cell sample or percent of telomeric DNA present in one sample relative to another. To measure mean telomere length, genomic DNA is first digested with a restriction enzyme or a cocktail of restriction enzymes followed by electrophoretic separation through an agarose gel. It is essential that DNA concentration be equivalent in each lane. The gel is Southern blotted and hybridized to a TTAGGG(n) probe labeled with a radionuclide or a fluorochrome producing a smear of fragments. Densitometry readings taken at a number of locations along the smear are summed and averaged. Mean telomere length is defined as $\sum(OD_i)/\sum(OD_i/L_i)$ where OD_i is the densitometer output and L_i is the length of the DNA at position i. Sums are calculated over the range of lengths covered by the smear of TTAGGG-hybridized DNA (Harley *et al.*, 1990, Swanberg and Delany, 2003).

In order to measure percent telomeric DNA present in one sample relative to a calibrator sample (Harley *et al.*, 1990), DNA is restricted, separated by gel electrophoresis, Southern blotted, and hybridized as with the determination of mean TRF length. However, rather than taking densitometry readings at discrete locations along the length of the smear of telomeric DNA, total telomeric DNA is measured by calculating the total integrated signal $(\sum OD_i)$ over the same range of fragment sizes used for mean TRF analysis. Total integrated signal in this range is measured in each lane of any given gel, and results are expressed as a percentage of the signal from the earliest passage (Harley *et al.*, 1990; Swanberg and Delany, 2003). The measurement of TRFs reveals a high degree of variability within cell lines prepared from single embryos of a highly inbred line, and mean TRF measurements are also subject to variability resulting from drift in the subpopulations within a culture. Therefore it is advisable to assay using more than one method to obtain a biologically relevant picture of telomere attrition or erosion (Swanberg and Delany, 2003).

FISH

Telomere arrays have been examined in a wide sampling of avian species, including chicken, using fluorescence *in situ* hybridization (FISH) (Nanda and Schmid, 1994; Nanda *et al.*, 2002). While the Nanda study was not quantitative, the existence of large telomere arrays in birds was quite apparent using traditional FISH techniques. Telomere quantitative fluorescence *in situ* hybridization (telomere Q-FISH), a variation of this method, has been utilized effectively in several organisms. Using Q-FISH, telomere length is expressed as a ratio of telomere fluorescence in cells that have undergone erosion to telomere fluorescence in cells in the same tissue section with intact telomeres. The inherent disadvantage of Q-FISH is that only a small subset of telomeres can be examined at any one time relative to the bulk methods (e.g., TRF analysis) (Nakagawa *et al.*, 2004 and references therein).

PCR-BASED METHODS FOR TELOMERE LENGTH MEASUREMENT

A technique that addresses some of the limitations of Q-FISH is single telomere length analysis (STELA). Using STELA, a 20-mer noncomplementary oligonucleotide with a TTAGGG tail is linked to the G-rich 3′ overhang of the telomere. The TTAGGG tail is then ligated to the complementary 5′ strand of the telomere. PCR is performed using one primer for the linked oligo and a second primer recognizing unique subtelomeric sequence. Use of this technique requires identification of subtelomeric sequences, which has not yet been accomplished in avian species, but should be possible in chicken now that the genome is sequenced (Nakagawa *et al.*, 2004 and references therein). Edges of telomeric DNA were identified in the draft sequence for the macrochromosomes (ICGSC, 2004, see supplementary information).

A second PCR-based technique that can be used to compare the abundance of telomere repeats is quantitative real-time PCR (Q-PCR). This technique quantifies the fold-difference between telomere-repeat copy number in an experimental sample compared to a reference DNA sample. Disadvantages of this method are that it does not determine absolute telomere length and that interstitial telomere sequences, present in avian species, will be measured as well as terminal repeats (Nakagawa *et al.*, 2004 and references therein). This should not be a problem if telomere shortening is being measured, because the number of interstitial repeats should not change relative to terminal repeats unless dramatic genome reorganization such as a breakage-fusion-bridge cycle is occurring.

TRAP ASSAY

The telomerase repeat amplification protocol (TRAP) assay, first described by Kim *et al.* (1994), relies upon primer extension of an oligonucletide by telomerase. Cells are lysed and cellular protein extracts are incubated with an oligonucletide to which a series of TTAGGG repeats will be added when telomerase is present in the cell extract. Variations of the TRAP assay exist, including radioactive or nonradioactive gel-based detection, ELISA-based detection and semiquantitative or quantitative protocols. For an excellent review of the TRAP assay and many of its iterations, see Saldanha *et al.* (2003).

GENE EXPRESSION ANALYSIS

Real-time fluorescence-based PCR and RT-PCR have emerged as powerful methods for examining gene expression patterns in many contexts. In traditional PCR, an amplicon which accumulates after a predetermined number of cycles is analyzed by gel electrophoresis. In real-time PCR, reactions are characterized by the PCR cycle at which amplification of a target molecule is first detected by release of a fluorescent signal in real time. The greater the quantity of the target molecule in the reaction mix, the earlier a significant increase in fluorescence will be measured. Quantitation is accomplished with reference to a threshold cycle, (C_t), defined as the fractional cycle number at which fluorescence, generated by the increase in PCR product, exceeds a set threshold above the baseline. For an excellent treatise on fluorescence-based real-time PCR, refer to Bustin *A Z of Quantitative PCR* (2004).

Recently, real-time quantitative TaqMan PCR was utilized to look at expression of genes involved in chicken telomere maintenance pathways. Chicken primers and fluorescent probes were developed for seven target genes (tankyrase 1, tankyrase 2, TRF1, TRF2, cTERT, cTR and c-myc) as well as for three housekeeping genes for normalization purposes. In cell culture, chicken GAPDH mRNA levels were found to show the least standard deviation for all samples examined, and therefore GAPDH values were used to normalize the target gene values.

Analysis of mRNA expression patterns of the target genes in CEFs, DT40, the gastrula embryo and cES cells revealed up-regulation of tankyrase 2, TRF1, TRF2, c-myc, cTERT and cTR in DT40 cells, with c-myc levels up-regulated 184-fold in DT40 relative to the gastrula and 282-fold in DT40 relative to CEFs and cES cells. Telomerase holoenzyme components (cTERT and cTR) were present, although at low levels, in CEFs and were up-regulated in DT40, cES cells and the gastrula relative to CEFs. Down-regulation of TRF1, c-myc, cTERT and cTR appeared to be a feature of senescing CEFs that had survived an average of 30.5 PD (Swanberg *et al.*, 2004; Swanberg and Delany, 2005). For a detailed discussion of these expression patterns as well as primer and probe sets, for target and housekeeping genes, see Swanberg *et al.* (2004) and Swanberg and Delany (2005).

ELECTROPORATION, RNAi AND MORPHOLINOS

One of the requirements for a good model system is the ability to do gain- and loss-of-function experiments. Techniques exist to perform such experiments in chicken. A number of investigators utilize electroporation to introduce exogenous DNA into the chicken embryo *in ovo* (Muramatsu *et al.*, 1997). For an excellent review of electroporation techniques *in ovo*, see Krull (2004). Loss-of-function experiments can be conducted by introducing short, interfering RNAs (siRNAs) or morpholinos into the chick embryo.

Double-stranded RNA-mediated interference (RNAi), a naturally occurring mechanism which results in the silencing of gene expression, has become a very powerful tool for experimental gene suppression in a number of organisms. The phenotypes observed with RNAi silencing of gene expression range from knockdown to knockout (Agrawal *et al.*, 2003). RNAi was successfully exploited in chicken (*in ovo*) for gene silencing (Bourikas and Stoeckli, 2003; Pekarik *et al.*, 2003; Krull 2004; Sato *et al.*, 2004). In addition to siRNAs, RNAi morpholinos were used in loss-of-function studies in chicken. For example, Sheng *et al.* (2003) used morpholino oligonucleotides to knock down expression of genes in the future neural plate of the chicken embryo.

GENOMIC TOOLS

Information regarding web-based tools for sequence and bioinformatics analysis of avian species, BAC and cDNA libraries, chicken gene chips and a number of other websites of interest to researchers are contained in Table 29.5. For further detail on cDNA arrays for chicken gene expression analysis, see Burnside *et al.* (2005). Tutorials oriented toward the biologist new to bioinformatics can be found in Antin and Konieczka (2005). Both Antin and Konieczka (2005) and Dequeant and Pourquie (2005) describe additional resources for the study of chicken genomics.

TELOMERES AS A TOOL FOR AGE DETERMINATION IN BIRDS

Estimating age in unmarked bird populations is of primary interest to many disciplines. The relationship between telomere shortening and chronological age was studied recently by determination of the telomere rate of change (TROC) or "telomere clock" in a number of bird species. Measuring the length of TRFs in DNA from erythrocytes and plotting mean telomere length against the maximum lifespan in years for each species, a correlation between TROC and lifespan was indicated.

TABLE 29.5
Internet resources for researchers in avian telomere biology

Genomic Resources	*URL*
ArkDB Chicken database	http://www.thearkdb.org/browser?species=chicken
Avian Sciences Net-Purdue	http://ag.ansc.purdue.edu/poultry/
AvianNET	http://www.chicken-genome.org
BBSRC ChickEST Database	http://chick.umist.ac.uk/
Chick FPC Database-Wageningen University	http://www.animalsciences.nl/ChickFPC/
ChickBASE	http://www.genome.iastate.educ/chickmap/dbase.html
Chicken genome mapping database of the Animal Sciences Group (Wageningen Universtiy)	https://acedb.asg.wur.nl/
Chicken Genome White Paper	http://genome.wustl.edu/projects/chicken/Chicken_Genome.pdf
Chicken SAGE Website	http://www.cgmc.univ-lyon1.fr/Grandrillon/chicken_SAGE.php
CHORI-261 Chicken BAC Library, Children's Hospital Oakland Research Institute	http://bacpac.chori.org/chicken261.htm
Ensemble Chicken Genome Browser	http://www.ensembl.org/Gallus_gallus/
Gallus gallus EST and in situ hybridization analysis database	http://geisha.biosci.arizona.edu/
Gallus gallus Trace Archive	http://www.ncbi.nih.gov/Traces/trace.cgi
GENEfinder Genomic Resources (Red Jungle and Chicken BAC Libraries) TAMU	http://hbz.tamu.edu/bacindex.html
NCBI Clone Registry	http://www.ncbi.nlm.nih.gov/genome/clone/query.cgi?EXPR=chicken
NCBI's compendium of chicken genomic resources	http://www.ncbi.nlm.nih.gov/projects/genome/guide/chicken/
NetVet	http://netvet.wustl.edu/birds.htm
Sanger Institute Chicken Genome Sequencing Project	http://www.sanger.ac.uk/Projects/G_gallus/
UD Chicken EST Database	http://www.chickest.udel.edu/
US Poultry Genome Website	http://poultry.mph.msu.edu/
Chicken Genome Array (Affymetrix)	http://www.affymetrix.com/products/arrays/specific/chicken.affx
Stocks, Lines and Cell Lines	
Poultry and Avian Research Resources: Living Stock Populations	http://animalscience.ucdavis.edu/AvianResources/
American Type Culture Collection (ATCC)	http://www.atcc.org
Husbandry	
CSREES – USDA Animal Breeding, Genetic and Genomics	http://www.csrees.usda.gov/ProgView.cfm?prnum=4030
USDA Animal Welfare Information Center	http://www.nal.usda.gov/awic/
USDA Bibliography on Poultry Production	http://www.nal.usda.gov/afsic/AFSIC_pubs/livestock/srb0406ch6.pdf
USDA Agricultural Research Service-Poultry Research Publications	http://www.lpsi.barc.usda.gov/gblab/research/poultryindex.html
USDA Housing, Husbandry, and Welfare of Poultry	http://netvet.wustl.edu/species/birds/QB9415.HTM
Poultry Science Association	http://www.poultryscience.org/

In most of the species studied, telomeres appeared to shorten more slowly in long-lived birds than short-lived birds. Interestingly, in a particularly long-lived bird, Leach's storm petrel, telomeres did not shorten with age, but lengthened (Vleck *et al.*, 2003, Haussmann *et al.*, 2003).

In another study examining DNA from erythrocytes, it was found that while telomere length in blood cells declined between the chick stage and the adult in two species of long-lived seabirds, telomere length in adults was not related to age. This study cautioned that rates of telomere loss were not constant with age and that there was a great deal of interindividual variation in the magnitude of telomere loss (Hall *et al.*, 2004). It should be noted that avian erythrocytes are the product of erythroid progenitor cells capable of extended self-renewal (Beug *et al.*, 1994) and therefore are likely to possess a significantly different telomere-length maintenance pathway than the majority of somatic cells whose telomeres typically demonstrate division-dependent shortening. It would not, therefore, be surprising to find that telomere shortening profiles in this renewable cell population would bear a greater resemblance to the profiles of other renewable tissues than to the telomeres of nonrenewable cell populations such as fibroblasts.

Research Resources: Stocks and Lines, Cells and Cell Lines

A variety of avian stocks and lines are available to the investigator of telomere biology. Genetic stocks and mutant lines are listed in an Avian Stocks Database linked to the Poultry and Avian Research Resources: Living Stock Populations website of the Animal Science Department, University of California, Davis (see Table 29.5 for URL). In addition, a selection of transformed and nontransformed avian cells and cell lines are available through the American Type Culture Collection (see Table 29.5 for URL). Protocols for primary culture of isolated chicken tissues can be found in Fresheny, *Culture of Animal Cells: A Manual of Basic Technique* (2000).

Husbandry

A number of excellent resources on basic chicken biology and husbandry are available including Sturkie's *Avian Physiology* (2000) and Scanes' *Poultry Science* (2004). In addition, the United States Department of Agriculture and several other agencies or associations provide both web-based and written materials on poultry husbandry and animal welfare. Table 29.5 contains web-based resources on poultry husbandry and related topics.

Conclusions

The study of telomere biology and telomere maintenance pathways has provided and will continue to provide a great deal of insight into the processes of replicative senescence, the relationship between cellular senescence and organismal aging, the genesis of cancer, and the regenerative potential of embryonic stem cells. Use of *in vivo* and *in vitro* avian systems to facilitate research in these fields can only add to our body of knowledge. With the 6.6X draft sequence of the chicken genome now available, the chicken is a much more powerful model.

Investigation of telomere maintenance pathways in the chicken and other birds establishes, among other things, that nonrenewable cells and tissues exhibit little or no telomerase activity accompanied by division-dependent telomere shortening; that embryonic cells and tissues as well as transformed cells exhibit high levels of telomerase; and that many telomere-associated genes are expressed differentially in pluripotent, differentiated and transformed cell systems, much as is seen in human systems. TERT and TR genes are transcribed in at least one telomerase-negative cell type, which suggests that the regulation of telomerase activity is more complex than merely switching the genes for telomerase enzyme components on and off. While telomere shortening profiles are unlikely to be the equivalent of rings on a tree for the determination of chronological age, comparisons of telomere status in pluripotent vs. differentiated, transformed vs. nontransformed and early passage vs. senescent cells are informative. Considerable work is necessary to fill in gaps, but the chicken model for telomere biology offers the opportunity to study a vertebrate system free from many of the issues inherent in the murine model. Chickens, therefore, have the potential to become the new "lab rat" for aging research.

REFERENCES

Agrawal, N., Dasaradhi, P.V., Mohmmed, A., Malhotra, P., Bhatnagar, R.K., Mukherjee, S.K. (2003). RNA interference: Biology, mechanism, and applications. *Microbiol Mol Biol Rev 67*, 657–685.

Austad, S.N. (1997). Birds as models of aging in biomedical research. *ILAR J 38*, 137–141.

Baker, S.J., Pawlita, M., Leutz, A., Hoelzer, D. (1994). Essential role of c-myc in ara-C-induced differentiation of human erythroleukemia cells. *Leukemia 8*, 1309–1317.

Baumann, P., Cech, T.R. (2001). Pot1, the putative telomere end-binding protein in fission yeast and humans. *Science 292*, 1171–1175.

Beug, H., Mullner, E.W., Hayman, M.J. (1994). Insights into erythroid differentiation obtained from studies on avian erythroblastosis virus. *Curr Opin Cell Biol 6*, 816–824.

Bianchi, A., Smith, S., Chong, L., Elias, P., de Lange, T. (1997). TRF1 is a dimer and bends telomeric DNA. *EMBO J 16*, 1785–1794.

Blackburn, E.H. (2001). Switching and signaling at the telomere. *Cell 106*, 661–673.

Bourikas, D., Stoeckli, E.T. (2003). New tools for gene manipulation in chicken embryos. *Oligonucleotides 13*, 411–419.

Broccoli, D., Smogorzewska, A., Chong, L., de Lange, T. (1997). Human telomeres contain two distinct Myb-related proteins, TRF1 and TRF2. *Nat Genet 17*, 231–235.

Burnside, J., Neiman, P., Tang, J., Basom, R., Talbot, R., Aronszajn, M., Burt, D., Delrow, J. (2005). Development of a cDNA array for chicken gene expression analysis. *BMC Genomics 6*, 13.

Bustin, S.A. (2004). *A–Z of Quantitative PCR*. International University Line, La Jolla.

Caldwell, R.B., Kierzek, A.M., Arakawa, H., Bezzubov, Y., Zaim, J., Fiedler, P., *et al.* (2005). Full-length cDNAs from chicken bursal lymphocytes to facilitate gene function analysis. *Genome Biol 6*, R6.

Cheong, C., Hong, K.U., Lee, H.W. (2003). Mouse models for telomere and telomerase biology. *Exp Mol Med 35*, 141–153.

Cristofalo, V.J., Lorenzini, A., Allen, R.G., Torres, C., Tresini, M. (2004). Replicative senescence: A critical review. *Mech Ageing Dev 125*, 827–848.

Delany, M.E., Daniels, L.M., Swanberg, S.E., Taylor, H.A. (2003). Telomeres in the chicken: Genome stability and chromosome ends. *Poult Sci 82*, 917–926.

Delany, M.E., Krupkin, A.B., Miller, M.M. (2000). Organization of telomere sequences in birds: Evidence for arrays of extreme length and for in vivo shortening. *Cytogenet Cell Genet 90*, 139–145.

Dequeant, M.L., Pourquie, O. (2005). Chicken genome: New tools and concepts. *Dev Dyn 232*, 883–886.

De Rycker, M., Venkatesan, R.N., Wei, C., Price, C.M. Vertebrate tankyrase domain structure and sterile alpha motif (SAM)-mediated multimerization. *Biochem J 372 (Pt 1)*, 87–96.

Du, X., Shen, J., Kugan, N., Furth, E.E., Lombard, D.B., Cheung, C., *et al.* (2003). Telomere shortening exposes functions for the mouse Werner and Bloom syndrome genes. *Mol Cell Biol 24*, 8437–8446.

Ellis, N.A., Groden, J., Ye, T.Z., Straughen, J., Lennon, D.J., Ciocci, S., Proytcheva, M., German, J. (1995). The Bloom's syndrome gene product is homologous to RecQ helicases. *Cell 83*, 655–666.

Eyal-Giladi, H., Kochav, S. (1976). From cleavage to primitive streak formation: A complementary normal table and a new look at the first stages of the development of the chick. I. General morphology. *Dev Biol 49*, 321–337.

Feng, J., Funk, W.D., Wang, S.S., Weinrich, S.L., Avilion, A.A., Chiu, C.P., *et al.* (1995). The RNA component of human telomerase. *Science 269*, 1236–1241.

Forsyth, R.N., Wright, W.E., Shay, J.W. 2002. Telomerase and differentiation in multicellular organisms: Turn it off, turn it on, and turn it off again. *Differentiation 69*, 188–197.

Fresheny, R.I. (2000). *Culture of Animal Cells: A Manual of Basic Technique* Wiley-Liss, New York.

Gray, M.D., Shen, J.C., Kamath-Loeb, A.S., Blank, A., Sopher, B.L., Martin, G.M., *et al.* (1997). The Werner Syndrome protein is a DNA helicase. *Nat Genet 17*, 100–103.

Greider, C.W., Blackburn, E.H. (1989). A telomeric sequence in the RNA of Tetrahymena telomerase required for telomere repeat synthesis. *Nature 337*, 331–337.

Greider, C.W. (1999). Telomeres do D-Loop-T-loop. *Cell 97*, 419–422.

Griffith, J.D., Comeau, L., Rosenfield, S., Stansel, R.M., Bianchi, A., Moss, H., de Lange, T. (1999). Mammalian telomeres end in a large duplex loop. *Cell 97*, 503–514.

Hall, M.E., Nasir, L., Daunt, F., Gault, E.A., Croxall, J.P., Wanless, S., Monaghan, P. (2004). Telomere loss in relation to age and early environment in long-lived birds. *Proc Biol Sci 271*, 1571–1576.

Hamburger, V., Hamilton, H. (1951). A series of normal stages in the development of the chick embryo. *J Morphol* 88, 49–92 reprinted *Dev Dyn (1992) 195*, 231–272.

Harley, C.B., Futcher, A.B., Greider, C.W. (1990). Telomeres shorten during ageing of human fibroblasts. *Nature 345*, 458–460.

Harris, L.L., Talian, J.C., Zelenka, P.S. (1992). Contrasting patterns of c-myc and N-myc expression in proliferating, quiescent, and differentiating cells of the embryonic chicken lens. *Development 115*, 813–820.

Haussmann, M.F., Winkler, D.W., O'Reilly, K.M., Huntington, C.E., Nisbet, I.C., Vleck, C.M. (2003). Telomeres shorten more slowly in long-lived birds and mammals than in short-lived ones. *Proc Biol Sci 270*, 1387–1392.

Hemann, M.T., Strong, M.A., Hao, L.Y., Greider, C.W. (2001). The shortest telomere, not average telomere length, is critical for cell viability and chromosome stability. *Cell 107*, 67–77.

International Chicken Genome Sequencing Consortium (ICGSC) (2004). Sequence and comparative analysis of the chicken genome provide unique perspectives on vertebrate evolution. *Nature 432*, 695–716.

Kaminker, P.G., Kim, S.H., Taylor, R.D., Zebarjadian, Y., Funk, W.D., Morin, G.B., *et al.* (2001). TANK2, a new TRF1-associated poly(ADP-ribose) polymerase, causes rapid induction of cell death upon overexpression. *J Biol Chem 276*, 35891–35899.

Karlseder, J., Smogorzewska, A., de Lange, T. (2002). Senescence induced by altered telomere state, not telomere loss. *Science 295*, 2446–2449.

Karlseder, J. (2003). Telomere repeat binding factors: Keeping the ends in check. *Cancer Lett 194*, 189–197.

Kim, H., You, S., Farris, J., Kong, B.W., Christman, S.A., Foster, L.K., Foster, D.N. (2002). Expression profiles of p53-, p16(INK4a)-, and telomere-regulating genes in replicative senescent primary human, mouse, and chicken fibroblast cells. *Exp Cell Res 272*, 199–208.

Kim, N.W., Piatyszek, M.A., Prowse, K.R., Harley, C.B., West, M.D., Ho, P.L., *et al.* (1994). Specific association of human telomerase activity with immortal cells and cancer. *Science 266*, 2011–2015.

Konrad, J.P., Mills, W., Easty, D.J., Farr, C.J. (1999). Cloning and characterization of the chicken gene encoding the telomeric protein TRF2. *Gene* 239, 81–90.

Kos, R., Tucker, R.P., Hall, R., Duong, T.D., Erickson, C.A. (2003). Methods for introducing morpholinos into the chicken embryo. *Dev Dyn 226*, 470–477.

Krull, C.E. (2004). A primer on using in ovo electroporation to analyze gene function. *Dev Dyn 229*, 433–439.

Levy, M.Z., Allsop, R.C., Futcher, A.B., Greider, C.W., Harley, C.B. (1992). Telomere end-replication problem and cell aging. *J Mol Biol 225*, 951–960.

Lima, L., Macieira-Coelho, A. (1972). Parameters of aging in chicken embryo fibroblasts cultivated in vitro. *Exp Cell Res 70*, 279–284.

Lima, L., Malaise, E., Macieira-Coelho, A. (1972). Aging in vitro. Effect of low dose irradiation on the division potential of chick embryonic fibroblasts. *Exp Cell Res 73*, 345–350.

Lingner, J., Hughes, T.R., Shevchenko, A., Mann, M., Lundblad, V., Cech, T.R. (1997). Reverse transcriptase motifs in the catalytic subunit of telomerase. *Science 276*, 561–567.

Macieira-Coelho, A., Azzarone, B. (1988). The transition from primary culture to spontaneous immortalization in mouse fibroblast populations. *Anticancer Res 8*, 660–676.

Muramatsu, T., Mizutani, Y., Ohmori, Y., Okumura, J. (1997). Comparison of three nonviral transfection methods for foreign gene expression in early chicken embryos in ovo. *Biochem Biophys Res Commun 230*, 376–380.

Nakagawa, S., Gemmell, N.J., Burke, T. (2004). Measuring vertebrate telomeres: Applications and limitations. *Mol Ecol 13*, 2523–2533.

Nakamura, T.M., Morin, G.B., Chapman, K.B., Weinrich, S.L., Andrews, W.H., Lingner, J., *et al.* (1997). Telomerase catalytic subunit homologs from fission yeast and human. *Science 277*, 955–959.

Nanda, I., Schmid, M., (1994). Localization of the telomeric (TTAGGG)n sequence in chicken (*Gallus domesticus*) chromosomes. *Cytogenet Cell Genet 65*, 190–193.

Nanda, I., Schrama, D., Feichtinger, W., Haaf, T., Schartl, M., Schmid, M. (2002). Distribution of telomeric (TTAGGG)(n) sequences in avian chromosomes. *Chromosoma 111*, 215–227.

Nikitina, T., Woodcock, C.L. (2004). Closed chromatin loops at the ends of chromosomes. *J Cell Biol 166*, 161–165.

Ohki, R., Ishikawa, F., (2004). Telomere-bound TRF1 and TRF2 stall the replication fork at telomeric repeats. *Nucleic Acids Res 32*, 1627–1637.

Pekarik, V., Bourikas, D., Miglino, N., Joset, P., Preiswerk, S., Stoeckli, E.T. (2003). Screening for gene function in chicken embryo using RNAi and electroporation. *Nature Biotechnol 21*, 93–96.

Piedra, M.E., Delgado, M.D., Ros, M.A., Leon, J. (2002). c-Myc overexpression increases cell size and impairs cartilage differentiation during chick limb development. *Cell Growth Differ 13*, 185–193.

Prowse, K.R., Greider, C.W. (1995). Developmental and tissue-specific regulation of mouse telomerase and telomere length. *Proc Natl Acad Sci USA 92*, 4818–4822.

Romanoff, A.L. (1960). *The Avian Embryo, Structural and Functional Development*. Macmillan Company, New York.

Saldanha, S.N., Andrews, L.G., Tollefsbol, T.O. (2003). Analysis of telomerase activity and detection of its catalytic subunit, hTERT. *Anal Biochem 315*, 1–21.

Sato, F., Nakagawa, T., Ito, M., Kitagawa, Y., Hattori, M-A. (2004). Application of RNA interference to chicken embryos using small interfering RNA. *J Exp Zoolog A Comp Exp Biol 301*, 820–827.

Shenge, G., dos Reis, M., Stern, C. D. (2003). Churchil, a zinc finger transcriptional activator, regulates the transition between gastrulation and neurulation. *Cell 115*, 603–613.

Skerka, C., Zipfel, P.F., Siebenlist, U. (1993). Two regulatory domains are required for downregulation of c-myc transcription in differentiating U937 cells. *Oncogene 8*, 2135–2143.

Smith, S., de Lange, T. (2000). Tankyrase promotes telomere elongation in human cells. *Curr Biol 10*, 1299–1302.

Smogorzewska, A., de Lange, T. (2002). Different telomere damage signaling pathways in human and mouse cells. *EMBO J 21*, 4338–4348.

Smorgorzewska, A., van Steensel, B., Bianchi, A., Oelmann, S., Schaefer, M.R., Schnapp, G., de Lange, T. (2000). Control of human telomere length by TRF1 and TRF2. *Mol Cell Biol 20*, 1659–1668.

Stansel, R.M., de Lange, T., Griffith, J.D. (2001). T-loop assembly in vitro involves binding of TRF2 near the 3′ telomeric overhang. *EMBO J 20*, 5532–5540.

Swanberg, S.E., Delany, M.E. (2003). Dynamics of telomere erosion in transformed and non-transformed avian cells in vitro. *Cytogenet Genome Res 102*, 318–325.

Swanberg, S.E., Delany, M.E. (2005). Differential expression of genes associated with telomere length homeostasis and oncogenesis in an avian model. *Mech Ageing Dev 126*, 1060–1070.

Swanberg, S.E., Payne, W.S., Hunt, H.D., Dodgson, J.B., Delany, M.E. (2004) Telomerase activity and differential expression of telomerase genes and c-myc in chicken cells in vitro. *Dev Dyn 231*, 14–21.

Tan, M., Wei, C., Price, C.M. (2003). The telomeric protein Rap1 is conserved in vertebrates and is expressed from a bidirectional promoter positioned between the Rap1 and KARs genes. *Gene 323*, 1–10.

Taylor, H.A., Delany, M.E. (2000). Ontogeny of telomerase in chicken: Impact of downregulation on pre- and postnatal telomere length in vivo. *Dev Growth Differ 42*, 613–621.

Tickle, C. (2004). The contribution of chicken embryology to the understanding of vertebrate limb development. *Mech Dev 121*, 1019–1029.

van Steensel, B., de Lange, T. (1997). Control of telomere length by the human telomeric protein TRF1. *Nature 385*, 740–743.

Vleck, C.M., Haussmann, M.F., Vleck, D. (2003). The natural history of telomeres: Tools for aging animals and exploring the aging process. *Exp Gerontol 38*, 791–795.

Wadhwa, R., Deocaris, C.C., Widodo, N., Taira, K., Kaul, S.C. (2005). Imminent approaches towards molecular interventions in ageing. *Mech Ageing Dev 126*, 481–490.

Watt, R., Stanton, L.W., Marcu, K.B., Gallo, R.C., Croce, C.M., Rovera, G. (1983). Nucleotide sequence of cloned cDNA of human c-myc oncogene. *Nature 303*, 725–728.

Wei, C., Price, C.M. (2003). Protecting the terminus: t-loops and telomere end-binding proteins. *Cell Mol Life Sci 11*, 2283–2294.

Wei, C., Price, C.M. (2004). Cell cycle localization, dimerization and binding domain architecture of the telomere protein cPot1. *Mol Cell Biol 24*, 2091–2102.

Wright, W.E., Shay, J.W. (2002). Historical claims and current interpretations of replicative aging. *Nat Biotechnol 20*, 682–688.

Wu, K.J., Grandori, C., Amacker, M., Simon-Vermot, N., Polack, A., Lingner, J., Dalla-Favera, R. (1999). Direct activation of TERT transcription by c-myc. *Nat Genet 21*, 220–224.

Zhong Z., Shiue, L., Kaplan, S., de Lange, T. (1992). A mammalian factor that binds telomeric TTAGGG repeats in vitro. *Mol Cell Biol 12*, 4834–4843.

30

Domestic and Wild Bird Models for the Study of Aging

D.J. Holmes and M.A. Ottinger

Comparative gerontologists now recognize that birds as a group are exceptionally long-lived for their body sizes, especially given their lifetime energy expenditures, and that domestic and wild avian models hold significant potential for understanding basic aging processes. Some domestic birds, including chickens, pigeons, quail and small cage bird species, are actually already well developed as laboratory models, and have been used for years in studies of neurobiology, reproductive biology, and developmental biology, as well as other disciplines. Avian models have already yielded a significant body of information about aging-related changes in fertility, neuroendocrinology and reproduction, as well as adult neuroregeneration and the basis of cellular resistance to oxidative damage. Field ornithologists have gathered a wealth of demographic data relevant to senescence in wild bird populations, which represent excellent systems for monitoring and developing biomarkers of aging—including changes in immune function—in outbred wild vertebrates subject to natural evolutionary forces. The slow aging of birds is accompanied by exceptionally slow or even negligible reproductive aging in many species, including wild seabirds. While the development of molecular resources for carrying out aging studies with birds lags behind that for classical mammalian and invertebrate laboratory models, the past decade has seen an increase in the use of birds in the field of aging. The development of promising, long-lived avian biogerontological models will require judicious use of the comparative method, adaptation of standard aging biomarkers for use in new domestic and wild bird models, and vigorous and creative interdisciplinary collaboration.

Introduction

The class Aves consists of around 9,000 bird species with an enormous range of body sizes, habits and life histories (Sibley and Monroe, 1990, 1993; Gill, 1995; Bennett and Owens, 2002). As in mammals, there is overall a reliable, inverse correlation between species life spans and body size for birds. As a rule, however, birds are significantly longer-lived and age more slowly than mammals of similar size. Many avian species routinely live up to three times longer than mammals of equivalent body mass. Even some of the tiniest birds, like the broad-tailed hummingbird (*Selasphorus platycercus*, body weight approximately 5 g), have reliably documented life spans in the wild of over 10 years. Songbirds often survive over five years in the wild; small cage parrots, like the budgerigar "parakeet" (*Melopsittacus undulatus*), regularly live over 15 years under favorable conditions in captivity. Some migratory seabirds survive for over 50 years; even the small (90 g) common tern, *Sterna hirundo*, lives up to 25 years or more in the wild. The slow aging rates seen in birds are correlated with delays in onset and a slower progression of aging-related pathologies, including cardiovascular disease, infertility, neoplasia, osteoarthritis and diabetes.

Over the past decade we and others have emphasized the potential utility of avian models for aging studies (see, for example, Holmes and Austad, 1995a,b, 2004; Austad, 1997; Holmes *et al.*, 2001; Holmes, 2003; Holmes and Ottinger, 2003). Comparative gerontologists now recognize that birds are exceptionally long-lived, and could be used to address key questions about basic aging processes. Less generally acknowledged, however, is the fact that certain bird species–wild *and* domestic–are *already* quite well developed as models for some key correlates of aging, including declines in fertility, neuroendocrine changes, and potential defenses against the aging-related damage thought to be caused by reactive oxygen species.

In this chapter we review recent progress in the application of avian models for aging and aging-related physiological and biochemical processes, and we revisit reasons we believe that birds have special potential for modeling aging in long-lived animals like humans (Table 30.1). We review the advantages, disadvantages and pitfalls of extending aging studies to include domestic and wild bird models, and we make some recommendations for developing avian models for aging studies over the next decade.

TABLE 30.1
Advantages and drawbacks of avian models for studies of basic aging processes

Advantages:

1. Birds are in general significantly longer-lived than mammals of comparable body size and lifetime energy expenditures
2. A growing body of evidence suggests that birds have special adaptations for resisting or slowing oxidative damage to cells and tissues
3. Many cage and domestic bird species are feasible and economical to maintain for aging studies, and some are already well developed as biomedical models
4. Genome sequencing has been completed for the domestic chicken, for which there are well-characterized strains with distinct physiological properties
5. Additional data are now emerging on the genetics underlying important physiological differences between highly specialized strains of domestic poultry
6. Many birds exhibit extremely slow or even negligible reproductive aging
7. Wild birds provide excellent systems for monitoring aging in outbred wild vertebrates subject to natural evolutionary pressures
8. Birds are already being utilized in aging studies, and reliable biomarkers of avian aging have been identified

Drawbacks:

1. Long-lived animals like birds can be costly to maintain for longitudinal aging studies
2. The best-developed domestic avian laboratory models for aging studies are galliforms (e.g., chicken, quail), which are relatively short-lived
3. Genetic resources are currently limited for non-poultry avian models of aging; isogenic inbred laboratory strains of any bird are currently unavailable
4. Studies utilizing songbird models in the laboratory have focused primarily on neuroethology or nutrition rather than aging
5. Studies of aging biomarkers in wild bird populations require monitoring of variables that are difficult to control or monitor over individuals' life spans
6. The development of good avian aging models and biomarkers, including wild species, requires adequate funding and interdisciplinary collaboration

Birds as Exceptionally Long-lived Animal Models

Like mammals, birds have a wide range of aging patterns, life spans, and patterns of reproductive decline. In general, however, birds are long-lived, slowly aging animals, and some species age even more slowly for their body sizes than humans and other primates. Even small songbirds, seabirds and hummingbirds enjoy surprisingly long life spans in the wild under natural mortality pressure, despite extremely high metabolic rates (often several times higher than similar-sized mammals) and total lifetime energy expenditures (5 or more times higher) (Table 30.2) (for earlier reviews, see Austad, 1993; Holmes and Austad, 1995a,b; Holmes *et al.*, 2001; Holmes and Ottinger, 2003).

Some avian longevities are more comparable to those of humans and other primates than those of the short-lived rodents and invertebrates typically used as laboratory aging models. This means that avian aging processes may in some respects be more relevant than those of standard animal models for understanding basic aspects of human aging. Since birds, like mammals, are homeotherms, or "warm-blooded" animals. Therefore, any antiaging mechanisms they possess could be expected to generalize well to specific mechanisms underlying longevity in mammals. In particular, it has been suggested that birds may model specific adaptations for combating oxidative and glycoxidative processes thought to be primary causes of aging-related cellular damage (Harman, 1956; Del Maestro, 1980; Cerami, 1985; Monnier *et al.*, 1991, 1999; Kristal and Yu, 1992; Barja, 1998).

AVIAN LONGEVITY IS CONSISTENT WITH EVOLUTIONARY PREDICTIONS

Why do birds live so long? In the past, it was often argued that life spans and aging rates in warm-blooded vertebrates were constrained by the "rate of living" (Pearl, 1928; Rose, 1991). This argument was based on a robust, positive correlation between animals' body size and longevity, and an equally strong, inverse association between life spans and basal metabolic rates. This generalization is clearly refuted, however, when the long life spans of birds and bats are compared with those of nonflying relatives of similar size. These disproportionately long-lived animals are particularly interesting to comparative gerontologists, especially considering the higher metabolic rates and lifetime oxygen expenditures

TABLE 30.2
Life spans and approximate lifetime energy expenditures in mice, humans and some typical birds
(c = from records of captive individuals)

Species	Maximum documented longevity (years)	Body mass (g)	Estimated lifetime energy expenditure (kcal)
Mouse			
(*Mus domesticus*)	6 (c)	20	250
Human			
(*Homo sapiens*)	122 (c)	50,000	800
Japanese Quail			
(*Coturnix japonica*)	6	90	460
American Robin			
(*Turdus migratorius*)	14	77	1,336
Budgerigar			
(*Melopsittacus undulatus*)	19 ± (c)	40	1,440
Raven			
(*Corvus corax*)	69 (c)	1,200	1,400
Starling			
(*Sturnus vulgaris*)	21	71	2,100
Canary			
(*Serinus canaria*)	24 (c)	22	3,200
Broad-tailed Hummingbird			
(*Selasphorus platycercus*)	5	14	8,834

Data from Lasiewski and Dawson, 1967; Altman and Dittmer, 1972; Gavrilov and Dolnik, 1982; Carey and Judge, 2000. Records for most wild birds are based on banding records from the field, and probably underestimate potential life span in captivity. Most longevities were validated using similar values from more than one large sample for a given species. Lifetime energy expenditures were calculated using published estimates of basal or resting metabolic rates.

of long-lived fliers (Finch, 1990; Austad and Fischer, 1991; Partridge and Barton, 1993). Evolutionary senescence theory predicts that organisms subject to natural selection in the form of high natural mortality rates from predation, disease, or accident will evolve life-histories characterized by rapid maturation, early reproductive investment, and relatively high fecundity (Medawar, 1952; Williams, 1957; Edney and Gill, 1968; Rose, 1991). Short life spans are a correlate of this evolutionary scenario, in which there is no long-term reproductive or genetic advantage to delayed or slow aging. Conversely, in the absence of high mortality rates and intense selection for reproductive investment early in life, natural selection should favor delayed maturity, repeated but smaller episodes of reproductive investment, and long-term somatic maintenance. In the latter scenario, organisms with effective defenses against predators and other sources of mortality, including the ability to fly, will also be expected to evolve long life spans and the molecular mechanisms supporting long-term somatic maintenance. In other words, effective antiaging adaptations—including, presumably, the ability to combat oxidative and glycoxidative damage—are most likely to be exhibited by organisms with naturally long life spans, including vertebrates like bats, mole-rats, and birds. A substantial amount of comparative data supports the idea that slow aging has accompanied the evolution of flight, in both birds and mammals (for reviews see Pomeroy, 1990; Partridge and Barton, 1993; Holmes and Austad, 1995b).

BIRDS MAY HAVE SPECIAL CELLULAR AND MOLECULAR ADAPTATIONS FOR DELAYING AGING

Avian defenses against ROS damage

There is growing experimental evidence that birds have unusually effective defenses against aging-related damage to specific tissues, cells, and molecules. Reactive oxygen species (ROS) are now implicated in a growing assortment of aging-related deteriorative processes. Since they are a normal by-product of oxidative metabolism, ROS theoretically should be generated at higher rates by organisms, like birds, with high metabolic rates. But data collected over the past decade using birds from several different orders, including canaries, pigeons, budgerigars and starlings, suggest that birds have better defenses against oxidative damage than short-lived laboratory rodents (see, for example, Barja *et al.*, 1994a,b; Pamplona *et al.*, 1996; Barja, 1998; Barja and Herrero, 1998; Herrero and Barja, 1998; Ogburn *et al.*, 1998, 2001; Perez-Campo *et al.*, 1998; Pamplona *et al.*, 1999a,b; Jaensch, 2001; Ku and Sohal, 1994; Chapter 16, "Estimation of the Rate of Production of Oxygen Radicals by Mitochondria," by Sanz and Barja). These defenses probably involve a complex array of mechanisms, including more efficient mitochondrial metabolism, as well as superior protection against—and repair of—damage by prooxidant molecules to DNA and other cellular components. They may include inducible defenses, like antioxidant enzymes, as well as constitutive or structural defenses, such as lower levels of saturated fatty acids in cell or mitochondrial membranes.

Avian defenses against glycosylative and glycoxidative damage

Data from the veterinary clinical literature on a wide taxonomic range of bird species show that healthy birds' blood glucose levels are typically two to three times higher than those of normal mammals. Glucose interacts with proteins, nucleic acids, and other molecules through a series of nonenzymatic reactions called "glycosylation" and "glycoxidation" (for reviews, see Monnier, 1990; Monnier *et al.*, 1991, 1999). These reactions can produce a plethora of harmful compounds referred to as "AGEs," or advanced glycosylation end-products, which are thought to contribute to the functional declines associated with aging. Without specialized defenses against AGEs or their formation, particularly in light of their high metabolic rates, birds would be expected to be more susceptible to these compounds than their mammalian counterparts (Monnier, 1990; Monnier *et al.*, 1991, 1999; Holmes and Austad, 1995a; Holmes *et al.*, 2001). Some recent studies suggest that birds produce lower amounts of particular AGEs, or may have adaptations for preventing AGE-related damage (see, for example, Iqbal *et al.*, 1999; Monnier, 1999).

Avian aging, telomere length, and telomerase activity

Telomeres, conserved nucleotide sequences on the ends of linear chromosomes that are essential for replication, have been shown to shorten with age in somatic cells of humans, and are implicated in cellular senescence in mice (Harley, 1995; Granger *et al.*, 2002). There is also interest in a possible relationship between telomere length, telomerase activity, and animal aging and life span. So far, neither telomere length nor telomerase activity has been shown to correlate consistently with species-specific aging rates or life spans, either in birds or mammals. Some recent studies focusing on wild bird populations of species with a range of longevities have reported associations between maximum documented species life span, individual age, and telomere length and telomerase activity (Hausmann *et al.*, 2003; Vleck *et al.*, 2003); others have failed to show a correlation (Delany, 2000; Hall *et al.*, 2004; Chapter 29, "Telomeres in Aging: Birds," by Swanberg and Delaney). As more data on the relationships between avian life span, individual age, and measures of telomere length and telomerase activity are collected using a range of cell and tissues types, the apparent conflict should be reconciled.

Domestic Bird Models for Aging Studies

Although mainstream gerontologists have come to recognize the merit of adapting avian models, there have been relatively few full-fledged life-span studies using birds. Birds, however, actually have been used in many recent studies generating data applicable to basic aging processes, as well as in other biomedical disciplines with direct relevance to the biology of aging. Many cage and domestic bird species are feasible and economical to maintain, and some of these have long served as laboratory models for developmental and reproductive biology (chickens and quail), neuroendocrinology (quail, zebra finches and canaries), cardiovascular disease (pigeons and quail), and bone physiology (turkeys and quail). Since birds are egg-layers, avian embryonic cells and tissues are readily harvested for cell-culture or other in-vitro studies. Furthermore, classic embryology studies of the domestic chick provide the foundation for studies in research areas of emerging concern—specifically, the developmental basis for many adult diseases, including diseases of aging. Any maternal influences on avian embryonic development act before the egg is laid, hence these influences can be separated from other effects by experimental manipulation of parent or embryo.

We and our colleagues have found birds to be hardy, economical and very useful laboratory animals for studies of cellular resistance to oxidative damage, relationships between telomere length and life span, neuroendocrine aging and plasticity, and basic mechanisms of fertility loss in females. The genome has been sequenced for the domestic chicken, and chicken microarrays are now commercially available and readily applicable to studies of the closely related Japanese quail. A number of laboratories are now applying these and other state-of-the-art molecular methods for addressing the genetic basis for neurobiological, reproductive and other physiological traits in domestic poultry, as well as in laboratory songbird models (see, for example, Kaiser *et al.*, 2003; LaMont, 2003; Cheeseman *et al.*, 2004; Clayton, 2004; Mott and Ivarie, 2004; Hillier *et al.*, 2004; Wade *et al.*, 2004; Wong *et al.*, 2004; Smith *et al.*, 2005).

AVIAN MODELS FOR REPRODUCTIVE AND NEUROENDOCRINE AGING

Domestic poultry models are particularly well-developed for studies of relatively rapid reproductive and neuroendocrine aging. Although their life spans have been documented at over 15 years, domestic chickens (*Gallus domesticus*) are short-lived for their size, and hens typically undergo reproductive aging during the first two years of egg production. The smaller, and substantially shorter-lived, domestic Japanese quail (*Coturnix japonica*) is in many ways an ideal bird model for studies of rapid reproductive and neuroendocrine aging, since its life history is very similar to that of a laboratory rodent. Quail maintained on long days (15L:9D) mature in 8 weeks, maintain peak production for about 10 months, and show fertility declines (30–50%) by 70 weeks of age, with complete ovulatory failure as early as 18 months. Aging females exhibit irregular egg production associated with diminished hypothalamic response to ovarian steroids (Ottinger and Bakst, 1995; Ottinger, 1996). Reproductive aging is relatively rapid (1–2 yrs) in quail hens, yet they have a substantially longer documented postreproductive life span (2–4 yrs) than that of rodents. Quail can be maintained inexpensively and bred in large numbers. The Ottinger lab has used an outbred domestic quail strain for two decades in studies of reproductive physiology and neuroendocrine aspects of aging in male birds (Ottinger *et al.*, 1997; Panzica *et al.*, 1996; Ottinger, 1998; Ottinger, 2001; Ottinger *et al.*, 2004).

Avian reproductive anatomy lends itself well to studies of basic mechanisms controlling female fertility and reproductive aging (Johnson, 2000; Holmes *et al.*, 2003). Most adult female birds have only one functional ovary. Unlike the mammalian ovary, however, in which developing follicles are contained in a capsule, the avian ovary has a lobular structure like a bunch of grapes, with a yolky hierarchy of large preovulatory follicles readily accessible on the outside. This arrangement makes it practical to measure or administer hormones, growth factors or other substances directly from or into individual follicles.

Birds adapted to temperate zones, including poultry and some small cage birds, like finches, often use photoperiod as the primary cue for the timing and onset of reproduction. In these species, manipulation of the photoperiod is a convenient, noninvasive means of shutting down the reproductive neuroendocrine axis. Since some photoperiodic regulation of reproduction occurs in the hypothalamus, the manipulation of photoperiod avoids the experimental confound of elevated GnRH and gonadotropins that accompany surgical castration.

In captivity under hospitable conditions, some birds (e.g., quail, budgies) have postreproductive life spans of one-third or more of the total life span (Woodard and Aplanalp, 1971; Holmes *et al.*, 2001). Zebra finch hens exhibit significant declines in egg production after several years (Holmes, unpublished data). Female birds and mammals both produce the vast majority of their primary oocytes, or developing eggs, before or shortly after birth (Tokarz, 1978; Guraya, 1989). This fundamental reproductive trait sets birds and mammals apart from most female fishes, amphibians and reptiles, in which new oocytes are produced as needed throughout reproductive life. For this reason, avian models are particularly relevant for studying the role the finite oocyte pool plays in the timing of reproductive aging. In mammals, fertility loss is generally thought to be correlated with age-related declines in stores of viable primary oocytes. Another advantage of egg-laying is that it facilitates studies of early gonadal development and the examination of primordial oocytes early in life. Domestic birds are excellent models for exploring the effects of early manipulation of embryonic development on health later in life and during aging.

Surprisingly little research has focused on natural variability in ovarian aging in birds of different orders or divergent life-history patterns. Studies of reproductive aging in domestic poultry, however, usually focusing on the heavier poultry breeds, have shown striking differences between strains in fertility, and some aspects of ovarian aging are well documented. For example, Leghorn chickens, referred to as "layers," have been bred for very high, consistent egg production levels (nearly one egg per day). In contrast, the heavier "broiler" poultry strains, bred for meat production, may lay under 200 eggs per year. There has been no systematic comparison of ovarian aging in long- and short-lived species in the class Aves as a whole. Moreover, there has been no concerted effort to establish whether common physiological, biochemical or genetic mechanisms are responsible for fertility loss in birds and mammals.

We have begun studies comparing reproductive aging in female quail, budgerigars, and wild terns in an attempt to determine the relative contributions of declining primordial oocyte stores, steroid hormones, gonadotropins and GnRH (gonadotropin-releasing hormone) in short- and long-lived bird species. These bird models are all diurnal, with highly stereotypical, easily identifiable courtship behaviors; egg production and fertility are also readily and noninvasively quantified.

Quail and budgerigars both have a high incidence of ovarian cancers, presumably resulting from the breakdown of normal apoptotic signaling. In species which ovulate frequently, the avian ovary is potentially an excellent model for the "rupture and repair" mechanisms implicated in ovarian cancer formation (Giles *et al.*, 2004). To our knowledge, there have been no studies of the molecular basis of aging-related dysregulation of healthy ovarian cellular signaling in longer-lived, non-poultry bird species.

The bones of female birds generally serve as a repository for calcium and other minerals needed for egg production. Female quail develop increasingly fragile bones as they age; these birds are a well-characterized model for the effects of hormones, vitamins and other factors on osteoporosis (see, for example, Keatzel and Soares, 1985).

Reproductive aging in the domestic hen

The domestic chicken is one of the classical models for developmental and reproductive biology, and many fundamental physiological correlates of ovarian aging in hens are thoroughly documented (Johnson *et al.*, 1986; Bahr and Palmer, 1989; Ottinger and Bakst, 1995). As egg production declines (between about 30 to 90 weeks of age), the normal recruitment of small white follicles into the preovulatory hierarchy slows, as does follicular maturation. Yolky preovulatory follicles become less sensitive to the surge of luteinizing hormone (LH) that normally stimulates ovulation. Administration of LH or gonadotropin-releasing hormone (GnRH), has been shown to stimulate arian response in aged hens, with older hens responding more slowly than young ones (Ottinger and Soares, 1988; Wu and Ottinger, unpublished data). Old hens are also less sensitive to progesterone and may require more to trigger a preovulatory LH surge (Williams and Sharp, 1978; Ottinger and Soares, 1988). Granulosa cells from old hens have been shown to have more follicle-stimulating hormone (FSH) receptors and to produce more progesterone (P4) in response to FSH administration than those of younger hens (Johnson *et al.*, 1986; Bahr and Palmer, 1989; Johnson, 2000a, 2000b). This has been attributed to membrane-level changes, rather than actual P4 secretion in response to the cyclic AMP stimulation that normally triggers P4 production.

Estrogen production in birds occurs primarily in small white prehierarchal follicles, and therefore may play a minor role in loss of ovulatory competence. While estrogen is less dominant in the bird than in the mammal ovary, declines in estrogen may be partly responsible for declining follicular responsiveness. Decreased responsiveness of granulosa cells of hierarchal follicles could be attributable to lower estrogen secretion by a declining pool of small follicles, as well as altered responsiveness to gonadotropins and GnRH (Bahr and Palmer, 1989). The proportion of the original follicular pool that is required for ovulation to occur, however, is unknown.

While age-related changes in follicular populations have not been quantified over the reproductive life span of any bird, follicular atresia rates have been shown to increase with age in domestic hens. Approximately 20 percent of smaller ($\leq$8 mm) prehierarchal follicles undergo atresia in younger hens; this rate increases as fertility declines. Atresia rate increases have been attributed to declines in FSH, which normally inhibits atresia. Atresia and its regulation, however, may be expected to vary a great deal between poultry and exotic bird species.

Apoptosis, the programmed cell death that is a normal part of development and aging, has been intensively studied in the ovary of the chicken and, to a lesser extent, in the Japanese quail (Yak *et al.*, 1998; Volentine *et al.*, 1998; Johnson, 2000a,b; Bridgham and Johnson, 2001; Johnson *et al.*, 2002). Changes in populations of mitotic and apoptotic cells in prehierarchal follicles have been quantified during chicken development and during a significant portion of the reproductive life of chickens and quail (Waddington *et al.*, 1985; Waddington and Walker, 1988; Kitamura *et al.*, 2002; Johnson, 2000). Many of the same molecules involved in mammalian apoptotic signaling and follicular development have also been shown to function in the ovaries of chickens and quail.

The Japanese quail as a model for male neuroendocrine aging and neuroplasticity

Over the past 20 years, the Ottinger laboratory has used the Japanese quail extensively as a model for aging-related declines in reproduction, focusing on a variety of changes in behavioral, gonadal, metabolic, sensory and central neuroendocrine function (for reviews, see Ottinger, 1991; 1996; 1998; 2001). Male quail mirror many aspects of mammalian neuroendocrine aging, but they offer some important advantages over laboratory rodent models. Unlike that of most mammals studied, the male hypothalamic–gonadal system retains plasticity during aging. This plasticity is most obvious in the recovery of male courtship and mating behavior in studies in which males were given exogenous testosterone (Ottinger *et al.*, 1997; Ottinger, 1998). Even very aged, infertile males respond to testosterone replacement and recover full reproductive behavior, including restored immunoreactivity of cells containing aromatase enzyme (AROM-ir) in the preoptic region of the hypothalamus. Furthermore, the critical role of AROM-ir for the expression of male courtship and mating behavior is seen in aging males that remain reproductively active without exogenous testosterone treatment. These males have significantly larger AROM-ir cells in the preoptic region (Ottinger *et al.*, 2004). Age-related declines in male reproductive function are also reflected in the function of the GnRH-1 system, including reduced hypothalamic GnRH-1 content, fewer GnRH-1 immunoreactive cells, and lower-amplitude GnRH-1 pulses in vitro (Ottinger *et al.*, 2004). These age-related hypothalamic changes provide a platform for identifying the sequence of neuroendocrinological events eventually culminating in loss of reproductive function. The retention of neuroplasticity in quail hypothalamic systems also offers the opportunity to examine and manipulate age-sensitive signals that appear to decline selectively during reproductive senescence.

Caloric restriction improves reproductive performance in poultry

Caloric restriction (CR) is a well-established experimental paradigm in biogerontology, and the beneficial effects of long-term CR have been documented for a broad range of animal taxa, including invertebrates. Reliable effects of CR typically include extended life span, delayed onset of aging-related diseases, sustained healthy metabolic and endocrine function, and delayed loss of reproductive capacity (for reviews, see Weindruch and Walford, 1988; Finch, 1990; Masoro, 1993, 2001). Shorter-term caloric

TABLE 30.3
Effects of caloric restriction on reproductive and hormonal parameters in adult male Japanese quail after 8 weeks of treatment

Treatment Group	Mean body weight (g)	Mean testes weight (g)	LH (ng/ml plasma)	Androgen (pg/ml plasma)	Corticosterone (ng/ml plasma)
Ad lib-fed controls	$115^a \pm 1.8$	$3.1^a \pm 0.2$	$7.2^a \pm 0.5$	$2828^a \pm 317$	$3.1^a \pm 0.6$
20% restriction	$97^b \pm 1.8$	$3.3^a \pm 0.2$	$4.7^b \pm 0.5$	$1392^b \pm 304$	$1.8^a \pm 0.6$
40% restriction	$75^c \pm 1.8$	$2.2^b \pm 0.2$	$2.5^c \pm 0.5$	$266^c \pm 304$	$7.2^b \pm 0.6$

^{a,b,c}: Different letters denote values that are significantly different within a column (1-way ANOVA (d.f. 1,2; $p < 0.05$) with Student-Newmann-Keuls test post hoc). $n = 6$ for each treatment group. References: Mobarak, 1990; Ottinger *et al.*, 2005.

or food restriction has also been routinely used by the poultry industry for many years to improve egg production and extend the reproductive life span of laying hens (see, for example, McDaniel, 1983; Sexton, 1989; Miles and Leeson, 1990; Zuidhof *et al.*, 1995; Walsh and Brake, 1999). While poultry biologists have not generally employed the standardized experimental protocols currently used by biogerontologists, in which CR is begun in young animals and continued for the natural life span, there is a wealth of published studies of effects of chronic or short-term food restriction on poultry. The levels of proteins, fatty acids, and other nutrients required for optimizing productivity in domestic egg- and meat-producing birds have been precisely determined, and micronutrients have been adjusted in the feed of "restricted" birds to compensate for their reduced calorie intake.

Results of avian feed-restriction studies are consistent on the whole with the antiaging effects of moderate (10–25 percent) CR on laboratory rodents and primates. CR initiated before full maturation slows the onset of puberty in chickens. Restricted hens are generally healthier, have lower mortality rates, and hatch more chicks over their life spans than controls (Joseph *et al.*, 2002). CR of 30 percent or more impairs or prevents reproduction in these birds, as in mammals (McDaniel, 1983; Bronson, 1989; Ottinger and Soares, 1988). Unlike in mammals, severe restriction followed by resumption of control feeding and restoration of the appropriate photoperiod, however, reinstates reproduction at relatively high levels, even in breeders previously exhibiting aging-related reproductive declines (Walsh and Brake, 1999). This procedure termed "forced molting" is often used to prolong reproduction.

The Ottinger lab has conducted CR experiments to determine the level of caloric intake needed for optimal reproductive performance and long-term health in a strain of heavy broiler chickens (bred for meat rather than egg production) (Byerly *et al.*, 1984; Ottinger and Soares, 1988; Holmes and Ottinger, 2003). In these studies, control birds became reproductive earlier than 10- and 20-percent CR hens when CR was initiated before complete maturity, with females producing eggs and males beginning sperm production earlier than either CR group. But fertility in controls declined relatively quickly, thereafter, and control birds developed other health problems. Both CR groups in this study matured more slowly and were reproductive longer, producing more chicks during the reproductive life span than controls. Hence many of the responses of chickens to CR were similar to those observed in short-lived laboratory rodents (for reviews, see Merry and Holehan, 1979; Bronson, 1989; Nelson *et al.*, 1995).

Ottinger and colleagues have also tested the effects of moderate, short-term CR on reproduction in male Japanese quail, and examined some of the neuroendocrine mechanisms involved in this effect (Mobarak *et al.*, 1988; Mobarak, 1990; Holmes and Ottinger 2003; Ottinger *et al.*, 2005) (Table 30.3). Twenty- and 40-percent CR quail both matured more slowly than controls and exhibited lower levels of plasma LH. The effects of 40-percent restriction were quite severe, and included reduced testes weight, low plasma testosterone, and elevated plasma corticosterone. However, when injected with GnRH, males in both CR treatment groups had sufficient LH stores to release measurable levels of LH, suggesting that CR had suppressed gonadotropin release at the hypothalamic level, rather than suppressing LH production. This effect is consistent with that seen in food-restricted rodents (Bronson, 1989; Nelson *et al.*, 1995). Subsequently, another experiment subjected male quail to an identical CR treatment protocol, but castrated them at two weeks of age, prior to diet treatment. When CR males were later subjected to LHRH pituitary challenge, all exhibited a normal LH response. In a third study, hypothalamic content and turnover of catecholamines were quantified in adult male quail that had been raised on CR. Twenty-percent CR altered only dopamine (DA) content in the ventromedial hypothalamus. More severe (40-percent) CR reduced both DA and norepinephrine (NE) content in the ventromedial hypothalami. In addition, DA and NE turnover (determined after treatment with alpha-methyl-paratyrosine) were reduced (Ottinger *et al.*, 2005). These results indicate that, in birds, CR may exert its effect through altered levels of catecholamines, which in turn stimulate GnRH-1 release and regulate normal reproduction in both sexes.

No full-length, classical biogerontological study of the effects of caloric restriction on molecular, cellular or pathological aging processes has yet been conducted using an avian model. But the beneficial effects of shorter-term CR on health and reproduction in poultry are likely to act through central-nervous-system effects on neuroendocrine and metabolic regulatory systems, as in mammals. Recent research supporting a central role of the IGF-1 pathway in aging and its modulation in invertebrates and vertebrates alike illustrates the need for more comparative studies of the neurophysiological effects of CR in vertebrates. Since CR also appears to protect animals against aging-related oxidative damage, and birds seem unusually resistant to this type of damage, long- and short-lived birds would make very interesting animal models for full-scale caloric restriction studies.

NON-POULTRY DOMESTIC AVIAN MODELS FOR AGING STUDIES

Avian models for learning and neuroregeneration

Small songbirds, including canaries, zebra finches, and sparrows, as well as small parrots and pigeons, have been used for decades in neurobiology, particularly in studies of song learning and reproductive and courtship behavior. More recently, these laboratory bird models have also become the focus of research on the potential for regeneration of certain brain regions. Male canaries normally change their songs each new breeding season as they come into reproductive readiness. This seasonal change is correlated with the death and subsequent regrowth of neurons located in song centers in the brain (see, for example, Kim *et al.*, 1994; Nottebohm *et al.*, 1994; Doetsch and Scharff, 2001). This type of adult neurogenesis has no direct counterpart in laboratory rodent neurobiological models. Studies of the molecular basis of avian neuroregeneration could be critically important for expanding the potential for therapeutic brain repair in humans.

The potential for neuroregeneration has also been demonstrated in other bird models. Japanese quail have been shown to exhibit a reduction in ganglion cells during aging (Ryals and Westbrook, 1988). Interestingly, however, quail retain the ability to regenerate hair cells in the inner ear, even after damage that has been inflicted throughout the life span (Ryals and Westbrook, 1990, 1994). Furthermore, selected brain regions show an age-related decline in neurogenesis in aging male quail (Lauay *et al.*, unpublished data).

Other promising domestic avian laboratory models

Longer-lived, non-galliform bird models are also poised for development for comparative aging studies. These include small domestic cage birds, like the budgerigar (*Melopsittacus undulatus*) (a small parrot with a maximum life span $\geq$20 years). There is a great deal of clinical veterinary information available for small parrots, captive husbandry practices are well established, and maintenance costs are comparable to those for laboratory rodents. We (in collaboration with Steven Austad) have found budgies to be economical and feasible laboratory animals for aging studies. We have used these birds, as well as quail, in comparative studies of cellular resistance to oxidative damage (Ogburn *et al.*, 1988, 2001).

In earlier reviews we have evaluated several other domestic birds with special potential as new laboratory models for aging studies, including small finches, pigeons, and sparrows (Table 30.4; Holmes and Austad, 1995a; Holmes and Ottinger, 2003; see also Austad, 1997). The most promising avian laboratory models are rodent-sized, outbred, relatively long-lived species which are commercially available. They are also economical to maintain and breed, and have husbandry practices which are well established. They include popular pet birds, like budgerigars (order Psittaciformes; maximum life span 20 years), canaries and zebra finches (order Fringillidae; maximum life span 25 and 9 years, respectively). Lifetime energy expenditures for all these birds exceed those of comparably-sized rodents. The lifetime oxidative liability of the 15-g zebra finch, for example, has been calculated at about twice that of humans. The white-crowned sparrow, a migratory North American songbird, is also a good laboratory bird model, and has been used for years in studies of neuroethology, migration, nutrition and physiology (see, for example, Murphy and King, 1990).

Wild Birds as Models for Aging Studies

Wild birds in nature, as well as more traditional domestic laboratory birds, have a great deal of potential for aging studies. Field biologists have now been banding and gathering data on wild bird populations for decades, generating a wealth of information relevant to the basic biology of aging, including evolutionary aging and life-history theory. Mark-recapture studies have now accumulated decades worth of demographic data for many other wild bird species, and the quality of much of these data is excellent (see, for example, Newton, 1989). Bird studies have other advantages for studies of aging and life-history trade-offs: because birds lay eggs, the effect of reproductive investment on subsequent aging can be experimentally manipulated by transferring or removing eggs or nestlings.

Changes in mortality rates and reproductive success consistent with aging have been documented for many bird populations (Holmes and Austad, 1995; Holmes *et al.*, 2001). Other indications of avian aging in the wild include higher parasite loads in older birds, as well as reduced fitness of offspring produced by aging parents.

TABLE 30.4
Avian laboratory model species with special potential for aging studies

Species and order	Body weight	Maturation time and MLS*	Qualifications and advantages	Drawbacks and special considerations
Japanese Quail (*Coturnix japonica*): Galliformes	100 g	6 yrs (C)	Fully domesticated. Excellent breeder. Extensive literature on behavior, reproduction, neuroendocrinology, and aging. Short-lived, but longer than laboratory rodents; very rapid reproductive aging.	Very short-lived for a bird; reproductive declines at 1 year. Sexes distinguishable.
Budgerigar (*Melopsittacus undulatus*): Psittaciformes	45 g	5–6 mos; 15–20 yrs (C)	Domesticated. Very good breeder. Extensive pet-husbandry and clinical literature including aging-related pathologies; some research on neurobiology. Some published studies of resistance to oxidative damage. Moderately long-lived with moderately slow reproductive aging. Prone to tumors, obesity, diabetes.	Longer-lived than laboratory rodents. Sexes distinguishable.
Canary (*Serinus canaria*): Passeriformes	30 g	15–20 yrs (C)	Domesticated. Good captive breeder. Extensive research and clinical literature including behavior, neurobiology, husbandry and including aging-related pathologies. Moderately long-lived with moderately slow reproductive aging. Less tumor-prone than budgies.	More difficult to breed than zebra finches or budgies. Longer-lived than laboratory rodents. Sexes distinguishable by song.
Zebra Finch (*Taeniopygia guttata*): Passeriformes	15 g	2–3 mos; 9 yrs (C)	Domesticated. Excellent captive breeder. Extremely high lifetime energy expenditures. Good husbandry information available; less clinical literature. Used extensively in behavior, physiology and neurobiology research.	Less clinical and pathological information available. Small body size makes blood and tissue collection difficult; longer-lived than laboratory rodents. Sexes distinguishable.
Pigeon (*Columba livia*): Columbiformes	250 g	4–6 mos; 35 yrs	Domesticated. Breeds well in captivity; husbandry information available. Large clinical, behavioral physiological and neurobiological literature. Free-radical production and oxidant status have been studied. Strains are available that are prone to special aging-related condition, e.g. cardiovascular disease.	Longer-lived than smaller pet bird species. Sexes not distinguishable.
White-crowned Sparrow (*Zonotrichia leucophrys*): Passeriformes	20–25 g	10–11 mos; approx 9 yrs (W)	Wild stock only, but captives can be maintained in substantial numbers. Extensive research literature on nutrition, physiology, neurobiology and behavior.	Not commercially available. Breeding difficult in captivity. Sexes similar.

*MLS = maximum reliably documented life span. "C" denotes longevity record from captive representatives; "W" denotes record from mark-recapture records from wild populations.

References: National Research Council, 1981; Murphy and King, 1990; Ku and Sohal, 1993; Nottebohm *et al.*, 1994; Holmes, *et al.*, 2001; Holmes and Austad 1995a; Austad, 1997; Ottinger, 2001; D. Nelson, pers. comm.; F. Nottebohm, pers. comm.

In addition, several teams of field ornithologists have published reports of aging-related declines in immunity in wild birds (for an earlier review, see Holmes and Austad, 2004).

AVIAN IMMUNOSENESCENCE IN THE WILD

The physiological declines associated with senescence, including declines in both innate and acquired immune defenses against parasites and pathogenic microorganisms, have been thoroughly documented in laboratory animals and humans (Wollscheid-Lengeling, 2004). But the fitness deficits associated with advancing age in the wild, where animals experience a full range of natural hazards, stresses and diseases, are far less well understood (Miller, 1996). Recently, reliable aging-related declines in aspects of either cellular or humoral immunity have been reported in wild populations of several bird species, including barn swallows (*Hirundo rustica*), collared flycatchers (*Ficedula hypoleuca*), and ruffs (*Philomachus pugnax*) (Saino *et al.*, 2003; Cichoń *et al.*, 2003; Lozano and Lank, 2003).

Lozano and Lank measured cell-mediated immunity in the ruff, a shorebird, using a measure of delayed hypersensitivity to phytohemagglutinin, a nonspecific mitogen foreign to the avian immune system. Males showed a marginally significant age-related decline in cellular immune response; this effect was more pronounced in nonbreeding than in breeding males, which probably expend significant amounts of energy defending territories. In a study focusing on the humoral immune response of barn swallows by Saino *et al.* (2003), banded swallows were immunized repeatedly against Newcastle disease virus. Breeding individuals showed declining antibody responses with advancing age (barn swallows live 5 to 7 years in the wild), and this trend was more likely to be statistically significant for females. Secondary humoral responses were considerably lower overall in females than males, as were initial antibody titers prior to secondary vaccination. This finding is consistent with the greater parental investment typical of females in this species. Cichoń *et al.* (2003) challenged the immune systems of nesting female flycatchers with sheep red blood cells, another nonspecific antigen. Older females mounted an antibody response only about half that shown by younger breeders. This result was correlated with a trend for older females to fledge offspring of lower body mass than those of young and middle-aged birds.

It remains unclear what contribution such age-related changes in immune responses actually make to senescence-related mortality in the wild, where environmental factors may be more important physiological stressors than the effects of aging. Studies like these, however, represent an exciting effort by ecologists and field zoologists to begin incorporating reliable biomarkers of aging into studies of population biology and mating systems, life-history evolution, or other aspects of avian behavioral ecology.

AVIAN MODELS OF EXTREMELY SLOW TO NEGLIGIBLE REPRODUCTIVE AGING

Patterns of reproductive aging vary even more widely among birds than among mammals studied to date. As predicted by evolutionary aging and life-history theory, the slower aging of birds relative to mammals is generally reflected in slower reproductive aging in birds of both sexes (for reviews, see Holmes *et al.*, 2003; Holmes and Ottinger, 2003; 2004). Bird species that mature and reproduce extremely slowly, including seabirds (e.g., albatrosses, terns, and gulls) and large raptors (e.g., condors), tend also to be among the longest-lived, with some species holding longevity records of 50 years or more.

Even shorter-lived wild birds exhibit much slower aging than mammals of equivalent body size. Many small (under 50 grams) passerine songbirds have average life spans of over several years in the wild, and exhibit steady declines in reproductive aging. Reproductive declines in these birds are often more than twice as slow as those of similar-sized captive rodents (McCleery and Perrins, 1988; Newton, 1989; Gustafsson and Pärt, 1991; Clum, 1995; Newton and Rothery, 1997). For example, the rat-sized (110 g) American Kestrel (maximum recorded life span of over 10 years), a small raptor, shows little reproductive aging for up to 7 years or so.

Wild seabirds, including gulls, albatrosses, fulmars and terns, typically exhibit little or no loss of reproductive fitness even at the end of their natural life spans in nature ($>$50 yrs for some fulmars), and even when rising mortality rates suggest significant deterioration of other physiological systems. Since few seabirds have been maintained in captivity, it remains unclear how long the postreproductive life spans might be for these species if their natural life spans could be prolonged in captivity. Terns (order Charadriiformes), for example, have an extreme life-history strategy typical of pelagic seabirds, characterized by slow sexual maturation, low lifelong reproduction rates (2–3 chicks fledged per year), long life spans, and very slight to negligible declines in reproductive success after peak fledging success is reached at about 15 yrs (Nisbet *et al.*, 1999; Nisbet, 2002a,b). This kind of very sustained reproductive investment is thought to have evolved only in animal populations with extremely low adult mortality rates ($<$10 percent per year). The extremely slow to negligible aging typical of seabirds is rare in wild bird or mammal populations, and its physiological basis merits additional study.

Long-lived animals with exceptionally slow reproductive aging likely have physiological or molecular mechanisms for prolonging fertility, and basic reproductive aging processes may differ significantly between long- and short-lived species (Finch, 1990; Austad, 1993; Martin *et al.*, 1996; Austad and Holmes, 1999; vom Saal *et al.*, 1994). With the exception of primates, however, few long-lived animal models have been developed for exploring basic mechanisms of delayed fertility loss. Studies of the physiological correlates of avian reproductive aging have largely been limited to short-lived poultry species (for exceptions, see Clum, 1995; Ottinger *et al.*, 1995; Nisbet *et al.*, 1999, 2002a). We have emphasized the potential of wild bird populations for studies of exceptionally slow—or even negligible—reproductive aging under natural conditions in earlier reviews (Holmes *et al.*, 2003; Holmes and Ottinger, 2003).

PITFALLS OF AVIAN AGING STUDIES IN THE WILD

Good studies of basic aging patterns and processes in wild animals in nature depend on the ability to quantify and repeatedly measure reliable biomarkers of aging in substantial numbers of individuals. The statistical approaches currently used by avian demographers are in many cases robust and sophisticated, taking into account potential biases inherent in this type of data. As we have illustrated above, bird studies have other advantages as well. On the other hand, studies of the effects of aging in wild animal populations have some drawbacks for investigating basic mechanisms of aging. The natural habitat of a wild bird is far removed from the pampered and protected environment enjoyed by inbred rodents, and carefully controlled longitudinal studies of aging in wild animals are much more difficult. Intrinsic causes of mortality (endogenous aging-related physiological declines) in these studies will be in many cases indistinguishable from extrinsic causes, like predation, disease, and other environmental stressors.

Wild bird populations are outbred and genetically variable. As in aging studies employing mammalian models (including humans), wild birds that live to older ages and survive repeated measurement of biomarkers may not be genetically representative of the population as a whole. Even in laboratory studies, the longest-lived animals in the population have passed through a significant selective "bottleneck"; this effect may be even more pronounced in the wild under natural selective regimes. Nonetheless, studies of exceptionally and naturally long-lived animals in the wild can contribute in important ways to our understanding of basic aging processes, providing important links between biogerontology, evolutionary and population biology, and natural history.

Birds as Models for Aging Studies: Special Challenges and Recommendations

Until recently, the selection of animal models in biogerontology has been driven primarily by economy, feasibility, and simplicity. Most key advances in our understanding of fundamental molecular and cellular aging processes have resulted either from the use of short-lived, rapidly aging species—inbred laboratory rodents, roundworms, flies—or highly specialized cell lines. But the most popular biogerontological animal models not only have life histories quite dissimilar to those of humans and most domestic animals, they also lack the very trait biologists most wish to understand and emulate: the ability to resist aging. The vertebrate animal models currently best developed for studies of aging, laboratory rats and mice, are highly suitable for use in controlled experiments, but, ironically, are poorly adapted for aging. As the field of aging has evolved, so has our understanding of the promise of carefully selected "nontraditional" vertebrate models for aging, including certain primate species, exceptionally long-lived animals like naked mole-rats, bats and birds.

Other recent reviews have emphasized the importance of a judiciously applied comparative approach to selecting animal models for aging studies, employing a variety of distantly related animal species, and identifying a range of potential molecular "solutions" to the problem of long-term somatic maintenance and repair (Finch, 1990; Austad, 1993; Austad and Holmes, 1999). As we have illustrated in this chapter, a number of bird species are poised for use as the kind of exceptionally long-lived laboratory models needed to apply this approach.

There are additional, obvious challenges to the development of avian aging models. Although some cage birds have been domesticated for over a century, and some basic genetic information is available on the species we have highlighted here, genetic resources for experimental bird models (including information about genetic variability, commercially inbred or isogenic strains, genetic markers and gene sequence libraries) lag far behind those available for use with traditional laboratory animals. It requires a concerted effort by the biogerontological research community and funding agencies to direct resources toward developing new animal models. Since birds typically are significantly longer-lived than laboratory rodents, well-conceived, longitudinal avian aging studies will inevitably take longer and require substantial financial investment if they are to be worthwhile. Accepted techniques for the measurement of standard aging biomarkers will need to be adapted and calibrated for new avian models. This effort will require careful collaboration and communication between biogerontologists and other zoologists, as well as a synthetic and interdisciplinary dialog among scholars in the field who are well versed in accepted methodologies in the field of aging, as well as evolutionary principles and comparative zoology.

ACKNOWLEDGMENTS

D. Holmes acknowledges the support of INBRE grant P20RR16454-01 (National Institutes of Health) to the University of Idaho during the preparation of this paper. M.A. Ottinger acknowledges National Science Foundation grant #9817024. A. Bressler assisted with the preparation of the manuscript.

REFERENCES

Altman, P.L., and Dittmer, D.S. (1972). *Biology Data Book*, Vol. 1. Federation of the American Sciences for Experimental Biology, Bethesda, MD.

Austad, S. (1997). Birds as models of aging in biomedical research. *ILAR J. Online 38(3)*.

Austad, S.N. (1993). The comparative perspective and choice of animal models in aging research. *Aging* (*Milano*) *5*, 259–267.

Austad, S.N., and Fischer, K.E. (1991). Mammalian aging, metabolism, and ecology: Evidence from the bats and marsupials. *J. Gerontol.: Biol. Sci. 46*, B47–B53.

Bahr, J.M., and Palmer, S.S. (1989). The influence of aging on ovarian function. *Crit. Rev. Poult. Biol. 2*, 103–110.

Barja, G. (1998). Mitochondrial free radical production and aging in mammals and birds. *Ann. N. Y. Acad. Sci. 854*, 224–238.

Barja, G., and Herrero, A. (1998). Localization at complex I and mechanism of the higher free radical production of brain nonsynaptic mitochondria in the short-lived rat than in the longevous pigeon. *J. Bioenerg. Biomemb. 30*, 235–243.

Barja, G., Cadenas, S., Roja, C., Perez-Campo, R., and Lopez-Torres, M. (1994). Low mitochondrial free radical production per unit of O_2 consumption can explain the simultaneous presence of high longevity and high aerobic metabolic rate in birds. *Free Rad. Res. 21*, 317–328.

Barja, G., Cadenas, S., Roja, C., Lopez-Torres, M., and Perez-Campo, R. (1994). A decrease in free radical production near critical targets as a cause of maximum longevity in animals. *Comp. Biochem. Physiol. Biochem. Molec. Biol. 108*, 501–512.

Bennett, P.M., and Owens, I. P. F. (2002). *Evolutionary Ecology of Birds. Life Histories, Mating Systems and Extinction*, Oxford University Press, Oxford.

Bridgham, J.T., and Johnson, A.L. (2001). Expression and regulation of Fas antigen and tumor necrosis factor receptor type 1 in hen granulosa cells. *Biol. Reprod. 65*, 733–739.

Bronson, F.H. (1989). *Mammalian Reproductive Biology*, University of Chicago Press, Chicago, IL.

Byerly, R.C., Soares, J.H.J., and Ottinger, M.A. (1984). Severe vs. moderate restrictions of feed intake: Effects on body weight, egg production, energetic efficiency and male development of broiler breeders. Proceeding of XVII—World's Poultry Congress.

Carey, J.R., and Judge, D.S. (2000). *Longevity Records: Life Spans of Mammals, Birds, Amphibians, Reptiles, and Fish.* Odense Monographs on Population Aging 8, Odense University Press, Odense, Denmark.

Cerami, A. (1985). Hypothesis: Glucose as a mediator of aging. *J. Amer. Geriatr. Soc. 33*, 626–634.

Cichoń, M., Sendecka, J., and Gustafsson, L. (2003). Age-related decline in humoral immune function in Collared Flycatchers. *J. Evol. Biol. 16*, 1205–1210.

Cheeseman, J.H., Kaiser, M.G., and Lamont, S.J. (2004). Genetic line effect on peripheral blood leukocyte cell surface marker expression in chickens. *Poult. Sci. 83*, 911–916.

Clum, N.J. (1995) Effects of aging and mate retention on reproductive success of captive female peregrine falcons. *Amer. Zool. 35*, 329–339.

Del Maestro, R.F. (1980). An approach to free radicals in medicine and biology. *Acta Physiol. Scand. 492*, 153–168.

Delany, M.E., Krupkin, A.B., and Miller, M.M. (2000). Organization of telomere sequences in birds: Evidence for arrays of extreme length and for in vivo shortening. *Cytogenet. Cell Genet. 90*, 139–145.

Doetsch, R., and Scharff, C. (2001). Challenges for brain repair: Insights from adult neurogenesis in birds and mammals. *Br. Behav. Evol. 58*, 306–322.

Edney, E.B., and Gill, R.W. (1968). Evolution of senescence and specific longevity. *Nature 220*, 281–282.

Finch, C.E. (1990) *Longevity, Senescence, and the Genome*, University of Chicago Press, Chicago, IL.

Gavrilov, V.M., and Dolnik, V.R. (1982). Basal metabolic rate, thermoregulation and existence energy in birds: World data. In Ilyichev, V.D., and Gavrilov, V.M. (Eds.). *Acta XVIII. Congress Internationalis Ornithologici*. Academy of Sciences of the USSR, Moscow, pp. 421–466.

Giles, J.R., Shivaprasad H.L., and Johnson, P.A. (2004). Ovarian tumor expression of an oviductal protein in the hen: a model for human serous ovarian aenocarcinoma. *Gynecologic Oncology 95*, 530–533.

Gill, F.B. (1995). *Ornithology*, W.H. Freeman, New York.

Granger, M.P., Wright, W.E., and Shay, J.W. (2002). Telomerase in cancer and aging. *Crit. Rev. Oncol. Hematol. 41*, 29–40.

Guraya, S.S. (1989). *Ovarian Follicles in Reptiles and Birds*, Springer-Verlag, Heidelberg.

Gustafsson, L., and Pärt, T. (1991). Acceleration of senescence in the collared flycatcher *Ficedula albicollis* by reproductive costs. *Nature 347*, 279–281.

Hall, M., Nasir, L., Daunt, F., Gault, E., Croxall, J., Wanless, S., and Monaghan, P. (2004). Telemere loss in relation to age and early environment in long-lived birds. *Proc. R. Soc. Lond. B. Biol. Sci. 271*, 1571–1576.

Harley, C.B. (1995). Telomeres and aging. In *Telomeres* (Blackburn, E.H., and Greider, C.W., eds.) pp. 247–263, Cold Spring Harbor Laboratory Press, Cold Spring Harbor.

Harman, D. (1956). Aging: A theory based on free radical and radiation chemistry. *J. Gerontol. 11*, 289–300.

Haussmann, M.F., Winkler, D.W., O'Reilly, K.M., Huntington, C.E., Nisbet, I.C.T., and Vleck, C.M. (2003). Telomeres shorten more slowly in long-lived birds and mammals than in short-lived ones. *Proc. Roy. Soc. Lond. B Biol. Sci. 70*, 1387–1392.

Herrero, A., and Barja, G. (1998). H_2O_2 production of heart mitochondria and aging rate are slower in canaries and parakeets than in mice: Sites of free radical generation and mechanisms involved. *Mech. Age. Devel. 103*, 133–146.

Hillier, L., Miller, W., Birney, E., Warren, W., Hardison, R., Ponting, C., *et al.* (2004). Sequence and comparative analysis of the chicken genome provide unique perspectives on vertebrate evolution. *Nature 432*, 695–716.

Holmes, D.J., and Austad, S.N. (1995). The evolution of avian senescence patterns: Implications for understanding primary aging processes. *Amer. Zool. 35*, 307–317.

Holmes, D.J., and Austad, S.N. (1995). Birds as animal models for the comparative biology of aging: A prospectus. *J. Gerontol. Biol. Sci. 50A*, 59–66.

Holmes, D.J., and Ottinger, M.A. (2003). Birds as long-lived animal models for the study of aging. *Exp. Gerontol. 38*, 1365–1375.

Holmes, D.J., and Austad, S.N. (2004). Declining Immunity with Age in the Wild? Evidence from Bird Populations. *Science of Aging Knowledge Environment (SAGE KE), Science Online 21*, pe22.

Holmes, D.J., Fluckiger, R., and Austad, S.N. (2001). Comparative biology of aging in birds: An update. *Exp. Gerontol. 36*, 869–883.

Holmes, D.J., Thomson, S.L., Wu, J., and Ottinger, M.A. (2003). Reproductive aging in female birds. *Exp. Gerontol. 38*, 751–756.

Iqbal, M., Probert, L.L., Alhumadi, N.H., and Klandorf, H. (1999). Protein glycosylation and advanced glycosylated endproducts (AGEs) accumulation: an avian solution? *J. Gerontol.: Biol. Sci. 54*, B171–B176.

Jaensch, S., Cullen, L., Morton, L., and Raidal, S.R. (2001). Normobaric hyperoxic stress in budgerigars: Nonenzymic antioxidants. *Comp. Biochem. Physiol. Part C Pharmacol. Toxicol. Endocrinol. 128*, 181–187.

Johnson, A.L. (2000a). Reproduction in the female. In *Sturkie's Avian Physiology* (Whittow, G.C., ed.), Academic Press, New York.

Johnson, A.L. (2000b). Granulosa cell apoptosis: Conservation of cell signaling in an avian ovarian model system. *Biol. Sig. Receptors 9*, 96–101.

Johnson, A.L., Langer, J.S., and Bridgham, J.T. (2002). Survivin as a cell cycle-related and antiapoptotic protein in granulosa cells. *Endocrinology 143*, 3405–3413.

Johnson, P.A., Dickerman, R.W., and Bahr, J.M. (1986). Decreased granulosa cell luteinizing hormone sensitivity and altered thecal estradiol concentration in the aged hen (*Gallus domesticus*). *Biol. Reprod. 5*, 641–646.

Kaetzel, D.M., and Soares, J.H. (1985). Effect of dietary calcium stress on plasma vitamin D3 metabolites in the egg-lying Japanese quail. *Poult. Sci. 64*, 1121–1127.

Kaiser, M.G., Lakshmanan, N., Arthur, J.A., O'Sullivan, N.P., and Lamont, S.J. (2003). Experimental population design for estimation of dominant molecular marker effect on egg-production traits. *Anim. Genet. 34*, 334–338.

Kim, J., O'Laughlin, B., Kasparian, S., and Nottebohm, F. (1994). Cell death and neuronal recruitment in the high vocal center of adult male canaries are temporally related to changes in song. *Proc. Nat. Acad. Sci. USA 91*, 7844–7848.

Kitamura, A., Yoshimura, Y., and Okamoto, T. (2002). Changes in the populations of mitotic and apoptotic cells in white follicles during atresia in hens. *Poult. Sci. 81*, 408–413.

Kristal, B.S., and Yu, B.P. (1992). An emerging hypothesis: Inductions of aging of free radicals and Maillard reactions. *J. Gerontol. Biol. Sci. 47*, B107–B114.

Ku, H., and Sohal, R.S. (1993). Comparison of mitochondrial pro-oxidant generation and anti-oxidant defenses between rat and pigeon: Possible basis of variation in longevity and metabolic potential. *Mech. Age. Devel. 72*, 67–76.

Lamont, S.J. (2003). Unique population designs used to address molecular genetics questions in poultry. *Poult. Sci. 82*, 882–884.

Lasiewski, R.C., and Dawson, W.R. (1967). A re-examination of the relation between standard metabolic rate and body weight in birds. *Condor 69*, 13–23.

Lozano, G., and Lank, D. (2003). Seasonal trade-offs in cell-mediated immunosenescence in ruffs (*Philomachus pugnax*). *Proc. Roy. Soc. Lond. B Biol. Sci. 270*, 1203–1208.

Martin, G.M., Austad, S.N., and Johnson, T.E. (1996). Genetic analysis of aging: Role of oxidative damage and environmental stresses. *Nat. Genet. 13*, 25–34.

Masoro, E.J. (1993). Dietary restriction and aging. *J. Amer. Geriatr. Soc. 41*, 994–999.

Masoro, E.J. (2001). Dietary restriction: An experimental approach to the study of biology and aging. In *Handbook of the Biology of Aging* (Masoro, E.J., and Austad, S.N., eds.), pp. 396–422, Academic Press, New York.

McCleery, R.H., and Perrins, C.M. (1988). Lifetime reproductive success in the Great Tit. In *Reproductive Success: Studies of Individual Variation in Contrasting Breeding Systems* (Clutton-Brock, T.H., ed.), pp. 136–153, University of Chicago Press, Chicago.

McDaniel, G.R. (1983). Factors affecting broiler breeder performance. 5. Effects of preproduction feeding regime on reproductive performance. *Poult. Sci. 62*, 1949–1953.

Medawar, P.B. (1952). *An Unsolved Problem of Biology*, H.K. Lewis, London.

Merry, B.J., and Holehan, A.M. (1979). Onset of puberty and duration of fertility in rats fed a restricted diet. *J. Reprod. Fret. 57*, 253–259.

Miles, S.A., and Leeson, S. (1990). Effects of feed restriction during the rearing period and age at photostimulation on the reproductive performance of turkey hens. *Poult. Sci. 69*, 1522–1528.

Miller, R. (1996). The aging immune system: Primer and prospectus. *Science 273*, 70–74.

Mobarak, M. (1990). *Effect of Dietary-Endocrine Interactions on Reproduction in Male Japanese Quail.* Thesis, University of Maryland.

Mobarak, M., Mench, J.A., and Ottinger, M.A. (1988). Effect of feed restriction on reproductive development of male Japanese quail. *Poult. Sci. 67*, 121.

Monnier, V.M. (1990). Nonenzymatic glycosylation: The Maillard reaction and the aging process. *J. Gerontol.: Biol. Sci. 45*, B105–B111.

Monnier, V.M., Sell, D.R., Ramanakoppa, H.N., and Miyata, S. (1991). Mechanisms of protection against damage mediated by the Maillard reaction in aging. *Gerontol. 37*, 152–165.

Monnier, V.M., Fogarty, J.F., Monnier, C.S., and Sell, D.R. (1999). Glycation, glycoxidation, and other Maillard reaction products. In *Methods in Aging Research* (Yu, B.P., ed.) pp. 657–681, CRC, Boca Raton, FL.

Murphy, M., and King, C.E. (1990). Diurnal changes in tissue glutathione pools of molting white-crowned sparrows: The influence of photoperiod and feeding schedule. *Physiol. Zool. 63*, 1118–1140.

Nelson, J.F., Karelus, K., Bergman, M.D., and Felicio, L. (1995). Neuroendocrine involvement in aging: Evidence from studies of reproductive aging and caloric restriction. *Neurobiol. Aging 16*, 837–843.

Newton, I., ed (1989). *Lifetime Reproduction in Birds*, Academic Press, London.

Newton, I., and Rothery, P. (1997). Senescence and reproductive value in sparrowhawks. *Ecology 78*, 1000–1008.

Nisbet, I., Apanius, V., and Friar, M.S. (2002). Breeding performance of very old common terns. *J. Field Ornithol. 73*, 117–124.

Nisbet, I., Finch, C.E., Thompson, N., Russek-Cohen, E., Proudman, J.A., and Ottinger, M.A. (1999). Endocrine patterns during aging in the common tern (*Sterna hirundo*). *Gen. Comp. Endocrinol. 114*, 279–286.

Nisbet, I.C.T. (2002). Common tern (*Sterna hirundo*). In *The Birds of North America* (Poole, A., and Gill, F.B., eds.), Vol. 618, pp. 1–40, The Birds of North America, Philadelphia, PA.

Nottebohm, F., O'Laughlin, B., Gould, K., Yohay, K., and Alvariez Buylla, A. (1994). The life span of new neurons in a song control nucleus of the adult canary brain depends on time of year when these cells are born. *Proc. Nat. Acad. Sci. USA 91*, 7849–7853.

Ogburn, C.E., Carlberg, K., Ottinger, M.A., Holmes, D.J., Martin, G.M., and Austad, S.N. (2001). Exceptional cellular resistance to oxidative damage in long-lived birds requires active gene expression. *J. Gerontol.: Biol. Sci. 56A*, B468–B474.

Ogburn, C.E., Austad, S.N., Holmes, D.J., Kiklevich, J.V., Gollahon, K., Rabinovitch, P.S., and Martin, G.M. (1998). Cultured renal epithelial cells from birds and mice: Enhanced resistance of avian cells to oxidative stress and DNA damage. *J. Gerontol.: Biol. Sci. 53A*, B287–B292.

Ottinger, M.A. (1991). Neuroendocrine and behavioral determinants of reproductive aging. *Crit. Rev. Poult. Biol. 3*, 131–142.

Ottinger, M.A. (1996). Aging in the avian brain: Neuroendocrine considerations. *Seminars in Av. Exot. Pet Med. 5*, 172–177.

Ottinger, M.A. (1998). Male reproduction: Testosterone, gonadotropins, and aging. In *Functional Endocrinology of Aging* (Mobbs, C.V., ed.), Vol. 29, pp. 105–126, Karger, Basel.

Ottinger, M.A. (2001). Quail and other short-lived birds. *Exp. Gerontol. 36*, 859–868.

Ottinger, M.A., and Soares, J.H. (1988). Comparative aspects of reproductive failure in aging male quail and broiler breeder chickens. *Proc. 11th Internat. Congr. Anim. Reprod. Art. Insem.*

Ottinger, M.A., and Bakst, M.R. (1995). Endocrinology of the avian reproductive system. *J. Av. Med. Surg. 9*, 242–250.

Ottinger, M.A., Thompson, N., Fan, Y., Panzica, G.C., Viglietti-Panzica, C., and Li, Q. (1997). Gonadotropin-releasing hormone (cGnRh-1) and neuropeptide systems reflect endocrine and behavioral changes during reproductive aging. In *Perspectives in Avian Endocrinology* (Harvery, S., and Etches, R.J., eds.), pp. 91–100, J.W. Arrowsmith, Ltd, Bristol.

Ottinger, M.A., Abdelnabi, M., Li, Q., Chen, K., Thompson, N., Harada, N., Viglietti-Panzica, C., and Panzica, G.C. (2004). The Japanese quail: A model for studying reproductive aging of hypothalamic systems. *Exp. Gerontol. 39*, 1679–1693.

Ottinger, M.A., Mobarak, M., Abdelnabi, M. Roth, G., Proudman, J., and Ingram, D.K. (2005). Effects of calorie restriction on reproductive and adrenal systems in Japanese quail: Are responses similar to mammals, particularly primates? *Mech. Aging Develop. 126*, 967–975.

Pamplona, R., Portero-Ótin, M., Requena, J.R., Thorpe, S.R., Herrero, A., and Barja, G. (1999). A low degree of fatty unsaturation leads to lower lipid peroxidation and lipoxidation-derived protein modification in heart mitochondria of the longevous pigeon than in the short lived rat. *Mech. Age. Devel. 106*, 283–296.

Pamplona, R., Prat, J., Cadenas, S., Roja, C., Perez-Campo, R., Lopez-Torres, M., and Barja, G. (1996). Low fatty acid unsaturation protects against lipid peroxidation in liver mitochondria from long-lived species: The pigeon and human case. *Mech. Age. Dev. 86*, 53–66.

Pamplona, R., Portero-Ótin, M., Riba, D., Ledo, F., Gredilla, R., Herrero, A., and Barja, G. (1999). Heart fatty acid unsaturation and lipid peroxidation, and aging rate, are lower in the canary and the parakeet than in the mouse. *Aging (Milano) 11*, 44–49.

Panzica, G.C., Garcia-Ojeda, E., Viglietti-Panzica, C., Thompson, N.E., and Ottinger, M.A. (1996). Testosterone effects on vasotocinergic innervation of sexually dimorphic medial preoptic nucleus and lateral septum during aging in male quail. *Br. Res. 712*, 190–198.

Partridge, L., and Barton, N.H. (1993). Optimality, mutation and the evolution of ageing. *Nature 362*, 305–311.

Pearl, R. (1928). *The Rate of Living*, Alfred A. Knopf, New York.

Pomeroy, D. (1990). Why fly? The possible benefits for lower mortality. *Biol. J. Linn. Soc. 40*, 53–65.

Rose, M.R. (1991). *Evolutionary Biology of Aging*, Oxford University Press, New York.

Ryals, B.M., and Westbrook, E.W. (1988). Ganglion cell and hair cell loss in Coturnix quail associated with aging. *Hear. Res. 36*, 1–8.

Ryals, B.M., and Westbrook, E.W. (1990). Hair cell regeneration in senescent quail. *Hear. Res. 50*, 87–96.

Ryals, B.M., and Westbrook, E.W. (1994). TEM analysis of neural terminals on autoradiographically identified regenerated hair cells. *Hear. Res. 72*, 81–88.

Saino, N., Ferrari, R., Romano, M., Rubolini, D., and Møller, A. (2003). Humoral immune response in relation to senescence, sex and sexual ornamentation in the barn swallow (*Hirundo rustica*). *J. Evol. Biol. 16*, 1127–1134.

Sexton, K.J., Renden, J.A., Marple, D.N., and Kempainen, R.J. (1989). Effects of dietary energy on semen production, fertility, plasma testosterone, and carcass composition of broiler-breeder males in cages. *Poult. Sci. 68*, 1688–1694.

Sibley, C.G., and Monroe, B.L.J. (1990). *Distribution and Taxonomy of Birds of the World*, Yale University Press, New Haven, CT.

Sibley, C.G., and Monroe, B.L.J. (1993). *A Supplement to Distribution and Taxonomy of Birds of the World*, Yale University Press, New Haven, CT.

Smith, E.J., Kamara, D., Pimentel, G., Geng, T., Guan, X., Lin, K., and Hartman, S. (2005). Avian genomes: Important resources for understanding vertebrate biology. *Curr. Genom. 6*, 75–80.

Tokarz, R.R. (1978). Oogonial proliferation, oogenesis, and folliculogenesis in nonmammalian vertebrates. In *The Vertebrate Ovary: Comparative Biology and Evolution* (Jones, R.E., ed.), pp. 145–179, Plenum Press, New York.

Vleck, C.M., Haussmann, M.F., and Vleck, D. (2003). The natural history of telomeres: Tools for aging animals and exploring the aging process. *Exp. Gerontol. 38*, 791–795.

Volentine, K.K., Yao, H.H., and Bahr, J.M. (1998). Epidermal growth factor in the germinal disc and its potential role in follicular development in the chicken. *Biol. Reprod. 59*, 522–526.

vom Saal, F.S., Finch, C.E., and Nelson, J.F. (1994). Natural history and mechanisms of reproductive aging in humans, laboratory rodents, and other selected vertebrates. In *The Physiology of Reproduction* (Knobil, E., and Neill, J.D., eds.), pp. 1213–1314, Raven Press, New York.

Waddington, D., and Walker, M.A. (1988). Distribution of follicular growth, atresia and ovulation in the ovary of the domestic hen (*Gallus domesticus*) at different ages. *J. Reprod. Fert. 84*, 223–230.

Waddington, D., Perry, M.M., Gilbert, A.B., and Hardie, M.A. (1985). Follicular growth and atresia in the ovaries of hens (*Gallus domesticus*) with diminished egg production rates. *J. Reprod. Fert. 74*, 399–405.

Wade, J., Peabody, C., Coussens, P., Tempelman, R.J., Clayton, D.F., Liu, L., Arnold, A.P. and Agate, R. (2004). A cDNA microarray from the telencephalon of juvenile male and female zebra finches. *J. Neurosci. Meth. 138*, 199–206.

Walsh, T.J., and Brake, J. (1999). Effects of feeding program and crude protein intake during rearing on fertility of broiler breeder females. *Poult. Sci. 78*, 827–832.

Weindruch, R., and Walford, R.L. (1988). *The Retardation of Aging and Disease by Dietary Restriction*, Charles C. Thomas, Springfield, IL.

Williams, G.C. (1957) Pleiotrophy, natural selection and the evolution of senescence. *Evolution 11*, 398–411.

Williams, J.B., and Sharp, P.J. (1978). Age-dependent changes in the hypothalamo-pituitary-ovarian axis of the laying hen. *J. Reprod. Fertil. 53*, 141–146.

Wollscheid-Lengeling, E., Müller, R.-J., R. Balling, R., and K. Schugart, K. (2004). Maintaining your immune system—one method for enhanced longevity. *Sci. Aging Knowl. Environ.* pe2 (2004).

Woodard, A.E., and Abplanalp, H. (1971). Longevity and reproduction in Japanese quail maintained under stimulatory lighting. *Poult. Sci. 50*, 688–692.

Wong, G.K, Liu, B. Wang, J., Zhang, Y., Yang, X., Meng, Q., *et al.* (2004). A genetic variation map for chicken with 2.8 million single–nucleotide polymorphisms. *Nature 432*, 717–722.

Zuidhof, M.J., Robinson, F.E., Feddes, J.J., Hardin, R.T., Wilson, J.L., McKay, R.I., and Newcombe, M. (1995). The effects of nutrient dilution on the well-being and performance of female broiler breeders. *Poult. Sci. 74*, 441–456.

31

A Transgenic Mini Rat Strain as a Tool for Studying Aging and Calorie Restriction

Isao Shimokawa

Mini rats, a transgenic strain of rats whose somatotropic axis was suppressed by overexpression of the antisense growth hormone gene, were shown to live longer than nontransgenic wild-type rats (−/−), when heterozygous for the transgene (tg/−); homozygous (tg/tg) rats died slightly earlier due to neoplastic causes. As observed in (tg/−) rats, moderate suppression of the somatotropic axis produced some phenotypes similar to those in (−/−) rats subjected to caloric restriction (CR), a well-known experimental intervention favoring longevity in animals. Thus, comparative studies using (tg/−) rats with the CR paradigm will help us understand the role of the somatotropic axis in regulation of lifespan and aging. Furthermore, the level of suppression of the somatotropic axis in (tg/−) rats was not as severe as in other mice models, and thus, experiments can be performed within physiological ranges.

Introduction

In the last decade, since Ames dwarf mice with spontaneous mutation of the prop-1 gene were reported to live longer than their wild-type counterparts (Brown-Borg *et al.*, 1996), over 10 rodent longevity models, in which a single gene has been spontaneously mutated or genetically engineered, have been reported (Miskin and Masos, 1997; Migliaccio *et al.*, 1999; Coschigano *et al.*, 2000; Flurkey *et al.*, 2001; Mitsui *et al.*, 2002; Shimokawa *et al.*, 2002; Bluher *et al.*, 2003; Holzenberger *et al.*, 2003). Many of the mice used show a reduction in growth hormone (GH)-insulin-like growth factor (IGF)-1 signaling or insulin signaling (Liang *et al.*, 2003). The importance of these models can be stressed in two ways. First, the DAF-2- AGE-1 pathway in nematodes increases lifespans when the signal input is reduced (Hekimi and Guarente 2003). These two molecules are orthologues of mammalian insulin or IGF receptor (Kimura *et al.*, 1997) and phosphatidylinositol 3-kinase (PI3K; (Morris *et al.*, 1996)), respectively. In fruit flies, mutation of the "Chico" gene, an orthologue of mammalian insulin receptor substrates, in the insulin-like pathway is also known to result in an extended lifespan (Clancy *et al.*, 2001). These findings suggest that insulin or IGF-1 signaling is an evolutionarily conserved pathway that controls longevity in animals. Second, calorie restriction (CR), a well-known experimental intervention for lifespan extension in a wide range of organisms, also suppresses GH-IGF-1/insulin signaling (Masoro, 2003), suggesting that CR increases animal lifespans partly through a reduction in the signaling pathway (Shimokawa *et al.*, 2003).

In the following chapter, a transgenic strain of mini rats whose somatotropic axis was suppressed by overexpression of the antisense GH gene (Matsumoto *et al.*, 1993) is described and compared with CR rats in terms of lifespan, pathology, and selected biomarkers potentially related to the effect of CR.

Mini Rats and Their Husbandry

The transgenic rats were produced from founders created by introducing fusion genes into rat embryos (Matsumoto *et al.*, 1993); their genetic background was Jcl: Wistar (Japan Clea, Inc., Tokyo, Japan). The transgene consisted of four copies of thyroid hormone response elements, rat GH promoter, and antisense cDNA sequences for rat GH. Transgenic offspring expressed the rat GH antisense transgene in the pituitary gland, and exhibited dwarfism as early as 3 weeks of age. Antisense GH-mRNA expression was detected by RT-PCR in the pituitary gland, spleen, and thymus in transgenic rats at 6 months of age, but not in the lungs, liver, heart, kidneys or testis (Shimokawa *et al.*, 2002).

Male and female transgenic rats showed a reduced growth rate but almost normal reproduction function, although maturation seemed to be slightly delayed and the fecundity in female transgenic rats was slightly lower than in control female Wistar rats.

F1 hybrid rats (Jcl:Wistar-TgN (ARGHGEN)1Nts × Jcl:Wistar) were also generated at our laboratory animal center to moderate the reduced level of suppression of the somatotropic axis. The experimental animals were referred to as (tg/tg), (tg/−), and (−/−) with respect to the presence of the transgene.

At 4 weeks of age, weanling male rats were transferred to a barrier facility (temperature, 22 to 25°C; 12-h light/dark cycle), housed separately, and maintained under specific pathogen-free (SPF) conditions. The procedure for monitoring the SPF status was fully described elsewhere (Shimokawa *et al.*, 2002) and has been maintained since 1997 when the rat colony was established.

Rats were provided with a CR-LPF diet (Oriental Yeast, Tsukuba, Japan) based on the formula of Charles River (CRF-1), but with a protein fraction of 18.2%; the original CRF-1 diet contains 22.6% protein on a weight basis. All rats were fed a CR-LPF diet and water ad libitum (AL) after weanling. At 6 weeks of age, rats were divided into two diet groups: one group (AL) continued to receive food ad libitum, while the other (CR) was provided every other day with 140% of the mean daily food intake of the AL group in each rat group 30 min before the lights were turned off. This regimen successively restricted the food intake of the CR rats by 30% that of the AL group during the entire experimental period. However, it also yielded a 2-day cycle in the pattern of food intake in the CR group, with most of the allotted food being ingested within the first 24-h. When the food intake pattern confounded serum insulin and other hormones, the CR group was subdivided into CR1 and CR2, rats sacrificed within the first 24-h after feeding and within the following 24-h, respectively. Consequently, when sacrificed in the CR1 phase, the CR group consumed the similar amount of food as each AL group before sacrifice.

The body weights and food intake of rats in each group during the lifespan study are illustrated in Figure 31.1.

It should be noted that both the body weight and food intake of (−/−)-CR rats were similar to those of (tg/−)-AL rats for a considerable period of the experiment. Thus, comparative studies using (tg/−)-AL and (−/−)-CR rats could give insight into the role of the GH-IGF-1 axis in CR.

Pulsatile secretion of GH has yet to be analyzed in all rat groups; however, an immunohistochemical study revealed that the number of GH-positive cells was markedly reduced in (tg/tg) rats compared with (−/−) rats (Shimokawa *et al.*, 2002). Plasma IGF-1 concentrations at 6 months of age are provided in Table 31.1. The IGF-1 concentration decreased by 43% in (tg/−)-AL rats and by 74% in (tg/tg)-AL rats compared with (−/−)-AL rats. CR further decreased the IGF-1 concentration in each rat group; values in the CR2 phase were slightly lower than in the CR1 phase. It should be noted that the IGF-1 level was slightly lower in (tg/−)-AL rats than (−/−)-CR rats.

Lifespan and Pathology

The survival curves of (−/−), (tg/−), and (tg/tg) rats fed ad libitum and the effect of CR on (−/−) and (tg/−) rats were published previously (Shimokawa *et al.*, 2002; Shimokawa *et al.*, 2003). At the 25th percentile survival point, the lifespan was increased by 10% in (tg/−)-AL rats compared with (−/−)-AL rats (Table 31.2). In contrast, the lifespan of (tg/tg)-AL rats was diminished by 9%. CR increased the lifespans of (−/−), (tg/−), and (tg/tg) rats by 11, 10, and 19%, respectively.

Postmortem examinations were performed to determine the prevalence of selected diseases and analyze probable causes of death. Prevalence of pituitary adenoma did not differ between (−/−)-AL and (tg/−)-AL rats, but was significantly decreased in (tg/tg)-AL rats (Table 31.3). CR reduced the prevalence of pituitary adenoma compared to the AL group in (tg/−) rats, while statistically insignificant in (−/−) and (tg/tg) rats. Prevalence of chronic nephropathy was also significantly reduced in (tg/−) and (tg/tg) rats, and similarly, CR also decreased the prevalence. Although the number of rats

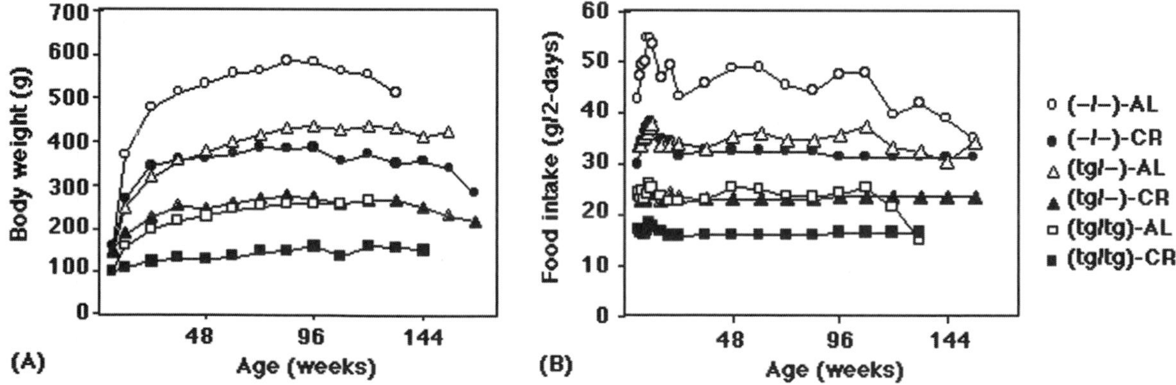

Figure 31.1. (A) Mean body weights of each rat group in the longevity study; $n = 30$ for each group at the start of the study, except the (tg/tg)-CR group ($n = 10$). Data are not depicted when the number of rats was below five, because of spontaneous death. (B) Mean food intake (g/rat/2 days) of the rat groups in the longevity study ($n = 10$, respectively). Data are not depicted when the number of rats was below five.

TABLE 31.1
Circulating concentrations of IGF-1, insulin, and glucose in not-fasting rats at 6-months of age

	(−/−)			(tg/−)			(tg/tg)		
	AL	CR1	CR2	AL	CR1	CR2	AL	CR1	CR2
IGF-1 (ng/ml)	1094 ± 119	864 ± 79[b]	773 ± 60[b, c]	627 ± 90[a]	346 ± 40[b] n/a	n/a	266 ± 23[a]	170 ± 11[b]	n/a
Insulin (ng/ml)	102 ± 49	15 ± 10[b]	18 ± 10[b]	22 ± 18[a]	20 ± 26	28 ± 30	21 ± 19[a]	n/a	m/a
Glucose (mg/dL)	126 ± 34	112 ± 12	102 ± 4	106 ± 18	90 ± 16	91 ± 12	106 ± 17	n/a	n/a

Data represent means ± SD ($n = 3$ to 6). [a]$p < 0.05$ vs (−/−)-AL group, [b]$p < 0.05$ vs the group AL in each rat group, [c]$p < 0.05$ vs the group CR1 in each rat group by a post hoc test (Fisher's protected least significant difference test) for multiple comparisons after 1-factor ANOVA. AL, groups of rats fed ad libitum. CR1 and CR2, groups of rats subjected to 30% calorie restriction, while sacrificed in the first day and the second day of 2-day feeding cycle, respectively (see the rat husbandry for the CR regimen, a modified alternate-day-feeding, used in the present study).

TABLE 31.2
Summary of lifespans

Survival points (percentile)	(−/−)		(tg/−)		(tg/tg)	
	AL	CR	AL	CR	AL	CR
50th	126 ± 7	142 ± 12	138 ± 14	157 ± 4	118 ± 1	145 ± 3
25th	140 ± 3	155 ± 10	154 ± 5	169 ± 6	127 ± 2	151 ± 4

Values represent the age (weeks) of each survival point of lifespan (±SE). $n = 30$ for (−/−) and (tg/−) rats at the start of the study, while 55 in (tg/tg)-AL rats and 35 in (tg/tg)-CR rats. A part of the data was published elsewhere (Shimokawa *et al.*, 2002; Shimokawa *et al.*, 2003). The survival rates were estimated using Kaplan–Meier product limit estimates. Although the survival curves are not shown in this chapter, the effect of CR was confirmed to be statistically significant in each rat group by the logrank test using the software "StatView 5.0" (SAS Institute, Cary, NC).

TABLE 31.3
Prevalence of selected diseases in rats dying spontaneously

	−/−		tg/−		tg/tg	
	AL	CR	AL	CR	AL	CR
n	30	26	30	30	39	17
Pituitary adenoma	20	13	22	8[a, b]	8[a]	2[a]
Chronic nephropathy						
Total	25	2[a]	8[a]	0	0	0
Mild	17	2	7	0	0	0
Moderate	5	0	1	0	0	0
Severe	3	0	0	0	0	0
Cardiac thrombus	6	0	3	0	0	0

n, the number of rats examined. [a]$p < 0.05$ versus −/− (AL) rats. [b]$p < 0.05$ versus tg/− (AL) rats. The total number of chronic nephropathy is statistically analyzed, but not the frequency of nephropathy by severity.

TABLE 31.4
Probable causes of death

	−/−		tg/−		tg/tg	
	AL	CR	AL	CR	AL	CR
Neoplastic (*subtotal*)	15	18	22	14	37[a]	11
Pituitary adenoma	5	8	11[c]	2[b]	1[c]	0
Tumor of subcutis or bone	5	3	4	2	5	0
Brain tumor	0	3	1	5	2	1
Tumor of visceral organs	1	2	2	2	4	2
Leukemia or lymphoma	0	1	2	3	21[d]	8
Others	4	1	2	0	4	0
Non-neoplastic (*subtotal*)	15	8	8	16	2	6
Cardiac thrombus	6	0	3	0	0	0
Prostatitis/lower urinary tract obstraction	1	3	1	5	0	0
Others (determined)	1	0	0	2	0	3
Undetermined	7	5	4	9	2	3

Data represent the number of rats. The proportion of each category or disease was analyzed by χ^2 test or Fisher exact test. $^a p < 0.05$ and $^c p < 0.10$ versus −/− (AL) rats. $^{b,d} p < 0.05$ versus tg/− (AL) rats.

that suffered from cardiac thrombi was limited, the prevalence was reduced in (tg/tg) rats; this was also seen in CR rats.

Probable causes of death differed among the three rat groups (Table 31.4). The (tg/tg) rats died mostly of neoplastic diseases, particularly leukemia, which was never observed in (−/−) rats. To assess the contribution of neoplastic causes of death to the shortened lifespan of (tg/tg) rats, conditional survival curves for neoplastic causes of death were generated (Figure 31.2).

In this analysis, nonneoplastic causes of death were considered to be the same censorship as random sacrifice of rats (see Shimokawa *et al.*, 1991 for details). Analysis confirmed that (tg/tg)-AL rats died earlier than other rats from neoplasms. The survival curve of (tg/−)-AL rats did not differ from that of (−/−)-AL rats, suggesting that the increased survival of (tg/−) rats is mostly due to delayed nonneoplastic causes of death. The proportion of pituitary adenoma as the cause of death increased in (tg/−)-AL rats compared with (−/−) rats, although the prevalence of pituitary adenoma was similar between the two groups. It is possible therefore that, in (tg/−)-AL rats, the reduced incidence of lethal nonneoplastic disorders contributes to lifespan extension, and thus, pituitary adenoma as a cause of death increased even though the onset and progression of pituitary tumors was not affected. In contrast, CR significantly decreased the prevalence of pituitary adenoma and the proportion of related deaths, suggesting that CR suppresses pituitary tumorigenesis. CR seemed to delay the occurrence of neoplastic causes (data not shown) as well as non-neoplastic causes of death in (−/−) and (tg/−) rats as

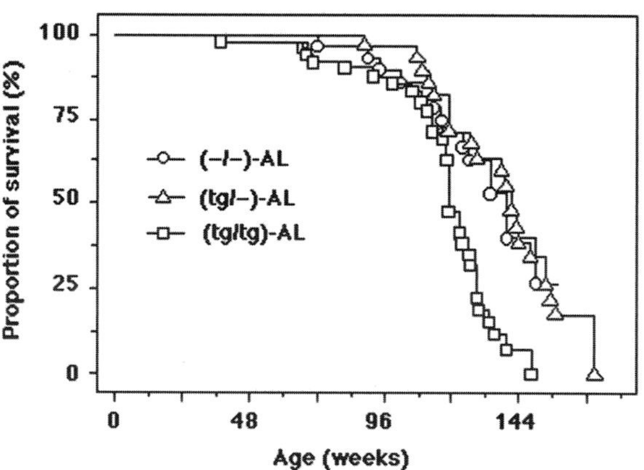

Figure 31.2. Conditional survival curves of the neoplastic causes of death. Non-neoplastic deaths were considered to be the same censorship as random sacrifice of rats. Survival curves were produced using Kaplan–Meier product limit estimates and compared using the log rank test (Shimokawa *et al.*, 1991).

seen in the inhibited prevalence of cardiac thrombi and proportion of related deaths.

At present, pathologic analyses of long-lived mice are limited; however, it has been reported that the occurrence of neoplastic causes of death is delayed in Ames mice (Ikeno *et al.*, 2003). Because GH and IGF-1 are anabolic hormones that might increase the risk of several cancers (Ibrahim and Yee, 2004), the reduced GH-IGF-1 axis was expected to reduce the occurrence or progression of neoplastic diseases, thus delaying neoplastic causes of death.

TABLE 31.5
Fasting blood glucose and insulin concentrations in the transgenic rats

	(−/−)		(tg/−)		(tg/tg)	
	AL	CR	AL	CR	AL	CR
Glucose (mg/dL)						
Young	109 ± 14	112 ± 7	105 ± 21	108 ± 10	94 ± 5	94 ± 6
Old	116 ± 9	106 ± 6	108 ± 3	109 ± 14	72 ± 10	83 ± 13
Insulin (ng/ml)						
Young	7.3 ± 4.5	4.5 ± 2.0	3.7 ± 1.6	2.4 ± 1.6	n/a	n/a
Old	41.6 ± 39.3	43.5 ± 37.5	29.4 ± 22.3	19.7 ± 24.6	n/a	n/a

Blood samples were drawn from the tail vein without anesthesia between 9:00 and 12:00 after overnight fasting. "Young" represents the age between 6 and 8 months; "Old" represents the age between 24 and 25 months. Data represent means ± SD of 4 to 7 rats. 3-f ANOVA analyzed the main effects of rat group, diet, and age.

Immunological analysis of transgenic rats demonstrated that the proportion and activity of NK cells in splenocytes were reduced significantly in (tg/tg) rats compared with (−/−) and (tg/−) rats (Shimokawa *et al.*, 2002). NK cells are known to protect animals from neoplastic processes (Lotzova, 1993); thus in Wistar rats, severe suppression of the GH-IGF-1 axis might promote neoplastic processes due to dysfunction of the immune system, because GH and IGF-1 are required for normal development of the immune system (Dorshkind and Horseman, 2000). In this regard, however, it is intriguing that Snell mice, which show the same phenotypes as Ames mice, including a lengthened lifespan, achieve normal immune responsiveness even if GH is almost deficient (Cross *et al.*, 1992).

Glucose, Insulin and Related Parameters

A distinctive feature of long-lived mice, in which the somatotropic axis is suppressed, is a reduced serum insulin concentration (Hsieh *et al.*, 2002; Shimokawa *et al.*, 2003). As noted above, diminished insulin-like signaling by reduction-of-function mutations favors longevity in invertebrates, in which insulin and IGF-1 signal pathways are not clearly separated. Similar manipulations of insulin signal genes in mammals, however, resulted in metabolic disorders and shortened lifespans; there was only one exception, a strain of mice whose insulin receptor gene was disrupted exclusively in white fat tissues (Bluher *et al.*, 2003).

SERUM GLUCOSE AND INSULIN UNDER NOT-FASTING AND FASTING CONDITIONS

During the feeding cycle in our laboratory, blood glucose levels did not statistically differ among (−/−)-AL, (tg/−)-AL, and (tg/tg)-AL groups, although the number of rats examined was limited (Table 31.1). In the CR groups, (−/−) and (tg/−) rats, blood glucose levels tended to be slightly decreased, although this difference was statistically insignificant. Serum insulin concentrations were significantly decreased in (tg/−)-AL and (tg/tg)-AL rats compared with (−/−)-AL rats (Table 31.1). In the CR groups, serum insulin was not significantly increased even in the CR1 phase even though (−/−)-CR and (tg/−)-CR rats consumed the same amount of food as each AL group overnight.

Data on fasting blood glucose and insulin concentrations were obtained by glucose tolerance tests. The blood glucose concentration in the tail vein after overnight fasting did not differ between (−/−) and (tg/−) rats, although it was slightly reduced in (tg/tg) rats, particularly at the age of 24 or 25 months (Table 31.5). Neither CR nor age affected blood glucose levels. Serum insulin concentrations were slightly, but significantly, lower in (tg/−) rats than (−/−) rats. This concentration significantly increased in the old group, but was insignificantly altered in the CR group. These data indicate that insulin resistance is already apparent in (−/−) and (tg/−) rats at old age, even if subjected to CR. It remains to be elucidated whether CR delays the occurrence of insulin resistance in middle age.

GLUCOSE TOLERANCE

At a young age, time-dependent alterations in blood glucose in the glucose tolerance test (GTT) were similar among (−/−), (tg/−), and (tg/tg) rats when fed ad libitum (Figure 31.3A).

In (−/−) rats, aging impaired glucose tolerance, particularly in the AL group (Figure 31.3B); in the CR group, it was mostly inhibited. In (tg/−) rats, glucose intolerance was also observed in the AL group at old age (Figure 31.3C); CR inhibited aging-related impairment. In (tg/tg) rats, time-dependent changes in blood glucose did not differ between young and old or AL and CR groups (Figure 31.3D).

Serum insulin concentrations during the GTT were measured in (−/−) and (tg/−) rats using samples drawn

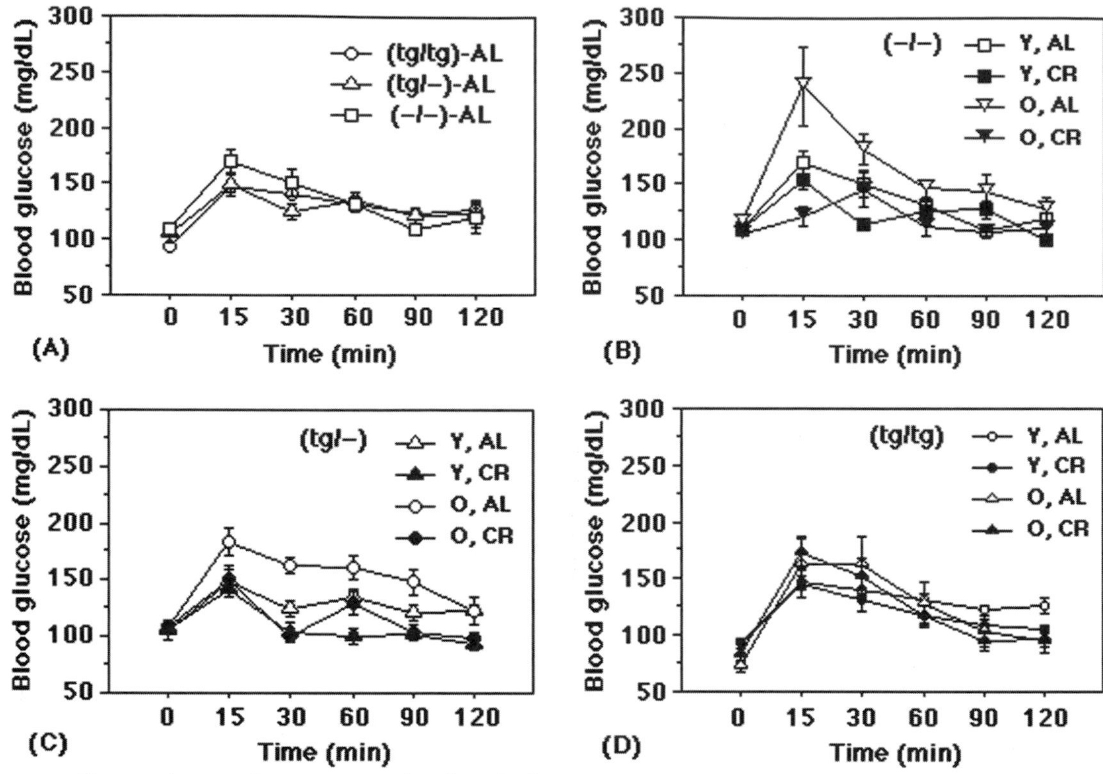

Figure 31.3. Glucose tolerance of transgenic rats; the effect of calorie restriction and aging. Values represent the mean ± SE of 4 to 7 rats. Y represents an age of 6 to 7 months, and O represents an age of 24 months. 2-f ANOVA was used to analyze the main effects of rat group and time and their interaction (A) or age and time and their interaction (B–D) on blood glucose tolerance.

from the tail vein (Yamaza *et al.*, 2004). Serum insulin concentrations were transiently elevated at 15 min in (−/−) rats at young age (Figure 31.4A); there was no insulin surge during the GTT in (tg/−)-AL, (tg/−)-CR or (−/−)-CR rats.

If serum samples were prepared from trunk blood after decapitation, insulin levels at 15 min after glucose load were increased in (−/−)-CR and (tg/−)-AL rats as in (−/−)-AL rats, but the level was significantly lower by 75–80% in (−/−)-CR and (tg/−)-AL rats (Figure 31.4B), although values fluctuated. Serum insulin concentrations during the GTT fluctuated largely in old rats (data not shown, but refer to Shimokawa (2005)) and no transient increases were detected. On a whole, however, serum insulin levels were greater in (−/−)-AL rats compared with (tg/−)-AL and (−/−)-CR rats.

The data described here indicate that in transgenic rats, glucose is effectively transported into tissues with lower concentrations of insulin as in CR rats, and the islet cell insulin response to a rise in blood glucose is blunted in transgenic and CR rats. Similarly, this suggests that CR modulates glucose metabolism and insulin responses through a reduction in the GH-IGF-1 axis.

Glucose disposal occurs as a result of both insulin-mediated and non–insulin-mediated glucose uptake (IMGU and NIMGU, respectively (Baron *et al.*, 1988)). By definition, IMGU can occur only in insulin-sensitive tissues, such as skeletal muscles and fat tissues, while, in the absence of insulin, NIMGU can occur in both insulin-sensitive and non-insulin-sensitive tissues including the central nervous system, peripheral nerves, visceral organs, and blood cells (Ferrannini *et al.*, 1985). A study conducted by Wetter *et al.* (1999) demonstrated that glucose uptake during the period before feeding, at which point serum insulin levels are lowered, is not reduced in most tissues of CR rats; in contrast, white and brown fat tissues showed increased glucose uptake rates. In the period after feeding—that is, postprandially, at which point the serum insulin concentration is increased—insulin-sensitive tissues such as skeletal muscles and fat tissues displayed an increase in glucose uptake in the AL and CR groups, while in some skeletal tissues and mesenteric fat, the glucose uptake tended to be greater in CR rats. GLUT4, the predominant glucose transporter expressed by skeletal muscle, seems to account for most of the insulin-stimulated glucose transport in muscles (Rodnick *et al.*, 1992). In the epitrochlearis muscle, CR increases the amount of cell surface GLUT-4 in response to insulin (Dean *et al.*, 1998). In human placental GH-overexpressing mice that exhibit severe insulin resistance, insulin-stimulated GLUT-4 translocation to the plasma membrane was shown to be reduced (Barbour

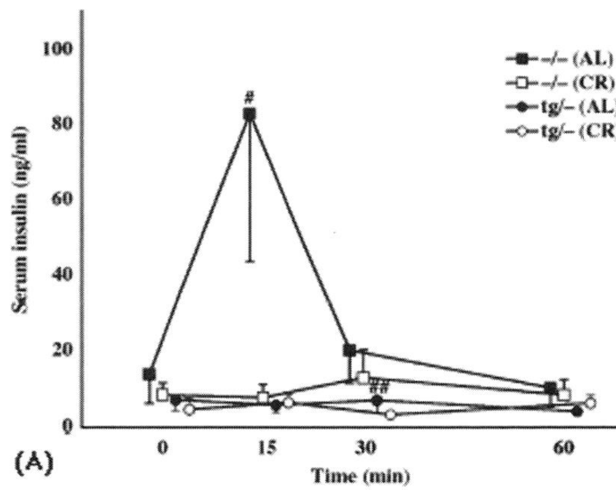

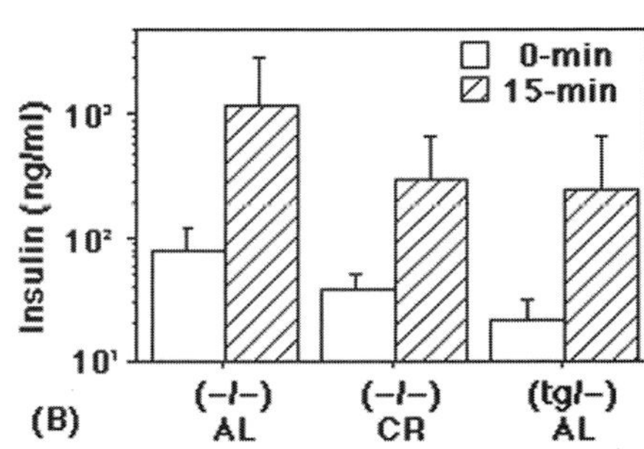

Figure 31.4. (A) Serum insulin concentrations during the glucose tolerance test. Serum samples were prepared from blood drawn from the tail vein. Values represent the mean ± SD of 3 to 6 rats. Reproduced from (Yamaza *et al.*, 2004) by copyright permission of Elsevier. (B) Blood glucose concentrations after glucose load using the same amount of glucose as in the glucose tolerance test. Blood glucose was measured in serum samples prepared from trunk blood at decapitation. Values represent the mean ± SD of 4 to 5 rats. 2-f ANOVA was used to analyze the main effects of rat group and time and their interaction. (C) Serum insulin concentrations after glucose load. Serum samples were the same as those in (B). Values represent the mean ± SD of 4 to 5 rats. 2-f ANOVA was used to analyze the main effects of rat group and time and their interaction.

et al., 2004), suggesting that the somatotropic axis has an inhibitory effect on cell surface translocation of GLUT4. Therefore, we speculate that CR enhances the GLUT4 translocation machinery in insulin-sensitive tissues by reducing the inhibitory effect of the GH-IGF-1 axis. The effect of the reduced GH-IGF-1 axis and CR on non–insulin-mediated mechanisms of glucose uptake remains to be assessed.

Glucose is the prime modulator of insulin secretion, although the precise mechanisms and factors involved in the insulin secretion process are not fully understood. The findings described above suggest that CR and the reduced GH-IGF-1 axis suppress the islet insulin response to a blood glucose rise. The mechanisms of glucose rises and the islet response in long-lived rodents remain to be elucidated.

Body Fat, the Blood Lipid Profile, Leptin and Adiponectin

GH deficiency affects lipid as well as carbohydrate metabolism, resulting in fat accumulation in the body (Gola *et al.*, 2005) and inducing insulin resistance and related disorders. As described above, the transgenic rats exhibited a number of characteristics indicating increased insulin sensitivity. The following section describes selected parameters related to fat metabolism in transgenic rats.

BODY FAT CONTENT AND BLOOD LIPID PROFILES

The fat content, when normalized by body weight, was slightly but significantly reduced in (tg/tg) rats, but there was no difference between (−/−) and (tg/−) rats (Figure 31.5A).

Aging tended to increase the fat content of the AL groups; however, when subjected to CR, the fat content was expectedly reduced. The aging-related increase was therefore prohibited in CR groups, but not in transgenic rat groups fed ad libitum.

The serum triacylglycerol (TG) concentration was reduced in (tg/tg) rats, but statistically insignificant between (−/−) and (tg/−) rats. CR reduced the serum TG concentration, but there was no difference between the CR1 and CR2 groups. Total serum cholesterol levels did not differ among rat groups, although CR resulted in a slight reduction (Table 31.6). HDL-cholesterol was greatest in (tg/tg) rats followed by (tg/−) and (−/−) rats, respectively. Correspondingly, serum concentrations of LDL-cholesterol were slightly greater in (−/−) rats compared with (tg/−) and (tg/tg) rats. HDL-cholesterol levels were slightly but significantly greater in CR1 compared to CR2 phase rats. As a result, LDL-cholesterol levels were particularly reduced in CR1 phase rats. The serum free fatty acid concentration did not differ among rat groups, but was reduced in CR1 phase rats and elevated in CR2 phase rats. Thus, transgenic rat strains, either (tg/−) or (tg/tg), exhibited no deleterious lipid metabolism profile; rather, the slightly lower concentration of total cholesterol and higher concentration of HDL-cholesterol in (tg/tg) rats suggested that a suppressed GH-IGF-1 axis yields some beneficial effects in animals.

PLASMA LEPTIN

Plasma leptin concentrations are known to reflect body fat content (Niswender and Schwartz, 2003). At the age between 6 and 8 months, plasma concentrations did not significantly differ among rat groups, although the fat content was slightly lower in (tg/tg) rats compared with

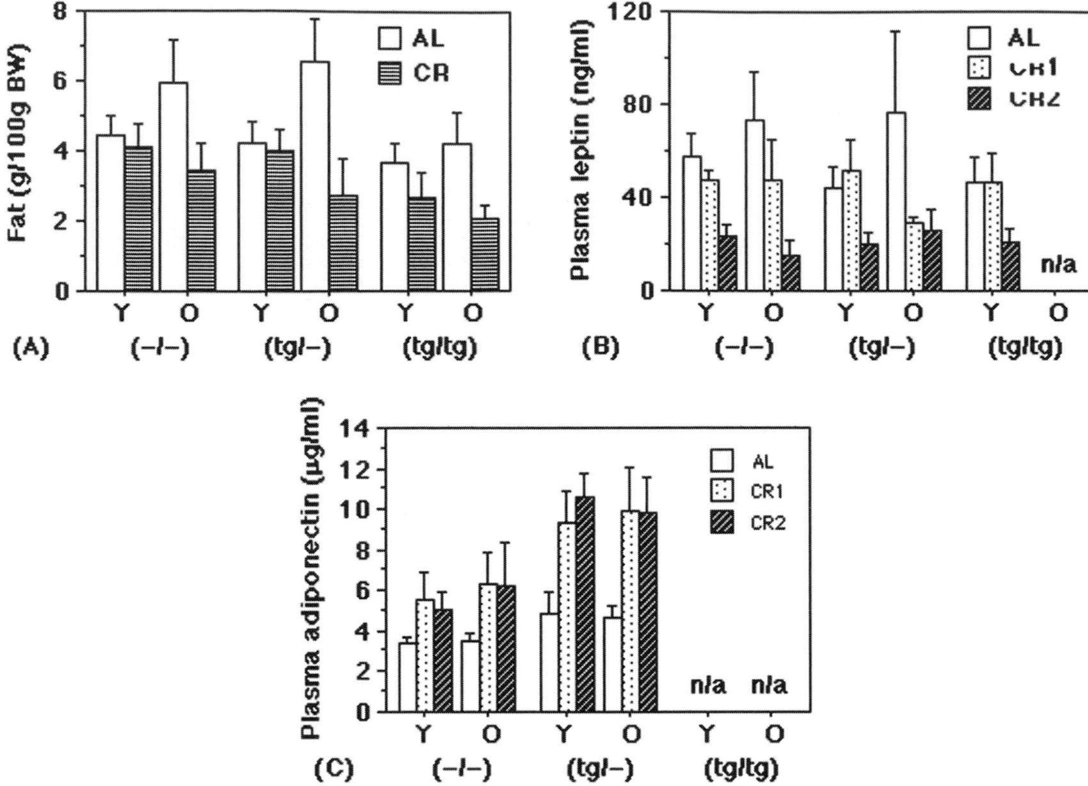

Figure 31.5. (A) Body fat content, and (B) plasma leptin and (C) adiponectin concentrations. The body fat content represents the combined wet weights of perirenal and epididymal fat normalized by body weight (g/100 g body weight (BW)). Fat content did not significantly differ between the CR1 and CR2 phase rats; thus data were combined into the CR group. Plasma samples were prepared from trunk blood collected at decapitation. Plasma leptin and adiponectin data was unavailable for (tg/tg) rats. "Young" represents an age of 6 to 8 months, while "Old" represents an age of 24 to 25 months. The numbers of rats examined were 7 to 24 for body fat content, 3 to 8 for plasma leptin, and 3 to 7 for plasma adiponectin. 3-f ANOVA was used to analyze the main effects of rat group, diet, and age and their interaction.

(−/−) and (tg/−) rats (Figure 31.5B). The CR regimen in the present study reduced plasma leptin levels only in the CR2 phase rats. However, in our previous study using F344 rats, leptin levels were consistently lower in the CR group during the 2-day feeding cycle (Shimokawa and Higami 1999). The plasma leptin findings paralleled the altered fat content resulting from CR.

With aging, plasma leptin concentrations were slightly increased in the AL group, staying constant or slightly decreased in the CR group. These aging-dependent changes were also comparable with the changes in fat content.

PLASMA ADIPONECTIN

Plasma adiponectin concentrations are inversely correlated with body fat content (Havel, 2004); that is, they are lowered in obese patients and animals. Adiponectin exerts an antidiabetic effect by sensitizing insulin action and augmenting fatty acid oxidation in the muscles. It also exhibits an antiatherosclerotic effect by attenuating inflammatory insults in the vascular wall. These metabolic and anti-inflammatory effects are also thought to be some of the beneficial effects of CR (Masoro, 2003). Indeed, recent reports demonstrated a higher plasma concentration of adiponectin in CR animals (Berg *et al.*, 2001; Combs *et al.*, 2003; Zhu *et al.*, 2004), and in long-lived dwarf animal models, plasma adiponectin concentrations have been shown to be increased (Berryman *et al.*, 2004).

In this study, plasma adiponectin levels were increased in (tg/−) rats, when fed ad libitum (Figure 31.5C). Levels were also increased in (−/−)-CR rats. In addition, CR of (tg/−) rats additively increased plasma adiponectin concentrations. The increased concentration with CR was slightly greater in (tg/−) rats.

This increased adiponectin concentration might be linked to the increased sensitivity of insulin or lower concentration of plasma insulin after glucose load. Recent studies have indicated that adiponectin could facilitate glucose uptake into skeletal muscle and adipocytes independent of insulin action, through activation of AMP-activated protein kinase (AMPK) (Tomas *et al.*, 2002; Wu *et al.*, 2003). The adiponectin-AMPK pathway might act as the insulin-independent pathway for glucose metabolism in long-lived dwarf and CR animals. The level of phosphorylated AMPK, the active form of the enzyme, is increased in GHRKO mice (Al-Regaiey *et al.*, 2005),

TABLE 31.6
The serum lipid profile in the transgenic rats at 6 or 7 months of age

	(−/−)			(tg/−)			(tg/tg)		
	AL	CR1	CR2	AL	CR1	CR2	AL	CR1	CR2
Triacylglycerol	329 ± 106	137 ± 57	144 ± 90	229 ± 79	146 ± 44	143 ± 28	144 ± 47	91 ± 20	87 ± 28
Total cholesterol	93 ± 6	84 ± 11	82 ± 4	94 ± 7	84 ± 6	38 ± 4	102 ± 4	81 ± 5	89 ± 6
HDL-cholesterol	30 ± 3	41 ± 8	32 ± 4	36 ± 3	47 ± 4	41 ± 6	47 ± 2	52 ± 3	49 ± 4
LDL-cholesterol	11 ± 1	7 ± 2	8 ± 1	10 ± 1	7 ± 1	8 ± 2	8 ± 1	8 ± 1	7 ± 1
Free fatty acid	0.66 ± 0.20	0.35 ± 0.16	0.74 ± 0.20	0.75 ± 0.34	0.39 ± 0.13	0.79 ± 0.51	0.79 ± 0.24	0.30 ± 0.05	0.89 ± 0.19

Serum samples were prepared from trunk blood at decapitation between 9:00 and 12:00. Data represent means ± SD (mg/dL) of 3 to 7 rats. 2-f ANOVA analyzed the main effects of rat group and diet and their interaction. AL, groups of rats fed ad libitum. CR1 and CR2, groups of rats subjected to 30% calorie restriction, while sacrificed in the first day and the second day of 2-day feeding cycle, respectively (see the rat husbandry for the CR regimen, a modified alternate-day-feeding, used in the present study).

while not in CR rats. Our preliminary experiment did not confirm the upregulation of phosphorylated AMPK in transgenic rats (data not shown).

Stress response

Stress resistance is linked to retardation of aging and an extended lifespan. CR rodents exhibit resistance to many types of stressors including toxic substances, inflammatory stimuli, ambient temperature, and surgery (Masoro, 2003). Some long-lived mice also show high survival rates after intraperitoneal injection of paraquat, a herbicide that generates reactive oxygen species (ROS) (Migliaccio *et al.*, 1999; Holzenberger *et al.*, 2003).

We therefore examined the resistance of the transgenic mice included here to lipopolysaccharide (LPS)-induced inflammatory challenge, which causes cellular injury by generating ROS and reactive nitrogen species (RNS). Six-month-old male Wistar (−/−), (tg/−), and (tg/tg) rats fed ad libitum were administered LPS (1.6 mg/ kg body weight) through the tail vein, then sacrificed 0-, 1-, 4-, and 8-h later. A preliminary study indicated that this dose of LPS induced necrotic foci in the liver at 8-h in 50% of (−/−) rats. Serum aspartate aminotransferase (AST) levels, an index of LPS-induced tissue damage, were consequently measured. The preliminary results at 4- and 8-h (Figure 31.6) indicated that serum AST levels were greater in (−/−) rats compared with (tg/−) and (tg/tg) rats, with no difference between (tg/−) and (tg/tg) rats.

Our previous study using a similar experimental protocol with F344 rats showed that CR rats resisted LPS-challenge (Tsuchiya *et al.*, 2005). Thus, common stress response machinery is thought to be elicited with reduced GH-IGF-1 and CR, respectively.

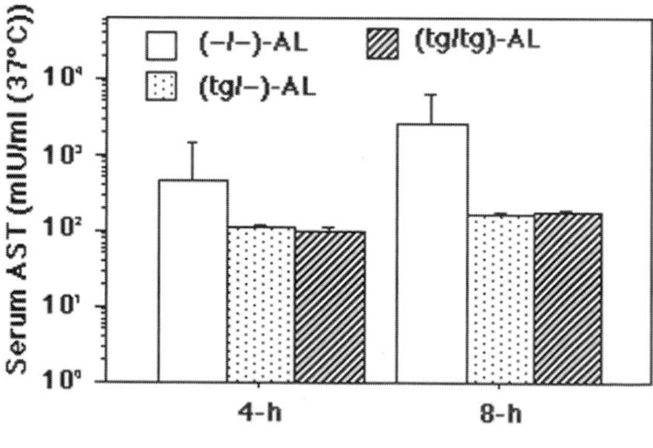

Figure 31.6. Stress response to lipopolysaccharide (LPS)-induced inflammation. Rats were sacrificed 0-, 1-, 4-, and 8-h after intravenous injection of 1.6 mg/kg body weight (BW) of LPS. Serum aspartate aminotransferase (AST) levels were measured as an index of LPS-induced tissue injury. Values represent the mean ± SD of 3 to 10 rats. AST levels at 0- and 1-h are not shown because levels were not significantly elevated. 2-f ANOVA was used to analyze the main effects of rat group and time and their interaction on AST levels.

Conclusions

When fed ad libitum, transgenic (tg/−) rats displayed several phenotypes similar to those of wild-type rats subjected to CR. For example, profiles of blood glucose, insulin and other hormones during the feeding cycle or after glucose load and an enhanced stress response were seen in both. These findings suggest that this rat model is suitable for analyses of the mechanisms underlying the effect of CR, particularly with regard to the role of the somatotropic axis in the regulation of lifespans and aging. Another merit of this model is that the reduced level of the GH-IGF-1 axis was moderate and less severe than in Ames or GHR/BP-KO mice whose GH-IGF-1 signaling was almost totally deficient. Thus, experiments using the transgenic mini rats can be conducted within physiological ranges.

The (tg/tg)-AL rats resembled (tg/−)-AL rats as well as (−/−)-CR rats with regard to glucose and insulin levels and the stress response. However, these (tg/tg) rats died earlier of neoplastic diseases. Although immunological dysfunction was noted in (tg/tg) rats, further studies are needed to determine whether severe suppression of the somatotropic axis results in negative effects on aging and longevity, because mice models with deficient GH signals were shown to live longer.

REFERENCES

Al-Regaiey, K.A., Masternak, M.M., Bonkowski, M., Sun, L. and Bartke, A. (2005). Long-lived growth hormone receptor knockout mice: Interaction of reduced insulin-like growth factor i/insulin signaling and caloric restriction. *Endocrinology 146*, 851–860.

Barbour, L.A., Shao, J., Qiao, L., Leitner, W., Anderson, M., Friedman, J.E. and Draznin, B. (2004). Human placental growth hormone increases expression of the p85 regulatory unit of phosphatidylinositol 3-kinase and triggers severe insulin resistance in skeletal muscle. *Endocrinology 145*, 1144–1150.

Baron, A.D., Brechtel, G., Wallace, P. and Edelman, S.V. (1988). Rates and tissue sites of non-insulin- and insulin-mediated glucose uptake in humans. *Am. J. Physiol. 255*, E769–E774.

Berg, A.H., Combs, T.P., Du, X., Brownlee, M. and Scherer, P.E. (2001). The adipocyte-secreted protein Acrp30 enhances hepatic insulin action. *Nat. Med. 7*, 947–953.

Berryman, D.E., List, E.O., Coschigano, K.T., Behar, K., Kim, J.K. and Kopchick, J.J. (2004). Comparing adiposity profiles in three mouse models with altered GH signaling. *Growth Horm. IGF Res. 14*, 309–318.

Bluher, M., Kahn, B.B. and Kahn, C.R. (2003). Extended longevity in mice lacking the insulin receptor in adipose tissue. *Science 299*, 572–574.

Brown-Borg, H.M., Borg, K.E., Meliska, C.J. and Bartke, A. (1996). Dwarf mice and the ageing process. *Nature 384*, 33.

Clancy, D.J., Gems, D., Harshman, L.G., Oldham, S., Stocker, H., Hafen, E., Leevers, S.J. and Partridge, L. (2001). Extension of life-span by loss of CHICO, a *Drosophila* insulin receptor substrate protein. *Science 292*, 104–106.

Combs, T.P., Berg, A.H., Rajala, M.W., Klebanov, S., Iyengar, P., Jimenez-Chillaron, J.C., *et al.* (2003). Sexual differentiation, pregnancy, calorie restriction, and aging affect the adipocyte-specific secretory protein adiponectin. *Diabetes 52*, 268–276.

Coschigano, K.T., Clemmons, D., Bellush, L.L. and Kopchick, J.J. (2000). Assessment of growth parameters and life span of GHR/BP gene-disrupted mice. *Endocrinology 141*, 2608–2613.

Cross, R.J., Bryson, J.S. and Roszman, T.L. (1992). Immunologic disparity in the hypopituitary dwarf mouse. *J. Immunol. 148*, 1347–1352.

Dean, D.J., Brozinick, J.T., Jr., Cushman, S.W. and Cartee, G.D. (1998). Calorie restriction increases cell surface GLUT-4 in insulin-stimulated skeletal muscle. *Am. J. Physiol. 275*, E957–E964.

Dorshkind, K. and Horseman, N.D. (2000). The roles of prolactin, growth hormone, insulin-like growth factor-I, and thyroid hormones in lymphocyte development and function: Insights from genetic models of hormone and hormone receptor deficiency. *Endocr. Rev. 21*, 292–312.

Ferrannini, E., Smith, J.D., Cobelli, C., Toffolo, G., Pilo, A. and DeFronzo, R.A. (1985). Effect of insulin on the distribution and disposition of glucose in man. *J. Clin. Invest. 76*, 357–364.

Flurkey, K., Papaconstantinou, J., Miller, R.A. and Harrison, D.E. (2001). Lifespan extension and delayed immune and collagen aging in mutant mice with defects in growth hormone production. *Proc. Natl. Acad. Sci. USA 98*, 6736–6741.

Gola, M., Bonadonna, S., Doga, M. and Giustina, A. (2005). Clinical Review: Growth hormone and cardiovascular risk factors. *J. Clin. Endocrinol. Metab. 90*, 1864–1870.

Havel, P.J. (2004). Update on adipocyte hormones: Regulation of energy balance and carbohydrate/lipid metabolism. *Diabetes 53 Suppl. 1*, S143–S151.

Hekimi, S. and Guarente, L. (2003). Genetics and the specificity of the aging process. *Science 299*, 1351–1354.

Holzenberger, M., Dupont, J., Ducos, B., Leneuve, P., Geloen, A., Even, P.C., *et al.* (2003). IGF-1 receptor regulates lifespan and resistance to oxidative stress in mice. *Nature 421*, 182–187.

Hsieh, C.C., DeFord, J.H., Flurkey, K., Harrison, D.E. and Papaconstantinou, J. (2002). Implications for the insulin signaling pathway in Snell dwarf mouse longevity: A similarity with the *C. elegans* longevity paradigm. *Mech. Ageing Dev. 123*, 1229–1244.

Ibrahim, Y.H. and Yee, D. (2004). Insulin-like growth factor-I and cancer risk. Growth Horm. *IGF Res. 14*, 261–269.

Ikeno, Y., Bronson, R.T., Hubbard, G.B., Lee, S. and Bartke, A. (2003). Delayed occurrence of fatal neoplastic diseases in Ames dwarf mice: Correlation to extended longevity. *J. Gerontol. A Biol. Sci. Med. Sci. 58*, 291–296.

Kimura, K.D., Tissenbaum, H.A., Liu, Y. and Ruvkun, G. (1997). daf-2, an insulin receptor-like gene that regulates longevity and diapause in *Caenorhabditis elegans. Science 277*, 942–946.

Liang, H., Masoro, E.J., Nelson, J.F., Strong, R., McMahan, C.A. and Richardson, A. (2003). Genetic mouse models of extended lifespan. *Exp. Gerontol. 38*, 1353–1364.

Lotzova, E. (1993). Definition and functions of natural killer cells. *Nat. Immun. 12*, 169–176.

Masoro, E.J. (2003). Subfield history: Caloric restriction, slowing aging, and extending life. *Sci. Aging Knowledge Environ.* 2003, RE2.

Matsumoto, K., Kakidani, H., Takahashi, A., Nakagata, N., Anzai, M., Matsuzaki, Y., *et al.* (1993). Growth retardation in rats whose growth hormone gene expression was suppressed by antisense RNA transgene. *Mol. Reprod. Dev. 36*, 53–58.

Migliaccio, E., Giorgio, M., Mele, S., Pelicci, G., Reboldi, P., Pandolfi, P.P., *et al.* (1999). The p66shc adaptor protein controls oxidative stress response and life span in mammals. *Nature 402*, 309–313.

Miskin, R. and Masos, T. (1997). Transgenic mice overexpressing urokinase-type plasminogen activator in the brain exhibit reduced food consumption, body weight and size, and increased longevity. *J. Gerontol. A Biol. Sci. Med. Sci. 52*, B118–B124.

Mitsui, A., Hamuro, J., Nakamura, H., Kondo, N., Hirabayashi, Y., Ishizaki-Koizumi, S., *et al.* (2002). Overexpression of human thioredoxin in transgenic mice controls oxidative stress and life span. Antioxid. *Redox Signal 4*, 693–696.

Morris, J.Z., Tissenbaum, H.A. and Ruvkun, G.. (1996). A phosphatidylinositol-3-OH kinase family member regulating longevity and diapause in *Caenorhabditis elegans. Nature 382*, 536–539.

Niswender, K.D. and Schwartz, M.W. (2003). Insulin and leptin revisited: Adiposity signals with overlapping physiological and intracellular signaling capabilities. *Front. Neuroendocrinol. 24*, 1–10.

Rodnick, K.J., Henriksen, E.J., James, D.E. and Holloszy, J.O. (1992). Exercise training, glucose transporters, and glucose transport in rat skeletal muscles. *Am. J. Physiol. 262*, C9–C14.

Shimokawa, I. (2005). Rodent models for the study of the role of GH-IGF-1 or the Insulin axis in aging and longevity: Special reference to a transgenic dwarf rat strain and calorie restriction. In *The Somatotrophic Axis in Brain Function* (F. Nyberg, ed.), Elsevier, Amsterdam (in press).

Shimokawa, I. and Higami, Y. (1999). A role for leptin in the antiaging action of dietary restriction: A hypothesis. *Aging (Milano) 11*, 380–382.

Shimokawa, I., Higami, Y., Tsuchiya, T., Otani, H., Komatsu, T., Chiba, T. and Yamaza, H. (2003). Life span extension by reduction of the growth hormone-insulin-like growth factor-1 axis: Relation to caloric restriction. *Faseb J. 17*, 1108–1109.

Shimokawa, I., Higami, Y., Utsuyama, M., Tuchiya, T., Komatsu, T., Chiba, T. and Yamaza, H. (2002). Life span extension by reduction in growth hormone-insulin-like growth factor-1 axis in a transgenic rat model. *Am. J. Pathol. 160*, 2259–2265.

Shimokawa, I., Yu, B.P. and Masoro, E.J. (1991). Influence of diet on fatal neoplastic disease in male Fischer 344 rats. *J. Gerontol. 46*, B228–B232.

Tomas, E., Tsao, T.S., Saha, A.K., Murrey, H.E., Zhang Cc, C., Itani, S.I., *et al.* (2002). Enhanced muscle fat oxidation and glucose transport by ACRP30 globular domain: Acetyl-CoA carboxylase inhibition and AMP-activated protein kinase activation. *Proc. Natl. Acad. Sci. USA 99*, 16309–16313.

Tsuchiya, T., Higami, Y., Komatsu, T., Tanaka, K., Honda, S., Yamaza, H., *et al.* (2005). Acute stress response in calorie-restricted rats to lipopolysaccharide-induced inflammation. *Mech. Ageing Dev. 126*, 568–579.

Wetter, T.J., Gazdag, A.C., Dean, D.J. and Cartee, G.D. (1999). Effect of calorie restriction on in vivo glucose metabolism by individual tissues in rats. *Am. J. Physiol. 276*, E728–E738.

Wu, X., Motoshima, H., Mahadev, K., Stalker, T.J., Scalia, R. and Goldstein, B.J. (2003). Involvement of AMP-activated protein kinase in glucose uptake stimulated by the globular domain of adiponectin in primary rat adipocytes. *Diabetes 52*, 1355–1363.

Yamaza, H., Komatsu, T., Chiba, T., Toyama, H., To, K., Higami, Y. and Shimokawa, I. (2004). A transgenic dwarf rat model as a tool for the study of calorie restriction and aging. *Exp. Gerontol. 39*, 269–272.

Zhu, M., Miura, J., Lu, L.X., Bernier, M., DeCabo, R., Lane, M.A., Roth, G.S. and Ingram, D.K. (2004). Circulating adiponectin levels increase in rats on caloric restriction: The potential for insulin sensitization. *Exp. Gerontol. 39*, 1049–1059.

32

Rat Models of Age-Related Cognitive Decline

Jennifer L. Bizon and Michelle M. Nicolle

Naturally occurring rat models can be useful for studying age-related cognitive decline. Long–Evans rats trained on the Morris water maze have been used to model individual differences in cognitive abilities that depend on the medial temporal lobe system. This approach has yielded a great deal of new information including the unexpected lack of neuronal loss in the hippocampus in aged rats with pronounced cognitive impairment. Despite this absence of neuron death, aged rats with impaired memory can be distinguished from those with intact memory at the neurobiological level. Cellular and molecular changes include alterations in the electrophysiological properties involved in synaptic plasticity, alterations in gene and protein expression, and efficacy of cell signaling pathways.

The prefrontal cortex and cognitive abilities supported by this brain region are also subject to age-related decline. The rat prefrontal cortex performs certain aspects of what is conventionally known as "executive function" in primates. This includes the ability to alter behavior in the face of changing environmental contingencies. Recently, an attentional set-shifting task has been designed for assessing executive function in rats. Individual differences in attentional set shifting have been described in aged rats, and this task is currently being combined with neurobiological studies to yield information regarding the underlying causes of behavioral impairment. The use of these two tasks assessing age-related cognitive impairment and the general approaches described in this chapter should yield informative data regarding our understanding of the neurobiology of age-related cognitive decline and should be useful for guiding therapeutic approaches targeting such deficits in humans.

Introduction

Age-related cognitive decline is a substantial problem, particularly based on the growing population of elderly in the United States and in other developed nations. The number of people over 65 living in the United States is expected to increase from 35 million in 2000 to 71.5 million by the year 2030, comprising almost 20% of the U.S. population (U.S. Census Bureau, 2004). It has further been estimated that 7–8% of individuals in the United States have severe cognitive impairment (Freedman *et al.*, 2002). This cognitive disability contributes a significant burden with regard to reduced individual quality of life as well as financial strain on the healthcare system and society—a burden that can only be expected to escalate. Understanding neurobiological factors that contribute to cognitive decline with aging is the initial step in combating this health problem. Animal models of aging complement human studies and can be advantageous for investigating the neurobiological changes that underlie age-related cognitive decline. Ultimately, the use of animal models will contribute to the discovery of efficacious treatment options for humans with cognitive impairment.

Using Rats to Model Aging

THE UTILITY OF A RAT MODEL

Rats provide an excellent and reproducible system in which to study age-related cognitive decline. There are surprising similarities between rodents and humans in the anatomy of brain systems, including those that are particularly vulnerable to cognitive decline during aging (e.g., the medial temporal lobe system). In addition, the availability of rodent subjects, as well as ethical concerns regarding the invasive procedures necessary for neurobiological research in humans, necessitates the use of animal models. Rats afford particular advantages because researchers can employ relatively large sample sizes and tightly controlled experimental conditions. Rats can also be used for invasive procedures that are important for uncovering the neurobiology responsible for age-related cognitive decline. In contrast to transgenic or knock-out mouse models of cognitive impairment and dementia, many aged rats strains provide a naturally occurring model of age-related impairment in which some rats demonstrate cognitive decline, whereas others have mnemonic abilities on a par with young rats. Making use of such naturally occurring rat models circumvents some of the challenges associated with transgenic mouse studies, including developmental abnormalities, thereby providing a rich model for uncovering the neurobiological factors responsible for age-related cognitive loss.

COMPARABILITY TO HUMAN AGE-RELATED COGNITIVE DECLINE

There is substantial evidence that specific factors that adversely impact cognition in rat models also correlate with age-related cognitive impairment in primates, including humans. For example, assessment of the degree of atrophy of the medial temporal lobe in humans is an effective predictor for the development of dementia in patients with mild cognitive impairment (Korf *et al.*, 2004), and medial temporal lobe atrophy in stroke patients predicts poor cognitive performance (Jokinen *et al.*, 2004). Likewise, lesions of medial temporal lobe structures induce memory impairments in rodents (reviewed by Jarrard, 1993). Moreover, age-related changes such as alterations in the glucocorticoid system and increases in oxidative stress are found among aged rat and human populations (Bizon *et al.*, 2001; Nicolle *et al.*, 2001; de Quervain *et al.*, 1998; Roozendaal, 2002; de Quervain *et al.*, 2003; Lupien *et al.*, 2005).

Finally, as discussed in more detail below, the absence of frank neural loss among aged rats with memory impairment has now been replicated in aged monkeys and humans. It should be emphasized that although parallels exist between behavioral deficits observed in the rat models of aging discussed here and both rodent experimentally induced brain lesions and human age-related disease, the models we employ are not intended to represent human neurodegenerative disease such as Alzheimer's or Parkinson's disease. Rather, we consider these naturally occurring rat models a tool for understanding the normal aging process in the absence of disease. Some have suggested that the cognitive decline seen in these rat models is akin to what is referred to as nonprogressive mild cognitive impairment in humans, although additional research on neuronal atrophy and other defining characteristics in both rats and humans are needed to support the use of this terminology (Gallagher *et al.*, 2003).

RAT AGING MODELS—STRAIN SELECTION

There is a plethora of rat strains commonly used in neurobiological research today, but special considerations need to be taken into account when choosing a rat strain in which to conduct cognitive aging research. The most popular strains used for aging research include Sprague Dawley, Fisher 344 (F344), Long–Evans, Brown Norway, and F344 × Brown Norway F1 (Bizon and Gallagher, 2005; Merrill *et al.*, 2003; Drapeau *et al.*, 2003; Kasckow *et al.*, 2005; Lichtenwalner *et al.*, 2001). Some critical factors to consider when selecting a rat strain include variability in health and lifespan inherent to the strain, strain-specific and sex-specific differences in cognition, and supplier availability. For example, certain strains may be more prone to tumors of the pituitary gland, a factor that can cause variability in circulating hormone levels and blindness through compression of the optic nerve. Such factors can impact cognitive performance and neurobiological data if behavioral tests are not carefully designed and aged rats are not properly screened for such tumors at sacrifice. Another consideration is the sex of rats chosen; the endocrine system certainly can influence memory and brain function, and it is well established that the endocrine system in rats, as in humans, is modified with aging. When using aged female rats one must therefore take into consideration circulating hormone levels in young and aged rats, as the estrous cycle in females is cyclic in young rats, becomes erratic at middle ages, and ceases at later ages (Savonenko and Markowska, 2003). Finally, availability must be a consideration for those wishing to conduct cognitive aging research. Indeed only three rat strains (F344, Brown Norway and F344 × Brown Norway F1 hybrids) are currently available for funded research from the National Institutes for Aging at the National Institutes of Health. Although we use the Long–Evans strain, which must be purchased as retired breeders (10–12 months of age) and then housed in the home institution, the latter can be an expensive and time-consuming option, as *per diem* expenses and long-term health monitoring for pathogens can become costly. Nevertheless, if the weaknesses of each strain are known (tendency for tumors, etc.), the behavioral characterization is soundly conducted, and aged rats are properly excluded due to poor health, the approach we describe below with Long–Evans rats should hold across strains.

THE LONG–EVANS HOODED RAT

As mentioned above, we have chosen male Long–Evans rats for our cognitive aging research. This strain has good visual acuity even at advanced ages and is out-bred, such that genetic variability is consistently introduced into the population. Thus their general physical health and eyesight tend to be excellent well into old age, and we find very few pituitary tumors (<5%) in these animals upon sacrifice. Our animals are obtained as retired breeders from Charles River Laboratories, Inc., Cambridge, MA at approximately 10–12 months of age and are individually housed for another 12 months before behavioral testing. During this time, water and food intake assessments and frequent screenings for pathogens are conducted to constantly monitor their health. Extreme measures are taken to maintain a healthy and pathogen-free colony for our Long–Evans rat model of cognitive aging. Individual differences in cognitive decline described in detail below are routinely observed in this model in rats 24–25 months of age.

Aging and the Medial Temporal System

ANATOMY AND FUNCTION

One brain system that is particularly vulnerable to age-related decline is the medial temporal lobe system (Barnes, 1979; Barnes and McNaughton, 1985; Gallagher *et al.*, 1993). The anatomy of this system can be contrasted in human versus rat brain, seen shaded in light blue in Figure 32.1.

As can be observed in the circuit diagram shown in Figure 32.1, information flow in the system is multi-directional. Memory processing involves the hippocampal formation and entorhinal cortex, and information flows bi-directionally between these structures. Both of these brain regions receive direct projections from other brain areas, including the neocortical regions and subcortical structures. Communication with the hippocampus to other cortical regions is through the entorhinal cortex that receives input from and sends output to the para-hippocampal gyrus (which includes the perirhinal and postrhinal cortices). Cellular regions of the hippocampus can be observed in the lower diagram (Figure 32.1), which highlights circuitry in a coronal section of rat hippocampus. The entorhinal cortex provides input to the dentate gyrus granule cells via the perforant path. The subgranular zone is a site of new neuron generation throughout the lifespan, a phenomenon that is the focus of considerable current aging research (Bizon and Gallagher, 2003; Bizon *et al.*, 2004; Merrill *et al.*, 2003; Litchenwalner *et al.*, 2001; Cameron and McKay, 1999). Granule cells project to the pyramidal neurons of CA3 and CA1 in turn. Finally, information is sent out of the hippocampus via projections through the subiculum to neocortical regions. This interaction of the medial temporal system with the neocortex underlies specific types of learning, consolidation, and retrieval of memories. This system is specifically important for processing explicit or declarative memory in humans, including conscious memories of events, people and places. Compromised function of the medial temporal system has been extensively studied across species, and contributes to specific memory deficits in normal aging, as well as in neurodegenerative conditions such as Alzheimer's disease.

AGE-RELATED IMPAIRMENT

Individual differences in age-related decline of the medial temporal lobe system have been observed in both humans and rodents (Gallagher *et al.*, 1993; Bizon and Gallagher, 2005; Wilson *et al.*, 2002). Across species, some aged subjects maintain mnemonic abilities well into advanced ages, whereas others experience loss of cognitive capacities relative to younger individuals. The basis for these individual differences in age-related cognition is a compelling focus of neurobiological research. Indeed, focusing on such variability among aged populations allows the investigator to compare neurobiological changes in the brain not only between young and aged subjects but also among aged rats that differ with respect to cognitive ability. For many years, we have used male Long–Evans rats trained on the widely used Morris water maze task to model individual variability in the function of the medial temporal lobe system among the aged human population.

MODEL FOR THE AGE-IMPAIRED MEDIAL TEMPORAL SYSTEM

The Morris water maze is a hippocampus-dependent task that has been described in detail in numerous publications (e.g., Morris, 1984; Gallagher *et al.*, 1993; Bizon *et al.*, 2001). Rodents use visual cues around a circular pool in order to learn the location of a platform submerged 2 cm below the surface of the water's surface (see Figure 32.2).

In our training procedure, rats receive three trials each day for eight consecutive days. All cognitive testing occurs during the light cycle. At each training trial, rats are placed in the water and permitted to swim until they locate the platform, or for 90 seconds, at which time they are placed on the platform. Animals remain there for 30 seconds, and then they are removed from the maze area. The next trial begins again after a 60-second interval.

For spatial learning assessment, the platform stays in one maze quadrant with a randomized starting position for each trial. On every sixth trial, the platform is retracted to the bottom of the pool (probe trial) for the first 30 seconds of the 90-second trial. Our primary measures of hippocampal function are obtained by proximity measures both on the training trials and interpolated probe trials described in detail below. Very importantly, on the ninth day of training, we test sensorimotor skills and escape motivation independent of spatial learning by giving the rats a training session with six trials of cued training. During cued training trials, rats are trained to escape to a visible platform that protrudes above the water and that varies in position on each trial. On each trial, a rat is started in a novel location and has 30 seconds to reach the platform at which point it remains there briefly prior to a 30-second intertrial interval. Cue training is an extremely important control to conduct when characterizing aged rats. It can identify those subjects that are ill (and perhaps not motivated to swim), that have physical impairments that hinder swimming ability, or that have visual acuity problems. Each of these concerns can be alleviated with a proper cue training session incorporated into the water maze protocol. Any rat that fails cue training (i.e., performs worse than the young rat distribution of scores) is eliminated from further experimentation in our model.

Accuracy of performance in the water maze is assessed using a cumulative search error calculated from training

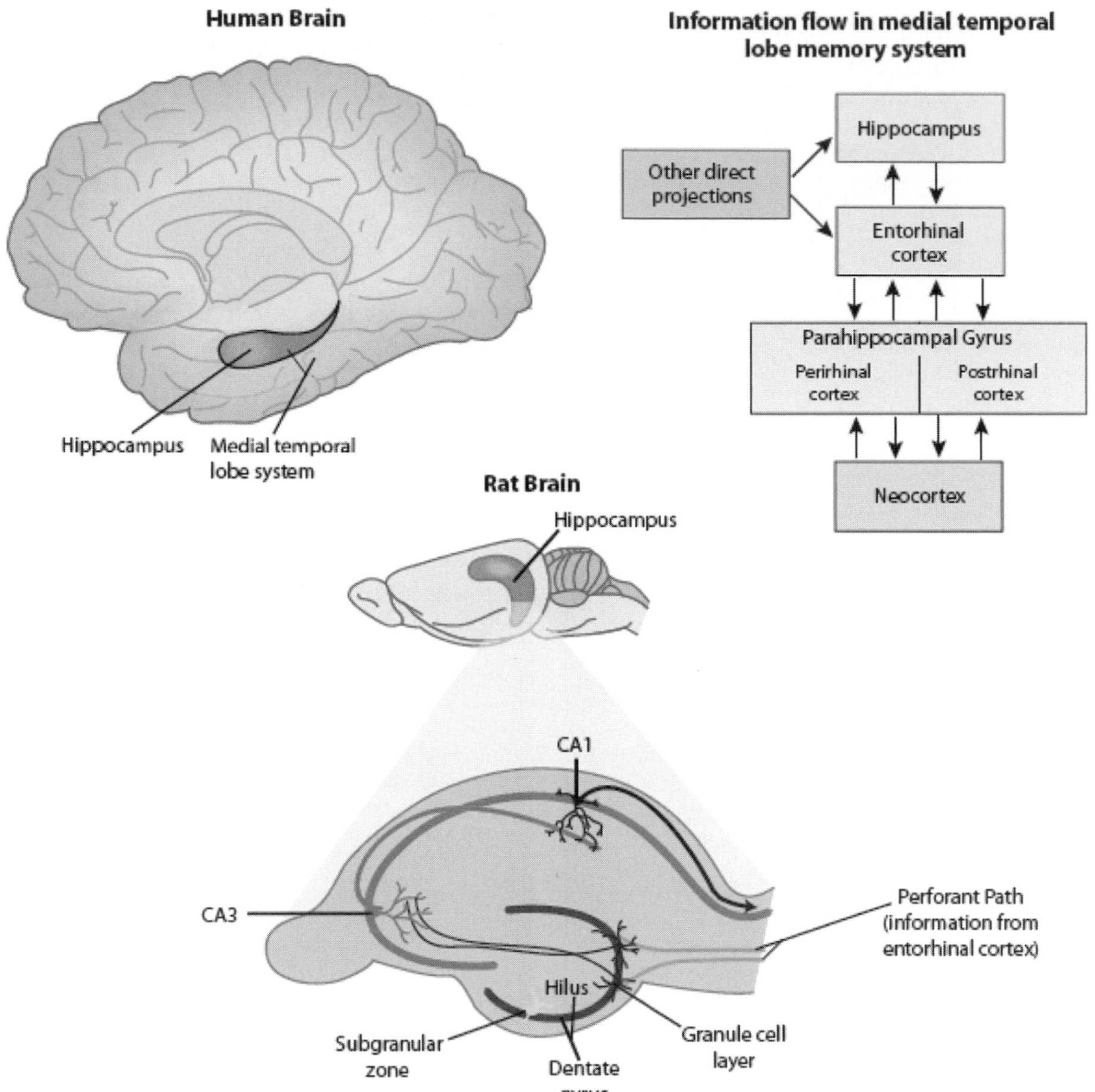

Figure 32.1 Schematic of the medial temporal lobe system, including the hippocampus and associated structures in human and rat brain. The top left diagram shows a mid-sagittal view of the human brain. The general area of the medial temporal lobe is identified and the hippocampal formation is shaded dark gray. The top right panel shows a circuit diagram, and demonstrates the flow of information within this system. Structures that are part of the medial temporal lobe in this system are seen in light gray boxes. Generally, the neocortex sends afferent projections to the hippocampus from the entorhinal cortex via parahippocampal structures. Other subcortical structures (e.g., cholinergic projections from the basal forebrain) also project to hippocampus and entorhinal cortex. The lower diagram shows the rat brain, with the hippocampus highlighted in dark gray. An enlarged coronal section through hippocampus illustrates the basic cellular circuitry within this region. Projections from entorhinal cortex (perforant path) carry information to the granule cell layer (thick black line in C-shape). The hilus is the region encompassed on either side by the granule cell layer of the dentate gyrus. General information flow in the hippocampus entails granule cell projections to the pyramidal neurons of hippocampus proper (i.e., CA3 and CA1, in turn), before exiting the structure via the subiculum and sending information back to the neocortex.

trials and a learning index score calculated from probe trials. This method was originally described and is detailed in Gallagher *et al.*, 1993. Specifically, these proximity measures take into account deviation from an optimal search (i.e., a search that leads the rat directly to the platform). Using computer tracking (HVS Image, UK), the rat's location relative to the platform is sampled in the maze 10 times per second, which gives

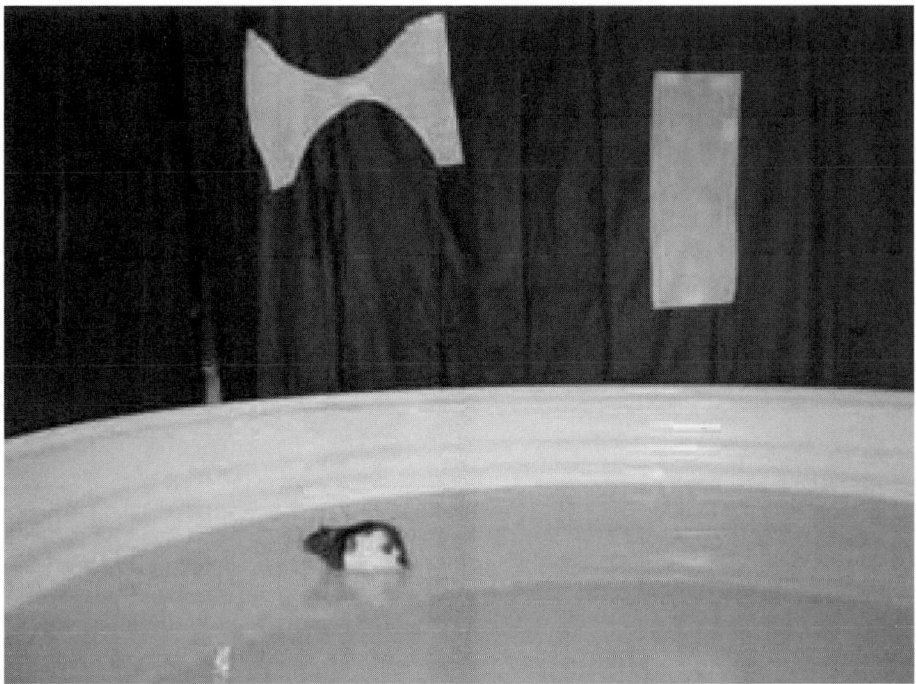

Figure 32.2 This figure shows a photograph of a young male Long–Evans rat in the Morris water maze standing on a submerged atlantis platform (HVS Image, UK). Distal visual cues, used to locate the hidden platform, are placed around the periphery of the pool (white geometric figures). Performance in this task is a well-established indicator of medial temporal lobe and, specifically, hippocampal function.

a measurement of the rat's distance from the platform in one second averages. For both probe and training trials, a correction is made for the optimal path based on any given start position, to alleviate bias on trial performance created by variations in the distance to the platform from the different start locations. After this correction is made, the cumulative distance for training trial performance can be summed across trials (see large panel on Figure 32.3) and the average distance from the goal calculated on probe trials (see inset panel of individual Learning Index Scores on Figure 32.3).

Search error has some advantages over traditional measures of water maze like latency (i.e., time to reach platform) or path length (i.e., distance swum to reach platform), particularly for aged rats. By considering the proximity of the rat during the entire trial, one can assume that the most accurate measure of spatial bias is being achieved. For example, one rat may be swimming in close proximity to the platform for 25 seconds, while another rat may be swimming randomly throughout the maze for 25 sec. Although the first rat in the aforementioned example apparently had some appreciation of the platform's location, neither a latency nor path length measure would detect it.

It is also noteworthy that probe trials are critical for the spatial learning assessment of aged rats. Aged rats have a tendency to develop a strategy of "circling" the pool at a given distance from the wall, which might result in short latencies and path lengths that are based entirely upon a nonhippocampal dependent strategy. Probe trials are therefore a better means by which to test rats' spatial knowledge, as rats with a good memory of the spatial location will consistently search in the area where the platform had been for at least 30 sec. Probe trials longer than this included throughout the protocol could lead to some extinction of learning. To minimize this problem, we employ an HVS atlantis platform (HVS Image, UK) that can be lowered to the bottom of the tank for the first 30 seconds of the probe trial and then raised again for the last 60 seconds of the trial. We find that this approach minimizes extinction that could be a concern with interpolated probe trials.

The data from these four interpolated probe trials are our main source of individual scores of spatial learning ability. The spatial learning index score is calculated from performance on all four of the interpolated probe trials. Performance on these trials is summed and weighted such that earlier trials receive greater weight (as age differences are generally larger earlier in training). As such, the Spatial Learning Index Score is an individual measure of spatial learning performance that takes acquisition and total spatial performance into account, and provides a single number that can be used to correlate with individual neurobiological data.

Figure 32.3 shows representative data from animals trained in this protocol. Note that as a whole, aged male

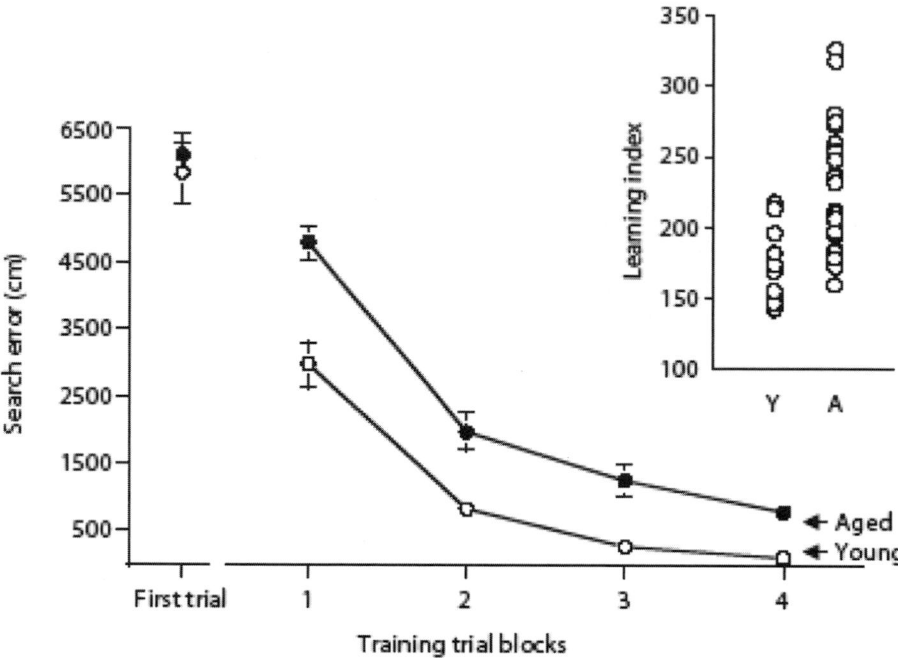

Figure 32.3 This graph shows typical performance in the Morris water maze of young (6-month-old) and aged (25-month-old) male Long–Evans rats. Note that both young (open circles) and aged rats (closed circles) performed comparably on the very first trial, demonstrating similar sensorimotor and motivational abilities. As shown in the large panel, both groups learn over the course of time, but the aged rats were significantly impaired in this task in comparison to young adult rats. However, the inset graph in the upper right corner shows that despite an overall impairment in the aged group compared to young, there was substantial individual variability among aged rats such that some aged rats performed on par with young rats and others performed outside the range of young, demonstrating impairment on this task. Note that a higher Learning Index Score indicates poorer performance. About half of the aged rats (A) performed outside the range of the young rats (Y) and were considered aged-impaired, and about half of the aged rats performed as well as the young rats and were considered aged-unimpaired.

Long–Evans rats are consistently impaired relative to young subjects; however, when individual performance (spatial learning index) is calculated, notice that there is much greater variability among aged rats than in young. About half of the aged rats perform on a par with young, and about half perform outside the distribution of young subjects. Assuming that these latter animals are healthy and perform comparably to young rats on cue training, we may interpret that this latter subset of rats is spatially impaired.

MEDIAL TEMPORAL LOBE-BASED COGNITION: CORRELATIONS WITH NEUROBIOLOGICAL CHANGES

Using the derived spatial Learning Index Score, one is then able to correlate a variety of neurobiological and neuroanatomical data with spatial learning performance among aged rats. Figure 32.4 shows data obtained using the behavioral model described above. In this study, the total number of neurons in the hippocampal region was assessed in behaviorally characterized rats using quantitative unbiased stereology, as many theories of age-related memory loss at the time regarded cell loss as the endpoint for age effects on cognition. However, as shown in Figure 32.4, Rapp and Gallagher (1996) found that frank neural loss in the hippocampal formation is not pervasive in the Long–Evans rat model, even though a considerable number of rats included in that study were spatially impaired.

This finding now has been documented for the principal neurons of the hippocampal formation, the entorhinal cortex, and the parahippocampal region, including the perirhinal and postrhinal cortices (Rapp *et al.*, 1996; Rapp *et al.*, 2002; Figure 32.1). The lack of frank neurodegeneration in normal aging has also been confirmed in other rodent models and primates, including humans (Merrill *et al.*, 2003; Rasmussen *et al.*, 1996; West *et al.*, 1994). Additional data supporting the lack of pervasive neurodegeneration in this model are provided by the absence of hypertrophied astrocytes (personal observation; Bizon and Rapp) and other markers such as OX-6 (Nicolle *et al.*, 2001), which are generally associated with widespread degeneration. These data challenge the long-standing view that neurodegeneration is a necessary condition of age-related cognitive impairment, and warrant further consideration.

Certainly, this absence of frank neuronal death has redirected our thinking about age-related neural impairment and focused our efforts toward identifying changes

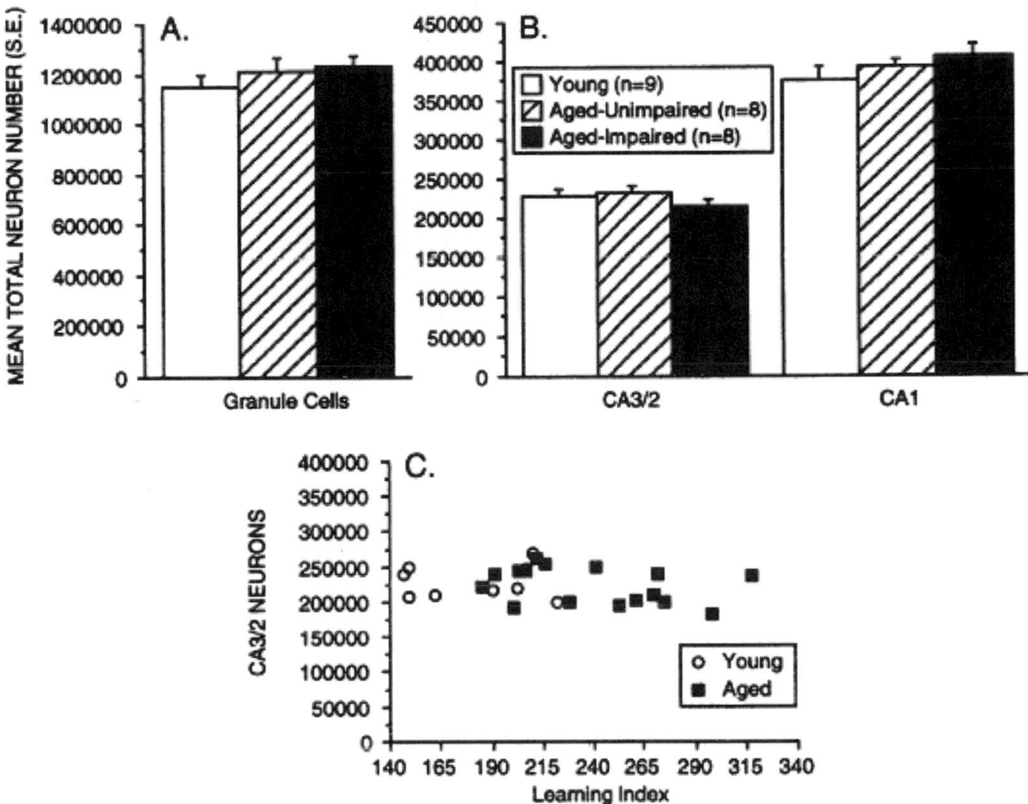

Figure 32.4 These graphs demonstrate a stereological analysis of neuronal number in all subfields of dentate gyrus and hippocampus proper in young and aged Long–Evans rats previously characterized on the Morris water maze task. Note in panels A and B that the total neuron number is not significantly different between young, aged-unimpaired, and aged-impaired animals for the granule cell layer (A), CA3/2 and CA1 (B). Moreover, no correlation between individual learning index (higher scores indicate greater impairment) and number of neurons in CA3/2 is observed (lower graph). This finding was consistent in both young (open circle) and aged (closed square) animals in hippocampus proper shown here and for the granule cells of the dentate gyrus (data not shown).

within and communication between neurons that are associated with neuronal plasticity as the main contributors to cognitive deficits. In other words, our current hypotheses are that suboptimal cell functioning and connectivity, rather than frank neuronal death, are likely to underlie the decline of many cognitive abilities that occur with age. Such cellular deficits have in fact been identified in the Long–Evans rat model. For example, differences have been found in the neurophysiological properties of place cells in aged-impaired rats versus young and aged unimpaired (see Chapter 33 by Nancy L. Nadon). Other findings, including changes in gene and protein expression and deficits in certain cell signaling pathways have been revealed using the Long–Evans rat model.

For example, using young and old Long–Evans rats behaviorally characterized on the Morris water maze as described above, our group has found that metabotropic glutamate receptor (mGluRs) and muscarinic cholinergic receptor signaling in the hippocampus is dysfunctional in the aged, learning-impaired rat (Nicolle *et al.*, 1999; Chouinard *et al.*, 1995). Both mGluR and muscarinic M1 receptor stimulation of phosphoinositide (PI) turnover is blunted in aged rats, and the magnitude of the decrease in signaling correlates with the severity of cognitive impairment. Figure 32.5 shows a correlation between the Learning Index and the PI turnover response that occurred as a consequence of stimulating Type 1 mGluR receptors with the agonist 1S,3R ACPD.

The magnitude of this deficit in PI turnover significantly correlated with the decline in age-related spatial memory ($R = -.67$, $p < .01$ when young and aged grouped together; $R = -.53$, $p < .05$ when the aged are considered alone). This study illustrates the general approach and power of using naturally occurring rat models to identify age-related neurobiological changes that could underlie memory impairment in the medial temporal lobe system. Further work in this rat model and in aged primates should help confirm that this signaling pathway is a contributor to age-related mnemonic impairment and whether therapeutic interventions directed at this pathway would be beneficial in the reversal of such deficits.

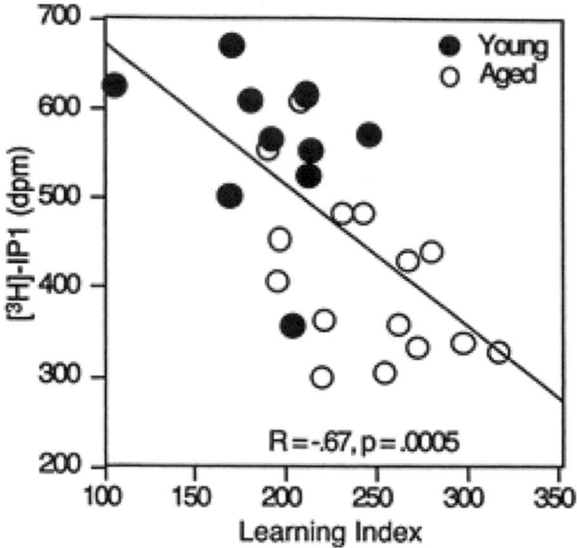

Figure 32.5 This graph shows the relationship of mGluR-mediated phosphoinositide (PI) turnover in the hippocampus in relation to spatial learning ability. Data points represent individual values for young and aged rats. The Learning Index is on the X-axis and the 1S,3R ACPD *EMAX*, a measure of PI turnover, on the Y-axis. The linear regression between PI turnover and the Learning Index for young and aged rats grouped together can be seen (solid line). A significant negative correlation was observed ($R = -0.67$, $p < .01$), with more impaired learning (higher learning index value) related to decreased turnover (lower disintegrations per minute [dpm] of [^{3}H]-IP1). Overall, mGluR-mediated PI turnover decreased with increasing chronological age and was most blunted in the aged rats with the most severe cognitive impairment, indicated by a significant correlation in the aged group alone ($R = -.53$, $p < .05$).

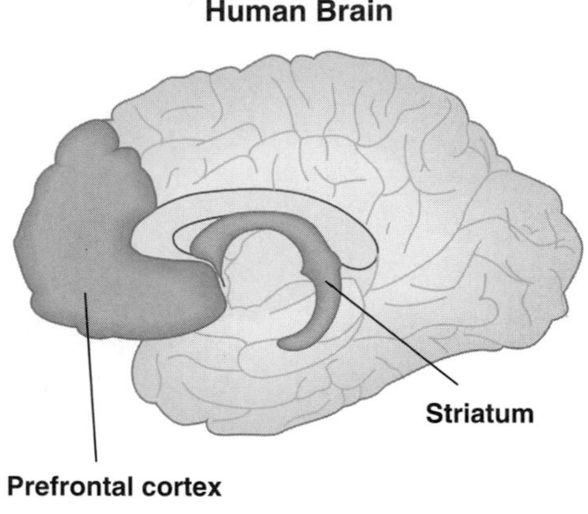

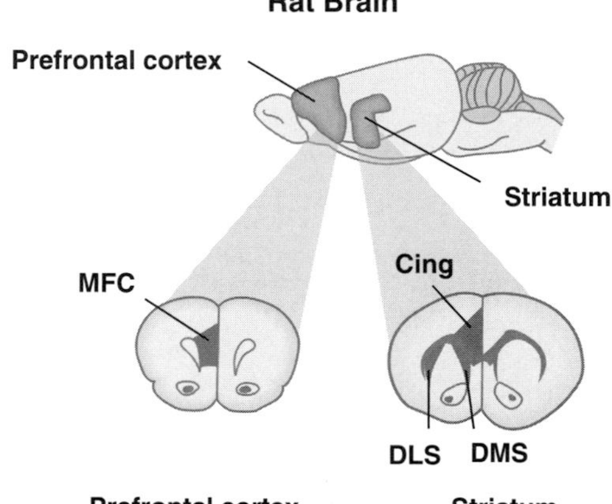

Figure 32.6 Schematic showing the prefrontal cortex and striatum in human (top) and rat brain. In both instances, these regions are shades in dark gray and labeled respectively. The bottom sections show coronal sections through rat brain in which medial prefrontal cortex (MFC), cingulate cortex (Cing), and dorsolateral and dorsomedial striatum (DLS and DMS, respectively) are highlighted in dark gray. Although there is behavioral and molecular evidence to suggest the diagrammed circuitry is critical for executive function in rodents, clarification of the precise functional system in rats that supports cognition associated with "executive function" in humans is the subject of ongoing experiments.

Aging and the Frontal Cortical–Striatal System

ANATOMY AND FUNCTION

Although a large body of literature has focused on the medial temporal lobe and the well-described age-related deficits in explicit or declarative memory that are dependent on this system, it is notable that other brain systems are also affected at advanced ages and contribute to losses in cognitive function. Frontal cortical and/or striatal circuitry is strongly affected in both normal aging and in pathological conditions associated with the aging process (i.e., Alzheimer's and Parkinson's disease). Subjects with prefrontal dysfunction are deficient in their ability to alter a behavioral response in the face of changing contingencies. This type of cognitive deficit may be caused by a disruption of striatal outflow resulting in frontal cortex dysfunction in circuitry connecting the prefrontal cortex, striatum and thalamus.

Figure 32.6 highlights the frontal cortex and striatum in the human and rat brain.

The frontal cortex (including infralimbic, prelimbic and anterior cingulater cortices) sends its major output to terminate throughout the striatum (McGeorge and Faull, 1989). Subregions of the striatum have been shown to have different functions in learning and memory. In particular, the dorsomedial striatum (DMS) has been implicated as a necessary structure to enable behavioral flexibility (Ragozzino *et al.*, 2002). The anterior cingulate cortex, highlighted in the coronal section of the rat brain, receives afferents from the subiculum (Finch *et al.*, 1984) and subsequently sends efferents to the striatum (Wang and Pickel, 2000).

The prefrontal cortex mediates executive function, cognitive processes particularly vulnerable to the effects of aging. Executive function is complex; it can be defined as choosing and implementing a strategy to achieve goal-directed behavior, coordinating the execution of the strategy, and disabling it afterwards (Band *et al.*, 2002). This combination of factors enables one to effectively alter one's behavior in response to changing environmental contingencies. Hence, executive function can be evaluated using tasks designed to assess a subject's ability to inhibit a previously learned rule in order to replace it with a new, more effective rule. Attentional set shifting is such a task. Set shifting is the ability to shift attention (attentional "set") from one perceptual feature of a stimulus (e.g., shape) to another, previously irrelevant and disregarded feature of a stimulus (e.g., color). The Wisconsin Card Sort Test (WCST) is often used to evaluate set shifting in humans. During the shift phase of the WCST, Positron Emission Tomography (PET) imaging has demonstrated an increase in activity of the prefrontal cortex (Nagahama *et al.*, 1997). Older adults display more perseverative behavior in the WCST and also show reduced prefrontal activation in response to task demands (Ridderinkhof *et al.*, 2002; Nagahama *et al.*, 1997). In a similar test, aged Rhesus monkeys were also impaired in set shifting, reflected by an increase in perseverative errors (Moore *et al.*, 2003).

AGE-RELATED IMPAIRMENT

The prefrontal cortex is particularly susceptible to the effects of aging at the morphological and molecular level. Although the neurons within the prefrontal cortex of primates are resistant to cell death with aging (O'Donnell *et al.*, 1999; Peters *et al.*, 1994), morphological evidence indicates that these cells may be effectively disconnected from communication due to a loss of synapses, dendritic reduction and a loss of insulating myelin. Decreases in the density of synapses and dendrites in the prefrontal cortex in aged monkeys have been reported, particularly in layer 1. The decrease in synapses in layer 1 may be due to the loss of subcortical cholinergic and dopaminergic projections to the prefrontal cortex (Herzog *et al.*, 2003; Stemmelin *et al.*, 2000; Kaasinen and Rinne, 2002). In addition to a loss in synaptic connections, degeneration of myelin sheaths of nerve fibers also occurs in the prefrontal cortex of aged monkeys, and this loss significantly correlates with the magnitude of cognitive impairment in the aged group (Peters *et al.*, 2002). Although the prefrontal cortex, particularly the dorsolateral prefrontal cortex in primates, has been most strongly implicated in executive functions, some data indicate that the dorsomedial striatum may also factor in this ability (Ragozzino *et al.*, 2002).

MODEL OF AGE-RELATED FRONTAL CORTICAL–STRIATAL IMPAIRMENT

Although the existence of a prefrontal cortex in rats analogous to the primate prefrontal cortex is a matter of controversy, it is generally accepted that the rat medial frontal cortex (infralimbic and prelimbic subregions) performs functions that are typically referred to as executive function in primates (Uylings *et al.*, 2003). Birrell and Brown (2000) adapted an attentional set shifting task used in monkeys and humans (Owen *et al.*, 1991; Dias *et al.*, 1996) for use in rats. This task was subsequently used to investigate the effects of aging on prefrontal function in the same study population as that used for the investigation of medial temporal lobe function described above (Barenese *et al.*, 2002).

The rat version of the attentional set shifting task involves digging in a pot for a food reward (see Figure 32.7).

Two perceptual dimensions vary: the odor of the pot (e.g., lemon vs. cinnamon) and the digging medium that is contained within the pot (e.g., confetti vs. gravel). By manipulating the combinations of the dimensions, several types of discriminations can be evaluated, including simple discriminations, compound discriminations, reversals of both simple and compound discriminations, and intra- and extradimensional shifts. The simple

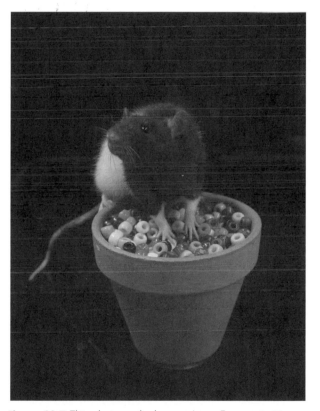

Figure 32.7 This photograph shows a Long–Evans rat sitting on a pot used for digging in the attentional set-shifting task. This task that is detailed in the text has been shown to be sensitive to cortical regions believed to be analogous to human dorsolateral prefrontal cortex. Individual differences in cognitive abilities that are supported by this system have been observed among aged male Long–Evans rats. As shown in this figure, rats are trained to dig in pots containing different types of media (such as the beads shown here) and different odors (e.g., lemon) for a food reward. Throughout the course of training, the rule required to successfully find the food is altered, and the ability of the rats to switch to the new rule is evaluated. *Photo credit:* Steve Kim, laboratory of Dr. Mark Baxter.

discriminations (SD) require identifying the rewarded pot that contains only a single relevant perceptual dimension (e.g., odors are relevant, and the digging medium is the same in both pots). The compound discriminations (CD) present combinations of both perceptual dimensions (the pots contain both a unique odor and a unique digging medium; either the odor or medium can be the relevant, rewarded stimulus). The reversal discriminations change the valence of the previously rewarded stimulus; e.g., the previously unrewarded pot (−) becomes rewarded (+). Discrimination reversals can occur with both compound (CD-Rev) and simple (SD-Rev) discriminations. An intradimensional (IDS) shift is a new discrimination using the same perceptual dimension as what was previously relevant; for example, if the previous discrimination consisted of a relevant odor stimulus (e.g., lemon and cinnamon), the IDS would be a comparison between two new odors (e.g., peppermint and sage). The extradimensional (EDS) shift requires changing the rule that was used previously and shifting attention to the previously irrelevant stimulus. For example, if the previous comparison was between a lemon/sawdust pot and a cinnamon/confetti pot and the subject had learned that the odor, in this case lemon, was the positive exemplar, then EDS would require inhibiting the "odor" rule and creating the "digging medium" rule, e.g., the subject now needs to pay attention to the digging medium in order to accurately identify the pot containing the reward.

The set shifting task described above has advantages in that it contains within-subject measurements that can be used for control data. The ability of the animal to perform simple discriminations to an equal degree across dimensions (e.g., for odors and for digging media) is crucial, and pilot studies must be performed to assure comparable trials to criterion using different odor or medium pairs and/or to eliminate stimuli that cause a natural aversion. Performance on the simple discrimination must be at a baseline level prior to beginning the subsequent phases of the task, and this may vary depending on species (rat or mouse) and even strain.

Because of the neuropsychological and neurobiological evidence that the prefrontal cortex is vulnerable to the effects of normal aging, Dr. Mark Baxter's group (Oxford, UK) examined attentional set shifting using the Birrell and Brown task in young and aged Long–Evans rats (Barense *et al.*, 2002). Performance of the aged rats on the EDS phase was significantly impaired compared to the young rats: the aged rats required significantly more trials to criterion to learn this discrimination (Figure 32.8).

The individual differences in EDS ability in the aged rats were not correlated with impaired spatial learning ability in the Morris water maze. These results indicate that the effects of age may be different in individuals not only within a specific brain region but also across brain regions that subserve different functions. The rat data obtained by Barense *et al.* (2002) parallels

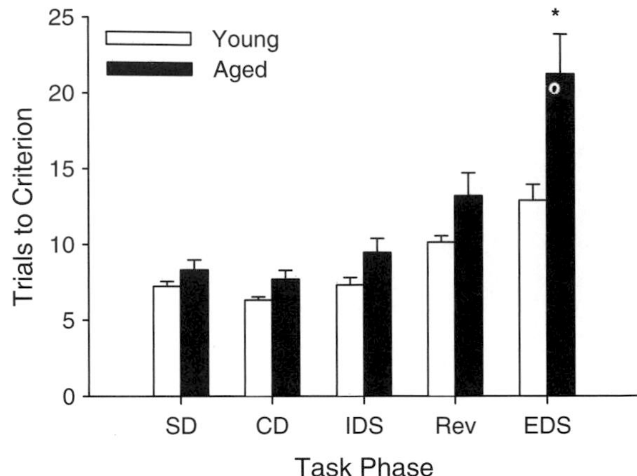

Figure 32.8 This graph shows the performance of both young and aged animals on the attentional set-shifting task. The aged rats require more trials than young rats to be proficient at the extradimensional phase (EDS) of the task ($p < 0.05$), while performing comparably to young on other discriminations in this task (SD = simple discrimination, CD = compound discrimination, IDS = intradimensional shift, REV = reversal). Extradimensional shifts are those that are most directly related to performance on human tasks that identify subjects with cognitive deficits and damage to the prefrontal cortex.

a neuropsychological study in healthy aged humans that also demonstrated a lack of correlation between deficits on tests traditionally associated with prefrontal function (including the WCST) and deficits on tasks traditionally associated with hippocampal/medial temporal lobe dysfunction (delayed cued recall) (Glisky *et al.*, 1995).

FRONTAL CORTICAL–STRIATAL-BASED COGNITION: CORRELATING AGE-RELATED DIFFERENCES

Attentional set shifting appears to be sensitive to the effects of aging on the prefrontal cortex, analogous to the sensitivity of spatial learning in the water maze to medial temporal lobe dysfunction in aging. Investigations of the neurobiological basis of age-related deficits in attentional set shifting are just beginning but have proven informative. For example, an analysis of ionotropic glutamate receptor binding in the aged Long–Evans rats assessed for attentional set shifting and spatial learning (described above) revealed that a decrease in binding to a glutamate-receptor subtype (kainate receptors) in the cingulate region of the prefrontal cortex was significantly correlated with poor performance in the EDS phase (Figure 32.9, top panel) but not spatial learning (Figure 32.9, bottom panel) (Nicolle and Baxter, 2003).

In that same study, decreases in NMDA receptor binding in the dorsomedial striatum of the aged group were shown to correlate with preserved memory ($R = +.79$, $p < .05$), perhaps indicating a neurobiological response that is compensatory in nature (Nicolle and Baxter, 2003). We hope that this model of age-related

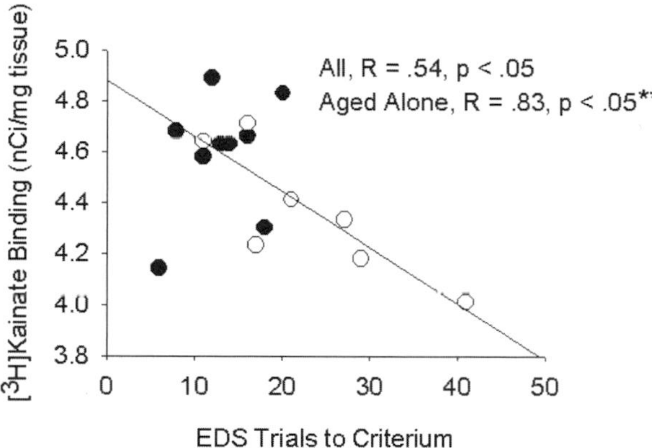

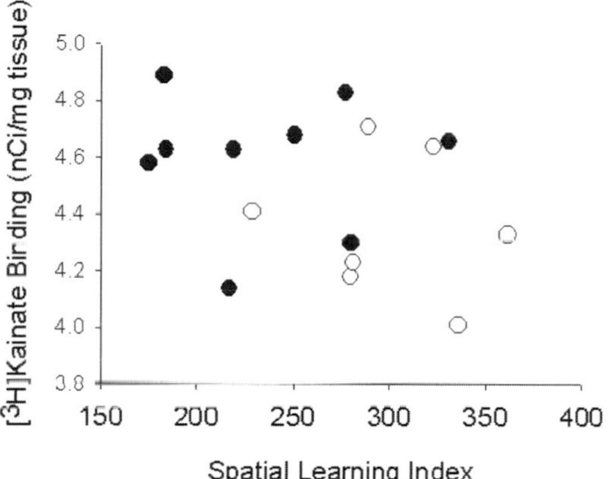

Figure 32.9 This graph shows the correlation between high-affinity [^{3}H]kainate binding in the cingulate cortex and trials to criterion on the extradimensional shift (EDS) phase of the attentional set-shifting task (top panel) or the spatial Learning Index (bottom panel) in young and aged Long–Evans rats. Lower levels of [^{3}H]kainate binding significantly correlated with more trials to criterion (poorer learning) in the cingulate cortex of the aged rats, $R = -.83$, $p < .05$. There was no correlation between [^{3}H]kainate binding in cingulate cortex with spatial learning index.

cognitive impairment will provide a rich source of neurobiological data that will be revealing as to the nature of frontal–cortical cognitive deficits in aging.

Conclusion

Overall, these studies demonstrate that rodent models of cognitive aging can provide a rich resource for uncovering neurobiological alterations associated with age-related cognitive deficits. Findings that some aged rat populations naturally differ in their maintenance of cognitive function with age affords the opportunity to model individual differences in cognitive abilities in the human population. Importantly, rat models are convenient and can be easily manipulated, and the results from such models have broadly paralleled findings observed in humans and nonhuman primates.

As described, there is now an extensive literature using spatial learning ability as a functional measure of the output of the hippocampus/medial temporal system in aged rats. This individual variability in spatial learning in the aged population has been capitalized upon by using subsequent neurobiological assessments to identify the cellular and molecular contributors to age-related impairments. Neurobiological alterations continue to be identified in this model, and it remains a challenge to integrate the current and future findings so that they can provide a comprehensive picture of the range and complexity of alterations that occur during aging. The complexity of normal aging is illustrated by consideration of two different neural systems, the medial temporal lobe and the frontal cortical–striatal system, and how these each relate overall to cognitive function in aging. Individual vulnerability may exist (and probably does) that predisposes some subjects to frontal dysfunction and others to medial temporal lobe dysfunction. There may also be a subpopulation of aged individuals that are vulnerable to deficits in cognitive decline associated with both brain systems. How to identify and how to push these findings to the next level will depend upon sensitive behavioral assessment of these neural systems that are vulnerable to the effects of aging.

The newly devised attentional set shifting task developed for rats shows real promise as a behavioral measure of the integrity of the frontal cortical system, a brain system that is adversely affected by normal age and in numerous pathological age-related diseases. As this model is further developed and refined, the hope is to yield data regarding both molecular and cellular contributors to cognitive impairments associated with frontal cortical–striatal circuitry. In this latter case, the specific circuitry responsible for "executive functions" is not yet fully elucidated, and we are just beginning to uncover the neurobiological underpinnings of the widely reported age-related deficits associated with this brain system in the human population. Over the next several years, refinement of this protocol along with a gained understanding of the neural and molecular circuitry should garnish important new data in this arena. This approach will be necessary to identify the neurobiological etiology of individual differences in cognitive deficits in the aged population and will be necessary when trying to reverse age-related cognitive deficits in the human population.

The general approach described here in terms of relating neurobiological changes to individual differences in cognitive abilities among aged rodents should help uncover the underlying brain mechanisms responsible for age-related deficits. Ultimately, this combination of behavioral and neurobiological assessment in the same animals will help direct future therapeutic approaches to combating cognitive decline in the human aged population.

Recommended Resources

Barense M.D., Fox M.T., and Baxter M.G. (2002). Aged rats are impaired on an attentional set-shifting task sensitive to medial frontal cortex damage in young rats. *Learn. Mem. 9*, 191–201.

Birrell J.M. and Brown V.J. (2000). Medial frontal cortex mediates perceptual attentional set shifting in the rat. *J. Neurosci. 20*, 4320–324.

Gallagher M. (1993). Severity of spatial learning impairments in aging: development of a learning index for performance in the Morris water maze. *Behavioral Neurosci. 107(4)*, 618–626.

Morris R. (1984). Developments of a water-maze procedure for studying spatial learning in the rat. *J. Neurosci. Methods 11*, 47–60.

http://www.hvsimage.com/

ACKNOWLEDGMENTS

We gratefully acknowledge Drs. Michela Gallagher, Mark Baxter, and Peter Rapp for their generosity in allowing us to include figures from their previously published work. We would further like to acknowledge Dr. Alisa Woods for editorial and intellectual contributions and Dr. Barry Setlow for helpful comments on this chapter.

REFERENCES

Band G.P., Ridderinkhof K.R., and Segalowitz S. (2002). Explaining neurocognitive aging: Is one factor enough? *Brain Cogn. 49*, 259–267.

Barense M.D., Fox M.T., and Baxter M.G. (2002). Aged rats are impaired on an attentional set-shifting task sensitive to medial frontal cortex damage in young rats. *Learn. Mem. 9*, 191–201.

Barnes C.A. and McNaughton B.L. (1985). An age comparison of the rates of acquisition and forgetting of spatial information in relation to long-term enhancement of hippocampal synapses. *Behav. Neurosci. 99*, 1040–1048.

Barnes C.A. (1979). Memory deficits associated with senescence: A neurophysiological and behavioral study in the rat. *J. Comp. Physiol. Psychol. 93*, 74–104.

Birrell J.M. and Brown V.J. (2000). Medial frontal cortex mediates perceptual attentional set shifting in the rat. *J. Neurosci. 20*, 4320–4324.

Bizon J.L., Helm K.A., Han J.S., Chun H.J., Pucilowska J., Lund P.K., and Gallagher M. (2001). Hypothalamic-pituitary-adrenal axis function and corticosterone receptor expression in behaviourally characterized young and aged Long-Evans rats. *Eur. J. Neurosci. 14*, 1739–1751.

Bizon J.L. and Gallagher M. (2003). Production of new cells in the rat dentate gyrus over the lifespan: Relation to cognitive decline. *Eur. J. Neurosci. 18*, 215–219.

Bizon J.L. and Gallagher M. (2005). More is less: Neurogenesis and age-related cognitive decline in long-evans rats. *Sci. Aging Knowledge Environ. 16*, 2.

Bizon J.L., Lee H. J., and Gallagher M. (2004). Neurogenesis in a rat model of age-related cognitive decline. *Aging Cell 3*, 227–234.

Cameron H.A. and McKay R.D. (1999) Restoring production of hippocampal neurons in old age. *Nat. Neurosci. 2*, 894–897.

Chouinard M.L., Gallagher M., Yasuda R.P., Wolfe B.B., and McKinney M. (1995). Hippocampal muscarinic receptor function in spatial learning-impaired aged rats. *Neurobiol. of Aging 16*, 955–963.

de Quervain D.J., Henke K., Aerni A., Treyer V., McGaugh J.L., Berthold T., *et al.* (2003). Glucocorticoid-induced impairment of declarative memory retrieval is associated with reduced blood flow in the medial temporal lobe. *Eur. J. Neurosci. 17*, 1296–1302.

de Quervain D.J., Roozendaal B., and McGaugh J.L. (1998). Stress and glucocorticoids impair retrieval of long-term spatial memory. *Nature 394*, 787–790.

Dias R., Robbins T.W., and Roberts A.C. (1996). Dissociation in prefrontal cortex of affective and attentional shifts. *Nature 380*, 69–72.

Drapeau E., Mayo W., Aurousseau C., Le Moal M., Piazza P.V., and Abrous D.N. (2003). Spatial memory performances of aged rats in the water maze predict levels of hippocampal neurogenesis. *Proc. Natl. Acad. Sci. USA 100*, 14385–14390.

Finch D.M., Derian E.L., and Babb T.L. (1984). Excitatory projection of the rat subicular complex to the cingulate cortex and synaptic integration with thalamic afferents. *Brain Res. 301*, 25–37.

Freedman V.A., Martin L.G., and Schoeni R.F. (2002). Recent trends in disability and functioning among older adults in the United States: A systematic review. *JAMA 288*, 3137–3146.

Gallagher M., Burwel R., and Burchinal M. (1993). Severity of spatial learning impairments in aging: Development of a learning index for performance in the Morris water maze. *Behavioral. Neurosci. 107(4)*, 618–626.

Gallagher M., Bizon J.L., Hoyt E.C., Helm K.A., and Lund P.K. (2003). Effects of aging on the hippocampal formation in a naturally occurring animal model of mild cognitive impairment. *Exp. Gerontol. 38*, 71–77.

Glisky E.L., Polster M.R., and Routhieaux B.C. (1995). Double dissociation between item and source memory. *Neuropsychol. 9*, 229–235.

Herzog C.D., Nowak K.A., Sarter M., and Bruno J.P. (2003). Microdialysis without acetylcholinesterase inhibition reveals an age-related attenuation in stimulated cortical acetylcholine release. *Neurobiol. Aging 24*, 861–863.

Jarrard L.E. (1993). On the role of the hippocampus in learning and memory in the rat. *Behav. Neural. Biol. 60*, 9–26.

Jokinen H., Kalska H., Ylikoski R., Hietanen M., Mantyla R., Pohjasvaara T., *et al.* (2004). Medial temporal lobe atrophy and memory deficits in elderly stroke patients. *Eur. J. Neurol. 11*, 825–832.

Kasckow J.W., Segar T.M., Xiao C., Furay A.R., Evanson N.K., Ostrander M.M., and Herman J.P. (2005). Stability of neuroendocrine and behavioral responsiveness in aging fischer 344/Brown-Norway hybrid rats. *Endocrinology 146*, 3105–3112.

Kaasinen V. and Rinne J.O. (2002). Functional imaging studies of dopamine system and cognition in normal aging and Parkinson's disease. *Neuroscience & Biobehav. Rev. 26*, 785.

Korf E.S., Wahlund L.O., Visser P.J., and Scheltens P. (2004) Medial temporal lobe atrophy on MRI predicts dementia in patients with mild cognitive impairment. *Neurology 63*, 94–100.

Lichtenwalner R.J., Forbes M.E., Bennett S.A., Lynch C.D., Sonntag W.E., and Riddle D.R. (2001). Intracerebroventricular infusion of insulin-like growth factor-I ameliorates the age-related decline in hippocampal neurogenesis. *Neuroscience 107*, 603–613.

Lupien S.J., Fiocco A., Wan N., Maheu F., Lord C., Schramek T., and Tu M.T. (2005). Stress hormones and human memory function across the lifespan. *Psychoneuroendocrinol. 30*, 225–242.

McGeorge A.J. and Faull R.L. (1989). The organization of the projection from the cerebral cortex to the striatum in the rat. *Neuroscience 29*, 503–537.

Merrill D.A., Karim R., Darraq M., Chiba A.A., and Tuszynski M.H. (2003). Hippocampal cell genesis does not correlate with spatial learning ability in aged rats. *J. Comp. Neurol. 459*, 201–207.

Moore T.L., Killiany R.J., Herndon J.G., Rosene D.L., and Moss M.B. (2003). Impairment in abstraction and set shifting in aged Rhesus monkeys. *Neurobiol. Aging 24*, 125–134.

Nagahama Y., Fukuyama H., Yamauchi H., Katsumi Y., Magata Y., Shibasaki H., and Kimura J. (1997). Age-related changes in cerebral blood flow activation during a Card Sorting Test. *Exp. Brain Res. 114*, 571–577.

Nicolle M.M., Colombo P.J., Gallagher M., and McKinney M. (1999). Metabotropic glutamate receptor-mediated hippocampal phosphoinositide turnover is blunted in spatial learning impaired aged rats. *J. Neurosci. 19*, 9604–9610.

Nicolle M.M., Gonzalez J., Sugaya K., Baskerville K.A., Bryan D., Lund K., *et al.* (2001). Signatures of hippocampal oxidative stress in aged spatial learning-impaired rodents. *Neuroscience 107*, 415–431.

Nicolle M.M. and Baxter M.G. (2003). Glutamate receptor binding in the frontal cortex and dorsal striatum of aged rats with impaired attentional set-shifting. *Eur. J. Neurosci. 18*, 3335 3342.

O'Donnell K.A., Rapp P.R., and Hof P.R. (1999). Preservation of prefrontal cortical volume in behaviorally characterized aged macaque monkeys. *Exp. Neurol. 160*, 300–310.

Owen A.M., Roberts A.C., Polkey C.E., Sahakian B.J., and Robbins TW. (1991). Extra-dimensional versus intra-dimensional set shifting performance following frontal lobe excisions, temporal lobe excisions or amygdalo-hippocampectomy in man. *Neuropsychologia 29*, 993–1006.

Peters A., Leahu D., Moss M.B., and McNally K.J. (1994). The effects of aging on area 46 of the frontal cortex of the rhesus monkey. *Cereb. Cortex 4*, 621–635.

Peters A. and Sethares C. (2002). Aging and the myelinated fibers in prefrontal cortex and corpus callosum of the monkey. *J. Comp. Neurol. 442*, 277–291.

Ragozzino M.E., Ragozzino K.E., Mizumori S.J., and Kesner R.P. (2002). Role of the dorsomedial striatum in behavioral flexibility for response and visual cue discrimination learning. *Behav. Neurosci. 116*, 105–115.

Rapp P.R. and M. Gallagher (1996). Preserved neuron number in the hippocampus of aged rats with spatial learning deficits. *Proc. Natl. Acad. Sci. USA 93*, 9926–9930.

Rapp P.R., Burwell R.D., and West M.J. (1996). Individual differences in aging: Implications for stereological studies of neuron loss. *Neurobiol. Aging 17*, 495–496.

Rapp P.R., Deroche P.S., Mao Y., and Burwell R.D. (2002) Neuron number in the parahippocampal region is preserved in aged rats with spatial learning deficits. *Cereb. Cortex. 12*, 1171–1179.

Rasmussen T., Schliemann T., Sorensen J.C., Zimmer J., and West M.J. (1996). Memory impaired aged rats: No loss of principal hippocampal and subicular neurons. *Neurobiol. Aging 17*, 143–147.

Ridderinkhof K.R., Span M.M., and van der Molen M.W. (2002). Perseverative behavior and adaptive control in older adults: Performance monitoring, rule induction, and set shifting. *Brain Cogn. 49*, 382–401.

Roozendaal B. (2002). Stress and memory: Opposing effects of glucocorticoids on memory consolidation and memory retrieval. *Neurobiol. Learn. Mem. 78(3)*, 578–595.

Savonenko A.V. and Markowska A.L. (2003). The cognitive effects of ovariectomy and estrogen replacement are modulated by aging. *Neuroscience 119*, 821–830.

33

Aged Rodents for Biogerontology Research

Nancy L. Nadon

Studies in animal models have provided much of our understanding of the changes that occur in normal aging and in age-related diseases that humans encounter in their journey through life. Even lower organisms such as flies and worms have contributed to our understanding of human aging. But the rodent has been the most valuable model for biogerontology research because of the similarity between rodent physiology and that of humans and the low cost to maintain them. This chapter will discuss the advantages of the rodent model for aging research, provide some examples of the types of investigations made possible with the rodent model, discuss the special issues and concerns to be considered when using aged rodents, and describe resources available to facilitate studies with rodents.

Introduction

Human aging is the result of a complex interaction between biological changes and environmental/social influences. Healthcare throughout life, diet, and habits such as smoking, alcohol consumption and physical activity can all impact the rate of biological aging and complicate the study of the biology of aging in human populations. The rodent provides a venue for modeling the biological changes with age and investigating the genetic and physiological basis of aging and age-related diseases while controlling intrinsic and extrinsic influences. The genetic background, diet, environment, and health status of the rodent can be strictly controlled. Rodents are similar to humans in much of their physiology, cellular function, and to a lesser degree, even their anatomy. The musculoskeletal system, immune and endocrine systems, and gastrointestinal tract are very similar in both function and architecture between rodents and humans. Cardiac function has been modeled in rodents, as have age-related changes in the liver. While the rodent brain is more primitive than the human brain on the organ level, at the cellular level there are many similarities between rodent and human central nervous systems that can be exploited.

Rodents provide a good model for testing potential therapeutics, combining the value of a mammalian system with a low-cost test subject. Longitudinal studies are more feasible in a short-lived rodent model than in a human population. The ability to analyze tissue at all stages of the process, be it normal aging or disease development, is one of the major benefits of working with the rodent model. In addition, the rodent model is amenable to manipulation at the genetic level, allowing us to test the role of gene products and pathways in age-related changes.

An example of an area of current emphasis where the rodent has made a vital contribution is the interaction of obesity with normal aging and age-related diseases. Obesity has become a serious public health concern—one that is the product of both biological and environmental/social contributions. It is a polygenic trait, with multiple genetic pathways contributing to the phenotype. Rodent studies allow for the dissection of the genetic contributions and the role of the environmental/behavioral contributions, and also the testing of potential therapeutic interventions. Many chromosomal regions (quantitative trait loci or QTL) have been identified as influencing obesity, and each contributes only a small percent of the overall phenotype (reviewed in Brockmann and Bevova, 2002). There are not only additive effects of different genes but also gene–gene interactions and gene–environment interactions, demonstrating the complexity of this phenotype.

Insulin resistance is a problem common to aging and obesity, and there are strain differences that can be exploited for studies in rodent models. Figure 33.1 compares the insulin resistance response to a high-fat diet in DBA/2J and C3H/HeJ mice, illustrating not only strain differences but also gender differences in the response by DBA/2J mice.

There are also many mutant and genetically engineered rodent models that address one or more aspects of obesity and the role of insulin resistance in aging, reviewed elsewhere (Tschop and Heiman, 2001; Mauvais-Jarvis *et al.*, 2002; Carroll *et al.*, 2004). One mutant mouse model of obesity, the leptin-deficient (ob/ob) mouse, exhibits obesity and increased insulin resistance. When leptin deficiency (ob/ob) was combined with the knockout of the adipocyte fatty acid binding protein aP2 gene,

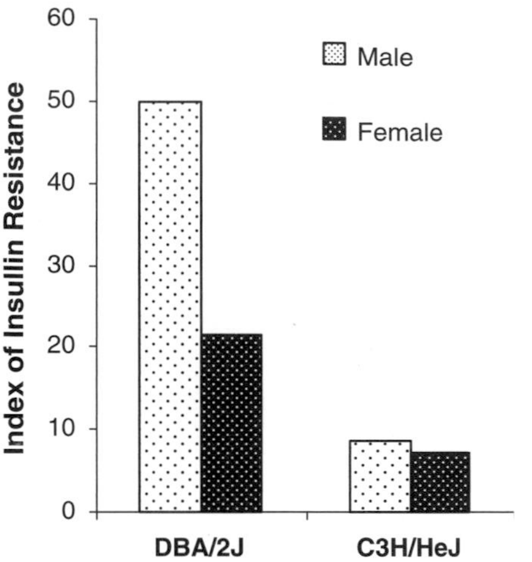

Figure 33.1 Homeostasis model assessment of insulin resistance at 6 months of age, after 18 weeks on an atherogenic diet. These findings illustrate both strain differences and gender differences (Naggert *et al.*, 2003).

to create ob/ob, aP2−/− mice, these mice showed an even greater obesity than ob/ob mice, but had significantly less insulin resistance (Uysal *et al.*, 2000). This finding suggests that aP2 functions in the insulin pathway independent of adiposity and hints at the complexity of the interactions leading to the altered physiological state in obese and aged individuals.

Sarcopenia, degeneration of the skeletal musculature with resulting weakness, is another serious problem in the elderly population being studied with the aid of rodent models. Investigations with the rodent model have illuminated some of the mechanisms behind age-related muscle loss and pointed to potential pathways for therapeutic interventions. For example, one cause of age-related muscle loss is the decreased ability of the muscle progenitor cells, the satellite cells, to divide and differentiate. Satellite cells in young muscle respond to cell death or injury by proliferating and differentiating into myoblasts, but in aged muscle that response is blunted. One involved pathway identified through rodent studies is the Notch pathway, a key signal pathway in muscle development and regeneration (Conboy *et al.*, 2002). The ability to regenerate muscle was restored in aged mice by directly activating Notch expression, suggesting that this is a candidate pathway for therapeutic interventions (Conboy *et al.*, 2003).

And one last example, Alzheimer's Disease (AD) provides a vivid illustration of both the potential of the rodent model and the challenges of modeling human disease in rodents. Rodents do not get AD, but do show decreases in cognition and memory that reflect changes seen in much of the aged human population (reviewed in Ingram *et al.*, 1994). There have been many attempts to make transgenic mouse models of the neuropathology of AD (plaques and tangles), too numerous to recount, but very few have successfully recapitulated even a portion of the disease process (reviewed in Ashe, 2001; Phinney *et al.*, 2003; Lee *et al.*, 2005). Simply engineering in the mutations found in familial AD is not sufficient to recreate the disease. Tg2576 carries the Swedish mutation of APP and shows early-onset learning deficits, but not the morphological hallmarks of the disease (Hsiao *et al.*, 1996). TgCRND8 has a double mutant form of APP and shows plaque formation and some cognitive deficits, but no tangles (Chishti *et al.*, 2001). Modeling AD has required combining mutant amyloid precursor protein (APP) genes with other components of the neuronal pathways involved in the disease, and the most faithful recapitulation of AD pathology is found in a triple transgenic mouse carrying mutant forms of three genes involved in AD, amyloid precursor protein, presenilin-1 and tau protein (Oddo *et al.*, 2003). The ability to make multiple genetic alterations in a mouse holds promise for modeling complex diseases.

Genetic Background

INBRED STRAINS

One of the most important considerations in choosing a rodent model is the genetic background. There are advantages and disadvantages of different genetic backgrounds that must be weighed equally. Inbred strains have the advantage that all individuals of the strain are genetically identical, providing a uniform population for study. Small sample sizes are sufficient for most studies because of the genetic homogeneity. Care must be taken to note the substrain being used, as there can be genetic differences between substrains, particularly those that diverged a long time ago. Most laboratory strains of mice originated 80 to 100 years ago, and because embryo cryopreservation is a relatively new technology, for most of their existence they were maintained by constant breeding. Roderick *et al.* (1985) illustrate the pitfalls of breeding the strains in different laboratories for many generations, describing the many substrains of BALB/c mice in existence now. For example, BALB/cJ and BALB/cByJ share most alleles, but there are some genetic differences and some biological differences between them. BALB/cJ mice are more aggressive than BALB/cByJ, have larger brain weights, and different susceptibility to induced diabetes. While these differences are minor considerations for most studies, they illustrate the need to understand the genetic background.

While no one strain is a perfect model for all aspects of human aging, different strains have characteristics valuable for modeling specific aspects of human physiology or disease, and the use of inbred strains allows the investigator to choose a model with characteristics pertinent to the questions at hand. For example, DBA/2 mice are useful for modeling epilepsy and related seizure disorders, as they are very sensitive to audiogenic and electrogenic seizures, while C57BL/6 mice are resistant to both audiogenic and electrogenic seizures (Seyfried *et al.*, 1986). F344 female rats have very low femoral bone strength compared to other inbred rat strains and have been used to model age-associated bone loss (Turner *et al.*, 2001).

There are also disadvantages to using inbred strains, notably strain-specific pathologies that can reach very high levels of incidence, confounding interpretation of results. F344 rats, for example, develop tumors in a large proportion of the population by old age, as well as a high incidence of nephropathy (Lipman *et al.*, 1999). Some strains of mice, particularly the albino strains, experience degeneration of visual acuity with age, as reported for 129 mice by Hengemihle *et al.* (1999), rendering them unsuitable for studies requiring the use of visual cues, such as maze training. And some strains have extremely short lifespans due to susceptibility to specific diseases. AKR mice develop T cell lymphoma and die by about a year of age, because of interactions between retroviruses that the strain carries (Brayton *et al.*, 2001). Clearly this strain would not be useful for aging studies.

Other strain-specific pathologies are unrelated to the biology of aging but nevertheless may impact aging studies by causing losses in the study population. One commonly encountered problem is the ulcerative dermatitis found in C57BL/6 mice, one of the most popular strains for aging research. Many factors play a role in the development of this pathology, including genetics, diet and husbandry. The etiology of this problem has been reported to be an immune complex-induced vasculitis (Andrews *et al.*, 1994). While the incidence of ulcerative dermatitis is low in young C57BL/6 mice, it increases with age. Andrews *et al.* analyzed 300 C57BL/6NNia mice that were barrier-raised and negative for ectoparasites and bacterial and fungal diseases. They found an incidence of ulcerative dermatitis of about 20% in the aged mice, with an average age of onset of 20 months. Males and females were affected approximately equally. It is important to take this condition into consideration when using C57BL/6 for aging studies because severe cases require euthanasia, and sample sizes must be large enough to allow for such losses. Aggression is another factor that can lead to losses in group-housed rodents, such as with BALB/c males where fighting leads to some losses in the population due to serious wounds requiring euthanasia.

HYBRID STRAINS

Hybrid mice and rats are the offspring of two dissimilar parents and tend to be more robust than the parental strains, with longer lifespan and fewer, or lower incidence of, strain-specific pathologies. F1 hybrid rodents are the first generation bred from two inbred strains, and like the inbred strains, F1 hybrids still have the advantage that all individuals in the population are the same at the genetic level, allowing small sample sizes to represent the population. The genetic variation contributed by the two different parental alleles at many loci produces the pay-off of improved health. Tables 33.1 and 33.2 compare the median lifespan and the average maximum body weight of some of the inbred and hybrid mouse and rat strains included in the NIA's aged rodent colonies.

TABLE 33.1
Median lifespan in days for selected rodent strains[a]

Strain	Males	Females
C57BL/6	850	800
DBA/2	800	680
B6D2F1	950	880
F344	740	780
BN	950	950
F344BNF1	1000	900

[a]From Turturro *et al.* (1999).

TABLE 33.2
Peak body weight of selected rodent strains[a]

Strain	Males	Females
C57BL/6	42 gm	32 gm
DBA/2	33 gm	24 gm
B6D2F1	47 gm	32 gm
F344	470 gm	320 gm
BN	480 gm	250 gm
F344BNF1	640 gm	350 gm

[a]From Turturrro *et al.* (1999).

Genetically heterozygous (HET) mice are another alternative to inbred strains. HET mice are mixtures of four (F2 generation) or eight (F3 generation) strains of mice. They have more genetic diversity, with individuals in the population differing from each other at a portion of the loci. That genetic diversity makes the population more reflective of the human population than an inbred strain, but also necessitates use of larger sample sizes due to the differences between individuals. HET mice are a valuable resource for mapping and identifying genes that influence or modify traits, by exploiting differences in characteristics specific to the parental strains. For example, Lipman *et al.* (2004) identified genetic regions that influence the types and prevalence of pathologies present at death. HET mice were also used to identify QTLs that influence the severity of age-related cataracts (Wolf *et al.*, 2004). Mice are a good model for age-related cataracts, as the timing and location of cataracts in mice are similar to what is observed in elderly humans. QTLs were identified on three chromosomes, and statistical analysis indicated that the effects of the three QTLs were additive—the more at-risk alleles a mouse had, the greater its risk for severe cataracts. Further description of HET mice can be found in Chapter 4 of this book and other references (Miller and Nadon, 2000; Miller and Chrisp, 2002).

Genetic Manipulations

The genetic makeup of rodents is easily manipulated by selective breeding and by genetic engineering. Table 33.3 summarizes types of rodent models produced by standard breeding protocols, selecting at each generation for chromosomal markers or phenotypic traits. They exploit strain-specific characteristics and are listed in descending order from the least amount of recombination between the strains to the most recombination between the strains. An example of the use of selective breeding models is found in Mountz *et al.* (2001), a review of recombinant inbred strains derived from a cross between C57BL/6 and DBA/2 mice that were used to identify genomic regions influencing immune response in young and aged mice.

Genetically engineered models have become an essential tool for identifying biochemical and genetic pathways involved in disease processes (summarized in Table 33.4). Transgenic mice are valuable for studying the effects of increased expression of a protein, expression of dominant-negative proteins, and replacement of defective proteins. Transgenic rats are also produced, but they have not caught on as well as mice as they are more costly and difficult to produce. Knockout mice are used to model diseases based on deficiency and to study the function of individual gene products in a pathway. A good review of both selective breeding models and genetically engineered models is provided in Brockmann and Bevova (2002). Genetic background is just as important when working with genetically engineered models as it is when working with inbred strains, because the phenotype of the genetic alteration can vary on different backgrounds. For example, the expression of an amyloid precursor protein transgene in FVB mice showed unexpected phenotypes, including premature death and seizures, not observed when the same transgene was expressed on other genetic backgrounds (Ashe, 2001).

Mutations, whether spontaneous or induced, have also contributed greatly to our understanding of aging. The Snell Dwarf mouse, first identified in the 1950s, was the first mutant to show an extended lifespan. There have been over 100 publications on the Snell Dwarf since then,

TABLE 33.3
Rodent models produced by selective breeding

Model	Description
Chromosome Substitution Strain (CSS)	An entire chromosome is moved to a different genetic background.
Congenic strain	One region of one chromosome is moved onto a different genetic background by backcrossing an F1 hybrid to one parental strain to inbreed.
Recombinant Congenic Strain (RCS)	Large regions of chromosomes moved onto another background by backcrossing an F1 hybrid to one parental strain for a few generations and inbreeding by brother–sister matings.
Recombinant Inbred Strain (RIS)	Large number of smaller recombination units made by creating an F2 hybrid and inbreeding by brother–sister matings.
Advanced Intercross Lines (AIL)	Multiple (F10 or more) intercrosses between two strains. They are not inbred, hence are heterozygous at many loci.

TABLE 33.4
Genetically engineered rodent models

Model	Description
Transgenic	A genetic element is added through DNA injection into the embryo, resulting in a gain-of-function at the genome level.
Inducible transgenic	Expression of a transgene is induced by exogenous compounds.
Knockout	Expression of a genetic element is eliminated by homologous recombination with a construct that prevents transcription of intact mRNA.
Knock-in	Homologous recombination creates a change in the mouse genome, replacing the wild-type mouse sequence with a mutation, human gene sequence, etc.
Conditional Knockout	Knockout of a genetic element is controlled in a temporal, developmental, or tissue-specific manner.

reporting on various aspects of aging in this mutant (reviewed in Bartke and Brown-Borg, 2004). It has been a key player in studies that demonstrate the importance of the insulin-signaling pathway in aging. The Ames Dwarf mouse is another spontaneous mutation with increased lifespan and a reduction in both total neoplastic load and total disease burden at death (Ikeno *et al.*, 2003). An in-depth discussion of the dwarf mouse models is presented in Chapter 34 of this book.

Liang *et al.* (2003) review seven mouse models with extended lifespan, three mutations (Snell and Ames Dwarf mice and Little mice [$Ghrhr^{lit/lit}$]), and four gene knockouts ($GHR/BP^{-/-}$, $p66^{shc-/-}$, $Igf1R^{+/-}$, and FIRKO). All of the models are loss-of-function changes at the genetic level. Six of the seven models (with the exception of $p66^{shc-/-}$) share many characteristics in spite of involving different genes: growth retardation and reduced body weight, altered metabolism, and alterations in the insulin signaling pathway. This concordance of phenotypes speaks to the importance of metabolism and the insulin-signaling pathway in lifespan determination.

There is some difference of opinion on the value of mutations that shorten lifespan rather than extend it. There are now several mouse mutants that have shortened lifespans, many of them based on mutations identified in human diseases. Clearly it is important when using models that shorten lifespan to distinguish between those that cause premature death due to a specific disease, such as cancer, and those that accelerate many aspects of the aging phenotype. Hasty and Vijg (2004) provide a good discussion of the pros and cons of the mutant rodent models with accelerated aging.

Caloric Restriction

An exciting field in biogerontology research is the emphasis on finding interventions that delay the onset of aging phenotypes or slow the process of aging. While many compounds have some beneficial effects in lower organisms or cell culture, the only intervention proven to extend lifespan and health span in mammals is caloric restriction (CR). When rodents are fed a nutritionally complete diet limited to 60–70% of their ad libitum food intake, they generally live longer, have a reduced disease burden, and show delayed onset of many of the common phenotypes of aging (reviewed in Masoro, 2000). Understanding the mechanisms by which CR extends lifespan and health span will likely lead to new therapeutic interventions to delay the negative aspects of aging. The insulin-signaling pathway is clearly one candidate pathway, as CR reduces age-associated insulin resistance. The action of CR appears to be independent of body weight reduction, as mice subjected to every-other-day fasting did not reduce their total food intake or body weight, yet still experienced the beneficial effect on glucose and insulin levels as seen in standard CR protocols (Anson *et al.*, 2003).

TABLE 33.5
Effect of caloric restriction on lifespan of selected mouse strains[a]

Mouse Strain	Median Lifespan	Maximal Lifespan
C57BL/6	+24%	+24%
DBA/2	−7%	−9%
B6D2F1	+26%	+31%

[a]Data is presented as percent increase (+) or decrease (−) in lifespan of caloric restricted mice as compared to ad libitum fed mice. From Forster *et al.*, 2003.

The CR effect is not universal, however, and different strains show different levels of response to CR. Table 33.5 shows the survival response to CR by male C57BL/6 mice, DBA/2 mice, and the F1 hybrid between them (Forster *et al.*, 2003). Note that while C57BL/6 showed a robust response to CR, with a 24% increase in both median and maximum lifespan, DBA/2 mice showed the opposite response, with a decrease in both median and maximum lifespan. The F1 hybrid, which lived longer than either parental strain under ad libitum (AL) feeding, showed a response to CR similar to the C57BL/6 parental strain. Willott *et al.* (1995) also reported that CR decreased lifespan in DBA/2 mice while increasing it in C57BL/6 mice, and Turturro *et al.* (1999) reported a similar result with male DBA/2 mice showing a 5% increase in lifespan. In the latter study, female DBA/2 showed a 30% increase in lifespan, illustrating a potent gender difference in this strain. In Turturro *et al.*'s study, both male and female C57BL/6 mice showed a similar increase in lifespan of about 40%. While these three studies gave similar results, the differences in lifespan changes due to CR (for example, 24% increase versus 40% increase for C57BL/6) illustrate that other factors, such as substrain, health status, diet formulation and environment, can affect experimental outcomes even when using inbred mice.

Most CR protocols are maintained from young adulthood through the rest of life, and there are conflicting reports on the benefits of CR when it is initiated later in life. Weindruch and Walford (1982) reported that CR initiated in mice in midlife produced beneficial results, while Forster *et al.* (2003) found that when CR was initiated at old age (22–25 months of age), mortality in the first 3 months was actually increased over that seen in the AL controls in 3 strains of mice studied (C57BL/6, DBA/2, B6D2F1). A study in F344BNF1 rats found no significant effect on lifespan and tumor burden when CR was initiated at midlife (17 months) or old age (24 months) (Lipman *et al.*, 1998). However, a study in B6C3F1 hybrid mice, in which CR was initiated at 19 months, produced a 4-month increase in median lifespan over the AL controls (Dhahbi *et al.*, 2004). While CR and AL groups had the same incidence of neoplasms, there was a delay in the onset in the CR group. These findings suggest that CR, or therapeutic targeting of the pathways altered by CR, may have potential for improving health in old age, even when the intervention is begun at midlife.

The effect of long-term CR on health varies by strain and also by pathology. While the general trend is that CR reduces the incidence of, or delays the onset of, most age-related pathologies, there are exceptions to the rule. For example, pancreatic atrophy is common in aged F344 and Brown Norway (BN) rats under AL feeding. Under CR, the incidence of pancreatic atrophy decreases in F344 rats but increases in BN rats (Lipman *et al.*, 1999). CR delays the onset of cataracts in BN rats, but by old age, the incidence of cataracts was the same in CR and AL controls (Wolf *et al.*, 2000). In F344 rats, the age of onset was the same in CR and AL but as the rats aged, the incidence of cataracts increased more in the AL rats than in the CR rats, so that the CR F344 rats showed a reduction in the incidence of cataracts at old age. And CR does not appear to moderate age-related hearing loss in most strains of mice (Willott *et al.*, 1995). These findings serve to illustrate the complexity of biological aging and also the importance of genetic background on the rate of aging and the modulation of the rate of aging through interventions such as caloric restriction.

Husbandry and Environment

One of the advantages of the rodent model is that the health, housing and environment of the colony can be strictly controlled. This is an important consideration because diseases in the experimental population could confound interpretation of results or give misleading results. Specific pathogen-free (SPF) barriers are the norm for commercial rodent breeders for research purposes, but investigators should be aware of the health status of their institution's vivariums, as exposure to new pathogens could affect the immune status and physiological responses. Susceptibility to infectious diseases varies greatly. Mites pose only a minor problem in some strains, but in C57BL/6 mice, mites exacerbate the ulcerative dermatitis common in this strain (Andrews *et al.*, 1994). *Helicobacter* species, first identified in the early 1990s and still endemic in some commercial colonies, cause little or no response in most strains of mice, but can cause inflammatory bowel disease, hepatitis, and hepatocellular cancer in some strains (Brayton *et al.*, 2001). Ward *et al.* (1994) examined 20 strains of mice for *Helicobacter hepaticus*-induced pathology and found only six strains that showed susceptibility to liver disease, with BALB/c mice highly susceptible and C57BL/6 resistant. Hepatic lesions increased with age in both incidence and severity in susceptible strains, and the chronic hepatitis is very persistent. While rats are believed to be resistant to most *Helicobacter* species, there may be effects that surface with more rigorous study.

The aged rodent has special health concerns unrelated to infectious disease, and extra vigilance is required even when they are raised under barrier conditions. Many strains of rodents are prone to developing tumors as they age. Tumors on the feet, jaw and joint areas may cause pain, loss of ambulatory function or difficulty eating even when they are relatively small (Nadon, 2004). Malocclusion, overgrown teeth, resulting from the lack of hard substrates on which to chew, is another problem in aged rodents (Nadon, 2004). Aged rodents should be checked weekly for evidence of tumors or other problems such as malocclusion.

Another consideration is the housing configuration. Rodents are social animals, and most do better in group housing because of the social enrichment. However, group housing can cause stress in rodents due to territorial behavior and aggression. Long-term group housing may lead to some losses due to fight wounds, so this should be taken into consideration when determining sample sizes. Aggression is quite variable between strains, and males are usually more aggressive than females. In the NIA aged rodent colonies, significant aggression is only found in the male BALB/cBy and DBA/2 mice. DBA/2 mice responded with a significant reduction in aggression when provided with Shepherd Shacks®, pressed paper huts that provide a nest environment. Male BALB/cBy mice did not respond favorably to the introduction of Shepherd Shacks®—they shredded them and went back to fighting. This experience illustrates the differences between strains, in that even a basic behavior like aggression has different causes and different solutions. Rats tend to be less aggressive than mice in general, and male F344 rats can even be group housed after being retired from a breeding program.

There are many forms of environmental enrichment available for rodents, including huts, tunnels, chew sticks, and nesting materials. The inclusion of some sort of enrichment appears beneficial under any circumstances, and there is abundant literature that shows that rodents prefer an enriched environment (reviewed by Olsson and Dahelborn, 2002). However, it is important to house experimental and control groups under the same conditions to avoid confounding the interpretation of experimental results. For example, environmental enrichment has positive effects on the brain, including increased plasticity and neuroprotective effects, so in studies of brain aging and cognitive changes it is essential that all groups are housed in identical environments to ensure that changes observed are due to the experimental protocol and not to differences in the environment.

One last concern must be noted when using rodents in biogerontology studies. There are important decisions to be made regarding the appropriate ages to be used, the number of time points required to accurately define age-related changes, and sample sizes that will provide

TABLE 33.6
Resources for studies with aged rodents

Resource	URL
Web portal to NIA-sponsored animal models resources	http://www.nia.nih.gov/ResearchInformation/ScientificResources/
Handbook for information on the NIA aged rodent colonies	http://www.nia.nih.gov/ResearchInformation/ScientificResources/AgedRodentColoniesHandbook/
Handbook for information on the NIA aged rodent tissue bank	http://www.nia.nih.gov/ResearchInformation/ScientificResources/AgedRodentTissueBankHandbook/
NIA aged rodent tissue arrays	http://www.nia.nih.gov/ResearchInformation/ScientificResources/AgedRodentTissueBankHandbook/TissueArrays/
NIA nonhuman primate tissue bank information	http://www.nia.nih.gov/ResearchInformation/ScientificResources/NHPTissueBankHandbook.htm
NIA aged cell bank	http://locus.umdnj.edu/nia
NIA microarray facility	http://www.daf.jhmi.edu/microarray/
Mouse genome informatics	http://www.informatics.jax.org/
Mouse phenome database	http://www.jax.org/phenome
Rat genome database	http://rgd.mcw.edu

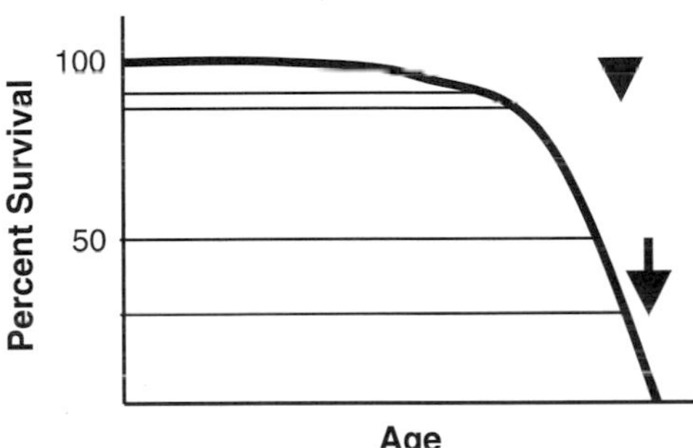

Figure 33.2 A typical survival curve for rodents.

statistical power and allow for expected mortality during the experiment (reviewed in Miller and Nadon, 2000). Figure 33.2 illustrates the need for excess animals when an experiment will require the animals to be maintained for some time. If the age of the animals puts them near the top of the mortality phase of the survival curve (arrowhead), few will die during the experimental period. But if the age of the animals puts them in the middle of the mortality phase (arrow), significantly more animals are needed to allow for the anticipated mortality. It is also important when comparing two different strains to compare biological age instead of chronological age. F344 × BN F1 male rats have a median lifespan of 34 months while F344 male rats have a median lifespan of 24 months. Comparing 24-month-old rats of the two strains would have them in very different points in their biological age. These concerns are covered in more detail in Chapter 4 of this book.

Resources

Getting started in the use of animal models to study biogerontology can be challenging, but there are many resources available to assist in this endeavor. The NIA supports many resources designed to provide the raw materials for studies into the process of normal aging and the prevention, progression and treatment of age-related diseases. Table 33.6 provides web URLs for NIA resources relating to animal models, as well as three informational resources: the Mouse Genome Informatics site, the Mouse Phenome Database, and the Rat Genome Database. The latter resources are valuable repositories of information crucial to deciding on the optimal strain for experimental purposes.

ACKNOWLEDGMENTS

The author deeply appreciates the critical review of the manuscript by Dr. Huber Warner and his support of the development of the NIA resources program, and the helpful discussions with Dr. Richard Miller.

REFERENCES

Andrews, A.G., Dysko, R.C., Spilman, S.C., Kunkel, R.G., Brammer, D.W., and Johnson, K.J. (1994). Immune complex vasculitis with secondary ulcerative dermatitis in aged C57BL/6/NNia mice. *Vet. Pathol. 31*, 293–300.

Anson, R.M., Guo, Z., de Cabo, R., lyun, T., Rios, M., Hagepanos, A., Ingram, D.K., Lane, M.A., and Mattson, M.P. (2003). Intermittent fasting dissociates beneficial effects of dietary restriction on glucose metabolism and neuronal resistance to injury from calorie intake. *Proc. Nat. Acad. Sci.* (USA) *100*, 6216–6220.

Ashe, K.H. (2001). Learning and memory in transgenic mice modeling Alzheimer's disease. *Learning and Memory 8*, 301–308.

Bartke, A., and Brown-Borg, H. (2004). Life extension in the dwarf mouse. *Current Topics Dev. Biol. 63*, 189–225.

Brayton, C., Justice, M., and Montgomery, C.A. (2001). Evaluating mutant mice: Anatomic pathology. *Vet. Pathol. 38*, 1–19.

Brockmann, G.A., and Bevova, M.R. (2002). Using mouse models to dissect the genetics of obesity. *Trends in Genetics 18*, 367–376.

Carroll, L., Voisey, J., and Dall, A.V. (2004). Mouse models of obesity. *Clinics in Dermatology 22*, 345–349.

Chishti, M.A., Yang, D.S., Janus, C., Phinney, A.L., Horne, P., Pearson, J., *et al.* (2001). Early-onset amyloid deposition and cognitive deficits in transgenic mice expressing a double mutant form of amyloid precursor protein 695. *J. Biol. Chem. 276*, 21562–21570.

Conboy, I.M., Conboy, M.J., Smythe, G.M., and Rando, T.A. (2003). Notch-mediated restoration of regenerative potential to aged muscle. *Science 302*, 1575–1577.

Conboy, I.M., and Rando, T.A. (2002). The regulation of Notch signaling controls satellite cell activation and cell fate determination in postnatal myogenesis. *Dev. Cell 3*, 397–409.

Dhahbi, J.M., Kim, H.J., Mote, P.L., Beaver, R.J., and Spindler, S.R. (2004). Temporal linkage between the phenotypic and genomic responses to caloric restriction. *Proc. Nat. Acad. Sci.* (USA) *101*, 5524–5529.

Forster, M.J., Morris, P., and Sohal, R.S. (2003). Genotype and age influence the effect of caloric intake on mortality in mice. *FASEB J. 17*, 690–692.

Hasty, P., and Vijg, J. (2004). Accelerating aging by mouse reverse genetics: A rational approach to understanding longevity. *Aging Cell 3*, 55–65.

Hengemihle, J.M., Long, J.M., Betkey, J., Jucker, M., and Ingram, D.K. (1999). Age-related psychomotor and spatial learning deficits in 129/SvJ mice. *Neurobiol. Aging 20*, 9–18.

Hsiao, K., Chapman, P., Nilsen, S., Eckman, C., Harigaya, Y., Younkin, S., *et al.* (1996). Correlative memory deficits, Aß elevation, and amyloid plaques in transgenic mice. *Science 274*, 99–103.

Ikeno, Y., Bronson, R.T., Hubbard, G.B., Lee, S., and Bartke, A. (2003). Delayed occurrence of fatal neoplastic diseases in Ames dwarf mice: Correlation to extend longevity. *J. Gerontol. 58A*, B291–B296.

Ingram, D.K., Spangler, E.L., Iijima, S., Kou, H.I.H, Greig, N.H., and London, E.D. (1994). Rodent models of memory dysfunction in Alzheimer's Disease and normal aging: Moving beyond the cholinergic hypothesis. *Life Sci. 55*, 2037–2049.

Lee, V. M.-Y., Kenyon, T.K., and Trojanowski, J.Q. (2005). Transgenic animal models of tauopathies. *Biochemica et Biophysica Acta 1739*, 251–259.

Liang, H., Masoro, E.J., Nelson, J.F., Strong, R., McMahan, C.A., and Richardson, A. (2003). Genetic mouse models of extended lifespan. *Exp. Gerontol. 38*, 1353–1364.

Lipman, R.D., Smith, D.E., Blumberg, J.B., and Bronson, R.T. (1998). Effects of caloric restriction or augmentation in adult rats: Longevity and lesion biomarkers of aging. *Aging (Milano) 10*, 463–470.

Lipman, R.D., Dallal, G.E., Bronson, R.T. (1999). Effects of genotype and diet on age-related lesions in ad libitum fed and calorie-restricted F344, BN and BNF3F1 rats. *J. Gerontol. 54A*, B478–B491.

Lipman, R., Galecki, A., Burke, D.T., and Miller, R.A. (2004). Genetic loci that influence cause of death in a heterogeneous mouse stock. *J. Gerontol. 59A*, B977–B983.

Masoro, E.J. (2000). Caloric restriction and aging: An update. *Exp. Gerontol. 35*, 299–305.

Mauvais-Jarvis, F., Kulkarni, R.N., and Kahn, C.R. (2002). Knockout models are useful tools to dissect the pathophysiology and genetics of insulin resistance. *Clinical Endocrinol. 57*, 1–9.

Miller, R.A., and Nadon, N.L. (2000). Principles of animal use for gerontological research. *J. Gerontol. 55A*, B117–B123.

Miller, R.A., and Chrisp, C. (2002). T cell subset patterns that predict resistance to spontaneous lymphoma, mammary adenocarcinoma, and fibrosarcoma in mice. *J. Immunol. 169*, 1619–1625.

Mountz, J.D., Van Zant, G.G., Zhang, H.G., Grizzle, W.E., Ahmed, R., Williams, R.W., and Hsu, H.C. (2001). Genetic dissection of age-related changes of immune function in mice. *Scand. J. Immunol. 54*, 10–20.

Nadon, N.L. (2004). Maintaining aged rodents for biogerontology research. *Lab Animal 33*, 36–41.

Naggert, J.K., Paigen, B., Svenson, K.L., and Peters, L.L. (2003). Diet effects on bone mineral density and content, body composition, and plasma glucose, leptin, and insulin levels. Mouse Phenome Database, the Jackson Laboratory, http://www.jax.org/phenome, MPD143, analyzed 12/13/04.

Oddo, A., Caccamo, A., Kitazawa, M., Tseng, B.P., and LaFerla, F. (2003). Amyloid deposition precedes tangle formation in a triple transgenic model of Alzheimer's disease. *Neurobiol. Aging 24*, 1063–1070.

Olsson, I.A., and Dahlborn, K. (2002). Improving housing conditions for laboratory mice: A review of "environmental enrichment." *Lab Animal 36*, 243–270.

Phinney, A.L., Horne, P., Yang, J., Janus, C., Bergeron, C., and Westaway, D. (2003). Mouse models of Alzheimer's disease: The long and filamentous road. *Neurol. Res. 25*, 590–600.

Roderick, T.H., Langley, S.H., and Leiter, E.H. (1985). Some unusual genetic characteristics of BALB/c and evidence for genetic variation among BALB/c substrains. *Current Topics in Microbiology and Immunology 122*, 9–18.

Seyfried, T.N., Glaser, G.H., Yu, R.K., and Palayoor, S.T. (1986). Inherited convulsive disorders in mice. *Adv. Neurol. 44*, 115–133.

Tschöp, M., and Heiman, M.L. (2001). Rodent obesity models: An overview. *Exp. Clin. Endocrinol. Diabetes 109*, 307–319.

Turner, C.H., Roeder, R.K., Wieczorek, A., Foroud, T., Liu, G., and Peacock, M. (2001). Variability in skeletal mass, structure, and biomechanical properties among inbred strains of rats. *J. Bone Miner. Res. 16*, 1532–1539.

Turturro, A., Witt, W.W., Lewis, S., Hass, B.S., Lipman, R.D., and Hart, R.W. (1999). Growth curves and survival characteristics of the animals used in the biomarkers of aging program. *J. Gerontol. 54A*, B492–B501.

Uysal, K.T., Scheja, L., Wiesbrock, S.M., Bonner-Weir, S., and Hotamisligil, G.S. (2000). Improved glucose and lipid metabolism in genetically obese mice lacking aP2. *Endocrinology 141*, 3388–3396.

Ward, J.M., Anver, M.R., Haines, D.C., and Benveniste, R.E. (1994). Chronic active hepatitis in mice caused by helicobacter hepaticus. *Am. J. Pathol. 145*, 959–968.

Weindruch, R., and Walford, R.L. (1982). Dietary restriction in mice beginning at 1 year of age: Effect on life-span and spontaneous cancer incidence. *Science 215*, 1415–1418.

Willott, J.F., Erway, L.C., Archer, J.R., and Harrison, D.E. (1995). Genetics of age-related hearing loss in mice. II. Strain differences and effects of caloric restriction on cochlear pathology and evoked response thresholds. *Hearing Res. 88*, 143–155.

Wolf, N.S., Li, Y., Pendergrass, W., Schmeider, C., and Turturro, A. (2000). Normal mouse and rat strains as models for age-related cataract and the effect of caloric restriction on its development. *Exp. Eye Res. 70*, 683–692.

Wolf, N., Galecki, A., Lipman, R., Chen, S., Smith-Wheelock, M., Burke, D., and Miller, R. (2004). Quantitative trait locus mapping for age-related cataract severity and synechia prevalence using four way cross mice. *Investigative Ophthalmology & Visual Science 45*, 1922–1929.

34

Life Extension in the Dwarf Mouse

Andrzej Bartke

Dwarf mice are remarkably long-lived. Congenital deficiency of growth hormone (GH), prolactin, and thyroid-stimulating hormone (TSH) due to mutations at the Pit1 or Prop1 loci, as well as GH resistance due to targeted disruption of the GH receptor gene lead to major increase in both average and maximal lifespan. Prolonged longevity of Snell dwarf (Pit1dw), Ames dwarf (Prop1df), and GHRKO mice is associated with a major extension of "health span" and multiple symptoms of delayed aging. Suspected mechanisms of prolonged longevity of hypopituitary and GH resistant mice include reduced peripheral levels of IGF-1 and insulin, enhanced sensitivity to insulin actions, reduced generation of reactive oxygen species, enhanced anti-oxidant defenses and stress resistance, and delayed onset of fatal neoplastic and nonneoplastic disease. Although negative correlation of body size and longevity applies to genetically normal mice and to other species, it remains to be determined whether reduced GH signaling delays aging in all mammals. However, the ability of reduced IGF-1/insulin signaling to prolong longevity applies broadly and perhaps universally.

Introduction

The realization that growth hormone (GH), insulin-like growth factor 1 (IGF-1), and insulin play important roles in the control of mammalian aging is a relatively recent development. In 1996, it was reported that hypopituitary Ames dwarf mice live significantly longer than their normal siblings (Brown-Borg *et al.*, 1996). These animals have primary deficiency of GH, prolactin (PRL), and thyroid-stimulating hormone (TSH) with secondary suppression of circulating levels of IGF-1, insulin, and thyroid hormones (details and references in the next section of this chapter). Soon afterwards, Kimura *et al.* (1997) demonstrated that mammalian IGF-1 receptor and insulin receptor genes exhibit significant homology to the daf-2 gene in a round worm, *Caenorhabditis elegans* (*C. elegans*), a key gene in the signaling pathway that controls aging and longevity in this species. Research results reported during the next few years provided evidence for prolonged longevity in another mouse mutant deficient in GH, PRL, and TSH, and in mice with various spontaneous or induced mutations affecting only the somatotropic (GH/IGF-1) axis. Moreover, several genes involved in the control of aging in yeast, *C. elegans* and the fruit fly *Drosophila melanogaster* were shown to be homologous to genes related to IGF-1 and insulin signaling in mammals (reviews in Guarente and Kenyon, 2000; Tatar *et al.*, 2003). The picture that emerges from these studies is that an ancient pathway widely conserved during evolution is involved in the control of aging in organisms from distant taxonomic groups and that in mammals this pathway is represented by IGF-1 and insulin, by their receptors, and by proteins that become activated after these receptors bind the corresponding ligands.

In this chapter, we will list key characteristics of mice in which mutation of a single gene related to GH synthesis or action is associated with a significant extension of longevity. We will also review mechanisms which are suspected of mediating the effects of altered somatotropic signaling on aging and longevity, and briefly discuss controversies surrounding the relationship of GH to aging. Finally, we will provide some information on the husbandry and breeding of long-lived mutant dwarf mice.

Origin and Characteristics of Snell Dwarf and Ames Dwarf Mice

In laboratory stocks of house mice (*Mus musculus*), several spontaneous mutations cause hereditary dwarfism. The first mutation with a major impact on growth and adult body size was described by George Snell three quarters of a century ago (Snell, 1929). This mutation was originally named dwarf, genetic symbol dw, but subsequently was referred to by various names including Snell–Bagg dwarf mice and Snell–Smith mice and is now known as Snell dwarf, Snell dwarf mouse or Snell dwarf (dw) mutant of the Pituitary factor1 (Pit1) gene, $Pit1^{dw}$. Snell dwarfism is due to a recessive autosomal mutation of the Pit1 gene located on chromosome 16 (Li *et al.*, 1990). Animals homozygous for this mutation appear to be normal at birth, but their growth soon begins to lag behind their normal +/+ and dw/+ siblings and they reach approximately 1/3 of the adult body weight of normal mice. Early studies of Snell dwarf mice demonstrated that these animals lack GH-and TSH-producing cells in the pituitary, are GH deficient and hypothyroid, and readily grow in response to injected GH (reviewed in Grüneberg, 1952; Bartke, 1979a). Reciprocal transplants of anterior pituitaries between dwarf and normal animals provided clear evidence that hormonal deficits and reduced growth in these animals are due to inherited anomalies in the pituitary rather than to altered hypothalamic control of pituitary function (Carsner and Rennels, 1960). Subsequent studies resulted in the demonstration that in addition to deficiency of GH and TSH, Snell dwarf mice also lack PRL (Bartke, 1965; reviewed in Bartke, 1979b).

Homozygous expression of $Pit1^{dw\text{-}J}$ (Jackson dwarf mouse), a mutation that independently arose at the same (Pit1) locus, produces the same phenotype as Snell dwarfism (Eicher and Beamer, 1980). Compound heterozygotes $Pit1^{dw}/Pit1^{dw\text{-}J}$ are dwarf, do not seem to differ from homozygous $Pit1^{dw}$ mice, and have been used in research on aging (Flurkey *et al.*, 2001).

Another autosomal recessive mutation producing dwarfism in the mouse was described in 1961 by Schaible and Gowen. It was shown to be genetically unrelated to Snell dwarfism and located on a different chromosome, and was named Ames dwarf, genetic symbol df (Schaible and Gowen, 1961). After cloning of the affected gene on chromosome 11, Ames dwarf became known also as a mutant of the Prophet of Pit1 (Prop1), $Prop1^{df}$ (Sorenson *et al.*, 1996). Mice homozygous for the Ames dwarf mutation that appear identical to Snell dwarfs and similar to Snell dwarf mice are GH, TSH, and PRL deficient (Bartke, 1979a, 1979b). Although the primary hormonal deficits and the resulting phenotype of Snell and Ames dwarf mice appear to be identical, detailed comparisons of the effects of these mutations expressed on the same genetic background have not been made, and subtle differences may exist. For example, the time course of postnatal changes in the number of hypothalamic (tuberoinfundibular) dopaminenergic neurons was recently shown to differ between Snell and Ames dwarf mice (Phelps, 2004).

Studies of the genetic control of development and cytodifferentiation of the anterior pituitary in fetal mice lead to the demonstration that the Prop1 and Pit1 genes, which are mutated in the Ames and Snell dwarfs, respectively, are normally sequentially expressed during days 12.5–15.5 of embryonic development. The Prop1 gene controls differentiation of Pit1 producing cells that give rise to cell lineages that eventually develop into somatotrophs, lactotrophs and thyrotrophs, i.e., adenohypophyseal cells that produce GH, PRL, and TSH (Li *et al.*, 1990; Sorenson *et al.*, 1996). In the adult, the normal product of the Pit1 gene controls expression of GH, PRL, and β subunit of TSH by binding to promoters of the corresponding genes. Mutations of either of these genes block normal pathways of the differentiation of GH, PRL and TSH producing cells (Sornson *et al.*, 1996) and thus produce primary deficiency of these hormones. Recent study of early postnatal development of the pituitary in Ames dwarfs revealed enhanced apoptosis and reduced proliferation (Ward *et al.*, 2005).

Failure to synthesize and secrete GH, PRL and TSH from the pituitary leads to a host of secondary hormonal deficits and phenotypic alterations, including reductions in hepatic expression of IGF-1, circulating IGF-1 levels, growth and adult body size, hypothyroidism, reduced body temperature and spontaneous locomotory activity, reduced circulating insulin and glucose levels, altered regulation of carbohydrate metabolism, delayed puberty, and female sterility due to luteal failure (reviewed in Bartke and Brown-Borg, 2004). Other characteristics of Snell and Ames dwarf mice include alterations in the profiles of gene expression, body composition, immune function, fibroblast responses to cytotoxic stress, and also significantly extended longevity, which is the subject of this chapter. For more detailed review of the characteristics of Snell and Ames dwarf mice and references to the corresponding studies, the reader is referred to recent reviews (Bartke, 2000; Bartke *et al.*, 2001a; Bartke and Brown-Borg, 2004).

Longevity of Dwarf Mice

Although Ames and Snell dwarf mice are now used in many laboratories to study the mechanisms of extended longevity, the evidence that they have increased lifespan was obtained only recently. Curiously, one of the first studies to address this issue concluded that Snell dwarf mice are extremely short lived because they are immunodeficient and succumb to infectious diseases at a very early age (Fabris *et al.*, 1972). These findings must have been unique to this particular population or to the husbandry conditions, because shortly afterwards other investigators working with Snell dwarf mice reported that they did not encounter early mortality of the dwarfs (Shire, 1973; Schneider, 1976). However, these reports did not provide any information on the average or maximal longevity of the dwarf mice. In contrast to the study of Fabris *et al.* (1972), in a paper published in the same year, Silberberg (1972) referred to Snell dwarf mice as having an "unusually long lifespan" and reported data from dwarfs that were killed at the ages ranging up to 41 months. Although no data on longevity or survival plots were provided or referenced, this was the first mention of extended longevity of these mutants. Moreover, this report included important evidence for delayed aging of joint cartilage in Snell dwarf as compared to normal mice and absence of osteoarthrosis in the dwarfs (Silberberg, 1972).

In 1996, Brown-Borg *et al.* reported that Ames dwarf mice live significantly longer than their normal siblings with the increase in average lifespan being over 45% in males and over 60% in females (Brown-Borg *et al.*, 1996). The survival plot included in this report suggests that the maximal lifespan of Ames dwarf mice was similarly increased and that there was a delayed onset of age-related mortality in the dwarfs with little change in the slope of the survival curve. Delayed longevity of Ames dwarf, compared to normal mice, was replicated in subsequent studies and in animals fed different diets (Bartke *et al.*, 2001b, 2004).

Flurkey *et al.* (2001) reported significantly extended longevity of Snell dwarf mice with an increase of average lifespan of 42%. The same report contained important evidence for delayed aging of the immune system and collagen in Snell dwarf as compared to normal mice (Flurkey *et al.*, 2001). The conclusion that the biological process of aging is delayed and/or slowed down in both Snell and Ames dwarf mice compared to normal animals received further support from the studies of cognitive function (Kinney *et al.*, 2001a) and incidence and severity of neoplastic and nonneoplastic disease (Ikeno *et al.*, 2003; Vergara *et al.*, 2004) in these animals. Extension of both the average and the maximal lifespan in Ames and Snell dwarf mice is also consistent with this conclusion. Thus prolonged longevity of Snell dwarf ($Pit1^{dw}$), Ames dwarf ($Prop1^{df}$), and GHRKO mice is associated with a major extension of "health span" and multiple symptoms of delayed aging.

Studies in Snell and Ames dwarf mice provided clear evidence that, similar to what was discovered earlier in yeast, worms, and flies (reviewed in Guarente and Kenyon, 2000; Tatar *et al.*, 2003), mutations of a single gene can produce a delay of aging and significant increase in life expectancy in a mammal. Similar extension of mean and maximal longevity in two types of dwarfism which are due to mutations of different genes located on different chromosomes but result in essentially identical defects in endocrine function indicates that prolonged longevity is due to these endocrine deficits rather than to some other unknown effects of Prop1 and or Pit1 mutations. Results obtained in mice with mutations or targeted disruption of genes related specifically to somatotropic (GH/IGF-1) signaling suggest that deficiency of GH is an important and probably the main cause of prolonged longevity of Ames and Snell dwarf mice. These results are discussed below.

Growth Hormone Receptor Knockout Mice

The first animal model of GH resistance was produced by Zhou *et al.* (1997) by targeted disruption of the GH receptor/GH binding protein gene in the mouse. GHR/GHBP knockout mice (hereafter referred to as GHRKO) lack functional GH receptor and therefore exhibit GH resistance manifested by a dramatic decrease in circulating IGF-1 levels, reduced growth, and approximately 60% reduction in adult body weight. GHRKO mice are of nearly normal size at birth, exhibit profound growth deficits starting before weaning, but thrive under standard laboratory conditions and most of them are fertile. Plasma GH levels are elevated presumably due to lack of negative GH feedback. In addition to reduced IGF-1 and diminutive size, GHRKO animals exhibit greatly reduced insulin levels, small reduction in circulating levels of thyroxine and 3′,3,5-triiodothyronine, hyperprolactinemia, reduced levels of follicle stimulating hormone (FSH), delayed puberty, and various deficits in reproductive function (Zhou *et al.*, 1997, Hauck *et al.*, 2001; Chandrashekar *et al.*, 2004).

In 2000, Coschigano *et al.* reported that the GHRKO (−/−) mice live significantly longer than both normal (+/+) and heterozygous (+/−) animals from the same population. The increase in average lifespan ranged from 38 to 55%, depending on the gender and genotype of the control (−/− or +/−) (Coschigano *et al.*, 2000). The observation of prolonged longevity of the GHRKO as compared to normal mice was replicated in subsequent studies of the same author (Coschigano *et al.*, 2003) as well as in another laboratory in animals with different genetic background (Bartke, 2002). Importantly, Coschigano *et al.* (2003) reported significantly extended lifespan of GHRKO mice backcrossed to the long-living C57BL/6 strain. Studies of cognitive function (Kinney *et al.*, 2001b; Kinney-Forshee *et al.*, 2004) and end of life pathology in GHRKO mice (Ikeno and Bartke, unpublished) suggest that these animals, similar to Snell and Ames dwarf mice, experience delayed aging.

Roughly comparable life extension in GHRKO mice with isolated GH resistance and in dwarf mice deficient in GH, PRL, and TSH suggests that reduced somatotropic (GH/IGF-1) signaling is an important determinant of delayed aging and prolonged longevity in each of these mutants.

Other Mutations Affecting the Somatotropic Axis

Evidence for prolonged longevity of mice with reduced activity of the somatotropic axis is not limited to results obtained in GHRKO, $Pit1^{dw}$ and $Prop1^{df}$ mice. Flurkey and his colleagues reported that "little" mice with a mutation of the GH releasing hormone (GHRH) receptor and the resulting GH deficiency live approximately 25% longer than normal mice if fed a low-fat diet (Flurkey *et al.*, 2001). "Little" ($GHRHR^{lit}$) mice exhibit profound, although not complete, suppression of circulating GH levels and reduced rate of postnatal growth. Body weight of young adults is reduced to about 50% of normal. Afterwards, this difference in body weight gradually diminishes due to a combination of slow growth and progressive development of obesity in little mice. If this mutation is maintained on the C57BL/6 background and the animals are fed a standard diet that contains 7% fat, the obesity of "little" mice is very pronounced, and their lifespan tends to be comparable to that of normal mice. Reducing fat content of the diet to 4% prevents extreme obesity of these mutants and uncovers their propensity to outlive their normal siblings (Flurkey *et al.*, 2001).

Targeted disruption of IGF-1 or IGF-1 receptor (IGF1R) genes produces animals with profoundly suppressed fetal growth, low birth weight, and high perinatal mortality. However, animals heterozygous for the "knock out" of the IGF1R gene (IGF1R+/−) exhibit a fairly small reduction in postnatal growth, are healthy and fertile, and have increased resistance to the lethal oxidative stress-related effects of paraquat. Female IGF1R +/− mice live 33% longer than normal females from the same stock (Holzenberger *et al.*, 2003). Males tend to live longer, but the 50% difference in lifespan between IGF1R +/− and normal animals were smaller and not statistically significant. A 50% reduction in the levels of IGF-1 receptors in various organs of IGF1R +/− mice suggests that these animals are partially resistant to IGF-1. Important implications of these findings include support for the role of IGF-1 signaling in the control of mammalian longevity and a demonstration that a modest reduction of somatotropic signaling that does not lead to overt dwarfism or compromised fertility can be sufficient to increase stress resistance, slow down aging, and increase lifespan. Although the role of IGF-1 in the control of aging was strongly suggested by the results obtained in GHRKO "little" and hypopituitary dwarf mice, the potential role of GH actions not mediated by IGF-1 could not be evaluated in these animals. Although the interpretation of the exciting findings of extended longevity of IGF1R+/− mice is somewhat complicated by a short lifespan of normal females of the employed stock, this work stands out as the first report that specifically associates reduced IGF-1 signaling with extended longevity in a mammal.

Studies in other types of genetically altered mice provide further support for the role of IGF-1 in the control of aging. Preliminary evidence suggests that lifespan is increased in mice with reduced IGF-1 levels due to a hypomorphic mutation of the IGF-1 gene (C. Sell; personal communication). Association of prolonged longevity with reduced plasma IGF-1 levels was also described in transgenic mice expressing urokinase-type plasminogen activator in the brain (Miskin and Masos, 1997). In these animals, suppression of IGF-1 may be due to reduced food consumption, thus resembling the situation in genetically normal animals subjected to caloric restriction (Masoro, 2001).

In contrast to numerous examples of extended longevity in animals with reduced levels of GH and/or IGF-1 or with GH or IGF-1 resistance, lifespan was not increased in transgenic mice overexpressing a GH antagonist (Coschigano *et al.*, 2003). In these animals, the action of endogenous GH is compromised as evidenced by reduced postnatal growth and adult body size, but lifespan is not affected. GH antagonist transgenic mice become extremely obese, resembling the phenotype of GH deficient GHRHR^{lit} mice, and it can be speculated that obesity masks or counteracts the effects of reduced GH signaling on longevity. Examining the effects of reduced dietary fat intake on longevity of GH antagonist transgenic mice would be of considerable interest.

Data concerning the relationship of somatotropic signaling to aging in other mammalian species will be discussed later in this chapter.

Cognitive Function of Ames Dwarf Mice; Possible Role of Hippocampal IGF-1 Expression

As mentioned earlier in this chapter, hypopituitary mouse mutants live much longer than their normal siblings and also exhibit various symptoms of delayed aging. In Ames dwarf mice this includes maintenance of youthful levels of cognitive function into a very advanced age. Studies conducted by Kinney (Kinney *et al.*, 2001a) using inhibitory avoidance task and other behavioral tests resulted in two striking and largely unexpected observations. First, learning and memory as measured by these tests did not differ between young adult dwarf mice and normal animals from the same stock. Second, the examined measures of cognitive function in old (22–29 months old) dwarf mice did not differ from values measured in young dwarf or normal mice. This was in contrast to results obtained in old normal mice that exhibited the expected age-related significant decline in learning and memory. These results were surprising and indeed opposite to what might have been expected in animals with profound suppression of circulating IGF-1 and thyroid hormone levels (details and references in Sun *et al.*, 2005a,b). The role of thyroid hormones in the development of the central nervous systems (CNS) and in adult brain function is very well documented. Perhaps Ames dwarfs benefit from exposure to maternal thyroid hormones via placental circulation and milk and from the amounts of thyroid hormones that can be produced in the absence of TSH stimulation. Coexistence of normal (and in aging animals, superior) cognitive function with the absence of GH and the resulting suppression of hepatic IGF-1 expression and IGF-1 deficiency is more difficult to explain. IGF-1 has major and very well documented neurostimulatory and neuroprotective effects. Eliminating IGF-1 production by targeted disruption of the IGF-1 gene in the mouse leads to severe defects in brain development (Cheng *et al.*, 2003). Deletion of the IGF-1 gene in the human is associated with mental retardation (Woods *et al.*, 1996). This discrepancy led Liou Sun in our laboratory to examine IGF-1 expression in the hippocampus of Ames dwarf mice, a brain region critically involved in learning and memory. His studies resulted in the demonstration that in both young adult and aging dwarf mice the levels of IGF-1 mRNA in the hippocampus do not differ from the levels measured in the hippocampus of normal animals of the same age (Sun *et al.*, 2005a). Moreover, IGF-1 protein levels in the same tissues were significantly higher in dwarfs than in normal mice (Sun *et al.*, 2005a). In keeping with the elevation of hippocampal IGF-1 levels, and the role of IGF-1 in the control of neuronal proliferation, the number of proliferating cells in the granular cell layer and the subgranular zone of the dentate gyrus in the hippocampus was greater in young adult Ames dwarfs than in normal animals of the same age (Sun *et al.*, 2005b). Results of labeling with specific neuronal and glial markers suggested that most of the proliferating cells in this region were neurons (Sun *et al.*, 2005b).

Although association of different phenotypic characteristics cannot prove causality, we strongly suspect that normal cognitive function in Ames dwarfs and its preservation during aging are related to enhanced IGF-1 expression in the hippocampus. These findings also indicate that Ames dwarf mice cannot be regarded simply as "IGF-1 deficient" in spite of undetectable levels of IGF-1 in peripheral circulation, because local IGF-1 levels in the various organs may be biologically significant or even elevated. This conclusion is consistent with prior evidence that IGF-1 expression is GH-dependent only in some tissues, and IGF-1 levels in the brain are either unrelated or only weakly related to peripheral levels of GH (Lupu *et al.*, 2001). The etiology of the elevation of IGF-1 protein levels in the dwarf hippocampus is unknown, and we can only suspect that some compensatory mechanisms or local (CNS) expression of GH or other regulatory factors are involved in the presumably altered post-transcriptional control of biosynthesis of IGF-1.

These observations pertain also to some broader issues concerning organ-specific or, more likely, cell type–specific mechanisms that may account for the phenotypic characteristics of animals expressing various "longevity assurance genes." Overexpression of antioxidant enzymes limited to the CNS was reported to extend the life of fruit flies (Phillips *et al.*, 2000), and longevity of two fruit fly mutants, with altered insulin-like signaling, was recently linked to the action of the corresponding genes in the heart (Wessells *et al.*, 2004). Without additional data, we can only speculate about the relative roles of the absence of GH action in the liver, adipose tissue, pancreatic beta cells and other targets, the reduction of IGF-1 levels in peripheral circulation, and maintenance of IGF-1 biosynthesis in the brain of long-lived mutant mice.

Altered Insulin Signaling as a Potential Mechanism of Extended Longevity

The mechanism or, more likely, mechanisms linking reduced somatotropic signaling with delayed aging remain to be identified. Our laboratory is interested in the possibility that alterations in insulin signaling, control of blood glucose levels, and expression of insulin-related genes are among the mechanisms involved. In Ames and Snell dwarf mice, levels of both insulin and glucose in peripheral circulation are significantly reduced (Borg *et al.*, 1995; Hsieh *et al.*, 2002). In GHRKO mice, insulin levels are dramatically suppressed while glucose levels are modestly reduced (Coschigano *et al.*, 2003). Coexistence of reduced insulin and low glucose levels in the long-lived mutant mice implies enhanced insulin sensitivity. In support of this conclusion, administration of insulin was shown to cause significantly greater suppression of plasma glucose levels in GHRKO and Ames dwarf mice than in age- and sex-matched normal animals from the same stock (Dominici *et al.*, 2002; Liu *et al.*, 2004).

There is considerable indirect evidence to support the view that these changes in the insulin control of glucose metabolism may contribute to extended longevity. Reduced levels of insulin and glucose, and enhanced insulin sensitivity, are found in genetically normal mice and rats subjected to caloric restriction, a dietary intervention that reliably delays aging and extends longevity in laboratory stocks of these rodents (Masoro, 2001). A contrasting phenotype of hyperinsulinemia and insulin resistance is associated with reduced lifespan and various symptoms of accelerated aging in transgenic mice overexpressing GH (Bartke, 2003). Insulin resistance represents an important risk factor for major age-related diseases in the human (Facchini *et al.*, 2001).

Chronic elevation of insulin levels and hyperglycemia are believed to promote aging (Parr, 1999). Insulin effects are likely mediated by its action on mitochondrial function (Lambert *et al.*, 2004), while elevated glucose levels can lead to formation of advanced glycation products (AGE) and damage of proteins (particularly those with a low turnover) by nonenzymatic glycation (Baynes and Monnier, 1989). There is recent evidence that this type of damage to hemoglobin, as measured by the levels of HbA1c, is a risk factor for cardiovascular disease and all-cause mortality in nondiabetic individuals (Khaw *et al.*, 2004).

In contrast to increased insulin sensitivity of Ames dwarf and GHRKO mice, the ability of these animals to dispose of an injected glucose load is reduced rather than increased (Dominici *et al.*, 2002; Liu *et al.*, 2004). This is presumably due to reduced ability to release insulin in response to an increase in plasma glucose levels. Diminished insulin responses to exogenous glucose and also to re-feeding after a fast (Bonkowski and Bartke, unpublished) may, in turn, reflect reduced mass of insulin-secreting β cells in the GHRKO mouse (Liu *et al.*, 2004) and reduced number of large islets in the pancreas of Ames dwarfs (Parsons *et al.*, 1995). Reduced responses of the skeletal muscle to insulin represent another factor likely to contribute to the counterintuitive association of improved insulin sensitivity and reduced glucose tolerance in these mutants. Acute effects of exogenous insulin on the early steps of insulin signaling are enhanced in the liver of Ames dwarf and GHRKO mice, but reduced in the skeletal muscle of these animals (Dominici *et al.*, 2000, 2002, 2003, and unpublished data). We suspect that the increased responses of the liver to insulin in Ames dwarf and GHRKO mice may account for the enhanced ability of insulin to suppress glucose levels while reduced insulin responsiveness of the skeletal muscle may contribute to the limited ability of these animals to dispose of glucose.

Reduced insulin/IGF-1/GH signaling in the liver of Snell dwarf mice is associated with decreased activity of the translational initiation pathway presumably leading to down-regulation of protein synthesis (Hsieh and Papaconstantinou, 2004).

Studies of gene expression in different insulin target organs and measurements of plasma adipokine levels suggest some possible mechanisms of altered insulin signaling in Ames dwarf and GHRKO mice. In the liver of 18-month-old Ames dwarfs, the levels of PPARγ mRNA and proteins, as well as the levels of insulin receptor, IRS-1, and IRS-1 proteins, were higher than the corresponding values measured in normal mice (Masternak *et al.*, 2004). PPARγ is an important regulator of insulin sensitivity and a target of antidiabetic drugs: IRS1 and 2 play a key role in transduction of insulin signals.

In the liver of GHRKO mice of similar age, the levels of phosphorylated (active) Akt were reduced, presumably reflecting reduced strength of the insulin signal in these profoundly hypoinsulinemic mice (Al-Regaiey *et al.*, 2005). The expression of a PPAR coactivator, PGC-1α, was increased in the liver of GHRKO mice with marked elevations of both PGC-1α mRNA and PGC-1α protein (Al-Regaiey *et al.*, 2005). PGC-1α is a key mediator of the effects of energy intake on metabolism and an activator of the gluconeogenetic pathway, and there is increasing evidence for its involvement in the regulation of lifespan and mediating the antiaging actions of caloric restriction (Rodgers *et al.*, 2005). Consistent with reduced insulin signaling and increased expression of the PGC-1α, expression of genes related to gluconeogenesis (PEPCK, G6Pase) was elevated in GHRKO as compared to normal mice (Al-Regaiey *et al.*, 2005). Microarray analysis of the broad profile of hepatic gene expression in Ames dwarf mice provided evidence that gluconeogenesis and β-oxidation of fatty acids are increased in these animals similar to the situation described in GHRKO mice. Results of this study also suggested that improved insulin sensitivity of Ames dwarfs may be related to reduced Gas6 and PTEN signaling in the liver (Tsuchiya *et al.*, 2004).

Recent studies suggest that secretory products of the adipocytes, collectively referred to as adipokines, have major effects on insulin sensitivity and that visceral fat is particularly important in this regard. In both Ames dwarf and GHRKO mice, the levels of adiponectin, an adipokine known to sensitize the animal to the actions of insulin, are significantly elevated (Al-Regaiey *et al.*, 2005).

Moreover, expression of IL-6 and TNF-α, adipokines that promote insulin resistance, was reduced in the adipocytes of Ames dwarfs as compared to adipocytes of normal mice, while plasma levels of adiponectin were increased (Wang and Bartke, unpublished data). The increase in adiponectin and decrease in IL-6 and TNF-α presumably contribute to increased insulin sensitivity of long-lived mutant mice and imply that the secretory profile of their adipocytes is different from the values encountered in normal animals. Obesity is normally associated with reduced adiponectin levels, and yet in GHRKO mice, adiponectin levels are elevated in spite of increased adiposity (Berryman *et al.*, 2004). In Ames dwarfs, percent of body fat is somewhat greater in young adults than in the corresponding normal mice and increases with age. In older adult dwarfs it is relatively lower than in normal animals due to greater age-related increases in adiposity of normal mice (Heiman *et al.*, 2003). Increased plasma adiponectin levels in Ames dwarf as compared to normal mice were detected at the age of 18 months when percentage of body fat presumably did not differ between the genotypes (Heiman *et al.*, 2003). We do not know whether the unexpected association of normal or increased percent body fat, with significantly increased circulating levels of adiponectin in Ames dwarf and GHRKO mice, may be related to different distribution of the adipocytes among different (e.g., visceral vs. subcutaneous) fat depots.

Other Mechanisms of Prolonged Longevity of Dwarf Mice

While reduced insulin release and enhanced responsiveness of the liver (and possibly other organs) to insulin appear to be important in mediating the effects of hypopituitarism and GH resistance on longevity, related and possibly unrelated mechanisms are undoubtedly also involved.

Reduced insulin signaling combined with reduced IGF-1 levels and hypothyroidism (which is modest in GHRKO and profound in Ames and Snell dwarf mice) is expected to lead to reduced oxidative metabolism. Oxygen consumption in Snell dwarf mice was reported to be reduced (Grüneberg, 1952), and body core temperature is slightly reduced in GHRKO (Hauck *et al.*, 2001) and markedly suppressed in Ames dwarf mice (Hunter *et al.*, 1999). Reductions in oxidative metabolism and reduced action of insulin on mitochondria would also be expected to result in reduced generation of hydrogen peroxide and a decrease in the total levels of reactive oxygen species (ROS). In support of this hypothesis, reduced H_2O_2 generation was observed in the mitochondria isolated from livers of Ames dwarf mice (Brown-Borg *et al.*, 2001).

There is also evidence that in addition to reduced levels of ROS, Ames dwarf mice have improved ability to eliminate free radicals and thus may be protected from ROS-induced oxidative damage. A series of studies by Brown-Borg and her colleagues provided evidence that the levels of antioxidant enzymes, including catalase, two forms of superoxide dismutase (SOD1 and SOD2), and glutathione peroxidase, are generally increased in various organs of Ames dwarf mice including the liver, kidney, heart and brain (Brown-Borg and Rakoczy, 2000, 2005; Brown-Borg *et al.*, 2001). Consistent with reduced generation of ROS and improved antioxidant defenses, oxidative damage to proteins, lipids, nuclear and mitochondrial DNA is smaller in Ames dwarfs than in normal mice (Brown-Borg *et al.*, 2001; Sanz *et al.*, 2002). There is also evidence for improved antioxidant defenses in GHRKO mice, although alterations in the activity of antioxidant enzymes were less consistent in these animals than in Ames dwarf mice (Hauck *et al.*, 2002).

Since oxidative damage is believed to represent a key mechanism of aging, these findings provide a very plausible explanation for extended longevity of hypopituitary and GH-resistant mice. Reduced generation of ROS and improved antioxidant defenses are likely acting downstream from reduced IGF-1 and insulin signaling and provide a final effector pathway for the life-extending actions of these hormonal alterations.

In further support of the role of improved antioxidant defenses in the longevity of dwarf mice, fibroblasts isolated from these animals are more resistant to oxidative cytotoxic stress than fibroblasts derived from normal mice (Murakami *et al.*, 2003; Salmon *et al.*, 2005). Other mechanisms that could contribute to delayed aging and prolonged longevity of dwarf mice include altered activity and responses of the hypothalamic–pituitary–adrenal axis (Hauck *et al.*, 2001; Al-Regaiey *et al.*, 2005), delayed sexual maturation (Chandrashekar *et al.*, 2004 and unpublished data), reduced activity of the hypothalamic–pituitary–gonadal axis (reviewed in Bartke, 2000; Bartke and Brown-Borg, 2004; Chandrashekar *et al.*, 2004), and/or some presently undefined characteristics that correlate with reduced postnatal growth and diminutive body size. Early sexual development and fecundity are, in general, negatively correlated with lifespan, even though many important exceptions are also known to exist (Partridge *et al.*, 2005). However, the importance of hypogonadism in the ethiology of longevity of mutant mice discussed in this chapter is unlikely. Comparable relative extension of lifespan was detected in Snell dwarf mice which are severely hypogonadal and sterile, and in GHRKO mice which exhibit relatively minor deficits in gonadal function and can successfully reproduce (Zhou *et al.*, 1997; Chandrashekar *et al.*, 2004). Recently Vergara *et al.* (2004) reported that longevity of male Snell dwarf mice was not reduced by a regimen of hormone replacement therapy that promoted testicular development and induced fertility.

Suppressed transcription of genes related to cholesterol biosynthesis (Boylston *et al.*, 2004) and increased expression of PPARα regulated genes (Stauber *et al.*, 2005) in the liver of Snell dwarf mice may also contribute to extension of longevity in these animals.

Although it appears very unlikely that diminutive body size per se is conferring any important advantages in terms of survival, negative correlation of adult body weight and lifespan in mice was consistently found in studies of various natural and experimentally produced mutants as well as different stocks of genetically normal animals (Rollo, 2002) and individuals within a genetically heterogeneous population (Miller *et al.*, 2002). We suspect that these associations are due to the relationship of growth and adult body size to somatotropic signaling.

Somatotropic Signaling and Aging in Other Species

Negative correlation of body size and longevity, which was demonstrated in numerous studies in laboratory stocks of mice and in recent meta-analysis (Rollo, 2002), applies also to rats (Rollo, 2002) and to other species. Probably the most striking data are derived from the study of different breeds of domestic dogs as well as mixed-breed individuals from this species (Patronek *et al.*, 1997). Small dogs live longer than large dogs, and in several studies differences in body size and longevity were related to differences in peripheral IGF-1 levels (Eigenmann *et al.*, 1988). Negative correlation of height and longevity was shown in various cohorts of human subjects (Samaras *et al.*, 2003). There are also anecdotal reports of exceptional longevity of miniature breeds of horses and donkeys. Controversies concerning relationship of GH to human aging will be discussed later in this chapter.

In rats, suppression of GH signaling by hemizygous expression of GH missense transgene produced a modest but statistically significant extension of longevity (Shimokawa *et al.*, 2002). Unexpectedly, animals homozygous for the expression of this transgene had a reduced rather than increased lifespan (Shimokawa *et al.*, 2002). Genetically GH-deficient mutant dwarf rats have normal lifespans. However, when these animals were treated with GH during the period that normally encompasses rapid postnatal growth to create a model of adult GH deficiency, they lived longer than vehicle treated mutant controls or genetically normal rats (Sonntag *et al.*, 2005).

There is considerable evidence that in invertebrates, specifically in a worm, *Caenorhabditis elegans*, and a fly, *Drosophila melanogaster*, cellular signaling pathways homologous to IGF-1 and insulin signaling in mammals are important in the regulation of aging and longevity (Guarente and Kenyon, 2000; Tatar *et al.*, 2003). Numerous mutations that reduce IGF-1/insulin-like signaling in these species cause an impressive increase of lifespan. Most intriguingly, homology of genes related to these signaling pathways and to aging extends also to unicellular yeast (Jazwinski, 1996). These homologies, extending across organisms that are taxonomically very distant and have enormous differences in physiology, life history, modes of reproduction, and life expectancy, strongly suggest, the existence of a fundamental relationship of IGF-1/insulin (or homologous) signaling to aging that is prevalent and likely universal in the animal kingdom and thus is almost certain to apply also to our own species.

Controversies Surrounding Relationship of Somatotropic Signaling to Human Aging

Congenital absence of GH signaling in the human, in addition to preventing normal postnatal growth, is believed to constitute an important risk factor for cardiovascular disease (Rosen and Bengtsson, 1990; Besson *et al.*, 2003). Unfavorable serum lipid profiles in these individuals likely represent secondary consequences of obesity that develops in the absence of GH signal. Increased risk of cardiovascular disease would obviously lead to reduced rather than increased life expectancy in sharp contrast to the situation in hypopituitary and GH resistant mice. Comparisons are further complicated by cardiovascular disease being a major cause of mortality in humans but not in mice, and by the relatively greater importance of cancers in mortality of mice.

In humans, absence of anti-insulinemic actions of GH improves insulin signaling, but obesity related to GH deficiency leads to insulin resistance. Potentially opposing effects of stimulation of the biosynthesis of IGF-1 and the IGF-1 binding proteins by GH may have to be completely elucidated before we reach a good understanding of all consequences of GH deficiency.

Individual human subjects with hypopituitarism due to a mutation of the Prop1 gene (the same gene that is mutated in the Ames dwarf mouse) or Laron dwarfism (homologous to the endocrine deficits in GHRKO mice) can survive to a very advanced age (Krzisnik *et al.*, 1999; Laron, 2005), but available data do not allow meaningful evaluation of their average or maximal lifespan. However, individuals with dwarfism due to congenital GH deficiency were recently reported to live significantly shorter than normal individuals from the same region (Besson *et al.*, 2003). Recent analysis of the relationship between height, survival, and polymorphisms of genes related to GH, IGF-1 and insulin in the human revealed that in, women, reduced activity of the insulin/IGF-1 signaling pathway was associated with improved old-age survival (van Heemst *et al.*, 2005). Carriers of a variant GH1 allele were shorter and had significantly reduced mortality (van Heemst *et al.*, 2005).

In contrast to these controversies, mitogenic and anti-apoptotic effects of IGF-1 have been linked to promoting cancer in both rodents and humans (Yu and Rohan, 2000). Height and plasma IGF-1 levels represent risk factors for several types of cancer (Tretli, 1989; Rosen and Pollak, 1999; Yu and Rohan, 2000). Pathological hypersecretion of GH from the pituitary tumor of acromegalic patients is associated with reduced life expectancy (Clayton, 2003) similar to the findings in transgenic mice overexpressing GH (reviewed in Bartke, 2003).

In the human, as in other mammalian species, GH secretion by the pituitary and circulating GH levels decline with age. Because many age-related changes in body composition including loss of muscle mass and increase in adiposity resemble symptoms of adult GH deficiency and can be at least partially reversed by GH administration, GH therapy has been and continues to be widely promoted as an "anti-aging treatment." Potential difficulties in extrapolating the findings in young or middle-aged adults with GH deficiency to endocrinologically normal elderly subjects and the issues related to the risk-benefit ratios of GH therapy are outside the scope of this chapter. However, it should be emphasized that from the available data it is not possible to determine whether GH therapy can influence the rate of aging or life expectancy in the human in either direction.

Pertinent to the studies of Snell and Ames dwarf mice that are TSH-deficient and hypothyroid, experimentally-induced hypothyroidism increased the lifespan of rats (Ooka *et al.*, 1983), and a recent study in humans over 85 years of age suggested an association of subclinical hypothyroidism with reduced rate of mortality (Gussekloo *et al.*, 2004).

Breeding and Husbandry of Long-lived Dwarf Mice

As was mentioned earlier in this chapter, Snell dwarfism and Ames dwarfism are caused by autosomal recessive mutations. Targeted disruption of the GHR/GHBP gene is also transmitted as an autosomal recessive trait. Consequently, homozygous Snell dwarf (dw/dw), Ames dwarf (df/df) and GHRKO (−/−) mice can be readily produced by mating heterozygous carriers of these mutations. Since homozygosity for these mutations appears to have no effect on prenatal mortality, matings of heterozygous carriers (e.g., dw/+ × dw/+) produce 25% of dwarf (dw/dw) progeny, 25% of progeny carrying only wild-type alleles at this locus (+/+), and 50% of heterozygotes (dw/+). Heterozygous and +/+ animals can be distinguished by DNA analysis (Dolle *et al.*, 2001; Chandrashekar *et al.*, 1999) or by breeding tests.

Since nearly all GHRKO (−/−) males are fertile, they can be bred to +/− females to produce equal

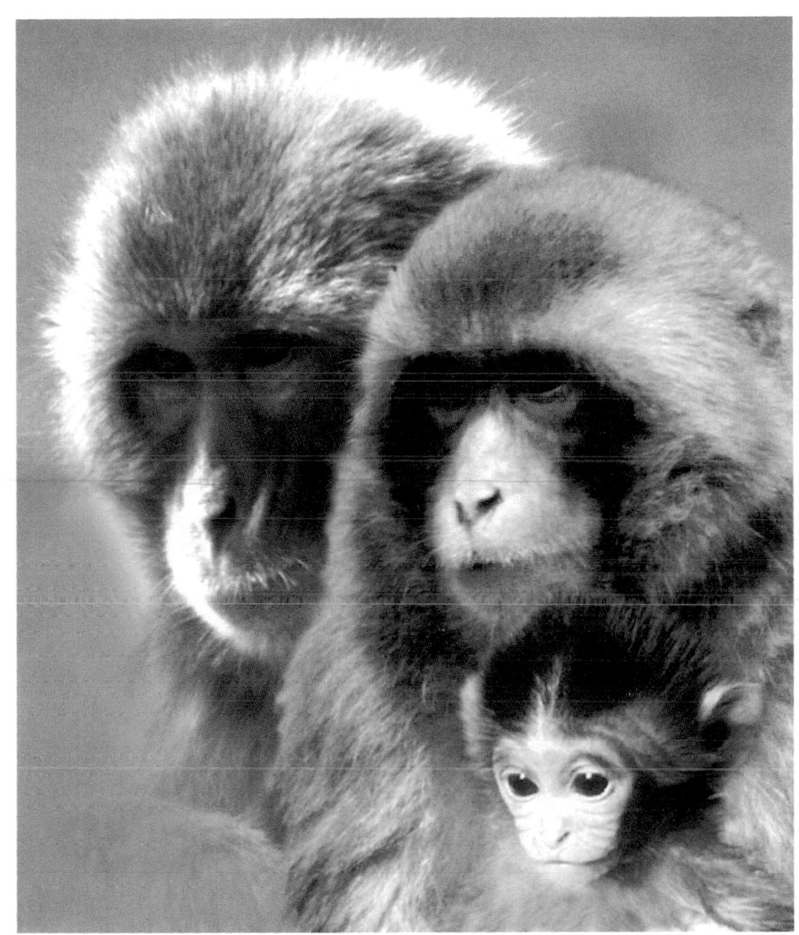

Plate 1

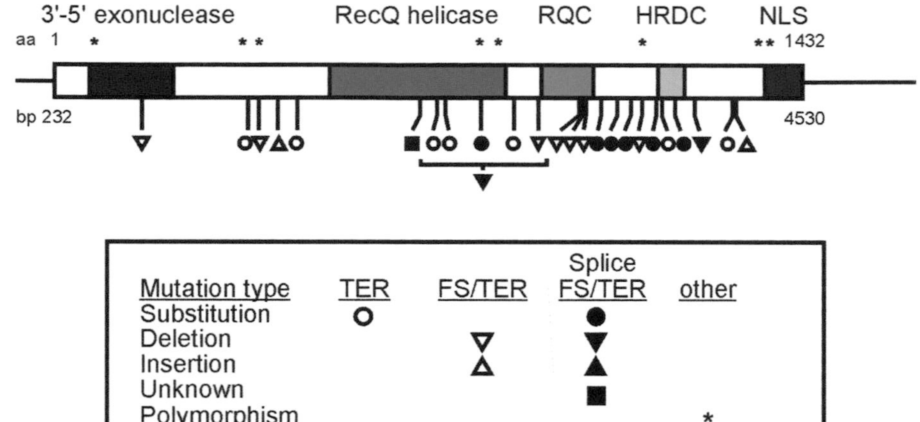

Plate 2

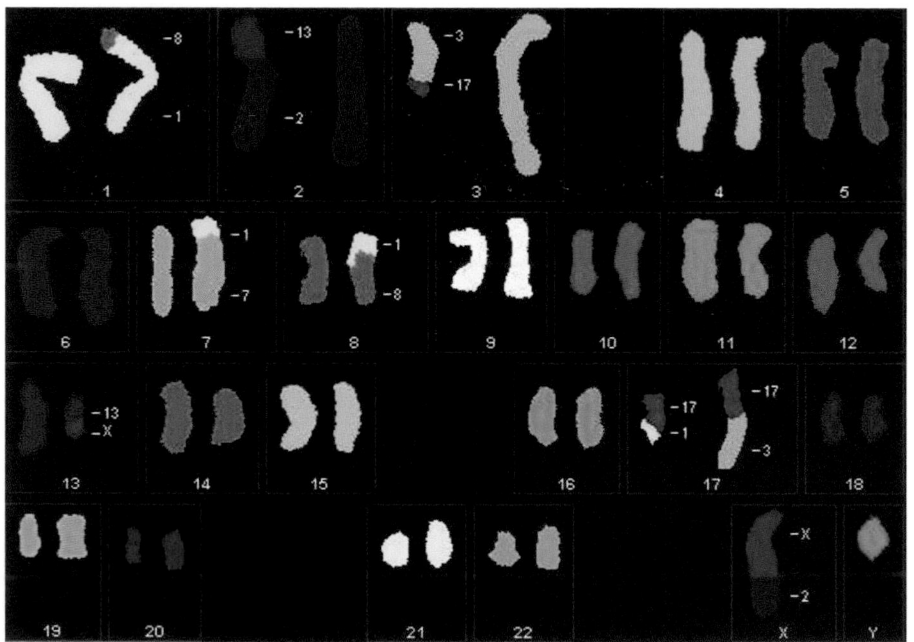

Plate 3

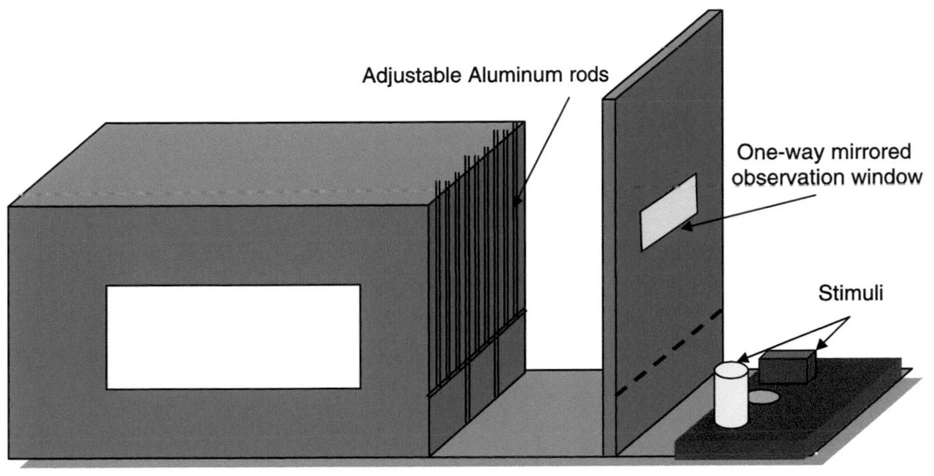

Plate 4

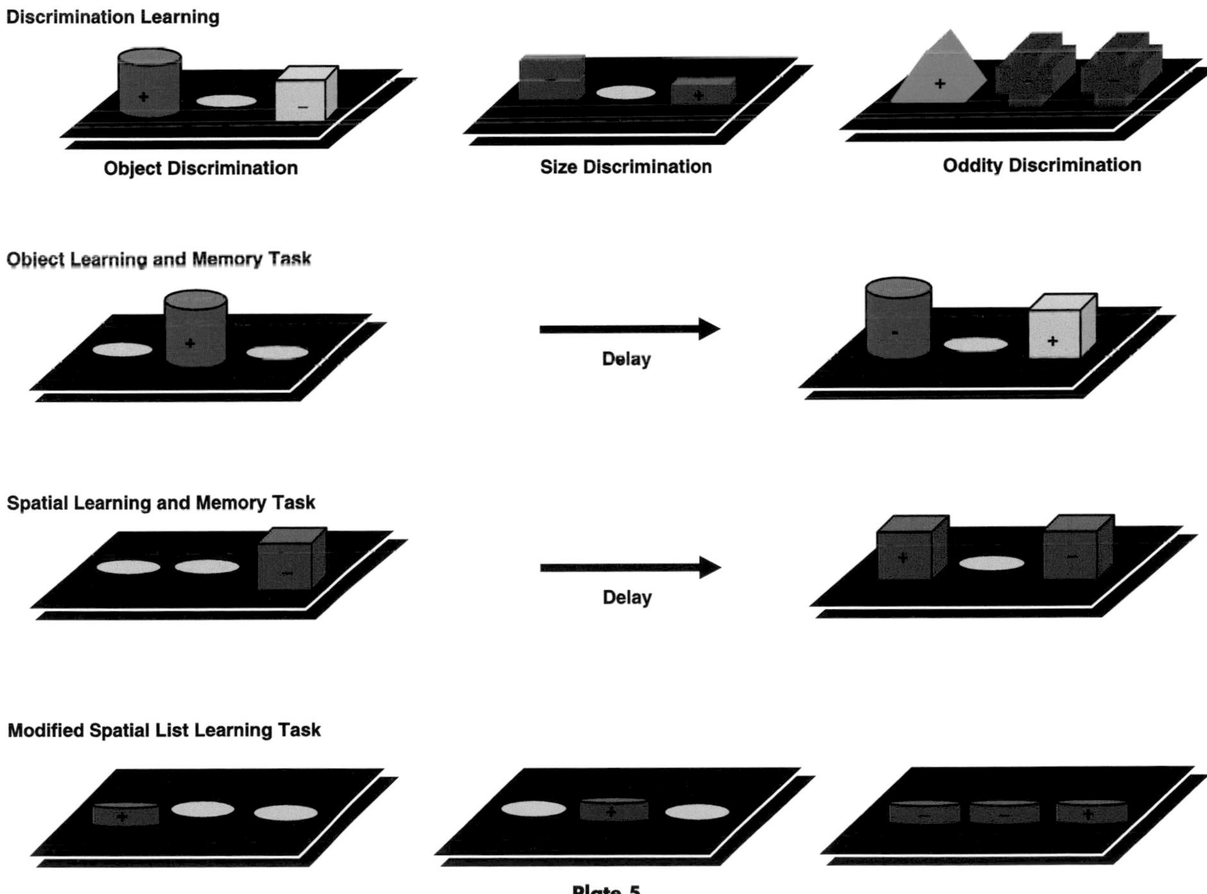

Plate 5

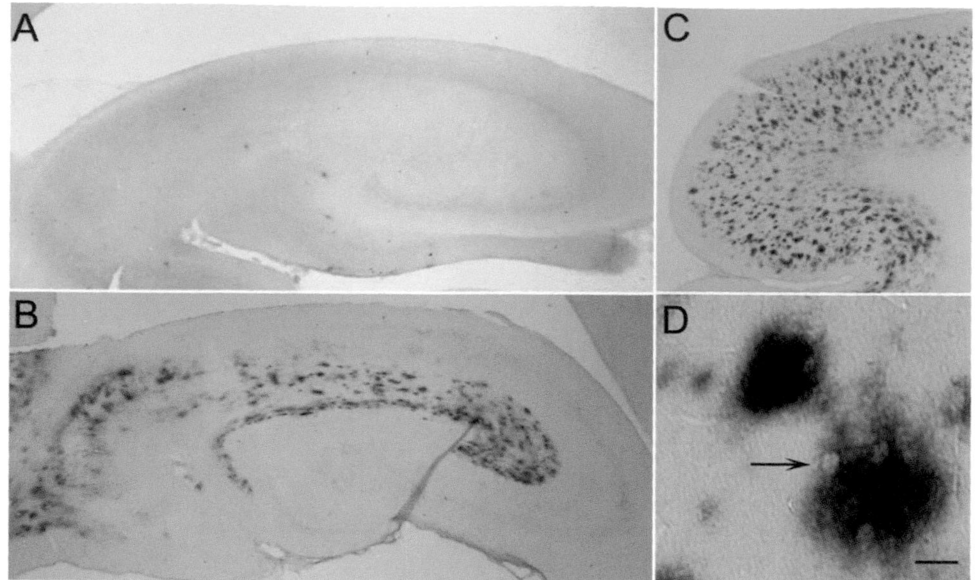

Plate 6

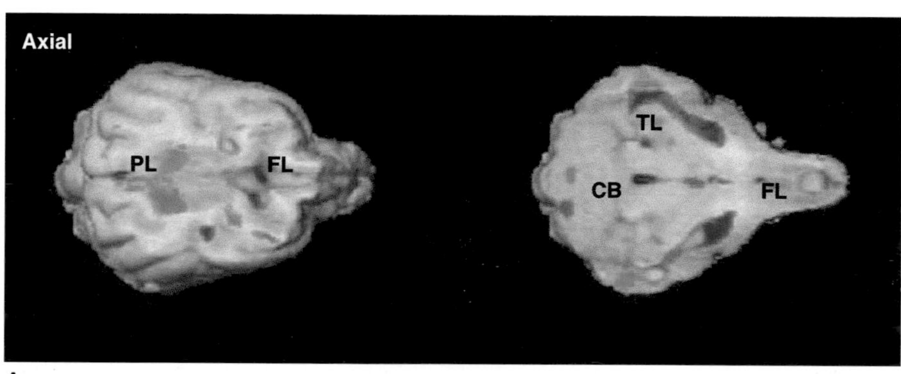

A

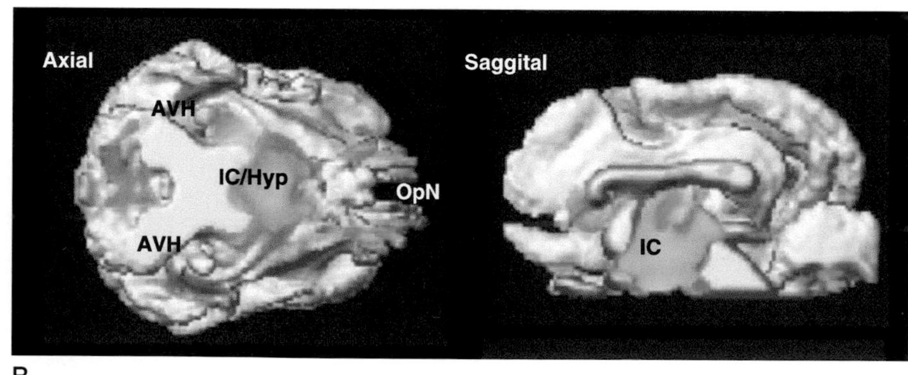

B

Plate 7

numbers of −/− and +/− progeny. Fertility of male Snell and Ames dwarfs depends on the genetic background, and most Ames dwarf males in the author's colony are fertile, although they attain puberty later than normal males. In stocks in which dwarf males are not fertile, fertility can be induced by treatment with thyroxine, GH, PRL, or combinations of these hormones (reviewed in Bartke, 1979a, 1979b, 2000; Bartke and Brown-Borg, 2004). The obvious advantages of using homozygous dwarf (dw/dw, df/df, GHRKO −/−) as breeders is that mating them with heterozygous females produces 50% rather than 25% of dwarf progeny. Moreover, in this breeding system all of the phenotypically normal animals are heterozygous carriers of these mutations and thus can be used as breeders without the need for genotyping or genetic testing. The only disadvantage of this breeding system is that it does not produce homozygous normal (+/+) animals. Using heterozygotes as normal controls is justified by lack of any obvious phenotypic differences between heterozygous and +/+ mice, except for a small reduction in body weight in young adult GHRKO +/− as compared to +/+ females. However, one must be cognizant of the possibility that any parameter under study might be influenced by heterozygous expression of the dwarfing genes.

Transplantation of anterior pituitary glands from normal mice under the kidney capsule of Snell or Ames dwarfs provides continued release of PRL and induces fertility in both males and females (Bartke, 1965, 1979b, 2000). Induction of female fertility in these mutants allows production of all-dwarf litters. This eliminates the need for genotyping individual animals in studies of the effects of these mutations during prenatal or early postnatal development. Fertile females can be used to provide placental tissue of purely mutant genotype (Soares *et al.*, 1984).

In contrast to their normal siblings, Snell and Ames dwarf mice often fail to thrive when they are weaned at 21 days of age. At this age, they may have difficulties in chewing pelleted diet and in reaching the food hopper and the water sipper in standard mouse cages. It is recommended to leave them with the dam (or both dam and sire) for a minimum additional 2–3 weeks. This is particularly beneficial if the dam becomes pregnant from postpartum estrus and is nursing her next litter during this period. After weaning, dwarfs should be housed in groups with other dwarfs or with normal females. Some laboratories consistently use normal female companions to house the dwarfs, and some provide them with readily accessible food in the bottom of the cage and use longer sipper tubes and/or thicker layer of bedding. Using a diet with high fat content (e.g., mouse breeder chow with 6.5 or 7.0% fat) is very important and probably essential. In the author's breeding colony of Ames dwarf mice, normal pups are weaned at 21 days of age, while dwarf pups are weaned 3–4 weeks later and housed in groups of 5 dwarfs per cage (or, occasionally, in groups comprised of dwarfs and normal females) but otherwise receive the same care as normal mice. GHRKO −/− mice can be weaned at the age of 21 days and require no special housing conditions, care or diet.

ACKNOWLEDGMENTS

Contributions of numerous colleagues, fellows, and students to the progress of our work on this topic are gratefully acknowledged. Recent and current studies of dwarf mice in our laboratory are supported by NIA (NIH) AG019899 and U19 AG023122 and by the Ellison Medical Foundation. We apologize to those whose work pertinent to this topic is not mentioned due to limitations of space or inadvertent omissions.

REFERENCES

Al-Regaiey, K.A., Masternak, M.M., Bonkowski, M., Sun, L., and Bartke, A. (2005). Long-lived growth hormone receptor knockout mice: Interaction of reduced insulin-like growth factor 1/insulin signaling and caloric restriction. *Endocrinology 146*, 851–860.

Bartke, A. (1965). Influence of luteotrophin on fertility of dwarf mice. *J. Reprod. Fertil. 10*, 93–103.

Bartke, A. (1979a). Genetic models in the study of anterior pituitary hormones. In *Genetic Variation in Hormone Systems*, Shire, J.G.M. (ed). Boca Raton: CRC Press, pp. 113–126.

Bartke, A. (1979b). Prolactin-deficient mice. In *Animal Models for Research on Contraception and Fertility*. Alexander, N.J. (ed). Hagerstown: Harper & Row, pp. 360–365.

Bartke, A. (2000). Delayed aging in Ames dwarf mice. Relationships to endocrine function and body size. In *The Molecular Genetics of Aging*. Vol. 29. Hekimi, S. (ed). Berlin, Heidelberg: Springer-Verlag, pp. 181–202.

Bartke, A., Coschigano, K., Kopchick, J., Chandrashekar, V., Mattison, J., Kinney, B., and Hauck, S. (2001a). Genes that prolong life: Relationships of growth hormone and growth to aging and lifespan. *J. Gerontol.: Biol. Sci. 56A*, B340–B349.

Bartke, A., Wright, J.C., Mattison, J., Ingram, D.K., Miller, R.A., and Roth, G.S. (2001b). Extending the lifespan of long-lived mice. *Nature 414*, 412.

Bartke, A., Chandrashekar, V., Bailey, B., Zaczek, D., and Turyn, D. (2002). Consequences of growth hormone (GH) overexpression and GH resistance. *Neuropeptides 36*, 201–208.

Bartke, A. (2003). Can growth hormone (GH) accelerate aging? Evidence from GH-transgenic mice. *Neuroendocrinology 78*, 210–216.

Bartke, A., and Brown-Borg, H. (2004). Life extension in the dwarf mouse. *Curr Top Developmental Biology 63*, 189–225.

Bartke, A., Peluso, M.R., Moretz, N., Wright, C., Bonkowski, M., Winters, T.A., *et al.* (2004). Effects of Soy-derived diets on plasma and liver lipids, glucose tolerance, and longevity in normal, long-lived and short-lived mice. *Horm. Metab. Res. 36*, 550–558.

Baynes, J.W., and Monnier, V.M. (1989). *The Maillard Reaction in Aging, Diabetes and Nutrition*. New York: Alan R. Liss.

Berryman, D.E., List, E.O., Coschigano, K.T., Behar, K., Kim, J.K., and Kopchick, J.J. (2004). Comparing adiposity profiles in three mouse models with altered GH signaling. *Growth Hormone & IGF Research 14*, 309–318.

Besson, A., Salemi, S., Gallati, S., Jenal, A., Horn, R., Mullis, P.S., and Mullis, P.E. (2003). Reduced longevity in untreated patients with isolated growth hormone deficiency. *J. Clin. Endocrinol. Metab. 88*, 3664–3667.

Borg, K.E., Brown-Borg, H.M., and Bartke, A. (1995). Assessment of the primary adrenal cortical and pancreatic hormone basal levels in relation to plasma glucose and age in the unstressed Ames dwarf mouse. *Proc. Soc. Exp. Biol. Med. 210*, 126–133.

Boylston, W.H., Gerstner, A., DeFord, J.H., Madsen, M., Flurkey, K., Harrison, D.E., and Papaconstantinou, J. (2004). Altered cholesterologenic and lipogenic transcriptional profile in livers of aging Snell dwarf (Pit1dw/dwJ) mice. *Aging Cell 3*, 283–296.

Brown-Borg, H.M., Borg, K.E., Meliska, C.J., and Bartke, A. (1996). Dwarf mice and the ageing process. *Nature 384*, 33.

Brown-Borg, H.M., and Rakoczy, S.G. (2000). Catalase expression in delayed and premature aging mouse models. *Exp. Gerontol. 35*, 199–212.

Brown-Borg, H., Johnson, W., Rakoczky, S., and Romanick, M. (2001). Mitochondrial oxidant generation and oxidative damage in Ames dwarf and GH transgenic mice. *Amer. Aging Assoc. 24*, 85–96.

Brown-Borg, H.M., and Rakoczy, S.G. (2005). Glutathione metabolism in long-living Ames dwarf mice. *Exp. Gerontol. 40*, 115–120.

Carsner, R.L., and Rennels, E.G. (1960). Primary site of gene action in anterior pituitary dwarf mice. *Science* 18:131:829.

Chandrashekar, V., Zaczek, D., and Bartke, A. (2004). The consequences of altered somatotropic system on reproduction. *Biol. Reprod. 71*, 17–27.

Chandrashekar, V., Bartke, A., Coschigano, K.T., and Kopchick, J.J. (1999). Pituitary and testicular function in growth hormone receptor gene knockout mice. *Endocrinology 140*, 1082–1088.

Cheng, C.M., Mervis, R.F., Niu, S.L., Salem, N., Witters, L.A., Tseng, V., *et al.* (2003). Insulin-like growth factor 1 is essential for normal dendritic growth. *Journal of Neuroscience Research 73*, 1–9.

Clayton, R.N. (2003). Cardiovascular function in acromegaly. *Endocr. Rev. 24*, 272–277.

Coschigano, K.T., Clemmons, D., Bellush, L.L., and Kopchick, J.J. (2000). Assessment of growth parameters and lifespan of GHR/BP gene-disrupted mice. *Endocrinology 141*, 2608–2613.

Coschigano, K.T., Holland, A.N., Riders, M.E., List, E.O., Flyvbjerg, A., and Kopchick, J.J. (2003). Deletion, but not antagonism, of the mouse growth hormone receptor results in severely decreased body weights, insulin, and insulin-like growth factor I levels and increased lifespan. *Endocrinology 144*, 3799–3810.

Dolle, M.E.T., Snyder, W.K., and Vijg, J. (2001). Genotyping the Prop-1 mutation in Ames dwarf mice. *Mech. Ageing Dev. 122*, 1915–1918.

Dominici, F.P., Arostegui Diaz, G., Bartke, A., Kopchick, J.J., and Turyn, D. (2000). Compensatory alterations of insulin signal transduction in liver of growth hormone receptor knockout mice. *J. Endocrinol. 166*, 579–590.

Dominici, F.P., Hauck, S., Argentino, D.P., Bartke, A., and Turyn, D. (2002). Increased insulin sensitivity and upregulation of insulin receptor, insulin receptor substrate (IRS)-I and IRS-2 in liver of Ames dwarf mice. *J. Endocrinol. 173*, 81–94.

Dominici, F.P., Argentino, D.P., Bartke, A., and Turyn, D. (2003). The dwarf mutation decreases high dose insulin responses in skeletal muscle, the opposite of effects in liver. *Mech. Ageing Dev. 124*, 819–827.

Eicher, E., and Beamer, W. (1980). New mouse dw allele: Genetic location and effects on lifespan and growth hormone levels. *Journal Heredity* May–Jun; *71*, 187–190.

Eigenmann, J.E., Amador, A., and Patterson, D.F. (1988). Insulin-like growth factor I levels in proportionate dogs, chondrodystrophic dogs and in giant dogs. *Acta Endocrinol. 118*, 105–108.

Facchini, F.S., Hua, N., Abbasi, F., and Reaven, G.M. (2001). Insulin resistance as a predictor of age-related diseases. *J. Clin. Endocrinol. Metab. 86*, 3574–3578.

Fabris, N., Pierpaoli, W., and Sorkin, E. (1972). Lymphocytes, hormones, and ageing. *Nature 240*, 557–559.

Flurkey, K., Papaconstantinou, J., Miller, R.A., and Harrison, D.E. (2001). Lifespan extension and delayed immune and collagen aging in mutant mice with defects in growth hormone production. *Proc. Nat. Acad. Sci., USA 98*, 6736–6741.

Grüneberg, H. (1952). *The Genetics of the Mouse*. Martinus Nijhoff, The Hague, pp. 122–129.

Guarente, L., and Kenyon, C. (2000). Genetic pathways that regulate ageing in model organisms. *Nature 408*, 255–262.

Gussekloo, J., van Exel, E., de Craen, A.J., Meinders, A.E., Frolich, M., and Westendorp, R.G. (2005). Thyroid status, performance, and survival in old age. *JAMA 292*, 2591–2599.

Hauck, S.J., Hunter, W.S., Danilovich, N., Kopchick, J.J., and Bartke, A. (2001). Reduced levels of thyroid hormones, insulin, and glucose, and lower body core temperature in the growth hormone receptor/binding protein knockout mouse. *Exp. Biol. Med. 226*, 552–558.

Hauck, S.J., Aaron, J.M., Wright, C., Kopchick, J.J., and Bartke, A. (2002). Antioxidant enzymes, free-radical damage, and response to paraquat in liver and kidney of long-living growth hormone receptor/binding protein gene-disrupted mice. *Horm. Metab. Res.* 481–486.

Heiman, M., Tinsley, F., Mattison, J., Hauck, S., and Bartke, A. (2003). Body composition of prolactin-, growth hormone-, and thyrotropin-deficient Ames dwarf mice. *Endocrine 20*, 149–154.

Holzenberger, M., Dupont, J., Ducos, B., Leneuve, P., Geloen, A., Evens, P., Cervera, P., and LeBouc, Y. (2003). IGF-1 receptor regulates lifespan and resistance to oxidative stress in mice. *Nature 421*, 182–187.

Hsieh, C.C., DeFord, J.H., Flurkey, K., Harrison, D.E., and Papaconstantinou, J. (2002). Effects of the Pit 1 mutation on the insulin signaling pathway: Implications on the longevity of the long-lived Snell dwarf mouse. *Mech. Ageing Dev. 123*, 1244–1255.

Hsieh, C.-C., and Papaconstantinou, J. (2004). Akt/PKB and p38 MAPK signaling, translational initiation and longevity in Snell dwarf mouse livers. *Mech. Ageing Dev. 125*, 785–798.

Hunter, W.S., Croson, W.B., Bartke, A., Gentry, M.V., and Meliska, C.J. (1999). Low body temperature in long-lived Ames dwarf mice at rest and during stress. *Physiol. Behav. 67*, 433–437.

Ikeno, Y., Bronson, R.T, Hubbard, G.B, Lee, S, Bartke, A. (2003). Delayed occurrence of fatal neoplastic diseases in Ames dwarf mice: Correlation to extended longevity. *J. Gerontol. A Biol. Sci. Med. Sci. 58A*, 291–296.

Jazwinski, S.M. (1996). Longevity, genes, and aging. *Science* 273, 54–59.

Khaw, K.T., Wareham, N., Bingham, S., Luben, R., Welch, A., and Day, N. (2004). Association of hemoglobin A1c with cardiovascular disease and mortality in adults: The European prospective investigation into cancer in Norfolk. *Ann. Intern. Med. 141*, 413–420.

Kimura, K.D., Tissenbaum, H.A., Liu, Y., and Ruvkun, G. (1997). daf-2, an insulin receptor-like gene that regulates longevity and diapause in *Caenorhabditis elegans*. *Science 277*, 942–946.

Kinney, B.A., Meliska, C.J., Steger, R.W., and Bartke, A. (2001a). Evidence that Ames dwarf mice age differently from their normal siblings in behavioral and learning and memory parameters. *Horm. Behav. 39*, 277–284.

Kinney, B.A., Coschigano, K.T., Kopchick, J.J., and Bartke, A. (2001b). Evidence that age-induced decline in memory retention is delayed in growth hormone resistant GH-R-KO (Laron) mice. *Physiol. Behav. 72*, 653–660.

Kinney-Forshee, B., Kinney, N., Steger, R., and Bartke, A. (2004). Could a deficiency in growth hormone signaling be beneficial to the aging brain? *Physiol. Behav. 80*, 589–594.

Krzisnik, C., Kolacio, Z., Battelino, T., Brown, M., Parks, J.S., and Laron, Z. (1999). The "Little People" of the island of Krk—revisited. Etiology of hypopituitarism revealed. *The Journal of Endocrine Genetics 1*, 9–19.

Lambert, A.J., Wang, B., and Merry, B.J. (2004). Exogenous insulin can reverse the effects of caloric restriction on mitochondria. *Biochemical and Biophysical Research Communications 316*, 1196–1201.

Laron, Z. (2005). Do deficiencies in growth hormone and insulin-like growth factor-1 (IGF-1) shorten or prolong longevity? *Mech. Ageing Dev. 126*, 305–307.

Li, S., Crenshaw, B.E., Rawson, E.J., Simmons, D.M., Swanson, L.W., and Rosenfeld, M.G. (1990). Dwarf locus mutants lacking three pituitary cell types result from mutations in the POU-domain gene pit-1. *Nature 347*, 528–533.

Liu, J.-L., Coschigano, K.T., Robertson, K., Lipsett, M., Guo, Y., Kopchick, J.J., Kumar, U., and Liu, Y.L. (2004). Disruption of growth hormone receptor gene causes diminished pancreatic islet size and increased insulin sensitivity in mice. *Am. J. Physiol. Endocrinol. Metab. 287*, E405–413.

Lupu, F., Terwilliger, J.D., Lee, K., Segre, G.V., and Efstratiadis, A. (2001). Roles of growth hormone and insulin-like growth factor I in mouse postnatal growth. *Develop. Biol. 229*, 141–162.

Masoro, E.J. (2001). Dietary restriction: An experimental approach to the study of the biology of aging. In *Handbook of the Biology of Aging* (5th ed.). Masoro, E.J. and Austad, S.N. (eds). San Diego: Academic Press, pp. 396–420.

Masternak, M., Al-Regaiey, K., Bonkowski, M., Panici, J., Sun, L., Wang, J., *et al.* (2004). Divergent effects of caloric restriction on gene expression in normal and long-lived mice. *Journal of Gerontology: A Biol. Sci. Med. Sci. 59*, 784–788.

Miller, R.A., Harper, J.M., Galecki, A., and Burke, D.T. (2002). Big mice die young: Early life body weight predicts longevity in genetically heterogeneous mice. *Aging Cell 1*, 22–29.

Miskin, R., and Masos, T. (1997). Transgenic mice overexpressing urokinase-type plasminogen activator in the brain exhibit reduced food consumption, body weight and size, and increased longevity. *J. Gerontol. 52A*, B118–B124.

Murakami, S., Salmon, A., and Miller, R. (2003). Multiplex stress resistance in cells from long-lived dwarf mice. *FASEB 17*, 1565–1566.

Ooka, H., Fujita, S., and Yoshimoto, E. (1983). Pituitary-thyroid activity and longevity in neonatally thyroxine-treated rats. *Mech. Ageing Dev. 22*, 113–120.

Parr, T. (1996). Insulin exposure controls the rate of mammalian aging. *Mech. Ageing Dev. 88*, 75–82.

Parsons, J.A., Bartke, A., and Sorenson, R.L. (1995). Number and size of islets of langerhans in pregnant, human growth hormone-expressing transgenic, and pituitary dwarf mice: Effect of lactogenic hormones. *Endocrinology 136*, 2013–2021.

Partridge, L., Gems, D., and Withers, D.J. (2005). Sex and death: What is the connection? *Cell 120*, 461–472.

Patronek, G.J., Waters, D.J., and Glickman, L.T. (1997). Comparative longevity of pet dogs and humans: Implications for gerontology research. *J. Gerontol. 52A*, B171–B178.

Phelps, C.J. (2004). Postnatal regression of hypothalamic dopaminergic neurons in prolactin-deficient snell dwarf mice. *Endocrinology 145*, 5656–5664.

Phillips, J.P., Parkes, T.L., and Hilliker, A.J. (2000). Targeted neuronal gene expression and longevity in *Drosophila*. *Exp. Gerontol. 35*, 1157–1164.

Rodgers, J.T., Lerin, C., Haas, W., Gygi, S.P., Spiegelman, B.M., and Puigserver, P. (2005). Nutrient control of glucose homeostasis through a complex of PGC-1[alpha] and SIRT1. *Nature 434*, 113–118.

Rollo, C.D. (2002). Growth negatively impacts the lifespan of mammals. *Evol. Dev. 4*, 55–61.

Rosen, T., and Bengtsson, B.A. (1990). Premature mortality due to cardiovascular disease in hypopituitarism. *Lancet 336*, 285–288.

Rosen, C.J., and Pollak, M. (1999). IGF-I and aging: A new perspective for a new century. *Trends Endocrinol. Metab. 10*, 136–142.

Salmon, A.B., Murakami, S., Bartke, A., Kopchick, J., Yasumura, K., and Miller, R.A. (2005). Fibroblast cell lines from young adult mice of long-lived mutant strains are resistant to multiple forms of stress. *Am. J. Physiol. Endocrinol. Metab. 10*, 1152.

Samaras, T., Elrick, H., and Storms, L. (2003). Is height related to longevity? *Life Science 72*, 1781–1802.

Sanz, A., Bartke, A., and Barja, G. (2002). Long-lived Ames dwarf mice: Oxidative damage to mitochondrial DNA in heart and brain. *J. Am. Aging Assoc. 25*, 119–122.

Schaible, R., and Gowen, J.W. (1961). A new dwarf mouse. *Genetics 46*, 896.

Schneider, G.B. (1976). Immunological competence in Snell-Bagg pituitary dwarf mice: Response to the contact-sensitizing agent oxazolone. *Am. J. Anat. 145*, 371–394.

Shimokawa, I., Higami, Y., Utsuyama, M., Tuchiya, T., Komatsu, T., Chiba, T., and Yamaza, H. (2002). Lifespan extension by reduction of the growth hormone-insulin-like growth factor-1 axis: Relation to caloric restriction. *Am. J. Pathol. 160*, 2259–2265.

Shire, J.G.M. (1973) Growth hormone and premature ageing. *Nature 245*, 215–216.

Silberberg, R. (1972) Articular aging and osteoarthrosis in dwarf mice. *Path. Miocrobiol. 38*, 417–430.

Snell, G.D. (1929) Dwarf, a new mendelian recessive character of the house mouse. *Proc. Natl. Acad. Sci. USA 15*, 733–734.

Soares, M.J., Bartke, A., Colosi, P., and Talamantes, F. (1984) Identification of a placental lactogen in pregnant Snell and Ames dwarf mice. *Soc. Exp. Biol. Med. 175*, 106–108.

Sonntag, W.E., Carter, C.S., Ikeno, Y., Ekenstedt, K., Carlson, C.S., Loeser, R.F., *et al.* (2005) Adult-onset growth hormone and IGF-1 deficiency reduces neoplastic disease, modifies age-related pathology and increases lifespan. *Endocrinology 146*, 2920–2932.

Sornson, M.W., Wu, W., Dasen, J.S., Flynn, S.E., Norman, D.J., O'Connell, S.M., *et al.* (1996) Pituitary lineage determination by the prophet of pit-1 homeodomain factor defective in Ames dwarfism. *Nature 384*, 327–333.

Stauber, A.J., Brown-Borg, H., Liu, J., Waalkes, M.P., Laughter, A., Staben, R.A., *et al.* (2005) Constitutive expression of peroxisome proliferator-activated receptor α-regulated genes in dwarf mice. *Mol. Pharmacol. 67*, 681–694.

Sun, L.Y., Al-Regaiey, K., Masternak, M.M., Wang, J., and Bartke, A. (2005a) Local expression of GH and IGF-1 in the hippocampus of GH-deficient long-lived mice. *Neurobiol. Aging 26*, 929–937.

Sun, L.Y., Evans, M.S., Hsieh, J., Panici, J., and Bartke, A. (2005b) Increased neurogenesis in dentate gyrus of long-lived Ames dwarf mice. *Endocrinology 146*, 1138–1144.

Tatar, M., Bartke, A., and Antebi, A. (2003) The endocrine regulation of aging by insulin-like signals. *Science 299*, 1346–1351.

Tretli, S. (1989) Height and weight in relation to breast cancer morbidity and mortality. A prospective study of 570,000 women in Norway. *Int. J. Cancer 44*, 23–30.

Tsuchiya, T., Dhahbi, J.M., Cui, X., Mote, P.L., Bartke, A., and Spindler, S.R. (2004) Additive regulation of hepatic gene expression by dwarfism and caloric restriction. *Physiol. Genomics 17*, 307–315.

van Heemst, D., Beekman, M., Mooijaart, S.P., Heijmans, B.T., Brandt, B.W., Zwaan, B.J., *et al.* (2005) Reduced insulin/IGF-1 signaling and human longevity. *Aging Cell 4*, 79–85.

Vergara, M., Smith-Wheelock, M., Harper, J.M., Sigler, R., and Miller, R.A. (2004) Hormone-treated Snell dwarf mice regain fertility but remain long lived and disease resistant. *J. Gerontol. A Biol. Sci. Med. Sci. 59*, 1244–1250.

Ward, R.D., Raetzman, L.T., Suh, H., Stone, B.M., Nasonkin, I.O., and Camper, S.A. (2005) Role of PROP1 in pituitary gland growth. *Mol. Endocrinol. 19*, 698–710.

Wessells, R.J., Fitzgerald, E., Cypser, J.R., Tatar, M., and Bodmer, R. (2004) Insulin regulation of heart function in aging fruit flies. *Nat. Genet. 36*, 1275–1281.

Woods, K.A., Camacho-Hubner, C., Savage, M.O., and Clark, A.J.L. (1996) Intrauterine growth retardation and postnatal growth failure associated with deletion of the insulin-like growth factor I gene. *N Engl. J. Med. 335*, 1363–1367.

Yu, H., and Rohan, T. (2000) Role of the insulin-like growth factor family in cancer development and progression. *Journal of National Cancer Inst. 20*, 1472–1489.

Zhou, Y., Xu, B.C., Maheshwari, H.G., He, L., Reed, M., Lozykowski, M., *et al.* (1997) A mammalian model for Laron syndrome produced by targeted disruption of the mouse growth hormone receptor/binding protein gene (The Laron mouse). *94*, 13215–13220.

35

The Canine Model of Human Brain Aging: Cognition, Behavior, and Neuropathology

P. Dwight Tapp and Christina T. Siwak

Dogs develop age-dependent cognitive deficits that parallel declines observed in normal and pathological aging in humans. Like humans, some dogs show no decline, some show mild decline, and others of the same age develop severe cognitive impairments. Aged dogs show decreases in locomotion and changes in other behaviors but continue to display appropriate responses, just to a lesser extent compared to young dogs. Impaired dogs by contrast, show abnormal responses. These dogs are hyperactive, unresponsive to social stimuli or toys, and often engage in stereotypical behaviors. The aged dog is also well suited for investigation of the initial stages of plaque formation in the aging brain. Beta-amyloid deposition in the form of diffuse plaques is a prominent feature of the aged dog brain. Oxidative damage and neuron loss are also features of the canine brain while neurofibrillary tangles are absent. MRI procedures also reveal commonalities between the aging dog and human brains, including shrinkage, spontaneous lesion formation, and reduced blood flow. These findings suggest that the dog can be used to model the earliest phases of cognitive, behavioral and neuropathological changes associated with brain aging in humans. The existence of dogs that maintain cognitive function with age may provide insight into promoting successful aging in humans.

Improvements in medical care for animals enable dogs to live longer; subsequently they may be at risk for developing age-related behavioral disorders comparable to the aging human. Clinically diagnosed as canine cognitive dysfunction syndrome, impairments include decreased activity, altered social interactions or responsiveness, disturbances of the sleep–wake cycle, disorientation, and a loss of prior house training (Landsberg, 1995). The aged dog develops more than 400 diseases that are phenotypically the same as the human, including reduced metabolic function, cardiovascular disease, inflammatory arthritis, decreased kidney function, cancer, visual and auditory impairments, and immunodeficiencies (Committee on Animal Models for Research on Aging, 1981). These similarities make the dog a practical model for investigating the biological bases of human aging and disease.

For over a decade, our laboratory has been investigating brain aging in the dog. We adopted a clinical–neuropathological approach to empirically investigate cognitive processes and concomitant neuropathological changes in aging dogs. This approach involved the development of neuropsychological tests to evaluate cognitive function and correlate these measures with behavioral and neuropathological analyses to assess brain aging in the dog. There are several advantages in using the dog to study brain aging, including (1) the ability to study large populations of aging dogs at reasonable costs, (2) the highly gregarious nature of dogs which makes them easy to work with, (3) the sophisticated repertoire of cognitive functions and behaviors innate to dogs, (4) analogous patterns of cognitive decline, behavioral alterations, and neuropathology in dogs and humans, (5) the ability to control intervals between cognitive testing and neuropathological analyses, (6) the critical 3–5 year period of age-dependent neuropathology, which makes longitudinal investigations practical, and (7) common environments shared between dogs and humans, which exposes dogs to the same environmental stressors present in human aging.

Although our initial work involved dogs of various breeds, most of our research has primarily focused on the beagle dog. We selected a single breed to control for differences in physiological aging between breeds (Patronek *et al.*, 1997). Although studying multiple breeds is useful to examine genetic influences on behavior, differences in the life span of dogs of different sizes result in dogs that age at different physiological rates. Thus, a large dog of the same chronological age as a small dog will differ in physiological age. For example, a 10-year-old Beagle is equivalent to a 66.6-year-old human, while a 10-year-old Great Dane would equal 76.3. Our age-related classifications of Beagle dogs attempted to equate physiological age to humans in the same category: young dogs were adults equal to the chronological age of humans considered to be young adults.

The utility of the dog as a model of brain aging will be presented in three sections, each summarizing one major research area. The first section will review findings from the neuropsychological tests our laboratory developed to evaluate the effects of age on different cognitive domains (learning, memory, and executive function) in the dog. The second section will describe changes in behaviors other than cognition such as locomotor activity, social responses, and exploratory behaviors in dogs. In the third section, the underlying neuropathology correlated with age-related cognitive and behavioral impairments in the dog will be presented. The objective of each section is to demonstrate that many aspects of aging empirically studied in the dog are consistent with functional and neuropathological markers of human aging, making the dog a practical model to study human brain aging.

Cognitive Function and Aging in the Dog

Interest in the cognitive abilities of dogs can be traced as far back as the late 1800s, with anecdotal reports of dogs displaying long-distance navigational memory and associative learning (Romanes, 1884). Although subsequent studies under controlled laboratory conditions supported these early observations, the effect of age on cognitive function in dogs did not gain scientific appeal until the 1970s, focusing primarily on the developmental stages (Fox, 1971).

The single most comprehensive research program to examine cognitive aging in the dog, however, is the work conducted in the Beagle dog by N.W. Milgram and colleagues. Using a modified version of the Wisconsin General Test Apparatus (Figure 35.1), dogs are tested on a number of standard tasks (Figure 35.2) designed to measure changes in learning, memory, and executive processes as a function of age.

Over a decade of research using these testing procedures has revealed that cognitive aging in the dog, like humans, is complex and nonlinear; striking individual differences are more the rule than the exception (Adams *et al.*, 2000a,b; Head *et al.*, 1995, 2001). Like elderly humans, some dogs show very little cognitive decline with age (i.e., successful agers) and perform at levels comparable to young animals (Figure 35.3).

Others exhibit a mild decline frequently observed in normal human aging. In certain cases, some dogs exhibit severe impairment corresponding to features of dementia observed in humans. Our studies have also revealed that learning and memory impairments can occur independently of one another and that executive dysfunction may be the earliest hallmark of cognitive decline in aging dogs.

IMPAIRED LEARNING IN THE AGED DOG

We developed a number of tests to investigate age-related changes in canine learning. Specific tests were designed to examine procedural learning, associative learning, and more complex types of learning.

Procedural learning

The procedural learning task, designed to assess skill acquisition in the dog, consists of two learning phases: reward-approach and object-approach learning (Milgram *et al.*, 1994). Procedural learning is well preserved in normal human aging (Vakil and Agmon-Ashkenazi, 1997) and Alzheimer's disease (Almkvist, 1996). In dogs, however, procedural learning depends on previous rearing experience. Aged dogs raised as pets, having diverse and varied life experiences, perform as well as or better than young dogs. Conversely, old kennel-reared dogs with limited experiences in the environment are slower than

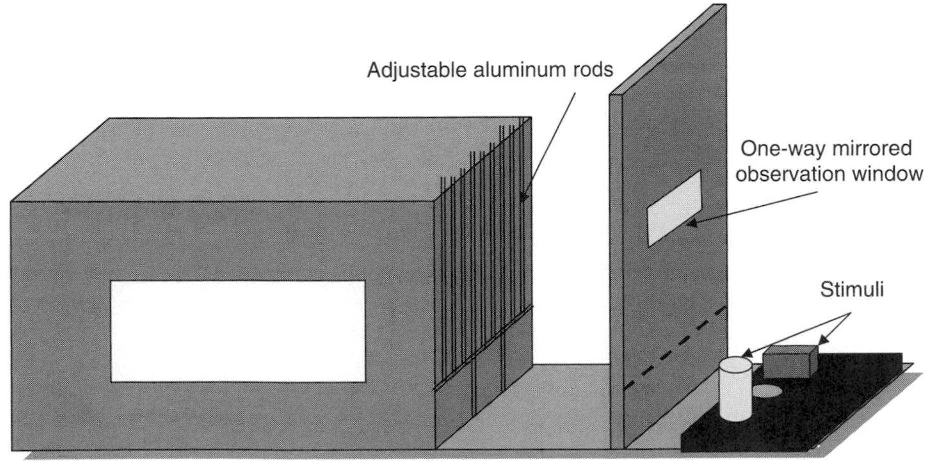

Figure 35.1 Toronto General Test Apparatus (TGTA) used to assess cognitive function in the Beagle dog. See the color plate section.

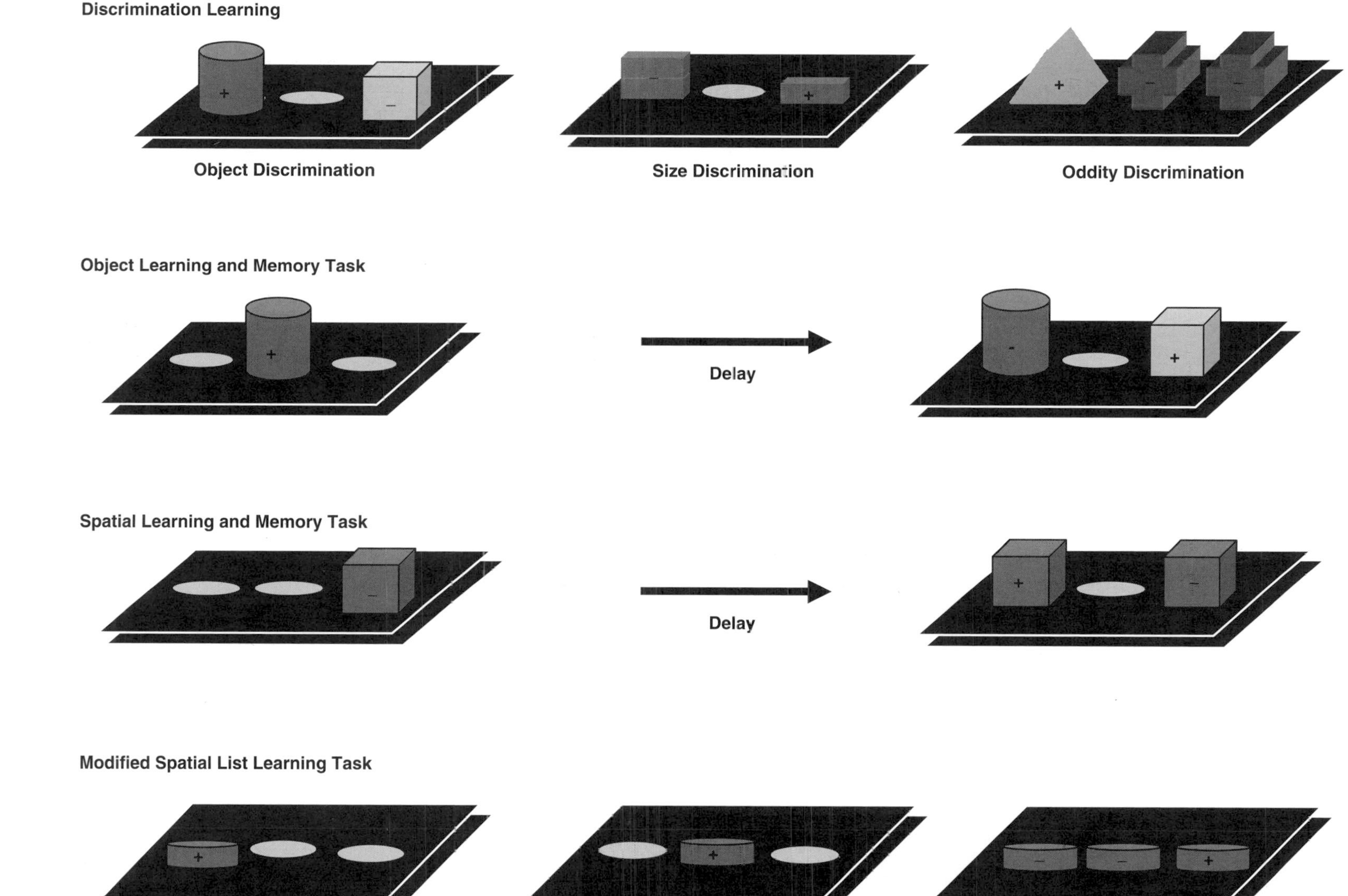

Figure 35.2 Example of tasks developed to assess cognitive function in dogs. Shown are tests of discrimination learning (object, size, and oddity discrimination), object and spatial learning and memory, and complex working memory (modified spatial list learning task). See the color plate section.

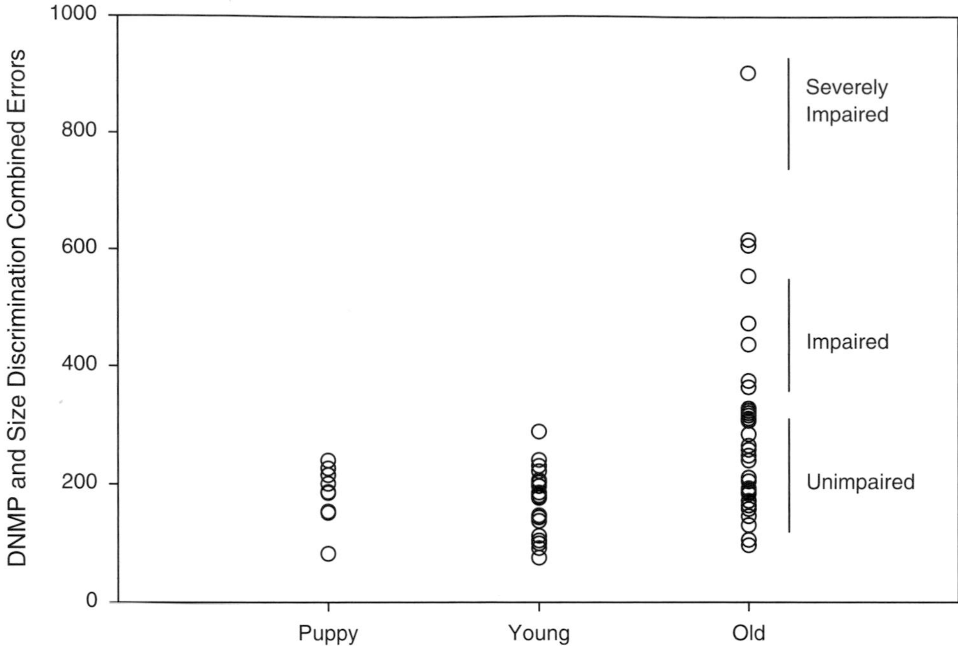

Figure 35.3 The combined sum of errors required to learn a delayed nonmatching-to-position task and an object discrimination and reversal task are plotted by age group. Aged dogs with scores greater than 2 standard deviations from the mean of the young dogs are considered impaired.

young dogs to acquire the procedural learning tasks (Milgram *et al.*, 1994). Thus, dogs with enriched experiences show a pattern similar to human learning, but having access to animals with restricted environments also revealed a dependency of learning ability on rearing history.

Discrimination learning

A common measure of learning used in animals is the discrimination task—an associative learning problem in which subjects must attend to the relevant stimulus feature(s) and acquire an association between the stimulus parameters and a food reward (Sutherland and Mackintosh, 1971). In the object discrimination task, an animal must learn that one object is associated with food reward. The two objects used differ on multiple stimulus dimensions (i.e., size, color, brightness, shape). Studies in nonhuman primates (Voytko, 1999) and dogs (Head *et al.*, 1998; Milgram *et al.*, 1994) indicate that simple discrimination learning tasks, like the object discrimination, are insensitive to age. The discrimination learning task can be made more difficult when the differences between the objects are reduced. In the size discrimination task, the two objects are identical in appearance but differ only in size (Figure 35.2). The task now becomes more complex and age differences appear (Tapp *et al.*, 2003a).

The importance of task complexity in evaluating discrimination learning in dogs is further demonstrated using an oddity discrimination task. In this task, the number of object choices is increased to make the task more difficult (Milgram *et al.*, 2002b). The animal is presented with three objects, two identical and one different. To obtain reward, the animal is required to respond to the odd object. After reaching criterion, the animal is presented with three new oddity tasks where the odd object progressively becomes more similar in features to the other two identical objects, until four problems are solved. Old dogs are not only impaired at this task, but the number of total errors increases with each successive oddity problem, suggesting a lack of ability to learn the rule of selecting the odd object. Young animals, less than 6 years old, show rapid learning after the initial problem relative to old dogs, 9 to 13 years old, despite the increasing similarities in the appearance of the objects.

Object recognition learning

Object recognition learning, the ability to classify and register the identity of objects, is examined using a delayed nonmatching to sample (DNMS) paradigm (Figure 35.2; Callahan *et al.*, 2000). Originally developed by Mishkin and Delacour (1975) for nonhuman primates, the DNMS paradigm begins by presenting the dog with a single stimulus object located over the center food well. A response to the object is followed by a delay interval, after which, two objects are presented over the two lateral wells—the original object and a novel discriminandum. The correct response for the dog is to choose the novel stimulus. The location of the novel stimulus is randomized across trials, and different stimuli selected from a large pool of objects are used for each trial.

Initial attempts to test dogs on the DNMS task suggested that dogs were impaired at object recognition learning (Milgram *et al.*, 1994). Using a weak criterion, only 4 of 10 young animals were successfully able to learn the task. Moreover, when tested on increasing delays, young dogs were able to respond with only 63% accuracy. None of the aged dogs could learn how to solve the problem. These results were initially interpreted as evidence that the canine visual system was not well suited for visual object recognition performance. A subsequent study, however, reported substantial improvements in object recognition learning in the dog when two important task-specific factors were modified (Callahan *et al.*, 2000). The first was to control for the dogs' visual near point, the shortest distance from the dog's face for an object to be in focus, which is 25–30 cm. This ensured that objects were distinctly visible to the dog before making a choice on the nonmatch phase of the task. The second was to increase the visual processing time for the dog by introducing a 5-second pause between presenting the objects and allowing dogs to respond. Aged human subjects tested on delayed matching-to-sample tasks perform less accurately than young adults, but the level of performance in both groups improves when the sample stimulus duration is increased (Oscar-Berman and Bonner, 1985). With these two modifications, most young and some old dogs were able to solve the DNMS task at over 80% accuracy, but aged dogs generally performed more poorly than young animals (Callahan *et al.*, 2000). A small proportion of severely impaired dogs, however, continued to fail the task, consistent with the strong DNMS impairments observed in Alzheimer's patients (Swainson *et al.*, 2001).

Spatial learning

One of the most consistent cognitive deficits in old dogs is the ability to acquire and use spatial information. In humans, spatial learning impairments are a common feature of aging and become more severe in neurodegenerative disorders (Freedman and Oscar-Berman, 1989). Spatial learning, the ability to locate objects in space, can be accomplished in two ways: (1) by reference to the observer's body position (egocentric learning) or (2) by reference to the position of an external referent or landmark (allocentric learning).

In the dog, we have assessed egocentric spatial learning with a delayed nonmatching to position (DNMP) task. Two versions of this task were developed, a 2-choice DNMP (Head *et al.*, 1995) and 3-choice DNMP (Chan *et al.*, 2002). In the 2-choice DNMP (2cDNMP) task (Figure 35.2), dogs are presented with a single object located over one of two lateral food wells, the sample phase. After a brief delay, a second identical object is presented over the remaining lateral food well, the match phase. Only responses to the nonmatch location are rewarded with food. Some old dogs perform as well as young dogs on this task while others show marked impairments.

The 3-choice DNMP (3cDNMP) task uses three food wells (two lateral and one medial) instead of two to prevent the use of positional strategies in solving the 2cDNMP. Similar age-related deficits were obtained using the 3cDNMP task, but this version of the DNMP procedure is much more difficult for all dogs (Chan *et al.*, 2002). Compared to only 18% of old dogs that failed the 2cDNMP (Adams *et al.*, 2000 a,b; Head *et al.*, 1995), 83% were unable to complete the 3cDNMP task. Young dogs never failed the 2cDNMP, but 12% were unable to solve the 3cDNMP.

Allocentric spatial learning in the dog is assessed with a landmark discrimination test originally developed in nonhuman primates (Pohl, 1973). In this task, subjects are rewarded for selecting one of the two identical objects that is closest to an external landmark. Solving the task relies solely on the use of allocentric spatial cues, because information about the correct response is provided only by the location of the landmark. Tests of allocentric learning in the dog indicate that landmark discrimination is far more difficult for both young and old dogs compared to the DNMP tasks. Initial attempts to train dogs on the landmark task were unsuccessful. The only way dogs could learn this task was to teach them to attend to the landmark. This was achieved by placing the landmark on top of one of the two identical objects and progressively move the landmark away from the object. Once the animals learned to attend to the landmark, allocentric spatial learning was observed in young and old dogs with age-related decrements in performance. Performance on this task declines in the old dogs as the distance between the landmark and the rewarded discriminanda increase (Milgram *et al.*, 1999; 2002a).

More recently, our lab developed an egocentric discrimination learning task to assess spatial learning where dogs were rewarded for responding to an object farthest to the left or right side of the tray (Christie *et al.*, 2005). Acquisition of the initial discrimination did not depend on age but the reversal task produced age-dependent declines in performance and correlated with performance on the landmark task. Thus, although the egocentric discrimination is similar to a visual discrimination, there is a common component with the allocentric spatial task suggesting that egocentric and allocentric based learning share some common neural substrates but are also subserved by unique brain regions.

Together, these results suggest that: (1) dogs in general may be predisposed to spatial learning based on an egocentric frame of reference, and (2) both egocentric and allocentric spatial learning are impaired with age.

AGE-RELATED MEMORY IMPAIRMENTS IN THE DOG

A gradual decline in memory occurs with normal aging and is relatively benign, but more extensive and selective memory loss may signal a transition into dementia. For example, mild cognitive impairment (MCI) is characterized by a selective impairment in memory and is thought to represent early or prodromal Alzheimer's disease. In the dog, we have developed two protocols for assessing age-related changes in memory function. One involves measuring task performance as a function of increasing the amount of information to be used in working memory. The second involves increasing the amount of time that information must be held in working memory. Learning deficits can be dissociated from memory deficits in the dog, revealing that a dog may be learning impaired but its memory is excellent, or that a dog can learn quickly but have a poor memory.

Spatial memory

Aged humans and patients with neurodegenerative diseases are often impaired on tests of spatial memory (Freedman and Oscar-Berman, 1989). Old dogs that do not exhibit spatial learning deficits may exhibit impairments when the memory demands of the task are increased. We developed two protocols for the DNMP task to study spatial memory in the dog. The first involves a variable delay paradigm in which the delay between the sample and match phases of each trial is varied between 20, 70, or 110 seconds. Both young and old dogs perform less accurately as the delay increases, but there is significant variability within the aged group of animals. Like young dogs, some old dogs continue to perform well as the delay interval increases. For others, accuracy decreases as the interval is increased from 20 seconds to longer delays (Adams *et al.*, 2000b; Head *et al.*, 1995). For these dogs, performance decrements do not represent impaired spatial learning since the animals successfully acquire the learning phase of the task (i.e., at 5-second delays). Rather, the deficit represents a working memory impairment—the inability to retain spatial information in memory during the delay interval.

The second protocol for studying memory uses a maximal memory paradigm in which the delay interval is progressively increased until the dog is unable to satisfy the pre-established task criterion or a preset number of sessions is attained. On the 2cDNMP, young dogs can perform this task at delays of 210–300 seconds. By contrast, old dogs generally reach delays of only 30–50 seconds (Adams *et al.*, 2000b), suggesting they cannot hold information in working memory for as long as young animals. When the maximal memory procedure is used on the 3cDNMP task, spatial memory for both young and old dogs is attenuated reflecting the greater complexity of this task. On the 3cDNMP, only 10% of young dogs achieve delays of 110 seconds or longer. Fewer than 10% of old dogs complete the 3cDNMP memory task at delays of 30 seconds; most (80%) are unable to complete the task at delays longer than 5 seconds. This suggests that while most old dogs can acquire the more difficult 3cDNMP, few can retain spatial information on this task at delays longer than 5 seconds (Chan *et al.*, 2002).

Nonspatial memory impairments

In the dog, object recognition memory is examined using a delayed nonmatching to sample (DNMS) paradigm with either the variable delay or progressive delay protocols, comparable to the DNMP task (Callahan *et al.*, 2000). Most young and some old dogs can perform the DNMS task at over 80% accuracy, but performance declines with longer delay intervals. The progressive delay protocol indicates that dogs are capable of responding accurately with delays up to 5 minutes. Spatial and nonspatial memory may be subserved by independent neural pathways that are differentially disrupted in aging (Courtney *et al.*, 1996).

EXECUTIVE DYSFUNCTION IN THE AGING CANINE

Absent from many early investigations of cognitive aging in the dog were measures of complex cognitive processes. Higher-order cognitive processes, often characterized as executive functions, include categorical abstraction, set maintenance and manipulation, shifting of set, and inhibitory control (West, 1996). Largely controlled by the frontal lobes (Fuster, 1999), tests of executive function are some of the most sensitive measures of aging; they indicate that executive function deficits precede many cognitive impairments in human aging (West, 1996). This final section on canine cognitive aging will describe the effects of age on executive functions in the Beagle dog.

Inhibitory control in aging dogs

Inhibitory control and performance monitoring are executive functions that show decreased efficiency during normal aging (McDowd *et al.*, 1995). According to the inhibitory deficit hypothesis of aging, the inability to maintain attention to relevant task features and to inhibit interfering information or previously activated cognitive processes is the single greatest factor affecting age-related cognitive decline (Hasher and Zacks, 1988). Deficits on tests of sensory processing, memory, and reading comprehension are often attributed to a lack of inhibitory control with age (McDowd *et al.*, 1995).

Although not exclusively designed to measure executive function, the nature of errors on discrimination reversal tasks provide evidence of inhibitory control deficits. Discrimination reversal tasks require subjects to inhibit prepotent responses to previously correct stimuli and shift responses to a new stimulus–reward contingency within the same perceptual dimension. In humans, reversal deficits correlate with dementia severity. For example, perseverative responding, a measure of impaired inhibitory control, is more severe in Alzheimer's patients than demented Parkinson's patients or normal controls

(Freedman and Oscar-Berman, 1989). Similar deficits are observed in aged nonhuman primates (Voytko, 1999) and rodents (Means and Holsten, 1992).

Reversal learning in the dog was previously examined using an object discrimination task (Milgram *et al.*, 1994). Aged dogs were impaired relative to young dogs on the object discrimination reversal task but not the initial object discrimination. Although this study found that aged dogs required more sessions for the initial phase of the reversal task, it did not determine whether this was an inhibitory control deficit or a stimulus–reward association deficit. More recently, the types of errors made during a size discrimination reversal learning task were examined to dissociate inhibitory control deficits from stimulus–reward learning deficits (Tapp *et al.*, 2003a). After learning an initial size discrimination (Figure 35.2) in which dogs were rewarded for responding to one of two identical stimuli that differed only in size (i.e., height), the reward contingencies were reversed. Reversal learning errors were categorized by stages based on previously published criteria (Duel *et al.*, 1971). Stage I errors were defined as seven or more errors per 10-trial test session and represented perseverative responding. Stage II and III errors were defined as four to six or less than 3 errors per 10-trial test session respectively, and represented a stimulus–reward deficit. Overall, old dogs made more errors than young dogs on both the size and size reversal tasks. Qualitative analysis of errors on the reversal task however, suggested that separate cognitive processes were responsible for the learning deficits in two subgroups of old dogs (Figure 35.4).

Most errors made by old dogs (aged 8–11 years) were Stage II, reflecting a deficit in learning a new stimulus–reward contingency. By contrast, senior dogs (aged 11.5–14 years) made significantly more Stage I, or perseverative errors. The old dogs were separated into old and senior dogs based on neuropathological and neuropsychological information. Senior dogs are over 11.5 years of age, equivalent to approximately 74 human years. Executive function deficits in humans commonly occur in people over the age of 70, and we wanted to isolate this age population in our dogs (Tapp *et al.*, 2003a, 2004b). Dogs over the age of 11.5 also show particular vulnerability to reduced frontal lobe volume and beta-amyloid deposition (Tapp *et al.*, 2004a; Head *et al.*, 1998), which warrants a distinction in the aged group. These data suggest that inhibitory control deficits are a characteristic of aging in very old dogs and, like aging humans and patients with dementia, may underlie patterns of cognitive or executive dysfunction in aging dogs.

Maintenance and manipulation impairments in aging dogs

Working memory incorporates a system for temporary storage and a mechanism for on-line manipulation of stored information during a wide variety of cognitive activities (Baddeley, 2001). In this context, maintenance is defined as the transferring, maintaining, and matching of

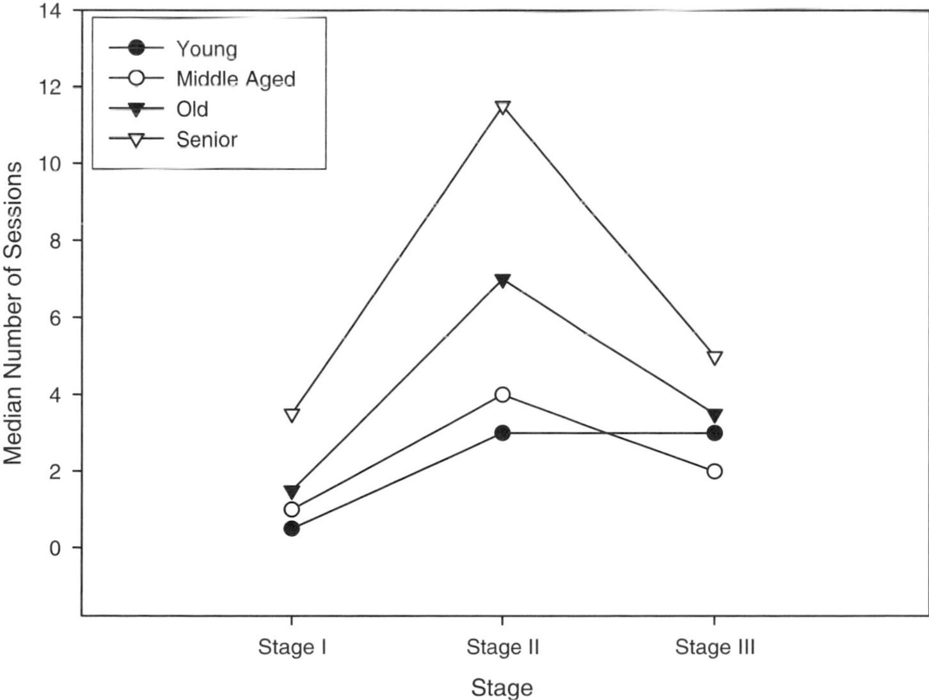

Figure 35.4 Median number of sessions spent at Stage I, II, and III during reversal learning by young, middle-aged, old, and senior Beagle dogs. Compared to young and old dogs, senior dogs exhibited greater perseveration and stimulus–reward learning deficits. Reprinted with permission from Cold Spring Harbor Laboratory Press. Copyright 2003, *Learning and Memory 10(1)*, p. 68.

information actively held in working memory, whereas manipulation is viewed as the additional reorganization or dynamic updating of information in a memory set. Both maintenance and manipulation functions in working memory may be differentially vulnerable to aging.

Tasks that require subjects to reorganize or manipulate information held in working memory before that information is recalled place greater demands on subjects' working memory processes. Alzheimer's and Parkinson's patients are particularly sensitive to tasks that place greater demands on working memory, especially those that elicit active processes (i.e., manipulation) during a working memory task (Belleville *et al.*, 2003).

The standard tests used to assess working memory in the dog are the DNMP and DNMS tasks. Working memory demands on these tasks are manipulated by changing the delay interval between the sample and non-match phases of the task. As mentioned previously, dogs do not perform as well with longer delays. An alternate method for changing working demands is to increase the amount of information that must be monitored or manipulated in memory during a task. In a recent study, the spatial list learning (SLL) paradigm was developed to examine this component of working memory in aging dogs (Tapp *et al.*, 2003b). Comparable to the delayed recognition span task used in primates (Herndon *et al.*, 1993), a key component of the SLL paradigm is that each response cannot be made in isolation, but must be made with reference to earlier responses and information in the trial. Thus, success on this task depends on the ability to maintain and continually up-date an on-line record of which locations were previously selected, and which were not.

In the original design the dog is presented with a single red disc randomly located over one of three food wells during the first phase of a trial (Figure 35.2). After a response is made, a brief delay interval occurs, followed by the second phase of the trial in which two identical red discs are presented, one in the original location and a second in one of the two remaining spatial locations. Only responses to the novel location are rewarded on the second phase. After a second delay period, the third phase of the task occurs in which the dog is presented with three identical red discs, two in the familiar locations and a third in the final novel location. Only responses to the novel location are rewarded. Locations of each object are randomized across trials.

This task proved to be much more difficult than the 3cDNMP task. Half of the young dogs tested on this task reached delays of 50 seconds, but only one-third of the old dogs successfully completed the 10-second delay. This was particularly surprising since the old dogs included in this study represented successful agers—dogs that performed the 3cDNMP task as well as young dogs. Impaired performance among the successful agers suggested that age-related impairments in spatial list learning reflect deficits in executive functions (i.e., manipulation), rather than maintenance processes. To further explore this finding, a modified version of the SLL task (mSLL) was developed (Figure 35.2).

The original SLL task design was such that positional strategies could be adopted for solving the task. The mSLL task minimizes nonmnemonic strategies and maximizes the cognitive demands on working memory by presenting the first and second discriminandum separately, rather than concurrently. This modification proved to be much more difficult for the old dogs. Only one old dog completed the learning stage of the task (i.e., a 5-second delay) but was unable to complete the task at the 10-second delay. All young dogs however, learned the task at the shortest delay and achieved the highest delay used of 50 seconds.

The results from both SLL tasks suggest that in the Beagle dog, working memory processes of maintenance and on-line monitoring are differentially affected by age. Specifically, executive processes associated with manipulating or updating information appear to be impaired relative to low-level processes required for actively holding information in working memory. These dissociative effects may represent differential rates of aging in distinct neuroanatomical regions specific to maintenance and executive functions.

Rule induction and concept abstraction in aging dogs

One of the most commonly observed executive deficits in aging is the inability to categorize or sort objects based on a conceptual dimension. In human studies, the most common paradigm to assess this deficit is the Wisconsin Card Sort Test (WCST; Berg, 1948). On the WCST subjects are required to sort stimuli according to an unknown principle, which the subject must deduce from feedback provided by the clinician. Elderly subjects frequently make more perseverative errors and complete fewer sorting categories on this task, which may reflect impaired rule induction, inhibitory control, performance monitoring, or set shifting abilities (Ridderinkhoff *et al.*, 2002).

Animal studies have also examined concept learning in a range of species, but few have explored the effect of age on this ability. We recently developed a size concept task to examine the effects of age on concept learning in the Beagle dog (Tapp *et al.*, 2004b). The protocol consisted of training dogs on several 2-choice and 3-choice size discrimination tasks, using the same sets of blocks, to teach the animals to attend to size. Subsequently, novel stimuli differing only in size were introduced to determine if dogs learned that size could also be used conceptually to solve this new task. Young dogs were the only age group successfully able to acquire the size concept and transfer this knowledge to the concept tests. Old and senior dogs were not able to transfer the information and approached the concept tests as new tasks without using the previously learned information. The results suggest that executive functions such as rule induction and concept abstraction decrease with age and may begin as early as 8–10 years of age in the dog.

SUMMARY

Dogs develop a variety of age-dependent cognitive deficits that parallel declines observed in normal and pathological aging in humans. Our studies revealed a large amount of variability in cognitive aging in the dog. Like humans, cognitive aging in the Beagle dog is complex and nonlinear, and striking individual differences are common. In both humans and dogs, some individuals show little decline (successful agers), some show mild decline, and others of the same age develop severe cognitive impairments. The earliest signs of cognitive decline observed in the dog appear to include executive functions.

Noncognitive Functions and Aging in the Dog

Although cognitive decline is the most common and frequently studied hallmark of aging and dementia, a number of noncognitive impairments are observed in elderly and demented subjects. The term *noncognitive* will refer to a range of diverse behaviors that do not explicitly involve testing for learning and memory but could be related to cognitive status. Such behaviors include general activity, social interaction, and psychotic and aggressive behaviors. A similar distinction is made in the case of humans (Folstein and Blysma, 1999). Using the dog as a model system to study aging, we have reported several noncognitive behavioral changes, which correlate with changes in cognitive functioning. The specific noncognitive behaviors examined include locomotor activity, activity rhythms, social interactions, and exploratory behavior.

LOCOMOTOR ACTIVITY

Physical movement or motor activity significantly declines with advancing age in humans (Bennett, 1998). Changes in physical activity become more severe in neurodegenerative disorders and can take several forms including ceaseless walking, trailing and checking, and wandering (Folstein and Bylsma, 1999). We have observed similar changes in locomotor activity in the dog, which vary with cognitive impairment (Siwak *et al.*, 2001, 2003). Locomotor activity in the dog is assessed with three different tests: the open field test (Siwak *et al.*, 2001, 2002; Head *et al.*, 1997), the home cage test (Siwak *et al.*, 2002); and the Actiwatch® activity monitoring system (Siwak *et al.*, 2003). The general finding is that locomotor activity decreases with age in the dog (Figure 35.5), but is dependent upon several factors including test situation, cognitive status, and previous experiences.

First, the environmental testing situation influences motor activity in dogs. In a novel environment, such as the open field arena, young and old dogs are aroused and responsive to the change in surroundings. Measures of locomotor activity are affected such that age-related decreases in activity are not observed. As the open field becomes familiar, locomotion declines in both young and aged dogs (Siwak *et al.*, 2001, 2002). Familiar home cage environments may reflect more spontaneous activity, and age-related decreases in motor activity are more easily observed (Siwak *et al.*, 2002).

Second, motor activity is related to cognitive impairment. When aged dogs are divided into cognitively impaired and unimpaired subgroups, robust differences in locomotor activity are observed (Siwak *et al.*, 2001; Head *et al.*, 1997). Aged dogs that are severely impaired on tests of cognitive function tend to be hyperactive compared to unimpaired aged dogs. This is consistent with studies in humans showing a relationship between hyperactivity and several disorders including dementia, autism, and attention deficit disorder (Folstein and Blysma, 1999; Castellanos *et al.*, 2001). These increased levels of activity in impaired dogs may be a manifestation of neurodegenerative changes that contribute to cognitive impairment.

Third, previous rearing history or possible genetic factors may affect locomotion. Dogs born and raised in a laboratory are hyperactive compared to dogs reared outside of the laboratory (Fox, 1971; Siwak *et al.*, 2003). Thus, environmental enrichment during the lifespan of the dog may interact with genetic factors and contribute to the severity of locomotor decline and cognitive dysfunction in aging (Siwak *et al.*, 2001; Head *et al.*, 1997).

ACTIVITY RHYTHMS

Approximately 40–70% of elderly people suffer from some type of sleep disorder such as increased waking at night or frequent napping during the day (Van Someren, 2000). These effects are exacerbated in subjects with dementia (Satlin *et al.*, 1991). We have assessed the circadian pattern of locomotor activity in dogs with the Actiwatch® actigraph monitoring system (Siwak *et al.*, 2003). Dogs exhibit clear activity–rest rhythms in which activity levels are high during the day and low at night. Moreover, circadian patterns of locomotor activity in dogs exhibit age-related alterations, which vary with cognitive status and housing environment.

Cognitively impaired aged dogs display higher levels of activity and fewer periods during the day where they exhibit no activity compared to unimpaired aged dogs. Peak activity for impaired dogs was shifted to later in the day, an observation consistent with findings in demented patients (Satlin *et al.*, 1991). The timing mechanism could be compromised due to neuropathology in both demented patients and impaired dogs.

Housing environment also influenced activity levels. Aged dogs housed indoors had shorter bouts of activity, required more time to become active after the lights came on, and exhibited extended periods of rest during the day compared to young dogs. These age-related differences

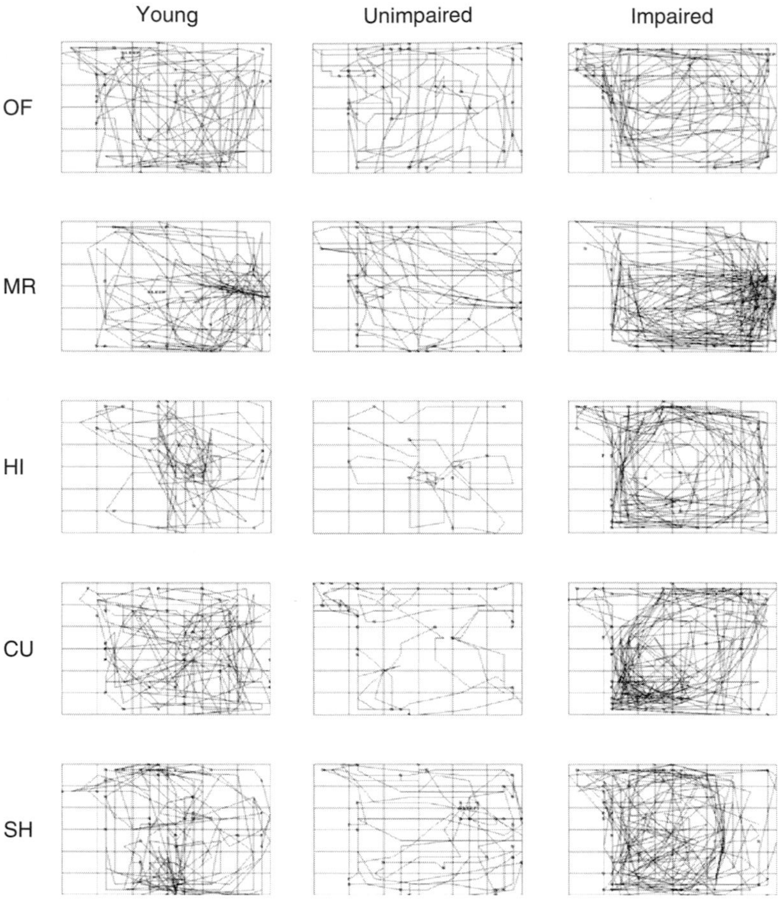

Figure 35.5 Tracings of the movement patterns of a representative dog from each group in the testing room. More lines reflect more movement. The activity patterns of the age-impaired dogs did not change with the different tests. This group showed the same pattern with all the stimuli except the mirror. The young and age-unimpaired showed similar responses and modified their behavior according to the test situation. OF = open field, MR = mirror, HI = human interaction, CU = curiosity, SH = silhouette. Reprinted with permission from Cold Spring Harbor Laboratory Press, copyright 2001, *Learning and Memory* 8(6) p. 321.

were not present in dogs housed outdoors exposed to the bright sunlight, suggesting that exposure to bright light is effective in synchronizing and consolidating the activity rhythm.

SOCIAL RESPONSIVENESS IN AGING DOGS

Like humans, dogs are highly social creatures. Dogs interact with other dogs and humans and share common environments with both species. In humans, demented individuals undergo several abnormal changes in social behavior. In the early stages of Alzheimer's disease, patients become withdrawn in social settings. As the disease progresses to within 4–7 years of disease onset, social function declines. Disruptive behaviors including agitation, restlessness, and aggression become more common. Gradually, patients neglect personal grooming, demonstrate poor table manners, and engage in socially inappropriate behaviors. In the final advanced stage of the disease, patients are completely withdrawn and unresponsive to their social surroundings (Folstein and Blysma, 1999).

We adapted a series of behavioral tests to assess social responsiveness in the aging dog (Siwak *et al.*, 2001; Head *et al.*, 1997). These tests include the mirror test, the human interaction test, the silhouette test, and the model dog test. Changes in social behavior varied with age and correlated with the severity of cognitive decline.

Human interaction test

In the human interaction test, the amount of time during a 10-minute session the dog spends near or physically in contact with a person seated in the center of the observation room is recorded (Siwak *et al.*, 2001). In this test, active social responses such as initiating physical contact, climbing, sniffing, and licking were more common in younger dogs. Age-unimpaired dogs preferred more passive responses like sitting or lying quietly beside the person. Both groups were significantly different from cognitively impaired dogs who exhibited very little interest in the person.

Mirror test

In the mirror test, dogs are placed in an enclosed arena with a mirror secured to one wall of the room. Reactions to the reflection in the mirror depend on the dogs' ability to recognize its own species (Fox, 1971). Consistent with Gallup (1968), the reactions of the dogs toward the mirror reflection were initially *other-directed*. Responses included jumping at, barking at, trying to play with the dog in the mirror as well as attempts to look behind the mirror to find the other dog. Differences between cognitively impaired and unimpaired aged dogs were very prominent in this test (Siwak *et al.*, 2001). Unimpaired old and young dogs habituated to the reflected image rapidly. Old impaired dogs spent significantly more time reacting to the reflection in the mirror, suggesting a deficit in habituation.

The silhouette and model dog tests

To further explore social responses to conspecifics, we used the silhouette and model dog tests (Fox, 1971). In the silhouette test, a black laminated cardboard-dog figure is attached to one wall of the open field test room and dogs are observed for their interactions (i.e., sniffing) with this object for 10 minutes. Dogs treated the cardboard cutout as a real dog by targeting sniffing in the facial and anal regions as is typical when dogs meet. Initially, all dogs sniffed the object with the same frequency, but young and old-unimpaired dogs habituated to the silhouette. When retested on the silhouette task two weeks later, young and old-unimpaired dogs paid little attention to the silhouette. The old-impaired dogs spent much more time sniffing the silhouette, probably reflecting a deficit in habituation or stimulus recognition.

We subsequently modified the procedure to make the conspecific more realistic by using a 3-dimensional model dog that more closely resembles a real living dog. In this test, beagle dogs are observed for their interactions with a life-sized sand-cast model of a Golden Retriever. Young dogs spent more time sniffing and interacting with the model than old-impaired and unimpaired dogs. Old-impaired and unimpaired dogs did not differ in the amount of time spent sniffing the model dog.

Together, the results from the four tests indicate that as in humans, social behaviors change with age in dogs. Old dogs, like elderly people, continue to be social creatures with age but become more passive in their social interactions compared to young dogs. As cognitive functions become increasingly impaired, however, social behaviors change from normal, appropriate responses to disrupted and inappropriate reactions.

EXPLORATORY BEHAVIOR

Reduced novelty seeking, curiosity, and exploratory behaviors are common hallmarks of normal aging (Daffner *et al.*, 1994). The decrement in exploratory behavior is more severe in demented patients (Daffner *et al.*, 1999). The curiosity test in the dog was intended to measure changes in exploratory behavior with age. Dogs were placed in an observation room with seven novel commercially available toys distributed throughout the room. Total time spent playing with or sniffing objects was recorded. Results from this task revealed a pattern of behavioral change consistent with other noncognitive measures. Specifically, young dogs spent more time playing with and sniffing objects than either group of old dogs. Old-unimpaired dogs showed similar reactions as young dogs but spent less time exploring objects. Exploratory behavior also varied with cognitive status. Old-impaired dogs generally avoided the toys and expressed no interest in investigating the objects (Siwak *et al.*, 2001).

SUMMARY

Taking all noncognitive tests into account, young and aged dogs exhibit distinct behavioral profiles. Young dogs exhibit higher levels of activity and more interest in interacting with toys, people, and artificial dogs, which modifies their movement pattern as shown in Figure 35.5. Aged dogs show decreases in locomotion and other behaviors but continue to display appropriate responses, just to a lesser extent than young dogs. Impaired dogs by contrast show abnormal responses. These dogs are hyperactive, unresponsive to social stimuli or toys, and often engage in stereotypical behaviors. These impaired subjects display atypical social responses on tests of human and mirror-image interactions. The profile of the impaired dogs is consistent with behavioral disruptions that occur in demented people.

Neuropathology

In parallel with our work on characterizing cognitive and behavioral changes in aging dogs, a third strategy in developing the canine as a model system of human brain aging involves identifying pathological brain changes related to age-associated cognitive-behavioral dysfunction in the dog. Specifically, we have examined beta-amyloid deposition, neuron loss, oxidative damage, and structural anatomy in the aging canine brain. These studies reveal that brain aging in dogs begins as early as middle age, varies across brain regions, and correlates with cognitive and behavioral impairments; dogs develop some of the pathological hallmarks found in Alzheimer's disease. This final section will summarize current knowledge on neuropathological and neuroanatomical markers of brain aging in the canine.

BETA-AMYLOID DEPOSITION

One of the hallmarks of Alzheimer's disease is the development of senile plaques. Dogs do not develop all

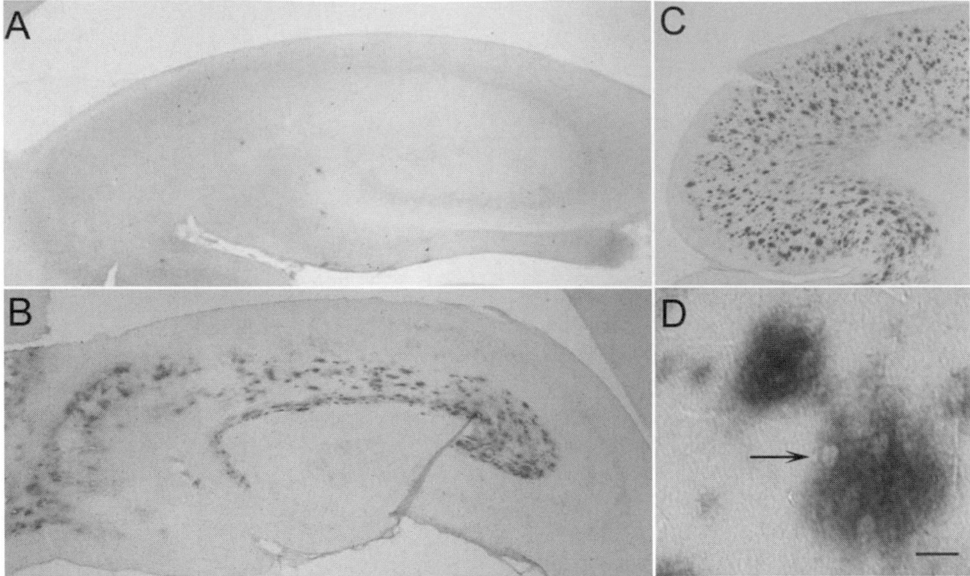

Figure 35.6 Beta-amyloid immunostaining in the hippocampus of a 5-year-old dog (A) and a 12-year-old dog (B) and in the temporal cortex of a 12 year-old-dog (C). Higher magnification in the 12-year-old (D) illustrates the presence of intact neurons (arrow) in the diffuse plaques. Bar in D is 20 μm. See the color plate section.

of the hallmarks of Alzheimer's disease, but the aged dog is particularly well-suited for studying early stages of beta-amyloid deposition in the aging brain. Plaque morphology in the dog is generally diffuse and cloud-like (Figure 35.6) and deposits are thioflavine-S negative, suggesting a lack of β-pleated sheets formation (Satou *et al.*, 1997).

In addition, dogs accumulate the longer, more toxic and less soluble form of $A\beta_{1-42}$ prior to the shorter more soluble $A\beta_{1-40}$ type, consistent with human brain aging (Cummings *et al.*, 1996). Beta-amyloid builds up initially in and around neurons and is present within apical and basal dendrites. Furthermore, beta-amyloid is deposited uniformly in select synaptic terminal fields, such as the terminal zone of the perforant pathway, that show a predilection for extensive plaque formation in Alzheimer's disease.

The regional pattern of beta-amyloid deposition in the dog parallels human brain aging. In the dog, the earliest and most consistent distribution of beta-amyloid plaques occurs in the prefrontal cortex beginning around 8 years of age (Head *et al.*, 1998). Early prefrontal beta-amyloid deposition is also common in nondemented (Bussière *et al.*, 2002) and preclinical Alzheimer's disease subjects (Yamaguchi *et al.*, 2001). By 14 years of age, beta-amyloid deposition progresses to the entorhinal and parietal regions of the canine cerebral cortex equally, leaving the cerebellum relatively unaffected. Further, our studies reveal a strong correlation between regional beta-amyloid deposition and cognitive decline in aging dogs (Head *et al.*, 1998; Tapp *et al.*, 2004a).

NEUROFIBRILLARY TANGLES

In humans, abnormal hyperphosphorylation of the microtubule protein tau leads to the development of neurofibrillary tangles (NFTs), which are linked to cognitive decline in aging (Duyckaerts *et al.*, 1997). In the dog, the role of neurofibrillary tangle formation is unclear. Although dogs exhibit early stages of tangle formation characterized by tau phosphorylation and an intracellular punctuate distribution, the morphology is distinct from the human brain and does not progress into thioflavine-S or silver positive NFTs (Cummings *et al.*, 1996). Using AT8, a marker for early neurofibrillary tangle formation, Head *et al.* (2001) observed hyperphosphorylated tau in select neuronal populations in middle-aged but not old dogs. This is consistent with earlier studies of cytoskeletal abnormalities (Cumming *et al.*, 1996), distended neurites (Wisniewski *et al.*, 1970), and tau positive neurons (Uchida *et al.*, 1993) in the dog.

One explanation for the absence of NFTs in the dog is that the tau protein in the dog is different from human tau protein and thus dogs are not predisposed to develop full NFTs with age (Head *et al.*, 2001). The implication of this finding is that beta-amyloid and not tau pathology may be sufficient to lead to cognitive and behavioral dysfunction in the aging dog. In the absence of NFTs, cognitive dysfunction increases proportionately with beta-amyloid deposition in the dog. All old dogs develop pathology, but old animals with extensive beta-amyloid deposition are more impaired than those with less beta-amyloid deposition (Head *et al.*, 1998). This suggests that beta-amyloid deposition may influence neuronal function and may lead to impaired cognition.

NEURONAL LOSS

Neuron loss is another potential morphological correlate of cognitive decline in normal and pathological aging in humans. Stereological studies have revealed regionally specific neuron loss in the hilus and subiculum of the hippocampus (West, 1993), the islands of the entorhinal cortex (Simic *et al.*, 2005), and mild loss in the neocortex including the frontal, temporal, parietal and occipital cortices (Pakkenberg *et al.*, 1997) in humans with age. In Alzheimer's disease the extent of neuron loss is even greater, occurring in the same regions as normal aging, hilus and subiculum, but extending into additional areas including area CA1 (West *et al.*, 1994). Age-related neuron loss in the canine brain occurs in the cingulate gyrus, superior colliculus, and claustrum (Ball *et al.*, 1983; Morys *et al.*, 1994). Calbindin-positive GABAergic neurons in the prefrontal cortex of the canine brain are also lost with age (Pugliese *et al.*, 2004). Our own stereological studies in the canine hippocampus reveal a reduction in the number of hilar neurons in aged dogs (Siwak *et al.*, 2005a).

OXIDATIVE DAMAGE

Another biological correlate of cognitive and behavioral dysfunction in dogs is the progressive accumulation of oxidative damage with age. Neurons in the brain are highly vulnerable to oxidative damage, which accumulates with age due to the high respiratory demands of the central nervous system. Generation of reactive oxygen species in the brain damages proteins, lipids, and nucleotides, which contribute to neuronal dysfunction and neurodegeneration in aging (Floyd *et al.*, 2001).

The brains of aged dogs accumulate oxidative damage to lipids and proteins (Head *et al.*, 2002). Beginning around 8 years of age, levels of malondialdehyde (MDA), a marker of lipid peroxidation, progressively increase in the prefrontal cortex and serum in the dog. In parallel with increased MDA, glutamine synthetase activity, an endogenous antioxidant, decreases with age in the prefrontal cortex. These age-related changes in oxidative damage coincide with increased beta-amyloid deposition in the prefrontal cortex and together may impair neuronal function.

If oxidative damage is a key contributor to cognitive dysfunction, then antioxidant supplementation may ameliorate these deficits. In Alzheimer's patients, antioxidant supplementation can improve cognitive function (Morris *et al.*, 2005) and delay institutionalization (Sano *et al.*, 1997). We hypothesized that if brain aging and the progressive accumulation of oxidative damage are related to cognitive and behavioral decline in the dog as well, then dogs treated with dietary antioxidants or mitochondrial cofactors should exhibit less cognitive decline with age relative to controls. This hypothesis was examined in a 4-year longitudinal study from 1999 to 2002 involving the collaborative participation of three laboratories in Canada and the United States. In this study, 48 aged dogs received either a control diet or a diet enriched with antioxidants and mitochondrial cofactors (to promote mitochondrial health). The antioxidant diet was enriched with vitamin E, vitamin C, l-carnitine, dl-alpha lipoic acid, and a 1% inclusion of spinach flakes, tomato pomace, grape pomace, carrot granules, and citrus pulp. Every six months after the start of the study, all dogs were routinely tested on an extensive battery of cognitive tasks (Milgram *et al.*, 2005, 2004) to evaluate the efficacy of antioxidant therapies on cognitive and behavioral function in aging. At the completion of the study, the effect of antioxidant treatment on beta-amyloid deposition was examined in the brains of half of the old dogs.

Cognitive function was significantly improved and maintained with dietary treatment. Old dogs performed more poorly than young dogs on many of the complex discrimination tasks, but old dogs given the enriched antioxidant diet performed significantly better than old dogs fed the control diet (Milgram *et al.*, 2002a,b; Siwak *et al.*, 2005b). The antioxidant diet had little effect in young dogs. In addition, old dogs fed an antioxidant diet improved on a number of noncognitive behavioral measures including recognition, interaction, agility, and compulsive behaviors (Dodd *et al.*, 2003).

Treatment with the antioxidant-enriched diet also reduced beta-amyloid deposition in old dogs, but the effects were brain-region specific. The extent of beta-amyloid, measured by loads, was lower in the parietal, entorhinal, and occipital cortices, but not the prefrontal cortex in aged treated dogs compared to control dogs (Pop *et al.*, 2003). The age at which dogs were provided with the antioxidant diet was previously established to be a time when prefrontal beta-amyloid deposition had begun (Head *et al.*, 1998). The absence of an effect in the prefrontal cortex therefore suggests that treatment with a broad spectrum antioxidant diet may prevent beta-amyloid deposition but does not reverse existing beta-amyloid deposition.

Collectively, the results from this study indicate that combinations of antioxidants and mitochondrial cofactors work together synergistically to improve age-related cognitive and behavioral decline. The mechanisms for this improvement may reflect a decrease in oxidative damage and beta-amyloid deposition, but our data suggest that a critical window exists for reducing beta-amyloid deposition in the brain; the earlier the treatment begins, the greater the benefits.

BRAIN IMAGING IN THE DOG

Recent advances in brain imaging technology permit noninvasive analyses of metabolic, vascular, and structural changes associated with normal and pathological aging. In addition to improved image acquisition devices, computer technology and software development have also advanced, producing more sophisticated methods for analyzing brain imaging data. Techniques such as manual-based region of interest (ROI) planimetry and voxel-based morphometry (VBM), widely used in humans, indicate that biological characteristics such as age, sex, and underlying pathology contribute significantly to the variability in brain aging.

In addition to *in vitro* neuropathological measures, we have used several imaging protocols to examine brain aging in the dog model. In the remaining section, the application of MRI to study structural, pathological, and cerebrovascular markers of aging in the dog brain will be discussed.

Age-related changes in global and focal brain volume

Our initial work with MRI involved using manual ROI planimetry to evaluate changes in brain and ventricular volume as a function of age. Standard quantitative procedures involved meticulously tracing brain regions of interest on multiple slices to compare differences in brain volume across subject cohorts (Figure 35.7).

This revealed that aged dog brains show increased cortical atrophy, ventricular dilation, decreased total brain volume, and decreased frontal lobe volume (Su *et al.*, 1998; Tapp *et al.*, 2004a). Age-related decreases in frontal lobe volume were associated with increased beta-amyloid deposition and impaired executive function (Tapp *et al.*, 2004a).

An alternate method of assessing volumetric brain changes in aging is VBM. VBM permits rapid voxel-by-voxel comparisons of local gray and white matter brain regions without the need for a priori selection of ROIs and is highly sensitive to volumetric differences in normal and pathological aging (Tisserand *et al.*, 2004). Despite its popularity in human brain imaging, application of VBM for mapping brain aging in animal models is less common. We recently developed a VBM procedure for analyzing regional brain aging in the dog (Tapp *et al.*, 2005b). The initial steps of this procedure are time consuming and require the creation of standardized dog brain templates and a priori probability maps; but once

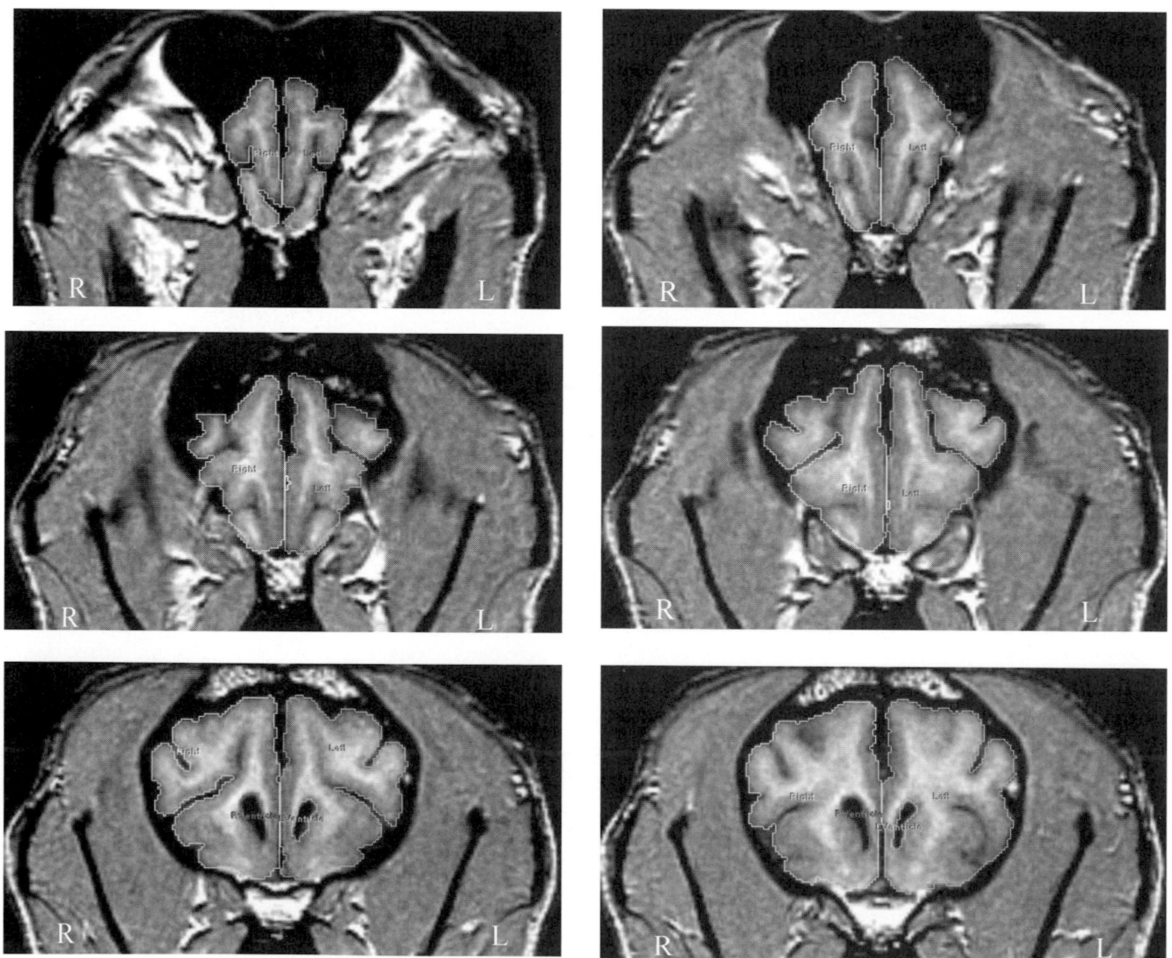

Figure 35.7 Coronal MRI slices through the frontal cortex of the dog brain. Images are presented rostrocaudally (front to back) top to bottom, left to right. Hemispheric and regional differences in brain volume were performed using manual planimetry to trace each region of interest.

complete, rapid voxel-by-voxel comparisons of gray and white matter volumetric changes in the aging dog brain are possible. Using this technique, we found a number of age and sex dependent changes in gray and white matter volume in the dog (Figure 35.8).

Age-related reductions in gray matter volume were observed bilaterally in the frontal gyrus, orbitalis gyrus, ectosylvian gyrus, olfactory bulb, and superior olivaris nucleus in the brainstem. Unilaterally, gray matter loss occurred in the proreal gyrus, sylvian gyrus, suprasylvian gyrus, cerebellum, and brainstem nuclei with advancing age. The effects of age on brain volume, however, differed in male and female dogs; decreased frontal lobe volume was more predominant in males, and decreased temporal lobe volume was more common in females. Similar patterns were observed in white matter brain regions as well. Age-related white matter loss was largely bilateral and included the internal capsula (including a small portion of the genu of the corpus callosum), white matter tracts of the anterior cingulate (anterior fascia cinguli), and the alveus of the hippocampus. Decreases in the volume of the internal capsula were more frequent in males, whereas atrophy of the alveus of the hippocampus occurred primarily in female dogs. The VBM results not only validated earlier findings of frontal lobe atrophy in aging dogs but extended these findings and suggested that brain aging in the dog, like humans, varies regionally and differs between males and females.

Progressive lesion formation in the aging dog brain

A second useful application of MRI is the ability to monitor longitudinal changes in the brain of aging dogs. Serial MRI (sMRI) techniques allow images collected longitudinally to be quantified at the individual level instead of using cross-sectional images to compare differences between young and old groups. In sMRI, images are co-registered using a goodness-of-fit function to align images collected at different time points into a unified stereotaxic space. In humans, sMRI studies are difficult to conduct due to attrition rates and long intervals required to observe significant changes in brain morphology—problems not encountered with dogs. sMRI procedures used in the dog to monitor lesion formation revealed that aging is associated with an increased frequency of a specific type of lesion resembling small lacunes (Su *et al.*, 2005). The majority of lesions observed in the dog brain were located in the frontal cortex and caudate nucleus (Figure 35.9). This is consistent with other evidence that

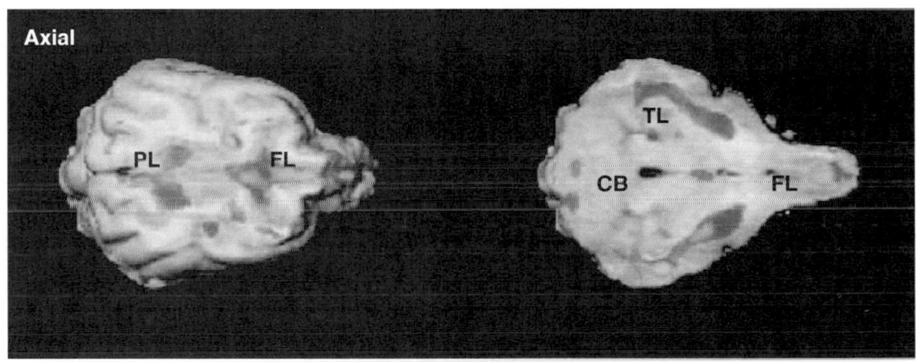

A

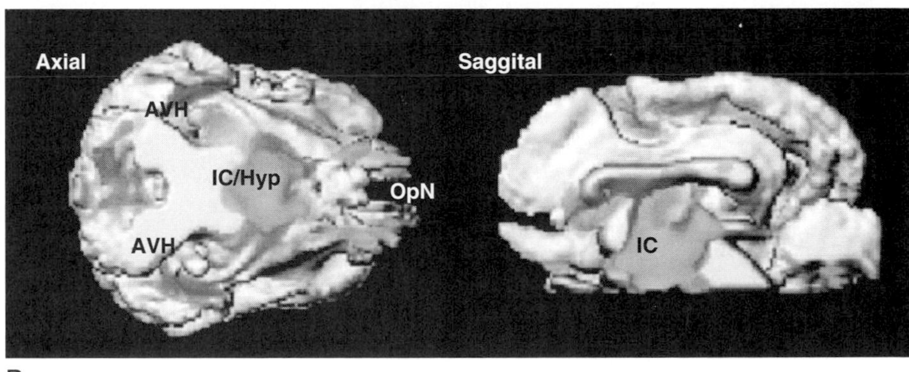

B

Figure 35.8 3-dimensional rendering of brain regions showing a significant age-related reduction in gray (A) and white matter (B) brain regions. Regional atrophy for males and females is shown in green and red, respectively. Areas of overlap for old males and females are shown in yellow. Brain renderings are presented in saggital and axial orientations. (Abbreviations: FL = frontal lobe, PL = parietal lobe, TL = temporal lobe, CB = cerebellum, IC = internal capsula, AVH = alveus of the hippocampus, OpN = optic nerve bundle, IC/Hyp = internal capsula/hypophysis.) See the color plate section.

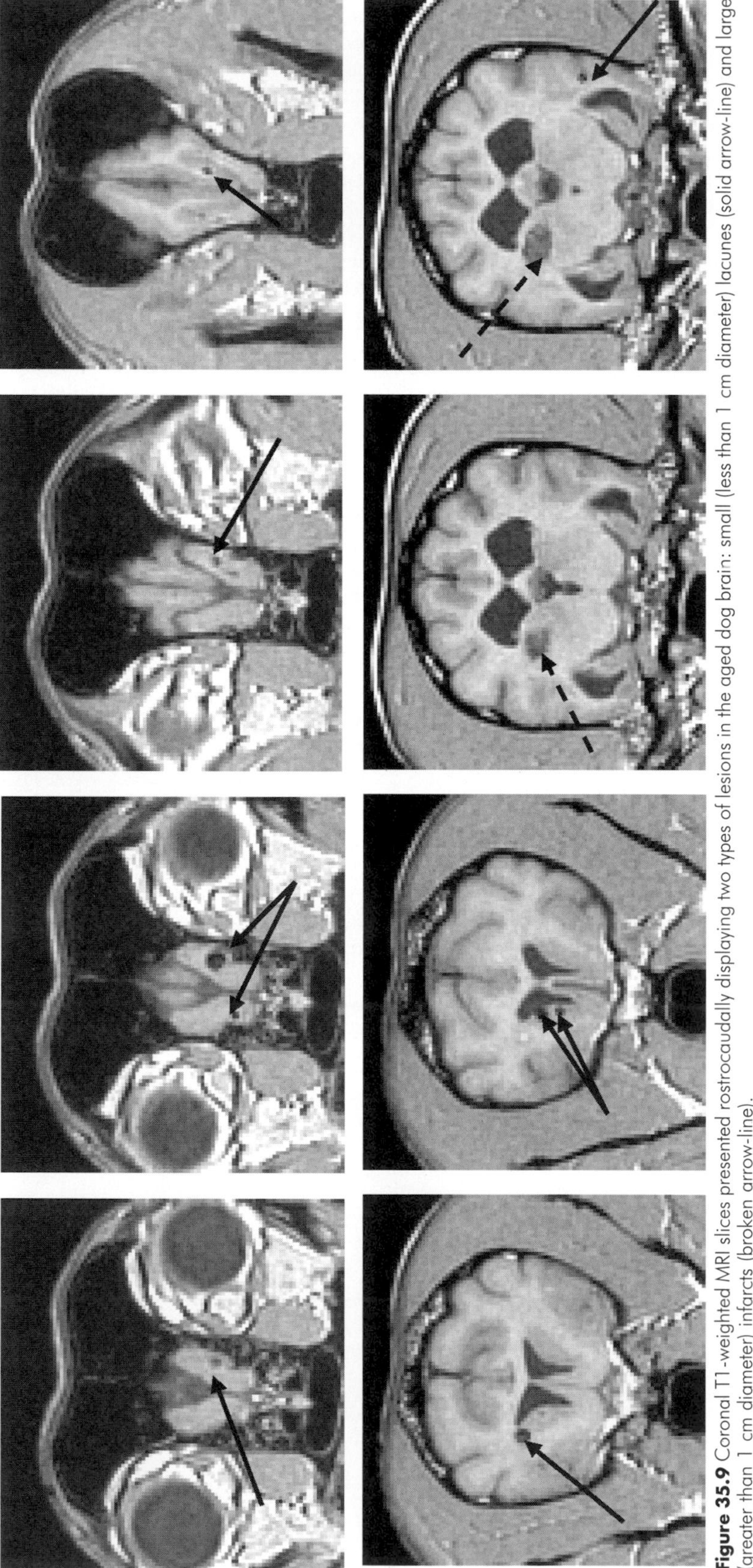

Figure 35.9 Coronal T1-weighted MRI slices presented rostrocaudally displaying two types of lesions in the aged dog brain: small (less than 1 cm diameter) lacunes (solid arrow-line) and large (greater than 1 cm diameter) infarcts (broken arrow-line).

the frontal lobes are especially vulnerable to aging in the dog (Head *et al.*, 1998; Tapp *et al.*, 2004a).

Cerebrovascular changes in the aging dog brain

MRI is also used to assess hemodynamic changes in the dog by combining high-resolution MRI and paramagnetic intravascular susceptibility contrast agents (e.g., Gd-DTPA) to derive measures of cerebrovascular volume, flow, and blood brain barrier integrity. In humans, dynamic susceptibility contrast enhanced (DSC)-MRI is sensitive to decreases in blood volume in temporoparietal brain regions in AD and MCI patients relative to healthy age-matched controls (Harris *et al.*, 1998). In a study of 18 dogs aged 4–15 years of age, a significant correlation was found between blood–brain barrier (BBB) permeability, beta-amyloid deposition, and ventricular dilation (Su *et al.*, 1998). Further, this increased BBB leakage occurred in the absence of cortical atrophy, suggesting that changes in BBB integrity precede cortical atrophy and may be an early consequence of aging.

Reduced blood flow and volume are frequently associated with age-related cognitive decline in humans. DSC-MRI studies performed in dogs have illustrated that impaired hemodynamics also contribute to brain aging (Tapp *et al.*, 2005a). First, gray matter regional cerebral blood volume (rCBV) was consistently higher than white matter rCBV in young and old dogs. Second, gray and white matter rCBV declined with age. Third, age-related changes in rCBV were largest in white matter brain regions compared to gray matter brain regions. Moreover, decreased rCBV and increased BBB permeability occurred in tandem with regional gray and white matter cortical atrophy.

SUMMARY

The aged dog is particularly well-suited to investigate the initial stages of plaque formation in the aging brain. Beta-amyloid deposition in the form of diffuse plaques is a prominent feature of the aged dog brain. The morphology of beta-amyloid exhibited in the dog is almost identical to the early plaque pathology reported in nondemented and demented human subjects and Down's syndrome individuals. Oxidative damage and neuron loss are also features of the canine brain even though NFTs are absent.

MRI procedures commonly used in humans offer a viable, noninvasive, and reproducible method for evaluating brain changes in vivo in the aging dog. Structural and vascular changes as well as spontaneous pathology can easily be monitored and show many similarities to observations in humans. Aged dogs show reduced brain volume, increased ventricles, spontaneous lesions, and reduced blood flow.

Conclusion

The canine is an innovative model for studying cognitive, behavioral, and brain aging. Aging in dogs leads to the manifestation and development of many hallmarks characteristic of human aging. Dogs exhibit cognitive decline with the same general patterns as well as individual variability that occurs in humans. Behavioral consequences are also common to both human and canine aging with parallel changes in locomotion, social responsiveness and exploration. Neuropathological investigations reiterate the similarities between canine and human conditions. In aged dogs there is a strong association between beta-amyloid deposition and cognitive dysfunction but other morphological correlates exist including oxidative damage and neuron loss. The canine is clearly a valuable model of aging to examine the relationship between cognitive function, behavior, and neuropathology, given the many demonstrated similarities to observations in human aging and dementia.

ACKNOWLEDGMENTS

This research was supported by the National Institute on Aging (NIA AG12694, AG17066) and by the United States Army Medical Research and Material Command under Contract No. DAMD17-98-1-8622. Additional support was provided by the Natural Sciences and Engineering Research Council of Canada.

REFERENCES

Adams, B., Chan, A., Callahan, H., and Milgram, N.W. (2000a). The canine as a model of human cognitive aging: recent developments. *Prog. Neuropsychopharmacol. Biol. Psychiatry 24(5)*, 675–692.

Adams, B., Chan, A., Callahan, H., Siwak, C., Tapp, D., Ikeda-Douglas, C., *et al.* (2000b). Use of a delayed non-matching to position task to model age-dependent cognitive decline in the dog. *Behav. Brain Res. 108*, 47–56.

Almkvist, O. (1996). Neuropsychological features of early Alzheimer's disease: Preclinical and clinical stages. *Acta Neurol. Stand. Suppl. 165*, 165–171.

Baddeley, A.D. (2001). Levels of working memory. In Perspectives on human and Cognitive Aging: Essays in honor of Fergus Craik (M. Naveh-Benjamin, M. Moscovitch, and H.L. Roediger III, eds.), pp. 11–123. Psychology Press, New York.

Ball, M.J., MacGregor, J., Fyfe, I.M., Rapoport, S.I., and London, E.D. (1983). Paucity of morphological changes in the brains of ageing beagle dogs: Further evidence that Alzheimer lesions are unique for primate central nervous system. *Neurobiol. Aging 4*, 127–131.

Belleville, S., Rouleau, N., Van der Linden, M., and Collette, F. (2003). Effect of manipulation and irrelevant noise on working memory capacity of patients with Alzheimer's dementia. *Neuropsychology 17*, 69–81.

Bennett, KM., (1998). Gender and longitudinal changes in physical activities in later life. *Age Ageing* 27(Suppl 3), 24–28.

Berg, E.A. (1948). Simple objective technique for measuring flexibility in thinking. *J. Gen. Psychol. 39*, 15–22.

Bussière, T., Friend, P.D., Sadeghi, N., Wicinski, B., Lin, G.I., Bouras, C., *et al.* (2002). Stereological assessment of the total cortical volume occupied by amyloid deposits and its relationship with cognitive status in aging and Alzheimer's disease. *Neuroscience 112*, 75–91.

Callahan, H., Ikeda-Douglas, C., Head, E., Cotman, C.W., and Milgram, N.W. (2000). Development of a protocol for studying object recognition memory in the dog. *Prog. Neuropsychopharmacol. Biol. Psychiatry 24(5)*, 693–707.

Castellanos, F.X., Giedd, J.N., Berquin, P.C., Walter, J.M., Sharp, W., Tran, T., *et al.* (2001). Quantitative brain magnetic resonance imaging in girls with attention-deficit/hyperactivity disorder. *Arch Gen Psychiatry 58(3)*, 289–295.

Chan, A.D., Nippak, P.M., Murphey, H., Ikeda-Douglas, C.J., Muggenburg, B., Head, E., *et al.* (2002). Visuospatial impairments in aged canines (*Canis familiaris*): The role of cognitive-behavioral flexibility. *Behav. Neurosci. 116(3)*, 443–454.

Christie, L.A., Studzinski, C.M., Araujo, J.A., Leung, C.S., Ikeda-Douglas, C.J., Head, E., *et al.* (2005). A comparison of egocentric and allocentric age-dependent spatial learning in the beagle dog. *Prog. Neuropsychopharmacol. Biol. Psychiatry 29(3)*, 361–369.

Committee on Animal Models for Research on Aging. (1981). *Carnivores*. pp. 180–242. National Academy Press, Washington, DC.

Courtney, S.M., Ungerleider, L.G., Keil, K., and Haxby, J.V. (1996). Object and spatial visual working memory activate separate neural systems in human cortex. *Cerebral Cortex 6*, 39–49.

Cummings, B.J., Head, E., Ruehl, W., Milgram, N.W., and Cotman, C.W. (1996). The canine as an animal model of human aging and dementia. *Neurobiol. Aging 17(2)*, 259–268.

Daffner, K.R., Scinto, L.F., Weintraub, S., Guinessey, J.E., and Mesulam, M.M. (1999). Diminished curiosity in patients with probable Alzheimer's disease as measured by exploratory eye movements. *Neurology 42(2)*, 320–328.

Daffner, K.R., Scinto, L.F., Weintraub, S., Guinessey, J., and Mesulam, M.M. (1994). The impact of aging on curiosity as measured by exploratory eye movements. *Arch. Neurol. 51(4)*, 368–376.

Dodd, C.E., Zicker, S.C., Jewell, D.E., Fritsch, D.A., Lowry, S.R., and Allen, T.A. (2003). Can a fortified food affect the behavioral manifestations of age-related cognitive decline in dogs? *Vet. Med.* May, 396–408.

Duel, R.K., Mishkin, M., and Semmes, J. (1971). Interaction between the hemispheres in unimanual somesthetic learning. *Experimental Neurology 30*, 123–138.

Duyckaerts, C., Bennecib, M., Grignon, Y., Uchihara, T., He, Y., Piette, F., and Hauw, J.J. (1997). Modeling the relation between neurofibrillary tangles and intellectual status. *Neurobiol. Aging 18(3)*, 267–273.

Floyd, R.A., West, M., and Hensley, K. (2001). Oxidative biochemical markers; clues to understanding aging in long-lived species. *Exp. Gerontol. 36(4–6)*, 619–640.

Folstein, M.F., and Bylsma, F.W. (1999). Noncognitive symptoms of Alzheimer's disease. In *Alzheimer's Disease*, 2nd ed. (R.D. Terry, R. Katzman, K.L. Bick, and S.S. Sisodia, eds.), pp. 25–37. Lippincott Williams & Wilkins, Philadelphia.

Fox, M.W. (1971). *Integrative Development of Brain and Behavior in the Dog*. The University of Chicago Press, Chicago.

Freedman, M., and Oscar-Berman, M. (1989). Spatial and visual learning deficits in Alzheimer's and Parkinson's disease. *Brain Cogn. 11(1)*, 114–126.

Fuster, J.M. (1999). Cognitive functions of the frontal lobes. In *The Human Frontal Lobes* (B.L. Miller and J.L. Cummings eds.), pp. 187–195. Guilford Press, New York.

Gallup, G.G. Jr. (1968). Mirror-image stimulation. *Psychol. Bull. 70(6)*, 782–793.

Harris, G.J., Lewis, R.F., Satlin, A., English, C.D., Scott, T.M., Yurgelun-Todd D.A., and Renshaw, P.F. (1998). Dynamic susceptibility contrast MR imaging of regional cerebral blood volume in Alzheimer disease: A promising alternative to nuclear medicine. *Am. J. Neuroradiol. 19(9)*, 1727–1732.

Hasher, L., and Zacks, R.T. (1988). Working Memory, comprehension, and aging: A review and a new view. *Psychology of Learning and Motivation 22*, 122–149.

Head, E., Callahan, H., Cummings, B.J., Cotman, C.W., Ruehl, W.W., Muggenburg, B.A., and Milgram, N.W. (1997). Open field activity and human interaction as a function of age and breed in dogs. *Physiol. Behav. 62(5)*, 963–971.

Head, E., Callahan, H., Muggenburg, B.A., Cotman, C.W., and Milgram, N.W. (1998). Visual-discrimination learning ability and beta-amyloid accumulation in the dog. *Neurobiol. Aging 19(5)*, 415–25.

Head, E., Liu, J., Hagen, T.M., Muggenburg, B.A., Milgram, N.W., Ames, B.N., and Cotman, C.W. (2002). Oxidative damage increases with age in a canine model of human brain aging. *J. Neurochem. 82(2)*, 375–381.

Head, E., Mehta, R., Hartley, J., Kameka, M., Cummings, B.J., Cotman, C.W., *et al.* (1995). Spatial learning and memory as a function of age in the dog. *Behav. Neurosci. 109(5)*, 851–858.

Head, E., Milgram, N.W., and Cotman, C.W. (2001). Neurobiological models of aging in the dog and other vertebrate species. In *Functional Neurobiology of Aging* (P.R. Hof and C.V. Mobbs, eds.), pp. 457–465. Academic Press, San Diego.

Herndon, J.G., Killiany, R.J., Rosene, D.L., and Moss, M.B. (1993). The recognition span memory capacity of intermediate aged (19–24 years old) rhesus monkeys. *Society for Neuroscience Abstracts 19*, 600.

Landsberg, G. (1995). The most common behavior problems of older dogs. *Vet. Med.* S16–S24.

McDowd, J.M., Oseas-Kreger, D.M., and Filion, D.L. (1995). Inhibitory processes in cognition and aging. In *Interference and Inhibition in Cognition* (F.N. Dempster and C.J. Brainerd, eds.), pp. 363–400. Academic Press, San Diego.

Means, L.W., and Holsten, R.D. (1992). Individual aged rats are impaired on repeated reversal due to loss of different behavioral patterns. *Physiol. Behav. 52(5)*, 959–963.

Milgram, N.W., Adams, B., Callahan, H., Head, E., Mackay, B., Thirlwell, C., and Cotman, C.W. (1999). Landmark discrimination learning in the dog. *Learn. Mem. 6(1)*, 54–61.

Milgram, N.W., Head, E., Muggenburg, B., Holowachuk, D., Murphey, H., Estrada, J., *et al.* (2002a). Landmark discrimination learning in the dog: Effects of age, an antioxidant fortified food, and cognitive strategy. *Neurosci. Biobehav. Rev. 26(6)*, 679–695.

Milgram, N.W., Head, E., Weiner, E., Thomas, E. (1994). Cognitive functions and aging in the dog: Acquisition of nonspatial visual tasks. *Behav. Neurosci. 108(1)*, 57–68.

Milgram, N.W., Head, E., Zicker, S.C., Ikeda-Douglas, C.J., Murphey, H., Muggenburg, B., *et al.* C.W. (2005). Learning ability in aged beagle dogs is preserved by behavioral enrichment and dietary fortification: a two-year longitudinal study. *Neurobiol. Aging 26(1)*, 77–90.

Milgram, N.W., Head, E., Zicker, S.C., Ikeda-Douglas, C., Murphey, H., Muggenburg, B.A., *et al.* (2004). Long-term treatment with antioxidants and a program of behavioral enrichment reduces age-dependent impairment in discrimination and reversal learning in beagle dogs. *Exp. Gerontol. 39(5)*, 753–765.

Milgram, N.W., Zicker, S.C., Head, E., Muggenburg, B.A., Murphey, H., Ikeda-Douglas, C.J., and Cotman, C.W. (2002b). Dietary enrichment counteracts age-associated cognitive dysfunction in canines. *Neurobiol. Aging 23(5)*, 737–745.

Mishkin, M., and Delacour, J. (1975). An analysis of short-term visual memory in the monkey. *J. Exp. Psychol. Anim. Behav. Process 1(4)*, 326–334.

Morris, M.C., Evans, D.A., Tangney, C.C., Bienias, J.L., Wilson, R.S., Aggarwal, N.T., and Scherr, P.A. (2005). Relation of the tocopherol forms to incident Alzheimer disease and to cognitive change. *Am. J. Clin. Nutr. 81(2)*, 508–514.

Morys, J., Narkiewicz, O., Maciejewska, B., Wegiel, J., and Wisniewski, H.M. (1994). Amyloid deposits and loss of neurons in the claustrum of the aged dog. *Neuroreport 5*, 1825–1828.

Oscar-Berman, M., and Bonner, R.T. (1985). Matching- and delayed matching-to-sample performance as measures of visual processing, selective attention, and memory in aging and alcoholic individuals. *Neuropsychologia 23(5)*, 639–651.

Pakkenberg, B., and Gundersen, J.G. (1997). Neocortical neuron number in humans: effect of sex and age. *J. Comp. Neurol. 384*, 312–320.

Patronek, G.J., Waters, D.J., and Glickman, L.T. (1997). Comparative longevity of pet dogs and humans: Implications for gerontology research. *J. Gerontol. Biol. Sci. Med. Sci. 52A(3)*, 171–178.

Pohl, W. (1973). Dissociation of spatial discrimination deficits following frontal and parietal lesions in monkeys. *J. Comp. Physiol. Psychol. 82(2)*, 227–239.

Pop, V., Head, E., Nistor, M., Milgram, N.W., Muggenburg, B.A., and Cotman, C.W. (2003). Reduced Aβ deposition with long-term antioxidant diet treatment in aged canines. *Society for Neuroscience Abstracts*, 525.4.

Pugliese, M., Carrasco, J.L., Geloso, M.C., Mascort, J., Michetti, F., and Mahy, N. (2004). Gamma-aminobutyric acidergic interneuron vulnerability to aging in canine prefrontal cortex. *J. Neurosci. Res. 77(6)*, 913–920.

Ridderinkhof, K.R., Span, M.M., and van der Molen, M.W. (2002). Perseverative behavior and adaptive control in older adults: Performance monitoring, rule induction, and set shifting. *Brain Cogn. 49*, 382–401.

Romanes, G.J. (1884). *Mental Evolution in Animals.* D. Appleton and Company, New York.

Sano, M., Ernesto, C., Thomas, R.G., Klauber, M.R., Schafer, K., Grundman, M., *et al.* (1997). A controlled trial of selegiline, alpha-tocopherol, or both as treatment for Alzheimer's disease. The Alzheimer's Disease Cooperative Study. *N. Engl. J. Med. 336(17)*, 1216–1222.

Satlin, A., Teicher, M.H., Lieberman, H.R., Baldessarini, R.J., Volicer, L., and Rheaume, Y. (1991). Circadian locomotor activity rhythms in Alzheimer's disease. *Neuropsychopharmacology 5(2)*, 115–126.

Satou, T., Cummings, B.J., Head, E., Nielson, K.A., Hahn, F.F., Milgram, N.W., *et al.* (1997). The progression of beta-amyloid deposition in the frontal cortex of the aged canine. *Brain Res. 774(1–2)*, 35–43.

Simic, G., Bexheti, S., Kelovic, Z., Kos, M., Grbic, K., Hof, P.R., and Kostovic, I. (2005). Hemispheric asymmetry, modular variability and age-related changes in the human entorhinal cortex. *Neuroscience 130*, 911–925.

Siwak, C.T., Head, E., Muggenburg, B.A., Milgram, N.W., and Cotman, C.W. (2005a). Region specific neuron loss in the aged canine hippocampus and the effects of an antioxidant diet and behavioral enrichment. *Society for Neuroscience Abstracts*. Program No. 91.

Siwak, C.T., Murphey, H.L., Muggenburg, B.A., and Milgram, N.W. (2002). Age-dependent decline in locomotor activity in dogs is environment specific. *Physiol. Behav. 75(1–2)*, 65–70.

Siwak, C.T., Tapp, P.D., Head, E., Zicker, S.C., Murphey, H.L., Muggenburg, B.A, *et al.* (2005b). Chronic antioxidant and mitochondrial cofactor administration improves discrimination learning in aged but not young dogs. *Prog Neuropsychopharmacol Biol. Psychiatry 29(3)*, 461–469.

Siwak, C.T., Tapp, P.D., and Milgram, N.W. (2001). Effect of age and level of cognitive function on spontaneous and exploratory behaviors in the beagle dog. *Learn. Mem. 8(6)*, 317–325.

Siwak, C.T., Tapp, P.D., Zicker, S.C., Murphey, H.L., Muggenburg, B.A., Head, E., *et al.* (2003). Locomotor activity rhythms in dogs vary with age and cognitive status. *Behav. Neurosci. 117(4)*, 813–824.

Su, M.Y., Head, E., Brooks, W.M., Wang, Z., Muggenburg, B.A., Adam, G.E., *et al.* (1998). Magnetic resonance imaging of anatomic and vascular characteristics in a canine model of human aging. *Neurobiol. Aging 19(5)*, 479–485.

Su, M.Y., Tapp, P.D., Vu, L., Chen, Y.F., Chu, Y., Muggenburg, B., *et al.* (2005). A longitudinal study of brain morphometrics using serial magnetic resonance imaging analysis in a canine model of aging. *Prog. Neuropsychopharmacol. Biol. Psychiatry 29(3)*, 389–397.

Sutherland, N.S. and MacKintosh, N.J. (1971). *Mechanisms of Animal Discrimination Learning*. Academic Press, New York.

Swainson, R., Hodges, J.R., Galton, C.J., Semple, J., Michael, A., Dunn, B.D., *et al.* (2001). Early detection and differential diagnosis of Alzheimer's disease and depression with neuropsychological tasks. *Dement. Geriatr. Cogn. Disord. 12*, 265–280.

Tapp, P.D., Chu, Y., Araujo, J.A., Chiou, J.Y., Head, E., Milgram, N.W., and Su, M.Y. (2005a). Effects of scopolamine challenge on regional cerebral blood volume. A pharmacological model to validate the use of contrast enhanced magnetic resonance imaging to assess cerebral blood volume in a canine model of aging. *Prog. Neuropsychopharmacol. Biol. Psychiatry 29(3)*, 399–406.

Tapp, P.D., Head, K., Head, E., Milgram, N.W., Muggenburg, B.A., and Su, M-Y. (2005b). Application of an automated voxel-based morphometry technique to assess regional gray and white matter brain atrophy in a canine model of aging. *Neuroimage* (in press). Available online November 7, 2005.

Tapp, P.D., Siwak, C.T., Estrada, J., Head, E., Muggenburg, B.A., Cotman, C.W., and Milgram, N.W. (2003a). Size and reversal learning in the beagle dog as a measure of executive function and inhibitory control in aging. *Learn. Mem. 10(1)*, 64–73.

Tapp, P.D., Siwak, C.T., Estrada, J., Holowachuk, D., and Milgram N.W. (2003b). Effects of age on measures of complex working memory span in the beagle dog (*Canis familiaris*) using two versions of a spatial list learning paradigm. *Learn. Mem. 10(2)*, 148–160.

Tapp, P.D., Siwak, C.T., Gao, F.Q., Chiou, J.Y., Black, S.E., Head, E., *et al.* (2004a). Frontal lobe volume, function, and beta-amyloid pathology in a canine model of aging. *J. Neurosci. 24(38)*, 8205–8213.

Tapp, P.D., Siwak, C.T., Head, E., Cotman, C.W., Murphey, H., Muggenburg, B.A., *et al.* (2004b). Concept abstraction in the aging dog: Development of a protocol using successive discrimination and size concept tasks. *Behav. Brain Res. 153(1)*, 199–210.

Tisserand, D.J., van Boxtel, M.P., Pruessner, J.C., Hofman, P., Evans, A.C., and Jolles, J. (2004). A voxel-based morphometric study to determine individual differences in gray matter density associated with age and cognitive change over time. *Cerebral Cortex 14(9)*, 966–973.

Uchida, K., Okuda, R., Yamaguchi, R., Tateyama, S., Nakayama, H., and Goto, N. (1993). Double-labeling immunohistochemical studies on canine senile plaques and cerebral amyloid angiopathy. *J. Vet. Med. Sci. 55*, 637–642.

Vakil, E., and Agmon-Ashkenazi, D. (1997). Baseline performance and learning of procedural and declarative memory tasks: Younger versus older adults. *J. Gerontol. B Psychol. Sci. Sot. Sci. 52(5)*, 220–234.

Van Someren, E.J. (2000). Circadian and sleep disturbances in the elderly. *Exp. Gerontol. 35(9–10)*, 1229–1237.

Voytko, M.L. (1999). Impairments in acquisition and reversal of two-choice discriminations by aged rhesus monkeys. *Neurobiol. Aging 20*, 617–627.

West, M.J. (1993). Regionally specific loss of neurons in the aging human hippocampus. *Neurobiol. Aging 14*, 287–293.

West, M.J., Coleman, P.D., Flood, D.G., and Troncoso, J.C. (1994). Differences in the pattern of hippocampal neuron loss in normal ageing and Alzheimer's disease. *Lancet 344*, 769–772.

West, R.L. (1996). An application of prefrontal cortex function theory to cognitive aging. *Psychol. Bull. 120*, 272–292.

Wisniewski, H., Johnson, A.B., Raine, C.S., Kay, W.J., and Terry, R. D. (1970). Senile plaques and cerebral amyloidosis in aged dogs: A histochemical and ultrastructural study. *Lab. Invest. 23*, 287–296.

Yamaguchi, H., Sugihara, S., Ogawa, A., Oshima, N., and Ihara, Y. (2001). Alzheimer beta amyloid deposition enhanced by apoE epsilon4 gene precedes neurofibrillary pathology in the frontal association cortex of nondemented senior subjects. *J. Neuropath. Exp. Neurol. 60(7)*, 731–739.

36

Bats as a Novel Model for Aging Research

Anja K. Brunet-Rossinni and Rocco E. Rossinni

Despite small body size and high metabolic rate, bats are exceptionally long-lived mammals. This longevity, the ecological, behavioral and morphological diversity, and the unique life history traits of this multispecied order of mammals make bats well-suited as model systems for aging research. Including bats in comparative investigations may provide insight into universal mechanisms of senescence as well as reveal mechanisms that confer resistance to expected senescent processes. In this chapter we provide a general description of this extraordinary order of mammals within the context of their potential use for aging research. We describe general methodologies including captive care, capturing and aging techniques as well as some of the health precautions researchers should observe when working with bats. We conclude with a brief summary of the current state of longevity and senescence research on bats and potential future lines of research. Probably most useful is a list of resources we have included, which can provide initial information and direction for researchers interested in using bats as a model system.

Introduction

Over the past several decades, biologists have assembled a long list of lifespan records for several species of bats providing clear evidence of the exceptional longevity of this order of mammals (Chiroptera). In fact, after accounting for body size and metabolic rate, bats are among the longest-lived mammals (Austad and Fischer, 1991). Despite our knowledge of this exceptional longevity, very few studies have examined the questions of why and how bats live so long. This is surprising considering the extensive literature available describing the ecology, behavior, physiology and anatomy of certain bat species, as well as some of the unique traits of Chiroptera, which may provide insight into universal mechanisms of aging.

This paucity in research is likely due to some of the logistical difficulties of working with bats, and a disconnect between the community of researchers on aging and that of bat biologists. With this chapter we hope to bridge that gap and promote interest in pursuing future research that includes bats. We will first describe the general characteristics of the order Chiroptera, focusing on traits that we feel make bats an excellent model system for aging research. We then discuss some of the advantages and disadvantages of using bats as model systems and summarize the limited research completed to date on bat senescence and longevity. We present methods and resources for the study, captive care, and age determination of bats, and finally, we finish the chapter by presenting some potential future lines of research.

General Characteristics and Life History Traits of the Order Chiroptera

With over 1100 species of bats worldwide, the order Chiroptera is the second most multispecied among mammals, accounting for almost one-fourth of all mammalian species. The order is divided into two suborders. The Megachiroptera is a group of just under 200 species, which includes the flying foxes and fruit bats of the Old World. The Microchiroptera with over 900 species includes all the bats of the New World and some Old World species. The two suborders differ in sensory and feeding characteristics. Megachiroptera are fruit- and nectar-feeding bats with a binocular visual pathway and rely on olfaction and vision to find food. Species of Microchiroptera consume a broad range of food including insects, fruit, nectar, small vertebrates, and blood. They have a monocular visual pathway but rely on echolocation to forage and navigate (Simmons and Conway, 2003). Despite the differences between the two suborders, the order Chiroptera is believed to be a single evolutionary lineage, and this monophyly is supported by extensive morphological and molecular evidence (Simmons, 2000).

Chiroptera are incredibly diverse in regards to ecology, behavior, and morphology. Bats can be found on every continent except Antarctica. They inhabit deserts, stone beaches, temperate forests, rainforests, and cities. They roost in caves, under tree bark, in tree hollows, among foliage, under rocks, and in buildings. Behaviorally, several bat species are solitary, others form harems, and still others form colonies that can include several millions of individuals.

Body sizes of bats vary from the hog-nosed or bumble bee bat (*Craseonycteris thonglangyai*), which weighs only 2 g, to the large flying fox (*Pteropus vampyrus*), weighing in at 1200 g. Their size is probably restricted by flight, as are several other anatomical and physiological traits. For example, females of most species have one reduced ovary and uterine horn likely to reduce body mass for flight (Barclay and Harder, 2003; Jones and MacLarnon, 2001), and juveniles have to achieve almost full adult size before fledging because full bone ossification is necessary to withstand twisting stresses and maintain the wing shape during flight (Barclay, 1994, 1995).

These flight-imposed restrictions translate into very unique life history traits. Mammals can be placed along a continuum of life history traits. At one extreme are small mammals with high metabolic rates, high reproductive rate, rapid maturation, and short lifespan. At the other extreme are typically large mammals with lower metabolic rates and long lifespan, which produce few, large offspring that mature slowly (Read and Harvey, 1989). Bats are paradoxical in that despite being relatively small and having high metabolic rate, they lie on the latter end of the continuum. The majority of species have one offspring per litter, and newborns weigh 15–30% of the body mass of the postpartum mother (Barclay and Harder, 2003; Tuttle and Stevenson, 1982). The gestation period in bats is long, and after birth, offspring take relatively long to reach full adult size (3–4 months in many species; Tuttle and Stevenson, 1982) and typically even longer to achieve sexual maturation (Jones and MacLarnon, 2001). Finally, on average, bats live three times longer than expected based on their body size and metabolic rate (Austad and Fischer, 1991). The oldest longevity record to date is 38 years from a 7-g Brandt's bat (*Myotis brandtii*). A small sample of bat longevities is listed in Table 36.1, and a more extensive list can be found in the appendix of Wilkinson and South (2001) and in Gaisler *et al.* (2003). Bat lifespan records come from the fortuitous recapture of wild individuals who were tagged at birth. Therefore, records likely are underestimates of actual maximum longevity (Wilkinson and South, 2002).

Bats have very high metabolic rates and many species are thermolabile. Ultimately, the thermoregulatory strategy of a species is determined by body size, habitat, diet, roosting choice, and social behavior. Because each of these traits varies greatly among species, bats exhibit a broad spectrum of thermoregulatory strategies. Species in the higher latitudes, where temperature varies seasonally, are heterothermic and use hibernation to survive cold winters without food and torpor during the remainder of the year to reduce energy expenditure while roosting. During hibernation, a bat will reduce its body temperature to a few degrees above ambient temperature, and its metabolic rate may drop to one-hundredth of waking rate. The extent of metabolic suppression during torpor depends on ambient temperature. Species living in tropical areas or which migrate to warmer latitudes during the winter do not hibernate and therefore are considered homeothermic. However, the extent of homeothermy varies among species from true homeothermy in Megachiroptera to different degrees and frequency of torpor (Speakman and Thomas, 2003).

TABLE 36.1
Maximum lifespan records of selected bat species (Geisler, 2004; Wilkinson and South, 2002)

Species	Body mass (g)	Maximum lifespan record (yrs)
Myotis brandti	7	38
Myotis lucifugus	8	34
Rhinolophus ferrumequinum	23.5	30.5
Pteropus rodricensis	400	30
Myotis daubentonii	9	28
Rosettus aegyptiacus	146	22.9
Desmodus rotundus	30	19.5
Eptesicus fuscus	22	19
Tadarida brasiliensis	11	10
Vespertilio murinus	16	12

Bats as Models for Aging Research: Advantages and Disadvantages

Uncovering differences and similarities in patterns of aging among various organisms from a broad phylogenetic spectrum is likely to yield insight into universal mechanisms of senescence. The inclusion of out-groups in aging research would allow investigators to assess whether these mechanisms or traits are unique to a given study species or shared by a broader taxonomic group (Austad, 1997). Bats may be an excellent out-group because they share life history traits with primates and other long-lived organisms, such as slow reproductive output and slow maturation.

Another advantage is that bats can be maintained in captivity (see following sections), which allows a researcher to carefully monitor individuals and eliminate several environmental factors that may confound results. Additionally, because some species exhibit high fidelity to roosting areas, it is possible to find a permanent wild colony where results from a captive colony can be tested (Brunet-Rossinni and Austad, 2004).

Heterothermic bats are metabolically malleable. A researcher can increase or decrease the metabolic rate of a bat by exposing it to lower or higher temperatures and, with the appropriate environmental cues, a bat may even enter torpor or hibernation. This plasticity makes bats an ideal system to study the role of metabolism and metabolic pathways in determining longevity and rates of senescence. Researchers will find extensive information in the literature on the physiology and metabolism of bats, though it should be noted that studies have focused on only a few bat families and not all species within a family can enter torpor. On the other hand, this prompt flexibility may pose a problem for studies where metabolic state should remain constant, especially caloric restriction studies, as bats may enter torpor in response to food scarcity (Brunet-Rossinni and Austad, 2004).

The extreme longevity of bats is both an advantage and a disadvantage. Studying an organism that naturally lives long should give insight to the physiological mechanisms that underlie its extended lifespan. However, long-term studies on bats that live 20–30 years are logistically difficult. This is exacerbated by the fact that unless a bat is tagged upon birth, there is currently no robust method to precisely estimate chronological age of an adult bat (see following sections). Nonetheless, there are a number of studies that have been tagging and monitoring bat colonies for over 10 years, and cellular mechanisms underlying extended longevity should be present in young adults (Brunet-Rossinni and Austad, 2004).

A final disadvantage is that only segments of nuclear and mitochondrial DNA of bats have been sequenced. This is, however, changing quickly as researchers continue to sequence new segments of both genomes.

Aging Research on Bats

Few studies have examined bat longevity, and due to continually improving lifespan data, it is not surprising that some of these studies have reached contradictory conclusions. Some of the earliest work that considered the question of *why* bats live so long was a comparative survey of lifespans by Bourliere (1958). Addressing the question from the standpoint of the rate of living theory (Pearl, 1928; Sacher, 1959), Bourliere described the extreme longevity of bats as a simple consequence of reduced metabolism during hibernation. This explanation, of course, neglects the long lifespan of homeothermic bats, which do not hibernate. In fact, Herreid (1964) and Austad and Fischer (1991) found no difference in maximum lifespan between hibernating and tropical bats. Jürgens and Prothero (1987) found that after accounting for torpor and hibernation, lifetime energy consumption and body mass predict maximum lifespan reasonably well in hibernating species, but fail to do so in nonhibernating species. The most recent survey study on bat longevity, which included an extensively updated dataset, found that the average longevity of hibernating species is about 6 years longer than that of nonhibernating species (Wilkinson and South, 2002).

Hibernation does appear to contribute to lifespan extension by concealing bats from predators, protecting them from inclement weather, and retarding physiological deterioration (Barclay and Harder, 2003). However, it does not account for the fact that *all* known bat longevity records exceed those of similar sized nonflying mammals, including those that hibernate (Austad and Fischer, 1991). In its original formulation, the rate of living theory predicts the existence of a constant mass-specific lifetime energy expenditure for all mammals (Sacher, 1959). Bats exceed the lifetime energy expenditure of nonflying placental mammals by two-fold (Austad and Fischer, 1991), contradicting the rate of living theory. Another formulation of the rate of living theory describes an inverse correlation between maximum lifespan and metabolic rate or body size. Austad and Fischer (1991) calculated that on average bats live over three times longer than expected based on body size, again contradicting the rate of living theory. There is ambiguous evidence regarding a possible correlation between body mass and longevity within the order Chiroptera. Two studies found no correlation (Austad and Fischer, 1991; Jones and MacLarnon, 2001), yet a third found a correlation when using a phylogentic analysis method which accounts for relationships among the species analyzed (Wilkinson and South, 2002).

From an evolutionary perspective, the exceptional longevity of bats is consistent with the evolutionary theory and the disposable soma theory of aging. The evolutionary theory of aging attributes senescence to the decreasing strength of natural selection with increasing age (Williams, 1957). This predicts that organisms that excel at escaping extrinsic mortality such as starvation, predation, disease, and accidents evolve to be long lived. Bats have terrestrial and aerial predators (e.g., snakes, opossums, owls, hawks) and are vulnerable to climate; however, the exposure is low relative to nonflying mammals. Like birds, which also exhibit exceptionally long lifespan, bats are able to escape predation by flying, and many species will migrate or adjust body temperature and metabolic rate to avoid adverse food and weather conditions (Wilkinson and South, 2002; Barclay and Harder, 2003).

The disposable soma theory of aging describes an inevitable evolutionary tradeoff between using limited resources and energy for somatic maintenance or to increase reproductive output (Kirkwood, 1977). An organism that experiences high extrinsic mortality is likely to die prior to the next reproductive season and would do well to invest in high and quick reproductive output instead of in somatic maintenance. The opposite would be true for an organism that experiences low extrinsic mortality as it can spread out reproductive output over a longer lifespan. Bat species with high reproductive rates and early sexual maturation exhibit shorter longevity (Rachmatulina, 1992; Wilkinson and South, 2002). Even within a species, females who delay breeding to a later age have higher survival rates than females who breed early in life (Ransome, 1995).

Very little is known about the physiological and molecular mechanisms underpinning the exceptional longevity of bats. Röhme (1981) included a bat (*Vespertilio murinus*) in a comparative study, which found a positive correlation between organism maximum lifespan and replicative lifespan of fibroblasts cultured from eight mammalian species. The involvement of cellular replicative lifespan in aging is still disputed (Cristofalo and Pignolo, 1995), and several laboratories are in the process of evaluating this correlation using fibroblast cell cultures from other species of bats (Brunet-Rossinni and Austad, 2004).

Baudry *et al.* (1986) examined a potential correlation between calpain activity and species maximum lifespan. The calpains are a family of calcium-dependent cystein proteases that have been implicated in age-related pathologies of kidneys, heart, and brain tissue deterioration, as calpain activity increases with age likely due to impaired inhibitory mechanisms. Based on a negative correlation between calpain activity and brain size, and a positive correlation between brain size and maximum longevity, Baudry *et al.* hypothesized that brain calpain activity should be inversely correlated with maximum longevity. By quantifying degraded proteins in the presence of calcium, the study compared calpain activity in brain tissues of two bat species to that of mice and found significantly lower calpain activity in the bat tissues. It should be noted, however, that bat brain size is not consistent with the reputed correlation between lifespan and brain size.

A more recent study tested the free radical theory of aging (Harman, 1956) as an explanation for the extreme longevity of bats. In a comparative study, Brunet-Rossinni (2004) measured mitochondrial hydrogen peroxide production in heart, kidney and brain tissue of the little brown bat, *Myotis lucifugus*, the short-tailed shrew, *Blarina brevicauda*, and the white-footed mouse, *Peromyscus leucopus*. Hydrogen peroxide production per unit of oxygen consumed was significantly lower in the bat tissues than in the two nonflying mammals. Brunet-Rossinni also measured activity of superoxide dismutase, a key enzyme in the antioxidant defense system of mammalian tissues. Activity of this enzyme did not differ between the three species. Though not an all-inclusive assessment of antioxidant defenses, this study suggests that free radical production is a better predictor of bat longevity than metabolic rate and antioxidant activity. Similar results have been found in birds and other mammals (Herrero and Barja, 1998; Ku, *et al.*, 1993).

Methods for the Study of Bats

WILD BAT POPULATIONS: MONITORING AND CATCHING

Bat roost selection varies considerably; they will roost in caves, mines, occupied and unoccupied buildings, trees, under leaves, under bark, under rocks and in cliff crevices (Kunz, 1982). Usually, roosts occupied by colonial species are easier to find because of the number of bats present and because some of these species exhibit high fidelity to their roosts. This is especially the case for species that form nursery colonies, as roosts that provide adequate climatic environment for fetal and neonatal development are at a premium. Most researchers conducting long-term monitoring of wild bat colonies identify a permanent roost like a cave or a building, which they then visit regularly. The composition of the colony varies from year to year as bats are very vagile, likely moving repeatedly among roosts, but the presence of the species is consistent over time. An excellent way of finding areas that are used by bats is to listen for vocalizations or look for evidence of foraging (such as guano or dropped fruit). With microchiroptera, researchers can listen for echolocation calls with an ultrasonic detector. These "bat detectors" slow down the ultrasonic calls emitted by bats as they fly, making them audible to the human ear. High echolocation activity may indicate the area is a good foraging site or a roost is nearby. Furthermore, specific patterns of echolocation frequencies have been used to identify the species of bats found in an area.

There are several techniques for capturing bats, and success with any requires knowledge of the roosting and foraging behavior of bats, as well as their emergence and dispersal patterns (Kunz and Kurta, 1988). Regardless of technique, three critical pieces of equipment for capturing bats are a light source, gloves, and "bat bags." Because bats are nocturnal, most capture sessions take place at dusk or at night when they emerge for foraging. Headlamps with halogen bulbs and battery packs are ideal for this work as they are reliable and keep a researcher's hands free for handling bats and manipulating equipment. Leather gloves should be used when handling bats to prevent bites and reduce stress to the animal. Lightweight leather gloves (e.g., baseball batter gloves) can be used for juveniles and smaller species, but heavier leather will be necessary for larger and more aggressive species, especially vampire bats and the large megachiroptera. The gloves should be soft and pliable to allow for improved dexterity and loose-fitting because sometimes it helps to let a bat chew on part of a glove during handling. "Bat bags" are simple drawstring bags made of muslin or nylon mesh that are used to temporarily hold bats after capture. We typically carry 50–100 bags for a trapping session so that each bat captured can be kept individually in a bag. However, this might not be practical if large numbers of bats are captured, and Kunz and Kurta (1988) describe several alternative temporary holding devices.

The most commonly used devices for capturing bats are mist nets and harp traps. It is possible to capture bats within a roost using hand nets, but this can be very disruptive and cause bats to abandon the roost. Mist nets are practical because they are lightweight, compact, easily erected, and commercially available in several lengths.

They can be erected on the ground or raised up into tree canopies, thereby targeting bats that fly at different heights. The preferred mist nets for capturing bats have four shelves formed by mesh made of 50 or 70 denier/2 ply nylon (Kunz and Kurta, 1988) that is tiered with shelving cords. The nets should be erected on 10-ft poles that are sunk into the ground and/or secured with rope. While lightweight aluminum mist net poles are commercially available, bamboo, small trees, electrical conduit and paint poles are also effective. Unable to detect the net, bats fly into the mesh and drop into a pocket formed by the netting and the shelving cords. There they usually become entangled as they try to escape the mesh. Researchers should continually monitor the mist net so that trapped bats can be removed as quickly as possible because the longer they remain in the net the more difficult it becomes to disentangle them. Removing a bat from a mist net takes some practice. It should be done from the side of the net the bat entered, and one should take particular care with wings as they can become damaged if handled roughly.

Harp traps are often used to capture bats that elude mist nets. Harp traps consist of one or two large frames holding banks of fine wires or monofilament fishing line that run vertically along the length of the frame. A large bag attached to the base of the trap serves to collect falling bats that have lost momentum after flying into the bank of filaments. Current harp trap designs are collapsible and portable and have the advantage that they do not require constant attendance as the bats do not become entangled in the filaments but are held in the trap bag. It should be noted, however, that bats in the trap bag are susceptible to predators and aggressive interspecies interactions, so bats should not be left in the trap bag for too long (Kunz and Kurta, 1988).

Placement of a mist net or harp trap will influence the capture success. The most successful locations can be identified by sighting flying bats or listening for vocalizations and are usually near roosts, near sources of water such as streams and lakes, and along clearings used as flyways. Other factors that may influence capture success are amount of moonlight, rain, wind, the visual and acoustic resolution and flight behavior of the bats (Kunz and Kurta, 1988). A few cautionary notes regarding netting or trapping bats at the entrance or in large roosts such as caves, mines or attics: (a) It is not uncommon to catch large numbers of bats at one time as they emerge together from a roost. This can damage the net and distress both bats and handlers as the bats become increasingly tangled in the mesh. (b) Bats may abandon a site where they are caught and handled so it is recommended to capture bats away from roosts and keep handling to a minimum (Barclay and Bell, 1988; Kunz and Kurta, 1988).

If a study requires multiple observations on the same individual, markings will be necessary. Several methods for marking bats have been use, and the choice of method will depend on the species of bat, how long the marking must last, how visible the marking needs to be, and how often the marking can be checked or renewed. It is also very important to ensure that the object used to mark a bat weighs less than 5% of the bat's body mass as the excess weight will impact flight.

Short-term marking of bats can be achieved by clipping patches of fur down to the skin, which can take up to four months to grow back if the bat is not molting. Obviously, this technique requires close handling of the bat for identification and should not be used during hibernation as the loss of fur can interfere with a bat's thermoregulation. Alternatively, livestock markers can be used to identify individuals. The nontoxic, lead-free paint of these markers adheres well to fur, comes in a variety of colors, and is safer to use than nail polish and dyes. In our experience, a colorful spot drawn between a bat's shoulder blades will last several weeks, depending on how often the individual grooms.

Long-term marking is most commonly done by wing banding. Metallic, aluminum or plastic bands are placed on the forearm of a bat, and identification is based on a unique number and/or a unique combination of colors. Reflective colored tape may be applied to the bands to permit identification of individuals during flight and while roosting. Wing bands should be used with caution as they can cause injury and infection. The band should be loose enough to slide freely along the forearm but tight enough to not slide onto the wrist and elbow joints, which can result in severe injury and immobility (Barclay and Bell, 1988). The opening of plastic split bands should be filed down to widen the gap and to smooth the edges that touch the wing as they will otherwise tear the thin wing membrane (Lollar and Schmidt-French, 1998) causing severe wounds likely to become infected. Some bats may chew at bands to the point of self-mutilation. In such instances, researchers should consider alternative methods. For example, neck collars made of bead-clasp chain or rachet-style plastic ties have been successfully used to mark some bats (Barclay and Bell, 1988; Issac *et al.*, 2003). It is important that the collar fit properly. Wounds and infection can result from tight collars, and small bats can trap their wrist under a loose collar. We do not recommend the use of either wing bands or neck collars for juveniles that have not yet achieved adult size as the markers can interfere with proper development.

Other banding techniques used for bats include radiotransmitters and chemiluminescent light tags which are glued to a bat's back, skin tattoos, and radioactive tags. We refer the reader to Barclay and Bell (1988) for more details, advantages and disadvantages of these techniques. Toe-clipping, ear-notching, or ear-tagging, which are routinely used to mark other mammals, should not be used with bats because toes are essential for perching and grooming and ears are critical for echolocation in microchiroptera (Barclay and Bell, 1988; Lollar and Schmidt-French, 1998).

CARE OF CAPTIVE BAT POPULATIONS

Several species of bats have been maintained in captivity, and there is ample information available regarding the proper care of captive bats. The following is a brief summary of some basic considerations for the captive care of bats. We refer readers to books listed in the Resources section of this chapter for more detailed information. Generally, a researcher interested in maintaining a captive colony must consider roosting and flight needs, climate and lighting needs, nutritional needs, and social needs. How these needs are met depends on the species of bat.

Flight cages and roosting cages

Bats need exercise and may lose the ability to fly if deprived of flight space for over a month (Wilson, 1988). Flight cages can be made of a variety of materials to meet the particular needs of the research, but good visibility, easy cleaning, and plenty of perching sites are important considerations. If the cage is made of wire mesh, it is important that the gaps in the mesh are small enough that wings and feet will not get trapped. Also, wire mesh can cause irritation to the wrist and ankle area of the bat as well as tear wing tissue, so it should be coated with a Teflon spray. Alternatively, one could use softer materials such as nylon or rubberized mesh (Lollar and Schmidt-French, 1998). While mesh provides good perching sites, toenails may grow excessively and require clipping. Therefore, it is recommended to provide branches which the bats can use to file their toenails. Other good perching materials include burlap, cork board, bark, plywood with small holes and textured plaster (Wilson, 1988). Lollar and Schmidt-French (1998) provide detailed instructions for well-designed flight cages.

Smaller roosting cages can be placed inside the flight cage to either isolate individuals, provide a location where mothers can keep their young, or accommodate specific roosting needs. There are a variety of different roosting cages ranging from small aquaria with mesh tops to plywood and mesh cages such as those described by Lollar and Schmidt-French (1998). The key is to meet the roosting needs of the species in question. For example, crevice-dwelling bats like to roost in tight, dark spaces. Many bat rehabilitators attach small padded pouches to the walls of roosting cages that bats can crawl into (for patterns see Lollar and Schmidt-French, 1998). Tree-dwelling bats like to roost among foliage typically in relatively high areas. One can tie branches or leaves of the foliage preferred by the species in question to the upper corners of a cage.

Climate and lighting conditions

Temperature, relative humidity, and light cycles play key roles in the digestive and reproductive function of bats (Heideman, 2000; Wilson, 1988). The optimal climate and lighting conditions are likely those experienced by the particular species naturally. For example, heterothermic bats in temperate areas experience warm roost temperatures with high relative humidity and long days in the summer but then require low temperatures and short days in the winter for torpor or hibernation. Digestion is most efficient at thermoneutral temperatures, and photoperiod and seasonal temperature changes are critical for reproduction in many bat species. In many species mating takes place in the fall, but fertilization of the ovum or implantation of the zygote occurs in spring. Also, spermatogenesis is likely influenced by photoperiod (Heideman, 2000). Many people working with captive bat colonies mimic natural conditions, while others keep their colonies within sites that bats might normally pick for roosting, such as old barns or attics. This way, the colony experiences natural cycles in temperature, relative humidity and light.

Providing climatic and light cycles that imitate natural conditions may not always be possible. Another option is to use a space heater, heating pad, or a lamp with a 25-W red light bulb to create a temperature gradient in the cage so individuals can choose the temperature they prefer (Lollar and Schmidt-French, 1998; Wilson, 1988). Generally, bats should be kept at a temperature between 24 and 35°C and a relative humidity between 50 and 90% (Lollar and Schmidt-French, 1998; Wilson, 1988), but determining a good climate regime may take some trial and error. Researchers establishing a new colony should consult the literature to find data on the thermoneutral temperature range of the species in question. If breeding is desired, researchers should investigate mating behavior and physiology and determine the ideal conditions for mating and proper fetal and neonatal development (Heideman, 2000).

Nutritional requirements

The dietary requirements of bats are easily accommodated in captivity, though at times training may be necessary so bats will accept the offered food. Regardless of the diet, vitamin, mineral, protein and fatty acid supplements should be provided when necessary. Vitamin and mineral supplements may be added by dusting food with vitamin/mineral powder or fortifying water with liquid vitamins. One should supplement vitamins and minerals with caution as overdoses may result in medical problems (Lollar and Schmidt-French, 1998). Linatone, a veterinary product for birds, dogs and cats, is an excellent source of additional fatty acids for bats.

The most common diet for insectivorous bats is mealworms, the larvae of *Tenebrio molitor*. Mealworms should be raised on a mixture of bran and oats enriched with a high protein cereal. Wedges of apple or potato provide the moisture mealworms need. Most insectivorous bats will need to be taught to eat the mealworms, and the speed with which they learn varies among species. To train a bat, one should offer a mealworm with a pair of tweezers. Sometimes it may be necessary to decapitate the mealworm to expose viscera but once bats recognize mealworms as food, they will feed independently on mealworms in a bowl. In lieu of live mealworms, bat handlers may use "bat glop," a blended mixture of mealworms and other ingredients such as baby food and veterinary vitamin/mineral supplements. Lollar and Schmidt-French (1998) provide excellent recipes for blended mealworm mixtures which can be frozen in ice cube trays and then thawed for a meal.

Suggested food items for carnivorous bats include chunks of beef, rabbit meat, chicken meat, birds, lizards, white mice, rats, bats, chicks, quail, papaya, mango, melon and banana. Piscivorous bats will readily accept small pieces of fish supplemented with red meat and enriched mealworms.

Frugivorous bats will eat several fruits and vegetables including banana, figs, apples, orange, guava, passion fruit, grapes, pineapple, papaya, mango, pear, tomato, lettuce, cooked sweet potato, cooked carrots. This diet should be supplemented with canned feline diet or New World primate diet. Nectivorous bats can be fed instant nectar combinations, though one should ensure that the used combination is properly supplemented and balanced (Wilson, 1988).

The common vampire bat (*Desmodus rotundus*) does well on a diet of 50 mg of fresh blood per day, which can usually be obtained from a local slaughterhouse. The blood must be defibrinated by stirring or by treatment with sodium citrate or oxalate and is usually served in a shallow dish or ice cube trays. While fresh blood is preferable, frozen citrated blood has been used successfully for extended periods of time (Dickson and Green, 1970).

Different bat species have variable needs for water, depending on the diet provided. However, water should always be provided *ad libitum* in multiple containers placed throughout a cage. Some bats can be trained to lick water from drinking bottles but all bats will readily drink from open containers. Water in open containers is easily fouled by food and feces, so it is critical to change the water at least twice a day. Also, deep water dishes should be filled with marbles to prevent bats from falling in the container and aspirating water (Lollar and Schmidt-French, 1998).

It is important to keep a systematic record of the health condition of every bat in a captive colony. Individuals should be weighed regularly to assess for weight loss, which may be a sign of illness, as well as hyperphagia, though it is important to remember that hibernating bats will gain weight in preparation for hibernation. Other clinical signs to assess include diarrhea, vomiting, loss of pigmentation and/or dryness of the skin, hair loss, and lethargy. Several of the books listed in the Recommended Resources section of this chapter have helpful information on diagnosing common medical conditions.

Sociality

Bats should be housed in accordance to their natural social behavior (Johnston, 1997). Solitary bats should always be caged separately except for a mother and her pups. Upon weaning, however, the pups should be separated from their mother. Colonial bats should always be housed with roost mates, as they often practice allo-grooming and may thermoregulate by clustering. For most colonial species, the sexes should be kept separate. Species that normally form harems may be housed in groups of multiple females with one male, though regardless of the social system researchers should continually look for signs of aggressive behavior and redistribute individual animals to minimize aggressive interactions.

HEALTH PRECAUTIONS FOR RESEARCHERS HANDLING BATS

Rabies

Rabies is a significant concern for researchers handling bats, not because bats exhibit a higher incidence of rabies infection than other wild mammals, but because without prompt treatment rabies is nearly always fatal in humans. The virus is most commonly transmitted via contact with infected saliva through a bite, but other means of transmission include contact of infected saliva and nervous tissue with mucous membranes of the mouth, nose and eyes. There have also been two cases of transmission by aerosolized rabies virus in a Texas cave (Constantine, 1988), but no other cases have been reported since. A bat infected with rabies is not aggressive, but rather lethargic and incapacitated as the virus spreads through its nervous system causing paralysis. Thus, the main source of rabies infection from bats is inappropriate handling of the sick animal which bites in self defense.

Symptoms of rabies usually develop 10–14 days after exposure and include pain, burning and numbness at the site of infection, headaches, insomnia, fever, and difficulty swallowing. However, usually by the time the symptoms are apparent, the progression of the disease can no longer be prevented, ultimately resulting in fatal inflammation of the brain and spinal cord. Therefore, it is imperative that a person seek immediate medical attention after any potential exposure. People handling bats should obtain pre-exposure immunization, which is conferred by 3 doses of vaccine, and check their titers regularly. Additionally, they should simply avoid exposure. Bats captured to establish a captive colony should be quarantined for at least 6 months to assess possible sickness. Always wear gloves when handling bats and avoid rapid and unpredictable movements which increase the chance of bites.

Histoplasmosis

Histoplasmosis is a respiratory infection caused by the fungus *Histoplasma capsulatum*, which develops well in organic materials such as bat and bird feces. Fungal spores become airborne when dry guano is disturbed and can be inhaled resulting in infection. Greatest likelihood of infection is in caves and mines with large guano accumulations where warmth and humidity enhance growth of the fungus, though cases of infection in buildings with large bat populations have also been reported (Smith, 1955). Symptoms of histoplasmosis usually appear one or two weeks after exposure and range from a dry-cough, chest pain and labored breathing to fever, nightsweats, weight loss and even blood-stained sputum. Histoplasmosis can be fatal. Persons entering a potentially contaminated roost should wear respirators with 2 micron filters and should bathe soon after departing the roost.

Hazardous atmospheric gases

Caves, mines, and other underground spaces are poorly ventilated, which can result in the accumulation of noxious gases and/or dangerously low concentrations of oxygen. These gases include irritants such as ammonia and sulfur dioxide, asphyxiants such as nitrogen, methane and carbon dioxide, and toxic asphyxiants such as carbon monoxide and hydrogen sulfide (Constantine, 1988). Several of these gases are odorless, and the concentration of others may increase due to the presence of large amounts of guano. One of the authors (ABR) has experienced respiratory distress and nausea from nitrogenous fumes emitting from vampire bat guano. A researcher should always obtain as much information as possible about a cave or mine prior to entering it and may wish to use portable toxic gas detectors during exploration.

Methods of Age Determination in Bats

Bats are difficult to age once they reach adulthood, and the currently available methods of age determination have several limitations. To begin with, bats show no visible markers of aging, and the few traits that have been correlated with age to establish reference standards show significant variation due to genetic structuring of populations and environmental variation which impacts development. Additionally, available reference standards lack data from very old bats, likely because the oldest individuals are few and seldom caught. Finally, several of the more robust methods are invasive, making repeated measures impossible, and their accuracy is questionable (Anthony, 1988).

Undoubtedly, the best method for age determination is capturing and tagging individuals during their birth year. Thereby, at every subsequent recapture exact chronological age can be easily calculated. However, long-term monitoring of marked individuals can be very time consuming, and recapture rates are often low. A researcher must assess the level of estimate precision necessary for his or her investigations. If exact chronological age is necessary, then permanently marking individuals is the appropriate method. Otherwise, one of the following methods may suffice.

After birth, bats grow quickly, achieving almost full adult size prior to fledging (Barclay, 1994; Jones and MacLarnon, 2001). During this time, long bones grow linearly and many researchers use forearm length measured with calipers to determine age of growing juveniles. In fact, this method provides very accurate estimates of age (Anthony, 1988). Its usefulness, however, is restricted to the first 2 to 6 weeks after birth, depending on species (Brunet-Rossinni and Wilkinson, *in review*). During this growth phase, the cartilaginous epiphyseal growth plates of the phalanges in the wing first expand to generate the phalangeal growth necessary for wing development and then become increasingly calcified. This process results in a linear increase and subsequent linear decrease in total length of the cartilaginous region between the boney diaphysis of a metacarpal and the boney diaphysis of the proximal phalanx (a.k.a. total gap). Epiphyseal growth plates are easily visualized by trans-illuminating the wing with a light source, as cartilaginous tissue allows more light to pass through than bone. Calipers can be used to measure total gap, though many researchers use a dissecting microscope with an ocular micrometer and a sub-stage light source to increase measurement accuracy (Kunz and Anthony, 1982). This linear change in total gap is a robust and accurate method for determining age of juveniles well beyond the valid age estimates provided by forearm length. The ease of obtaining measurements and the minimal equipment requirement are advantages of this aging method. However, once the epiphyseal growth plates are calcified, age estimates are no longer possible.

Nonetheless, the presence of cartilage in and the shape of phalangeal joints can be used to classify bats into general age categories such as infant, juvenile, and adult. If when trans-illuminating a wing cartilage is visible, the bat is a juvenile. Once the epiphyseal plate calcifies, one can still distinguish juveniles from adults as juvenile phalangeal joints are more tapered and less knobby than adult joints (see Figure 1 in Anthony, 1988). External reproductive traits can also be used to distinguish adults and juveniles. The presence of scrotal testes and well-developed teats are characteristic of reproducing adults (Racey, 1988).

The methods of age determination for adult bats involve assessing tooth wear and counting incremental dentin and cementum lines in teeth. Both methods are based on traits that vary tremendously and are difficult to measure, so researchers should exercise caution when using them for age estimations.

Bats have a permanent set of teeth by the time they can fly and feed independently, and mastication over a lifetime results in tooth cusps wearing down and becoming dull. Assessing the extent of tooth wear can be used to place bats into relative age categories, and standards have been developed for a few species (Brunet-Rossinni and Wilkinson, *in review*). However, noticeable differences in tooth wear occur over long time periods, which necessarily results in broad age categories. Additionally, scrutiny of some established reference standards attests to the limited predictive power of this method due to extensive variation in tooth wear associated with diet and behavior (Hall *et al.*, 1957). Due to this variation, it is critical that estimates be based on reference standards developed for the particular study population and that these estimates be made by investigators with extensive experience and knowledge about tooth wear patterns in the particular species.

Dental incremental lines or "annuli" have been used to determine age of adult bats under the assumption that one new layer of dentine and cementum is laid on pre-existing dental tissue each year (Klevezal' and Kleinenberg, 1967). Thus, by extracting and sectioning a tooth, the lines can be visualized and counted under a microscope, giving an estimate of a bat's age in years. However, incremental lines may be difficult to count, especially in small species, the number of incremental lines counted may depend on the tooth extracted, and several factors can result in nonannual cycles of deposition (Batulevicius *et al.*, 2001; Cool *et al.*, 1994; Phillips *et al.*, 1982). The aforementioned problems put in question the accuracy of this method. An additional drawback is the laborious process of preparing the sectioned tooth, which can only be extracted from a dead specimen, making repeated measures impossible.

Future Lines of Research

Future research using the bat as a model for the study of aging may reveal mechanisms that confer resistance to expected senescent processes observed in other long-lived mammals. Elucidation of the physiological mechanisms that give rise to the exceptional longevity observed in bats may provide insight into the development of novel treatments and therapies of degenerative diseases associated with senescence in humans. Chien and Karsenty (2005) describe the typical manifestation of the aging phenotype in long-lived mammals as development of osteoporosis, reduction in body weight, lean-reduced fat tissue, loss of hair or alopecia, cardiomyopathy, early loss of fertility in females, anemia with extramedullary hematopoiesis, reduction in physical activity, and lack of obvious cause of death. Following is a brief review of potentially heuristic lines of research using the bat as a model for the study of aging.

CARDIOVASCULAR RESILIENCE

The capabilities of the cardiovascular system of the typical bat are exceptional. Heart rates vary from as few as 10 beats per minute during hibernation up to 700–1000 beats per minute during flight (Brunet-Rossinni and Austad, 2004; Pauziene *et al.*, 2000). Given the exceptional longevity of bats, one would expect that a cardiovascular system exposed to such extremes in hemodynamic demand would exhibit a decline in cardiac function over time. One would also expect to observe ischemic cardiomyopathy associated with potentially low availability of oxygen during arousal from hibernation. The mammalian heart is composed of distinct cardiomyocyte lineages that give rise to the various anatomical components such as the atrium, ventricles and conduction systems (Chien and Karsenty, 2005). Examination of the mechanisms responsible for the development and maintenance of these cell lineages using techniques such as cell fate mapping should help to elucidate the mechanisms by which bats mediate the expected cardiovascular senescent processes seen in other long-lived mammals. For example, humans exhibit a stereotypic reduction in cardiac ventricular ejection fraction, pacemaker function and electrophysiological conduction fidelity over time (Schwartz and Zipes, 2005). A potentially heuristic line of research would be to determine if these same senescent processes are exhibited in old bats. Cell lineage fate mapping may reveal protective mechanisms, potentially at the genetic level, that staves off expected decline in cardiovascular function. For example, Wallace (2001) has proposed that gradual accumulation of mutations in mitochondrial DNA over time might explain observed senescent processes in long-lived organisms. No studies have focused on the burden of mitochondrial DNA mutations in aged bats.

NEUROPHYSIOLOGICAL RESISTANCE

Bats exhibit an unusual ability to tolerate potentially ischemic conditions in both the cardiovascular and neurophysiological systems during arousal from hibernation and/or daily torpor. Lee *et al.* (2002) reported that oxygen consumption during arousal thermogenesis increased from near zero to 11.9 ml/kg/h. They also reported a rise in body temperature from 7 to 35°Celsius, suggesting potentially ischemic conditions in the heart, brain and other vital organs and tissues. Glucose related proteins (GRPs), which are oxidative stress signaling molecules, were also observed to increase in the brain of the bat. One potentially valuable line of research might be to determine whether expression of the GRPs change over time in the bat and if a similar mechanism prevent cardiac damage due to hypoxia.

The auditory system of Microchiropteran bats is highly refined and potentially represents the single most valuable sensory system inherent to their survival as they rely in echolocation to forage and navigate. Kirkegaard and Jørgensen (2000) report that adult Daubenton's bats exhibit both innervated hair cells and apoptotic hair cells, suggesting a continuous turnover in their postembryonic life. This is contrary to what is observed in humans and mice where the number of innervated hair cells continuously declines with age. Research into the mechanisms underlying regeneration of innervated hair cells might provide a useful model for potential therapeutic applications in humans.

SKELETAL CHANGES

Osteoarthritis and osteoporosis are stereotypically observed in aged long-lived mammals (Cooper and Melton, 1996). Strong bones are critical for bats to handle the physical stresses of flight (Barclay, 1994), and bone remodeling and formation is typically observed during the summer months in bats; however, sex differences have been observed. Kwiecinski *et al.* (1987) report that lactating bats exhibit significant bone loss over the summer months. A compensatory bone resorption mechanism via osteocytic osteolysis exists that alleviates observed bone loss over time. It is not known whether this mechanism declines with age. Conversely, males show continual bone accretion over the summer months. Elucidation of the mechanisms underlying bone resorption and remodeling in bats may provide novel insight into a therapy for osteoporosis in humans.

A critical future line of research will be the establishment of a robust and well-tested method for the determination of chronological age in adult bats. Efforts are currently underway to assess the utility of mitochondrial DNA mutation accumulation and advanced glycation end product accumulation (Wilkinson, G.S., pers. comm.) to estimate age in bats. A great part of developing such methods will be uncovering the actual manifestation of senescence in bats. Research to date on bats has focused on determinants of longevity, yet, aside from tooth wear, we know nothing about the physical decay of bats with age. What do old bats die of? Do they get cancer? Do they develop cardiac disease? Given the high sugar-content in the diet of nectar-feeding bats, do they develop hyperglycemia or diabetes with age? This is a small sample of questions that if answered have the potential to contribute significantly to our understanding of universal mechanisms of senescence. We hope that this chapter will serve to promote the utility of bats in furthering aging research and expose the truly unique qualities of Chiropterans.

Recommended Resources

The following is a list of books and webpages that may be of use to researchers working with bats. Most of the books provide a survey of bat research and can direct a person in their exploration of the literature.

PHYSIOLOGY, ANATOMY, REPRODUCTION, ECOLOGY, AND EVOLUTION OF BATS

The Biology of Bats, Vols. 1–3. 1970. W.A. Wimsatt, ed. Academic Press, New York.

Ecology of Bats. 1982. T.H. Kunz, ed. Plenum Press, New York, 425 pp.150.

Communication in the Chiroptera. 1985. M.B. Fenton. Indiana University Press, Bloomington, Indiana.

Recent Advances in the Study of Bats. 1987. M.B. Fenton, P.A. Racey, and J.M.V. Rayner, eds. Cambridge University Press, Cambridge.

The Natural History of Hibernating Bats. 1990. R. Ransome. Christopher Helm, London.

Walker's Bats of the World. 1994. R.M. Nowak. Johns Hopkins University Press, Baltimore.

Bat Biology and Conservation. 1998. T.H. Kunz and P.A. Racey, eds. Smithsonian Instititution Press, Washington, DC.

The Biology of Bats. 2000. G. Neuweiler (Ellen Covey, translator). Oxford University Press, New York.

Bat Ecology. 2003. T.H. Kunz and M.B. Fenton, eds. University of Chicago Press, Chicago.

METHODS FOR THE STUDY OF BATS

Captive Care and Medical Reference for the Rehabilitation of Insectivorous Bats. 1998. A. Lollar and B. Schmidt-French. Bat World Publications, Mineral Wells, Texas.

Ecological and Behavioral Methods for the Study of Bats. 1988. T.H. Kunz, ed. Smithsonian Institution Press, Washington. *Note:* T.H. Kunz and S. Parsons are in the process of compiling an updated and greatly enhanced 2nd edition of this book.

Zoo and Wild Animal Medicine, 5th ed. 2003. M.E. Fowler and R.E. Miller, eds. W.B. Saunders Company, Philadelphia.

The Animal Welfare Information Center of the United States Department of Agriculture has compiled an extensive bibliography on bats covering topics from anatomy to nutrition, zoonotic diseases, physiology and captive care. The bibliography is available on-line at www.nal.usda.gov/awic/pubs/bats/

REFERENCES

Anthony, E.L.P. (1988). Age determination in bats. In *Ecological and Behavioral Methods for the Study of Bats* (T.H. Kunz, ed.), pp. 47–58. Smithsonian Institution Press, Washington.

Austad, S.N. (1997). Comparative aging and life histories of mammals. *Exp. Gerontol. 32*, 23–38.

Austad, S.N., and Fischer, K.E. (1991). Comparative aging and life histories of mammals. *J. Comp. Physiol. B 119*, 141–154.

Barclay, R.M.R. (1994). Constraints on reproduction by flying vertebrates: Energy and calcium. *Am. Nat. 144*, 1021–1031.

Barclay, R.M.R. (1995). Does energy or calcium availability constrain reproduction by bats? *Symp. Zool. Soc. Lond. 67*, 245–258.

Barclay, R.M.R., and Bell, G.P. (1988). Marking and observational techniques. In *Ecological and Behavioral Methods for the Study of Bats* (T.H. Kunz, ed.), pp. 59–76. Smithsonian Institution Press, Washington.

Barclay, R.M.R., and Harder, L.D. (2003). Life histories of bats: Life in the slow lane. In *Bat Ecology* (T.H. Kunz and M.B. Fenton, eds.), pp. 209–253. University of Chicago Press, Chicago.

Batulevicius, D., Pauziene, N., and Pauza, D.H. (2001). Dental incremental lines in some small species of the European vespertilionid bats. *Acta Theriol. 46*, 33–42.

Baudry, M., DuBrin, R., Beasley, L., Leon, M., and Lynch, G. (1986). Low levels of calpain activity in Chiroptera brain: Implications for mechanisms of aging. *Neurobiol. Aging 7*, 255–258.

Bourliere, M.D. (1958). The comparative biology of aging. *J. Gerontol. 13*, 16–24.

Brunet-Rossinni, A.K. (2004). Reduced free-radical production and extreme longevity in the little brown bat (*Myotis lucifugus*) versus two non-flying mammals. *Mech. Ageing Dev. 125*, 11–20.

Brunet-Rossinni, A.K., and Austad, S.N. (2004). Ageing studies on bats: A review. *Biogerontol. 5*, 211–222.

Brunet-Rossinni, A.K., and Wilkinson, G.S. *in review*. Methods for age determination and the study of senescence in bats. In *Ecological and Behavioral Methods for the Study of Bats*, 2nd ed. (T.H. Kunz and S. Parsons, eds.). Johns Hopkins University Press, Baltimore.

Chien, K.R., and Karsenty, G. (2005). Longevity and lineages: Toward the integrative biology of degenerative diseases in heart, muscle and bone. *Cell 120*, 533–544.

Christofalo, V.J., and Pignolo, R.J. (1995). Cell culture as a model. In *Handbook of Physiology* Sect. 11: Aging (E.J. Masoro, ed.), pp. 53–82. American Physiological Society, New York.

Constantine, D.G. (1988). Heath precautions for bat researchers. In *Ecological and Behavioral Methods for the Study of Bats* (T.H. Kunz, ed.), pp. 491–528. Smithsonian Institution Press, Washington.

Cool, S.M., Bennett, M.B., and Romaniuk, K. (1994). Age estimation of pteropodid bats (Megachiroptera) from hard tissue parameters. *Wildl. Res. 21*, 353–364.

Cooper, C., and Melton, L.J.I. (1996). Magnitude and impact of osteoporosis and fractures. In *Osteoporosis*. (J. Kelsey, ed.), pp. 419–434. Academic Press, San Diego.

Dickson, J.M., and Green, D.G. (1970). The vampire bat (*Desmodus rotundus*): Improved methods of laboratory care and handling. *Lab. Anim. 4*, 37–44.

Gaisler, J., Hanák, V., Hanzal, V., and Jarksy, V. (2003). Results of bat banding in the Czech and Slovak republics, 1948–2000. *Vespertilio 7*, 3–63. (In Czech, English summary).

Hall, J.S., Cloutier, R.J., and Griffin, D.R. (1957). Longevity records and notes on tooth wear of bats. *J. Mammal. 38*, 407–409.

Harman, D. (1956). Aging: A theory based on free radical radiation chemistry. *J. Gerontol. 11*, 298–300.

Heideman, P.D. (2000). Environmental regulation of reproduction. In *Reproductive Biology of Bats* (E.G. Crichton and P.H. Krutzsch, eds.), pp. 469–500. Academic Press, London.

Herreid, C.F. (1964). Bat longevity and metabolic rate. *Exp. Gerontol. 1*, 1–9.

Herrero, A., and Barja, G. (1998). H_2O_2 production of heart mitochondria and aging rate are slower in canaries and parakeets than in mice: Sites of free radical generation and mechanisms involved. *Mech. Ageing Dev. 103*, 133–146.

Issac, S., Balasingh, J., Nathan, P.T., Doss, D.P., Sudhakaran, M.R., and Kunz, T.H. (2003). An improved, beaded, polymer necklace for marking bats. *Bat Res. News. 44*, 87–89.

Johnston, D.S. (1997). Social and behavioral well-being of captive bats. *J. Wildl. Rehab. 20*, 15–18.

Jones, K.E., and MacLarnon, A. (2001). Bat life histories: Testing models of mammalian life-history evolution. *Evol. Ecol. Res. 3*, 465–476.

Jürgens, K.D., and Prothero, J. (1987). Scaling of maximal lifespan in bats. *Comp. Biochem. Physiol. A 88*, 361–367.

Kirkegaard, M., and Jørgensen, J.M. (2000). Continuous hair cell turnover in the inner ear vestibular organs of a mammal, the Daubenton's bat (*Myotis daubentonii*). *Naturwissenschaften. 87*, 83–86.

Kirkwood, T.B.L. (1977). Evolution of ageing. *Nature 270*, 301–304.

Klevezal', G.A., and Kleinenberg, S.E. (1967). Age determination of mammals from annual layers in teeth and bones. Israel Program for Scientific Translations, Jerusalem, TT 69–55033 (1969). (Translated from Russian).

Ku, H.-H., Brunk, U.T., and Sohal, R.S. (1993). Relationship between mitochondrial superoxide and hydrogen peroxide production and longevity of mammalian species. *Free Radic. Biol. Med. 15*, 621–627.

Kunz, T.H. (1982). Roosting ecology. In *Ecology of Bats* (T.H. Kunz, ed.), pp. 1–55. Plenum Press, New York.

Kunz, T.H., and Anthony, E.L.P. (1982). Age estimation and post-natal growth in the bat *Myotis lucifugus*. *J. Mammal. 63*, 23–32.

Kunz, T.H., and Kurta, A. (1988). Capture methods and holding devices. In *Ecological and Behavioral Methods for the Study of Bats* (T.H. Kunz, ed.), pp. 1–29. Smithsonian Institution Press, Washington.

Kurta, A., and Kunz, T.H. (1987). Size of bats at birth and maternal investment during pregnancy. *Symp. Zool. Soc. Lond. 57*, 79–106.

Kwiecinski, G.G., Krook, L., and Wimsatt, W.A. (1987). Annual skeletal changes in the little brown bat, *Myotis lucifigus*, with particular reference to pregnancy and lactation. *Am. J. Anat. 178*, 410–420.

Lee, M., Choi, I., and Park, K. (2002). Activation of stress signaling molecules in bat brain during arousal from hibernation. *J. Neurochem. 82*, 867–873.

Lollar, A., and Schmidt-French, B. (1998). *Captive Care and Medical Reference for the Rehabilitation of Insectivorous Bats.* Bat World Publications, Mineral Wells, Texas.

Pauziene, N., Pauza, D.H., and Stropus, R. (2000). Morphological study of the heart innervation of bats *Myotis daubentonii* and *Eptesicus serotinus* (Microchiroptera:Vespertilionidae) during hibernation. *Eu. J. Morphol. 38*, 195–205.

Pearl, R. (1928). *The Rate of Living*. A.A. Knopf, New York.

Phillips, C.J., Steinberg, B., and Kunz, T.H. (1982). Dentin, cementum, and age determination in bats: A critical evaluation. *J. Mammal 63*, 197–207.

Racey, P.A. (1982). Ecology of bat reproduction. In *Ecology of Bats* (T. H. Kunz, ed.), pp. 57–104. Plenum Press, New York.

Racey, P.A. (1988). Reproductive assessment in bats. In *Ecological and Behavioral Methods for the Study of Bats* (T.H. Kunz, ed.), pp. 31–46. Smithsonian Institution Press, Washington.

Rachmatulina, I.K. (1992). Major demographic characteristics of populations of certain bats from Azerbaijan. In *Prague Studies in Mammalogy* (J. Horacek and V. Vohralik, eds.), pp. 127–141. Charles University Press, Prague.

Ransome, R.D. (1995). Earlier breeding shortens life in female greater horseshoe bats. *Phill. Trans. Soc. Lond. B 350*, 153–161.

Read, A.F., and Harvey, P.H. (1989). Life-history differences among the eutherian radiations. *J. Zoo. Lond. 219*, 329–353.

Röhme, D. (1981). Evidence for a relationship between longevity of mammalian species and lifespans of normal fibroblasts *in vitro* and erythrocytes *in vivo*. *Proc. Natl. Acad. Sci. USA 78*, 5009–5013.

Sacher, G.A. (1959). Relation of lifespan to brain weight and body weight in mammals. *Ciba Found. Coll. 5*, 115–141.

Schwartz, J.B., and Zipes, D.P. (2005). Cardiovascular disease in the elderly. In *Braunwald's Heart Disease, A Textbook of Cardiovascular Medicine* (D.P. Zipes and E. Braunwald, eds.), pp. 1925–1949. Elsevier Saunders, Pennsylvania.

Simmons, N.B. (2000). Bat phylogeny: An evolutionary context for comparative studies. In *Ontogeny, Functional Ecology, and Evolution of Bats* (R.A. Adams and S.S. Pedersen, eds.), pp. 9–58. Cambridge University Press, Cambridge.

Simmons, N.B., and Conway, T.M. (2003). Evolution of ecological diversity in bats. In *Bat Ecology* (T.H. Kunz and M.B. Fenton, eds.), pp. 493–535. University of Chicago Press, Chicago.

Smith, R.T. (1955). Histoplasmosis: A review with an epidemiological and clinical study of an outbreak occurring in Minnesota. *J. Lancet 75*, 83–100.

Speakman, J.R., and Thomas, D.W. (2003). Physiological ecology and energetics of bats. In *Bat Ecology* (T.H. Kunz and M.B. Fenton, eds.), pp. 209–253. University of Chicago Press, Chicago.

Tuttle, M.D., and Stevenson, D. (1982). Growth and survival of bats. In *Ecology of Bats* (T.H. Kunz, ed.), pp. 105–150. Plenum Press, New York.

Wallace, D.C. (2001). A mitochondrial paradigm for degenerative diseases and ageing. *Novartis Found. Symp.* 235, 247–263.

Wilkinson, G.S., and South, J.M. (2002). Life history, ecology and longevity in bats. *Aging Cell 1*, 124–131.

Williams, G.C. (1957). Pleiotropy, natural selection and the evolution of senescence. *Evol. 11*, 398–411.

Wilson, D.E. (1988). Maintaining bats for captive studies. In *Ecological and Behavioral Methods for the Study of Bats* (T.H. Kunz, ed.), pp. 247–263. Smithsonian Institution Press, Washington.

37

Memory in the Aging Hippocampus: What Can Place Cells Tell Us?

Iain A. Wilson

Spatial memory impairments in normal aged individuals are associated with changes in hippocampal connectivity and plasticity. Electrophysiological recordings of single-cell activity while an animal is freely behaving allow us to see the brain in action and compare how young and aged individuals process information differently. Specifically, as a rat explores an environment, hippocampal neurons referred to as place cells show location-specific activity. Because the same network of cells is activated for repeated visits to one environment whereas a completely different network is used to represent a second environment, place cells provide a promising window into how the hippocampus forms and uses memories. Studies have found that place cells of aged rats, while showing robust spatial selectivity, do not encode or recall environmental landmark information as well as those of young rats. These weakened processing capabilities may be closely related to the spatial memory impairments suffered by aged individuals. The view from the place cell window is particularly revealing towards age-related memory impairments when placed in the context of known neurobiological changes to the normal aging brain. For these reasons, hippocampal place cells have been and will continue to be a useful tool to investigate memory disabilities of the aged and to evaluate potential preventive measures.

Introduction

Aged people often seem to maintain strong memories of childhood places, but sometimes have difficulties making new memories of new places. My great-grandmother, for example, would tell stories of her childhood, bringing us all vividly back to explorations of her favorite red-brick house, but after the story, she would wonder how we got to the living room of the nursing home.

Indeed, normal aging is associated with diminished memory capacity in both humans and animals (Gallagher and Rapp, 1997). How can we study why the aging brain has trouble making memories? This chapter will address how we can gain insight into the mechanisms underlying age-associated memory impairment. Memories are believed to be formed by strengthening some connections between neurons, while weakening others. Accordingly, encoding a memory involves binding a network of neurons together so that later the same neuronal network will be recalled into activity. The chapter will focus on one technique: recording electrophysiological signals from single cells in rats that are freely behaving. By recording action potentials of single neurons, researchers can ask how networks of neurons store information in their patterns of activity. Although this technique is far from explaining all questions of the aging brain, it does provide powerful insight into its information processing capabilities, especially when considered alongside well-documented neurobiological changes to the aging brain.

Why Study Spatial Memory and the Aging Hippocampus?

Because age-associated memory impairment occurs only in specific systems of learning, it is important to focus on a kind of memory that is impaired similarly in both humans and in animals. The learning and memory of places is particularly appropriate for investigations into the mechanisms of cognitive aging for four reasons. First, diminished spatial memory capacity is associated with aging in humans and in animals (for review, see Gallagher and Rapp, 1997). Second, spatial learning and memory play significant roles in the daily functioning of both humans and other species of mammals, and memories of places are easily tested in many different species. These tests can be arranged to compare the strength of memories for well-learned places with memories for novel places, a distinction relevant to aging (for review, see Hedden, 2004). Third, the mechanisms of spatial memory appear largely conserved between animals and humans, and these have been and continue to be well-studied in young individuals. Much research in young animals has shown that the hippocampus region of the brain is intimately linked with spatial cognition. Fourth, the hippocampus of rats, like that of humans, undergoes specific age-associated degenerations to its circuits.

As discussed in Chapter 32 by Bizon and Nicolle in this book, rats provide a useful model for studying the mechanisms underlying age-associated impairments in spatial memory. The spatial water maze task, which requires the use of spatial landmarks to navigate in an open field (described in detail by Bizon and Nicolle), is abnormally difficult both for aging rats (Gallagher *et al.*, 1993) and for aging humans on dry land and virtual versions (Moffat and Resnick, 2002; Newman and Kaszniak, 2000). Spatial learning and memory are critically dependent upon the hippocampus region of the brain (O'Keefe and Nadel, 1978), and indeed many of cognitive impairments suffered by aged individuals are similar to disabilities caused by lesions to the hippocampus, both in humans and in animals (Gallagher and Rapp, 1997). This has inspired researchers to focus on the hippocampus as a possible source of age-associated memory impairments.

The hippocampus receives highly processed multimodal information from the association cortices (Amaral and Witter, 1995). This information from all the sensory modalities—vision, hearing, touch, and so on—flows in a circuit through the hippocampal formation where relationships can be rapidly bound together, perhaps into a memory of an event, place, or context (Eichenbaum *et al.*, 1999; O'Keefe and Nadel, 1978; Redish, 2001). Information flow within the hippocampus is classically described as a tri-synaptic circuit, signifying a cascade of processing (Amaral, 1993; Amaral and Witter, 1995). Information flow in the tri-synaptic circuit cascades from the entorhinal cortex to the dentate gyrus (1) to the CA3 (2) and to the CA1 (3). The principal cells that provide the output of each subregion are arranged in tightly packed layers (see Figure 37.1). To complete the circuit, the entorhinal cortex receives the output of the CA1 (via the subiculum).

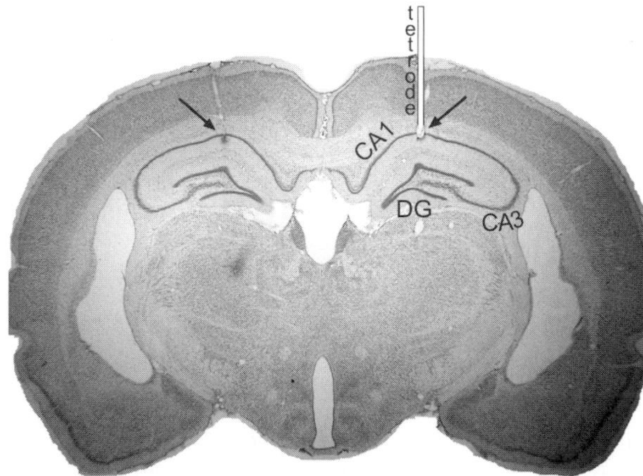

Figure 37.1 A histological section showing the recording sites of hippocampal place cells. Tetrodes (drawn in the right hemisphere) were advanced through the overlying cortex to the CA1 pyramidal cell layer. The actual recording sites in both hemispheres are marked with lesions and indicated with arrows. The cell layers of the CA1, CA3 and dentate gyrus (DG) subregions of the hippocampus are highlighted by the Nissl staining.

Why Measure Neuronal Activity?

In order to understand how the hippocampus processes the information it receives, and to compare how the aged hippocampus does this differently from the young one, one useful technique has been to study brain in action. The brain represents information by activating networks of neurons, and each piece of information will be represented by a different network of neurons. It is therefore keenly interesting to identify which neurons are active at which times. By placing extracellular electrodes near the soma of cells inside the brain, it is possible to record the action potentials of neurons as they communicate with one another through changes in electric potentials. The great advantage of this technique is that we can monitor cell activity while the animal is awake and even performing a task. By providing a window to *when* neurons are active, single cell recordings have given unique insight into *what* information is processed within particular brain regions. In other words, by knowing when action potentials occur (to the nearest tenths of a millisecond), we can ask how this activity relates to what the animal was doing at that particular time. Much of our understanding of the function of a particular brain region has come from this window into the brain's activity. For example, single-cell recordings have made enormous contributions to our understanding of how each region of the visual cortex contributes to vision—from responses in the primary visual cortex to precisely oriented lines to responses in the inferior temporal cortex to particular classes of objects.

Neuronal Activity of the Young Hippocampus: What Are Place Cells?

Because single-cell recordings can be done while an animal is exploring an environment, the technique provides researchers with a view of the neurons of the hippocampus in action as it is processing spatial information in the rat (O'Keefe and Dostrovsky, 1971), the monkey (Rolls, 1999), and the human (Ekstrom *et al.*, 2003). The best-researched of these is the freely moving rat. The pyramidal cells of the CA1 and CA3 hippocampus fire action potentials when the rat occupies particular places (for review, see Muller, 1996). "Place cells" have high firing rates in a particular area of an environment, referred to as the place field; outside this place field the cells are nearly silent (see examples of Figure 37.2).

In typical place cell experiments, the rat is placed into an environment, either an open field or a linear track. The rat then explores the arena, often with the encouragement of randomly placed food rewards. In the top row of the example (Figure 37.2) the rat is shown exploring cylindrical and square environments, which contain three distinct landmarks on the walls that the rat

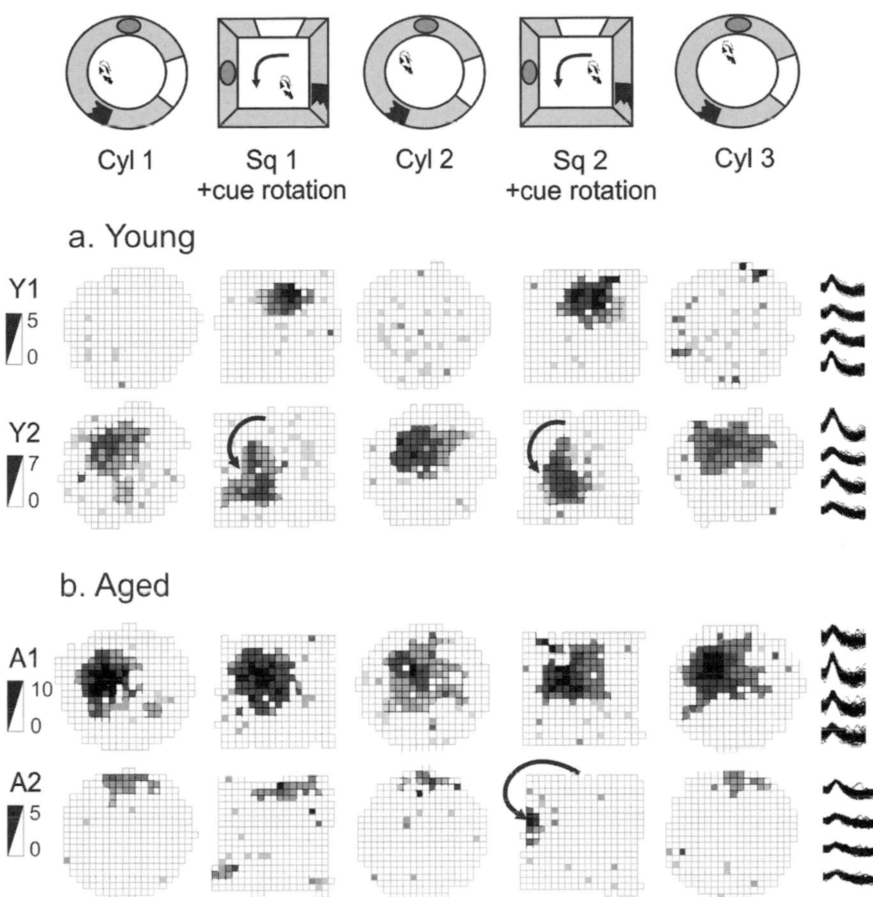

Figure 37.2 Place fields of hippocampal cells in young and aged rats. The top row depicts the experimental setup with the rats exploring a familiar cylindrical arena (Cyl) and a novel square arena (Sq). Each subsequent row represents the activity of one cell over the entire experiment. Firing rate scales are provided on the left of the figure, such that darker pixels indicate areas in which more action potentials occurred. Sample tetrode waveforms of each cell are shown on the right side. Data are shown (a) for two place cells of two young rats and (b) for two cells of two aged, memory-impaired rats. Cell Y1 is an example of the generation of new spatial representations by cells of young rats. Cell Y2 shows a place cell whose field rotated, following the landmarks in the square. Cell A1 shows an example of rigid place fields of aged memory-impaired rats despite changes in the environment. Cell A2 is rigid in response to the first exposure to the novel-square, but then rotates with the square's landmarks in the second trial (Figure adapted from Wilson *et al.*, 2003).

can use for orientation. As the rat explores, the action potentials of pyramidal cells from the hippocampus are recorded. Each row in the figure depicts the activity of one neuron throughout the manipulations of the experiment. Each grid represents the floor space where the rat was moving. Dark pixels show high firing rates for a particular cell, whereas white pixels indicate no action potentials but that the rat did visit the area. The dark areas are referred to as the place field for that cell. Each time the rat passes through the place field, the place cell fires action potentials; outside the field the place cell is silent.

With thousands of cells active within an environment and each cell with its own place field, these neurons could compute the rat's spatial location and reflect elements of a rat's "cognitive map" (O'Keefe and Nadel, 1978). Wilson and McNaughton (1993), recording simultaneously from as many as 141 pyramidal cells, were able to estimate the rat's position to 1-cm accuracy even with only this number of cells. It is clear that these cells participate in a broad system of spatial processing that is important for navigation (Redish and Touretzky, 1997). The cells may also participate in a broader spectrum of memories; alternatives to the cognitive map theory posit that these cells could represent places where significant events occur within episodic memories (Eichenbaum *et al.*, 1999) or participate in associations of contexts within memories (O'Reilly and Rudy, 2001; Redish, 2001).

Regardless of what they imply for hippocampal theory, place cells possess four characteristics that make them a useful window into how the hippocampus stores information, especially spatial information. The first property of place cells that attracts memory researchers is that they are *not simply sensory neurons*. The hippocampus receives multimodal information, so it is not a surprise that place fields are controlled by contributions from all the sensory modalities. Rats navigate by vision, smell, touch, hearing, and self-motion information; all of these have influence over place cell firing patterns (Muller, 1996). This characteristic means that researchers can study how the sensory modalities interact to control stored patterns of activity.

The second property of place cells that makes them attractive as a model of memory is their remarkable *stability* across time. Place cells are active in the same location with respect to each other and to the environment both within a continuous session in an environment and when the rat reenters the same environment after an absence (Muller and Kubie, 1987; Thompson and Best, 1990). This is clearly illustrated in cell Y1 in Figure 37.2. The cell is silent in the cylinder 1 environment. The rat is then removed from the arena and placed in a holding bucket while the arena is changed to a square out of the rat's sight. The rat is lifted back to the arena, and this process is repeated several times. Each of the three times that the rat explored the cylinder, this cell fired very few action potentials. The two exposures to the square arena, though, had distinct place fields in the same location; hence, the place fields were stable. This appears to be a function of memory recall because different environments are represented by different sets of place cells (discussed later), and reentering the original environment primes the retrieval of the original spatial representation. This characteristic of place cells indicates that a representation of the environment is stored in the hippocampus, and place cells allow researchers easy access to explore the mechanisms of these memories.

The third important feature of place cells is that they are largely controlled by visual landmarks, and therefore the place cells *rotate with rotations of the visual landmarks*. When the rat is removed from an arena and the visual landmarks of an arena are then rotated by 90°, upon reentry the place cells follow the landmark rotation by almost exactly 90° (Muller and Kubie, 1987; O'Keefe and Conway, 1978). This effect is shown in the cell Y2 of Figure 37.2. The place fields in the square environment have simply followed the 90° rotation of the landmarks (in this experiment the landmarks were the same in both environments, but rotated by 90°). Because tests of spatial memory, such as the water maze, rely upon use of the visual landmarks, the fact that place cells rotate with visual cues strengthens the link between hippocampal cells and spatial navigation. The rotations provide a simple way to test how well the cues of a particular environment control the hippocampal spatial representations.

The fourth attraction of place cells for memory researchers is the creation of *new spatial representations* in new environments. When a rat enters a visually new arena from a familiar one, the place cells drastically alter their place field firing patterns, quickly forming completely new firing patterns in the relation of the cells to each other and to the visual landmarks (Frank *et al.*, 2004; Hill, 1978; Wilson and McNaughton, 1993). For two environments, two different sets of hippocampal neurons are active. Cell Y1 of Figure 37.2 illustrates a cell that is silent in one environment (the cylinder) and active in the other (the square). Alternatively, the cell may use two different place field locations to represent two environments. Each environment recalls into activity the unique network of neurons bound to it, much resembling a stored memory. The learning of a new environment and the creation of new spatial representation are not always rapid. When two environments are similar, place cells may initially use the same representation but with additional exposure may slowly (over as many as twenty days) develop distinct representations for each (Lever *et al.*, 2002). Place cells, therefore, provide researchers the perfect opportunity to study the storage of a memory from its creation in the hippocampus.

In support of these assertions, several experiments have found that successful spatial navigation to a goal requires place fields consistent with that goal (Lenck-Santini *et al.*, 2001; Lenck-Santini *et al.*, 2002; O'Keefe and Speakman, 1987; Rosenzweig *et al.*, 2003). For example, in a study by Lenck-Santini and colleagues (2001) rats performed a continuous spatial alternation task in a 3-armed Y-maze. After a series of landmark rotations, some place fields became out-of-register with the goal arm, and for these rats, performance on the task was poor. Place fields of other rats maintained their correct relationship with the goal arm, and for these rats, performance on the task remained accurate. These studies strongly suggest that a consistent place field-goal relationship is essential for finding goals that require spatial navigation.

How Can Place Cells Be Useful for the Study of Memory and Aging?

CA1 and CA3 pyramidal cells reflect how spatial information is processed and stored in the hippocampus. Because place cells are not simply sensory neurons, because place cells are stable over time and repetition, because place cells clearly use the visual landmarks, and because place cells form new spatial representations of new environments, they provide an intriguing window into the formation of memories by the brain. Furthermore, consistent spatial representations are necessary for correct performance on spatial tasks and serve as a likely step in the mechanisms of spatial navigation and memory. Because these are precisely the behavioral impairments from which some aged individuals suffer, researchers have turned to place cells in order to tighten the connection between the behavioral deficits of aged animals and information processing capabilities within the hippocampus region. Hence, comparing the information processing of place cells of young and aged rats can yield unique insight into what goes wrong in the hippocampus of aged memory-impaired individuals.

Technical Challenges and Advances – What Are Tetrodes and Microdrives?

Action potentials of single cells are recorded by bringing small-diameter wires close to the soma of neurons (see Figure 37.1). Because the pyramidal cells of the hippocampus are so tightly packed, a single 13-micron diameter electrode will detect action potentials from many neurons. This is good, except that with a single electrode, one cannot differentiate action potentials from individual neurons. To solve this problem, hippocampal researchers twist several electrodes together into a tetrode with four electrodes (Gray *et al.*, 1995; McNaughton *et al.*, 1983). Tetrodes bring four electrode tips to the hippocampal pyramidal cell layer, and therefore triangulation can be used to discriminate between active cells. The amplitudes of the waveforms that the wires record are largest for cells that are nearest to a particular electrode tip. More distant electrodes will have waveforms of smaller amplitude for that cell. This is illustrated in the waveforms of Figure 37.2. The action potentials of each neuron produce their own unique signature of tetrode waveforms. This allows researchers to distinguish between different neurons that are recorded simultaneously. With this technological advance, it is now possible to record simultaneously from ten or more well-isolated neurons from one tetrode.

Another important technological development has been the ability to advance many tetrodes individually down to the cell layers. Because the position of the electrodes must be precisely in the pyramidal cell layer during recordings, the electrodes are not advanced to the hippocampal layers when the rat is anesthetized during surgery. Instead, the tetrodes are implanted to the overlying cortex and slowly advanced (50 microns/day) so that the rat is awake and potentially ready for recordings when the cell layer is found (see Figure 37.1). To do this, each tetrode is attached to its own microdrive, enabling precise adjustments in recording location to be made so that each tetrode will find the ideal layer and stay there for stable recordings over at least several days. Using these demanding techniques, today laboratories are able to record from twelve tetrodes simultaneously, which allows recordings to distinguish between as many as 100 cells at a time. Recording from such a network of activity with stable cells over one week allows investigation of the information processing of neurons during the formation and retrieval of memories.

What Have We Learned So Far from Aging Place Cell Research?

Although aged rats are certainly impaired in hippocampal-dependent spatial memory, the hippocampus of aged rats does possess place cells with firing properties similar to those of young rats. Most importantly, the hippocampal cells of even the most spatially-impaired aged rats have place fields that are equally as crisp as those of young rats (see examples A1 and A2 of Figure 37.2; for a review of these data, see (Barnes, 1998)). The difficulties of cognitive aging, therefore, do not lie in simply a lack of spatial processing by the hippocampus. Instead, research has consistently shown that differences between the spatial representations of young and aged rats are brought out when the hippocampus is challenged to encode changes in the environment. In order to illustrate how place cells can be used as an effective tool in aging research, I will highlight three experiments that demonstrated these differences in hippocampal information processing and tied them to age-related memory impairments.

The experiment shown in Figures 37.2 and 37.3 was designed to draw a closer association between hippocampal encoding of a new environment and the degree of age-related memory impairments in individual rats (Wilson *et al.*, 2003). The spatial learning abilities of young and aged rats were determined by the water maze task; the young rats and some aged rats performed well, whereas other aged rats were significantly impaired (see Figure 37.3, the Y-axis).

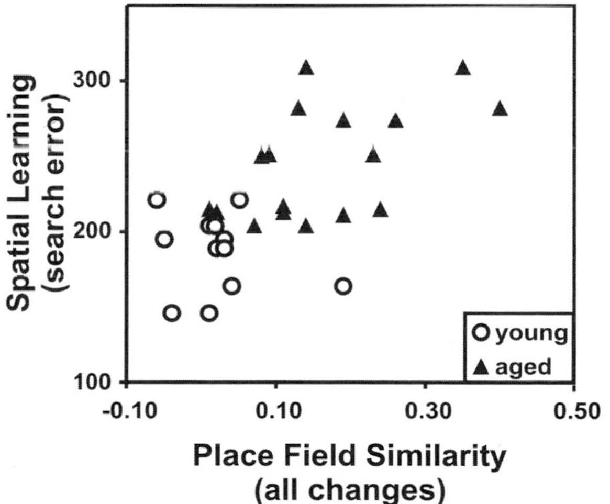

Figure 37.3 The degree of place cell rigidity predicts the magnitude of spatial learning impairment. Similarity in place fields between exposures to the familiar cylinder and novel square are plotted against spatial learning performance in the water maze. Poor spatial memory is indicated by high spatial learning search error scores. Similarity scores (rigidity) correlated strongly with spatial memory performance of all groups combined ($r(29) = 0.63$, $p < 0.001$), and within the group of nine aged rats ($r(17) = 0.55$, $p < 0.05$). (Figure adapted from Wilson *et al.*, 2003.)

Subsequently, hippocampal place cells were recorded as the rats explored a familiar environment (the cylinder) and a geometrically altered version of the environment (the square; see Figure 37.2, top row). Place fields of young and aged memory-intact rats changed upon exposure to the altered environment (Figure 37.2, cells Y1 and Y2). In contrast, many place fields of aged memory-impaired rats were unaffected by the environmental alteration (Figure 37.2, cells A1 and A2).

One possibility that must always be considered with aged rats is that the aged memory-impaired rats fail to use the visual landmarks in the water maze and place cell recordings because their vision is poor. The example in Figure 37.2, cell A2, illustrates why poor vision appears unlikely to account for the rigidity in the place cells in this experiment. The field was rigid during the first exposure to the square arena (Sq 1), but during the second exposure the field rotated with the landmarks (Sq 2). This indicates that the visual information could at least reach the hippocampus, but on some occasions it was not encoded properly.

To quantify this place field rigidity of aged rats, pixel-by-pixel correlation comparisons were done between the firing rate maps of the two environments. Place cells with different place fields in the cylinder and square environments had correlations near 0.0 (Figure 37.1, young cells Y1 and Y2), whereas place fields that are similar between the two environments had higher correlations approaching 1.0 (aged cells A1 and the first three trials of A2). These place cell characteristics of aged rats were then related to the abilities of the same rats on the spatial water maze. As Figure 37.3 shows, the degree of the rigidity in spatial representation predicted the magnitude of the spatial memory impairment. Thus, the heterogeneity of the spatial memory capacity with aging may be due to differential information encoding capacities by the young and aged hippocampus.

In a complement to these encoding difficulties, Barnes *et al.* (1997) have shown that, under other conditions, aged rats do not retrieve place cell representations properly. In an elegantly simple experiment, place cells were recorded in a familiar environment, and then the rats were taken on a tour of several new environments. When the rats were placed back into the familiar environment, the authors performed a correlation analysis between the place fields used initially in the familiar environment and those used after the new exposures. The young rats used the same place fields to represent both sessions in the familiar environment. The aged rats, on the other hand, recalled the former place fields correctly only about 70% of the time. On 30% of the occasions the aged rats used a completely novel arrangement of place fields to represent the familiar environment, suggesting a multistability of spatial representations in aged rats. As a control, the authors compared the place cell activity within uninterrupted sessions; in this case the aged rats, as well as the young, maintained the same spatial representations throughout the sessions. These results suggest that the aged rats had no difficulties maintaining a consistent representation during uninterrupted exposure to an environment, but that new experiences could interfere with successful recall of even a highly familiar environment.

To test how this place cell retrieval deficit related to spatial navigation abilities, the authors (Barnes *et al.*, 1997) compared water maze data from 98 young and 93 aged rats (these rats were different individuals than those recorded). After four days of training, the young rats quickly found the hidden platform almost every time, whereas the aged rats sometimes found it and sometimes had much longer search paths. The variability of the aged rats was not due to between-rat differences, but rather each aged rat had good performances and bad performances. Together these data suggest that the aged rats sometimes got lost; that is, their place cells failed to recall the correct spatial representation, and this caused them to search incorrectly for the water maze platform.

In addition to difficulties encoding and retrieving place cell memories, aged rats are not as capable as young rats at making appropriate updates to their place cell representations during a continuous experience. Rosenzweig *et al.* (2003) recorded place cells of young and aged rats as they were actually performing a spatial navigation task. This cleverly designed experiment manipulated the relationship between external cues and self-motion cues. The goal location on a linear track remained constant with respect to the external visual cues, but the start box was shifted for each trial causing the walking distance to the goal location to vary. On each trial place fields were initially determined by the self-motion cues, and successful performance entailed a switch in the control of place fields from self-motion cues to external landmark cues well before the goal area was reached (Gothard *et al.*, 1996). Young rats successfully updated their spatial representations, whereas many aged rats failed to update their representation to the relevant spatial information and therewith failed on the task. Furthermore, the learning of a goal location correlated strongly with how readily the place fields of the rats were adjusted into control by spatial cues.

This chapter has been intended to provide only examples of how place cells can be a useful tool for aging research; for more complete reviews of the aging place cell literature, please see Rosenzweig and Barnes (2003) and Wilson (2005). The experiments discussed here do serve to illustrate a rising theme from the literature: the hippocampus of aged rats is impaired in the processing of external environmental information. Under different demands on memory processing, this manifests itself in different forms (Wilson *et al.*, 2004). Aged place cells that fail to change despite new environments allow us to see failures during encoding. The multistability of aged place cells upon return to a familiar environment allows us to see failures during recall. Aged place cells that do not readily adjust from self-motion to external landmark control allow us to see failures during updating of the representation. Place cells, therefore, provide a powerful window into the workings of memory in the aged hippocampus.

What Are the Limitations to Place Cell Research?

Single-cell recordings allow the study of information processing by individual neurons of a particular region within the brain with enough temporal precision to correlate activity of individual neurons with particular behaviors. The power of single-cell recordings is limited, however, by the facts that the electrodes sample a very small selection of the neurons from only one subregion of the brain, monitoring numerous brain regions simultaneously is difficult (but see Lee *et al.*, 2004), and the anatomical locations and connections of the recorded neurons can be defined only in general terms. For example, the CA1 hippocampus contains roughly 400,000 pyramidal cells (Rosenzweig and Barnes, 2003); even the published "world record" for number of place cells recorded simultaneously of 141 cells (Wilson and McNaughton, 1993) manages only a small sample of the hippocampus. Furthermore, single-cell recordings are highly invasive and cannot be done in human subjects (although see Ekstrom *et al.*, 2003).

Electrophysiological recording of single-cells is not the only means of studying neuronal activity. For example, the fMRI technique is a noninvasive way to study activation over the entire human brain, while the subject thinks about a computer screen (for applications relevant to aging, see Chapter 12 by Small). However, the spatial precision of fMRI is far from individual neurons, the trials must be averaged, which reduces temporal precision, and the subjects are restricted in behavior. Recently in animal research, gene activation studies have proved capable of studying the activity of single neurons simultaneously across many brain regions. cFos, Arc, and Homer are genes whose expression is induced immediately following neuronal activity. Through immunostaining, these genes provide a marker for which neurons have been activated during a particular time period prior to sacrifice of the rat. A drawback of the immediate–early gene technique to study neuronal activation is that the rat must be sacrificed in order to get the information. This means that one cannot measure changes in activity across different behavioral settings or across learning, as one can do with *in vivo* electrophysiology.

Monitoring of place cells contributes one piece to our understanding of cognitive aging through their insight into spatial memory, but there is convincing evidence that the hippocampus handles more than just spatial information (reviewed by Eichenbaum *et al.*, 1999). Important studies have, therefore, examined the activity of single cells during a nonspatial task in aged rabbits (for example, McEchron *et al.*, 2001). Moreover, to reap the full benefit of the single-cell recording technique, place cell results must be placed in the context of well-researched age-related behavioral impairments and deteriorations to hippocampal connectivity and plasticity (for reviews of this, see Foster, 1999; Wu *et al.*, 2002; Rosenzweig and Barnes, 2003; Wilson, 2005). Many of these neuroanatomical changes to the aging brain are discussed in Chapter 32 by Bizon and Nicolle. Each technique provides its own insight into the mechanisms underlying age-related memory impairments; by putting many technique pieces together, we can begin to understand why the aging brain is sometimes impaired.

What Can Future Research with Place Cells Tell Us about Cognitive Aging?

Neurobiological investigations on aging have repeatedly stressed the subtlety and the regional specificity of changes within the hippocampus, affecting synaptic connections, physiology, and plasticity (for review, see Barnes, 1994). These changes may cause subtle shifts in how information is processed by the aging brain. In accordance with this view, age-related changes to hippocampal place cells are also subtle. Spatial information is certainly reaching and being processed by the aged hippocampus since location-specific activity is equally robust in both young and aged rats. Nevertheless, place cell studies have shown that aged rats have behaviorally significant deficits in encoding and recall of spatial information within the hippocampal region.

In the near future hippocampal place cells may, therefore, serve as a useful tool for investigating three specific aspects of age-related memory impairments. First, it will be important to understand how aged rats fail to encode and recall spatial goals. Researchers have found that weakened processing of external landmarks by place cells during a spatial task predicts performance of the aged rats on that task (Rosenzweig *et al.*, 2003), and the next step may be to measure the activity of hippocampal cells as the rat is actually learning spatial goals and recalling them.

Second, recent technological advances, such as recordings from twelve independently-movable tetrodes, have made it possible to record cells from several regions of the brain simultaneously. With a better understanding of the particular contributions each region makes to the formation and recall of memories (such as Lee *et al.*, 2004), the way has recently been paved for information processing studies to match the well-documented subregional specificity of age-related changes to hippcampal neurobiology. These advances may prove important as we aim towards prevention of age-related memory impairments with specifically-targeted pharmacological interventions. Third, place cells of aged rats provide a window for evaluation of these potential drugs. Place cells are already in common use to evaluate effects on memory of receptor-blocking drugs (for example, Kentros *et al.*, 1998) and mutations of specific genes in mice (Cho *et al.*, 1998). With respect to normal aging, therapies that reinstate normal encoding and recall to place cells of aged animals will be particularly promising.

Conclusion

What have hippocampal place cells told us about why my great-grandmother maintained strong memories of her childhood but failed to make to new memories in her old age? When people are young, spatial environments are fully encoded by hippocampal cells and probably eventually become cortical memories, no longer requiring the hippocampus (Squire and Alvarez, 1995). As people age, new spatial environments are encoded more weakly by hippocampal cells, and they are less able to prompt later recall. Hippocampal place cells, thus, provide a clear window for investigating age-related impairments in the formation and retrieval of memories and may serve as a powerful tool for evaluating potential preventive measures.

Recommended Resources

Eichenbaum, H., Dudchenko, P., Wood, E., Shapiro, M., and Tanila, H. (1999). The hippocampus, memory, and place cells: is it spatial memory or a memory space? *Neuron* 23, 209–226.

This article presents an overview of how place cells could contribute to the episodic memory theory of hippocampal function.

Gallagher, M., and Rapp, P.R. (1997). The use of animal models to study the effects of aging on cognition. *Annu. Rev. Psychol.* 48, 339–370.

This excellent review explores the functions of the medial temporal lobe and the frontal lobes and then examines how each system is affected by aging in humans and in animals.

Hargreaves, E.L. Page O' Neuroplasticity. http://homepages.nyu.edu/~eh597/.

This webpage provides a comprehensive introduction to many aspects of hippocampal neuroplasticity. This is an excellent introduction to place cell technique, complete with descriptive photos, references, and links to scientists who do place cell research.

Hedden, T., and Gabrieli, J.D. (2004). Insights into the ageing mind: A view from cognitive neuroscience. *Nat. Rev. Neurosci.* 5, 87–96.

This review presents an elegant overview of normal human aging and relates it to findings from animal research.

O'Keefe, J., and Nadel, L. (1978). *The Hippocampus as a Cognitive Map*. Clarendon, Oxford.

This influential book drew the connection between spatial navigation and the hippocampus, arguing that hippocampal place cells represent elements of the rat's cognitive map. It has spawned a great deal of research into the spatial nature of the hippocampus. Furthermore, the book distinguished between two systems of navigation learning, one based on routes and guidances and another based on the cognitive map of spatial information.

Rosenzweig, E.S., and Barnes, C.A. (2003). Impact of aging on hippocampal function: Plasticity, network dynamics, and cognition. *Prog. Neurobiol.* 69, 143–179.

This article comprehensively reviews age-related changes to the hippocampus from behavioral, neurobiological, and place cell perspectives. This provides an outstanding review of age-related changes to synaptic plasticity.

Wilson, I.A. (2005). *Hippocampal place cells as a window into cognitive aging*. Ph.D. thesis, University of Kuopio, Finland.

This dissertation ties together spatial memory impairments, neurobiological deteriorations in the hippocampus, and weakened processing by hippocampal place cells associated with normal aging.

ACKNOWLEDGMENTS

This work was carried out at the University of Kuopio, Finland in the laboratory of Heikki Tanila, who made this research possible and contributed invaluable discussions to this chapter. The author greatly appreciates the collaborative contributions of Howard Eichenbaum, Michela Gallagher, and Sami Ikonen to this aging research project. The author is grateful to Silvia Gratz for critical editing comments on this chapter. This work was supported by the National Institute on Aging, grant AG09973, by the Academy of Finland, grant 46000, by the Northern Savo Cultural Foundation, and by the Research and Science Foundation of Farmos.

REFERENCES

Amaral, D.G. (1993). Emerging principles of intrinsic hippocampal organization. *Curr. Opin. Neurobiol. 3*, 225–229.

Amaral, D.G. and Witter, M.P. (1995). Hippocampal formation. In *The Rat Nervous System*, 2nd ed. (G. Paxinos, ed.), pp. 443–493. Academic Press, San Diego.

Barnes, C.A. (1994). Normal aging: Regionally specific changes in hippocampal synaptic transmission. *Trends Neurosci. 17*, 13–18.

Barnes, C.A. (1998). Spatial cognition and functional alterations of aged rat hippocampus. In *Handbook of the Aging Brain*. (E. Wang and D.S. Snyder, eds.), pp. 52–67. Academic Press, New York.

Barnes, C.A., Suster, M.S., Shen, J., and McNaughton, B.L. (1997). Multistability of cognitive maps in the hippocampus of old rats. *Nature 388*, 272–275.

Cho, Y.H., Giese, K.P., Tanila, H., Silva, A.J., and Eichenbaum, H. (1998). Abnormal hippocampal spatial representations in alphaCaMKIIT286A and CREBalphaDelta-mice. *Science 279*, 867–869.

Eichenbaum, H., Dudchenko, P., Wood, E., Shapiro, M., and Tanila, H. (1999). The hippocampus, memory, and place cells: Is it spatial memory or a memory space? *Neuron 23*, 209–226.

Ekstrom, A.D., Kahana, M.J., Caplan, J.B., Fields, T.A., Isham, E.A., Newman, E.L., and Fried, I. (2003). Cellular networks underlying human spatial navigation. *Nature 425*, 184–188.

Foster, T.C. (1999). Involvement of hippocampal synaptic plasticity in age-related memory decline. *Brain Res. Brain Res. Rev. 30*, 236–249.

Frank, L.M., Stanley, G.B., and Brown, E.N. (2004). Hippocampal plasticity across multiple days of exposure to novel environments. *J. Neurosci. 24*, 7681–7689.

Gallagher, M., Burwell, R., and Burchinal, M. (1993). Severity of spatial learning impairment in aging: Development of a learning index for performance in the Morris water maze. *Behav. Neurosci. 107*, 618–626.

Gallagher, M., and Rapp, P.R. (1997). The use of animal models to study the effects of aging on cognition. *Annu. Rev. Psychol. 48*, 339–370.

Gothard, K.M., Skaggs, W.E., and McNaughton, B.L. (1996). Dynamics of mismatch correction in the hippocampal ensemble code for space: Interaction between path integration and environmental cues. *J. Neurosci. 16*, 8027–8040.

Gray, C.M., Maldonado, P.E., Wilson, M., and McNaughton, B. (1995). Tetrodes markedly improve the reliability and yield of multiple single-unit isolation from multi-unit recordings in cat striate cortex. *J. Neurosci. Methods 63*, 43–54.

Hedden, T., and Gabrieli, J.D. (2004). Insights into the ageing mind: A view from cognitive neuroscience. *Nat. Rev. Neurosci. 5*, 87–96.

Hill, A.J. (1978). First occurrence of hippocampal spatial firing in a new environment. *Exp. Neurol. 62*, 282–297.

Kentros, C., Hargreaves, E., Hawkins, R.D., Kandel, E.R., Shapiro, M., and Muller, R.V. (1998). Abolition of long-term stability of new hippocampal place cell maps by NMDA receptor blockade. *Science 280*, 2121–2126.

Lee, I., Rao, G., and Knierim, J.J. (2004). A double dissociation between hippocampal subfields: Differential time course of CA3 and CA1 place cells for processing changed environments. *Neuron 42*, 803–815.

Lenck-Santini, P.P., Muller, R.U., Save, E., and Poucet, B. (2002). Relationships between place cell firing fields and navigational decisions by rats. *J. Neurosci. 22*, 9035–9047.

Lenck-Santini, P.P., Save, E., and Poucet, B. (2001). Evidence for a relationship between place-cell spatial firing and spatial memory performance. *Hippocampus 11*, 377–390.

Lever, C., Wills, T., Cacucci, F., Burgess, N., and O'Keefe, J. (2002). Long-term plasticity in hippocampal place-cell representation of environmental geometry. *Nature 416*, 90–94.

McEchron, M.D., Weible, A.P., and Disterhoft, J.F. (2001). Aging and learning-specific changes in single-neuron activity in CA1 hippocampus during rabbit trace eyeblink conditioning. *J. Neurophysiol. 86*, 1839–1857.

McNaughton, B.L., O'Keefe, J., and Barnes, C.A. (1983). The stereotrode: A new technique for simultaneous isolation of several single units in the central nervous system from multiple unit records. *J. Neurosci. Methods. 8*, 391–397.

Moffat, S.D., and Resnick, S.M. (2002). Effects of age on virtual environment place navigation and allocentric cognitive mapping. *Behav. Neurosci. 116*, 851–859.

Muller, R. (1996). A quarter of a century of place cells. *Neuron 17*, 813–822.

Muller, R.U., and Kubie, J.L. (1987). The effects of changes in the environment on the spatial firing of hippocampal complex-spike cells. *J. Neurosci. 7*, 1951–1968.

Newman, M.C., and Kaszniak, A.W. (2000). Spatial memory and aging: Performance on a human analog of the Morris water maze. *Aging Neuropsychol. Cogn.* 86–93.

O'Keefe, J., and Conway, D.H. (1978). Hippocampal place units in the freely moving rat: Why they fire where they fire. *Exp. Brain Res. 31*, 573–590.

O'Keefe, J., and Dostrovsky, J. (1971). The hippocampus as a spatial map. Preliminary evidence from unit activity in the freely-moving rat. *Brain Res. 34*, 171–175.

O'Keefe, J., and Nadel, L. (1978). *The Hippocampus as a Cognitive Map*. Clarendon, Oxford.

O'Keefe, J., and Speakman, A. (1987). Single unit activity in the rat hippocampus during a spatial memory task. *Exp. Brain Res. 68*, 1–27.

O'Reilly, R.C., and Rudy, J.W. (2001). Conjunctive representations in learning and memory: Principles of cortical and hippocampal function. *Psychol. Rev. 108*, 311–345.

Redish, A.D. (2001). The hippocampal debate: Are we asking the right questions? *Behav. Brain Res. 127*, 81–98.

Redish, A.D., and Touretzky, D.S. (1997). Cognitive maps beyond the hippocampus. *Hippocampus 7*, 15–35.

Rolls, E.T. (1999). Spatial view cells and the representation of place in the primate hippocampus. *Hippocampus*. 9, 467–480.

Rosenzweig, E.S., and Barnes, C.A. (2003). Impact of aging on hippocampal function: Plasticity, network dynamics, and cognition. *Prog. Neurobiol. 69*, 143–179.

Rosenzweig, E.S., Redish, A.D., McNaughton, B.L., and Barnes, C.A. (2003). Hippocampal map realignment and spatial learning. *Nat. Neurosci. 6*, 609–615.

Squire, L.R., and Alvarez, P. (1995). Retrograde amnesia and memory consolidation: A neurobiological perspective. *Curr. Opin. Neurobiol. 5*, 169–177.

Thompson, L.T., and Best, P.J. (1990). Long-term stability of the place-field activity of single units recorded from the dorsal hippocampus of freely behaving rats. *Brain Res. 509*, 299–308.

Wilson, I.A. (2005). *Hippocampal place cells as a window into cognitive aging*. Ph.D. thesis, University of Kuopio, Finland.

Wilson, I.A., Ikonen, S., Gureviciene, I., McMahan, R.W., Gallagher, M., Eichenbaum, H., and Tanila, H. (2004). Cognitive aging and the hippocampus: How old rats represent new environments. *J. Neurosci. 24*, 3870–3878.

Wilson, I.A., Ikonen, S., McMahan, R.W., Gallagher, M., Eichenbaum, H., and Tanila, H. (2003). Place cell rigidity correlates with impaired spatial learning in aged rats. *Neurobiol. Aging. 24*, 297–305.

Wilson, M.A., and McNaughton, B.L. (1993). Dynamics of the hippocampal ensemble code for space [see comments] [published erratum appears in Science 1994 Apr 1;264(5155):16]. *Science 261*, 1055–1058.

Wu, W.W., Oh, M.M., and Disterhoft, J.F. (2002). Age-related biophysical alterations of hippocampal pyramidal neurons: implications for learning and memory. *Ageing Res. Rev. 1*, 181–207.

38

The Rhesus Macaque as a Model of Human Aging and Age-Related Disease

Mary Ann Ottinger, Julie A. Mattison, Mary B. Zelinski, Julie M. Wu, Steven G. Kohama, George S. Roth, Mark A. Lane, and Donald K. Ingram

*The rhesus monkey (*Macaca mulatta*) offers an advantageous model for biomedical research because of the close relatedness of this species to humans. As in humans, the rhesus monkey experiences deteriorating function of multiple physiological systems during aging, as well as an increasing incidence of pathologies and other health issues. These health issues are generally considered part of "normal" aging. However, there are health problems that arise, which contribute to disease states that become more prevalent in aging populations, such as osteoporosis and metabolic disorders, including diabetes. In addition, the rhesus female provides a valuable experimental model for understanding the biological changes that accompany the process of ovarian aging and the perimenopausal transition, which is an area of high visibility and intense research at this time. Rhesus males also experience age-related increases in health issues despite the fact that they do not have the precipitous hormonal changes seen in females. Moreover, evaluation of cognitive performance and other behavioral changes in rhesus monkeys has proven useful for understanding age-related changes and developing clinically relevant interventions and treatments. Once the elements of the biology and endocrinology of age-related changes are well documented, then there is the opportunity for evaluating other potential interventions that may impact aging processes, including dietary or pharmaceutical regimens. The marked advantage of the rhesus macaque as an experimental model is the similarity and parallel changes to aging in humans. However, this advantage is accompanied by other considerations, including the fact that the rhesus macaque is also long-lived with a lifespan that may be 30–40 years. Therefore, studies utilizing this species for investigating the fundamental biology of aging require the inclusion of aged animals in the study or sufficient time for a study to be completed, especially for research on the consequences of early exposures or long-term treatments. Nonetheless, the rhesus macaque is unparalleled for obtaining insights into the complexities of aging processes, especially for alterations in cognitive, sensory, and physiologic changes relevant for biomedical applications. In addition, there is growing recognition of the long-term consequences of environmental and health factors on later successful aging as well as the variability among individuals in their lifetime responses. We will provide an overview of the utility of the rhesus macaque as a biomedical model for the study of aging, with emphasis on studies of behavior and on the biology of aging in the female. We will also review some recent research conducted in our laboratories on the potential impact of interventions such as calorie restriction on successful aging.*

Introduction

The search for an ideal system for elucidating biological changes that accompany aging and relate to processes in humans has led to the development of a variety of invertebrate and vertebrate models. More recently, fundamental processes have been examined across a number of vertebrate classes to determine if these mechanisms occur more generally and if there are some species that show resistance to these age-related challenges that contribute to the demise of the animal. Invertebrates (including *Drosophila*, nematodes), avian models, and mammalian (rodent) models provide significant contributions to our understanding of aging processes. These models provide essential data that greatly extend the knowledge base to increase understanding of mechanisms of aging. These studies supply the background to facilitate testing of more sophisticated hypotheses. However, the rodent model and other mammalian models do not replace the requirement for subsequent investigations in the nonhuman primate.

In particular, aging is accompanied by increasing incidence of disease and health issues. In some cases, spontaneous disease arises as the physiological condition of the individual worsens. In addition, metabolic and reproductive endocrine systems decline during aging, resulting in a suite of age-related changes that have global impacts, including altered cognitive function. In particular, female rhesus monkeys experience a true menopause, characterized by the cessation of endometrial sloughing (menstruation). A true menopause is one of the most distinct differences between the nonhuman primate model and other mammalian models. These differences include not only the obvious difference of a lack of a menstrual cycle in rodents, but also differences in neuroendocrine and endocrine events leading to menopause. For example, rodents experience a transitional period of constant estrus, which is associated with declining ovarian function. Although primates also experience a transitional phase in which ovarian function declines with fewer luteal phases, this unopposed estrogen exposure is not as pronounced as in the rodent. In addition, there are a number of high visibility issues associated with the perimenopausal transition that include metabolic, cognitive, and overall health changes. These aspects of the perimenopausal transition require investigations in nonhuman primates, especially relative to development and testing potential interventions for clinical applications.

Therefore, the close relatedness and similarity of physiological systems of the rhesus macaque with humans is a major advantage of this model. In addition, the rhesus monkey has been studied extensively at all stages of the life cycle. This species is considered a long-lived species, with a lifespan of about 1/3 that of humans. However, their long lifespan does present a challenge for researchers because studies on the biology of aging must be long term or utilize retired breeders or other aged individuals. Nonetheless, the complexity of human physiology requires elucidation of fundamental mechanisms operating in the process of aging as well as studies in nonhuman primates to provide definitive data to verify the relevance of these mechanisms to humans.

ADVANTAGES AND DISADVANTAGES OF THE MODEL

The major advantage of the rhesus macaque as a research model is its similarity to humans. With 92.5 to 95% genetic homology to humans, rhesus macaques are a closely related, well-characterized animal. The use of rhesus monkeys in biomedical studies spans questions from molecular and cellular biology to physiology and onto behavior. This interest has created an extensive literature and knowledge of this species and its relation to human health and biology. The long lifespan of this species (approximately 40 years) means that age-related changes more closely reflect that of humans than shorter-lived species, and the rate of aging can be compared at an approximately 1:3 ratio.

However, the longevity of this species also presents a challenge for researchers. There are few opportunities to study an individual over the entire lifespan. Most often, intervention studies are more similar to a human clinical trial looking only at specific variables for a preset length of time, with lifespan rarely used as an endpoint. In addition, due to the high costs of procuring monkeys, sample sizes are generally small, with significant individual variation. Thus, unlike rodent studies where strains are inbred and similar, monkeys are as different as humans. Additionally, monkeys are costly to maintain and require individualized animal care.

Overall, the many advantages of rhesus monkeys for aging studies are also their disadvantages. Yet, no other animal model comes as close to resembling human systems. Furthermore, because there is a generalized recognition of the value of each individual animal, the nonhuman primate aging research community has developed into a collaborative effort to better understand and further characterize the aging process.

Characteristics of the Rhesus Macaque Model

NONHUMAN PRIMATE MODELS

Several macaque species have been routinely used for studies on aging, including rhesus (*M. mulatta*), cynomolgus (*M. fasicularis*), pigtail (*M. nemestina*), stump-tail (*M. arctoides*), and bonnet (*M. radiata*). Obtaining sufficient numbers of aging animals is difficult, and estimating age in wild-caught individuals is a challenge. Some investigators have estimated age by tooth wear, but this is often inaccurate. Age of young animals may be estimated based on maturity, stature, and pubertal status. However, birth records are really the only reliable data.

In the rhesus macaque, there are Chinese- and Indian-derived monkeys, with the latter being most represented in the literature. These monkeys may be considered subspecies in that they differ somewhat in their physical characteristics. There have been some studies that have attempted to identify characteristics that differ between these subspecies to determine if they can both be used in a single study. An excellent study was conducted to compare the subspecies and to evaluate their growth characteristics (for review, see Clarke and O'Neill, 1999). Chinese-origin adult males were larger than their Indian-origin counterparts, whereas the Chinese-derived females were generally larger as young animals. Interestingly, the Indian-derived females caught up and surpassed the Chinese-origin females as adults. To further complicate this issue, there is evidence that individuals born in the laboratory were larger as adults compared to those monkeys caught in the wild. In addition, there are some data that suggest differences in immune response between these subspecies (Messaoudi and Nicolich-Zugich, personal communication). Clearly, the distribution of individuals of these subspecies must be considered when developing an experimental design in which there are limitations in the number of animals and availability of these subspecies.

HUSBANDRY OF THE RHESUS MACAQUE

There are extensive data on the maintenance of the rhesus macaque in laboratory conditions as well as in outdoor pens. The type of housing may vary with the experimental paradigm and the objectives of the study. In the case of studies in which diet or other interventions are used to determine effects during aging, animals are likely to be housed individually in standard primate caging that meet the NIH Guide for the Care and Use of Laboratory Animals. Studies in which social behavior and family groups are investigated will often utilize field stations with outdoor enclosures and pens within the area. These field stations may include opportunities for individuals to opt out of threatening situations and find areas removed from more dominant animals.

Although the daily routine will vary with the primate facility, there are animal care guidelines that standardize the level of care and husbandry for the rhesus monkey. The diet should meet the National Research Council Guidelines for nonhuman primates with essential nutrients and vitamins in concentrations that insure the monkeys receive appropriate nutrients and energy. Environmental conditions also will vary with the facility. For example, a controlled laboratory environment might have the monkey rooms maintained on a 12-hour photoperiod (12 hr light/12 hr dark), with room temperature at 78 ± 2°F and humidity at 60 ± 5%.

Aging: General Characteristics

Aging in the rhesus monkey has many similarities to human aging. The incidence of cancer, type 2 diabetes, and other diseases increase in the rhesus monkey similar to humans. In addition, diseases and clinical conditions, such as osteoporosis, that occur in aging women also occur in the rhesus female. Changes that occur during aging fall into two categories: those associated with declining physiological function and those contributing to a disease state (Hadley *et al.*, 2005). Obvious signs of aging in nonhuman primates and humans include loss of posture due to muscle loss (sarcopenia). Recent evidence has directed new attention to the important role of immune system function as a central element in a possible range of health-related issues and disease states that emerge as the individual ages (Nikolich-Zugish and Messaoudi, 2005). In addition, visual and auditory systems undergo an age-related decline, similar to humans (Torre and Fowler, 2000; Roth *et al.*, 2004). Similarly, there is declining motor function, activity level, and cognitive performance (Moscript *et al.*, 2000; Zhang *et al.*, 2000). Metabolic function slows, similar to humans, and is accompanied by increasing insulin insensitivity and ultimately diabetes. In males, there is a gradual decline in reproductive endocrine function, whereas females experience the perimenopausal transition leading to menopause. In females, these age-related changes include evidence of declining performance on learning and memory with aging (Voytko, 2000, 2002). Furthermore, in females, the perimenopausal transition presents some additional heath challenges, especially as the individual becomes postmenopausal. Thus, it is important to understand the progression of events and to attempt to characterize these age-related changes in endocrine and physiological states.

Aging and Spontaneous Development of Diseases

METABOLIC CHANGES, CARDIOVASCULAR DISEASE, AND OTHER EVIDENCE OF CHANGING PHYSIOLOGY

Metabolic endocrine systems show age-related changes that are similar to those experienced in humans, with increasing risk of prediabetic symptoms and changing metabolic function. Body composition in rhesus also parallels changes observed in humans. Fat mass, particularly abdominal fat, increases with age while lean body mass declines (Schwartz and Kemnitz, 1992). As in humans, rhesus can develop diet-dependent obesity and diabetes, thereby providing an excellent model for testing antiobesity and antidiabetic treatments. Other studies have shown the potential therapeutic value of antidiabetic and antiobesity drugs in obese or insulin-resistant rhesus monkeys (Roth *et al.*, 1995; Oliver *et al.*, 2001; Bodkin *et al.*, 2003). Metabolic Syndrome includes several characteristics known to be associated with increased cardiovascular risk (Scuteri *et al.*, 2005). Studies of the characteristics associated with Metabolic Syndrome in nonhuman primates will provide crucial information about efficacy of potential interventions and the age at which they are most effective. Furthermore, early preventive measures may be identified and then tested in nonhuman primates to attenuate or prevent cardiovascular disease.

Cardiovascular disease poses a major threat to aging individuals. The rhesus monkey has been used extensively in the development of diagnostic methods for cardiovascular disease (Neemen *et al.*, 2004). In women, there is increased incidence of heart disease after the age of 50, presumably associated with the loss of estradiol in postmenopause (Campos *et al.*, 1988). The other suspected problem contributing to the onset of this condition is altered lipoprotein profiles, with increased (10–15%) low density lipoproteins (LDL) in menopausal women. Research in monkeys has shown that hormone replacement therapy (HRT) decreased the severity of atherosclerosis in controlled experiments in monkeys (Mikkola and Clarkson, 2002). Once the data are gathered in the monkey, then it will be important to establish if HRT administered during the perimenopausal transition decreases the risk of cardiovascular disease in women (Speroff and Fritz, 2005).

The resilience of the skin also declines during aging, partially due to glycation, which occurs in a similar manner in rhesus skin proteins to that in humans (Sell *et al.*, 1996). Another evidence of the loss of resilience of the skin is that there is an age-related decrease in wound healing ability (Roth *et al.*, 1997).

OSTEOPOROSIS, OSTEOARTHRITIS, AND FRAILTY

Similar to humans, postural and structural changes occur associated with diminished bone mineral density in aging rhesus monkeys (Black *et al.*, 2001). In addition, there are age-related changes in cartilage as the space between vertebrae becomes reduced, resulting in a condition similar to osteoarthritis in humans (Kramer *et al.*, 2002). Taken together, these changes contribute to an overall frailty in which the individual becomes more vulnerable to bone breakage, exhibits poor appetite, reduced activity level, and possibly behavioral changes. As such, frailty is becoming recognized as a serious condition for the elderly.

Postmenopausal women are also at risk for developing osteoporosis due to increased osteoclast activity (Riggs *et al.*, 2002; Riggs, 2004). While calcium supplements, exercise and weight-lifting help, bone loss with estrogen loss appears inevitable. Selective estrogen receptor modulators may ameliorate bone loss (Cranney *et al.*, 2002; Robertson *et al.*, 2004). Often there is loss of muscle that accompanies increasing bone fragility, and together they contribute to overall frailty (Vanitallie, 2003). Moreover, both estrogen and androgens affect bone, muscle, and metabolic function, which in turn contribute to the risk of fractures (Joseph *et al.*, 2005).

ENDOMETRIOSIS

Steroids produced by the ovary stimulate uterine endometrial cells. In endometriosis, cells that have escaped from the uterus grow in the peritoneal cavity, resulting in clinical symptoms that include tumors, obstructions, painful menses, and disrupted GI tract function. In women the incidence of endometriosis increases with age and has been estimated to be 10–20% in young reproductive women and up to 35% in women with menstrual difficulties.

Endometriosis in captive colonies of female rhesus monkeys can occur in relatively high incidence ($\sim$26%). The causes of endometriosis appear to be varied and range from surgery to radiation exposure (Fanton and Golden, 1991). One of the major issues of endometriosis, especially in rhesus macaques, is diagnosis at a treatable stage of the disease. As observed by a number of laboratories, endometriosis is difficult to diagnose until relatively advanced (Rippy *et al.*, 1996). Use of indicators, such as plasma levels of CA-125, have been examined as a possible indicator of endometriosis (Rippy *et al.*, 1996). The condition is accompanied by lesions, cyst formation, adhesions to organs, anorexia, and abdominal masses (Fanton and Golden, 1991). The disease progresses in a manner similar to that observed in women (Osteen *et al.*, 2005). Similarly, the escaped endometrial cells retain their responsiveness to ovarian steroids and proliferate vigorously outside of the uterine environment, especially in response to 17β-estradiol (E_2). This leads to more advanced disease, categorized according to clinical characteristics and gross and histological evaluation of the lesions and cysts (Fanton *et al.*, 1986). These lesions often occur on the serosal surface of the uterus and proliferate to associated regions of the peritoneal cavity (Rippy *et al.*, 1996). Although women do not generally have this disease progression due to earlier diagnosis, endometriosis does present a clinical issue for many young women. However, little is really understood about the etiology of this disease and interventions that may limit the disease and minimize the trauma associated with surgical treatment.

Aging and the Hypothalamic–Pituitary–Gonadal (HPG) Axis

Both males and females experience an age-related decline in the HPG axis. However, aging in the male system is a more gradual process in humans and in other species. Nonetheless, data show an age-related decline in testis function and decreased circulating androgen levels (for review, see Ottinger 1998). A recent study showed that circadian patterns in adrenal steroids were maintained in aging males for cortisol (Urbanski *et al.*, 2004). Similarly, levels of dehydroepiandrosterone sulfate (DHEAS) also had a circadian pattern and did show an age-related decline.

AGING OF THE REPRODUCTIVE SYSTEM IN FEMALES

The rhesus monkey (*Macaca mulatta*) has been a biomedical model for reproductive studies in women since the early 1900s (Heape, 1900). Female rhesus monkeys are pubertal by 2.5 to 3.5 years of age and exhibit menstrual cycles approximately 28 days in length, similar to humans. Furthermore, rhesus monkeys experience a reproductive decline much like that of human menopause around 24 years (Gilardi *et al.*, 1997; Bellino and Wise, 2003). Urinary hormone profiles demonstrated that, like women, menopause in rhesus monkeys is associated with amenorrhea, low urinary estrogen conjugates, and irregular patterns of urinary concentrations of progesterone metabolites (Gilardi *et al.*, 1997). Urinary FSH levels also increase in postmenopausal rhesus monkeys (Shideler *et al.*, 2001).

Key components of the reproductive decline

Human fecundity declines rapidly after age 40, with a decrease in the follicular "ovarian reserve" and increased abnormalities in oocyte quality. However, little is known about the mechanism that initiates menopause. Age alone is not a reliable predictor of menopause, but endocrine disturbances often precede noticeable irregularities in menstrual cyclicity. Few longitudinal studies have addressed these endocrine aspects of ovarian senescence; morphologic studies, when performed, are derived from ovarian specimens obtained retrospectively from aging women of unknown endocrine status. Thus, the rhesus monkey is an ideal model for investigating the mechanisms underlying menopause beacuse females display similar neuroendocrine mechanisms in the menstrual cycle.

There has been extensive research on the hypothalamic changes that accompany ovarian decline in multiple species. In humans, pituitary gonadotropins show age-related changes with a transient increase in plasma luteinizing hormone (LH) and a dramatic increase in follicle stimulating hormone (FSH). Isolating age-related changes in hypothalamic response from ovarian aging is difficult; however, a number of studies have been conducted using the rodent model. Previous studies have examined the response of the HPG axis at various stages in the life cycle of the female as well as the functional changes of the hypothalamus and pituitary gland with aging. Wise (1991) reported decreased amplitude and frequency in LH secretion in older rats and a decline in the number of activated GnRH neurons, despite normal cycles (Scarbrough and Wise, 1990; Lloyd *et al.*, 1994). These papers by Wise and colleagues and many others point to alterations in the systems that modulate GnRH as key elements of the reproductive decline. Overall, these studies indicate that hypothalamic response decreases, potentially in tandem with declining ovarian function (Wise, 1991; Mills *et al.*, 2002; Micevych *et al.*, 2003). In addition, ovarian secretion of inhibin is beginning to be studied and may emerge as an important element of the aging process (Groome *et al.*, 1994; 1996; Welt *et al.*, 1999). Data collected in female nonhuman primates and in humans suggest that there are similar mechanisms operating during the perimenopausal transition (Klein *et al.*, 1996; Bellino and Wise, 2003).

The perimenopausal transition: A time of changing hormones

As the perimenopausal transition progresses, there is declining function of the hypothalamic–pituitary–gonadal axis (HPG axis), ultimately resulting in cessation of ovarian function and menopause. The average age of menopause in women is approximately 51 years, resulting in a postreproductive period that extends for nearly 1/3 of their lives (Treolar *et al.*, 1981). If menopause merely affected fertility, the study of ovarian aging would likely not be of such high priority. As mentioned earlier, a number of other physiological systems are also affected by the sudden withdrawal of hormonal support associated with menopause, including bone density, cardiovascular health, cognition and possibly some cancers (Gosden, 1985; Prior, 1998; Sherwin, 2003).

Characterization of perimenopausal transition

Rhesus monkeys that have been observed at the Oregon National Primate Research Center (ONPRC) indicate that the frequency of regular menstrual cyclicity declines with age (Wu *et al.*, 2004; Zelinski-Wooten, unpublished data). Approximately 70% of rhesus females between the ages of 20 and 22 years did not exhibit the onset of irregular cycles, but by 23–25 years of age, 50% of females did have irregular cycles. The data from ONPRC agrees with that published by Gilardi and colleagues (1997) at the California Regional Primate Research Center, where the mean age of old animals displaying regular cycles was 22 years, those displaying irregular cycles (i.e., perimenopausal) was 24 years, and postmenopausal monkeys of 29 years as compared to normal cycles observed in young adult females (Zelinski-Wooten *et al.*, 1999).

Brain Aging and Cognitive Function

AGE-RELATED NEUROPATHOLOGY

Among other age-related changes in neural anatomy and function, rhesus monkeys also develop pathological characteristics of Alzheimer's disease (AD), specifically regional deposition of amyloid-β (Aβ) plaques similar to aged humans (Gearing *et al.*, 1996). These Aβ plaques are associated with angiopathy. Although Aβ accumulates in rhesus brains, neurofibrillary tangles, another hallmark AD pathology, are not formed (Nelson *et al.*, 1996). Paralleling success in mice, current interest is emerging for producing transgenic monkeys in which AD can be accurately modeled.

Studies have also examined age-related changes in rhesus brain. While brain mass does not decline with age (Herndon *et al.*, 1998), reductions have been observed in specific regional volumes, for example, the basal ganglia (Matochik *et al.*, 2000). The age-related decline in fine motor behavior has been associated with diminished nigrostriatal system function and was not improved in aging female monkeys given ethinyl estradiol treatment (Lacreuse and Herndon, 2003). Interestingly, males showed greater slowing of fine motor function; both males and females had age-related decreases in normalized caudate and putamen volumes (Lacreuse *et al.*, 2005). Furthermore, the age-related decrease in delay-match-to-sample and nonmatch-to-sample cognitive performance was linked to prefrontal cortex activity on fMRI (Lamar *et al.*, 2005).

Also similar to humans, no significant age-related loss of hippocampal or neocortical neurons is observed in rhesus monkeys (Duan *et al.*, 2003; Keuker *et al.*, 2003). Rather, behavioral deficits associated with hippocampal dysfunction appear to result from neurophysiological deficits in interneuronal signaling rather than cell death

(Small *et al.*, 2004). Cerebral blood volume decreases with age in hippocampal dentate gyrus (Small *et al.*, 2004). Cerebral cortex loses dendrites and arbors with advancing age (Duan *et al.*, 2003). Neurotransmitter receptor and transporter binding in specific regions, including post-synaptic dopamine receptors and presynaptic vesicular acetylcholine transporters (Voytko, 2000, 2002; Tinkler and Voytko, 2005), show age-related loss in basal ganglia. Hippocampal cholinergic fibers are also lost with age (Calhoun *et al.*, 2004) as well as changes in the integrity of white matter (Peters *et al.*, 1996).

MRI

CLINICAL STUDIES

Magnetic resonance imaging (MRI) is frequently used to document *in vivo* neuropathology in humans, such as stroke, multiple sclerosis and Alzheimer's disease. However, this imaging technology has also been applied to human aging studies, in both cross-sectional and longitudinal designs. The utility of repeated imaging is that each individual serves as his or her own baseline, avoiding many of the pitfalls of cross-sectional studies (secular trends). In general, these studies have concentrated on the evaluation of dual-echo or 3-dimensional scans generated by MRI sequences (SPGR, MPRAGE), which yield high-resolution images that can be used to measure total brain volume or segmented into various tissue compartments (gray, white, cerebrospinal fluid) or specific anatomical regions.

The results of these clinical studies have, in general, revealed age-related declines in overall brain volume or gray and white matter, with a concomitant increase of the volume of cerebrospinal fluid (CSF). For example, a significant trend for an age-related loss of total brain volume (and increased CSF) was observed in elderly (66–90 years) men and women, which correlated with cognitive deficits (Coffey *et al.*, 2001). Examination of a broader age range (1–80 yrs) confirmed that the volume of gray matter decreased in the oldest adults (Courchesne *et al.*, 2000, Good *et al.*, 2001), while another study of men and women (20–86 years) demonstrated decreases in overall volumes of both gray and white matter with age (Ge *et al.*, 2002). However, in a study with good representation of men and women in their 60s and 70s, white matter loss was more evident (Guttman *et al.*, 1998). Age-related volumetric loss was also observed in sub-regions of the brain, including the hippocampus, cortical and cerebellar gray and white matter (Jernigan *et al.*, 2001). It is also important to note that these recent studies concentrate on healthy subjects, prescreened for general health and free of neuropathology, and as such represent normative aging.

Longitudinal studies of the effects of aging on brain structure have revealed results similar to reports using a cross-sectional design. An earlier report, looking at the effect of aging on the size of the hippocampus, used repeated annual scans across almost four years in the oldest-old (>84 years) and found a progressive diminution in volume (Kaye *et al.*, 1997). Another study examined a broad range of subject (14–77 years) and reported a longitudinal decrease in white matter and hippocampal volume in older subjects at a second timepoint of 3.5 years (Liu *et al.*, 2003). Resnick *et al.* (2000) reported a cross-sectional difference in brain volume utilizing subjects (59–85 years) from the Baltimore Longitudinal Study, in which after one year, the subjects experienced a further increase in CSF volume. A follow-up study four years after baseline also revealed a significant loss of both gray and white matter with an increase in the volume of CSF (Resnick *et al.*, 2003).

MRI has also more recently been utilized to examine the underlying chemical nature of modifications in the white matter as a function of age (Bartzokis *et al.*, 2004, Davatzikos *et al.*, 2002). Similarly, documentation of age-related volumetric losses in brain sub-regions has provided a functional-anatomical basis for behavioral changes, including the cortex (Bartzokis *et al.*, 2004; Covit *et al.*, 2001)], and striatum (Raz *et al.*, 2003). Clinical data have also shown age by sex differences in brain volume (Raz *et al.*, 2004a), with hormone replacement having a significant protective effect on the maintenance of cortical volume (Raz *et al.*, 2004b). Thus, clinical MR imaging studies of normative brain aging have revealed volumetric and neurochemical changes that are related to behavioral and physiological manifestations of senescence.

MONKEY STUDIES

In parallel to the MRI aging studies of the human brain, there have been similar monkey-based reports of global volumetric changes with age, with decreases in gray matter, compensatory increases in CSF, but stability in white matter volume (Andersen *et al.*, 1999). Age-related changes in the monkey brain were analyzed in another MRI-based study and linked cognitive deficits to white matter loss (Lai *et al.*, 1995; reviewed in Peters *et al.*, 1996; Wisco *et al.*, 2001). A more recent study on the effects of aging in squirrel monkeys also showed cognitive deficits with age, but with an increase in white matter content in the anterior half of the brain (Lyons *et al.*, 2004). However, it is important to note that the other studies cited above used rhesus monkeys and examined a wider range of older animals. Evaluations of subcortical structures have also been published, such as the report on the decrease in overall volume with age in the male rhesus monkey striatum (Matochik *et al.*, 2000). This age-related striatal change was recently confirmed in both sexes, although it was noted that only the aged male rhesus monkeys performed worse than young controls on fine motor tasks (Lacreuse *et al.*, 2005). In the monkey hippocampus, cerebral blood volume, as assessed with MRI, suffered from an age-related decline that correlated with cognitive deficits (Small *et al.*, 2004). Neurochemical studies in monkeys using proton magnetic resonance spectroscopy are limited (Herndon *et al.*, 1998), but have disclosed effects of aging on various neurochemical parameters of neuronal function.

Few manipulations on monkeys as they relate to MRI-based brain studies have been performed. A recently published study (Matochik *et al.*, 2004) examined the effects of age and calorie restriction (CR) on the caudate and putamen of monkeys, but revealed differential effects of treatment on these subregions. Indeed, acute CR was found not to globally protect against the age-related volumetric loss in male rhesus brain. Additional research will address whether long-term CR is protective against both the structural changes in the brain with age and if cognitive function is preserved in a parallel manner.

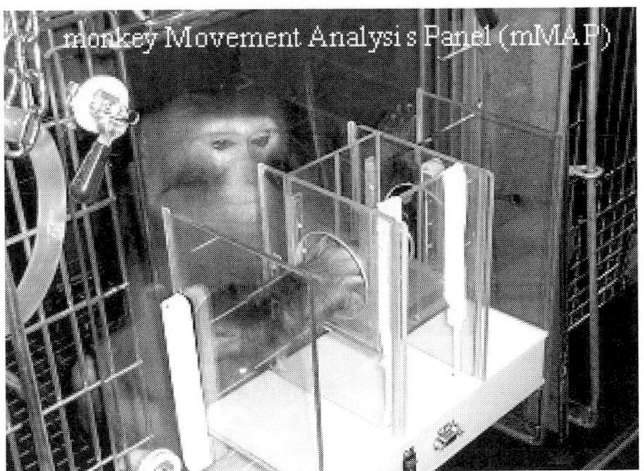

Figure 38.1 This photograph shows a rhesus monkey retrieving a food reward in the mMAP apparatus. This test allows for assessment of motor control.

Tests of Cognitive Function and Brain Regions Important for Cognitive Function

One of the most controversial issues pertaining to management of the perimenopausal transition is that of neuroprotection and maintenance of cognitive function. The rhesus macaque provides a highly useful model for performing tasks that provide specific information on neural systems. This allows for characterization of age-related changes in cognitive function with females during the perimenopausal transition and with surgical removal of ovarian steroids. Moreover, selected interventions may be tested for their efficacy in enhancing cognitive performance in aging individuals. A few of these tests will be briefly described below because these tests provide methods for assessment of age-related changes in motor capabilities and cognitive function.

MOVEMENT ANALYSIS PANEL (mMAP)

Several behavioral studies have been conducted in monkeys, including assessments of general locomotor activity, motor performance, and simple cognitive tasks. Regarding general locomotor activity, two studies have been published indicating age-related declines in activity of male and female rhesus monkeys measured by an infrared/ultrasonic apparatus placed on the home cage of the monkeys (Weed *et al.*, 1997; Moscript *et al.*, 2000). Monkeys may be assessed for motor performance in the Movement Analysis Panel (mMAP), which has proven to be age-sensitive in rhesus monkeys. This task evaluates the response time required to retrieve a food reward from different manipulanda located in a box mounted to the home cage of the monkey. The simplest task is a flat platform; the next most difficult is a straight rod, and the most difficult is hook. Figure 38.1 shows an apparatus with an individual performing the task using the mMAP (Ingram *et al.*, unpublished data).

Tasks on visual–motor skill have been demonstrated to be age-sensitive (Bachevalier *et al.*, 1991; Grondin 2003) and involve deficits in the nigral–striatal pathways. The prefrontal cortex is involved with working memory/executive function, whereas the temporal lobe-hippocampal region is involved in spatial memory (Bartus, 1978; Rapp, 1989). It is clear that consistent with a recent report (Lacreuse *et al.*, 1995) female rhesus monkeys are faster in this task than males.

SPATIAL-DELAYED RECOGNITION SPAN TEST (SPATIAL-DRST)

Spatial-DRST is a memory test that depends on the integrity of the hippocampus (Beason-Held *et al.*, 1999). It requires the subject to identify, trial-by-trial, the new location of a stimulus among an increasing array of serially presented identical stimuli. Different versions of this test have been used in normal aged humans and in a variety of neurologic patient populations. In monkeys, the spatial-DRST has been used to examine age-related impairments of rhesus macaques, to examine sex differences in young and old rhesus monkeys (Lacreuse *et al.*, 1999) and to compare the performance of aged OVX and age-matched intact female rhesus monkeys (Lacreuse *et al.*, 2000). This test appears to be useful in detecting memory loss during aging.

OBJECT-DELAYED RECOGNITION SPAN TEST (OBJECT-DRST)

Object-DRST follows the same rules as spatial-DRST, but the stimuli are different objects instead of identical disks. The objects are randomly drawn from a pool of 3000 color clipart objects. On each trial, the position of the stimuli changes in a random fashion so that the monkey is able to identify the new stimulus based only on visual, rather than spatial cues. The mean number of objects that the monkey is able to correctly identify before making an error and the mean response times will be recorded. The object-DRST is a task of visual recognition memory that is sensitive to hippocampal lesions in monkeys (Beason-Held *et al.*, 2005).

Calorie Restriction: An Effective Intervention in the Rhesus Model

Calorie restriction (CR) has been long recognized for its benefits to health and aging in a variety of species (Weindruch and Walford, 1988). These benefits have been demonstrated in numerous studies of invertebrate and vertebrate models, which have shown that CR is a robust method for slowing aging as evidenced by reduced incidence and delayed onset of age-related diseases, extension of mean and maximum lifespan, increased stress resistance, and improved function (Bordone and Guarente, 2005). However, longitudinal CR studies are difficult in nonhuman primates due to their long lifespan and availability of sufficient numbers of animals to conduct this type of a study (Roth *et al.*, 2004). Long-term studies have focused on obesity and diabetes (University of Maryland Medical School), and on the impact of a nutritious, low calorie diet (30% CR) on aging processes, survival, and longevity (Wisconsin National Primate Research Center and NIA). The NIA and WNPRC studies represent the first experiments to evaluate effects of CR on aging processes in a primate species. Moreover, the genetic heterogeneity in these primates provides an excellent view of the range of responses likely to occur in the human population with CR. A number of parameters have been examined over the course of these studies, including those shown on Table 38.1. It is clear that new information pertinent to aging processes will emerge from these studies in rhesus monkeys that document parallels to human aging. A range of variables have been considered in both studies, including reproductive, metabolic, sensory, gene expression, and health parameters (Ramsey *et al.*, 2000; Mattison *et al.*, 2003; Roth *et al.*, 2004). Interestingly, CR did not affect bone density in the younger animals (Black *et al.*, 2001). As many of these animals are currently middle-aged, we may still observe differences associated with diet with advancing age.

Because CR was initiated in some of these animals around the time of puberty, it was possible to assess the effects of the diet during sexual maturation and in young adults. Interestingly, a shift appeared to occur in young animals on CR from growth and reproduction to a life maintenance strategy. This was observed in a delay in maturation in some individuals. However, once balance was achieved, these animals became reproductive, with reproductive endocrine function similar to control

TABLE 38.1
Measurements conducted in females over the course of the long-term CR Study at the NIA, ages/age range at measurement, intervals between repeated assessments, and investigators

Variable assayed	Assay used	When measured	Measurement intervals	Investigators
Ovarian steroids•	Radioimmunoassay (RIA)	2003–2005	N/A	Zelinski-Wooten, Wu, Mattison & Ottinger
Ovarian reserve•	Clomid challenge	2003–2005	N/A	Zelinski-Wooten, Wu, Mattison & Ottinger
Gonadotropins•	RIA	2003–2005	N/A	Zelinski-Wooten, Wu, Mattison & Ottinger
Evidence of menses•	Visual inspection	Entire study	daily	NIA studies
Inhibin/activin•	RIA	2004–2005	N/A	Zelinski-Wooten, Wu, Mattison & Ottinger
GH	RIA			NIA studies
Insulin	RIA			NIA studies
Thyroid hormones	RIA			NIA studies
Cortisol	RIA			NIA studies
Osteoarthritis•	X-ray	2003–2006		Kramer
Bone density	DEXA scan	Entire study	5 years	Poolesville staff
Ocular health•+	Imaging	2 times	5 years	Neuringer
Cognition/memory•	Behavioral tests	2001–2005	Scheduled	Ingram/Young
Health checks•+	Visual inspection	Entire study	3X/day	Ingram/Mattison
Immune status•+	T cell status	2001–2007	Scheduled	Nikolich-Zugich
Volume of selected brain regions	MRI		3–5 yr intervals	NIA-Poolesville staff, Matochik, & Kohama

•denotes measures that are currently ongoing. + denotes measures that are routinely collected by the NIA-Poolesville staff or by other investigators (Matochik, Nikolich-Zugich, Neuringer).

monkeys. Interestingly, males and females on the NIA study appear to exhibit normal reproductive function in both control and CR groups, suggesting that moderate CR likely does not have a detrimental impact on reproductive function. Further, the shift associated with the CR dietary regimen is associated with a drop in body temperature consistent with increased protective mechanisms against various insults and pathologies, slower rate of tissue deterioration, and more reserve capacity (Roth *et al.*, 1995, 2004).

Conclusions

Use of the primate as a model for aging is increasing, and the *in vivo* MRI-based studies enjoy the advantage of repeated measures, with each subject serving as its own baseline control. A controlled longitudinal study of the nonhuman primate, a moderately long-lived species with close phylogenetic ties with humans, could contribute to the brain-aging field in better defining age-related changes in gray and white matter, which are still somewhat controversial in the clinical literature. For example, with about a third of the maximum lifespan of humans, it would be feasible to compare repeat scans of individual monkeys at the critical middle-age to old and old to oldest-old transitions. In addition, with the increased usage of the monkey model and simultaneous evolution of MRI technology, the ability to explore anatomical loci with increasing sensitivity is rapidly evolving. Moreover, the generation of sophisticated neurochemical analysis and physiological measures by MRI will substantially augment existing behavioral and neurophysiological analyses in describing the neurobiological underpinnings of brain function in the nonhuman primate model.

Compared to the rhesus monkey, there is no other well-characterized animal model with such extensive similarity to humans across a wide range of physiological responses. Rhesus monkeys share a significant portion of the genetic information found in humans and are more closely related to humans than rodents. This species has been extensively used in biomedical research and is among the best characterized of the nonhuman primates, particularly with respect to normal aging. Finally, these *in vivo* assays, coupled with neurochemical and histological approaches, will make a powerful approach to addressing aging of the brain, enable a more comprehensive assay of potential interventions, and translate well to the clinic.

REFERENCES

Anderson, A.H., Zhang, Z., Zhang, M., Gash, D., and Avison, M.J. (1999). Age-associated changes in rhesus CNS composition identified by MRI. *Brain Research 829*, 90–98.

Bachevalier, J., Landis, L.S., Walker, L.C., Brickson, M., Mishkin, M., Price, D.L., and Cork, L.C. (1991). Aged monkeys exhibit behavioral deficits indicative of widespread cerebral dysfunction. *Neurobiol. Aging* Mar–Apr; *12(2)*, 99–111.

Bartus, R.T., Fleming, D., and Johnson, H.R. (1978). Aging in the rhesus monkey: Debilitating effects on short-term memory. *J Gerontol. 33(6)*, 858–871.

Bartzokis, G., Beckson, M., Lu, P.H., Neuchterlein, K.H., Edwards, N., and Mintz, J. (2001). Age-related changes in frontal and temporal lobe volumes in men. *Archive of General Psychiatry 58*, 461–465.

Bartzokis, G., Sultzer, D., Lu, P.H., Nuechterlein, K.H., Mintz, J., and Cummings, J.L. (2004). Heterogenous age-related breakdown of white matter structural integrity: Implications for cortical disconnection in aging and Alzheimer's disease. *Neurobiology of Aging 25*, 843–851.

Beason-Held, L.L., Rosene, D.L., Killiany, R.J., and Moss, M.B. (1999). Hippocampal formation lesions produce memory impairment in the rhesus monkey. *Hippocampus 9(5)*, 562–574.

Beason-Held, L.L., Golski, S., Kraut, M.A., Esposito, G., and Resnick, S.M. (2005). Brain activation during encoding and recognition of verbal and figural information in older adults. *Neurobiol. Aging 26(2)*, 237–250.

Bellino, F.L., and Wise, P.M. (2003). Nonhuman primate models of menopause workshop. *Biol. Reproduction 68*, 10–18.

Black, A., Allison, D.B., Shapses, S.A., Tilmont, E.M., Handy, A.M., Ingram, D.K., *et al.* (2001). Calorie restriction and skeletal mass in rhesus monkeys (*Macaca mulatta*): Evidence for an effect mediated through changes in body size. *J. Gerontol. A. Biol. Sci. Med. Sci. 56(3)*, B98–B107.

Bodkin, N.L., Pill, J., Meyer, K., and Hansen, B.C. (2003). The effects of K-111, a new insulin-sensitizer, on metabolic syndrome in obese prediabetic rhesus monkeys. *Horm. Metab. Res. 35*, 617.

Bordone, L., and Guarente, L. (2005). Calorie restriction, SIRT1 and metabolism: Understanding longevity. *Nature Rev. Mol. Cell Biol. 6*, 298–305.

Calhoun, M.E., Mao, Y., Roberts, J.A., and Rapp, P.R. (2004). Reduction in hippocampal cholinergic innervation is unrelated to recognition memory impairment in aged rhesus monkeys. *J. Comp. Neurol. 475(2)*, 238–246.

Campos, H., McNamara, J.R., Wilson, P.W., Ordovas, J.M., and Schaefer, E.J. (1988). Differences in low density lipoprotein subfractions and apolipoproteins in premenopausal and postmenopausal women. *J. Clin. Endocrinol. Metab. 67*, 30–36.

Clark, M.R., and O'Neill, J.A.S. (1999). Morphometric comparison of Chinese-origin and Indian derived rhesus monkeys (*Macaca mulatta*). *Am. J. Primatol. 47*, 335–346.

Coffey, C.E., Ratcliff, G., Saxton, J.A., Bryan, R.N., Fried, L.P., and Lucke, J.F. (2001). Cognitive correlates of human brain aging: A quantitative magnetic resonance imaging investigation. *Journal of Neuropsychiatry and Clinical Neurosciences 13*, 471–485.

Courchesne, E., Chisum, H.J., Townsend, J., Cowles, A., Covington, J., Egaas, B., *et al.* (2000). Normal brain development and aging: Quantitative analysis at in vivo MRI imaging in healthy volunteers. *Radiology 216*, 672–682.

Covit, A., Wolf, O.T., deLeon, M.J., Patalinjug, M., Kandil, E., Caraos, C., *et al.* (2001). Volumetric analysis of the prefrontal regions: Findings in aging and schizophrenia. *Psychiatry Research: Neuroimaging Section 107*, 61–73.

Cranney, A., Tugwell, P., Zytaruk, N., Robinson, V., Weaver, B., Adachi, J., *et al.* (2002). The Osteoporosis Methodology Group, and The Osteoporosis Research Advisory Group. IV. Meta-analysis of raloxifene for the prevention and treatment of postmenopausal osteoporosis. *Endocrine Rev. 23*, 524–528.

Davatzikos, C., and Resnick, S.M. (2002). Degenerative age changes in white matter connectivity visualized *in vivo* using Magnetic Resonance Imaging. *Cerebral Cortex 12*, 767–771.

Duan, H., Wearne, S.L., Rocher, A.B., Macedo, A., Morrison, J.H., and Hof, P.R. (2003). Age-related dendritic and spine changes in corticocortically projecting neurons in macaque monkeys. *Cereb. Cortex 13*, 950.

Fanton, J.W., Yochmowitz, M.G., Wood, D.H., and Salmon, Y.L. (1986). Surgical treatment of endometriosis in 50 rhesus monkeys. *Am. J. Vet. Res. 47(7)*, 1602–1604.

Fanton, J.W., and Golden, J.G. (1991). Radiation-induced endometriosis in *Macaca muatta. Radiat. Res. 126*, 141–146.

Ge, Y., Grossman, R.I., Babb, J.S., Rabin, M.L., Mannon, L.J., and Kolson, D.L. (2002). Age-related total gray and white matter changes in normal adult brain. Part I: Volumetric MR imaging analysis. *Am. J. Neuroradiol. 23*, 1327–1333.

Gearing, M., Tigges, J., Mori, H., and Mirra, S.S. (1996). A beta 40 is a major form of beta-amyloid in non human primates. *Neurobiol. Aging 17(6)*, 903–908.

Gilardi, K.V. K., Shideler, S.E., Valverde, C.R., Roberts, J.A., and Lasley, B.L. (1997). Characterization of the onset of menopause in the rhesus macaque. *Biol. Reprod. 57*, 335–340.

Good, C.D., Johnsrude, I.S., Ashburner, J., Henson, R.N.A., Friston, K.J., and Frackowiak, S.J. (2001). A voxel-based morphological study of ageing in 465 normal adult human brains. *Neuroimage 14*, 21–36.

Gosden, R.G. (1985). *The Biology of Menopause: The Causes and Consequences of Ovarian Aging*. Academic Press, New York.

Grondin, R., Cass, W.A., Zhang, Z., Stanford, J.A., Gash, D.M., and Gerhardt, G.A. (2003). Glial cell line-derived neurotrophic factor increases stimulus-evoked dopamine release and motor speed in aged rhesus monkeys. *J. Neurosci. 123(5)*, 1974–1980.

Groome, N.P., Illingworth, P.J., O'Brien, M., Cooke, I., Ganesan, T.S., Baird, D.T., and McNeilly, A.S. (1994). Detection of dimeric inhibin throughout the human menstrual cycle by two-site enzyme immunoassay. *Clin. Endocrinol. 40*, 717–723.

Groome, N.P., Illingworth, P.J., O'Brien, M., Pai, R., Rodger, F.E., Mather, J.P., and McNeilly, A.S. (1996). Measurement of dimeric inhibin B throughout the human menstrual cycle. *J. Clin. Endocrinol. Metab. 81*, 1401–1405.

Guttmann, C.R. G., Jolesz, F.A., Kikinis, R., Killiany, R.J., Moss, M.B., Sandor, T., and Albert, M.S. (1998). White matter changes with normal aging. *Neurology 50*, 972–978.

Hadley, E.C., Lakatta, E.G., Morrison-Bogorad, M., Warner, H.R., and Hodes, R.J. (2005). The future of aging therapies. *Cell 120*, 557–567.

Heape, W. (1900). The sexual season of mammals. *Quarterly J. Microsc. Sci. 44*, 1–70.

Herndon, J.G., Tigges, J., Klumpp, S.A., and Anderson, D.C. (1998). Brain weight does not decrease with age in adult rhesus monkeys. *Neurobio. Aging 19(3)*, 267–272.

Herndon, J.G., Constantinidis, I., and Moss, M.B. (1998). Age-related brain changes in rhesus monkeys: A magnetic resonance spectroscopic study. *Neuro. Report 9*, 2127–2130.

Jernigan, T.L., Archibald, S.L., Fennema-Notestine, C., Gamst, A.C., Stout, J.C., Bonner, J., and Hesselink, J.R. (2001). Effects of age on tissues and regions of the cerebrum and cerebellum. *Neuro. Aging 22*, 581–594.

Joseph, C., Kenny, A.M., Taxel, P., Lorenzo, J.A., Duque, G., and Kuchel, G.A. (2005). Role of endocrine-immune dysregulation in osteoporosis, sarcopenia, frailty and fracture risk. *Molec. Aspects of Medicine 26*, 181–201.

Kaye, J.A., Swihart, T., Howieson, D., Dame, A., Moore, M.M., Karnos, T., *et al.* (1997). Volume loss of the hippocampus and temporal lobe in healthy elderly persons destined to develop dementia. *Neurology 48*, 1297–1304.

Keuker, J.I., Luiten, P.G., and Fuchs, E. (2003). Preservation of hippocampal. neuron numbers in aged rhesus monkeys. *Neurobio. Aging 24*, 157–165.

Klein, N.A., Illingworth, P.J., Groome, N.P., McNeilly, A.S., Battaglia, D.E., and Soules, M.R. (1996). Decreased inhibin B secretion is associated with the monotropic FSH rise in older, ovulatory women: A study of serum and follicular fluid levels of dimeric inhibin A and B in spontaneous menstrual cycles. *J. Clin. Endocrinol. Metab. 81*, 2742–2745.

Kramer, P.A, Newell-Morris, L.L., and Simkin, P.A. (2002). Spinal degenerative disk disease (DDD) in female Macaque monkeys: Epidemiology and comparison with women. *J. Orthop. Res. 20*, 399.

Lacreuse, A., and Herndon, J.G. (2003). Effects of estradiol and aging on fine manual performance in female rhesus monkeys. *Horm. Behav. 43(3)*, 359–366.

Lacreuse, A., Herndon, J.G., Killiany, R.J., Rosene, D.L., and Moss, M.B. (1999). Spatial cognition in rhesus monkeys: Male superiority declines with age. *Horm. Behav. 36(1)*, 70–76.

Lacreuse, A., Herndon, J.G., Moss, M.B. (2000). Cognitive function in aged ovariectomized female rhesus monkeys. *Behav. Neurosci. 114(3)*, 506–513.

Lacreuse, A., and Herndon, J.G. (2003). Effects of estradiol and aging on fine manual performance in female rhesus monkeys. *Horm. Behav. 43*, 359–366.

Lacreuse, A., Diehl, M.M., Goh, M.Y., Hall, M.J., Volk, A.M., Chhabra, R.K., and Herndon, J.G. (2005). Sex differences in age-related motor slowing in the rhesus monkey: behavioral and neuroimaging data. *Neurobiol. Aging 26*, 543–551.

Lai, Z.C., Rosene, D.L., Killiany, R.J., Pugliese, D., Albert, M.S., and Moss, M.B. (2001). Age-related changes in the rhesus monkey: MRI changes in the forebrain white matter but not gray matter. *25th Annual Meeting Society for Neuroscience* Abstract 614.7.

Lamar, M., Yousem, D.M., and Resnick, S.M. (2004). Age differences in orbitofrontal activation: An fMRI investigation of delayed match and nonmatch to sample. *Neuroimage 21*, 1368–1376.

Liu, R.S., Lemieux, L., Bell, G.S., Sisodiya, S.M., Shorvon, S.D., Sander, J.W., and Duncan, J.S. (2003). A longitudinal study of brain morphometrics using quantitative magnetic resonance imaging and difference image analysis. *Neuroimage 20*, 22–33.

Lloyd, J.M., Hoffman, G.E., and Wise, P.M. (1994). Decline in immediate early gene expression in gonadotropin-releasing hormone neurons during proestrus in regularly cycling, middle-aged rats. *Endocrinology 134*, 1800–1805.

Matochik, J.A., Chefer, S.I., Lane, M.A., Woolf, R.I., Morris, E.D., Ingram, D.K., *et al.* (2000). Age-related decline in striatal volume in monkeys as measured by magnetic resonance imaging. *Neurobiology of Aging 21*, 591–598.

Matochik, J.A., Chefer, S.I., Lane, M.A., Roth, G.S., Mattison, J.A., London, E.D., and Ingram, D.K. (2004). Age-related decline in striatal volume in rhesus monkeys: Assessment of long-term caloric restriction. *Neurobiology of Aging 25*, 193–200.

Mattison, J.A., Lane, M.A., Roth, G.S., and Ingram, D.K. (2003). Calorie restriction in rhesus monkeys. *Exp. Gerontol. 38*, 35–46.

Micevych, P., Sinchak, K., Mills, R.H., Tao, L., LaPolt, P., and Lu, J.K. (2003). The luteinizing hormone surge is preceded by an estrogen-induced increase of hypothalamic progesterone in ovariectomized and adrenalectomized rats. *Neuroendocrinol. 78*, 29–35.

Mills, R.H., Romeo, H.E., Lu, J.K., and Micevych, P.E. (2002). Site-specific decrease of progesterone receptor mRNA expression in the hypothalamus of middle-aged persistently estrus rats. *Brain Res. 955*, 200–206.

Mikkola, T.S., and Clarkson, T.B. (2002). Estrogen replacement therapy, atherosclerosis, and vascular function. *Cardiovasc. Res. 53*, 605–619.

Moscrip, T.D., Ingram, D.K., Lane, M.A., Roth, G.S., and Weed, J.L. (2000). Locomotor activity in female rhesus monkeys: Assessment of age and calorie restriction effects. *J. Gerontol. A Biol. Sci. Med. Sci. 55*, B373–B380.

Neeman, Z., Hirshberg, B., Tal, M.G., Wood, B.J., and Harlan, D.M. (2004). Pulmonary angiography for the diagnosis of thromboembolic events in the non-human primate. *Transplantation 15*, 1025–1029.

Nelson, P.T., Stefansson, K. Gulcher, J. and Saper, C.B. (1996). Molecular evolution of tau protein: Implications for Alzheimer's disease. *J. Neurochem. 67(4)*, 1622–1632.

Nikolich-Zugish, J., and Messaoudi, I. (2005). Mice and flies and monkeys too: Caloric restriction rejuvenates the aging immune system of non human primates. *Exper. Gerontol. 40(11)*, 884–893.

Oliver, W.R. Jr. Shenk, J.L., Snaith, M.R., Russell, C.S., Plunket, K.D., Bodkin, N.L., *et al.* (2001). A selective peroxisome proliferator-activated recptor delta agonist promotes reverse cholesterol transport. *Proc. Natl. Acad. Sci. USA 98*, 5306.

Osteen, K.G., Bruner-Tran, K.L., and Eisenberg, E. (2005). Endometrial biology and the etiology of endometriosis. *Fertility Sterility. 84(1)*, 33–34.

Ottinger, M.A. (1998). Male reproduction: Testosterone, gonadotropins, and aging. In *Functional Endocrinology of Aging* (C.V. Mobbs, P.R. Hof, eds.), Vol. 29, 105–126. Karger Press.

Ottinger, M.A., Abdelnabi, M., Li, Q., Chen, K., Thompson, N., Harada, N., *et al.* (2004). The Japanese quail: A model for studying reproductive aging of hypothalamic systems. *Exp. Geront. 39*, 1679–1693.

Peters, A., Rosene, D.L., Moss, M.B., Kemper, T.L., Abraham, C.R., Tigges, J., and Albert, M. (1996). Neurobiological bases of age-related cognitive decline in the rhesus monkey. *J. Neuropathol. Exp. Neurol. 55*, 861–974.

Prior, J.C. (1998). Perimenopause: The complex endocrinology of the menopausal transition. *Endocrine Rev. 19*, 397–428.

Ramsey, J.J., Colman, R.J., Binkley, N.C., Christensen, J.D., Gresl, T.A., Kemnitz, J.W., and Weindruch, R. (2000). Dietary restriction and aging in rhesus monkeys: The University of Wisconsin study. *Exp. Gerontol. 35*, 1131–1149.

Rapp, P., and Amara, I.D. (1989). Evidence for task-dependent memory dysfunction in the aged monkey. *J. Neuroscience 9*, 3568–3576.

Raz, N., Rodrique, K.M., Kennedy, K.M., Head, D., Gunning-Dixon, F., and Acker, J.D. (2003). Differential aging of the human striatum: Longitudinal evidence. *Amer. J. Neuroradiology 24*, 1849–1856.

Raz, N., Gunning-Dixon, F., Head, D., Rodrique, K.M., Williamson, A., Acker, J.D. (2004a). Aging, sexual dimorphism, and hemispheric asymmetry of the cerebral cortex: replicability of regional differences in volume. *Neurobiology of Aging 25*, 377–396.

Raz, N., Rodrigue, K.M., Kennedy, K.M., and Acker, J.D. (2004b). Hormone replacement therapy and age-related brain shrinkage: Regional effects. *Neuroreport 15*, 2531–2534.

Resnick, S.M., Goldszal, A.F., Davatzikos, C., Golski, S., Kraut, M.A., Metter, E.J., *et al.* (2000). One-year age changes in MRI brain volumes in older adults. *Cereb Cortex. 10*, 464–472.

Resnick, S.M., Pham, D.L., Kraut, M.A., Zonderman, A.B., and Davatzikos, C. (2003). Longitudinal magnetic resonance imaging studies of older adults: A shrinking brain. *J. Neurosci. 23(8)*, 3295–3301.

Riggs, B.L., Khosla, S., and Melton, III, L.J. (2002). Sex steroids and the construction and conservation of the adult skeleton. *Endocrine Rev. 23*, 279–302.

Rippy, M.K., Lee, D.R., Pearson, S.L., Bernal, J.C., and Kuchi T.J. (1996). Identification of rhesus macaques with spontaneous endometriosis. *J. Med. Primatol. 25*, 346–355.

Robertson, J.F.R. (2004). Selective oestrogen receptor modulators/new antioestrogens: A clinical perspective. *Cancer Treatment Rev. 30*, 695–706.

Roth, G.S., Ingram, D.K. and Lane, M.A. (1995). Slowing aging by caloric restriction. *Nature Medicine 1*, 414–415.

Roth, G.S., Lane, M.A., Ball, S.S., and Ingram, D.K. (1997). Multiple "anti-aging" mechanisms of caloric restriction: Maintenance of serum DHEAS levels in rhesus monkeys, *Journal Clinical Endocrinology and Metabolism 82*, 2093–2096.

Roth, G.S., Mattison, J.A., Ottinger, M.A., Chachich, M.E., Lane, M.A., and Ingram, D.K. (2004). Aging in rhesus monkeys: Relevance to human health interventions. *Science 305(5689)*, 1423–1426.

Scarbrough, K. and Wise, P.M. (1990). Age-related changes in pulsatile luteinizing hormone precede acyclicity and depend upon estrous cycle history. *Endocrinol. 126*, 884–890.

Schwartz, S.M., and Kemnitz, J.W. (1992). Age- and gender-related changes in body size, adiposity, and endocrine metabolic parameters in free-ranging rhesus macaques. *Am. J. Phys. Anthropol. 89*, 109–121.

Scuteri, A., Najjar, S.S., Morrell, C.H., and Lakatta, E.G. (2005). The metabolic syndrome in older individuals: Prevalence and prediction of cardiovascular events. *Diabetes Care 28(4)*, 882–887.

Sell, D.R., Lane, M.A., Johnson, W.A., Masoro, E.J., Mock, O.B., Reiser, K.M., *et al.* (1996). Longevity and the genetic determination of collagen glycoxidation kinetics in mammalian senescence. *Proc. Natl. Acad. Sci. USA 93*, 485.

Sherwin, B.B. (2003). Estrogen and cognitive functioning in women. *Endocrinol. Rev. 24*, 133–151.

Shideler, S.E., Gee, N.A., Chen, J., and Lasley, B.L. (2001). Estrogen metabolites and follicle-stimulating hormone in the aged macaque female. *Biol. Reprod. 65*, 1718–1725.

Small, S.A., Chawla, M.K., Bunocore, M., Rapp, P.R., and Barnes, C.A. (2004). Imaging correlates of brain function in monkeys and rats isolates a hippocampal subregion differentially vulnerable to aging. *Proc. Natl. Acad. Sci. USA 101*, 7181.

Soules, M.R., Battaaglia, D.E., and Klein, N.A. (1998). Inhibin and reproductive aging in women. *Maturitas 30*, 193–204.

Tinkler, G.P. and Voytko, M.L. (2005). Estrogen modulates cognitive and cholinergic processes in surgically menopausal monkeys. *Prog. Neuropsychopharmacol. Biol. Psychiatry 29(3)*, 423–431.

Torre, III, P., and Fowler, C.G. (2000). Age-related changes in auditory function of rhesus monkeys (*Macaca mulatta*). *Hear. Res. 142*, 131.

Treolar, A.E. (1981). Menstrual cyclicity and the pre-menopause. *Maturitas 3*, 49–64.

Urbanski, H.F., Downs, J.L., Garyfallou, V.T., Mattison, J.A., Lane, M.A., Roth, G.S., and Ingram, D.K. (2004). Effect of caloric restriction on the 24-hour plasma DHEAS and cortisol profiles of young and old male rhesus macaques. *Ann. NY Acad. Sci. 1019*, 443–447.

Vanitallie, T.B. (2003). Frailty in the elderly: Contributions of sarcopenia and visceral protein depletion. *Metabolism 52(10), suppl 2*, 22–26.

Voytko, M.L. (2000). The effects of long-term ovariectomy and estrogen replacement therapy on learning and memory in monkeys (*Macaca fascicularis*). *Behav. Neurosci. 114(6)*, 1078–1087.

Voytko, M.L. (2002). Estrogen and the cholinergic system modulate visuospatial attention in monkeys (*Macaca fascicularis*) *Behav. Neurosci. 116(2)*, 187–197.

Wahlund, L-O., Almkvist, O., Basun, H., and Julin, P. (1996). MRI in successful aging, a 5 year follow-up study from the eighth to ninth decade of life. *Magnetic Resonance Imaging 6*, 601–608.

Weed, M.R., Paul, I.A., Dwoskin, L.P., Moore, S.E., and Woolverton, W.L. (1997). The relationship between reinforcing effects and in vitro effects of D1 agonists in monkeys. *J. Pharm. Exp. Ther. 283(1)*, 29–38.

Weindruch, R., and Walford, R. (1988). *The Retardation of Aging and Disease by Dietary Restriction* (Charles C. Thomas, Springfield).

Welt, C.K., McNicholl, J. Taylor, A.E., and Hall, J.E. (1999). Female reproductive aging is marked by decreased secretion of dimeric inhibin. *J. Clin. Endocrinol. Metab. 84(1)*, 105–111.

Wisco, J.J., Guttman, C.R.G., Warfield, S.K., Wells, W.M., Killian, R.J., Rosene, D.L., and Moss, M.B. (2001). An MRI investigation of age-realted structural changes in the rhesus monkey brain. *31st Annual Meeting Society for Neuroscience* Abstract 550.15.

Wise, P.M. (1991). Neuroendocrine influences on aging of the female reproductive system. Front. *Neuroendocrinol. 12*, 323–356.

Wu, J.M., Mattison, J., Lawson, M.S., Takahashi, D.L., Pau, F., Ingram, D., Roth, G., *et al.* (2004). Dynamic changes in follicle-stimulating hormone and inhibin B during perimenopause in rhesus monkeys. *37th Annual Meeting, Society for the Study of Reproduction*, Special Issue, page 100, Abstract 33.

Zelinski-Wooten, M.B., Hutchison, J.S., Chandresekher, Y.A., and Stouffer, R.L. (1999). Duration, amplitude and specificity of the gonadotropin surge in a nonhuman primate model. In *Ovulation: Evolving Scientific and Clinical Concepts* (E. Y. Adashi, ed.), pp. 98–109. Serono Symposium, New York: Springer-Verlag, Inc.

Zhang, Z., Andersen, A., Smith, C., Grondin, R., Gerhardt, G., and Gash, D. (2000). Motor slowing and parkinsonian signs in aging rhesus monkeys mirror human aging. *J. Gerontol. A Biol. Sci. Med. Sci. 55*, B473–B480.

39

Nonhuman Primates as Models for Reproductive Aging and Human Infertility

Barry D. Bavister and Carol A. Brenner

Nonhuman primates are invaluable models for a wide range of basic and applied studies related to human health. In vitro production (IVP) of preimplantation embryos makes them available in significant numbers for embryo manipulations and research aimed at a variety of biomedical applications. Rhesus monkeys (Macaca mulatta) *are well established models for many biomedical research studies into diseases affecting humans. Their basic physiology and reproductive endocrinology are very similar to those of humans, and they are relatively easy to breed and manage in captivity. The rhesus monkey exhibits an approximately 28-day menstrual cycle, like that of humans. It is also a long-lived species, living up to 30 years, so that age-related diseases similar to those in humans are likely to appear. In these major respects, rhesus monkeys are a much more appropriate model for humans than rodents or other nonprimates that differ markedly in their susceptibility to human-related diseases and in their reproductive physiology. In particular, macaque monkeys are appropriate for research into primate infertility and for effects of aging on this disease. In this chapter, we review some of the key areas for which the rhesus monkey is an ideal transitional model between laboratory animals and humans, and we discuss some of the basic research questions and technologies underlying studies with this animal. Special attention is given to the roles of mitochondria in infertility and aging because anomalies in these key organelles may underlie many of the defects that have been reported in embryos and in embryonic stem cells.*

Introduction

FREQUENCY OF INFERTILITY

Infertility is common in humans. It is estimated that about 15% of couples have difficulty in conceiving or are outright infertile. There are numerous contributing factors, some of which can be helped by resorting to Assisted Reproductive Technology or ART, which comprises artificial insemination, in vitro maturation (IVM) of oocytes, in vitro fertilization (IVF), embryo culture and embryo transfer. For presumptively infertile women aged up to about 37, the outcome of clinical "IVF" (in this general context meaning IVF together with embryo culture and transfer) is good, with an average of about 32% of treatment cycles in the United States resulting in a live birth (Wright *et al.*, 2003). But for women approaching 40 or over, the efficiency of IVF drops sharply, to only about 5% after the age of 42 (Wright *et al.*, 2003). Similarly, the incidence of natural conceptions falls progressively towards the age of 40, prior to overt menopause. The reasons for this precipitous drop in fertility are not well understood, but a decline in the ability of the uterus to support pregnancy does not seem to be a primary factor, in view of the number of births to women over 40 carrying a surrogate embryo made with oocytes from younger women. The quality of oocytes and/or ovarian factors appear to be much more likely contributors to the low pregnancy success in older women.

QUALITY OF HUMAN OOCYTES AND IMPACT ON FERTILITY

The quality or health of human oocytes is progressively diminished with age due to (i) inherent or genetic factors as part of the natural aging process; and (ii) epigenetic factors such as nutrition, smoking and environmental effects. While reduced fertility in women derives in large part from diminished oocyte quality or "health," there is currently no reliable way to measure this attribute, nor any real understanding of why it happens.

We need ways to measure oocyte quality that could improve selection of oocytes/embryos in ART clinics, which would increase pregnancy success rates, especially in low-outcome patients such as women aged 40 or over. Such methods will come from better understanding of the cellular and molecular properties of oocytes. A key component of all cells including oocytes is the mitochondrion, which provides energy and possesses its own DNA for encoding protein production. Defects in either of these functions could lead to loss of oocyte competence in the short term (failure of fertilization or embryo development) or long term (nonviable fetuses or incompetent placentas, leading to pregnancy loss, or possibly postnatal health defects). Human oocytes would be the optimal subjects for undertaking studies on oocyte quality and the embryos derived from them; however, practical and ethical constraints preclude intensive studies with human oocytes and embryos, so suitable animal models must be used.

For investigating oocyte quality, it is important that some studies are conducted with animals closely related to humans, because of the wide diversity in cellular, molecular and endocrine mechanisms used by different mammals in their reproductive strategies. A strong case can be made for using nonhuman primates as the most appropriate models for human reproduction, especially mtDNA studies (see below). In our laboratory, current studies with rhesus monkeys focus on mitochondria as potential markers for oocyte quality and competence, and these efforts may help explain defects in low-quality oocytes.

In higher primates (humans and, for example, macaque monkeys), high extrinsic gonadotropin stimulation in ART cycles produces inherent variations in oocyte quality and competence, possibly by recruiting defective oocytes from potentially atretic follicles. Even in natural human and rhesus menstrual cycles, it is estimated that only about 25% of potential conceptions support clinical pregnancies; most likely, defects in oocytes and anomalies of fertilization are major contributors to this loss. This inefficiency is in marked contrast to natural cycles in some rodents, where 98% of ovulated oocytes develop into blastocysts and almost all of these become viable fetuses (Gonzales and Bavister, 1995). It can be estimated that in infertile patients, human ART efficiency *on average* is only about 15% or less per embryo transferred, or less than 5% per cleaved embryo or oocyte inseminated (Bavister and Brenner, 2004), although some clinics report much higher success rates.

One component of low fertility with increased reproductive age is "ovarian senescence," which is marked by a rise in circulating Follicle Stimulating Hormone (FSH) levels due to decreasing negative hormone feedback from the ovary, and by declining numbers of competent ovarian follicles (Wright *et al.*, 2003). Concomitant with this condition is an increase in oocyte anomalies, especially aneuploidies but also including mitochondrial defects. Aneuploidy in oocytes of older women is a well-recognized condition, but defects in mitochondria are not so obvious because they are harder to detect. However, considering that mitochondria not only carry their own genomes but also provide most of the energy for cell functions, defects in mitochondria are likely to have serious consequences for oocyte competence.

ANIMAL MODELS FOR STUDYING INFERTILTY

It is very difficult to study the etiology of chromosomal or mitochondrial defects in humans, or to relate such deficiencies to developmental outcomes, simply because the principal focus in humans is to help infertile women to become pregnant and have healthy babies. This goal is antithetical to basic research because the latter usually involves destructive analysis of oocytes and embryos. Human oocytes and embryos that are surplus to clinical needs and available for research are scarce, and may not be representative of developmentally competent oocytes and embryos. As a result, it is not surprising that the majority of research on oocyte and embryo function has been done with animal material, usually from rodents although sometimes with suitable domesticated animals, such as cattle and pigs. The problem with this approach, though it is logical, is that gamete physiology and even basic reproductive strategies can vary considerably in different mammals, so that it may be difficult to extrapolate from an experimental animal to humans. This is strikingly so in the case of mice, which have been used in the vast majority of studies into mammalian gamete biology, fertilization, embryo development and implantation. However, in all these respects, mice are not appropriate as models for humans. In contrast, nonhuman primates, especially higher primates such as the macaques, are highly suitable models for human reproduction.

Rhesus monkeys (*Macaca mulatta*) are well established models for many kinds of biomedical research studies into diseases affecting humans. The basic physiology of these monkeys is very similar to that of humans, and they are easy to breed and manage in captivity. The rhesus monkey exhibits an approximately 28-day menstrual cycle, and its reproductive endocrinology is very similar to that of humans. Accordingly, rhesus monkeys have been especially used as models to study human infertility and effects of aging thereon. Because of their long lifespan, we should expect that rhesus monkeys would exhibit age-related declines in fertility and ovarian reserve, which is discussed in the next section. By using ovarian stimulation regimens similar to those used for infertile women, rhesus monkeys can provide adequate, although not large, numbers of eggs for embryology studies. Such studies, together with those performed with human embryos, have shown that the basic biology of preimplantation embryology in primates is significantly different from that of rodents. A striking example is the derivation of the centrosome, which is the microtubule organizing center for fertilization: in most mammals studied, including primates, this structure is provided by the fertilizing spermatozoon, whereas in rodents it is maternally derived (Hewitson *et al.*, 2002). The marked similarities in oocyte maturation, fertilization, embryo metabolism, the timing of embryonic genome activation, the endocrinology of reproduction, and the modes of implantation and pregnancy underscore the need to study nonhuman primate models to obtain information relevant to human infertility and its treatment.

AVAILABILITY OF MONKEYS FOR RESEARCH

In spite of their great value as models for studying mechanisms of infertility in primates, macaque monkeys suffer from one major drawback: they are not readily available in substantial numbers for this purpose. This is ironic, because the United States has the largest nonhuman primate research infrastructure in the world, in the form of the eight National Primate Research Centers supported by the NIH. Each of these centers has several thousand nonhuman primates, and rhesus monkeys comprise a large proportion of the total. However, the great demand for this species for AIDS-related research means that few animals are available for other kinds of research, including infertility studies. It may be time to ask if priorities for allocation of monkeys to research studies should be reassessed.

Evidence for Ovarian Senescence in Rhesus Monkeys

The number of potentially viable oocytes available to the reproducing female depends on the size of the primordial follicle population within the ovary. In humans, primarily due to follicular atresia and secondarily because of follicular recruitment, the numbers of primordial follicles decrease dramatically from birth to the onset of menopause. At the end of the reproductive lifespan, the "ovarian reserve" of viable follicles and oocytes is essentially depleted, and the ovary is said to be senescent (Faddy and Gosden, 1996). Concomitantly, ovulatory activity ceases and levels of estrogen decrease markedly. As a result, FSH secretion increases strikingly because of diminished negative feedback from estrogen (Walker, 1995). Bioactive FSH retrieved from postmenopausal women's urine was in high demand for a number of years as a means to stimulate ovaries of infertile women to produce large numbers of follicles and oocytes. However, such ovarian stimulation for ART becomes ineffective once the ovarian reserve is seriously depleted and oocyte quality is reduced (Hansen *et al.*, 2003). Female rhesus macaques are excellent models for studying the loss of reproductive capacity with increasing age. They are reproductively active over about 20 years starting at about age 5, and undergo similar pathological and hormonal changes to human females nearing the end of their reproductive lifespan (Shideler *et al.*, 2001). Although there have been several reports on ovarian changes in macaques, including oocyte numbers, most studies examined younger females and did not study older animals (ages 15–25) that would be expected to show ovarian senescence. In view of this, our laboratory conducted a study of the ovarian reserve in rhesus macaque females across a wide age range (ages ~1–25), covering the entire reproductive lifespan of this species. Histological examination of ovarian sections showed clear evidence of follicular depletion with increasing age, especially in the older age groups (Nichols *et al.*, 2005).

Ovaries were collected over a 5-year period at the Tulane National Primate Research Center (Covington, LA) and archived for later examination. These ovaries (64 pairs total) were divided into several groups by age (<5, >5–10, >10–15, >15–20 and >20 years old) to examine age-related changes in ovarian morphology. A representative histological section from each ovary was examined for the number of primordial, primary or antral follicles it contained (Figure 39.1).

We found that, while the percentage of antral follicles remained nearly unchanged across age groups, the percentages of primary and primordial follicles changed significantly with age (Figure 39.2).

This change reflects the degenerative processes occurring within the ovary. Similarly, the *total numbers* of follicles in each of the three classes significantly decreased with increasing age of the female. Because growth of

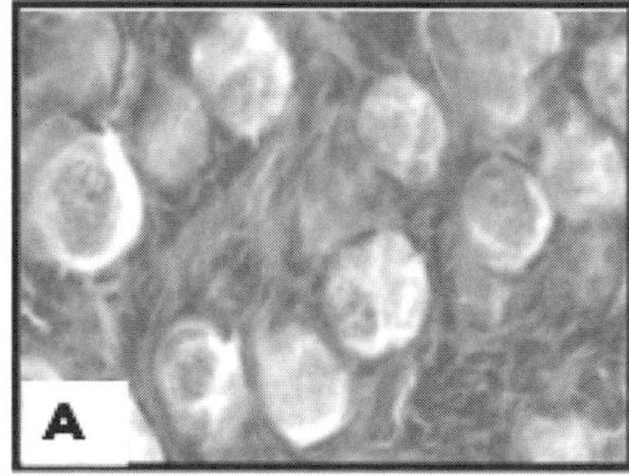

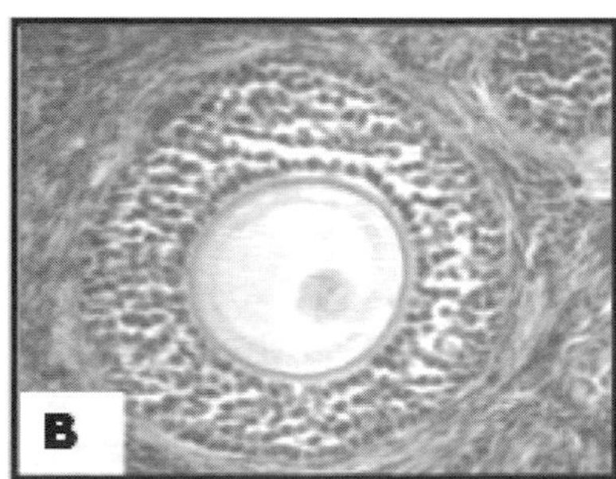

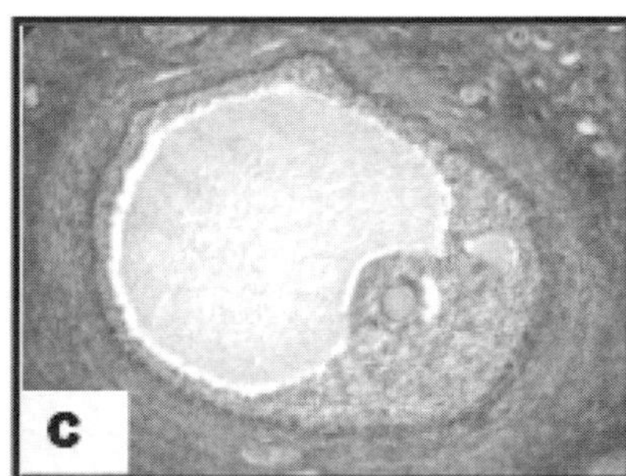

Figure 39.1 Follicles representing various stages of development in the rhesus ovary. Primordial follicles (A) are characterized by a flattened granulosa cell border. The representative primary follicle (B) demonstrates several layers of granulosa cells surrounding the oocyte and a developed zona pellucida. Antral follicles (C) contain a well-developed antrum. Reproduced from Nichols *et al.* (2005) *Hum. Reprod.* 20:79–83 ©European Society of Human Reproduction and Embryology. Reproduced by permission of Oxford University Press/Human Reproduction.

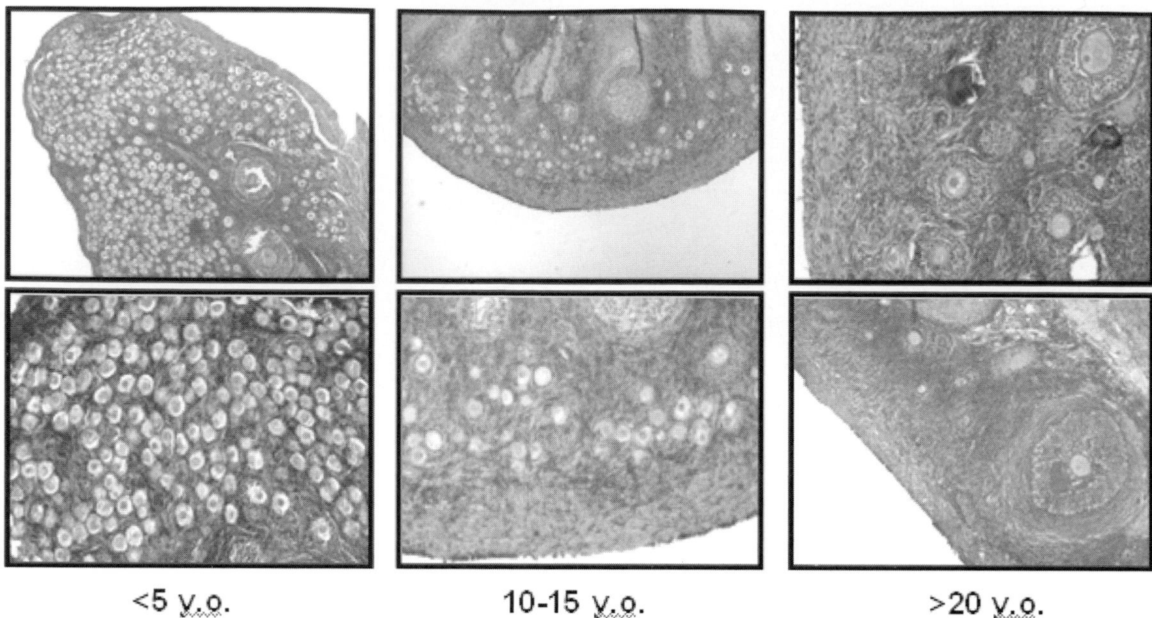

Figure 39.2 Ovarian sections illustrating changing follicle populations with increasing age. Reproduced from Nichols *et al.* (2005) *Hum. Reprod.* 20:79–83 ©European Society of Human Reproduction and Embryology. Reproduced by permission of Oxford University Press/Human Reproduction.

primary follicles is gonadotropin-dependent (Macklon and Fauser, 1999), many of the newly formed primary follicles in older females cease development or become atretic, possibly due to lack of FSH receptors on the surrounding follicular cells. Loss of ovarian reserve was most obvious in females undergoing the perimenopausal and menopausal transition (age group 20–25 y.o.), with scattered and atretic follicles, occasional primordial follicles and reduced amounts of stromal tissue. Interestingly, the number of births within each female was significantly correlated with the proportion of primordial and primary follicles independent of her age, with the mean percentage of primordial follicles decreasing and the percentage of primary follicles increasing. This was likely because females who give birth to a large number of offspring are pregnant or lactating for much of their reproductive lifespan. The menstrual cycle stops during pregnancy/lactation, because of continued production of progesterone, which blocks FSH production and secretion from the pituitary gland (Pohl *et al.*, 1982). As a result, recruitment and growth of primary follicles are halted, while recruitment and loss of the primordial follicles continues unabated throughout life because they are independent of gonadotropins.

This study (Nichols *et al.*, 2005) illustrates that in several important respects, the rhesus monkey is an appropriate model for studying age-related loss of fertility in human females. However, it is not a perfect model because some details of human menopause are not shared by macaque females. For example, in humans there is a subtle and gradual onset of menopause-related changes before irregular cycling begins (Santoro, 2002), whereas macaques appear to undergo abrupt changes at the onset of irregular cycles (Shideler *et al.*, 2001). Also, in this study we did not observe any age-related differences in sex hormone or gonadotropin levels in the rhesus females. However, this is not surprising because we had only one time point measurement for each female from a single blood sample drawn at the time of necropsy, so no comparative data during the reproductive lifespan of each female were available. Additional studies with the rhesus macaque model could be useful for understanding mechanisms underlying reproductive aging, so that it might be possible to devise ART strategies to address this phenomenon.

Nonhuman Primates as Models for Developing ART

Because the rhesus monkey is a good model for obtaining information about reproduction in primates, the use of ART procedures in this species might reveal details about preimplantation events, including age-related phenomena, that could be relevant to the problem of "IVF" failure in older human females. Ovarian stimulation, IVF and embryo culture, collectively known as "in vitro production" (IVP) are well-established techniques for a variety of species (Bavister and Boatman, 1993; Bavister, 1995). These ARTs are useful and even commercially viable in domesticated animals, and have long been employed in research with rodents and other species. The success of

ART in addressing infertility problems in humans, though not as efficient as it could be, is well known (Olivennes and Frydman, 1998). In contrast, ART has been employed far less frequently or effectively with nonhuman primates, in spite of the huge potential benefits for biomedical and reproductive research. The techniques for nonhuman primate embryo IVP are well established and have been used for more than 20 years for in vitro studies on embryos (Boatman and Bavister, 1984; Bavister *et al.*, 1983, 1984; Bavister and Boatman, 1993). Protocols for IVP of macaque embryos are quite efficient, with approximately 60% of IVF ova becoming blastocysts (Schramm and Bavister, 1996); however, the total number of offspring born from transfer of IVP embryos for all nonhuman primate species is very small. This is because only a small proportion of the total ART research effort in animals has involved monkeys, and because most of the nonhuman primate studies have focused on developing protocols for producing IVP embryos. Relatively little attention has been paid to embryo transfer strategies for producing offspring, and almost none to studying the effectiveness of other ART techniques such as preimplantation genetic diagnosis. Nevertheless, ART in nonhuman primates is successful (Bavister, 2004), and paying more attention to the use of these animals for providing basic information about primate embryology could be very rewarding.

OVARIAN STIMULATION

Initially, we used PMSG and subsequently human menopausal gonadotropins for stimulating rhesus monkey ovaries (Bavister *et al.*, 1983; Boatman *et al.*, 1986), but these biological preparations were very immunogenic, so that females could only be stimulated once (Bavister *et al.*, 1986). This restriction on use of animals seriously limited the numbers of macaque oocytes previously obtainable, and this is a major reason why nonhuman primate embryo research lagged behind work with many other species. However, this difficulty was overcome when recombinant human gonadotropins were used for nonhuman primate research. Using these gonadotropins, female macaques have been stimulated successfully up to five times each, before refractoriness becomes apparent.

Limitations of this approach are that IVP embryos most likely have inherent defects such as anomalies of gene expression. Although this has not been examined in monkey embryos, such anomalies including abnormal expression of imprinted genes have been clearly documented in cattle and mouse embryos (Morgan *et al.*, 2005). We may infer that IVP primate embryos, both human and monkey, are likely to exhibit a high incidence of such defects. In that case, it is difficult to ascertain exactly what constitutes a "normal" embryo, and this detracts from our ability to understand defects in oocytes and embryos that may contribute to age-related loss of fertility. It would clearly be valuable to examine putatively normal embryos flushed from the reproductive tract. For example, it is not known what the inner cell mass (ICM) and trophectoderm cell numbers are in naturally-occurring primate blastocysts. Reduced ICM cell counts in IVP embryos compared with in vivo blastocysts would indicate a reason for their lower average viability. The cell counts of normal, in vivo–produced blastocysts could serve as a benchmark for evaluating the quality of IVP blastocysts. Although embryo flushing was done in one small study with humans, the flushed embryos were immediately transferred to infertile patients (Buster *et al.*, 1985), and no useful information was produced about the characteristics of viable embryos. This approach is very unlikely to be repeated for ethical reasons. Again, the nonhuman primate could serve as a useful model for obtaining information on in vivo produced embryos, but this approach has rarely been exploited.

SUPEROVULATION OF RHESUS MONKEYS AND FLUSHING EMBRYOS FROM THE REPRODUCTIVE TRACT

The term "superovulation" is used liberally in human clinical IVF, but in that context it implies ovarian stimulation with gonadotropins to recruit large numbers of follicles, which are then aspirated prior to ovulation to recover oocytes. In animal studies, superovulation usually means allowing or inducing gonadotropin-stimulated follicles to ovulate into the oviduct, followed by collection from the reproductive tract of oocytes for IVF or of embryos for further study in vitro. The U.S. cattle breeding industry has been transformed by the application of artificial insemination together with "Multiple Ovulation and Embryo Transfer" (MOET: Gearhart *et al.*, 1989), which results in the collection of perhaps 10 20 high-quality embryos for transfer to recipient females. Collection of flushed embryos from non-stimulated rhesus monkey females is feasible, as shown by years of effort at the Wisconsin National Primate Research Center (Wolfgang *et al.*, 2001). While these embryos are enormously valuable because they are almost certainly "normal," and no comparable human embryos are available, the effort involved in collecting them is huge. The application of the MOET principle to rhesus monkeys would be a considerable advantage for the collection of numerous in vivo produced embryos, but success has never been reported in nonhuman primates. Administration of human recombinant gonadotropins to monkeys should make the MOET approach more feasible. This in vivo approach would eliminate the need to culture embryos, which avoids introduction of IVP-induced gene expression anomalies. The embryos collected from superovulated rhesus monkeys (morulae and early blastocysts) would be expected to have high viability, which would benefit not only studies on age-related infertility but also production of better quality embryonic stem cells. Because of their immense value for embryological studies, the collection of nonhuman primate embryos produced in vivo should be strongly encouraged.

Methods for Detecting Chromosomal Abnormalities in Monkey Oocytes and Embryos

FREQUENCY OF CHROMOSOME ERRORS IN PRIMATES

It is well established that aneuploidy is common in human oocytes and IVF embryos, and that the frequency of these anomalies increases with age, especially after age 25 (Munne and Cohen, 1998; Munne *et al.*, 2002). Several studies have reported frequencies up to 50% for aneuploidy (Gras *et al.*, 1992) and as high as 48% for mosaicism (Munne *et al.*, 2002). In the latter study, as many as 84% of cells in "chaotic mosaic" embryos were abnormal. However, all the data are from oocytes and IVP embryos of infertile women, in which occurrence of chromosome anomalies may be especially marked compared with the general population, and may also be exacerbated by gonadotropin stimulation for IVF. Moreover, humans are not suitable experimental subjects for studying the etiology or frequency of aneuploidy in the general population. In order to study these questions, a suitable experimental model is needed, which clearly needs to be a nonhuman primate. However, no study has adequately examined the frequency of aneuploidies in monkey oocytes, either under natural conditions or following ovarian stimulation with gonadotropins.

Aneuploidy is defined as any deviation from the normal number of chromosomes, usually meaning a cell nucleus possessing too many or too few chromosomes. Aneuploidy generally results from nondisjunction events during meiosis, subsequent to "germinal vesicle" (GV) breakdown. About 85% of aneuploidy errors in mice derive from meiotic nondisjunction (Hunt and Hassold, 2002). Alternatively, aneuploidy can result from errors subsequent to meiosis, i.e., mitotic nondisjunction during embryo development. This represents about 15% of chromosomal anomalies. One study reported a significant relationship between maternal age and embryo mosaicism caused by mitotic nondisjunction (Munne and Cohen, 1998). In addition, embryos with impaired developmental competence had a higher frequency of chromosome abnormalities. Gross forms of aneuploidy such as polyploidy can also result from polyspermic fertilization or failure of second polar body extrusion. However, these gross errors are easily distinguishable from nondisjunction errors that are more prevalent in primate IVP embryos. It is important to understand the etiology of these high error rates so that more normal embryos can be produced, with consequent improvement in the success rates of human IVF, especially for older women for whom the aneuploidy rate is much higher. There are two main possibilities.

1. High rates of aneuploidy and associated mosaicism in embryos due to aberrant chromosome separation are inherent in humans and other "Old World" primates, and this frequency increases with age. If this is true, then little or nothing can be done to decrease the frequencies of these errors. This possibility seems unlikely, partly because such high error rates are not seen in oocytes or embryos from other species examined, such as laboratory or domestic animals. Another reason for doubting this explanation is the source of the information on aneuploidy/mosaicism rates in human oocytes and embryos, as discussed next.
2. The high aneuploidy/mosaicism rates reported in human IVP embryos may result from several factors. (i) The subjects are patients attending IVF clinics; many of these women are infertile, and thus, they are not representative of the general population; (ii) These patients are mostly in the 30–40 years age bracket, and it is likely that the frequency of aneuploidy (nondisjunction) and mosaicism errors in oocytes increases with age (Pellestor *et al.*, 2003); (iii) The patients are stimulated with gonadotropins which raise estradiol levels much higher than normal (Hughes *et al.*, 1990). This abnormal endocrine environment could adversely affect chromosome separation during meiosis. Recent data in mice indicate that estrogenic compounds that elevate blood estradiol levels greatly increase the nondisjunction frequency (Hunt *et al.*, 2003); (iv) The artificial culture conditions used for embryo production (IVP) may have an impact on genetic quality of embryos by influencing chromosomal segregation during early cleavage (Bean *et al.*, 2002). The mechanism of this effect is not known. Factors (iii) and (iv) may synergize to increase the overall rate of chromosome anomalies. If (iii) is true, then the high rate of aneuploidy/mosaicism seen in many infertile women is potentially treatable by designing new stimulation regimens, or even avoiding gonadotropin stimulation altogether. This may be especially important for older women who are at higher risk for chromosome anomalies. If (iv) is true, then new embryo culture media are needed to reduce mosaicism frequency.

Without reliable information on the cause(s) of high error rates during chromosomal segregation in humans, it is difficult to know how to proceed in order to ameliorate the condition to produce more normal IVF embryos. It is also entirely plausible that the conditions giving rise to chromosomal anomalies cannot be ameliorated, but again, this will not be elucidated without further studies. It would be useful to know the frequency of aneuploidy/mosaicism in the general human population, but this information is not available, nor is it likely to be. Alternatively, donor oocytes from young women could be examined, but this is not practical because chromosome analysis is destructive and thus precludes use of these oocytes for their primary purpose of embryo production and transfer. Information on oocytes from unstimulated, infertile patients would be helpful, but there are almost no data on this. Because of all these difficulties in obtaining relevant information from humans, the etiology of aneuploidy/mosaicism in primate oocytes and embryos remains a mystery.

The rhesus monkey should prove an ideal model for unraveling this mystery, for several reasons. First, destructive analysis can be done on rhesus oocytes and embryos because this is an experimental model, and complete analysis of all cells is needed to gauge the degree of mosaicism in embryos. Second, we can obtain oocytes from several sources to help determine the etiology of chromosome defects: in vivo matured oocytes from nonstimulated and from gonadotropin-stimulated monkeys, and IVP embryos from IVM or from in vivo matured oocytes. In effect, we can devise a 2×2 factorial study with stimulation vs. nonstimulation and in vivo vs. IVP embryos, which is impractical in humans. In these ways, we could compare aneuploidy and mosaicism frequencies, within and across age groups. We would expect to find substantial chromosomal error rates (perhaps 20% or more) in embryos derived from IVM oocytes due to errors in nondisjunction as a result of the artificial conditions during meiosis in vitro. This would help to account for the low developmental competence of primate (monkey and human) IVM oocytes, and help to determine whether the high frequency of aneuploidy observed in oocytes and embryos of older women is inherent or if their oocytes are more susceptible to ART procedures.

CYTOGENETIC ANALYSIS OF RHESUS MACAQUE OOCYTES AND EMBRYOS

Aneuploidy analysis can be done in two ways. First, standard karyotyping analysis can be performed on metaphase II oocytes exhibiting a first polar body. Karyotyping was previously used to examine age-related defects in rhesus monkey oocytes (Schramm *et al.*, 2002). In that study, no statistically significant difference was found between young vs. old rhesus monkeys in aneuploidy frequency of oocytes. However, the number of oocytes examined was very small, totaling only 30 oocytes for both groups. We need to reexamine the question of whether aneuploidy increases with age in rhesus oocytes, using much larger numbers of oocytes obtained from ovaries excised at necropsy. The rhesus chromosome number is 42, and the homologies to the human karyotype are simple. There are two homologues of human chromosome 2 (HSA2), HSA14 and 15 as well as HSA 7 and 21, and HSA 20 and 22 are fused. Rhesus macaque BAC clones have now been generated in the laboratory of Dr. Leslie Lyons at the School of Veterinary Medicine, University of California-Davis. In collaboration with Dr. Lyons, our laboratory is trying to develop a macaque whole chromosome paint set. Meanwhile, we are developing three or four chromosome probes simultaneously, either by chromosome painting with human probes or by FISH with human BAC clones. Dr. Lyons' laboratory is making progress in developing a series of rhesus macaque FISH probes that we plan to compare against simple karyotyping methodologies using rhesus blood cells.

Interestingly, we have found that the AneuVysion® Assay (CEP 18, X, Y-alpha satellite, LSI 13 and 21) Multi-color Probe Panel from Vysis does not work on rhesus blood cells. Since these human centromeric probes from Vysis do not hybridize with highly repeated human satellite DNA sequences usually located at the centromeric region of the chromosome, Dr. Lyons' laboratory is now comparing repeat sequences in the monkey genome to the human genome. We found that Vysis LSI probes that consist of DNA probe sequences homologous to specific human genes or unique sequence FISH probes do hybridize quite well with human, chimpanzee and baboon as well as rhesus blood cell chromosomes (Figure 39.3).

In summary, because the FISH probes for detecting rhesus chromosomes are not fully developed yet, we recommend using standard karyotyping to ensure results. In a well-designed experiment, half of the oocytes, selected at random, from each cohort should be examined by karyotyping, while the other half is fertilized to study chromosome error rates in the embryos derived from the oocytes. After adequate FISH probe analysis methods become available for rhesus oocytes, then some oocytes should be examined in this way, to find if this is more suitable for future, larger-scale studies. Alternatively, for karyotype analysis, oocytes or embryo blastomeres can be processed and chromosomes prepared using methods previously described (Schramm and Bavister, 1999). Metaphase spreads are performed on mature (metaphase II) oocytes as described by Kamiguchi et al. (1993).

Aneuploidy-Causing Mechanisms

Mosaicism is defined as differences in chromosome numbers among blastomeres of the same embryo, that is, nondisjunction errors occurring during mitosis. We might expect to find substantial frequencies of mosaicism within macaque embryos, because this has been the experience with human embryos produced in vitro (Munne *et al.*, 2002). For any single embryo, a chromosomal segregation error during second meiosis will result in all cells being aneuploid. However, an error

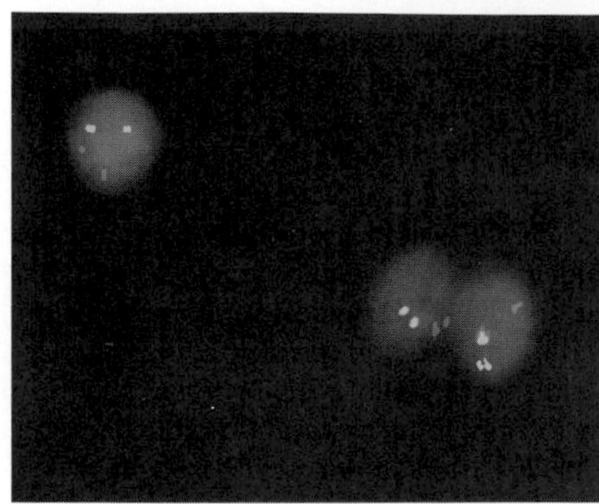

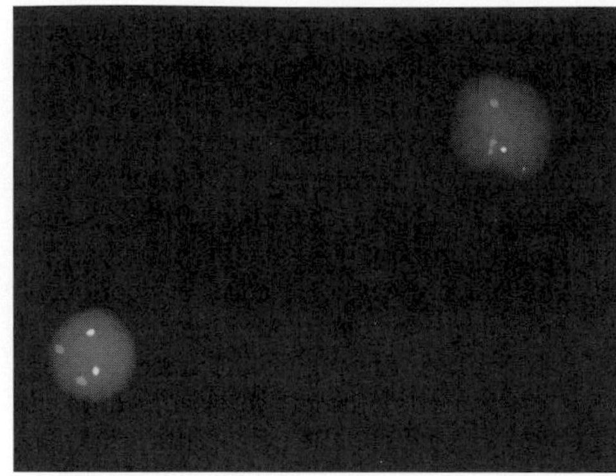

Figure 39.3 Human (left) and rhesus monkey (right) blood cell nuclei, stained with probes for LS12 and LS 21. From pilot experiments performed to determine if human probes can be used in fluorescent in situ hybridization (FISH) for monkey chromosomes. Unpublished data by Brenner *et al*.

during mitosis will result in mosaicism of varying levels depending upon the embryonic developmental level at which the error occurs. Therefore, if mosaicism is not present, any aneuploidies can be assumed to be due to meiotic nondisjunction. Since reports indicate that there is over 50% aneuploidy and 30% or more mosaicism in human embryos after IVF (Munne *et al*., 2002), we can expect that both anomalies will also be present in macaques. It is also likely that the frequency of aneuploidy increases with age of the animals. This was not found in the study reported by Schramm et al. (2002), but probably insufficient numbers of oocytes were examined in this study. Both higher numbers of oocytes need to be examined as well as using more animals to assess the true frequency of aneuploidy, and especially the effect of age on aneuploidy frequency needs to be examined more rigorously.

Cohorts of oocytes exhibiting high aneuploidy frequencies ought to produce embryos showing poor development, for two reasons: first, because from a logical viewpoint aneuploidy should be detrimental to normal embryo development; and second, because poor development of human embryos was correlated progressively with higher frequencies of chromosomal abnormalities in the embryos (Munne and Cohen, 1998). However, the logical expectation does not seem to always be correct. Some human embryos exhibiting chromosome defects can develop to the blastocyst stage and, it has been suggested, may even go to term after embryo transfer. We should be cautious about accepting the latter statement, because sampled aneuploid blastomeres may not faithfully represent the remaining cells in an embryo, due to mosaicism, while complete ploidy analysis requires destruction of the whole embryo, so how can aneuploidy be tightly correlated with embryo development? An advantage of using rhesus monkeys is that, following gonadotropin stimulation and oocyte collection, half of the oocytes can be randomly assigned to immediate chromosome analysis while the remainder are subjected to IVF and embryo culture, and then destructively analyzed for chromosome complements, as described above. This strategy, which is impractical in a human IVF clinic due to the primary goal of achieving pregnancy, allows the frequency of nondisjunction defects to be compared in meiosis vs. mitosis. In addition, the consequences of high aneuploidy frequency on embryo development can be evaluated. It is possible, however, that this experiment will show low frequencies of aneuploidy in stimulated oocytes and embryos derived from them, due to the fact that mostly young, fertile females are used, unlike the situation in human clinical patients. This outcome would indicate that monkeys are not a good model for assessing effects of aneuploidy on embryo development in infertile humans. This remains to be seen. However, monkeys could still be good models for investigating the etiology of aneuploidy in primate oocytes and embryos.

Another problem is that we should control for male aneuploidy because this can also contribute to chromosome defects in embryos. A high frequency in anomalies of the sex chromosomes was found in human spermatozoa (Martin *et al*., 1991). To control for this, we could assess spermatozoa, preferably from a known fertile male, in one of two ways. Using a variation of a technique used for analyzing human sperm aneuploidy rates (Martin *et al*., 1991), intracytoplasmic sperm injection (ICSI) could be used to inject monkey spermatozoa into zona-free hamster oocytes. The ooplasm will decondense chromatin and support formation of chromosomes for karyotyping. For this approach, ICSI is necessary because, unlike spermatozoa of many other species including humans, macaque spermatozoa do not readily fuse with the hamster oocyte membrane. In another approach, macaque spermatozoa could be chemically decondensed in vitro using established protocols (Spriggs *et al*., 1996). To avoid contributions from sperm chromosome defects when studying aneuploidy in oocytes, males should be rejected for IVF embryo production if their spermatozoa show more than 1 or 2% aneuploidy.

Mitochondria, Reproduction and Infertility

THE ROLE OF MITOCHONDRIA IN EMBRYO DEVELOPMENT

Mitochondria play a key role in the physiology of eukaryotic cells. They are important for mammalian oocyte and preimplantation embryo development, as well as for nuclear transplantation and stem cells (Bavister and Squirrell, 2000; Cummins, 2001a, 2002; Hiendleder and Wolf, 2003). This is not only due to the fundamental role of mitochondria in energy metabolism, but also because they are semi-autonomous organelles and each one contains one or several copies of its genome (mtDNA) that must be replicated during embryo development. In humans, the mitochondrial genome is a 16.6kb circular strand of DNA encoding 37 genes. These include 13 components of the oxidative phosphorylation (OXPHOS) pathway, two ribosomal RNAs and 22 transfer RNAs. The coding capacity of mtDNA is quite limited, because over 200 of the genes needed for mitochondrial function actually reside in the cell's nuclear genome (Cummins, 2001a). This indicates that most of the original mitochondrial genome has migrated to the cell nucleus, with only a small subset of genes remaining within the mitochondrion for OXPHOS control. Existence of this arrangement is verified by several mutations found either in the nuclear and/or mitochondrial genes that impair OXPHOS; potentially lethal disorders are often associated with these mutations (Thorburn and Dahl, 2001). As a result, we know that mitochondrial functions depend on cytoplasm–nucleus information exchange. This exchange is exerted through nuclear-encoded transcription factors, such as mitochondrial transcription factor A (TFAM), that regulate mitochondrial biogenesis and energy metabolic functions.

MIGRATION OF MITOCHONDRIA IN OOCYTES AND EMBRYOS

Data from our laboratory using hamsters and rhesus monkeys show that during fertilization, active mitochondria become unequally distributed in the oocyte cytoplasm. In general, active mitochondria relocate to surround the pronuclei (Barnett *et al.*, 1996, 1997; Squirrell *et al.*, 2003). In hamster oocytes, active mitochondria were homogeneously distributed in the oocyte cytoplasm before activation by spermatozoa, but a few hours later they began to translocate to the peripronuclear region (Squirrell, 2002; Squirrell *et al.*, 2003). This localization occurs naturally and is tightly correlated with embryo development competence in vitro, because culture conditions that disturb or block embryo development in vitro also disrupted the normal mitochondrial localization profile (Barnett *et al.*, 1997; Squirrell *et al.*, 2001; Ludwig *et al.*, 2001). Although we do not know whether this is a cause or effect relationship, the observation does suggest that caution is needed in designing culture conditions for IVP of embryos in ART.

We next studied rhesus monkey oocytes using multiphoton laser scanning microscopy (MPSLM; Squirrell *et al.*, 2003). During fertilization, oocytes exhibited a peripronuclear clustering of mitochondria, but this accumulation was not present throughout the entire period prior to syngamy. The duration ranged from <1 hr to 10 hr, with a mean of 3 hr. However, unlike in hamsters, the distribution of mitochondria became more homogeneous after fertilization. The localization profile of active mitochondria differed among oocytes from the same cohort. To understand possible relationships between mitochondrial distribution, especially pronuclear localization, and subsequent embryo development, macaque oocytes were labeled, then imaged, inseminated, imaged again and allowed to develop in separate culture drops. Mitochondrial localization in the oocytes was consistent with their competence to develop into blastocysts. Similar studies revealed a relationship between mitochondrial localization and competence in cattle oocytes (Krisher and Bavister, 1997, 1998). Mitochondria also relocalize to the perinuclear region in fertilized human oocytes, but data are insufficient to establish a link with development (Van Blerkom *et al.*, 2000; Sathananthan and Trounson, 2000).

IMPLICATIONS OF MITOCHONDRIAL ANOMALIES FOR ART

Mitochondrial dysfunction is suggested as a prime cause of low oocyte and embryo quality and hence the low efficiency of human ART on a per-embryo basis. Not surprisingly, attention has been drawn to possible effects of current ARTs on mitochondrial function. The coexistence of different mitochondrial genomes in the same cell is termed mitochondrial heteroplasmy. There is evidence that heteroplasmy in some infants resulted from "ooplasm transfer," a technique involving injection of ooplasm from oocytes from young women into oocytes from older women patients in an effort to improve their developmental competence (Cohen *et al.*, 1998). In this procedure, about 10% of the ooplasm from an oocyte of a presumptively fertile donor was microinjected into a recipient oocyte from an older, infertile patient with presumptively compromised oocyte quality (Cohen *et al.*, 1998). However, this transfer would introduce numerous cytoplasmic components into the recipient oocytes, including proteins and mRNAs as well as mitochondria and other organelles (Van Blerkom *et al.*, 1998). It is still unknown if injection of donor mitochondria can improve the quality of oocytes and embryos derived from them, although several babies were born after this procedure. The children resulting from IVF of these oocytes were found to be carrying mitochondria from both the donor and recipient, in varying proportions in different tissues.

Heteroplasmy also results from nuclear transfer—the fusion of somatic cells with enucleated oocytes (somatic cell nuclear transfer, SCNT)—in studies on cloned sheep, cattle and monkeys. All efforts to produce identical monkeys by SCNT have failed so far to produce cloned (identical) monkeys for biomedical research, but any success in this approach will have to contend with the problem of heteroplasmy. It may be that techniques such as ooplasm transfer, nuclear transfer and other approaches involving heteroplasmy perturb the normal interchanges between nuclear and mitochondrial genomes required for proper mtDNA replication, as described above. This could account for the low success of these technologies. Nevertheless, if ooplasm transfer or the reverse procedure, "pronuclear fusion" (see below), is ever to gain acceptance for treatment of infertility in the older patient, it seems that their safety as well as their efficacy must first be confirmed in monkeys.

Other approaches that may cause heteroplasmy or other mitochondrial problems include the transfer of oocyte nuclei (germinal vesicles) from oocytes of older women into enucleated oocytes of younger women, in efforts to allow older women to be the genetic mothers of their babies even though "oocyte donation" is used. In a related technique, the nucleus of an IVF oocyte is removed and injected into an enucleated donor oocyte ("pronuclear fusion"; Zhang *et al.*, 1999). Whether or not these techniques are effective for treatment of infertility in older patients, heteroplasmy is a concern, and possible effects of age on this condition cannot be discounted. In addition, because many of the genes required for mitochondrial function reside in the nucleus, mismatches between mitochondrial and nuclear genomes may cause problems in bioenergetics.

While mitochondria are strictly maternally inherited, paternally-derived mitochondrial are eliminated selectively during early fertilization and/or subsequent embryonic cell divisions (Sutovsky and Schatten, 2000; St. John, 2002). Nevertheless, there are some reports from human patients as well as in animals that occasionally paternal mitochondria escape the elimination process, which has sometimes resulted in severe pathologies (Cummins, 2001b). Because invasive techniques such as ICSI are becoming more prevalent in human ART, there is some concern that such techniques may increase the frequency of heteroplasmy. Paternal mitochondria can sometimes survive in abnormally fertilized embryos (St. John *et al.*, 1997). If spermatozoa carrying mitochondrial point mutations and deletions were introduced into an oocyte by ICSI, and mitochondria of such spermatozoa are not properly eliminated in the embryo, then there could be a possibility for inadvertent transmission of mitochondrial diseases and/or introduction of fertility problems. Because mechanisms of paternal mitochondrial elimination may differ across species, it is important that consequences of introducing sperm mtDNA mutations into embryos should be examined in an appropriate, nonhuman primate model such as the rhesus monkey using ICSI (Hewitson *et al.*, 2002).

Recently, transmission of paternal mitochondrial DNA into nonhuman primate offspring produced by embryonic cell nuclear transfer (ECNT) was described (St. John and Schatten, 2004). This process involves not only introduction of the blastomere nucleus but also a substantial volume of blastomere cytoplasm that includes remnants of mitochondria from the fertilizing spermatozoon. Thus, there is considerable risk of aberrant mtDNA transmission in ECNT. Nonhuman primate offspring produced by ECNT actually contained three mtDNA populations, derived from maternal mtDNA from the recipient oocyte, a different maternal mtDNA from the donor blastomere, and paternal mtDNA from the fertilizing spermatozoon. This outcome represents another example of multiparental mtDNA heteroplasmy.

Mitochondrial Point Mutations in the Control Region and Aging

RELATIONSHIP BETWEEN mtDNA MUTATIONS AND OOCYTE COMPETENCE

The origin and mechanism of mutant mtDNA accumulation (up to 99% in some tissues) in patients with mitochondrial diseases are still debatable. Several mutations of mitochondrial DNA occur either as sporadic large-scale rearrangements (deletions and duplications) or maternally inherited point mutations, which have been associated with defined clinical syndromes. Point mutations of mtDNA can occur in several different regions of the mitochondrial genome. Also, the severity of the clinical and biochemical phenotype correlates with the degree of mtDNA heteroplasmy in the somatic tissues. Mitochondrial mutations and rearrangements in oocytes and preimplantation embryos and resulting mitochondrial dysfunction may have important implications for embryo development. Numerous laboratories have detected a particular mtDNA mutation called the "common deletion," ΔmtDNA4977, in human oocytes at a frequency of 30 to 50% (Brenner *et al.*, 1998; Barritt *et al.*, 1999; Keefe *et al.*, 1995). In our laboratory, this mutation was found in 30 to 50% of human oocytes. Additionally, 23 novel mtDNA rearrangements have been identified in human oocytes and embryos (Barritt *et al.*, 1999). Using a nested PCR strategy, 51% of human oocytes and 32% of embryos exhibited mtDNA rearrangements, while multiple rearrangements were detected in 31% of oocytes and 14% of embryos. However, the important question is whether the mutational load actually reflects the quality of affected oocytes.

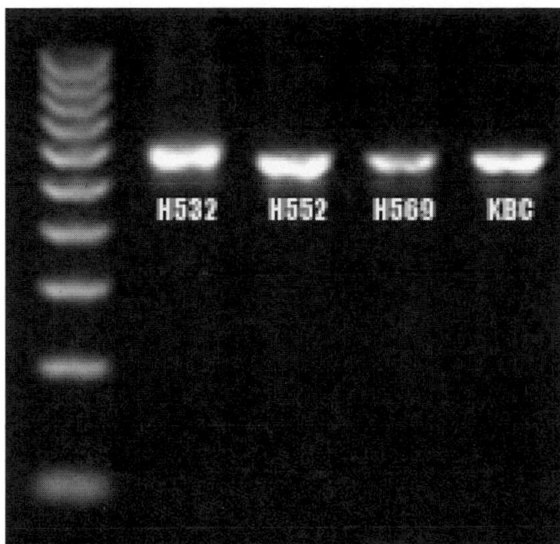

Figure 39.4 Mitochondrial hypervariable D-loop 600 bp PCR amplicon from 3 female and 1 male rhesus macaques. Samples were run on a 1.0% agarose gel at a constant voltage of 70V for 45 min. Initial primer sets have been designed, and preliminary PCR demonstrated positive amplification of a ~600 bp region of the mitochondrial D-loop of Indian origin rhesus macaques. We have now cloned and DNA sequenced the complete 1600 bp *M. mulatta* mitochondrial DNA, D-loop hypervariable region (see Figure 39.5). Unpublished data by Brenner *et al.*

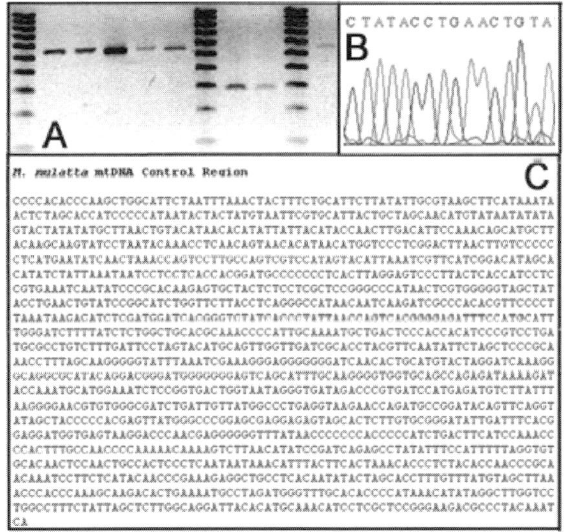

Figure 39.5 A. Mitochondrial hypervariable D-loop PCR amplicons from monkey, cat and bovine. Lanes 1, 7, 10: 100 bp ladder. Lanes 2-4: *M. mulatta*. Lanes 5, 6: M. nemestrina. Lanes 8, 9: *F. catus;* Lane 11: B. taurus. B. DNA chromatogram of *M. mulatta* mitochondrial control region. C. *M. mulatta* mitochondrial DNA, D-loop hypervariable region (1600 bp). Unpublished data by Brenner *et al.*

Since all embryonic stem (ES) cell lines are derived from fertilized oocytes, it is expected that such oocyte defects are also present in these cells, and because virtually all primate (monkey and human) oocytes used in research or IVF clinics come from females stimulated with gonadotropins, which may increase mtDNA error frequencies, we must be cautious about heavily investing in research using this source of material.

Several mtDNA mutations appear in somatic tissues at a higher frequency in older than in younger subjects. Some of these mutations are associated with overt pathologies while others are not. A key question is, Do mitochondrial DNA mutations affect oocyte quality and developmental capacity? This raises a related question: because mtDNA mutations accumulate in oocytes with increasing age of the patient, do these errors play a significant role in age-related loss of fertility? Our laboratory has investigated whether there is an age-dependent, oocyte-specific point mutation in the mtDNA control region of human oocytes. Preliminary data showed that a prevalent point mutation at bp position 414 in the mitochondrial genome may preferentially accumulate with age in human oocytes (Barritt *et al.*, 2000).

EVALUATION OF MITOCHONDRIAL COPY NUMBER, DELETIONS AND MUTATIONS AS MARKERS OF OOCYTE COMPETENCE

Accumulation of mtDNA mutations in the mitochondrial genome may be inherent in oocytes and in embryos derived from them, especially those derived using IVP (see above), and could contribute to impaired metabolic function and thus to developmental incompetence (Keefe *et al.*, 1995; Brenner *et al.*, 1998; Barritt *et al.*, 1999, 2000). Mutations may result in diminished ATP content, leading to defects such as slow or arrested cell division, apoptosis, numerical chromosomal abnormalities such as aneuploidy, and ultimately failure to develop or establish pregnancy (Barnett *et al.*, 1997; Van Blerkom *et al.*, 1995, 2001). But any adverse affect of mtDNA mutations associated with respiratory function would depend upon the magnitude of the mutant population (mutant load). This load could increase with each embryo cell division. Functional defects could also result from asymmetrical mitochondrial distribution following cell division, which could lead to disproportionate mitochondrial inheritance and perhaps thereby produce cells with diminished ATP-generating capacity. This type of error could be related to mitochondrial distribution in the cell (see Migration of Mitochondria in Oocytes and Embryos) (Van Blerkom *et al.*, 1995, 2000). Mitochondria are not only the major site of ATP production in cells but also an important source of reactive oxygen species (ROS) under certain pathological conditions. Because mitochondrial DNA (mtDNA) in the mitochondrial matrix is exposed to ROS that leak from the respiratory chain, this extranuclear genome is prone to mutations. Therefore, the mitochondrial genome is a rich site for both deletions and mutations.

MITOCHONDRIAL COPY NUMBERS IN PRIMATE OOCYTES

The number of mitochondrial genomes in human oocytes has been estimated by fluorescent rapid cycle DNA amplification, a highly sensitive technique for quantifying mtDNA copy numbers in individual cells (Steuerwald *et al.*, 2000). From the log–linear phase of amplification during real-time PCR, preliminary results showed 90,000–1,000,000 copies of mtDNA in each human oocyte (Steuerwald *et al.*, 1999, 2000). The average mtDNA copy number in over 70 human oocytes during maturation was 779,000 + 240,000 (range 240,000–1,550,000) (Barritt *et al.*, 2000). Age-related differences were not seen (Steuerwald *et al.*, 2000; Barritt, unpublished results). The relationship between copy number and function (ATP production) remains to be investigated. However, a minimum amount of mitochondrial activity must be necessary for normal cell functions (Barnett and Bavister, 1996; Van Blerkom *et al.*, 1995, 2000). Perhaps the total numbers of mitochondria are not as relevant as the proportion of functional mitochondria in the cell, indicative of ATP production, or their distribution profile. Such detailed analyses have not yet been conducted with monkey oocytes, and it will be informative to obtain this information to establish whether the monkey is a faithful model for the human in this respect. However, as mentioned previously, there are inherent differences between human and monkey IVP, since studies in humans are usually done with discarded oocytes or embryos, unlike in monkeys, while monkey embryo research generally uses fertile individuals vs. infertile humans.

MITOCHONDRIAL MUTATIONS IN PRIMATE OOCYTES

One of the most promising leads related to mitochondrial mutations in primate oocytes has been found in the control region of the mitochondrial genome. The main control region of mtDNA, or the D-loop, is adjacent to transcription promoters, is the most variable portion of the human mitochondrial genome, may contain heteroplasmic point mutations, and is responsible for DNA replication. Our laboratory showed that an oocyte-specific mtDNA point mutation occurs frequently in oocytes of some women (Barritt *et al.*, 2000; Michikawa *et al.*, 1999) and appeared to be more prevalent in the oocytes of women of advanced reproductive age. This point mutation represents a single base pair transversion of a thymine (T) to guanine (G) at base pair 414 (T414G) in the mitochondrial genome. DNA sequence analysis confirmed this mutation in only one oocyte from 11 patients aged 26 to 36 ($n = 23$), compared to 17 oocytes from 10 patients aged 37 to 42 ($n = 43$). The younger group exhibited this mtDNA point mutation in only 4% of oocytes compared to 40% from the older group ($p < 0.01$). Therefore, single human oocytes may contain the mtDNA T414G transversion point mutation, which accumulates with age. The potential significance of this point mutation may be its correlation with reproductive senescence or ovarian reserve. Furthermore, other oocyte-specific mutations may also be present in the mitochondrial control region and thus may be responsible for impaired transcription and replication regulation. If these potentially high copy number point mutations can be confirmed by more extensive studies in normal oocytes from aging primates, this could be an important and unrecognized factor in pregnancy outcome because mitochondrial replication is believed not to begin until after implantation. Therefore, replication defects would not be expected to compromise preimplantation development, but depending upon mutant load, could manifest as postimplantation death. These data imply that ES cell lines derived from embryos made with oocytes from older individuals (human or monkey) may exhibit impaired mitochondrial function.

ES Cells from Primate Blastocysts Produced in vivo vs. in vitro, and Aging

Thus far, we have discussed aging in the sense of changes occurring in the fertility of an individual female primate as she becomes older. But in another sense, aging is a property of individual cells, and this not only may underlie age-related events in the individual but also account for functional changes in a cell as it reaches the end of its life. In this context, aging is a key aspect of cultured cells, including ES cells. We believe that a major focus on mitochondria is warranted in ES cell studies. A sufficient number of normal mitochondria is required in somatic cells to support normal functions. A high frequency of genetically abnormal mitochondria (mutational load) could reduce the number of functional mitochondria, leading to poor cell performance, manifested as slow cell divisions, karyotypic anomalies, and/or perturbation of mitochondrial distribution profiles. Moreover, the presence of mtDNA anomalies may be increased in cell lines derived from in vitro produced embryos compared with embryos produced in vivo.

Mitochondria play a key role in early development, though one that is far from being fully understood (Barnett and Bavister, 1996; Van Blerkom *et al.*, 2000; Bavister and Squirrell, 2000; Barnett *et al.*, 1996; Ludwig *et al.*, 2001). By analogy with their fundamental metabolic roles in somatic cells (Yaffe, 1999), we can expect that mitochondria have similar importance in the inner cell mass (ICM) of blastocysts and in the ES cells derived from them, which are primordial somatic cells. Culture conditions that affect mitochondrial activity, such as providing oxidizable substrates, during oocyte maturation or early cleavage stages can profoundly alter embryo development in several species including nonhuman primates (McKiernan *et al.*, 1991; Rose-Hellekant *et al.*, 1998; Krisher and Bavister, 1999; Zheng *et al.*, 2001,

2002). Mitochondria sequester cytoplasmic calcium, and "uncoupling" them caused apoptotic cell death in embryos (Liu *et al.*, 2001). Moreover, mitochondrial structure and activity change strikingly during preimplantation development, suggesting an increasingly important role once differentiation (blastocele formation) occurs. Some somatic cells such as fibroblasts and neurons also exhibit a pronounced clustering of active mitochondria (Yaffe, 1999; Mattson and Partin, 1999). In some cells, the distribution of mitochondria is under genetic control (Yaffe, 1999). In fibroblasts, mitochondria cluster around the nucleus while peripheral cytoplasm is devoid of mitochondria, the same profile as in fertilizing oocytes and early preimplantation embryos (Yaffe, 1999; Barnett *et al.*, 1996; Squirrell *et al.*, 2003). In neurons, mitochondrial clustering is involved in establishing cell polarity and disrupting their distribution results in loss of polarity (Mattson and Partin, 1999).

In view of these observations on preimplantation embryos and on somatic cells, it seems very likely that clustering (nonrandom distribution) of mitochondria occurs in primate ES cells and thus may be important for their normal functions. If so, the distribution profile(s) could become a simple marker of ES cell competence, as well as an indicator of impending differentiation. We should examine primate (human and monkey) ES cells to determine this. Next, we should ascertain if mitochondrial localization patterns are different in ES cells from IVP vs. in vivo produced blastocysts, because most of the IVP embryos are nonviable, while we expect most blastocysts produced in vivo to be viable. This difference should be reflected in ES cell quality and functional competence. However, because of the complete lack of human embryos produced in vivo, this comparative study can only be done in a suitable nonhuman primate model, such as the rhesus monkey, in which protocols both for IVP and for flushing uteri of mated animals have been established (Schramm and Bavister, 1996; Wolfgang *et al.*, 2001). Once this study has been completed, we can move on to examination of effects of aging, in both senses of the term: (i) effects of age of the individual on mitochondrial localization (and other aspects such as mtDNA errors as described above) in ES cells from IVP and in vivo produced embryos, and (ii) effects of aging of the ES cells in culture (i.e., increasing passage numbers) on these parameters.

Conclusions

The reproductive physiology and embryology of the rhesus monkey make this species a good model for examining the etiology of reproductive failure in humans. In addition, because this is a long-lived species, we would expect that age-related impairment of infertility will have similar causes to that seen in humans. A great advantage of using rhesus monkeys is that it is possible, albeit with considerable difficulty, to collect normally-developing embryos from the female reproductive tract. These represent the most normal primate embryos available, and are thus invaluable for providing comparative data against which we can assess cellular and molecular parameters of IVP embryos. This advantage also applies to embryonic stem cells, both human and macaque, for which some kind of benchmark is greatly needed. Much attention has been focused on aneuploidy frequencies in human IVP embryos, both to explain the lack of viability in many human IVP embryos and to understand why the frequency of this anomaly appears to be so high. We propose that IVP macaque embryos are more suitable for addressing the latter question, because they can all be destroyed to obtain the maximum amount of information, whereas in humans, usually only discard oocytes and reject embryos are available for research. We believe that it is important to study mitochondria in oocytes and embryos, as well as in ES cells, because defects in these important organelles are likely to contribute to lack of developmental and functional competence. Both the bioenergetic function and the genomic aspects of mitochondria should be examined, in order to gain better understanding of infertility caused by oocyte incompetence, and we suggest that these two properties may be functionally linked. In conclusion, using rhesus monkeys for well-designed experimental studies is likely to provide insights into reasons for human infertility and age-related loss of fertility, and also to supply valuable information on embryonic stem cell culture and differentiation.

ACKNOWLEDGMENTS

We are grateful to the National Institutes of Health NCRR and NICHD for supporting parts of our studies mentioned in this chapter, through grants no. RR15395, HD046553 and HD04596.

REFERENCES

Barnett, D.K. and Bavister, B.D. (1996). What is the relationship between the metabolism of preimplantation embryos and their development *in vitro*? *Mol. Reprod. Dev. 43*, 105–133.

Barnett, D.K., Clayton, M.K., Kimura, J. and Bavister, B.D. (1997). Glucose and phosphate toxicity in hamster preimplantation embryos involves disruption of cellular organization, including distribution of active mitochondria. *Mol. Reprod. Dev. 48*, 227–237.

Barnett, D.K., Kimura, J. and Bavister, B.D. (1996). Translocation of active mitochondria during hamster preimplantation embryo development studied by confocal laser scanning microscopy. *Dev. Dynamics 205*, 64–72.

Barritt, J.A., Brenner, C.A., Willadsen, S. and Cohen, J. (2000). Spontaneous and artificial changes in human ooplasmic mitochondria. *Hum. Reprod. 15*, 207–217.

Barritt, J.A., Brenner, C.A., Cohen, J. and Matt, D.W. (1999). Mitochondrial DNA rearrangements in human oocytes and embryos. *Mol. Hum. Reprod. 5*, 927–933.

Barritt, J.A., Cohen, J. and Brenner, C.A. (2000). Mitochondrial DNA point mutation in human oocytes is associated with maternal age. *Reprod. Biomed. Online 1*, 96–100.

Bavister, B.D. (1995). Culture of pre-implantation embryos: Facts and artifacts. *Hum. Reprod. Update 1*, 91–148.

Bavister, B.D. (2004). ARTs in action in nonhuman primates: Symposium summary—Advances and remaining issues. *Reprod. Biol. Endocrinol. 2*, 43–50.

Bavister, B.D. and Boatman, D.E. (1993). IVF in non-human primates: Current status and future directions. In *In Vitro Fertilization and Embryo Transfer in Primates* (R.M. Brenner, D.P. Wolf and R.L. Stouffer, eds.), pp. 30–45. Springer-Verlag, New York.

Bavister, B.D., Boatman, D.E., Leibfried, M.L., Loose, M. and Vernon, M.W. (1983). Fertilization and cleavage of rhesus monkey oocytes *in vitro*. *Biol. Reprod. 28*, 983–999.

Bavister, B.D., Boatman, D.E., Collins, K., Dierschke, D.J. and Eisele, S.G. (1984). Birth of rhesus monkey infant after *in vitro* fertilization and non-surgical embryo transfer. *Proc. Natl. Acad. Sci. U.S.A. 81*, 2218–2222.

Bavister, B.D. and Brenner, C.A. (2004). How can basic science help human ART? *The Clinical Embryologist 7*, 6–11.

Bavister, B.D., Dees, H.C. and Schultz, R.D. (1986). Refractoriness of rhesus monkeys to repeat ovarian stimulation by exogenous gonadotropins is caused by non-precipitating antibodies. *Am. J. Reprod. Immunol. Microbiol. 11*, 11–16.

Bavister, B.D. and Squirrell, J. (2000). Mitochondrial distribution and function in oocytes and early embryos. *Hum. Reprod. 15*, 189–198.

Bean, C.J., Hassold, T.J., Judis, L. and Hunt, P.A. (2002). Fertilization *in vitro* increases non-disjunction during early cleavage divisions in a mouse model system. *Hum. Reprod. 17*, 2362–2367.

Boatman, D.E. and Bavister, B.D. (1984). Stimulation of rhesus monkey sperm capacitation by cyclic nucleotide mediators. *J. Reprod. Fertil. 77*, 357–366.

Boatman, D.E., Morgan, P.M. and Bavister, B.D. (1986). Variables affecting the yield and developmental potential embryos following superstimulation and *in vitro* fertilization in rhesus monkeys. *Gamete Res. 13*, 327–338.

Brenner, C.A., Wolny, Y.M., Barrit, J.A., Matt, D.W., Munne, S. and Cohen, J. (1998). Mitochondrial DNA deletions in human oocytes and embryos. *Mol. Hum. Reprod. 4*, 887–892.

Buster, J.E., Bustillo, M., Rodi, I.A., Cohen, S.W., Hamilton, M., Simon, J.A., *et al.* (1985). Biologic and morphologic development of donated human ova recovered by nonsurgical uterine lavage. *Am. J. Obstet. Gynecol. 153*, 211–217.

Cohen, J., Scott, R., Alikani, M., Schimmel, T., Munne, S., Levron, J., *et al.* (1998). Ooplasmic transfer in mature human oocytes. *Mol. Hum. Reprod. 4*, 269–280.

Cummins, J. (2001a). Mitochondria: potential roles in embryogenesis and nucleocytoplasmic transfer. *Hum. Reprod. Update 7*, 217–228.

Cummins, J.M. (2001b). Cytoplasmic inheritance and its implications for animal biotechnology. *Theriogenology 55*, 1381–1399.

Cummins, J.M. (2002). The role of maternal mitochondria during oogenesis, fertilization, and embryogenesis. *Reprod. Biomed. Online 4*, 176–182.

Faddy, M.J. and Gosden, R.G. (1996). A model confirming the decline in follicle numbers to the age of menopause in women. *Hum. Reprod. 11*, 1484–1486.

Gearheart, W.W., Smith, C. and Teepker, G. (1989). Multiple ovulation and embryo manipulation in the improvement of beef cattle: Relative theoretical rates of genetic change. *J. Anim. Sci. 67*, 2863–2871.

Gonzales, D.S. and Bavister, B.D. (1995). *Zona pellucida* escape by hamster blastocysts *in vitro* is delayed and morphologically different compared with zona escape in vivo. *Biol. Reprod. 52*, 470–480.

Gras, L., McBain, J., Trounson, A. and Kola, I. (1992). The incidence of chromosomal aneuploidy in stimulated and unstimulated (natural) uninseminated human oocytes. *Hum. Reprod. 7*, 1396–1401.

Hansen, K.R., Morris, J.L., Thyer, A.C. and Soules, M.R. (2003). Reproductive aging and variability in the ovarian antral follicle count: Application in the clinical setting. *Fertil. Steril. 80*, 577–583.

Hewitson, L., Simerly, C.R. and Schatten, G. (2002). Fate of sperm components during assisted reproduction: Implications for infertility. *Hum. Fertil. 5*, 110–116.

Hiendleder, S. and Wolf, E. (2003). The mitochondrial genome in embryo technologies. *Reprod. Domest. Anim. 38*, 290–304.

Hughes, E.G., Robertson, D.M., Handelsman, D.J., Jayward, S., Healy, D.L. and de Kretser, D.M. (1990). Inhibin and estradiol responses to ovarian hyperstimulation: Effects of age and predictive value for *in vitro* fertilization outcome. *J. Clin. Endocrinol. Metab. 70*, 358–364.

Hunt, P.A. and Hassold, T.J. (2002). Sex matters in meiosis. *Science 296*, 2181–2183.

Hunt, P.A., Koehler, K.E., Susiarjo, M., Hodges, C.A., Ilagan, A., Voigt, R.C., *et al.* (2003). Bisphenol A exposure causes meiotic aneuploidy in the female mouse. *Curr. Biol. 13*, 546–553.

Kamiguchi, Y., Rosenbusch, B., Sterzik, K. and Mikamo, K. (1993). Chromosomal analysis of unfertilized human oocytes prepared by a gradual fixation-air drying method. *Hum. Genet. 90*, 533–541.

Keefe, D.L., Niven-Fairchild, T., Powell, S. and Buradagurna, S. (1995). Mitochondrial deoxyribonucleic acid deletion in oocytes and reproductive aging in women. *Fertil. Steril. 64*, 577–583.

Krisher, R.L. and Bavister, B.D. (1997). Correlation of mitochondrial organization with developmental competence in bovine oocytes matured *in vitro*. *Biol. Reprod. 556*, 602.

Krisher, R.L. and Bavister, B.D. (1998). Responses of oocytes and embryos to the culture environment. *Theriogenology 49*, 103–114.

Krisher, R.L. and Bavister, B.D. (1999). Enhanced glycolysis after maturation of bovine oocytes *in vitro* is associated with increased developmental competence. *Molec. Reprod. Dev. 53*, 19–26.

Liu, L., Hammar, K., Smith, P.J., Inoue, S. and Keefe, D. (2001). Mitochondrial modulation of calcium signaling at the intiation of development. *Cell Calcium 30*, 423–433.

Ludwig, T.E., Squirrell J.M., Palmenberg, A.C. and Bavister, B.D. (2001). Relationship between development, metabolism and mitochondrial organization in 2-cell hamster embryos in the presence of low levels of phosphate. *Biol. Reprod. 65*, 1648–1654.

Macklon, N.S. and Fauser, B.C. (1999). Aspects of ovarian follicle development throughout life. *Horm. Res. 52*, 161–170.

Martin, R.H., Ko, E. and Rademaker, A. (1991). Distribution of aneuploidy in human gametes: Comparison between human sperm and oocytes. *Am. J. Med. Genet. 39*, 321–331.

Mattson, M.P. and Partin, P. (1999). Evidence for mitochondrial control of neuronal myopathy. *J. Neurosci. Res. 56*, 8–20.

McKiernan, S.H., Bavister, B.D. and Tasca, R.J. (1991). Energy substrate requirements for in-vitro development of hamster 1- and 2- cell embryos to the blastocyst stage. *Hum. Reprod. 6*, 64–75.

Michikawa, Y., Mazzucchelli, F., Bresolin, N., Scarlato, G. and Attardi, G. (1999). Aging-dependent large accumulation of point mutation in the human mtDNA control region for replication. *Science 286*, 774–779.

Morgan, H.D., Santos, F., Green, K., Dean, W. and Reik, W. (2005). Epigenetic reprogramming in mammals. *Hum. Mol. Genet. 14 Suppl. 1*, R47–R58.

Munne, S. and Cohen, J. (1998). Chromosome abnormalities in human embryos. *Hum. Reprod. Update 4*, 842–855.

Munne, S., Sandalinas, M., Escudero, T., Marquez, C. and Cohen, J. (2002). Chromosome mosaicism in cleavage-stage human embryos: Evidence of a maternal age effect. *Reprod. Biomed. Online 4*, 223–232.

Nichols, S.M., Bavister, B.D., Brenner, C.A., Didier, P.J., Harrison, R.M. and Kubisch, H.M. (2005). Ovarian senescence in the rhesus macaque (*Macaca mulatta*). *Hum. Reprod. 20*, 79–83.

Olivennes, F. and Frydman, R. (1998). Friendly IVF: The way of the future? *Hum. Reprod. 13*, 1121–1124.

Pellestor, F. Andreo, B., Arnal, F., Humeau, C. and Demaille, J. (2003). Maternal aging and chromosomal abnormalities: New data drawn from *in vitro* unfertilized human oocytes. *Hum. Genet. 112*, 195–203.

Pohl, C.R., Richardson, D.W., Marshall, G. and Knobil, E. (1982). Mode of action of progesterone in the blockade of gonadotropin surges in the rhesus macaque. *Endocrinology 110*, 1454–1455.

Rose-Hellekant, T.A., Libersky-Williamson, E.A. and Bavister, B.D. (1998). Energy substrates and amino acids provided during *in vitro* maturation of bovine oocytes alter acquisition of developmental competence. *Zygote 6*, 285–294.

Santoro, N. (2002). The menopause transition: An update. *Hum. Reprod. 8*, 155–160.

Sathananthan, A.H. and Trounson, A.O. (2000). Mitochondrial morphology during preimplantational human embryogenesis. *Hum. Reprod. 15*, 148–159.

Schramm, R.D. and Bavister, B.D. (1996). Development of *in vitro* fertilized primate embryos into blastocysts in chemically-defined, protein-free culture medium. *Hum. Reprod. 11*, 1690–1697.

Schramm, R.D. and Bavister, B.D. (1999). A macaque model for studying mechanisms controlling oocyte development and maturation in primates. *Hum. Reprod. 14*, 2544–2555

Schramm, R.D., Paprocki, A.M. and Bavister, B.D. (2002). Features associated with reproductive aging in female rhesus monkeys. *Hum. Reprod. 17*, 1597–1603.

Shideler, S.E., Gee, N.A., Chen, J. and Lasley, B.L. (2001). Estrogen and progesterone metabolites and follicle-stimulating hormone in the aged macaque female. *Biol. Reprod. 65*, 1718–1725.

Spriggs, E.L., Rademaker, A.W. and Martin, R.H. (1996). Aneuploidy in human sperm: the use of multicolor FISH to test various theories of nondisjunction. *Am. J. Hum. Genet. 58*, 356–362.

Squirrell, J.M. (2002). Multiphoton microscopy for imaging mammalian embryos. In *Assessment of Mammalian Embryo Quality: Invasive and Non-Invasive Techniques* (A. Van Soom, M.L. Boerjan eds.), pp. 195–217. Kluwer Academic Press, Dordrecht, The Netherlands.

Squirrell, J.M., Lane, M. and Bavister, B.D. (2001). Altering intracellular pH disrupts development and cellular organization in preimplantation hamster embryos. *Biol. Reprod. 64*, 1845–1854.

Squirrell, J., Schramm, R.D., Paprocki, A.M., Wokosin, D.L. and Bavister, B.D. (2003). Imaging mitochondrial organization in living primate oocytes and embryos using multiphoton microscopy. *Microsc. Microanal. 9*, 190–201.

St. John, J.C. (2002). The transmission of mitochondrial DNA following assisted reproductive techniques. *Theriogenology 57*, 109–123.

St. John, J.C., Cooke, I.D. and Barratt, C.L. (1997). Mitochondrial mutations and male infertility. *Nature Med. 3*, 124–125.

St. John, J.C. and Schatten, G. (2004). Paternal mitochondrial DNA transmission during nonhuman primate nuclear transfer. *Genetics 167*, 897–905.

Steuerwald, N., Cohen, J., Herrera, R.J. and Brenner, C.A. (1999). Analysis of gene expression in single oocytes and embryos by real-time rapid cycle fluorescence monitored RT-PCR. *Mol. Hum. Reprod. 5*, 1034–1039.

Steuerwald, N., Cohen, J., Herrera, R.J. and Brenner, C.A. (2000). Quantification of mRNA in single oocytes and embryos by real-time rapid cycle fluorescence monitored RT-PCR. *Mol. Hum. Reprod. 6*, 448–453.

Sutovsky, P. and Schatten, G. (2000). Paternal contributions to the mammalian zygote: Fertilization after sperm-egg fusion. *Intl. Rev. Cytol. 195*, 1–65.

Thorburn, D.R. and Dahl, H.H. (2001). Mitochondrial disorders: Genetics, counseling, prenatal diagnosis and reproductive options. *Am. J. Med. Genet. 106*, 102–114.

Van Blerkom, J., Davis, P. and Alexander, S. (2000). Differential mitochondrial distribution in human pronuclear embryos leads to disproportinate inheritance between bloastomeres: Relationship to microtubular organization, ATP content and competence. *Hum. Reprod. 15*, 2621–2633.

Van Blerkom, J., Davis, P. and Alexander, S. (2001). A microscopic and biochemical study of fragmentation phenotypes in stage-appropriate human embryos. *Hum. Reprod. 16*, 719–729.

Van Blerkom, J., Davis, P. and Lee, J. (1995). ATP content and developmental potential and outcome after in-vitro fertilization and embryo transfer. *Hum. Reprod. 10*, 415–424.

Van Blerkom, J., Sinclair, J. and Davis, P. (1998). Mitochondrial transfer between oocytes: Potential implications of mitochondrial donation and the issue of heteroplasmy. *Hum. Reprod. 13*, 2857–2868.

Walker, M.L. (1995). Menopause in female rhesus monkeys. *Am. J. Primatol. 35*, 59–71.

Wolfgang, M.J., Eisele, S.G., Knowles, L., Browne, M.A., Schotzko, M.L. and Golos, T.G. (2001). Pregnancy and live birth from nonsurgical transfer of *in vivo*- and *in vitro*-produced blastocysts in the rhesus monkey. *J. Med. Primatol. 30*, 148–155.

Wright, V.C., Schieve, L.A., Reynolds, M.A. and Jeng, G. (2003). Assisted reproductive technology surveillance—United States, 2000. *MMWR Surveill. Summ. 52*, 1–16.

Yaffe, M.P. (1999). The machinery of mitochondrial inheritance and behavior. *Science 283*, 1493–1497.

Zhang, J., Wang, C.W., Krey, L., Liu, H., Meng, L., Blaszczyk, A., *et al.* (1999). In vitro maturation of human preovulatory oocytes reconstructed by germinal vesicle transfer. *Fertil. Steril. 71*, 726–731.

Zheng, P., Bavister, B.D. and Ji, W. (2001). Energy substrate requirements for *in vitro* maturation of oocytes from unstimulated adult rhesus monkeys. *Mol. Reprod. Dev. 58*, 348–355.

Zheng, P., Si, W., Bavister, B.D. and Ji, W. (2002). Amino acid requirements for maturation of rhesus monkey oocytes in culture. *Reproduction 124*, 515–522.

40

Neurobiology of the Aging Brain

Carlo Bertoni-Freddari, Patrizia Fattoretti, Tiziana Casoli, and Giuseppina Di Stefano

Different anatomical, histological, cellular, and subcellular alterations occur in the human brain during aging. Because of this wide variety of changes, often masked by compensating reactions, the identification of clear-cut decays due to age may constitute a difficult task. In the elderly, brain volume and weight decrease because of an insignificant loss of neurons, dendritic atrophy, and glial cells degeneration. Damage of blood vessels, due to atherosclerosis and amyloid angiopathy, by reducing brain blood perfusion, may play a role in neuronal, glial, and dendritic degenerative phenomena. Impaired cellular membrane turnover leads to accumulation of age pigments or lipofuscin. Loss of synapses, paired with an imbalance of neurotransmitter systems, occurs in physiological and, to a higher degree, pathological aging.

Brain energy metabolism also declines in aging, which involves a decay in the mitochondrial metabolic competence that can be considered an unfavorable condition affecting several other processes such as calcium homeostasis and the development of SP and NFT. Nonhuman primates and transgenic mice, presently adopted as animal models to investigate human brain aging and AD, may further our understanding of the mechanisms underlying the formation of Alzheimer-like alterations, and may help to set up intervention strategies leading to an increase of the percent of cognitive intact and successfully aged subjects.

Introduction

A well-accepted definition of aging is that it is a time-related progressive loss in the cell capacity to maintain homeostasis. With advancing age, somatic changes come into being because the persistent action of stress conditions is not fully counteracted by cellular repair functions, thus resulting in alterations of organ and system functions. A typical inherent feature of aging is heterogeneity; that is, in addition to genetic individual variability vs. physiological values, vitality is markedly influenced by different lifestyles (Rowe and Kahn, 1987). Thus some elderly individuals age successfully since their aging parameters fall within the adult range; others typically show marked declines of some functions. With specific reference to the brain, the heterogeneity existing among individuals and the different groups of neurons must also be considered when looking for the potential factors and/or the causative events leading to age-related alterations. In this context, it must be stressed that brain aging represents a condition in which pathological changes exist without clinically evident manifestations. At variance with other organs, where the functional and structural units are repeated, the brain is a composite assembly of groups of cells with different metabolic features and functional tasks. Deterioration of function occurs when the number of neurons or their connections decreases below a critical reserve level, and coping with environmental stimulation is seriously hampered. Moreover, the well-documented brain's plastic condition plays a critical role in the balance between deteriorative events and compensating reactions, thus contributing to mask significant changes and to delay decline of function.

In this chapter, we will consider the age-related alterations occurring in the brain on different systems, at cellular and subcellular levels, with the aim to provide a comprehensive view of the many factors and interdependent mechanisms involved in such a multifactorial process.

Brain Atrophy and Neuron Loss

A significant decrease in brain weight is a widely documented sign of aging. In neurologically normal elderly individuals, it has been estimated that this decrease begins at the age of 60 years and proceeds at a rate of 2 to 3 grams/year. Considering the average brain weights of adult men (1400 g) and women (1250 g), by the age of 80, an overall reduction of about 3 to 5% has occurred. In addition to brain weight another more reliable measurement of the extent of the brain macroscopic decline in elderly subjects is the ratio between brain and skull volume, which is reported to remain constant around the value of 95% up to the age of 60, but decreases to 80% beyond 90 years of age. Widening of sulci and enlargement of ventriculi are also estimations accounting for an age-related brain atrophy and are reported to progress according to the reduction in brain weight. It has been estimated that the average volume of the lateral and third ventricles undergoes a fourfold increase in elderly over 60 when compared with young subjects between 13 and 19.

Studies in vivo by imaging methodologies have confirmed this data obtained from autopsy studies, and have shown a great individual variability, suggesting that age-related changes, at least at macroscopic level, may be significantly influenced by genetic determinants and environmental factors, first of all the very specific lifestyle of each individual. During the past two decades, neuron loss has been supported to occur at a significant extent in the aging brain (it commonly was accepted that adults lose as many as 100,000 neurons a day). As reported by an extensive review by Coleman and Flood (1987), some early papers on this research topic documented that most neocortical areas and hippocampal subfields lose 25 to 50% of their neurons, and they were able to influence successive investigations that substantially confirmed a consistent and widespread neuronal death in aging, although these data were reporting different degrees of neuronal loss. The common feature of these studies is that, as a morphometric parameter, they took into account the density of neurons within a given structure and not the total neuron number. Thus, although all these studies agreed in supporting an extensive neuron loss in aging, over the past several years it was increasingly evident that confounding factors might have influenced neuron counting and led to obtaining erroneous results. Namely, tissue processing, method of sampling, strain differences, and the specific anatomy of the area of the central nervous system (CNS) where neuronal counts were performed have been reported to represent sources of potential mistakes in estimating the number of neurons. Contrary to the previously held conviction that with advancing age there is a progressive neuron loss, the development of more accurate counting procedures produced more reliable estimations and led to the conclusion that normal aging does not involve a significant neuronal numeric decrease through neuron death. Unbiased stereological analyses (i.e., the disector; see the section, "Age-related Alterations of Synaptic Structural Dynamics") have shown that, across the overall lifespan, the loss of neurons is around 10%, but this cannot be interpreted as a specific time-related significant impairment since sex has been found to be more important than age in modulating the total neuron number in a given brain region, for example, the neocortex (Pakkenberg and Gundersen, 1997). The marked heterogeneity of the whole brain and even of specific brain regions makes it difficult to interpret any decrease of neuron number from a functional standpoint, thus only those studies conducted in localized CNS zones with clearly demonstrated functions and connections have provided useful information on age-related impairments in which neuron loss may play a role. In this context, because of their documented direct implication in memory, enthorinal cortex and hippocampus have been investigated in different animal models and in human beings. In these CNS areas from old rodents, old nonhuman primates, as well as old human beings, there is no significant neuron loss that may account for the known decay in memory functions due to age (Gomez-Isla *et al.*, 1997). However, these CNS areas show a significant neuron loss in Alzheimer's disease (AD), and this lends support to the assumption that the severity of neuronal death is different in physiological aging and age-related pathological conditions, and that selected areas of the CNS are preferentially affected by age and pathology-related changes (West *et al.*, 1994). It must be stressed that neuronal loss reflects the cumulative tissue damage accrued with age (and, eventually, an age-related neuropathological status). Thus even if the lack of significant neuron loss cannot be considered as the main causative alteration of a manifest functional decline, the neuronal circuits on which the specific function, for example, memory, relies may undergo a progressive damage leading to a subtle deterioration and resulting in impaired brain performances.

Summarizing the results on neuron number and changes in brain size in aging, at present, the well-documented brain shrinkage due to age does not appear to be due to the numeric loss of neurons that has been demonstrated to be far less significant than previously thought and occurs in localized CNS regions, whereas other zones are not affected at all. Atrophy of neurons and of their connections is reported to be the main causative event responsible for the age-related reduction in brain volume, and this provides a rationale for interventional strategies to repair dysfunctional neuronal networks.

Glia Alterations

Glial cells are very numerous and in some parts of the brain they outnumber the nerve cells by 10 to 1. The well-known classification of this type of cells into astrocytes, oligodendrocytes, and microglia in addition to referring to their morphological features also categorizes their specific functions that include providing structural support for nerve cells, isolation and grouping of nerve fibers and terminals, participating in metabolic pathways that modulate the ions, transmitters, and metabolites involved in nerve cell functions. The function of oligodendrocytes is to form the myelin around axons in the CNS; microglia are small cells scattered throughout the nervous system that play a central role in injury and degeneration; that is, these cells proliferate, move to the site where damage has occurred, and transform into large macrophages that remove and phagocytize the debris, thus defending the CNS against inflammation and infection. Glial cells and neurons interact intensely; thus many alterations of this type of cells occurring with advancing age may be secondary to neuronal damage and not regarded as primary glial changes. Given the many functions in which glial cells are involved, it appears difficult to rule out the early different changes affecting these cells in aging. An improved characterization of primary glial changes occurring in the aging CNS has been achieved by the use of recently developed immunohistochemical and silver impregnation methods that enabled the revelation of new aspects on time-related glial degeneration. As an example, paired helical filaments (PHF), long believed to occur only in neurons, were also demonstrated in astrocytes from AD patients (Nakano *et al.*, 1992). In glial cells, the demonstration of variegated abnormal argyrophilic structures immunoreactive with ant-tau antibodies is supporting the concept that glial cytoskeletal abnormalities are related to the specific pathological condition in which they occur. With specific reference to physiological aging, reactive gliosis, probably occurring as a consequence of neuronal damage, is the most common of all glial changes. It has been found that in the eighth decade there is an age-associated increase in the number of cerebral cortical astrocytes immunoreactive for glial fibrillary acid protein (GFAP) (Hansen *et al.*, 1987). This reaction is directly connected with the essential function of astrocytes that play important roles both in nutritional supply, via glucose transfer to neurons, and in the metabolism of glutamic acid, used as neurotransmitter. The early step of gliosis is represented by a consistent swelling of the nucleus followed by proliferation of astrocytes and hypertrophy of a strongly GFAP-positive cytoplasm. In the human cerebral cortex, these activated astrocytes are reported to be immunoreactive for a neurotrophic cytokine (S100β), which is involved in the development of neuritic senile plaques (SP) in AD. In normal aging, S100β-immunoreactive astrocytes increase in number together with the tissue level of S100β protein and S100β mRNA, thus supporting that with advancing age the appearance of SP may predispose to the development of an AD pathological condition (Sheng *et al.*, 1996). Over 60 years, microglia also show changes due to age in the human brain: in addition to an altered morphology, the increased number of activated microglia express the immunomodulatory cytokine interleukin-1, which is paired by increased tissue levels of interleukin-1 mRNA (Mrak *et al.*, 1995), an alteration implicated in AD pathogenesis. On the basis of these data, in addition to the age-related neuronal damage and loss, glial degenerative phenomena also must seriously be taken into account in studying brain aging. A better understanding of glial alterations and of neuron-glia interactions may help in identifying the precocious signs of degenerative phenomena and dysfunction.

Vascular Changes

The consistent damage of blood vessels documented with advancing age in the body also affects the cerebral arteries with the outcome of a significant reduction of blood supply to the brain. As a consequence, selective loss of nerve cells and infarcts may occur and these alterations may lead to the aggravating dementing process of multinfarct dementia. Since atherosclerosis and amyloid angiopathy are reported to represent the most important changes responsible for the age-related progressive decay in blood cerebral perfusion, they were thoroughly investigated in the brain of both humans and experimental animal models. The results have provided detailed information on mechanisms, determinants, and the many causative events involved in these alterations of the aging brain.

ATHEROSCLEROSIS

Atheroma is the term used to define the caseous material, containing high amounts of lipids, found in plaque-like thickenings of the interior portion of the vessel wall. Accordingly, the term *atherosclerosis* reflects the fibrous character of these pathologic alterations affecting large and small peripheral arteries in aging. Atherosclerosis begins as a disease of the innermost layer of the vessel wall (the intima), where the main lesions responsible for its development have been categorized as fatty streaks, fibrous plaques, and complicated lesions.

Fibrous streaks consist mainly of monocyte-derived macrophages that have entered the intima from the blood stream. The abundant presence of lipid droplets, mainly cholesterol ester, within the cytoplasm transforms these macrophages into foam cells. In advanced fatty streaks, lipid infiltration may proceed to fill smooth muscle cells in the tunica media of the blood vessel wall.

The fibrous plaque is a dense fibrous cap at the inner surface of the atherosclerotic lesion that contains a connective tissue matrix rich in collagen that surrounds smooth muscle cells and macrophages on the side of the vessel wall, and is covered by endothelial cells on the side of the lumen. The complicated lesion is supposed to represent a calcification of a fibrous plaque, with the serious possibility of developing cracks, ulcerations, hemorrhages, and thrombosis. In turn, these changes may lead to a cerebral infarction. Specifically in hypercholesterolemic subjects, foam cells are particularly abundant in the area where a complicated lesion occurs in addition to the presence of several muscle cells and macrophages containing lipids that are localized beneath the dense fibrous cap. In advanced lesions, necrotic changes may be found, which results in consistent amounts of extracellular debris and caseous material. The frequent occurrence of cracks and fissures constitutes a further complication of these lesions and results in secondary intramural hemorrhages in large arteries leading to stenosis and thrombosis that obliterate the vessel. As mentioned earlier, these changes affect the intima, but are responsible for secondary damage to the tunica media that may progress to the lamina elastica interna with a final conclusion of a breakdown of the vessel wall.

As it appears from this description, atherogenesis is a very dynamic process involving not only the cells of the arterial blood vessel, but also circulating blood cells, that is, macrophages, monocytes, platelets, and lymphocytes. With the aim of repairing cell and tissue damage, various growth factors are produced by these cells, and their combined action serves to maintain or remodel the function of the vascular system. In this context, injuries to endothelial cells induce to express mitogens such as platelet-derived growth factor (PDGF) and interleukin-1. Activated macrophages are also capable of forming fibroblast growth factor (FGF), which plays a significant role in capillary formation and in secreting transforming growth factor (TGF-alpha) responsible for epithelial migration and proliferation and transforming growth factor (TGF-beta) that inhibits cell proliferation and induces collagen synthesis. The macrophages themselves may be responsible for further tissue injury and play a role in maintaining the progression of atherogenesis by acting as scavenger cells that oxidize ingested lipids through free radicals formation. Namely, secretion of oxidized material and hydrolytic enzymes may cause damage in the still healthy cells located close to the initial lesion. Activated platelets secrete an epidermal growth factor-like substance (TGF-beta) and play a major role in the coagulation and thrombosis process. In turn, proliferation of smooth muscle cells within the thrombi induces the deposition of connective tissue that is stimulated by many growth factors released by platelet aggregation and degranulation.

The many risk factors able to trigger the atherogenetic process have been revealed by several epidemiological studies. As primary determinants, these include hypercholesterolemia and hypertension, but several other causes and causative changes, such as diabetes and cigarette smoking, are reported to be seriously involved. A defective metabolism of lipoproteins is responsible for a high cholesterolemia that may be specifically due to a deficient cholesterol removal or overproduction, or to a combination of both these processes. Monogenic or polygenic hyperlipidemias also play a significant role in atherogenesis, as demonstrated by epidemiological studies reporting a clear correlation between these diseases and the incidence and severity of atherosclerosis. The mechanisms leading to cellular changes involved in atherogenesis are not known in hypertensive patients; however, an acceleration of the atherogenetic process resulting in an increased incidence of cerebrovascular and coronary heart disease has been documented by epidemiological studies. It is suggested that increased monocyte adherence and the localization of monocyte-derived macrophages at the intima, associated with changes in humoral mediators of blood pressure (e.g., angiotensin and renin), as well as drugs and poisons and hemodynamic parameters may result in an overall unfavorable condition predisposing to the development of atherosclerosis.

Several hypotheses have been proposed to give a tenable interpretation of the different deteriorating phenomena participating in atherogenesis. Considering the many proposed assumptions, a unifying concept is represented by the fact that the organism responds to the initial injury of an atherogenetic process. Namely, any damage to the endothelium lining triggers a sequence of events leading to a migration, accumulation, and proliferation of intimal muscle cells. The very early step of this process may be represented by a functional change due to different factors such as side-effects of drugs or radiation injury. As a consequence, monocytes and lymphocytes adhere to the endothelium and trigger an accelerated endothelial turnover with the induction of the gene expression of growth factors that accelerate the smooth muscle cell proliferation up to the formation of a typical atherosclerotic plaque.

Cerebral atrophy is responsible for secondary changes of the artery wall that lead to pathological alterations of the aging brain. Narrowing or obliteration of the vessel lumen as well as the formation of thrombi with the consequence of disturbances of the blood circulation in the specifically irrigated cerebral zones are the unfavorable outcomes of atherosclerosis that frequently result in cerebral infarctions. Although the clinical manifestations due to a cerebral infarction are the consequences of the destroyed structures in the brain area where the lesion has occurred, further pathological development of damaged tissue may cause additional symptoms (e.g., multinfarct dementia). Multiple microinfarctions, or lacunar infarcts (diameter: 3–20 mm) are lesions most common and most severe in hypertensive patients, although they also have been found in normotensive subjects. The frequency of lacunar infarcts increases in the fifth and sixth decade, but thereafter they become less common. This type of lesion affects the deeper neocortical parts of the brain and brainstem (basal ganglia, thalamus, pons) and is due to the occlusion of penetrating branches of the larger cerebral arteries. In addition to hypertension, vascular hyalinosis, and atheromatous degeneration of the vessels are reported to represent predisposing conditions in the development of a lacunar state. Cortical granular atrophy (CGA) is another development of cerebral infarcts. Namely, reactive gliosis substitutes the lesions of small cortical infarctions, resulting in multiple gliotic micro scars; this, in turn, results in multiple small shrinkages appearing as granuli on the surface of the gyri. In the majority of cases, CGA occurs at the territorial border zones of irrigation between the anterior, medial, and posterior cerebral arteries.

Thickening, hyalinosis, and fibrosis are responsible for the degeneration of arterioles with the consequence of perivascular demielinating lesions affecting axons and the cerebral white matter, specifically in frontal and occipital areas. Arteriolopathy due to hypertension is considered as the causative event of this pathological condition of the white matter (vasculogenic leukoencephalopathy: Binswanger disease), although lacunar changes are found in several patients.

AMYLOID ANGIOPATHY

The deposition of amyloid in the wall of cerebral blood vessels is a well-documented change found in physiological and pathological (AD) aging of the human brain. Amyloid fibrils are deposited extracellularly and are derived from soluble circulating proteins that have undergone partial proteolysis and polymerization resulting in insoluble aggregates. Different components take part in the final composition of amyloid deposits and include, in addition to the straight, nonbranching protein fibrils (diameter: 7–10 nm), a serum glycoprotein (P-component) showing a structural homology with c-reactive protein (an acute phase reactant) and sulphated proteoglycans. Since amyloid fibrils have an affinity for Congo red stain, show a green birefringence in polarized light and a β-plated sheet pattern at X-ray diffraction analysis, they have been reliably identified and precisely localized in selected areas of the brain tissue. The favorite sites of amyloid deposition are the outer surface of the endothelial basement membrane of the capillaries, the basement membrane of pericytes, and the basement membrane surrounding the smooth muscle cells of veins and arteries (see Figure 40.1).

The basement membranes of astrocytes surrounding the perivascular space are also favorite sites of amyloid deposition. Not all regions are affected by amyloid angiopathy, but capillaries, veins, and arteries may be involved. White matter is reported to be free of amyloid deposits, whereas gray matter regions (cerebral and cerebellar cortex) and leptomeninges may show consistent amyloid angiopathy with advancing age. The progressive accumulation of amyloid around capillaries results in the occlusion of lumen; the same process affecting the smooth muscle cells of arteries and veins leads to degenerative alterations and necrotic lesions of the tunica media of the blood vessel wall, and, as a consequence, the formation of small aneurysms, focal thrombosis, and hemorrhages may occur. Amyloid angiopathy is particularly severe in temporal and occipital regions, and in these CNS areas the clinical manifestation of a spontaneous intracerebral mass hemorrhage constitutes the first symptom of a pathological condition (Haan *et al.*, 1994). Specifically in generalized amyloidoses, amyloidogenic proteins may come from the blood and their deposition begins at the inner surface of the tunica media, whereas in primary cerebral amyloidoses, the outer side of the same location of the vessel wall is the target of amyloid deposition: a finding supporting that amyloidogenic proteins diffuse from outside into the vessel wall.

More than 30 types of amyloidoses, differentiated according to their location and distribution in the human body, have been classified. With specific reference to brain aging and age-related neurodegenerative diseases, the most common and important is βA4 amyloidosis. The amyloid precursor protein (APP), a protein spanning the cellular membrane, is secreted by nerve and other types of cells. The spontaneous aggregation of short fragments of APP in the extracellular space is one of the early steps in the formation of insoluble fibrillar amyloid deposits. In the brain, nerve cells and their dendrites are the main sources of APP and are responsible for its metabolism; then APP is transported along the perivascular spaces to the subarachnoid space and may deposit in external regions of the blood vessel walls. Although βA4 amyloid angiopathy may occur without evident clinical signs, it is almost frequently combined with the presence of amyloid deposits, in the form of SP in the cerebral parenchyma (hippocampus, frontal cortex, and amigdala) of AD patients.

Age Pigments

The accumulation of age pigments, or lipofuscin, is a distinctive feature of nerve cells (both neurons and glia) in aging. At the light microscope, lipofuscin can be seen as granules diffused throughout the cytoplasm, aggregated at one pole of the cell or clustered around the nucleus (see Figure 40.2).

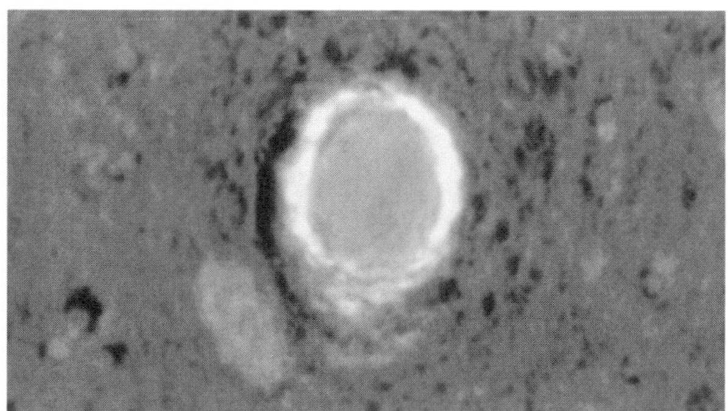

Figure 40.1 Amyloid angiopathy. Transverse section of a human cerebral vessel infiltrated with amyloid. The deposit of amyloid appears white and compact on the vessel wall. Thioflavin S staining.

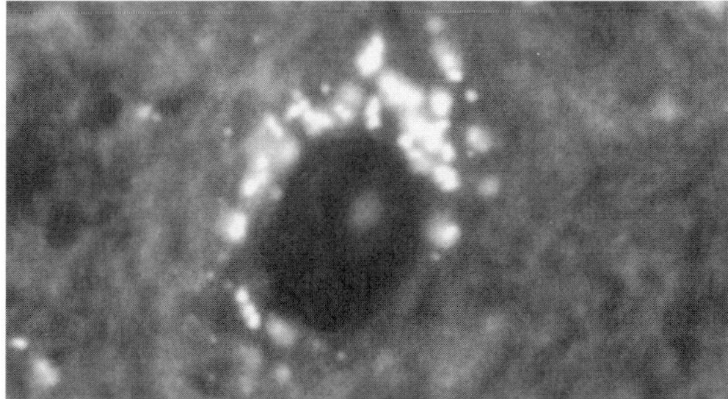

Figure 40.2 Lipofuscin granules clustered around the nucleus of a pyramidal cell. Because of the autofluorescence of the lipofuscin granules, no staining is needed to evidence this alteration in the aging neuron.

Since lipofuscin forms during adult life and increases with age, it has been suggested that it represents the morphological outcome of "wear and tear" cellular function. Lipofuscin is a by-product of lipid peroxidation and originates from secondary lysosomes that transform into lipopigment granules. In neurons, the membranes undergo a continuous turnover with the involvement of lysosomal degradation of proteins and lipids. The interaction between the products of the peroxidation of polyunsaturated fatty acids and other biological molecules leads to the formation of these pigments, which are difficult to digest, and accumulate as residual bodies within the cytoplasm. Any type of biological molecule may become a constituent of lipofuscin, and this finds a well-grounded support in the documented ultrastructural heterogeneity of neuronal pigments reported in the aging human brain (Boellaard and Schlote, 1986). Autofluorescence is the most consistent property of lipofuscin. Under stimulation by visible or near-ultraviolet light, lipofuscin granules appear as yellow, yellowish-green, and orange deposits. Most of the lipofuscin lipid constituents (20 to 50%) are phospholipids (75%), and the protein fraction (30 to 50%) shows a high lipid-binding capacity and an amount of enzymes and enzymatic activity similar to intact tissues.

Lipofuscin accumulates in neurons throughout the CNS and is particularly abundant in cranial and spinal motor nuclei, in large neurons of the precentral gyrus, and in cortical pyramidal cells. Within neurons the lipofuscin mass is reported to displace the nucleolus; however, it is not yet proven whether this is due to the excessive accumulation of the pigment or whether the cell first undergoes impairment of function and lipofuscin granules are formed as a consequence of cell deterioration. Although the significance of lipofuscin accumulation in neuronal function is not clear, as a reasonable interpretation, it may be hypothesized that the lipofuscin masses within the neuron may be able to decrease the plastic capacity of the nerve cells to adapt to environmental stimulation. Lipofuscin accumulation has been proposed to be a function of cellular metabolic activity rather than of chronological age and, in this context, repetitive metabolic accidents may lead to the accumulation of a nonfunctional by-product of cellular metabolism. This assumption finds support in the fact that caloric restricted animals (i.e., that have undergone a reduction in metabolic rate) show less lipofuscin accumulation associated with a longer lifespan than age-matched normally fed littermates (Moore *et al.*, 1995).

Dendritic Changes

An age-related reduction in the number of dendrites and dendritic spines has been reported in normal aging, and this results in an overall decrease of dendritic complexity. The regressive changes occurring at the dendrite tree affect mainly frontal and temporal cortex and the limbic system in the human brain. The first step in the age-related alterations of dendrites is the loss of spines followed by changes in shape and size of basilar dendrites and then of the branches of the apical shaft (Scheibel *et al.*, 1975). Dendrites are receptor membranes of the neurons, and their spines amplify this function and have been reported to isolate increases of synaptic calcium transport utilized for information storage (Koch *et al.*, 1992). As a consequence, the age-related loss of dendrites and dendritic spines isolates neurons and leads to disturbances in cell-to-cell communication. Because of its dynamic condition, the old CNS is capable of a significant compensating response to the age-related loss of neurons and dendritic retraction by increasing the dendritic growth to fill the neuropil space left by the dendritic trees of dead neurons. In parahippocampal pyramidal cells of cognitively normal individuals the continual growth of dendrites occurs well into the eighth decade of life, whereas in pathological brain aging, for example, AD, this compensating reaction has not been found (Buell and Coleman, 1979).

The dendritic changes due to age have been demonstrated by the Golgi method—an old neurohistological procedure that is still in use. In Golgi-impregnated tissue, staining reveals the complete contours of the cells and of their processes. Nerve cells can be seen against the background because only a small fraction (2 to 5%) of the cells are impregnated, but the reasons of this selective positivity are not known. In the original Golgi method, fresh tissue is hardened in a dichromate solution and impregnated in 1% silver nitrate. In the rapid version of this procedure, the tissue pieces are hardened in 4 parts of potassium dichromate (3.5%) and 1 part of osmic acid (1%) for 2 to 7 days, and then they are transferred to 0.75% silver nitrate for 1 to 2 days. In double and triple impregnations, the tissue samples are returned to osmium-dichromate and then impregnated in the same silver nitrate solution. Although this version of the Golgi method is called rapid, all these steps take long periods of time and several laboratory preparations before obtaining a sample to be analyzed: this increases the possibility to damage the tissue and to see unspecific precipitates.

Several modifications of the original Golgi procedure have been introduced with the aim of reducing the extent and frequency of tissue artifacts. In the Golgi-Cox method, tissue hardening and impregnation take place in a simple bath of potassium dichromate and potassium chromate to which sublimate is added. When the tissue blocks or sections are alkalized, the original yellow compound with divalent mercury is transformed into a black substance. The Golgi-Cox version is more rapid than the original procedure, but the impregnation is rather coarse and never occurs in axons. In the Golgi-Kopsch version the animals are perfused with a freshly prepared mixture of potassium dichromate and formalin (or glutaraldehyde); then the hardened brain is sectioned and impregnated in silver nitrate (0.75%). Perfusion, as the first step of the Golgi-Kopsch procedure, limits its use to studies to be conducted on laboratory animals. Large sampling of tissue, impregnated with different modifications of the Golgi method, have enabled the collection of several data converging on the common conclusion from different laboratories that in the aging brain basal arborizations are lost in selected areas of the CNS.

Age-related Alterations of Synaptic Structural Dynamics

It is well demonstrated that the nervous system is capable of consistent structural adaptive changes throughout the individual's lifespan. Specifically, the synaptic terminal regions are in a very dynamic condition responsible for continuous remodeling interventions to optimize the critical role of the synaptic junctional areas in signal transduction and information processing. Synaptic plasticity is the commonly used term defining such a function-driven adaptive response of the synaptic contact zones, and its meaning includes the many different morphological, biochemical, molecular, and genetic changes occurring at synapses as a consequence of environmental stimulation.

During the last decades, the significant advancement in the accuracy and reliability of the investigative procedures has contributed to a better identification and to an improved quantitative analysis of function-related synaptic parameters, thus furthering our understanding of the basic mechanisms contributing to the fine tuning of synaptic transmission. From a morphological point of view, synaptic junctional areas undergo significant rearrangements of their ultrastructural features that mirror the functional status of the neural network where they are located, thus enabling an estimation of the adaptive capacities (i.e., plasticity) of selected CNS zones. In performing any quantitative morphological, or morphometric, study in a given biological tissue, collection of the data is a laborious time-consuming procedure since several histological sections, and perhaps zones within the tissue samples, must be analyzed and measured in order to obtain statistically comparable pools of findings between the experimental groups. Thus, until the late 1980s, analysis and measurement of tissue sections was a significant limiting step in performing these investigations.

The subsequent introduction in laboratory routine procedures of modern computer-assisted image analyzers, though facilitating and objectifying the morphometric procedures, resulted in a marked acceleration of data collection. The application of these procedures to the study of the aging nervous system has provided novel information on the modulation of synaptic architecture to respond to the changing functional needs (Bertoni-Freddari *et al.*, 1996). It is consistently documented that the staining procedures used in conventional electron microscopy to prepare the tissue samples for qualitative and quantitative analyses enable a better visualization of the whole cellular architecture. This is due to the fact that the traditionally used staining reagents bind ubiquitously to the biological molecules (namely, proteins and lipids), leaving the background completely unstained or faintly stained. The more or less dark and sharp contrast of the cellular structures depends on various factors and, besides the concentration and incubation time of the contrasting reagents (Miquel and Bertoni-Freddari, 2000), also includes the chemical composition of the cellular structure where the staining reaction occurs. In this context, the synaptic contact zones are functionally differentiated areas of the neuronal membrane where polyunsaturated fatty acids are abundant because of the presence of several double bonds between carbon atoms. This very specific feature, although constituting the chemical basis of their plastic condition for adequate functional tasks, is also the reason why pre- and postsynaptic membranes abundantly bind osmium tetroxide and, subsequently other contrasting compounds (namely, uranyl acetate and lead citrate), resulting in being markedly darker than any other zone of the neuronal membrane. These specific properties have favored the conduction of several morphometric studies of synaptic ultrastructure on tissue samples conventionally stained by osmium tetroxide, uranyl acetate, and lead citrate, but they have also prompted the development of various preferential cytochemical techniques with the aim of evidencing selectively fine structural details reporting on specific functional aspects of synaptic morphology. Among the different staining techniques to evidence synaptic junctions, the ethanol phosphotungstic acid (E-PTA) procedure originally was developed to analyze synapse formation and maturation in cultured neurons, and then it was applied to tissue sections. The E-PTA staining enables visualization of the pre- and postsynaptic membranes against a very faint background that is almost completely unstained (see Figure 40.3). This is due to the fact that the fixed tissue pieces are stained in a 1% ethanolic solution of PTA at 60°C for 1 hour, and the nonpositive structures are degraded substantially during this step.

Although the reasons for the specificity of the synapses to this staining technique are still under investigation, it has been clearly demonstrated that PTA binds to the basic amino acid residues of the proteins as also supported by the E-PTA positivity of the chromatin due to the presence of histones. Whatever the mechanisms or reasons of the E-PTA preferential staining of the synapses, the big molecule of the PTA does not penetrate easily into the tissue. Thus in order to obtain good samples for quantitative analysis it is important that very thin sections must be used for incubation in the E-PTA solution. Because of the sharp precipitate due to the

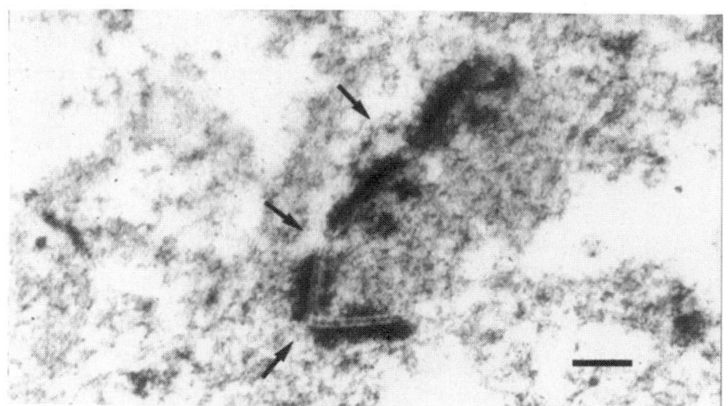

Figure 40.3 Perforated E-PTA stained synaptic junction from the human cerebral cortex. The postsynaptic density appears as a continuous dark line. The presynaptic apposition can be seen as a dotted line. Arrows indicate the perforations. Bar: 0.5 μm.

E-PTA cytochemical staining, no further contrasting procedure is needed, thus avoiding the risk of staining artifacts. Accordingly, the synapses may be easily identified as two parallel black lines or as a range of dark peaks and a black sharp line representing the pre-and postsynaptic membrane appositions, respectively. At the electron microscope, in the tissue samples stained by the E-PTA procedure, the identification of the synapses is greatly facilitated and the semiautomatic measurement of ultrastructural parameters with a defined functional meaning may be reliably carried out by applying morphometric formulas with the use of computerized image analysis systems.

SYNAPTIC NUMERIC DENSITY

As points of communication between neurons, the synapses play different roles and are characterized by various degrees of efficacy at different locations; accordingly, their number represents the amount of neural inputs to the neurons of a CNS region. The size of the postsynaptic potential is influenced by the density of the synapses in a given tissue area or volume (Nv), and this, in turn, may significantly modulate information processing. Overproduction of synapses occurs in early developmental periods; then the synapses are pruned through competitive interactions and activity-based mechanisms in order to set up the best topographical map of synaptic connections adapted to environmental stimulations. In the fully-differentiated adult CNS, the synaptic pattern can still be modified by the growth of novel connections as a consequence of the experiential framework of each individual. In aging, loss of synaptic contacts has been reported to occur, although the extent and the statistical significance of the age-related reduction of Nv depends both on the specific vulnerability to aging of the CNS area taken into account and on the method of counting. Namely, despite the fact that the early investigations on synaptic number in aging were carried out about 25 years ago (Cotman and Scheff, 1979; Bertoni-Freddari and Giuli, 1980), there is still no consensus on the criteria for counting them unbiasedly, and this has yielded a consistent amount of sometimes contradictory data (Genisman *et al.*, 1995). Profile counts, assumption-based methods, serial reconstructions, and stereological methods are the procedures that have been used to estimate the number of synapses in tissue sections, and the criteria for these methods are different, thus resulting in a marked variability of data.

In the early 1980s, the introduction of the disector as a sterological procedure for counting objects in tissue sections (Sterio, 1984) resulted in a complete break from the previous methods of counting; now this procedure is becoming the method of choice in the estimation of synaptic number because it is unbiased and easy to use. The dissector may be defined as a three-dimensional stereological probe composed of pairs of sections: the reference section and a serial section called the look-up section. The volume of the disector is determined by the area of the sections and the distance between them. Objects are considered to be in the disector and counted if they can be identified in the look-up section, but not in the reference one. In order to detect all the objects to be counted, the distance between reference and look-up sections must be less than the shortest dimension of the objects; with specific reference to synaptic counts, adjacent sections can be used, and they must be located randomly within a given neural region (Bertoni-Freddari *et al.*, 2002). It must be considered that several data on synaptic numeric density have been collected according to methods used prior to the introduction and the frequent use of the unbiased stereological technique of the disector. Thus, these results cannot be compared with those obtained by the disector; however, they may be useful to estimate ratios as, for instance, synapse-to-neuron, and the conclusions drawn must be referred to the portion of the structure from which samples were obtained.

On the basis of these concepts, a decrease of synaptic number in aging has been documented by several authors in different CNS zones from different animal species and human beings, thus supporting the fact that this alteration is a ubiquitous feature of the aging brain. Reliable support to this assumption is given by relating the number of neurons to the number of synapses estimated in the same CNS zone. The synapse-to-neuron ratio is a parameter independent from artifacts of tissue processing (e.g., shrinkage) or the physiological decrease of the overall volume of a given CNS zone, thus providing reliable information on the real situation of the analyzed tissue area from a morphofunctional standpoint.

In a study conducted in CNS samples from adult, old, and demented (AD) patients at autopsy, the synapse-to-neuron ratio estimated in the cerebellum (glomerular areas in the granular layer) and hippocampus (dentate gyrus supragranular layer) showed different findings

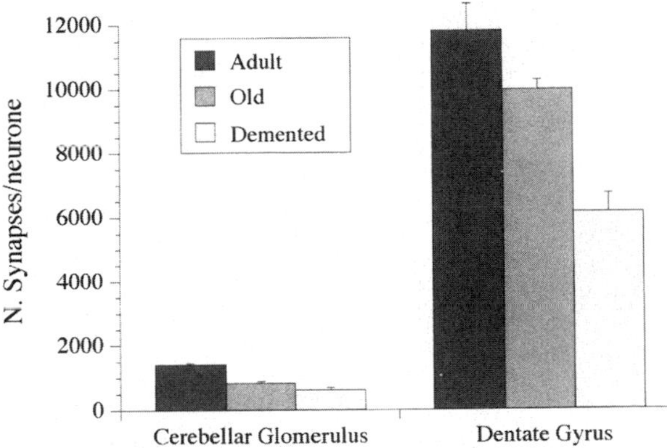

Figure 40.4 Synapse-to-neuron ratio in the cerebellum and hippocampus of adult, old, and demented (AD) patients. No significant difference can be seen in the cerebellar granular layer. This parameter shows a significant (52%) decrease in the hippocampal dentate gyrus of demented vs. normal old patients of the same age. This result suggests that synaptic loss per se is a prominent alteration of the demented brain in selected CNS areas.

according to the CNS zone and the health condition of the patients (see Figure 40.4). Namely, in the cerebellum there was no significant difference between adult, old, and demented subjects although a reduction of this parameter was clearly evident between the adult group and the other two groups of patients.

In the hippocampal dentate gyrus, the synapse-to-neuron ratio decreased insignificantly between adult and old patients, whereas between adult and AD patients a significant decrease of more than 50% was found. Since in both the areas investigated the number of neurons was almost unchanged with aging, these results suggest that the loss of synapses per se is a prominent and early alteration in physiological brain aging and may represent a sustainable pathological marker in AD.

SYNAPTIC AVERAGE SIZE

A growing number of reports from the current literature documents that synaptic size is a very sensitive ultrastructural parameter undergoing significant changes as a consequence of different environmental stimulations. Reasonably, it can be assumed that the size of the synaptic contact area may influence the amount of transmitter released and also the extent of trafficking of the many substances involved in information processing, thus strengthening the transmission of the nervous impulse among neurons. As a consequence, enlargement or reduction in synaptic size supposedly may lead to changes in function. On the other hand, the possibility to modulate the extension of the junctional zones may be considered a means to carry out a significant structural intervention on the plastic condition of the synapses. The awareness of the biological significance of changes in synaptic size has prompted the development of several methods to estimate this parameter by applying conventional morphometric formulas since the early investigations performed around the late 1970s to early 1980s (Dyson and Jones, 1976; Bertoni-Freddari and Giuli, 1980; Hillman and Chen, 1984) up to the present application of the disector (Mayhew, 1996; Bertoni-Freddari *et al.*, 2002). Synaptic size has been frequently estimated by measuring the profile length of the postsynaptic apposition (L) in tissue samples prepared according to both the conventional osmium tetroxide method and to the E-PTA preferential technique. Some authors have considered L as the cord of circular disk (assumed to be the shape of the synaptic contact) and have calculated mathematically the radius and the area (S) of the synaptic disks. In E-PTA processed samples the postsynaptic membrane appears always sharply contrasted, which facilitates the identification and measurement of L by semiautomatic computerized procedures. In the brain of old laboratory animals and human beings it has been found that the size of the synapses is increased. Although not all the data obtained from different laboratories in old subjects are statistically significant vs. the adult values, the synaptic contact zones appear to enlarge with advancing age, and this alteration, in addition to being a feature occurring in different zones of the CNS, has also been documented in the CNS of patients suffering from AD (Bertoni-Freddari *et al.*, 1990; DeKosky and Scheff, 1990). The percent distribution of S showed that the complement of larger synapses increases in physiological aging and AD (see Figure 40.5). This occurs both in zones reported to be very vulnerable to aging and age-related pathologies (e.g., the hippocampus) and in zones documented to be less sensitive to time-related damage (e.g., the cerebellar cortex), thus supporting that this modification in the composition of the synaptic population is a ubiquitous feature of the aging CNS.

In looking for a tenable interpretation of the age- and pathology-related increased complement of enlarged synapses, some current concepts on the mechanism(s) and steps supposed to be involved in synaptic structural remodeling must be taken into account. Along with their dynamic condition, it has been clearly demonstrated that the synaptic junctional areas undergo continuous rearrangements of their ultrastructural features, and, accordingly, some papers report studies proposing mechanisms and suggesting sequential steps occurring during the functional modulation of synapses (Carlin and Siekevitz, 1983; Wolff *et al.*, 1995; Bertoni-Freddari *et al.*, 1996). Although some differences exist in the interpretation of the single steps by different authors, at present, a concept that can be reasonably sustained is that, as a consequence of repeated stimulations, the synaptic size (0.2–0.3 μm) may increase two- to threefold and up to more than 1 μm. These megasynapses can perforate and split into smaller junctional areas that may again increase in size, perforate, and split (see Figure 40.6).

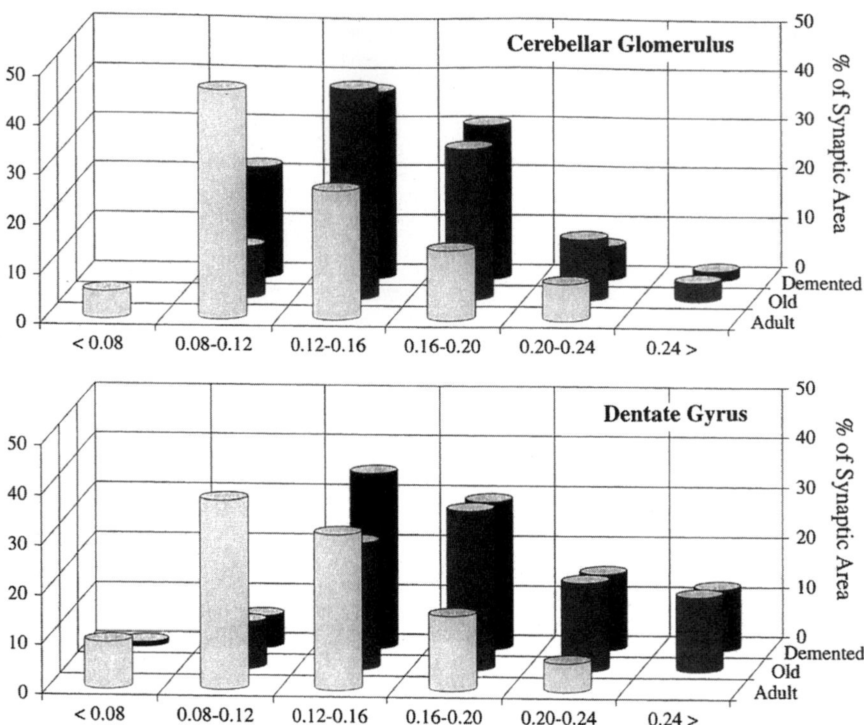

Figure 40.5 Percent distribution of the synaptic average size (area: S) in the cerebellum and hippocampus of adult, old, and demented (AD) patients. An increased complement (%) of synapses of larger size is present in the hippocampal dentate gyrus of old and demented patients. The same change can be envisaged also in the cerebellum, although at a lesser degree.

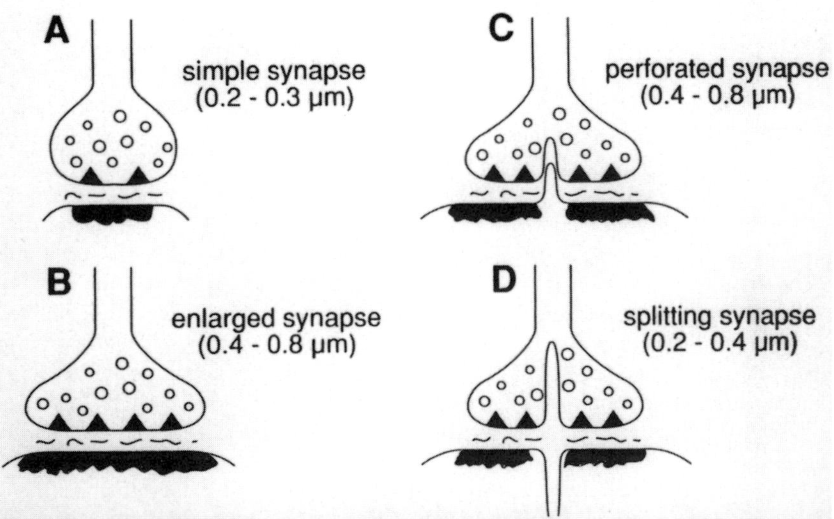

Figure 40.6 Proposed steps of synaptic remodeling. Each diagram reports the cross-section of a synapse. A: simple synapse reported to measure 0.2–03. μm. B: on stimulation, synapse length may increase two- or threefold and even more. C: if synaptic size attains a still undefined limit, perforations may appear. D: the holes in the enlarged synapse cause a break into smaller synaptic clods that, in turn, may give rise to daughter junctions or undergo regression with disconnection of the interested area. (Reproduced with permission from *Gerontology 42*, 170–180, 1996).

The reasons why larger contact zones should divide are not known; however, since they have been found to be associated with a decrease in synaptic number, it has been proposed that synaptic enlargement is carried out as a compensating reaction to balance the lost contacts. Thus, interpreting the results reported in aging, it can be supposed that the preceding proposed cycle of events occurring in synaptic remodeling is halted at the early step of synaptic enlargement, thus resulting in only a partial compensation for the reduced number of junctions. Whatever mechanism(s) are activated in synaptic remodeling, the consistent presence of larger contacts in the aging CNS may be considered, at the same time, a sign of impairment and of the CNS plastic reaction to unfavorable conditions as supported by studies conducted on malnourished laboratory animals (Chen and Hillman, 1980).

SYNAPTIC VOLUME DENSITY

The overall area of the synaptic contact zones present in a defined tissue volume (usually 1 μm^3) accounts for the response capacities of the neural circuitries of a given discrete CNS area. The morphometric term to define such a parameter is surface density (Sv), and, as any other morphological feature of the synaptic junctional areas, it may undergo relevant changes as a consequence of several modulating actions including electrical stimulation, behavioral conditioning, and trophic factors. The Sv value may also be influenced by the intensity and the duration of the stimulus as well as the level of plasticity of the specific CNS zone analyzed (Desmond and Levy, 1986). Over the past two decades, the reliability of the results obtained in estimating the Sv value in different experimental models has been continuously challenged by the progressive advancements in the accuracy of the morphometric methods that are presently applied by computer-assisted image analyzers. Namely, sampling and counting of synapses have been refined repeatedly, both by improved staining methods as well as unbiased procedures, which resulted in a better estimation of the Sv value. Several converging data are now supporting that in a given CNS zone, an adequate-to-function value of Sv is maintained according to the experiential framework of each individual. During the maturation of the CNS, an optimal Sv value is attained through a balance between selective pruning of the redundant synaptic contacts and the reinforcement of those junctional areas that have undergone frequent stimulation and physiological response adaptation (Purves and Lichtman, 1980). Although the adult, fully differentiated CNS retains a high level of plasticity, significant modifications of the experience-stabilized neural circuits do not easily occur since the maintenance of Sv constancy constitutes an important prerequisite to preserve the experience-driven fine tuning of select neuronal networks representing the structural basis of acquired skills (Hillman and Chen, 1984). Memory and learning abilities also rely on adequate Sv values, since an extended network of contacts provides a micro-anatomical structural basis of these important functions. Different physiological mechanisms and biological determinants contribute to maintain constant Sv value by modulating number and size of the synaptic contact zones present in selected CNS areas, and this has led to propose the reasonable assumption of the existence of a close relationship among these three parameters of the synaptic ultrastructure. Namely, although quantitatively measured by independent methodological approaches and analysis procedure, it appears that S and Nv are inversely correlated and that the final outcome of this balance is the Sv value. Thus, while each of these parameters provides specific information on single aspects of synaptic morphology, when taken together per experimental sample, they constitute a reliable index of synaptic plasticity from a morpho-functional point of view. Accordingly, functional decay may result from an imbalance among Nv, S, and Sv leading to altering the maintenance of the synaptic ultrastructural homeostasis. In humans, Sv has been found to be significantly decreased in the old hippocampus, whereas an age-related, not significant reduction of Sv affects the cerebellar cortex. In AD patients a further decrease of Sv occurs only in the hippocampus, probably in connection with the consistent presence in this CNS zone of senile plaques, a typical hallmark of this disease (Bertoni-Freddari *et al.*, 1990, 1996). The Sv decline in physiological aging and AD appears to be due to the numeric loss of contacts (Nv) since the average area (S) of the surviving contacts is significantly enlarged. Although it can reasonably be supported that synaptic enlargement strengthens information processing by the release of more neurotransmitters and the activation of more receptors, this reinforcement of the surviving contacts appears to be less functional than the fine-tuning of the neural networks provided by the higher density of smaller junctional areas typically found in adult individuals.

Neurotransmitter Systems

Neurotransmitters play a central role in neuron-to-neuron information processing and in transferring information from neurons to target cells. Classical neurotransmitters include acetylcholine, the catecholamines (norepinephrine, epinephrine, and dopamine), and serotonine. In addition, neurotransmission may be accomplished and/or modulated by amino acids, such as glycine, glutamate, and gamma aminobutyric acid (GABA), as well as peptides (e.g., enkephalin, substance P, and cholecystokinin), gas (nitric oxide and carbon dioxide), and metals, acting as neuromodulators (zinc). Nitric oxide and carbon dioxide originally were viewed as toxic, but it has been demonstrated that they can act as biological messengers in mammals. It is important to consider that different neurotransmitters may coexist within the same neuron, and this implies a vast expansion of the potential for synaptic communication. This coexistence of multiple neurotransmitters results in a reciprocal modulation of the specific action of these substances aimed at providing the adequate response from neurons to environmental stimuli by a fine balance of the inhibitory and excitatory effect of classical neurotransmitters and their neuromodulators. Turnover, release, and binding of neurotransmitter substances constitute important steps in the mechanisms involved in signal transduction between adjacent nerve cells; therefore changes in any of them may result in functional alterations. It is well known that many synapses are identified by the neurotransmitter released, thus at terminal regions of different synapses very specific mechanisms are operating to work out these processes, and these include, in addition to the synthesis of neurotransmitters, the activity of degrading and synthesizing enzymes. Complete and reliable analysis to detect neurotransmitter changes occurring at synaptic regions should take into account studies aimed at testing proper functioning at different levels. Thus, precursor availability, synthesis of enzymes, degradation of neurotransmitters, their storage, reuptake, and ionic regulation refer to the presynaptic area, and free neurotransmitters as well as the enzymes of their degradation pertain to transynaptic events. Receptor binding, enzyme degradation, ionic regulation, and the induction of second messengers refer to the postsynaptic zone. On the basis of this high complexity of the mechanisms of neurotransmission, the knowledge accumulated on age differences regarding this function is still fragmentary and incomplete, particularly with specific reference to human studies. In humans, the measurement of neurotransmitter substances or their metabolites is carried out in urine, blood, or cerebrospinal fluid or, recently, by using labeled probes and imaging techniques. It is clearly understandable that all these methods enable an indirect and remote analysis of the neurotransmitter substance, and any subtle alteration in the physiological condition may not be identified. Despite these difficulties, a general consensus can be envisaged among the different scientific reports; that is, during physiological aging the levels and activity of neurotransmitters and related enzymes decline in many brain regions, and the corresponding receptors may or may not respond to these changes by increasing their number and/or affinity. In details, with reference to human beings, it has been found that brain acetylcholine transferase levels as well as muscarinic binding decrease in aging (Perry, 1980). The levels of striatal dopamine uptake sites, dopamine and dopamine transporters show an age-associated decline (Kish *et al.*, 1992) as do serotonin binding sites, $\alpha 2$ and $\beta 1$ adrenoceptors, and cortical GABAergic innervation (Allen *et al.*, 1983; Kalaria *et al.*, 1989). Alterations due to age in tissue levels of glutamate and aspartate are distributed in different brain areas (Banay-Schwartz *et al.*, 1992). Studies in different discrete zones of the CNS of laboratory animals (rats) have shown that while the concentration of serotonine is constant throughout the lifespan, dopamine and norepinephrine progressively decease starting from adulthood. Thus, in the aging rat brain the ratio of serotonin to catecholamines progressively increases, but the functional manifestation of this imbalance may be due to the impairment of only one of these three neurotransmitters. It must be stressed that different neurotransmitter systems show a differential rate of aging that may be responsible for an imbalance as an early event before the appearance of changes affecting a specific neurotransmitter. In summary, although several data have been obtained from animal studies, it may be assumed that alteration of function in aging may result from an imbalance among the many neurotransmitter substances and neuromodulators that could be due to deteriorative event(s) affecting any of them, rather than to specific focal impairments affecting a single neurotransmitter system.

Energy Metabolism: The Critical Role of Mitochondrial Function Decay

The human brain, representing less than 2% of the body weight, receives about 16 to 17% of the cardiac output and accounts for about 20% of the total oxygen consumption in resting conditions. From these data it can easily be inferred that routine brain functions are critically dependent on the synthesis of high energy intermediates by neurons and glia, although these two types of nerve cells have different energy requirements and, of course, there are marked differences between their energy demands.

Cerebral energy metabolism in aging has been investigated in animal models and human beings by measuring different parameters, such as cerebral blood flow (CBF) and cerebral metabolic rate for glucose (CMRGlc) or oxygen ($CMRO_2$). Noninvasive techniques have been developed during the past decades beginning in the early 1960s to measure these important parameters. Positron emission tomography (PET) is one of these currently used methods and is based on principles of computerized tomography and radioisotope imaging. Specifically in emission tomography, the image is generated by differences in the distribution in the tissue of injected or inhaled isotopes that are constituents of important biological molecules. The radiation emitted by the isotopes can be detected, analyzed, and used by a computer to visualize the zones where a specific biological molecule is metabolized. In PET, the isotopes of elements that decay after minutes or hours are normally used and emit positrons (positive charged particles similar in mass to electrons). With the exception of severe injury, such as stroke and head trauma, CBF is coupled to cerebral metabolism since neural mechanisms that need energy to be accomplished are also able to modulate the brain's blood perfusion. PET has been used to estimate local rates of CBF and the results obtained documented that in human aging a decrease in this parameter occurs in the limbic system and association areas. This is probably due to the changes that occur with aging in cognitive functions. Other areas of the old human brain appear to be differently affected by a decrease in CBF, but the most commonly observed age-related impairment has been found in the frontal lobes bilaterally. Moreover it has been found that in aging there is a decrease of CBF in gray, but not in white, matter (Leenders *et al.*, 1990). The quantitative estimations of CBF may easily be affected by physiological, psychological, and environmental factors. However, the regional values estimated in each individual are normalized to the whole brain blood flow with the aim of eliminating variations in the measurements of absolute flow. Multiple factors may be responsible for the age-related changes in CBF, and these include a decline in the mechanisms that regulate CBF, alterations of the cerebral blood vessels due to age (e.g., mild amyloid angiopathy), and a decrease of neuron function leading to brain atrophy. The 18F-deoxyglucose is the most commonly used radiopharmaceutical for PET imaging to investigate CMRGlc or $CMRO_2$. In aging, CMRGlc decreases in temporal, parietal, and frontal regions of the brain. $CMRO_2$ also is reported to decrease with advancing age, particularly in the gray matter in subjects over 51 years of age (Takada *et al.*, 1992). The reliability of the results on cerebral metabolism from PET analysis is challenged by measurements of brain atrophy since PET data are the outcome of an average of signals from the brain tissue and CSF spaces (i.e., the spaces occupied by the cerebrospinal fluid), and a marked atrophy may result in a lower PET value. A reasonable suggestion for a correct interpretation of PET data is that changes in brain volume must be considered. Atrophy correction of cerebral metabolism has been carried out in AD studies, and it has been documented that the AD hypometabolism is related to the loss of tissue, whereas the still existing tissue does not show metabolic differences vs. controls. Age-related brain damage and the appearance of potential neuropathological signs may depend on causative events leading to an impaired metabolism affecting different groups of neurons in which reduction of energy may result from the decay of the cell's metabolic machinery, that is, from subtle, though significant, mitochondrial dysfunctions.

IMPAIRMENT OF MITOCHONDRIAL STRUCTURAL DYNAMICS IN AGING

In order to accomplish their peculiar task, consisting of the coupling of respiration to ATP synthesis, mitochondria have a unique and peculiar morphology: namely, an outer membrane surrounding an inner membrane (the cristae) that surrounds an internal matrix. The ordered architecture of this topologically closed bilayered system represents a critical topographic arrangement for the mitochondrial mechanisms involved in the synthesis of adenosinetriphosphate (ATP) from adenosine diphosphate and inorganic phosphate via oxidative phosphorylation. During this process protons are pumped into the intermembrane space by the respiratory chain located at the inner mitochondrial membrane; therefore all the reactions of the oxidative phosphorylation process (OXPHOS) significantly rely on the structural features of the organelles. Mitochondrial morphology is known to be heterogeneous and may be quite different from cell to cell of the same organ or from one cellular compartment to another within the same cell. In addition, select mitochondrial pools are in a very dynamic condition and may undergo significant ultrastructural remodeling to tailor the cellular energy providing machinery to the functional energy requirements of the actual environmental conditions (Bertoni-Freddari *et al.*, 1993; Bereiter-Hahn and Voth, 1994; Bertoni-Freddari *et al.*, 2001). Quantitative estimations of these mitochondrial structural dynamics may be carried out, in semiautomatic mode, applying morphometric procedures by computer-assisted image analyzers. Namely, volume and numeric densities (i.e., the mitochondrial volume fraction and number/μm^3 of tissue) as well as the average size and/or shape of the mitochondria are the ultrastructural parameters currently investigated and reported to be significantly modulated by actual energy demands. It has been documented that these parameters provide information on discrete aspects of mitochondrial ultrastructure; however, they are dependent on each other. Thus the overall quantitative estimation of their reciprocal changes may represent an index of the mitochondrial functional plasticity. The clear awareness that this function-driven dynamic condition of discrete pools of mitochondria is continuously challenged by any cellular activity requiring an adequate ATP supply has led to several investigations on the many factors potentially able to modulate the mitochondrial morphological features and, in turn, the bioenergetic competence in specific cellular compartments where the organelles are located.

In agreement with this knowledge on the plastic condition of the mitochondrial morphology, the aging process has been considered as a very critical, though physiological, condition able to exert a subtle and significant modulating action on the mitochondrial structural dynamics. Several studies conducted in different organs and types of cells from various animal species and human beings document the notion that a general trend can be clearly envisaged: in old organisms mitochondria decrease in number, but increase in size; the final outcome of these balanced changes is that the overall mitochondrial volume density (i.e., the mitochondrial fraction/μm^3 of tissue) is constant during the individual's lifespan (Bertoni-Freddari *et al.*, 1993; Solmi, 1994; Walter *et al.*, 1999) (see Figure 40.7).

An impaired duplicative capacity, due to age, may account for mitochondrial numeric loss, whereas the enlargement in the average mitochondrial volume has been considered as a compensating reaction aimed at

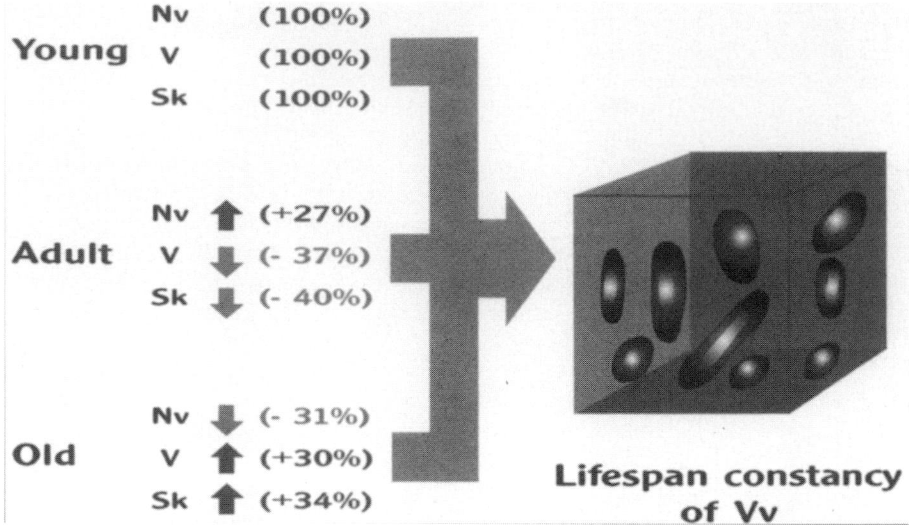

Figure 40.7 Age-related ultrastructural alterations of rat synaptic mitochondria. The cytoplasmic volume fraction occupied by mitochondria (volume density: Vv) appears to be constant throughout the whole lifespan. With regard to the numeric density (Nv), the average mitochondrial volume (V), and the skeleton (Sk: an estimation of mitochondrial elongation), if the values of these parameters are considered 100%, in the adult rats the increase of Nv (+27%) is paired by a decrease of V (-37%) and Sk (-40%). In old rats opposite changes can be observed; that is, a 31% decrease of Nv is paired by an increase of V (+30%) and Sk (+34%).

increasing the mitochondrial area involved in cellular respiration (see Figure 40.8).

Specifically, at the synaptic terminals of old animals the percent of oversized organelles is reported to be markedly increased. Oversized organelles, also referred to as megamitochondria (MM), have been found in some adverse conditions, sometimes representing a serious threat for cell survival; therefore a positive interpretation of the consistent presence within the cell of MM is questioned. The conventional staining procedures adopted to carry out electron microscopic investigations, though enabling a better visualization of all the cellular constituents by increasing ubiquitously their contrast against the background, do not provide detailed information from a functional point of view. Thus, in order to obtain a better insight into the biological significance of any estimated ultrastructural change, specific cytochemical techniques have been developed to visualize arrays of molecules with well-defined and reliable functional meaning.

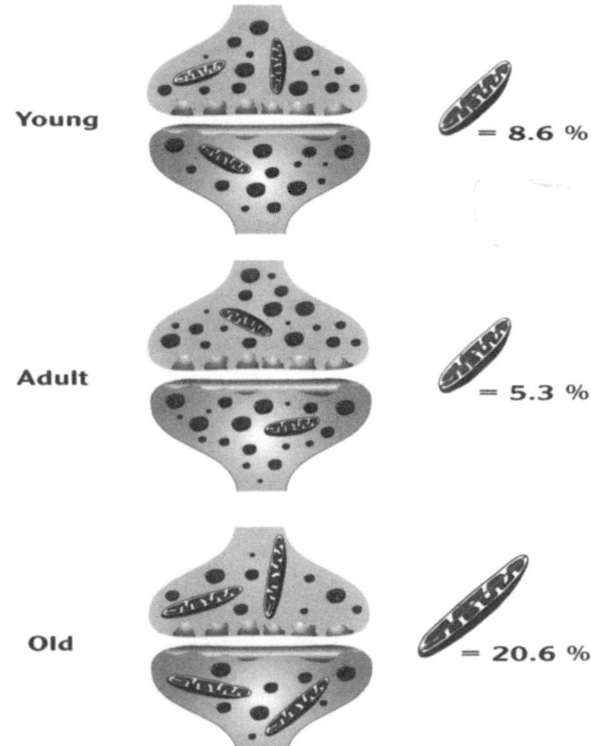

Figure 40.8 Reactive plasticity of mitochondrial size at synaptic terminals in aging. The complement of oversized mitochondria was estimated by considering a Feretratio value threshold of ≤ 0.2. (Feretratio is obtained by dividing the shorter by the longer diameter of each mitochondrion). At the synaptic terminals of old rats, the percent of megamitochondria accounts for 20.6% vs. 8.6% and 5.3% found at the synaptic regions of young and adult animals, respectively.

CYTOCHEMISTRY OF SUCCINIC DEHYDROGENASE ACTIVITY IN THE AGING BRAIN

It is currently supported that the generation of reactive oxygen species (ROS) during the physiological process of cellular respiration is not properly controlled in old cells, and this may be responsible for significant damage to mitochondrial DNA (mtDNA) and membranes resulting, with increasing mtDNA mutation and membrane deterioration load, in alterations of mitochondrial morphology and in a progressive impairment of mitochondrial

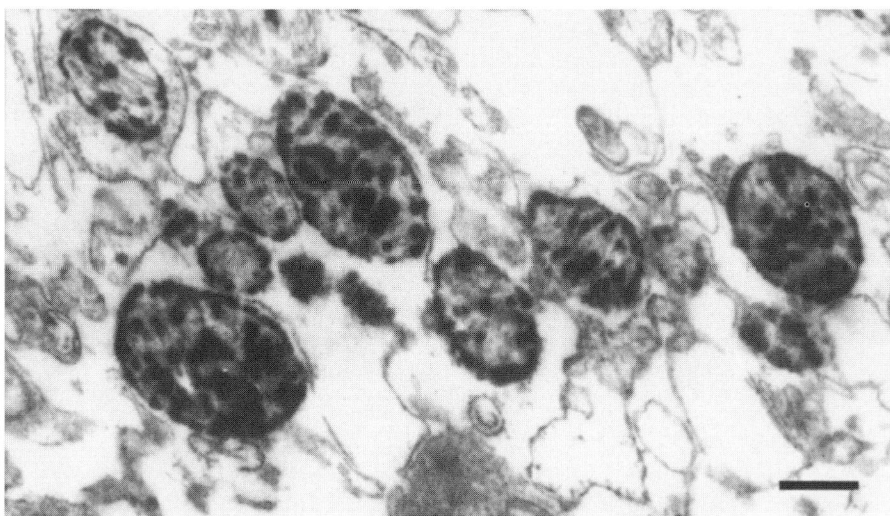

Figure 40.9 SDH-positive mitochondria in the perykaryon of a CA1 pyramidal cell. The dark precipitate due to the reaction of copper ferrocyanide with the enzyme molecules is localized at the inner mitochondrial membrane. Bar: 0.5 μm.

functions. This concept has been concisely expressed and convincingly stressed in an important paper by Linnane *et al.* (1989) reporting that in aging the mitochondrial population present in a given cell (or cellular compartment) is composed of a mosaic of units with different metabolic competence because of the different mutation load accumulated with advancing age. This concept particularly applies to the old nerve cells that accumulate mtDNA mutations both as a consequence of ROS attacks during cellular respiration and because of the number of replications of their mtDNA. Namely, in the postmitotic nerve cells, considering that the half-life of neuronal mitochondria is about four weeks (Menzies and Gold 1971), mtDNA replicates at the rate of once a month, thus in 80 to 85 year-old human beings, mtDNA has undergone replication about 1000 times, at variance with the nuclear genome that does not replicate (Toescu *et al.*, 2000). Considering the Linnane mitochondrial mosaic concept, it appears reasonable to hypothesize that the fraction of impaired or less functional mitochondria should increase with advancing age in postmitotic nerve cells, which can play an early significant role in the progressive decay in specific neuronal functional tasks (e.g., memory and learning capacities). In this context, the activity of succinic dehydrogenase (SDH) may represent a reliable parameter to verify the functional state of a given mitochondrial population. SDH, complex II of the oxidative phosphorylation (OXPHOS) process, constitutes a secondary entrance of the electron transport chain and has been reported to play a critical role when mitochondrial oxidative capacity is high. SDH is the only mitochondrial enzyme common both for electron and carbon fluxes, thus representing the unique molecule for cross control between cellular respiration and the Krebs cycle. Frequent burst of activity requiring adequate ATP amounts is an almost physiological condition of nerve cells; thus the activity of SDH reasonably may be considered as a reliable marker of the efficiency of ATP provision in neurons when energy demand is high. SDH activity can clearly be evidenced within single organelles by the preferential cytochemical reaction of copper ferrocyanide. As originally documented in the mid-1960s by Ogawa *et al.* (1968), the ferricyanide readily accepts electrons from the respiratory chain and is reduced to ferrocyanide that is captured by copper at the site of the enzyme activity. In turn, this molecule is trapped at mitochondrial cristae in the form of insoluble, electron opaque precipitate (see Figure 40.9).

SDH-positive mitochondria are easily identified at the electron microscope, and their ultrastructural features can be estimated reliably by conventional morphometric methods. In performing the preferential staining of SDH by the copper ferrocyanide method, only fresh samples can be used since the tissue must not be fixed to preserve SDH activity. Although this limits these studies to laboratory animals or human bioptic material, the data obtained may be considered as a reliable estimation of the actual oxidative capacity of the mitochondrial population analyzed. Studies conducted in old rats have shown that the volume density of SDH-positive mitochondria (i.e., the fraction of organelles/μm^3 of cytoplasm or neuropil) is significantly decreased in the perykaria of large-sized neurons, such as cerebellar Purkinje cells and hippocampal CA1 pyramidal cells. In both these types of cells, this decrease is due to a significant numeric loss of the SDH-positive organelles, even though their average volume does not change significantly. Because of their large size, Purkinje and CA1 cells are reliable neuronal models to investigate cellular bioenergetics in aging since their extended dendritic trees and lengthy projections need high amounts of energy for normal maintenance and function, thus being particularly sensitive to any change in ATP supply. Considering the previously mentioned SDH functional features, these data support the idea that, in aging, neuronal mitochondria may not be able to match the energy needs for proper function when ATP demand is high.

CYTOCHEMISTRY OF CYTOCHROME OXIDASE ACTIVITY IN THE AGING BRAIN

On the basis of the age-related constancy of the mitochondrial volume density (Vv), reported by many investigations using conventional electron microscopic methods, ATP supply is supposed to be adequate to the physiological housekeeping processes of the neuron in resting conditions. Namely, because of the known dynamic condition of mitochondrial morphology, the ultrastructural features of a given population of organelles (i.e., size, number, and volume density) appear to be modulated according to actual physiological stimulations reasonably to facilitate the provision of adequate ATP amounts needed for the cell's proper response to environmental challenges. An obvious question is whether the age-related rearrangements in mitochondrial morphology have any functional significance. According to Linnane *et al.*'s mosaic concept, the heteroplasmic status of a given mitochondrial population implies that each organelle is characterized by its own functional efficiency. This very specific and functional mitochondrial metabolic feature, defined as mitochondrial metabolic competence (MMC) (Bertoni-Freddari *et al.*, 2003, 2005), has been tested in aging by preferential cytochemistry of cytochrome oxidase (COX) activity measured in single organelles by computer-assisted image analyzers and morphometric programs. COX, an integral transmembrane protein of the inner mitochondrial membrane, is the terminal enzyme of the electron transport chain (complex IV) and represents a reliable endogenous marker of neuronal metabolism (Wong-Riley, 1989). By using diaminobenzidine (DAB) as electron donor, COX activity can be preferentially evidenced at the inner mitochondrial membranes as dark reaction deposits (see Figure 40.10).

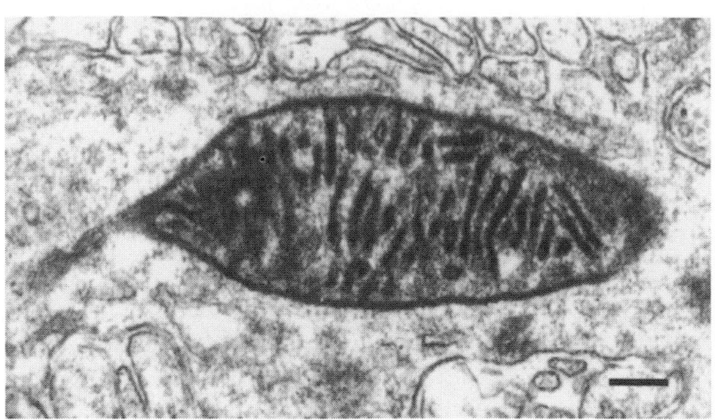

Figure 40.10 COX-positive mitochondrion at synaptic terminals in the rat cerebellar cortex (glomerular areas in the granular layer). The cristae and the inner mitochondrial membrane appear preferentially stained by the reaction of diaminobenzidine with the enzyme molecules and subsequent osmium staining. The overall area of the reaction deposits (that can be easily measured by an image analyzer) accounts for the fraction (%) of the surface of the inner mitochondrial membrane involved in cellular respiration. Bar: 0.5 μm.

The overall area of the DAB-COX cytochemical precipitate, measured within each mitochondrion by computer-assisted quantitative methods, represents the surface fraction of the inner membrane of the mitochondria directly involved in cellular respiration, and it also accounts for COX activity. Namely, to observe an accumulation of the cytochemical precipitate, the continuous oxidation of cytochrome c by COX is needed. Therefore the overall area of the dark deposits at the inner membranes of the mitochondria is proportional to the functional and actual activity of the enzyme and the ratio (R) between the area of the precipitate, and the overall area of the mitochondrion may be considered as a reliable MMC estimation (Bertoni-Freddari *et al.*, 2003, 2005). A recent investigation carried out on synaptic mitochondria in the cerebellum of adult and old rats has compared the age-related MMC vs. size of each mitochondrion. In old animals the MMC of small and medium-sized organelles was significantly decreased by 31.6 and 26.4%, respectively (see Figure 40.11), but in both adult and old rats the fraction of enlarged mitochondria appeared to show the same capacity for ATP provision (the value of R was 0.30 in adult rats and 0.29 in old rats).

Most of the mitochondria of a given population (80 to 95%) is represented by small and medium-sized organelles. The provision of ATP required for cellular metabolic needs is in charge of this fraction of organelles, and the enlarged ones are suggested to represent an intermediate ultrastructural feature in the genesis of new mitochondria or in the functional remodeling of the existing mitochondria following fusion. Conceivably, the complement of smaller mitochondria appear to be of critical importance from a functional standpoint since the decreased numeric density of mitochondria found at the aging synaptic terminals is due to a significant loss of the organelles of this size. On the other hand, the age-related increase in the fraction of the enlarged mitochondria, according to their lower value of R, appears to represent a weak compensating reaction.

By taking together the age-related alterations in mitochondrial ultrastructure as well as SDH and COX activities, it appears that the decay of MMC may play an early and critical role in the development and progression of synaptic pathology associated with physiological and pathological brain aging.

Calcium Homeostasis

Several physiological processes ranging from cell division to muscle contraction to secretion and neurotransmission

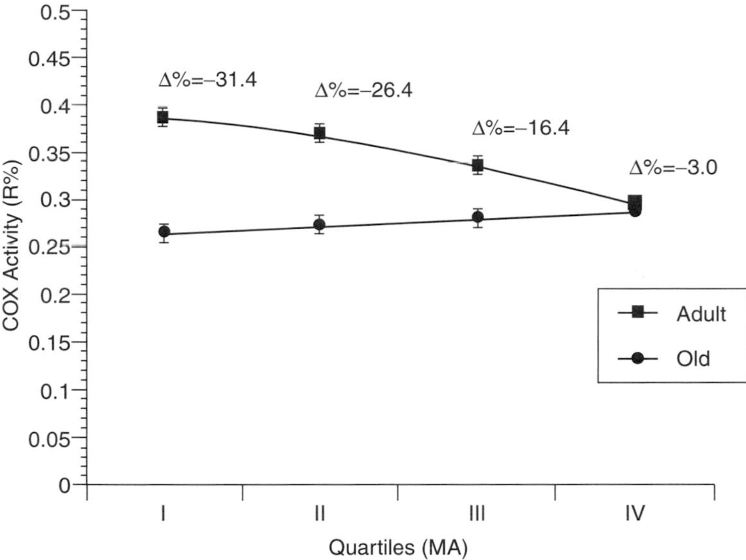

Figure 40.11 Age-based comparison of the quartile values of R (area of the COX cytochemical precipitate/overall area of each mitochondrion). The quartile values are the respective means of the I, II, III, and IV groups of data ordered by increasing values of the area of synaptic mitochondria (from the rat cerebellar cortex). In adult animals there is a progressive decrease in R (quartiles I–II: −4.7%, quartiles II–III: −9.3%, quartiles III–IV: −11.5%); in old rats an increasing trend can be envisaged (quartiles I–II: +2.6%, quartiles II–III: +3.0%, quartiles III–IV: +2.7%). The paired-quartile decreases in R due to aging were: I (−31.6%), II (−26.4%), III (−16.4%), IV (−3.0%). As clearly shown by the intersection point of the two lines, the very large mitochondria showed almost the same values of R (adult animals 0.30, old animals 0.29). (Reproduced with permission from *Naturwissenschaften* 92, 82–85, 2005.)

are accomplished through proper movements of calcium ions. In aging most of these processes decline, and this has suggested the hypothesis that a defective calcium homeostasis may represent an early change responsible for functional decay. The nervous system appears to be very vulnerable to an altered calcium homeostasis since many brain functions depend on many calcium-regulated processes. Within the cell, calcium can be found as bound and free (ionized) and its concentration is maintained at around 10^{-7} M by complex processes. Intracellular organelles, such as endoplasmic reticulum and mitochondria, sequester calcium that can be extruded across the plasma membrane by energy-dependent transport systems. The equilibrium between uptake and efflux mechanisms across the plasma and organelle membranes balances the set point for calcium concentration within the cell or a given cellular compartment. Specific calcium binding proteins (calmodulin, calbindin, troponin, and vitamin D-dependent protein) as well as negatively charged residues within or at the surface of the cell membranes (sialic acid) can bind calcium and modulate the free cytosolic calcium concentration $[Ca^{2+}]_i$. Changes in any of these aspects of calcium homeostasis may alter calcium-dependent processes. In looking for age-dependent changes in calcium regulation leading to cellular dysfunction, very subtle alterations in the cell's ability to respond to normal stimuli must be investigated since the changes may be so subtle that they are clearly manifest only when cells are severely stressed, for example, by adverse conditions or excessive stimulation. By taking into account the multiple roles that calcium plays in neurotransmission and intracellular signaling, it appears reasonable to suppose that minor changes in calcium-regulating processes in neurons may result in the alterations affecting cognition and behavior reported in aging. Because of the complexity of the overall cellular calcium regulation, the identification of alterations due to age in calcium-handling systems is a rather difficult task. Direct measurement of intracellular calcium is possible only in isolated cells or tissue slices that do not mirror exactly the actual situation present in the living tissue; therefore, this enables data to be obtained on very discrete aspects of intracellular calcium regulation. Moreover, Ca^{2+} relays the signals elicited by the first messengers to their omnidirectional destinations: this Ca^{2+} dynamic signaling involves $[Ca^{2+}]_i$ fluctuations within very short time frames (fraction of millisecond) that add further complications in measuring basal levels of calcium even in isolated cells (Chen and Fernandez, 1999). Despite these difficulties, several reports document that in the aging nerve terminals calcium handling is slower and less effective than in terminals from younger laboratory animals. Namely, in aged rats presynaptic Ca^{2+} signals are prolonged or Ca^{2+} clearance is slowed; that is, following stimulation the kinetics of the buffering or the clearing of Ca^{2+} are altered in aging, thus Ca^{2+} remains elevated for a longer period of time. Considering that calcium regulates metabolic pathways and serves important functions as second messenger, reasonably $[Ca^{2+}]_i$ must be tightly regulated.

In agreement with this assumption, the age-related changes in Ca^{2+} homeostasis just described are supposed to underlie a decline in brain function; however, the complexity of the dynamics of Ca^{2+} regulation does not allow the interpretation of a prolonged elevation of $[Ca^{2+}]_i$ at the old nerve terminals as necessarily deleterious for neuronal function.

Alzheimer-like Alterations

The brain of AD patients is characterized by the consistent presence of SP and NFT, two hallmarks of structural protein precipitation occurring in neuronal aging. SP and NFT are also found, but to a lesser degree, in the brain of elderly, cognitive intact individuals. SP are focal and irregular alterations of the neuropil ranging in size from 30 to 30,000 μm^2 or more according to the age of the subject, brain size, and neuronal size distribution in the brain cortex. SP appear as a lattice of altered neurites containing at the center of the lesion, amyloid deposits (see Figure 40.12).

Shape size and composition of SP vary according to the age of the patients: younger individuals are characterized by large SP with diffuse neurites and poorly defined shape; in middle-aged subjects SP have a more regular circular shape, and in elderly patients SP show increasing amounts of amyloid and cellular debris. Beta amyloid protein (βA), derived from the large precursor (APP), is the major constituent of SP amyloid. βA is composed of 4–8 fibrils with a β-pleated sheet molecular conformation, a feature that provides amyloid with birefringence after Congo red staining and fluorescence after thioflavine treatment. In classical SP, amyloid fibrils are intermingled with a large number of degenerating neuronal processes that may also surround the whole SP. In addition to βA, other proteins, lipids, and carbohydrates participate in SP formation. NFT are bundles of fibrillary material observed in the perikarya where they can partially accumulate or completely fill the nerve cell soma and the axon hillock (see Figure 40.13).

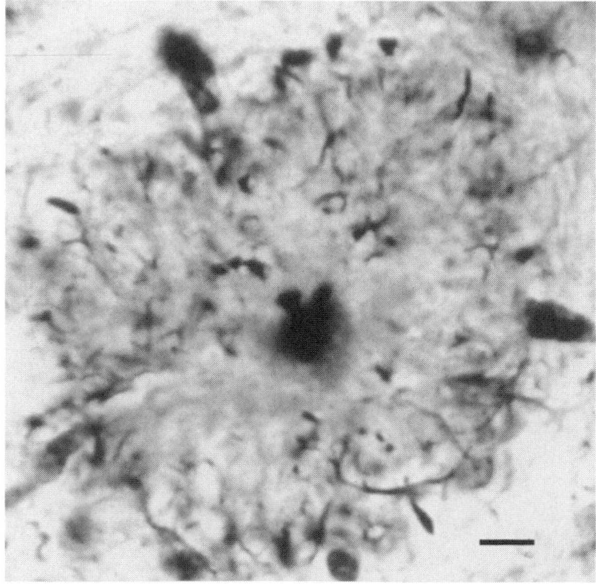

Figure 40.12 Classical type of SP stained by a silver impregnation technique. The central dark spot representing the focal deposition of βA is surrounded by dystrophic neurites. Bar: 10 μm.

At the electron microscope, NFT appear morphologically heterogeneous since they contain mainly straight and paired helical filaments (PHF) in addition to other elements. PHF are composed by the microtubule associated protein tau derived from alternative splicing of a single tau gene. PHF width alternates between 8 and 20 nm with an apparent period of 80 nm. There is a wide range of NFT size and aspect that is particularly apparent in NFT located outside the cytoplasm where they look enlarged and less compact. If they look diffuse, it is difficult to differentiate them from SP. Studies conducted in post-mortem human samples have shown that an increasing tendency to develop SP and NFT is typical of some groups of neurons of larger size—that is, the pyramidal neurons found in layers III and V of the neocortex and subiculum and layer II of the enthorinal cortex. By means of a recently introduced silver impregnation procedure (Reusche, 1991), extensive quantitative analyses have shown that SP and NFT incidences increase exponentially with age and increasing neuronal size. It has been hypothesized that SP and NFT may represent different phases of the same neurodegenerative process: the formation of SP is suggested to be a primary neuronal damage affecting neurites that progresses to the onset of NFT in the perykarion (Dani and Weiss, 1994).

Models of Brain Aging and Age-related Pathologies

The studies on aging of the human brain are hampered by the obvious difficulties of carrying out investigations on fresh samples. On the other hand, post-mortem material may provide erroneous information because of the different circumstances and factors that can affect the reliability of the data obtained. These include, first of all, the agonal state of the patient and the post-mortem delay in performing autopsy. Neurobiological, genetic, and molecular studies conducted in laboratory rodents or *in vitro* systems, have documented the vulnerability of selected pools of neurons and the changes occurring in several neural systems and molecular processing with advancing age. However, in order to get results matching as much as possible those that potentially can be found in the old human brain, some animal models have been developed. These models, though constituting abundant sources of fresh brain samples to be investigated, may be helpful in better delineating the mechanisms of

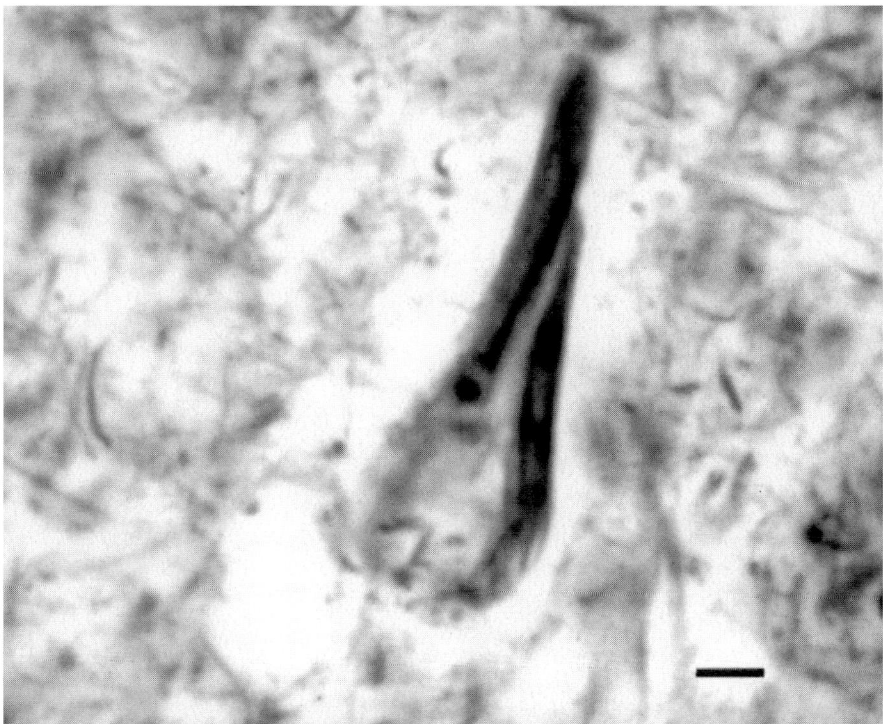

Figure 40.13 NFT in a pyramidal neuron from an AD patient. The neuronal body and the axon hillock are completely filled in with NFT. Bar: 10 μm.

physiological brain aging as well as the early pathogenic determinants of age-related diseases. In turn, testing of new therapeutic approaches to treat neurodegenerative diseases, such as AD, can be carried out on these models.

AGED NONHUMAN PRIMATES

Nonhuman primates, for example, different monkey strains, develop age-related behavioral and brain alterations similar to those found in humans. Monkeys (e.g., *Macaca mulatta*) have an estimated lifespan of more than 35 years and are the best available model to study AD pathology. Behavioral testing has shown that memory and cognition decline in the second decade of the monkey life and are particularly evident in the mid- to late twenties. In old monkeys, dystrophic neurites, amyloid deposition, and alterations of specific neurotransmitter systems are similar, although less severe, than those reported in the old human brain and AD patients. Namely, slightly enlarged neurites and pre-amyloid deposits constitute the earliest lesions found in the parenchyma of the cortex of the animals around 20 years of age. In addition to the classical alterations found in the human brain (i.e., neurites containing membranous elements, degenerating mitochondria, lysosomes, APP, phosphorylated neurofilaments) in the neuronal perikarya, axons, and neurites within SP containing βA of old monkeys, an APP-like immunoreactivity has been found. This implies that neurons may serve as a source of some βA deposits. As in humans, in the old monkey brain nonneuronal cells may participate in the formation of βA as shown by the proximity of this peptide to reactive astrocytes, microglia, and vascular cells. On the basis of these features, nonhuman primates appear to represent a reliable animal model of aging to investigate the many alterations occurring in the old human brain.

TRANSGENIC MICE

Transgenic mouse models have been developed through the expression of mutated APP (or the overexpression of its wild type) to study the involvement of βA-containing fragments in AD-type abnormalities. Among the many transgenic mice, the PDAPP mouse is one of the best characterized since it develops βA accumulation in neocortex and hippocampus after 12 months of age. These mice show consistent pathological symptoms before βA accumulates, thus suggesting that neuronal pathology may come from developmental abnormalities or that soluble βA is responsible for these alterations. Namely, loss of dendritic arborizations leading to a reduction in the volume of the dentate gyrus is apparent as early as three months of age.

As in AD, the initial accumulation of βA occurs in the enthorinal cortex and dentate gyrus, but in PDAPP mice a minimal neuronal death occurs, at variance with AD. In a mouse model with mutations of APP and presenilin 1, neuronal death is significant, and the selective vulnerability of neurons (e.g., the hippocampal CA1 pyramidal cells) is similar to the results found in AD patients. In this model, at variance with the PDAPP one, loss of neurons close to and in zones devoid of βA deposits is the same, which suggests that aggregation of βA into plaques does not necessarily imply neuron loss. Conceivably, it is clearly apparent that comparison of the results obtained from different transgenic mice may help to envisage the sequential events involved in age- and pathology-related alterations of the brain.

Conclusion

The process of aging is characterized by a marked heterogeneity among individuals, a hallmark that is reflected also by the different groups of brain cells accomplishing different tasks. Although composed by fully differentiated postmitotic cells, the brain retains a consistent potential for adaptive response even in old individuals. Compensating reactions are actively counteracting age-related alterations, thus masking the decay of specific functions until a critical threshold of impairment is attained. Several determinants are reported to play a role in brain aging, and these may affect interdependent processes that, in turn, compromise the proper efficiency of selected neural network. As a final outcome, coping with environmental stimuli becomes increasingly difficult, particularly under excessive stimulation or stress, and impairment of function becomes clearly apparent. Current literature data support the idea that early disturbances occur on synaptic and mitochondrial functions both in physiological aging and in the progressive pathogenesis of age-related neurodegenerative diseases. This suggests that both synapses and mitochondria may constitute reliable targets for early therapeutic interventions at least to decrease the severity of the alterations occurring in human brain aging.

Recommended Resources

Bereiter-Hahn, J., and Voth, M. (1994). Dynamics of mitochondria in living cells: shape changes, dislocations, fusion and fission of mitochondria. *Microsc. Res. Tech. 27*, 198–219.

Bertoni-Freddari, C., Fattoretti, P., Paoloni, R., Caselli, U., Galeazzi, L., and Meier-Ruge, W. (1996). Synaptic structural dynamics and aging. *Gerontology 42*, 170–180.

Bertoni-Freddari, C., Fattoretti, P., Paoloni, R., Caselli, U., Giorgetti, B., and Solazzi, M. (2003). Inverse correlation between mitochondrial size and metabolic competence: a quantitative cytochemical study of cytochrome oxidase activity. *Naturwissenschaften 90*, 68–71.

Bertoni-Freddari, C., Fattoretti, P., Giorgetti, B., Spazzafumo, L., Solazzi, M., and Balietti, M. (2005). Age-related decline in metabolic competence of small and medium-sized synaptic mitochondria. *Naturwissenschaften 92*, 82–85.

Boellaard, J.W., and Schlote, W. (1986). Ultrastructural heterogeneity of neuronal lipofuscin in the normal brain cerebral cortex. *Acta Neuropathol. 71*, 285–294.

Buell, S.J., and Coleman, P.D. (1979). Dendritic growth in the aged brain and failure of growth in senile dementia. *Science 206*, 854–856.

Carlin, R.K., and Siekevitz, P. (1983). Plasticity in the central nervous system: Do synapses divide? *Proc. Natl. Acad. Sci. USA 80*, 3517–3521.

Chen, M., and Fernandez, H.L. (1999). Ca^{2+} signaling downregulation in ageing and Alzheimer's disease: why is Ca^{2+} so difficult to measure? *Cell Calcium 26*, 149–154.

Coleman, P.D., and Flood, D.G. (1987). Neuron number and dendritic extent in normal aging and Alzheimer's disease. *Neurobiol. Ageing 8*, 521–545.

Geinisman, Y., deToledo-Morrel, L., Morrel, F., and Heller, R.E. (1995). Hippocampal markers of age-related memory dysfunction: behavioral, electrophysiological and morphological perspectives. *Progr. Neurobiol. 45*, 223–252.

Hillman, D.E., and Chen, S. (1984). Reciprocal relationship between size of postsynaptic densities and their number. Constancy in contact area. *Brain Res. 295*, 325–343.

Linnane, A.W., Marzuky, S., Ozawa, T., and Tanaka, M. (1989). Mitochondrial DNA mutations as an important contributor to aging and degenerative diseases. *The Lancet 1*, 642–645.

Mayhew, T.M. (1996). How to count synapses unbiasedly and efficiently at the ultrastructural level: proposal for a standard sampling and counting protocol. *J. Neurocytol. 25*, 793–804.

Sterio, D.C. (1984). The unbiased estimation of number and size of arbitrary particles using the dissector. *J. Microsc. 134*, 127–136.

Toescu, E.C., Myronova, N., and Verkhratsky, A. (2000). Age-related structural and functional changes of brain mitochondria. *Cell Calcium 28*, 329–338.

Wong-Riley, M.T.T. (1989). Cytochrome oxidase: an endogenous metabolic marker for neuronal activity. *Trends Neurosci. 12*, 94–101.

REFERENCES

Allen, S.J., Benton, J.S., Goodhardt, M.J. (1983). Biochemical evidence of selective nerve cell changes in the normal ageing human and rat brain. *J. Neurochem. 41*, 256–265.

Banay-Schwartz, M., Lajtha, A., Palkovitz, M., and Nathan, S. (1992). Regional distribution of glutamate and aspartate in adult and old human brain. *Brain Res. 594*, 343–346.

Bereiter-Hahn, J., and Voth, M. (1994). Dynamics of mitochondria in living cells: shape changes, dislocations, fusion and fission of mitochondria. *Microsc. Res. Tech. 27*, 198–219.

Bertoni-Freddari, C., and Giuli, C. (1980). A quantitative morphometric study of synapses of rat cerebellar glomeruli during aging. *Mech. Ageing Dev. 12*, 127–136.

Bertoni-Freddari, C., Fattoretti, P., Casoli, T., Meier-Ruge, W., and Ulrich, J. (1990). Morphological adaptive response of the synaptic junctional zones in the human dentate gyrus during aging and Alzheimer's disease. *Brain Res. 517*, 69–75.

Bertoni-Freddari, C., Fattoretti, P., Casoli, T., Spagna, C., Meier-Ruge, W., and Ulrich, J. (1993). Morphological plasticity of synaptic mitochondria during aging. *Brain Res. 628*, 193–200.

Bertoni-Freddari, C., Fattoretti, P., Paoloni, R., Caselli, U., Galeazzi, L., and Meier-Ruge, W. (1996). Synaptic structural dynamics and aging. *Gerontology 42*, 170–180.

Bertoni-Freddari, C., Fattoretti, P., Casoli, T., Di Stefano, G., Solazzi, M., Meier-Ruge, W. (2001). Quantitative cytochemical mapping of mitochondrial enzymes in rat cerebella. *Micron 32*, 405–410.

Bertoni-Freddari, C., Fattoretti, P., Ricciuti, R., Vecchioni, S., Casoli, T., Solazzi, M., *et al.* (2002). Morphometry of E-PTA stained synapses at the periphery of pathological lesions. *Micron 33*, 447–451.

Bertoni-Freddari, C., Fattoretti, P., Paoloni, R., Caselli, U., Giorgetti, B., and Solazzi, M. (2003). Inverse correlation between mitochondrial size and metabolic competence: a quantitative cytochemical study of cytochrome oxidase activity. *Naturwissenschaften 90*, 68–71.

Bertoni-Freddari, C., Fattoretti, P., Giorgetti, B., Spazzafumo, L., Solazzi, M., and Balietti, M. (2005). Age-related decline in metabolic competence of small and medium-sized synaptic mitochondria. *Naturwissenschaften 92*, 82–85.

Boellaard, J.W., and Schlote, W. (1986). Ultrastructural heterogeneity of neuronal lipofuscin in the normal brain cerebral cortex. *Acta Neuropathol. 71*, 285–294.

Buell, S.J., and Coleman, P.D. (1979). Dendritic growth in the aged brain and failure of growth in senile dementia. *Science 206*, 854–856.

Carlin, R.K., and Siekevitz, P. (1983). Plasticity in the central nervous system: Do synapses divide? *Proc. Natl. Acad. Sci. USA 80*, 3517–3521.

Chen, M., and Fernandez, H.L. (1999). Ca^{2+} signaling down-regulation in ageing and Alzheimer's disease: why is Ca^{2+} so difficult to measure? *Cell Calcium 26*, 149–154.

Chen, S., and Hillman, D.E. (1980). Giant spines and enlarged synapses induced in Purkinje cells by malnutrition. *Brain Res. 187*, 487–493.

Coleman, P.D., and Flood, D.G. (1987). Neuron number and dendritic extent in normal aging and Alzheimer's disease. *Neurobiol. Ageing 8*, 521–545.

Cotman, C.W., and Scheff, S.W. (1979). Compensatory synapses growth in aged animals after neuronal death. *Mech. Ageing Dev. 9*, 103–117.

Dani, S.U., and Weiss, S. (1994). Looking for histological correlates of dementia: the neurodegeneration progression rate (NDPR). *Clin. Neuropathol. 5*, 240–241.

DeKosky, S.T., and Scheff, S.W. (1990). Synapses loss in frontal cortex biopsies in Alzheimer's disease: Correlation with cognitive severity. *Ann. Neurol. 27*, 457–464.

Desmond, N.L., and Levy, W.B. (1986). Changes in the numerical density of synaptic contacts with long-term potentiation in the hippocampal dentate gyrus. *J. Comp. Neurol. 253*, 466–475.

Dyson, S.E., and Jones, D.G. (1976). The morphological categorization of developing synaptic junctions. *Cell Tissue Res. 167*, 363–371.

Geinisman, Y., deToledo-Morrel, L., Morrel, F., and Heller, R.E. (1995). Hippocampal markers of age-related memory dysfunction: behavioral, electrophysiological and morphological perspectives. *Progr. Neurobiol. 45*, 223–252.

Gomez-Isla, T., Hollister, R., West, H., Mui, S., Growdon, J.H., Petersen, R.C., Parisi, J.E., and Hyman, B.T. (1997). Neuronal loss correlates with but exceeds neurofibrillary tangles in Alzheimer's disease. *Ann. Neurol. 41(1)*, 17–24.

Haan, J., Maat Schieman, M.L., and Roos, R.A. (1994). Clinical aspects of cerebral amyloid angiopathy. *Dementia 5*, 210–213.

Hansen, L.A., Armstrong, G.,M., and Terry, R.D. (1987). An immunohistochemical quantification of fibrous astrocytes in the aging human cerebral cortex. *Neurobiol. Ageing 8*, 1–6.

Hillman, D.E., and Chen, S. (1984). Reciprocal relationship between size of postsynaptic densities and their number. Constancy in contact area. *Brain Res. 295*, 325–343.

Kalaria, R.N., Andorn, A.C., Tabaton, M., Whitehouse, P.J., Harik, S.I., and Unnerstall, J.R. (1989). Adrenergic receptors in aging and Alzheimer's disease: Increased beta 2-receptors in prefrontal cortex and hippocampus. *J. Neurochem. 53*, 1772–1782.

Kish, S.J., Shannak, K., Rajput, A., Deck, J.H., and Hornykiewicz, O. (1992). Aging produces a specific pattern of striatal dopamine loss: Implications for the etiology of idiopathic Parkinson's disease. *J. Neurochem. 58*, 642–648.

Koch, C., Zador, A., and Brown, T.H. (1992). Dendritic spines: convergence of theory and experiment. *Science 256*, 973–974.

Leenders, K.L., Perani, D., Lammertsma, A.A., Heather, J.D., Buckingham, P., Healy, M.J., Gibbs, J.M., Wise, R.J., Hatazawa, J., Herold, S., *et al.* (1990). Cerebral blood flow, blood volume, and oxygen utilization—normal values and effects of age. *Brain 113*, 27–47.

Linnane, A.W., Marzuky, S., Ozawa, T., and Tanaka, M. (1989). Mitochondrial DNA mutations as an important contributor to aging and degenerative diseases. *The Lancet 1*, 642–645.

Mayhew, T.M. (1996). How to count synapses unbiasedly and efficiently at the ultrastructural level: proposal for a standard sampling and counting protocol. *J. Neurocytol. 25*, 793–804.

Menzies, R.A., and Gold, P.H. (1971). The turnover of mitochondria in a variety of tissues of young, adult and aged rats. *J. Biol. Chem. 246*, 2425–2429.

Miquel, J., and Bertoni-Freddari, C. (2000). Causes and consequences of damage to mitochondria. In Y.A. Barnett and R.C. Barnett, *Methods in Molecular Medicine* (vol. 38): Aging Methods and Protocols (pp. 221–235). Totowa, NJ: Humana Press Inc.

Moore, W.A., Davey V.A., Weindruch, R., Walford, R., and Ivy, G.O. (1995). The effect of caloric restriction on lipofuscin accumulation in mouse brain with age. *Gerontology 41(2)*, 173–185.

Mrak, R.E., Sheng, J.G., and Griffin, W.S.T. (1995). Glial cytokines in Alzheimer's disease: Review and pathogenic implications. *Human Pathol. 26*, 816–823.

Nakano, I., Iwatsbuo, T., Otsuka N., Kamei M., Matsumura, K., and Mannen, T. (1992). Paired helical filaments in astrocytes: electron microscopy and immunohistochemistry in a case of atypical Alzheimer's disease. *Acta Neuropathol. 83(3)*, 228–232.

Ogawa, K., Saito, T., and Mayahara, H. (1968). The site of ferrocyanide reduction by reductases within mitochondria as studied by electron microscopy. *J. Histochem. Cytochem. 16*, 49–57.

Pakkenberg, B., and Gundersen, H.J. (1997). Neocortical neuron number in humans: effect of sex and age. *J. Comp. Neurol. 384*, 312–320.

Perry, E.K. (1980). The cholinergic system in old age and Alzheimer's s disease. Age *Ageing 9*, 1–8.

Purves, D., and Lichtman, J.W. (1980). Elimination of synapses in the developing nervous system. *Science 210*, 153–157.

Rowe, J.W., and Khan, R.L. (1987). Human aging: usual and successful. *Science 237*, 143–149.

Reusche, E. (1991). Silver staining of senile plaques and neurofibrillary tangles in paraffin sections. A simple and effective method. *Pathol. Res. Pract. 187*, 1045–1049.

Scheibel, M.E., Lindsay, R.D., Tomiyasu, U., and Scheibel, A.B. (1975). Progressive dendritic changes in the human cerebral cortex. *Exp. Neurol. 47*, 392–403.

Sheng, J.G., Mrak, R.E., Rovnaghi, C.R., Kozlowska, E., Eldik, L.J., and Griffin, W.S.T. (1996). Human brain S100β and S100β mRNA expression increases with age: Pathogenic implications for Alzheimer's disease. *Neurobiol. Ageing 17*, 359–363.

Solmi, R., Pallotti, F., and Rugolo, M. (1994). Lack of major mitochondrial bioenergetic changes in cultured skin fibroblasts from aged individuals. *Biochem. Mol. Biol. Int. 33*, 477–484.

Sterio, D.C. (1984). The unbiased estimation of number and size of arbitrary particles using the disector. *J. Microsc. 134*, 127–136.

Takada, H., Nagata, K., Hirata, Y., Satoh, Y., Watahiki, Y., Sugawara, J., *et al.* (1992). Age-related decline of cerebral oxygen metabolism in normal population detected with positron emission tomography. *Neurol. Res. 14*, 128–131.

Toescu, E.C., Myronova, N., and Verkhratsky, A. (2000). Age-related structural and functional changes of brain mitochondria. *Cell Calcium 28*, 329–338.

Walter, P.B., Beckman, K.B., and Ames, B.N. (1999). The role of iron and mitochondria in aging. In E. Cadenas and I. Packer (Eds.), *Understanding the process of aging: the role of mitochondria, free radicals and antioxidants* (pp. 203–227). New York: Marcel Dekker.

West, M.J., Coleman, P.D., Flood, D.G., and Troncoso J.C. (1994). Differences in the pattern of hippocampal neuronal loss in normal ageing and Alzheimer's disease. *Lancet 344*, 769–772.

Wolff, J.R., Laskawi, R., Spatz, W.B., and Missler, M. (1995). Structural dynamics of synapses and synaptic components. *Behav. Brain Res. 66*, 13–20.

Wong-Riley, M.T.T. (1989). Cytochrome oxidase: an endogenous metabolic marker for neuronal activity. *Trends Neurosci. 12*, 94–101.

41

Mitochondrial DNA and Aging

Mikhail F. Alexeyev, Susan P. LeDoux, and Glenn L. Wilson

The goal of this chapter is to introduce the reader to the current state of the mitochondrial theory of aging as it pertains to mitochondrial DNA (mtDNA). Several aspects will be covered, including a basic biology of mitochondrial DNA, the experimental evidence supporting the mitochondrial theory of aging, and the experimental data that appear to contradict this theory. Finally, an overview of experimental approaches used to study mtDNA in aging will be presented, and weaknesses of each approach will be discussed.

Introduction

Aging can be defined as a multifactorial phenomenon characterized by a time-dependent decline in physiological function (Mandavilli *et al.*, 2002). This physiological decline is believed to be associated with an accumulation of defects in metabolic pathways. It has been almost 50 years since Harman first put forward his free radical theory of aging (Harman, 1956). Over the years it has been refined to include not only free radicals, but also other reactive species, such as hydrogen peroxide. Another important development was the identification by Harman, in 1972, of mitochondria as a biological clock. Despite its intellectual simplicity, this theory was as universally rejected initially as it is universally accepted today. RNA, proteins, and other cellular macromolecules that are turned over rapidly are poor candidates for progressive accumulation of damage over a lifetime. Therefore, even early studies on the mechanisms of aging focused on DNA (e.g. Price *et al.*, 1971). In mammalian cells, mitochondria and the nucleus are the only organelles that possess DNA. However, until recently the mitochondrial genome has received less attention than its nuclear counterpart in the context of aging.

Today we have at our disposal an overwhelming body of evidence in support of the mitochondrial theory of aging, yet the amount of discordant data continues to grow as well. The controversial nature of the experimental results appears to be rooted in both the intrinsic complexity of the aging process and the imperfection of experimental tools available today. Here, we will review both the role played by mitochondrial DNA (mtDNA) in the aging process and experimental approaches used to study mtDNA.

Basic mtDNA Biology

Human mtDNA is a circular double-stranded molecule that is 16,569 bp long (other sequenced mammalian mitochondrial genomes have similar lengths; see Figure 41.1).

It carries 37 genes, of which two encode rRNAs, 22 encode tRNAs, and 13 encode polypeptides. All 13 mitochondrially encoded polypeptides represent components of the electron transfer chain (ETC). Of these, seven are subunits of complex I (NADH dehydrogenase), three are subunits of complex IV (cytochrome c oxidase), two are subunits of complex V (ATP synthase), and cytochrome b (a subunit of complex III). The inheritance of mtDNA is almost exclusively maternal, although instances of paternal inheritance have been reported in humans, mice, and birds. mtDNA is present in one to several thousand copies per cell and is *encapsulated* into mitochondria between 1 and 11 copies per mitochondrion, with the mean being two genomes per organelle. Mitochondria are dynamic structures that, in different cell types and under different physiological conditions, can assume a variety of conformations, the two extremes being *reticular* (all mitochondria in a cell are fused to form a network) and *particular* (each mitochondrion exists as a separate entity). In both conformations, mitochondria perpetually undergo the processes of fission and fusion. Therefore, the earlier definitions of reticulate and particulate mitochondrial conformations are relative terms referring to a snapshot of the mitochondrial network in a cell. Nevertheless, these terms are useful as they describe the prevalence of either mitochondrial fission (particulate conformation) or fusion (reticulate conformation) in a given cell under given physiological conditions. In this light, the average number of mtDNA copies per mitochondrion may simply reflect the extent of mitochondrial fragmentation under the assay conditions, which is defined by two factors: a) the mitochondrial conformation inside the cell, and b) the extent of mitochondrial fragmentation during isolation for the analysis of mtDNA content.

The two mtDNA strands can be separated by denaturing CsCl gradient centrifugation. Most of the information is encoded in the heavy (purine-rich) strand

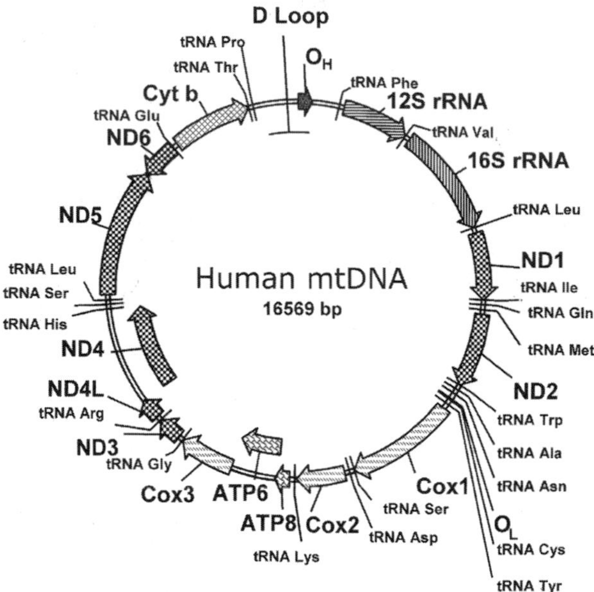

Figure 41.1 The map of human mitochondrial DNA. OH and OL, origins of heavy and light strand replication, respectively; ND1-ND6 NADH dehydrogenase (ETC complex I) subunits 1 through 6; Cox1-Cox3, cytochrome oxidase subunits 1 through 3 (ETC complex IV), ATP6 and ATP8, subunits 6 and 8 of mitochondrial ATPase (complex V), Cyt b, cytochrome b (complex III).

(2 rRNA, 14 tRNA, and 12 polypeptides). The light (pyrimidine-rich) strand contains genetic information for only one polypeptide and eight tRNAs. Mitochondrial genes have no introns, and intergenic sequences are absent or limited to a few bases. Some genes overlap, and, in some instances, termination codons are not encoded but are generated post-transcriptionally by polyadenylation (Ojala *et al.*, 1981). mtDNA is totally dependent upon proteins encoded in the nuclear genome for its maintenance and transcription. In fact, although the mitochondrial proteome consists of an estimated 1500 polypeptides, only 13 of those are encoded by mtDNA. The mitochondrial proteome is dynamic; that is, both the precise polypeptide composition and the relative abundance of a given polypeptide may vary in mitochondrial proteomes of different tissues as well as in the same tissue over time. mtDNA replication is conducted by the heterodimeric DNA polymerase gamma. The current paradigm states that replication of mammalian mtDNA continues throughout the lifespan of an organism in both proliferating and post-mitotic cells. It occurs bidirectionally, initiated at two spatially and temporally distinct origins of replication, O_H and O_L, for the heavy and light strand origins of replication, respectively (for review, see Taanman, 1999). However, this paradigm recently has been challenged, and evidence has been presented for bidirectional θ-like replication initiated over a fairly wide zone (Yang *et al.*, 2002). With the discovery of mitochondrial diseases caused by mutations of mtDNA, it has been found that wild-type (WT, normal) and mutated mtDNA may coexist in the same cell, a condition called *heteroplasmy*.

mtDNA Damage and the Mitochondrial Theory of Aging

Despite the fact that in animal cells mtDNA comprises only 1 to 3% of the genetic material, it has been argued that its contribution to cellular physiology could be much greater than would be expected from its size alone. For instance:

1. It mutates at higher rates than nuclear DNA, which may be a consequence of its close proximity to the electron transfer chain (ETC).
2. It encodes either polypeptides of ETC or components required for their synthesis. Therefore, any coding mutations in mtDNA will affect the ETC as a whole. This could affect both the assembly and/or function of the products of numerous nuclear genes in ETC complexes.
3. Defects in the ETC can have pleiotropic effects because they affect cellular energetics as a whole.

Several lines of evidence indirectly implicate mtDNA in longevity. The Framingham Longevity Study of Coronary Heart Disease has indicated that longevity is more strongly associated with age of maternal death than that of paternal death, suggesting that mtDNA inheritance might be involved. On the other hand, longevity was shown to be associated with certain mtDNA polymorphisms. For instance, Italian male centenarians have an increased incidence of mtDNA haplogroup J, whereas French and Japanese centenarians have increased incidences of G to A transition at mt9055 and C to A transversion at mt5178, respectively. However, a study of an Irish population failed to link longevity to any particular mitochondrial haplotype, suggesting that factors other than mtDNA polymorphism also may play a role in aging (Ross *et al.*, 2001).

Mitochondria have been shown to accumulate high levels of lipophilic carcinogens such as polycyclic aromatic hydrocarbons. When cells are exposed to some of these compounds, mtDNA is damaged preferentially. Other mutagenic chemicals, such as chromium (VI), N-methyl-N′-nitro-N-nitrosoguanidine (MNNG), 4-nitroquinoline 1-oxide (4NQO), and aflatoxin B1 also have been shown to preferentially target mtDNA. Therefore, it is conceivable that life-long exposure to certain environmental toxins could result in a preferential accumulation of mtDNA damage and accelerate aging. However, perhaps the most relevant kind of insult to which mtDNA is exposed is oxidative damage. The lack of protective histones and close proximity to the ETC, whose complexes I and III are believed to be the predominant sites for the reactive

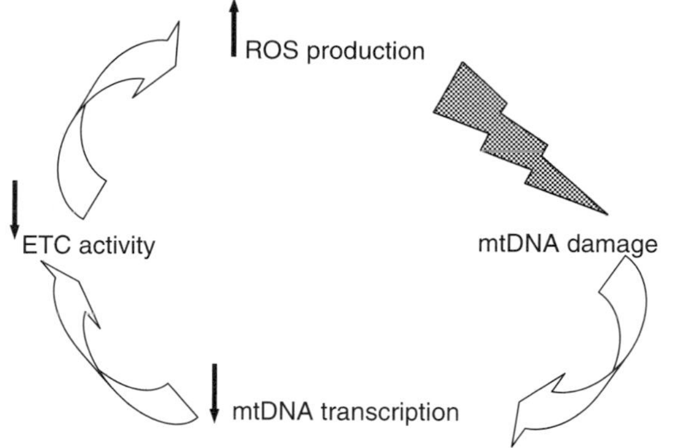

Figure 41.2 "Vicious cycle" during which ROS produced in ETC lead to the inhibition of mtDNA transcription and ETC activity, resulting in even higher levels of ROS production.

oxygen species (ROS) production inside the cell, make mtDNA extremely vulnerable to oxidative stress. Indeed, the free radical theory of aging states that it is the mitochondrial production of ROS and the resulting accumulation of damage to macromolecules that causes aging. Cumulative damage to biological macromolecules was proposed to overwhelm the capacity of biological systems to self-repair, resulting in an inevitable functional decline. The mitochondrial theory of aging can be considered as an extension and refinement of the free radical theory. Its major premise is that mtDNA mutations accumulate progressively during life, and are directly responsible for a measurable deficiency in cellular oxidative phosphorylation (OXPHOS) activity, leading to enhanced ROS production. In turn, increased ROS production results in an increased rate of mtDNA damage and mutagenesis, thus causing a "vicious cycle" of exponentially increasing oxidative damage and dysfunction that ultimately culminates in death (see Figure 41.2).

Since Miquel *et al.* first suggested that mtDNA might be damaged in aging (Miquel *et al.*, 1980), numerous studies over the past two decades have provided a wealth of information consistent with the predictions of the free radical/mitochondrial theory of aging.

OXIDATIVE DAMAGE IN CELLS, AND IN PARTICULAR, IN mtDNA, IS UBIQUITOUS, SUBSTANTIAL, AND, LIKE MORTALITY RATES, INCREASES EXPONENTIALLY WITH AGE (SOHAL AND WEINDRUCH, 1996)

Exhalation of ethane and n-penthane, indicators of ROS-mediated lipid peroxidation, increase with age. mtDNA was shown to accumulate oxidative damage in an age-dependent manner in skeletal muscle, the diaphragm, cardiac muscle, and the brain. Additionally, an age-related increase in oxidative damage to mtDNA appears to be more substantial than oxidative damage to nuclear DNA in houseflies. In rodents, an age-related increase in 7,8-dihydro-8-oxoguanine (8-oxodG), a mutagenic DNA base lesion caused by oxidative stress, was observed in mtDNA isolated from the livers of both rats and mice (Hamilton *et al.*, 2001). Dietary restriction, which is known to retard aging and increase the lifespan in rodents, has been found to significantly reduce the age-related accumulation of 8-oxodG levels in nDNA in all tissues of male B6D23F1 mice and in most tissues of male F344 rats. This study also showed that dietary restriction prevented the age-related increase in 8-oxodG levels in mtDNA isolated from the livers of both rats and mice (Hamilton *et al.*, 2001). Another study found that the activities of the DNA repair enzymes for 8-oxoguanine, hypoxanthine, and uracil increase in liver extracts of Wistar and OXYS rats with age. In both strains, 8-oxoguanine DNA glycosylase (OGG1) activities were about 10 times greater in nuclear extracts than in mitochondrial extracts (Ishchenko *et al.*, 2003). However, although OGG1 activity in nuclear extracts remained relatively constant throughout the study, this activity increased with age in mitochondrial extracts. Importantly, in OXYS rats, which are characterized by the overproduction of ROS, high levels of lipid peroxidation, protein oxidation, and decreased life span, the levels of mitochondrial OGG1 activity were greater than in normal Wistar rats, and an increase in this activity began earlier (Ishchenko *et al.*, 2003). The increase in 8-oxodG levels in mtDNA with aging appears to be a general phenomenon and has been reported by several groups (Hudson *et al.*, 1998; de Souza-Pinto *et al.*, 2001). The steady-state concentration of 8-oxodG in mitochondrial DNA was shown to be inversely correlated with maximum lifespan (MLSP) in the heart and brain of mammals, such that slowly aging mammals show lower 8-oxodG levels in mtDNA than rapidly aging ones (Barja and Herrero, 2000). Furthermore, these authors show that this inverse relationship is restricted to mtDNA, due to the fact that 8-oxodG levels in nuclear DNA were not significantly correlated with MLSP. The correlation between 8-oxodG and MLSP was better in the heart and in the brain, possibly in part because these organs are composed predominantly of postmitotic cells (Barja and Herrero, 2000).

LONGER LIFE EXPECTANCY IN ORGANISMS BELONGING TO THE SAME COHORT GROUP IS ASSOCIATED WITH RELATIVELY HIGHER LEVELS OF ANTIOXIDANTS AND LOWER CONCENTRATIONS OF THE PRODUCTS OF OXYGEN FREE RADICAL REACTIONS

All houseflies lose the ability to fly prior to death. Therefore, in an aging population, shorter-lived flies can be identified as flightless "crawlers" in contrast to their longer-lived cohorts, the "fliers." The average lifespan of crawlers is about one-third shorter than the fliers. Levels of antioxidant defenses (superoxide dismutase (SOD), catalase (CAT), and glutathione) and products of oxygen free radical reactions (inorganic peroxides and thiobarbituric acid [TBA]-reactants) were compared between crawlers and fliers. The fliers showed greater SOD and CAT activities and glutathione concentrations than crawlers, whereas the amount of inorganic peroxides (H_2O_2) and TBA-reactants was higher in the crawlers than in fliers (Sohal *et al.*, 1986).

AN EXPERIMENTALLY INDUCED DECREASE IN OXIDATIVE STRESS RETARDS AGE-ASSOCIATED DETERIORATION AT THE ORGANELLE AND ORGANISMIC LEVELS AND EXTENDS CHRONOLOGICAL AND METABOLIC LIFE SPAN

Simultaneous overexpression of Cu, Zn SOD, and CAT in *Drosophila* was shown to increase the maximum and average lifespan by one-third, to retard the age-related accumulation of oxidative damage to DNA and protein, to increase resistance to the oxidative effects of X-ray exposure, to attenuate the age-related increase in the rate of mitochondrial H_2O_2 generation, to increase the speed of walking, and to increase the metabolic potential defined as the total amount of oxygen consumed during the adult life per unit body weight (Orr and Sohal, 1994). Moreover, others have been able to extend the *Drosophila* lifespan by overexpressing either Mn–SOD or Cu,Zn–SOD in motor neurons. Very recently, it became possible to modestly increase longevity in mice by overexpressing mitochondrially targeted catalase (Schriner *et al.*, 2005). However, Schriner's report is somewhat vulnerable to technical criticisms on the grounds of the experimentally observed mosaic expression of the transgene and nonphysiological targeting of the enzyme (mitochondria in transgenic vs. peroxisomes in WT animals). In *Drosophila*, overexpression of Cu,Zn–SOD or CAT alone failed to extend lifespan (Orr *et al.*, 2003). Additionally, overexpression of Cu,Zn–SOD failed to increase longevity in mice (Gallagher *et al.*, 2000).

VARIATIONS IN LONGEVITY AMONG DIFFERENT SPECIES CORRELATE INVERSELY WITH THE RATES OF MITOCHONDRIAL GENERATION OF SUPEROXIDE ANION RADICAL ($O_2^{\bullet -}$) AND H_2O_2

As has been mentioned earlier, a longer lived subpopulation of *Drosophila* was found to have a lower rate of mitochondrial $O_2^{\bullet -}$ and H_2O_2 generation (Sohal *et al.*, 1986). Similar results were observed in a recent cross-species study of bats, shrews, and mice, where mitochondria from long-lived bats were found to produce half to one-third the amount of hydrogen peroxide per unit of oxygen consumed compared to mitochondria from shrews and mice, respectively (Brunet-Rossinni, 2004).

RESTRICTION OF CALORIC INTAKE LOWERS STEADY-STATE LEVELS OF OXIDATIVE STRESS AND DAMAGE, RETARDS AGE-ASSOCIATED CHANGES, AND EXTENDS THE MAXIMUM LIFE-SPAN IN MAMMALS

Reducing dietary intake has been shown to be the most effective means for modulating the aging processes in laboratory rodents (Weindruch *et al.*, 1986). Dietary restriction also has been shown to be a modulator of membrane lipid peroxidation and cytosolic antioxidant status. Lee *et al.* studied the anti-ROS action of dietary restriction by quantifying the formation of the $O_2^{\bullet -}$, $OH^{\bullet}$, and H_2O_2 by liver microsomes from rats of various ages. The results show that the *ad libitum*-fed group maintained a higher production of $O_2^{\bullet -}$ and $OH^{\bullet}$ radicals when compared to the food-restricted group of the same age. H_2O_2 formation followed the same trend but was statistically greater only at three and six months of age. The food-restricted group displayed higher SOD activity in both cytosolic and mitochondrial fractions compared to *ad libitum*-fed controls (Lee and Yu, 1990). These data indicate that the ROS activity observed in liver microsomes of *ad libitum*-fed rats can be attenuated by dietary restriction, thereby providing a possible mechanism for its life-extending action.

MTDNA MUTATIONS ARE PATHOGENIC AND CAN INCREASE ROS PRODUCTION BY MITOCHONDRIA

The discovery, in 1988, that mtDNA mutations can be pathogenic has provided a major support for the mitochondrial theory of aging. That year, several groups reported that both mtDNA point mutations and deletions could be the underlying cause of defined human pathologies. Moreover, being heteroplasmic, these diseases have revealed that not all the mtDNA copies in a cell need to be mutated in order to achieve a disease state. The last decade produced an explosive growth of the number of mtDNA mutations implicated in human disease. The recent release of the Mitomap database lists almost 200 pathogenic point mutations, single nucleotide deletions and insertions (Brandon *et al.*, 2005). Not only have mitochondrial diseases revealed a causative link between mtDNA mutations and pathology, but they also have displayed, in agreement with the predictions of the mitochondrial theory of aging, an increased oxidative burden in patients suffering from these diseases (Kunishige *et al.*, 2003; Lu *et al.*, 2003).

mtDNA Repair and Aging

It appears obvious that the physiological integrity of the cell must critically depend upon the integrity of its genome, which is maintained by DNA repair machinery. However, although the organization, synthesis, and repair of nuclear DNA have been the focus of intense studies, mitochondrial DNA has received much less attention until recently.

In the nucleus, the steady state or induced levels of mutagenesis are determined by a balance between mutagenic insult and DNA repair. In contrast, early studies revealed that mammalian cells could not repair UV-induced mtDNA damage (Clayton *et al.*, 1974). Also, Miyaki *et al.* (1977) suggested that repair of mtDNA after exposure to N-methyl-N′-nitro-N-nitrosoguanidine or 4-nitroquinoline-1 oxide was absent or very slow. These findings led to the belief that damaged mtDNA was destroyed and replaced with replicated undamaged DNA. However, through the use of technical advances in the analysis of DNA repair in specific sequences (Bohr *et al.*, 1985) and the treatment of the whole mitochondrial genome as simply a unique 16.5 kb DNA sequence, it was possible to show that some types of mtDNA damage can be efficiently repaired (Pettepher *et al.*, 1991; LeDoux *et al.*, 1992; LeDoux *et al.*, 1999; LeDoux and Wilson, 2001). Currently, it is believed that mitochondria possess DNA Base Excision Repair (BER) machinery, while lacking the Nucleotide Excision Repair (NER) capacity.

Mitochondrial DNA accumulates high levels of the mutagenic 8-oxodG, arguably the most important base damage caused by ROS, and it is widely believed to play a major role in the aging process (Hamilton *et al.*, 2001). The important role played by DNA repair enzymes in the accumulation of this lesion is underscored by the fact that the liver mtDNA from knockout mice for 8-oxoguanine DNA glycosylase (OGG1, the glycosylase that recognizes this lesion) accumulates 20 times as much 8-oxodG as the mtDNA from WT control mice (de Souza-Pinto *et al.*, 2001). Interestingly, several studies have indicated that OGG1 activity in mitochondrial extracts from old rats is higher compared to extracts from young animals, which is apparently at odds with the observed accumulation of 8-oxodG in mtDNA from older animals (Hudson *et al.*, 1998; de Souza-Pinto *et al.*, 2001). The theory that explains this apparent discrepancy was put forward by Szczesny *et al.*, who have shown that in both hepatocytes from old mice and in senescent human fibroblasts, mitochondrial import of OGG1β, the predominantly mitochondrial isoform of OGG1, is impaired and that a significant fraction of this enzyme remains localized in the outer membrane and intermembrane space in the precursor form (Szczesny *et al.*, 2003). Because UNG, another BER enzyme, has shown a similar age-dependent impairment in mitochondrial import, these authors conclude that there appears to be a general deficiency in the import of BER enzymes into mitochondria from senescent animals and cells. Therefore, although age-related impairment in mitochondrial protein import does not necessarily extend beyond some DNA repair enzymes, it can explain the simultaneous accumulation of 8-oxodG and increased *in vitro* OGG1 activity in mitochondria from senescent animals in some settings. However, a recent report from Bohr and colleagues has demonstrated that purified OGG1β is not enzymatically active and that mitochondrial OGG1 activity can be accounted for by traces of OGG1α, a predominantly nuclear isoform (Hashiguchi *et al.*, 2004). These findings may present a challenge to the theory of Szczesny *et al.* or may simply indicate the existence of a yet unknown cofactor required for OGG1β activity in mitochondria. It should also be noted that other studies point out that the ability of mitochondria to import proteins is a dynamic function that can be modulated by various stimuli, such as thyroid hormone (Craig *et al.*, 1998), which may provide an alternative explanation for the observed phenomena. Consistent with this notion is the observation that the rate of mitochondrial import of matrix chaperonins GRP75 and HSP60, which are essential for the import of precursor proteins, increases with age (Craig and Hood, 1997). Also, there is an apparent lack of consensus in the literature regarding the increase in mitochondrial OGG1 activity with aging in both senescent cells and animals. Some groups have reported a decline in both activity and expression of several key mitochondrial repair enzymes, including OGG1 (e.g., S Shen *et al.*, 2003). One of the possible explanations for this lack of consensus is in the intrinsic variability between cell types and tissues with respect to their reliance on antioxidant defenses vs. DNA repair for the maintenance of structural integrity of mtDNA. Results from our laboratory suggest that the differential susceptibility of glial cell types to oxidative damage and apoptosis does not appear related to cellular antioxidant capacity but rather to differences in their ability to repair oxidative mtDNA damage (Hollensworth *et al.*, 2000), and that different glial cell types differ in their capacity to repair oxidative damage (Druzhyna *et al.*, 2003)

Experimental Evidence that Is not Readily Explained by the Mitochondrial Theory of Aging

Despite the wealth of experimental evidence in support of the mitochondrial theory of aging, there is a very significant and growing body of data that appear to be at odds with it. Thus, the rate of ROS generation by mitochondria under physiological conditions, which is a cornerstone of the mitochondrial theory of aging, has been recently critically reexamined by several groups. Hansford *et al.* have found that active H_2O_2 production (an indirect measure of $O_2^{\bullet -}$ generation) requires both a high fractional reduction of complex I (indexed by NADH/NAD+ + NADH ratio) and a high membrane potential, $\Delta\Psi$. These conditions are achieved only with supraphysiological concentrations of succinate. With physiological concentrations of NAD-linked substrates, rates of

H_2O_2 formation are much lower (less than 0.1% of respiratory chain electron flux). This H_2O_2 production may be stimulated by the complex III inhibitor antimycin A, but not by myxothiazol (Hansford *et al.*, 1997). Staniek and Nohl further reported that mitochondria respiring on complex I and complex II substrates generate detectable H_2O_2 only in the presence of the antimycin A. They also suggested that the rates of mitochondrial H_2O_2 production reported by others are artificially high due to flaws in experimental design (Staniek and Nohl, 2000). Martin Brand's group capitalized on these findings and used an improved experimental design to show that mitochondria do not release measurable amounts of superoxide or hydrogen peroxide when respiring on complex I or complex II substrates, but release significant amounts of superoxide from complex I when respiring on palmitoyl carnitine (St-Pierre *et al.*, 2002). However, even at saturating concentrations of palmitoyl carnitine, in their estimation only 0.15% of the electron flow gives rise to H_2O_2 under resting conditions with a respiration rate of 200 nmol of electrons/min/mg mitochondrial protein. Under physiological conditions, this rate should be even lower due to a) lower partial oxygen pressure, b) lower concentration of palmitoyl carnitine, and c) lower mitochondrial membrane potential. Therefore, under physiological conditions in cells with uncompromised antioxidant defenses, ROS are produced by ETC in quantities that should be efficiently scavenged by mitochondrial antioxidant systems. As a consequence, no significant oxidative damage can be expected in mtDNA due to an electron leak from ETC, provided that cells have normal levels of antioxidants. This conclusion is in agreement with the observations of Orr *et al.* (2003), who recently have reexamined their earlier findings and those of others on the effect of overexpression of antioxidant enzymes on extension of *Drosophila* lifespan. They have found that significant increases in the activities of both CuZn-SOD and CAT had no beneficial effect on survivorship in relatively long-lived yw mutant flies, and were associated with slightly decreased life spans in WT flies of the Oregon-R strain. The introduction of additional transgenes encoding Mn-SOD or thioredoxin reductase in the same genetic background also failed to cause life span extension. These authors conclude that increasing the activities of major antioxidative enzymes above WT levels does not decrease the rate of aging in long-lived strains of *Drosophila*, although there may be some effect in relatively short-lived strains (Orr *et al.*, 2003). In line with this conclusion, Van Remmen *et al.*, in their study of mice heterozygous for the MnSOD gene knockout, have found that although life-long reduction of MnSOD activity leads to increased levels of oxidative damage to mitochondrial and nuclear DNA and increased cancer incidence, it does not appear to affect aging (Van Remmen *et al.*, 2003).

As mentioned earlier, accumulation of 8-oxodG in mtDNA correlates with mitochondrial dysfunction in aging. In addition, mtDNA 8-oxodG levels inversely correlate with mammalian life span. 8-OxodG-induced mutagenesis is prevented by removal of the lesion from mtDNA via base excision repair (BER), which involves recognition and incision of the modified base by OGG1. MtDNA from mice deficient for OGG1 accumulates 8-oxodG to 20-fold higher levels than WT controls by six months of age (de Souza-Pinto *et al.*, 2001). This elevation of 8-oxodG levels in the mtDNA of Ogg1−/− mice is almost an order of magnitude greater than is observed in old mice. One can predict, in line with mitochondrial theory of aging, that these mice would accumulate mutations in their mtDNA, which would result in the production of defective subunits for and decline in activity of mitochondrial respiratory complexes (especially complexes I and IV, to which most of mitochondrially encoded polypeptides cater), which in turn would result in accelerated aging. However, these mice are not reported to age prematurely, nor do they show any decline in mitochondrial respiratory function in the heart and liver, or signs of oxidative stress as judged by protein carbonyl content (Stuart *et al.*, 2005).

Rasmussen *et al.* assayed 13 different enzyme activities using optimized preparation techniques and found that the central bioenergetic systems, including pyruvate dehydrogenase, tricarboxylic acid cycle, respiratory chain, and ATP synthesis, appeared unaltered with age (Rasmussen *et al.*, 2003). Maklashina and Ackrell have recently critically examined the literature regarding the role of ETC dysfunction in aging (Maklashina and Ackrell, 2004). They conclude that the evidence for age-related inactivation of the respiratory chain can be challenged on the grounds of preparation purity and the use of inadequate assay procedures, and that recent experimental evidence does not support the mitochondrial theory of aging (Maklashina and Ackrell, 2004).

In contrast, Jacobs does not challenge experimental evidence supporting the mitochondrial theory of aging but rather points out that all the evidence available to date is indirect in its nature (Jacobs, 2003). He argues that studies performed so far do not address the critical issue of cause and effect; that is, does the somatic mutation of mtDNA result in OXPHOS dysfunction and increased oxidative stress? Does increased oxidative stress promote mtDNA mutagenesis? Finally, he points out that the results from his own lab suggest that, at least in a tissue culture model, progressive accumulation of mtDNA mutations due to expression of mutant DNA polymerase gamma (Polγ) does not lead to significant phenotypic changes despite the accumulation of mtDNA mutations at a level three times greater than that found in aged tissues.

Very recently, however, Nils-Göran Larsson and colleagues reported the generation of a homozygous knock-in mice that express a proofreading-deficient catalytic subunit of Polγ, the only DNA polymerase found in mammalian mitochondria (Trifunovic *et al.*, 2004).

These mice develop a mtDNA mutator phenotype with a three- to five-fold increase in the levels of mtDNA point mutations, as well as increased amounts of deleted mtDNA. This increase in somatic mtDNA mutations is associated with reduced lifespan and the premature onset of age-related phenotypes such as weight loss, reduced subcutaneous fat, alopecia (hair loss), kyphosis (curvature of the spine), osteoporosis, anemia, reduced fertility, and heart enlargement. Thus results of this study provide the best evidence so far for a causative link between mtDNA mutations and aging phenotypes in mammals.

However, as these authors concede, the detailed kinetics of the accumulation of somatic mtDNA mutations remains to be elucidated. The mutation load in the brain of mutator mice at two months of age is already two- to three-fold greater than in six-month old WT littermates. This, and the rather uniform mutation loads between tissues, suggests that much of the accumulation of mutations may occur during embryonic and/or fetal development. Also, the onset of premature aging in this model is not accompanied, temporally, by a large *de novo* accumulation of mtDNA mutations around six months. Therefore, it appears plausible that the premature onset of aging in this model may be the result of the cumulative physiological damage caused by the high mutation load present during adult life and/or to segregation or clonal expansion of specific mutations. This is supported by the observed mosaicism for the respiratory chain deficiency found in the heart. However, since the effects of high mutational burden in mtDNA during embryonic and fetal development are poorly understood, and since very substantial mutation loads were observed in the mtDNA at the earliest time point tested in this study, we have to consider the possibility that premature aging in this model could be predetermined at the prenatal, rather than postnatal, stage (developmental programming; Cameron and Demerath 2002).

As Aubrey de Grey (2004) has pointed out recently, the only tissues directly affected by the elevated mtDNA mutation rate in these mice are those that are mitotically active. This suggests that embryonic development can be compromised by high mtDNA mutational loads, as embryonic tissues undergo active mitosis. If this holds true, then the issue of a causative relationship between mtDNA mutations and normal aging is likely to remain open, since, in normal aging, accumulation of mtDNA mutations is not observed during embryonic development. Thus, a substantial mutational load in mtDNA during embryonic development might be an important limitation of this model, and a model with an inducible mtDNA mutator phenotype should help to resolve this and other outstanding issues. Finally, mtDNA mutations in this study are generated by a mutator Polγ rather than by oxidative DNA damage. Therefore, this study does not address one of the central premises of the mitochondrial theory of aging, namely, that oxidative mtDNA damage is the driving force behind the accumulation of mtDNA mutations.

Earlier we discussed the support provided for the mitochondrial theory of aging by the discovery of mitochondrial disease. We might then reasonably expect, based on the mitochondrial theory of aging, that mitochondrial ROS would be causative in a significant fraction of pathogenic mtDNA mutations. We have analyzed 188 pathogenic mtDNA point mutations (Brandon *et al.*, 2005) and found that the mutagenic effect of 8-oxodG, widely regarded as a prime lesion resulting from an oxidative insult to DNA, can be implicated in the etiology of only a few mutations. Indeed, unrepaired 8-oxodG in mtDNA can pair with both C and A with almost equal efficiency resulting in G to T (and C to A on complementary strand) transversions, which account for only 5.9% of pathogenic mtDNA mutations. Even when the potentially mutagenic pool of 8-oxo deoxyguanosine triphosphate (8-oxo-dGTP, the product of cytoplasmic/matrix dGTP pool oxidation) is taken in consideration (T to G and A to C transversions), the cumulative impact of both types of mutation is still only 8.5%. For comparison, 82% (almost 10 times as many) of the pathogenic point mutations in mtDNA can be attributed to deamination of adenine and cytosine. Similarly, it was found that 8-oxodG-mediated transversions can account for only about 25% of mutations detected in both frontal cortex and substantia nigra of old subjects (Simon *et al.*, 2004). The efficient repair of 8-oxodG by BER pathways in mitochondria (Thorslund *et al.*, 2002) explains these phenomena and argues against it being the prime mutagenic lesion. Transversions, the type of mutations caused by 8-oxodG, are rare events in both nuclear and mitochondrial DNA, which also argues against 8-oxodG being the prime mutagenic lesion. Thus, the exact factors required for the accumulation of point mutations in mtDNA are yet to be fully defined. Oxidative DNA damage can produce a variety of base lesions whose mutagenic potential has not been fully elucidated (Evans *et al.*, 2004). Therefore, it is possible that other, at present unidentified, lesions are responsible for the bulk of ROS-mediated mutagenesis. Alternatively, it can be postulated that ROS do not play a major role in mtDNA mutagenesis.

Experimental Approaches to Studying mtDNA in Aging

DETECTION OF AGING-ASSOCIATED LARGE DELETIONS IN mtDNA

The first evidence that implicated mtDNA in aging came from the studies of mtDNA deletions (Corral-Debrinski *et al.*, 1992). Specific mtDNA deletions (e.g., "common" 5kb deletion) can be relatively easily detected by using PCR with primers that flank deletion breakpoints. The selectivity and sensitivity of the assay can be enhanced by employing a second round of PCR with nested primers. When detecting large deletions, using short extension times in PCR reaction helps avoid amplification of large WT fragments and increases sensitivity. The tradeoff of this approach is that it does not allow for the determination of the cellular content of deleted mtDNA. However, it was possible to perform semiquantitative evaluations by conducting PCR on multiple serial dilutions of samples to normalize DNA content (Cortopassi *et al.*, 1992).

DETECTION OF OXIDATIVE DNA BASE DAMAGE

Electron leak from the ETC results in the formation of ROS, which may cause oxidative damage to mtDNA. To date, 24 major products of oxidative damage to DNA bases have been identified (Evans *et al.*, 2004), of which 8-oxodG has received the most attention as marker of oxidative DNA damage because it can readily be detected by various techniques. However, wide discrepancies in the reported basal levels (over two orders of magnitude) of 8-oxodG in DNA recently have prompted the establishment of the European Standards Committee on Oxidative DNA Damage (ESCODD), which consists of 27 member laboratories who will examine critically the different approaches to measuring base oxidation in DNA, in particular 8-oxodG. It is now widely recognized that the guanine in DNA is readily oxidized during sample preparation. Techniques that utilize gas chromatography followed by mass spectrometry (GC-MS) are particularly susceptible to this artifact if the derivatization step is carried out at high temperature in the presence of oxygen. Therefore, protocols currently in use address this problem by the inclusion of antioxidants and metal chelators during sample preparation. Several techniques were evaluated by ESCODD: HPLC with electrochemical detection (HPLC-ECD), GC-MS, and HPLC followed by tandem mass spectrometry-mass spectrometry (HPLC-MS/MS). Laboratories that employ HPLC-ECD were able to detect induced 8-oxodG with similar efficiencies with very similar dose response profiles whereas GC-MS and HPLC-MS/MS, employed in three laboratories, failed to detect a dose response. Median values for 8-oxodG in untreated cells were determined to be 4.01 per 10^6 guanines. However, approximately a 10-fold difference was observed between the highest and the lowest values of background mtDNA damage (ESCODD 2003). Overall, it can be concluded that because of this high variability in the background damage determined by different labs using the same techniques and starting material, any published quantitative data on the 8-oxodG content in mtDNA should be interpreted with caution.

DETECTION OF mtDNA DAMAGE

Quantitative Southern blot analysis can be used for the quantitation of oxidative damage to mtDNA. This method is based on the detection of strand breaks within linearized mtDNA. These strand breaks can be generated by oxidative stress or by treatment of DNA containing oxidative base lesions with either FPG (recognizes oxidized purines) or *E. coli* endonuclease III (EndoIII, recognizes oxidized pyrimidines) followed by alkaline agarose gel electrophoresis. Under the alkaline conditions, the two mtDNA strands separate and single strand breaks occur at abasic sites created by the activity of FPG or EndoIII, which results in a decreased hybridization signal from the damaged DNA (LeDoux *et al.*, 1999).

An alternative approach for the detection of mtDNA damage was developed by Bennett van Houten. This method, QPCR, is based on the ability of the lesions present in mtDNA to block the progression of thermostable DNA polymerase on a template, resulting in a decrease of DNA amplification in the damaged template when compared to undamaged DNA (Yakes and Van Houten, 1997). The QPCR actually measures the fraction of undamaged template, which decreases with increased number of lesions.

The successful outcome of experiments with both quantitative Southern blot and QPCR is heavily dependent upon the ability to accurately measure the amount of DNA used. Spectrophotometric methods (A_{260}) appear to be inappropriate for this purpose because of the intrinsic difficulties associated with controlling the quantity and spectrum of contaminants in DNA preparations. Fluorescence-based methods (PicoGreen and Hoechst33258 dyes), unlike spectrophotometric techniques, show little sensitivity to such contaminants as proteins, single-stranded DNA, RNA, and so on, which are common to genomic DNA preparations and therefore are deemed methods of choice. Also, when using QPCR, one has control for changes in the mtDNA copy number. Indeed, reduction in mtDNA copy number will manifest itself as DNA damage because of the reduction in the number of amplifiable mtDNA genomes in the template. To control for this problem, amplification of a short (about 300bp) fragment of the gene under the study is performed. The rationale is that encountering DNA damage in such a short fragment is an event with a very low probability, and therefore profiles of amplification of such a fragment should be essentially identical between damaged and undamaged DNA. Therefore, variations in the degree of amplification are assumed to be the result of fluctuations in mtDNA copy number, and the results of small fragment amplification are used for the normalization of the data obtained for the large (15 kb) mtDNA fragments.

mtDNA SEQUENCING

The total burden of mtDNA point mutations in tissues can be quantified using mtDNA sequencing. This approach measures consequences of oxidative stress and other mutagenic insults on the integrity of mtDNA. The protocol includes PCR amplification of specific DNA regions, cloning of the PCR fragments, and sequencing either resulting plasmid DNA or PCR template amplified from it (Simon *et al.*, 2004). The high sensitivity of this technique raises several technical concerns. The first is that PCR errors might be misinterpreted as somatic mtDNA mutations. The use of a high-fidelity PCR system limits this possibility. However, the fidelity of DNA polymerase can be affected by experimental conditions, and therefore the spectrum and the level of contaminants in DNA preparations can affect the level of PCR-induced mutations. The fidelity of this approach was experimentally tested by amplifying a single clone followed by a repeat cloning step. The lack of identification of any mutations out of 107 clones and nearly 98,000 base pairs of sequencing demonstrates the high fidelity of this method. A second concern is that oxidative damage to the original template DNA might lead to the induction of mutations due to replication errors in the early precloning PCR cycles. This possibility is not ruled out by the preceding control study, since cloned DNA would not necessarily have the same oxidative damage as the original DNA. However, a control study failed to detect a significant difference in mutation frequencies when the template DNA was exposed *ex vivo* to high levels of oxidative stress (Lin *et al.*, 2002). The third concern is that it remains possible that some other form of template damage that differs between DNA derived from different brain regions or from subjects of different ages may lead to PCR errors. The fourth concern is inadvertent amplification of nuclear *pseudogenes*. There are 612 independent integrations of mtDNA sequences evenly distributed over the nuclear genome. Our observations indicate that nuclear insertions of mitochondrial sequences occurred independently in human and mouse lineages after their separation from a common ancestor (see Figure 41.3).

Interestingly, no integration of the D-loop region into the nuclear DNA has occurred in either human or mouse genomes, which makes studies focused on mutations in this region free of potential artifacts introduced by amplification of pseudogenes. The interference from nuclear pseudogenes is generally pertinent only to large-scale studies because mtDNA present in the cell in a great molar excels over the nuclear DNA. Additionally, most regions of homology are relatively small and will not interfere if the experimental design involves amplification and sequencing of large mitochondrial fragments. Finally, because of the accumulation of mutations in nuclear pseudogenes, it is often possible to design primers that would specifically amplify mtDNA.

MEASURING THE CHANGES IN THE LEVELS OF DNA REPAIR ENZYMES

We already have mentioned that mutagenic lesions can only become a mutation if DNA repair systems fail to repair the damage. Mitochondria appear to possess a limited repertoire of DNA repair pathways, and therefore are incapable of repairing certain types of DNA damage. However, they are proficient in BER, which operates on oxidatively damaged mtDNA. Measurements of the age-related changes in the activity of BER enzymes were used to infer mechanisms of accumulation of mtDNA mutations in aging. The methods used to evaluate activity of these enzymes are described in great detail by Nyaga and Bohr (2002) and will not be discussed here.

Earlier we mentioned the lack of consensus regarding the age-related trend in mitochondrial content of DNA-repair enzymes, with some groups reporting an increase and others reporting a decrease. Both increase and decrease in the activity of DNA-repair enzymes in mitochondria appear to be consistent with increased oxidative stress and an increased number of oxidative mtDNA lesions with aging, phenomena on which a consensus does exist. Therefore, decreased expression of DNA repair enzymes is believed to result in a decreased ability of mitochondria to repair oxidative lesions, which leads to their accumulation. On the other hand, increased expression of DNA repair enzymes was interpreted to represent an adaptive response to increased oxidative stress. The magnitude of this response is believed to be insufficient to completely protect mtDNA when oxidative stress overwhelms antioxidant and DNA-repair systems, resulting in the net accumulation of oxidative DNA lesions. This ambiguity in interpretation somewhat reduces the value of measuring changes in mtDNA repair pathways as end-point assay in studies of aging. Despite this drawback, measurements of DNA repair enzyme activities remain an invaluable component of global evaluation of mtDNA-related parameters in aging.

Conclusion

Aging is a complex multifactorial process that we are only beginning to understand. Although the current evidence strongly suggests that mitochondria play a role in this process, there appears to be a wide range of opinions as to the exact nature of the involvement of mtDNA in aging. Contradictory data make it difficult to reach a consensus on the rates and precise mechanisms of ROS generation with aging. Unavailability of experimental tools that allow for the discrimination of the effects resulting from oxidative damage to mtDNA from the consequences of oxidative damage to other mitochondrial components adds another layer of difficulty. The lack of validated animal models of mitochondrial aging further complicates progress in this area of aging research. However, a recent report on the generation of mice with a mitochondrial mutator phenotype (Trifunovic *et al.*, 2004) may represent an important advance. Clearly, more research must be done to fully elucidate how oxidative damage to mtDNA contributes to the aging process. It is possible that the seemingly contradictory results of different studies will be reconciled or explained through the use of integrative approaches and unified model systems.

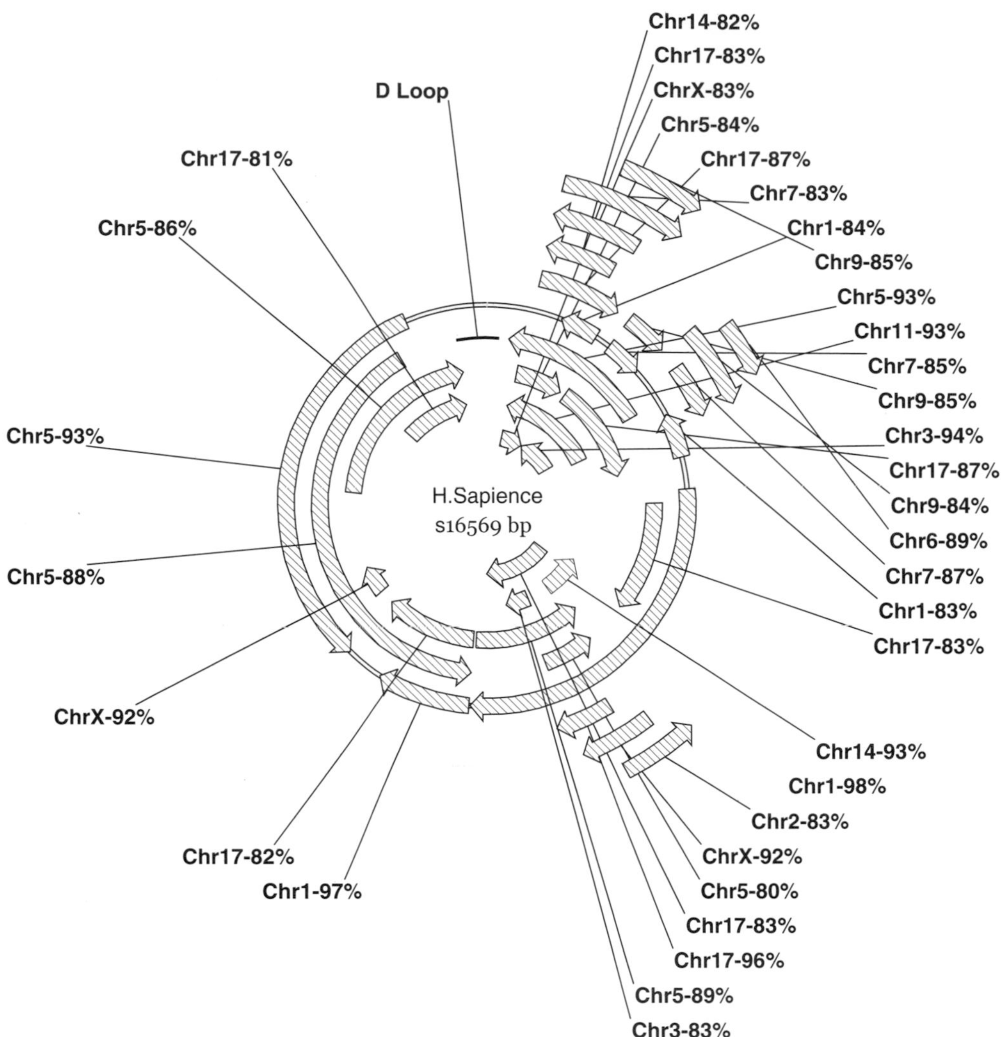

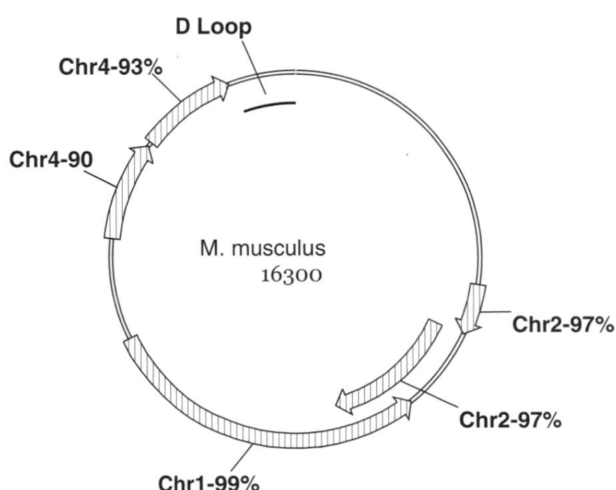

Figure 41.3 Distribution of regions of nuclear DNA homology over human and mouse mitochondrial genomes. Arrows indicate the orientation of insert, and Chr#A-#B% indicate the site of integration (chromosome #A) and the extent of homology (B%).

Recommended Resources

http://www.mitage.org/ Home page for EU MitAGE project devoted to experimentally testing the mitochondrial theory of aging.

http://www.answers.com/topic/dna-repair General information on DNA damage and repair, and its relevance to aging.

Copeland, W.C. (2002) *Mitochondrial DNA. Methods and protocols.* Totowa, NJ: Humana Press. Series, Methods in molecular biology. vol.197, specifically devoted to methods for studying mtDNA.

ACKNOWLEDGMENTS

M.A. is supported by the grant from the United Mitochondrial Disease Foundation; G.L.W. is supported by AG19602 and ES03456; and S.P.L is supported by ES05865 and NS047208.

REFERENCES

Barja, G., and Herrero, A. (2000). Oxidative damage to mitochondrial DNA is inversely related to maximum life span in the heart and brain of mammals. *Faseb J 14(2)*: 312–318.

Bohr, V.A., Smith, C.A., Okumoto, D.S., and Hanawalt, P.C. (1985). DNA repair in an active gene: Removal of pyrimidine dimers from the dhfr gene of cho cells is much more efficient than in the genome overall. *Cell 40(2)*: 359–369.

Brandon, M.C., Lott, M.T., Nguyen, K.C., Spolim, S., Navathe, S.B., Baldi, P., and Wallace, D.C. (2005). Mitomap: A human mitochondrial genome database—2004 update. *Nucleic Acids Res. 33*(Database issue): D611–D613.

Brunet-Rossinni, A.K. (2004). Reduced free-radical production and extreme longevity in the little brown bat (*myotis lucifugus*) versus two non-flying mammals. *Mech. Ageing Dev. 125(1)*: 11–20.

Cameron, N. and Demerath, E.W. (2002). Critical periods in human growth and their relationship to diseases of aging. *Am. J. Phys. Anthropol. Suppl. 35*: 159–184.

Clayton, D.A., Doda, J.N., and Friedberg, E.C. (1974). The absence of a pyrimidine dimer repair mechanism in mammalian mitochondria. *Proc. Natl. Acad. Sci. USA 71(7)*: 2777–2781.

Corral-Debrinski, M., Horton, T., Lott, M.T., Shoffner, J.M., Beal, M.F., and Wallace, D.C. (1992). Mitochondrial DNA deletions in human brain: Regional variability and increase with advanced age. *Nat. Genet. 2(4)*: 324–329.

Cortopassi, G.A., Shibata, D., Soong, N.W., and Arnheim, N. (1992). A pattern of accumulation of a somatic deletion of mitochondrial DNA in aging human tissues. *Proc. Natl. Acad. Sci. USA 89(16)*: 7370–7374.

Craig, E.E., Chesley, A., and Hood, D.A. (1998). Thyroid hormone modifies mitochondrial phenotype by increasing protein import without altering degradation. *Am. J. Physiol. 275(6 Pt 1)*: C1508–C1515.

Craig, E.E., and Hood, D.A. (1997). Influence of aging on protein import into cardiac mitochondria. *Am. J. Physiol. 272(6 Pt 2)*: H2983–H2988.

de Grey, A.D. (2004). Mitochondrial mutations in mammalian aging: An over-hasty about-turn? *Rejuvenation Res. 7(3)*: 171–174.

de Souza-Pinto, N.C., Eide, L., Hogue, B.A., Thybo, T., Stevnsner, T., Seeberg, E., Klungland, A., and Bohr, V. A. (2001). Repair of 8-oxodeoxyguanosine lesions in mitochondrial dna depends on the oxoguanine dna glycosylase (oggl) gene and 8-oxoguanine accumulates in the mitochondrial dna of oggl-defective mice. *Cancer Res. 61(14)*: 5378–5381.

de Souza-Pinto, N.C., Hogue, B.A., and Bohr, V.A. (2001). DNA repair and aging in mouse liver: 8-oxodg glycosylase activity increase in mitochondrial but not in nuclear extracts. *Free Radic. Biol. Med. 30(8)*: 916–923.

Druzhyna, N.M., Hollensworth, S.B., Kelley, M.R., Wilson, G.L., and Ledoux, S.P. (2003). Targeting human 8-oxoguanine glycosylase to mitochondria of oligodendrocytes protects against menadione-induced oxidative stress. *Glia 42(4)*: 370–378.

ESCODD (2003). Measurement of DNA oxidation in human cells by chromatographic and enzymic methods. *Free Radic. Biol. Med. 34(8)*: 1089–1099.

Evans, M.D., Dizdaroglu, M., and Cooke, M.S. (2004). Oxidative DNA damage and disease: Induction, repair and significance. *Mutat Res. 567(1)*: 1–61.

Gallagher, I.M., Jenner, P., Glover, V., and Clow, A. (2000). Cuzn-superoxide dismutase transgenic mice: No effect on longevity, locomotor activity and 3h-mazindol and 3h-spiperone binding over 19 months. *Neurosci. Lett. 289(3)*: 221–223.

Hamilton, M.L., Van Remmen, H., Drake, J.A., Yang, H., Guo, Z.M., Kewitt, K., Walter, C.A., and Richardson, A. (2001). Does oxidative damage to DNA increase with age? *Proc. Natl. Acad. Sci. USA 98(18)*: 10469–10474.

Hansford, R.G., Hogue, B.A., and Mildaziene, V. (1997). Dependence of h2o2 formation by rat heart mitochondria on substrate availability and donor age. *J Bioenerg. Biomembr. 29(1)*: 89–95.

Harman, D. (1956). Aging: A theory based on free radical and radiation chemistry. *J. Gerontol. 11(3)*: 298–300.

Hashiguchi, K., Stuart, J.A., de Souza-Pinto, N.C., and Bohr, V. A. (2004). The c-terminal alphao helix of human oggl is essential for 8-oxoguanine DNA glycosylase activity: The mitochondrial beta-oggl lacks this domain and does not have glycosylase activity. *Nucleic Acids Res. 32(18)*: 5596–5608.

Hollensworth, S.B., Shen, C., Sim, J.E., Spitz, D.R., Wilson, G. L., and LeDoux, S.P. (2000). Glial cell type-specific responses to menadione-induced oxidative stress. *Free Radic. Biol. Med. 28(8)*: 1161–1174.

Hudson, E.K., Hogue, B.A., Souza-Pinto, N.C., Croteau, D.L., Anson, R.M., Bohr, V.A. *et al.* (1998). Age-associated change in mitochondrial DNA damage. *Free Radic. Res. 29(6)*: 573–579.

Ishchenko, A., Sinitsyna, O., Krysanova, Z., Vasyunina, E.A., Saparbaev, M., Sidorkina, O. *et al.* (2003). Age-dependent increase of 8-oxoguanine-, hypoxanthine-, and uracil-DNA glycosylase activities in liver extracts from oxys rats with inherited overgeneration of free radicals and wistar rats. *Med. Sci. Monit. 9(1)*: BR16–BR24.

Jacobs, H.T. (2003). The mitochondrial theory of aging: Dead or alive? Aging Cell *2(1)*: 11–17.

Kunishige, M., Mitsui, T., Akaike, M., Kawajiri, M., Shono, M., Kawai, H. *et al.* (2003). Overexpressions of myoglobin and antioxidant enzymes in ragged-red fibers of skeletal muscle from patients with mitochondrial encephalomyopathy. *Muscle Nerve 28(4)*: 484–492.

LeDoux, S.P., Driggers, W.J., Hollensworth, B.S., and Wilson, G.L. (1999). Repair of alkylation and oxidative damage in mitochondrial DNA. *Mutat. Res. 434(3)*: 149–159.

LeDoux, S.P., and Wilson, G.L. (2001). Base excision repair of mitochondrial DNA damage in mammalian cells. *Prog. Nucleic Acid Res. Mol. Biol. 68*: 273–284.

LeDoux, S.P., Wilson, G.L., Beecham, E.J., Stevnsner, T., Wassermann, K., and Bohr, V.A. (1992). Repair of mitochondrial DNA after various types of DNA damage in chinese hamster ovary cells. *Carcinogenesis 13(11)*: 1967–1973.

Lee, D.W., and Yu, B.P. (1990). Modulation of free radicals and superoxide dismutases by age and dietary restriction. *Aging 2(4)*: 357–362.

Lin, M.T., Simon, D.K., Ahn, C.H., Kim, L.M., and Beal, M. F. (2002). High aggregate burden of somatic mtdna point mutations in aging and Alzheimer's disease brain. *Hum. Mol. Genet. 11(2)*: 133–145.

Lu, C.Y., Wang, E.K., Lee, H.C., Tsay, H.J., and Wei, Y.H. (2003). Increased expression of manganese-superoxide dismutase in fibroblasts of patients with cpeo syndrome. *Mol. Genet. Metab. 80(3)*: 321–329.

Maklashina, E. and Ackrell, B.A. (2004). Is defective electron transport at the hub of aging? *Aging Cell 3(1)*: 21–27.

Mandavilli, B.S., Santos, J.H., and Van Houten, B. (2002). Mitochondrial DNA repair and aging. *Mutat. Res. 509(1–2)*: 127–151.

Miquel, J., Economos, A.C., Fleming, J., and Johnson, J.E., Jr. (1980). Mitochondrial role in cell aging. *Exp. Gerontol. 15(6)*: 575–591.

Miyaki, M., Yatagai, K., and Ono, T. (1977). Strand breaks of mammalian mitochondrial DNA induced by carcinogens. *Chem. Biol. Interact 17(3)*: 321–329.

Nyaga, S.G., and Bohr, V.A. (2002). *Characterization of specialized mtdna glycosylases. Mitochondrial DNA: Methods and protocols.* W.C. Copeland. Totowa, NJ, Humana Press: 227–244.

Ojala, D., Montoya, J., and Attardi, G. (1981). tRNA punctuation model of RNA processing in human mitochondria. *Nature 290(5806)*: 470–474.

Orr, W.C., Mockett, R.J., Benes, J.J., and Sohal, R.S. (2003). Effects of overexpression of copper-zinc and manganese superoxide dismutases, catalase, and thioredoxin reductase genes on longevity in *Drosophila melanogaster. J. Biol. Chem. 278(29)*: 26418–26422.

Orr, W.C., and Sohal, R.S. (1994). Extension of life-span by overexpression of superoxide dismutase and catalase in *Drosophila melanogaster. Science 263(5150)*: 1128–1130.

Pettepher, C.C., LeDoux, S.P., Bohr, V.A., and Wilson, G. L. (1991). Repair of alkali-labile sites within the mitochondrial DNA of rinr 38 cells after exposure to the nitrosourea streptozotocin. *J. Biol. Chem. 266(5)*: 3113–3117.

Price, G.B., Modak, S.P., and Makinodan, T. (1971). Age-associated changes in the DNA of mouse tissue. *Science 171(974)*: 917–920.

Rasmussen, U.F., Krustrup, P., Kjaer, M., and Rasmussen, H. N. (2003). Experimental evidence against the mitochondrial theory of aging. A study of isolated human skeletal muscle mitochondria. *Exp. Gerontol. 38(8)*: 877–886.

Ross, O.A., McCormack, R., Curran, M.D., Duguid, R.A., Barnett, Y.A., Rea, I.M. *et al.* (2001). Mitochondrial DNA polymorphism: Its role in longevity of the irish population. *Exp. Gerontol. 36(7)*: 1161–1178.

Schriner, S.E., Linford, N.J., Martin, G.M., Treuting, P., Ogburn, C.E., Emond, M. *et al.* Extension of murine life span by overexpression of catalase targeted to mitochondria. *Science. 380(5730)*: 1909–1911.

Shen, G.P., Galick, H., Inoue, M., and Wallace, S.S. (2003). Decline of nuclear and mitochondrial oxidative base excision repair activity in late passage human diploid fibroblasts. *DNA Repair (Amst) 2(6)*: 673–693.

Simon, D.K., Lin, M.T., Zheng, L., Liu, G.J., Ahn, C.H., Kim, L.M. *et al.* (2004). Somatic mitochondrial DNA mutations in cortex and substantia nigra in aging and Parkinson's disease. *Neurobiol. Aging 25(1)*: 71–81.

Sohal, R.S., Toy, P.L., and Allen, R.G. (1986). Relationship between life expectancy, endogenous antioxidants and products of oxygen free radical reactions in the housefly, *Musca domestica. Mech. Ageing Dev. 36(1)*: 71–77.

Sohal, R.S., and Weindruch, R. (1996). Oxidative stress, caloric restriction, and aging. *Science 273(5271)*: 59–63.

St-Pierre, J., Buckingham, J.A., Roebuck, S.J., and Brand, M.D. (2002). Topology of superoxide production from different sites in the mitochondrial electron transport chain. *J. Biol. Chem. 277(47)*: 44784–44790.

Staniek, K., and Nohl, H. (2000). Are mitochondria a permanent source of reactive oxygen species? *Biochim. Biophys. Acta 1460(2–3)*: 268–275.

Stuart, J.A., Bourque, B.M., de Souza-Pinto, N.C., and Bohr, V.A. (2005). No evidence of mitochondrial respiratory dysfunction in ogg1-null mice deficient in removal of 8-oxodeoxyguanine from mitochondrial DNA. *Free Radic Biol. Med. 38(6)*: 737–745.

Szczesny, B., Hazra, T.K., Papaconstantinou, J., Mitra, S., and Boldogh, I. (2003). Age-dependent deficiency in import of mitochondrial DNA glycosylases required for repair of oxidatively damaged bases. *Proc. Natl. Acad. Sci. USA 100(19)*: 10670–10675.

Taanman, J.W. (1999). The mitochondrial genome: Structure, transcription, translation and replication. *Biochim. Biophys. Acta 1410(2)*: 103–123.

Thorslund, T., Sunesen, M., Bohr, V.A., and Stevnsner, T. (2002). Repair of 8-oxog is slower in endogenous nuclear genes than in mitochondrial DNA and is without strand bias. *DNA Repair (Amst) 1(4)*: 261–273.

Trifunovic, A., Wredenberg, A., Falkenberg, M., Spelbrink, J. N., Rovio, A.T., Bruder, C.E. *et al.* (2004). Premature ageing in mice expressing defective mitochondrial DNA polymerase. *Nature 429(6990)*: 417–423.

Van Remmen, H., Ikeno, Y., Hamilton, M., Pahlavani, M., Wolf, N., Thorpe, S.R. *et al.* (2003). Life-long reduction in MnSOD activity results in increased DNA damage and higher incidence of cancer but does not accelerate aging. *Physiol. Genomics 16(1)*: 29–37.

Weindruch, R., Walford, R.L., Fligiel, S., and Guthrie, D. (1986). The retardation of aging in mice by dietary restriction: Longevity, cancer, immunity and lifetime energy intake. *J. Nutr. 116(4)*: 641–654.

Yakes, F.M., and Van Houten, B. (1997). Mitochondrial DNA damage is more extensive and persists longer than nuclear DNA damage in human cells following oxidative stress. *Proc. Nat.*l *Acad. Sci. USA 94(2)*: 514–519.

Yang, M.Y., Bowmaker, M., Reyes, A., Vergani, L., Angeli, P., Gringeri, E. *et al.* (2002). Biased incorporation of ribonucleotides on the mitochondrial l-strand accounts for apparent strand-asymmetric DNA replication. *Cell 111(4)*: 495–505.

42

Models for Apoptosis: From Newborn to Adult

Christiane Charriaut-Marlangue and Sylvain Renolleau

Neurodegenerative diseases are characterized by progressive impairment of brain function as a consequence of ongoing neuronal cell death. Apoptotic mechanisms have been implicated in this process, but the immature brain differs from the adult brain in its sensitivity. To better understand the pathogenesis and developmental variations of hypoxic-ischemic neuronal death, several models have been developed and investigated to characterize cell death features in the developing brain. Involvement of apoptosis-related proteins such as Bax/Bcl-2 and caspases is overviewed during development and hypoxic-ischemic injury in various models.

Introduction

Ischemic stroke results from a transient or permanent reduction in cerebral blood flow that is restricted to the territory of a major brain artery. The reduction in blood flow in a specific region is, in most cases, caused by the occlusion of a cerebral artery either by an embolus or by local thrombosis. With an incidence of approximately 250 to 400 in 100,000 head of population aged 45 to 89 (Warlow, 1998) and a mortality rate around 30%, stroke remains the third leading cause of death in major industrialized countries. Hypoxic-ischemic and stroke injury to the perinatal brain is also a major clinical problem causing death in a large number of affected infants, recognized in about 1 per 4000 live term birth (Vannucci, 2000; Nelson and Lynch, 2004). More than 95 percent of infants who have a stroke survive to adulthood, and many have residual motor or cognitive disabilities (permanent neuropsychological handicaps including mental retardation, cerebral palsy, epilepsy, or learning disability) (Nelson and Lynch, 2004).

The immature brain has long been considered to be resistant to the damaging effects of hypoxia and hypoxia-ischemia (HI). However, it is now recognized that there are specific periods of increased vulnerability related to the developmental stage at the time of the insult. Much of our knowledge of the pathophysiology of cerebral HI is based on extensive experimental studies using *in vitro* and *in vivo* models relevant to mechanisms seen in humans. The major pathogenic mechanisms of brain injury following cerebral HI include excitotoxicity, inflammation, and apoptosis. This chapter will summarize most of the commonly used models in rodents (rat, mouse) and some of the recent data on developmental differences in the immature brain that create periods of selective vulnerability to hypoxia-ischemia, and are quite distinct from the responses in adult hypoxia-ischemia.

Models in Immature Animals

It is generally accepted that neurons in the immature brain tolerate a longer period of oxygen deprivation and/or ischemia than those in the adult (Towfighi *et al.*, 1997). However, there are conflicting reports, showing that the immature brain is less resistant to hypoxic-ischemic brain damage than its adult counterpart (Yager *et al.*, 1996). This is supported by other studies after HI or excitotoxic injury (McDonald *et al.*, 1988; Ikonomidou *et al.*, 1989; Marret *et al.*, 1995). Furthermore, clinical data suggest that outcome and mortality after acute brain injury are age-dependent, with more severe injuries in infants than in adults (Adelson and Kochanek, 1998).

Precise correlations with human brain development are difficult, in particular because of the fact that rodents present an arrhinencephalic brain. However, brains of 7-day-old rats and 10-day-old mice are similar to third-trimester (34 to 35 weeks of gestation) human fetuses (and thus premature human newborns), in terms of cellular proliferation, cortical organization, synapse number, neurochemical indices such as neurotransmitter synthetic enzymes, and electrophysiology (Hagberg *et al.*, 1994; Marret *et al.*, 1995). Cortex of the 10- to 12-day-old rats (18–35 g) could correspond to term newborn with myelination of the fiber tract beginning on approximately day 11 in the rat (Rice *et al.*, 1981). Based on these considerations, postnatal day 1 (P1) could be equivalent to 18 to 20 weeks gestation and P3 of 24 to 28 weeks gestation in humans.

NEONATAL MODELS OF HYPOXIA

In these models, 10 to 24 hours after birth, rat pups were placed in a thermostated Plexiglas chamber flushed with

100% nitrogen for 20 min (see Table 42.1). The temperature inside the chamber was adjusted to 36°C, to maintain body temperature within the physiologic range. Under these conditions, the final rates of mortality were less than 10%. After exposure to gas, rats were allowed to recover for 20 min in normoxic conditions, and then returned to their mothers (Grojean *et al.*, 2003). Similar procedure could be performed with 7-day-old rats, but the N2 duration was only of 8 min (Grojean *et al.*, 2003). A very small number of laboratories used the piglet as an animal model for hypoxia. Newborn piglets aged 2 to 5 days were ventilated with an FiO_2 of 5 to 7% for one hour (Ravishankar *et al.*, 2001). In these models, apototic and/or necrotic features were shown depending on the age of the animal (Daval and Vert, 2004; Delivoria-Papadopoulos and Mishra, 2004).

NEONATAL MODELS OF HYPOXIA-ISCHEMIA

Until now, the most commonly used model to study hypoxic-ischemic injury in the newborn has been the Rice-Vannucci model in 7-day-old (P7, 12–20 g) rats (Rice *et al.*, 1981), adapted on the Levine procedure (Levine, 1960). The left or right common carotid artery (CCA) was cut between double ligatures of prolene sutures (see Figure 42.1A).

After the surgical procedure the wounds were infiltrated with a local anesthetic, and the pups were allowed to recover for one to two hours. The litters were placed in a chamber perfused with a humidified gas mixture (8% oxygen in nitrogen) for 1.5 hour. The temperature in the incubator, and the temperature of the water used to humidify the gas mixture, were kept at 36°C. After hypoxic exposure the pups were returned to their biological dam to recover for several hours or days (see Figure 42.1). The damage usually is restricted to the hemisphere ipsilateral to the ligation and is observed primarily in the cerebral cortex, subcortical and periventricular white matter, striatum/thalamus, and hippocampus. Such neuropathological damage is rarely seen in the contralateral hemisphere and never in pups rendered hypoxic without ligation (Towfighi *et al.*, 1995; Vannucci and Vannucci, 1997). However, it suffers from a certain degree of variability (animals with an infarct score ranging from 0, no infarct, to 3, very large infarct). Therefore, authors have modified two variables (FiO_2 and hypoxia duration) to decrease this variability and obtain a more or less reproducible lesion in most of all animals (see Table 42.1). For example, such a model performed in Hagberg's laboratory with a standardized 7.7% O_2 for 55 min gives a total infarct volume of 42.3 ± 15.4 mm^3 (Zhu *et al.*, 2003). Many investigators have used this technique to study neonatal asphyxia in several newborn species (rat pups, piglets, dogs, kittens) (Roohey *et al.*, 1997). This model was also recently extended to the immature mouse (Sheldon *et al.*, 1998), with 10% oxygen (see Table 42.1). However, it was found that some strains (CD1) are

TABLE 42.1
Differential hypoxic and hypoxic-ischemic insults in rat, mouse, and piglet depending on the age, strain, percentage, and duration of O_2, and left or right CCA occlusion or ligation

Rodent	Age Strain	Hypoxic insult	Reference
Rat	P0 (8–24 h) Sprague-Dawley	100% N_2 for 20 min	Daval *et al.*, 2004
Rat	P1 Sprague-Dawley	Right CCA ligation + 6% O_2 for 3.5 h	Sheldon *et al.*, 1996
	P3 Wistar	Right CCA coagulated + 6% O_2 for 30 min	Sizonenko *et al.*, 2003
	P3 Sprague-Dawley	Left CCA coagulated + 6% O_2 for 15 min	Stadlin *et al.*, 2003
Rat	P7 Wistar	Right CCA coagulated + 8% O_2 for 2 h	Vannucci *et al.*, 1999
	P7 Wistar	permanent bilateral CCA ligation + 6.5 % O_2 for 1 h	Pulera *et al.*, 1998
	P7 Sprague-Dawley	Left CCA coagulated + 8% O_2 for 2.5 h	Cheng *et al.*, 1998
	P7 Wistar F	Left CCA coagulated + 7.7% O_2 for 65 min	Puka-Sundvall *et al.*, 2000
	P7 Wistar	Left CCA coagulated + 7.7% O_2 for 70 min	Gill *et al.*, 2002
Mouse	P7 CD-1	Right CCA coagulated + 10% O_2 for 50 min	Hagberg *et al.*, 2004
Piglet	P2–P5	5–7% FiO_2 for 1 h	Ravishankar *et al.*, 2001

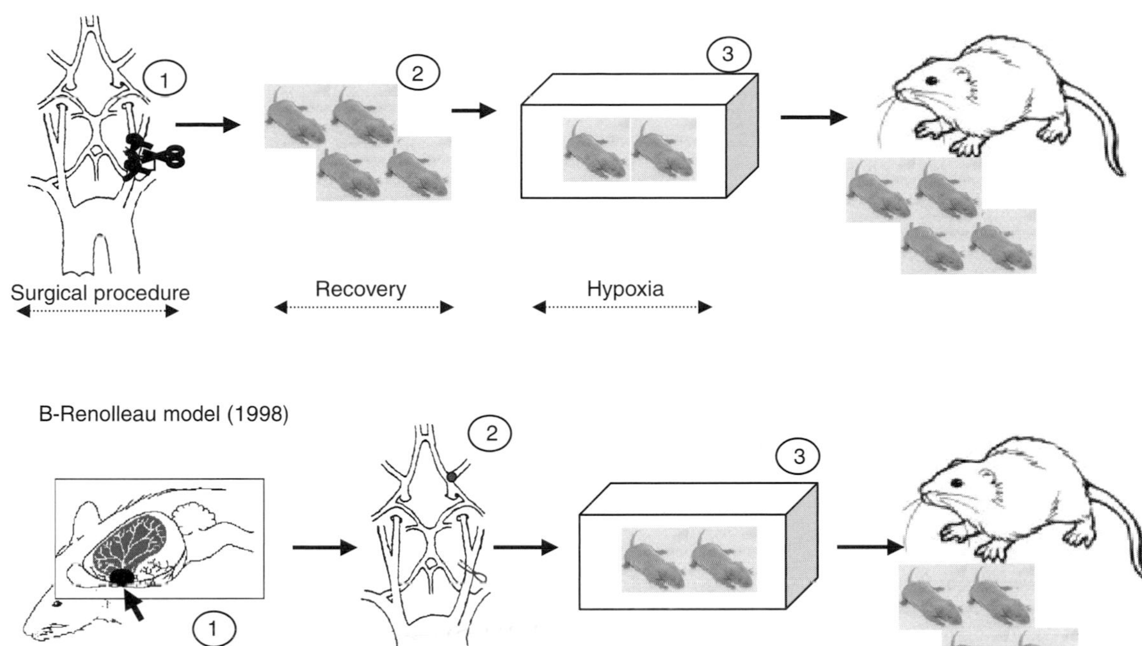

Figure 42.1 Schematic representation of Rice-Vannucci (hypoxia-ischemia, A) and Renolleau (stroke, B) models. **A**: Left, blood supply to the chest and the base of the brain. Position of the two ligatures on the common carotid artery followed by its cutting (1). Rat pups were then allowed for recovery (2). The litters were placed in a thermostated and humidified chamber perfused with a low oxygen percentage for several hours (3). At the end of hypoxic exposure, the pups returned to their biological dam. **B**: Left, MCA branching pattern with electrocoagulation site (arrow in (1)). Right, position of the vascular clip to occlude the left common carotid artery (2). Removal of the clip occurred between 50 and 60 min. After overnight recovery in a thermostated incubator (3), the pups returned to their biological dam.

particularly susceptible to brain damage in this model, whereas others (129Sv) are resistant (Sheldon *et al.*, 1998). In addition, to obtain similar extent of injury in C57/Bl6 mice whatever their postnatal age, Zhu and coauthors adjusted the duration of the hypoxia (10% O_2) time from 65 min (P5) to 60 min (P9), 50 min (P21) or 40 min (P60) (Zhu *et al.*, 2005).

The Rice-Vannucci model has recently been adapted to the P1 (Sheldon *et al.*, 1996) and P3 (Sizonenko *et al.*, 2003; Stadlin *et al.*, 2003) rat. However, the model performed in P1 was not so easily performed in other laboratories because survival was not possible. In the P3 rat pups, the mortality rat decreased from 33 to 0% with decreasing hypoxia duration (45 to 10 min, respectively).

NEONATAL MODELS OF STROKE

These models generally require a permanent occlusion of one of the two major cerebral arteries in association with a transient occlusion of the other one to produce low cerebral blood flow, because of the presence of the Circle of Willis. In the Renolleau model (Renolleau *et al.*, 1998) (see Figure 42.1B), anaesthetized rats were positioned on their backs, and a median incision was made in the neck to expose the left common carotid artery. Rats were then placed on the right side, and an oblique skin incision was made between the ear and the eye. After excision of the temporal muscle, the cranial bone was removed from the frontal suture to a level below the zygomatic arch. Then, the left middle cerebral artery (MCA), exposed just after its appearance over the rhinal fissure, was coagulated at the inferior level of the cerebral vein (see Figure 42.1B). After this procedure, a clip was placed to occlude the left common carotid artery. Rats were then placed in an incubator to avoid hypothermia. After 50 minutes, the clip was removed. Carotid blood flow restoration was verified with the aid of a microscope. Both neck and cranial skin incisions were then closed. During the surgical procedure, body temperature was maintained at 37 to 38°C. After recovery, pups were transferred to their mothers. Such an ischemic procedure leads to damage in the frontoparietal cortex, and in 20% of animals the head of the caudate putamen was also injured. The mean infarct volume is 58 ± 6 mm^3 (24.3 ± 2.2% of ipsilateral hemisphere) at 48 hours of

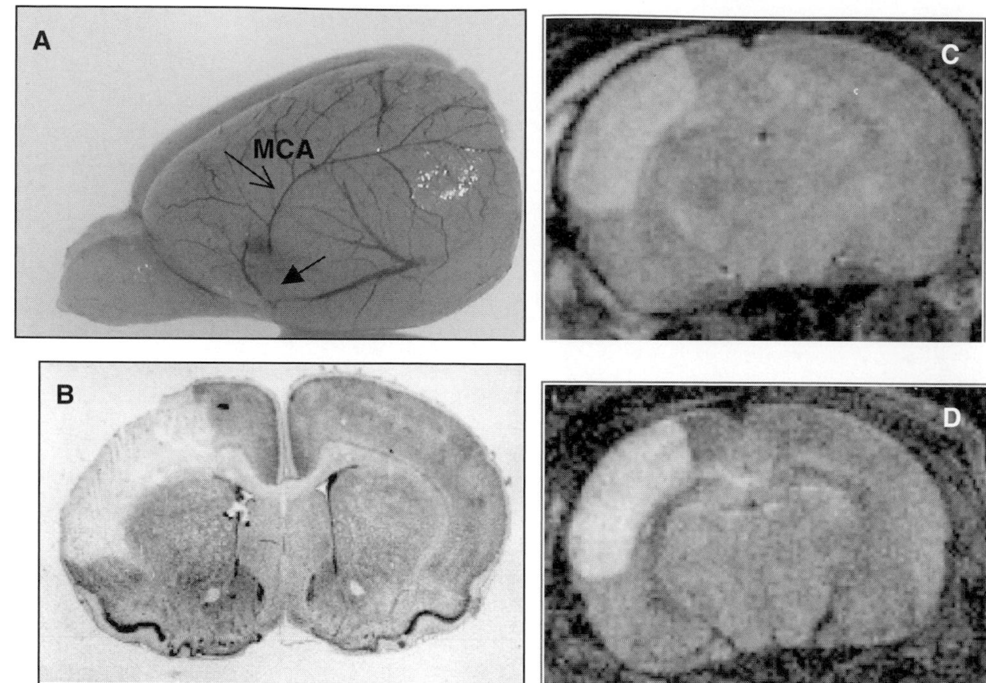

Figure 42.2 Presence of a cortical infarct in a model of neonatal stroke in 7-day-old rat (P7), 24 hours after reperfusion. **A**: Reperfusion was detected in the MCA territory (MCA, open black arrow, with its different branches and anastomoses), after methylene blue injected in the jugular vein, except at the low level of the MCA (little black arrow). **B**: representative Cresyl violet-stained coronal section. Note the cortical ill-defined pale area. **C–D**: T2 and ADC IRM images (7 Tesla) on 1 mm slice thickness, respectively, demonstrated the presence of a cortical infarct.

reperfusion, with only 5 to 10% animals dying in the first few hours after the clip removal (Ducrocq *et al.*, 2000; Joly *et al.*, 2004). This model evolves in a cystic infarct three weeks post-ischemia (see Figure 42.2).

More recently several groups have adapted to the newborn the filament technique of transient middle cerebral artery occlusion (MCAo) that is preferentially used in adult animal models of stroke. This includes the P7 (Derugin *et al.*, 1998) and the SHR P14 to P18 (35 g) Wistar rat (Ashwal *et al.*, 1995). Duration of endovascular nylon filament (6-0, 0.07 mm) occlusion varied from approximately 90 to 180 min MCAo. The volume of infarct involving cortical and caudoputamenal regions observed in these rat pup models is similar to that in adult models (infarct volume was of 180 $\pm$ 29 mm^3 corresponding to 49 $\pm$ 7% of the left hemisphere). However, reliably using such a model of reversible newborn MCAo without craniectomy is technically challenging, and the survival rate was very poor during the occlusion period or within the first hours of reperfusion.

In conclusion, the different models of cerebrovascular neonatal injury at one specific age (P7, for example) can be considered complementary since they analyze different types of cerebral insults (hypoxia-ischemia versus stroke), but no single model can ever replicate the human condition. All these models exhibited apoptotic features as demonstrated by electron microscopy (Pulera *et al.*, 1998; Renolleau *et al.*, 1998; Puka-Sundvall *et al.*, 2000), DNA cleavage in high molecular weight fragments and laddering (Ferrer *et al.*, 1994b; Hill *et al.*, 1995; Cheng *et al.*, 1998; Charriaut-Marlangue *et al.*, 1999) and TUNEL-positive nuclei (see Figure 42.3A, B).

Models in Adult Rodents

Various animal models have been developed to study cerebral ischemia, and they can be broadly classified as either focal or global. Focal ischemia models try to mimic a human stroke situation, whereas global models try to replicate the consequences of global ischemia following situations such as cardiac arrest or drowning. There is no doubt that such animal studies represent only certain aspects of the complex human cerebral ischemia.

FOCAL MODEL OF ISCHEMIA

The most stringent model of stroke or focal ischemia is permanent occlusion of the MCA via coagulation or using a suture threaded into the MCA via the internal carotid artery. Permanent MCA occlusion using the coagulation method is used mostly in rats, whereas permanent or transient MCA occlusion (pMCAo or tMCAo) can be used in mice (Benchoua *et al.*, 2001) and rats (Margaill *et al.*, 1996). Focal ischemia results in a necrotic core that is surrounded by a salvageable penumbra in which

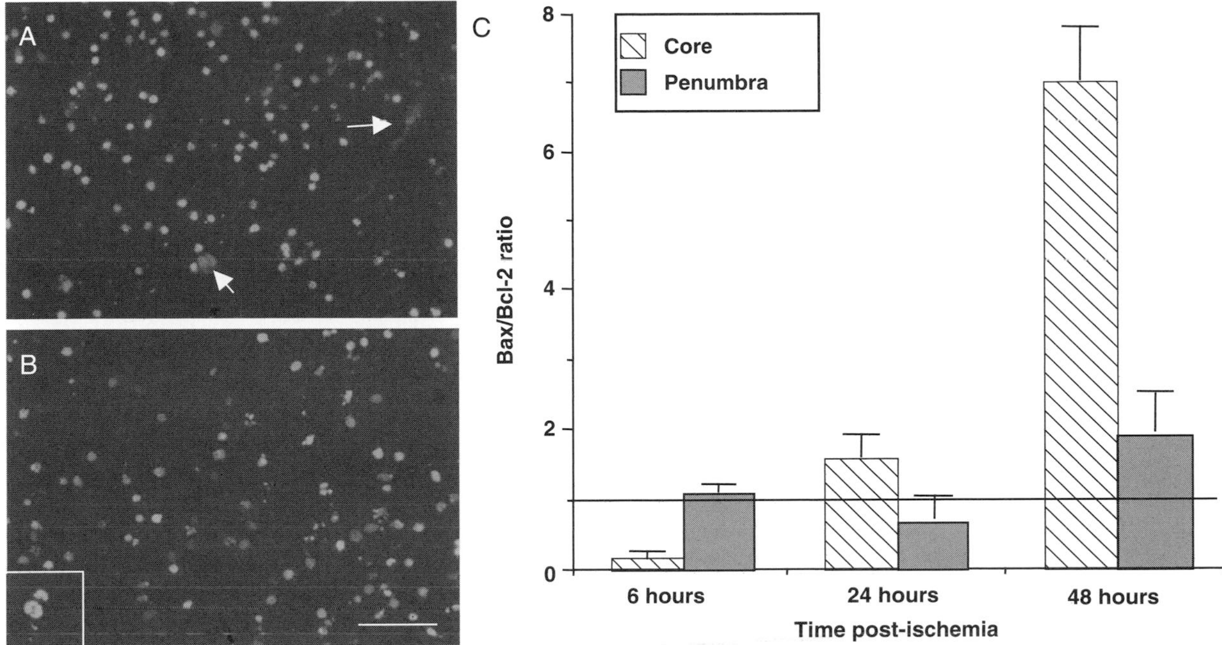

Figure 42.3 Apoptosis in the ipsilateral cortex after neonatal stroke in 7-day-old rat. **A-B**: Typical illustration of DNA fragmentation by the TUNEL assay in the core (A) and penumbra (B), 24 hours post-ischemia. Note the presence of a few necrotic neurons (white arrows in A) near apoptotic nuclei in the core and numerous apoptotic bodies in both the core and penumbra (insert in B). Bar represents 50 (A, B) and 25 μm (insert in B). **C**: Evolution of the Bax/Bcl-2 positive cell ratio in the cerebral cortex. Immunohistochemical studies were performed at 6, 24, and 48 h post-ischemia. No Bcl-2 positive cells and a few (2 to 4) Bax positive cells were detected in controls. The data represent mean values ± S.D. obtained from three separate experiments. Note a rapid Bax/Bcl-2 ratio increase in the core during time of reperfusion. In contrast, the Bax/Bcl-2 ratio evolution was delayed in the penumbra.

DNA fragmentation and apoptotic bodies could be detected by the TUNEL assay (Charriaut-Marlangue *et al.*, 1995; Charriaut-Marlangue *et al.*, 1996a; Charriaut-Marlangue *et al.*, 1996b; Du *et al.*, 1996; MacManus *et al.*, 1997; Fujimura *et al.*, 1999; Benchoua *et al.*, 2001).

GLOBAL MODEL OF ISCHEMIA

The global models of cerebral ischemia consist of a brief period of ischemia (5–15 min), during which complete arrest of cerebral blood flow to the brain is achieved, followed by reperfusion. The common models used are bilateral occlusion of the carotid arteries in gerbils (Cho *et al.*, 2003), occlusion of vertebral arteries and carotid arteries (four-vessel occlusion, 4VO) for 10 to 20 min (Pulsinelli and Brierley, 1979) and occlusion of the carotid arteries (two-vessel occlusion, 2VO) with concomitant hypotension to 50 mm Hg for 5 to 15 min in rats (Gill *et al.*, 2002). Global ischemia tends to result in delayed neuronal death in the hippocampus, cortex, and striatum. In general, this delayed degeneration is also believed to be necrotic (Petito *et al.*, 1997), although DNA laddering and TUNEL-positive nuclei have been reported (Heron *et al.*, 1993; MacManus *et al.*, 1993; Ferrer *et al.*, 1994b; MacManus *et al.*, 1994). Prominent apoptotic cell death occurs following global ischemia in neuronal groups that are interconnected with selectively vulnerable populations of neurons and also in nonneuronal cells (Martin *et al.*, 1998).

Differential Expression of Apoptotic Proteins during Development and Aging

Many of the key elements of apoptosis have been demonstrated to be strongly up-regulated in the immature brain, such as caspase-3 (Hu *et al.*, 2000; Blomgren *et al.*, 2001), apoptotic protease-activating factor-1 (Apaf-1) (Ota *et al.*, 2002), Bcl-2 (Merry *et al.*, 1994), and Bax (Vekrellis *et al.*, 1997), and could be expected to have a prominent role in pathological situations such as HI.

BAX/BCL-2 PROTEINS

A differential and unique expression of apoptosis-regulating Bcl-2 family proteins has been demonstrated in the rat brain during the course of development and aging. Bcl-2 is expressed highly during embryonic development but is downregulated after birth (as early as one week) (Min *et al.*, 2003). During naturally occurring cell death (NOCD) in the rat cerebral cortex, neurons expressing Bcl-2 may determine whether a neuron dies or survives, as over-expression of Bcl-2 in transgenic mice protects neurons from NOCD (Martinou *et al.*, 1994). Low levels of Bcl-2 protein are still present in the adult and aged brain. The sustained expression of this protein may protect neurons from various injuries or neurodegeneration. In contrast, Bcl-x_L expression is maintained at a high level postnatally in the brain, suggesting that it may play an important role in the regulation of neuronal survival in the adult and aged brain (Gonzalez-Garcia *et al.*, 1995). Bax, Bak, and Bad promote apoptosis, probably by forming heterodimers with Bcl-2 or Bcl-x, and abolishing their protective function (Davies, 1995; Yang *et al.*, 1995). Bax and Bad expression decrease from embryonic to two to four weeks postnatal age (Vekrellis *et al.*, 1997; Shimohama *et al.*, 1998; Polster *et al.*, 2003), but little is known during the development and aging of the brain. In the brain of mice, Bax is highly expressed between embryonic day 19 and one-week postnatal age of early development, but thereafter the expression dramatically declines (Min *et al.*, 2003). In an immunochemical study, Obonai *et al.* showed that Bak expression in the cerebrum and cerebellum is high in the human fetuses and elderly subjects, but low in those of young adults, and suggested that Bak regulates neuronal death associated with the development and aging (Obonai *et al.*, 1998).

CASPASE PROTEINS

The expression of each caspase is differentially regulated during the development and aging of the brain. One of the most studied was caspase-3, a typical pro-apoptotic executioner protease. A profound downregulation of caspase-3 transcription has been reported between postnatal day 1 (P1) and 12 (P12) (de Bilbao *et al.*, 1999). Developmental regulation of pro-caspase-3 translation has also been reported with high and low or even undetectable levels in the newborn and adult brain, respectively (Krajewska *et al.*, 1997; Ni *et al.*, 1997; Hu *et al.*, 2000). Caspase-3 expression displays an inverse correlation with cytochrome c, as demonstrated in the rat brain (Blomgren *et al.*, 2001; Zhu *et al.*, 2003). It has also recently been demonstrated that procaspase-3 in the neonatal P7 rat cortex exists as a complex of molecular weight of 170 kDa (Kurosu *et al.*, 2004). Caspase-7, -8, and -10 are also highly expressed during embryonic and early postnatal development, but are downregulated after birth (Hu *et al.*, 2000; Shimohama *et al.*, 2001; Yakovlev *et al.*, 2001; Kurosu *et al.*, 2004). Naturally occurring cell death in the development rat cerebral cortex, which increases during the first postnatal week and decreases thereafter, disappearing by the end of the first month, displays the characteristic of apoptosis and is associated with endonuclease activation (Ferrer *et al.*, 1994a). During this process, neurons expressing caspase-3, -7, -8, and -10 may determine whether a neuron dies or survives. In contrast, cytosolic caspase-2, -6, -9, and Apaf-1 are maintained at a high level postnatally in the brain, and both caspase-9 and Apaf-1 are constitutively expressed in the rat brain from E19 to 96 weeks of age (Shimohama *et al.*, 2001). Although the mechanism remains unknown, continued expression of caspase-2, -6, -9, and Apaf-1 after the downregulation of caspase-3, -7, -8, and -10 may require the maintenance of cell homeostasis during development and aging.

Apoptotic Protein Activation Following Cerebral Ischemia: Newborn versus Adult

It is now well accepted that immature neurons may be more prone to apoptotic death, whereas terminally differentiated neurons exhibit pyknosis or die by necrosis. Both neuronal apoptosis and necrosis have repeatedly been observed in neonatal HI (Pulera *et al.*, 1998; Renolleau *et al.*, 1998; Nakajima *et al.*, 2000), whereas neuronal degeneration in the adult cerebral nervous system exists as a continuum between apoptosis and necrosis (Charriaut-Marlangue *et al.*, 1996a; Liu *et al.*, 2004). This morphological continuum is defined as the occurrence of classic apoptosis and necrosis at opposite ends of the spectrum of cell death, with many possible variant forms of cell death residing between these classic endpoints (Martin *et al.*, 1998). These different forms of cell death may explain the presence or absence of apoptosis-associated proteins upregulation in newborn and adult, respectively.

BAx/Bcl-2 REGULATION

In models of hypoxia, a significant elevation of the Bax/Bcl-2 protein ratio was determined between 6 and 13 days following injury in the P0-1 rat brain (Daval and Vert, 2004). In contrast, the lack of significant variations of the expression of Bax and Bcl-2 proteins appeared to be in good agreement with the absence of detectable levels of apoptosis as a consequence of the hypoxic insult in P7 rats (Grojean *et al.*, 2003). In the newborn piglet (P2–P5), the ratio of Bax to Bcl-2 proteins increased more than twofold during hypoxia as compared to normoxia (Ravishankar *et al.*, 2001). Similarly, we observed a sixfold significant elevation of Bax/Bcl-2 protein ratio in our neonatal model of stroke in the P7 rat in the core at 48 hours postreperfusion but not in the penumbra (see Figure 42.3C). High levels of Bax immunoreactivity in many neurons undergoing apoptosis were found in one study on global ischemia (Krajewski *et al.*, 1995).

CASPASE REGULATION

Caspase-3 is markedly activated after HI in the immature rat brain (Zhu *et al.*, 2000; Wang *et al.*, 2001; Benjelloun *et al.*, 2003) compared to ischemia in the adult brain (Namura *et al.*, 1998). In P7 rat brain, caspase-3 activation contributes substantially to cell death after ischemia with reperfusion not only in the penumbra but also in the core (Benjelloun *et al.*, 2003; Manabat *et al.*, 2003), and cells with the cleaved active form of caspase-3 colocalize with markers of DNA fragmentation in injured brain regions (Zhu *et al.*, 2000). There is also a good correlation between the downregulation of procaspase-3 expression and a decline of procaspase-3 activation in the maturing rat brain (Hu *et al.*, 2000; Blomgren *et al.*, 2001) as well as for Apaf-1 and caspase-3 genes (Yakovlev *et al.*, 2001). Considering these results together, it has been proposed that, in the brain, the cytochrome c-dependent mitochondrial pathway is abrogated within two to four weeks after birth, whereas this pathway is still observed in other adult tissues such as the liver (Ota *et al.*, 2002). Caspase-3 activity was the most repeatedly detected enzyme activation after synthetic acetyl-Asp-Glu-Val-Asp-7-amino-4-trifluoromethyl-coumarin (ac-DEVD-AMC) substrate cleavage. As shown in Table 42.2, caspase-3 activity was reported in several but not all studies following ischemia in the adult rats or mice, but sometimes authors were unable to detect it. In contrast, DEVDase activity was found in all the studies in neonatal HI, peaking at 24 hours. This DEVDase activity appeared to be 10- to 20-fold higher in the P7 compared to adult rat and 31- and 25-fold in P5 and P9 mice, respectively, whereas it increases by only about 40% in P21 and P60 mice (Zhu *et al.*, 2005). In the mitochondrial apoptotic pathway, caspase-9 activity precedes caspase-3 activity as reported in the P7 rat brain, after stroke (Benjelloun *et al.*, 2003). Caspase-9 activity was reported only in two studies in adult rodents, but the peak of its activity was shown to follow, and not to precede, that of caspase-3 activity. In addition, caspase-9 activity was demonstrated in the penumbra and not in the core of the infarct (Benchoua *et al.*, 2001).

POLY (ADP-RIBOSE) POLYMERASE (PARP) CLEAVAGE

PARP is a nuclear protein used for DNA repair. It is one of the prototype substrates for caspase-3-mediated cleavage and has been used in many systems to indicate the presence of activated caspase-3. Disappearance of the full-length (116 kDa) PARP and appearance of the cleavage product 89 kDa allow identification of caspase-3-mediated apoptosis (Duricz and Shah, 1997; Casiano *et al.*, 1998). PARP cleavage into the 89 kDa protein was identified in adult and neonatal models of cerebral hypoxia-ischemia, in studies that demonstrated caspase-3 activation (see Table 42.2).

CASPASE INHIBITION

The pharmacology of caspase inhibition is a rapidly expanding field, and effectiveness of blocking caspase activity is still largely debated (Loetscher *et al.*, 2001). Small peptides that irreversibly inactivate the active enzyme site by alkylating the cysteine residue in the consensus sequence QACXG have recently been synthesized, and block caspases and apoptosis *in vitro* as well as *in vivo*. Initially, the involvement of caspases in ischemia-induced cell death was inferred from studies demonstrating that administration of zVAD-fmk, Boc-aspartyl-(Ome)fluoromethyl-ketone (BAF) or z-DEVD-fmk, which are broad-spectrum caspase-inhibitors, before ischemia were neuroprotective in animal models of focal and global ischemia (Loddick *et al.*, 1996; Adachi *et al.*, 2001; Gill *et al.*, 2002). However, the efficacy of these inhibitors in focal ischemia was less clear in later studies. z-DEVD-fmk also has been tested in a transient ischemic model, and, although some reduction in neuronal death was observed, impairment of motor function and long-term potentiation was not prevented (Gillardon *et al.*, 1999), suggesting that caspase inhibition alone does not preserve neuronal function. Intracerebroventricular injections of the same caspase-3 inhibitor promoted cell survival when administered 30 minutes before or two hours after transient ischemia in adult mice (Fink *et al.*, 1998). Another pan-caspase inhibitor, benzyloxycarbonyl-Asp-CH2-dichlorobenzene (zD), also was shown to have neuroprotective effects in a transient ischemia model in gerbils (Himi *et al.*, 1998). The discrepancy between these results may, in part, be due to the different models of ischemia used (global or focal) and the severity of the insult (mild or severe). Administration of a *broad-spectrum* inhibitor BAF was significantly neuroprotective in P7 rat pups subjected to HI (Rice-Vannucci model) when given by intracerebroventricular injection three hours after cerebral hypoxia-ischemia. In addition, systemic injection of BAF significantly protected brain tissue (Cheng *et al.*, 1998). A combination of systemic hypothermia and BAF produced a strong protective effect against neuronal damage in the same model used (Adachi *et al.*, 2001). These results were not confirmed in the previous model used (Zhu *et al.*, 2003) and in a model of unilateral focal ischemia with reperfusion in 7 day-old-rats, in which systemic BAF administration did not induce a significant reduction in infarct volume (see Figure 42.4A).

However, two populations of animals were found, one of which had no apparent infarct (Joly *et al.*, 2004). A general trend to reduce size lesion was observed after a delayed second dose of BAF administration (Joly *et al.*, 2004). Very recently, a potent nontoxic (due to its carboxy-terminal O-phenoxy group) pan-caspase inhibitor with enhanced cell-permeant properties (due to its amino-terminal quinoline), quinoline-Val-Asp(Ome)-CH2-O-Phenoxy (Q-VD-OPh), was shown to significantly reduce neuronal damage and conferred long-lasting neuroprotection (see Figure 42.4B) and appears as a wider caspase inhibitor than BAF, especially against caspases 2 and 6 (Charriaut-Marlangue *et al.*, 2004). These data were in agreement with a role of mitochondrially derived cytochrome c and pro-caspase-3 activation in ischemia-induced cell death in neonatal but not in adult brain (Gill *et al.*, 2002; Blomgren *et al.*, 2003).

It is now well known that distinct mechanisms of cell protection (i.e., anti-excitotoxic and anti-apoptotic) may be effective in animal models of stroke, suggesting that, when combined, these treatments could act in synergy.

TABLE 42.2
Caspase-9 and –3 activation and PARP cleavage in the different models of hypoxia-ischemia or stroke in adult and neonatal rodent brains. Caspase-9 and caspase-3 activities were determined by fluorogenic LEDH and DEVD substrate cleavage, respectively. The presence of the 89 kDa of the PARP, poly (ADP-ribose) polymerase, a caspase-3 substrate, was described to be an apoptotic feature.

Model	Animal	LEDHase activity (Caspase-9)	DEVDase activity (Caspase-3)	PARP cleavage (89 kDa)	Reference
tMCAo	Rat	–30%/control activity at 24 h	+ 58%/control activity at 6–12 h	6 to 48 h	Cho *et al.*, 2003
2 VO	Gerbil	N.D.	+ 30%/control activity at 12 h		Cho *et al.*, 2003
pMCAo	Rat	N.D.	No induction	N.D.	Gill *et al.*, 2002
t2VO + hypotension	Rat		No induction		Gill *et al.*, 2002
tMCAo	Mouse		No induction		Gill *et al.*, 2002
4VO	Rat	N.D.	28 Units/mg at 24 h	72 h	Chen *et al.* 1998
pMCAo	Rat (SHR)	N.D.	150 pmoles/mg/min at 24 h	N.D.	Rabuffetti *et al.* 2000
tMCAo	Mouse	N.D.	18 pmoles/mg/min at 30–60 min	N.D.	Namura *et al.*, 1998
pMCAo	Mouse	566 pmoles/mg/h at 3 h	116 pmoles/mg/h at 1 h	N.D.	Benchoua *et al.*, 2001
		536 pmoles/mg/h at 24 h	100 pmoles/mg/h at 12 h		Benchoua *et al.*, 2001
1 CCA ligated + 8% O2 for 2.5 h	Rat (P7)	N.D.	150 FU/mg/h	18 h	Cheng *et al.* 1999
1 CCA ligated + 7.7% O2 for 65 min	Rat (P7)	N.D.	95 pmoles/mg/min at 24 h	N.D.	Puka-Sundvall *et al.*, 2000
1 CCA ligated + 7.7% O2 for 70 min	Rat (P7)	N.D.	2500–3000 pmoles/mg/h at 24 h	N.D.	Gill *et al.*, 2002
1 CCA ligated +	Rat (P7)				Manabat *et al.*, 2003
tMCAo		N.D.	90 pmoles/mg/min at 24 h	N.D.	Manabat *et al.*, 2003
pMCAo			38 pmoles/mg/min at 11 h		Manabat *et al.*, 2003
pMCAo + tCCAo	Rat (P7)	15 pmoles/mg/min at 6 h	21 pmoles/mg/min at 24 h	24 h to 7 days	Benjelloun *et al.*, 2003
–1 CCA ligated + 10% O2 for 65 min	Mouse (P5)	N.D.	430 pmoles/mg/min at 24 h	N.D.	Zhu *et al.*, 2005
–1 CCA ligated + 10% O2 for 60 min	Mouse (P9)	N.D.	240 pmoles/mg/min at 24 h	N.D.	Zhu *et al.*, 2005

FU, Fluorescence unit; N.D. not determined.

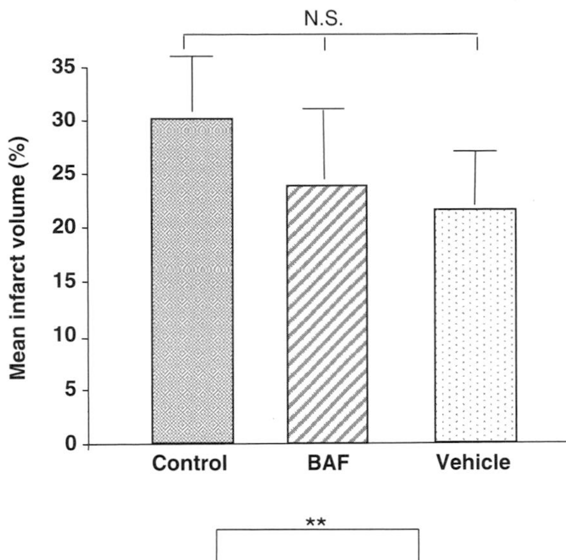

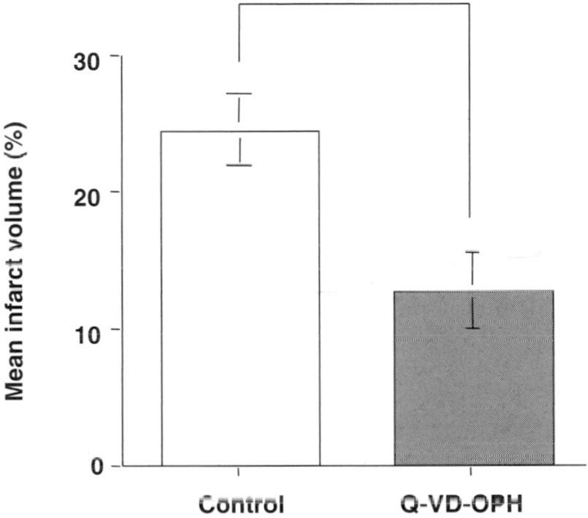

Figure 42.4 Effect of pan-caspase inhibitors on infarct volume measured 48 hours after neonatal ischemia in P7 rat brain (neonatal stroke model). The drug was given five minutes before clip removal and consisted of a single intraperitoneal injection of either BAF in 10% DMSO (n = 16) or vehicle (10% DMSO, n = 15) (A) or Q-VD-OPH (B, see text). Control ischemic rats (n = 14 and 16, respectively) also were studied. Data are mean ± SEM (bar). BAF did not induce a significant reduction of infarct volume (N.S., not significant) as compared to Q-VD-OPH (p = 0.04, Mann-Whitney test).

Pretreatment with subthreshold doses of the NMDA receptor antagonist MK-801 and delayed treatment with subthreshold doses of zVAD-fmk provided synergistic protection compared with each treatment alone (Schulz *et al.*, 1998). Moreover, both treatments extended the therapeutic window for caspase inhibition for an additional two to three hours. Further, pretreatment with subthreshold doses of zVAD-fmk extended the therapeutic window for MK-801 by two hours (Ma *et al.*, 1998; Schulz *et al.*, 1998). These data suggest the potential value of combining treatment strategies to reduce side effects and extend the treatment window in cerebral ischemia.

THE ROLE OF GENDER

Importantly, data from sex-stratified preclinical studies indicate that stroke sensitivity, which means the damage resulting when an ischemic insult occurs, is sexually dimorphic in adults, with less damage tissue in females versus males. It is less clear if ischemic injury in the developing brain is different in males and females. However, provocative new evidence from cells cultured directly from fetal or newborn brain suggests that mechanisms of cell death are not identical in cells that are genetically male (XY) or female (XX). After cytotoxic challenge, programmed cell death proceeded predominately via an apoptosis-inducing factor-dependent pathway in XY neurons versus a cytochrome c-dependent pathway in XX neurons (Du *et al.*, 2004). Recently, deletion of Bax was shown to eliminate sex differences in the mouse forebrain (Forger *et al.*, 2004).

Conclusion

The importance of apoptosis was found to be dependent on brain immaturity and/or delayed development of tissue injury after mild cerebral ischemia in experimental models. Brain injury is a diffuse process with a range of developmental outcomes. Understanding the characteristics, strengths, and limitations of each of the relevant animal models will enable future studies to address mechanistic issues in smaller species such as rodents, and apply the information obtained to larger animals. In addition, these mechanistic issues will allow the development of new therapeutic strategies to provide long-term efficiency of this protection in terms of functional recovery in both the immature and mature brain.

REFERENCES

Adachi, M., Sohma, O., Tsuneishi, S., Takada, S., and Nakamura, H. (2001). Combination effect of systemic hypothermia and caspase inhibitor administration against hypoxic-ischemic brain damage in neonatal rats. *Pediatr Res 50*, 590–595.

Adelson, P.D., and Kochanek, P.M. (1998). Head injury in children. *J Child Neurol 13*, 2–15.

Ashwal, S., Cole, D.J., Osborne, S., Osborne, T.N., and Pearce, W.J. (1995). A new model of neonatal stroke: reversible middle cerebral artery occlusion in the rat pup. *Pediatr Neurol 12*, 191–196.

Benchoua, A., Guegan, C., Couriaud, C., Hosseini, H., Sampaio, N., Morin *et al.* (2001). Specific caspase pathways are activated in the two stages of cerebral infarction. *J Neurosci 21*, 7127–7134.

Benjelloun, N., Joly, L.M., Palmier, B., Plotkine, M., and Charriaut-Marlangue, C. (2003). Apoptotic mitochondrial pathway in neurones and astrocytes after neonatal hypoxia-ischaemia in the rat brain. *Neuropathol Appl Neurobiol 29*, 350–360.

Blomgren, K., Zhu, C., Hallin, U., and Hagberg, H. (2003). Mitochondria and ischemic reperfusion damage in the adult and in the developing brain. *Biochem Biophys Res Commun 304*, 551–559.

Blomgren, K., Zhu, C., Wang, X., Karlsson, J.O., Leverin, A.L., Bahr, B.A. *et al.*(2001). Synergistic activation of caspase-3 by m-calpain after neonatal hypoxia-ischemia: a mechanism of "pathological apoptosis"? *J Biol Chem 276*, 10191–10198.

Casiano, C.A., Ochs, R.L., and Tan, E.M. (1998). Distinct cleavage products of nuclear proteins in apoptosis and necrosis revealed by autoantibody probes. *Cell Death Differ 5*, 183–190.

Charriaut-Marlangue, C., Aggoun-Zouaoui, D., Represa, A., and Ben-Ari, Y. (1996a). Apoptotic features of selective neuronal death in ischemia, epilepsy and gp 120 toxicity. *Trends Neurosci 19*, 109–114.

Charriaut-Marlangue, C., Joly, L.M., Chauvier, D., Jacotot, E., Renolleau, S., and Mariani, J. (2004). Caspase inhibition following neonatal ischemia. *34th Annual Meeting of the SFN*, Abstract 1019.1015.

Charriaut-Marlangue, C., Margaill, I., Plotkine, M., and Ben-Ari, Y. (1995). Early endonuclease activation following reversible focal ischemia in the rat brain. *J Cereb Blood Flow Metab 15*, 385–388.

Charriaut-Marlangue, C., Margaill, I., Represa, A., Popovici, T., Plotkine, M., and Ben-Ari, Y. (1996b). Apoptosis and necrosis after reversible focal ischemia: an in situ DNA fragmentation analysis. *J Cereb Blood Flow Metab 16*, 186–194.

Charriaut-Marlangue, C., Richard, E., and Ben-Ari, Y. (1999). DNA damage and DNA damage-inducible protein Gadd45 following ischemia in the P7 neonatal rat. *Brain Res Dev Brain Res 116*, 133–140.

Cheng, Y., Deshmukh, M., D'Costa, A., Demaro, J.A., Gidday, J.M., Shah, A. *et al.* (1998). Caspase inhibitor affords neuroprotection with delayed administration in a rat model of neonatal hypoxic-ischemic brain injury. *J Clin Invest 101*, 1992–1999.

Cho, S., Liu, D., Gonzales, C., Zaleska, M.M., and Wood, A. (2003). Temporal assessment of caspase activation in experimental models of focal and global ischemia. *Brain Res 982*, 146–155.

Daval, J.L., and Vert, P. (2004). Apoptosis and neurogenesis after transient hypoxia in the developing rat brain. *Semin Perinatol 28*, 257–263.

Davies, A.M. (1995). The Bcl-2 family of proteins, and the regulation of neuronal survival. *Trends Neurosci 18*, 355–358.

de Bilbao, F., Guarin, E., Nef, P., Vallet, P., Giannakopoulos, P., and Dubois-Dauphin, M. (1999). Postnatal distribution of cpp32/caspase 3 mRNA in the mouse central nervous system: an in situ hybridization study. *J Comp Neurol 409*, 339–357.

Delivoria-Papadopoulos, M., and Mishra, O.P. (2004). Nuclear mechanisms of hypoxic cerebral injury in the newborn. *Clin Perinatol, 31*, 91–105.

Derugin, N., Ferriero, D.M., and Vexler, Z.S. (1998). Neonatal reversible focal cerebral ischemia: a new model. *Neurosci Res 32*, 349–353.

Du, C., Hu, R., Csernansky, C.A., Hsu, C.Y., and Choi, D.W. (1996). Very delayed infarction after mild focal cerebral ischemia: a role for apoptosis? *J Cereb Blood Flow Metab 16*, 195–201.

Du, L., Bayir, H., Lai, Y., Zhang, X., Kochanek, P.M., Watkins, S.C. *et al.* (2004). Innate gender-based proclivity in response to cytotoxicity and programmed cell death pathway. *J Biol Chem 279*, 38563–38570.

Ducrocq, S., Benjelloun, N., Plotkine, M., Ben-Ari, Y., and Charriaut-Marlangue, C. (2000). Poly(ADP-ribose) synthase inhibition reduces ischemic injury and inflammation in neonatal rat brain. *J Neurochem 74*, 2504–2511.

Duriez, P.J., and Shah, G.M. (1997). Cleavage of poly(ADP-ribose) polymerase: a sensitive parameter to study cell death. *Biochem Cell Biol 75*, 337–349.

Ferrer, I., Tortosa, A., Blanco, R., Martin, F., Serrano, T., Planas, A. *et al.* (1994a). Naturally occurring cell death in the developing cerebral cortex of the rat. Evidence of apoptosis-associated internucleosomal DNA fragmentation. *Neurosci Lett 182*, 77–79.

Ferrer, I., Tortosa, A., Macaya, A., Sierra, A., Moreno, D., Munell, F. *et al.* (1994b). Evidence of nuclear DNA fragmentation following hypoxia-ischemia in the infant rat brain, and transient forebrain ischemia in the adult gerbil. *Brain Pathol 4*, 115–122.

Fink, K., Zhu, J., Namura, S., Shimizu-Sasamata, M., Endres, M., Ma, J. *et al.* (1998). Prolonged therapeutic window for ischemic brain damage caused by delayed caspase activation. *J Cereb Blood Flow Metab 18*, 1071–1076.

Forger, N.G., Rosen, G.J., Waters, E.M., Jacob, D., Simerly, R.B., and de Vries, G.J. (2004). Deletion of Bax eliminates sex differences in the mouse forebrain. *Proc Natl Acad Sci USA 101*, 13666–13671.

Fujimura, M., Morita-Fujimura, Y., Kawase, M., Copin, J.C., Calagui, B., Epstein, C.J. *et al.* (1999). Manganese superoxide dismutase mediates the early release of mitochondrial cytochrome C and subsequent DNA fragmentation after permanent focal cerebral ischemia in mice. *J Neurosci 19*, 3414–3422.

Gill, R., Soriano, M., Blomgren, K., Hagberg, H., Wybrecht, R., Miss, M.T. *et al.* (2002). Role of caspase-3 activation in cerebral ischemia-induced neurodegeneration in adult and neonatal brain. *J Cereb Blood Flow Metab 22*, 420–430.

Gillardon, F., Kiprianova, I., Sandkuhler, J., Hossmann, K.A., and Spranger, M. (1999). Inhibition of caspases prevents cell death of hippocampal CA1 neurons, but not impairment of hippocampal long-term potentiation following global ischemia. *Neuroscience 93*, 1219–1222.

Gonzalez-Garcia, M., Garcia, I., Ding, L., O'Shea, S., Boise, L.H., Thompson, C.B. *et al.* (1995). Bcl-x is expressed in embryonic and postnatal neural tissues and functions to prevent neuronal cell death. *Proc Natl Acad Sci USA 92*, 4304–4308.

Grojean, S., Pourie, G., Vert, P., and Daval, J.L. (2003). Differential neuronal fates in the CA1 hippocampus after hypoxia in newborn and 7-day-old rats: effects of pre-treatment with MK-801. *Hippocampus 13*, 970–977.

Hagberg, H., Gilland, E., Diemer, N.H., and Andine, P. (1994). Hypoxia-ischemia in the neonatal rat brain: histopathology after post-treatment with NMDA and non-NMDA receptor antagonists. *Biol Neonate 66*, 205–213.

Heron, A., Pollard, H., Dessi, F., Moreau, J., Lasbennes, F., Ben-Ari, Y. *et al.* (1993). Regional variability in DNA fragmentation after global ischemia evidenced by combined histological and gel electrophoresis observations in the rat brain. *J Neurochem 61*, 1973–1976.

Hill, I.E., MacManus, J.P., Rasquinha, I., and Tuor, U.I. (1995). DNA fragmentation indicative of apoptosis following unilateral cerebral hypoxia-ischemia in the neonatal rat. *Brain Res 676*, 398–403.

Himi, T., Ishizaki, Y., and Murota, S. (1998). A caspase inhibitor blocks ischaemia-induced delayed neuronal death in the gerbil. *Eur J Neurosci 10*, 777–781.

Hu, B.R., Liu, C.L., Ouyang, Y., Blomgren, K., and Siesjo, B.K. (2000). Involvement of caspase-3 in cell death after hypoxia-ischemia declines during brain maturation. *J Cereb Blood Flow Metab 20*, 1294–1300.

Ikonomidou, C., Mosinger, J.L., Salles, K.S., Labruyere, J., Olney, J.W. (1989). Sensitivity of the developing rat brain to hypobaric/ischemic damage parallels sensitivity to N-methyl-aspartate neurotoxicity. *J Neurosci 9(8)*, 2809–2818.

Joly, L.M., Mucignat, V., Mariani, J., Plotkine, M., and Charriaut-Marlangue, C. (2004). Caspase inhibition after neonatal ischemia in the rat brain. *J Cereb Blood Flow Metab 24*, 124–131.

Krajewska, M., Wang, H.G., Krajewski, S., Zapata, J.M., Shabaik, A., Gascoyne, R. *et al.* (1997). Immunohistochemical analysis of in vivo patterns of expression of CPP32 (Caspase-3), a cell death protease. *Cancer Res 57*, 1605–1613.

Krajewski, S., Mai, J.K., Krajewska, M., Sikorska, M., Mossakowski, M.J., and Reed, J.C. (1995). Upregulation of bax protein levels in neurons following cerebral ischemia. *J Neurosci 15*, 6364–6376.

Kurosu, K., Saeki, M., and Kamisaki, Y. (2004). Formation of high molecular weight caspase-3 complex in neonatal rat brain. *Neurochem Int 44*, 199–204.

Levine, S. (1960). Anoxic-ischemic encephalopathy in rats. *Am J Pathol 36*, 1–17.

Liu, C.L., Siesjo, B.K., and Hu, B.R. (2004). Pathogenesis of hippocampal neuronal death after hypoxia-ischemia changes during brain development. *Neuroscience 127*, 113–123.

Loddick, S.A., MacKenzie, A., and Rothwell, N.J. (1996). An ICE inhibitor, z-VAD-DCB attenuates ischaemic brain damage in the rat. *Neuroreport 7*, 1465–1468.

Loetscher, H., Niederhauser, O., Kemp, J., and Gill, R. (2001). Is caspase-3 inhibition a valid therapeutic strategy in cerebral ischemia? *Drug Discov Today 6*, 671–680.

Ma, J., Endres, M., and Moskowitz, M.A. (1998). Synergistic effects of caspase inhibitors and MK-801 in brain injury after transient focal cerebral ischaemia in mice. *Br J Pharmacol 124*, 756–762.

MacManus, J.P., Buchan, A.M., Hill, I.E., Rasquinha, I., and Preston, E. (1993). Global ischemia can cause DNA fragmentation indicative of apoptosis in rat brain. *Neurosci Lett 164*, 89–92.

MacManus, J.P., Hill, I.E., Huang, Z.G., Rasquinha, I., Xue, D., and Buchan, A.M. (1994). DNA damage consistent with apoptosis in transient focal ischaemic neocortex. *Neuroreport 5*, 493–496.

MacManus, J.P., Rasquinha, I., Tuor, U., and Preston, E. (1997). Detection of higher-order 50- and 10-kbp DNA fragments before apoptotic internucleosomal cleavage after transient cerebral ischemia. *J Cereb Blood Flow Metab 17*, 376–387.

Manabat, C., Han, B.H., Wendland, M., Derugin, N., Fox, C.K., Choi, J. *et al.* (2003). Reperfusion differentially induces caspase-3 activation in ischemic core and penumbra after stroke in immature brain. *Stroke 34*, 207–213.

Margaill, I., Parmentier, S., Callebert, J., Allix, M., Boulu, R.G., and Plotkine, M. (1996). Short therapeutic window for MK-801 in transient focal cerebral ischemia in normotensive rats. *J Cereb Blood Flow Metab 16*, 107–113.

Marret, S., Mukendi, R., Gadisseux, J.F., Gressens, P., and Evrard, P. (1995). Effect of ibotenate on brain development: an excitotoxic mouse model of microgyria and posthypoxic-like lesions. *J Neuropathol Exp Neurol 54*, 358–370.

Martin, L.J., Al-Abdulla, N.A., Brambrink, A.M., Kirsch, J.R., Sieber, F.E., and Portera-Cailliau, C. (1998). Neurodegeneration in excitotoxicity, global cerebral ischemia, and target deprivation: A perspective on the contributions of apoptosis and necrosis. *Brain Res Bull 46*, 281–309.

Martinou, J.C., Dubois-Dauphin, M., Staple, J.K., Rodriguez, I., Frankowski, H., Missotten, M. *et al.* (1994). Overexpression of BCL-2 in transgenic mice protects neurons from naturally occurring cell death and experimental ischemia. *Neuron 13*, 1017–1030.

McDonald, J.W., Silverstein, F.S., and Johnston, M.V. (1988). Neurotoxicity of N-methyl-D-aspartate is markedly enhanced in developing rat central nervous system. *Brain Res 459*, 200–203.

Merry, D.E., Veis, D.J., Hickey, W.F., and Korsmeyer, S.J. (1994). Bcl-2 protein expression is widespread in the developing nervous system and retained in the adult PNS. *Development 120*, 301–311.

Min, S.H., Hwang, D.Y., Kang, T.S., Hwang, J.H., Lim, C.H., Lee, S.H. *et al.* (2003). Differential expression of proteins of caspases and Bcl-2 families in the brain of mice. *Int J Mol Med 12*, 181–183.

Nakajima, W., Ishida, A., Lange, M.S., Gabrielson, K.L., Wilson, M.A., Martin, L.J. *et al.* (2000). Apoptosis has a prolonged role in the neurodegeneration after hypoxic ischemia in the newborn rat. *J Neurosci 20*, 7994–8004.

Namura, S., Zhu, J., Fink, K., Endres, M., Srinivasan, A., Tomaselli, K.J. *et al.* (1998). Activation and cleavage of caspase-3 in apoptosis induced by experimental cerebral ischemia. *J Neurosci 18*, 3659–3668.

Nelson, K.B., and Lynch, J.K. (2004). Stroke in newborn infants. *Lancet Neurol 3*, 150–158.

Ni, B., Wu, X., Du, Y., Su, Y., Hamilton-Byrd, E., Rockey, P.K. *et al.* (1997). Cloning and expression of a rat brain interleukin-1beta-converting enzyme (ICE)-related protease (IRP) and its possible role in apoptosis of cultured cerebellar granule neurons. *J Neurosci 17*, 1561–1569.

Obonai, T., Mizuguchi, M., and Takashima, S. (1998). Developmental and aging changes of Bak expression in the human brain. *Brain Res 783*, 167–170.

Ota, K., Yakovlev, A.G., Itaya, A., Kameoka, M., Tanaka, Y., and Yoshihara, K. (2002). Alteration of apoptotic protease-activating factor-1 (APAF-1)-dependent apoptotic pathway during development of rat brain and liver. *J Biochem (Tokyo) 131*, 131–135.

Petito, C.K., Torres-Munoz, J., Roberts, B., Olarte, J.P., Nowak, T.S., Jr., and Pulsinelli, W.A. (1997). DNA fragmentation follows delayed neuronal death in CA1 neurons exposed to transient global ischemia in the rat. *J Cereb Blood Flow Metab 17*, 967–976.

Polster, B.M., Robertson, C.L., Bucci, C.J., Suzuki, M., and Fiskum, G. (2003). Postnatal brain development and neural cell differentiation modulate mitochondrial Bax and BH3 peptide-induced cytochrome c release. *Cell Death Differ 10*, 365–370.

Puka-Sundvall, M., Gajkowska, B., Cholewinski, M., Blomgren, K., Lazarewicz, J.W., and Hagberg, H. (2000). Subcellular distribution of calcium and ultrastructural changes after cerebral hypoxia-ischemia in immature rats. *Brain Res Dev Brain Res 125*, 31–41.

Pulera, M.R., Adams, L.M., Liu, H., Santos, D.G., Nishimura, R.N., Yang, F. *et al.* (1998). Apoptosis in a neonatal rat model of cerebral hypoxia-ischemia. *Stroke, 29*, 2622–2630.

Pulsinelli, W.A., and Brierley, J.B. (1979). A new model of bilateral hemispheric ischemia in the unanesthetized rat. *Stroke 10*, 267–272.

Ravishankar, S., Ashraf, Q.M., Fritz, K., Mishra, O.P., and Delivoria-Papadopoulos, M. (2001). Expression of Bax and Bcl-2 proteins during hypoxia in cerebral cortical neuronal nuclei of newborn piglets: effect of administration of magnesium sulfate. *Brain Res 901*, 23–29.

Renolleau, S., Aggoun-Zouaoui, D., Ben-Ari, Y., and Charriaut-Marlangue, C. (1998). A model of transient unilateral focal ischemia with reperfusion in the P7 neonatal rat: morphological changes indicative of apoptosis. *Stroke 29*, 1454–1460; discussion 1461.

Rice, J.E., 3rd, Vannucci, R.C., and Brierley, J.B. (1981). The influence of immaturity on hypoxic-ischemic brain damage in the rat. *Ann Neurol 9*, 131–141.

Roohey, T., Raju, T.N., and Moustogiannis, A.N. (1997). Animal models for the study of perinatal hypoxic-ischemic encephalopathy: a critical analysis. *Early Hum Dev 47*, 115–146.

Schulz, J.B., Weller, M., Matthews, R.T., Heneka, M.T., Groscurth, P., Martinou, J.C. *et al.* (1998). Extended therapeutic window for caspase inhibition and synergy with MK-801 in the treatment of cerebral histotoxic hypoxia. *Cell Death Differ 5*, 847–857.

Sheldon, R.A., Chuai, J., and Ferriero, D.M. (1996). A rat model for hypoxic-ischemic brain damage in very premature infants. *Biol Neonate 69*, 327–341.

Sheldon, R.A., Sedik, C., and Ferriero, D.M. (1998). Strain-related brain injury in neonatal mice subjected to hypoxia-ischemia. *Brain Res 810*, 114–122.

Shimohama, S., Fujimoto, S., Sumida, Y., and Tanino, H. (1998). Differential expression of rat brain bcl-2 family proteins in development and aging. *Biochem Biophys Res Commun 252*, 92–96.

Shimohama, S., Tanino, H., and Fujimoto, S. (2001). Differential expression of rat brain caspase family proteins during development and aging. *Biochem Biophys Res Commun 289*, 1063–1066.

Sizonenko, S.V., Sirimanne, E., Mayall, Y., Gluckman, P.D., Inder, T., and Williams, C. (2003). Selective cortical alteration after hypoxic-ischemic injury in the very immature rat brain. *Pediatr Res 54*, 263–269.

Stadlin, A., James, A., Fiscus, R., Wong, Y.F., Rogers, M., and Haines, C. (2003). Development of a postnatal 3-day-old rat model of mild hypoxic-ischemic brain injury. *Brain Res 993*, 101–110.

Towfighi, J., Mauger, D., Vannucci, R.C., and Vannucci, S.J. (1997). Influence of age on the cerebral lesions in an immature rat model of cerebral hypoxia-ischemia: a light microscopic study. *Brain Res Dev Brain Res 100*, 149–160.

Towfighi, J., Zec, N., Yager, J., Housman, C., and Vannucci, R.C. (1995). Temporal evolution of neuropathologic changes in an immature rat model of cerebral hypoxia: a light microscopic study. *Acta Neuropathol (Berl) 90*, 375–386.

Vannucci, R.C. (2000). Hypoxic-ischemic encephalopathy. *Am J Perinatol 17*, 113–120.

Vannucci, R.C., and Vannucci, S.J. (1997). A model of perinatal hypoxic-ischemic brain damage. *Ann N Y Acad Sci 835*, 234–249.

Vekrellis, K., McCarthy, M.J., Watson, A., Whitfield, J., Rubin, L.L., and Ham, J. (1997). Bax promotes neuronal cell death and is downregulated during the development of the nervous system. *Development 124*, 1239–1249.

Wang, X., Karlsson, J.O., Zhu, C., Bahr, B.A., Hagberg, H., and Blomgren, K. (2001). Caspase-3 activation after neonatal rat cerebral hypoxia-ischemia. *Biol Neonate 79*, 172–179.

Warlow, C.P. (1998). Epidemiology of stroke. *Lancet 352 Suppl 3*, SIII1–SIII4.

Yager, J.Y., Shuaib, A., and Thornhill, J. (1996). The effect of age on susceptibility to brain damage in a model of global hemispheric hypoxia-ischemia. *Brain Res Dev Brain Res 93*, 143–154.

Yakovlev, A.G., Ota, K., Wang, G., Movsesyan, V., Bao, W.L., Yoshihara, K. *et al.* (2001). Differential expression of apoptotic protease-activating factor-1 and caspase-3 genes and susceptibility to apoptosis during brain development and after traumatic brain injury. J *Neurosci 21*, 7439–7446.

Yang, E., Zha, J., Jockel, J., Boise, L.H., Thompson, C.B., and Korsmeyer, S.J. (1995). Bad, a heterodimeric partner for Bcl-XL and Bcl-2, displaces Bax and promotes cell death. *Cell 80*, 285–291.

Zhu, C., Qiu, L., Wang, X., Hallin, U., Cande, C., Kroemer, G. *et al.* (2003). Involvement of apoptosis-inducing factor in neuronal death after hypoxia-ischemia in the neonatal rat brain. *J Neurochem 86*, 306–317.

Zhu, C., Wang, X., Hagberg, H., and Blomgren, K. (2000). Correlation between caspase-3 activation and three different markers of DNA damage in neonatal cerebral hypoxia-ischemia. *J Neurochem 75*, 819–829.

Zhu, C., Wang, X., Xu, F., Bahr, B.A., Shibata, M., Uchiyama, Y. *et al.* (2005). The influence of age on apoptotic and other mechanisms of cell death after cerebral hypoxia-ischemia. *Cell Death Differ 12*, 162–176.

43

Age-related Changes in Hormones and Their Receptors in Animal Models of Female Reproductive Senescence

Jacqueline A. Maffucci and Andrea C. Gore

Traditionally, the onset and progression of menopause in humans has been attributed to ovarian follicular decline. Because the follicles are the primary source of circulating estrogens, these age-related changes lead to a number of symptoms such as hot flashes, mood swings, irritability, and depression, as well as increased risk of osteoporosis, cardiovascular disease, and age-associated diseases. Recent research indicates that along with the ovarian changes at menopause, the hypothalamic and pituitary levels of the reproductive axis also undergo significant changes during reproductive aging. Indeed, current research suggests a neural, as well as hormonal, mechanism involved in the menopausal process. A number of animal models are available to study these processes, most commonly the nonhuman primates and rodents, and to a lesser extent, avian systems. Here, we will discuss Old and New World monkey models, rats, mice (wild type, transgenic, and genetically modified), and birds as models for reproductive aging. An overview of the reproductive aging process will be discussed for each model, along with their advantages, disadvantages, and biomedical relevance. In addition, we will present recent findings pertaining to the mechanisms for the onset of reproductive aging in all of these models, focusing on the hypothalamic-pituitary-gonadal axis, and emphasizing molecular changes and hormonal output.

Introduction

Reproductive senescence is a natural and inevitable part of the aging process in the female life cycle. In humans, this process is referred to as *menopause*. Menopause is defined as the permanent cessation of menstruation and is an immediate consequence of the loss of ovarian follicular activity (World Health Organization, 1996). This depletion results in a decrease in estrogen levels, leading to a number of symptoms including sleep disturbances, vasomotor symptoms, mood swings, irritability, depression, memory loss, urogenital symptoms, osteoporosis, and cardiovascular morbidity. Menopause is divided into two stages, *perimenopause* and *postmenopause*, as defined by the STRAW panel (Soules *et al.*, 2001). Perimenopause begins when the first symptoms of menopause appear (including increases in menstrual cycle variability, decreases in fecundity, and changes in hormonal status) and continues until one year following the final menstrual period. Once menstruation is absent for a year or more, the female is considered to be postmenopausal. The average age at which perimenopause begins is at 47.5 years, and it lasts for an average of four to six years. However, peak follicular degeneration may occur as early as 38 years old, with declines in fertility occurring between 30 and 35 years (Zapantis *et al.*, 2003).

Despite the universality of menopause among women, its mechanism remains largely unclear, and treatment to ease its symptoms is uncertain. Currently, the most commonly used treatment is estrogen replacement therapy, which has been met with considerable controversy. It is critical that we understand the mechanism by which menopause occurs and the effects of estrogen depletion during menopause in order to evaluate the advantages of estrogen replacement therapy in women and to determine other possible treatments for menopausal symptoms. Animal models are an essential part of uncovering these mechanisms, as studies in humans are often constrained.

Traditionally, menopause and its resulting symptoms have been attributed to the decline of the ovarian follicle. Although this is clearly the proximal event leading to ovarian failure, recent research using animal models has revealed an interaction of both neuroendocrine and ovarian events that lead to the transition to acyclicity (Wise *et al.*, 1999). Studies on humans are often difficult due to the limitations on invasive procedures and difficulties encountered when trying to normalize the subject population. Animal models are much more useful in these endeavors, each with its strengths and weaknesses. For studies in reproductive aging, primates are commonly used, as they mimic the human menstrual cycle and therefore provide an excellent model for studying the role of ovarian hormones in this process. However, aged primates are limited in number, extremely expensive, and undergo the menopausal transition far later in the life cycle than women. By contrast, rodents do not undergo extensive follicular decline, but do show changes in gonadotropin-releasing hormone (GnRH) neurons and the central regulatory factors influencing these neurons, making them a relevant model for studying the neural component of this process. Additionally, the use of transgenic or knockout mice has made it possible to understand the role of specific genes in the aging process. Finally, nonmammalian animal models, particularly birds, have been used to shed light on other mechanisms by which senescence occurs. This chapter will examine these animal models in detail.

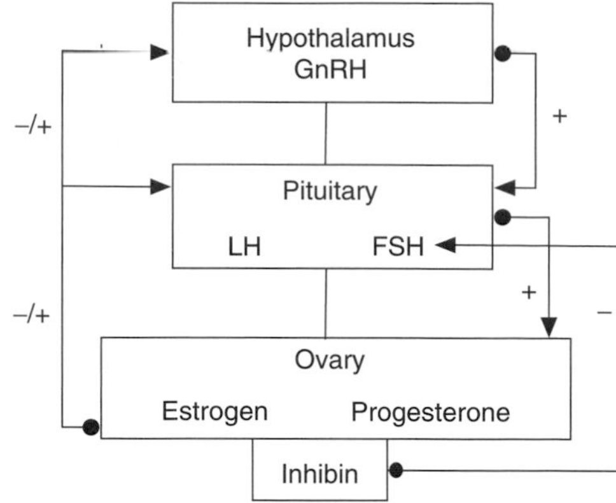

Figure 43.1 A summary of the hypothalamic-pituitary-gonadal axis of females. GnRH stimulates gonadotropin release (LH and FSH), which then stimulates ovarian steroid hormone release (estrogen and progesterone). Estrogen either has positive (just prior to ovulation) or negative feedback actions on the hypothalamus and pituitary. Inhibin is also released by the ovary and inhibits FSH release. In rats, the "estropause" is characterized by continued high estrogen levels and a persistent estrus vaginal cytology until much later in life. On the arrows, the circle refers to the initiator of the signal, and arrows indicate the termination of the signal.

The Hypothalamic-Pituitary-Gonadal (HPG) Axis and Age-related Changes

Understanding the mechanisms influencing the onset of reproductive senescence first requires familiarity with the HPG axis that controls reproduction in all vertebrates. The hypothalamus is located at the base of the brain and contains approximately 1000 neurons that release the neuropeptide, GnRH. GnRH is transported to the anterior pituitary gland via a capillary portal system. At the pituitary, it stimulates the synthesis and release of the gonadotropin luteinizing hormone (LH) and follicle-stimulating hormone (FSH), which are released into the systemic blood system. At the ovary, LH and FSH are responsible for the growth, maturation, and release of ovarian follicles, and steroidogenesis. The release of GnRH, and subsequently LH, are pulsatile in all mammals, in which pulse amplitude and frequency are important determinants of reproductive function. Additionally, the HPG axis of females is regulated both by negative and positive feedback from circulating estrogens and progestins onto the pituitary and hypothalamus (see Figure 43.1). Although feedback regulation by steroid hormones is negative throughout most of the cycle, increasing preovulatory estrogen concentrations trigger transient positive feedback. This process is referred to here as the preovulatory GnRH/LH surge, and is crucial for ovulation in all animals with spontaneous ovulatory cycles (see Figure 43.2).

Research investigating the mechanisms of estrogen's positive feedback upon GnRH and LH release has localized few estrogen or progestin receptors within GnRH neurons, which express low levels of the estrogen receptor (ER) β but not α (Herbison and Pape, 2001). This surprising finding suggests that estrogen exerts many of its feedback actions via *inputs* to GnRH neurons. Studies have shown that, indeed, many neurotransmitters and neuropeptides regulate GnRH neurons, and that their receptors are localized to GnRH cells. For example, glutamate, γ-aminobutyric acid (GABA), catecholamines, neuropeptide Y (NPY), neurotensin, and vasoactive intestinal polypeptide (VIP) contact GnRH neurons and also express estrogen receptors, making them targets at which estrogen can indirectly regulate the GnRH neuron (reviewed in Gore, (2002)). Additionally, some of these neurotransmitters and their receptors, such as GABA and glutamate, change expression in the brains of aging rats (reviewed in Gore, (2002)), suggesting that these neurotransmitters play a role in mediating age-related changes observed in GnRH output during the onset of reproductive senescence. Therefore, it is important to consider age-associated changes in these neuromodulators as well as direct changes to the HPG axis to understand neural changes affecting the onset of reproductive senescence.

Nonhuman Primate Models

OLD WORLD MONKEYS

Nonhuman primates (NHP) are classified as Old World monkeys, New World monkeys, and Great Apes. The Old World monkeys (OWM) are most commonly used in biomedical research, and, of these, the Asian macaques and the baboons of Africa are most frequently used. OWMs have a genetic makeup approximately 92.5 to 95% similar to humans and undergo similar reproductive processes as humans. The NHP reproductive cycle is approximately 28 to 30 days, with a follicular, proliferative, and luteal phase that results in a hormonal milieu similar to that in humans (Hendrickx *et al.*, 1995) (see Figure 43.2). Additionally, in aging OWMs, as in humans, a decrease in fertility and changes in HPG hormone levels are accompanied by the onset of irregular menstrual cycles and finally, cessation of menses. However, OWMs spend a much shorter period (15–23%) of their

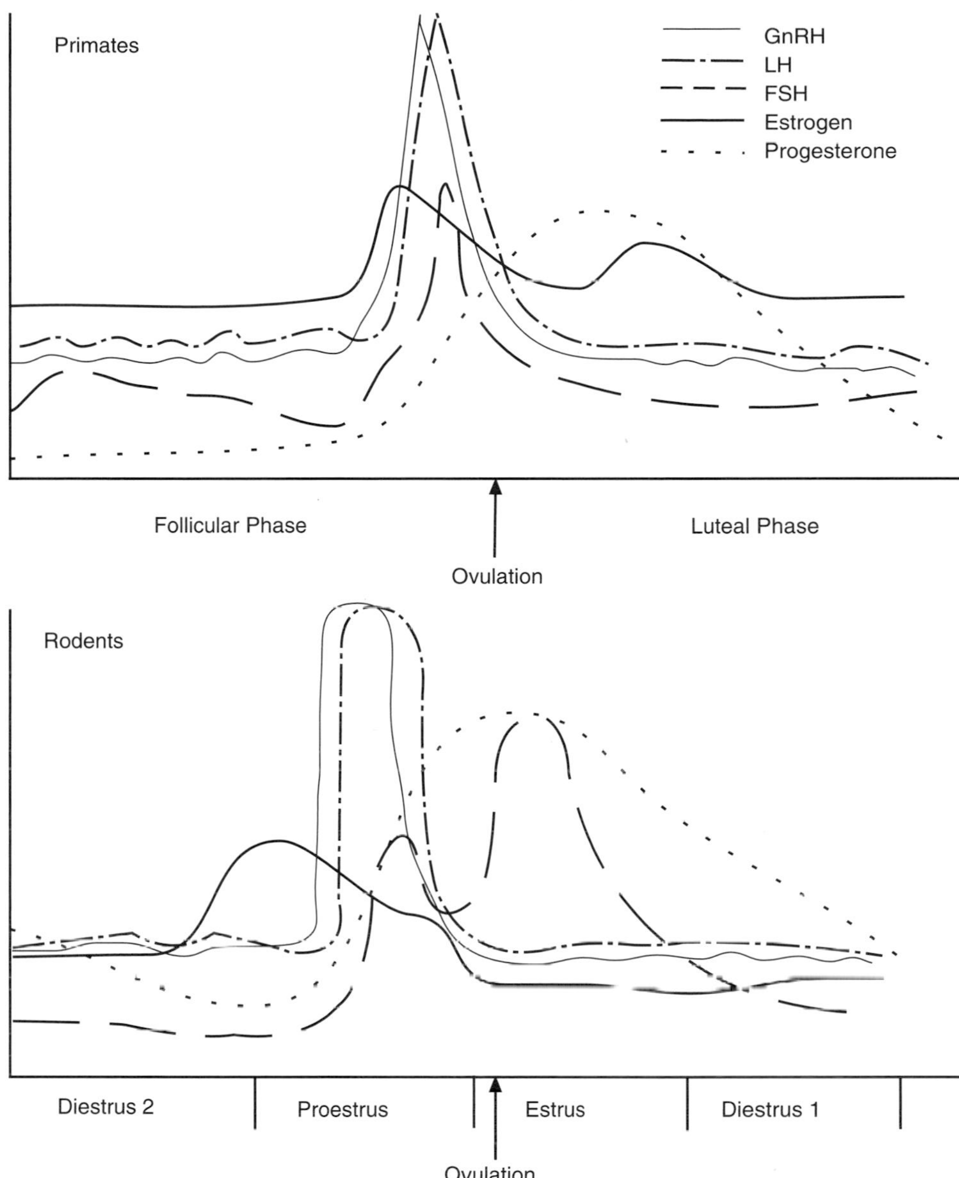

Figure 43.2 Hormonal changes accompanying the primate (human and nonhuman primates) and rodent normal reproductive cycles. In both primates and rodents, an increase in estrogen occurs immediately prior to the GnRH/LH surge, followed by a slight surge in FSH. A gradual increase in progesterone occurs just prior to ovulation. Levels of progesterone are elevated during the luteal phase of primates, and during diestrus in rodents.

lifespan in an anovulatory state, as compared to humans (50%) (Tardif *et al.*, 1992; Bellino and Wise, 2003), making it difficult to study postmenopausal changes. Additionally, researchers face high costs to obtain and care for these animals (expensive due to the cost involved in maintaining them for 20+ years), the supply is limited, and there is a higher risk of loss of data due to age-related illness or death. Thus, two models have been developed to alleviate these challenges: the intact, aged, and the ovariectomized, young monkey.

The intact, aged model, though costly, provides a natural model of studying hormonal and neural changes associated with aging. Researchers can use this model to look toward modifications in brain structures as well as ovarian hormones when considering reproductive aging. Thus, differences in neuronal morphology, neuronal populations, and receptor density in the aging brain can be observed. Additionally, studies examining age-associated genetic alterations and relations to neural changes, and age-associated diseases, such as osteoporosis, cardiovascular diseases, and vasomotor symptoms (e.g., hot flash) can be undertaken in this model. These factors make the aged OWM a favored model for studies of reproductive senescence.

Studies in intact, aged macaques and baboons focus primarily on the perimenopausal period, when menstrual cycle variability increases, fecundity decreases, and hormonal status first changes. Humans and OWMs show very similar changes in urinary estrogen and progestin profiles once they begin perimenopause. However, there are a few differences in the timing of the hormonal transition to perimenopause: middle-aged women show a period of increase in FSH and decrease in inhibin A along with a cyclically high level of estrogen prior to onset, whereas rhesus monkeys do not (Bellino and Wise, 2003). Hence rhesus monkeys show a more immediate transition to perimenopause, whereas the human transition is more gradual. In both humans and OWMs, the onset of perimenopause is accompanied by declines in estrogen and progesterone levels, and a shorter follicular phase is observed during the menstrual cycle. In accordance with this, LH/FSH levels increase, partly due to the release from negative feedback associated with estrogen release (Bellino and Wise, 2003). Although this transition in macaques may occur as early as 18 to 20 years of age, it has been noted that rhesus monkeys may not show this transition until 25 years of age or later, an age equivalent to 65 to 90 years in humans (Gore *et al.*, 2004). It is for this reason that the intact, aged monkey model has yet to meet its research potential, as these animals undergo reproductive senescence so late in their life cycle that they are difficult both to attain and maintain.

Activity of the HPG axis of intact, aged monkeys has been assessed in two studies. First, Woller *et al.* (2002) demonstrated changes in LH pulsatile activity in late perimenopausal and postmenopausal rhesus monkeys, showing not only increases in mean LH amplitude, but also increases in pulse amplitude and higher baseline LH levels when compared to young animals. Estrogen levels of the aged monkeys were also lower; no differences were observed in progesterone. Gore *et al.* (2004) used push-pull perfusion to measure changes in GnRH levels in peri- and postmenopausal monkeys and recorded increases in mean GnRH concentrations and higher pulse amplitudes compared to young monkeys. These latter data are consistent with the observed changes in LH pulses (Woller *et al.*, 2002) and suggest a novel mechanism by which hormonal changes may affect the onset of reproductive aging. Taken together, the age-associated increases in pulsatile GnRH and gonadotropin, even prior to complete ovarian senescence, indicate a role of the hypothalamus and the pituitary, respectively, in reproductive senescence in a NHP model. Moreover, the observations of age-related changes in pulsatility and accompanying neural changes promise to enhance our understanding of the finer mechanism of reproductive decline.

Even though intact, aging animals provide some advantages for studying age-associated neural changes, researchers often turn to the young, ovariectomized (OVX) animal as a substitute. Ovariectomized animals have a negligible level of circulating estrogen and cessation of menses. Thus, these monkeys model changes that occur during reproductive aging. It is important to remember that these are not aged animals, and that the loss of estrogen in a young monkey by OVX does not necessarily mimic natural, age-related changes in estrogen in the aged brain. However, they have proven to be effective for studying at least some of the neural changes associated with estrogen loss and replacement, including changes to hormone receptor densities and neuronal morphology and populations of neuropeptides and neuromodulators associated with the HPG axis. Concurrently, researchers can uncover the benefits of estrogen replacement therapy (ERT) and the acute and chronic treatment effects of ERT on diseases and symptoms associated with menopause.

As discussed earlier, aged animals show an increase in GnRH and LH levels, and estrogen loss may contribute to these observed increases (Woller *et al.*, 2002; Bellino and Wise, 2003; Gore *et al.*, 2004). The OVX, young monkey model has extended these results to show inhibitory effects of estrogen on GnRH release (Chongthammakun and Terasawa, 1993), GnRH mRNA expression (El Majdoubi *et al.*, 1998; Krajewski *et al.*, 2003), and circulating LH concentrations (El Majdoubi *et al.*, 1998). Parallel results have been reported in humans, in which estrogen replacement for postmenopausal women diminishes LH and FSH levels as compared to nontreated women (Gill *et al.*, 2002), and decreases in GnRH mRNA occur following estradiol replacement (Rance and Uswandi, 1996). Additionally, effects of estrogen on hypothalamic neuropeptides associated with GnRH pulsatility have been suggested for norepinephrine and neuropeptide Y. Both of these neuromodulators demonstrate pulsatile release, and increase just prior to the GnRH surge associated with ovulation. Estrogen replacement in OVX females upregulates norepinephrine release and increases the sensitivity of GnRH release to neuropeptide Y, suggesting that neuromodulators playing a role in reproductive aging undergo changes with the age-associated decline in estrogen levels (Terasawa, 1998).

Estrogen receptor expression in neuroendocrine and other brain regions is important to consider in the aging model. In recent years, estrogen has been found to be responsible not only for feedback actions upon the hypothalamus, but also other neurophysiological functions such as cognition and neuroprotection. Two nuclear estrogen receptors, ERα and ERβ, have been localized in mammalian brain tissue, each showing unique expression patterns in subregions of the hypothalamus (Chakraborty and Gore, 2004). The roles of ERα and ERβ, as well as the interplay between these two receptors in reproductive aging (i.e., whether they are modulatory, inhibitory, or reciprocal) remain undetermined. It is important to understand the changing dynamics of these receptors in the aging hypothalamus, so as to uncover the potential roles that these play in endocrine function as well as endocrine aging. One study by Gundlah *et al.* (2000)

reported that administration of estrogen followed by progesterone in OVX macaque monkeys decreases ERα mRNA and protein expression in the ventromedial hypothalamus, an area associated with sexual behavior, but has minimal effects on ERβ. Age-associated decreases in ER populations in various nuclei of the hypothalamus very likely contribute to declines in sexual behavior, ovulation, and fecundity as well as observed changes in HPG hormone levels. Additionally, cognitive decline, onset of stroke, osteoporosis, and other age-related diseases may be in close correlation with such decreases. Studies to this effect have not been extensively pursued in NHPs to determine the presence or absence of these changes, but the finding of Gundlah *et al.* (2000) and those in other animal models (discussed elsewhere) suggest that this warrants further examination. Understanding the distribution and activation of estrogen receptors and their collective role in reproduction and other physiological processes will prove important in future studies of disease and reproductive aging.

NEW WORLD MONKEYS

The New World monkeys share some similarities in reproductive aging with their Old World counterparts, such as decreased follicular numbers, reduced numbers of steroid receptors, and lower levels of estrogen and progesterone with higher LH levels in anovulatory females (Tardif *et al.*, 1992). However, these animals do not undergo menstruation; rather, they have an estrous cycle (Hendrickx *et al.*, 1995). Additionally, these animals appear to have moderate levels of estrogen and progesterone in the anovulatory phase of life (see Figure 43.3), as compared to the low levels seen in Old World monkeys, and exhibit a shorter life span.

Evidence of active luteal cell masses on the ovaries of these anovulatory females has been reported, distinguishing them from their Old World counterparts (Tardif *et al.*, 1992) and suggests this as a possible source of these hormones. This difference in hormone levels probably relates to the ability of NWMs to maintain bone mass into the later stages of life, and may provide a unique mechanism for studying the role of estrogen in age-related diseases and disease resistance. Furthermore, their small size and tractability, combined with the absence of susceptibility to pathogens such as Herpes B, which are infectious to humans, make these an attractive model for biomedical studies (Abbott *et al.*, 2003).

Rodents

The rodent model is used in a majority of research laboratories due to their high availability, relatively lower cost of care, and less demanding housing needs. Additionally, though not as genetically similar as the primate model, they retain 90% homology with humans, and their shortened reproductive cycle and gestation period affords them a larger number of offspring each year. The rat and mouse models are most common to the laboratory setting, and each species offers unique benefits to research in reproductive aging.

Rats and mice undergo estrous cycles, as opposed to menstrual cycles in humans. Thus the process by which reproductive aging occurs in rodents is sometimes called estropause, and it shares some similarities, as well as some differences, with human menopause. The rodent estrous cycle is four to five days long, consisting of four phases: proestrus, estrus, diestrus I (sometimes referred to as metestrus), and diestrus II (see Figure 43.2). In rodents, estrous cyclicity can be tracked by observing daily vaginal cytology. Through this methodology, researchers have determined that rodents begin to show irregular cycles at middle age (9–12 months), as defined by prolonged cycles, most commonly with additional days of cornified vaginal cells, interspersed with the normal four- to five-day rhythm. As aging occurs, these animals transition into an acyclic, anestrus status, in which persistent estrus is observed and ovulation has ceased (Rubin, 2000). In accordance with humans, rodents begin to show reproductive decline in middle-age. Prior to the loss of regular estrous cycles, rats show increased FSH and estrogen levels accompanied by an attenuation and delay of the LH surge (Rubin, 2000), similar to humans (Wise *et al.*, 2002). As irregular cycles set in and progress to anestrus, progesterone levels decline, with estrogen levels remaining moderately elevated in rats (see Figure 43.3). This latter phenomenon is dissimilar to that in humans and mice, in which estrogen levels decline (Rubin, 2000).

Age-related changes to the pituitary have also been noted in rodents, with decreased sensitivity to GnRH stimulation, decreased GnRH receptor mRNA during the

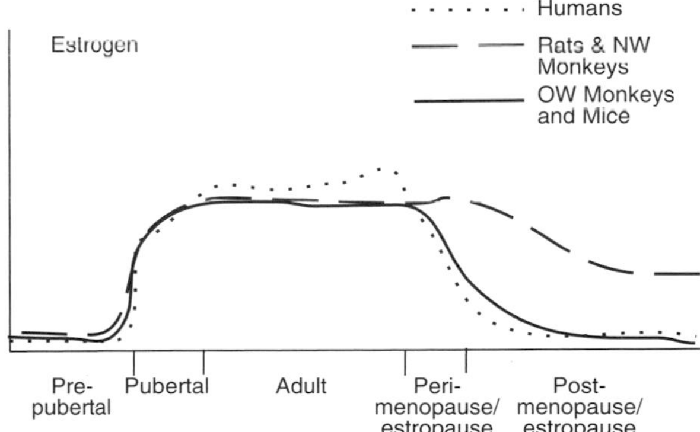

Figure 43.3 A summary of estrogen release across the life cycle in humans, nonhuman primates, rats, and mice. Please note that avians are excluded due to the variability within their group. In these species, estrogen concentrations increase during the pubertal period and are at high levels in adulthood. Declines in estrogen are precipitous in humans, monkeys, and mice, although they occur at different relative times in the life cycle. In rats, the *estropause* is characterized by continued high estrogen levels and a persistent estrus vaginal cytology until much later in life.

preovulatory surge, and decreases in LHβ subunit mRNA expression during the GnRH/LH surge and following OVX (Rubin, 2000; Wise *et al.*, 2002). However, evidence for hypothalamic involvement in rodents is by far the most compelling reason for using this model of reproductive aging. Transplantation of ovarian tissue from acyclic, aged rats into young females showed that these ovaries can support regular estrous cycling, whereas transference of young ovarian tissue into aged animals showed no resumption of cyclicity. A similar experiment confirmed this for mice as well (Rubin, 2000). Taken together, these studies provide evidence for an age-dependent change in the hypothalamic-pituitary axis that causes a disruption in the normal estrous cyclicity, and suggests that this mechanism may supersede the observed changes in ovarian morphology. Additionally, electrophysiological stimulation of the acyclic, female rat hypothalamus is able to restore function to the reproductive axis (Rubin, 2000), providing strong evidence that a neural aspect contributes to the onset of estropause. Thus, the rodent model has become an important contributor to studies of neuroendocrine influences on reproductive function.

RATS

Rats have a maximal lifespan of approximately 2.5 to 3.5 years, and they experience reproductive decline beginning at 9 to 12 months of age. Follicular degeneration is complete by two years, and the animal enters persistent diestrus. However, unlike humans, monkeys, and mice, the aged rat retains a much larger number of primary oocytes, resulting in higher estrogen levels at the onset of persistent diestrus (Holmes *et al.*, 2003b; Chakraborty and Gore, 2004). Thus, the OVX rat model is often used to mimic the natural, low estrogen levels found in humans, whereas the intact, aged model is utilized for studying natural changes to the HPG axis. In rodents, the OVX model is also used for research into the role of estrogen manipulation on reproductive aging, effects of estrogen therapy, or to study changes at the level of the hypothalamus or pituitary during the GnRH/LH surge or ovulation (achieved via controlled steroid priming). This differs from the monkey, where ovariectomy and steroid treatment are used as a cost-effective way to mimic a menopausal animal.

When using the OVX animal model, the following parameters must be taken into consideration for data interpretation: (1) Age at OVX: young animals have a more robust response to OVX than older animals. Ovarian hormones clear and gonadotropin levels increase within one week post-OVX in young rats, whereas middle-aged and aged rats take up to four weeks for total clearance of ovarian hormones and for the gonadotropin rise to occur. (2) Duration of steroid replacement: young animals need a shorter duration of estradiol replacement (approximately two days) to reach physiological estrogen levels, whereas older animals may take a minimum of four days. (3) Steroid hormone responsiveness: in younger animals, effects of steroid negative feedback onset are faster and greater than those of older animals, and positive feedback is also achieved sooner. Additionally, the GnRH/LH surge can occur earlier in the day in younger rather than in older animals, and the amplitude of the surge itself is greater (Chakraborty and Gore, 2004).

Hypothalamic changes: GnRH

To uncover the mechanisms of hypothalamic regulation of reproductive senescence, it is important to observe changes to GnRH neuronal function, as well as changes in neuronal morphology. The former can be done using a number of methods, most commonly through GnRH gene expression, protein expression, and neuropeptide release. The resultant data are controversial due to differences in methodology, hormonal treatments, and animal model (intact versus OVX and rat strain). Overall, there are data supporting age-related increases, decreases, and no change to GnRH expression. Unfortunately, due to the complexity of this field, as well as the variables just mentioned, such contradictions are common. The following will attempt to present these data from a critical viewpoint (summarized in Table 43.1).

Studies in the rat examining changes to GnRH focus on the GnRH/LH surge, since there is a known attenuation and delay of this surge in middle-aged animals in the estropause transition period (Scarbrough and Wise, 1990; Wise *et al.*, 2002). Expression of GnRH mRNA in OVX, steroid-primed as well as in intact females shows age-related differences, with young animals undergoing a decline in gene expression just prior to the GnRH/LH surge followed by an increase thereafter. By contrast, middle-aged rats fail to show any significant fluctuation (Rubin *et al.*, 1997; Gore *et al.*, 2000a). Measurements of GnRH gene expression are interpreted as an index of biosynthesis. A parallel study examining GnRH protein expression preceding and following the proestrus GnRH/LH surge in intact rats demonstrates similar results (Rubin, 2000). These findings suggest specific changes to the hypothalamus in animals transitioning to senescence, with a loss of drive on the GnRH/LH surge by middle age.

The aforementioned studies on the preovulatory GnRH/LH surge also examined overall mRNA expression in the hypothalamus of young, middle-aged, and aged rats. Gore *et al.* (2000a) found an overall increase in hypothalamic GnRH mRNA expression associated with aging in intact females, and Rubin *et al.* (1997), using the OVX, steroid-treated model, reported a decline. These differences are possibly due to the different animal models used (intact vs. OVX), or differing techniques used to quantify mRNA. The latter group used in situ hybridization, excellent for determining specific populations of gene expression, whereas the former group used RNase protection assays, useful in quantifying overall

TABLE 43.1
Representative studies and methods used to determine GnRH expression in the aging rat hypothalamus

Technique	OVX duration before steroid treatment	Steroid hormone treatment	Effect on GnRH gene or protein expression	Citation
Gene expression				
in situ hybridization	3 wks	EB 4 ug/100 g s.c.⇒ P 0.8 mg/100 g 2d later	Temporal fluctuation in GnRH mRNA during proestrus surge in Y, not MA; overall decline in GnRH mRNA in OVLT-POA of MA	Rubin *et al.*, 1997
RNase protection assay	1 or 6 mos	17β-E2 (10% capsule) for 2d or 2 wks	No significant effects of age or estrogen replacement	Gore *et al.*, 2002
RNase protection assay	Intact	None	↑ GnRH mRNA from Y to MA to A; fluctuation in GnRH during proestrus surge in Y, but not MA	Gore *et al.*, 2002
Protein levels				
IHC: GnRH	4 wks	None	Aged rats show decreases compared to Y rats in GnRH cell numbers in Septum-DBB, OVLT, POA, SON, Rch with more extreme declines in rostral regions	Funabashi *et al.*, 1995
IHC: co-expression of GnRH and c-fos	Intact	None	Decline in c-fos and c-jun co-expression with GnRH in hypothalamus of regularly cycling MA vs. Y during proestrus surge	Lloyd *et al.*, 1994
IHC: co-expression of GnRH and c-fos	3–4 wks	EB 4 ug/100 g s.c. ⇒ P 0.8 mg/100 g 2d later	Higher proportion of GnRH co-expression of c-fos in Y vs. MA	Rubin *et al.*, 1994
IHC: co-expression of GnRH and c-fos	Intact	None	Age-related, region-specific differences of co-expression during varying time intervals on proestrus	Rubin *et al.*, 1994
Peptide release				
Push-pull perfusion	3 wks	EB 4ug/100g s.c. ⇒ P 0.8mg/100g 2d later	Mean GnRH levels and pulse amplitudes are lower in MA than Y animals	Rubin *et al.*, 1989

Abbreviations: Y, young; MA, middle-aged; A, aged; d, days; DBB, diagonal band of broca: EB: estradiol benzoate; 17β-E2, 17-beta estradiol; s.c., subcutaneously; OVLT, organum vasculosum of the lamina terminalis; P, progesterone; POA, preoptic area; SCN, supraoptic nucleus; Rch, retrochiasmatic nucleus; IHC, immunohistochemistry.

hypothalamic mRNA. It is noteworthy that a study of mRNA expression in human subjects, both pre- and postmenopausal, also supported on overall increase in GnRH mRNA with age (Rance and Uswandi, 1996), in agreement with the findings of Gore *et al.* (2000a). However, it should be noted that the nuclei examined by Rubin *et al.* (1997) are thought to correspond to GnRH neurons involved in maintenance of the GnRH/LH surge (Blake and Sawyer, 1974). Thus, localized decreases may occur in these nuclei, whereas an overall increase in GnRH gene expression occurs more generally in the aging hypothalamus, suggesting a mechanism of decline specific to the GnRH/LH surge generator.

Changes to GnRH mRNA expression are often, although not always, reflected by changes to protein expression. Immunohistochemistry can be used to detect the specific protein of interest, such as GnRH, or changes in the coexpression of GnRH protein with the immediate early genes c-jun and c-fos, thought to be markers of gene activation (discussed in the next paragraph). Several studies have compared GnRH cell numbers in young, middle-aged, and/or aged animals, the majority of which report no or very slight decreases in the aged hypothalamus (reviewed in Gore, (2001)). There have, however, been reports of age-associated changes in the distribution of GnRH neurons throughout the hypothalamus. In middle-aged animals undergoing the transition to irregularity, a decline of GnRH neurons in the medial septum was seen in irregularly cycling, middle-aged, proestrus females. No differences were seen in other nuclei such as OVLT, POA, or diagonal brand of Broca (Gore, 2001). Taken together with data suggesting specific roles of different subpopulations of GnRH neurons, with more caudal regions associated with LH pulsatility and more rostral with the GnRH/LH surge (Blake and Sawyer, 1974; Soper and Weick, 1980), researchers are beginning to examine these areas for specific age-related changes. This will enhance our understanding of the age-associated neuronal changes driving alterations of pituitary and gonadal output. Localized adjustments to GnRH neuronal populations would support a mechanism by which age-related changes to gonadotropin release and maintenance of pulsatility occur, and may explain the inconsistencies seen in studies reporting changes to hypothalamic GnRH neuronal expression.

Immediate early genes are transcription factors that are commonly used to measure the activity of a particular cell. Previously, c-fos activity has been correlated with GnRH neuronal activity during the preovulatory GnRH/LH surge in young animals. Studies extending these findings to either intact, or OVX, steroid-treated middle-aged animals reported a decline in the coexpression of c-fos within GnRH neurons compared to young rats (see Table 43.1). Similar results were observed using the immediate early gene c-jun (Rubin, 2000). These findings support a decline in GnRH neuronal activity during the transition to anestrus.

In support of these observed molecular declines in GnRH activity, push-pull perfusion was used to sample the level of neuropeptide released. GnRH levels were lower in OVX, steroid-treated middle-aged versus young animal, and there was an overall decline in pulse frequency as well as amplitude (Rubin, 2000; Table 43.1). This result is in contrast to the report in the monkey showing an age-related *increase* in pulsatile GnRH release, measured by push-pull perfusion (Gore *et al.*, 2004) as well as studies in humans showing age-related *increases* in gonadotropins (Gharib *et al.*, 1990). This species difference highlights a shortcoming of the rat model, in which push-pull perfusion measurements may simply lack the sensitivity of that in monkeys. Nevertheless, taken together, these results show age-associated differences in GnRH gene expression, protein levels, activity, and release. Now we must focus on the mechanisms driving these changes.

GnRH neurons are regulated by a number of neurotransmitters, including (but not limited to) GABA, glutamate (GLU), catecholamines, and neuropeptide Y (NPY). Both protein and mRNA expression of receptors for these and other neurotransmitters have been colocalized to GnRH neurons (Smith and Jennes, 2001; Wise *et al.*, 2002). Moreover, many of the neuromodulators synapsing onto GnRH neurons are colocalized with a large population of ERs (Smith and Jennes, 2001; Chakraborty *et al.*, 2004). We propose that the modification of these inputs may be responsible for some of the age-associated differences in the HPG axis. Although there has been no indication of changes to synaptic input onto GnRH neurons in intact female aged rats, Romero *et al.* (1994) noted a decrease in the number of rough endoplasmic reticulum and Golgi apparati, suggestive of a decrease in GnRH biosynthesis. Additionally, long-term OVX (performed at 10 months of age and observed eight months following) resulted in a greater density of synaptic inputs. These data are suggestive of a role for aging, estrogen, and their possible interactions in GnRH synaptic input. These findings suggest that changes in activation of these estrogen sensitive cells may result in the observed changes to synaptic input onto GnRH neurons.

Following is a brief overview of some age-related changes in a few select neurotransmitters known to regulate GnRH neurons (GLU, GABA, catecholamines, and NPY, summarized in Table 43.2). Greater coverage of this subject can be found in (Gore, 2001; Smith and Jennes, 2001; Gore, 2002; Wise *et al.*, 2002).

1. Glutamate: The most abundant excitatory neurotransmitter in the brain and probably the best-studied neurotransmitter with respect to age-related changes in the regulation of GnRH neurons. Glutamate agonists potentiate, and antagonists attenuate, GnRH/LH release, and this is modulated by estrogen (Gore, 2001; Smith and Jennes, 2001;

TABLE 43.2
Summary of the actions of select neuromodulators on the GnRH system

	Glutamate (+)	GABA (−)	NE/E (+)	NPY (+)
Agonist action	Potentiates GnRH/LH release; enhances mRNA and protein expression.	Attenuates GnRH/LH release; may inhibit preovulatory LH surge.	Stimulates pulsatile and preovulatory GnRH/LH release.	Potentiates GnRH/LH release.
Antagonist action	Attenuates GnRH/LH release; decreases mRNA and protein expression.	Potentiates GnRH/LH release; may cause early preovulatory LH surge.	Alpha-adrenergic receptor antagonists prevent preovulatory LH surge.	Inhibition of gene expression with antisense oligonucleotides or protein with immunoneutralization inhibits the LH surge.
Input onto HPG axis	Direct synapse at GnRH cell bodies and presence of receptor on GnRH perikarya and terminals.	Direct action on GnRH neurons via synapses and presence of receptors.	Neurons project in the vicinity of GnRH neurons (indirect input). Presence of α1B- and α2A-adrenergic receptors on GnRH neurons.	Synaptic contacts with GnRH cell bodies and processes in POA and median eminence.
Estrogen regulation	Glutamate receptors and ERα and β are coexpressed in hypothalamus and POA.	GABA cells in hypothalamus are colocalized with ERα.	A2 NE neurons express ERs; all E cell types express ERs.	ERα coexpression with NPY cells in arcuate nucleus.
Age-related changes	Decline of NMDAR sensitivity and effects in the aging hypothalamus.	Declines in GABA synthesis in POA with aging.	Decreased NE turnover with aging.	Decreased NPY hypothalamic gene expression with age.

Table modified from Smith *et al.* 2001. Specific aging-related citations: Glutamate (Gore 2002); GABA (Cashion *et al.*, 2004); NE (Wise *et al.*, 1997); NPY (Wise *et al.*, 1997). Abbreviations: NE, norepinephrine; E, epinephrine; NPY, neuropeptide Y; ER, estrogen receptor; GABA, gamma-aminobutyric acid; NMDAR; N-methyl-D-aspartate receptor; POA, preoptic area

Gore, 2002). Although all classes of glutamate receptors may be involved, the NMDA receptor (NMDAR) is most strongly implicated in this role. NMDARs, made up of heteromeric subunits, undergo age-related changes in subunit expression, both on GnRH neurons as well as in the surrounding hypothalamus-POA. A possible decline in NMDAR sensitivity to GLU has been reported with aging (Gore *et al.*, 2000b). Finally, both ERα and ERβ are colocalized with NMDAR subunits (Chakraborty *et al.*, 2003b), indicating that estrogen and GLU can act upon the same target cells to exert their effects.

2. GABA: The main inhibitory neurotransmitter in the central nervous system, which interacts with GnRH neurons to suppress the preovulatory GnRH/LH surge. Like glutamate, the GABA influence on GnRH function is estrogen-sensitive and GABA receptors are colocalized with ERs in the hypothalamus (Smith and Jennes, 2001). Changes in GABA synthesis in the POA accompany changes in age and estrous cycle stage (Cashion *et al.*, 2004).
3. Catecholamines: Epinephrine and norepinephrine release strongly correlate with or are even causal to GnRH/LH pulse frequency and amplitude, and both are found in axons juxtaposed to GnRH neurons in the septum and diagonal band of Broca. Additionally, the A2 cell group of noradrenergic neurons and all cell groups of the adrenergic neurons express ERs, suggestive of direct action of estrogen on these neurons (Smith and Jennes, 2001). Wise *et al.* (1997) noted decreased norepinephrine (NE) turnover rates in middle-aged females in a number of hypothalamic nuclei. Middle-aged animals also lose diurnal rhythms of NE activity, suggesting a mechanism by which declines in NE activity are related to declines in the pulsatile regulation of GnRH release.
4. NPY: NPY gene expression and secretion are decreased in middle-aged compared to young animals, and pulsatile release of NPY is also associated with GnRH/LH release (Rubin, 2000). Again, these effects are modulated by estrogen (Smith and Jennes, 2001).

5. Together, these alterations are suggestive of changes to the pulsatile regulation of GnRH by its neurotransmitter inputs. We believe that age-related changes to these and other neuromodulatory systems are key factors contributing to the age-related dysregulation of GnRH function.

Steroid hormones

ERα: The effects of gonadal steroid hormones in the brain are mediated by the hormone receptors, which are expressed at high levels in a number of rat hypothalamic regions associated with reproduction. With regard to the two nuclear ERs, some regions express only one receptor, and others have overlapping expression. In general, these regions of overlap are most strongly implicated in the control of reproductive behavior and physiology (Chakraborty and Gore, 2004). Studies on the role of changing ovarian steroid feedback in aging rats have quantified hypothalamic ERα using a number of techniques, including estradiol binding assays, *in situ* hybridization, and protein expression by immunohistochemistry. Rubin *et al.* (1986) reported age-related, region-specific (preoptic area and medial basal hypothalamus) decreases in estradiol binding in the OVX, middle-aged rat. Wise and Parsons (1984) reported a similar finding in OVX, steroid-treated animals and Brown *et al.* (1990) extended this, finding similar results in aged animals as compared to young and middle-aged. More recent studies using *in situ* hybridization of ERα gene expression are summarized in Table 43.3, and in general, they demonstrate little to no changes in mRNA expression in the observed regions in aging rats. However, this technique does not take into account possible post-transcriptional or translational changes to ERα expression. Experiments using immunohistochemistry to examine protein expression in the hypothalamus show no age-related changes to ERα cell number in the medial preoptic nucleus (MPN) of intact (Madeira *et al.*, 2000) or OVX, steroid-treated (Chakraborty *et al.*, 2003a) females at young, middle-aged, and aged stages. Chakraborty *et al.* (2003a) also extended their studies to include the anteroventral periventricular nucleus and ventromedial nucleus, and showed an increase in ERα cell number from middle-age to aged animals in these regions. Thus, there are nuclei-specific changes in ERα expression in the aging rat hypothalamus, and uncovering the roles of these nuclei in reproductive aging will be vital to understanding the mechanism behind senescence. Effects of estrogen on expression of its ER have been studied in an age-related context. In the previous study by Chakraborty *et al.* (2003a), estrogen had little effect on overall ER expression in OVX rats of any age in the anteroventral periventricular nucleus, medial preoptic nucleus, arcuate nucleus, and ventromedial nucleus. Wise and Parsons (1984), when examining ERα nuclear DNA expression, found that estrogen treatment did have effects on ERα expression, with a two-day treatment causing decreases in OVX, middle-aged females in the preoptic area and medial basal hypothalamus. This effect was no longer apparent after four days of estrogen treatment. The techniques used in these studies differed in that the former study examined protein expression and the latter studied gene expression. This suggests a mechanism for posttranscriptional or translational changes to ERα mRNA that may compensate for the observed down-regulation of gene expression with estrogen treatment. Additionally, the ER may undergo age-related changes to protein expression, but only in very specific subpopulations. For example, a study

TABLE 43.3
Representative *in situ* hybridization studies of ERα expression in aging rat hypothalamus

Rat strain	OVX duration before steroid treatment	Steroid hormone treatment	Effect on ERα
Fischer 344	Immediate	17β-E2 (50% capsule) for 2 weeks.	⇓ ERα in POA with E2 treatment. No age effects (Y, MA, A).
Fischer 344	10 days	17β-E2 (5% capsule) for 4 days.	⇓ ERα in VMN and ARC in E2-treated Y; in POA of MA compared to Y.
Sprague-Dawley	1 week	17β-E2 capsules [180 mg/ml; 20 (Y) or 30 (MA) mm)], for 2 days.	⇑ ERα in PePOA in A compared to Y and MA rats. No differences in MPN, ARC, VMN.

Modified from Chakraborty and Gore (2004).

Abbreviations: ER: estrogen receptor; 17β-E2: 17-beta estradiol; Y: young; MA: middle-aged; A: aged; POA: preoptic area; VMN: ventromedial nucleus; ARC: arcuate nucleus; PePOA: periventricular preoptic area.

examining ERα protein coexpression with the NR1 subunit of the NMDAR showed hypothalamic changes as a result of estrogen treatment (Chakraborty *et al.*, 2003b). Since ERs are coexpressed with a number of known neuromodulators to GnRH neurons, this may be an alternate mechanism by which age-related changes of feedback occur in the hypothalamus.

ERβ: Studies examining age-related changes to ERβ are not as numerous as those on ERα, as this receptor was more recently discovered and thus has not been studied as extensively. However, it is important to note that ERβ has repeatedly been colocalized to GnRH neurons (Herbison and Pape, 2001) albeit at low levels, whereas ERα has not, suggesting a mechanism by which ERβ may directly regulate GnRH neurons. An *in situ* hybridization study in young, middle-aged, and aged OVX, steroid-treated rats showed a decline in mRNA expression in the supraoptic nucleus of the hypothalamus of middle-aged as compared to young females, with no declines in other hypothalamic nuclei observed (Wilson *et al.*, 2002; Chakraborty and Gore, 2004). A study that extended this to examine protein expression found a decrease in middle-aged and aged as compared to young OVX, estrogen-treated females in the anteroventral periventricular nucleus (Chakraborty *et al.*, 2003a), an area in which earlier studies reported increases in ERα (Chakraborty and Gore, 2004). These findings suggest a possible interplay of the two ERs, in which differential expression of these receptors in various hypothalamic nuclei at different ages could alter the outcome of estrogen activation and effect on the HPG axis. To our knowledge, no studies on effects of estrogen replacement on specific populations of ERβ within GnRH neurons or upon GnRH neuromodulators have been reported in aging animals, but this is an important area that warrants future study.

Progesterone receptor (PR): Progesterone levels fluctuate throughout the reproductive cycle, with highest levels reported during proestrus and lowest during diestrus (see Figure 43.2). Age-related changes in circulating progesterone concentrations are first observed well before the onset of irregular cyclicity, with delayed release occurring in middle-aged, regularly cycling animals when compared to young. Once the transition to irregular cycles begins, progesterone levels in rats decrease as compared to young animals. However, persistent diestrus animals show relatively high levels of progesterone, demonstrating the persistence of this hormone in aged animals (reviewed in Chakraborty and Gore, 2004).

Progesterone effects are influenced by the presence or absence of estrogen. Progesterone cannot induce a GnRH/LH surge on its own, but when administered at the proper timing following estrogen priming, the hormonal treatment will facilitate a maximal GnRH/LH surge (Attardi *et al.*, 1997). Therefore, the progesterone response is mediated by the presence of estrogen, in large part due to induction of the PR by estradiol (Chakraborty and Gore, 2004). Interestingly, middle-aged animals treated with chronic estrogen are eventually unable to generate a GnRH/LH surge. However, administration of progesterone within a certain time period will reverse these effects and generate a surge. As the transition to persistent estrus occurs, the hypothalamus is thought to lose its responsiveness to estrogen, followed by a decline in progesterone responsiveness, but these findings show a small time window in which administration of estrogen and progesterone may reinstate the preovulatory surge. Once that window has passed, without hormone treatment, sensitivity is lost and cannot be recovered (Tsai *et al.*, 2004). This suggests that a temporal change occurs within the hypothalamic axis, supporting the supposition that hormone replacement therapy, if it is to work in humans, must be given in the perimenopausal stages, as once the transition to acyclicity occurs (postmenopause), it may not be effective in treating symptomology.

Few studies have observed the effect of aging on PR expression in the hypothalamus, and those few show differing results, most probably due to different assay methodologies and animal treatments. A summary of these can be found in Table 43.4. In brief, the results range from no age-related change observed in PR mRNA in specific hypothalamic nuclei (Funabashi *et al.*, 2000) to decreases of PR gene expression localized to specific nuclei (Wise and Parsons, 1984). A study of intact females showed decreases in PR expression in specific nuclei in middle-aged (12–15 mos.) animals (Mills *et al.*, 2002), in agreement with Wise and Parsons (1984). Interestingly, the effects were seen in long-term persistent estrus (PE) females, but not in short-term PE, reinforcing the fact that the intact and gonadectomized models both contribute important information when studying age-related declines in reproductive function. It is likely that PR as well as ER expression declines with aging in the mammalian brain, yet more studies must be done to verify this. In these studies researchers must be sure to meticulously monitor and record animal reproductive status and experimental treatments, as these methodologies can play a large role in the reported outcomes of these experiments. Additionally, as is indicated for ERs, any age-associated changes in PRs are more likely to be region-specific.

Overall, the rat is an excellent model for studying neuroendocrine mechanisms of reproductive senescence, as they experience predominantly neural changes in relation to reproductive function, and are relatively inexpensive, easy to attain and care for. The literature on changes in hormone receptors that mediate feedback effects of estradiol and progesterone onto GnRH neurons is also expanding. The number of manipulations

TABLE 43.4
Effects of aging and hormone treatment on progesterone receptor (PR) expression in the hypothalamus of aging rats

Rat strain	OVX duration before steroid treatment	Steroid hormone treatment	Technique	Effect on progesterone receptor (PR)
Sprague-Dawley	7 d	17β-E2 capsule 2 d ⇒ P 0.2 mg/kg s.c. 17β-E2 4 d ⇒P 0.2 mg/kg s.c.	Nuclear exchange assay to determine DNA content of POA, MBH, and AMYG of Y and MA.	E2 (2d): ⇑ PR binding sites in POA and MBH in Y vs. MA. E2 (4d): No age-related change.
Sprague-Dawley	17 d	17β-E2, 3 d	Binding assay in POA, PVP, BNST, VMN, ARC, AMYG of Y, MA, or A.	No age-related differences in induction of PR binding by E2 in any of the observed structures.
Fischer 344	10 d	17β-E2, 4 d	*in situ* hybridization in POA and MBH of Y, MA, A.	No differences among any age groups.
Long-Evans	Intact	None	*in situ* hybridization in AVPV, POA, ARC, VMN of Y and MA (early and late PE).	POA: no age difference. VMN/ARC: PR mRNA lower in long-term PE versus early PE and young, proestrus. AVPV: lower PR mRNA in early and long-term PE compared to young.

Modified from Chakraborty and Gore 2004.

Abbreviations: P, Progesterone; POA, Preoptic area; MBH, medial basal hypothalamus; AMYG, amygdala; PVP, periventricular preoptic area; BNST, bed nucleus of the stria terminalis; ARC, arcuate nucleus; VMN, ventromedial nucleus; AVPV, anteroventral periventricular nucleus; d, days; Y, young; MA, middle-aged; A, aged; PE, persistent estrus; 17β-E2 17-beta estradiol.

and treatments that can be used with these animals warrant careful consideration when constructing a study focusing on effects of age-related changes on reproductive function.

MICE

Normal wild-type mice

Studies examining age-related changes to the mouse HPG axis have demonstrated similar findings to those of the rat, and thus only the highlights and differences will be presented in this section. The mouse lifespan is similar to that of the rat. In mice, the mean maximal life-span is 30 months, during which persistent estrus appears at approximately 12 months, followed by exhaustion of oocytes at 24 months (Finch *et al.*, 1984). Unlike rats, estrogen levels in mice transitioning from persistent estrus to anestrus are low, as is seen in humans and OWMs (Finch *et al.*, 1984). As in rats, mice show a transition from a four- to five-day cycle to longer cycles and delayed onset and attenuation of the GnRH/LH surge in later stages of life (Finch *et al.*, 1984; Nelson *et al.*, 1995).

Changes in ER expression and binding have been studied in depth in mouse models. Overall, age-related decreases in hypothalamic ER expression and receptor binding, and a decrease in the duration of binding have all been reported (Nelson *et al.*, 1995). Bergman *et al.* (1991) suggested that there is an age-associated delay in cytosolic ER replenishment in the hypothalamus, which causes the observed decrease in nuclear ER in middle-aged animals. This, accompanied by a decreased amount of time estrogen is spent bound to the receptor, possibly interferes with the positive feedback mechanism associated with ovulation, thus causing eventual delays in estrous cyclicity.

Because the mouse is more similar to humans in ovarian steroid levels and follicular function later in life, this model has been used predominantly for studies into ovarian changes. The few reports examining numbers of GnRH neurons in the hypothalamus showed little or no loss with aging (reviewed in Gore, 2001). Age-related losses in pituitary GnRH receptors were not detected in mice, but increases in GnRH and gonadotropins were, suggesting age-related changes in reproductive status may result from a mechanism independent of GnRH receptor activation (reviewed in Gore, 2001). The latter hormonal increases are similar to those in human and nonhuman primates, and suggestive of a loss of estrogen-negative feedback. Finally, attenuation of the estrogen-induced GnRH/LH surge begins to occur prior to the onset of irregular cyclicity in rodents (Nelson *et al.*, 1995).

Ovarian grafting experiments have been used to examine ovarian versus extra-ovarian influences on reproductive changes occurring in aging animals. Mice have most commonly been used for such studies. Young ovaries implanted into middle-aged animals prior to cessation of cycling extended the period of cyclicity beyond that of intact controls. This is suggestive of ovarian influences. However, this did not restore cycle frequency to the expected four-day cycle of young animals, suggestive of hypothalamic-pituitary influences. Additionally, the preovulatory estrogen and progesterone levels were restored, but the overall amplitude of these surges was not (Nelson *et al.*, 1995). Further transplantation studies showed these results to be age sensitive, as 17-month old, short-term OVX females showed a shorter period of recovered cyclicity (3 mos. of cyclicity was restored in 25% of the young controls) and 25-month-old females showed a very small recovery (30% of 17-month-old) (Felicio *et al.*, 1983). Together, these studies demonstrate the complexity of the reproductive system, as it suggests different but complementary roles of the ovary and the hypothalamus in the regulation of cycle duration and frequency.

As aging occurs, ovarian morphology changes, and the mouse model has been used to examine these changes in detail. Studies in mice have revealed that there is a similar number of oocytes in middle-aged as in aged animals, clutches of ova continue to be released, follicles do mature (albeit in lower number), and administration of hormones can stimulate normal ovulation (Finch *et al.*, 1984). Recent studies also have led to a challenge of one of the main doctrines of female reproduction. It has remained a firm belief that a female is supplied with a certain number of follicles at birth, and as this supply dwindles, the female enters perimenopause. However, Johnson *et al.* (2004) recently provided evidence for replenishment of ovarian follicles in adult female mice. This group discovered active germ cells in the ovary that seem to replenish the follicular pool. They theorize that there is a fine balance in young adults in which the number of follicles undergoing atresia is matched or surpassed by the number of germ cells undergoing meiosis and forming replacement follicles. As animals age, the number of atretic follicles increases and eventually surpasses the number being replaced, causing an overall decline in the population of ovarian follicles (Johnson *et al.*, 2004). This theory is very new but makes sense. Underlying the old doctrine, in which females were believed to be endowed with a set number of follicles for life, was the question of reproductive survival. It is a basic tenet of biology that the main purpose of all living beings is to reproduce. Hence, where the body is very efficient in most areas, the supposition of a set number of ovarian follicles seems very inefficient. These findings, though extremely recent, pose a new method for looking at follicular decline and may lead to a new arena of research into reproductive aging. Molecular examination of follicular pools may lead to new technologies by which menopause can be treated.

Transgenics

With the publication of the mouse genome, the mouse model has become first and foremost a means by which genetic manipulation can be used to study the role that each gene plays in the system as a whole. There are a number of transgenic and other mice that are used in studying the reproductive system and its component parts, and these animals can also prove useful in the study of mechanisms of reproductive senescence. This section will cover those mutations or knockouts directly affecting the HPG axis. We will not include those that target neuromodulatory systems of this axis, such as the NMDA receptor, GABA receptor, and dopamine-beta-hydoxylase (a biosynthetic enzyme important in catecholamine synthesis) knockouts, but these, too, may play an important role in examining mechanisms influencing the onset of reproductive aging.

The follitropin receptor knockout mouse (FORKO) is deficient of the FSH receptor (FSH-R). Recall that one of the main indices of the onset of menopause in women and estropause in rodents is an increase in FSH prior to the onset of irregular menstrual cycles. FSH is thought to mediate the apoptosis of follicles, but requires the proper interaction with its receptor to do so (Simoni *et al.*, 1997). Thus, it is possible that changes to the number of FSH-Rs trigger the onset of age-associated ovarian disruption. The FORKO knockout provides one model in which to study this hypothesis.

The FORKO homozygous null (−/−) mouse shows estrogen deficiency, sterility, and acyclicity. Histology of the ovary demonstrates that the follicles cannot proceed past the preantral stage and thus cannot completely mature (Danilovich *et al.*, 2004). The heterozygous null mutant shows a reduction in fertility in adulthood, but can still produce offspring. By seven to nine months, these animals no longer breed, thus demonstrating an earlier onset of senescence (see Table 43.5; Danilovich *et al.*, 2004). In aging heterozygotes (+/−) testosterone levels and gonadotropins are higher than those of the wild types. Estrogen, progesterone, and inhibin are lower. Measured ovulation rate, number of ova released, and presence of corpora lutea are all lower (with no corpora lutea by 12 months in heterozygotes). Finally, there is a greater change in binding to FSH-R in heterozygotes than wild types (Danilovich *et al.*, 2002) (for a summary, see Table 43.5). These characteristics are similar to that of aging women, and are accompanied by acyclicity, skeletal abnormalities, and obesity, all common to menopausal women (Danilovich *et al.*, 2004).

Danilovich *et al.* (2004) have used these mice to begin investigating changes to the central nervous system accompanied by reproductive senescence, as well as the use of hormone replacement therapy to treat symptoms associated with this condition. They assert that the use of a genetically altered, intact model that does not need surgical manipulation will add to the evaluation of drugs useful for treating menopausal symptoms. Thus far, they

TABLE 43.5
Follitropin receptor (FORKO) heterozygous mouse (+/−) and wild type (+/+) reproductive aging characteristics at 3, 7, and 12 months

	Age	Wild Type (+/+)	Heterozygous FORKO (+/−)
% reproductive success	3 mos.	96%	85%
	7 mos.	83%	49%
	12 mos.	73%	12%
Litter size	3 mos.	9.4 ± 1.1	6.3 ± 1.0
	7 mos.	~7.9 ± 0.8	~3.0 ± 1.0
	12 mos.	4.5 ± 2.0	0.5 ± 0.3
% regular estrous cycles	3 mos.	92%	84%
	7 mos.	78%	49%
	12 mos.	62%	0%
Oocyte numbers	3 mos.	–	–
	7 mos.	Reduced by 40%	Reduced by 75%
	12 mos.	<2%	Decreased by 67%
Atretic numbers	All age groups	NA	Show larger number than WT
Ovarian histology	3 mos.	NA	Atretic pockets at histological levels
	7 mos.	NA	Abnormal antral follicles, sparse corpora lutea
	12 mos.	NA	Advanced regression

Adapted from Danilovich *et al.* 2002.
Abbreviations: WT, wild type; mos, months; NA, not applicable.

have used these animals to examine the status of the ER signaling system and have found that the decrease in estrogen had no impact on ER gene transcription or translation, nor on functional activation of ERs in the uterus, vagina, or adipose tissue of mice (Danilovich *et al.*, 2004). Hypothalamic tissue has yet to be studied. Their initial findings suggest that treatment of these estrogen-deficient animals with estrogen is successful in producing target-specific results, supporting the use of hormone replacement therapy.

Inactivation of luteinizing hormone (LH) receptors results in a mouse that shows acyclicity (and hence infertility), smaller ovaries, and a smaller reproductive tract overall. Ovulation does not occur, and follicular maturation cannot be recovered even with estrogen/progesterone treatment. Hormonally, these animals have increased gonadotropin levels with detectable, but low levels of ovarian steroid hormones. This appears to be accompanied by decreased ERα and increased ERβ ovarian mRNA, suggestive of effects of LH on ER gene expression (Rao and Lei, 2002). Interestingly, the heterozygotes are virtually indistinguishable from their wild-type littermates, with the exception of a modest increase in FSH and decrease in estrogen levels. As in the FORKO heterozygotes, these animals appear to undergo reproductive senescence earlier than wild types, becoming obese and showing bone loss by one year (Rao and Lei, 2002). As of yet, mechanisms of aging have not been examined in detail in the female heterozygotes, but they offer an alternative model for studying the role of LH in reproduction and on the onset of reproductive aging. Additionally, changes in hypothalamic morphology would be interesting to observe in these knockouts.

The estrogen receptor knockouts (ERKOs) have played a large role in expanding our understanding of the role of estrogen in reproduction. These include the alpha-ERKO (αERKO), beta-ERKO (βERKO), and the double $\alpha\beta$ERKO. There is also an aromatase knockout (ArKO) mouse that lacks the enzyme converting testosterone to estradiol. Table 43.6 summarizes the reproductive phenotypes associated with these mutants. The ArKO is an interesting model, in that the animals have complete expression of both ERs, but are lacking aromatase activity, and thus endogenous ovarian estrogens are not synthesized. Because this has not been examined in the context of aging, it will not be discussed in detail here, but a recent study by Britt *et al.* (2005) observed uterine and ovarian weight and morphology as well as gonadotropin levels resulting from treatment of wild type and ArKO mice fed soy-free, soy, or the isoflavine genistein (a phytoestrogen) diets from two weeks prenatally to 16 weeks of age. Overall, they found estrogenic effects of

TABLE 43.6
Reproductive characteristics of the female estrogen receptor knockout alpha (αERKO), estrogen receptor knockout beta (βERKO), estrogen receptor alpha and beta double knockout (αβERKO), and aromatase knockout (ArKO) mouse

	Cyclicity	Fertility	Ovarian histology	Folliculogenesis	Gonadotropin levels	Ovarian hormones
αERKO	Acyclic	Infertile	Hemorrhagic cyst with no corpora lutea	Occurs, but fewer oocytes released	Elevated LH	Elevated estradiol
βERKO	Cycles	Decreased fertility	Small ovaries w/ few corpora lutea	Arrested	Normal	Normal
αβERKO	Acyclic	Infertile	Degenerating oocytes, loss of granulosa cells; no corpora lutea	NA	Elevated LH	Elevated estrogen
ArKO	Acyclic	Infertile	No corpora lutea	Arrested at antral stage	Elevated	Undetectable estrogen

Adapted from Hewitt *et al.* 2005 and Britt *et al.* 2005.

phytoestrogens in the ArKO mice. It would be worthwhile to extend these studies to an aging context.

The progesterone receptor knockout (PRKO) has been useful in determining progesterone's importance in the regulation of ovulation. Even with administration of superovulatory LH levels, these animals do not ovulate. Histological analysis of the follicles showed development through the luteal formation, but progesterone was needed to actually rupture the follicle. These animals also show impaired sexual behavior and gonadotropin regulation, anovulation, and uterine dysfunction (Conneely *et al.*, 2002). The development of the PRAKO and PRBKO now allows researchers to determine the function of the two PR isoforms, A and B, respectively. In PRAKO mice, there are severe abnormalities in ovarian and uterine function that lead to female infertility, whereas the PRBKO shows changes to mammary gland morphogenesis. These differential changes suggest that the two isoforms have differential activities, with studies suggesting PR-A is responsible for the progesterone-dependent responses necessary for female fertility and PR-B for generating the progesterone-induced proliferative response of the mammary gland, It has also been suggested that PR-A may be the dominant of the two isoforms, and exerts a dominant effect over PR-B (Conneely *et al.*, 2002).

To date, we are unaware of any studies characterizing aging in the aforementioned knockout models (excluding the FORKO and the LH receptor knockout mouse). Future research looking at these phenotypes in an age-related context may help to further uncover the roles of these various receptors in the aging mouse model.

Nonconditional knockouts, such as those described above, have an "incomplete" or altered genome from development, and observations generated for these animals must be considered carefully, as developmental effects may influence the interpretations generated for these animals. Conditional knockouts, when available, may be preferable to nonconditional, as the animals mature with their genome intact, and the researcher may then temporarily inactivate the gene of interest to conduct experiments, and then reactivate it when appropriate. This technology also allows selective areas to be knocked out. Currently, we do not know of any conditional knockouts for the hypothalamic or pituitary levels of the HPG axis, nor have existing lines been used for studies of reproductive aging. However, it is important to note that there are a number of lines that currently exist, which may help to uncover the roles of the neuromodulators of the HPG system, including the NPY receptor, the NMDAR, and the GABAR conditional knockouts. These have not yet been used for studies of reproductive aging, but hold potential for future examination into this system. Finally, this section did not go into detail about the transgenic strains available that *overexpress* genes. These, too, can offer valuable information as to the function of the many components feeding into the reproductive system, and eventually may prove useful in examining the mechanisms of reproductive aging.

Altered mouse strains

Although rodents are a popular animal model to use for reproductive aging, and are far less expensive than the non-human primate, it is still costly for a researcher to house these animals for the necessary one to three years in order to establish an aging colony. Additionally, mice often need to be kept in a barrier facility to maintain a pathogen-free environment, and the onset of old age also makes these animals more susceptible to age-related decline and death. An additional consideration is the strain of mouse used in these studies, as often they exhibit strain-specific traits. These strains are inbred for homozygosity, a trait useful for controlling genetic variations in animals, but also disadvantageous because of its artificiality. One way to avoid this is to use F1 crosses between inbred strains (Sprott and Ramirez, 1997).

The development of a senescence-accelerated mouse (SAM) is an alternative available for researchers interested in reproductive aging. To date, there exist 12 lines of mice, nine senescence-prone (SAMP) and three senescence-resistant (SAMR). These mice arose while inbreeding pairs of mice from the strain AKR/J (Takeda *et al.*, 1997). The SAMP animals have a lifespan of approximately 9.7 months; the SAMR have approximately 13.3 months (Takeda *et al.*, 1997). These animals have been used to examine deficits in learning and memory, joint disease, cataracts, and other age-related diseases. They show signs of osteoporosis, but to the authors' knowledge, no reproductive studies have yet been conducted. It would be interesting to extend research with these animals to the reproductive level, and with new technologies to compare their genotypes with those of wild-type AKR/J mice, to begin examination of genetic differences that might have resulted in their age-accelerated phenotype.

Birds

Until this point, we have focused on mammalian models of female reproductive senescence, but there are also a few nonmammalian models worth noting, among them, birds. Some birds, including chickens, are continuous breeders, breeding throughout the year, whereas others, such as parrots or songbirds, are opportunistic or seasonal breeders, having a distinct breeding season dictated most often by environmental conditions and other external cues. All of these animals, however, follow a similar reproductive cycle, with activation of GnRH neurons causing release of gonadotropins, followed by ovarian hormone release, resulting in ovulation. It is important to note that, in contrast to mammals, the majority of avian species have only one functional ovary and oviduct, with the right ovary regressing during embryonic development. The developing follicles are visible on the external surface of the ovary, in contrast to the mammalian ovary, in which they are hidden within connective-tissue capsules. These avian follicles show a graded size hierarchy, allowing researchers to directly determine reproductive status without having to histologically prepare the ovary, and of course, these cells are different in appearance, with a yolky membrane developing as they mature (Holmes *et al.*, 2003b).

Birds serve as an interesting model of aging, and the study of reproductive aging is slowly becoming more prevalent. Compared to mammals, birds have a much longer overall life span when body size is taken into account. The adaptation of flight causes these animals to have a much higher overall energy expenditure and an extremely fast metabolism, which is thought to keep oxidative and glycoxidative cellular damage to a minimum, causing slower cellular aging (Holmes and Ottinger, 2003a). Additionally, the avian brain has proven to be highly plastic through adulthood, including the reproductive axis (although this is best studied in males) (Holmes *et al.*, 2003b).

Overall, class *Aves* is composed of females with a slower onset of reproductive aging, with a division of this class into three general reproductive groups (see Table 43.7). Theme 1 includes most *Galliformes*, including quail, chicken, and, pheasant so on, and is composed of the rapid breeders. These show rapid declines in reproductive success and shorter life spans (6 years or under). Theme 2, consisting mostly of the *Passerine* songbirds, raptors, and parrots, show moderately slow declines in reproductive aging and moderately long life spans. The final theme, consisting mostly of seabirds, shows

TABLE 43.7
The three themes of avian reproduction

	Theme 1: Galliformes	Theme 2: Passerine songbirds, parrots, raptors	Theme 3: Sea birds
Commonly studied species	Japanese quail	Zebra finch, canary, white-crowned sparrow, budgerigar	Common Tern
Onset of reproductive decline (measured by reproductive success)	Rapid	Moderately slow: characterized by increased reproductive success followed by gradual decline	Very slow or nonexistent
Life span	Short (under 6 years)	Moderately long (on average 20–30 years, but up to 100 years)	Very long (more than 50 years); maturation delayed and clutch sizes small
Postreproductive life span	Reproductive decline begins by 2–3 years, noted by captive studies	Varies, but documented in some captive species	No captive data available and not documented in wild populations

Modified from Holmes *et al.* 2003b.

very slow to negligible reproductive aging, with very long lifespans (greater than 50 years) (Holmes *et al.*, 2003b). The information on the latter two groups has been collected predominantly in the wild, and as such, observations of reproductive success in later stages of life remain incomplete.

In bird species, declines in reproductive success are noted by decreases in egg production and clutch size, slowed or absent responses to outside cues inducing ovulation, and reduction in the viability and survival rate of the egg, as well as survival of the fledgling (Holmes *et al.*, 2003b). Often this is the only means by which reproductive declines can be measured in wild populations. Studies in wild populations are often difficult, due to a number of factors. Most wild species live 20 years or more and unless the researcher tags them early into development, the exact age of these animals is not known, making senescence studies difficult. Often there is migration in and out of colonies, identification bands may be lost, and most commonly, wild populations of animals often have skewed distributions of younger animals versus older, making longitudinal studies very challenging. Very little to date is known about these populations. The common tern, a long-lived seabird (Theme 3 in Table 43.7), appears to be the only seabird with any data available concerning reproductive status and aging.

The common tern does not seem to show age-related declines in reproductive performance except in the very oldest birds, which make up a negligible percentage of the wild population (Nisbet *et al.*, 1999). Nisbet *et al.* (1999) noted that there may be a very slight decline in reproductive performance by 12 years, but senescence is not evident until 16 years of age. Hormonal studies on these animals indicate an increase in LH levels with age, but the authors note that this might be due either to age, or to the onset of early breeding in older animals, as age and breeding schedule were found to be inversely related. These studies are often useful for environmental research concerning specific populations, but limited results can be obtained purely for the understanding of neuroendocrine correlates of reproductive aging. For this, researchers turn to the captive model.

Birds are extremely hardy animals, are not very costly, are easy to maintain, and many breed well in a laboratory setting. Birds from the order *Galliformes*, specifically the Japanese quail, are often used for captive studies on reproductive aging. Sex differences during the aging process have been reported, the most prevalent being that of the timing of the onset of reproductive senescence. Females age much faster than males, with a decline in fertility noted by 1.5 to 2 years, accompanied by irregular egg production and shorter clutch length due to decreased ovarian function and response of hypothalamus to progesterone. The females generally reach senescence by three years of age (Ottinger, 2001). Aged females show a decrease in plasma progesterone and FSH along with decreased follicular growth and decline in primary oocyte numbers. A decline in the preovulatory response has also been noted (Holmes *et al.*, 2003b).

Neural changes to the female avian hypothalamus have not been examined in many studies, but Ottinger *et al.* (2004) have reported a significant decline of GnRH-I protein in median eminence of aged laying hens. No difference in expression was observed in the preoptic area of young and aged laying hens, but the authors noted a trend toward increases in GnRH pulse amplitude recorded in hypothalamic slices *in vitro* (Ottinger *et al.*, 2004). This trend is consistent with mammalian studies discussed earlier.

The unique ability of many avians to age at a slower rate compared to mammals, as well as their unique bone structure specific for flight, make these animals an intriguing model to pursue in reproductive aging research. Osteoporosis is a prevalent concern in the aging human population, especially in women. In female birds, their bones act as a repository for the minerals and calcium important for egg production, and as they age, the skeletons become more fragile, providing an avian model for osteoporosis (Holmes and Ottinger, 2003a). The three classes of avian reproductive aging (see Table 43.7) provide a way to compare brain regions and gene expression in these regions among different avian models, which may shed light on specific anatomical and molecular changes in the brain that may delay or even hinder the onset and development of reproductive aging, and specifically, osteoporosis. Research to this point has been limited in that many of the longer lived species can be studied only in the wild, and even this provides limitations, as long-term funding and researcher consistency is difficult. However, establishment of captive populations for some of these longer lived species may prove useful in the long term for further studies into mechanisms of reproductive aging.

Conclusion

In this chapter, we have discussed several important models of female reproductive aging: the nonhuman primate (Old and New World monkeys), rodents (rat and mouse, including genetically altered mice), and birds, with a presentation of some of the strengths and weaknesses of these models for reproductive aging research. A summary of the reproductive lifespans of the mammalian species is shown in Figure 43.3. Although reproductive aging has been studied in other animals not mentioned here, these models represent the bulk of the literature available on this topic, with other studies providing anecdotal data showing similar changes in fecundity, fertility, and hormonal levels during aging.

Recent findings by the Women's Health Initiative (Anderson *et al.*, 2004) have raised concerns about the use of estrogen replacement therapy as a treatment for menopausal symptoms. Therefore, it is important now more than ever that researchers focus on the mechanisms contributing to the onset of menopause, and the accompanying symptoms that are typical to this condition. With the increase in average human lifespan, thereby ensuring that the majority of women will spend approximately half of their life in the menopausal state, the development of alternative therapies and the clarification of the use of current therapies are vital for the improvement of female quality of life. Additionally, information as to the mechanisms of reproductive aging may contribute critical information to therapy for infertile females.

Recommended Resources

WEB SITES

National Institute for Aging, www.nia.nih.gov

Provides health and research information on aging-related studies, and a great source of funding for age-related research.

The North American Menopause Society, http://www.menopause.org/

A scientific organization presenting information and current research on menopause and its management.

The Endocrine Society, www.endo-society.org

An international scientific organization, consisting of basic researchers and clinicians, that supports research in all areas of endocrinology, including menopause.

JOURNAL ARTICLES AND REVIEWS

Bellino, F.L. and Wise, P.M. (2003). Nonhuman primate models of menopause workshop. *Biol Reprod 68(1)*, 10–18.

A summary of neuroendocrine studies of reproductive aging in Old World monkeys.

Burger, H.G., Dudley, E.C., Robertson, D.M., and Dennerstein, L. (2002). Hormonal changes in the menopause transition. *Rec Prog Horm Res 57*, 257–275.

A comprehensive review of human studies encompassing hormonal changes that accompany the onset and progression of menopause.

Tsien, J.Z., Chen, F.C., Gerber, D., Tom, C., Mercer, E.H., Anderson D.J. *et al.* (1996). Subregion and cell type restricted gene knockout in mouse brain. *Cell 87(7)*, 225–238.

Provides a summary of the use of the *Cre/lox P* recombination system to produce mouse knockout animals.

Wise, P.M., Smith, M.J., Dubal, D.B., Wilson, M.E., Rau, S.W., Cashion, A.B. *et al.* (2002). Neuroendocrine modulation and repercussions of female reproductive aging. *Rec Prog Horm Res 57*, 235–256.

Reviews studies (in rats) suggesting that changes in the coordination of neuromodulators influencing the preovulatory GnRH/LH surge due to age-associated changes in estrogen concentrations contribute to the onset of reproductive senescence. Also reviews more global repercussions of age-related declines in estrogen.

BOOKS

Gore, A.C. (2002). *GnRH: The Master Molecule of Reproduction.* Norwell: Kluwer Academic Publishers.

Provides background into studies of reproductive neuroendocrinology, encompassing laboratory and applied research, focusing on the role of GnRH in reproduction. Includes coverage of the role of GnRH neurons in menopause and aging.

Dixson, A.F. (1999). *Primate Sexuality: Comparative Studies of the Prosimians, Monkeys, Apes, and Humans.* Cary: Oxford University Press.

A comprehensive work covering primate sexuality in detail. A chapter on the ovarian cycle and sexual behavior (11) is suggested for reproductive aging information.

ACKNOWLEDGMENTS

Supported by NIH AG16765 (ACG) and Glenn/AFAR (JAM).

REFERENCES

Abbott, D.H., Barnett, D.K., Colman, R.J., Yamamoto, M.E. and Schultz-Darken, N.J. (2003). Aspects of common marmoset basic biology and life history important for biomedical research. *Comp Med 53(4)*, 339–350.

Anderson, G.L., Limacher, M., Assaf, A.R., Bassford, T., Beresford, S.A., Black, H. *et al.* (2004). Effects of conjugated equine estrogen in postmenopausal women with hysterectomy: the Women's Health Initiative randomized controlled trial. *Jama 291(14)*, 1701–1712.

Attardi, B., Klatt, B., Hoffman, G.E., and Smith, M.S. (1997). Facilitation or inhibition of the estradiol-induced gonadotropin surge in the immature rat by progesterone: regulation of GnRH and LH messenger RNAs and activation of GnRH neurons. *J Neuroendocrinol 9(8)*, 589–599.

Bellino, F.L. and Wise, P.M. (2003). Nonhuman primate models of menopause workshop. *Biol Reprod 68(1)*, 10–18.

Bergman, M.D., Karelus, K., Felicio, L.S., and Nelson, J.F. (1991). Age-related alterations in estrogen receptor dynamics are independent of cycling status in middle-aged C57BL/6J mice. *J Steroid Biochem Mol Biol 38(2)*, 127–133.

Blake, C.A. and Sawyer, C.H. (1974). Effects of hypothalamic deafferentation on the pulsatile rhythm in plasma concentrations of luteinizing hormone in ovariectomized rats. *Endocrinology 94(3)*, 730–736.

Britt, K.L., Simpson, E.R., and Findlay, J.K. (2005). Effects of phytoestrogens on the ovarian and pituitary phenotypes of estrogen-deficient female aromatase knockout mice. *Menopause 12(2)*, 174–185.

Brown, T.J., MacLusky, N.J., Shanabrough, M., and Naftolin, F. (1990). Comparison of age- and sex-related changes in cell nuclear estrogen-binding capacity and progestin receptor induction in the rat brain. *Endocrinology 126(6)*, 2965–2972.

Cashion, A.B., Smith, M.J., and Wise, P.M. (2004). Glutamic acid decarboxylase 67 (GAD67) gene expression in discrete regions of the rostral preoptic area change during the oestrous cycle and with age. *J Neuroendocrinol 16(8)*, 711–716.

Chakraborty, T.R. and Gore, A.C. (2004). Aging-related changes in ovarian hormones, their receptors, and neuroendocrine function. *Exp Biol Med (Maywood) 229(10)*, 977–987.

Chakraborty, T.R., Hof, P.R., Ng, L., and Gore, A.C. (2003a). Stereologic analysis of estrogen receptor alpha (ER alpha) expression in rat hypothalamus and its regulation by aging and estrogen. *J Comp Neurol 466(3)*, 409–421.

Chakraborty, T.R., Ng, L. and Gore, A.C. (2003b). Colocalization and hormone regulation of estrogen receptor alpha and N-methyl-D-aspartate receptor in the hypothalamus of female rats. *Endocrinology 144(1)*, 299–305.

Chongthammakun, S. and Terasawa, E. (1993). Negative feedback effects of estrogen on luteinizing hormone-releasing hormone release occur in pubertal, but not prepubertal, ovariectomized female rhesus monkeys. *Endocrinology 132(2)*, 735–743.

Conneely, O.M., Mulac-Jericevic, B., DeMayo, F., Lydon, J.P., and O'Malley, B.W. (2002). Reproductive functions of progesterone receptors. *Recent Prog Horm Res 57*, 339–355.

Danilovich, N., Javeshghani, D., Xing, W., and Sairam, M.R. (2002). Endocrine alterations and signaling changes associated with declining ovarian function and advanced biological aging in follicle-stimulating hormone receptor haploinsufficient mice. *Biol Reprod 67(2)*, 370–378.

Danilovich, N., Maysinger, D., and Sairam, M.R. (2004). Perspectives on reproductive senescence and biological aging: studies in genetically altered follitropin receptor knockout [FORKO] mice. *Exp Gerontol 39(11–12)*, 1669–1678.

El Majdoubi, M., Sahu, A., and Plant, T.M. (1998). Effect of estrogen on hypothalamic transforming growth factor alpha and gonadotropin-releasing hormone gene expression in the female rhesus monkey. *Neuroendocrinology 67(4)*, 228–235.

Felicio, L.S., Nelson, J.F., Gosden, R.G., and Finch, C.E. (1983). Restoration of ovulatory cycles by young ovarian grafts in aging mice: potentiation by long-term ovariectomy decreases with age. *Proc Natl Acad Sci USA 80(19)*, 6076 6080.

Finch, C.E., Felicio, L.S., Mobbs, C.V., and Nelson, J. F. (1984). Ovarian and steroidal influences on neuroendocrine aging processes in female rodents. *Endocr Rev 5(4)*, 467–497.

Funabashi, T., Kleopoulos, S.P., Brooks, P.J., Kimura, F., Pfaff, D.W., Shinohara, K. *et al.* (2000). Changes in estrogenic regulation of estrogen receptor alpha mRNA and progesterone receptor mRNA in the female rat hypothalamus during aging: an in situ hybridization study. *Neurosci Res 38(1)*, 85–92.

Gharib, S.D., Wierman, M.E., Shupnik, M.A., and Chin, W. W. (1990). Molecular biology of the pituitary gonadotropins. *Endocr Rev 11(1)*, 177–199.

Gill, S., Sharpless, J.L., Rado, K., and Hall, J.E. (2002). Evidence that GnRH decreases with gonadal steroid feedback but increases with age in postmenopausal women. *J Clin Endocrinol Metab 87(5)*, 2290–2296.

Gore, A.C. (2001). Gonadotropin-releasing hormone neurons, NMDA receptors, and their regulation by steroid hormones across the reproductive life cycle. *Brain Res Brain Res Rev 37(1–3)*, 235–248.

Gore, A.C. (2002). *GnRH: The Master Molecule of Reproduction.* Norwell: Kluwer Academic Publishers.

Gore, A.C., Oung, T., and Woller, M.J. (2002). Age-related changes in hypothalamic gonadotropin-releasing hormone and N-methyl-D-aspartate receptor gene expression, and their regulation by oestrogen, in the female rat. *J. Neuroendocrinol 14(4)*, 300–309.

Gore, A.C., Oung, T., Yung, S., Flagg, R.A., and Woller, M.J. (2000a). Neuroendocrine mechanisms for reproductive senescence in the female rat: gonadotropin-releasing hormone neurons. *Endocrine 13(3)*, 315–323.

Gore, A.C., Windsor-Engnell, B.M., and Terasawa, E. (2004). Menopausal increases in pulsatile gonadotropin-releasing hormone release in a nonhuman primate (*Macaca mulatta*). *Endocrinology 145(10)*, 4653–4659.

Gore, A.C., Yeung, G., Morrison, J.H., and Oung, T. (2000b). Neuroendocrine aging in the female rat: the changing relationship of hypothalamic gonadotropin-releasing hormone neurons and N-methyl-D-aspartate receptors. *Endocrinology 141(12)*, 4757–4767.

Gundlah, C., Kohama, S.G., Mirkes, S.J., Garyfallou, V.T., Urbanski, H.F., and Bethea, C.L. (2000). Distribution of estrogen receptor beta (ERbeta) mRNA in hypothalamus, midbrain and temporal lobe of spayed macaque: continued expression with hormone replacement. *Brain Res Mol Brain Res 76(2)*, 191–204.

Hendrickx, A. and Dukelow, W. (1995). Reproductive Biology. In B.T. Bennet, C.R. Abee, R. Henrickson, (Eds.), *Nonhuman Primates in Biomedical Research: Biology and Management.* (pp. 147–191) San Diego: Academic Press.

Herbison, A.E. and Pape, J.R. (2001). New evidence for estrogen receptors in gonadotropin-releasing hormone neurons. *Front Neuroendocrinol 22(4)*, 292–308.

Hewitt, S.C., Harrell, J.C., and Korach, K.S. (2005). Lessons in estrogen biology from knockout and transgenic animals. *Annu Rev Physiol 67*, 285–308.

Holmes, D.J. and Ottinger, M.A. (2003a). Birds as long-lived animal models for the study of aging. *Exp Gerontol 38(11–12)*, 1365–1375.

Holmes, D.J., Thomson, S.L., Wu, J., and Ottinger, M.A. (2003b). Reproductive aging in female birds. *Exp Gerontol 38(7)*, 751–756.

Johnson, J., Canning, J., Kaneko, T., Pru, J.K., and Tilly, J. L. (2004). Germline stem cells and follicular renewal in the postnatal mammalian ovary. *Nature 428(6979)*, 145–150.

Krajewski, S.J., Abel, T.W., Voytko, M.L., and Rance, N.E. (2003). Ovarian steroids differentially modulate the gene expression of gonadotropin-releasing hormone neuronal subtypes in the ovariectomized cynomolgus monkey. *J Clin Endocrinol Metab 88(2)*, 655–662.

Madeira, M.D., Andrade, J.P., and Paula-Barbosa, M.M. (2000). Hypertrophy of the ageing rat medial preoptic nucleus. *J Neurocytol 29(3)*, 173–197.

Mills, R.H., Romeo, H.E., Lu, J.K., and Micevych, P.E. (2002). Site-specific decrease of progesterone receptor mRNA expression in the hypothalamus of middle-aged persistently estrous rats. *Brain Res 955(1–2)*, 200–206.

Nelson, J.F., Karelus, K., Bergman, M.D., and Felicio, L.S. (1995). Neuroendocrine involvement in aging: evidence from studies of reproductive aging and caloric restriction. *Neurobiol Aging 16(5)*, 837–843; discussion 855–856.

Nisbet, I.C., Finch, C.E., Thompson, N., Russek-Cohen, E., Proudman, J.A., and Ottinger, M.A. (1999). Endocrine patterns during aging in the common tern (*Sterna hirundo*). *Gen Comp Endocrinol 114(2)*, 279–286.

Ottinger, M.A. (2001). Quail and other short-lived birds. *Exp Gerontol 36(4–6)*, 859–868.

Ottinger, M.A., Abdelnabi, M., Li, Q., Chen, K., Thompson, N., Harada, N. *et al.* (2004). The Japanese quail: a model for studying reproductive aging of hypothalamic systems. *Exp Gerontol 39(11–12)*, 1679–1693.

Rance, N.E. and Uswandi, S.V. (1996). Gonadotropin-releasing hormone gene expression is increased in the medial basal hypothalamus of postmenopausal women. *J Clin Endocrinol Metab 81(10)*, 3540–3546.

Rao, C.V. and Lei, Z.M. (2002). Consequences of targeted inactivation of LH receptors. *Mol Cell Endocrinol 187(1–2)*, 57–67.

Romero, M.T., Silverman, A.J., Wise, P.M., and Witkin, J.W. (1994). Ultrastructural changes in gonadotropin-releasing hormone neurons as a function of age and ovariectomy in rats. *Neuroscience 58(1)*, 217–225.

Rubin, B.S. (2000). Hypothalamic alterations and reproductive aging in female rats: evidence of altered luteinizing hormone-releasing hormone neuronal function. *Biol Reprod 63(4)*, 968–976.

Rubin, B.S., Fox, T.O., and Bridges, R.S. (1986). Estrogen binding in nuclear and cytosolic extracts from brain and pituitary of middle-aged female rats. *Brain Res 383(1–2)*, 60–67.

Rubin, B.S., Lee, C.E., Ohtomo, M., and King, J.C. (1997). Luteinizing hormone-releasing hormone gene expression differs in young and middle-aged females on the day of a steroid-induced LH surge. *Brain Res 770(1–2)*, 267–276.

Scarbrough, K. and Wise, P.M. (1990). Age-related changes in pulsatile luteinizing hormone release precede the transition to estrous acyclicity and depend upon estrous cycle history. *Endocrinology 126(2)*, 884–890.

Simoni, M., Gromoll, J., and Nieschlag, E. (1997). The follicle-stimulating hormone receptor: biochemistry, molecular biology, physiology, and pathophysiology. *Endocr Rev 18(6)*, 739–773.

Smith, M.J. and Jennes, L. (2001). Neural signals that regulate GnRH neurones directly during the oestrous cycle. *Reproduction 122(1)*, 1–10.

Soper, B.D. and Weick, R.F. (1980). Hypothalamic and extra-hypothalamic mediation of pulsatile discharges of luteinizing hormone in the ovariectomized rat. *Endocrinology 106(1)*, 348–355.

Soules, M.R., Sherman, S., Parrott, E., Rebar, R., Santoro, N., Utian, W. *et al.* (2001). Executive summary: Stages of Reproductive Aging Workshop (STRAW). *Climacteric 4(4)*, 267–272.

Sprott, R.L. and Ramirez, I. (1997). Current inbred and hybrid rat and mouse models for gereontological research. *Ilar J 38(3)*, 104–109.

Takeda, T., Higuchi, K., and Hosokawa, M. (1997). Senescence-accelerated Mouse (SAM): With special reference to development and pathological phenotypes. *Ilar J 38(3)*, 109–118.

Tardif, S.D. and Ziegler, T.E. (1992). Features of female reproductive senescence in tamarins (*Saguinus spp.*), a New World primate. *J Reprod Fertil 94(2)*, 411–421.

Terasawa, E. (1998). Cellular mechanism of pulsatile LHRH release. *Gen Comp Endocrinol 112(3)*, 283–295.

Tsai, H.W., LaPolt, P.S., Olcott, A.P., and Lu, J.K. (2004). Temporal changes occur in the neuroendocrine control of gonadotropin secretion in aging female rats: role of progesterone. *Biol Reprod 71(3)*, 845–852.

Wilson, M.E., Rosewell, K.L., Kashon, M.L., Shughrue, P.J., Merchenthaler, I., and Wise, P.M. (2002). Age differentially influences estrogen receptor-alpha (ERalpha) and estrogen receptor-beta (ERbeta) gene expression in specific regions of the rat brain. *Mech Ageing Dev 123(6)*, 593–601.

Wise, P.M., Kashon, M.L., Krajnak, K.M., Rosewell, K.L., Cai, A., Scarbrough, K. *et al.* (1997). Aging of the female reproductive system: a window into brain aging. *Recent Prog Horm Res 52*, 279–303; discussion 303–305.

Wise, P.M. and Parsons, B. (1984). Nuclear estradiol and cytosol progestin receptor concentrations in the brain and the pituitary gland and sexual behavior in ovariectomized estradiol-treated middle-aged rats. *Endocrinology 115(2)*, 810–816.

Wise, P.M., Smith, M.J., Dubal, D.B., Wilson, M.E., Krajnak, K.M., and Rosewell, K.L. (1999). Neuroendocrine influences and repercussions of the menopause. *Endocr Rev 20(3)*, 243–248.

Wise, P.M., Smith, M.J., Dubal, D.B., Wilson, M.E., Rau, S. W., Cashion, A.B. *et al.* (2002). Neuroendocrine modulation and repercussions of female reproductive aging. *Recent Prog Horm Res 57*, 235–256.

Woller, M.J., Everson-Binotto, G., Nichols, E., Acheson, A., Keen, K.L., Bowers, C.Y. *et al.* (2002). Aging-related changes in release of growth hormone and luteinizing hormone in female rhesus monkeys. *J Clin Endocrinol Metab 87(11)*, 5160–5167.

World Health Organization (1996). Research on the menopause in the 1990s. Report of a WHO scientific group. World Health Organization Technical Report Series 866. Geneva, Switzerland, World Health Organization: 1–107.

Zapantis, G. and Santoro, N. (2003). The menopausal transition: characteristics and management. *Best Pract Res Clin Endocrinol Metab 17(1)*, 33–52.

44

Model of Chaperones in Aging

J. Krøll and J.O. Nehlin

The molecular chaperones or heat shock proteins (Hsp) are constitutive and stress-induced proteins participating in "housekeeping" functions such as proofreading and folding of other polymers (proteins, RNA, DNA), preventing the aggregation of polymers, disgregation of misfolded molecules, facilitation of the transport of polymers across biological membranes, and participation in the degradation of ubiquitinated molecules. The decrease in the constitutive expression and inductivity of the chaperones with age—possibly caused by progressive silencing of the chaperone genes—probably contributes decisively to the phenotype of aging, as illustrated also from the progeric syndromes caused by mutational defects of the RecQ protein/DNA chaperones. Conversely, high levels of chaperone expression is a common denominator in conditions or procedures leading to an increase in cellular and species longevity as well as in the process of cellular immortalization, the inherent immortality of the embryonic stem cells, and the inhibition of cellular apoptosis.

The inherent immortality of the embryonic stem cells implies that replicative senescence as possibly the aging of species are epigenetic phenomena. The involvement of RNA chaperones in the process of cellular immortalization and mutational DNA chaperones in the progeric syndromes suggests that RNA/DNA-chaperones are of major importance for the definition of cellular and species longevity. Accordingly, evidence has been presented to suggest that the evolution of longevity depends on alterations in the expression of relatively few regulatory genes. Possibly the molecular chaperones are evolution facilitators, contributing to the definition of the life span of differentiated cells as well as the longevity of species.

Introduction

The term *replicative senescence* describes the observation that normal eukaryotic cells cultured *in vitro* can attain a maximal number of population doublings proportional to the life span of the species and inversely proportional to the age of the individual (Handbook chapter 4). Cells can transgress this *Hayflick limit* to immortalization by viral transformation, for example, by transfection with the SV40 T protein. Analysis of the T protein showed that the immortalizing effect specifically could be ascribed to the C-terminal ATPase module. Hypothetically it was suggested that this ATPase module somehow could replace—or by transactivation of the ATP-synthase gene—compensate for a functional defect of the beta-subunit of the mitochondrial F1-ATPase: the master of ATPases serving the reverse function of producing ATP, the universal currency of free energy (Krøll, 1994). Support for this suggestion was gained from observations of exposure of the catalytic beta-subunit of the ATP synthase on the surface of different tumor cell lines, indicating an overexpression of this ATPase module in some immortalized cell lines (Krøll, 1996).

The ATPase module is an important subunit also in other essential cellular machines such as the membrane pumps and the heat shock proteins/molecular chaperones. That the SV40 T-protein was recognized as a molecular chaperone gave rise to the suggestion that this property might contribute to the general increased *in vitro* life span and occasional immortalization observed in cells transfected with the SV40 T-protein. This suggestion gained support from the observation that a similar increase in cellular life span *in vitro* could be obtained by transfection with other chaperones or by heat shock or hormetic procedures raising the cellular level of expression of the heat shock proteins. The probable importance of the molecular chaperones for the process of cellular immortalization also appears from the observation that an increase in the level of expression of molecular chaperones is a common feature of the various procedures used to attain immortalization of primary cells *in vitro*, as well as from the frequent hyper-expression of various chaperones in immortal cancer cell lines, as in the inherently immortal primary cell lines from catfish (Krøll, 2002). The recognition that the SV40 T-protein as the human homologue p68 are DEAD box RNA-chaperones and the Werner Protein WRN probably is a RecQ DNA-chaperone places some emphasis on the importance of the RNA/DNA-chaperones in the definition of cellular longevity (Krøll, 2004). Accordingly evidence has been presented to suggest that the evolution of longevity depends on alterations in the expression of relatively few regulatory genes (Krøll, 2005). This chapter presents evidence on the probable importance of the molecular chaperones as antagonists of the aging process and for the evolution of cellular and species longevity.

Functions and Classes of the Molecular Chaperones

HOUSEKEEPING FUNCTIONS

The molecular chaperones are a highly conserved class of proteins expressed constitutively or synthesized in response to stressful physiological conditions such as heat shock (cf. the term Heat Shock Proteins, or Hsp). The chaperones are essential for viability even under normal temperatures by assisting in housekeeping functions such as proofreading and correct folding of other proteins, RNA and DNA, preventing the aggregation of polymers and disgregation of misfolded molecules, facilitation of the transport of polymers across biological membranes, and participation in the degradation of ubiquitinated molecules.

PROTEIN CHAPERONES

During evolution, the number, size, and complexity of chaperones increase from the small Hsp/crystallins, prefoldins, and chaperonins forming the minimal protein-folding system of the hyperthermophilic archaea (Laksanalamai *et al.*, 2004) to the families of larger chaperones Hsp40/DnaJ, Hsp60, Hsp70, Hsp90, and Hsp110 cooperating in the complex chaperone machines of the eucarya (Young *et al.*, 2004).

RNA/DNA CHAPERONES

The DEAD box proteins (e.g., the viral SV40 T-protein and the mammalian homolog p68) are RNA chaperones, as probably the RecQ proteins are DNA chaperones (Krøll, 2004). Hsp90 is unique among the protein chaperones due to its unconventional highly conserved Bergerat ATP-binding fold shared by the DNA gyrases and DNA-mismatch-repair enzymes. Probably the Hsp90 machinery includes DNA in its chaperoning activity; possibly serving as a chaperone for the reverse transcription of telomeric DNA, in analogy to its requirement for the hepatitis B virus reverse transcriptase function (Hu *et al.*, 2004).

CHAPERONES OF THE CELLULAR COMPARTMENTS

Molecular chaperones have been described across tissues and subcellular compartments (see Table 44.1 and Figure 44.1).

Cytoplasmic chaperones

The HSP70 and HSP90 families are found mainly in the cytoplasmic compartment. Hsp90 and Hsp70 refold proteins in an ATP-dependent way, where Hsp90 is dedicated to specific substrates and Hsp70 refolds more general substrates (Young *et al.*, 2004).

The super-family of mammalian small heat shock or stress proteins (sHsp) in humans consists of the known members HSP27, αB-crystallin, αA-crystallin, Hsp20, HspB2, HspB3, and cvHsp. sHsp's have the ability to form supra-molecular structures, either homo-oligomeric or hetero-oligomeric complexes, ranging in molecular weight from 50 to 1000 kDa depending on the degree of stress. The basic structural units of sHsp complexes are dimers that are formed by interaction of segments of the α-crystallin domain. The sHsp's can bind and prevent aggregation of denatured proteins, but usually they cannot refold them. They may help target their substrate for proteolysis, or they may store it for subsequent refolding by the Hsp70 chaperone system (Laksanalamai *et al.*, 2004).

Whereas unfolded cytoplasmic proteins evoke the heat shock response, other cellular organelles also can evoke appropriate protective mechanisms.

Chaperones of the endoplasmic reticulum

During protein synthesis, nascent proteins are processed within the endoplasmic reticulum (ER), where a subset of chaperones and folding enzymes form multiprotein complexes. The lectins calnexin and calreticulin and the oxidoreductase Erp57 are involved in ER-quality control, which prevents aggregation and export along the secretory pathway of misfolded and incompletely assembled proteins. Appropriate folding of polypeptides requires chaperone proteins such as Bip/Grp78 and calreticulin. Overexpression of proteins or abnormally folded nascent proteins can lead to protein accumulation and aggregation in cells, causing ER stress, which in severe cases could trigger cell death. A cellular protective mechanism known as the unfolded protein response (UPR) evolved to induce the expression of various genes including molecular chaperones and to activate ER-associated protein degradation (ERAD). The ER-chaperones relay a signal that temporarily induces a general slow-down in cellular division to prioritize the expression of proteins required for the appropriate synthesis of the nascent protein. Cells with high secretory capacity such as the ones found in endocrine glands or immunoglobulin-producing cells often require high ER-chaperone usage. The 47-kDa heat shock protein 47 (HSP47) is an ER-resident, collagen-specific molecular chaperone that has been shown to play a major role during the processing and/or secretion of procollagen in, for example, fibroblasts (Miyaishi *et al.*, 1995; Castro-Fernandez *et al.*, 2005).

Mitochondrial chaperones

Mitochondria contain several members of the major chaperone families that have important functions in maintaining this organelle's function. Changes in the energy status of the cells require adaptations in the protein import machinery such as the induction of cytosolic molecular chaperones that transport precursors to the matrix, the up-regulation of outer membrane import receptors, and the increase in matrix chaperonins (e.g., Hsp60) that facilitate the import and proper folding of the protein for subsequent compartmentation in

TABLE 44.1
Classes of molecular chaperones

Chaperone	Function and subcellular localization
αA-crystallin	Small hsp—Stabilization against aggregation during heat shock. Localization: Post-Golgi membranes
αB-crystallin	Small hsp—Stabilization against aggregation during heat shock. Localization: Post-Golgi membranes
BBS6/MKKS	McKusick-Kaufman syndrome—Homology to chaperonin
Calnexin	Interacts and assists with the folding of new proteins that carry monoglucosylated N-linked glycans; retains incompletely folded proteins in the ER. Localization: ER membrane
Calreticulin/Grp95	Folding of glycosylated proteins in the ER in coperation with glucosyltransferase; similar to calnexin. Localization: ER lumen
Clusterin/XIP8/apo-J	ERP29 endoplasmic reticulum protein 29. Localization: ER
Erdj4/MDG1	DnaJ family member. Localization: ER
GRP78 (BIP)	Ca2+-binding—Hsp70 family member. Localization: ER
Grp94/gp96	Hsp90 ER luminal homolog—Possible role in the antigen presentation pathway. Localization: ER
GRP170	Localization: ER
Hsp20/25/27 HspB2, HSPB3, cvHsp	Small hsp's—Stabilization against aggregation during heat shock. Localization: Multiple
Hsp40/Erdj1-5/DnaJ	Stimulates BIP ATPase activity; binds nascent polypetides. Localization: ER
Bind unfolded proteins, interact with matching hsp70's	
Hdj1: human dnaJ homologue abundant in neurons	
Hsp47	Processing and secretion of collagen. Localization: ER
Hsp56/FKBP59	FK506 binding protein 59 induced by cardiotrophin; cardiac hypertrophy. Localization: ER
Hsp60/Hsp10	Folding of imported proteins (known as chaperonins in bacteria). Localization: Mitochondria
Hsp70 family	ATP-dependent stabilization of hydrophobic regions in extended polypeptide segments; role in the ubiquitin-proteasome system; binding of nascent polypetides; maintains translocation-competent ER and mitochondrial precursor proteins in the cytosol Hsp72: stress inducible, Hsc73, binds to nascent chains, constitutive Mortalins mot-1, mot-2/mthsp70/GRP75

(Continued)

TABLE 44.1
Continued

Chaperone	Function and subcellular localization
Hsp90	Mitochondrial Hsp70 (hsc70) alias Survivin—Conformational maturation of steroid hormone receptors and signalling kinases. Localization: Cytoplasm/Nucleus
Hsp100	ATP-dependent disaggregation and unfolding for degradation. Localization: Cytoplasm
Hsp104	
Hsp105α	Suppresses formation of aggregates; found in nuclear inclusions formed by androgen receptor. Localization: Cytoplasm/nucleus
Peptidyl-prolyl	Cyclophilins (A,B) and FK506-binding proteins. Localization: ER Isomerases (PPIases)
Pre-senilins	Localization: ER
Protein disulphide	Protein processing Isomerase A3-PDI/CaBP1. Localization: ER
Thiol-disulphide	Protein processing Oxidoreductases. Localization: ER
PDI, Erp72, Erp57, p5	
SDF2-L1	
TCP-1	t-complex-polypeptide-1. Localization: Cytoplasm
UDP-glucosyltransferase (UDP-GT)	
DEAD box proteins	RNA-Chaperones. Localization: Nucleom
RecQ proteins	DNA-Chaperones. Localization: Nucleom

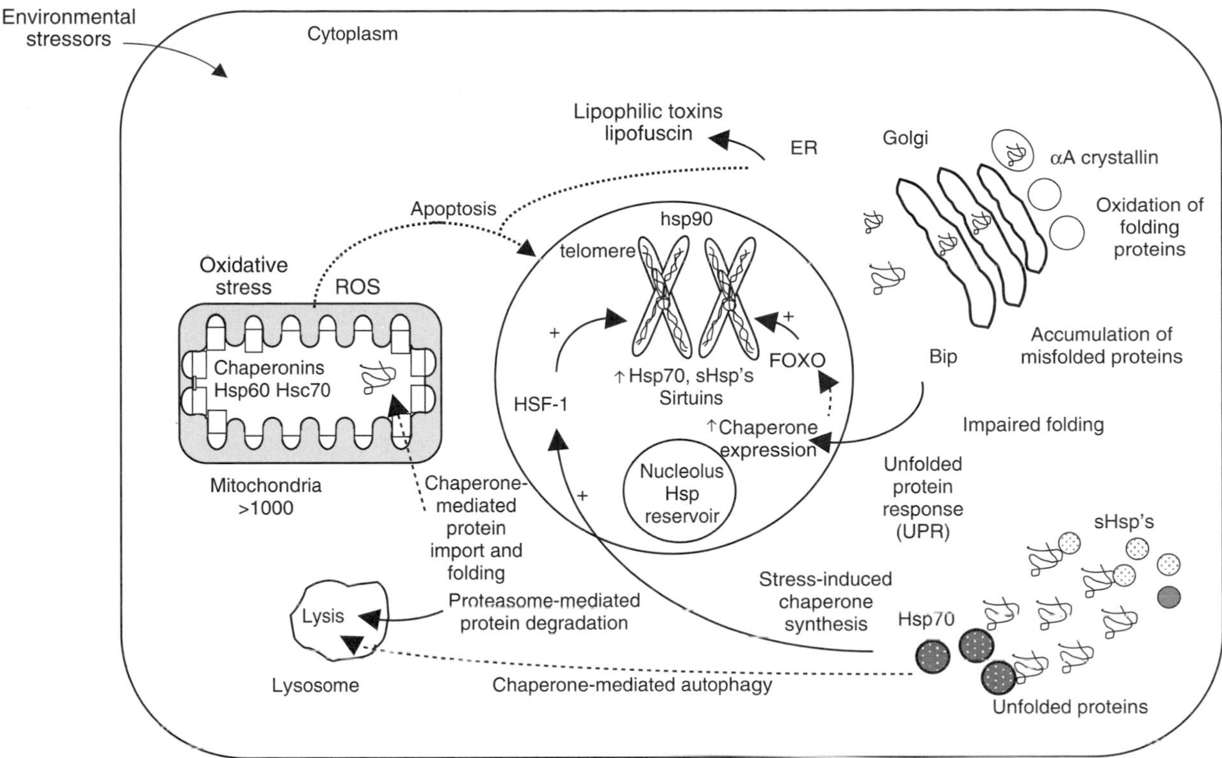

Figure 44.1 Roles of subcellular chaperones during aging. Various environmental stressors lead to protein damage and misfolded proteins that bind to chaperones within the various cellular compartments. Irreversibly damaged proteins are targeted for degradation. If degradation is impaired and if there is an increase in protein damage, the chaperone systems might be overwhelmed, compromising the cell's ability to function properly. Also, chaperones might be damaged, leading to their removal and subsequent up-regulation. These events might trigger the senescent phenotype, and consequently, gradual tissue dysfunction.

the matrix or inner membrane. The physiological importance of these changes is an increased capacity for import into the organelle at any given precursor concentration. Defects in the protein import machinery components have been associated with mitochondrial disorders (Hood and Joseph, 2004) During synthesis of ATP in mitochondria, reactive oxygen species (ROS) are generated that are detrimental to mitochondrial and cellular function that with time contributes to the aging process. Chaperone species within the mitochondria could slow down the damage caused by ROS and participate in mitochondrial protein biogenesis (Voos and Röttgers, 2002).

Lysosomal chaperones

Physiological stresses such as prolonged starvation lead to chaperone-mediated autophagy (CMA) whereby a lysosomal pathway of proteolysis is activated (Majeski and Dice, 2004).

Chaperones Aging and Longevity

The decrease in the constitutive expression and inductivity of the chaperones with age probably contributes to the phenotype of aging, as an involvement in the definition of longevity can be assumed from high levels of chaperone expression as a common denominator in conditions or procedures leading to an increase in cellular and species longevity as well as in the process of cellular immortalization. The inherent immortality of the embryonic stem cells implies that replicative senescence as possibly aging are epigenetic phenomena, possibly influenced by the progressive age-related epigenetic changes in promoter methylation that have the potential to permanently silence gene expression (Krøll, 2005).

AGING AND LONGEVITY OF CELLS

Aging and longevity of differentiated cells in vitro

That replicative senescence—the model of aging *in vitro*—probably is related to a chaperone deficit can be assumed from the increase in life span obtained by transfection with protein-chaperones, as well as from the attainment of cellular immortalization by heat shock procedures or transfection with RNA-chaperones (Krøll, 2004).

Aging and longevity of differentiated cells in vivo

The great variability in the life span of differentiated cells in the organism shows a direct correlation to the constitutive expression of the molecular chaperones. Thus, compared with the short-lived epithelial cells, the basal expression of chaperones is relatively high in the long-lived post-mitotic cells as, for example, the neurons of the brain and the stromal cells of the eye lens. Thus, in the brain, the constitutive unstressed level of expression of Hsp70, Hsp90, and Hsp100 resembles that of heat-stressed somatic cells. In the stromal cells of the eye lens, the dominant chaperone is alpha-crystallin, which constitutes 40% of total cellular protein and assures the preservation of lifelong transparency of the lens in the absence of structural protein turnover. Chaperone dysfunction leads to protein aggregation, lens opacity and cataracts (Krøll, 2005).

The inducibility of Hsp70 by heat shock is reduced to approximately 50% in old rat hepatocytes, suggesting that a reduced ability to express hsp70 in response to stress may be a common phenomenon underlying the aging process. This age-related decline in the Hsp70 stress response was reversed by caloric restriction (Heydari *et al.*, 1996). There is a functional link between age-related decrements in Hsp70 expression and pathophysiological responses to heat stress leading to tissue injury and dysfunction (Kregel, 2002). Efficient removal of oxidized proteins depends on chaperone-mediated autophagy (see the section on lysosomal chaperones). This mechanism is severely impaired during aging demonstrated by the accumulation of oxidized proteins in old age (Kiffin *et al.*, 2004).

Cells derived from older people show a very low heat response in terms of Hsp47 expression, and there is a gradual down-regulation of Hsp47 expression with age, regulated by transcriptional mechanisms. Hsp47 induction is markedly attenuated in high PDL cells, showing an age-related decrease in response to pro-collagen retention in the ER (Miyaishi *et al.*, 1995). Polyphenol-rich Salix alba extracts can obviate this decrease in HSP47 expression (Nizard *et al.*, 2004).

Damage to the ER organelle and its subsequent impaired functionality may be involved in the process of aging, judging by increased ER-chaperone expression, preferential oxidation of ER-resident proteins, and altered calcium homeostasis (van der Vlies *et al.*, 2003).

Old cells show a greater sensitivity to ER stress than young cells, suggesting a link between stress resistance and longevity (Li and Holbrook, 2004).

Experimental procedures increasing the life span of differentiated cells

Experimental procedures increasing the level of expression of various chaperones have been shown to increase cellular life span and resistance against apoptosis. Thus, intermittent mild heat stress (hormesis) increases the level of various chaperones and improves cellular resistance against noxious agents. Further, an *in vitro* model of caloric restriction (CR) demonstrates an increase in Hsp70 expression and cellular resistance obtained by cell culture in CR-sera, possibly contributing to the effect of CR on cellular longevity. Also, the anti-apoptotic effect of nitric oxide is associated with an increase in the expression of Hsp70 as well as of the RNA-chaperone p68. The anti-apoptotic effect of nicotine could possibly relate to activation of the heat shock factor (Krøll, 2005).

AGING AND LONGEVITY OF SPECIES

Reference conditions

An involvement of the molecular chaperones in the definition of species longevity can be assumed from the observed influences of genotypes, levels of Hsp expression, and mutational defects. Thus, a modifier of life span linked to chromosome 4 has been identified as a haplotype marker within the microsomal transfer protein complex comprising the chaperone protein disulfide isomerase (PDI). An influence of genotype can be supposed also from the observation that for Hsp70 the TT polymorphic variant was observed to be significantly increased within a healthy aged Irish population, while conversely the TC genotype was significantly decreased. Also correlations have been observed between a polymorphism in the Hsp70-A1 gene promoter and low self-rated health in aged Danish twins (Singh *et al.*, 2004) as well as impaired longevity in women (Altomare *et al.*, 2003).

A relationship between the level of chaperone expression and the longevity of species can be assumed from the observation that the constitutional expression of Hsp70 in human pancreatic islets is about five times higher than in the islets of mice or rats. Also, the basal level of expression of Hsp70 in the human brain has been observed to be about 50 fold higher than in rat brain. Modifications of chaperone expression caused by hormonal factors may also influence life span. Thus, in humans, the estrogen-induced higher levels of expression of Hsp72 and Hsp90 alpha might contribute to the difference in longevity between genders. Concerning the circulating levels of chaperones, regression analysis has revealed a progressive decline with age in the serum levels of Hsp60 and Hsp70, probably a consequence of the age-related reduced ability to respond to stress (Krøll, 2005).

Possibly, the level of expression or the stress response of selected chaperones could be used for the estimation of a biological age index (Krøll and Saxtrup, 2000).

That not only the protein chaperones but also the DNA chaperones are probably important modifiers of longevity can be assumed from the consequences of inborn errors of the RecQ protein/DNA-chaperones. Thus, various mutations in these proteins shorten life span as observed in the mosaic progeric syndromes of Werner, Blooms, and Rothmund-Thomson (Krøll, 2004).

The increasing awareness of the possible significance of the functional decline of the molecular chaperones for age-related disorders has initiated the development of a mathematical model to explore the chaperone system and its possible implications in aging (Proctor *et al.*, 2005).

Experimental procedures influencing the life span of species

An increase in the level of expression of the molecular chaperones is a common denominator for the experimental procedures so far known to cause an increase of life span in species.

Transgenic modulation of chaperone expression. Transgenic overexpression of chaperones has been shown to extend the life span of a number of experimental organisms as e.g., for Hsp104 in yeast (Shama *et al.*, 1998), Hsp16 in *C. elegans*, Hsp70 in *Drosophila* (Tatar *et al.*, 1997), hsp26 and hsp27 in *Drosophila* (Krøll, 2005). Heat shock proteins normally decrease in expression as a function of age, as judged from individual cases to whole-genome transcriptional profiles in *C. elegans* (Lund *et al.*, 2002).

Overexpression of the transcription factor HSF-1 that controls stress-inducible gene expression and protein folding homeostasis, extends life span in *C. elegans* daf-2-insulin/IGF-1 receptor mutants (Hsu *et al.*, 2003), as down-regulation of HSF-1 shortens life span of the mutants. Down-regulation of the individual molecular chaperones decreased longevity of the mutants to a lesser extent and did not affect life span in wild-type animals, probably due to the redundancy of chaperone function (Morley and Marimoto, 2004).

The Ames mouse model of longevity also showed an up-regulation of a heat shock protein, suggesting a contribution of a chaperone to extended life in a hormone model (low levels of human growth hormone releasing hormone) (Dozmorov *et al.*, 2001).

Hormesis. Intermittent mild heat stress (hormesis) increases the level of expression of the molecular chaperones and has been observed to give rise to life span extension in *Drosophila* (Hercus, 2003) and in yeast (Shama *et al.*, 1998). For the possible benefits of exposure to stress in humans, we need to consider that chaperone expression and function might not be the same in all individuals. This reflects the levels of genetic variation in the human population that are expressed as heritable phenotypic variation during periods of environmental change. This phenotypic variation results in differential modulation of chaperone and target function in response to stress. The availability of free chaperones correlated with the type and degree of stress confers the organism a level of protection that ultimately regulates survival fitness (Rutherford, 2003). Thus, exposure to stress in itself might not be beneficial if the response of the organism towards stress is deficient or inappropriate. A competitive edge might be found in organisms whereby stress can induce a good protective response of properly working molecular chaperones that can help achieve improved life conditions at an advanced age without risk for chaperone overload (Söti *et al.*, 2005).

The extraordinary capacity of centenarians to achieve exceptional old age is due to some extent to their ability to counter the increased cellular stress normally associated with aging. Hsp70 protein induction by heat is reduced in the cells of most aged humans but not in centenarians. This effect is likely due to potent HSF-1 activity. As a matter of fact, HSF-1 has auxiliary factors that contribute to its activation, and could be involved in the age-associated attenuation in the response to stress (Shamovsky and Gershon, 2004). Another study reported that low circulating serum levels of Hsp70 in centenarians could well correlate with the absence of a disease state, since damage to tissues or organs as observed in cardiovascular disease or autoimmune diseases would result in high serum levels of Hsp70 (Krøll, 2005).

Caloric restriction. The best experimental intervention so far, which can extend life span in rodents and in multiple invertebrate species and reliably retard aging and age-related degenerative diseases, is dietary caloric restriction (CR). Gene and protein expression profiles are profoundly altered as a consequence of dietary CR. In particular, several molecular chaperones are induced to protect cells from stress, by preserving not only protein structures but also general cellular structure, increasing the levels of GSH, inhibiting apoptotic death, and maintaining a pool of vital proteins (Li *et al.*, 2004). Life-span studies due to CR in nonhuman primates have not yet been completed, but recent data indicate the beneficial effects of CR on a number of physiological markers. The effects of CR on human metabolism are various, but the specific mechanism(s) that lead to its positive effect on life span are not completely understood, but they might coincide with other well-described mechanisms known to regulate life span. Possibly the observed increase in the expression of Hsp70 caused by CR contributes to the positive effect on life span (Ingram *et al.*, 2004).

Interference with histone acetylation. The recently discovered histone deacetylase (HDAC) inhibitors (i.e., tricostatin A and phenylbutyrate) can induce the expression of heat shock proteins hsp22 and hsp70, resulting in extended life span in *Drosophila*. In particular, hsp22, a mitochondrial chaperone, has been linked to decreased survival when absent. Life extension has also been shown in cells exposed to polyphenolic compounds capable of activating the sirtuins (family of NAD+ dependent deacetylases) in a manner comparable to CR (Lamming *et al.*, 2004). Evidence that sirtuin activators might slow down aging by inducing chaperone function has not yet been presented. However, it is likely that organisms in nature responding to signals such as the ones elicited by sirtuin activators might prepare in advance to a deteriorating environment. Such stress-signaling molecules might enhance chaperone function prior to forthcoming insults (Lamming *et al.*, 2004). Sirt1, the mammalian analog of yeast Sir2, recently has been shown directly to modify chromatin and silence transcription (Vaquero *et al.*, 2004). The question is open whether Sirt1, in addition to silencing transcription, also influences the aging of mammals by suppression of recombination and genomic instability (Lombard *et al.*, 2005) in possible association with histone chaperones (Prado *et al.*, 2004). Thus, the positive effect of the sirtuins on life span might depend less on gene-silencing than on genomic stabilization—a scenario obviating the apparent contradiction that deacetylases as well as deacetylase inhibitors contribute to longevity (Krøll, 2005).

Chemical chaperones. Future intervention studies are aimed at inducing the heat shock response with chemical mimicry, that is, with synthetic compounds—chemical chaperones or nonspecific agents—that could imitate the effect of environmental stressors without the damaging effects they might carry (Castro-Fernandez *et al.*, 2005), and in clinical studies follow up the up-regulation of the heat shock response (e.g., by epigenetic derepression or specific reactivation of Hsf-1). Also, the functional promiscuity of the molecular chaperones opens for the possibility of an increase in chaperone capacity by transfection with individual chaperones (Krøll, 2005).

Conclusion

The housekeeping functions of the chaperones tend to antagonize the phenotype of aging. Thus, aging is characterized by a progressive decrease in the expression and stress-inductivity of the chaperones, whereas an increase in chaperone expression is a common denominator in conditions or procedures leading to an increase of cellular and species longevity, for example, by providing chaperonic protection of the disposable soma.

The inherent immortality of the embryonic stem cells implies that replicative senescence, as possibly the aging of species, are epigenetic phenomena.

The involvement of RNA chaperones in the process of cellular immortalization and defective DNA-chaperones in the progeric syndromes place emphasis on the RNA/DNA-chaperones as contributors to the definition of cellular and species longevity. Accordingly, evidence is given that the evolution of longevity is governed by changes in the expression of relatively few regulatory genes.

Possibly, the molecular chaperones are evolution facilitators participating in the definition of life span of differentiated cells as well as for the evolution of longevity in species.

Future Developments

The correlation between chaperones and aging/longevity should be further examined with focus on the chaperone matrix of the inherently immortal embryonic stem cells.

With emphasis on DAN/RNA-chaperones it is proposed:

- To consider a more comprehensive characterization of the differences in the constitutive level of chaperone expression in relation to the life span of different species.
- To further investigate the effect on species life span of a constitutive increase in the expression of the various chaperones with emphasis on p68 (the putative mammalian analogue to the SV40 T-protein).
- To investigate means for a specific reactivation of chaperone genes silenced during aging as well as to stop the progressive silencing of chaperone genes during normal aging.
- To investigate the redundancy of function of the molecular chaperones to approach a definition of a minimal polymer folding system.
- To identify the chaperone of the large heat shock proteins (autonomous small Hsp's).

REFERENCES

Altomare, K., Greco, V., Bellizzi, D., Berardelli, M., Dato, S., DeRango, F. *et al.* (2003). The allele (A)(-110) in the promoter region of the HSP70-1 gene is unfavourable to longevity in women. *Biogerontology 4*, 4, 215–220.

Castro-Fernandez, C., Maya-Nunez, G., and Conn, M. (2005). Beyond the signal sequence: Protein routing in health and disease. *Endocrine Reviews*, in press.

Dozmorov, I., Bartke, A., and Miller, R.A. (2001). Array-based expression analysis of mouse liver genes: effect of age and of the longevity mutant Prop1df. *Journals of Gerontology Series A, Biological Sciences and Medical Sciences 56*, 2, B72–B80.

Hercus, M.J., Loeschcke, V., and Rattan, S.I. (2003). Lifespan extension of *Drosophila melanogaster* through hormesis by repeated mild heat stress. *Biogerontology 4*, 3, 149–156.

Heydari, A.R., You, S., Takahashi, R., Gutsmann, A., Sarge, K.D., and Richardson, A. (1996). Effect of caloric restriction on the expression of heat shock protein 70 and the activation of heat shock transcription factor 1. *Developmental Genetics 18*, 2, 114–124.

Hood, D.A., and Joseph, A.M. (2004). Mitochondrial assembly: protein import. *Proceedings of the Nutrition Society 63*, 2, 293–300.

Hsu, A.L., Murphy, C.T., and Kenyon, C. (2003). Regulation of aging and age-related disease by DAF-16 and heat-shock factor. *Science 300*, 5622, 1142–1145.

Hu, J., Flores, D., Toft, D., Wang, X., and Nguyen, D. (2004). Requirement of heat shock protein 90 for human hepatitis B virus reverse transcriptase function. *Journal of Virology 78*, 23, 13122–13131.

Ingram, D.K., Anson, R.M., de Cabo, R., Mamczarz, J., Zhu, M., Mattison, J. *et al.* (2004). Development of calorie restriction mimetics as a prolongevity strategy. *Annals of the New York Academy of Sciences 1019*, 412–423.

Kiffin, R., Christian, C., Knecht, E., and Cuervo, A.M. (2004). Activation of chaperone-mediated autophagy during oxidative stress. *Molecular Biology of the Cell 15*, 11, 4829–4840.

Kregel, K.C. (2002). Heat shock proteins: modifying factors in physiological stress responses and acquired thermotolerance. *J Appl Physiol 92*, 5, 2177–2186.

Kroll, J. (1994). The mitochondrial F1-ATPase and the aging process. *Medical Hypotheses 42*, 6, 359–396.

Kroll, J. (1996). The ATPase module and the process of cellular immortalization [Review]. *Annals of the New York Academy of Sciences 786*, 57–61.

Kroll, J. (2002). Molecular chaperones and the process of cellular immortalization in vitro. *Biogerontology 3*, 3, 183–185.

Krøll, J. (2004). The Molecular Chaperones and the Phenomena of Cellular Immortalization and Apoptosis in vitro. *Annals of the New York Academy of Sciences 1019*, 568–571.

Krøll, J. (2005). Chaperones and longevity. *Biogerontology, 6*, 1–5.

Kroll, J., and Saxtrup, O. (2000). On the use of regression analysis for the estimation of human biological age. *Biogerontology 1*, 4, 363–368.

Laksanalamai, P., Whitehead, T.A., and Robb, F.T. (2004). Minimal protein-folding systems in hyperthermophilic archaea. *Nat Rev Microbiol 2*, 4, 315–324.

Lamming, D.W., Wood, J.G., and Sinclair, D.A. (2004). Small molecules that regulate lifespan: evidence for xenohormesis. *Molecular Microbiology 53*, 4, 1003–1009.

Li, D., Sun, F., and Wang, K. (2004). Protein profile of aging and its retardation by caloric restriction in neural retina. *Biochemical and Biophysical Research Communications 318*, 1, 253–258.

Li, J., and Holbrook, N.J. (2004). Elevated gadd153/chop expression and enhanced c-Jun N-terminal protein kinase activation sensitizes aged cells to ER stress. *Experimental Gerontology 39*, 5, 735–744.

Lombard, D.B., Chua, K.F., Mostoslavsky, R., Franco, S., Gostissa, M., and Alt, F.W. (2005). DNA repair, genome stability, and aging. *Cell 120*, 4, 497–512.

Lund, J., Tedesco, P., Duke, K., Wang, J., Kim, S.K., and Johnson, T.E. (2002). Transcriptional profile of aging in *C. elegans*. *Current Biology 12*, 18, 1566–1573.

Majeski, A.E., and Dice, J.F. (2004). Mechanisms of chaperone-mediated autophagy. *International Journal of Biochemistry and Cell Biology 36*, 12, 2435–2444.

Miyaishi, O., Kozaki, K., Saga, S., Sato, T., and Hashizume, Y. (1995). Age-related alteration of proline hydroxylase and collagen-binding heat shock protein (HSP47) expression in human fibroblasts. *Mechanisms of Ageing and Development 85*, 1, 25–36.

Morley, J.F., and Morimoto, R.I. (2004). Regulation of longevity in *Caenorhabditis elegans* by heat shock factor and molecular chaperones. *Mol Biol Cell 15*, 657–664.

Nizard, C., Noblesse, E., Boisdé, C., Moreau, M., Faussat, A.M., Schnebert, S. *et al.* (2004). Heat shock protein 47 expression in aged normal human fibroblasts: modulation by Salix alba extract. *Annals of the New York Academy of Sciences 1019*, 223–227.

Prado, F., Cortés-Ledesma, F., and Aguilera, A. (2004). The absence of the yeast chromatin assembly factor Asf1 increases genomic instability and sister chromatid exchange. *EMBO Rep* 5, 5, 497–502.

Proctor, C.J., Soti, C., Boys, R.J., Gillespie, C.S., Shanley, D.P., Wilkinson, D.J. *et al.* (2005). Modelling the actions of chaperones and their role in ageing. *Mechanisms of Ageing and Development 126*, 1, 119–131.

Rutherford, S.L. (2003). Between genotype and phenotype: protein chaperones and evolvability. *Nat Rev Genet 4*, 4, 263–274.

Shama, S., Lai, C.Y., Antoniazzi, J.M., Jiang, J.C., and Jazwinski, S.M. (1998). Heat stress-induced life span extension in yeast. *Experimental Cell Research 245*, 2, 379–388.

Shamovsky, I., and Gershon, D. (2004). Novel regulatory factors of HSF-1 activation: facts and perspectives regarding their involvement in the age-associated attenuation of the heat shock response. *Mechanisms of Ageing and Development 125*, 10–11, 767–775.

Singh, R., Kølvraa, S., Bross, P., Gregersen, N., Andersen Nexø, B., Frederiksen, H. *et al.* (2004). Association between low self-rated health and heterozygosity for −110A > C polymorphism in the promoter region of HSP70-1 in aged Danish twins. *Biogerontology 5*, 3, 169–176.

Soti, C., Pál, C., Papp, B., and Csermely, P. (2005). Molecular chaperones as regulatory elements of cellular networks. *Current Opinion in Cell Biology 17*, 2, 210–215.

Tatar, M., Khazaeli, A.A., and Curtsinger, J.W. (1997). Chaperoning extended life [letter]. *Nature 390*, 6655, 30.

Van der Vlies, D., Woudenberg, J., and Post, J.A. (2003). Protein oxidation in aging: endoplasmic reticulum as a target. *Amino Acids 25*, 3–4, 397–407.

Vaquero, A., Scher, M., Lee, D., Erdjument-Bromage, H., Tempst, P., and Reinberg, D. (2004). Human SirT1 interacts with histone H1 and promotes formation of facultative heterochromatin. *Molecular Cell 16*, 1, 93–105.

Voos, W., and Röttgers, K. (2002). Molecular chaperones as essential mediators of mitochondrial biogenesis. *Biochimica et Biophysica Acta 1592*, 1, 51–62.

Young, J.C., Agashe, V.R., Siegers, K., and Hartl, F.U. (2004). Pathways of chaperone-mediated protein folding in the cytosol. *Nat Rev Mol Cell Biol 5, 10*, 781–791.

45

Therapeutic Potential of Stem Cells in Aging-Related Diseases

Shannon Whirledge, Kirk C. Lo, and Dolores J. Lamb

Stem cells are derived from embryonic as well as adult sources and vary in their potential for differentiation. Although obtaining stem cells from their natural source (an embryo or fetus) is controversial, they can also be generated in the research laboratory through somatic cell nuclear transfer. Embryonic stem cells can differentiate into a wide variety of cell types (hematopoietic, neural, muscle, germ, islet, and bone marrow), and provide the promise of new therapies for degenerative diseases of aging, tissue replacement, and organ transplantation. In addition, the more differentiated adult stem cells found in tissues, such as the testis, muscle, liver, hematopoietic system, and neural tissues, have considerable regenerative potential and may also have potential applications to rejuvenate failing organ function associated with aging.

Introduction

Embryonic and adult stem cells hold great promise for the treatment of disease and the rejuvenation of aging tissues—a concept that captures the imagination and hopes of the scientific and medical communities. No area of research focus since gene therapy evokes such enthusiasm among scientists and physicians but, nevertheless, raises ethical controversies as well. Proposed to be the ultimate cure for degenerative diseases of aging and a solution for the shortage of donated organs for transplantation, stem cells may even unlock the mysteries of early human development while providing the fountain of youth for an aging society. This chapter reviews the current state of knowledge, the controversies generated by stem cell research, and their application to diseases of aging.

Two basic types of stem cells exist: embryonic and adult. They are characterized by their ability to renew themselves for an indefinite period of time, as well as the ability to divide to create a differentiated cell type while remaining undifferentiated. In the adult, these self-renewing cell types are found in many tissues within a niche that provides a microenvironment that signals to renew the stem cell population or signals to induce unidirectional differentiation.

Depending upon the source of the stem cell, the differentiative potential of embryonic and adult stem cells varies. Fertilized oocytes and blastomeres (up to the eight-cell stage embryo) are described as being *totipotent* with the potential to differentiate and generate a complete organism. In contrast, embryonic stem cells (derived from the inner cell mass (ICM) of a blastocyte (see Figure 45.1) share the property of self-renewal and can differentiate into cells and tissues from any of the three germ layers. These cells are *pluripotent*, but not totipotent (these cells cannot form a placenta). As cells progress along the various steps of differentiation, they become less able to exhibit plasticity or to differentiate into cells of different lineages.

Thus, although the pluripotent embryonic stem cell has the capacity to become any cell type, adult stem cells are *multipotent* and persist into adulthood forming cells of the tissue in which they reside. These adult stem cells are responsible for the regenerative potential of the gastrointestinal, integumentary, spermatogenic, and hematopoietic systems. For example, spermatogonial stem cells (located near the basement membrane of the seminiferous tubules surrounded by Sertoli cells) can rejuvenate spermatogenesis following a gonadotoxic insult. Likewise, adult stem cells isolated from the liver, pancreas, kidney, and nervous system exhibit varying regenerative potential.

Embryonic Stem and Primordial Germ Cells Are Pluripotent

Methods to isolate stem cells were first developed using animal models more than 20 years ago (Evans *et al.*, 1981; Martin, 1981). Pluripotent stem cells are derived from either excess embryos (embryonic stem (ES) cells) or an aborted fetus (embryonic germ (EG) cells). To initiate an ES cell line, they must first be extracted from the inner cell mass (ICM) of a blastocyte (which contains about 30 cells with regenerative potential), cultured, passaged, and eventually maintained *in vitro* (see Figure 45.1). Similarly, primordial germ cells

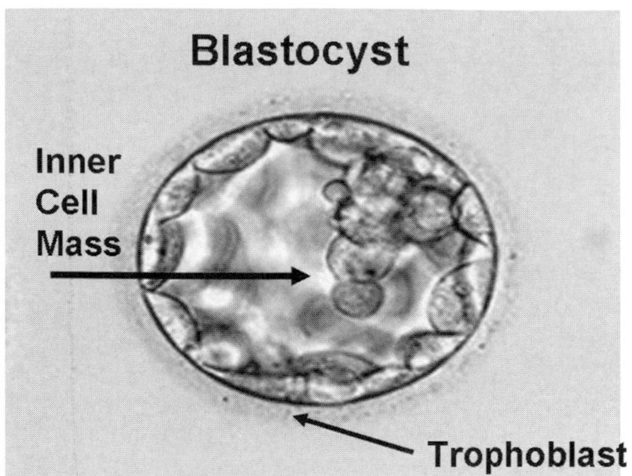

Figure 45.1 The Inner Cell Mass (ICM) of a human blastocyst is a source of embryonic stem cells. A blastocyst is derived from a embryo created by *in vitro* fertilization. The arrows denote the inner cell mass of the blastocyst found internal adjacent to the blastocoels (the hollow core). These 30 or so cells have the potential to become embryonic stem cells under proper culture conditions. If implanted into a receptive uterus, they have the potential to also become a fetus.

(obtained from a fetus) exhibit a similar developmental potential (Matsui *et al.*, 1992). Stem cell lines provide the tools for unique investigations into the intrinsic and extrinsic controls of cell growth and differentiation (Guan *et al.*, 2001; Wobus *et al.*, 1997), signaling molecules and transduction pathways and transcription factors (Burdon *et al.*, 2002) in stem cell biology. Stem cells have also been used to evaluate the cytotoxicity of drugs, and this may provide a unique approach to assessing the safety of pharmaceuticals (Rohwedel *et al.*, 2001).

New therapies are expected to be realized with the advent of ES cell culture that provides an unlimited source for stem cell therapy. The technology still has limitations in that transplantation of undifferentiated ES cells results in the formation of teratomas. Indeed, about 20% of the Parkinson rats developed teratoma-like tumors after transplantation of ES cells into the brain striatum of rats resulted in differentiation of domainergic cells improving motor asymmetry (Bjorklund *et al.*, 2002). ES cell culture may circumvent the tumorgenic problem; nevertheless, a few contaminating undifferentiated ES cells could be problematic. Not surprisingly, with the technology available today, the tumorgenic potential of undifferentiated ES cells limits its rapid translation to human cell therapy.

The molecular controls of ES cell differentiation are poorly understood, but are thought to require growth factors to control differentiation during development (Schuldiner *et al.*, 2000). The production of human ES and EG cells was reported in 1998 (Shamblott *et al.*, 1998; Thomson *et al.*, 1998). Culture of ES cells under conditions leading to the development of embryoid bodies (EB) induces the differentiation of neural, dopaminergic, and glial elements (Brustle *et al.*, 1999; Kim *et al.*, 2002; Schuldiner *et al.*, 2000), and insulin-secreting cells (Assady *et al.*, 2001; Lumelsky *et al.*, 2001), among others. Although the results in the mouse were not perfect (transplantation of the insulin-secreting cells did not produce a sustained correction of hyperglycemia in the engrafted animals), the islet-like clusters survive and secrete insulin *in vivo*. Other tissues generated from ES cell lines include mouse and human cardiomyocytes (Kehat *et al.*, 2001; Maltsev *et al.*, 1993; Wobus *et al.*, 1997), hematopoietic cells (Kaufman *et al.*, 2002; Nakano *et al.*, 1996; Wiles *et al.*, 1991), endothelial cells (Risau *et al.*, 1988; Yamashita *et al.*, 2000), skeletal muscles (Miller-Hance *et al.*, 1993; Rohwedel *et al.*, 1994), chondrocytes (Kramer *et al.*, 2000), liver (Hamazaki *et al.*, 2001), neural cells (Carpenter *et al.*, 2001; Reubinoff *et al.*, 2001; Zhang *et al.*, 2001), and adipocytes (Dani *et al.*, 1997). This will be discussed in detail later. Obviously, the potential for the development of new stem cell therapies is immense. Nevertheless, progress has been stymied by the availability of an insufficient number of fully functional cell lines.

Technical challenges remain concerning research using human ES cell lines. Although human ES cells and monkey ES cells are similar, there are significant differences between these primate models and their mouse counterparts. Some differences are as simple as their growth patterns (i.e., human ES cells grow in compact flat colonies, whereas murine ES cells form spherical colonies). Others include differences in protein expression. For example, human ES cells temporally express the embryonic antigens SSEA-3, SSEA-4, and SSEA-1 in a stage-specific manner upon differentiation; the order of expression is reversed in murine ES cells (Andrews *et al.*, 1996; McLaren, 2001; Thomson *et al.*, 1998). Due to these morphological and developmental differences, some investigators have called into question the applicability of murine models to human ES cell research.

Furthermore, after ES stem cell differentiation, transplantation of allogenic cells/tissues may be hindered by immunological incompatibility between the donor ES cells and the recipient. Admittedly, administration of immunosuppressive drugs prior to the transplantation is an option, but not without significant side effects. In the future, genetic alteration of histocompatibility gene expression may be an option, but presently research on this topic is sparse.

EMBRYONIC STEM CELLS AND CLONING

Therapeutic cloning or *somatic cell nuclear transfer* provides one alternative to the ethical dilemmas raised by ES cell research (see Figure 45.2).

With this technology, a somatic cell nucleus is fused to an enucleated egg and essentially reprogrammed to create ES cells. An artificial blastocyst forms, and the inner cell mass again provides the ES cells for subsequent

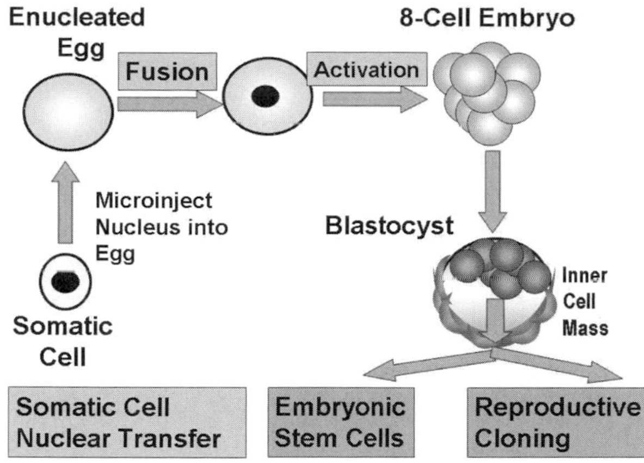

Figure 45.2 Somatic cell nuclear transfer provides an alternative to embryonic stem cells. Somatic cell nuclear transfer can create an artificial blastocyst for a source of embryonic stem cells. In this method, the somatic cell nucleus is transplanted into an enucleated egg. Upon activation, the early events in embryonic development are initiated and a blastocyst forms. This blastocyst can provide the source of embryonic stem cells without the necessity of destroying a human embryo. At this stage, the blastocyst can also be transferred into a receptive uterus to form a fetus (albeit at low efficiency). When transferred to a uterus, this is now termed *reproductive cloning*.

manipulation or alternatively reproductive cloning (discussed later). Culture conditions are developed to induce ES cells to differentiate into functional somatic tissues/cells and then transplanted. The technique requires a substantial number of donated eggs from an IVF laboratory and can be technically challenging. Infertile couples seeking to conceive a child by IVF face significant personal expense, and there is a high demand for oocyte donation to other infertile couples attempting to conceive. Thus, with current methodologies, these caveats are likely to limit this approach to the few privileged and capable of affording this technology.

As mentioned earlier, although the goal of somatic cell nuclear transplantation is to generate cells, tissues, or organs for transplantation, the success of reproductive cloning in animals (such as Dolly the lamb (Wilmut *et al.*, 1997)) brings new concerns regarding this technology. Prior to the cloning of Dolly, the rules governing stem cell research were nonspecific, limiting only federal funding of research on human embryos for *in vitro* fertilization (IVF). During this time, research funds were limited to those approved by a congressionally appointed ethics advisory board. In 1996, the Dicky Amendment completely banned the use of federal funds for any human embryo research.

Development of the first human embryonic stem cell line by Thomson *et al.* in 1998 pushed the debate over stem cell usage back into center court. In 1999, the National Institute of Health announced that current U.S. law did not ban federal support for the use of embryonic stem cells, instead stating that support could not be used for the isolation of stem cells but could be used on stem cells once obtained. This opened the floodgates for ethical debate over the issue of extraction versus research. The National Bioethics Advisory Committee released a statement supporting the federal funding for both the isolation and use of embryonic stem cells stating the inability to ethically separate the two.

In a report in *Science* in 1999, Pittenger *et al.* described the novel isolation of a multipotent cell derived from adult human tissue. This served only to reinforce the debate against embryonic stem cell research, arguing that adult stem cells (discussed later) are adequate for research purposes. The wavering under the Clinton administration was firmly halted when President Bush took office. On August 9, 2001, President Bush announced that federal funding would be allowed for research on human embryonic stem cells, but only on those lines that had been derived before the date of announcement. At that time more than 60 lines were estimated to be available for research; since then the number of NIH available lines has dropped to 22.

Although President Bush's policy does allow some research to proceed, it fails to address research in private or nonfederally funded sources. In November of 2004, California's voters passed Proposition 71, which authorizes $3 billion in state funds to support stem cell research in California. Other states are expected to follow, and currently, bills are continually being introduced in individual states regarding the legality of collaborations, with researchers using such funds and prohibiting one or all forms of cloning research. Funding and laws are not the only factors prohibiting stem cell research from advancing.

Of the 60 to 75 lines originally available for federally funded stem cell research in 2001, scientists have encountered several problems with their use. To date, as noted, there are actually only 22 lines available from the NIH. These cell lines are degrading with time, becoming more vulnerable to chromosomal abnormalities. Also, the cell lines lack the genetic diversity required for broad-spectrum disease treatment, and there is an absence of disease-specific lines. Within the private sector, these problems are being circumvented by creating a variety of new lines from wide genetic backgrounds, but limitations on the freedom of scientists in the United States to work and publish on these cell lines has hindered any real progression toward disease treatments. Not only do investigators have difficulty obtaining functional cell lines, but also the exact mechanism for cell culture has yet to be discovered. One of the vital components of ongoing work is determining the conditions required to sustain undifferentiated stem cells as well as differentiating them along defined pathways. Determining what the right signal is at the right time will better allow scientists to manipulate the stem cell fate, and controlling this is what ultimately leads to powerful medical therapy.

Indeed, the fear of human cloning (illegal in the United States and a number of other countries) has led to many countries banning research on this technology. Because of these restrictions over the use of ES and primordial germ cell lines, some researchers have focused their studies on adult stem cells, reexamining their potential regenerative potential and cell type plasticity.

Application of Stem Cell Technologies for Rejuventation of Aging Tissues: Embryonic and Adult Stem Cells

Unique cells with regenerative potential in the adult include spermatogonial and Leydig cells, stem cells in the testis, mesenchymal progenitors of muscle, neural stem cells, hematopoetic stem cells, bone, spleen, and those of the gastrointestinal system. These adult stem cells are described next, in more detail. We discuss the potential applications of both embryonic and adult stem cells to rejuvenate failing organ function associated with aging.

THE STEM CELLS OF THE HEMATOPOIETIC SYSTEM ARE USED THERAPEUTICALLY TODAY

Hematopoietic stem cells (HSC) are widely studied, well-characterized, and currently used for patient care. The studies of Till and McCullough (Till *et al.*, 1961), which provided the basis for subsequent studies, focused on the identification and enrichment of a population of bone marrow-derived cells capable of self-regeneration and repletion of the entire hematopoietic cell line (Blau *et al.*, 2001; Weissman, 2000).

A heterogeneous mix of stem cells exists in the bone marrow composed of HSC and mesenchymal stem cells (MSC). MSC are readily separated from the HSC based upon their characteristic adherence to plastic (Poulsom *et al.*, 2002). There are two types of HSCs: long term (LT-HSC) and short term (ST-HSC). The potential long-term cells offer is most important, defined by their ability to self-renew for life, and also to give rise to the short-term cells, which in turn self-renew for a period of about eight weeks. The short-term cells can give rise to differentiated or multipotent progenitors that subsequently differentiate into the various blood cell types (Morrison *et al.*, 1997).

Researchers focused on methods to enrich the HSC from bone marrow using protocols that rely on the presence of cell surface proteins and using this approach to remove cells expressing markers of maturity. First identified in a mouse model, human HSC are Thy-1 and CD34 positive, but Lin and CD38 negative (Uchida *et al.*, 1998). With current technologies, hematopoietic stem cells can be enriched about 10,000 fold (Morrison *et al.*, 1994). Despite stringent criteria for cell separation and great enrichment potential, some enriched cells cannot replete the blood cells, reinforcing the notion that stem cell markers are not completely identified or understood.

Transplantation of highly enriched, histocompatible HSC offers the potential of complete reconstitution of the entire hematopoietic system in patients after whole body radiation or chemotherapy. Not surprisingly, transplantation of allogeneic HSC induces a graft-versus-host (GVH) and tumor responses. Transplantation of enriched allogeneic HSC reduces the incidence of the GVH response because the transplant patient later develops tolerance to donated cells (Burdon *et al.*, 2002).

Hematopoietic stem cells: chemotherapy strategies for older patients

The application of standard-dose chemotherapy to elderly patients usually results in a higher rate of treatment-related deaths compared to that of their younger patient counterparts (Gaynor *et al.*, 1994). The mechanisms underlying the changes within the hematopoetic system that result in reduced tolerance to chemotherapy is unclear. Age-related changes of the hematopoietic system are probably irrelevant for normal aging function, but under several courses of chemotherapy, the stress becomes clinically evident. This suggests hematopoietic stem cell (HSC) exhaustion. In order to effectively treat older patients, the mechanisms by which this occurs and the strategies for HSC treatment and renewal must be discovered.

NEURAL STEM CELLS ARE PRESENT IN THE ADULT BRAIN

The ability of the central nervous system (CNS) to repair itself following injury or age-related disease is limited, and previous development of therapeutic approaches focused only on preserving at-risk neuronal populations. Yet these strategies are limited to patients where substantial neuronal loss has not already occurred. Hope for the targeting of new neurons into injured regions of the brain or expanded neural cells grafted into regions of degeneration has stemmed from the observation of endogenous generation of new neurons in the adult brain. Although once thought to be restricted to prenatal development, emerging evidence suggests that neurogenesis continues through adult life.

Researchers were surprised to learn that stem cells were present in the adult brain, an organ long thought to comprise nonrenewable neurons. The subventricular zone and the subgranular zone of the dentate gyrus of the hippocampus have the highest concentrations of dividing cells (Cameron *et al.*, 1994). Neuronal stem cells isolated from fetal and adult brains and then cultured were induced to differentiate into the three distinct neuronal cell types—astrocytes, oligodendrocytes, and neurons (Gage *et al.*, 2000). After transplantation, cultured stem cells engrafted into developing fetal and adult brains migrated throughout the nervous system and differentiated into tissues ranging from the hippocampus to the olfactory bulb (Gage *et al.*, 1995; Suhonen *et al.*, 1996). Neuronal stem cells are classified by their expression of a number of cell surface markers (CD133 positive, CD34 negative, and CD45 negative) (Uchida *et al.*, 2000). Following expansion of adult neuronal stem cells *in vitro*, transplantation, and engraftment into rat brains, neural function was apparent based upon the presence of synaptic electrical activity (Auerbach *et al.*, 2000).

Neural stem cells are defined by their ability to differentiate into the three major cell types of the CNS—neurons, astrocytes, and oligodendrocytes—*in vitro*. The mechanism by which this occurs *in vivo* has yet to be elucidated. Regulation of transcription, via Re1 silencing transcription factor mediated recruitment of histone deacetylases, is critical in the transition from neural stem cell to mature neuron (Ballas *et al.*, 2005). Cooperation between the Smad and STAT signaling pathways is involved in gene expression and suppression during astrocyte differentiation (Sun *et al.*, 2001). Oligodendrocytes, the myelinating glial cell type of the CNS, differentiate from a common neural-oligodendrocyte precursor through coexpression of Olig2, a basic helix-loop-helix transcription factor, and Nkx2.2 (Zhou *et al.*, 2001). It is through a delicate interplay of transcriptional activators and repressors that neuronal stem cell fate is decided. The therapeutic potential of neural stem cells for the aging brain makes determining these factors essential.

In vitro, neural stem cells have the potential to ubiquitously give rise to neurons. In the adult brain, neurogenesis is spatially restricted to two areas, the subventricular zone and the hippocampal dentate gyrus (Cameron *et al.*, 1994). Under normal conditions, newly generated neurons are restricted to defined pathways of migration followed by highly regulated, sequential steps to integration. Although these steps are equivalent to those undergone during early development, neurogenesis in the adult brain occurs in a less permissive environment, with new adult neurons having to integrate into preexisting circuits. The quest for producing an effective therapy from induced neurogenesis relies on the discovery of several factors. These include identifying the cellular cues that are responsible for a neurogenic niche becoming permissive for neurogenesis and how the proliferation of adult neural stem cells is regulated.

Neural stem cells as therapeutic agents for age-related brain repair

The prevalence of stem cells in the nervous system appears to decline with age, as is true for a number of organ systems. The aging brain also is characterized by reduced neurogenesis. Several diseases and injuries of the brain also consist of acute neuronal loss. Parkinson's disease is distinguished by progressive loss of dopaminergic neurons in the substantia nigra zona compacta. A leading cause of death and disability, acute ischemic stroke causes a loss of neurons, astrocytes, and oligodendroctyes. Decreased neurogenesis in the adult hippocampus has been genetically linked to Alzheimer's disease, a neurodegenerative disorder of the CNS. Alzheimer's has also been linked to age-related structural deterioration and cellular senescence of the neuroprotective microglia.

Though understanding the basis for age-related reduction of neurogenesis would be necessary to determine the functional contributions of newly generated neurons, preliminary studies suggest a link between neuronal replacement and phenotype recovery for disease models. In a rodent model of Parkinson's disease, treatment with TGFα and a mitogen for stem cells caused an improvement of behavioral deficits and the appearance of new neurons (Fallon *et al.*, 2000). In a study examining the combined effects of FGF-2 and EGF on a degenerative hippocampal model, the authors observed a significant number of new neurons believed to be integrated into the hippocampal circuitry (Nakatomi *et al.*, 2002). Behavior studies showed improved behavior recovery after growth factor treatment. Implantation of neural stem cells into the midbrains of aged mice was associated with reconstitution of neural depleted areas (Ourednik *et al.*, 2002). Not only did this study show that aged brains can support engraftment and extensive migration of neural stem cells, but also that neural stem cells migrate more readily in the aged mouse brain than in the intact young brain.

Neural stem cells may prove to be a useful pool for age-related brain injury or disease that could be recruited or expanded in culture for transplantation to repopulate regions of neuronal loss (see Figure 45.3).

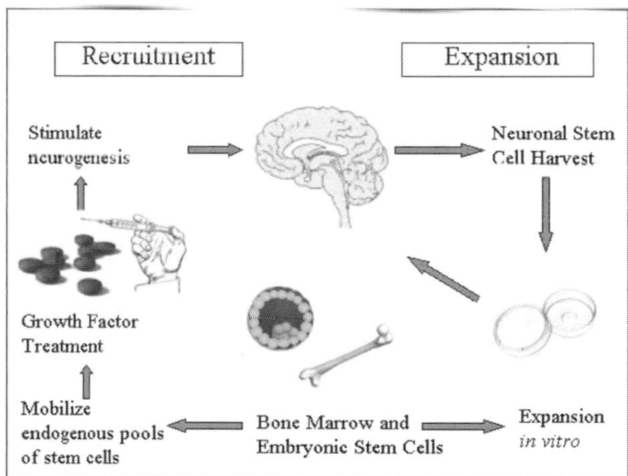

Figure 45.3 Approaches to stem cell therapy for age-related injury or disease. There are several defined therapeutic targets for using stem cells to treat age-related injury or disease. Strategies include the isolation or recruitment of stem cells (shown in this figure are models for neural and hematopoietic stem cells) as well as targeted differentiation of embryonic stem cells. Research needs include the development of techniques for the enrichment and expansion of the stem cells *in vitro*, control of differentiation and cell function, as well as methods to stimulate the growth of new neurons (i.e., for neurogenesis in the brain).

In order for a recruitment strategy to become a viable therapy, scientists must find a way to overcome age-related loss of progenitors. Recruitment strategies must also incorporate factors involved in guided migration of newly generated neuronal progenitors to areas of injury. The alternative method, expansion of neural stem cells *in vitro* with subsequent transplantation, is limited by the extent to which an aged brain can tolerate grafting surgeries. Another challenge is discovering the environmental cues necessary for successful survival, differentiation, and functional integration. Certainly the field of neural stem cell research has many obstacles to overcome, but with the promise of potential therapies for neurodegenerative diseases that affect many, the light at the end of the tunnel remains a driving force.

THE LIVER HAS REGENERATIVE CAPACITY: HEPATIC STEM CELLS

The liver is an organ that exhibits significant regenerative capacity; the entire organ can regrow from as little as a third of its original tissue (Vessey *et al.*, 2001). The resting hepatocytes can undergo cell division—up to 12 to 16 divisions per cell providing the basis for this regenerative capacity (Sell, 2001). Evidence of liver stem cells capable of forming both hepatocytes and bile ducts has been demonstrated in a rodent model. Administration of a hepatotoxic agent (carbon tetrachloride) to rats pretreated with N-2-acetylaminofluorene (an agent used to block hepatocyte proliferation) creates hepatocellular injury, simultaneously blocking the normal hepatocyte proliferative response following toxic injury (Petersen *et al.*, 1998).

Liver regeneration is believed to occur through three mechanisms: replication of existing hepatocytes, differentiation of oval cells, or hematopoietic stem cells. After a 70% hepatectomy, liver regeneration requires no more than two rounds of hepatocyte replication (Fausto, 2004). Hepatocytes have enormous proliferative potential, but there is evidence of diminished replicative activity with injury and disease. Due to the ability of liver regeneration to occur through fully differentiated hepatocytes, initial arguments were against the need or existence of a hepatic stem cell. Observations in the 1950s first indicated that another source of hepatocytes existed, termed oval cells (Farber, 1956). Oval cells refer to single cells or clusters of cells that form a ductule. They arise after toxic insult to the liver stem cells, located along the canal of Herring, and are identified based upon the expression of OV-6 (Thorgeirsson, 1996). These cells arise from an intrahepatic stem cell niche corresponding to the canals of Hering and terminal bile ductules of the adult liver.

Even though the term *oval cell* often is used synonymously with hepatic stem cell, whether or not they are one and the same remains in dispute. Certainly oval cells give rise to multiple cell lineages in the liver, but the oval cell may be an activated progeny of stem cells in the liver. One of the challenges facing researchers today is the lack of definitive markers of hepatic stem cells. Candidate markers include OV6, CD34, c-kit, cytokeratins CK 7 and CK-9, chromogranin-A, and the cell adhesion molecule N-CAM (Dunsford *et al.*, 1989; Roskams *et al.*, 1998). Improved protocols are continuously emerging for the purification and culture of hepatic stem cells (Lazaro *et al.*, 1998).

Some markers expressed by oval cells are also hematopoietic stem cell markers. This suggests a relationship between a liver-derived stem cell population and a circulating bone marrow-derived stem cell fraction. In fact, in sex-mismatched bone marrow transplantation experiments, oval cells and hepatocytes were found from bone marrow origin (Petersen *et al.*, 1999). Similar findings revealed the interchangeability of tissue stem cells after transplanted bone marrow side population cells, stem cells purified on the basis of their ability to efflux Hoechst 33342 dye, could be isolated in hepatic side population cells and were recruited to repair liver damage (Wulf *et al.*, 2003). Although there is clear evidence of cells originating from the bone marrow contributing to the formation of hepatocytes, this transformation is a rare event. Much of this work supports the phenotypic plasticity of stem cells in response to a microenvironment, but it has yet to be seen if these relatively rare events could play a noteworthy part in human liver or tissue damage repair.

Hepatic stem cells: hope for liver transplantation

The immense regenerative potential of the liver makes the resident stem cells a target for cell-based therapies for a variety of liver diseases. Hepatocyte transfusion may provide a short-term solution for patients awaiting liver transplantation (Strom *et al.*, 1997). Transfusion of cultured hepatocytes has realized some success for the treatment of metabolic conditions such as ornithine carbamoylase deficiency (Strom *et al.*, 1997), homozygous familial hypercholesterolemia (Raper *et al.*, 1996), and Crigler-Najjar syndrome type I (Fox *et al.*, 1998).

Hepatic stem cells and aging

Although the rate of liver regeneration declines with age, the regenerative capacity remains unchanged. The aged liver is more vulnerable to injury from toxins, viruses, and ischemia. A decline in hepatic clearance of certain drugs leads to a marked increase in the frequency of adverse drug reactions in geriatric patients. The development of cell therapy strategies for liver failure and metabolic diseases has become a necessity due to limitations on rates of regeneration in the aged population as well as shortage of donor livers. The availability of *in vitro* expandable progenitors would facilitate studies on cell engraftment and serve as a model for clinical applications.

Currently, cell transplantation for the treatment of liver failure is restricted to the transplantation of primary hepatocytes. Due to shortage of donor human hepatocytes, liver stem cell research must be aimed at expanding a progenitor population *in vitro*. Another potential avenue for cell-based therapies includes discovering a potential functional role for bone marrow-derived cells in hepatic tissue transplant. Human fetal tissue remains a promising source of bipotential stem cells. Providing this tissue type remains accessible, these cells could be more efficient than adult hepatocytes for the repair of liver damage. At the present rate of progress, transplantation is a goal achievable within the foreseeable future.

MUSCLE STEM CELLS

Muscle satellite cells, located in the periphery between the muscle fiber sarcolemma and the surrounding basement membrane, provide the basis for the repair and regeneration of muscle tissue (Goldring *et al.*, 2002; Mauro, 1961). These cells are rare, accounting for only 5% of the nuclei present in muscle fiber (Schultz *et al.*, 1982). Muscle satellite cells are critical to understanding the role of adult stem cells in myogenic growth and regeneration. Of note, stem cells of other tissue origins, bone marrow (Lipton *et al.*, 1979; Wakitani *et al.*, 1995), neural (Galli *et al.*, 2000), or even skin (Pyc *et al.*, 2001) can contribute to muscle regeneration. Muscle progenitors offer great hope for the treatment of primary muscle diseases such as muscular dystrophy, and these may reach clinical reality in the future.

Muscle stem cells: Regeneration for primary muscle diseases and maintenance of blood vessels

Cardiovascular disease is the number one cause of death in the United States. Although many risk factors associated with cardiovascular disease can be managed, the aging process and hereditary predisposition cannot be changed. Current pharmacological agents fail to address the cell loss associated with heart failure. Cardiac muscle of the adult heart is unable to repair itself following loss of cardiac function due to severe disease or injury. Although once thought to be a post-mitotic organ, recent support for the regeneration of myocytes shows cardiac muscle replenished with newly generated cells. A resident cardiac stem cell population is thought to be capable of limited repair, but may be ineffective for thorough restoration of function after severe injury. Adult as well as embryonic stem cells have been shown to differentiate into cardiomyocytes, providing a new type of treatment for patients. Evidence suggests that adult stem cells of the bone marrow and adipose tissue can be a source of *de novo* cardiomyocyte population. In fact, when GFP expressing hematopoietic stem cells were purified and injected directly into the myocardium of infracted mouse hearts, over 50% of all new myocytes, confirmed as maturing and functional, expressed GFP (Orlic *et al.*, 2001). The transplanted bone marrow stem cells were able to acquire a cardiomyocyte phenotype and regenerate considerable amounts of contractile myocardium. Though bone marrow stem cells are the most widely studied source of stem cells, they are by no means the only source or the most abundant. The large volume of adipose tissue makes it an attractive alternative to study stem cell plasticity as it relates to cardiac failure. Rangappa *et al.* showed differentiation into cardiomyocytes from adipose derived cells in 2003. Coculture and the addition of the proper signaling molecules relay the external cues required for differentiation of human mesenchymal stem cells into cardiomyocytes. These studies suggest that extra cardiac stem cells can repopulate the myocardium and participate in myocardial repair, but considerable controversy exists regarding the rate at which this occurs *in vivo*.

Increasing the number of functional cardiomyocytes has obvious therapeutic potential. Circulating multipotent and resident cardiac stem cells have demonstrated the potential to contribute to cardiac repair and recovery, but this does not preclude the importance and promise of embryonic stem cell-derived cardiomyocytes. ES cells can easily be genetically manipulated through fusion gene transfection to produce a highly differentiated, 99% pure cardiomyocyte culture (Klug *et al.*, 1996). The ES-derived cardiomyocytes exhibit normal contractile sensitivity to calcium and display many of the physical attributes observed in endogenous populations (Metzger *et al.*, 1994). Upon grafting into adult mice hearts, ES-derived cardiomyocytes formed suitable intracardiac grafts for as long as seven weeks. Embryonic stem cells hold promise for cellular engraftment and tissue engineering. Through simple genetic manipulation, relatively pure cultures of cardiomyocytes from ES cells can be used for successful intracardiac grafts. If this therapy can be translated to patients through the generation of cardiogenic human ES cell lines, the factor that limits the number of heart failure patients from receiving life-saving procedures would be nearly eliminated.

TESTICULAR STEM CELLS

Spermatogonial stem cells are a unique population of stem cells due to their ability to genetically contribute to the next generation. In 1994, Brinster and Zimmerman described a novel method to isolate and transplant the spermatogonial stem cell. Stem cells are isolated from the testes of mice carrying the β-galactosidase transgene. This allows transplantation and colonization to be followed by visualizing blue staining cells; donor cells of fluorescently labeled mice, such as GFP, could also be used. The isolated cells are then microinjected into a germ cell deficient host via efferent duct or rete testes. After an incubation period equivalent to the time needed to undergo normal mouse spermatogenesis, the testes are harvested and stained with β-gal to identify the presence of spermatogenesis and blue staining seminiferous tubules, indicative of transplanted spermatogonial stem cells. The development of this technique and the ability to successfully repeat it, including by our own lab, have opened the door to a range of therapeutic possibilities. Xenogenic transplants are possible and are looking at the complex relationship between the Sertoli cells and the resident stem cell (Franca *et al.*, 1998). The development of male mouse spermatogonial stem cell long-term culture conditions by Konatsu-Shinohara *et al.* in 2004 will allow scientists to determine the signals that regulate the self-renewal division of spermatogonial stem cells along with those factors that signal differentiation.

Leydig cells are the steroid-producing cells of the interstitial tissue of the testis. Their primary function, the production of androgen, is essential for spermatogenesis and development of the male phenotype. Throughout development the lineage of Leydig cells changes; five classifications of Leydig cells have been identified. Although the population of progenitors is relatively small, Leydig cell turnover is maintained with age, and therefore, the ability to isolate this population offers a novel technique to restore androgen synthesis.

Leydig cell progenitors can be isolated from adult testes as shown by Lo *et al.* in 2004. Making use of a technique developed by Goodell *et al.* with hematopoietic stem cells, Leydig progenitors are enriched through flow cytometry analysis of the Hoechst dim side population (see Figure 45.4).

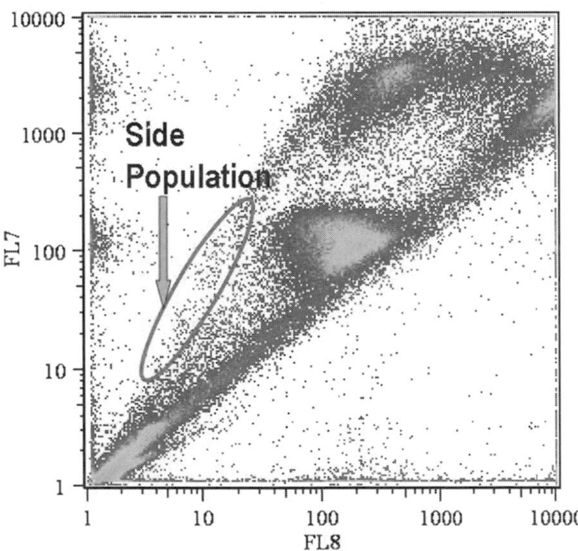

Figure 45.4 Enrichment of Leydig cell progenitors by flow cytometry analysis of the Hoechst dim side population. Goodell and colleagues reported the use of Hoechst dye exclusion to select for a population of stem cells based upon their ability to exclude the dye via the multidrug resistance transporter protein. The cells are sorted into SP (side-population), which extrudes the dye, and non-SP which retains the dye. The SP fraction represents about 0.9% of the total population. Briefly, after the Hoechst dye staining, the cell solution is excited with the UV laser at 350 nm. Duo-wavelength filters in the flow cytometer are used to detect the resulting fluorescence (Dakocytomation, Carpinteria, California).

Lo *et al.* were able to identify successful transplantation of Leydig stem cells by restoration of spermatogenesis and a significant increase in the levels of circulating testosterone in infertile mice. The ability to isolate Leydig progenitor offers a powerful method to study the adult testicular Leydig stem cell, characterize the phenotype, and discover what signals regulate differentiation, which will ultimately lead to human reproductive therapies.

Recent work by Davidoff *et al.* describes the progenitors of Leydig cells as vascular smooth muscle cells (VSMCs) and pericytes (PCs). Using an *in vivo* model of EDS treatment, Leydig cell regeneration was preceded by a proliferation of VSMCs and PCs and their subsequent conversion into steriodogenic Leydig cells. As advances in reproductive technology allow us to isolate and transplant testicular stem cells into infertile men and cancer patients, the ethical responsibility to the patient and society cannot be disregarded. Considerations for all involved parties, including unborn children, must be in place before human therapies can be implemented.

Testicular stem cells and andropause

Aging is described as "the progressive loss of function accompanied by decreasing fertility and increasing mortality with advancing age" (Kirkwood *et al.*, 2000). Androgen secretion by the testis progressively declines with age. Currently, a variety of drugs are on the market for replacement of testosterone in hypogonadal aging men (Androgel, Androderm). Similarly, loss of fertility due to chemotherapy or radiotherapy (as well as other infertility problems) is a deficiency that cannot be corrected with any available treatment, but recent work with testicular stem cells has given hope for therapies. Specifically, the findings of Atala and colleagues (Machluf *et al.*, 2003) that encapsulated transplanted Leydig cells or granulosa cells (Yoo *et al.*, 2000) can provide the basis for natural hormone replacement in aging. Similarly, germ cell transplantation may allow for restoration of fertility.

BONE MARROW STEM CELLS

The vast majority of bone mass is achieved in the human adult by the age of 18, with a small amount accumulated up to the age of 30. In a healthy adult, bone remodeling is a balance between bone resorption, via osteoclasts, and bone formation, by osteoblasts. Changes in levels of endogenous hormone and mechanical load, due to age-related changes in physical activity, determine the extent of bone remodeling.

The prospect of bone repair and prevention

Reduced activity of osteoblasts observed with aging is due in part to estrogen and progesterone deficiency. Loss of bone mass, also attributed to reduced activity of osteoblasts, is responsible for enhanced risk or fractures and reduced bone fracture repair. Of those over the age of 70, only 31 to 36% are predicted to have normal bone mass. Many people in the aging population are affected by hip fractures: up to 20% of hip fracture patients die within the first year, and only 30% ever regain prefracture function (Akesson *et al.*, 2003). A major consequence of the aging population is the inability to replace or repair aging tissue. The bone marrow contains stem cells that are progenitors for osteoblasts, capable of forming bone cartilage and other connective tissue. Osteoprogenitor cells may provide a potential therapy for bone repair, reconstructing bone tissue in the area of injury.

Mending broken or damaged bones through bone grafts is a common practice performed by doctors in the United States every year. Although not all patients are eligible for this commercial process, including aged patients whose quality and quantity of bone are not sufficient, there is hope for these patients. Bone engineering has made great strides in developing therapies that colonize damaged areas and form new bone. A group in China has recently shown that engraftment of bone marrow stem cells was capable of repairing segmental bone defects in sheep metatarsus (Li *et al.*, 2005). Bone marrow stem cells were enriched over a Percoll density gradient and implanted with porous-TCP in a sheep metatarsus defect. Compared to controls, the stem cell implants healed the bone defect more efficiently and quicker. The use of a biological scaffold, a hydrogel, in concert with bone marrow stem cell cultures also provided new bone formation when transplanted into a region of bone defect (Srouji *et al.*, 2004). A three-dimensional hydrogel scaffold that contained an osteogenic subpopulation of bone marrow stem cells was transplanted into rat tibia and examined six weeks postimplantation. Due to the decrease in skeletal bone formation and rate of fracture repair seen with aging, the fact that the scaffold and stem cells induced bone repair is promising as a potential therapy. If bone tissue could be engineered to interchange senescent or apoptosing cells with a fresh supply from stem cells, the effects of aging on bone could be mitigated.

STEM CELLS OF THE SPLEEN

Diabetes is an insulin insufficiency disease that affects over 6% of the U.S. population. People with diabetes are at higher risk for heart disease, blindness, kidney failure, and other chronic conditions. Diabetes cost the United States an estimated $132 billion in 2002 in direct medical and indirect expenditures (Hogan *et al.*, 2003). Pancreatic β-cell death directly leads to Type I diabetes, causing a misregulation of glucose homeostasis. Patients with Type I, insulin-dependent diabetes require exogenous insulin therapy to regulate glucose levels. Neogenesis of β-cells could lead to an important mechanism of islet cell repopulation and restoration of normoglycemia. Two strategies for producing human islet cells have made significant advances in the past few years: the transformation of pancreatic cells into new islet cells and the isolation and development of stem cells into insulin-producing islet cells. Acquiring renewable sources of cells, either from embryonic or adult stem cells, may overcome problems related to obtaining sufficient numbers of islets for transplant. Specifically, stem cells of the spleen, an organ previously not thought to harbor pancreatic stem cells, have been demonstrated to mature into fully functional islet cells (Kodama *et al.*, 2003). Islet replacement, via adult and embryonic stem cells, represents a promising cure for diabetes.

Regeneration of islet cells for the treatment of diabetes

Although the onset and progression of Type I diabetes can be managed through intensive insulin therapy, this type of therapy does not liberate the patient from insulin dependence. Restoring β-cell function through regenerating β-cells from islet cell precursors is an attractive alternative to transplantation of exogenous β-cells. Problems with scarcity of material and immunological rejection are circumvented by the use of embryonic stem (ES) cells, which can differentiate into a variety of cell lineages *in vitro*. Soria *et al.* made use of a cell-trapping system to generate an insulin-secreting cell clone from undifferentiated ES cells (Soria *et al.*, 2000). ES-implanted animals reached a normalized weight by four weeks postimplantation, and implantation led to correction of hyperglycemia within one week. ES-derived insulin-containing cells are able to normalize blood glucose in diabetic mice, but using this technology in human therapies involves first solving problems with ES cell use, including overcoming political obstacles and potential tumor development.

Kodama *et al.* identified endogenous adult precursor cells of the spleen that can reconstitute functional islets and restore normoglycemia in the pancreas (Kodoma *et al.*, 2003). By utilizing flow cytometry sorting against CD45, a surface marker absent on precursor cells, treatment of prediabetic mice with splenic precursor cells prevents diabetic onset, whereas their untreated littermates became diabetic. The donor precursor splenocytes contributed to *de novo* islet regeneration and rescue of damaged islets. These findings implicate the endogenous adult population of stem cells in therapies to reverse diabetes without the ethical issues associated with the use of ES cells.

CONTROVERSY: POTENTIAL PLASTICITY OF ADULT STEM CELLS

The idea that adult stem cell lineage is restricted to their resident tissue has recently been challenged. The transplantation of a single hematopoeitic stem cell resulted in reconstitution of hematopoeitic tissue and the generation of epithelial cells in the liver, skin, lungs, and gastrointestinal tracts (Krause *et al.*, 2001). The plasticity of several known adult stem cells is being questioned along with the possibility of resident stem cells in every human tissue. It is such possibilities that show promise for tissue repair and regeneration using adult stem cells from the patient.

Using adult stem cells to screen drugs represents another potential use that could drastically reduce the time it takes to get a drug to market. Embryonic stem cells represent a more promising source of therapies due to their pluripotent nature. These cells represent a novel approach to exploring human development. By being able to discover how cells become differentiated, the potential for cell-based therapies becomes real. Human embryonic stem cells have been grown into heart muscle, nerves, pancreas, liver, bone, cartilage, and several other tissue types. With the knowledge of how to send stem cells along the path toward differentiated tissue, there is great possibility to prevent and treat several diseases including Alzheimer's, heart disease, diabetes, arthritis, Parkinson's, and numerous others. The potential for stem cells is immense, but several obstacles must first be overcome in order to make stem cell-based therapy a reality.

Conclusion

As of yet, we do not know what causes aging, but we do know that the rate at which aging occurs can be altered through nature and intervention. Cell turnover and replacement is routine in many tissues and does not cause tissue dysfunction when cells are adequately replaced. Changes in aging tissue include cellular senescence and apoptosis, which results in reduced numbers of fully functional cells. The use of stem cells to replace or renew these populations could lead to the treatment of several aging-related diseases; the fate lies in the hands of the scientists. The explosion of information on stem cells and their newly emerging potential holds great promise for the understanding and treatment of many diseases; however, the excitement requires tampering with careful and detailed examination of the data as well as adherence to strict criteria to form a solid basis for future work. The message from the stem-cell research community has been a resounding call for more research on both adult and ES cells in animal models of human disease. It will be years before human therapies emerge from the stem cell research, but the potential is undeniable.

REFERENCES

Andrews, P.W., Casper, J., Damjanov, I., Duggan-Keen, M., Giwercman, A., Hata, J. *et al.* (1996). Comparative analysis of cell surface antigens expressed by cell lines derived from human germ cell tumours. *Int.J.Cancer 66(6)*:806–816.

Assady, S., Maor, G., Amit, M., Itskovitz-Eldor, J., Skorecki, K.L., and Tzukerman, M. (2001). Insulin production by human embryonic stem cells. *Diabetes 50(8)*:1691–1697.

Auerbach, J.M., Eiden, M.V., and McKay, R.D. (2000). Transplanted CNS stem cells form functional synapses in vivo. *Eur. J. Neurosci. 12(5)*:1696–1704.

Bjorklund, L.M., Sanchez-Pernaute, R., Chung, S., Andersson, T., Chen, I.Y., McNaught, K.S. *et al.* (2002). Embryonic stem cells develop into functional dopaminergic neurons after transplantation in a Parkinson rat model. *Proc. Natl. Acad. Sci. USA 99(4)*:2344–2349.

Blau, H.M., Brazelton, T.R., and Weimann, J.M. (2001). The evolving concept of a stem cell: entity or function? *Cell 105(7)*:829–841.

Brustle, O., Jones, K.N., Learish, R.D., Karram, K., Choudhary, K., Wiestler, O.D. *et al.* (1999). Embryonic stem cell-derived glial precursors: a source of myelinating transplants. *Science 285(5428)*:754–756.

Burdon, T., Smith, A., and Savatier, P. (2002). Signalling, cell cycle and pluripotency in embryonic stem cells. *Trends Cell Biol. 12(9)*:432–438.

Cameron, H.A. and Gould, E. (1994). Adult neurogenesis is regulated by adrenal steroids in the dentate gyrus. *Neuroscience 61(2)*:203–209.

Carpenter, M.K., Inokuma, M.S., Denham, J., Mujtaba, T., Chiu, C.P., and Rao, M.S. (2001). Enrichment of neurons and neural precursors from human embryonic stem cells. *Exp.Neurol. 172(2)*:383–397.

Dani, C., Smith, A.G., Dessolin, S., Leroy, P., Staccini, L., Villageois, P. *et al.* (1997). Differentiation of embryonic stem cells into adipocytes in vitro. *J.Cell Sci. 110(Pt 11)*: 1279–1285.

Evans, M.J. and Kaufman, M.H. (1981). Establishment in culture of pluripotential cells from mouse embryos. *Nature 292(5819)*:154–156.

Fox, I.J., Chowdhury, J.R., Kaufman, S.S., Goertzen, T.C., Chowdhury, N.R., Warkentin, P.I. *et al.* (1998). Treatment of the Crigler-Najjar syndrome type I with hepatocyte transplantation. *N. Engl. J. Med. 338(20)*:1422–1426.

Franca, L.R., Ogawa, T., Avarbock, M.R., Brinster, R.L., and Russell, L.D. (1998). Germ cell genotype controls cell cycle during spermatogenesis in the rat. *Biol. Reprod. 59(6)*:1371–1377.

Gage, F.H. (2000). Mammalian neural stem cells. *Science 287(5457)*:1433–1438.

Gage, F.H., Coates, P.W., Palmer, T.D., Kuhn, H.G., Fisher, L.J., Suhonen, J.O. *et al.* (1995). Survival and differentiation of adult neuronal progenitor cells transplanted to the adult brain. *Proc. Natl. Acad. Sci. USA 92(25)*:11879–11883.

Galli, R., Borello, U., Gritti, A., Minasi, M.G., Bjornson, C., Coletta, M. *et al.* (2000). Skeletal myogenic potential of human and mouse neural stem cells. *Nat. Neurosci. 3(10)*:986–991.

Goldring, K., Partridge, T., and Watt, D. (2002). Muscle stem cells. *J. Pathol. 197(4)*:457–467.

Guan, K., Chang, H., Rolletschek, A., and Wobus, A.M. (2001). Embryonic stem cell-derived neurogenesis. Retinoic acid induction and lineage selection of neuronal cells. *Cell Tissue Res. 305(2)*:171–176.

Hamazaki, T., Iiboshi, Y., Oka, M., Papst, P.J., Meacham, A.M., Zon, L.I. *et al.* (2001). Hepatic maturation in differentiating embryonic stem cells in vitro. *FEBS Lett. 497*(1):15–19.

Kaufman, D.S. and Thomson, J.A. (2002). Human ES cells–haematopoiesis and transplantation strategies. *J. Anat. 200(Pt 3)*:243–248.

Kehat, I., Kenyagin-Karsenti, D., Snir, M., Segev, H., Amit, M., Gepstein, A. *et al.* (2001). Human embryonic stem cells can differentiate into myocytes with structural and functional properties of cardiomyocytes. *J. Clin. Invest. 108(3)*:407–414.

Kim, J.H., Auerbach, J.M., Rodriguez-Gomez, J.A., Velasco, I., Gavin, D., Lumelsky, N., Lee, S.H. *et al.* (2002). Dopamine neurons derived from embryonic stem cells function in an animal model of Parkinson's disease. *Nature 418(6893)*:50–56.

Kramer, J., Hegert, C., Guan, K., Wobus, A.M., Muller, P.K., and Rohwedel, J. (2000). Embryonic stem cell-derived chondrogenic differentiation in vitro: activation by BMP-2 and BMP-4. *Mech. Dev. 92(2)*:193–205.

Lazaro, C.A., Rhim, J.A., Yamada, Y., and Fausto, N. (1998). Generation of hepatocytes from oval cell precursors in culture. *Cancer Res. 58(23)*:5514–5522.

Lipton, B.H. and Schultz, E. (1979). Developmental fate of skeletal muscle satellite cells. *Science 205*(4412):1292–1294.

Lumelsky, N., Blondel, O., Laeng, P., Velasco, I., Ravin, R., and McKay, R. (2001). Differentiation of embryonic stem cells to insulin-secreting structures similar to pancreatic islets. *Science 292(5520)*:1389 1394.

Machluf, M., Orsola, A., Boorjian, S., Kershen, R., and Atala, A. (2003). Microencapsulation of Leydig cells: a system for testosterone supplementation. *Endocrinology 144(11)*:4975–4979.

Maltsev, V.A., Rohwedel, J., Hescheler, J., and Wobus, A.M. (1993). Embryonic stem cells differentiate in vitro into cardiomyocytes representing sinusnodal, atrial and ventricular cell types. *Mech. Dev. 44(1)*:41–50.

Martin, G.R. (1981). Isolation of a pluripotent cell line from early mouse embryos cultured in medium conditioned by teratocarcinoma stem cells. *Proc. Natl. Acad. Sci. USA 78(12)*:7634–7638.

Matsui, Y., Zsebo, K., and Hogan, B.L. (1992). Derivation of pluripotential embryonic stem cells from murine primordial germ cells in culture. *Cell 70(5)*:841–847.

Mauro, A. (1961). Satellite cell of skeletal muscle fibers. *J. Biophys. Biochem. Cytol. 9*:493–495.

McLaren, A. (2001). Ethical and social considerations of stem cell research. *Nature 414(6859)*:129–131.

Miller-Hance, W.C., LaCorbiere, M., Fuller, S.J., Evans, S.M., Lyons, G., Schmidt, C. *et al.* (1993). In vitro chamber specification during embryonic stem cell cardiogenesis. Expression of the ventricular myosin light chain-2 gene is independent of heart tube formation. *J. Biol. Chem. 268(33)*:25244–25252.

Morrison, S.J., Wandycz, A.M., Hemmati, H.D., Wright, D.E., and Weissman, I.L. (1997). Identification of a lineage of multipotent hematopoietic progenitors. *Development 124(10)*:1929–1939.

Morrison, S.J. and Weissman, I.L. (1994). The long-term repopulating subset of hematopoietic stem cells is deterministic and isolatable by phenotype. *Immunity 1(8)*:661–673.

Nakano, T., Kodama, H., and Honjo, T. (1996). In vitro development of primitive and definitive erythrocytes from different precursors. *Science 272(5262)*:722–724.

Petersen, B.E., Zajac, V.F., and Michalopoulos, G.K. (1998). Hepatic oval cell activation in response to injury following chemically induced periportal or pericentral damage in rats. *Hepatology 27(4)*:1030–1038.

Poulsom, R., Alison, M.R., Forbes, S.J., and Wright, N.A. (2002). Adult stem cell plasticity. *J. Pathol. 197(4)*:441–456.

Pye, D. and Watt, D.J. (2001). Dermal fibroblasts participate in the formation of new muscle fibres when implanted into regenerating normal mouse muscle. *J. Anat. 198(Pt 2)*:163–173.

Raper, S.E., Grossman, M., Rader, D.J., Thoene, J.G., Clark, B.J., III, Kolansky, D.M. *et al.* (1996). Safety and feasibility of liver-directed ex vivo gene therapy for homozygous familial hypercholesterolemia. *Ann. Surg. 223(2)*:116–126.

Reubinoff, B.E., Itsykson, P., Turetsky, T., Pera, M.F., Reinhartz, E., Itzik, A. *et al.* (2001). Neural progenitors from human embryonic stem cells. *Nat. Biotechnol. 19(12)*:1134–1140.

Risau, W., Sariola, H., Zerwes, H.G., Sasse, J., Ekblom, P., Kemler, R. *et al.* (1988). Vasculogenesis and angiogenesis in embryonic-stem-cell-derived embryoid bodies. *Development 102(3)*:471–478.

Rohwedel, J., Guan, K., Hegert, C., and Wobus, A.M. (2001). Embryonic stem cells as an in vitro model for mutagenicity, cytotoxicity and embryotoxicity studies: present state and future prospects. *Toxicol. In Vitro 15(6)*:741 753.

Rohwedel, J., Maltsev, V., Bober, E., Arnold, H.H., Hescheler, J., and Wobus, A.M. (1994). Muscle cell differentiation of embryonic stem cells reflects myogenesis in vivo: developmentally regulated expression of myogenic determination genes and functional expression of ionic currents. *Dev. Biol. 164(1)*:87 101.

Roskams, T., De, V.R., Van, E.P., Myazaki, H., Van, D.B., and Desmet, V. (1998). Hepatic OV-6 expression in human liver disease and rat experiments: evidence for hepatic progenitor cells in man. *J. Hepatol. 29(3)*:455–463.

Schuldiner, M., Yanuka, O., Itskovitz-Eldor, J., Melton, D.A., and Benvenisty, N. (2000). Effects of eight growth factors on the differentiation of cells derived from human embryonic stem cells. *Proc. Natl. Acad. Sci. USA 97(21)*:11307–11312.

Schultz, E. and Lipton, B.H. (1982). Skeletal muscle satellite cells: changes in proliferation potential as a function of age. *Mech. Ageing Dev. 20(4)*:377–383.

Sell, S. (2001). Heterogeneity and plasticity of hepatocyte lineage cells. *Hepatology 33(3)*:738–750.

Shamblott, M.J., Axelman, J., Wang, S., Bugg, E.M., Littlefield, J.W., Donovan, P.J. *et al.* (1998). Derivation of pluripotent stem cells from cultured human primordial germ cells. *Proc. Natl. Acad. Sci. USA 95(23)*:13726–13731.

Strom, S.C., Fisher, R.A., Thompson, M.T., Sanyal, A.J., Cole, P.E., Ham, J.M. *et al.* (1997). Hepatocyte transplantation as a bridge to orthotopic liver transplantation in terminal liver failure. *Transplantation 63(4)*:559–569.

Suhonen, J.O., Peterson, D.A., Ray, J., and Gage, F.H. (1996). Differentiation of adult hippocampus-derived progenitors into olfactory neurons in vivo. *Nature 383(6601)*:624–627.

Thomson, J.A., Itskovitz-Eldor, J., Shapiro, S.S., Waknitz, M.A., Swiergiel, J.J., Marshall, V.S. *et al.* (1998). Embryonic stem cell lines derived from human blastocysts. *Science 282(5391)*:1145–1147.

Thorgeirsson, S.S. (1996). Hepatic stem cells in liver regeneration. *FASEB J. 10(11)*:1249–1256.

Till, J.E. and McCulloch, E.A. (1961). A direct measurement of the radiation sensitivity of normal mouse bone marrow cells. *Radiat. Res. 14*:213–222.

Uchida, N., Buck, D.W., He, D., Reitsma, M.J., Masek, M., Phan, T.V. *et al.* (2000). Direct isolation of human central nervous system stem cells. *Proc. Natl. Acad. Sci. USA 97(26)*:14720–14725.

Uchida, N., Tsukamoto, A., He, D., Friera, A.M., Scollay, R., and Weissman, I.L. (1998). High doses of purified stem cells cause early hematopoietic recovery in syngeneic and allogeneic hosts. *J. Clin. Invest. 101(5)*:961–966.

Vessey, C.J. and de la Hall, P.M. (2001). Hepatic stem cells: a review. *Pathology 33(2)*:130–141.

Wakitani, S., Saito, T., and Caplan, A.I. (1995). Myogenic cells derived from rat bone marrow mesenchymal stem cells exposed to 5-azacytidine. *Muscle Nerve 18(12)*:1417–1426.

Weissman, I.L. (2000). Stem cells: units of development, units of regeneration, and units in evolution. *Cell 100(1)*:157–168.

Wiles, M.V. and Keller, G. (1991). Multiple hematopoietic lineages develop from embryonic stem (ES) cells in culture. *Development 111(2)*:259–267.

Wilmut, I., Schnieke, A.E., McWhir, J., Kind, A.J., and Campbell, K.H. (1997). Viable offspring derived from fetal and adult mammalian cells. *Nature 385(6619)*:810–813.

Wobus, A.M., Kaomei, G., Shan, J., Wellner, M.C., Rohwedel, J., Ji, G. *et al.* (1997). Retinoic acid accelerates embryonic stem cell-derived cardiac differentiation and enhances development of ventricular cardiomyocytes. *J. Mol. Cell Cardiol. 29(6)*:1525–1539.

Yamashita, J., Itoh, H., Hirashima, M., Ogawa, M., Nishikawa, S., Yurugi, T. *et al.* (2000). Flk1-positive cells derived from embryonic stem cells serve as vascular progenitors. *Nature 408(6808)*:92–96.

Yoo, J.J. and Atala, A. (2000). Tissue engineering applications in the genitourinary tract system. *Yonsei Med J. 41(6)*:789–802.

Zhang, S.C., Wernig, M., Duncan, I.D., Brustle, O., and Thomson, J.A. (2001). In vitro differentiation of transplantable neural precursors from human embryonic stem cells. *Nat. Biotechnol. 19(12)*:1129–1133.

46

Nuclear Transfer and Cloning: Preservation or Expansion of Proliferative Lifespan?

Keith E. Latham

Cloning of animals by somatic cell nuclear transfer has provided the potential for undertaking therapeutic cloning to produce stem cells that can be used to treat human disease. This chapter considers limitations in the ability of the oocyte to restore replicative potential to adult somatic cell nuclei. Specifically, questions related to somatic mutation load and aneuploidy, mitochondrial replacement, and telomere restoration are considered. Additionally, the feasibility of therapeutic cloning in humans is addressed.

Introduction

Complex organisms are comprised of two fundamental lineages, the germ cell lineage and the somatic lineage. The germ cell lineage produces during each generation the gametes that are required for reproduction, and thus must be immortal. This lineage must undergo meiotic recombination but remains genetically intact, and must retain full replicative potential, reflected, for example, in elongated telomeres and robust mitochondria, so that each new generation begins at the same starting point. A general feature of development of most animals, marking its unique place in the life cycle, is that the germ line forms quite early, often before the major differentiative milestones of the soma.

The somatic lineage, by contrast, is required to grow and develop in order to form the vessel for carrying the germ line, provide the mechanical means for accomplishing reproduction, and provide some measure of early support to the resulting progeny. The multitude of sizes, morphologies, and behaviors seen among organisms comprise specific adaptations to enable the soma to complete its mission. Once its reproductive mission has been accomplished, the soma becomes evolutionarily expendable, to a degree that varies with the degree of support of the offspring early in their lives. The endurance of the soma is affected by a variety of factors, primarily disease, environmental factors, and the genetically programmed onset of senescence as individuals age.

For most organisms, maximum lifespan is established at birth, being determined by the individual genotype. For the first time in history, however, *Homo sapiens*, unique among all other organisms, may possess the potential to modify an individual's maximum lifespan, by manipulating the long-term fate of the somatic component, effectively overcoming the preordained limits imposed by the individual genotype. This potential has arisen out of the new and exciting technology known as mammalian somatic cell nuclear transfer (SCNT), wherein nuclei from somatic cells are transplanted into oocytes, followed by the activation and development of the resulting construct. With this technology, it is now possible, in theory at least, to derive stem cells that are genetically identical to any individual. These stem cells can be manipulated in culture to correct genetic defects, and made to differentiate along specific pathways in order to produce cells for tissue repair.

This exciting new technology has raised a myriad of ethical and moral issues. These will not be addressed here. Instead, this review will address the question: To what degree can stem cells derived by the SCNT method and associated technologies modulate the lifespan of an individual? In addressing this question, three fundamental restrictions of cellular proliferative lifespan will be evaluated, namely, somatic mutation load, mitochondrial fitness, and replicative potential of the genome as reflected in telomere length.

Overview of SCNT Method

The cloning method requires the substitution of a somatic cell genome in place of a normal embryonic genome (see Figure 46.1).

Early efforts to accomplish this using fertilized 1-cell cytoplasts as recipients failed to produce advanced development. It is now clear that the oocyte possesses a myriad of activities that mediate important early events that normally prepare the incoming sperm-derived nucleus for function. One such activity is the ability to disrupt the nuclear envelope (nuclear envelope breakdown, or NEB) (Latham, 1999). Another is the ability to exchange chromatin proteins. Normally, protamines must be removed and replaced with histones.

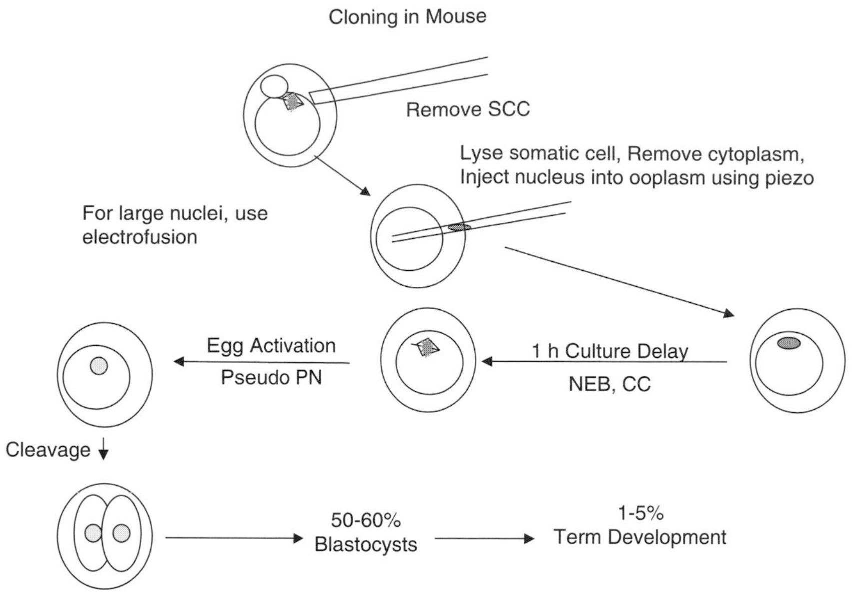

Figure 46.1 Basic steps of cloning in mice. The MII stage oocyte genetic material is first removed along with the second meiotic spindle. A donor nucleus is lysed with a narrow bore pipet and the nucleus injected into the oocyte using a piezo pipet drill to assist. If donor cells are larger and have larger nuclei, electrofusion can be employed. During the following hour, the nuclear envelope breaks down, chromosomes condense, and a new spindle forms. The oocyte is then activated to initiate cleavage development. As indicated, development to term remains somewhat inefficient.

Additionally, oocyte-specific chromatin proteins typically are assembled onto the incoming sperm DNA (e.g., oocyte-specific histones; Latham (1999); Gao and Latham (2004)). Another activity is the ability to direct nuclear envelope formation and DNA decondensation, leading ultimately to the transcriptional activation of the genome (Latham, 1999). All these activities are developmentally regulated, and essentially lost within a few hours of oocyte activation (Latham, 1999).

Somatic cell nuclei need to recapitulate the same sequence of events as does the incoming sperm nucleus, but when zygote stage recipients are employed, these activities are no longer present, the corresponding processes do not occur, and embryos fail to develop. For this reason, oocytes are most often employed for nuclear transfer, and this typically involves the use of metaphase II (MII) stage oocytes. The first step in the procedure is to remove the oocyte genome, typically by aspirating the spindle-chromosome complex (SCC) into a small glass micropipette. This can be accomplished by a variety of means, each particularly suited to a given species. It should be noted that this procedure eliminates not only the oocyte DNA, but also other factors that are specifically associated with the SCC. After SCC removal, the donor cell nucleus can be introduced. There are three basic kinds of methods employed for nuclear transfer to MII stage oocytes. One involves fusion of the entire donor cell to the oocyte. Fusion is accomplished most often by electrofusion, wherein one or more electrical pulses are delivered in order to induce membrane fluidity changes that lead to fusion. Some alternative fusion methods involve the use of inactivated Sendai virus, or chemicals such as polyethylene glycol coupled with the use of phytohemagluttin. Fusion methods have the advantage of being somewhat noninvasive, but the disadvantages are that the entire contents of the donor cell are transferred to the oocyte, and that the efficiency of cell fusion is reduced by smaller donor cell size, which reduces physical contact between donor cell and oocyte. The second method of nuclear transfer involves simple injection of the nucleus into the oocyte. This works with some species, but not with all (e.g., rodents), due to an increased propensity for the oocyte to lyse after injection. The third method, first applied in rodents, is to employ a piezo-assisted pipette driver, which permits microinjection of nuclei, for example, into rodent oocytes, without lysis. With the injection methods, the donor cell can be lysed and repeatedly aspirated and expelled in order to remove the bulk of the cytoplasm before injection.

Once the nuclear transfer has been accomplished, typically one hour or more is permitted for the ooplasm to act upon the nucleus, bringing about NEB and then condensation of chromosomes (CC) and their assembly on a newly formed spindle. Then, the nuclear transfer construct is activated to begin development, whereupon pseudo-pronuclei form and the embryo eventually undergoes cleavage. Activation can be accomplished either as a result of electrical pulses (in some cases delivered at the time of fusion) or the use of chemical treatments, such as the use of ionophores, cycloheximide, 6-dimethylaminopurine (DMAP), or strontium chloride in calcium-free medium. Recent studies in fertilized embryos revealed a potentially important role for sperm-induced calcium oscillations in long-term embryo viability, with particular relevance on the amplitude, number, and frequency of such oscillations (Ducibella *et al.*, 2002). As such oscillations likely are not recapitulated during artificial oocyte activation, cloned embryos may be initially disadvantaged relative to fertilized embryos due to an absence of correct calcium signaling and downstream events.

Once the cloned constructs are activated, they must be cultured *in vitro* for some period before being returned to the reproductive tract of a suitable foster mother for continued gestation. Recent studies reveal that cloned embryos have radically different culture medium requirements as compared with fertilized embryos (Latham, 2004). This is most likely the result of continued expression of genes from the donor cell nucleus. Reprogramming of gene expression appears to be a rather prolonged process, possibly continuing until just before the time of gastrulation. As a result, when gene transcription commences in the early cloned embryo, many somatic cell-expressed genes will be aberrantly expressed in the embryo. The products of these aberrantly expressed genes likely alter basic processes of osmoregulation, homeostasis, and metabolism (these processes differ substantially between somatic cells and normal fertilized embryos). Thus, although traditional embryo culture media have been most widely employed for culturing cloned embryos, such media are likely to be grossly suboptimal. In fact, somatic cell formulations have produced superior results in several instances (Latham, 2004). The cloning technique is thus faced with a fundamental problem: in order to achieve continued development, embryos must be returned to the reproductive tract, and yet the environment there is likely optimized for fertilized embryos and thus poorly suited to cloned embryos. If we accept the possibility that nuclear reprogramming continues up through the time of gastrulation, then it is likely that the exposure of the cloned embryos to a suboptimal environment, either *in vitro* or *in vivo*, inhibits the reprogramming process and reduces clone viability.

The overall outcome of the cloning procedure is that only about 1 to 5% of all nuclear transfer constructs develop to term. About half of all constructs can complete preimplantation development, and then there are additional waves of loss during the peri-implantation period, and around the time of gastrulation (Yanagimachi, 2002). From the standpoint of contemplating therapeutic uses for cloning, it is fortunate that a substantial number of constructs can form blastocysts and eventually give rise to an inner cell mass population, from which can be derived embryonic stem cells (ESCs).

The Question of Donor Cell State

One theoretical uncertainty that besets all cloning studies is the precise phenotypic state of the donor cells from which the rare surviving clones are obtained. Typically, adult or fetal tissues are dissociated into single-cell suspensions. Various enrichment procedures might be employed to favor isolation of a particular cell type. The operator then selects from that suspension cells of a particular type. For example, the operator might select the smallest size cells present, presumably because such cells should be in the G1 stage of the cell cycle, if MII stage oocytes are employed as recipients and polar body extrusion is prevented during oocyte activation. Alternatively, G2/M phase cells may be selected if polar body extrusion is to be permitted. The cell cycle status of cultures can be manipulated (e.g., by serum starvation/stimulation) to enrich for cells of particular cell cycle stages. If no further enrichment methods are applied, the donor cells are thus selected from a population that is to some degree heterogeneous. Within that population of cells may reside somatic stem cells. Whether such rare stem cells in fact contribute preferentially to live clone births has not been thoroughly studied. There are two circumstances in which the presence of stem cells probably does not contribute to cloning outcome. First, differentiated cells expressing specific molecular markers can be employed. In such cases, cloning success rates are about an order of magnitude lower than observed with primary cell sources (Hochedlinger and Jaenisch, 2002), an outcome that could reflect the differentiated state, absence of stem cells, or simply a differential response of clones made with those particular cell types to the *in vitro* cloned embryo culture system. The second circumstance wherein stem cell contamination would not affect outcome would be in cases where clonally selected cell lines are established following genetic manipulation (e.g., gene knockout or transgenesis).

Whether stem cells contribute preferentially to the production of clones that develop to term could affect conclusions derived from the study of cloned progeny. Stem cells can differ from differentiated cells in fundamental respects such as the number of past rounds of cell division, telomere length, and telomerase expression. Because reprogramming is slow, these phenotypic differences between stem cells and differentiated cells will likely persist to some degree in cloned embryos. Thus, conclusions regarding somatic mutation load, mitochondrial fitness, and replicative potential of the genome as reflected in telomere length in the context of cloned embryo and cloned stem cell derivation need to account for possible effects of donor cell state.

Somatic Mutations and Effects on SCNT

ANEUPLOIDY AND POLYPLOIDY ARISING DURING CLONING

Recent studies reveal that a large proportion of cells in cloned blastocysts are aneuploid or polyploid (Nolen *et al.*, 2005; Booth *et al.*, 2003; Shi *et al.*, 2004). Thus, although a large proportion of cloned constructs can attain blastocyst stage and be used to generate ESCs, the genetic integrity of the ESCs obtained must initially be suspect. This places obvious restrictions and requirements on plans to employ clone-derived ESCs for therapy.

When does this aneuploidy arise? We might argue that this most likely occurs during the early cleavage divisions of the cloned constructs, on the premise that the somatic cells should initially be predominantly euploid. In a recent study of aneuploid in cloned bovine embryos, completely euploid constructs comprised only 22% of the total blastocyst population based on the analysis of two chromosomes; the remaining embryos were either polyploid or mixoploid (Booth *et al.*, 2003). A significant rate of polyploidy/aneuploidy was also observed in mouse cloned blastocysts, although less than the rate seen in the bovine study (Nolen *et al.*, 2005). If we assume that at most only a small fraction of somatic cells would be aneuploid or polyploid, then these results suggest that aneuploidy/polyploidy in cloned embryos likely arises due to mitotic errors during cleavage.

It has been suggested that cloning in primate species may be hindered by the removal of proteins associated with the SCC (Simerly *et al.*, 2003, 2004). Studies in mice reveal spindle defects in SCNT embryos (Miyara *et al.*, 2006). Other studies reveal that removal of the SCC likely depletes the embryo of factors that otherwise could modulate its phenotypes (i.e., tetraploid constructs prepared by SCNT without SCC removal appear more like fertilized embryos than do diploid clones) (Gao and Latham, 2004).

It is also possible that aneuploidy in clones is the result of aneuploidy in the donor cells. In a study of developing brain, one-third of neuroblasts were aneuploid (Rehen *et al.*, 2001). Aneuploidy was also detectable in adult neurons, which displayed more than 1% aneuploidy for sex chromosomes.

With respect to producing ESCs for therapy, it appears likely that a stringent selection may operate, such that clones with a greater degree of aneuploidy/polyploidy tend to have smaller numbers of cells (Booth *et al.*, 2003), and thus may be less likely to form a healthy inner cell mass from which to derive an ESC line. This may account for why the one clone-derived human ESC line is euploid (Hwang *et al.*, 2004), despite evidence from bovine clones of a high rate of aneuploidy.

SOMATIC MUTATIONS IN CLONING

Somatic mutation and somatic recombination following DNA damage and repair could affect the outcome of cloning procedures. Exposure to mutagenic chemicals and radiation can obviously damage somatic cells. Nondividing stem cells within adult tissues could be less susceptible to damage by transient exposures. Cloning with somatic cells bearing *de novo* mutations would then give rise to cloned embryos displaying either lethality or aberrant phenotypes later in life. Recombination-based repair of DNA damage, as well as aberrant mitoses can lead to loss of heterozygosity or uniparental disomy for entire chromosomes or chromosome regions. Loss of heterozygosity could lead to phenotypic exposure of recessive traits, whereas uniparental disomy could lead to abnormal phenotypes associated with imprinted regions of the genome.

CLONING WITH CANCER CELLS

Cancer cells display characteristics of continued cell growth, lack of crisis or senescence in culture, altered growth properties (e.g., anchorage independence), and an arrest or reversion of cellular differentiation. These characteristics can arise through a combination of somatic oncogenic mutations and loss of genomic integrity, including gene duplication/amplification and loss of heterozygosity. An obvious question made approachable by the SCNT method is whether the oocyte can reprogram the nuclei of such cells to an embryonic state. Additionally, we can ask whether the oncogenic mutations in particular cancer cells would predispose the cloned animal to only a single form of cancer, or to cancer in multiple tissues.

Cloning with cancer cells recently has been reported. Hochedlinger *et al.* (2004) reported that cloning with several types of cancer cells (leukemia, lymphoma, breast cancer) led to the formation of blastocysts, but not to development of inner cell masses (ICMs), the early progenitor of the embryo proper and ESCs. However, ESCs were established from clones made with nuclei from a RAS-inducible melanoma cell line, and these were subsequently used to produce chimeric mice using the tetraploid complementation method. The chimeric mice were predisposed to cancer, with an expanded spectrum of tumorigenesis. This result reveals that, although developmental pluripotency can be conferred upon cancer cell nuclei by the cloning method, the genetic factors that originally induced carcinogenesis predispose the clone to develop tumors of the same type as the donor, as well as other cell types that can respond to that genetic defect.

It is interesting that cloning by SCNT provides a novel means of exploring the transforming potential of various carcinogenic genetic changes by providing a situation in which the effects of those genetic lesions can be examined during the formation of all the cell lineages of the body. Blelloch *et al.* (2004) produced ESCs from clones made with embryonal carcinoma cell nuclei. These ESCs behaved much like the embryonal carcinoma cells themselves, with respect to developmental potential, a result that appears to be related to specific genetic lesions in the embryonal carcinoma cells. Shi *et al.* (2003) found that bovine immortalized cell nuclei were unable to support clone development to the blastocyst stage, even following a number of treatments applied in order to try to expand developmental potential. Sheep clones made with nuclei from nontransformed fibroblasts immortalized with the human telomerase (hTERT) gene can display significant postimplantation development (Cui *et al.*, 2003).

Although elevated telomerase expression maintained telomere length and prevented senescence in the donor cell cultures, no term development was achieved (Cui *et al.*, 2003). This could reflect a cell-line specific or insertion site-specific defect, or could reflect an inhibitory effect of immortalization and elevated hTERT expression on development. It is interesting that fetal development was achieved in the study of Cui *et al.* (2003) but not that of Shi *et al.* (2003). This may reflect the activity of additional genetic lesions in the cells employed by Shi *et al.* (2003), rather than an effect of immortalization specifically. Species-specific differences also must be considered. Further studies defining the effects of various immortalizing or transforming mutations on the ability to establish pluripotency should prove interesting.

Mitochondrial Fitness

MITOCHONDRIAL CHANGES DURING AGING

The preceding section illustrates that genetic alterations in the somatic cells employed as nuclear donors for SCNT exert effects on cloned embryo phenotypes. What of the mitochondrial genome? The mitochondrial theory of aging holds that mitochondria accumulate mutations as a result of damage by reactive oxygen species they generate, and that the accumulation of defective mitochondria leads ultimately to cellular senescence and tissue degeneration. The rate of repair relative to the incidence of DNA damage would affect the overall rate of accumulation of damaged mitochondrial genomes.

MITOCHONDRIAL FATE AFTER SCNT

If cells harboring these mutant mitochondria are selected for SCNT, several possible fates might await them. As "foreign" (i.e., not oocytic) mitochondria, they might actively be eliminated, much as sperm mitochondria typically are eliminated. They might fail to replicate and thus be eliminated by attrition. They might persist in the embryo, leading to mitochondrial heteroplasmy. Last, they might experience a replicative advantage over endogenous ooplasmic mitochondria, and thus become the predominant mitochondria in the cloned animal.

In one study, a mouse model was employed in which mitochondrial dysfunction was associated with telomere shortening and genomic instability (Liu *et al.*, 2002). Using nuclear transfer to transfer nuclei from cells with defective mitochondria to oocytes with normal mitochondria alleviated these defects. This suggests that mitochondrial defects related to aging might be eliminated by nuclear transfer. To what extent replacement of "aged" mitochondria by "young" ooplasmic mitochondria would occur is not clear. A variety of nuclear transfer studies have described diverse results concerning the fate of mitochondria after various micromanipulations involving oocytes.

Oocytes are designed to eliminate the mitochondria that are transmitted via the sperm (Kaneda *et al.*, 1995). These paternal mitochondria carry ubiquitin tags that seem to target them for elimination by the ooplasm (Sutovsky *et al.*, 2000). Interestingly, with interspecies crosses, paternal mitochondria can avoid elimination (Kaneda *et al.*, 1995), indicating that there exists species specificity to the recognition of the sperm ubiquitinated proteins by the ooplasm. Cell type specificity also exists. Injection of *Mus spretus* spermatid or liver mitochondria into oocytes of *Mus domesticus* revealed that the liver mitochondria persisted to birth, whereas spermatid mitochondria were gradually eliminated and then were not detected in progeny (Shitara *et al.*, 2000). It is therefore unlikely that donor cell mitochondria would be eliminated in cloned embryos by the same mechanism that eliminates sperm mitochondria, as the donor cell mitochondria would not be expected to carry the appropriate ubiquitinated tags.

If not actively eliminated, then to what degree might donor cell mitochondria in SCNT embryos be eliminated by attrition, persist at a low level, or assume a replicative advantage over endogenous mitochondria? Mitochondrial heteroplasmy was not observed in sheep clones (Evans *et al.*, 1999). In SCNT embryos made with *Bos indicus*, donor nuclei transferred to *Bos taurus* oocytes, donor cell mitochondria were nearly undetectable in cloned fetuses (Hiendler *et al.*, 2003) and calves (Meirelles *et al.*, 2001). However, donor cell mitochondria were not eliminated in monkey-to-rabbit or panda-to-rabbit NT embryos (Chen *et al.*, 2002; Yang *et al.*, 2003). Mitochondrial heteroplasmy was also reported for nuclear transfers made between Holstein and Luxi Yellow cow (Han *et al.*, 2004), and in other studies involving bovine species (Takeda *et al.*, 2003; Steinborn *et al.*, 2002). Embryonic blastomere nuclear transfer in *Macaca mullatta* produces offspring with mitochondria from both the recipient oocyte and the donor blastomere (St. John and Schatten, 2004). In this case, both maternal and paternal mitochondria derived from the donor embryonic blastomere were detected, indicating that the sperm mitochondria were not eliminated as expected, revealing a possible defect in the process of paternal mitochondrial elimination in cloned constructs. Similarly, with ooplasm transfer approaches in human infertility treatment, mitochondrial heteroplasmy can be detectable in the resulting children (Barritt *et al.*, 2001). Collectively, the results obtained to date indicate that mitochondrial heteroplasmy is likely to accompany the application of SCNT methods in the human.

The persistence of mitochondrial heteroplasmy to birth indicates that the donor cell mitochondria replicate following SCNT. In some cases, the donor cell mitochondria may actually have a replicative advantage. In the panda-to-rabbit NT embryos, donor cell mitochondria, in fact, can become the predominant organelle by fetal life (Chen *et al.*, 2002). In bovine NT studies, donor cell mitochondria can account for as much as 40% of the total (Takeda *et al.*, 2003), again indicating a replicative advantage over recipient mitochondria at some point during development. It is worth noting that, although it is often assumed that donor cell mitochondria might be eliminated due to incompatibilities with recipient cell nuclear genomes, these observations indicate that this need not always be the case. It is thus of interest that mitochondria carrying mutated genomes can be unevenly distributed within adult tissues, consistent with a clonal expansion (both intracellular and cellular) during aging (Khrapko *et al.*, 2003). The ability of such mutated mitochondria from aging cells to expand within adult tissues might also result in their expansion, and possibly a replicative advantage, in SCNT embryos.

Replicative Potential

TELOMERE LENGTH CHANGES DURING DEVELOPMENT AND *IN VITRO* CULTURE

With the exception of stem cells, the replicative potential of somatic cells is limited due to the eventual onset of cellular senescence. It is widely thought that progressive shortening of telomeres during DNA replication contributes to the aging process, so that after a sufficient number of rounds of replication, the telomeres shorten below a critical point needed to maintain genomic integrity. Overexpression of telomerase can be associated with cellular immortalization and may contribute to cancer, although other events leading to uncapped, shortened telomeres are also associated with cancer (Cui *et al.*, 2003; Wai, 2004). During normal development, telomerase activity may decline with age. Shorter lived species display a rapid loss of telomerase activity during development, whereas longer lived species delay this decrease in telomerase activity (Haussman *et al.*, 2004). Increased telomere length in *Caenorhabditis elegans* correlates with increased life span (Joeng *et al.*, 2004). Oxidative DNA damage from reactive oxygen species, irradiation, and various forms of stress are believed to shorten telomeres prematurely, leading to accelerated aging (Kawanishi *et al.*, 2004; Liu *et al.*, 2002).

SERIAL NUCLEAR TRANSFER

One striking result to come from SCNT studies is the apparent extension of replicative potential that accompanies the process. This is most apparent where serial nuclear transfer has been undertaken. This is the process of producing cloned embryos or progeny, recloning using donor cells from that cloned individual, and repeating the process for a number of generations. This has been performed in both cattle (Stice and Keefer, 1993; Puera and Trounson, 1998) and mice (Wakayama *et al.*, 2000). An additional type of serial NT indicative of expanded replicative potential involves not repeated rounds of NT, but rather the derivation of NT ESCs, which are then employed as nuclear donors for cloning. Thus, with nuclear transplantation, it is possible to entice adult somatic cell genomes to undergo extensive replication, illustrating an expanded replicative potential relative to the original donor cells.

PRESERVATION VERSUS ELONGATION OF TELOMERE LENGTH IN CLONED ANIMALS

The expanded replicative potential demonstrated by serial NT indicates that progressive diminishment of telomere length may be halted following the initial NT step in order to permit an expanded replicative potential. It is also possible that telomere lengths become expanded during cloning, under the influence of reactivated expression of telomerase, thus restoring an authentic embryonic cellular replicative potential. A third possibility relates to the inherent uncertainties about donor cell origins, and the low efficiency of success of the cloning procedure; specifically, that the rare donor cell nuclei that give rise to the rare surviving clones represent stem cell contaminants in the donor cell population. Stem cells would likely possess longer telomeres than differentiated cells, and yet this greater telomere length would be undetectable by typical Southern blot hybridization of the whole cell population. Stem cells may also possess a greater capacity to activate telomerase expression after SCNT and restore telomere length to counter aging effects evident in differentiated cells (Allsopp *et al.*, 2003). The first of these two possibilities have been examined extensively in a variety of studies of clones of many different species, but the third possibility related to stem cell donor nuclei remains to be examined.

The Wilmut laboratory reported that nuclear transfer can lead to telomere elongation of late-passage donor cells (fibroblasts) used for cloning in sheep, but that the telomeres do not become fully restored relative to early passage cells (Clark *et al.*, 2003). Dolly was reported to have shorter than normal telomeres (Shiels *et al.*, 1999), consistent with incomplete restoration of telomere length (Clark *et al.*, 2003). Observations in cattle indicated that cloned calves could be obtained from senescent fibroblasts, suggesting an ability to elongate telomeres and thus restore replicative potential (Lanza *et al.*, 2000). Other studies (Tian *et al.*, 2000; Betts *et al.*, 2001) reported cloned calves made using fibroblast nuclei possessed telomeres that were not different from those of control calves, indicating restoration of telomere length relative to donor nuclei. Kato *et al.* (2000) reported that the observed telomere lengths of clones depended on the cell type assayed; telomere length in ear cells of cloned calves were similar to those of ear cells of the nuclear donor animal, but that telomere length was shorter in white blood cells of clones. Miyashita *et al.* (2002) reported that donor clones made with muscle and fibroblast cell nuclei had telomeres longer than those of the donor animal, but similar to control calves, whereas clones made with cumulus, mammary epithelial, and oviductal cell nuclei had telomeres shorter than those of control animals. Clones made with embryonic stem cell nuclei appeared to have expanded telomeres. Thus, a donor cell type effect on subsequent telomere length appeared to occur.

The results of Miyashita *et al.* (2002) may reflect the continued expression of the donor cell program in the early cloned embryo, so that different nuclear donor cell types may direct different levels of expression of telomerase and other factors required for telomere elongation. An alternative explanation for the apparent effect of donor cell type is that the different populations contain different proportions of some form of undifferentiated stem cell. If the donor cell gene expression program continues after nuclear transfer, and includes telomerase expression, then such a donor cell nucleus could direct the expression of telomerase and expansion of its own telomeres. The variability seen among different tissues of cloned animals bears further study. Additionally, species-dependent differences in replicative potential, which varies with adult size (Haussmann *et al.*, 2003), could contribute to diversity in observations obtained with different model organisms. Overall, it appears that cloning by SCNT can lead to telomere expansion, but the degree of that expansion is affected by a variety of factors, most notably donor cell type.

GENETIC MANIPULATION OF TELOMERE LENGTHS OF DONOR NUCLEI

One approach that has been applied recently to cloning in animals is to try to manipulate genetically the donor cell genome so that it becomes more efficient for SCNT. Cui *et al.* (2003) performed SCNT with telomerase-immortalized cells. The nuclei from these cells supported significant development, but were unable to support term development. It is thus not clear whether such genetic manipulation of telomerase expression confers sufficient advantage to offset the risk associated with mutagenesis of the genome.

Conclusion

Cloned animals that are born and survive beyond the neonatal period and appear generally of good health seem to be capable of lifespans that are normal for the species. Dolly was born in mid-1996 and died in 2003. A majority of cloned mice of otherwise apparently normal phenotypes display normal lifespans (Yanagimachi, 2002). These results illustrate that reproductive cloning is possible, without profound restrictions on lifespan. Serial NT studies further illustrate the ability of SCNT to drive somatic cell genomes to extended replicative potential. It seems clear, therefore, that SCNT methods can expand the proliferative lifespan of the donor cell genome. The degree to which this occurs, however, appears to be affected by such parameters as the donor age, the donor cell type, and the differentiated state of the donor cell. In a broader context, SCNT may provide the means necessary for preserving individual lifespan as well.

The potential for SCNT to be employed to derive ESCs for therapeutic purposes has been demonstrated in both animal models and in humans (Rideout *et al.*, 2002; Hwang *et al.*, 2004; review, Latham, 2004). Additionally, the ability of cloned ESCs to rescue phenotypic defects has been shown in mice, effectively illustrating the principle of therapeutic cloning (Rideout *et al.*, 2002). In moving forward with devising strategies for therapeutic cloning, several pertinent questions arise. One is the issue of mutation load. It may be advantageous to restrict donor cell types to those that may experience the least risk of somatic mutation or aneuploidy. Of course, two kinds of mutations must be considered: mutations that affect donor cell phenotype, and thus may be detectable using methods that could permit the exclusion of mutant cells, and "silent" or "masked" mutations that do not immediately affect the donor cell phenotype because they arise in unexpressed genes, or because additional mutations would be needed to allow penetrance. In the latter case, ESCs derived by therapeutic cloning might bear some measurable increase in risk of cancer development if they harbor oncogenic mutations. Selection for stem cells from adult tissues may be worth considering, because stem cells may have less risk of accumulating genetic mutations, as a result of active DNA replication and associated expression of DNA repair proteins, selective partitioning of newly replicated DNA strands (Potten *et al.*, 2002; Merok *et al.*, 2002), and apoptosis of cells with damaged DNA. Additionally, stem cells may confer advantages with respect to mitochondrial phenotype and telomerase expression.

Another consideration is whether the age of the donor individual/patient affects the likely outcome of therapeutic cloning. Will cells from older versus younger individuals display differences in the quality of ESCs that can be produced? Might there arise analytical methods to enrich for the appropriate population of cells, making it possible to avoid such an age effect? Might cells from older individuals require serial NT procedures in order to eliminate defective mitochondria or to achieve suitable telomere lengths? Will younger recipients/patients require higher quality or "younger equivalent" ESCs to be produced, with respect to mitochondria or telomere lengths?

Epigenetic changes may also be problematic, as cloned embryos often display defects in DNA methylation and regulation of imprinted genes (Latham, 2004). During cloning in animals, clones with severe epigenetic changes are likely to die during gestation, and thus be eliminated.

Cloning to produce ESCs, however, would not require this level of selection, because the embryos are converted to ESCs before this is likely to happen. It may thus be necessary to characterize ESCs thoroughly with respect to methylation state and expression of imprinted genes before using in therapeutic applications.

Given that cloning has been successful in so many different mammalian species, it seems likely that therapeutic cloning should be feasible in humans. However, recent studies indicate that cloning may be more difficult in primates and may not be possible using the protocols described to date. Cloned rhesus monkeys were produced using blastomere nuclei (Meng *et al.*, 1997), and an additional advanced pregnancy was again achieved later (Mitalipov *et al.*, 2002). Cloned rhesus monkeys have not been produced successfully using adult or fetal somatic cell nuclei (Mitalipov *et al.*, 2002; Simerly *et al.*, 2003). It appears that this limitation may reflect an inability of adult somatic cell components, in particular the centrosome, to substitute for authentic sperm-derived components, as indicated in studies by Simerly *et al.* (2003, 2004) and Miyara *et al.* (2006). This deficiency could lead to incorrect mitotic segregation of chromosomes and aneuploidy, which would account for the failure to obtain live progeny. The use of cloned human embryos to produce ESCs (Hwang *et al.*, 2003) was clearly a milestone with respect to illustrating the feasibility of the approach. Further research will be needed to identify, and hopefully correct, potential pitfalls in applying this technology in medicine.

ACKNOWLEDGMENTS

The author thanks Carmen Sapienza for critical comments on the manuscript. The work in the author's laboratory is supported in part by grants from the NIH/NICHD (HD38381, HD43092).

REFERENCES

Allsopp, R.C., Morin, G.B., DePinho, R., Harley, C.B., and Weissman, I.L. (2003). Telomerase is required to slow telomere shortening and extend replicative lifespan of HSCs during serial transplantation. *Blood 102*, 517–520.

Barritt, J.A., Brenner, C.A., Malter, H.E., and Cohen, J. (2001). Mitochondria in human offspring derived from ooplasmic transplantation. *Hum. Reprod. 16*, 513–516.

Betts, D., Bordignon, V., Hill, J., Winger, Q., Westhusin, M., Smith, L., and King, W. (2001). Reprogramming of telomerase activity and rebuilding of telomere length in cloned cattle. *Proc. Natl. Acad. Sci. USA. 98*, 1077–1082.

Blelloch, R.H., Hochedlinger, K., Yamada, Y., Brennan, C., Kim, M., Mintz, B. *et al.* (2004). Nuclear cloning of embryonal carcinoma cells. *Proc. Natl. Acad. Sci., USA 101*, 13985–13990.

Booth, P.J., Viuff, D., Tan, S., Holm, P., Greve, T., and Callesen, H. (2003). Numerical chromosome errors in day 7 somatic nuclear transfer bovine blastocysts. *Biol. Reprod. 68*, 922–928.

Chen, D.Y., Wen, D.C., Zhang, Y.P., Sun, Q.Y., Han, Z.M., Liu, Z.H. *et al.* (2002). Interspecies implantation and mitochondria fate of panda-rabbit cloned embryos. *Biol. Reprod. 67*, 637–642.

Clark, A.J., Ferrier, P., Aslam, S., Burl, S., Denning, C., Wylie, D. *et al.* (2003). Proliferative lifespan is conserved after nuclear transfer. *Nat. Cell. Biol. 5*, 495–496.

Cui, W., Wylie, D., Aslam, S., Dinnyes, A., King, T., Wilmut, I. *et al.* (2003). Telomerase-immortalized sheep fibroblasts can be reprogrammed by nuclear transfer to undergo early development. *Biol. Reprod. 69*, 15–21.

Ducibella, T., Huneau, D., Angelichio, E., Xu, Z., Schultz, R.M., Kopf, G.S. *et al.* (2002). Egg-to-embryo transition is driven by differential responses to Ca(2+) oscillation number. *Dev. Biol. 250*, 280–291.

Evans, M.J., Gurer, C., Loike, J.D., Wilmut, I., Schnieke, A.E., and Schon, E.A. (1999). Mitochondrial DNA genotypes in nuclear transfer-derived cloned sheep. *Nat. Genet. 23*, 90–93.

Gao, S, and Latham, K.E. (2004). Maternal and environmental factors in early cloned embryo development. *Cytogenet. Genome Res. 105*, 279–284.

Han, Z.M., Chen, D.Y., Li, J.S., Sun, Q.Y., Wan, Q.H., Kou, Z.H. *et al.* (2004). Mitochondrial DNA heteroplasmy in calves cloned by using adult somatic cell. *Mol. Reprod. Dev. 67*, 207–214.

Haussmann, M.F., Winkler, D.W., Huntington, C.E., Nisbet, I.C., and Vleck, C.M. (2004). Telomerase expression is differentially regulated in birds of differing life span. *Ann. N.Y. Acad Sci. 1019*, 186–190.

Hiendleder, S., Zakhartchenko, V., Wenigerkind, H., Reichenbach, H.D., Bruggerhoff, K., Prelle, K. *et al.* (2003). Heteroplasmy in bovine fetuses produced by intra- and inter-subspecific somatic cell nuclear transfer: neutral segregation of nuclear donor mitochondrial DNA in various tissues and evidence for recipient cow mitochondria in fetal blood. *Biol. Reprod. 68*, 159–166.

Hochedlinger, K., Blelloch, R., Brennan, C., Yamada, Y., Kim, M., Chin, L. *et al.* (2004). Reprogramming of a melanoma genome by nuclear transplantation. *Genes Dev. 18*, 1875–1885.

Hochedlinger, K., and Jaenisch, R. (2002). Monoclonal mice generated by nuclear transfer from mature B and T donor cells. *Nature 415*, 1035–1038.

Hwang, W.S., *et al.* (2004). Evidence of a pluripotent human embryonic stem cell line derived from a cloned blastocyst. *Science 303*, 1669–1674.

Joeng, K.S., Song, E.J., Lee, K.J., and Lee, J. (2004). Long lifespan in worms with long telomeric DNA. *Nat. Genet. 36*, 607–611.

Kaneda, H., Hayashi, J., Takahama, S., Taya, C., Lindahl, K.F., and Yonekawa, H. (1995). Elimination of paternal mitochondrial DNA in intraspecific crosses during early mouse embryogenesis. *Proc. Natl. Acad. Sci. USA 92*, 4542–4546.

Kato, Y., Tani, T., and Tsunoda, Y. (2000). Cloning of calves from various somatic cell types of male and female adult, newborn and fetal cows. *J. Reprod. Fertil. 120*, 231–237.

Kawanishi, S., and Oikawa, S. (2004). Mechanism of telomere shortening by oxidative stress. *Ann. N.Y. Acad. Sci. 10192*, 278–284.

Khrapko, K., Nekhaeva, E., Kraytsberg, Y., and Kunz, W. (2003). Clonal expansions of mitochondrial genomes: implications for in vivo mutational spectra. *Mutat. Res. 522*, 13–19.

Lanza, R.P., Cibelli, J.B., Blackwell, C., Cristofalo, V.J., Francis, M.K., Baerlocher, G.M. *et al.* (2000). Extension of cell lifespan and telomere length in animals cloned from senescent somatic cells. *Science 288*, 586–587.

Latham, K.E. (1999). Mechanisms and control of embryonic genome activation in mammalian embryos. *Int. Rev. Cytol. 193*, 71–124.

Latham, K.E. (2004). Cloning: questions answered and unsolved. *Differentiation 72*, 11–22.

Liu, L., Trimarchi, J.R., Smith, P.J., and Keefe, D.L. (2002). Mitochondrial dysfunction leads to telomere attrition and genomic instability. *Aging Cell 1*, 40–46.

Meirelles, F.V., Bordignon, V., Watanabe, Y., Watanabe, M., Dayan, A., Lobo, R.B. *et al.* (2001). Complete replacement of the mitochondrial genotype in a *Bos indicus* calf reconstructed by nuclear transfer to a *Bos taurus* oocyte. *Genetics 158*, 351–356.

Meng, L., Ely, J.J., Stouffer, R.L., and Wolf, D.P. (1997). Rhesus monkeys produced by nuclear transfer. *Biol. Reprod. 57*, 454–459.

Merok, J.R., Lansita, J.A., Tunstead, J.R., and Sherley, J.L. (2002). Cosegregation of chromosomes containing immortal DNA strands in cells that cycle with asymmetric stem cell kinetics. *Cancer Res. 62*, 6791–6795.

Mitalipov, S.M., Yeoman, R.R., Nusser, K.D., and Wolf, D.P. (2002). Rhesus monkey embryos produced by nuclear transfer from embryonic blastomeres or somatic cells. *Biol. Reprod. 66*, 1367–1373.

Miyara, F., Han, Z., Gao, S., Vassena, R., and Latham, K.E. (2006). Non-equivalence of embryonic and somatic cell nuclei affecting spindle composition in clones. *Dev. Biol.* (in press).

Miyashita, N., Shiga, K., Yonai, M., Kaneyama, K., Kobayashi, S., Kojima, T. *et al.* (2002). Remarkable differences in telomere lengths among cloned cattle derived from different cell types. *Biol. Reprod. 66* 1649–1655.

Nolen, L., Gao, S., Han, Z., Chung, Y.G., Bartolomei, M., and Latham, K.E. (2005) X chromosome reactivation and regulation in cloned embryos. *Dev. Biol.*, in press.

Potten, C.S., Owen, G., and Booth, D. (2002). Intestinal stem cells protect their genome by selective segregation of template DNA strands. *J. Cell Sci. 115*, 2381–2388.

Peura, T.T., and Trounson, A.O. (1998). Recycling bovine embryos for nuclear transfer. *Reprod. Fertil. Dev. 10*, 627–632.

Rehen, S.K., McConnell, M.J., Kaushal, D., Kingsbury, M.A., Yang, A.H., and Chun, J. (2001). Chromosomal variation in neurons of the developing and adult mammalian nervous system. *Proc. Natl. Acad. Sci. USA 98*, 13361–13366.

Rideout, W.M., 3rd, Hochedlinger, K., Kyba, M., Daley, G.Q., and Jaenisch, R. (2002). Correction of a genetic defect by nuclear transplantation and combined cell and gene therapy. *Cell 109*, 17–27.

Shi, W., Dirim, F., Wolf, E., Zakhartchenko, V., and Haaf, T. (2004). Methylation reprogramming and chromosomal aneuploidy in in vivo fertilized and cloned rabbit preimplantation embryos. *Biol. Reprod. 71*, 340–347.

Shi, W., Hoeflich, A., Flaswinkel, H., Stojkovic, M., Wolf, E., and Zakhartchenko, V. (2003). Induction of a senescent-like phenotype does not confer the ability of bovine immortal cells to support the development of nuclear transfer embryos. *Biol. Reprod. 69*, 301–309.

Shiels, P.G., Kind, A.J., Campbell, K.H., Waddington, D., Wilmut, I., Colman, A. *et al.* (1999). Analysis of telomere lengths in cloned sheep. *Nature* 399, 316–317.

Shitara, H., Kaneda, H., Sato, A., Inoue, K., Ogura, A., Yonekawa, H. *et al.* (2000). Selective and continuous elimination of mitochondria microinjected into mouse eggs from spermatids, but not from liver cells, occurs throughout embryogenesis. *Genetics 156*, 1277–1284.

Simerly, C. *et al.* (2003). Molecular correlates of primate nuclear transfer failures. *Science 300*, 297.

Simerly, C. *et al.* (2004). Embryogenesis and blastocyst development after somatic cell nuclear transfer in nonhuman primates: overcoming defects caused by meiotic spindle extraction. *Dev. Biol. 276*, 237–252.

Steinborn, R., Schinogl, P., Wells, D.N., Bergthaler, A., Muller, M., and Brem, G. (2002). Coexistence of *Bos taurus* and *B. indicus* mitochondrial DNAs in nuclear transfer-derived somatic cattle clones. *Genetics 162*, 823–829.

Stice, S.L., and Keefer, C.L. (1993). Multiple generational bovine embryo cloning. *Biol. Reprod. 48*, 715–719.

St. John, J.C., and Schatten, G. (2004). Paternal mitochondrial DNA transmission during nonhuman primate nuclear transfer. *Genetics 167*, 897–905.

Sutovsky, P., Moreno, R.D., Ramalho-Santos, J., Dominko, T., Simerly, C., and Schatten G. (2000). Ubiquitinated sperm mitochondria, selective proteolysis, and the regulation of mitochondrial inheritance in mammalian embryos. *Biol. Reprod. 63*, 582–590.

Takeda, K., Akagi, S., Kaneyama, K., Kojima, T., Takahashi, S., Imai, H. *et al.* (2003). Proliferation of donor mitochondrial DNA in nuclear transfer calves (*Bos taurus*) derived from cumulus cells. *Mol. Reprod. Dev. 64*, 429–437.

Tian, X.C., Xu, J., and Yang, X. (2000). Normal telomere lengths found in cloned cattle. *Nat. Genet. 26*, 272–273.

Wai, L.K. (2004). Telomeres, telomerase, and tumorigenesis—a review. *Med. Gen. Med. 6*, 19.

Wakayama, T., Shinkai, Y., Tamashiro, K.L., Niida, H., Blanchard, D.C., Blanchard, R.J. *et al.* (2000). Cloning of mice to six generations. *Nature 407*, 318–319.

Wakayama, T., and Yanagimachi, R. (1999). Cloning the laboratory mouse. *Semin. Cell. Dev. Biol. 10*, 253–258.

Yanagimachi, R. (2002) Cloning: experience from the mouse and other animals. *Mol. Cell. Endocrinol. 187*, 241–248.

Yang, C.X., Han, Z.M., Wen, D.C., Sun, Q.Y., Zhang, K.Y., Zhang, L.S. *et al.* (2003). *In vitro* development and mitochondrial fate of macaca-rabbit cloned embryos. *Mol. Reprod. Dev. 65*, 396–401.

47

Human Models of Longevity

Thomas Perls

Centenarians, though rare at a prevalence of approximately one per 10,000 in industrialized countries, are among the fastest growing segment of our population. Familial studies indicate that exceptional longevity runs strongly in families, but as of yet, few genetic variations have been found to account for this survival advantage. It is likely that the prevalence of centenarians is increasing because achieving exceptional old age is multifactorial. A number of factors important to such longevity are becoming more prevalent with modern public health measures and interventions. Such a multiple trait model would predict that the more extreme the phenotype, the more likely discernible environmental and genetic characteristics are to be discovered that are important to achieving very old age, much of it disability-free. Thus studies of families highly clustered for longevity or studies of supercentenarains, people age 110 and older, hold promise of facilitating such discoveries.

Introduction

People vary a great deal in terms of how they age. Some seem to age relatively quickly and develop age-related illnesses such as heart disease or stroke in their 40s and 50s, whereas others appear to age very slowly, and if they do develop age-related illnesses it may only be toward the end of their very long lives. Within these two extremes are the majority of people who, at least in industrialized nations, have an average life expectancy in their late 70s. Much of the variation around this average appears to be due to differences in environment, behavior, and luck. As in the case of the Seventh Day Adventists, if one has good health habits, they are quite likely to live to an age that many humans appear to be capable of achieving, their late 80s (20 years beyond the age of 60!) (Fraser and Shavlik, 2001). Distinguishing themselves from most Americans, the behavioral traits that lead to such a survival advantage are regular exercise, a frugal vegetarian diet, not smoking, and perhaps having a religious faith is also helpful.

However, what does it take to live to even longer, beyond the nonagenarian years, to age 100 and older? First, it appears that a resistance to disability is necessary. One study retrospectively found that nearly 90% of centenarians were independently functioning at an average age of 92 years (Hitt, Young-Xu, Silver, and Perls, 1999). On the other hand, many of these very old individuals can live with age-related illness(es) for a long period of time (unlike many other older people who die of those diseases) (Evert, Lawler, Bogan, and Perls, 2003). Thus, achieving exceptional old age, with its compression of disability toward the relative end of life, would appear to be a true advantage to which most people would aspire. So, what does it take to live to 100?

Demographic Selection

There has been significant debate among demographers as to what happens to the rate of mortality at extreme old ages. The answer has important ramifications for deciphering the factors that are important to survival to extreme old age. An important possibility is that demographic selection occurs at very old age, yielding a select, relatively healthy cohort at even older ages. Demographic selection describes the process of old frail individuals dying, leaving behind a more fit surviving cohort (Vaupel *et al.*, 1998). The observation by some research groups that the incidence of AD plateaus at very old ages is consistent with this phenomenon. Ritchie and Kildea (1995) performed a meta-analysis of nine epidemiological studies, finding that the rate of increase in dementia prevalence fell off among octogenarians and plateaued at approximately 40% at age 95. In a longitudinal study of older people living in Cache County, Utah, the incidence of both dementia and AD increased almost exponentially until ages 85 to 90, but declined after age 93 for men and age 97 for women (Miech, 2002).

A genetic example of demographic selection is the decreased frequency of the apolipoprotein E epsilon-4 (ApoE ε-4) allotype in the oldest old. Individuals who are homozygous for ApoE ε-4 have 2.3 to 8.0 times greater risk of developing AD than the general Caucasian population (Corder, 1993). The allelic frequency of ApoE ε-4 drops off dramatically in the oldest age groups, presumably because of its association with AD and vascular disease (Schachter *et al.*, 1994). Interestingly, the effect of ApoE allotype upon AD incidence appears to decrease with age at these very old ages (Sobel, 1995).

These examples notwithstanding, the phenomenon of demographic selection occurring at extreme old ages remains controversial. Some argue that because of marked improvements in medical care and public health measures, such selection no longer occurs. In this case, decreased mortality due to improved health care could lead to an increased prevalence of frailty among older survivors because treatment of existing diseases simply postpones death to older ages (Carnes, 2001).

Gender Differences

Save for a very few exceptions, in most populations, the vast majority of centenarians are women and generally, in industrialized nations, they comprise 85% of centenarians. In Sardinia, Italy, Michel Poulain has reported that approximately 50% of centenarians, particularly those living in the mountainous region of the island, are male (Poulain, 2004). But again generally speaking, female centenarians outnumber males almost nine to one. Despite the fact that many more women achieve exceptional longevity than men, among centenarians the men generally have better functional status. One explanation for this may be that men must be in excellent health to achieve such extreme old age (Perls, 1998). Women on the other hand, may be better adept at living with age-associated illnesses, and thus they can achieve exceptional old age even with significant chronic disability, particularly compared to men of similar age.

These observations might indicate a demographic crossover in which women are better off than men in younger old age and men, although fewer in number, are functionally better off in extreme old age. The underlying reasons why women generally live longer than men and are, at least before menopause, significantly less likely to develop heart disease and stroke are unclear. Estrogen, which might be a powerful antioxidant, has been implicated as an important reason. However it has been noted that premenopausal women who undergo hysterectomy but not oophrectomy experience an increased risk for vascular disease that is similar to men (Kiechl, 1997). Another possible reason is that women, because of menses, are relatively iron-deficient compared to men for a 30- to 40-year period. Iron is a crucial catalyst in mitochondrial production of free radicals as a byproduct of metabolism. Perhaps a reduction in available iron leads to less free-radical production. For example, iron deficiency has been associated with significant reductions in levels of oxidized low-density lipoprotein (LDL) cholesterol, an essential component of atherosclerotic plaque production (Sullivan, 1989). In addition, diets high in heme have been associated with significantly increased risk of heart disease (van der A, 2005).

Another potential female advantage studied by scientists relates to the fact that males possess one X chromosome and women have two. Women thus have the prospect for somatic cell selection with advancing age where the more fit of two somatic cell population survives. Stem cell populations that give rise to highly proliferative cell populations (for example, intestinal and skin epithelium, leukocytes) would be particularly prone to such selection. Among the genes on the X chromosome that are of particular interest are those that affect telomere length, in part because those cell populations that resist oxidative stress better might have longer telomeres (Aviv, 2005). Increased telomere length has been associated with both improved proliferative capacity and decreased mortality.

The Familiality of Exceptional Longevity

HERITABILITY ESTIMATES

Twin studies have estimated the heritability of life expectancy to range between 25 and 30% (McGue, Vaupel, Holm, and Harvald, 1993). These twin studies cannot infer the heritability of living to extreme old age because the oldest subjects in these studies are only octogenarians. In contrast, centenarians who live an additional 15 to 20 years beyond average life expectancy may require more than an advantage in their habits and environment. They may require a genetic advantage that translates into a significant inherited component to exceptional longevity. Some estimates are higher when the phenotype is more specific, as in the case of cognitive function at very old age (McClearn, 1997). Centenarians and their family members may have or lack certain genetic characteristics that result in a significant survival advantage.

FAMILIALITY OF EXCEPTIONAL LONGEVITY

Perls, Wilmoth, and colleagues (2002) analyzed the pedigrees of 444 centenarian families in the United States that included 2,092 siblings of centenarians. Survival was compared to 1900 birth cohort survival data from the U.S. Social Security Administration. As shown in Figure 47.1, female siblings had death rates at all ages that were about one-half the national level; male siblings had a similar advantage at most ages, though diminished somewhat during adolescence and young adulthood.

The siblings had an average age of death of 76.7 for females and 70.4 for males compared to 58.3 and 51.5 for the general population born around the same time. Even after accounting for race and education, the net survival advantage of siblings of centenarians was found to be 16 to 17 years greater than the general population. Relative survival probabilities (RSP) for these siblings increased markedly at older ages, reflecting the cumulative effect of their mortality advantage throughout life (see Table 47.1). Compared to the U.S. 1900 birth cohort, male siblings of centenarians were 17 times more likely to attain age 100 themselves, and female siblings were 8.2 times more likely.

The analysis of death rates indicates that the siblings' mortality advantage does not grow as they get older. Rather, their relative probability of survival is a cumulative measure and reflects their life-long advantage

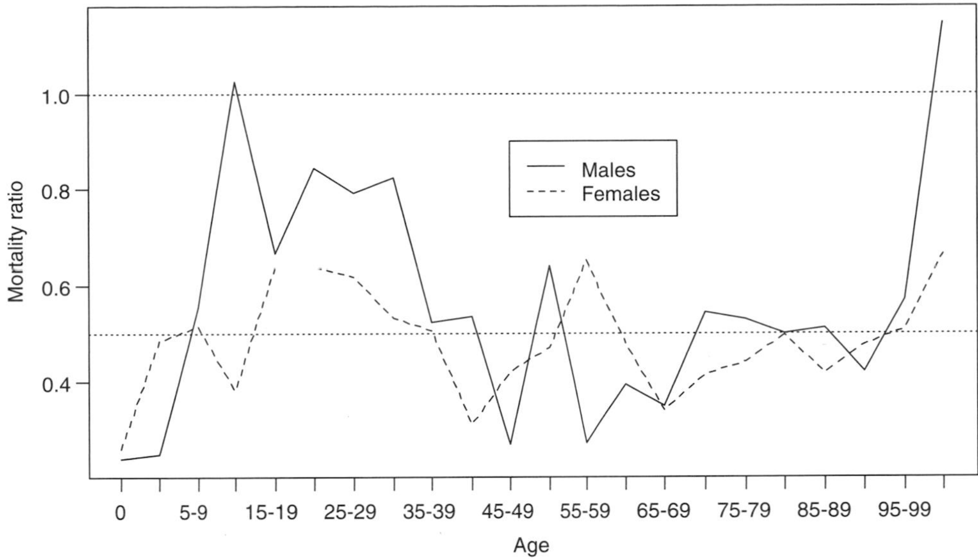

Figure 47.1 Relative mortality rate, siblings of centenarians compared with their 1900 birth cohort for ages 20 to 100.

TABLE 47.1
RSP with 95% confidence intervals (CI) of siblings of centenarians versus U.S. 1900 cohort

Age	MALES			FEMALES		
	RSP	Lower 5% CI	Upper 95% CI	RSP	Lower 95% CI	Upper 95% CI
20	1.00	1.00	1.00	1.00	1.00	1.00
25	1.00	0.99	1.01	1.01	1.00	1.02
60	1.18	1.15	1.21	1.12	1.09	1.14
65	1.29	1.25	1.33	1.16	1.13	1.19
70	1.48	1.42	1.53	1.24	1.21	1.28
75	1.68	1.60	1.77	1.36	1.31	1.41
80	2.03	1.90	2.16	1.54	1.47	1.60
85	2.69	2.47	2.91	1.83	1.73	1.93
90	4.08	3.62	4.54	2.56	2.39	2.74
95	8.35	6.98	9.71	4.15	3.73	4.57
100	17.0	10.8	23.1	8.22	6.55	9.90

over the general population born about the same time. Such elevated RSP values support the hypothesis that these family members have genetic variations in common that are important to achieving exceptional longevity. Furthermore, mortality rates of different groups (e.g., gender, race, education, physical activity, socioeconomic status) converge at very old age, and thus such a sustained advantage is unusual. The substantially higher RSP values for men at older ages might reflect the fact that male disease-specific mortality is significantly higher than for females at these older ages, and thus the males experience a greater relative advantage from beneficial genotypes compared with women. Another possibility could be that an even greater, and thus more rare combination of genetic and environmental factors are required for men to achieve extreme age compared to women. Either possibility could explain why men comprise only 15 percent of centenarians.

Richard Cutler, in what is now a classic paper in gerontology, proposed that persons who achieve extreme old age do so in part because they have genetic variations that affect the basic mechanisms of aging and that result in a uniform decreased susceptibility to age-associated diseases (Cutler, 1975). Persons who achieve extreme old age probably lack many of the variations (the "disease genes") that substantially increase risk for premature death by predisposing persons to various fatal diseases, both age-associated and non-age-associated. More controversial is the idea that genetic variations might confer protection against the basic mechanisms of aging or age-related illnesses (the "longevity-enabling genes"). Centenarians may be rare because a complex set of environmental and genetic variables must coexist for such survival to occur. Based upon studies of centenarian pedigrees, it appears that family members are more likely to have such combinations of factors in common than the general population.

CHILDREN OF CENTENARIANS

Offspring of centenarians have been found to have lipid profiles associated with lower risk for cardiovascular disease (Barzilai, Gabriely, Gabriely, Iankowitz, and Sorkin, 2001). Other findings show that middle-aged sons of long-lived parents had better systolic pressures, cholesterol levels, and decreased frequencies of the apoE ε-4 allele, compared to middle-aged sons of shorter-lived parents. Using a questionnaire-based cross-sectional study design, Terry and colleagues (2004) assessed the health histories of a nationwide sample of centenarian offspring (n = 176) and controls (n = 166). The controls consisted of offspring whose parents were born in the same years as the centenarians but at least one of whom died at age 73, the average life expectancy for that birth cohort. The average age at death of the other parent was 77 years, the same as the spouses of the centenarians. Centenarian offspring were found to have a 56% reduced relative prevalence of heart disease, a 66% reduced relative prevalence of hypertension, and a 59% reduced relative prevalence of diabetes in multivariate analyses that controlled for age, gender, years of education, annual income, IADL score, ethnicity, marital status, exercise, smoking, and alcohol use. There were no significant differences in the prevalence of a number of other age-related diseases including cancer, stroke, dementia, osteoporosis, cataracts, glaucoma, macular degeneration, depression, Parkinson's disease, thyroid disease, and COPD. The lack of differences for these diseases may be a function of the sample size, the choice of controls, or it may be that families with exceptional longevity do not have differential susceptibility to these diseases. For the offspring of centenarians who did report hypertension, the age of onset was significantly later when compared to controls. Similar delays were noted for the age of onset of coronary heart disease, diabetes, and stroke.

GENES PREDISPOSING TO EXCEPTIONAL LONGEVITY

The discovery of genetic variations that explain even 5 to 10% of the variation in survival to extreme old age could yield important clues about the cellular and biochemical mechanisms that affect basic mechanisms of aging and susceptibility to age-associated diseases. Until recently, only one genetic variation had been reproducibly associated with exceptional longevity, but even this might vary with ethnicity and other, as yet unknown sources of stratification. Schachter and colleagues (1994) from the French Centenarian Study noted that the Apolipoprotein E $\varepsilon4$ allele becomes markedly less frequent with advancing age. One of its counterparts, the $\varepsilon2$ allele, becomes more frequent with advancing age in Caucasians (Rebeck *et al.*, 1994).

Nir Barzilai and colleagues (2003), studying Ashkenazi Jewish centenarians and their families, recently investigated a cardiovascular pathway and gene that is differentiated between centenarians and controls. In this study, controls were spouses of the children of centenarians. Barzilai and colleagues noted that high-density lipoprotein (HDL) and low-density lipoprotein (LDL) particles were significantly larger among the centenarians and their offspring, and that particle size also differentiated between subjects with and without cardiovascular disease, hypertension, and metabolic syndrome. In a candidate-gene approach, the researchers then searched the literature for genes that affect HDL and LDL particle size, and hepatic lipase and cholesteryl ester transfer protein (CETP) emerged as candidates. Compared with a control group representative of the general population, centenarians were three times as likely to have a specific CETP gene variant (24.8% of centenarians had it vs. 8.6% of controls), and the centenarians' offspring were twice as likely to have it.

Discovering genes that could impart the ability to live to old age while compressing the period of disability toward the end of life should yield important insight into how the aging process increases susceptibility to diseases associated with aging, and into how this susceptibility might be modulated. Human longevity enabling genes are likely to influence aging at its most basic levels, thus affecting a broad spectrum of genetic and cellular pathways synchronously. The centenarian genome should also be an efficient tool for ferreting out disease genes. Comparing single nucleotide frequencies implicated in disease in centenarians with frequencies in persons with the disease should show clinically relevant polymorphisms. Another approach that researchers are in the early stages of understanding is differential gene expression in models suspected of slowing the aging process, such as caloric restriction. This might prove to be another potent tool for discovering longevity-enabling genes. The hope, of course, is that these gene discoveries will help in identification of drug targets and creation of drugs to allow persons to become more "centenarian-like" by maximizing the period of their lives spent in good health.

A Multifactorial Model for Exceptional Longevity

The fact that siblings maintain half the mortality risk of their birth cohort from age 20 to extreme age suggests a multifactorial model for achieving exceptional longevity. For example, socio-demographic advantages may play key roles at younger ages, whereas genetic advantages may distinguish the ability to go from old age to extreme old age. Undoubtedly exceptional longevity is much more complicated, with temporally overlapping roles for major genes, polygenic, environmental, and stochastic components. Such a scenario would be consistent with a *threshold model*, where predisposition for exceptional longevity can be measured on a quantitative scale. Figure 47.2 illustrates the standard threshold model proposed by Falconer (Falconer, 1965), where it is predicted that the proportion of affected relatives will be highest among the most severely affected individuals.

In the case of exceptional longevity, perhaps severity may be measured by additional years beyond a certain age (threshold) or in further years of delay in the case of exceptional survival phenotypes such as age of onset of disability or certain diseases.

Examples of phenotypes fitting the threshold model are early onset breast cancer or Alzheimer's disease (AD),

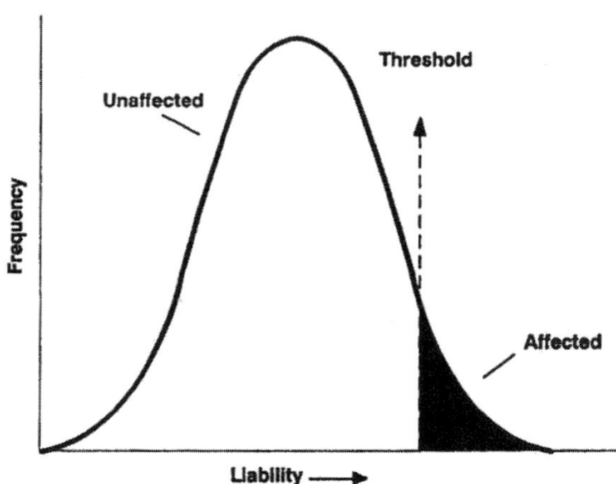

Figure 47.2 Threshold model of a multifactorial trait.

where relatives of patients who develop these diseases at unusually young ages are themselves at increased risk or liability. Thus, a 108-year-old's "liability" or predisposition for exceptional longevity is further beyond the threshold than someone more mildly affected, for example, a person who died at age 99 years. One interpretation of data indicating the higher RSP of male siblings of centenarians compared to female siblings is that the males carry a higher liability for the trait given the presence of the requisite traits. The model predicts that if a multifactorial trait is more frequent in one sex (as is the case with exceptional longevity, which is predominantly represented by females), the liability will be higher for relatives of the less susceptible sex (males, in the case of exceptional longevity) (Farrer, 1998). Although we have not yet looked at RSP of siblings of male versus female probands (something that certainly needs to be done), these elevated risks for male versus female siblings are interesting in this context. The model also predicts that the risk for exceptional longevity will be sharply lower for second-degree relatives compared to first-degree relatives, another observation we hope to test by having access to many expanded pedigrees.

Important questions to pursue in light of this proposed model are:

Are siblings of males with exceptional longevity (EL) more likely to achieve EL themselves compared to siblings of females with EL?

Does this risk for EL in siblings and offspring increase with the age of the proband of either sex? What are the quantitative differences of such liability with or without accounting for the gender of the proband?

The ramifications of this model holding true for EL include:

The older the subject, the better for discovering traits predisposing for EL.

There are gender-related differences in both relatives and probands in liability for EL given the presence of specific traits conducive to EL.

Conclusion

Genetic findings related to human longevity have primarily been related to vascular health. This is not surprising given that vascular disease is the number one killer among older people, including centenarians. We would expect that the oldest old would have to have some genetic advantages regarding a relative resistance to vascular disease in order to survive to their extreme ages. More elusive has been the search for genetic variations that impact upon the basic biology of aging that could impact upon the rate of aging and susceptibility to a broad range of age-related diseases. Discovering such so-called longevity-enabling genes might entail the study of the extreme of the extreme such as supercentenarians, those who live to 110 years old and older or those who achieve extreme old age despite habits that would otherwise be associated with high mortality and age-associated disease risk.

Recommended Resources

Barzilai, N., Atzmon, G., Schechter, C., Schaefer, E.J., Cupples, A.L., Lipton, R. *et al.* (2003). Unique lipoprotein phenotype and genotype in humans with exceptional longevity. JAMA 290, 2030–2040.

An important phenotypic discovery that led to a genetic association with exceptional longevity and a demonstration of the power of studying centenarian families for discovering phenotypes and genotypes that play important roles in survival to exceptional old age.

Hadley, E.C., and Rossi, W.K. (2005). Exceptional survival in human populations: National Institute on Aging perspectives and programs. *Mech Ageing Dev 126*, 231–234.

An excellent overview from the perspective of the National Institute on Aging.

Hagberg, B., Alfredson, B.B., Poon, L.W., and Homma, A. (2001). Cognitive Functioning in Centenarians: A Coordinated Analysis of Results from Three Countries. *J Gerontol B Psychol Sci Soc Sci 56*, P141–P151.

An important example demonstrating the importance of multinational studies to assesses reproducibility of findings across populations.

Hazzard, W.R. (2001). What heterogeneity among centenarians can teach us about genetics, aging, and longevity. *J Am Geriatr Soc 49*, 1568–1569.

An important perspective of how complicated and subtle studies of aging and longevity can be.

Herskind, A.M., McGue, M., Holm, N.V., Sorensen, T.I., Harvald, B., and Vaupel, J.W. (1996). The heritability of human longevity: a population-based study of 2872; Danish twin pairs born 1870-1900. *Hum Genet 97*, 319–323.

Among the most quoted studies regarding the heritability of how people age.

Perls, T. (1995). The Oldest Old. *Sci Amer 272*, 70–75.

An early review article redefining the oldest old as people living beyond the age of 100.

Perls, T., Silver, M., and Lauerman, J. (1999). *Living to 100: Lessons in maximizing your potential at any age.* New York: Basic Books.

A lay text about findings from the New England Centenarian Study and other aging research.

Kenneth W. Wachter and Caleb E. Finch, Eds. *Between Zeus and the Salmon, The Biodemography of Longevity.* Committee on Population, Commission on Behavioral and Social Sciences and Education, National Research Council. Washington, D.C.: National Academy Press.

An excellent text exploring numerous biodemographic aspects of longevity.

ACKNOWLEDGMENTS

The author received support from the National Institute on Aging (U01-AG023755), and he has no potential conflicts of interest to report.

REFERENCES

Aviv A, S.J., Christensen, K, and Wright, W. (2005). The Longevity Gender Gap: Are Telomeres the Explanation? *Sci Aging Knowl Environ 23*, pe16.

Barzilai, N., A.G., Schechter, C., Schaefer, E.J., Cupples, A.L., Lipton, R., Cheng, S. *et al.* (2003). Unique lipoprotein phenotype and genotype in humans with exceptional longevity. *JAMA 290(15)*, 2030–2040.

Barzilai, N., Gabriely, I., Gabriely, M., Iankowitz, N., and Sorkin, J.D. (2001). Offspring of centenarians have a favorable lipid profile. *J Am Geriatr Soc 49(1)*, 76–79.

Carnes, B.A., and Olshansky, S.J. (2001). Heterogeneity and its biodemographic implications for longevity and mortality. *Exp Gerontol 36*, 419–430.

Corder, E.H., S.A., Strittmatter, W.J., Schmechel, D.E., Gaskell, P.C., Small, G.W., Roses, A.D. *et al.* (1993). Gene dose of apolipoprotein E type 4 allele and the risk of Alzheimer's disease in late onset families. *Science 261*, 921–923.

Cutler, R. (1975). Evolution of Human Longevity and the Genetic Complexity Governing Aging Rate. *Proc Natl Acad Sci USA 72*, 4664–4668.

Evert, J., Lawler, E., Bogan, H., and Perls, T. (2003). Morbidity profiles of centenarians: survivors, delayers, and escapers. *J Gerontol A Biol Sci Med Sci 58(3)*, 232–237.

Falconer, D. (1965). The inheritance and liability to certain disease estimated from the incidence among relatives. *Ann Hum Genet 29*, 51–76.

Farrer, L., and Cupples, A. (1998). Determining the Genetic Component of a Disease. In J. Haines and M.A. Pericak-Vance, Eds., *Approaches to Gene Mapping in Complex Human Diseases.* New York: Wiley-Liss.

Fraser, G.E., and Shavlik, D.J. (2001). Ten years of life: Is it a matter of choice? *Arch Intern Med 161(13)*, 1645–1652.

Hitt, R., Young-Xu, Y., Silver, M., and Perls, T. (1999). Centenarians: the older you get, the healthier you have been. *Lancet 354(9179)*, 652.

Kiechl, S., Willeit, J., Egger, G., Poewe, W., and Oberhollenzer, F. (1997). Body iron stores and the risk of carotid atherosclerosis: Prospective results from the Bruneck study. *Circulation 96*, 3300–3307.

McClearn, G.E., Johansson, B., Berg, S., Pedersen, N.L., Ahern, F., Petrill, S.A. *et al.* (1997). Substantial Genetic Influence on Cognitive Abilities in Twins 80 or More Years Old. *Science 276*, 1560–1563.

McGue, M., Vaupel, J. W., Holm, N., and Harvald, B. (1993). Longevity is moderately heritable in a sample of Danish twins born 1870–1880. *J Gerontol 48(6)*, B237–B244.

Miech, R.A., Breitner, J.C., Zandi, P.P., Khachaturian, A.S., Anthony, J.C. *et al.* (2002). Incidence of AD may decline in the early 90s for men, later for women: The Cache County study. *Neurology 58*, 209–218.

Perls, T., Fretts, R. (1998). Why women live longer than men. *Sci Amer Pres*, 100–107.

Perls, T. T., Wilmoth, J., Levenson, R., Drinkwater, M., Cohen, M., Bogan, H. *et al.* (2002). Life-long sustained mortality advantage of siblings of centenarians. *Proc Natl Acad Sci USA 99(12)*, 8442–8447.

Poulain, M., Pes, G.M., Grasland, C., Carru, C., Ferrucci, L., Baggio, G. *et al.* (2004). Identification of a geographic area characterized by extreme longevity in the Sardinia island: the AKEA study. *Exp Gerontol 39*, 1423–1429.

Rebeck, G.W., Perls, T.T., West, H.L., Sodhi, P., Lipsitz, L.A., and Hyman, B.T. (1994). Reduced apolipoprotein epsilon 4 allele frequency in the oldest old Alzheimer's patients and cognitively normal individuals. *Neurology 44(8)*, 1513–1516.

Ritchie, K., and Kidea, D. (1995). Is senile dementia "age-related" or "ageing related" evidence from meta-analysis of dementia prevalence in the oldest old. *Lancet 346*, 931–934.

Schachter, F., Faure-Delanef, L., Guenot, F., Rouger, H., Froguel, P., Lesueur-Ginot, L., *et al.* (1994). Genetic associations with human longevity at the APOE and ACE loci. *Nat Genet, 6(1)*, 29–32.

Sobel, E., Louhija, J., Sulkava, R., Davanipour, Z., Kontula, K., Miettinen, H. *et al.* (1995). Lack of association of apolipoprotein E allele epsilon 4 with late-onset Alzheimer's disease among Finnish centenarians. *Neurology 45*, 903–907.

Sullivan, J. (1989). The iron paradigm of ischemic heart disease. *Am Heart J 117*, 1177–1188.

Terry, D., Wilcox, M., McCormick, M., and Perls, T. (2004a). Cardiovascular disease delay in the offspring of centenarians. *J Gerontol Med Sci 59(4)*, M385–M389.

Terry, D.F., Wilcox, M., McCormick, M., Pennington, J., Schoenhofen, E., Andersen, S. *et al.* (2004a). Reduced all-cause, cardiovascular and cancer mortality in centenarian offspring. *J Amer Geriatr Soc 52*, 2074–2076.

Van der A, D.L., Peeters, P.H., Grobbee, D.E., Marx, J.J., and van der Schouw, Y.T. (2005). Dietary heme iron and coronary heart disease in women. *Eur Heart J 26*, 257–262.

Vaupel, J.W., Carey, J.R., Christensen, K., Johnson, T.E., Yashin, A.I., Holm, N.V., *et al.* (1998). Biodemographic trajectories of longevity. *Science 280(5365)*, 855–860.

48

Computational Models of Mitochondrial DNA in Aging

David C. Samuels

In this chapter we present simulation methods for modeling the development of somatic mitochondrial DNA mutations over a human lifetime. The simulation method descriptions are intended for the advanced undergraduate, the graduate student, or the researcher planning to develop simulations in this field, and for the general biomedical reader. Different modeling methods that we have used are described, and their strengths and weaknesses are compared.

Introduction

In this chapter we will be using a different meaning of *model* than is used in the rest of this book. Here we discuss the use of *computational* models of mitochondrial DNA (mtDNA) applied to aging research. Computational models have unique advantages for investigating the aging process. With a simulation we can follow the changes over a full human lifetime in a single cell, or in a group of dividing cells. We can do this nondestructively, and we can do this down to the level of single DNA molecules or even to the level of individual genes on each DNA molecule. The computational model should be thought of as a way to determine the consequences of explicit assumptions and hypotheses. Given the long time scales involved in human aging, and the important role of random processes in mtDNA maintenance and mutation, these consequences are often nonintuitive. The primary use of our simulations has not been to calculate exact numerical values. Instead, we are more concerned with understanding the qualitative behavior of the system. Based on this increased understanding of the simulated system we can propose new hypotheses, which can then be tested in the lab, completing the circle between theory and experiment that is fundamental to the scientific method.

Our purpose in this chapter is to discuss the different simulation methods that we have used in our work on mtDNA dynamics (Chinnery and Samuels, 1999; Elson *et al.*, 2001; Chinnery *et al.*, 2002; Capps *et al.*, 2003). We will discuss two general methods of modeling: DNA-molecule level simulations and cell level simulations. Each method has its strengths and weaknesses, and each is suitable for investigating different types of questions about the dynamics of mtDNA.

Acquired mtDNA Mutations, Clonal Expansion, and Their Relationship with Aging

Dysfunctional mitochondria and mutated mtDNA are associated with the aging process in a wide range of species, from *C. elegans* to humans. A recent experiment showed that mice with a mutated mitochondrial polymerase had an increased rate of mtDNA mutation and suffered from accelerated aging (Trifunovic *et al.*, 2004). This was the first experiment to deliberately manipulate the rate of mutation of mtDNA in an organism and to show a direct effect on the rate of aging.

The general idea of the mitochondrial theory of aging is that mitochondrial dysfunction increases with time, causing a decreased rate of ATP production and the eventual loss of function of cells throughout the organism. Our work focuses on mitochondrial dysfunction due to mtDNA mutations. Mitochondrial DNA is not well protected against mutation and has few mutation repair mechanisms. Furthermore, mtDNA is located near the primary source of ROS in the cell, the electron transfer chain (ETC) in the mitochondrial inner membrane (for more on ROS production see Chapter 16). This combination of little mtDNA protection or repair in a high ROS environment causes a very high mutation rate in mtDNA, much higher than is found in the nuclear DNA.

For more on the relationship between mitochondrial DNA mutations and aging, refer to Chapter 41 and to several recent review papers (Alexeyev *et al.*, 2004; Barja 2004; Huang and Manton, 2004; Skulachev, 2004). However there is one feature of mtDNA that I must point out in preparation for the following discussion. Each mitochondrion contains several copies of mtDNA (roughly 5 to 10 copies). Therefore there are a large number of mtDNA molecules in just a single cell. This number depends on cell type and ranges from a few

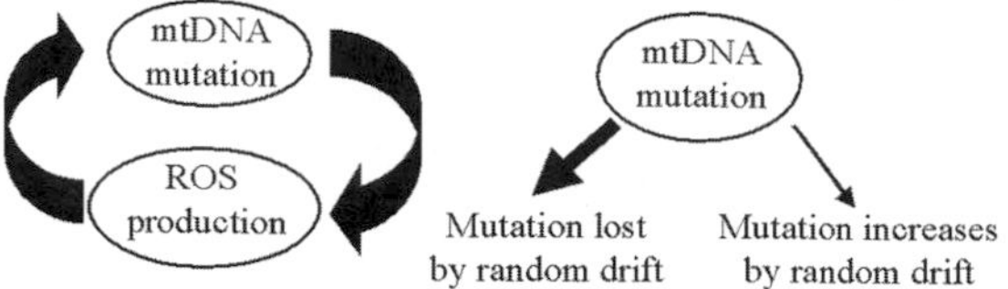

Figure 48.1 Two alternate mechanisms for the increase over time of the mutated mtDNA in the cell.

hundred in skin cells to 100,000 in oocytes. A typical number for our simulated cells is 1,000 to 10,000 mtDNA per cell. The purpose of our simulations is to model the dynamics of this population of mtDNA molecules within a cell. Generally we model the changes over time in the number of wild-type and mutant mtDNA molecules in a single simulated cell.

To design a simulation model of mtDNA mutation in aging we must first choose the hypotheses on which we will base the model. There are two basic hypotheses on this subject that you will find in the literature (see Figure 48.1).

By far the most commonly presented is the *error cascade hypothesis*. In this hypothesis, mutations of mtDNA cause a disruption of either the production or the function of one (or more) of the proteins that make up the ETC. This disruption slows the transfer of electrons through the ETC, increasing the risk that the electrons may be diverted to form ROS. The increased ROS production in the mitochondrion then raises the rate of mutation of mtDNA, resulting in a vicious cycle of increasing ROS production and increasing mtDNA mutation.

The error cascade hypothesis is reasonable, and there is little doubt that this process does actually occur in cells. However, there is doubt that this process plays a significant role in aging, at least in humans. The problem is that the error cascade process would result over time in the formation of a large number of *different* mutations in the mtDNA of a single cell. This is not what is observed in the cells of elderly humans. Instead, it is found in the elderly that cells with large numbers of mutated mtDNA generally contain many copies of a single mutation (Taylor *et al.*, 2001; Nekhaeva *et al.*, 2002), not the wide range of different mutations that would be expected from the error cascade mechanism. Different cells in the same tissue may contain different mtDNA mutations, so this effect is detectable only if measurements of mtDNA mutation are done at the single-cell level, not at the tissue sample level.

This observation that a single cell tends to have only one mtDNA mutation present in large numbers has led to the *clonal expansion hypothesis* (see Figure 48.1). In this hypothesis only a single mutation event is responsible for all of the identical mutated mtDNA found in the elderly cell. Over time this mutated mtDNA was copied more often than the other mtDNA molecules, either through some replicative advantage or simply through chance (genetic drift). Other mtDNA mutation events may have occurred, but those mutated mtDNA molecules were eventually lost from the population within the cell, again either though a replicative disadvantage or by random genetic drift.

Our simulation work began as a computational test of the random genetic drift version of the clonal expansion hypothesis (Chinnery and Samuels, 1999). The question was whether purely random drift, with no replicative advantage or disadvantage, could lead to clonal expansions of mutant mtDNA in a reasonable population size of 1,000 mtDNA per cell, within a reasonable timescale of 50 to 80 years. Therefore our modeled mechanisms and methods are aimed at this question, not at the error cascade hypothesis. This means that no model of ROS production is used in these particular simulations, as ROS production is not central to the clonal expansion hypothesis, and that, in general, we do not consider any replicative advantages to the mutant mtDNA molecules. Now we will discuss the mechanisms that are included in our mtDNA simulations and the computational techniques that we have used to model these mechanisms.

Modeling the Basic Processes: mtDNA Replication, Degradation, and Cell Division

The two fundamental mechanisms that must be included in all simulations of the population of mtDNA molecules within a cell are mtDNA replication and degradation. We begin with degradation, since this is the simplest process.

mtDNA DEGRADATION

Given the high ROS environment of the interior of the mitochondrion, it is no surprise that the lifetime of mtDNA is relatively short. A typical measurement of the half-life of mtDNA in mammals is approximately 10 days, with some reported values as high as 30 days. It is possible that this measured degradation actually reflects the degradation of the entire organelle. As is generally the case in simulations involving molecular degradation, we model this as a random process. Given a half-life of T_{half}, the probability that a given mtDNA molecule will degrade within a time Δt is

$$P_d = 1 - \exp(-\ln(2)\Delta t / T_{half}). \quad (1)$$

With a population of N mtDNA molecules in a cell, the number of degradation events, n_d, that would occur within a time span of Δt is given by a cumulative Poisson distribution.

$$n_d = Poisson(N \times P_d). \quad (2)$$

The quantity $N \times P_d$ is the mean number of degradation events expected, and the Poisson function returns a number that has random fluctuations about this mean. When $\Delta t \ll T_{half}$, the mean number of degradation events $\langle n_d \rangle$ is given by

$$\langle n_d \rangle = N \ln(2) \Delta t / T_{half}. \quad (3)$$

For details on the cumulative Poisson distribution and the binomial distribution used in the next section, I highly recommend the series of Numerical Recipes books (Press *et al.*, 1988), and refer you to the books for details on programming these functions. As a concrete example of the degradation rate, for a population of 10,000 mtDNA molecules with a half-life of 10 days, over a time Δt of one hour, the mean number of mtDNA molecules degraded would be 29. The actual number returned from the Poisson routine would fluctuate about that mean value.

mtDNA REPLICATION

To balance the loss of mtDNA molecules by degradation, mtDNA must be continually copied. This replication is independent of the cell cycle, and occurs in all cells, including postmitotic cells. The total number of mtDNA molecules replicated, n_{copy}, in a time span Δt must be equal to the mean number lost to degradation plus any additional growth, n_{grow}, which would be needed in dividing cells.

$$n_{copy} = \langle n_d \rangle + n_{grow} = N(\ln(2)\Delta t / T_{half}) + n_{grow} \quad (4)$$

Little is known about the control of the mtDNA replication rate, so for the modeling we generally choose the simplest possible model, a constant replication rate. For examples of simulations with a variable mtDNA replication rate, see Chinnery and Samuels (1999) and Capps *et al.* (2003).

Equation 4 gives the total mtDNA replication rate. We are usually simulating conditions where the cell contains a mixture of wild-type and mutant mtDNA. The total number of replicated mtDNA molecules is split into two parts,

$$n_{copy} = W_{copy} + M_{copy} \quad (5)$$

where W_{copy} is the number of wild-type mtDNA copied in the time Δt and M_{copy} is the number of mutant mtDNA copied. If more than one type of mutant mtDNA is being modeled in the simulation, then the term M_{copy} can be further subdivided into these mutation subtypes. Based on the assumption that there is no replicative advantage to the mutants, we model the number of wild-type and mutant copied as a binomial process. Let W be the number of wild-type mtDNA and M be the number of mutant, with the total number of mtDNA $N = W + M$. Then we can write

$$\begin{aligned} W_{copy} &= binomial(n_{copy}, W/N) \\ M_{copy} &= n_{copy} - W_{copy} \end{aligned} \quad (6)$$

where the notation $binomial(n_{copy}, W/N)$ means that a total of n_{copy} objects are being chosen from a population where a fraction W/N of the objects are wild-type mtDNA. The *binomial* function (Press *et al.*, 1988) returns the random number of wild-type mtDNA chosen to copy, with $W_{copy} \leq n_{copy}$. Note that only one call to the routine *binomial* is needed to calculate both W_{copy} and M_{copy}. By using a binomial routine, the values W_{copy} and M_{copy} will have natural random variations that are an important driving force behind the random genetic drift in the system.

CELL DIVISION

We model cell division by periodically dividing the mtDNA within the simulated cell into two subpopulations, representing the two daughter cells. Since the division will not be exactly even, we again use a Poisson model for the division of the mtDNA between the two daughter cells. We must determine separately the number of mutant and wild-type mtDNA that end up in each daughter cell. Let W_0 represent the number of wild-type mtDNA in the parent cell and W_1 and W_2 the number in the two daughter cells, with $W_0 = W_1 + W_2$. Similar definitions are made for the mutant mtDNA. Then we have the following.

$$\begin{aligned} W_1 &= Poisson(W_0/2) \\ W_2 &= W_0 - W_1 \\ M_1 &= Poisson(M_0/2) \\ M_2 &= M_0 - M_1 \end{aligned} \quad (7)$$

ACQUIRED mtDNA MUTATIONS

We have used two slightly different computational models to represent the somatic mutations that occur in mtDNA as part of the aging process. One method is to tie mutation to the replication process, to represent mutations that arise from replication errors. In this case, at every mtDNA replication event there is some probability P_{mut} that a new mtDNA mutation will be created. An alternative method is to model mutation formation independent of the mtDNA replication process. Then, over every time interval Δt there is a probability P_{mut} that a mtDNA molecule may be converted to a new mutation. Unless the replication rate is varying with time in the model, there is little significant difference between these two models for *de novo* mtDNA mutation formation. The parameter P_{mut} can also be made a function of time to represent changing mutation conditions, such as periods of increased radiation exposure, for example.

Models of acquired mtDNA mutations based on the mechanisms of mtDNA replication and degradation have a particular behavior that must be considered in the design of the simulation. Just after a new mutation forms, the population of mtDNA within the simulated cell will have only one copy of that mutation and about 1,000 other mtDNA molecules that are wild-type or different mutations. In simulated postmitotic cells (where the cellular mtDNA population is not growing with time) there is a 50% chance that this particular mutant mtDNA molecule will be degraded before it is copied, thus removing the new mutation relatively quickly from the cell. Even if the mutated mtDNA does manage to be copied, then you have only two copies of the new mutant and it is still very likely that you will lose both of those copies to degradation. So you should expect that the majority of *de novo* mutations will survive in the simulated cell for only a short time (Elson *et al.*, 2001), and the data structures and memory management of your simulation design should be made with this point in mind to avoid wasting memory on the many mutations that transiently appear in the simulated cell.

COMPLEMENTATION OF MUTATIONS

It can be useful to model the effect of mtDNA mutations at the level of individual genes, instead of just counting the number of mutated mtDNA molecules in the cell. To see why, consider a cell with 100% mutated mtDNA consisting of clonal expansions of two different mutations that have occurred on different genes. Call the mutants A and B. Mutant A may have a nonfunctional ND1 gene whereas mutant B has a nonfunctional tRNA-W gene. Even though all the mtDNA molecules in the cell are mutated in some way, all the mutant A mtDNA molecules contain functioning tRNA-W genes and all the mutant B molecules contain functioning ND1 genes, so the two mutant mtDNA molecules still complement each other and the cell function would be normal. To allow for this complementation of different mutant mtDNAs, we can assign to each mutation a profile indicating which genes, if any, are deleteriously affected by that mutation. We can do this with a logical vector with 37 elements (22 tRNAs, 13 protein genes, and 2 rRNAs). Table 48.1 gives an example of this for three specific mutations: the common deletion, the A3243G point mutation, and any silent point mutation. The columns of the table are arranged in the gene order on the human mtDNA genome, for simplicity in representing deletions that affect multiple genes. In the examples shown in Table 48.1, the common deletion removes a wide swath of genes, the relatively common A3243G point mutation affects only the L1 tRNA gene, and a neutral mutation affects no gene products.

The specification of the gene products affected by the simulated mutant will allow you to be more specific in the modeling of COX cells. COX staining is a very common laboratory method of detecting mitochondrial dysfunction in tissue samples. However, the COX staining only directly detects the presence of complex IV of the respiratory chain. This complex will be directly affected by mutations in the genes CO I, CO II, CO III, and also by any tRNA or rRNA mutation (see Table 48.1). This includes the majority of all known pathogenic point mutations and deletions, but not all. Specifying the gene products affected by the mutation allows the possibility of pathogenic mutations that will not produce COX- cells. By including this detail in your simulation you allow a very valuable comparison between the simulation and clinical data.

Choosing the Scale of Your Simulation Design

The design of every simulation begins with a choice of scale. What is the smallest level of detail that you will attempt to simulate, and what is the largest level of organization to be included? Biological questions often cover a wide range of scales, from the molecular to the organism level. This is also true of our mtDNA simulations. A list of the possible levels that can be included in these simulations is given in Table 48.2.

TABLE 48.1
Three examples for a data structure to represent mutations: a deletion (the common deletion), a point mutation (the 3243 mutation), and a neutral mutation. "1" indicates the gene product is not affected and "0" indicates that the gene product is defective or not produced. Single letter column headings denote the 22 tRNA genes

Mutation	F	12S	V	16S	L1	ND1	I	Q	M	ND2	W	A	N	C
Common Deletion	1	1	1	1	1	1	1	1	1	1	1	1	1	1
A3243G	1	1	1	1	0	1	1	1	1	1	1	1	1	1
Neutral	1	1	1	1	1	1	1	1	1	1	1	1	1	1

Mutation	Y	CO I	S	D	CO II	K	ATP8	ATP6	CO III	G	ND3
Common Deletion	1	1	1	1	1	1	0	0	0	0	0
A3243G	1	1	1	1	1	1	1	1	1	1	1
Neutral	1	1	1	1	1	1	1	1	1	1	1

Mutation	R	ND4L	ND4	H	S2	L2	ND5	ND6	E	CytB	T	P
Common Deletion	0	0	0	0	0	0	0	1	1	1	1	1
A3243G	1	1	1	1	1	1	1	1	1	1	1	1
Neutral	1	1	1	1	1	1	1	1	1	1	1	1

TABLE 48.2
The range of potential levels of complexity of simulations of mitochondrial DNA in aging

Levels of simulation
Base pairs
Mitochondrial genes
MtDNA molecules
Nucleoids
Mitochondrion
Cell level
Tissue or organ level
Organism level
Pedigree (maternal relatives)
Mitochondrial haplogroups

We have used almost all these levels in various simulations that we have created, but you can expect to cover no more than two or at most three levels of scale in any one simulation.

For aging simulations we have focused on the smaller scales given in Table 48.2, generally around the cellular level. However, this still leaves a wide range of scales to consider, too wide a range for a single simulation design to handle efficiently. We have dealt with this multiple-scale problem by developing two types of simulation. The *mtDNA Molecule Level simulation* can deal with the scales from the mtDNA molecule level to the cellular level. The *Cell Level simulation* deals with the scales from the cellular level only to the small tissue level. The practical upper limit (with the current computers) on the Cell Level simulation is a few tens of millions of simulated cells over a time span of 100 years. Each of these two simulations has its strengths and its limitations. In the following we describe the computational methods for each simulation model separately, and then we compare the computer requirements of each model.

THE mtDNA MOLECULE LEVEL SIMULATION

The lowest level represented in these simulations is the individual mtDNA molecule. The basic data structure is a vector of integer values, with each element of the vector representing a particular mtDNA molecule in the simulated cell. Call this data structure DNA(1, . . . , N). A typical simulation will have 1,000 to 10,000 mtDNA molecules (in one cell). The integer values of the vector are used to represent the mutation state of that mtDNA molecule. A value of "0" denotes a wild-type mtDNA molecule; higher integer values denote various mutations. The coding of the mutations depends on the particular application of the simulation, but for an aging simulation, typically "1" represents the first acquired mutation to appear and is carried by all the descendants of that molecule, the value "2" denotes the second mutation to appear, and so on.

If you wish to define any characteristics of each acquired mutation, such as the list of genes affected as in Table 48.1, then this can be handled by a separate data structure. The important design point is that these *mutation characteristics* should not be recorded directly in your data structure DNA(1, . . ., N), since we expect that many of the elements of this data structure will be clonal expansions of one or two separate mutation events, and that would waste memory space and slow the simulation. Instead the mutation characteristics should be stored in a separate array that can be indexed by the integer value stored in the vector DNA(1, . . ., N), recording the identity of the original mutation event.

One mutation characteristic that we have found very useful to record is the time of the original mutation event. With this data we were able to look at the mutations found in the simulated cell at age 80 years and determine the distribution of ages when the original mutation event occurred. The surprising result was that the majority of the mutations found in the simulated 80-year-old cell were acquired before the age of 20 years (Elson *et al.*, 2001). The ability to "tag" individual DNA molecules with information such as the mutation date allows you to gather data that is simply impossible to acquire in a real experiment.

The modeling of mtDNA replication, degradation, and cell divisions in the mtDNA level simulations is fairly simple. The number of each event occurring in a time-step of length Δt is calculated from Eqs. 1 through 7. Typically we use a time step of one hour (so that 100 years requires less than 1 million time steps, a reasonable amount). For example, say that in one time step 23 mtDNA molecules are destroyed and 27 are copied. First, we would randomly choose 23 elements of the data structure DNA(1, . . ., N) to remove, modeling degradation. The data structure is then compressed from N elements to N-23 elements, to remove the empty spaces. Then, 27 elements of the vector DNA(1, . . ., N) are chosen at random for replication. The new mtDNA molecules are added at the end of the vector, and their attributes such as the mutation value are copied from the parent mtDNA molecules. Any acquired mutations are calculated at this point, resulting in a change of the mutation state between the parent and offspring mtDNA molecules.

Note that there is no need to separate out the degradation or replication processes into mutant and wild-type mtDNA in this model. This occurs naturally through the random choice from the elements of the DNA(1, . . ., N) vector, which contains both the mutant and mtDNA molecules.

Since the mtDNA replication and degradation processes are fundamentally random, the results for any one simulated cell are also stochastic. Therefore simulating a single cell is not sufficient. One must simulate a number of cells, and take statistics over the set of simulated cells. For the mtDNA Level simulations, the practical limit of the simulations is on the order of 1,000 simulated cells, over a time scale of one century for aging studies.

THE CELL LEVEL SIMULATION

To model larger numbers of cells in a reasonable time requires a change in the level of the simulation. Details at the DNA molecule level must be sacrificed to allow the simulation to extend to higher levels of organization (see Table 48.2). For this we have designed simulations where the lowest level of detail represented is the level of a single cell (Capps *et al.*, 2003; Rajasimha *et al.*, 2004). In the most basic form of this model each simulated cell, is now represented by just two integer values. W is the number of wild-type mtDNA molecules in the cell, and M is the number of mutant mtDNA. Over a time step Δt the changes in the values W and M are given by the following integer difference equations.

$$\begin{aligned} W(t+\Delta t) &= W(t) - W_{loss}(t) + W_{copy}(t) \\ M(t+\Delta t) &= M(t) - M_{loss}(t) + M_{copy}(t) \end{aligned} \tag{8}$$

The number of wild-type and mutant mtDNA lost to degradation is calculated from the following equations.

$$\begin{aligned} W_{loss} &= Poisson(W \times P_d) \\ M_{loss} &= Poisson(M \times P_d) \end{aligned} \tag{9}$$

Acquired mutations are represented by decreasing W and increasing M. For example, if the probability of *de novo* mutation within a time step Δt is set at P_{mut}, then mutation terms are added to Eq. 8 to give the following.

$$\begin{aligned} N_{mut} &= Poisson(W(t) \times P_{mut}) \\ W(t+\Delta t) &= W(t) - W_{loss}(t) + W_{copy}(t) - N_{mut} \\ M(t+\Delta t) &= M(t) - M_{loss}(t) + M_{copy}(t) + N_{mut} \end{aligned} \tag{10}$$

This description of the Cell Level simulation lumps all mutant mtDNA together in a single category. To follow different mutations separately is more complicated in the Cell Level simulation than it was in the mtDNA Molecule Level model. To include more than one mutation type we must extend the basic data structure to $W(t)$, $M_1(t)$, $M_2(t)$, …, $M_n(t)$. Each variable $M_i(t)$ represents the number of mtDNA molecules with a specific mutation. The simulation may be set up to represent a set of predefined mutations, or each new mutation event may define a new mutation type. In the latter case, since we expect most mutations to appear only transiently in the cell before being lost to random drift, it is best to remove any data structure $M_i(t)$ that falls to zero and reuse that data structure for the next new mutation to occur. Otherwise you will end up with a large number of empty data structures. From our experimental and simulation work on human colon crypt cells we found that some crypt cells contained three mtDNA mutations at detectable levels (Taylor *et al.*, 2003), and most crypt cells contained fewer than three different mutations. These experimental results indicate that only a few different mutation data structures would be needed to simulate the range of mtDNA mutations found in a single aging human cell.

Comparison of the mtDNA Molecule Level Model and the Cell Level Model

When you are preparing to build a simulation model of mtDNA in aging, how do you choose the level of detail for the model? The ability to follow individual mtDNA molecules in the mtDNA Molecule Level model makes this approach flexible. It is easier to add new mechanisms to this model, and it is easier to make the characteristics of the mtDNA molecules variable, such as including a replicative advantage to a deletion mutation but not for a point mutation, for example. The price is that the mtDNA Molecule Level simulations require more computation resources than the Cell Level simulations. The mtDNA Molecule Level models are practically limited to simulating a few thousand cells over 100 years.

The Cell Level simulations can model up to a million cells over a time span of a century. This ability to model large numbers of cells is their main advantage. The disadvantage is that adding lower level detail, such as distinguishing between different mtDNA mutants, significantly increases the computational time required and is also difficult to implement. In my experience this type of model is less flexible than the mtDNA Molecule Level models. Also, the presentation of this type of model generally involves more mathematics, and that can be a barrier to communication with the intended biomedical audience.

The choice between the two levels of model often boils down to a practical consideration. Do you have enough computational power available to use the simple and flexible mtDNA Molecular Level model, or do you need the efficiency of the Cell Level simulations? As a guide in making this choice, we present some measurements of the computational time requirements of both models, as a function of the number of simulated cells and the average number of mtDNA molecules per cell. The simulation times were measured on a 2 GHz Pentium 4 CPU with 512 MB RAM running LINUX. Each simulation was run for 100 years, with approximately 1,000 mtDNA molecules in each cell (average value). For both simulation methods the computational time rises linearly with the number of simulated cells (see Figure 48.2).

However, the mtDNA Molecule Level simulation requires 54 seconds per cell per century, whereas the Cell Level model requires only 1.3 seconds per cell per century, a factor of 40 difference.

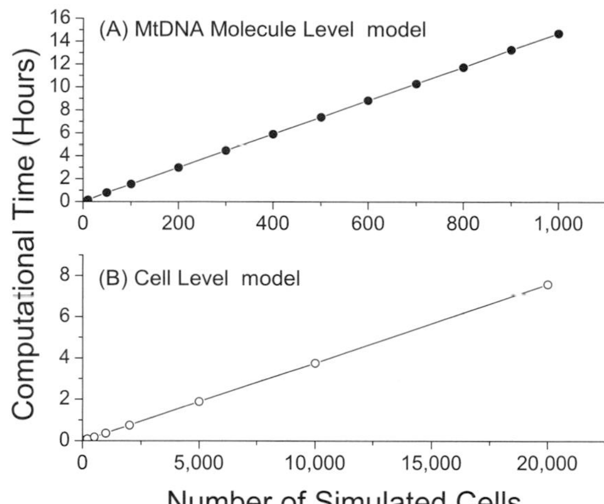

Figure 48.2 Computational time required as a function of the number of compartments simulated for the two simulation methods. Each simulated cell containing approximately 1,000 mtDNA molecules. Simulations were run for 100 years, with a time step of one hour.

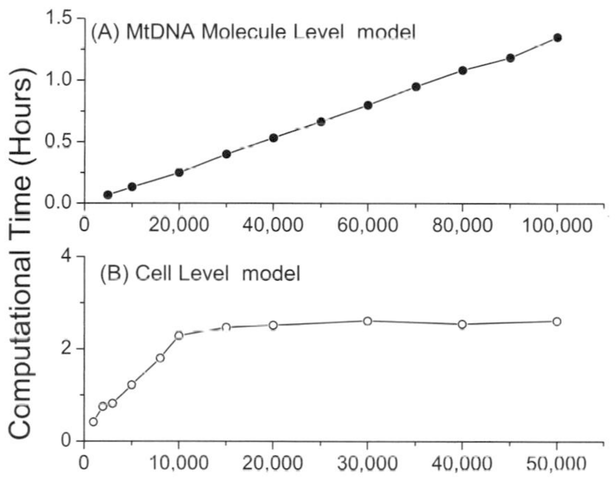

Figure 48.3 Computational time as a function of the number of mtDNA molecules per cell. (A) mtDNA Molecule Level simulation. One cell was simulated for 100 years. The computational time requirements for this method are approximately 48 seconds per cell per century per 1,000 mtDNA molecules. (B) Cell Level simulation. One thousand cells were simulated for 100 years. In the plateau region for more than 10,000 mtDNA molecules per cell, the simulation requirements are approximately nine seconds per simulated cell per century.

In Figure 48.3 we show the dependence of the computation time on the number of mtDNA molecules per compartment.

The mtDNA Molecule Level simulation shows a linear increase in computational time with increasing numbers of mtDNA molecules per cell. This is expected since each mtDNA molecule is modeled separately in this simulation. For the Cell Level simulation (see Figure 48.3B) the behavior is more complicated. The change in behavior from a linear increase up to 10,000 mtDNA per compartment to a relatively constant computation time for a higher number of mtDNA is due to a change in the numerical methods used to calculate the binomial and Poisson distributions (shifting from the direct method to the rejection method). This shift in methods is done automatically by the standard numerical methods described in detail in *Numerical Recipes in C* (Press *et al.*, 1988). The direct method is used when the number returned by the binomial or Poisson distribution subroutines is small, so the location of this switch in numerical methods depends on the time step used. The values in Figure 48.3 are for a time step of one hour. By coincidence, with this time step the computation time flattens out at about 10,000 mtDNA molecules per cell, so the computational requirements of this simulation method are insensitive to the number of mtDNA molecules per cell over an important physiological range (10,000 to 100,000 mtDNA molecules per cell).

Generally, the simulated cells do not interact with each other, and we are interested only in the statistics taken over a large number of independent cells. In this case I recommend that simulations of multiple cells be run sequentially, with each simulated cell run one at a time. Data may be saved at set time points along the simulation, and then statistics over the set of cells can be calculated at these time points after all simulated cells are run. By running the cells sequentially, instead of all at once, the RAM memory requirements of both simulation methods are negligible. However, in simulations where the cells interact in some way, the full set of simulated cells must be calculated simultaneously. For example, we have had to do this in simulations of cell cultures where the cell division rate depends on the number of cells in the simulated culture. In these cases, the Cell Level simulation is the only practical choice since less data must be stored per simulated cell in that method compared to the mtDNA Molecule Level models. On a PC with 512 MB RAM the memory requirements of the Cell Level simulation are not a limitation until the number of simulated cells reaches 8 million.

ADVICE ON THE CHOICE OF SIMULATION METHOD

If you need to simulate either a large number of cells, or cells with more than about 10,000 mtDNA molecules, then the most practical choice is the Cell Level simulation. However, for simplicity and flexibility the mtDNA Molecule Level simulations are the best choice, but you will be limited to simulations of approximately 1,000 cells in order to complete a simulation of 100 years duration in a single day.

Modeling mtDNA Mutations and Aging in Different Species

How do these computational models account for the radically different aging rates that occur in different species? Our simulations show that the time required for the clonal expansions of mtDNA mutations by random drift is proportional to the number of mtDNA molecules per cell, N, and the mtDNA half-life, T_{half} (Chinnery and Samuels, 1999). However, neither of these parameters is believed to vary significantly across mammalian species. The simulations indicate that there is no biologically reasonable way to speed up the process of clonal expansion of mtDNA mutations in short-lived species. The long time scale necessary for clonal expansion by random drift leads us to reconsider the two hypotheses illustrated in Figure 48.1. Although the clonal expansion hypothesis may be the best explanation for the increase in mtDNA mutations with age in the long-lived species, such as humans, for the short-lived species we have to return to the error-cascade hypothesis.

The relative importance of the clonal expansion and error cascade mechanisms in the mtDNA aging simulations is controlled by the parameter P_{mut}, the probability of *de novo* mutation formation in mtDNA. At low mtDNA mutation rates clonal expansions dominate (Taylor *et al.*, 2003), whereas at high mutation rates the error cascade mechanism of enhanced ROS production should be included in the simulations. There is good reason to believe that the mtDNA mutation rate is higher in short-lived species than it is in humans. This has been repeatedly observed in experiments on aging in rodents (Wang *et al.*, 1997; Herrero and Barja, 1999). Finally, our own analysis of the mtDNA sequences of mammals indicates that the mitochondrial genomes of the short-lived species are physically more susceptible to mutations than are those in the long-lived species (Samuels, 2004, 2005).

Conclusion

There are only a few other research groups that have recently worked on simulations of mtDNA dynamics and the aging process. The simulation research program of Tom Kirkwood (Kowald and Kirkwood, 1993; Kowald and Kirkwood, 2000; Sozou and Kirkwood, 2001; Kirkwood and Proctor, 2003) is based on a different general hypothesis than that of our modeling efforts. Their work uses the *delayed degradation* hypothesis, which assumes that mitochondria carrying a large fraction of mutated mtDNA suffer less damage and are thus degraded more slowly than the mitochondria with a larger proportion of wild-type mtDNA. This gives the mutant mtDNA a competitive advantage over the wild-type mtDNA. Another research group that is active in this area of simulation is headed by Konstatin Khrapko (Nekhaeva *et al.*, 2002; Kraytsberg, *et al.*, 2003). The simulations of this group follow the same general hypotheses as we do in our modeling.

For an idea of the future challenges to be dealt with in mtDNA simulations, take another look at Table 48.2. The simulation methods described in this chapter cover only a small range of the scales important to the role of mtDNA in the aging process. In particular, building on simulations of aging at the cellular level to develop an understanding of the aging process at the organism level is a grand challenge.

There are significant challenges to be faced even within the scale range covered by these simulations, between the mtDNA molecule level and the cell level. The complicated spatial organization of mtDNA in separate organelles, and even further into nucleoids (small groupings of 1–5 mtDNA molecules), is a challenge to simulation. The simulations described here do not deal with these intermediate levels of organization, though those of Kirkwood do include the organelle level.

Recommended Resources

Although there are many off-the-shelf simulation packages for biochemical models, there are few such packages available for the types of simulations described in this chapter. For this reason, the research in this area is still primarily done by writing original programs in either C or Fortran. Until a very flexible and general simulation package is available, I recommend that you write your own programs for this research. However, this does not mean writing every line of simulation code from scratch. Here are two excellent sources of code for basic simulation methods, such as the Poisson and Binomial routines used repeatedly in this chapter.

For advice on programming methods for simulation I recommend the very popular series of *Numerical Recipes* books (Press *et al.*, 1988), now available in Fortran, C, C++, and Fortran 90. These books take a very practical approach to numerical methods, not a theoretical one, describing routines that are both effective and relatively simple. The books contain example codes for each numerical method discussed. These codes can be used directly in your simulation for convenience, though often an expert programmer can improve on their efficiency.

For an alternative to the *Numerical Recipes* books, I recommend the GNU Scientific Library (or GSL), available for free download at www.gnu.org/software/gsl. This software library contains over 1000 routines, in C and C++, which can be used as basic building blocks for developing simulation code. The most effective approach may be to read the *Numerical Recipes* books for an understanding of the methods, and use the GSL code in your programs.

Finally, for cross-species comparisons of mitochondrial genomes, the National Center for Biotechnology Information (NCBI), a part of the National Institutes of Health, is the standard repository for all sequenced mitochondrial genomes. These genomes are available at www.ncbi.nlm.nih.gov/genomes/ORGANELLES/organelles.html, in a convenient taxonomic organization. As of this writing (mid-2005), this database contained complete mitochondrial genomes from 713 different species, including 639 metazoa species.

REFERENCES

Alexeyev, M.F., LeDoux, S.P., and Wilson, G.L. (2004). Mitochondrial DNA and aging. *Clin. Sci. 107*, 355–364.

Barja, G. (2004). Free radicals and aging. *Trends Neurosci. 27*, 595–600.

Capps, G.J., Samuels, D.C., and Chinnery, P.F. (2003). A model of the nuclear control of mitochondrial DNA replication. *J. Theor. Biol. 221*, 565–583.

Chinnery, P.F. and Samuels, D.C. (1999). Relaxed replication of mtDNA: A model with implications for the expression of disease. *Am. J. Hum. Genet. 64*, 1158–1165.

Chinnery, P.F., Samuels, D.C., Elson, J., and Turnbull, D.M. (2002). Accumulation of mitochondrial DNA mutations in ageing, cancer, and mitochondrial disease: Is there a common mechanism? *Lancet 360*, 1323–1325.

Elson, J.L., Samuels, D.C., Turnbull, D.M., and Chinnery, P.F. (2001). Random intracellular drift explains the clonal expansion of mitochondrial DNA mutations with age. *Am. J. Hum. Genet. 68*, 802–806.

Herrero, A. and Barja, G. (1999). 8-oxo-deoxyguanosine levels in heart and brain mitochondrial and nuclear DNA of two mammals and three birds in relation to their different rates of aging. *Aging-Clin. Exp. Res. 11*, 294–300.

Huang, H. and Manton, K.G. (2004). The role of oxidative damage in mitochondria during aging: A review. *Front. Biosci. 9*, 1100–1117.

Kirkwood, T.B.L. and Proctor, C.J. (2003). Somatic mutations and ageing in silico. *Mech. Ageing Dev. 124*, 85–92.

Kowald, A. and Kirkwood, T.B.L. (1993). Mitochondrial Mutations, Cellular-Instability and Aging—Modeling the Population-Dynamics of Mitochondria. *Mutat. Res. 295*, 93–103.

Kowald, A. and Kirkwood, T.B.L. (2000). Accumulation of defective mitochondria through delayed degradation of damaged organelles and its possible role in the ageing of post-mitotic and dividing cells. *J. Theor. Biol. 202*, 145–160.

Kraytsberg, Y., Nekhaeva, E., Bodyak, N.B., and Khrapko, K. (2003). Mutation and intracellular clonal expansion of mitochondrial genomes: two synergistic components of the aging process? *Mech. Ageing Dev. 124*, 49–53.

Nekhaeva, E., Bodyak, N.D., Kraytsberg, Y., McGrath, S.B., Van Orsouw, N.J., Pluzhnikov, A. *et al.* (2002a). Clonally expanded mtDNA point mutations are abundant in individual cells of human tissues. *Proc. Natl. Acad. Sci. USA 99*, 5521–5526.

Nekhaeva, E., Kraytsberg, Y., and Khrapko, K. (2002b;). mtLOH (mitochondrial loss of heteroplasmy), aging, and 'surrogate self'. *Mech. Ageing Dev. 123*, 891–898.

Press, W.H., Flannery, B.P., Teukolsky, S.A., and Vetterling, W.T. (1988). *Numerical Recipes in C.* Cambridge: Cambridge University Press.

Rajasimha, H.K., Samuels, D.C., and Nance, R.E. (2004). A simulation methodology in modeling cell divisions with stochastic effects. *Proc. 2004; Winter Sim. Conf.* 2032–2038.

Samuels, D.C. (2004). Mitochondrial DNA repeats constrain the life span of mammals. *Trends Genet. 20*, 226–229.

Samuels, D.C. (2005). Life span is related to the free energy of mitochondrial DNA. *Mech. Ageing. Dev., 126*, 1123–1129.

Skulachev, V.P. (2004). Mitochondria, reactive oxygen species and longevity: some lessons from the Barja group. *Aging Cell 3*, 17–19.

Sozou, P.D. and Kirkwood, T.B.L. (2001). A stochastic model of cell replicative senescence based on telomere shortening, oxidative stress, and somatic mutations in nuclear and mitochondrial DNA. *J. Theor. Biol. 213*, 573–586.

Taylor, R.W., Taylor, G.A., Durham, S.E., and Turnbull, D.M. (2001). The determination of complete human mitochondrial DNA sequences in single cells: implications for the study of somatic mitochondrial DNA point mutations. *Nucleic Acids Res. 29*, art. no.-e74.

Taylor, R.W., Barron, M.J., Borthwick, G.M., Gospel, A., Chinnery, P.F., Samuels, D.C. *et al.* (2003). Mitochondrial DNA mutations in human colonic crypt stem cells. *J. Clin. Invest. 112*, 1351–1360.

Trifunovic, A., Wredenberg, A., Falkenberg, M., Spelbrink, J. N., Rovio, A.T., Bruder, C.E. *et al.* (2004). Premature ageing in mice expressing defective mitochondrial DNA polymerase. *Nature 429*, 417–423.

Wang, E.D., Wong, A., and Cortopassi, G. (1997). The rate of mitochondrial mutagenesis is faster in mice than humans. *Mutat. Res.-Fundam. Mol. Mech. Mutagen. 377*, 157–166.

49

Mouse Models of Accelerated Aging

Jan Vijg and Paul Hasty

Mouse mutants displaying aging phenotypes much earlier in time than normal control animals offer the opportunity to develop and test interventions to reduce aging-related morbidity and mortality in humans. However, the few natural mouse mutants identified in the past as accelerated aging models have been criticized as less suitable for studying mechanisms of normal aging because neither the nature of the mutational defect nor the genetic background was accurately defined. A more general critique involved the perceived large variety of ways to reduce life span by causing pathologies similar to those normally occurring at late age. To address this problem one would ideally specifically design mouse models on the basis of known causes of aging. The validity of such models should then be demonstrated by showing that the genetic intervention accelerates a host of symptoms of normal aging rather than one or few.

Accumulation of DNA damage with age has been implicated as a major cause of aging, an hypothesis strongly supported by the discovery that most human segmental progeroid syndromes are caused by heritable mutations in genes involved in DNA repair and genome maintenance. There are now a number of mouse models, harboring engineered defects in various aspects of genome maintenance, which prematurely display a range of aging phenotypes. This strengthens the hypothesis that aging is driven by spontaneous DNA damage causing genomic instability and cellular stress responses, such as apoptosis and cellular senescence, eventually resulting in systems dysfunction at all levels. In this chapter we will review the recent developments in this field and discuss the validity of the aging phenotypes observed in the mouse models, with a focus on the possible implications with respect to DNA damage as a proximate cause of aging common to all mammals.

Introduction

Aging is poorly defined at the mechanistic level, even though in recent years much progress has been made by studying genetic mutations altering life span and the onset of age-related characteristics (Vijg and Suh, 2005). Subjects of these analyses include yeast (*Saccharomyces cerevisiae*), nematodes (*Caenorhabditis elegans*), fruit flies (*Drosophila melanogaster*), and mice (*Mus musculus*). Intriguingly, in all these species, mutations downregulating activities of growth, reproduction, or nutrient sensing significantly increase longevity, possibly by interfering in the generation of somatic damage or through the upregulation of mechanisms that protect against such damage.

Although the mechanisms underlying age-related degeneration and death in these and other species still need to be uncovered, a consensus as to why and how we age has begun to emerge. It is now generally accepted that the time-dependent decrease in fitness in most multicellular organisms is nonadaptive; that is, it is not controlled by a purposeful genetic program similar to the control of development. Aging provides no specific advantage to the individual and most researchers now accept that age-related degeneration and death is ultimately due to the greater relative weight placed by natural selection on early survival or reproduction than on maintaining vigor at later ages. This decline in the force of natural selection is largely due to the scarcity of older individuals in natural populations owing to mortality caused by extrinsic hazards (Kirkwood, 2005). Because resources are limited, this strategy would not allow a maximization of somatic maintenance and repair, which is not required for periods of time that greatly exceed the time needed to reproduce. Under conditions of lower extrinsic mortality, permitting reproduction at later ages, the allocation of resources would shift toward somatic maintenance, thereby increasing life span. However, maintenance of the soma is never maximized since, according to the nineteenth-century biologist August Weismann, the soma merely provides the housing for the germline, seeing to it that the germ cells are protected, nourished, and conveyed to the germ cells of the opposite sex to create the next generation (Kirkwood and Cremer, 1982). With the soma being dispensable, the trade-off between growth and reproduction on the one hand and somatic maintenance on the other, is biased toward reproduction.

This "disposable soma theory" not only provides a rationale for why we age, but also predicts the nature of its proximate cause; that is, the accumulation of unrepaired somatic damage (Kirkwood, 2005). This explanation, which is now supported by a large body of evidence, also explains the similarities in symptoms of aging, both within and across species, and the apparent universality of genetic pathways of life extension across different phyla. Indeed, rather than being programmed to age, animals are programmed to survive long enough to reproduce, possibly by using highly conserved cellular defense systems against somatic damage common to all or most species. Such damage may come from the environment e.g., radiation, infectious agents but also from inside the organism e.g., reactive oxygen species (ROS), normal by-products of metabolism.

Mouse Models of Aging

Although it is now clear that life span is highly plastic and can be manipulated by metabolic switches that can affect the levels of spontaneous somatic damage or the proportional effort that is devoted to somatic maintenance, we still have only limited insight into the mechanisms of aging in different animal species. To elucidate human aging, mice are a good model system for several reasons. First, mice are positioned close to humans on the evolutionary scale. Second, their relatively short life span and small size permit extensive life span studies on an economic basis. Third, mouse genetics has closely emulated the progress in human genetics and is now almost equally powerful. Fourth, although in mice a full phenotypic characterization of aging is still far from the systematic catalogue of signs and symptoms of old age presently available for humans, the species ranks a solid second with rapid improvements underway.

Indeed, in the wake of the current explosion in genetically engineered mouse models, major coordinated efforts have emerged to obtain standardized and comprehensive databases for morphologic, biochemical, physiologic, or behavioral characteristics of various mouse strains (e.g., the mouse phenome project; http://www.jax.org/phenome). More recently, patterns of age-related pathology of the mouse have been made computationally accessible using ontologies—controlled vocabularies of terms—in the context of a federated database (e.g., www.niehs.nih.gov/cmgcc/dbmouse.htm). Such progress greatly facilitates the development and use of mouse models of accelerated aging.

Mouse models of accelerated aging have been criticized in the past based on the argument that many of the degenerative phenotypes associated with aging could result from a variety of interventions and need not necessarily involve the same causes that underlie natural aging. Although this is a valid argument, it should be realized that the use of model systems to study natural phenomena is a generally accepted approach in biology. For example, human cancer has been studied extensively using laboratory rodents subjected to treatment with a variety of genotoxic agents. Although we were all well aware of the fact that natural human cancers normally were not caused by such treatments, this approach nevertheless allowed us to obtain valuable information about the etiology of this disease. Of note, such rodent models for studying human cancer were based on the rationale that cancer is caused by DNA damage—hence, the use of DNA damaging agents to generate these model systems. By the same token, the most recent series of mouse models for human cancer is based on highly specific genetic alterations, known to increase human susceptibility to cancer. Hence, a logical approach in generating animal models for human aging is to develop specific interventions based on our increased knowledge of what causes human aging.

What can we say about the proximate causes of aging? The disposable soma theory predicts that aging is caused by the accumulation of unrepaired somatic damage (Kirkwood, 2005). There are strong arguments that DNA damage is the most important type of age-accumulated damage and a likely cause of many aging-related phenotypes. Among biological macromolecules, the DNA of the genome is unique in view of its role in transferring genetic information from cell to cell and from generation to generation. A strong, logical argument to consider the DNA of the genome as the Achilles heel of an aging organism is the lack of a back-up template. This is in contrast to proteins, which at least in principle, can be easily replaced with the corresponding gene as template. Indeed, the maintenance of genomic DNA is of crucial importance to survival because its alteration by mutation is essentially irreversible and has the potential to affect all downstream processes. A logical approach for making mouse models for human aging, therefore, would be to inactivate genes involved in DNA repair and genome maintenance. Interestingly, nature itself has preceded us, in this respect, by creating natural human mutants displaying premature aging as a consequence of defects in DNA repair and genome maintenance. This is by itself a powerful argument that changes in DNA drive the aging process. Indeed, genetic defects in few, if any, other systems than DNA repair and genome maintenance have been associated with premature aging (Martin, 2005). The rationale for generating mouse models of human aging on the basis of genetic alterations in genome maintenance pathways is therefore strong but not without problems.

Next we will first discuss the validity of premature aging symptoms in such mouse models and then discuss a number of them in more detail.

Validity of Accelerated Aging Phenotypes

Aging differs from all human diseases by its complexity. It is the most complex phenotype currently known and the only example of generalized biological dysfunction. Its effects become manifest in all organs and tissues, it influences an organism's entire physiology, impacts function at all levels and increases susceptibility to all major chronic diseases. Nevertheless, typical symptoms of aging, often similar across species, can and have been defined.

For human aging, valuable information has been gleaned from a century of clinical observations. It was on this basis that, as mentioned earlier, a series of life-shortening genetic alterations in humans were described over a century ago that appeared to accelerate multiple signs of normal aging (Martin, 2005). These so-called segmental progeroid syndromes, already briefly discussed, were described by the medical community well before the discovery of DNA, and are therefore not biased toward a DNA-based hypothesis of aging. So it is remarkable that so many of these syndromes are defective in genome maintenance. The most striking of the human progeroid syndromes are Werner Syndrome (WS) (Epstein *et al.*, 1965) and Hutchinson-Gilford Progeria Syndrome (HGPS) (Pollex and Hegele, 2004). WS is caused by a defect in a gene that is a member of the RecQ helicase family (Yu *et al.*, 1996). The affected gene, WRN, encodes a RecQ homologue whose precise biological function remains elusive, but is important for DNA transactions, probably including recombination, replication, and repair.

HGPS is caused by a defect in the gene LMNA, which through alternative splicing encodes both nuclear lamins A and C (Eriksson *et al.*, 2003). Nuclear lamins play a role in maintaining chromatin organization. Less striking segmental progeroid syndromes include ataxia telangiectasia, caused by a heritable mutation of the gene ATM (ataxia telangiectasia mutated), a relay system conveying DNA damage signals to effectors (Shiloh, 2003), Cockayne syndrome and trichothiodystrophy, diseases based on defects in DNA repair and transcription (Lehmann, 2003), and Rothmund Thomson syndrome, like Werner syndrome, based on a heritable mutation in a RecQ gene (Lindor *et al.*, 2000). There is evidence that each of these genes when defective can also lead to aging symptoms in the mouse, sometimes in combination with other gene defects (see later, and Hasty *et al.*, 2003).

Although in both humans and mice cancer incidence increases exponentially with age, the tumor spectrum in the two species differs significantly, with sarcomas and lymphomas predominant in the mouse and epithelial cancers in older humans (DePinho, 2000). Likewise, the spectrum of normal age changes (other than cancer) in mice and humans is not exactly the same, which always needs to be kept in mind when using these models (Hasty and Vijg, 2004). Moreover, although cancer as a phenotype is generally undisputed, aging has diffuse characteristics, and includes cancer and a variety of degenerative phenotypes (see www.niehs.nih.gov/cmgcc/dbmouse.htm). Progeroid genotypes are associated with an early onset of some, but not all, characteristics of senescence and must therefore be interpreted with caution.

Loose criteria that help identify genuine mouse mutants of accelerated aging are (1) the phenotype should present after development and maturation are complete; (2) the phenotype should be demonstrable in control populations at a more or less similar point in their survival curve; and (3) the genetic alteration should accelerate multiple aging phenotypes (Hasty and Vijg, 2004). None of these criteria is written in stone. Indeed, accelerated aging can occur even before development is complete, as in the case of HGPS. Such cases, however, are more difficult to recognize as authentic models of aging and may not be as valid as those that exhibit aging phenotypes after maturation. It is also easily imaginable that a genetic alteration accelerates certain symptoms of aging much more than expected on the basis of the survival curve. Such so-called exaggerated aging would be expected if, rather than a quantitative, chronological master switch, the mutation would affect only one critical pathway for somatic maintenance leading to severe imbalance of the survival network.

Interestingly, the single-gene mutations that increase life span in worms, flies and mice may do so through the upregulation of cellular defense systems, including DNA repair and antioxidant defense. Candidate genes implicated in the control of such a survival response are FOXO and SIRT1, which have been demonstrated in nematodes and fruit flies to control downstream targets of the pro-longevity mutations affecting nutrient sensing, reproduction, and growth (Vijg and Suh, 2005). Downregulation of these effector genes could then conceivably lead to an acceleration of all possible aging phenotypes. FOXO3a and SIRT1 knockout mice do not display apparent signs of accelerated aging, although it is possible that a progeroid phenotype will become visible after a more quantitative downregulation of these genes (Cheng *et al.*, 2003; Hosaka *et al.*, 2004).

It should be noted that the mutations that lead to increased longevity in nematodes, flies or mice are likely to do so only at the cost of some selective disadvantage, often not obvious under laboratory conditions (Jenkins *et al.*, 2004). For some of the mouse longevity mutants, such as the growth hormone deficient Ames dwarf mice, fitness costs are readily apparent in the form of infertility and hypothyroidism (Bartke and Brown-Borg, 2004). However, for another longevity mutant in the mouse, $p66^{SHC}$, there is no obvious selective disadvantage

(Migliaccio *et al.*, 1999). At this time the only known consequence of deleting p66SHC is increased life span; thus, we presume the laboratory environment masks any disadvantage. For example, it is possible that p66SHC functions to increase cellular ROS to initiate cellular destruction as a part of our defense system against infectious agents. This potential disadvantage would be masked in the p66SHC-mutant mice since they are housed in a pathogen-free environment. We currently lack the detailed phenotypic comparisons to confirm that longevity-conferring mutations do so by retarding all possible symptoms of aging equally. Hence, though it is clear that mutations in single genes can activate survival pathways conferring increased longevity, the concept of master regulator genes to control the rate of aging is doubtful.

Defects in Genome Maintenance: Observations for Aging and Cancer

Embryonic stem cells and gene targeting technologies have been instrumental in confirming during the last decade the general prediction that genome maintenance systems are critical for suppressing tumor formation (Hoeijmakers, 2001). The data show that mutation of a single gene can increase genomic instability, leading to cancer. Of note, the cancer spectrum in such mutants, as in human cancer hereditary syndromes, is segmental even though these DNA repair pathways function in many cell types that are not predisposed to cancer. Importantly, while focused on cancer, several investigators have found that mutating some genome maintenance genes causes progeroid syndromes. Currently there are a number of mouse lines harboring specific genetic alterations that present with a shortened life span and precocious aging phenotypes (for an exhaustive listing, see Lombard *et al.* (2005)). In each of these mouse models some aspect of genome maintenance is affected. Next, we will briefly discuss the most prominent models with some details of the aging-related phenotypes they affect and their possible link to one or more causal factors. It should be noted that none of these models has been subjected to standardized, objective phenotyping, only some of them were compared side-by-side with littermate controls, and the genetic background may be different from model to model, making comparisons difficult.

THE p53 ANTI-TUMOR RESPONSE AS A CAUSE OF AGING

Defects in cell cycle control have been demonstrated to cause premature aging in mice, most notably mutations in the p53 gene. The p53 tumor suppressor is a transcription factor that controls a network of genes that regulates responses to DNA damage (Vogelstein *et al.*, 2000). The p53 protein inhibits cell cycle progression, facilitates DNA repair, and activates both cellular senescence and apoptosis pathways (Campisi, 2005). Two mutant alleles of p53 have been described, which, in combination with a wild-type allele, result in multiple symptoms of aging and a shortened life span. The p44 allele, a naturally occurring, splice varient first described in 1987, lacks the first transactivation domain (Maier *et al.*, 2004). The other mutant allele, termed M, is a deletion of the 5′ region of the p53 gene, lacking both transactivation domains (Tyner *et al.*, 2002). Both mutants display prominent signs of premature aging, but the two animal models differ, mainly in the severity of the symptoms. The first symptoms of aging in the M mutant become apparent only at 18 months, whereas the p44 animals already show aging-related mortality as early as five months. Severity is probably correlated with the expression level of the mutant allele, which is very low in the case of the M allele. In the p44 model it has been demonstrated that with increasing p44 expression symptoms become much more severe.

Both models display early osteoporosis and kyphosis, major forms of aging-related pathology in both mice and humans. The p44 mice show early fertility loss, to some extent caused by a breakdown of the reproductive axis (H. Scrable, personal communication). This loss of the hypothalamic pituitary gonadal axis is very similar to the situation in natural human and mouse aging (Wise *et al.*, 1997). This loss of fertility is not observed in the M mutant, but again, the symptoms in that model are generally much less severe. Both mouse models suffer from a typical aging-related redistribution of fat resulting in loss of subcutaneous fat. Other typical aging-related phenotypes in these mice are skin problems and various forms of atrophy.

Surprisingly, in both mutants cancer incidence was lower than in the controls. Of note, mice expressing additional copies of wild-type p53 under the control of its own promoter do not show signs of premature aging, but do show lower cancer incidence (Garcia-Cao *et al.*, 2002). In this case, the normal p53 gene dosage is minimally increased (i.e., by one additional copy), resulting in an increased response to DNA damage without affecting basal levels of p53. By contrast, in the two accelerated aging mutants, p53 may be constitutively activated through an interaction of a truncated p53 with a full-length polypeptide. This apparently results in postnatal growth impairment of the animals, possibly caused by a reduced cell proliferation rate as observed in cultured fibroblasts from these animals (Maier *et al.*, 2004). It is also supported by the observation of a two-fold increase of senescent cells in tissue sections of liver and spleen in the p53+/M mice, as compared to control animals (Dumble *et al.*, 2004), a modest rise in comparison to the increase in the number of senescent cells in both mutant and control animals during aging, which was more than ten-fold in these tissues. (Cellular senescence is the irreversible cessation of cell division, which can be observed with all normal mammalian cells in culture.

Senescent cells can be identified by staining for β-galactosidase at pH6.0.)

Of note, increased rates of apoptosis (programmed cell death) in these two mutant mouse models have not been observed (H. Scrable and L. Donehower, personal communication). Indeed, the hyperactive p53 protein most likely causes its effects through increased cell cycle arrest, leading to a general inhibition of cell proliferation. This may explain many of the premature aging phenotypes. For example, impairment of osteoblast proliferation, a likely natural cause of osteoporosis in the elderly, may cause the increased, premature osteoporosis in these mutant mice.

Overall, therefore, abnormally enhanced p53 activity appears to promote many aging-related phenotypes through the inhibition of normal regenerative processes that are essential for adult animals to survive and maintain organ function. As the guardian of the genome, p53 is supposed to inhibit cell growth and proliferation, but only in response to DNA damage, when extra time is needed for repair. Though cancer is also a major aging-related phenotype, enhanced p53 activity would be expected to greatly suppress tumor formation due to its inhibition of normal cell proliferative activities. It is conceivable that in normal mice p53 responses naturally increase with age due to the aforementioned increased load of DNA damage. This would then result in very similar phenotypes as in the p53 mutants, but later in life, as part of the normal aging process.

THE IMPORTANCE OF DNA DOUBLE-STRAND BREAK REPAIR

Double-strand breaks (DSBs) in DNA are highly toxic lesions that can be created through a variety of mechanisms, including effects of reactive oxygen species. Double-strand breaks are repaired by either of two mechanistically distinct DNA repair pathways, homologous recombination (HR) or nonhomologous end-joining (NHEJ) (van Gent *et al.*, 2001). A key factor of DSB repair by NHEJ is the DNA-end-binding Ku70/Ku80 heterodimer. Mice harboring a null mutation in the Ku80 gene have a significantly shorter life span and display a range of premature aging phenotypes (Vogel *et al.*, 1999). For this mouse model the age-related phenotypes have been compared to those of their littermate controls in a side-by-side study in an identical environment (same air, same food, same bedding, same cage). Figure 49.1 shows the survival curve of the Ku80 mutant mice, indicating a significantly shorter life span than their littermate controls.

One of the most prominent aging-related phenotypes occurring early in the mutants is lordokyphosis, the lateral curvature of the spine that is also present in the p53 mutants (see Figure 49.2). Lordokyphosis in these mice is likely due to osteoporosis because histology showed the older Ku80-mutant and control bones to exhibit osteopenia (thinning of the bone and reduced trabeculae). Figure 49.3 shows growth plate closure, a well-known age-related phenotype that is a part of maturation, not senescence, in humans. Mice are different

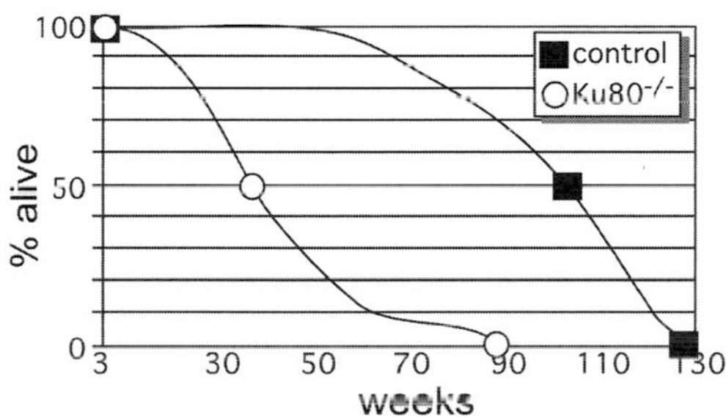

Figure 49.1 Life span and mortality of Ku80-mutant and control mice (Vogel *et al.*, 1999). The survival curve begins after weaning (three weeks), because ku80−/− pups are less able to compete than their bigger littermate controls for mother's milk, and often die within the first two weeks (Nussenzweig *et al.*, 1996). Symbols are shown at the points of 100%, 50%, and 0% survival. Number of mice observed: 47 control mice represented by a filled box and 89 ku80−/− mice represented by an open circle.

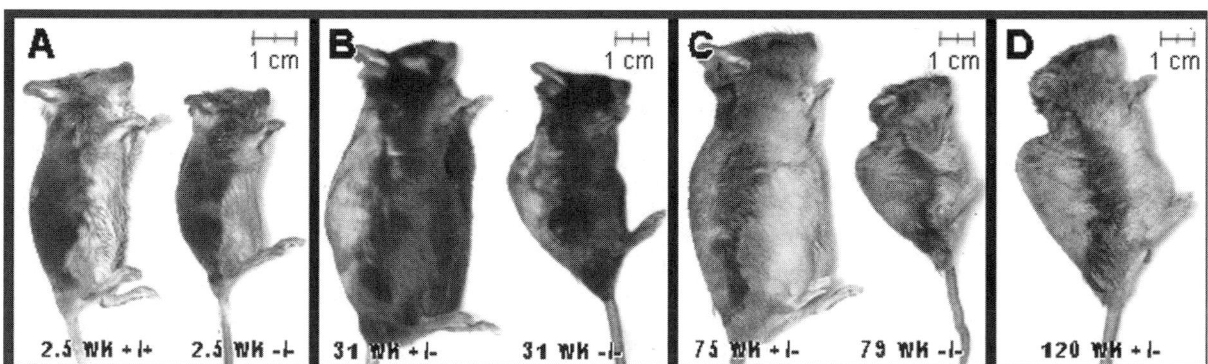

Figure 49.2 Lordokyphosis in control (+/+ and +/−) and ku80−/− (−/−) mice (Vogel *et al.*, 1999). **A**. Mice at 2.5 wk. No kyphosis. **B**. Mice at 31 wk. Kyphosis in only ku80−/− mouse. **C**. Mice at 75–79 wk. Kyphosis in only ku80−/− mouse. **D**. Control mice at 120 weeks (ku80−/− mice do not live this long). Kyphosis observed.

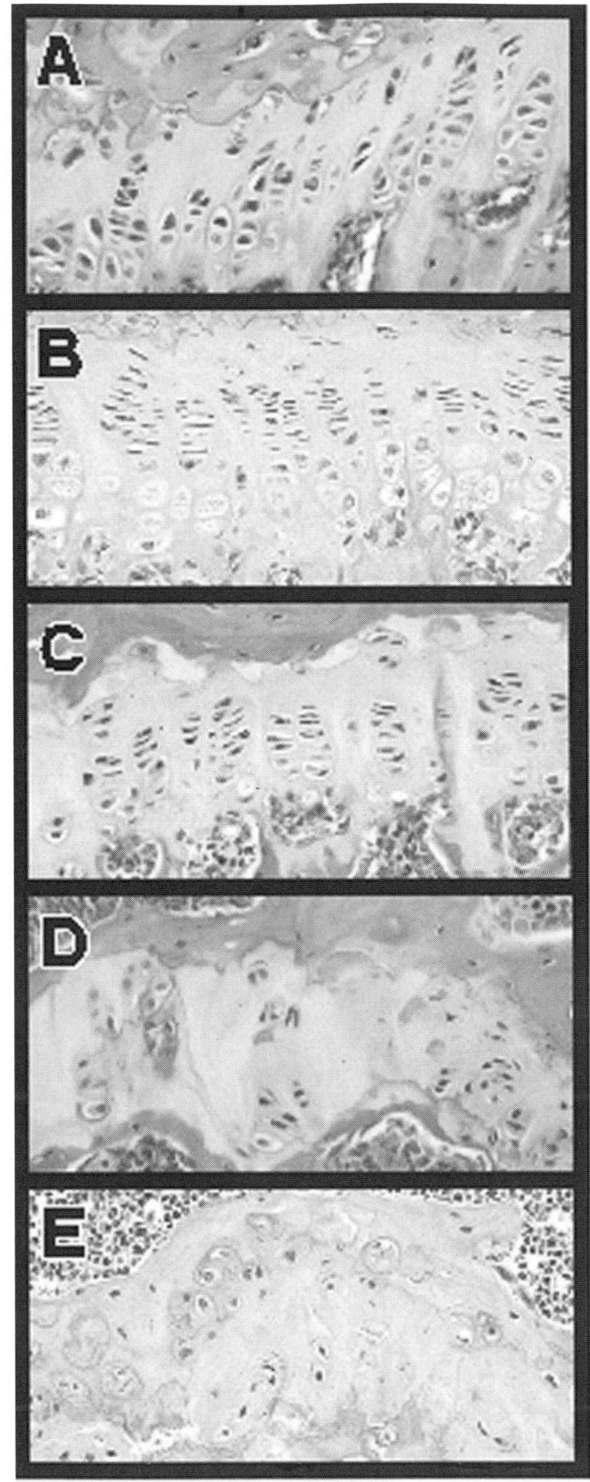

Figure 49.3 Growth plate closure (Vogel *et al.*, 1999). Growth plates look the same for both cohorts between 1 and 15 weeks. However, by 20–45 weeks, compared to controls, the number of chondrocytes is reduced, and the columnar organization of chondrocytes is lost for the ku80−/− epiphysis. This same phenotype is observed for control mice by 70 weeks. Section of epiphysis from control (**A, C, E**) and ku80−/− (**B, D**) mice. (**A, B**), 1–15 weeks (shown are one-week old growth plates). (**C, D**) 20–45 weeks (shown are 22-week-old growth plates). (**E**) Greater than 70 weeks of age. Only the control is shown because very few Ku80-mutant mice survive to this age.

from humans in that growth plates do not close until well after maturation. Here, growth plates close much earlier in Ku80-mutant mice than in control mice. Figure 49.4 illustrates skin atrophy, a well-described age-related phenotype in both mice and humans. Again, skin atrophy was observed earlier in Ku80-mutant mice than in their littermate controls. In addition, various other aging-related phenotypes were observed in Ku80-mutant mice, well before they appeared in their littermate controls (forms of liver degeneration, reactive immune responses). Even though these phenotypes occur earlier in Ku80-mutant mice than in the controls, they all occur at about the same point in their biological life spans (the latter half of their survival curve). Despite these similarities, there are differences; most obvious is the difference in cancer incidence (cancer incidence is much lower in Ku80-mutant mice than in their littermate controls).

The most straightforward explanation for the accelerated aging phenotypes in Ku80 null mice is increased genomic instability resulting from erroneous or inefficient repair of DNA double-strand breaks in the absence of NHEJ. Such increased genomic instability would trigger apoptosis and interfere with normal cell growth and tissue regeneration. Whereas increased genomic instability normally would be expected to promote tumor formation, the increased rate of apoptosis in the presence of an intact p53 checkpoint is likely to restrain tumor development. This scenario is supported by actual observations. Ku80 mutant mouse cells display growth impairment, increased susceptibility to apoptosis, and a marked increase in chromosomal aberrations, including breaks, translocations, and aneuploidy (Difilippantonio *et al.*, 2000). Results from our laboratories indicate increased genomic instability at a lacZ reporter locus in liver, and, especially, in spleen, already at five months of age. In liver of 10-month-old mice, increased numbers of TUNEL or caspase 3 positive cells were observed, indicating a higher rate of spontaneous apoptosis (Y. Suh and P. Hasty, unpublished results).

Hence, though the inability of the Ku80 mutant mouse to repair DNA damage leads to excessive genome rearrangements, the resulting increase in cell death or dysfunction becomes manifest as impaired proliferation and regeneration, resulting in diminished cancer and accelerated age-related organ and tissue degeneration. This situation may be very similar for two other mouse models with defects in double-strand break repair: mice with defects in DNA-PK_{CS}, the catalytic subunit of the Ku70/Ku80 complex, and mice harboring a hypomorphic mutation in the BRCA1 gene, a major player in HR. In DNA-PK_{CS} null mice the situation resembles the Ku80 null model: the absence of intact NHEJ promotes genomic instability leading to impaired tissue growth and regeneration (Espejel *et al.*, 2004). Complete loss of BRCA1 is embryonically lethal, and the same is true for the homozygous BRCA1 hypomorph, lacking exon 11. However, the homozygous hypomorph can be rescued completely in a p53 heterozygous background. In a p53-homozygous mutant background, these mice exhibit a high incidence of cancer. In the p53 heterozygous background, BRCA1 hypomorphic mice exhibit a long list of premature aging phenotypes and a significant reduction of life span, probably caused by the activity of the remaining p53 allele, which is triggered by genomic instability to prevent normal cell proliferation (Cao *et al.*, 2003).

Thus far, there is no evidence that inactivation of Ku80's partner in NHEJ (i.e. Ku70) is causing accelerated aging (Gu *et al.*, 1997). However, Ku70 null mice have never been studied as an aging cohort over longer periods of time in parallel with their littermate controls. Such studies are now underway and should soon reveal if there really is a difference between the Ku80 and Ku70 mutants. It is possible that each of these two key players in DSB repair has other, tissue-specific functions that confound their role in suppressing aging.

AGING, DNA REPAIR, AND TRANSCRIPTION

Another type of DNA repair defect associated with premature aging involves transcription-related nucleotide excision repair (NER). NER removes a broad range of helix-distorting lesions, from UV-induced DNA damage and numerous chemical adducts to oxidative damage produced by endogenous metabolism (Hoeijmakers, 2001). Within NER two subpathways are recognized, differing in damage recognition but sharing the same repair machinery: global genome NER (GG-NER) for the removal of distorting lesions anywhere in the genome and transcription-coupled NER (TC-NER) for the elimination of distorting DNA damage blocking transcription. Two mouse models with defects in NER have been reported to display premature aging symptoms: the Xpd hypomorph (de Boer *et al.*, 2002) and the Ercc1 knockout or hypomorph (Weeda *et al.*, 1997).

In humans, a heritable mutation in the XPD gene is responsible for the disorder trichothiodystrophy (TTD). TTD shows no predisposition to cancer, but leads to severely impaired physiological and neurological development, including retarded growth, cachexia, sensorineural hearing loss, retinal degeneration and its hallmark features of brittle hair, nails, and scaly skin (Lehmann, 2003). TTD patients have a strongly reduced life span, and the disease often is considered as a segmental progeroid syndrome. The helicase encoded by the XPD gene is one of the 10 subunits of basal transcription factor IIH (TFIIH), which is required for multiple processes: GG-NER, TC-NER of NER and non-NER lesions, as well as transcription initiation by RNA polymerase I and II.

An Xpd-deficient mouse model was generated by mimicking a human mutation that causes TTD (de Boer *et al.*, 1998). This mutation does not ablate but rather alters the normal activity of Xpd. These mice have impaired transcription and mildly impaired NER.

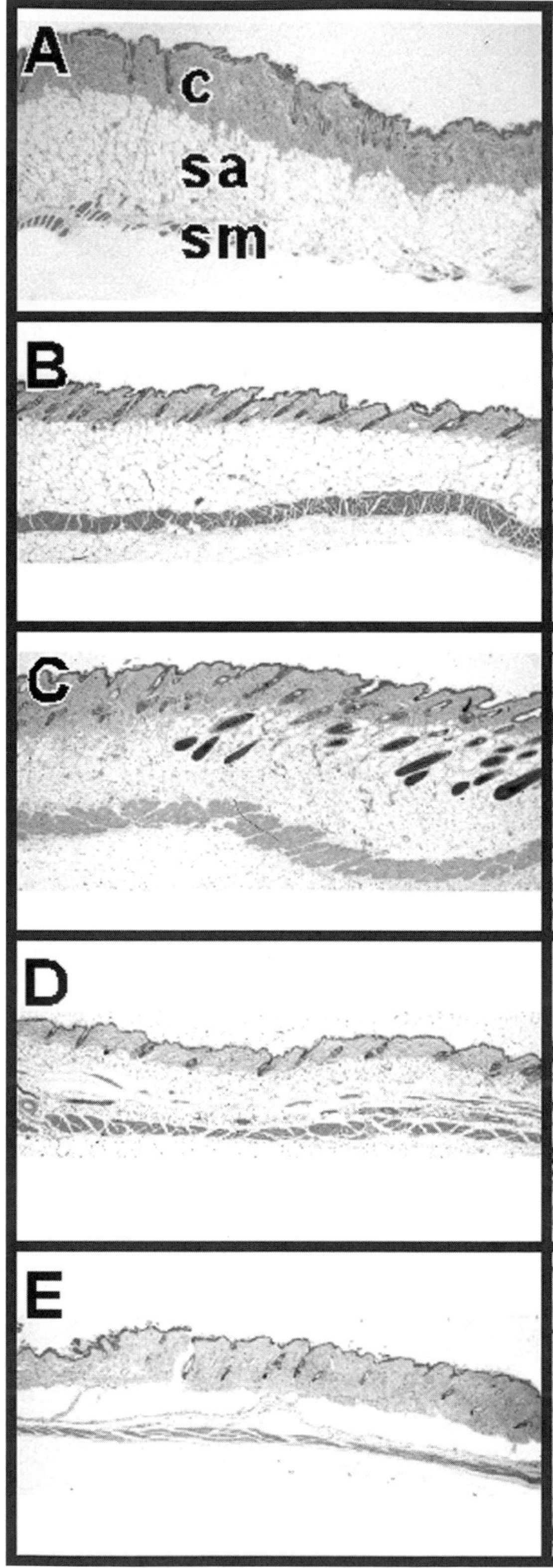

Figure 49.4 Skin atrophy (Vogel *et al.*, 1999). Section of skin (dorsal region over cranial to mid-thorax) from control (**A, C, E**) and ku80−/− (**B, D**) mice. Skin looks the same for both cohorts between 1 and 15 weeks. However, by 40 weeks, compared to control, all subcutaneous elements, including superficial collagen, subcutaneous adipose and skeletal muscle are atrophied for ku80−/− skin. This same phenotype is observed for control mice by 70 weeks.

TABLE 49.1
Aging-related phenotypes in *Xpd* mutants and C57BL/6 control mice (Wijnhoven *et al.*, 2005)

	C57BL/6		*XpdTTD*	
	Incidence	Severity	Incidence	Severity
Osteoporosis femur	88.2	3.3	97.1	4.1
Hepatic lipofuscin accumulation	85.0	1.6	97.1	3.1
Hepatic intranuclear inclusions	10.0	0.1	28.6	0.5
Hepatocellular atrophy	5.0	0.1	34.3	0.5
Renal karyomegaly	17.9	0.2	38.2	0.7
Renal tubular dilatation	30.8	0.5	85.3	2.2
Renal hyaline glomerulopathy	15.4	0.3	52.9	1.1
Aortic sarcopenia	5.6	0.1	87.9	2.0
Lymphoid depletion spleen	30.8	0.4	85.7	2.0
Lymphoid depletion thymus	82.8	2.6	100	3.7
Skin reduced hypodermal fat	18.9	0.5	85.7	2.9
Heart lipofuscin accumulation	100	1.9	100	2.3

These characteristics closely resemble those of humans with the disorder, including brittle hair. At this time, Xpd mice have been exhaustively characterized side-by-side with their littermate controls in a similar C57Bl/6 genetic background. The results indicate a host of premature aging symptoms (see Table 49.1), but also a limited number of TTD-specific phenotypes (Wijnhoven *et al.*, submitted). Life span was reduced in this model by about 10%.

Are the accelerated aging characteristics observed in the Xpd mutant mice due to defective DNA repair alone? Xpd is important for repairing DNA in association with transcription, so the exact way in which it delays age-related decline is difficult to determine. Complete abrogation of NER, accomplished by mutating Xpa, has not yet been shown to cause premature aging in mice (de Vries *et al.*, 1995). Thus, defective NER, which leads to an accumulation of DNA mutations, is unlikely to be the sole cause of early senescence in Xpd mutant mice. However, defective DNA repair apparently does contribute to premature senescence in these animals. This can be derived from the observation that a much more severe phenotype is obtained by crossing the Xpd mutants with an Xpa-knockout mouse (Jan Hoeijmakers, Harry van Steeg, personal communication).

It is conceivable that a response to stalled transcription at sites of DNA damage is responsible for early aging in the Xpd mutant mice. In this scenario, a defective TFIIH results in stalled transcription that decreases gene activity and leads to a mild accumulation of DNA damage. Cells respond by undergoing apoptosis, which may cause the early organismal senescence in these mice. In the absence of Xpa alone (with a fully functional Xpd protein), transcription from a damaged DNA template can still take place, possibly because the amount of spontaneous damage subject to NER is low. (Base excision repair, not NER, is the main pathway for removing the most abundant forms of spontaneous DNA damage, such as oxidative lesions.) In combination with the Xpd mutation, however, the complete absence of Xpa would exacerbate the suboptimal performance of TFIIH, leaving the DNA lesion exposed for a greater period of time; this would result in a further decline in gene activities and an enhanced response. Thus, the premature aging symptoms in the Xpd mutant mouse may be primarily the result of a cellular response to impaired TFIIH at the site of a spontaneous DNA lesion, rather than the accelerated accumulation of DNA damage or mutations. Indeed, mutation frequencies at a lacZ reporter locus in this mouse model were not elevated as compared to control animals of the same age (Dollé *et al.*, in press). The role of p53 responses as a possible causal factor in the aging phenotypes displayed by Xpd mutant mice is unknown.

Another NER-defective mouse model showing symptoms of premature aging involves the gene ERCC1. The ERCC1-XPF complex forms an endonuclease, which is required for the 5′ incision to remove the damage-containing oligonucleotide during NER, but also essential for interstrand crosslink repair (ICLR). Hence, Ercc1 knock-out ($Ercc1^{-/-}$) mice are deficient in GG-NER, TC-NER, and ICLR. These mice show a severe phenotype including runted growth, progressive neurological abnormalities, kyphosis, a short life span of about three weeks, and liver and kidney dysfunction (Weeda *et al.*, 1997). At the cellular level the Ercc1 defect leads to accelerated nuclear polyploidization. The combination of a knock-out allele with a truncated Ercc1 allele

($Ercc1^{-/m}$), resulting in a protein lacking the last seven amino acids, delays the onset of the premature aging phenotype and extends the maximal life span to about four to six months (Weeda *et al.*, 1997). Similar to the Xpd mutant, the premature appearance of aging symptoms is not caused by the defect in NER (which may contribute), but mainly to the defect in the removal of the highly toxic interstrand crosslinks. In the hypomorphic Ercc1 mutant mouse an increased level of genomic instability at a lacZ reporter locus was observed at four months of age (Dolle *et al.*, in press). Although this mouse model may ultimately appear as a valid model of accelerated aging, the fact that severe symptoms already appear before development is complete makes this less suitable for modeling aging phenotypes that normally appear only in adult animals.

WRN, ATM, AND TELOMERES IN MICE AND MEN

At least three other mouse mutants harboring defects related to DNA repair have been identified as models of accelerated aging. The first of these models that should be mentioned is the WRN-defective mouse. In most of the preceding cases the mouse mutants of genome instability were generated primarily for studying cancer, but the WRN gene defect was modeled on its own account as an accelerated aging model (Lebel and Leder, 1998; Lombard *et al.*, 2000). Human WS patients prematurely exhibit signs of senescence including atrophic skin, graying and loss of hair, osteoporosis, malignant neoplasms, diabetes, and shortened life span (Goto, 1997). Furthermore, increased genomic instability at the HPRT locus has been reported in peripheral blood lymphocytes from these patients (Fukuchi *et al.*, 1989). Mice deleted for Wrn exhibit no obvious phenotype, suggesting redundancy with another RecQ helicase or differences in threshold levels or nuclear localization (Lebel and Leder, 1998; Lombard *et al.*, 2000).

However, the fact that Wrn-mutant mice do not recapitulate WS as seen in humans does not diminish the potential importance of the human phenotype with regard to aging or the importance of mouse models. Similar cases, in which the mouse model failed to recapitulate the human phenotype, have been observed many times for genes that suppress cancer in humans. However, at a closer look, the proteins involved were found to perform remarkably similar biochemical functions with the same physiological significance in both species. For example, the retinoblastoma protein (pRb) is a tumor suppressor that in humans prevents the formation of tumors in the retina. However, in Rb-deficient mice, retinoblastoma does not occur. Instead, adenomas develop in the intermediate pituitary gland. However, retinoblastomas will develop in Rb mutant mice after reducing the expression of an Rb family member, p107 (Robanus-Maandag *et al.*, 1998). Thus, the difference in phenotype between mouse and human is due simply to different levels of expression of Rb family genes. Therefore, tumor suppressor genes perform remarkably similar functions in mice and humans at both the biochemical and physiological levels.

An important confounder of modeling human cancer and aging in the mouse involves telomere instability. Telomeres are the nucleoprotein complexes that occur at the ends of eukaryotic linear chromosomes. In the mammalian genome they consist of several kilobase pairs of repetitive DNA sequences (TTAGGG) that attract a number of sequence- and structure-specific binding proteins. These chromosomal caps prevent nucleolytic degradation and provide a mechanism for cells to distinguish natural termini from DNA double-strand breaks, which signal DNA damage, resulting in cell cycle arrest, senescence, or apoptosis. Telomeres terminate in 35-600 bases of single-stranded TTAGGG at the 3′ end (the 3′ overhang). This 3′ overhang folds back into the duplex TTAGGG repeat array forming a so-called t-loop. Telomeres are also thought to buffer the internal coding regions of the genome from the consequences of the end replication problem, that is, the inability to complete the 5′ end by lagging strand synthesis. Although this may temporarily protect the genome against attrition, cells would inevitably lose terminal DNA with each cell division. However, telomere attrition can be countered by elongation mechanisms. The most important of these elongation mechanisms is telomerase, a reverse transcriptase composed of a protein component and an RNA (complementary to the telomeric single-stranded overhang) that can synthesize telomeric DNA directly onto the ends of chromosomes. Telomerase is present in most fetal tissues, normal adult male germ cells, inflammatory cells, proliferative cells of renewable tissues, and in most tumor cells (for a recent review on telomeres and telomerase, see Blackburn (2005)).

Telomerase null mice have been made by ablation of the RNA component of the enzyme, Terc (Blasco *et al.*, 1997). The enzyme is less important in mice than in humans because mice have very long telomeres. This is thought to be the reason that mice are more prone to sarcomas and lymphomas whereas humans are more prone to epithelial tumors (DePinho, 2000). Indeed, late-generation (i.e., fifth to eighth generation) of telomerase knockout mice display a more human tumor spectrum (Artandi *et al.*, 2000). Progressive telomere erosion in Terc null mice of somewhat earlier generation has been found associated with premature aging symptoms, but these represented far from a full spectrum of classical pathophysiological symptoms of aging. In these mice, age-dependent telomere shortening and increased genetic instability were associated with shortened life span as well as a reduced capacity to respond to stresses such as wound healing and hematopoietic ablation (Rudolph *et al.*, 1999).

As mentioned earlier, the ataxia-telangiectasia mutated (ATM) gene, when defective, causes a segmental progeroid disorder in humans. ATM stimulates cell cycle responses to the highly toxic DNA double-strand breaks. One of its targets is actually p53, which can also be activated via ATM-independent mechanisms. Premature aging in ataxia telangiectasia is not that obvious (Chun and Gatti, 2004), and in its mouse counterpart progeroid symptoms are even less prominent (Xu *et al.*, 1996) unless they are bred into a Terc-deficient background. Against the background of eroding telomeres, the double null mice exhibited a general growth and cell proliferation defect, probably causing the extensive organ dysfunction observed in this mouse model (Wong *et al.*, 2003). In contrast to the p53 mutants, the cause of the problems in these mice is likely to be increased genomic instability and an elevated apoptosis rate. This is typically observed in the Atm and Terc mutants separately, but greatly accelerated by the combined defect. It results in diminished stem cell reserve in several organ systems, and, similar to the situation in the p53 mutants, this impairment in regenerative capacity results in premature aging, exemplified by lordokyphosis, reduced muscle and fat mass, and several other aging-related phenotypes. Hence, in the combined Terc/Atm mutants the accelerated aging phenotype is much more convincingly expressed than in each mutant separately.

Similar to the Atm mutants, bringing the Wrn defect into a Terc-deficient background dramatically uncovered an array of premature aging phenotypes reminiscent of the human syndrome (Chang *et al.*, 2004). After four to six generations, during which the initially long telomeres of these mice become progressively shorter, mice were obtained of shorter life span displaying premature aging symptoms at 12 to 16 weeks. Symptoms included hair loss, cataract formation and hypogonadism, osteoporosis, type II diabetes and lordokyphosis, which are typical for Werner syndrome patients. Since Werner syndrome patients display high levels of spontaneous genome instability in their peripheral blood lymphocytes, bone marrow metaphases in the late-generation double knockout mice were examined and showed similar, marked genomic instability. Increased genomic instability was also observed in embryonic fibroblasts from these mice as well as a reduction in their replicative life span. A marked increase in apoptosis rates was observed in intestinal crypt cells. Although not prominently cancer prone, the earlier generation Terc null mice succumbed to osteosarcomas and soft tissue sarcomas, typical for Werner syndrome patients but not for mice.

It is known that WRN, like ATM, plays a role in telomere maintenance, and the conclusion could easily be drawn that the Wrn mutation mainly reinforces the premature phenotype reported to be associated with the ablation of Terc alone. Conceivably, in mesenchymal tissues, which are mainly affected in the Terc/Wrn double knockouts, intact WRN is able to compensate for the lack of telomerase. It may be able to do that through its role (like ATM) in HR, a repair process known to be involved in the maintenance of eukaryotic telomeres (Tarsounas and West, 2005). Ultimately, the cause of the accelerated aging phenotypes is likely to be very similar to the one discussed for the Terc/Atm, Ku80, and Brca1 defective mice, namely, increased genomic instability resulting in impairment of cell proliferation. The same probably would apply to a third "accessory DNA repair"-defective mouse model, the topoisomerase IIIβ deficient mouse model.

It is known that topoisomerases interact with RecQ helicases (Laursen *et al.*, 2003). Even though there is virtually no phenotype in Wrn mutant mice, deletion of the helicase domain of Wrn increases the mutation frequency at the Hprt locus and reduces proliferation of embryonic fibroblasts from these mice. Both cellular phenotypes are exacerbated by inhibition of topoisomerase I (Lebel and Leder, 1998). The Wrn defect also increases tumor formation in a p53 defective background, much more than the p53 defect by itself (Lebel *et al.*, 2001; Lombard *et al.*, 2000). The combined defect also resulted in tumors, such as sarcomas, which do not normally develop in a p53 null mouse model. Based on the increased sensitivity to topoisomerase inhibition of cells from the Wrn defective mice (which has also been demonstrated for lymphoblastoid cells derived from Werner syndrome patients Poot *et al.*, 1999) it is possible that the Wrn defect is to some extent caused by impaired interaction with topoisomerases. This is supported by the observation of some aspects of premature aging in mice with a topoisomerase defect, that is, topoisomerase IIIβ null mice. Such mice develop normally but exhibit a shortened life span with an age-related phenotype that includes a marked increase in ulcerative dermatitis (Kwan and Wang, 2001). Analyses of yeast cells suggest that the topoisomerase IIIβ phenotype is influenced by RecQ helicase activity. Yeast cells deleted for the topoisomerase III homologue, TOP3, exhibit slow growth, hyper-recombination, genomic instability, impaired sporulation and increased sensitivity to genotoxic agents (Wallis *et al.*, 1989). Interestingly, this phenotype is suppressed by deletion of Sgs1, a RecQ helicase, indicating that Sgs1 creates a deleterious topological substrate that needs to be resolved by TOP3 (Gangloff *et al.*, 1994). Conceivably, ablating the Top3β gene may impair the RecQ family members causing the symptoms of aging, which Wrn inactivation alone, at least in the mouse, cannot accomplish.

NUCLEAR STRUCTURE

Attention was drawn to the importance of maintaining nuclear organization as a longevity assurance system once it was demonstrated that Hutchinson Gilford Progeroid Syndrome (HGPS) is caused by *de novo* mutations in the gene LMNA, encoding both lamin A and lamin B through alternative splicing (Eriksson *et al.*, 2003). A *de novo* mutation activates a cryptic splice site, effectively resulting in a protein with a 50 amino acid deletion near the C-terminus of lamin A. This deletion allows farnesylation but prevents proteolytic cleavage of the prelamin A to generate the final product. The resulting mutant lamin A acts in a dominant fashion (patients are heterozygous), and the aberrant protein is called progerin. Although mouse models accurately mimicking the human defect are now being generated in different laboratories, two potentially relevant mouse models deserve some discussion. The first is a null mouse for the gene Zmptse24 metalloproteinase, an enzyme involved in the proteolytic processing of prelamin A. Apart from nuclear abnormalities, this model shows growth retardation, alopecia, bone fractures, muscle weakness, and early cardiac dysfunction (Bergo *et al.*, 2002). More recently, accelerated aging in these mice has been linked to p53 signalling activation, supporting the concept that hyperactivation of the tumour suppressor p53 may cause accelerated ageing (Varela *et al.*, 2005). The second model originally was aimed at mimicking a mutation in LMNA that in humans normally results in Emery-Dreifuss muscular dystrophy (EDMD). (Heritable mutations in lamin A/C or lamin-binding proteins cause various diseases other than HGPS. For example, mutations in emerin, a lamin-binding protein, or LMNA cause EDMD, and mutations in LMNA can also cause Dunnigan-type partial lypodystrophy. The mutations that cause these diseases are nonoverlapping, and it is unclear as to how different mutations in the same gene can cause different diseases.) The homozygous EDMD mutation in the mouse causes death in four to six weeks. The mice develop severe growth retardation and a number of other symptoms reminiscent to HGPS patients (Mounkes *et al.*, 2003). In neither of the two mouse models have genomic instability, cell growth rate, or apoptosis rate been studied thus far. In interpreting these results, keep in mind that HGPS is an early-onset segmental progeroid syndrome that occurs before reproductive maturation. Hence, it is unrealistic to expect an adult-onset type of premature aging.

Is it possible to ascribe HGPS to a defect in genome maintenance? Lamins at the nuclear periphery and throughout the nucleoplasm are thought to maintain nuclear shape. However, they may also contribute to tissue-specific gene expression, through their role as key elements in nuclear architecture (Gruenbaum *et al.*, 2005). Regions of chromatin appear to be anchored to the lamina, and, at least *in vitro*, lamins have been demonstrated to bind directly to chromatin. In this respect, the actions of a gene are not only influenced by its position in the one-dimensional DNA sequence, relative to regulatory elements, but also by its particular location in the nucleus. Such position effects may include not only transcription, but also replication, repair, and recombination. For example, when DNA undergoes more than one double-strand break the spatial proximity of the broken ends is positively correlated with the probability of illegitimate joining. Hence, it is of the utmost importance to faithfully maintain lamin organization, defects that are likely to result in genomic instability. Indeed, it was recently found that Zmpste24-deficient mouse embryonic fibroblasts show increased DNA damage and chromosome aberrations and are more sensitive to DNA-damaging agents (Liu *et al.*, 2005).

MITOTIC SPINDLE CHECKPOINT AND THE ROLE OF ANEUPLOIDY

Before mitosis, the mitotic spindle checkpoint allows every chromosome to send a stop signal, arresting cell growth until all the chromosomes are appropriately distributed. Defects in this checkpoint provoke chromosome missegregation and aneuploidy (gain or loss of chromosomes), which can have adverse functional consequences, including cell death, but also cancer. For example, defects in different components of the mitotic spindle checkpoint have consistently been observed in cancer cells, characterized by chromosomal instability (Hanks and Rahman, 2005). Recently, a mouse model was made based on partial inactivation of the gene BubR1, encoding a spindle assembly checkpoint protein. These mice have a median life span of only six months and display a host of premature aging symptoms, including lordokyphosis, cataracts, and muscle atrophy (Baker *et al.*, 2004). They developed aneuploidy from the age of two months onward that increased as the mice aged further. There was a strong correlation between the degree and severity of the chromosome number instability and the onset and progression of the aging phenotypes. Increased apoptosis in several tissues from these animals at one year of age was not found. However, senescence-associated β-galactosidase activity was high as compared to control mice. This observation of increased cellular senescence *in vivo* was further supported by an accelerated rate of senescence of embryonic fibroblasts cultured from these mice, which also correlated with the degree of aneuploidy observed in these same cells. Hence, the progressive aneuploidy was assumed to be the underlying cause of both *in vitro* senescence and the premature aging symptoms *in vivo*. Interestingly, BubR1 expression declines in tissues of normal mice with age (Baker *et al.*, 2004). Hence, it is conceivable that increased aneuploidy, which has been observed in aging animals, contributes to normal aging as well.

A somewhat unexpected finding in this study was the virtual lack of spontaneous tumors in the mutants, in spite of the fact that aneuploidy is one of the hallmarks of cancer. In this respect, it is possible that the severity of the aneuploidy, while initially promoting the genesis of cancer cells, eventually prevents further tumor progression, similar to the situation in the aforementioned Atm/Terc mutant mice. This could be a direct effect of ongoing polyploidization or facilitated through the activation of an aneuploidy checkpoint.

BACK TO MITOCHONDRIA

Another example of a mouse model with a defect in genome maintenance especially designed to test the hypothesis that genomic instability is involved in aging is the PolgA proofreading-deficient mouse model. PolgA, the catalytic core of the mitochondrial DNA polymerase gamma (Polg), is a mtDNA polymerase, encoded in the nuclear genome. Hence, proofreading defects in this gene would be expected to lead to increased mutations in the mitochondrial genome. Mutations in both nuclear and mitochondrial DNA have been demonstrated to accumulate with age in a tissue-specific pattern (Arnheim and Cortopassi, 1992; Vijg and Dollé, 2002). Hence, in the PolgA deficient mouse we would expect to see the premature appearance of aging-related phenotypes, which turned out to be correct. Apart from a three- to five-fold increase in mtDNA mutations in brain, heart, and liver, and respiratory chain dysfunction in the heart, a host of premature aging symptoms was observed in this mutant, including osteoporosis, lordokyphosis, alopecia, a growth defect, reduced subcutaneous fat, hypertrophy of the heart, and anemia (Trifunovic *et al*., 2004). Life span was reduced by about 50%. Interestingly, the enhanced mitochondrial mutation load in these mtDNA mutator mice already was established at two months and did not dramatically increase thereafter. This suggests that once present, somatic mutations can continue to exert adverse physiological effects even without any further dramatic increases. It is possible that the premature aging phenotypes arise through increased ROS production as a consequence of respiratory chain dysfunction in these mice. However, in a more recent study, in which a similar mouse model was generated and studied, evidence for increased oxidative stress was not found. Instead, accumulation of mtDNA mutations was found to be associated with increased apoptosis (Kujoth *et al*., 2005).

Conclusion

We have reviewed a range of genetically engineered mouse models, harboring specific defects in genome maintenance and exhibiting a common array of aging-related phenotypes, even though the mutated genes represent a diverse range of pathways. As discussed, the most convincing models undergo normal development and then prematurely exhibit such an impressive array of common aging features that it is difficult to maintain that these mutants do not faithfully mimic aspects of the normal aging process. At this point in time, the question is no longer whether the premature aging phenotypes in these mice are genuine, but rather why different genetic defects in some aspect of the complex network of genome maintenance all lead to very similar endpoints in aging. To the best of our knowledge, genome maintenance is the only system in which such a wide variety of defects leads to such a recognizable pattern of phenotypic changes. Before discussing the most logical explanation of this phenomenon, we will first address two specific caveats of accelerated aging models.

The first caveat involves the lack of mouse models recapitulating all possible aging symptoms in an accelerated fashion. We could argue that only gene defects that accelerate all possible symptoms of normal aging are likely to truly intervene in its core mechanisms. In this respect, it is important to realize that it is unknown if some of the aforementioned mouse mutants do not display a full complement of aging characteristics, like their littermate controls. First of all, in a typical population of humans or mice, there is not a single individual displaying all possible symptoms of aging. Although it is indeed very likely that human progeroid disorders are in fact segmental (Martin, 2005), the number of patients is often too small to exclude the possibility that other aging-related phenotypes also are accelerated. In mice, the situation is seriously confounded due to the variation in genetic background. It is very possible that a particular phenotype that is associated with normal aging in one genetic background is not observed in others. However, the expectation of mutants accelerating or decelerating all aspects of normal aging is probably unrealistic.

We have already alluded to the lack of evidence for pacemaker genes orchestrating all the critical aspects of the fundamental mechanisms of normal aging. Because of its very nature as a byproduct of evolution, the postmaturational changes considered as aging are ill-defined, with major confounders in the form of genetic, environmental, and stochastic variation. It seems highly unlikely that the many different individual phenotypes of aging, which may be related and/or interact with each other, are controlled by one or few genes. Therefore, it is not to be expected that single-gene mutations accelerate all aging symptoms characteristic for the normal population. Indeed, if DNA damage would be the single most important cause of aging, the hundreds of genes directly involved in its metabolism immediately refute the possibility of a simple genetic control center specifying each and every aging-related phenotype. Mutations in only one of these genes may cause one or few aging symptoms, but will never accelerate all possible signs of aging that are characteristic for the population under study.

On the other hand, there is abundant evidence that multiple cellular defense systems can be upregulated in concert, to increase stress resistance and survival in a diverse range of organisms (Tatar *et al*., 2003). This is exemplified by the identification of a wealth of mutants in nematodes, flies, and mice, downregulating pathways of growth, reproduction, and energy metabolism, resulting in significant increases in life span as well as increased stress resistance, including resistance to oxidative stress. We do not know if in all these mutants, in different species, increased survival is controlled in the same way, by the same mechanism, but it is possible that in some way they all reflect the selective advantage of temporarily delaying reproduction and maximizing survival in times of famine, awaiting better times. There is no convincing evidence that this could also work the other way around, although, for example, growth hormone overexpressing mice have been found associated with at least some symptoms of accelerated aging (Bartke *et al.*, 2002). A logical conclusion therefore would be that DNA damage is a major proximate cause of aging and only direct interference at that level uncovers accelerated aging phenotypes. Any upstream interference would probably have too many side effects or require a much more sophisticated type of genetic engineering than we currently have available.

A second caveat in using mouse models of accelerated aging is the potential misinterpretation of a life-shortening effect of early diseases as signs of an acceleration of fundamental mechanisms of normal aging. It often is argued that mouse models with a mutation that accelerates aging simply are showing some disease that has nothing to do with normal aging. Based on the aforementioned evolutionary basis of aging we could say that all genetic variations that exclusively manifest after the age of first reproduction are by definition part of the aging phenotype. How likely is it that a random germline change would give rise to a phenotype that can superficially be diagnosed as aging (i.e., adversely affects postmaturation fitness)? The first results of mouse ENU mutagenesis programs in which the effects of many different randomly induced germline mutations are assessed suggest that aging phenotypes are rare. The phenotypes observed in ENU mutagenesis screens are, to a large extent, developmental, and very few if any have been defined as aging-related (Kile *et al.*, 2003). In addition, very few mouse knockouts exhibit aging phenotypes. Thus, genetic alterations rarely impact aging. In view of the convincing array of aging phenotypes in the genome maintenance mutants discussed, the point is probably moot, but it remains useful to point out the difference between a disease and an aging phenotype.

Consider the well-known genetic diseases, cystic fibrosis and sickle cell anemia. These genetic alterations reduce life span by impairing the function of a vital system independent of normal aging. The negative impact of both these diseases is apparent very early in life, and neither disease is observed in the elderly. On the other hand, arteriosclerosis and its sequelae, such as coronary and cerebrovascular disease, is an age-related disease process. Used by Williams as a theoretical example of the effect of a pleiotropic aging gene, late-life arteriosclerosis could be promoted by depositions of calcium in the arterial wall, a possible pleiotropic effect of a gene variant causing enhanced calcium deposition in the bones, offering a selective advantage at a young age (Williams, 1957). A similar reasoning could be applied to diseases, such as diabetes, osteoporosis, and cancer. Although none of these diseases occurs exclusive in the elderly, the high incidence in this segment of the population is compelling, and it is very difficult to argue that they are not genuine aging phenotypes. Hence, in interpreting accelerated aging symptoms it is critically important to correctly diagnose the phenotype. On this basis it should be possible to differentiate between genuine aging phenotypes and phenotypes related to disorders unrelated to aging.

How can so many clinical end points of aging undergo acceleration as a consequence of genetic defects in a set of functional pathways that superficially have no relationship to the original function that is impaired—for example, bone metabolism, functional skin mass, neuronal activity, growth? As already alluded to, this observation points toward a key role of the network of genome maintenance genes as the last line of defense against aging by removing damage induced by metabolism-related reactive oxygen species.

The key consideration here is that aging is characterized by progressive system dysfunction as a consequence of the loss of functional cells, ultimately driven by the accumulation of DNA damage. This could reflect two major underlying processes. First, organ and tissue dysfunction could be caused by cellular responses to DNA damage, including apoptosis and cellular senescence. Second, cells could degenerate by a process of intrinsic aging, possibly driven by increased genomic alterations. Although the former would mainly result in various forms of tissue atrophy and loss of regenerative capacity, increased genomic instability at old age is likely to contribute to the well-documented exponential increase in cancer during aging. Indeed, hyperplastic and neoplastic lesions can comprise as much as 50% of all pathological lesions observed at old age (Bronson and Lipman 1991). However, an increased load of genomic mutations, including sequence alterations and methylation changes, also could lead to a progressive increase in the number of dysfunctional cells, without causing them to die immediately or become transformed. We can call such cells *senescent* cells, and they may include permanently arrested cells, as a consequence of replicative senescence (for a discussion of the phenomenon of cell senescence and its implications for *in vivo* aging, see Campisi 2005). Similar to increased cell death, an increased fraction of dysfunctional cells would be expected to lead to organ dysfunction.

As we have seen, in all mouse models of premature aging, the genetic defect leads to increased impairment of growth and cellular proliferation, either through cell cycle arrest, or other elicited DNA damage responses, such as replicative senescence and apoptosis. In many of these mutants we also see an increase in mutations—irreversible changes in DNA sequence due to misreplication or misrepair. This increased genomic instability promotes the emergence of cancer cells but is so dramatic that it ultimately represses tumor progression, due to increased anti-cancer responses, such as apoptosis. Indeed, deletion of p53 rescues the accelerated aging mutants from the premature replicative senescence that is often observed in their tissue culture cells. This suggests that many of the premature aging phenotypes in mice with defects in genome maintenance are caused by cellular responses to DNA damage, including the activity of a p53-dependent cell cycle checkpoint.

Are these same cellular responses, identified in the mouse models as a likely cause of their accelerated aging, also responsible for normal aging? There can be no doubt that loss of cells per se contributes to normal aging and various forms of atrophy are common among older mice. Hence, part of normal aging is also likely to be due to the adverse effects of cellular responses to DNA damage. Of note, it has been demonstrated that SIRT1, the aforementioned candidate master regulator of life extension, is capable of deacetylating Foxo3a, the ortholog of the main longevity effector gene DAF16 in nematodes, increases its ability to induce cell cycle arrest, raises its resistance to oxidative stress, but inhibits its ability to induce cell death (Motta *et al.*, 2004). However, normal aging generally is not associated with the dramatic forms of growth reduction, tissue atrophy, and loss of organ functional mass as observed in many of the accelerated aging models. For example, Table 49.1 indicates symptoms of aging in the Xpd mouse model that are much more severe than would be expected from their biological age as derived from the survival curve. Indeed, these data were obtained by complete histopathology at the end of life. Hence, we would expect to see an incidence and severity level very similar to the control animals, but this is not the case. Hence, it is possible that accelerated aging in many of these models is caused mainly by excessive cellular responses to genomic stress, in contrast to normal aging, which is more likely due to a gradual accumulation of persistent DNA damage or mutations. Indeed, the bursts of DNA damage necessary to evoke, for example, an apoptosis response must be quite rare during normal aging, as can be derived from the extremely low number of apoptotic cells in tissues of normally aged animals.

Normal steady-state levels of DNA damage, such as 8-oxo-guanine, are extremely low (Hamilton *et al.*, 2001) and therefore also unlikely to directly cause aging-related degenerative defects. However, DNA damage can be turned into mutations by erroneous processing of DNA damage. Evidently, the frequency of such events is low, as exemplified by the normally low frequency of neoplastic transformation. However, it is likely that many mutations of different kinds (from point mutations to large genome rearrangements and aneuploidy) are needed to generate a tumor cell. Most of such mutations do not involve actual genes, but gene regulatory sequences. Indeed, rather than a catalog of useful genes interspersed with functionless DNA, each chromosome is now viewed as a complex information organelle with sophisticated maintenance and control systems. In this concept of a genome, each part has a function, even its nonprotein-coding parts. Such a holistic view of the genome would assign a variety of functions to noncoding DNA (e.g., structural maintenance, gene regulation). The continuous process of irreversible alteration of the DNA sequence organization of the genome would lead to a mosaic of cells, with each individual cell in a tissue bearing a different pattern of genomic scars (Vijg and Dollé, 2002). Rather than the inactivation of unique genes with unique functions, which has thus far been given primacy, a scenario of an initially tolerable loss of genome structural integrity is more likely. This could lead to increased loss of function, highly variable from cell to cell, thus contributing to increased organ dysfunction. Hence, whereas age-related systems dysfunction in premature aging may predominantly involve cellular responses evoking proliferation impairment and programmed cell death, normal aging could be due to the gradual accumulation of persistent genomic or epigenomic alterations, leading to a progressive increase of dysfunctional cells. Both scenarios would result in organ and tissue dysfunction. Figure 49.5 schematically depicts the hypothetical causes of aging as driven by DNA damage for (1) accelerated aging, mostly due to adverse effects of cellular responses to DNA damage; (2) normal aging, with a reduced role of cellular responses, and (epi)genomic alterations as the main cause of cell and organ dysfunction; and (3) delayed aging with reduced cellular responses as well as reduced accumulation of irreversible, (epi)genomic alterations.

It would be premature to consider DNA damage as the sole driving force of aging in all multicellular organisms. However, based on the model systems now available, it accounts for a significant number of the observations that have been made. Of note, DNA damage as the original driver of a universal process of aging

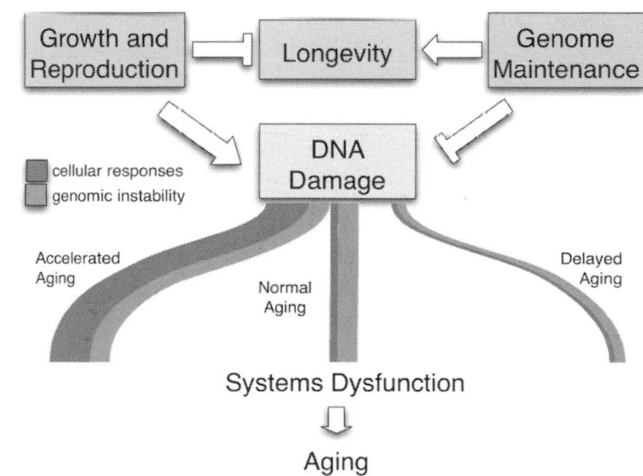

Figure 49.5 DNA damage, mainly resulting from oxidative stress, byproducts of normal growth and metabolism, as the hypothetical main driver of the aging process, in accelerated aging, normal aging, and delayed aging conditions. The trade-off between somatic maintenance and growth and reproduction is from Kirkwood (2005).

has some inherent logic. After all, damage to nucleic acids is the most ancient example of damage accumulation in the living world. Ever since the first replicators, genetic damage posed both a fundamental problem and an opportunity for living systems. This is a problem, because genetic damage essentially prevents the perpetuation of life, since it interferes with replication (and transcription); it is also an opportunity, because it allows the generation of genetic variation through errors in the replication of a damaged template, thereby facilitating evolutionary change. Genetic stability in somatic cells of metazoa has become part of the trade-off between the allocation of scarce resources to either reproduction or somatic maintenance and is not expected to be maximized. Though the concept of DNA damage as a main driver of aging is intuitively attractive, evolutionary logic dictates that other causes of aging would have emerged over evolutionary time. Indeed, it is likely that age-related deterioration and functional decline is synchronized across different organismal functions. This would imply that given a molecular machinery of limited endurance, all bodily functions would adapt, and under such conditions a variety of harmful physiological late-life effects, unrelated to DNA damage, can be expected to develop.

ACKNOWLEDGMENTS

The authors are grateful for support from NIH grants AG 17242, AG20438, ES11044 (JV), and R01 CA76317-05A1 (PH). We thank Drs. Yousin Suh, Judith Campisi, Jan Hoeijmakers, and Harry van Steeg for stimulating discussions, and John David Garza for creating Figure 49.5 and for his help with the manuscript.

REFERENCES

Arnheim, N. and Cortopassi, G. (1992). Deleterious mitochondrial DNA mutations accumulate in aging human tissues. *Mutat Res 275*, 157–167.

Artandi, S.E., Chang, S., Lee, S.-L., Alson, S., Gottlieb, G.J., Chin, L., and DePinho, R.A. (2000). Telomere dysfunction promotes non-reciprocal translocations and epithelial cancers in mice. *Nature 406*, 641–645.

Baker, D.J., Jeganathan, K.B., Cameron, J.D., Thompson, M., Juneja, S., Kopecka, A. *et al.* (2004). BubR1 insufficiency causes early onset of aging-associated phenotypes and infertility in mice. *Nat Genet 36*, 744–749.

Bartke, A. and Brown-Borg, H. (2004). Life extension in the dwarf mouse. *Curr Top Dev Biol 63*, 189–225.

Bartke, A., Chandrashekar, V., Bailey, B., Zaczek, D., and Turyn, D. (2002). Consequences of growth hormone (GH) overexpression and GH resistance. *Neuropeptides 36*, 201–208.

Bergo, M.O., Gavino, B., Ross, J., Schmidt, W.K., Hong, C., Kendall, L.V. *et al.* (2002). Zmpste24 deficiency in mice causes spontaneous bone fractures, muscle weakness, and a prelamin A processing defect. *Proc Natl Acad Sci USA 99*, 13049–13054.

Blackburn, E.H. (2005). Telomeres and telomerase: their mechanisms of action and the effects of altering their functions. *FEBS Lett 579*, 859–862.

Blasco, M.A., Lee, H.W., Hande, M.P., Samper, E., Lansdorp, P.M., DePinho, R.A. *et al.* (1997). Telomere shortening and tumor formation by mouse cells lacking telomerase RNA. *Cell 91*, 25–34.

Bronson, R.T. and Lipman, R.D. (1991). Reduction in rate of occurrence of age-related lesions in dietary restricted laboratory mice. *Growth, Development & Aging 55*, 169–184.

Campisi, J. (2005). Senescent cells, tumor suppression, and organismal aging: good citizens, bad neighbors. *Cell 120*, 513–522.

Cao, L., Li, W., Kim, S., Brodie, S.G., and Deng, C.X. (2003). Senescence, aging, and malignant transformation mediated by p53 in mice lacking the Brca1 full-length isoform. *Genes Dev 17*, 201–213.

Chang, S., Multani, A.S., Cabrera, N.G., Naylor, M.L., Laud, P., Lombard, D. *et al.* (2004). Essential role of limiting telomeres in the pathogenesis of Werner syndrome. *Nat Genet 36*, 877–882.

Cheng, H.L., Mostoslavsky, R., Saito, S., Manis, J.P., Gu, Y., Patel, P. *et al.* (2003). Developmental defects and p53 hyperacetylation in Sir2 homolog (SIRT1)-deficient mice. *Proc Natl Acad Sci USA 100*, 10794–10799.

Chun, H.H. and Gatti, R.A. (2004). Ataxia-telangiectasia, an evolving phenotype. *DNA Repair (Amst) 3*, 1187–1196.

de Boer, J., Andressoo, J.O., de Wit, J., Huijmans, J., Beems, R.B., van Steeg, H. *et al.* (2002). Premature aging in mice deficient in DNA repair and transcription. *Science 296*, 1276–1279.

de Boer, J., de Wit, J., van Steeg, H., Berg, R.J., Morreau, H., Visser, P. *et al.* (1998). A mouse model for the basal transcription/DNA repair syndrome trichothiodystrophy. *Mol Cell 1*, 981–990.

de Vries, A., van Oostrom, C.T., Hofhuis, F.M., Dortant, P.M., Berg, R.J., de Gruijl, F.R. *et al.* (1995). Increased susceptibility to ultraviolet-B and carcinogens of mice lacking the DNA excision repair gene XPA. *Nature 377*, 169–173.

DePinho, R.A. (2000). The age of cancer. *Nature 408*, 248–254.

Difilippantonio, M.J., Zhu, J., Chen, H.T., Meffre, E., Nussenzweig, M.C., Max, E.E. *et al.* (2000). DNA repair protein Ku80 suppresses chromosomal aberrations and malignant transformation. *Nature 404*, 510–514.

Dolle, M.E. and Vijg, J. (2002). Genome dynamics in aging mice. *Genome Res 12*, 1732–1738.

Dollé, M.E.T., Busuttil, R.A., Garcia, A.M., Wijnhoven, S., van Drunen, A., Niedernhofer, L.J., van der Horst, G., Hoeijmakers, J.H.J., van Steeg, H., and Vijg, J. Increased genomic instability is not a prerequisite for shortened life span in DNA repair deficient mice. *Mutation Research*, in press.

Dumble, M., Gatza, C., Tyner, S., Venkatachalam, S., and Donehower, L.A. (2004). Insights into aging obtained from p53 mutant mouse models. *Ann N Y Acad Sci 1019*, 171–177.

Epstein, C.J., Martin, G.M., and Motulsky, A.G. (1965). Werner's syndrome; caricature of aging. A genetic model for the study of degenerative diseases. *Trans Assoc Am Physicians 78*, 73–81.

Eriksson, M., Brown, W.T., Gordon, L.B., Glynn, M.W., Singer, J., Scott, L. *et al.* (2003). Recurrent de novo point mutations in lamin A cause Hutchinson-Gilford progeria syndrome. *Nature 423*, 293–298.

Espejel, S., Martin, M., Klatt, P., Martin-Caballero, J., Flores, J.M., and Blasco, M.A. (2004). Shorter telomeres, accelerated ageing and increased lymphoma in DNA-PKcs-deficient mice. *EMBO Rep 5*, 503–509.

Fukuchi, K., Martin, G.M., and Monnat, R.J., Jr. (1989) Mutator phenotype of Werner syndrome is characterized by extensive deletions. *Proc Natl Acad Sci USA 86*, 5893–5897.

Gangloff, S., McDonald, J.P., Bendixen, C., Arthur, L., and Rothstein, R. (1994) The yeast type I topoisomerase Top3 interacts with Sgs1, a DNA helicase homolog: a potential eukaryotic reverse gyrase. *Mol Cell Biol 14*, 8391–8398.

Garcia-Cao, I., Garcia-Cao, M., Martin-Caballero, J., Criado, L.M., Klatt, P., Flores, J.M. *et al.* (2002). "Super p53" mice exhibit enhanced DNA damage response, are tumor resistant and age normally. *Embo J 21*, 6225–6235.

Goto, M. (1997). Hierarchical deterioration of body systems in Werner's syndrome: implications for normal ageing. *Mech Ageing Dev 98*, 239–254.

Gruenbaum, Y., Margalit, A., Goldman, R.D., Shumaker, D.K., and Wilson, K.L. (2005). The nuclear lamina comes of age. *Nat Rev Mol Cell Biol 6*, 21–31.

Gu, Y., Seidl, K.J., Rathbun, G.A., Zhu, C., Manis, J.P., van der Stoep, N. *et al.* (1997). Growth retardation and leaky SCID phenotype of Ku70-deficient mice. *Immunity 7*, 653–665.

Hamilton, M.L., Van Remmen, H., Drake, J.A., Yang, H., Guo, Z.M., Kewitt, K. *et al.* (2001). Does oxidative damage to DNA increase with age? *Proc Natl Acad Sci USA 98*, 10469–10474.

Hanks, S. and Rahman, N. (2005). Aneuploidy-cancer predisposition syndromes: a new link between the mitotic spindle checkpoint and cancer. *Cell Cycle 4*, 225–227.

Hasty, P., Campisi, J., Hoeijmakers, J., van Steeg, H., and Vijg, J. (2003). Aging and genome maintenance: lessons from the mouse? *Science 299*, 1355–1359.

Hasty, P. and Vijg, J. (2004). Accelerating aging by mouse reverse genetics: a rational approach to understanding longevity. *Aging Cell 3*, 55–65.

Hoeijmakers, J.H. (2001). Genome maintenance mechanisms for preventing cancer. *Nature 411*, 366–374.

Hosaka, T., Biggs, W.H., 3rd, Tieu, D., Boyer, A.D., Varki, N.M., Cavenee, W.K. *et al.* (2004). Disruption of forkhead transcription factor (FOXO) family members in mice reveals their functional diversification. *Proc Natl Acad Sci USA 101*, 2975–2980.

Jenkins, N.L., McColl, G., and Lithgow, G.J. (2004). Fitness cost of extended lifespan in *Caenorhabditis elegans*. *Proc Biol Sci 271*, 2523–2526.

Kile, B.T., Hentges, K.E., Clark, A.T., Nakamura, H., Salinger, A.P., Liu, B. *et al.* (2003). Functional genetic analysis of mouse chromosome 11. *Nature 425*, 81–86.

Kirkwood, T.B. (2005). Understanding the odd science of aging. *Cell 120*, 437–447.

Kirkwood, T.B. and Cremer, T. (1982). Cytogerontology since 1881: a reappraisal of August Weismann and a review of modern progress. *Hum Genet 60*, 101–121.

Kujoth, G.C., Hiona, A., Pugh, T.D., Someya, S., Panzer, K., Wohlgemuth, S.E., Hofer, T., Seo, A.Y., Sullivan, R., Jobling, W.A., Morrow, J.D., Van Remmen, H., Sedivy, J.M., Yamasoba, T., Tanokura, M., Weindruch, R., Leeuwenburgh, C., and Prolla, T.A. (2005). Mitochondrial DNA mutations, oxidative stress, and apoptosis in mammalian aging. *Science 309*, 481–484.

Kwan, K.Y. and Wang, J.C. (2001). Mice lacking DNA topoisomerase IIIbeta develop to maturity but show a reduced mean lifespan. *Proc Natl Acad Sci USA 98*, 5717–5721.

Laursen, L.V., Bjergbaek, L., Murray, J.M., and Andersen, A.H. (2003). RecQ helicases and topoisomerase III in cancer and aging. *Biogerontology 4*, 275–287.

Lebel, M., Cardiff, R.D., and Leder, P. (2001). Tumorigenic effect of nonfunctional p53 or p21 in mice mutant in the Werner syndrome helicase. *Cancer Res 61*, 1816–1819.

Lebel, M. and Leder, P. (1998). A deletion within the murine Werner syndrome helicase induces sensitivity to inhibitors of topoisomerase and loss of cellular proliferative capacity. *Proc Natl Acad Sci USA 95*, 13097–13102.

Lehmann, A.R. (2003). DNA repair-deficient diseases, xeroderma pigmentosum, Cockayne syndrome and trichothiodystrophy. *Biochimie 85*, 1101–1111.

Lindor, N.M., Furuichi, Y., Kitao, S., Shimamoto, A., Arndt, C., and Jalal, S. (2000). Rothmund-Thomson syndrome due to RECQ4 helicase mutations: report and clinical and molecular comparisons with Bloom syndrome and Werner syndrome. *Am J Med Genet 90*, 223–228.

Liu, B., Wang, J., Chan, K.M., Tjia, W.M., Deng, W., Guan, X., Huang, J.D., Li, K.M., Chau, P.Y., Chen, D.J., Pei, D., Pendas, A.M., Cadinanos, J., Lopez-Otin, C., Tse, H.F., Hutchison, C., Chen, J., Cao, Y., Cheah, K.S., Tryggvason, K., and Zhou, Z. (2005). Genomic instability in laminopathy-based premature aging. *Nat Med 11*, 780–785.

Lombard, D.B., Beard, C., Johnson, B., Marciniak, R.A., Dausman, J., Bronson, R. *et al.* (2000). Mutations in the WRN gene in mice accelerate mortality in a p53-null background. *Mol Cell Biol 20*, 3286–3291.

Lombard, D.B., Chua, K.F., Mostoslavsky, R., Franco, S., Gostissa, M., and Alt, F.W. (2005). DNA repair, genome stability, and aging. *Cell 120*, 497–512.

Maier, B., Gluba, W., Bernier, B., Turner, T., Mohammad, K., Guise, T. *et al.* (2004). Modulation of mammalian life span by the short isoform of p53. *Genes Dev 18*, 306–319.

Martin, G.M. (2005). Genetic modulation of senescent phenotypes in *Homo sapiens*. *Cell 120*, 523–532.

Migliaccio, E., Giorgio, M., Mele, S., Pelicci, G., Reboldi, P., Pandolfi, P.P. *et al.* (1999). The p66shc adaptor protein controls oxidative stress response and life span in mammals. *Nature 402*, 309–313.

Motta, M.C., Divecha, N., Lemieux, M., Kamel, C., Chen, D., Gu, W. *et al.* (2004). Mammalian SIRT1 represses forkhead transcription factors. *Cell 116*, 551–563.

Mounkes, L.C., Kozlov, S., Hernandez, L., Sullivan, T., and Stewart, C.L. (2003). A progeroid syndrome in mice is caused by defects in A-type lamins. *Nature 423*, 298–301.

Nussenzweig, A., Chen, C., da Costa Soares, V., Sanchez, M., Sokol, K., Nussenzweig, M.C. *et al.* (1996). Requirement for Ku80 in growth and immunoglobulin V(D)J recombination. *Nature 382*, 551–555.

Pollex, R.L. and Hegele, R.A. (2004). Hutchinson-Gilford progeria syndrome. *Clin Genet 66*, 375–381.

Poot, M., Gollahon, K.A., and Rabinovitch, P.S. (1999). Werner syndrome lymphoblastoid cells are sensitive to camptothecin-induced apoptosis in S-phase. *Hum Genet 104*, 10–14.

Robanus-Maandag, E., Dekker, M., van der Valk, M., Carrozza, M.L., Jeanny, J.C., Dannenberg, J.H. *et al.* (1998). p107 is a suppressor of retinoblastoma development in pRb-deficient mice. *Genes Dev 12*, 1599–1609.

Rudolph, K.L., Chang, S., Lee, H.W., Blasco, M., Gottlieb, G.J., Greider, C. *et al.* (1999). Longevity, stress response, and cancer in aging telomerase-deficient mice. *Cell 96*, 701–712.

Shiloh, Y. (2003). ATM and related protein kinases: safeguarding genome integrity. *Nat Rev Cancer 3*, 155–168.

Tarsounas, M. and West, S.C. (2005). Recombination at mammalian telomeres: An alternative mechanism for telomere protection and elongation. *Cell Cycle 4*.

Tatar, M., Bartke, A., and Antebi, A. (2003). The endocrine regulation of aging by insulin-like signals. *Science 299*, 1346–1351.

Trifunovic, A., Wredenberg, A., Falkenberg, M., Spelbrink, J.N., Rovio, A.T., Bruder, C.E. *et al.* (2004). Premature ageing in mice expressing defective mitochondrial DNA polymerase. *Nature 429*, 417–423.

Tyner, S.D., Venkatachalam, S., Choi, J., Jones, S., Ghebranious, N., Igelmann, H. *et al.* (2002). p53 mutant mice that display early ageing-associated phenotypes. *Nature 415*, 45–53.

Van Gent, D.C., Hoeijmakers, J.H., and Kanaar, R. (2001). Chromosomal stability and the DNA double-stranded break connection. *Nat Rev Genet 2*, 196–206.

Varela, I., Cadinanos, J., Pendas, A.M., Gutierrez-Fernandez, A., Folgueras, A.R., Sanchez, L.M., Zhou, Z., Rodriguez, F.J., Stewart, C.L., Vega, J.A., Tryggvason, K., Freije, J.M., and Lopez-Otin, C. (2005). Accelerated ageing in mice deficient in Zmpste24 protease is linked to p53 signalling activation. *Nature 437*, 564–568.

Vijg, J. and Dollé, M.E. (2002). Large genome rearrangements as a primary cause of aging. *Mech Ageing Dev 123*, 907–915.

Vijg, J. and Suh, Y. (2005). Genetics of longevity and aging. *Annual Review of Medicine 56*.

Vogel, H., Lim, D.S., Karsenty, G., Finegold, M., and Hasty, P. (1999). Deletion of Ku86 causes early onset of senescence in mice. *Proc Natl Acad Sci USA 96*, 10770–10775.

Vogelstein, B., Lane, D., and Levine, A.J. (2000). Surfing the p53 network. *Nature 408*, 307–310.

Wallis, J.W., Chrebet, G., Brodsky, G., Rolfe, M., and Rothstein, R. (1989). A hyper-recombination mutation in *S. cerevisiae* identifies a novel eukaryotic topoisomerase. *Cell 58*, 409–419.

Weeda, G., Donker, I., de Wit, J., Morreau, H., Janssens, R., Vissers, C.J., *et al.* (1997). Disruption of mouse ERCC1 results in a novel repair syndrome with growth failure, nuclear abnormalities and senescence. *Curr Biol 7*, 427–439.

Wijnhoven, S.W., Beems, R.B., Roodbergen, M., van den Berg, J., Lohman, P.H., Diderich, K., van der Horst, G.T., Vijg, J., Hoeijmakers, J.H., and van Steeg, H. (2005). Accelerated aging pathology in ad libitum fed Xpd(TTD) mice is accompanied by features suggestive of caloric restriction. *DNA Repair 4*, 1314–1324.

Williams, G.C. (1957). Pleiotropy, natural selection, and the evolution of senescence. *Evolution 11*, 398–411.

Wise, P.M., Kashon, M.L., Krajnak, K.M., Rosewell, K.L., Cai, A., Scarbrough, K. *et al.* (1997). Aging of the female reproductive system: a window into brain aging. *Recent Prog Horm Res 52*, 279–303; discussion 303–305.

Wong, K.K., Maser, R.S., Bachoo, R.M., Menon, J., Carrasco, D.R., Gu, Y. *et al.* (2003). Telomere dysfunction and Atm deficiency compromises organ homeostasis and accelerates ageing. *Nature 421*, 643–648.

Xu, Y., Ashley, T., Brainerd, E.E., Bronson, R.T., Meyn, M.S., and Baltimore, D. (1996). Targeted disruption of ATM leads to growth retardation, chromosomal fragmentation during meiosis, immune defects, and thymic lymphoma. *Genes Dev 10*, 2411–2422.

Yu, C.E., Oshima, J., Fu, Y.H., Wijsman, E.M., Hisama, F., Alisch, R. *et al.* (1996). Positional cloning of the Werner's syndrome gene. *Science 272*, 258–262.

50

Models, Definitions, and Criteria of Frailty

David B. Hogan

This chapter will examine the current state of research on frailty. A number of competing and complementary models for its development will be described. This will be followed by a working definition of frailty. Finally, criteria for the identification of frailty in older individuals will be discussed. Promising future directions for research will be noted throughout the chapter. The aim is to provide useful background information about frailty for researchers interested in the field. It is an area of inquiry still early in its evolution.

Introduction

In a radio broadcast on October 3, 1939, Sir Winston Churchill said about Russia that, "It is a riddle, wrapped in a mystery, inside an enigma." The same can be said about frailty.

The term *frail elderly* is defined in the National Library of Medicine's MeSH database as "Older adults or aged individuals who are lacking in general strength and are unusually susceptible to disease or to other infirmity." The concept that aging is associated with declining resiliency goes back to the dawn of western medicine, and likely, before. The Hippocratic tradition held that aging was caused by a progressive loss of the body's store of heat, which resulted in a depletion of vitality and increased vulnerability (Thane, 1993). At birth it was assumed that we were granted a finite supply of energy. During childhood it was used for growth. At maturity we were to maintain a balance with our environment, but in old age we decayed as our remaining energy was spent. Benjamin Rush, a signer of the Declaration of Independence, stated that the loss of vitality led to a "predisposing debility." The older individual became unable to remain in balance with the world (Haber, 1986).

In this short overview of frailty I'll deal first with select models and mechanisms for the development of frailty. I'll then present a working definition followed by an examination of the currently favored criteria for the identification of frail older persons.

Models and Mechanisms

KNOWLEDGE DISCOVERY FROM DATASETS

Mathematical models can simulate and predict the behavior of systems. Many biomedical researchers, though, are more comfortable with verbal or visual models of complex phenomena. Various mathematical models for frailty have been reviewed elsewhere (Rockwood *et al.*, 2002). An example of the knowledge discovery from the dataset approach would be the work of Drs. Mitnitski and Rockwood. Using large databases, they developed a *frailty index* consisting of a number of variables including symptoms, attitudes, illnesses, and function that can be used to predict the likelihood of mortality (Mitnitski *et al.*, 2002).

This approach has been used to produce highly predictive models for certain outcomes associated with frailty but will not necessarily further our understanding of it. The most readably available outcomes for database research—death, disability, and institutionalization—do not arise solely from frailty and/or only capture a subset of all frail individuals. Although the presence of frailty makes death more likely, not all deaths in old age are "frail" deaths. Between 20 and 47% of deaths in old age have a *frail trajectory* (Lunney *et al.*, 2002, *et al.*, 2003). Likewise there is more than one pathway to disability. It can arise in a catastrophic or a progressive manner (Ferrucci *et al.*, 1997). Older individuals with frailty commonly show an insidious development of disability (Gill *et al.*, 2004). Ferrucci found that approximately half (51.6%) of older individuals who developed a severe disability over two to three years did so in a catastrophic manner (Ferrucci *et al.*, 1997). The risk factors and outcomes of the two modes of disability onset are different (Ferrucci *et al.*, 1997; Guralnik *et al.*, 2001). Although most residents in long-term care facilities are frail, only a subset of frail individuals reside in institutions. Defining frailty as being in a long-term care residence would be specific but not sensitive (Rockwood *et al.*, 1996).

SENESCENCE AND FRAILTY

Are frailty and aging (or more accurately senescence) the same? Senescence refers to the time-dependent changes seen in living organisms that have cumulative and deleterious effects (Yates, 1996). A senescent organism lacks resiliency, and, as will be seen later in this review, increased vulnerability is a hallmark of frailty. I feel that at some very advanced, but currently unspecified age, a degree of frailty will become universal. Others argue that frailty is not inevitable with aging but is due to a distinct biological pathway (Kolata, 2002). I would agree that few if any frail individuals currently develop the state *solely* because of senescence. Other factors (e.g., behaviors, life-styles, diseases) typically play a role. Even though very advanced age is arguably a sufficient cause of frailty, it isn't a necessary one.

ROLE OF GENES

Saying that the frailty phenotype arises from gene–environment interactions doesn't move us very far forward as these interactions are pervasive throughout biology. Nonetheless, the emerging work on the genetics of aging, age-associated diseases, and age-associated functional decline will become increasingly relevant to our understanding of frailty (Johnson *et al.*, 1996; Hamet *et al.*, 2003; Gurland *et al.*, 2004; Martin 2005; Hadley *et al.*, 2005). Although genes likely influence the development of frailty, environmental influences probably predominate. For example, a twin study of the genetic contribution to late-life disability found that although genetic factors did play a significant role, environmental factors were more important (Gurland *et al.*, 2004). Genetic influences will operate partially, if not primarily, through the mechanism of susceptibility to diseases.

A few studies about the potential relationship between genetic polymorphism and frailty have been published. The Apolipoprotein E (ApoE) gene has been referred to as a *frailty gene* (Gerdes *et al.*, 2000). Epislon 2 carriers are more likely to survive to extreme old age, but epsilon 4 carriers are less likely. The differential mortality rates for the various ApoE genotypes extend into extreme old age (Corder *et al.*, 2000). Genetic influences on immune and muscle function will likely be relevant to frailty research, but no consistent picture has emerged yet. Genetic variation in intraleukin-6 (IL-6) was not associated with frailty in older women (Walston *et al.*, 2005), but a significant genetic association with the IL-10 promoter gene has been found (van den Biggelaar *et al.*, 2004). In the latter study, those genetically predisposed to lower cytokine production seemed predisposed to frailty. As will be seen, this seems to go against the prevailing thinking about the pathogenesis of frailty. Polymorphism in the insulin-like growth factor-2 (IGF2) was modestly associated (only 1% of the variance was attributable to IGF2 genotype) with grip strength in men aged 64 to 74 (Sayer *et al.*, 2002). Those with the AA genotype were marginally stronger than those with the GG genotype. Angiotensin-converting enzyme (ACE) gene polymorphism is associated with response to physical training (Montgomery *et al.*, 1999). Low ACE activity was associated with a greater response to intensive physical training in young white male British Army recruits.

Interestingly, other studies have shown that the use of ACE-inhibitors for hypertension is associated with maintained muscle mass, muscle strength, and walking speed in older individuals (Onder *et al.*, 2002; Di Bari *et al.*, 2004). The issue of age-dependent regulation of gene expression requires study. Transcriptional profiling of human frontal cortex from individuals aged 26 to 106 showed both reduced expression of certain genes (e.g., involved with synaptic transmission and vesicular transport) and the induction of genes (e.g., involved with stress response and DNA repair) after the age of 40 (Lu *et al.*, 2004). The greatest diversity in gene expression was seen between 40 and 70 when a switch-over in genetic expression seems to occur. Middle and early old age may represent a critical period for the development of frailty in our later life.

ALLOSTATIC LOAD AND HORMESIS

The concepts of allostasis and hormesis deal with the relationship between an organism and its environment. They may have particular relevance to frailty and could explain how early life events could have late-life consequences. Allostasis (literally meaning "achieving stability through change") is a dynamic regulatory process that allows the organism to adapt to the challenges of its environment. It is an extension of the concept of homeostasis (the ability or tendency of an organism or a cell to maintain internal equilibrium by adjusting its physiological processes). Many physiologic parameters do not remain constant but vary significantly in response to perceived stress. The neuroendocrine, autonomic nervous, and immune system responses, though beneficial in the short run, can be damaging long term if not shut down when no longer needed. Allostatic load refers to the price of the chronic overactivation of these regulatory systems (McEwen, 2003; McEwen, 2004). Although there are no studies showing a direct association with frailty, a summary measure for allostatic load was found to be an independent predictor of functional decline in the MacArthur studies of successful aging (Karlamangla, *et al.*, 2002). Hormesis refers to the beneficial effects of low doses of potentially harmful substances. It is becoming apparent that environmental stress does more than "cull the herd" by eliminating the weakest individuals (Semenchenko *et al.*, 2004). A number of mild stresses (e.g., cold, heat, irradiation, caloric restriction) have been found to be associated with increased longevity in various animal models. The proposed mechanism is that the stress induces stimulation of maintenance and repair pathways (Tattan, 2004; Radek *et al.*, 2005). Frailty may be the long-term outcome of a complex interaction between the type, severity, and timing of environmental stresses and the nature (and consequences) of the response to these stresses.

SYSTEM DYSFUNCTION

Dysfunction of key organ systems might explain the phenomenon of frailty. This would include musculoskeletal abnormalities (e.g., sarcopenia) (Marcell 2003; Doherty 2003; Vanltallie 2003), endocrine deficiency states (e.g., gonadal hormones, DHEA, growth hormone/IGF-1) (Morley *et al.*, 2005), or immune dysfunction (e.g., high levels of inflammatory markers like TNF-α and IL-6) (Cohen 2000). It is not felt, though, that frailty arises from a single system problem (i.e., frailty $\neq$ sarcopenia). There is widespread agreement that a core feature of frailty is the dysfunction of *multiple* physiologic systems. Different investigators have proposed various combinations of the following abnormalities as underlying frailty: diminished aerobic capacity; abnormalities in the neurological system (e.g., cognition, balance, and gait); musculoskeletal problems; precarious or deficient nutritional states; endocrine-metabolic dysfunction; stimulation of the immune system; and cardiovascular concerns (Buchner *et al.*, 1992; Lipsitz *et al.*, 1992); Lipsitz, 2002; Bortz, 2002; Campbell *et al.*, 1997). Endocrine-immune dysregulation is a particularly favored partnering (Walston, 2004; Joseph *et al.*, 2005; Ferrucci *et al.*, 2003). At the present time there are no widely accepted animal models for frailty.

LIFE COURSE APPROACH

Life course epidemiology studies the long-term effects on later health- or disease-risk of physical or social exposures during gestation, childhood, adolescence, young adulthood, and later adult life (Kuh *et al.*, 2003). It allows the integration of biological, behavioral, clinical, psychological, and social processes that interact across a person's life (Ben-Shlomo *et al.*, 2002). This is not a new concept in aging research. Over 50 years ago Nathan Shock wrote, "In the broadest sense, problems of growth, development, and maturation are as much a part of gerontology as are those of atrophy, degeneration, and decline" (Baker *et al.*, 1992). He emphasized the need to examine aging over the entire life span.

The likelihood of developing certain chronic conditions (e.g., type 2 diabetes, ischemic heart disease) appears to depend in part on the early environment (Gluckman *et al.*, 2004). A noxious stimulus at a critical, sensitive period earlier in life may lead to permanent structural, physiologic, and/or metabolic changes (Godfrey *et al.*, 2001). These changes in the young organism might confer immediate survival advantages but at a subsequent cost, especially if there is a mismatch between the developmental and adult environments (e.g., constrained fetal growth followed by exposure to high-calorie foods after birth). This is not to deny the importance of adult risk factors—life course epidemiology allows the joint study of both early life and adult factors. Understanding the biological, clinical, psychological, lifestyle, and social factors that influence physical performance in midlife may provide clues to the origin of frailty in old age.

Whether frailty risk accumulates or there is a required chain of events is unknown (Kuh *et al.*, 2003). It is also unknown whether there are critical or sensitive periods for the development of frailty; middle-age might be a critical period (Lu *et al.*, 2004). Confounding, mediating, and modifying factors will require consideration. The very complexity of the life course approach in the study of frailty would be an attraction—it would allow the consideration of a mix of both early and late risk factors as well as biomedical and psychosocial influences.

The Alameda County Study looked at risk factors for frailty over the previous three decades in an older cohort (Strawbridge *et al.*, 1998). It was found that (listed alphabetically) depression, fair or poor self-rated health, heavy drinking, physical inactivity, prevalence of chronic conditions, prevalence of chronic symptoms, and smoking were adult risk factors that predicted the occurrence of what they defined as frailty (i.e., problems in two or more of the following domains—physical functioning, nutritional status, cognition, sensation).

Although we have no direct evidence linking early life factors and frailty, suggestive data are becoming available. Muscle weakness typically is included as one of its characteristics. Grip strength is often used in epidemiological studies to measure this attribute. The Medical Research Council National Survey of Health and Development found a positive relationship between birth weight and grip strength at the age of 53 (Kuh *et al.*, 2002). The Hertfordshire cohort study found that grip strength in the mid-60s was significantly associated with birth weight (Sayer *et al.*, 2004). A suggested mechanism for the association is that birth weight is related to the number of muscle fibers at birth. Because of the loss of muscle fibers with aging, a deficit in the number at birth could predispose an individual to sarcopenia later in life.

Other early life factors that may be associated with the development of late-life frailty include exposure to infections and chronic stress. The induction of chronic inflammation might explain the relationship between early-life infections and late-life morbidity and mortality. The reduction in lifetime exposure to infectious diseases and other sources of inflammation may be contributing to the decline we've seen throughout the developed world in late-life mortality (Finch *et al.*, 2004). As noted previously, activation of the immune system may play a role in the etiology of frailty. An interesting and potentially testable hypothesis is whether lifetime exposure to infectious diseases influences the incidence of frailty. A recent study found that chronic cytomegalovirus infection was associated with the presence of frailty (Schmaltz *et al.*, 2005). High IL-6 levels increased the strength of the association.

Challenging social conditions (e.g., having a relatively lower social standing) over the life course can be associated with chronic stress and increased susceptibility to various disease states (Brunner, 1997). When survivors of the Whitehall Study were resurveyed after a 29-year gap, men in clerical or manual jobs at middle age were four times more likely to report poor physical performance than senior administrators (Breeze *et al.*, 2001). It was estimated that at most 20% of this could be explained by baseline differences in cardio-respiratory disease and risk factors. Chronic stress has been shown to be associated with a variety of biological effects including increases in IL-6 levels (Kiecolt-Glaser *et al.*, 2003) and accelerated telomere shortening (Epel *et al.*, 2004).

PROPOSED MODEL

Figure 50.1 presents a descriptive model based on a life course approach for the development of frailty.

Genotype and prenatal environment will determine the birth phenotype. The specific nature of the prenatal environmental could lead to development plasticity, predictive adaptive responses, and developmental disruption (Gluckman *et al.*, 2004). When there is a mismatch between the prenatal and the predicted postnatal environment (e.g., predicted postnatal food restriction versus abundant postnatal food availability), the risk of problems down the road might be increased. After maturity is reached, aging, the physical and social environment, coping strategies, affect, lifestyle/behavioral choices, and the presence of disease(s) can contribute to the onset of frailty in the aged individual. In this model disability and healthcare utilization would be a consequence of frailty and modified by the relative assets and deficits of the individual. Although more complex, I think a life course approach will be required to comprehensively understand this entity.

Definition

CORE FEATURES

There is agreement that frailty is a syndrome encountered in older individuals that is marked by increased vulnerability to a number of adverse outcomes. Other hallmarks are the presence of multisystem impairment (see preceding section) and the concept of a gradient. Although vulnerability is present to a degree in all of us, frailty is marked by a greater than normal susceptibility. In studies we will likely continue to treat frailty as either a dichotomous value (frail/ not frail) or categorize it on a short ordinal frailty scale (e.g., not present, mild, moderate, and severe frailty) in order to make the data easier to manage and understand. There is likely a diverse mix of predisposing, precipitating, enabling, and reinforcing factors (see Table 50.1). It is hoped that a characteristic clustering of characteristics will allow for its accurate identification (see Table 50.2). The consequences of frailty in a given individual will depend on their particular balance of assets and deficits (see Table 50.3). The physical and social environment of the older person coupled with how they cope with their limitations will be modifiers of outcomes. As can be seen, there is some overlap between Tables 50.1 and 50.2 as well as between Tables 50.2 and 50.3. This arises because of our current uncertainty about the pathogenesis, manifestations, and consequences of frailty. Ultimately there should be a clear distinction between the three.

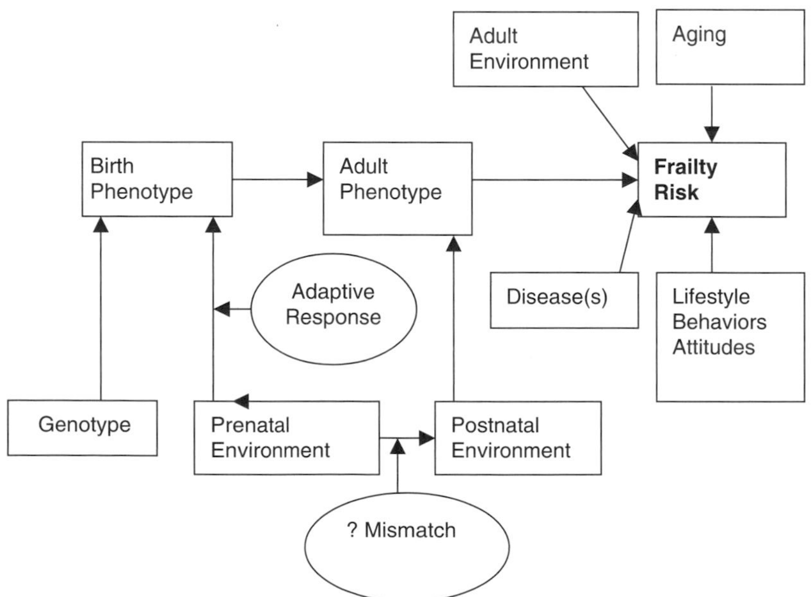

Figure 50.1 Life course model for frailty.

TABLE 50.1
Candidate predisposing, precipitating, enabling, and reinforcing factors

Socio-demographic
Age
Sex
Socioeconomic status
Social standing
Education
Social engagement/social network
Social support
Attitudes
Affect
Perceived degree of autonomy/control
Self-rated health/life satisfaction
Behaviors
Smoking
Alcohol intake
Activity level/exercise
Biological & environmental factors
Genetic endowment (e.g., ApoE)
Gene expression
Allostatic load (see text)
Hormesis (see text)
Environmental stressors (type, timing, duration and severity)
Organ system abnormalities (MSK, endocrine, immune, cardiovascular, and/or neurological)
Nutritional status
Diseases
Presence of co-morbidity (two or more conditions)
Specific conditions
Cardiovascular disease
Cerebrovascular disease
Chronic renal failure
Dementia (e.g., Alzheimer's disease)
Depression
Diabetes mellitus
Fractures (especially hip)/Osteoporosis
Osteoarthritis
Parkinson's disease
Renal failure

TABLE 50.2
Candidate manifestations or markers of frailty

Symptoms and clinical presentations
Chronic symptoms
Depressive symptoms
Anxiety
Stamina/energy/fatigue
Atypical presentations
Delirium
Falls
Physical findings and performance measures
Body composition/nutritional status
Blood pressure
Presence of postural hypotension
Muscle strength
Balance
Gait speed
Lower extremity function
Upper extremity function
Motor processing (coordination, movement planning, and speed)
Neurocognitive processing (alertness, attention, multitasking)
Cognition measures
Vision/hearing
Laboratory features
Albumin
Cholesterol
Hemoglobin/hematocrit
C-reactive protein
Factor VIII
D-dimer
Interleukin-6
Insulin-like growth factor I or IGF-I
Dehydroepiandrosterone sulfate or DHEA-S
Testosterone
Lutenizing hormone
Cortisol/DHEA-S ratio
Response to dexamethasone suppression
Plasma osmolality

SUBTYPES

Even though a consensus has not been achieved on a specific definition for frailty, a number of subtypes of frailty have been proposed (see Table 50.4). Darwin wrote, "Those who make many species are the 'splitters,' and those who make few are the 'lumpers'" (Gallagher, 2002). At this stage in its uncertain evolution, I would confess membership in the "lumpers" club and have reservations about "splitting" frailty into a number of "species" before we reach consensus on the defining features of frailty.

TABLE 50.3
Consequences of frailty

Consequences of frailty
Clinical problems and presentations
Delirium
Falls
Other atypical presentations for acute illnesses
Mortality
Activities of Daily Living (ADL) and leisure activities
Basic ADL
Instrumental ADL
Advanced ADL
Recreational/leisure activities
Health care utilization
Institutionalization
Medication use
Hospitalization
Community-based services
Physician visits
Access to care
Insurance coverage
Use of medical devices

RELATIONSHIP WITH DISABILITY AND DISEASES

Frailty was used initially as another term for disability (Hogan *et al.*, 2003). Although frailty has been disentangled from ADL disability (Fried *et al.*, 2004), there is considerable overlap between frailty and both instrumental ADL (IADL) limitations and mobility disability (Fried *et al.*, 2001). In the Cardiovascular Heart Study (CHS), 27.4% of those categorized as frail had an ADL, 59.7% had an IADL, and 71.7% had a mobility disability (Fried *et al.*, 2001). To further complicate the relationship, disability can be an outcome of frailty. If frailty is the cause of disability for an individual (Albert *et al.*, 2002), frailty doesn't disappear with the onset of the disability.

Diseases alone (e.g., subclinical cardiovascular disease (Newman *et al.*, 2001), chronic renal insufficiency (Shiplak *et al.*, 2004), or in combination (i.e., comorbidity)) are associated with frailty. In the CHS study, only 7.3% of frail subjects had no chronic disease compared to 23.2% in those who were not frail (Fried *et al.*, 2001). Sixty-eight percent of frail individuals had two or more chronic conditions compared to 40% in the not frail group (Fried *et al.*, 2001). It should be noted, though, that it was a small proportion of those with comorbidities (10.5%) who were also frail (Fried *et al.*, 2001). Nearly all frail individuals will have at least one chronic condition, and most will have two or more. The presence of comorbidities, though, is not specific for frailty.

Criteria

IDENTIFICATION OF FRAIL OLDER INDIVIDUALS

Over 30 criteria have been proposed for identifying frail older individuals (Hogan *et al.*, 2003). The set that has attracted the most interest is the one developed by Dr. Linda Fried and her colleagues (Fried *et al.*, 2004). They categorized older individuals as being frail if they have three or more of the following five characteristics: diminished grip strength (compared to peers); complaints of fatigue/exhaustion; limited physical activity (compared to peers); slow gait (compared to peers); and unintentional weight loss. In a validation study, both those who were frail by these criteria and those who were intermediate (presence of one or two of the characteristics) had worse outcomes than nonfrail subjects (those with none) (Fried *et al.*, 2001).

UNSETTLED QUESTIONS

Although an important step forward, there are questions about these criteria. First, were the components selected essential to the recognition of frailty? They are not specific for frailty. A number of chronic diseases can have similar manifestations. Chronic Obstructive Pulmonary Disease, for example, is associated with diminished grip strength (Rantanen *et al.*, 1998), complaints of fatigue (Walke *et al.*, 2004), limited physical activity (Garcoa-Aymerich *et al.*, 2004), slow gait speed (Butcher *et al.*, 2004), and weight loss (Schols, 2000). Fried and her colleagues recognized the nonspecific nature of their criteria. In their validation study, they excluded individuals with significant cognitive impairment/Alzheimer's disease, depression, and Parkinson's disease as "these conditions could potentially present with frailty characteristics as a consequence of a single disease" (Fried *et al.*, 2001). The late Pope John Paul II, because of his Parkinson's disease, would not have been considered frail in this study. In their subsequent writings they have suggested secondary frailty due to diseases as a subtype of frailty (see Table 50.4). Primary frailty, from their perspective, would arise from aging-associated processes such as changes in gene expression, oxidative DNA damage, and teleomere shortening (Walston, 2004). They theorize that there is substantial interaction between primary and secondary mechanisms in the development of frailty. Of the five characteristics proposed by Fried and her colleagues, weight loss seems the most problematic. Frailty is not necessarily a wasting condition. Obese seniors appear to have a high prevalence of frailty (Villareal *et al.*, 2004). The combination of sarcopenia and obesity (the sedentary obese) delineate a group at particularly high risk for functional decline (Pierson, 2003).

The second major question deals with what was not included as a component. It is debatable that the Fried criteria captured all the essential clinical characteristics of frailty. Cognition, depressive symptoms, psychological

TABLE 50.4
Subtypes of frailty (listed alphabetically)

Cognitive: The presence of demonstrable cognitive decline or being at risk for significant cognitive deterioration; it is the opposite of *cognitive vitality* (Fillit *et al.*, 2002).
Dynamic and Static: Dynamic frailty would be a significant worsening over time on one or more preselected marker(s) of frailty; static frailty occurs when subjects are found to be in the lowest quintile, at a point in time, on preselected frailty markers; dynamic frailty requires longitudinal data collection, whereas static frailty is based on cross-sectional data (Puts *et al.*, 2005).
Global and Intrinsic: Global frailty includes *intrinsic frailty* (see following) and *consequences* (i.e., changes in functional independence, social roles, psychosocial factors, and healthcare utilization) (Studenski *et al.*, 2004). Intrinsic is defined as "physiologically based organ system impairments and physical performance limitations, such as losses of strength, endurance, balance, body weight, and mobility" (Studenski *et al.*, 2004).
Physical: Defined as impairments in the physical abilities needed to live independently (Hogan *et al.*, 2003). Described as "a final common pathway, in which the effect of disease, disuse, and aging across organ systems contribute to further decline and adverse events or states" (Studenski *et al.*, 2004); operational criteria used to identify subjects with physical frailty range from looking at a single attribute (e.g., slow gait speed) (Hardy *et al.*, 2004) to utilizing a battery (e.g., manifesting 2+ of low-peak aerobic power, self-reported difficulty, or need for assistance with two instrumental activities of daily living or one basic activity of daily living, and modified Physical Performance Test score of 18 to 22) (Villareal *et al.*, 2001).
Physiologic: Incorporates the concepts of age-associated declines in physiological systems/reduced physiologic reserve and vulnerability (Farquharson *et al.*, 2001; Hawkes *et al.*, 1998; Katz *et al.*, 1994).
Primary and Secondary: Primary causes of frailty would be age-related mechanisms (e.g., changes in gene expression, oxidative DNA damage, telomere shortening) and secondary causes would be diseases (e.g., congestive heart failure, depression, hypothyroidism, malignancy) (Fried *et al.*, 2004; Walston, 2004).
Psychosocial: Equated to the presence of depressive symptoms; de Jonge wrote that "Subjects experiencing depressive symptoms before the onset of a somatic event may have fewer resources to deal with a stressful event... Depressive symptoms reported before by elderly people may thus signal psychosocial frailty" (de Jonge *et al.*, 2004); Katz elaborated upon this and stated that "(late-life) depression is a state associated with cognitive dysfunctions that interfere with coping, adaptation, and resilience" (Katz, 2004).

attributes (e.g., positive affect; Ostir *et al.* (2004)) and others are also candidate criteria (see Table 50.2). The origin of the factors included by Fried was a survey of like-minded individuals—academic geriatricians (Fried *et al.*, 2004). A more diverse group would have added other perspectives (Surowiecki, 2004). For example, older patients and their caregivers, when considering frailty, prioritized emotional and social factors higher than clinicians (Studenski *et al.*, 2004). Excluding cognitive and psychological attributes in the definition of frailty has been justified by stating that the inquiry is limited to "physical" frailty (see Table 50.4) (Hogan *et al.*, 2003; Studenski *et al.*, 2004; Hardy *et al.*, 2004; Villareal *et al.*, 2001; Gill *et al.*, 2002; Hadley *et al.*, 1993). The wisdom of proposing a Cartesian mind–body dualism is debatable. For example, predisposing or enabling factors underpinning physical frailty may also be associated with impaired cognition. Chronic inflammation is felt to play a central role in the pathogenesis of frailty, and increased inflammatory proteins have been found to be associated with an increased risk of developing dementia (Englehart *et al.*, 2004). A correlation between cognitive processing speed and physical performance measures has been shown (Binder *et al.*, 1999). A brief instrument for the identification of frailty, the Frailty Scale (that predicted both mortality and institutionalization), included cognition as an essential feature (Rockwood *et al.*, 1999). There are data linking depressive features and subsequent physical functioning. Depressive symptoms at baseline predicted a decline in physical performance measures (standing balance, walking speed, chair rises) in four years time (Pennix *et al.*, 1998). Compared to nondepressed individuals and those with transient symptoms, older subjects with persistent depressive symptoms were at an increased risk for a worsening of their functional abilities (Lenze *et al.*, 2005). Other instruments proposed for the identification of frailty, such as the Groningen Frailty Indicator (Schuurmans *et al.*, 2004), include cognition and affect as core characteristics.

FUTURE DIRECTIONS

The various criteria proposed for frailty should be examined and compared. Do they describe the same group of individuals? The answer is, "probably not." How do they compare in predicting the outcomes associated with aging? Can their components be linked to a common pathogenesis? The respective validity, reliability, sensitivity to change, and practicality of the available criteria should be examined and contrasted. I suspect we will move away from clinical characteristics to the use of biomarkers (alone or in combination with clinical features) in identifying frail older individuals.

The challenges in establishing criteria for frailty are analogous to those faced in establishing the diagnostic criteria for the metabolic syndrome (also known as syndrome X, the dysmetabolic syndrome, the insulin resistance syndrome, and the deadly quartet). This is a cluster of abnormalities (glucose intolerance, obesity, hypertension, dyslipidemia) that are well-documented risk factors for cardiovascular disease in themselves (Eckel *et al.*, 2005). The grouping of certain characteristics known to independently predict adverse outcomes can be justified only if they are synergistic in their effect or have a common etiology (Domanski *et al.*, 2004). This appears to be the case in the metabolic syndrome. Whether a similar synergistic effect on outcomes will be seen with the components of frailty requires confirmation.

Conclusion

There is potential harm in labeling an older person as frail. Although it is a term frequently used *about* seniors, it is rarely used *by* them when discussing their status. Labeling a person can adversely change how they view themselves and how others view them. Studies have shown that priming older individuals with stereotypes can influence decision-making about life-prolonging interventions (Levy *et al.*, 1999–2000), performance on memory testing (Levy, 1996), and gait speed (Hausdorff *et al.*, 1999). An examination of the underinvestigation and undertreatment of cancer in old age concluded that it could not be wholly explained by appropriate adjustments for the condition of individual patients (Turner *et al.*, 1999). The adjective "frail" was often used to describe older patients, but it was not clearly defined. Older patients must not be inappropriately denied (or prescribed) interventions on the basis of a specious diagnostic label.

Frailty is both one of the more exciting and frustrating research areas in clinical gerontology. What leads to it, how best to recognize frailty, and ultimately what we can do to prevent or treat it are uncertain. To date there has been a "Blind Men and the Elephant" quality to frailty research. In order to achieve clarity on frailty, a concerted effort to integrate concepts and disciplines will be required. Otherwise as John Godfrey Saxe wrote, we'll

Rail on in utter ignorance
Of what each other mean,
And prate about an Elephant
Not one of them has seen!

Recommended Resources

See the Web page of the Canadian Initiative on Frailty and Aging: http://www.frail-fragile.ca.

ACKNOWLEDGMENTS

I would like to thank Dr. Howard Bergman, Dr. Ken Rockwood, and my other colleagues in the Canadian Initiative on Frailty and Aging. To them goes all credit for useful insights; to me, all blame for any confusion is assigned.

REFERENCES

Albert, S.M., Im, A., and Raveis, V.H. (2002). Public health and the second 50 years of life. *Am J Pub Health 92*, 1214–1216.

Baker III, G.T., and Achenbaum, W.A. (1992). A historical perspective of research on the biology of aging from Nathan W. Shock. *Exp Gerontol 27*, 261–273.

Ben-Shlomo, Y., and Kuh, D. (2002). A life-course approach to chronic disease epidemiology: conceptual models, empirical challenges and interdisciplinary perspectives. *Int J Epidemiol 31*, 285–293.

Binder, E.F., Storandt, M., and Birge, S.J. (1999). The relation between psychometric test performance and physical performance in older adults. *J Gerontol A Biol Sci Med Sci 54*, M428–M432.

Bortz, W.M. (2002). A conceptual framework for frailty: A review. *J Gerontol A Biol Sci Med Sci 57*, M283–M288.

Breeze, E., Fletcher, A.E., Leon, D.A., Marmot, M.G., Clarke, R.J., and Shipley, M.J. (2001). Do socioeconomic disadvantages persist into old age? Self-reported morbidity in a 29-year follow-up of the Whitehall Study. *Am J Public Health 91*, 277–283.

Brunner, E. (1997). Socioeconomic determinants of health – Stress and the biology of inequality. *BMJ 314*, 1472–1476.

Buchner, D.M., and Wagner, E.H. (1992). Preventing frail health. *Clin Geriatr Med 8*, 1–17.

Butcher, S.J., Meshke, J.M., and Sheppard, M.S. (2004). Reductions in functional balance, coordination, and mobility measures among patients with stable chronic obstructive pulmonary disease. *J Cardiopulm Rehabil 24*, 274–280.

Campbell, A.J., and Buchner, D.M. (1997). Unstable disability and the fluctuations of frailty. *Age & Ageing 26*, 315–318.

Cohen, H.J. (2000). In search of the underlying mechanisms of frailty. *J Gerontol A Biol Sci Med Sci 55A*, M706–M708.

Corder, E.H., Basun, H., Fratiglioni, L., Guo, Z., Lannfelt, L., Viitanen, M. *et al.* (2000). Inherited frailty—ApoE alleles determine survival after a diagnosis of heart disease or stroke at ages 85+. *Ann NY Acad Sci 908*, 295–298.

de Jonge, P., Ormel, J., Slaets, J.P.J., Kempen, G.I., Ranchor, A.V., van Jaarsveld, C.H. *et al.* (2004). Depressive symptoms in elderly patients predict poor adjustment after somatic events. *Am J Geriatr Psychiatry 12*, 57–64.

Di Bari, M., van de Poll-Franse, L.V., Onder, G., Kritchevsky, S.B., Newman, A., Harris, T.B. *et al.* (2004). Antihypertensive medications and differences in muscle mass in older persons: The health, aging and body composition study. *J Am Geriatr Soc 52*, 961–966.

Doherty, T.J. (2003). Invited review: Aging and sarcopenia. *J Appl Physiol 95*, 1717–1727.

Domanski, M., and Proschan, M. (2004). The metabolic syndrome. *J Am Coll Cardiol 43*, 1396–1398.

Eckel, R.H., Grundy, S.M., and Zimmet, P.Z. (2005). The metabolic syndrome. *Lancet 365*, 1415–1428.

Englehart, M.J., Geerlings, M.I., Meijer, J., Kiliaan, A., Ruitenberg, A., van Swieten, J.C. *et al.* (2004). Inflammatory proteins in plasma and the risk of dementia: the Rotterdam Study. *Arch Neurol 61*, 668–672.

Epel, E.S., Blackburn, E.H., Lin. J., Dhabhar, F.S., Adlrer, N.E., Morrow, J.D. *et al.* (2004). Accelerated telomere shortening in response to life stress. *Proc Natl Acad Sci 101*, 17312 17315.

Farquharson, S.M., Gupta, R., Heald, R.J., and Moran, B.J. (2001). Surgical decisions in the elderly: the importance of biological age. *J R Soc Med 94*, 232–235.

Ferrucci, L., Guralnik, J.M., Pahor, M., Corti, M.C., and Havlik, R.J. (1997). Hospital diagnoses, Medicare charges, and nursing home admissions in the year when older persons become severely disabled. *JAMA 277*, 728–734.

Ferrucci, L., and Guralnik, J.M. (2003). Inflammation, hormones, and body composition at a crossroad. *Am J Med 115*, 501–502.

Finch, C.E., and Crimmins, E.M. (2004). Inflammatory exposure and historical changes in human life-spans. *Science 305*, 1736–1739.

Fillit, H.M., Butler, R.N., O'Connell, A.W., Albert, M.S., Birren, J.E., Cotman, C.W. *et al.* (2002). Achieving and maintaining cognitive vitality with aging. *Mayo Clin Proc 77*, 681–696.

Fried, L.P., Tangen, C.M., Walston, J., Newman, A.B., Hirsch, C., Gottdiener, J. *et al.* (2001). Frailty in older adults: Evidence of a phenotype. *J Gerontol A Biol Sci Med Sci 56*, M146–M156.

Fried, L.P., Ferrucci, L., Darer, J., Williamson, J.D., and Anderson, G. (2004). Untangling the concepts of disability, frailty, and comorbidity: Implications for improved targeting and care. *J Gerontol A Biol Sci Med Sci 59*, M255–M263.

Gallagher, R. (2002). One lumper or two. *The Scientist 16(22)*, 12.

Garcia-Aymerich, J., Felez, M.A., Escarrabill, J., Marrades, R.M., Morera, J., Elosua, R. *et al.* (2004). Physical activity and its determinants in severe chronic obstructive pulmonary disease. *Med Sci Sports Exerc 36*, 1667–1673.

Gerdes, L.U., Jeune, B., Ransberg, K.A., Nubo, H., and Vaupel J.W. (2000). Estimation of Apoliporotein E genotype-specific relative mortality risks from the distribution of genotypes in centenarians and middle-aged men: Apolipoprotein E gene is a "frailty gene," not a "longevity gene." *Genetic Epidemiology 19*, 202–210.

Gill, T.M., Baker, D.I., Gottschalk, M., Peduzzi, P.N., Allore, H., and Byers, A. (2002). A program to prevent functional decline in physically frail. Elderly persons who live at home. *N Engl J Med 347*, 1068–1074.

Gill, T.M., Allore, H., Holford, T.R., and Guo, Z. (2004). The development of insidious disability in activities of daily living among community-living older persons. *Am J Med 117*, 484–491.

Gluckman, P.D., and Hanson, M.A. (2004). Living with the past: Evolution, development, and patterns of disease. *Science 305*, 1733–1736.

Godfrey, K.M., and Barker, D.J. (2001). Fetal programming and adult health. *Public Health Nutr 4(2B)*, 611–624.

Guralnik, J.M., Ferrucci, L., Balfour, J.L., Volpato, S., and Di Iorio A. (2001). Progressive versus catastrophic loss of the ability to walk: implications for the prevention of mobility loss. *J Am Geriatr Soc 49*, 1463–1470.

Gurland, B.J., Page, W.F., and Plassman, B.L. (2004). A twin study of the genetic contribution to age-related functional impairment. *J Gerontol A Biol Sci Med Sci 59A*, 859–863.

Haber, C. (1986). Geriatrics: A specialty in search of specialists. In *Old Age in a Bureaucratic Society: The Elderly, the Experts, and the State in American History*, pp. 66–84. New York: Greenwood Press.

Hadley, E.C., Ory, M.G., Suzman, R., and Weindruch, R. (1993). Foreword to special issue on physical frailty. *J of Gerontol 48 (Special Issue)*: vii–viii.

Hadley, E.C., Lakatta, E.G., Morrison-Bogorad, M., Warner, H.R., and Hodes, R.J. (2005). The future of aging therapeutics. *Cell 120*, 557–567.

Hamet, P., and Tremblay, J. (2003). Genes of aging. *Metabolism 52 (10 Suppl 2)*, 5–9.

Hardy, S.E., and Gill, T.M. (2004). Recovery from disability among community-dwelling persons. *JAMA 291*, 1596–1602.

Hausdorff, J.M., Levy, B.R., and Wei, J.Y. (1999). The power of ageism on physical function of older persons: reversibility of age-related gait changes. *J Am Geriatr Soc 47*, 1346–1349.

Hawkes, K., O'Connell, J.F., Blurton Jones, N.G., Alvarez, H., and Charnov, E.L. (1998). Grandmothering, menopause, and the evolution of human life histories. *Proc Natl Acad Sci USA 95*, 1336–1339.

Hogan, D.B., MacKnight, C., and Bergman, H. (2003). Models, definitions, and criteria of frailty. *Aging Clin Exp Research 15* (*Suppl to No. 3*), 3–29.

Johnson, T.E., Lithgow, G.J., Murakami, S., and Shook, D.R. (1996). Genetics. In J.E. Birren, Editor-in-Chief, *Encyclopedia of Gerontology—Age, Aging and the Aged, Volume I*, pp. 577–586. San Diego: Academic Press.

Joseph, C., Kenny, A.M., Taxel, P., Lorenzo, J.A., Duque, G., and Kuchel, G.A. (2005). Role of endocrine-immune dysregulation in osteoporosis, sarcopenia, frailty and fracture risk. *Molecular Aspects of Medicine 16*, 181–201.

Karlamangla, A.S., Singer, B.H., McEwen, B.S., Rowe, J.W., and Seeman, T. (2002). Allostatic load as a predictor of functional decline—MacArthur studies of successful aging. *J Clin Epidemiol 55*, 696–710.

Katz, I.R., Parmelee, P.A., Beaston-Wimmer, P., and Smith B.D. (1994). Association of antidepressants and other medications with mortality in the residential-care elderly. *J Geriatr Psychiatry Neurol 7*, 221–226.

Katz, I.R. (2004). Depression and frailty—the need for multidisciplinary research. *Am J Geriatr Psychiatry 12*, 1–5.

Kiecolt-Glaser, J.K., Preacher, K.J., MacCallum, R.C., Atkinson, C., Malarkey, W.B., and Glaser, R. (2003). Chronic stress and age-related increases in the proinflammatory cytokine IL-6. *Proc Natl Acad Sci 100*, 9090–9095.

Kolata G. (2002). Is frailty inevitable? Experts say no. *New York Times, November 19, 5.*

Kuh, D., Bassey, J., Hardy, R., Aihie Sayer, A., Wadsworth, M., and Cooper, C. (2002). Birth weight, childhood size, and muscle strength in adult life: evidence from a birth cohort study. *Am J Epidemiol 156*, 627–633.

Kuh, D., Ben-Shlomo, Y., Lynch, J., Hallqvist, J., and Power, C. (2003). Life course epidemiology. *J Epidemiol Community Health 57*, 778–783.

Lenze, E.J., Schulz, R., Martire, L.M., Zdaniuk, B., Glass, T., Kop, W.J. *et al.* (2005). The course of functional decline in older people with persistently elevated depressive symptoms: Longitudinal findings from the cardiovascular health study. *J Am Geriatr Soc 53*, 569–575.

Levy, B. (1996). Improving memory in old age through implicit self-stereotyping. *J Pers Soc Psychol 71*, 1092–1107.

Levy, B., Ashman, O., and Dror, I. (1999–2000). To be or not to be: The effects of aging stereotypes on the will to live. *Omega (Westport) 40 (3)*, 409–420.

Lipsitz, L.A., and Goldberger, A.L. (1992). Loss of "complexity" and aging—Potential applications of fratuals and chaos theory to senescence. *JAMA 267*, 1806–1809.

Lipsitz, L.A. (2002). Dynamics of stability: the physiologic basis of functional health and frailty. *J Gerontol A Biol Sci Med Sci 57*, B115–B125.

Lu, T., Pan, S-Y., Li, C., Kohane, I., Chan, J., and Yankner, B.A. (2004). Gene regulation and DNA damage in the ageing human brain. *Nature 429*, 883–891.

Lunney, J.R., Lynn, J., and Hogan, C. (2002). Profiles of older Medicare decedents. *J Am Geriatr Soc 50*, 1108–1112.

Lunney, J.R., Lynn, J., Foley, D.J., Lipson, S., and Guralnik, J.M. (2003). Patterns of functional decline at the end of life. *JAMA 289*, 2387–2392.

Marcell, T.J. (2003). Sarcopenia: Causes, consequences, and preventions. *J Gerontol A Biol Sci Med Sci 58A*, 911–916.

Martin, G.M. (2005). Genetic modulation of senescent phenotypes in *Homo sapiens*. *Cell 120*, 523–532.

McEwen, B.S. (2003). Interacting mediators of allostasis and allostatic load: Towards an understanding of resilience in aging. *Metabolism 52 (10 Suppl 2)*, 10–16.

McEwen, B.S. (2004). Protective and damaging effects of the mediators of stress and adaptation: Allostasis and allostatic load. In J. Schulkin, Ed. *Allostasis, Homeostasis, and the Costs of Physiological Adaptation*, pp. 65–98. Cambridge: Cambridge University Press.

Mitnitski, A.B., Mogilner, A.J., MacKnight, C., and Rockwood, K. (2002). The mortality rate as a function of accumulated deficits in a frailty index. *Mechanisms of Aging and Development 123*, 1457–1460.

Montgomery, H., Clarkson, P., Barnard, M., Bell, J., Byrnes, A., Dollery, C. *et al.* (1999). Angiotensin-converting-enzyme gene insertion/deletion polymorphism and response to physical training. *Lancet 353*, 541–545.

Morley, J.E., Kim, M.J., and Haven, M.T. (2005). Frailty and hormones. *Reviews in endocrine and metabolic disorders 6*, 101–108.

Newman, A.B., Gottdiener, J.S., McBurnie, M.A., Hirsch, C.H., Kop, W.J., Tracy, R. *et al.* (2001). Associations of subclinical cardiovascular disease with frailty. *J Gerontol A Biol Sci Med Sci 56*, M158–M166.

Onder, G., Penninx, B.W.J.H., Balkrishnan, R., Fried, L.P., Chaves, P.H.M., Williamson, J. *et al.* (2002). Relation between use of angiotensin-converting enzyme inhibitors and muscle strength and physical function in older women: an observational study. *Lancet 359*, 926–930.

Ostir, G.V., Ottenbacher, K.J., and Markides, K.S. (2004). Onset of frailty in older adults and the protective role of positive affect. *Psychology and Aging 19*, 402–408.

Pennix, B.W.J.H., Guralnik, J.M., Ferrucci, L., Simonsick, E.M., Deeg, D.J.H., and Wallace, R.B. (1998). Depressive symptoms and physical decline in community-dwelling older persons. *JAMA 279*, 1720–1726.

Pierson, R.N. (2003). Body composition in aging: a biological perspective. *Current Opinion in Clinical Nutrition and Metabolic Care 6*, 15–20.

Puts, M.T.E., Lips, P., and Deeg, D.J.H. (2005). Sex differences in the risk of frailty for mortality independent of disability and chronic diseases. *J Am Geriatr Soc 53*, 40–47.

Radek, Z., Chung, Y., and Goto, S. (2005). Exercise and hormesis: oxidative stress-related adaptation for successful aging. *Biogerontology 6*, 71–75.

Rantanen, T., Masaki, K., Foley, D., Izmirlian, G., White, L., and Guralnik, J.M. (1998). Grip changes over 27 years in Japanese-American men. *J Appl Physiol 85*, 2047–2053.

Rockwood, K., Stolee, P., and McDowell, I. (1996). Factors associated with institutionalization of older people in Canada: testing a multifactorial definition of frailty. *J Am Geriatr Soc 44*, 578–582.

Rockwood, K., Stadnyk, K., MacKnight, C., McDowell, I., Hébert, R., and Hogan, D.B. (1999). A brief clinical instrument to classify frailty in elderly people. *Lancet 353*, 205–206.

Rockwood, K., Mitnitski, A.B., and MacKnight, C. (2002). Some mathematical models of frailty and their clinical implications. *Reviews in Clinical Gerontology 12*, 109–117.

Sayer, A.A., Syddall, H., O'Dell, S., Chen, X-H., Briggs, P.J., Briggs, R. *et al.* (2002). Polymorphism of the IGF2 gene, birth weight and grip strength in adult men. *Age and Ageing 31*, 468–470.

Sayer, A.A., Syddall, H.E., Gilbody, H.J., Dennison, E.M., and Cooper C. (2004). Does sarcopenia originate in early life? Findings from the Hertfordshire cohort study. *J Gerontol A Biol Sci Med Sci 59*, M930–M934.

Schmaltz, H.N., Fried, L.P., Xue, Q-L., Walston, J., Leng, S.X., and Semba, E.D. (2005). Chronic cytomegalovirus infection and inflammation are associated with prevalent frailty in community-dwelling older women. *J Am Geriatr Soc 53*, 747–754.

Schols, A.M. (2000). Nutrition in chronic obstructive pulmonary disease. *Curr Opin Pulm Med 6*, 110–115.

Schuurmans, H., Steverink, N., Lindenberg, S., Frieswijk, N., and Slaets, J.P.J. (2004). Old or frail: What tells us more? *J of Gerontol A Biol Sci Med Sci 59*, 962–965.

Semenchenko, G.V., Anisimov, V.N., and Yashin, A.I. (2004). Stressors and antistressors: how do they influence life span in HER-2/neu transgenic mice? *Exp Gerontol 39*, 1499–1511.

Shlipak, M.G., Stehman-Breen, C., Fried, L.F., Song, X., Siscovick, D., Fried, L.P. *et al.* (2004). The presence of frailty in elderly people with chronic renal insufficiency. *Am J Kidney Dis 43*, 861–867.

Strawbridge, W.J., Shema, S.J., Balfour, J.L., Higby, H.R., and Kaplan, G.A. (1998). Antecedents of frailty over three decades in an older cohort. *J Gerontol 53*, S9–S16.

Studenski, S., Hayes, R.P., Leibiwitz, R.Q., Bode, R., Lavery, L., Walston, J. *et al.* (2004). Clinical global impression of change in physical frailty: Development of a measure based on clinical judgment. *J Am Geriatr Soc 52*, 1560–1566.

Surowiecki, J. (2004). *The wisdom of crowds—Why the many are smarter than the few and how collective wisdom shapes business, economics, societies, and nations.* New York: Doubleday.

Tattan, S.I.S. (2004). Aging intervention, prevention, and therapy through hormesis. *J Gerontol A Biol Sci Med Sci 59A*, 705–709.

Thane, P. (1993). Geriatrics. In W.F. Bynum and R. Porter, Eds., *Companion Encyclopedia of the History of Medicine, Volume 2*, pp. 1092–1115. London: Routledge.

Turner, N.J., Haward, R.A., Mulley, G.P., and Selby P.J. (1999). Cancer in old age—Is it inadequately investigated and treated? *BMJ 319*, 309–312.

Van den Biggelaar, A.H.J., Huizinga, T.W.J., de Craen, A.J.M., Gussekloo, J., Heijmans, B.T., Frölich, M. *et al.* (2004). Impaired innate immunity predicts frailty in old age. *Exp Gerontol 39*, 1407–1414.

Vanltallie, T.B. (2003). Frailty in the elderly: contributions of sarcopenia and visceral protein depletion. *Metabolism 52 (10 Suppl 2)*, 22–26.

Villareal, D.T., Binder, E.F., Williams, D.B., Schechtman, K.B., Yarshehski, K.E., and Kohrt, W.M. (2001). Bone mineral density response to estrogen replacement in frail elderly women: A randomized controlled trial. *JAMA 286*, 815–820.

Villareal, D.T., Banks, M., Siener, C., Sinacore, D.R., and Klein, S. (2004). Physical frailty and body composition in obese elderly men and women. *Obesity Research 12*, 913–920.

Walke, L.M., Gallo, W.T., Tinetti, M.E., and Fried, T.R. (2004). The burden of symptoms among community-dwelling older persons with advanced chronic disease. *Arch Intern Med 164*, 2321 2324.

Walston, J. (2004). Frailty—The search for underlying causes. *Sci Aging Knowl Environ 4 (January 28)*, e4.

Walston, J., Arking, D.E., Fallin, D., Li, T., Beamer, B., Xue, Q. *et al.* (2005). IL-6 gene variation is not associated with increased serum levels of IL-6, muscle, weakness, or frailty in older women. *Exp Gerontol 40*, 344–352.

Yates, F.E. (1996). Theories of Aging: Biological. In J.E. Birren, Editor-in-Chief, *Encyclopedia of Gerontology—Age, Aging and the Aged, Volume II*, pp. 545–555. San Diego: Academic Press.

51

Fertility and Aging Men: An Introduction to the Male Biological Clock

Puneet Masson, Sarah M. Lambert, Peter N. Schlegel, and Harry Fisch

Data obtained in the past decade suggested a worldwide decline in male fertility. The increase in paternal age is both a personal problem for couples and a public health problem because of the simple fact that male fertility declines with age. Journal articles by Kidd and Ford demonstrate that men over the age of 35 are twice as likely to be infertile as men younger than 25. In addition, a study of couples undergoing fertility treatments found that the amount of time it takes for a man to achieve a pregnancy rises significantly with age.

The levels of sex hormones in men decline with age. The roughly 1% per year decline in testosterone levels after age 30 has been termed andropause, or "symptomatic hypogonadism in the aging male." Rhoden and Morgentaler estimate that between 2 and 4 million men in the United States alone suffer from hypogonadism, but only 5% of men are getting treatment for their symptoms.

Although increasing maternal age has long been known to be associated with an increased incidence of birth defects, new data show that the age of the male does matter and the genetic quality of sperm does decline with age. Several studies have demonstrated that older men are at higher risk of fathering a child with various genetic diseases such as schizophrenia and Down Syndrome, to name a few. Additionally, there has been an increased risk of miscarriage with increasing paternal age.

This review discusses the relationship between advanced paternal age and male infertility. Continuing this dialogue will improve the sexual and reproductive health of aging males.

Introduction

Say "biological clock," and most people immediately think, "women." Female fertility, after all, "strikes midnight" with the cessation of menses. This occurs in association with distinct—and dramatic—declines in estrogen production. And as women age, the genetic quality of their eggs declines and the subsequent increased proportion of genetically damaged embryos leads to an increased risk of genetic problems in their offspring. This triad of declining fertility, declining hormone levels, and increasing risk for genetic problems is what most people mean when they say "biological clock."

Until recently, that is. Although it is an idea that has not yet filtered down to the general public, we now know that men have biological clocks, too. And those clocks involve the same physiological triad experienced by women. Male fertility and male sex hormones *do* decline with age. And the genetic quality of sperm *does* decline, leading to an increased risk of genetic problems in offspring above and beyond any contributed by the female. The object of this review is to describe these features of male aging and, hence, to expand the notion of the "biological clock" to include *both* sexes.

Conceptions of Fertility

It is a well established fact that a reduction in fertility status happens with increasing age. In women, we recognize that a decline in oocyte production occurs in their late 30s to early 40s. Men, on the contrary, can continue to father children well beyond their 40s, and to date there is no significant limit with respect to spermatogenesis. As paternal age continues to increase, many investigators have explored the effect of age on seminal parameters with the central question: Is advanced paternal age associated with diminished semen quality and a higher risk of infertility?

In a mouse model, studies have demonstrated that aging is correlated with histologic changes in testes and a decline in semen quality. Tanemura *et al.* (1993) demonstrated that older mice (at the age of 18 months) have several age-related changes, including an increased number of vacuoles in germ cells and a thinner seminiferous epithelium. By the age of 30 months, extremely thin seminiferous epithelia with very few spermatocytes or spermatids were found. In another study, Wang *et al.* (1993) found that total sperm production was significantly reduced in 22- and 30-month-old rats. Further studies also documented an increased incidence of preimplantation losses, mutation frequencies, and anueploidy in the offspring of older male mice (Serre *et al.*, 1998; Walter *et al.*, 1998; Lowe *et al.*, 1995).

With the abundant evidence on the association between aging and male infertility in mice, the appropriate question is whether such a correlation exists in men. A comprehensive review by Kidd *et al.* (2001) evaluated the effects of male aging on semen quality in men; they looked at all studies in published literature between January 1 1980 and December 31 1999, and examined the outcome parameters of semen volume, sperm concentration, sperm motility, sperm morphology, pregnancy rate, and time to pregnancy/subfecundity (Kidd *et al.*, 2001).

The overall consensus in the stated literature demonstrated a decrease in semen volume with increasing age. There have been 16 major studies examining semen volume with respect to advanced age. Though individual studies have varied with respect to the setting in which they were conducted (i.e., infertility clinics versus sperm banks), Kidd's meta-analysis of the results provides a comprehensive overview of the effect of male age on seminal parameters. Out of the 16 studies analyzed, 11 reported decreases in semen quality with increasing age. Two of these studies adjusted for the confounder of duration of abstinence and found that a statistically significant correlation still exists between decreasing semen volume and increasing age; they reported decreases of 0.15 to 0.5% for each increase in year of age (Fisch *et al.*, 1996; Andolz *et al.*, 1999). The duration of abstinence has been correlated with semen volume in a time-dependent fashion (Mortimer *et al.*, 1982). Out of four studies showing no association between age and semen volume, only one study adjusted for duration of abstinence, and this study had a maximum patient age of 50 years (Schwartz *et al.*, 1983). One study reported a slight increase (0.01mL/year) in semen volume with increasing age; however, this effect disappeared when adjusted for year of birth. Therefore, there is abundant evidence linking decreased semen volume with increased age, which becomes more significant in men over 50 years of age. When comparing men under the age of 30 with men aged 50 or older, most of the studies document decreases of 20 to 30% in semen volume between the two groups (Kidd *et al.*, 2001). The correlation between advanced paternal age and semen volume suggests that age contributes to a decline in semen quality necessary for fertilization.

Unlike semen volume, the relationship between increasing age and sperm concentration was found to be inconclusive. Kidd *et al.* (2001) reviewed 21 studies examining the association between age and decreased sperm concentration and found no clear relationship between these parameters. Five studies documented decreasing sperm concentration with increasing age. However, only one study controlled for abstinence and year of birth as potential confounders; this study found a decrease in sperm concentration of 3.3% per year of age and also a 66% decrease in concentration from age 30 to 50 (Auger *et al.*, 1995). Six studies found little or no association between age and sperm concentration, and none of these studies adjusted for duration of abstinence. Eight studies documented that with increasing age, sperm concentration had linear increases from 0.03 to 3.3% per year of age. Only two of these studies adjusted for duration of abstinence as a confounder and, interestingly enough, the increase in sperm concentration per year of age was found to be minimal (Fisch *et al.*, 1996; Andolz *et al.*, 1999). Based on the review by Kidd *et al.* there is substantial inconsistency among the studies exploring the relationship between sperm concentration and age. Even the results of the studies adjusting for duration of infertility are conflicting, suggesting that there is no clear association between sperm concentration and increasing paternal age.

Sperm motility, on the other hand, was found to be strongly linked to age as a substantial decline in sperm motility went hand-in-hand with increasing age. Kidd *et al.* (2001) reviewed 19 studies examining the relationship between the percentage of motile sperm and age; the majority of these studies (17/19) used visual assessment of sperm motility by light microscopy. Thirteen of the 19 studies found a decrease in sperm motility with increasing age; five of these studies adjusted for duration of abstinence, and the observed changes were statistically significant (Fisch *et al.*, 1996; Rolf *et al.*, 1996; Schwartz *et al.*, 1983; Auger *et al.*, 1995; Henkel *et al.*, 1999). When these studies compared men age 50 or older to men under the age of 30, they reported a 3 to 37% decline in motility. Four studies reviewed by Kidd *et al.* found no association between age and sperm motility, and two studies reported a positive correlation; none of these studies adjusted for duration of infertility. Thus, the extensive body of evidence suggests that an inverse correlation exists between age and sperm motility: there is a decline in sperm motility with increasing male age.

Likewise, an adverse correlation exists between sperm morphology and age. Kidd *et al.* (2001) reviewed 14 studies examining the relationship between age and sperm morphology. There were nine studies documenting a decrease in the percent of normal sperm with increasing age, five of which were found to be statistically significant. Controlling for the potential confounders of duration of abstinence and year of birth, Auger *et al.* (1995) reported that the percent of normal sperm decreased by 0.9% per year of age, and Andolz *et al.* (1999) reported a decline of 0.2% per year of age. When studies utilized age as a categorical variable, there was an observable trend with increasing age group and decreasing percent normal sperm. Five studies found no association between percent normal sperm and age, and none of these studies were found to be statistically significant. Despite the variation among morphological criteria to assess sperm abnormalities, there was a substantial amount of evidence linking increasing age to decreasing percent normal sperm.

The associations between increasing age and decreasing semen volume, sperm motility, and sperm morphology suggest that semen quality diminishes in the aging male. Whether age is analyzed as a continuous or categorical variable, the body of evidence suggests that a trend exists between increasing male age and decreasing semen quality based on these parameters. Aging in the human male results in degenerative changes to the prostate, such as a decrease in protein and water content (Schneider, 1978); these may contribute to the decrease in seminal volume and sperm motility. Additionally, age-related degenerative changes to the germinal epithelium can impact sperm morphology (Johnson, 1986). Though we recognize that advanced paternal age affects semen quality, it is necessary to study the impact of increasing age on fertility itself.

In his extensive analysis, Kidd *et al.* (2001) also studied the impact of increasing age on pregnancy rate, defined as the percent of male subjects whose partners achieved a pregnancy over a period of time, and subfecundity, defined as the percent of couples remaining infertile at a defined time point. Kidd *et al.* (2001) reviewed nine studies that examined the association between male age and pregnancy rate. The study population consisted of participants from infertility and assisted conception clinics. Seven of these studies reported a correlation between decreasing pregnancy rates and increasing age, and five of them reached statistical significance. However, four of the seven studies did not adjust for female age in the analysis, and female age is a well-established independent predictor of achieving pregnancy. Two of the studies that controlled for female partner age found that, after stratifying the study population into men under 30 and men over 50, the pregnancy rate in the cohort of older men was 23 to 38% lower (Rolf *et al.*, 1996; Mathieu *et al.*, 1995). One study did not find an effect of male age on pregnancy rates when female age was less than 35 years (Dondero *et al.*, 1985), and another study reported lower pregnancy rates for couples where the man was over 30 years compared to those where the man was under 30 (van der Westerlaken *et al.*, 1998); neither study determined the statistical significance of these differences. Overall, we see that there is an extensive amount of evidence linking increased paternal age and decreased pregnancy rate, with more substantial declines in men over the age of 50.

Kidd *et al.* (2001) also reviewed 11 studies evaluating the association between male age and subfecundity. Nine of these studies found that the time to pregnancy increases with male age, and four of the nine studies employed a proportional hazard analysis, which adjusted for varying lengths of observation before pregnancy was achieved. Seven of the nine studies reporting a direct correlation between paternal age and time to pregnancy reached statistical significance. In these studies, the increased risks of subfecundity with older age groups ranged from 11 to 250%. Only one study by Mathieu *et al.* (1995) adjusted for duration of infertility and irregular ovulation; Mathieu *et al.* found that after stratifying men into cohorts of age 35 or greater and less than age 30, there was a 60% decrease in the chance of initiating a pregnancy for the older men. Since this study was conducted for couples undergoing intrauterine artificial insemination, female age was found to be a poor prognostic value in predicting risk of pregnancy. There were two studies that did not show an association between male age and time to pregnancy; neither of these studies showed statistically significant differences (Kidd *et al.*, 2001). Thus, the weight of the evidence suggests a strong correlation between paternal age and time required for a couple to achieve pregnancy.

A landmark study by Ford *et al.* (2000) explored the effect of paternal age on the likelihood of delayed conception. With a study population of 8515 planned pregnancies, the study found that older men were significantly less likely to impregnate their partners in less than six or less than 12 months, compared to their younger counterparts. After adjusting for various confounding factors such as age of the female partner, BMI, smoking, passive smoke exposure, education, duration of cohabitation, duration of oral contraceptive use, and paternal alcohol consumption, paternal age still remained highly significantly associated with conception within six or 12 months. If paternal age was treated as a continuous variable, there was a statistically significant linear relationship; the odds ratio for conception within six months decreased by 2% per year of age, and for conception within 12 months decreased by 3% per year of age. After comparing their study with the existent literature, Ford *et al.* concluded that the probability that a fertile couple will take greater than 12 months to conceive nearly doubles from approximately 8% when a man is less than 25 years old to approximately 15% when he is greater than age 35.

Kidd's review and Ford's study include a vast body of articles with variable evaluations and diverse patient populations. Additionally, the studies also vary in their adjustment of potential confounders as well as age-group stratifications. For these reasons, there can be no single conclusion about the linearity of the relationship between male age and semen parameters and/or fertility. Nevertheless, advanced paternal age is associated with a decline in semen quality and fertility status. As paternal age continues to increase in industrialist societies, it is worthwhile to continue engaging in a dialogue about the risks of infertility associated with a population of aging potential fathers.

Testosterone Decline

As with women, the levels of sex hormones in men decline with age (Harman *et al.*, 2001). The drop is not as steep or as sudden as that associated with menopause, but it can be equally significant for fertility and overall well-being. Recently, there has been a lot of interest in declining testosterone levels in men. The roughly 1% per year decline in testosterone levels after age 30 has been termed andropause and is associated with a plethora of congenital and acquired disease-syndromes (McLachlan, 2000).

Previous longitudinal studies have demonstrated that abnormally low testosterone levels are present in elderly men (Sparrow *et al.*, 1980; Harman *et al.*, 2001; Feldman *et al.*, 2002). Several large-scale studies in healthy, fertile men have evaluated mean values for serum testosterone (Ferrini *et al.*, 1998). Additionally, there have been numerous cross-sectional investigations documenting lower concentrations of total testosterone and/or free testosterone in older men (Vermeulen *et al.*, 1972; Gray *et al.*, 1991). Most recently, the Massachusetts Male Aging Study, a large population-based random-sample cohort, reported that in a cohort of 1,709 healthy men aged 40 to 70 with a mean age of 55.2 years, the mean total testosterone value was 520 ng/mL. In follow-up data approximately a decade later, another cohort of 1,156 healthy men with a mean age of 62.7 years had a mean total testosterone value of 450 ng/mL (Feldman *et al.*, 2002). This is a decline in testosterone in the same population of men sampled approximately 10 years later. Feldman *et al.* quantified the decreasing testosterone levels as a cross-sectional decline of 0.8%/year of age and a longitudinal decline of 1.6%/year within the follow-up data. Other aging studies also have reported a longitudinal decline in serum testosterone (Rodriguez-Rigau *et al.*, 1978; Morley *et al.*, 1997). Additionally, Feldman *et al.* reported that the rate of decline was the same in apparently healthy men as well as men reporting a chronic illness, obesity, alcoholism, prescription medication, or prostate problems.

The decline in testosterone with age puts a greater number of elderly men at risk for developing hypogonadism. Rhoden and Morgentaler estimated that between two and four million men in the United States alone suffer from hypogonadism (defined as serum total testosterone levels lower than 325 ng per deciliter) (Rhoden *et al.*, 2004). More alarmingly though, the same study reported that only 5% of these men are getting treatment for their symptoms, which include decreased libido and erectile dysfunction, loss of muscle mass and strength, weight gain, and declining cognitive function. Hypogonadism is also associated with type II diabetes, musculoskeletal frailty, cardiovascular disease, and the metabolic syndrome.

Because of the increasing prevalence of abnormally low levels of testosterone in elderly men, it is worthwhile to assess the relationship between hypogonadism and aging. The Baltimore Longitudinal Study on Aging, a large-scale study measuring total and free testosterone levels in 890 healthy men without any reported fertility or varicocele complications, found that using total testosterone, the frequency of detection of hypogonadal testosterone levels increased to about 20% of men over 60, 30% over 70, and 50% over 80 years of age (Harman *et al.*, 2001). The study also found that 78% of men identified as hypogonadal by a single testosterone determination had low total testosterone levels on all subsequent samples. Additionally, a multivariate analysis confirmed that age is an independent predictor of a longitudinal decline in both total and free testosterone. Testosterone also decreased with increasing body mass index (BMI), independent of age.

To rectify the increased prevalence of hypogonadism in the aging male, treatments such as exogenous testosterone replacement and stimulation of endogenous testosterone production are gaining tremendous popularity. Sales of prescription testosterone products have soared more than 500% since 1993 and continue to increase (Bhasin *et al.*, 2001). This enormous increase is not without risks; indiscriminate use of testosterone supplements can raise the risk of prostate problems, blood disorders, and infertility.

It has been established that there is a natural decline in serum testosterone as a process of aging; however, it demands to be explored if there are subsets of men with lower serum testosterone levels at an earlier age. Varicoceles are a well-established condition causing infertility. Varicoceles affect sperm function, and several studies suggest that they may contribute to testicular dysfunction and induce a subhypogonadal or hypogonadal state. Animal experiments have demonstrated an association between varicoceles and decreased serum testosterone biosynthesis (Rodriguez-Rigau *et al.*, 1978). However, such studies in humans have not shown as strong an association. Gorelick and Goldstein reported that infertile males with varicoceles have a mean serum testosterone level that is within the limits of normal (Gorelick *et al.*, 2000). Yet, Younes (2000) reported that mean serum testosterone was substantially decreased in male infertility patients with varicoceles compared to controls. Though there have been several further studies examining the testosterone profile of infertile men with varicoceles, results continue to be conflicting (Nagao *et al.*, 1986; Comhaire *et al.*, 1975).

At Columbia University Medical Center, we retrospectively reviewed testosterone levels of 237 men presenting with male factor infertility and clinical varicoceles between 1994 and 2004 who underwent varicocelectomy. For the entire cohort of men, the median age was 36.0 years, and the average testosterone level was 389.7 ng/mL. Out of our sample, 30.3% (72/237) patients were found to be hypogonadal (testosterone < 300 ng/mL). When stratified into groups, the student's t test of independent samples showed that infertile men with varicoceles under the age of 30 had a mean testosterone level of 420.3ng/mL and those age 50 or older had mean testosterone level of 342.1 ng/mL ($p = 0.05$); men between the ages of 30 and 49 had a mean testosterone level of 389.2 ng/mL (Shah *et al.*, 2005). This is the largest study to date reporting the testosterone profile of infertile men with varicoceles. Infertile men with varicoceles have a much lower serum testosterone level than was previously anticipated, with almost one-third being hypogonadal. With increasing age, we found a trend indicating that older men have even lower testosterone levels than younger men. A similar study by Su *et al.* (1995) confirmed this trend and demonstrated that correction of the varicocele can improve testosterone levels for infertile men with varicoceles.

The lower testosterone levels observed in older men compared to younger men in our study population may implicate progressive local damage of the varicocele on testicular function. Previous studies suggest that various mechanisms may account for the testicular dysfunction associated with varicoceles (Howards, 1995). Both intrascrotal and intratesticular temperatures are higher in men with varicoceles compared to controls (Zorgniotti *et al.*, 1979). However, not all investigators have found an association between higher intratesticular temperatures and varicoceles (Tessler *et al.*, 1966). As a result, nonthermal mechanisms have been suggested to account for the effect of a varicocele on testicular function; reflux of renal and adrenal metabolites from the renal vein, decreased blood flow, and hypoxia have all been postulated, and there is substantial evidence that smoking augments varicocele-induced testicular dysfunction (Comhaire *et al.*, 1974; Saypol *et al.*, 1981; Chakraborty *et al.*, 1985; Klaiber *et al.*, 1987). It is now accepted that infertility in the varicocele patient may be multifactorial, and the associated testicular dysfunction appears to worsen with age. Our data suggests this as well. Chehval and Purcell reported that varicoceles have a progressive effect on semen quality, which has also been reported by other studies (Chehval *et al.*, 1992). Though there is abundant evidence that varicoceles are associated with lower semen quality over time, there is limited data available discussing the progressive effect that clinical varicoceles have on testosterone status. For this reason, further studies need to explore this trend as it may lead to hypogonadism in a substantial population of men. Additionally, it is worthwhile to investigate whether repair of the varicocele can improve testosterone levels in these hypogonadal men.

Advanced Paternal Age and Reproductive Capacity

Population studies within the United States reveal a significant increase in paternal age, with many couples postponing childbearing until their mid-30s to mid-40s. According to the CDC birth statistics, the average maternal age in 2003 was 25.1, which represents an increase from the average maternal age of 21.4 years in 1974. A trend toward advanced parental age is simultaneously occurring in American men. The birth rate among men 25 to 44 years has been steadily increasing since the 1970s, whereas the birth rate of men less than 25 years has been decreasing (Hamilton *et al.*, 2003). An improved understanding of the effects of increased parental age on the developing fetus and newborn is imperative for counseling older couples preparing for childbearing. Advanced paternal age has been suggested to result in increased spontaneous abortions, autosomal dominant disorders, trisomy 21, and recently, schizophrenia.

Women aged 35 years or greater are at higher risk than younger women for adverse reproductive events including infertility, abortion, congenital abnormalities, and perinatal mortality. Paternal age often correlates with maternal age and can confound the effects of advanced maternal age. The first connection between spontaneous abortion and paternal age was raised during an analysis of fetal death certificates in 1939 (Yershalmy, 1939). Recent data confirms the association between advanced paternal age and the risk of spontaneous abortion. A prospective study of 5,121 American women revealed that the risk of spontaneous abortion increased with advanced paternal age (Slama *et al.*, 2005). A prospective analysis of 23,821 women from the Danish National Birth Cohort further demonstrated that pregnancies fathered by men 50 years or older had almost twice the risk of spontaneous abortion when compared with pregnancies with younger fathers after adjustment for maternal age, reproductive history, and maternal lifestyle during pregnancy (Nybo Andersen *et al.*, 2004). Although the correlation between advanced paternal age and spontaneous abortion is well demonstrated, there remains debate within the current literature regarding which trimester is at greatest risk with advanced paternal age. De La Rochebrochard and colleagues (2002) utilized the unique single variable "couple age" to elucidate the interaction between maternal and paternal age and the risk of spontaneous abortion. The retrospective data collected from this multicenter European study revealed that the effects of advanced paternal age and maternal age are cumulative; the risk of spontaneous abortion is highest if both partners are advanced in age. It is theorized that this increased risk of spontaneous abortions associated with advanced maternal or paternal age reflects chromosomal abnormalities in the developing fetus.

In this regard, advanced parental age is a recognized risk factor for many genetic abnormalities in the developing newborn. In men, advancing age decreases semen volume, percent normal sperm, and sperm motility (Rolf *et al.*, 1996). Though these factors adversely affect fertility, the genetic integrity of the sperm is also at risk. In contrast to oogenesis, spermatozoa are continuously produced and undergo lifelong replication, meiosis, and spermatogenesis (Evans, 1996). This continued replication allows for spontaneous mutations within the paternal cell line. Apoptosis of sperm with damaged DNA is an essential aspect of spermatogenesis that ensures selection of normal sperm DNA (Roosen-Runge, 1973). As men age, the rate of genetic abnormalities that occur during spermatogenesis increases. Investigation of advanced paternal age in the murine model reveals age-dependent effects on the meiotic and premeitotic phase of sperm development. These abnormalities in replication result in both aneuploidy and structural abnormalities in male germ cells (Lowe *et al.*, 1995). Additionally, the frequency of these numerical and structural aberrations in sperm chromosomes increases with increasing paternal age in humans (Sartorelli *et al.*, 2001). This age-related increase in sperm cells with highly damaged DNA results from both increased double-strand DNA breaks and decreased apoptosis during spermatogenesis (Singh *et al.*, 2003).

As a result, advanced paternal age is associated with many autosomal dominant disorders such as Apert syndrome, achondroplasia, osteogenesis imperfecta, progeria, Marfan syndrome, Waardenburg's syndrome, and thanatophoric dysplasia (Lian *et al.*, 1986). Apert syndrome results from an autosomal dominant mutation on chromosome 10, mutating the fibroblast growth factor receptor 2 (FGFR2). The incidence of sporadic Apert syndrome increases exponentially with paternal age, resulting in part from an increased frequency of FGFR2 mutations in the sperm of older men (Glaser *et al.*, 2003). Achondroplasia results from an autosomal dominant mutation on FGFR-3. Data from clinical achondroplasia registries reveal that 50% of affected children were born to men 35 years or older. In addition, the rate of achondroplasia increased exponentially with increasing paternal age (Orioli *et al.*, 2004). The Muenke-type craniosynostosis results from an autosomal dominant mutation in FGFR-3 resulting entirely from the paternal allele. The average paternal age of children with Muenke-type craniosynostosis has been reported as 34.7 years (Rannan-Eliya *et al.*, 2004). Therefore, men as young as 35 years are at higher risk for many autosomal dominant disorders, most notably costochondrodysplasias.

In addition to structural errors and resultant autosomal dominant disorders, aneuploidy errors in germ cell lines also occur at higher rates with advanced parental age. Trisomy 21 or Down syndrome is a common aneuploidy error that affects 1/800 to 1000 newborns (Cunningham *et al.*, 2001). The association of advanced maternal age and trisomy 21 was first documented as early as 1933 (Fisch *et al.*, 2001). Further amniocentesis data from the European collaborative study of Ferguson-Smith and Yates determined that the rate of trisomy 21 increases exponentially from a maternal age of 35 years (Ferguson-Smith *et al.*, 1984). Although the correlation between trisomy 21 and advanced maternal age is well documented, it is only recently that the affects of advanced paternal age have been elucidated. Investigation of the meiotic nondisjunctional error in trisomy 21 reveals the origin of the extra chromosome 21 to be paternal in 5 to 20% of cases (Antonarakis, 1991; Jyothy *et al.*, 2001). Despite this recognized paternal origin, to our knowledge no chromosomal studies evaluating parental origin of chromosomal defects in offspring and paternal age are available.

Early studies from the 1970s and 1980s failed to demonstrate a consistent effect related to advanced paternal age. Initial epidemiological studies utilizing city and state birth registries failed to show any correlation between trisomy 21 and advanced paternal age while confirming the effect of advanced maternal age (Erickson, 1978; Hook, 1987). In contrast, an evaluation of the Medical Birth Registry of Norway from 1967 to 1978 that included 685,000 total births and 693 cases of Down syndrome revealed an increased risk of Down syndrome with a paternal age of 50 years or greater (Erickson *et al.*, 1981). As parental age is increasing in the United States, recent studies provide more men of advanced age to evaluate. The New York State Department of Health congenital malformations registry containing 3,419 trisomy 21 births was analyzed from 1983 to 1997 and demonstrated a 111% and 60% increase in women and men over 35 years, respectively. This contemporary evaluation revealed no effect of parental age on trisomy 21 until 35 years. A paternal age effect was apparent in association with a maternal age of 35 years or greater and was most pronounced when maternal age was 40 years or greater. The rate of Down syndrome with a combined parental age greater than 40 years was 60/10,000 births that represents a six-fold increase compared with parents less than 35 years (Fisch *et al.*, 2003). Advanced paternal age in interaction with advanced maternal age significantly increases the risk of trisomy 21 and may possibly explain the exponential increase in trisomy 21 in women greater than 35 years.

In contrast to the effects of combined parental age in trisomy 21, schizophrenia is associated with spontaneous mutations arising in the paternal germ cells. Although schizophrenia is a complex disease of unclear etiology, there is substantial evidence for a genetic component (Kendler *et al.*, 1993). Since most individuals with schizophrenia are born to unaffected parents and have reduced reproductive activity, it is unclear how the disease is maintained within the population (Fananas *et al.*, 1991). Early studies from the 1960s and 1970s suggested an association between advanced paternal age and the development of schizophrenia (Hare *et al.*, 1979; Gregory, 1959). Recent studies have confirmed this association between advanced paternal age and schizophrenia in large population-based studies (Zammit *et al.*, 2003). A 12-year evaluation of the Jerusalem birth registry and the Israel psychiatric registry that included 658 individuals with schizophrenia revealed that the risk of schizophrenia increased monotonically with increasing paternal age. This increased risk culminated in a relative risk of 2.96 (95% confidence interval, 1.60–5.47) for offspring of men 50 years or greater (Malaspina *et al.*, 2001). Conversely, maternal age demonstrated no effect on the development of schizophrenia. A Swedish birth registry study revealed that the association between paternal age and schizophrenia was present in families without previous history of the disorder, but not in those with a family history. Based upon the stronger association between paternal age and schizophrenia in people without a family history, the authors suggested that accumulation of *de novo* mutations in paternal sperm contributed to the risk of schizophrenia (Sipos *et al.*, 2004).

Men of advanced paternal age, much like their female counterparts, are at greater risk for spontaneous abortion and genetic abnormalities. The continually replicating spermatogonia and the decreasing apoptotic rate are likely causes of the amplified meiotic and premeiotic errors in the male germ cell line. These chromosomal abnormalities increase in the aging male and potentially result in spontaneous abortion, autosomal dominant disorders, trisomy 21, and schizophrenia. In light of the trend toward delayed childbirth, the potential deleterious effects of advanced parental age become increasingly important. Therefore, appropriate prenatal counseling of older couples regarding the effects of advanced parental age on the developing fetus and newborn is imperative.

Conclusion

This brief discussion of the aging male demonstrates an unappreciated reality: men have biological clocks that affect their fertility, hormones levels, and the genetic quality of their sperm. This clock plays a role on a personal level (when couples must grapple with infertility or birth defects) and on a public health level (when society must decide policies governing, for instance, insurance coverage for advanced fertility treatments such as *in vitro* fertilization). Women should no longer be viewed as solely responsible for age-related fertility and genetic problems. Infertility is not just a woman's problem, and with the new awareness of a new male biological clock, couples and their physicians can much more accurately proceed with proper testing, diagnosis, and (if needed) treatment of the male. The field of male-factor infertility is still very young and much more research is needed to fully characterize risks and to find more effective treatments. We also need to better understand the cellular and biochemical mechanisms of "gonadal" aging in order to find safe, effective ways to delay this process and, in effect, "rewind" the male biological clock. Doing so will lessen the potential for adverse genetic consequences in offspring, improve the sexual and reproductive health of aging males, and increase a *woman's* chance of having healthy children by correcting defects in the *male* reproductive machinery (Fisch, 2005).

Recommended Resources

Harry Fisch, M.D.
Professor of Clinical Urology
Male Reproductive Center of Columbia University/
New York Presbyterian Hospital
944 Park Avenue, New York, NY 10028
212-879-0800
www.malebiologicalclock.com

Peter N. Schlegel, M.D.
Professor and Chairman
Urologist-in-Chief
Weill Medical College of Cornell University/
New York Presbyterian Hospital 525 East 68th Street, Starr 900, New York, NY 10021 212-746-5491 FAX: 212-746-8425

American Association of Sex Educators, Counselors, and Therapists
P.O. Box 5488, Richmond, VA 23220-0488
www.aasect.org

Sexual Function Health Council
American Foundation for Urologic Disease
1128 North Charles Street, Baltimore, MD 21201
800-433-4215 or 410-468-1800
impotence@afud.org
www.impotence.org

American Fertility Association
666 Fifth Avenue, Suite 278, New York, NY 10103
888-917-3777
www.theafa.org

American Society for Reproductive Medicine
1209 Montgomery Highway, Birmingham, AL 35216-2809
205-978-5000
www.asrm.org

Includes a "find a doctor" service for locating fertility specialists in your area.

American Urological Association
1120 North Charles Street, Baltimore, MD 21201
410-727-1100
aua@auanet.org
www.auanet.org

RESOLVE: The National Infertility Association
1310 Broadway, Somerville, MA 02144
888-623-0744
info@resolve.org
www.resolve.org

REFERENCES

Andolz, P., Bielsa, M., and Vila J. (1999). Evolution of semen quality in North-eastern Spain: A study in 22,759 infertile men over a 36 year period. *Hum Reprod 14*, 731–735.

Antonarakis, S. (1991). Parental origin of the extra chromosome in trisomy 21 as indicated by analysis of DNA polymorphisms. Down Syndrome Collaborative Group. *N Engl J Med 324*, 872–876.

Auger, J., Kunstmann, J., Czyglik, F., and Jouannet, P. (1995). Decline in semen quality among fertile men in Paris during the past 20 years. *N Engl J Med 332*, 281–285.

Bhasin, S., and Buckwalter, J. (2001). Testosterone supplementation in older men: a rational idea whose time has not yet come. *J Androl 22*, 718–731.

Chakraborty, J., Hikim, A., and Jhunjhunwala, J. (1985). Stagnation of blood in the microcirculatory vessels in the testes of men with varicocele. *J Androl 6*, 117–126.

Chehval, M., and Purcell, M. (1992). Deterioration of semen parameters over time in men with untreated varicocele: evidence of progressive testicular damage. *Fertil Steril 57*, 174–177.

Comhaire, F., and Vermeulen, A. (1975). Plasma testosterone in patients with varicocele and sexual inadequacy. *J Clinic Endocrinol Metab 40*, 824–829.

Comhaire, F., and Vermeulen, A. (1974). Varicocele sterility: Cortisol and catecholamines. *Fertil Steril 25*, 88–95.

Cunningham, F., MacDonald, P., Gant, N., Leveno, K., Gilstrap, C., Hankins, G., *et al. Williams Obstetrics, 21st ed.* New York: McGraw-Hill.

de La Rochebrochard, E., and Thonneau, P. (2002). Paternal age and maternal age are risk factors for miscarriage; results of a multicentre European study. *Human Repro 17*, 1649–1656.

Dondero, F., Mazzilli, F., Giovenco, P., Lenzi, A., and Cerasaro, M. (1985). Fertility in elderly men. *J Endocrinol Invest Suppl 8*, 87–91.

Erickson, J. (1978). Down syndrome, paternal age, maternal age and birth order. *Ann Hum Genet 41*, 289–298.

Erickson J., and Bjerkedal, T. (1981). Down syndrome associated with father's age in Norway. *J Med Genet 18*, 22–28.

Evans, H. (1996). Mutation and mutagenesis in inherited and acquired human disease. *Mutat Res 351*, 89–103.

Fananas, L., and Bertranpetit, J. (1991). Reproductive rates in families of schizophrenic patients in a case-control study. *Acta Psychiatr Scand 99*, 441–446.

Feldman, H., Longcope, C., Derby, C., Johannes, C., Araujo, A., Coviello, A. *et al.* (2002). Age trends in the level of serum testosterone and other hormones in middle-aged men: longitudinal results from the Massachusetts Male Aging Study. *J Clin Endocrinol Metab 87*, 589–598.

Ferguson-Smith, M., and Yates, J. (1984). Maternal age specific rates for chromosome aberrations and factors influencing them: report of a collaborative European study on 52,965 amniocenteses. *Prenat Diagn 4*, 5–44.

Ferrini R., and Barrett-Connor, E. (1998). Sex hormones and age: A cross-sectional study of testosterone and estradiol and their bioavailable fractions in community-dwelling men. *Am J Epidemiol 147*, 750–754.

Fisch, H. (2005). *The Male Biological Clock.* New York: Free Press.

Fisch, H., Golden, R., Libersen, G., Hyun, G., Madsen, P., New, M.I. *et al.* (2001). Maternal age as a risk factor for hypospadias. *J Urol 165*, 934–936.

Fisch, H., Goluboff, E., Olson, J., Feldshuh, J., Broder, S., and Barad, D. (1996). Semen analyses in 1,283 men from the United States over a 25-year period: No decline in quality. *Fertil Steril 65*, 1009–1014.

Fisch, H., Hyun, G., Golden, R., Hensle, T., Olsson, C., and Liberson, G. (2003). The influence of paternal age on Down syndrome. *J Urol 169*, 2275–2278.

Ford, W., North, K., Taylor, H., Farrow, A., Hull, M., and Golding J. (2000). Increasing paternal age is associated with delayed conception in a large population of fertile couples: Evidence for declining fecundity in older men. The ALSPAC Study Team (Avon Longitudinal Study of Pregnancy and Childhood). *Hum Reprod 15*, 1703–1708.

Glaser, R., Broman, K., Schulman, R., Eskenazi, B., Wyrobek, A., and Jabs, E. (2003). The paternal-age effect in Apert syndrome is due, in part, to the increased frequency of mutations in sperm. *Am J Hum Genet 73*, 939–947.

Gorelick, J., and Goldstein, M. (1993). Loss of fertility in men with varicocele. *Fertil Steril 59*, 613–616.

Gray, A., Berlin, J., McKinlay, J., and Longcope C. (1991). An examination of research design effects on the association of testosterone and male aging: results of a meta-analysis. *J Clin Epidemiol 44*, 671–684.

Gregory, I. (1959). An analysis of family data on 1000 patients admitted to a Canadian mental hospital. *Acta Genet Stat Med 9*, 54–56.

Hamilton, B., Martin, J., and Sutton, P. (2003). Births; Preliminary data for 2003. *National Vital Statistics Report 53.*

Hare, E., and Moran, P. (1979). Raised paternal age in psychiatric patients: evidence for the constitutional hypothesis. *Br J Psychiatry 134*, 169–177.

Harman, S., Metter, E., Tobin, J., Pearson, J., and Blackman M. (2001). Longitudinal effects of aging on serum total and free testosterone levels in healthy men. Baltimore Longitudinal Study of Aging. *J Clin Endocrinol Metab 86*, 724–31.

Henkel, R., Bittner, J., Weber, R., Huther, F., and Miska, W. (1999). Relevance of zinc in human sperm flagella and its relation to motility. *Fertil Steril 71*, 1138–1143.

Hook, E. Issues in analysis of data on paternal age and 47, +21: implication for genetic counseling for Down syndrome. *Hum Genet 77*, 303–306.

Howards, S. (1995). Treatment of male infertility. *N Engl J Med. 332*, 312–317.

Johnson, L. (1986). Spermatogenesis and aging in the human. *J Androl 7*, 331–354.

Jyothy, A., Kumar, K., Mallikarjuna, G., Babu Rao, V., Uma Devi, B., Sujatha, M. *et al.* (2001). Parental age and the origin of extra chromosome 21 in Down syndrome. *J Hum Genet 46*, 347–350.

Kendler, K., and Diehl, S. (1993). The genetics of schizophrenia: a current genetic-epidemiologica perspective. *Schizophr Bull 19*, 261–285.

Kidd, S., Eskenazi, B., and Wyrobek, A. (2001). Effects of male age on semen quality and fertility: a review of the literature. *Fertil Steril 75*, 237–248.

Klaiber, E., Broverman, D., Pokoly, T., Albert, A., Howard, P., and Sherer, J. (1987). Interrelationships of cigarette smoking, testicular varicoceles, and seminal fluid indexes. *Fertil Steril 47*, 481–486.

Lian, A., Zack, M., and Eriskson, J. (1986). Paternal age and the occurrence of birth defects. *Am J Hum Genet 39*, 648.

Lowe, X., Collins, B., Allen, J., Titenko-Holland, N., Breneman, J., van Beek, M. *et al.* (1995). Aneuploidies and micronuclei in the germ cells of male mice of advanced age. *Mutat Res 338*, 59–76.

Malaspina, D., Harlap, S., Fennig, S., Heiman, D., Nahon, D., Feldman, D. *et al.* (2001). Advancing paternal age and the risk of schizophrenia. *Arch Gen Psych 58*, 361–367.

Mathieu, C., Ecochard, R., Bied, V., Lornage, J., and Czyba, J. (1995). Cumulative conception rate following intrauterine artificial insemination with husband's spermatozoa: influence of husband's age. *Hum Reprod 10*, 1090–1097.

McLachlan, RI. (2000). The endocrine control of spermatogenesis. *Baillieres Best Pract Clin Endocrinol Metab 14*, 345–362.

Morley, J., Kaiser, F., Perry, H., Patrick, P., Morley, P., Stauber, P. *et al.* (1997). Longitudinal changes in testosterone, luteinizing hormone, and follicle-stimulating hormone in healthy older men. *Metabolism 46*, 410–413.

Mortimer, D., Templeton, A., Lenton, E., and Coleman, R. (1982). Influence of abstinence and ejaculation-to-analysis delay on semen analysis parameters of suspected infertile men. *Arch Androl 8*, 251–256.

Nagao, R., Plymate, S., Berger, R., Perin, E., and Paulsen C. (1986). Comparison of gonadal between fertile and infertile men with varicocele. *Fertil Steril 46*, 930–933.

Nybo Andersen, A., Hansen, KD., Andersen, P., and Davey Smith, G. (2004). Advanced paternal age and risk of fetal death: a cohort study. *Am J Epidemiol 160*, 1214–1222.

Orioli, I., Castilla, E., Scarano, G., and Mastroiacovo, P. (1995). *Am J Med Genet 59*, 209–217.

Rannan-Eliya, S., Taylor, I., De Heer, M., Van Den Ouweland, A., Wall, S., and Wilkie, A. (2004). Paternal origin of FGFr-3 mutation in Muenke-type craniosynostosis. *Hum Genet 115*, 200–207.

Rhoden, E., and Morgentaler, A. (2004). Risks of testosterone-replacement therapy and recommendations for monitoring. *N Engl J Med 350*, 482–492.

Rodriguez-Rigau, L., Weiss, D., Zukerman, Z., Grotjan, H., Smith, K., and Steinberger, E. (1978). A possible mechanism for the detrimental effect of varicocele on testicular function in man. *Fertil Steril 30*, 577–585.

Rolf, C., Behre, H., and Nieschlag, E. (1996). Reproductive parameters of older compared to younger men of infertile couples. *Int J Androl 19*, 135–142.

Roosen-Runge, EC. (1973). Germinal-cell loss in normal metazoan spermatogenesis. *Reprod Fertil 35*, 339–348.

Sartorelli, E., Mazzucatto, L., and de Pina-Neto, J. (2001). Effect of paternal age on human sperm chromosomes. *Fertil Steril 76*, 1119–1123.

Saypol, D., Howards, S., Turner, T., and Miller, E. (1981). Influence of surgically induced varicocele on testicular blood flow, temperature, and histology in adult rats and dogs. *J Clin Invest 68*, 39–45.

Schneider, E. (1978). *The Aging Reproductive System* New York: Raven Press.

Schwartz, D., Mayaux, M., Spira, A., Moscato, M., Jouannet, P., Czyglik, F. *et al.* (1983). Semen characteristics as a function of age in 833 fertile men. *Fertil Steril 39*, 530–535.

Serre, V., and Robaire, B. (1998). Paternal age affects fertility and progeny outcome in the Brown Norway rat. *Fertil Steril 70*, 625–631.

Shah, J., Masson, P., Schlegel, P., and Fisch H. 2005. Is there an association between varicoceles and hypgonadism in infertile men? *AUA*.

Singh, N., Muller, C., and Berger R. (2003). Effects of age on DNA double-strand breaks and apoptosis in human sperm. *Fertil Steril 80*, 1420–1430.

Sipos, A., Fasmussen, F., Harrison, G., Tynelius, P., Lewis, G., Leon, D., and Gunnell, D. (2004). Paternal age and schizophrenia: a population based cohort study. *BMJ 329*, 1070.

Slama, R., Bouyer, J., Windham, G., Fenster, L., Werwatz, A., and Swan, S. (2005). Influence of paternal age on the risk of spontaneous abortion. *Am J Epidemiol 161*, 816–823.

Sparrow, D., Bosse, R., and Rowe J. (1980). The influence of age, alcohol consumption, and body build on gonadal function in men. *J Clin Endocrinol Metab 51*, 508–512.

Su, L., Goldstein, M., and Schlegel, P. (1995). The effect of varicocelectomy on serum testosterone levels in infertile men with varicoceles. *J Urol 154*, 1752–1755.

Tanemura, K., Kurohmaru, M., Kuramoto, K., and Hayashi, Y. (1993). Age-related morphological changes in the testis of the BDF1 mouse. *J Vet Med Sci 55*, 703–710.

Tessler, A., and Krahn, H. (1966). Varicocele and testicular temperature. *Fertil Steril 17*, 201–203.

Van der Westerlaken, L., Naaktgeboren, N., and Helmerhorst F. (1998). Evaluation of pregnancy rates after intrauterine insemination according to indication, age, and sperm parameters. *J Assist Reprod Genet 15*, 359–364.

Vermeulen, A., Rubens, R., and Verdonck, L. (1972). Testosterone secretion and metabolism in male senescence. *J Clin Endocrinol Metab 34*, 730–735.

Walter, C., Intano, G., McCarrey, J., McMahan, C., and Walter R. (1998). Mutation frequency declines during spermatogenesis in young mice but increases in old mice. *Proc Natl Acad Sci USA 95*, 10015–10019.

Wang, C., Leung, A., and Sinha-Hikim, A. (1993). Reproductive aging in the male brown-Norway rat: a model for the human. *Endocrinology 133*, 2773 2781.

Yershalmy, J. (1939). Age of father and survival of offspring. *Hum Biol* 11, 342–356.

Younes, A. (2000). Low plasma testosterone in varicocele patients with impotence and male infertility. *Arch Androl 45*, 187–195.

Zammit, S., Allebeck, P., Dalman, C., Lundberg, I., Hemmingson, T., Owen, M. *et al.* (2003). Paternal age and risk for schizophrenia. *Br J Psych 183*, 405–408.

Zorgniotti, A., and MacLeod, J. (1979). Studies in temperature, human semen quality, and varicocele. *Fertil Steril 24*, 1979.

52

Benign Prostatic Hyperplasia

Peter Celec

Benign prostatic hyperplasia is a common disease of aged males. It is associated with low urinary tract syndrome and can result in serious complications including renal failure. The main pathophysiological factors, and consequently, therapeutic targets, are sex hormones and sympathetic activity. Testosterone, dihydrotestosterone, and estradiol play crucial roles, and their effects are influenced by several genetic factors.

The models of benign prostatic hyperplasia can be divided into in vivo and in vitro models. Animal models include spontaneous and hormonally or pharmacologically induced prostatic hyperplasia, as well as newly generated transgenic models. Cell cultures are simple and cost effective, but the research in vitro is difficult to interpret for human pathology.

The number of various models indicates that an ideal model of benign prostatic hyperplasia does not exist. Thus, further improvements are awaited to enhance the biomedical research with clinical outcome on this entity.

Introduction

Male aging is accompanied by several prostate diseases including prostate cancer and prostatitis. However, by far the highest incidence and prevalence is reached by benign prostatic hyperplasia (BPH). Despite huge scientific and clinical effort, this entity is still an important biomedical problem, as neither the understanding of pathophysiology nor the currently applied therapy are satisfying. Research focused on BPH, thus, clearly is needed and should be supported by appropriate models of BPH. Nevertheless, the wide spectrum of models indicates that there is no clear winner of the race—no ideal model of BPH.

Although the existence of a female prostate is more or less accepted (Zaviacic and Ablin, 1998, 2000), this chapter will focus on male prostate hyperplasia, as the incidence of diseases of female prostate seems to be low and no specific animal or cell culture models exist for research on female prostate.

The contemporary view on the pathophysiology of BPH is presented, as it implies several different internal as well as external factors that influence prostate growth. This divergence can also explain the number of different available BPH models and the related problems regarding the interpretation of the results of various studies, both clinical and experimental. There is a need for further development of new models that would be closer to human pathology.

Epidemiology

About 50% of men over 60 years have a pathologically increased prostate (see Figure 52.1).

The huge prevalence of BPH in men over the age of 80 years of more than 90% makes BPH "an inescapable phenomenon" for the male population if taking into account the contemporary rise of life expectancy in the developed world (Berry *et al.*, 1984; Lepor, 2005). The volume and weight of prostate tissue is increasing from 20 g in 40 years to 60 g in 80 years of age (Oesterling *et al.*, 1993). The hyperplasia of the prostate is not a life-threatening condition per se; however, BPH causes serious and dangerous complications. These include acute urinary retention as the most frequent complication, recurrent infections, chronic urinary retention, and even renal failure (Thorpe and Neal, 2003).

Most patients with BPH are asymptomatic and undiagnosed. The most prominent complication is so-called LUTS—low urinary tract syndrome (see Table 52.1). LUTS and bladder outlet obstruction bring the patient to the clinician, but although the prevalence of LUTS also increases with age, the relationship between BPH and LUTS is complex (see Figures 52.2 and 52.3).

The severity of LUTS, for example, does not depend linearly on prostate size, although further research is needed (Girman, 1998). To distinguish between BPH, obstruction syndrome, and LUTS is difficult in epidemiologic studies because the borders are unclear. However, this clinical feature is mostly not a part of the BPH models for research.

The mortality from BPH decreases steadily during the last 50 years. Bias caused by better diagnostics and differences in the inclusion criteria cannot be excluded. However, the increase in mortality in Eastern Europe and some other parts of the world is a warning signal that should not be overlooked (Levi *et al.*, 2003).

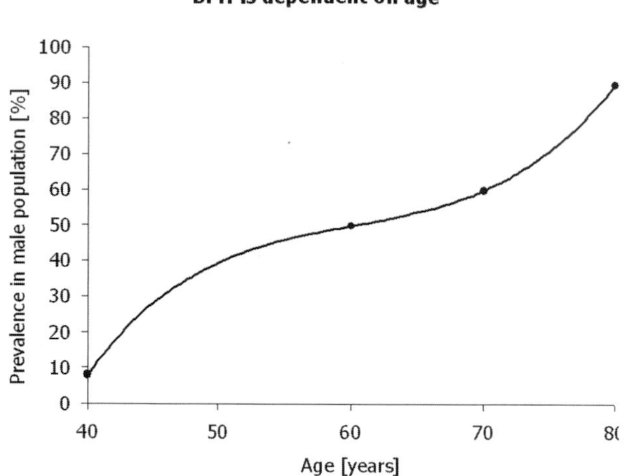

Figure 52.1 Prevalence of BPH in male population based on the results of several epidemiological studies.

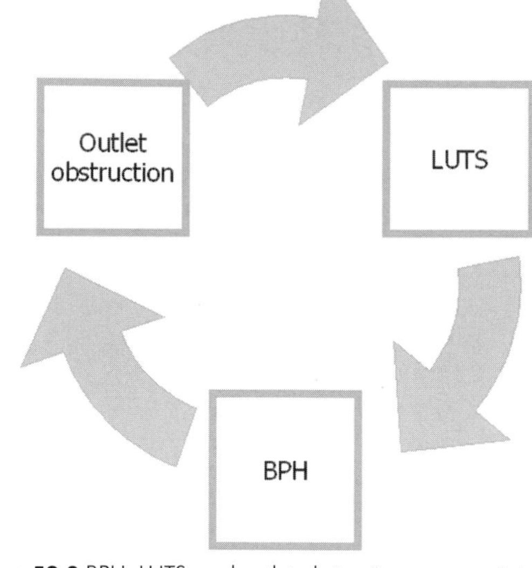

Figure 52.3 BPH, LUTS, and outlet obstruction are associated, and the relations are not linear.

TABLE 52.1
Low urinary tract syndrome—LUTS symptoms

Voiding
Prolonged urination
Post-micturation dribbling
Poor urinary flow
Incomplete bladder emptying
Delay in onset of micturation
Storage
Urge incontinence
Nocturia
Frequent urination

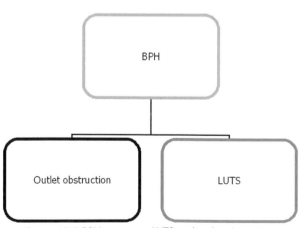

Figure 52.2 BPH is causing LUTS and outlet obstruction.

Pathophysiology

There are many factors influencing the so-called aging male. Androgens and other sex hormones that decrease in elderly men definitely belong to these factors; this condition is called PADAM—partial androgen deficiency of the aging male (Schulman and Lunenfeld, 2002). The role of androgens in the pathogenesis of BPH is common to their role in the prostatic carcinogenesis (Parnes *et al.*, 2005). The relationship between prostate cancer and BPH is a matter of debate, which is out of scope of this chapter. Nevertheless, it should be noted that the BPH does not represent a clear premalignancy and the pathogenesis of both entities is divergent, although androgens play an important role in both pathologies.

Androgens affect the static part of BPH pathophysiology—the size of the prostate. The other group of factors is related to the dynamic tension of prostatic smooth muscles (see Figure 52.4).

In general, currently used therapy of BPH involves antiandrogenic treatment (reducing the prostate size) and alpha adrenergic blockade (relaxing of smooth muscle inside the prostate). The finding that alpha adrenergic blockade improves the symptoms of patients three-fold in comparison to antiandrogenic treatment does not ultimately mean that the adrenergic stimulation is more important in the pathogenesis of BPH. Other studies have shown the opposite, if longer observation periods were chosen. Moreover, many clinically important symptoms might be caused by conditions other than BPH, including functional denervation or detrusor dysfunctions, and these conditions might be affected by the alpha adrenergic blockade (Skolarikos *et al.*, 2004).

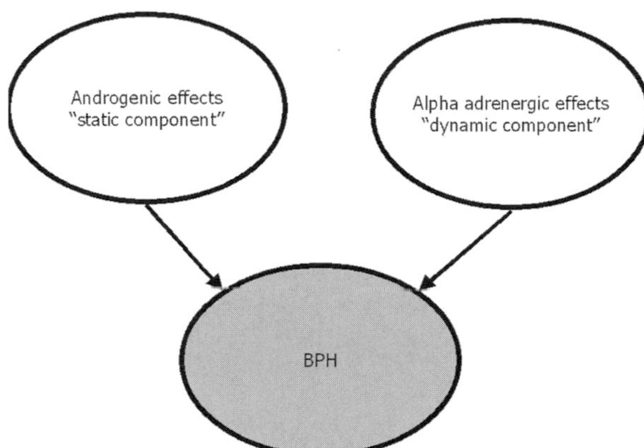

Figure 52.4 Two major factors participating in BPH pathogenesis. The static component is represented by the antiapoptotic and proliferative effects of androgens. The dynamic component is represented by the action of sympathomimetics on smooth muscle cells in the fibromuscular stroma of the prostate.

The hormonal influence on the pathogenesis of BPH is undoubted. Castrated males do not develop BPH. Sex hormones have been shown to be a major factor in normal physiological development of prostate, but also in the pathological hyperplasia. However, the detailed mechanism of their effects is not clear (Roberts *et al.*, 2004). Besides *androgens*, recently the role of estrogens in prostate growth is also discussed, although previously, *estrogens* were thought to act protectively against BPH.

A common precursor of steroids is cholesterol, and the specific precursor of androgens is dehydroepiandrosterone (Celec and Starka, 2003). The main metabolic pathways of androgens are shown in Figure 52.5.

Nevertheless, testosterone and dihydrotestosterone (DHT) seem to be of major importance. Both steroids are recognized by the intracellular androgen receptor, but the activation of this transcription factor via DHT is stronger by a factor of 10 in comparison to testosterone. The production of DHT from testosterone is mediated by the enzyme 5-alpha reductase. Inhibiting this catalytic activity pharmacologically is one of the major therapeutical approaches currently used in the treatment of BPH. The levels of testosterone slightly increase due to the inhibition of 5-alpha reductase, but the clinical outcome is clearly a reduction of prostate size, so it seems that testosterone plays a secondary role in BPH pathogenesis. It may be explained by the fact that only 1% of testosterone is bioavailable for the activation of androgen receptors. The rest is bound to plasma proteins, specifically to sex hormone binding globulin (SHBG), and nonspecifically to albumin. As the concentrations of SHBG rise with age, the proportion of bioavailable free

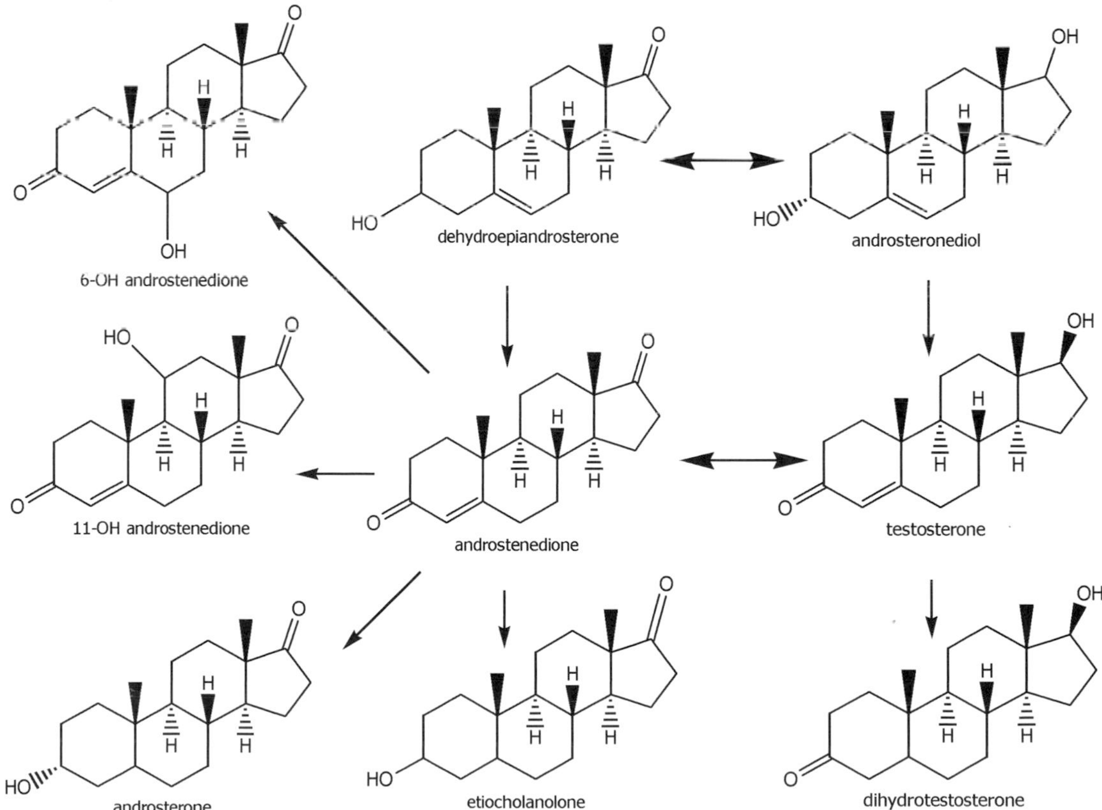

Figure 52.5 Metabolic pathways of androgens.

testosterone decreases. Moreover, the production of testosterone in Leydig cells in testes also decreases; thus, the absolute concentration of free testosterone decreases considerably. However, there are other receptors for testosterone than androgen receptor; some of them are membrane bound, and some of them even recognize testosterone bound to SHBG. Their role in prostate growth is currently unknown and is expected to be of less importance, but future research will make this clear.

An interesting question is the role of estrogens in the pathogenesis of BPH. Estradiol is produced from testosterone, and this one step–one direction reaction is catalyzed by *aromatase* (see Figure 52.6).

Although the presence of aromatase in the prostate tissue is a matter of discussion, and the results of molecular studies are divergent and puzzling, the production of estradiol affects prostate growth independently from the site of its production (Risbridger *et al.*, 2003). Estradiol increases the production of SHBG and thus decreases the free fraction of plasma testosterone available for the DHT production by 5-alpha reductase. This fact would explain a protective role of estrogens in BPH, but the last decade of research has shown that estrogens play the opposite role—they stimulate the growth of prostate tissue, particularly in a highly androgenic environment (Roberts *et al.*, 2004). The molecular aspects of estrogen action include the upregulation of androgen receptor expression. Thus, the sensitivity of the tissue to androgens is increased and the response to testosterone and also to DHT is enhanced. The effects of estradiol on prostate growth are age- and dose-dependent. The most prominent influence has been shown for low-dose estradiol during fetal life (vom Saal *et al.*, 1997). Interestingly, estrogens and androgens act synergistically in BPH pathogenesis (see Figure 52.7), even if some effects are contradictory if these hormones are applied alone (Fujimoto *et al.*, 2004).

There are several genetic factors that affect the actions of sex hormones in the prostate. The androgen receptor undergoes alternative splicing, and a longer version of the protein is more sensitive to DHT. Various polymorphisms have been associated with altered function of the androgen receptor. A CAG repeat in the first exon is the best described short tandem repeat (STR) in the androgen receptor gene. Normal number repeats is 10 to 40; a higher number is associated with a rare neurodegenerative Kennedy disease, and the activation of androgen receptor is weaker. Lower number of repeats is related to increased androgenity—increased response to androgens, and this condition is clinically associated with an increased risk of Alzheimer's, breast and prostate cancer, and BPH.

Similarly, the gene encoding 5-alpha reductase includes several polymorphisms important for the activity of the enzyme; best studied is the A49T polymorphism that increases the activity of 5-alpha reductase five-fold. Aromatase is encoded by a gene with a single nucleotide polymorphism C1558T and several STRs. Besides sex hormone receptors and metabolic enzymes, other genes and their polymorphisms are associated with BPH in humans, but their role in the etiology of BPH is unclear. It has been reported that the expression of a potential tumor suppressor protein p27Kip1 is very low or undetectable in BPH tissue in contrast to control prostate tissue (Cordon-Cardo *et al.*, 1998).

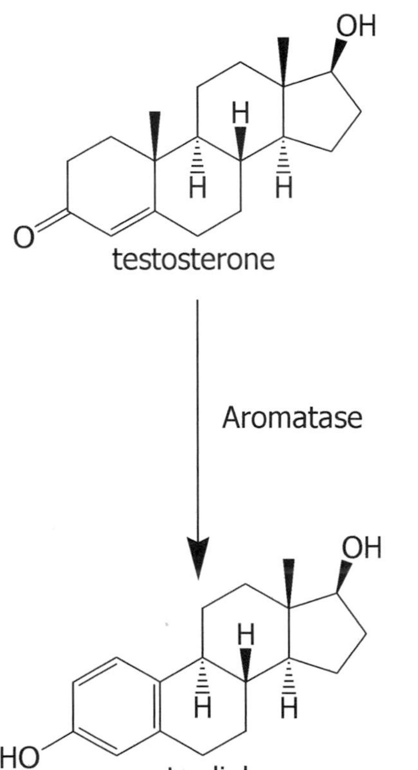

Figure 52.6 Aromatase catalyzes the aromatization of testosterone to estradiol.

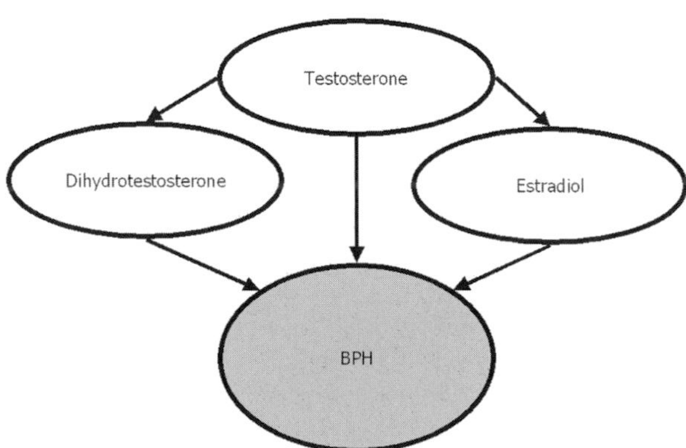

Figure 52.7 Androgens and estrogens act synergistically on the pathogenesis of BPH.

Although the prostate is an exocrine gland, BPH is caused mainly by proliferative changes of the fibromuscular stroma. The histological classification distinguishes stromal and epithelial origin of BPH. The stromal BPH accounts for cca 80% and is further divided into proliferative processes of the fibrous tissue (40%) and smooth muscle (40%). Cell culture studies have provided evidence for the hypothesis that on a molecular level an important role in the pathogenesis of BPH is played by several growth factors (see Figure 52.8).

These growth factors include fibroblast growth factors (FGF) 2 and 9, insulin-like growth factors (IGF) I and II, and also transforming growth factor beta 1 (TGF), although the latter affects stromal cells of the prostate differentially according to its concentrations—stimulatory at lower and inhibitory in higher concentrations (Eaton, 2003). The effects of TGF are especially interesting as it induces apoptosis in epithelial cells but the opposite in stromal cells. The influence of growth factors on prostate is dependent on the presence of appropriate receptors at the surface of cell membranes as well as on the intracellular response pathway. Molecular biology and its modern methodological improvements like microarray experiments will facilitate the detailed understanding of BPH pathophysiology (Prakash *et al.*, 2002).

In vivo Models

Best described and widely used *in vivo* models include rodent, canine, and primate models (see Table 52.2). These can be either spontaneous or induced using various hormonal application regimes. Modern genetic technologies allow the production of several new transgenic mice models. Another approach is to use transplantation of the prostate tissue, either embryonic or pathologically hyperplasic. Some of the aspects of BPH can be studied in alternative models, for example, in the phenylephrine-induced increase of intraurethral pressure (Akiyama *et al.*, 1999).

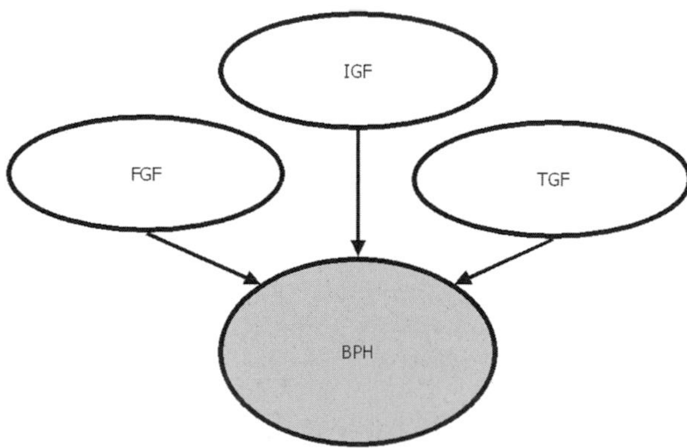

Figure 52.8 Several growth factors are participating on the growth regulation of prostate tissue.

TABLE 52.2
Comparison of animal species used in BPH models

Animal model	Similarity to human BPH		Availability	Costs
	Anatomy	Histology		
Rodent	+	+	Very good	Low
Canine	+	++	Fair	Moderate
Primate	+++	+++	Poor	High

SPONTANEOUS BPH MODELS

Dogs and chimpanzees are the only experimental animal species that develop BPH spontaneously. In both species the BPH occurs in an age-dependent manner, but there are important differences from the human BPH.

Nonhuman primates represent the best model for most human diseases when it comes to similarity to human pathology. BPH is not an exception. Chimpanzee prostate is anatomically very similar to the human prostate (Steiner *et al.*, 1999). It is divided into two lobes—caudal, which resembles the human transition and peripheral zone, and cranial, which resembles the central zone in the human prostate. The age dependence of BPH in chimpanzees does not differ from human BPH, and histological evaluation has shown that the epithelium/stroma ratio is also similar. Is chimpanzee BPH an ideal model? No, but it is currently the best available. The problems lie just in the availability, as primates are available for research use only in specialized primate research centers. Spontaneous BPH occurs in chimpanzees at their elderly age—cca 30 years. Furthermore, the prostate-specific antigen is present only in very low concentration; thus, to follow the development of BPH in primates biochemically is complicated. On the other hand, the presence of outlet obstruction enables functional evaluation.

Canine prostate lacks a capsule, and its growth is oriented not to the urethra, but to the pelvic cavity due to anatomical relations, including the lack of a fixation to symphysis. This explains why BPH in dogs does not result in LUTS but is mostly asymptomatic or it causes defecation problems due to rectal obstruction. Canine prostate is not divided into clear morphological subunits; similarly, canine BPH does not resemble the nodular pathogenesis of human BPH. Moreover, the histological picture of canine BPH involves epithelial proliferation in contrast to human BPH, where fibrostromal proliferation is usually present. This might be explained by the finding that the activity of 5-alpha reductase is higher in the epithelium than in the stroma. Several other biochemical differences have been described, including the expression of prostate-specific antigen and prostate-specific esterase. Nevertheless, canine spontaneous BPH is a widely used model of human BPH, and if differences are taken into account, pathophysiologic and therapeutic studies can make use of this model.

INDUCED BPH MODELS

Spontaneous models of BPH are closer to human pathology, but these models are difficult to obtain due to the slow aging process. BPH pathogenesis can be induced or accelerated in dogs, as well as in standard laboratory rodents like mice and rats. Dogs have an androgen responsive prostate tissue; thus the application of androgens can induce BPH. It has been experimentally shown that a regime involving androstanediol and estradiol application induced BPH. DHT and testosterone were not able to induce BPH in dogs if applied alone. Combinational treatment with DHT and estradiol applied subcutaneously daily usually during 14 or 28 days induces BPH in dogs (Yokota *et al.*, 2004). Similarly, eight-months-long daily treatment with testosterone and androstenedione induced a canine BPH even in young animals (Ito *et al.*, 2000). The problematic anatomy of canine prostate described earlier is still a problem in modeling the human BPH using hormonal induction. This problem can be overcome using a surgical approach, where the canine prostate is enveloped by a mesh that does not allow growth into the peritoneal cavity. This is currently the only way to induce BPH in dogs that is accompanied with urethral obstruction seen in human BPH.

The rodent prostate differs considerably from the human prostate in anatomy and physiology. Rodent prostate consists of anterior, ventral, and dorsolateral lobes. Only the dorsolateral lobe has been reported to be comparable to human prostate. The main factor in BPH induction is the long-term application of high doses of androgens and estrogens. Some studies report an induction of BPH using only chronic testosterone treatment, but this model suffers from several limitations (Mitra *et al.*, 1999). The response is strain specific; however, some rat strains do not develop BPH after this treatment, and classic strains like Wistar or Sprague-Dawley are responsive. Except for sex hormones, chronic applications of prolactin or sympathomimetic phenylephrine also lead to BPH in rodents (Van Coppenolle *et al.*, 2000; Marinese *et al.*, 2003). However, this model is used only sporadically as the use of sympathomimetic drugs affects not only the urogenital system, but notably other systems as well (Golomb *et al.*, 1998). Reports of spontaneous development of BPH in rodents are lacking; normal rodent prostate tissue even undergoes an age-dependent atrophy. Exceptions are the brown Norway rats (Banerjee *et al.*, 1998; Banerjee *et al.*, 2001) and spontaneously hypertensive rats (Zhang *et al.*, 2004). However, the mechanism of BPH etiology in these strains is specific and does not resemble the multifactorial origin of human BPH.

Besides hormonal treatment there is an additional approach for the induction of BPH—the so-called mouse prostate reconstitution model. Fetal urogenital tissue is transplanted into the prostate of an adult animal. Without androgen treatment only epithelial proliferation is induced, but additional androgen application results in BPH (Guo *et al.*, 2004). It can be expected that specific growth factors in the transplanted tissue are responsible for the induction of proliferation, but the identification of the active compounds is not complete. Nevertheless, previously mentioned growth factors like FGF, IGF, and TGF might be involved. Xenografting of human BPH tissue into immunodeficient mice or rats is also possible. However, the survival of this tissue is limited, and the use of such models is currently questionable, although biochemically the transplants produce prostate-specific enzymes. Another possibility is to implant prostate tissue cell lines ectopically (e.g., under the renal capsule) in recipient animals (Takao *et al.*, 2003). This model however, resembles *in vitro* more than *in vivo* models.

Transgenic Models

Transgenic animals present a totally new approach for modeling human diseases. They are very important for the study of the pathogenesis of diseases, mostly the role of specific genes and gene products. However, their use in finding and evaluating potential therapeutics is limited, and the results of such studies must be taken with caution. BPH, like most other so-called civilization diseases, has a multifactorial etiology and thus cannot be reduced to a deficiency or overexpression of one protein. Nevertheless, transgenic animals represent an invaluable tool for BPH research. Based on the known pathophysiology of BPH, these animals are genetically modified to overexpress growth factors like FGF and IGF in a more or less prostate-specific manner. The organ specificity of expression is guaranteed by the use of prostate-specific promoters. Interestingly, another endocrine factor can be added to the pathogenesis of BPH after research using transgenic mice—prolactin. Mice overexpressing prolactin have been shown to develop BPH with high histological similarity to human BPH (Dillner *et al.*, 2003). The role of prolactin in BPH remains uncertain, as its overproduction was associated with higher androgen levels and an altered expression of several metabolic genes in the transgenic rodents (Dillner *et al.*, 2002).

In vitro studies show that prolactin alone can have a proliferative or at least antiapoptotic effect on prostate tissue. As mentioned previously, the tumor suppressor protein p27Kip1 might be involved in the pathogenesis of BPH. This has been shown on p27Kip1 knock-out mice that develop an enlarged prostate. This model might also explain the puzzling relationship between BPH and prostate cancer (Cordon-Cardo *et al.*, 1998). Of the transgenic animals currently described as models of BPH prolactin, overexpressing mice seem to develop a histological picture that is closest to the human BPH, though with several shortcomings. The generation of mice with prolactin overexpression restricted to the prostate tissue has improved the potential of this model considerably (Kindblom *et al.*, 2003).

In vitro Models

In part due to the pressure from ecologic organizations, cell culture models are used more and more by researchers. It is difficult to study BPH in Petri dishes, but it is possible. The advantages are the generally assumed advantages of all cell culture models—easy reproducibility, virtually unlimited material for experiments, very good control over the cell growth conditions, no ethical problems. On the other side, cell cultures, especially in the case of BPH, are a very distant model. The biggest problem is the interaction between epithelial and stromal cells that plays a crucial role in the BPH pathogenesis *in vivo*. This interaction is lacking in classic pure cell culture models. Most cultures are derived from clinical specimens obtained during prostatectomy or transurethral resection. An important issue in the evaluation of cell cultures for research is the ability of the cells to express the androgen receptor, 5-alpha reductase, and the prostate-specific antigen. On the functional level, this means that the cells must retain their androgen responsiveness. Caution must be paid to cell cultures derived from prostate carcinoma. These tumor cell lines have a different phenotype, and research on these cells is difficult to interpret for BPH, although many studies have been published using these cell lines. Nontumorigenic cell cultures are few, and some of them are prepared from prostate tissue of various experimental animals. Similar to the *in vivo* models, cell cultures from rats or mice differ considerably from canine or primate cell lines.

Some problems of classic mono-layer cell cultures can be overcome by using a 3D histoculture—sponge-gel-supported or the so-called total-immersion histoculture (Olbina *et al.*, 1998). The problem of a lacking interaction between different cell types is partially solved by using a coculture model where primary cell lines of prostate fibroblasts and epithelial cells are cultured together, separated by a porous membrane that enables the diffusion of soluble factors produced by the one or the other cell type. It must be noted that this—although definitely an improvement—is still a virtual interaction that only partially resembles the situation *in vivo*. A detailed description of such a coculture model was published repeatedly (Bayne *et al.*, 1998; Habib *et al.*, 2000).

Conclusion

The wide spectrum of available models shows that there is still no ideal model for BPH research (see Figure 52.9 and Table 52.3).

On one site, there is the need to make the model as close as possible to the human pathology; this is true for the spontaneous model of BPH in chimpanzees. On the other site, there is a need for simple, reproducible, and relatively cheap models; this is true for some of the cell culture models. It is probable that an ideal model will never exist and the knowledge about BPH will be composed of numerous puzzle pieces from many studies on various models as is the case today. One possibility to get closer to the ideal is to generate transgenic animals

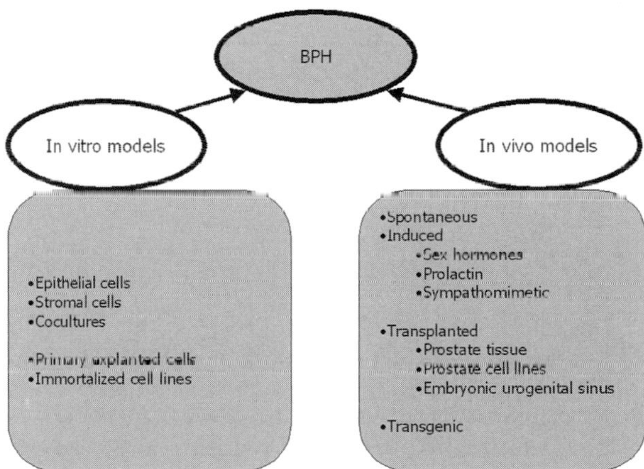

Figure 52.9 *In vivo* and *in vitro* models of BPH pathogenesis described in this chapter.

TABLE 52.3
Comparison of practical applications of BPH models

Model	Variability	Reproducibility	Availability	Costs	Similarity to human BPH	Applicability for research on	
						Pathogenesis	Therapy
Spontaneous	High	Poor	Fair	High	+++	++	+++
Induced	High	Moderate	Very good	Low	++	+	++
Xenografts	High	Poor	Poor	High	+	+	++
Transgenic	Low	Very good	Fair	High	+	+++	+
Cell culture	Low	Very good	Good	Low	–	+	++

with several genetic alternations. This would be at least closer to the real multifactorial etiology of BPH in humans. On the other hand, the clinically relevant biological variability of human BPH can be reached only in spontaneous animal models, but the species-related differences to human BPH should always be kept in mind (Mahapokai *et al.*, 2000). Tough major advances in this field of biomedical research are due to the cooperation of specialists—urologists, molecular biologists, and others. The hormonally induced BPH in rodent and canine animals will still be the most popular and most often used model at least for the next few years.

Recommended Resources

Bayne, C.W., Donnelly, F., Chapman, K., Bollina, P., Buck, C., and Habib, F. (1998). A novel coculture model for benign prostatic hyperplasia expressing both isoforms of 5 alpha-reductase. *J Clin Endocrinol Metab 83*, 206–213.

A description of an in vitro model using the coculture technique.

Eaton, C.L. (2003). Aetiology and pathogenesis of benign prostatic hyperplasia. *Curr Opin Urol 13*, 7–10.

A short review about the pathogenesis of BPH.

Kindblom, J., Dillner, K., Sahlin, L., Robertson, F., Ormandy, C., Tornell, J. *et al.* (2003). Prostate hyperplasia in a transgenic mouse with prostate-specific expression of prolactin. *Endocrinology 144*, 2269–2278.

Detailed analysis of one transgenic model of BPH using prostate-specific expression of prolactin.

Mahapokai, W., Van Sluijs, F.J., and Schalken, J.A. (2000). Models for studying benign prostatic hyperplasia. *Prostate Cancer Prostatic Dis 3*, 28–33.

A short review about available research models of BPH.

Shappell, S.B., Thomas, G.V., Roberts, R.L., Herbert, R., Ittmann, M.M., Rubin, M.A. *et al.* (2004). Prostate pathology of genetically engineered mice: Definitions and classification. The consensus report from the Bar Harbor meeting of the Mouse Models of Human Cancer Consortium Prostate Pathology Committee. *Cancer Res 64*, 2270–2305.

Histopathological review about transgenic mouse model for various prostate diseases.

Thorpe, A. and Neal, D. (2003). Benign prostatic hyperplasia. *Lancet 361*, 1359–1367.

Clinically oriented review about BPH.

ACKNOWLEDGMENTS

I would like to thank Assoc. Prof. Daniela Ostatníková, Dr. Michaela Príhodová, Dr. Július Hodosy and Children Hope's Club for continuous support.

REFERENCES

Akiyama, K., Hora, M., Tatemichi, S., Masuda, N., Nakamura, S., Yamagishi, R. *et al.* (1999). KMD-3213, a uroselective and long-acting alpha(1a)-adrenoceptor antagonist, tested in a novel rat model. *J Pharmacol Exp Ther 291*, 81–91.

Banerjee, P.P., Banerjee, S., and Brown, T.R. (2001). Increased androgen receptor expression correlates with development of age-dependent, lobe-specific spontaneous hyperplasia of the brown Norway rat prostate. *Endocrinology 142*, 4066–4075.

Banerjee, P.P., Banerjee, S., Lai, J.M., Strandberg, J.D., Zirkin, B.R., and Brown, T.R. (1998). Age-dependent and lobe-specific spontaneous hyperplasia in the brown Norway rat prostate. *Biol Reprod 59*, 1163–1170.

Bayne, C.W., Donnelly, F., Chapman, K., Bollina, P., Buck, C., and Habib, F. (1998). A novel coculture model for benign prostatic hyperplasia expressing both isoforms of 5 alpha-reductase. *J Clin Endocrinol Metab 83*, 206–213.

Berry, S.J., Coffey, D.S., Walsh, P.C., and Ewing, L.R. (1984). The development of human benign prostatic hyperplasia with age. *J Urol 132*, 474–479.

Celec, P. and Starka, L. (2003). Dehydroepiandrosterone—Is the fountain of youth drying out? *Physiol Res 52*, 397–407.

Cordon-Cardo, C., Koff, A., Drobnjak, M., Capodieci, P., Osman, I., Millard, S.S. *et al.* (1998). Distinct altered patterns of p27KIP1 gene expression in benign prostatic hyperplasia and prostatic carcinoma. *J Natl Cancer Inst 90*, 1284–1291.

Dillner, K., Kindblom, J., Flores-Morales, A., Pang, S.T., Tornell, J., Wennbo, H. *et al.* (2002). Molecular characterization of prostate hyperplasia in prolactin-transgenic mice by using cDNA representational difference analysis. *Prostate 52*, 139–149.

Dillner, K., Kindblom, J., Flores-Morales, A., Shao, R., Tornell, J., Norstedt, G. *et al.* (2003). Gene expression analysis of prostate hyperplasia in mice overexpressing the prolactin gene specifically in the prostate. *Endocrinology 144*, 4955–4966.

Fujimoto, N., Suzuki, T., Honda, H., and Kitamura, S. (2004). Estrogen enhancement of androgen-responsive gene expression in hormone-induced hyperplasia in the ventral prostate of F344 rats. *Cancer Sci 95*, 711–715.

Girman, C.J. (1998). Natural history and epidemiology of benign prostatic hyperplasia: relationship among urologic measures. *Urology 51*, 8–12.

Golomb, E., Kruglikova, A., Dvir, D., Parnes, N., and Abramovici, A. (1998). Induction of atypical prostatic hyperplasia in rats by sympathomimetic stimulation. *Prostate 34*, 214–221.

Guo, Q.L., Ding, Q.L., and Wu, Z.Q. (2004). Effect of baicalein on experimental prostatic hyperplasia in rats and mice. *Biol Pharm Bull 27*, 333–337.

Habib, F.K., Ross, M., and Bayne, C.W. (2000). Development of a new in vitro model for the study of benign prostatic hyperplasia. *Prostate Suppl 9*, 15–20.

Ito, K., Fukabori, Y., Shibata, Y., Suzuki, K., Mieda, M., Gotanda, K. *et al.* (2000). Effects of a new steroidal aromatase inhibitor, TZA-2237, and/or chlormadinone acetate on hormone-induced and spontaneous canine benign prostatic hyperplasia. *Eur J Endocrinol 143*, 543–554.

Kindblom, J., Dillner, K., Sahlin, L., Robertson, F., Ormandy, C., Tornell, J. *et al.* (2003). Prostate hyperplasia in a transgenic mouse with prostate-specific expression of prolactin. *Endocrinology 144*, 2269–2278.

Lepor, H. (2005). Pathophysiology of benign prostatic hyperplasia in the aging male population. *Rev Urol 7*, S3–S12.

Levi, F., Lucchini, F., Negri, E., Boyle, P., and La Vecchia, C. (2003). Recent trends in mortality from benign prostatic hyperplasia. *Prostate 56*, 207–211.

Mahapokai, W., Van Sluijs, F.J., and Schalken, J.A. (2000). Models for studying benign prostatic hyperplasia. *Prostate Cancer Prostatic Dis 3*, 28–33.

Marinese, D., Patel, R., and Walden, P.D. (2003). Mechanistic investigation of the adrenergic induction of ventral prostate hyperplasia in mice. *Prostate 54*, 230–237.

Mitra, S.K., Sundaram, R., Mohan, A.R., Gopumadhavan, S., Venkataranganna, M.V., Venkatesha, U. *et al.* (1999). Protective effect of Prostane in experimental prostatic hyperplasia in rats. *Asian J Androl 1*, 175–179.

Oesterling, J.E., Jacobsen, S.J., Chute, C.G., Guess, H.A., Girman, C.J., Panser, L.A. *et al.* (1993). Serum prostate-specific antigen in a community-based population of healthy men. Establishment of age-specific reference ranges. *JAMA 270*, 860–864.

Olbina, G., Miljkovic, D., Hoffman, R.M., and Geller, J. (1998). New sensitive discovery histoculture model for growth-inhibition studies in prostate cancer and BPH. *Prostate 37*, 126–129.

Parnes, H.L., Thompson, I.M., and Ford, L.G. (2005). Prevention of hormone-related cancers: Prostate cancer. *J Clin Oncol 23*, 368–377.

Prakash, K., Pirozzi, G., Elashoff, M., Munger, W., Waga, I., Dhir, R. *et al.* (2002). Symptomatic and asymptomatic benign prostatic hyperplasia: Molecular differentiation by using microarrays. *Proc Natl Acad Sci USA 99*, 7598–7603.

Risbridger, G.P., Bianco, J.J., Ellem, S.J., and McPherson, S.J. (2003). Oestrogens and prostate cancer. *Endocr Relat Cancer 10*, 187–191.

Roberts, R.O., Jacobson, D.J., Rhodes, T., Klee, G.G., Leiber, M.M., and Jacobsen, S.J. (2004). Serum sex hormones and measures of benign prostatic hyperplasia. *Prostate 61*, 124–131.

Schulman, C. and Lunenfeld, B. (2002). The ageing male. *World J Urol 20*, 4–10.

Skolarikos, A., Thorpe, A.C., and Neal, D.E. (2004). Lower urinary tract symptoms and benign prostatic hyperplasia. *Minerva Urol Nefrol 56*, 109–122.

Steiner, M.S., Couch, R.C., Raghow, S., and Stauffer, D. (1999). The chimpanzee as a model of human benign prostatic hyperplasia. *J Urol 162*, 1454–1461.

Takao, T., Tsujimura, A., Coetzee, S., Salm, S.N., Lepor, H., Shapiro, E. *et al.* (2003). Stromal/epithelial interactions of murine prostatic cell lines in vivo: a model for benign prostatic hyperplasia and the effect of doxazosin on tissue size. *Prostate 54*, 17–24.

Thorpe, A. and Neal, D. (2003). Benign prostatic hyperplasia. *Lancet 361*, 1359–1367.

Van Coppenolle, F., Le Bourhis, X., Carpentier, F., Delaby, G., Cousse, H., Raynaud, J.P. *et al.* (2000). Pharmacological effects of the lipidosterolic extract of *Serenoa repens* (Permixon) on rat prostate hyperplasia induced by hyperprolactinemia: Comparison with finasteride. *Prostate* 4I3, 49–58.

vom Saal, F.S., Timms, B.G., Montano, M.M., Palanza, P., Thayer, K.A., Nagel, S.C. *et al.* (1997). Prostate enlargement in mice due to fetal exposure to low doses of estradiol or diethylstilbestrol and opposite effects at high doses. *Proc Natl Acad Sci USA 94*, 2056–2061.

Yokota, T., Honda, K., Tsuruya, Y., Nomiya, M., Yamaguchi, O., Gotanda, K. *et al.* (2004). Functional and anatomical effects of hormonally induced experimental prostate growth: A urodynamic model of benign prostatic hyperplasia (BPH) in the beagle. *Prostate 58*, 156–163.

Zaviacic, M. and Ablin, R.J. (1998). The female prostate. *J Natl Cancer Inst 90*, 713–714.

Zaviacic, M. and Ablin, R.J. (2000). The female prostate and prostate-specific antigen. Immunohistochemical localization, implications of this prostate marker in women and reasons for using the term "prostate" in the human female. *Histol Histopathol 15*, 131–142.

Zhang, X., Na, Y., and Guo, Y. (2004). Biologic feature of prostatic hyperplasia developed in spontaneously hypertensive rats. *Urology 63*, 983–988.

53

Murine Models of Infectious Diseases in the Aged

Kevin P. High

Immune responses typically wane with age in both humans and mice. This phenomenon is termed immune senescence and renders older adults more susceptible to many infections and less likely to respond to vaccines. Murine models of immune senescence offer a window into the mechanisms that increase the incidence and severity of infection with advanced age and have furthered our understanding of host defenses. Strain differences between inbred mice and limited availability of genetically heterogeneous populations limit some of these findings, but overall, these models accurately reflect many human conditions and allow critical variables to be isolated by appropriate experimental design. In a few instances, older mice are actually more resistant to infection than are young mice, suggesting there may be immune mechanisms that remain intact or are even enhanced with advanced age. This might be exploited to improve vaccine responses and host defense in older adults.

Introduction

It is widely accepted that older adults are more susceptible to infectious diseases when compared to young adults, and infection is a major cause of morbidity and mortality in the elderly (High, 2004). Animal models are frequently used to assess the impact of age on infectious diseases, and to gather preclinical data on preventive strategies such as novel vaccine preparations. This chapter will focus on murine models of infection across the age spectrum, utilizing specific examples to illustrate general considerations when using these models.

Limitations of Murine Models in the Study of Infection in the Aged

Murine models of aging have distinct limitations for infectious diseases research that are important to recognize in order to place these models in the context of the human condition. The limitations outlined mandate that findings in murine models be validated in other animal model systems and, whenever possible, in humans. However, despite the limitations, murine models can be invaluable for studying infection in the aged by allowing manipulation of genes, diet, immune function, route of infection, and other control variables important in study design.

INBRED MOUSE STRAINS

There is a general waning of immunity with age, termed immune senescence. This phenomenon is discussed in depth in other chapters of this text. Although murine immune senescence is similar in many ways to the waning of immunity experienced by older humans, there are marked interspecies differences (Miller, 1996). A major difference between murine and human models is that most studies in mouse models utilize inbred strains or F1 crosses of inbred strains. Though there are human populations of relative genetic homogeneity (e.g., the Amish), the diversity of most human populations raises distinct issues as to whether inbred mouse strains can appropriately model human disease and host defense (Miller, Austad *et al.*, 1999; Miller, Harper *et al.*, 2002). Inbred strains were originally produced for rapid maturation and large body size, likely significantly changing the gene pool and selecting for mutations that might shorten life span. Outbred mice live longer and have fewer tumors than inbred strains, traits associated with lower levels of insulin growth factor-1 (IGF-1) in young adulthood (Miller *et al.*, 2002).

There are four inbred mouse strains (BALB/cBy, CBA, C57BL/6, DBA/2) and three F1 hybrid strains (CB6ByF1, B6C3F1, B6D2F1) available from the mouse colony of the National Institute of Aging (NIA) (www.nia.nih.gov/ResearchInformation/ScientificResources). All these strains have been widely used in infectious diseases research, but each inbred strain has a distinct median life span, markedly different Th-orientation of immune response, and varied susceptibility to specific infectious agents (see Table 53.1). This can lead to very different conclusions when aged mice of one strain are compared to others with regard to the influence of age on disease outcome. For example, an old female DBA/2 mouse may be only 16 to 18 months of age, whereas C57BL/6 mice of this age would still

TABLE 53.1
Comparison of the median life span, Th-orientation and susceptibility to selected infectious agents for four inbred mouse strains available from the National Institute of Aging's mouse colony (+ relatively resistant; ++ modestly susceptible; +++ susceptible; ++++ highly susceptible). Data summarized from www.informatics.jax.org/external/festing/mouse/docs

	BALB/cBy	CBA	C57BL/6	DBA/2
Median life span (months)	Males: 18 Females: 19	Males: 17.5 Females: 17.5	Males: 22.5 Females: 23	Males: 20.5 Females: 18
Th-orientation	Primarily Th2	Mixed (Th1 > Th2)	Primarily Th1	Mixed (Th2 > Th1)
Susceptibility to infection with:				
Influenza	+++	++++	+++	++++
Leishmania spp.	++++	++	+	++
Listeria monocytogenes	+++	+++	+	+++
Mycobacterium spp.	+++	+++	++	++++
Plasmodium bergheia	++	++++	+++	+++
Pseudomonas aeruginosab	++	No Information	+++	++++
Salmonella	++++	++	++	+++

[a]Relative susceptibility depends on outcome measured (e.g., *parasitemia* vs. cerebral symptoms).
[b]Lung infection susceptibility is shown; differences exist with regard to corneal and other sites of infection.

be considered middle-aged or mature; old C57BL/6 mice are usually in the 22- to 24-month range. The condition in which mice are housed also affects life span. Specific pathogen-free (SPF) conditions result in decreased life span in some (e.g., BALB/cBy), but increased life span in others (e.g., C57BL/6) (www.informatics.jax.org/external/festing/mouse/docs).

Strain-specific changes in immunity and life span may underlie much of the variability and contradictions in the literature. An excellent example of this is shown in Figure 53.1, demonstrating strain- and age-related changes of *B. microttii* parasitemia in murine models (Vannier *et al.*, 2004).

In the cited study, age-related differences of susceptibility were attributed to strain specificity (i.e., DBA/2 mice were assessed to experience an age-related decline in susceptibility to babesiosis, whereas C57BL/6 and BALB/c were not), and there are clearly strain-related differences with young DBA/2 mice showing greater susceptibility than the other two strains. However, as evidenced by the lower panels in Figure 53.1, outcomes in 18-month-old mice show some age-related changes in strains other than DBA/2, particularly in BALB/c mice. It is possible that age-associated declines in immunity render old C57BL/6 mice more susceptible to babesiosis as well, but that 18 months is not old enough for that particular strain to demonstrate statistically significant changes. Thus, it is important to try to match the stage of human life we are attempting to replicate in an inbred strain of mouse. This concept is illustrated in Figure 53.2 (Turnbull *et al.*, 2003).

PHYSIOLOGIC AGE VS. CHRONOLOGIC AGE

Although aging occurs in all organisms, the inter-individual variability of entering old age is marked. There are old 70-year-old humans and young 70-year-old humans. The same is undoubtedly true for animals, but there is no standard way to assess the physiologic age of mice. In older humans, frailty, disability, comorbidity, and other contributing factors to disease risk have been defined and their inclusion in infectious diseases research encouraged (High *et al.*, 2005). Correlates of these measures in animal studies would be a tremendous advance. There are some data in F1 hybrid rats that indicate reproducible physical and cognitive measures can predict survival in rodent models of aging (Carter *et al.*, 2002). There have not been any data published using murine models, but initial studies are being done in mice and should be forthcoming (personal communication, C.S. Carter).

STUDYING AGING VS. OBESITY/INACTIVITY

Aging mice in a caged environment is quite different from rodents aging in the wild. Apart from the obvious climate control, group housing, lack of predators, and so on, two major factors previously shown to impact age-related changes in physiology and life span are profoundly altered by the caged environment: diet and exercise. Caged animals have more fat, and many changes in immunity that are associated with obesity mimic immune senescence. Both states are associated with underlying constitutive activation of inflammatory pathways (most strikingly noted as an increase in NFκB

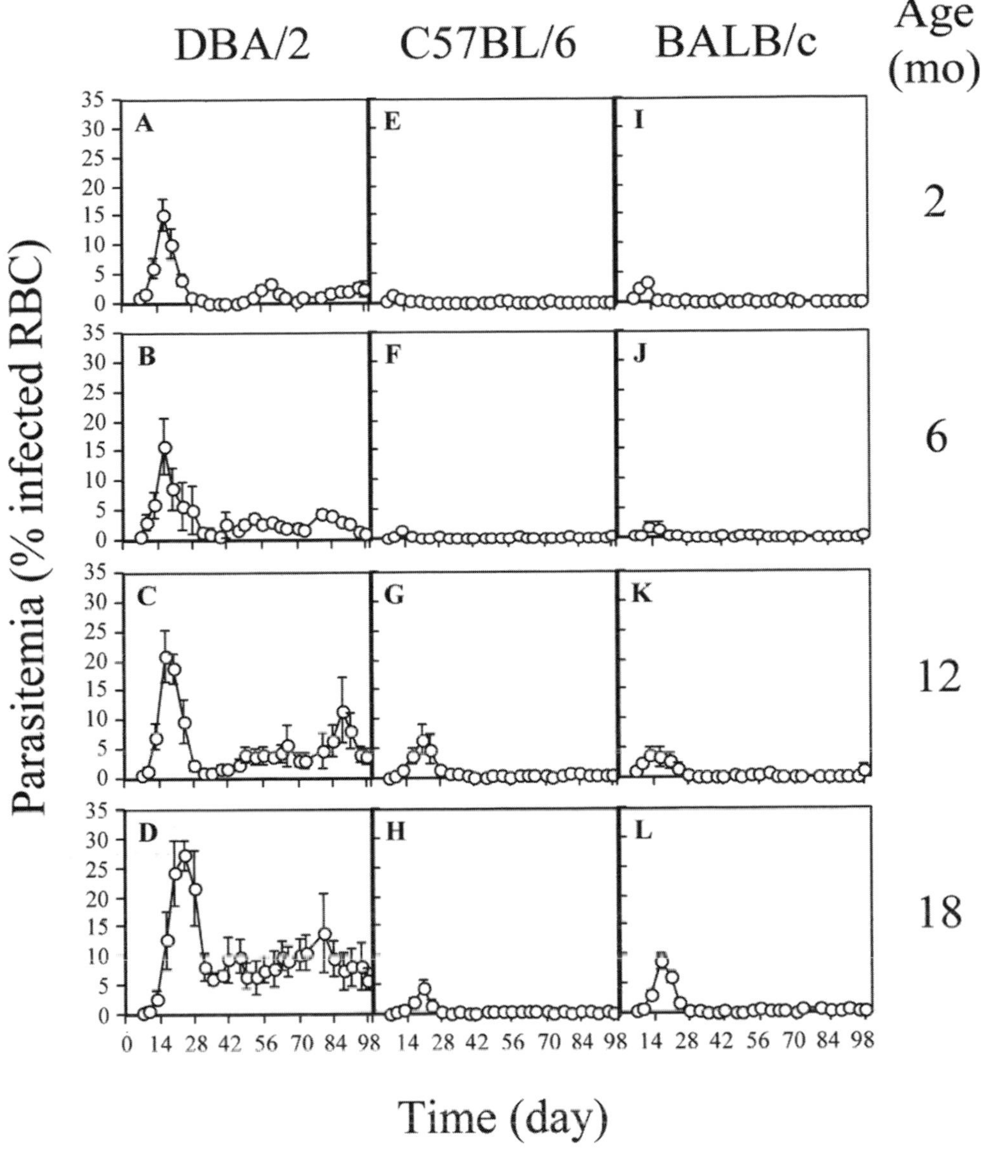

Figure 53.1 Parasitemia in DBA/2, C57BL/6 and BALB/c mice of various ages after experimental infection due to *Babesia microti* expressed as a percentage of red blood cells infected. Reprinted from Vannier (2004) with permission.

activation in the absence of any particular stimulus, i.e., constitutive activation), perhaps mediated by IGF-1 and its receptor (Quarrie, 2004). Caloric restriction extends life in virtually every species investigated to date, including mice, and reversal of suspected physiologic changes by caloric restriction is often viewed as confirmation of an age-related phenomenon (Quarrie, 2004). However, given the convergence of IGF-1, leptin, cortisol, and other hormones in both aging and obesity, investigators are cautioned that age-related alterations in host defense that reverse with caloric restriction may reflect body composition or activity level-dependent phenomena rather than age itself.

Age-related Differences in Common Infection Models

SEPSIS/OVERWHELMING INFECTION: MODELING CLINICALLY RELEVANT HUMAN PHENOMENA

Many investigators have determined that older mice are more likely to die from overwhelming infection and sepsis than are young adult mice. Two examples are shown to illustrate this fact and demonstrate important outcomes relevant to the study of infection in the aged. Sepsis can be induced by various methods, but direct injection of bacterial lipopolysaccharide (LPS) is most widely used

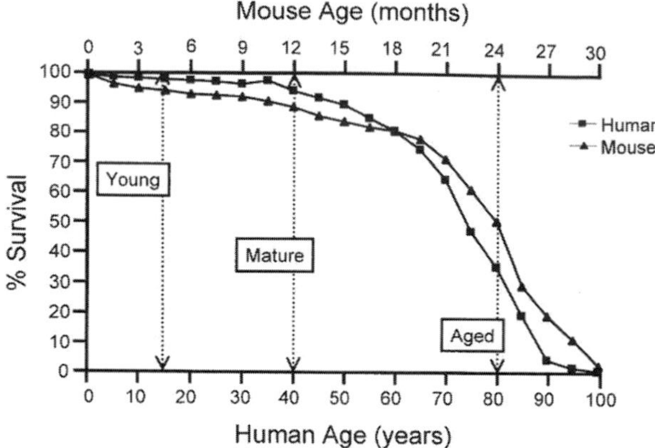

Figure 53.2 Human and murine (C57BL/6) survival curves by age expressed as years for humans and months for mice. Reprinted from Turnbull *et al.* (2003) with permission.

and cecal ligation and puncture (CLP) is used as a more physiologically relevant method to induce overwhelming bacterial infection. As shown in Figure 53.3, both LPS injection and CLP reveal markedly impaired host defense in older C57BL/6 mice when compared to young adult mice (Saito, 2003).

Based on these data, we might assume very advanced old age is a risk factor for increased mortality in sepsis. However, data from other investigators using the CLP method (Turnbull *et al.*, 2003) suggest the change in risk occurs sometime during mature adulthood, not merely in advanced age (see Figure 53.3B). A 12-month-old C57BL/6 mouse is roughly equivalent to a 40-year-old human (see Figure 53.1), and it is possible that the change in sepsis mortality risk occurs as early as six months (about age 20 years in humans). Further, whatever change occurs between four and 12 months, there appears to be no further decline in host defense after 12 months as assessed by this model since 12-month and 24-month-old mice appear to respond similarly. This illustrates a general tenet that studies of aging should investigate animals across the age spectrum. If we study only the extremes of age, the pattern of change over the entire life span of the organism is lost and may lead to erroneous conclusions.

The example of overwhelming sepsis also demonstrates that many physical exam and laboratory findings can efficiently replicate human phenomena in murine models. Older mice and humans demonstrate a lower baseline body temperature than young adults, and older humans admitted with infection have a much higher risk of mortality if hypothermia is present (Bender and Scarpace, 1997). Figure 53.4A shows that the CLP model can mimic this event and accurately predict survival in murine models. Further, hypothermia after LPS administration or CLP correlates with the degree of inflammation as measured by serum interleukin-6 (IL-6) (see Figure 53.4B), indicating that the CLP procedure is an excellent correlative model of human sepsis (Saito, 2003).

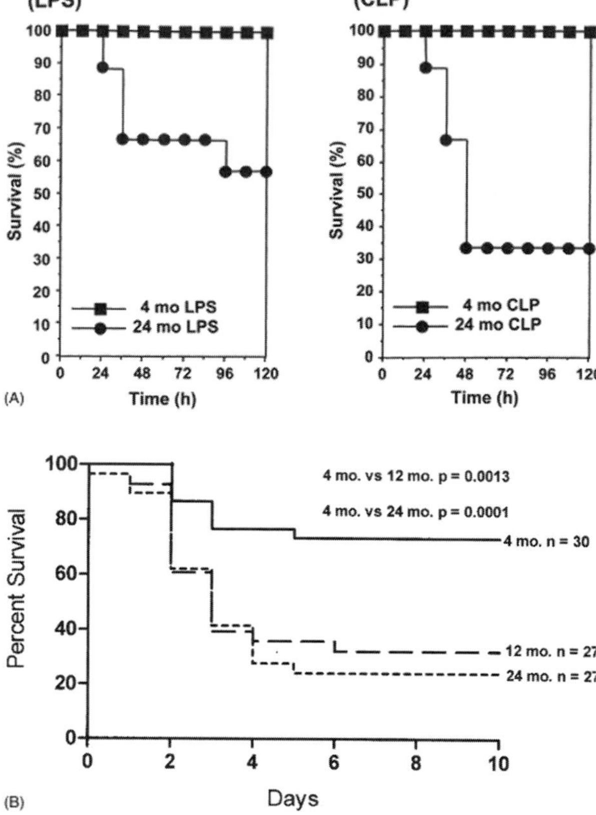

Figure 53.3 (A) Survival after injection of lipopolysaccharide (LPS) or cecal ligation and puncture (CLP) in C57BL/6 mice aged 4 or 24 months. Reprinted from Saito (2003) with permission. (B) Survival after CLP in 4-, 12-, and 24-month-old C57BL/6 mice. Reprinted from Turnbull *et al.* (2003) with permission.

TUBERCULOSIS: THE IMPORTANCE OF ROUTE OF INFECTION, USE OF MULTIPLE STRAINS, AND LIMITATIONS OF KNOCKOUT MODELS

Tuberculosis is one of the prototype infections in which the elderly are disproportionately affected (Rajagopalan, 2001). The enhanced disease rate in older adults is due to both reactivated and newly acquired *Mycobacterium tuberculosis*. The cohort of aged adults is more likely to have encountered the organism in childhood or young adulthood due to increased population prevalence at that time of their lives, but the risk is also greater for this group since older adults often reside in nursing homes or other domiciliary settings that increase exposure risk (Rajagopalan, 2001). Waning immunity with advanced age is also widely suspected of contributing to this risk, but the data are mixed. A series of elegant experiments by Orme and colleagues over 20 years has shed light on

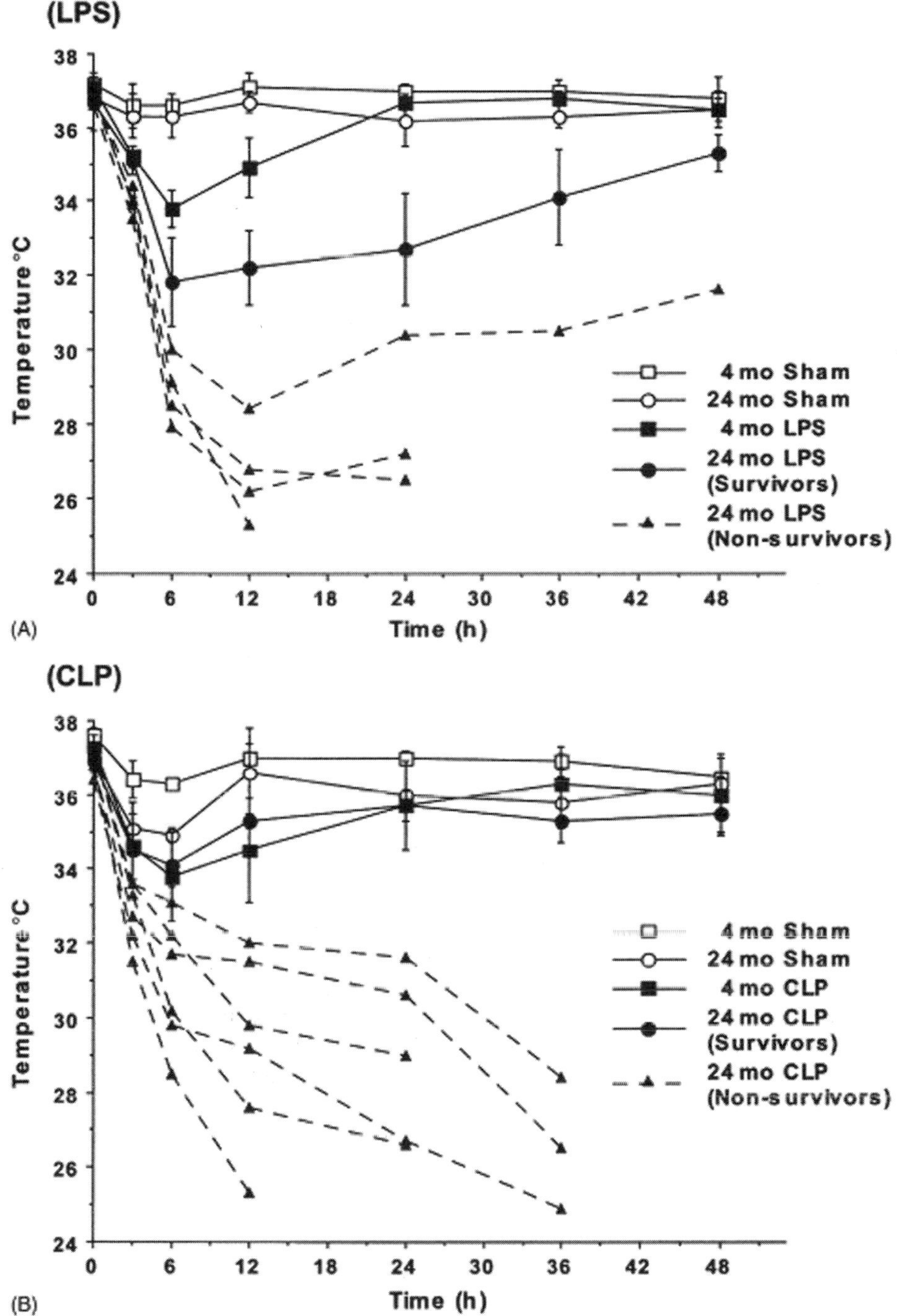

Figure 53.4 (A) Survival as a function of body temperature in 4- or 24-month-old C57BL/6 mice either injected with lipopolysaccharide (LPS), or (B) after cecal ligation and puncture (CLP) or Sham CLP. Temperature in C57BL/6 mice with sepsis induced by LPS or CLP as a function of serum IL-6. As serum IL-6 increases, body temperature declines. Reprinted from Saito (2003) with permission.

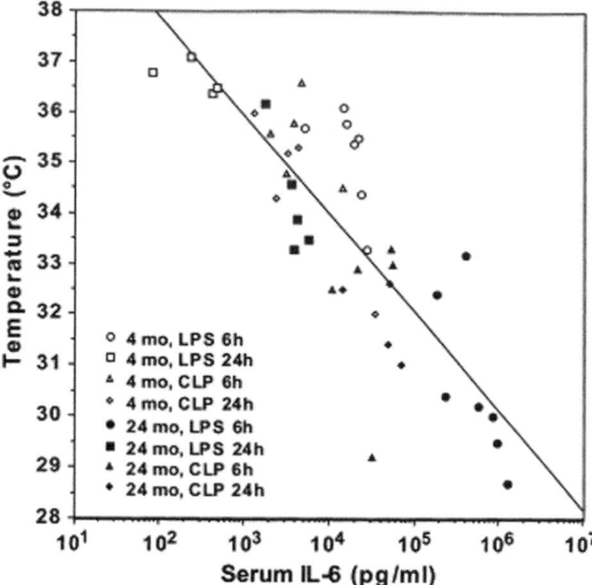

Figure 53.4 Continued.

this issue and provides an excellent example of how different infection models can be confusing but also complementary (Cooper *et al.*, 1995; Orme 1987; Turner *et al.*, 2002; Turner and Orme, 2004).

Early data suggested that older mice (F1 offspring of an A/Tru × C57BL/6) were more susceptible to a challenge with *M. tuberculosis* than were young adult mice (Orme, 1987). Transfer of splenocytes from young, infected mice was able to protect the old mice, suggesting a defect in adaptive immunity was responsible for the age-related decline in host defense. The model employed in those studies utilized intravenous administration of a high inoculum (10^5 organisms). However, intravenous injection is not a typical route of acquisition for *M. tuberculosis*, and Orme and colleagues later attempted to examine a more physiologic model using a low inoculum (50–100 organisms/lung) delivered via aerosol inhalation. In those studies, overall survival of old mice was comparable to that of young mice. However, older mice actually were found to have *increased* resistance early in mycobacterial infection when compared to young adult mice (Cooper *et al.*, 1995). Importantly, the investigators went on to demonstrate that this phenomenon was common to two different in-bred murine strains (C57BL/6, BALB/c) and an hybrid F1 strain (B57BL/6 × Cd8a) (Turner *et al.*, 2002). Old mice of a murine knockout strain that results in disruption of CD8+ T cells lost the enhanced capacity to control early tuberculosis infection (Turner *et al.*, 2002). Other knockout mouse models suggest this immune response is dependent upon interferon-γ, but not type I interferons (Miller *et al.*, 2002). In those studies knockout mice were aged until they reached very late adulthood, providing a powerful tool to examine specific mechanisms. However, a note of caution: a mouse aging throughout 18 to 24 months in the absence of a specific immune mechanism is likely to develop alternate immune responses (see Miyamoto *et al.* (2003) for an example), but it is possible, perhaps likely, that those mechanisms do not contribute to host defense to the same degree in wild-type mice in old age. Techniques currently in their infancy, such as whole animal siRNA (Buckingham *et al.*, 2004), may allow studies of old wild-type mice with silencing of genes just prior to experimental infection, which is likely to better model host defenses in the aged than are knockout models.

INFLUENZA AND RESPIRATORY SYNCYTIAL VIRUS (RSV): AGE-RELATED CHANGES IN Th PARADIGM AND VACCINE MODELS

Viral infections frequently cause morbidity and mortality in older adults, and winter-time illnesses including influenza and RSV bring annual threats that excessively affect the elderly (Thompson *et al.*, 2003). Since viruses are obligate intracellular pathogens, Th1-biased immunity (i.e., cell-mediated immunity) is critical for host defense. Th1 responses are characterized by reduced production of the cytokines IL-4, IL-10 and enhanced production of IFN-γ. Th2 responses show the opposite relationship. Immunoglobulin subtypes also indicate Th-specificity with IgG2a primarily associated with Th1 responses, IgG1 with Th2 responses, and the IgG1:IgG2a ratio is often used to assess the degree of Th1 vs. Th2 response. Although exceptions exist, aged mouse models generally reveal a shift of immune responses away from Th1 toward a mixed Th1/Th2 response in advanced age in response to viral infections such as RSV (Zhang *et al.*, 2002) or vaccines such as the influenza vaccine (Asanuma *et al.*, 2001). This shift is hypothesized to contribute to the increased susceptibility of older mice to viral infections when compared to young adult mice (Asanuma *et al.*, 2001; Bender and Small 1993; Hirokawa and Utsuyama 2002; Zhang *et al.*, 2002).

The shift in Th-bias may also underlie impaired vaccine responses found in older humans and animals; influenza vaccine is discussed in greater detail to illustrate this issue. Most data support efficacy of the currently available influenza vaccine for reducing infection-related death (Bridges *et al.*, 2002) and influenza-induced decompensation of underlying disease in older adult humans (Nichol *et al.*, 2003). However, other studies clearly show limited protection in the very old and frail vs. young, healthy adults, and have questioned the utility of influenza vaccine in older adults, particularly the frail elderly who need protection most (Simonsen *et al.*, 2005). Many other vaccines are less effective in older adults as well; thus, improved vaccine responses are a priority area of research for older adults, and influenza and RSV are specifically targeted organisms.

Murine models of both influenza and RSV, and vaccine strategies aimed at these organisms have been widely published. Vaccine strategies employed have included subunit vaccines, alternate routes of immunization, DNA vaccines, hybrid live-virus vaccines, and others. Recently, there has been great interest in new adjuvants. Only alum is currently FDA-approved as an adjuvant in humans, and this compound has minimal adjuvant activity in older adults. Adjuvant biology has been greatly advanced by the discovery of a strong link between Toll-like receptors (TLRs) and adaptive immunity (Pasare and Medzhitov, 2004). An extensive discussion of TLRs and their influence on vaccine responses is beyond the scope of this chapter; however, examples illustrate several key points.

Specific TLR agonists can modulate the aged immune response back toward Th1 responses (Ichinohe *et al.*, 2005; Manning *et al.*, 2001). For example, the addition of CpG, a TLR-9 agonist, can greatly enhance vaccine responses and induce mucosal immunity in older mice (Manning *et al.*, 2001). This boost is associated with a concomitant shift in the IgG1:IgG2a ratio from a clearly Th2-predominate 63:1 toward a Th-1/Th-2 mixed response ratio of 8:1 in older mice. The latter ratio closely reflects that seen in immunized young adult mice. Despite early success with TLR-agonists in murine models, it should be noted that TLR expression, regulation, and cellular distribution vary from mice to humans (Heinz *et al.*, 2003; Rehli 2002), and the road to human vaccines from murine models is littered with previous failures.

LEISHMANIASIS: ADVANCING AGE SOMETIMES LEADS TO IMPROVED HOST DEFENSE

Though many immune responses wane with age, some elements of host defense appear to actually be enhanced with advanced age. The resistance early in experimental tuberculosis noted earlier (Cooper *et al.*, 1995; Turner *et al.*, 2002; Turner and Orme, 2004) is one example, but others exist. The most clearly documented and mechanistically determined example is leishmaniasis (Ehrchen *et al.*, 2004). As previously outlined (see Table 53.1), BALB/c mice generally respond to immune challenges with a Th-2 response, whereas C57BL/6 mice are oriented toward a Th-1 response. Since Th1 immunity more effectively controls leishmaniasis, C57BL/6 mice have less severe disease than do BALB/c mice. However, as the mice age, BALB/c, but not C57BL/6, demonstrate an increased Th-1 response vs. *L. major* (see Figure 53.5) that leads to disease more closely resembling that of C57BL/6 with lower levels of parasites in the spleen and reduced footpad swelling (see Figure 53.6).

Further studies of the mechanism of enhanced host defense in old BALB/c mice demonstrated strong, age-related increases in IL-12 secretion in the absence of any stimulus. This spontaneous release of IL-12 by macrophages was present whether mice were raised in SPF or conventional conditions, but was augmented

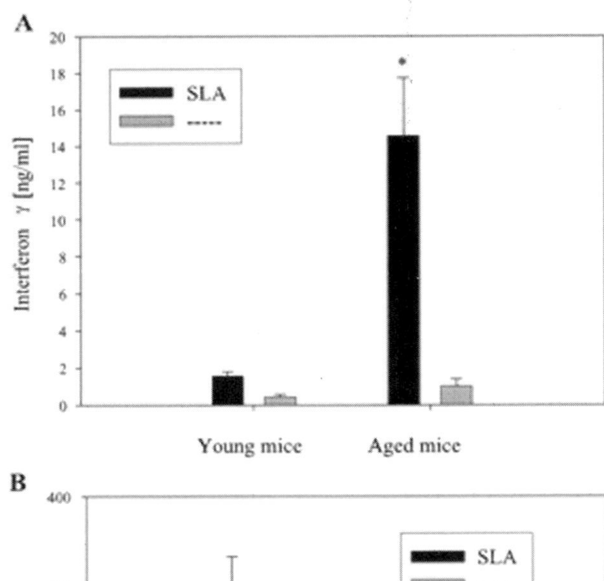

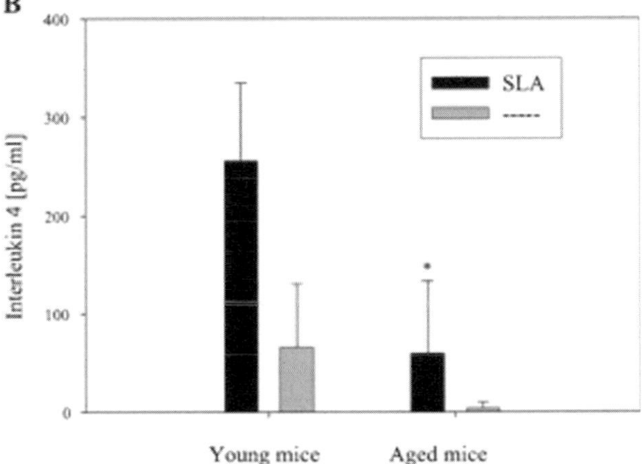

Figure 53.5 Production of the Th-1 cytokine interferon-γ and the Th-2 cytokine interleukin-4 by splenocytes isolated from young (8–10 weeks) or old (18 months) BALB/c mice stimulated with soluble leishmania antigen (SLA)12 weeks after infection with *Leishmania major*. Reprinted from Ehrchen *et al.* (2004) with permission.

if animals were exposed to pathogens throughout life (Ehrchen *et al.*, 2004). It is likely that C57BL/6 already have such a marked Th-1 orientation that the same age-related shift would have little effect on disease and be undetectable using measures employed even if present.

We have demonstrated that older DBA/2 mice have enhanced resistance to infection due to attenuated or fully virulent strains of *Brucella abortus* (unpublished observation), similar to the findings outlined for leishmaniasis. Although *Leishmania* spp., *Brucella* spp., *Salmonella* spp., *Mycobacteria* spp., and viruses are all intracellular pathogens, they have vastly different immune evasion strategies and intracellular survival mechanisms. The differences outlined earlier demonstrate that we cannot predict age-dependent susceptibility or resistance in the absence of specific data. Examining the immune responses active against organisms in which older mice have augmented resistance is likely to elucidate pathways that

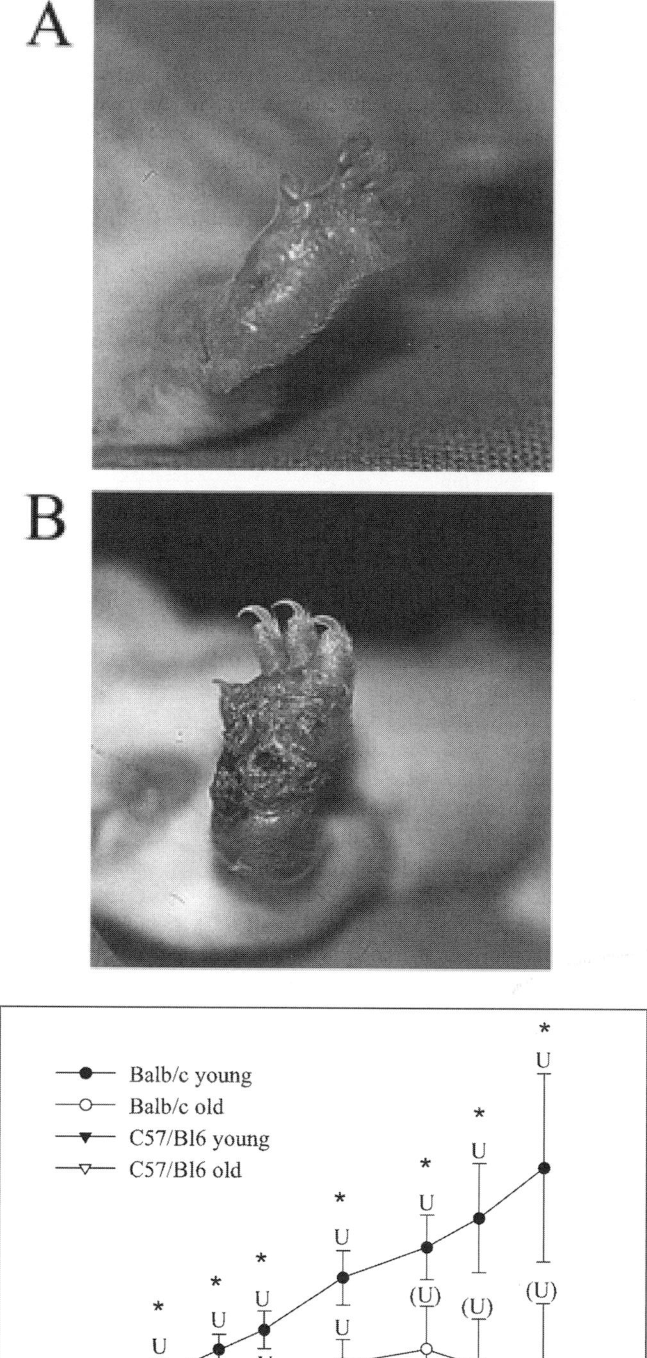

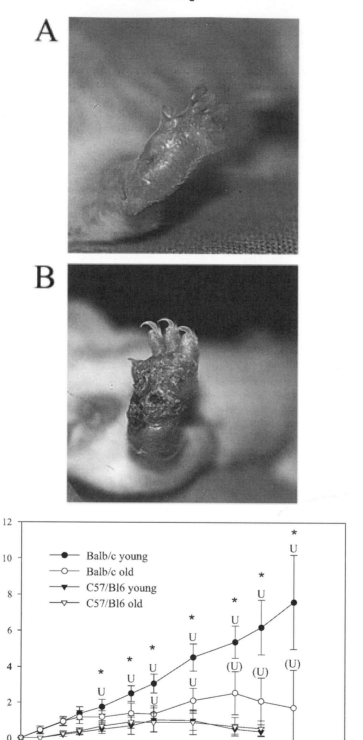

Figure 53.6 (A) Foot pad swelling 12 weeks after infection with *L. major* in old (18 months; top) or young (8–10 weeks; bottom) BALB/c mice. The old mouse demonstrates marked healing by 12 weeks whereas the young mouse shows a large crusted ulcer. (B) Foot pad swelling in young or old L. major infected BALB/c or C57BL/6 mice. No age-related difference is seen in C57BL/6 mice, but there are marked differences in BALB/c mice by age at time of infection. Reprinted from Ehrchen *et al*. (2004) with permission.

remain intact into advanced age. It may be possible to exploit these mechanisms to improve host defense and/or vaccine responses in seniors.

Senescence-Accelerated Murine Models of Chronic, Degenerative Infectious Diseases

Senescence accelerated-prone (SAMP) and -resistant (SAMR) mouse strains have been widely used to investigate a variety of disorders common with advancing age, and recent data suggest these may be relevant models for chronic infectious diseases such as prion disease (Carp *et al.*, 2000). SAMP and SAMR mice were derived from a cross between an unknown mouse strain and the AKR strain of mice known to be infected with an endogenous murine retrovirus called murine leukemia virus (MuLV). Interestingly, SAMP mice demonstrate infection with MuLV, typically with high viral titers in multiple organs including brain, whereas SAMR mice are MuLV negative or have extremely low MuLV titers (Carp *et al.*, 2000). SAMP mouse brains demonstrate changes that mimic scrapie-infection in non-SAM mice. Further, experimental scrapie infection in AKR, SAMP, and SAMR mice results in enhanced MuLV titers in AKR > SAMP, but not in SAMR mice. Brain pathology consistent with scrapie is eventually found in all three strains, but the incubation period is markedly different and parallels MuLV titer (i.e., the higher the MuLV titer, the shorter the incubation). This suggests there may be an interaction between microbes and the transmissible agents of prion disease. Senescence-accelerated mice may provide important insight into this relationship.

Conclusion

Murine models have greatly advanced the study of infectious diseases in the aged and can accurately model many human conditions. In general, immune responses shift from a Th1-predominate paradigm in young adulthood to a more mixed (Th1/Th2) model in advanced age, but exceptions to this general rule exist. In a few instances older mice are even more resistant to some pathogens than are young adult mice. When designing investigations of aging and infection, it is important when possible to include multiple murine strains, utilize physiologically relevant routes of infection, and assess underlying immune responses across the age spectrum to elucidate mechanisms. The growing field of TLR biology and the role of TLR agonists as vaccine adjuvants hold great promise for enhancing vaccine responses and protection in older adults, and murine models are likely to be the foundation for human studies.

REFERENCES

Asanuma, H., Hirokawa, K., Uchiyama, M., Suzuki, Y., Aizawa. C., Kurata, T. *et al.* (2001). Immune responses and protection in different strains of aged mice immunized intranasally with an adjuvant-combined influenza vaccine. *Vaccine 19*, 3981–3989.

Bender, B.S., and Scarpace, P.J. (1997). Fever in the Elderly. In P.A. Mackowiak, Ed., *Fever: Basic Mechanisms and Management*, pp. 363–373. New York: Lipincott–Raven.

Bender, B.S., and Small, P.A. Jr. (1993). Heterotypic immune mice lose protection against influenza virus infection with senescence. *J Infect Dis 168*, 873–880.

Bridges, C.B., Winquist, A.G., Fukuda, K., Cox, N.J., Singleton, J.A., and Strikas, R.A. (2000). Advisory Committee on Immunization Practices. Prevention and control of influenza: recommendations of the Advisory Committee on Immunization Practices (ACIP). *MMWR Recomm Rep 49(RR-3)*, 1–38.

Buckingham, S.D., Esmaeili, B., Wood, M., and Sattelle, D.B. (2004) RNA interference: From model organisms towards therapy for neural and neuromuscular disorders. *Hum Mol Genet 13 Spec No 2*, R275–R288.

Carp, R.I., Meeker, H.C., Kozlowski, P., and Sersen, E.A. (2000). An endogenous retrovirus and exogenous scrapie in a mouse model of aging. *Trends Microbiol 8*, 39–42.

Carter, C.S., Sonntag, W.E., Onder, G., Pahor, M. (2002). Physical performance and longevity in aged rats. *J Gerontol A Biol Sci Med Sci 57*, B193–B197.

Cooper, A.M., Callahan, J.E., Griffin, J.P., Roberts, A.D., and Orme, I.M. (1995). Old mice are able to control low-dose aerogenic infections with *Mycobacterium tuberculosis. Infect Immun 63*, 3259–3265.

Ehrchen, J., Sindrilaru, A., Grabbe, S., Schonlau, F., Schlesiger, C., Sorg, C. *et al.* (2004). Senescent BALB/c mice are able to develop resistance to Leishmania major infection. *Infect Immun 72*, 5106–5114.

Heinz, S., Haehnel, V., Karaghiosoff, M., Schwarzfischer, L., Muller, M., Krause, S.W. *et al.* (2003). Species specific regulation of Toll–like receptor 3 genes in men and mice. *J Biol Chem 278*, 21502–21509.

High, K.P., Bradley, S., Loeb, M., Palmer, R., Quagliarello, V., and Yoshikawa, T. (2005). A new paradigm for clinical investigation of infectious syndromes in older adults: Assessment of functional status as a risk factor and outcome measure. *Clin Infect Dis 40*, 114–122.

High, K.P. (2004). Infection as a cause of age–related morbidity and mortality. *Ageing Res Rev 3*, 1–14.

Hirokawa, K., and Utsuyama, M. (2002). Animal models and possible human application of immunological restoration in the elderly. *Mech Ageing Dev 123*, 1055–1063.

Ichinohe, T., Watanabe, I., Ito, S., Fujii, H., Moriyama, M., Tamura, S. *et al.* (2005). Synthetic Double-stranded RNA poly(I:C) combined with mucosal vaccine protects against influenza virus infection. *J Virol 79*, 2910–2919.

Manning, B.M., Enioutina, E.Y., Visic, D.M., Knudson, A.D., and Daynes, R.A. (2001). CpG DNA functions as an effective adjuvant for the induction of immune responses in aged mice. *Exp Gerontol 37*, 107–126.

Miller, R.A., Austad, S., Burke, D., Chrisp, C., Dysko, R., Galecki, A. *et al.* (1999). Exotic mice as models for aging research: Polemic and prospectus. *Neurobiol Aging 20*, 217–231.

Miller, R.A., Harper, J.M., Dysko, R.C., Durkee, S.J., and Austad, S.N. (2002). Longer life spans and delayed maturation in wild–derived mice. *Exp Biol Med 227*, 500–508.

Miller, R.A. (1996). The aging immune system: primer and prospectus. *Science 273*, 70–74.

Miyamoto, M., Emoto, M., Emoto, Y., Brinkmann, V., Yoshizawa, I., Seiler, P. *et al.* (2003). Neutrophilia in LFA-1-deficient mice confers resistance to listeriosis: possible contribution of granulocyte-colony-stimulating factor and IL-17. *J Immunol 170*, 5228–5234.

Nichol, K.L., Nordin, J., Mullooly, J., Lask, R., Fillbrandt, K., and Iwane, M. (2003). Influenza vaccination and reduction in hospitalizations for cardiac disease and stroke among the elderly. *N Engl J Med 348*, 1322–1332.

Orme, I. (1987). Aging and immunity to tuberculosis: increased susceptibility of old mice reflects a decreased capacity to generate mediator T lymphocytes. *J Immunol 138*, 4414–4418.

Pasare, C., and Medzhitov, R. (2004) Toll–dependent control mechanisms of CD4 T cell activation. *Immunity 21*, 733–741.

Quarrie, J.K., Riabowol. (2004). Murine models of life span extension. *Sci Aging Knowledge Environ 31*, re5.

Rajagopalan, S. (2001). Tuberculosis. In T.T. Yoshikawa and D.C. Norman, Eds. *Infectious Disease in the Aging: A Clinical Handbook*, pp. 67–77. Totowa, NJ: Humana Press.

Rehli, M. (2002). Of mice and men: Species variations of Toll–like receptor expression. *Trends Immunol 23*, 375–378.

Saito, H., Sherwood, E.R., Varma, T.K., and Evers, B.M. (2003). Effects of aging on mortality, hypothermia, and cytokine induction in mice with endotoxemia or sepsis. *Mech Ageing Dev 124*,1047–1058.

Simonsen, L., Reichert, T.A., Viboud, C., Blackwelder, W.C., Taylor, R.J., and Miller, M.A. (2005). Impact of influenza vaccination on seasonal mortality in the US elderly population. *Arch Intern Med 165*, 265–272.

Thompson, W.W., Shay, D.K., Weintraub, E., Brammer, L., Cox, N., Anderson, L.J. *et al.* (2003). Mortality associated with influenza and respiratory syncytial virus in the United States. *JAMA 289*, 179–186.

Turnbull, I.R., Wlzorek, J.J., Osborne, D., Hotchkiss, R.S., Coopersmith, C.M., and Buchman, T.G. (2003). Effects of age on mortality and antibiotic efficacy in cecal ligation and puncture. *Shock 19*, 310–313.

Turner, J., Frank, A.A., and Orme, I.M. (2002). Old mice express a transient early resistance to pulmonary tuberculosis that is mediated by CD8 T cells. *Infect Immun 70*, 4628–4637.

Turner, J, and Orme, I.M. (2004). The expression of early resistance to an infection with *Mycobacterium tuberculosis* by old mice is dependent on IFN type II (IFN-gamma) but not IFN type I. *Mech Ageing Dev 125*, 1–9.

Vannier, E., Borggraefe, I., Telford, S.R. 3rd, Menon, S., Brauns, T., Spielman, A. *et al.* (2004). Age-associated decline in resistance to *Babesia microti* is genetically determined. *J Infect Dis 189*, 1721–1728.

www.informatics.jax.org/external/festing/mouse/docs; accessed February 21, 2005.

Zhang, Y., Wang, Y., Gilmore, X., Xu, K., Wyde, P.R., and Mbawuike, I.N. (2002). An aged mouse model for RSV infection and diminished CD8(+) CTL responses. *Exp Biol Med 227*, 133–140.

54

Studying Infection in the Elderly: Physiopathology, Clinical Symptoms and Causative Agents of Pneumonia

Jean-Paul Janssens

Pneumonia is a major threat to older individuals, with a high mortality. Aging is associated with a high rate of atypical clinical presentations (delirium, falls, incontinence, absence of fever, or cough) that may delay diagnosis. In this chapter, pneumonia will be discussed as a model of infection in older subjects. The normal age-related changes in respiratory physiology (such as decrease in forced expiratory volumes, respiratory muscle performance, and mucociliary clearance efficacy) and their relevance for explaining the higher susceptibility of older subjects to infection of the lower respiratory tract are detailed.

The main mechanisms leading to community-acquired and nursing-home acquired pneumonia are reviewed, with an emphasis on the importance of micro-aspiration, on risk factors such as colonization of the oro-pharyngeal flora by pathogenic organisms, and risk associated with artificial enteral feeding (naso-gastric tube or percutaneous gastrostomy). Immunosenescence and its relevance to lower respiratory tract is discussed elsewhere, in Chapter 65. Particularities of the clinical presentation of pneumonia in this age group, as well as prognostic indicators as to short-term and long-term outcome, are described. The most important pathogenic organisms and their epidemiological and clinical characteristics are reviewed, as well as more unusual organisms and their specificities. Alternative diagnoses to be considered in the situation of nonresponsive pulmonary infiltrates are also discussed.

Introduction: Epidemiology of Pneumonia in the Very Old

The annual incidence of pneumonia increases with aging and is higher in institutionalized subjects than in community-dwellers. In noninstitutionalized older subjects, incidence of community-acquired pneumonia (CAP) is estimated at between 25 and 44 per 1000 population—up to four times that of patients less than 65 years of age. Incidence of nursing-home acquired pneumonia (NHAP) has been reported as high as 137 cases per 1000 population per year (Fein, 1994; Sund-Levander *et al.*, 2003). Mortality rates for older patients in hospital-based studies of CAP (up to 30%) are correlated with comorbidities, nutritional and functional status, and presence of cognitive disorders (delirium) (Kaplan *et al.*, 2002; Janssens *et al.*, 2004; Torres *et al.*, 2004). For NHAP, mortality rates may reach 57%. Hospitalization for community-acquired pneumonia (CAP) per se is associated with a high risk of hospital readmission and a high mortality within the following year (Bohannon *et al.*, 2004).

The diagnosis of pneumonia in this age group is often delayed because of the frequent absence of fever, the paucity or absence of cough, and changes in mental status (delirium), further contributing to the high morbidity and mortality. Cognitive impairment (dementia), present in 20% of subjects aged over 80, is a risk factor for nonspecific presenting symptoms of CAP or NHAP (such as weakness, falls, and delirium), and thus delayed diagnosis and poor prognosis (Johnson *et al.*, 2000; Morrison *et al.*, 2000; Sund-Levander *et al.*, 2003).

Age-related Changes in Respiratory Mechanics

IMPACT OF NORMAL AGING ON COMPLIANCE OF THE LUNG PARENCHYMA AND CHEST WALL, AND PERFORMANCE OF RESPIRATORY MUSCLES

Normal aging is associated with changes in the respiratory system that have important consequences on the ability of older subjects to cope with the decrease in lung compliance (infiltration by inflammatory cells related to infection) and increase in airway resistance (bronchial edema, secretions) caused by lower respiratory tract infection (LRTI).

When compared to younger individuals, elastic recoil of the lung, compliance of the chest wall, and strength of respiratory muscles are all decreased in older subjects.

Age-related alterations in lung parenchyma (enlargement of alveoli, also referred to as *ductectasia* or *senile emphysema*) explain the decline in elastic recoil of the lung and the resulting increase in functional residual capacity (FRC). Indeed, FRC (lung volume at the end of a quiet expiration) is determined by the equilibrium between two opposite forces: the elastic recoil of the lung parenchyma and that of the chest wall, the latter tending to expand the chest. Thus a decrease in elastic recoil of the lung increases the FRC: older patients breathe at higher lung volumes, increasing the workload imposed on respiratory muscles.

Decreased compliance of the chest wall (i.e., "stiffening" of the chest wall) is explained to some extent by calcifications and other structural changes within the rib cage and its articulations. Changes in the shape of the thorax as a result of osteoporosis and vertebral fractures, resulting in dorsal kyphosis and increased anteroposterior (AP) diameter (barrel chest), also affect chest wall compliance. Indeed, prevalence of vertebral fractures in the aged is high and increases with age: in Europe, for female subjects aged over 60, the prevalence of vertebral fractures is 17% in the 60 to 64 age group, increasing to 35% in the 75 to 79 age group (Cummings *et al.*, 2002). Males also have an increase in vertebral fractures with age, but rates are approximately half those of the female population. The increase in AP diameter of the chest decreases the curvature of the diaphragm and has a negative effect on its force-generating capabilities. Respiratory muscle performance in older subjects is thus limited by the increase in FRC, the decrease in chest-wall compliance, and geometric changes in the rib cage (Janssens *et al.*, 1999).

Respiratory muscle strength is also affected by nutritional status, often deficient in the elderly, and by the age-related decrease in muscle mass (sarcopenia) (Enright *et al.*, 1994; Tolep *et al.*, 1995; Polkey *et al.*, 1997). Indeed, normal values for maximal inspiratory pressure in subjects aged over 80 are below the threshold defined in an adult population for clinically relevant respiratory dysfunction (Enright *et al.*, 1994). Situations in which an additional load is placed on the respiratory muscles, such as decreased parenchymal compliance (pneumonia, congestive heart failure) or increased airway resistance (presence of tracheal or bronchial secretions and inflammation, asthma), may lead to hypoventilation and hypercapnic respiratory failure. Patients with preexisting structural changes in lung mechanics (such as COPD, interstitial lung disease, or Kyphoscoliosis) are, of course, at increased risk of hypercapnic respiratory failure.

Respiratory muscle function also depends on energy availability (i.e., blood flow, oxygen content); indeed, decreased respiratory muscle strength has been described in patients with chronic heart failure (CHF), a frequent occurrence in older subjects (Nishimura *et al.*, 1994; Evans *et al.*, 1995). Presence of CHF with a New York Heart Association (NYHA) functional class 3 or 4 was shown to be associated with a 30% decrease in maximal mouth inspiratory pressure (PI_{MAX}) compared to control subjects. Furthermore, a significant relationship was demonstrated between cardiac index (CI) and PI_{MAX}, the latter decreasing when CI decreased (Nishimura *et al.*, 1994). Other frequent clinical situations decreasing respiratory muscle function in the elderly include Parkinson's disease and sequelae of cerebral vascular disease. Indeed, in hemiplegic patients, limitation of thoracic excursions caused by weakness and uncoordination of the chest muscles may lead to decreased chest wall compliance and compromise respiratory muscle function (Annoni *et al.*, 1990).

AGING, FORCED EXPIRATORY VOLUMES, AND PEAK FLOW: IMPLICATIONS FOR COUGHING AND CLEARANCE OF AIRWAY SECRETIONS

Forced expiratory volumes and peak expiratory flow show an age-related linear decrease, probable reflecting structural changes, and chronic low-grade inflammation in peripheral airways (Enright *et al.*, 1993). Indeed, for a male subject with a height of 180 cm, between the ages of 25 and 75, forced expiratory volume in 1 sec (FEV1) drops by 32%, forced vital capacity (FVC), by 24%, and peak expiratory flow (PEF), by 22% (Quanjer *et al.*, 1993). In the very old, both the decrease in forced expiratory flow rates and in lung elastic recoil may compromise the efficacy of clearing airway secretions by coughing. Critical values for PEF have been reported, under which the risk of pneumonia markedly increases (Tzeng *et al.*, 2000). In patients with neuromuscular disorders, a PEF below 270 L/min is associated with an increase in risk of pulmonary infection, and at PEF values < 160 L/min, cough is ineffective for clearing secretions from the airways (predicted PEF for an 80-year-old woman, measuring 160 cm, is 300 L/min). Coughing requires a precise coordination of laryngeal and respiratory muscle function: after a rapid inspiration, airways are submitted to a compression phase in which active glottic closure and abdominal contraction are critical, before the "explosive" expiratory phase. A decrease in expiratory muscle strength may thus compromise the efficacy of the cough reflex. The efficacy of glottic closure depends on the integrity of laryngeal muscle function and complex integrated reflexes that may be altered in the elderly by transient or permanent neurological disorders (cerebro-vascular disorders, extra-pyramidal, or cerebellar disorders). Indeed, ischemic stroke increases markedly the risk of pneumonia: in a large series of 13440 patients, pneumonia was the most frequent and serious complication, causing 31% of all deaths (Heuschmann *et al.*, 2004). Glottal gap related to unilateral vocal cord paralysis is a potentially reversible sequel of acute cerebro-vascular events that may also increase the risk and frequency of aspiration (Fang *et al.*, 2004).

Mucociliary clearance (progression of mucus layer lining the tracheal and bronchial epithelium) is also affected by the aging process. Even in the healthy non-smoking aged population, mucociliary clearance rates are slowed in comparison with the young. Nasal mucociliary clearance and frequency of mucosal ciliary beat are decreased in older subjects; aging also is associated with ultrastructural changes in microtubules of ciliae of the respiratory epithelium. Indeed, both smoking and non-smoking elderly have reduced tracheal mucus velocity compared with younger individuals (Ho *et al.*, 2001). Dehydration, frequent in older debilitated subjects, may further compromise mucociliary clearance.

SENSITIVITY OF RESPIRATORY CENTERS AND CLINICAL SYMPTOMS

Lower sensitivity of respiratory centers to hypoxia or hypercapnia in older subjects results in a diminished ventilatory response in case of acute disease such as heart failure, infection, or airway obstruction, and thus delays important clinical symptoms and signs such as dyspnea and tachypnea, which are important for the diagnosis of pneumonia and appreciation of its severity (Kronenberg *et al.*, 1973; Peterson *et al.*, 1981). Aging is also associated with a decreased perception of added resistive loads, such as that induced by asthma or increased airway secretions. Indeed, older subjects have a lower perception of methacholine-induced bronchoconstriction when compared with younger subjects (Cuttitta *et al.*, 2001).

Pathogenesis of Infection of the Lower Airways

Mechanisms implicated in the pathogenesis of infection of the lower airways are essentially aspiration of oro-pharyngeal secretions or gastric contents, inhalation of pathogenic organisms (i.e., viral or mycobacterial infections), and hematogenous dissemination (either iatrogenic or from a distant infectious focus). Among these mechanisms, aspiration of oro-pharyngeal secretions is probably the most prevalent.

ASPIRATION

Approximately half of all healthy adults aspirate small amounts of oropharyngeal secretions during sleep. The low burden of virulent bacteria in normal pharyngeal secretions, together with forceful coughing, active ciliary transport, and normal humoral and cellular immune mechanisms, protect the airways from repeated clinical infection. However, defense of the airway is impaired in the elderly by decreased mucociliary clearance, alteration in respiratory mechanics, and, in some cases, concomitant illnesses that predispose to aspiration. Furthermore, normal aging is associated with impaired oro-pharyngeal deglutition. This has been attributed to an increased neural processing time (Tracy *et al.*, 1989). Indeed, there is a high incidence of silent aspiration in elderly patients who develop pneumonia: 71% of patients with CAP vs. 10% of the control subjects (Kikuchi *et al.*, 1994). Cough reflex sensitivity may also be altered in older subjects with recurrent pneumonia. Conversely, intensive oral care for one month has been shown to enhance cough reflex sensitivity, in a controlled randomized trial of older nursing home patients (Niimi *et al.*, 2003; Watando *et al.*, 2004).

As previously mentioned, aspiration pneumonia is a frequent complication of acute ischaemic stroke. Aspiration pneumonia was documented in 13.6% of 1455 patients during the three months following the acute event; associated risk factors were male gender, age, and diabetes; furthermore, pneumonia was associated with a higher mortality, and a lower functional status at three months (Barthel Index, Rankin scale) (Aslanyan *et al.*, 2004). In a large study of 13440 patients with ischemic stroke, in-hospital mortality was 4.9%; pneumonia accounted for 31% of all deaths (Heuschmann *et al.*, 2004).

UPPER AIRWAY COLONIZATION

Colonization of the upper respiratory tract by both Gram-negative (GNB: *Enterobacteriaceae, P. aeruginosa*) and Gram-positive bacteria (*S. aureus*) is more prevalent in the elderly and is related more to the severity of systemic illness and level of care than to age *per se* (Johanson *et al.*, 1969; Valenti *et al.*, 1978). Factors leading to colonization of the lower and upper respiratory tract include antibiotic therapy, endotracheal intubation, smoking, malnutrition, surgery, and any serious medical illness. Decreased salivation such as that induced by antidepressants, antiparkinsonian medications, diuretics, antihypertensives, and antihistamines also contributes to oropharyngeal GNB colonization.

Periodontal disease and dental plaque are clearly identified risk factors for the development of nursing-home acquired aspiration pneumonia. Recent studies have focused on the relationship between oral hygiene, colonization of dental plaques, and subsequent risk of pneumonia (El-Solh *et al.*, 2003; El-Solh *et al.*, 2004). A high plaque index and/or evidence of periodontal disease has been associated with presence of anaerobic bacteria in broncho-alveolar lavage (BAL) samples (Imsand *et al.*, 2002). In a study of 49 older patients from chronic long-term facilities requiring intensive care for a lower respiratory tract infection (LRTI), El-Solh *et al.* (2004) assessed dental status (plaque index, culture of dental plaques) upon admission to the ICU; BAL was performed in 14 subjects. The study showed a high rate of colonization of dental plaque by aerobic bacteria (*S. aureus*: 45%; *P. aeruginosa*: 13%; other GNB: 42%). Furthermore, pathogens recovered from BAL matched the micro-organisms recovered from dental plaques in

61% of subjects. Dental plaque colonization thus appears as a potential reservoir for LRTI. Indeed, earlier studies have shown the potential benefit of oral care to reduce the incidence of pneumonia in elderly nursing home residents (Terpenning *et al.*, 2002; Yoneyama *et al.*, 2002). The risk of aspiration pneumonia is also reduced in edentate subjects.

In summary, there is an increased number of pathogenic bacteria in the upper respiratory tract of sick and institutionalized elderly patients, which increases the risk of pneumonia following aspiration of oropharyngeal secretions.

ASPIRATION PNEUMONIA VS. ASPIRATION PNEUMONITIS

The term *aspiration pneumonia* has been used to define two different clinical conditions: aspiration of gastric contents into the lung (chemical injury with a subsequent inflammatory response), also referred to as *aspiration pneumonitis*, and aspiration of oropharyngeal content into the lung with resultant bacterial infection. Aspiration pneumonitis is not infectious in its initial stage, and many episodes of aspiration pneumonitis may resolve with supportive care, without antibiotherapy. It is frequently associated with naso-gastric tube feeding; in fact, tube feeding has been shown to be an independent predictor of gastric content aspiration (Marik, 2001). It is associated, however, with a high risk of secondary bacterial infection after more than 24 hours (Mylotte *et al.*, 2003).

ASPIRATION AND FEEDING TUBES

Feeding tubes do not protect from bronchoaspiration; this is true for naso-gastric tubes (NGT) and percutaneous enterogastric (PEG) tubes. In fact, feeding tubes are associated with an increased rate of pneumonia and death from pneumonia (Strong *et al.*, 1992; Croghan *et al.*, 1994; Marik, 2001).

The use of a NGT or a PEG tube appears to alter the oro-pharyngeal ecosystem, and increases upper airway colonization by *P. aeruginosa*, other GNB, and *S. aureus* (Leibovitz *et al.*, 2003a; Leibovitz *et al.*, 2003b; Leibovitz *et al.*, 2003c). In a study of 215 nursing-home patients (78 patients with a NGT, 57 with a PEG, and 80 patients fed orally), *P. aeruginosa* was recovered from the oropharyngeal flora of 31% of patients with NGT, and 10% of those with PEG, vs. 0% of controls; GNB were recovered from 71% of patients with NGT, 44% of those with PEG vs. only 7.5% of controls. Globally, the upper airways of 81% of patients with NGT were colonized by potential respiratory pathogens vs. 51% of patients with PEG, and 17.5% of controls. Decreased mechanical clearance of organisms by chewing and swallowing, and appearance of a bio-film on the NGT itself probably contribute to upper airway colonization by GNB. The biofilm may facilitate growth and colonization by *P. aeruginosa*. The reason for the important upper airway colonization by *S. aureus* and GNB in patients with PEG is unclear.

In summary, aspiration is an important pathogenic mechanism for pneumonia in the elderly; in patients with neurologic impairment of the glottic barrier, the use of a NGT or PEG does not abolish and may in fact increase the risk of pneumonia.

Prognostic Indicators and Outcome

Items associated with a higher risk of in-hospital or 30-day mortality for older patients hospitalized with pneumonia are NHAP vs. CAP, bedridden status, altered mental status, absence of fever ($<37°C$), absence of cough or chills, tachypnea (RR $>$ 30/min), systemic hypotension (SBP $<$ 90 mmHg), respiratory failure, CRP $>$ 100mg/L, multilobar involvement, pleural effusion, radiological signs of cavitation, suspicion of aspiration, presence of swallowing disorders, hypo-albuminemia, hyperphosphoremia, renal failure, liver disease, and Gram-negative pneumonia (Janssens *et al.*, 2004).

Factors associated with a prolonged length of hospital stay are age, delirium, NHAP vs. CAP, roentgenograms suggestive of aspiration, cyanosis, leucocytosis, and presence of band forms in blood smears (Janssens *et al.*, 2004).

Hospitalization for CAP is associated with a high rate of readmission (53–62%) and a high mortality in the year following discharge (24–41%) (Kaplan *et al.*, 2002; Bohannon *et al.*, 2004; Torres *et al.*, 2004). Aspiration pneumonia and total number of comorbidities were identified as predictive of readmission within a year of discharge. In the large study by Kaplan *et al.* (2003), 1-year mortality increased from 29% for patients without comorbidities to 57% in patients with $\geq$3 comorbidities. Factors reported as significantly related to death were Barthel Index scores (quantifying dependence in activities of daily life), peripheral muscle strength (handgrip), and absolute number of comorbidities.

A recent French prospective case-control study focused on risk factors for nosocomial pneumonia (NP) in a geriatric hospital; 75 cases were identified, with a complication rate of 58% and a 12% mortality (Rothan-Tondeur *et al.*, 2003). Most significant risk factors for NP were prior NP, oxygen therapy, NGT feeding, and malnutrition.

Clinical Presentation of CAP and NHAP

Among the most common symptoms of CAP and NHAP, cough (40–81%), sputum (37–66%), chills (8–58%), and pleural pain (9–43%) are reported less frequently in NHAP than in CAP; conversely, elderly patients present more often with altered mental status (delirium) when hospitalized for NHAP (53–77%) than CAP (12–45%) (Janssens *et al.*, 2004). Fever (12–76%) is frequently absent in elderly subjects with pneumonia.

Tachypnea (respiratory rate >20/min) and tachycardia (>100/min) is found in about two-thirds of elderly with pneumonia and may precede other clinical findings by three to four days (Fein *et al.*, 1991). The classical triad of cough, fever, and dyspnea was present in only 56% of 48 elderly veterans admitted for CAP, and 10% of patients had none of these symptoms (Harper *et al.*, 1989). Subtle clinical manifestations of CAP in the very old, such as unexplained falls, incontinence, failure to thrive, or sudden aggravation of a preexisting comorbidity (i.e., diabetes, congestive heart failure, Parkinson's disease) have to be actively sought after.

The regular (monthly) use of pulse oximetry has been suggested as a simple parameter to help detect pneumonia in nursing home patients. In a study of 67 older nursing home patients, an oxygen saturation (SaO_2) < 94% had a sensitivity for pneumonia of 80%, a specificity of 91% and a positive predictive value of 95%; a drop in SaO_2 of >3% had a sensitivity for pneumonia of 73%, but a specificity and positive predicitive value of 100% (Kaye *et al.*, 2002). Clearly, alternative diagnoses must also be considered in the presence of decreased SaO_2, but LRTI is probably the most frequent cause of desaturation in this setting.

Microbiology of Pneumonia in the Elderly

BACTERIAL PNEUMONIA

In recent clinical studies of older patients with either CAP or NHAP, the most frequently identified microorganisms were *S. pneumoniae*, *H. Influenzae*, Enterobacteriacae, and *S. aureus*.

S. pneumoniae is by far the predominant pathogen isolated in hospital-based studies of elderly patients with either CAP (up to 58%) or NHAP (up to 30%) (Riquelme *et al.*, 1996; Lieberman *et al.*, 1997; Marrie *et al.*, 1997; Riquelme *et al.*, 1997; Lim *et al.*, 2001; Kaplan *et al.*, 2002; Zalacain *et al.*, 2003). In older subjects treated in the ICU, *S. pneumoniae* reportedly causes 14% of CAP and 9% of NHAP (El-Solh *et al.*, 2001). The presence of *S. pneumoniae* is associated with coexisting lung disease, hepatic disorders, or alcohol abuse.

H. influenzae is reported in up to 14% of older patients with CAP or NHAP, and was identified in 7% of elderly subjects with severe pneumonia leading to admission to an ICU (El-Solh *et al.*, 2001). *H. influenzae* is frequently linked to exacerbations of COPD and bronchiectasis and thus should be considered as a potential pathogen in these patients.

Staphylococcus aureus was documented in up to 7% of patients with CAP and 4% of patients with NHAP. One study shows an even higher occurrence of *S. aureus*-related pneumonia. Of 104 elderly patients with severe CAP or NHAP admitted to an ICU, 17% had (mostly methicillin-sensitive) *S. aureus* as causative agent (El-Solh *et al.*, 2001). In this study, *S. aureus* was identified in 29% of the patients with severe NHAP (78% methicillin-sensitive) vs. 7% of those with CAP (all methicillin-sensitive). Because of the increasing rate of MRSA colonization in the nursing home population, and the relatively high probability for MRSA carriers of developing symptomatic infection, MRSA pneumonia is likely to become a more frequently encountered entity. *S. aureus* is associated with lung abscess, empyema, and secondary bacterial pneumonia after viral respiratory infection.

Enteric Gram-negative bacteria (GNB)

Both colonization by, and infection with, GNB is a function of the number and severity of comorbidities (Valenti *et al.*, 1978). The likelihood of GNB pneumonia increases in nursing home patients and in patients with decreased functional status. In a community setting, GNB infection occurs primarily in debilitated and chronically ill patients. The presence of *Pseudomonas* suggests bronchiectasis (Fein *et al.*, 1994). If appropriate, the presence of bronchiectasis should be investigated by high-resolution computed tomography; indeed, the presence of bronchiectasis warrants prolonged treatment for LTRI (14 to 21 days).

AGENTS OF ATYPICAL PNEUMONIA

M. pneumonia is seldom reported as a causative agent in CAP or LRTI in the very old (1–13%) (Janssens *et al.*, 1996; Marrie *et al.*, 1997; Riquelme *et al.*, 1997; Lim *et al.*, 2001; Kaplan *et al.*, 2002), and has not been identified in elderly patients admitted to the ICU for severe CAP (El-Solh *et al.*, 2001).

C. pneumoniae infection in the elderly generally is considered a mild disease and was reported in only 1% of patients admitted to ICU for CAP (El-Solh *et al.*, 2001). However, *C. pneumoniae* has been reported in up to 18% of NHAP and 28% of CAP. Occasional *C. pneumoniae* outbreaks in nursing homes have been associated with a high attack rate (44–68%) and high mortality (~35%) of confirmed cases (Troy *et al.*, 1997). *C. pneumoniae* has no specific clinical presentation but the combination of pharyngitis or hoarseness (laryngitis) and nonproductive cough should suggest *C. pneumoniae* infection. Duration of illness > 8 days before admission also increases the probability of *C. pneumoniae* infection (Socan *et al.*, 2004). A case-control study comparing older patients admitted for *C. pneumoniae* CAP vs. non-*C. pneumoniae* CAP, showed that residing in a nursing home vs. living at home was associated with a marked increase in the probability of *C. pneumoniae* infection. *C. pneumoniae* infection can be identified by direct fluorescent antibody staining, nasopharyngeal swabs (PCR or culture), or retrospectively by serology.

Prevalence of *L. pneumophilia* in CAP shows important geographic variations, being in the range of 1.8 to 24% in hospital-based studies (Janssens *et al.*, 1996). In Switzerland, 261 cases of definite *L. pneumophilia* infection were reported between 1999 and 2001 (incidence: 1.7 per 10^5 inhabitants). Median age of patients infected was 61 years; that of patients dying from the infection was 67 years; 34% of subjects infected were aged over 70 (OFSP, 2003). *Legionella sp.* infection was community-acquired in 60%, travel-related in 27%, and hospital- or nursing home-acquired in 10% and 3% of cases, respectively (OFSP, 2003). Colonization of potable water in long-term care institutions and geriatric hospitals is a potential hazard for *Legionella sp.* infection.

Because of a low to moderate sensitivity of diagnostic tests, the incidence of *Legionella* infection may be underestimated in clinical studies. Indeed, sensitivity of serology ranges from 40 to 60%; that of direct fluorescent antibody staining of sputum is 30 to 70% (specificity of 94–99%), and sputum culture has a sensitivity of approximately 80% (Stout *et al.*, 1997). The most useful test, namely dosage of urinary *Legionella* antigen is highly specific (100%), yet has a sensitivity of 79 to 83%, increasing to 94% if only *L. pneumophilia* serogroup 1 is considered (Stout *et al.*, 1997; Helbig *et al.*, 2001).

Infection by *Legionella* is frequently heralded by an abrupt onset of malaise, weakness, headaches, and myalgia (Bentley 1984). Most patients cough; hemoptysis occurs in one-third of patients. Mental status changes are reported in 25 to 75% of older patients. Other associated features are bradycardia, liver dysfunction, diarrhea, and hyponatriemia, but none of these features are specific and all may occur with severe pneumonia of other etiologies.

The probability of *L. pneumophilia* infection increases in severe CAP or NHAP and must definitely be considered in this setting (El-Solh *et al.*, 2001). Interestingly, in a study of older patients with pneumonia admitted to the ICU, *L. pneumophilia* infection was strongly associated with immunosuppression: 60% of patients had been under prolonged corticosteroid therapy. In up to 65% of patients, radiographic findings initially worsen after treatment has been started, and even after 10 weeks of therapy, only 50% of chest radiographs are normal (Macfarlane *et al.*, 1984).

VIRAL INFECTION

Viral infection (adenovirus, Respiratory Syncitial Virus (RSV), influenza, parainfluenza, rhinoviruses) may cause up to 42% of acute LRTI during the winter months in institutionalized elderly subjects, RSV being the most common viral pathogen in this setting (Falsey *et al.*, 1992; Falsey *et al.*, 1995). In community-acquired LRTI, a history of a familial flu-like illness, better functionality, and a lower leucocyte count ($<10^{10}$/L) are predictive of viral infection (Flamaing *et al.*, 2003). Among patients admitted to a hospital for CAP or NHAP, viruses are the causative agents in 2 to 32% of patients admitted, influenza, RSV, and parainfluenza being the most commonly implicated (Falsey *et al.*, 1995; Janssens *et al.*, 1996; El-Solh *et al.*, 2001; Fernandez-Sabe *et al.*, 2003; Zalacain *et al.*, 2003). In a recent prospective study of healthy elderly subjects, followed for up to two winter seasons, clinical RSV infection occurred in 3 to 7% of healthy elderly and 4 to 10% of high-risk elderly subjects. Although symptoms of RSV and Influenza A were similar, RSV led to less physician and emergency room visits than Influenza A and was associated with a lower use of antibiotics (Falsey *et al.*, 2005). Influenza A is reported in 1.5 to 26% of admissions for CAP or LRTI (Fernandez-Sabe *et al.*, 2003; Flamaing *et al.*, 2003; Saldias Penafiel *et al.*, 2003; Zalacain *et al.*, 2003; Torres *et al.*, 2004). Para-influenza and RSV were identified respectively in 1 to 1.3% and 0.6 to 3.6% of admissions (Fernandez-Sabe *et al.*, 2003; Flamaing *et al.*, 2003; Zalacain *et al.*, 2003).

MYCOBACTERIAL INFECTION

Older subjects are today the main reservoir of tuberculosis infection in the indigenous population of industrialized countries. The incidence of tuberculosis in patients aged over 65 is higher than in all other age groups, except for HIV-infected subjects. In Switzerland, the incidence of tuberculosis in patients aged over 70 ($20/10^5$ inhabitants) is 2.5 times that of the general population. Comorbidities, immunosenescence, malnutrition, and immunosuppressive therapy all contribute to the higher incidence of tuberculosis in this age group.

Clinical presentations of mycobacterial infection in the elderly are often atypical, leading to delayed diagnosis. Thus, mortality of tuberculosis is much higher than in younger age groups, and increases with age. When compared to younger adults, elderly patients with active tuberculosis have less cough, fever, hemoptysis, and night sweats. Their tuberculin skin test is more often negative (32% vs. 10% in younger subjects) (Katz *et al.*, 1987; Korzeniewska-Kosela *et al.*, 1994; Mathur *et al.*, 1994; Chan *et al.*, 1995). On chest roentgenograms, older subjects have more frequent lower or middle lobe involvement, miliary tuberculosis, and atypical presentations (solitary nodules, pseudo-masses, and infiltrates resembling bronchopneumonia), and a lower incidence of cavitary lesions (Korzeniewska-Kosela *et al.*, 1994; Chan *et al.*, 1995). Finally, tuberculostatic treatment is associated with an age-related increase in side-effects (mainly hepatotoxicity).

UNUSUAL ORGANISMS

Pulmonary cryptococcosis and nocardiosis have been reported in nonimmuno-compromised older patients (Laszlo *et al.*, 2001; Nadrous *et al.*, 2003). Chronic necrotizing pulmonary aspergillosis and actinomycosis must be considered in older patients with slowly evolving pulmonary infiltrates, malnutrition, weight loss, immunosuppressive therapy, and preexisting chronic pulmonary disorders. Atypical mycobacteria (mainly *Mycobacterium avium-intracellulare* complex) may cause a slowly evolving destructive pulmonary infection, occurring more frequently in nonsmoking women (80%), who present with a chronic cough (86%), fatigue (42%), prolonged fever (10–14%), progressive weight loss leading to cachexia (14–52%), and nonspecific pulmonary infiltrates (Prince *et al.*, 1989; Kennedy *et al.*, 1994). Over the past years, several reports have drawn attention to the possibility of opportunistic infections (i.e., *P. Carinii* pneumonia, unusual presentations of tuberculosis), revealing unsuspected HIV infection in older patients (McMeeking *et al.*, 1989; Rosenzweig *et al.*, 1992; Chen *et al.*, 1998; Cloud *et al.*, 2003; Laszlo *et al.*, 2003).

When the Pneumonia Doesn't Get Better

In patients who are poorly responsive to adequate antibiotic treatment, alternative diagnoses must be explored. Unusual pathogens and mycobacterial infection must be rapidly ruled out, whenever possible by fiberoptic bronchoscopy. Noninfectious disorders—which may mimic pneumonia—must be considered, such as pulmonary infarction, cryptogenic organizing pneumonia (previously referred to as idiopathic bronchiolitis obliterans organizing pneumonia, or BOOP), vasculitis (Wegener's granulomatosis, or Churg-Strauss Syndrome), bronchocentric granuloma, mucous plugging with infiltrates in allergic broncho-pulmonary aspergillosis, idiopathic acute eosinophilic pneumonia, chronic eosinophilic pneumonia, and carcinoma (mainly bronchoalveolar carcinoma). Cavitary lesions suggestive of pulmonary abscess in fact may be excavated primary pulmonary tumors, or vasculitis (Wegener's granulomatosis).

Conclusion

In this chapter, we focused on the pathogenic mechanisms leading to pneumonia in older individuals. Aging is associated with important changes in respiratory mechanics (decreased compliance of the respiratory system and strength of the respiratory muscles, increased work of breathing for a given level of ventilation), which increase the vulnerability of the very old to any further aggression to the respiratory tract. Higher rates of aspiration occur in this age group, with frequently occurring risk factors such as cerebro-vascular events, or extrapyramidal disorders. Efficacy of mucociliary clearance mechanisms, including cough, tends to decrease in the very old. Aspiration of oro-pharyngeal secretions is the most important cause of LRTI: oro-pharyngeal flora is influenced by dental status and comorbidities. Increasing morbidity leads to colonization of upper airways by pathogenic micro-organisms such as GNB and *S. aureus*. As in younger subjects, *S. pneumoniae* remains the most frequently identified pathogen. Atypical organisms play a minor role in CAP or NHAP, although the contribution of *C. pneumoniae* may be underestimated. Unusual organisms and alternative diagnoses must be rapidly considered and sought after in nonresolving pneumonia.

REFERENCES

Annoni, J.M., Ackermann, D., and Kesselring, J. (1990). Respiratory function in chronic hemiplegia. *Int Disabil Stud 12(2)*, 78–80.

Aslanyan, S., Weir, C.J., Diener, H.C., Kaste, M., and Lees, K.R. (2004). Pneumonia and urinary tract infection after acute ischaemic stroke: A tertiary analysis of the GAIN International trial. *Eur J Neurol 11(1)*, 49–53.

Bentley, D.W. (1984). Bacterial pneumonia in the elderly: Clinical features, diagnosis, etiology, and treatment. *Gerontology 30*, 297–307.

Bohannon, R.W., Maljanian, R., and Ferullo, J. (2004). Mortality and readmission of the elderly one year after hospitalization for pneumonia. *Aging Clin Exp Res 16(1)*, 22 25.

Chan, C.H.S., Woo, J., Or, K.K.H., Chan, R.C.Y., and Cheung, W. (1995). The effect of age on the presentation of patients with tuberculosis. *Tubercle and Lung Disease 76*, 290–294.

Chen, H.X., Ryan, P.A., Ferguson, R.P., Yataco, A., Markowitz, J.A., and Raksis, K. (1998). Characteristics of acquired immunodeficiency syndrome in older adults. *J Am Geriatr Soc 46(2)*, 153–156.

Cloud, G.C., Browne, R., Salooja, N., and McLean, K.A. (2003). Newly diagnosed HIV infection in an octogenarian: The elderly are not "immune." *Age Ageing 32(3)*, 353–354.

Croghan, J.E., Burke, E.M., Caplan, S., and Denman, S. (1994). Pilot study of 12-month outcomes of nursing home patients with aspiration on videofluoroscopy. *Dysphagia 9(3), 141–146.*

Cummings, S.R. and Melton, L.J. (2002). Epidemiology and outcomes of osteoporotic fractures. *Lancet 359(9319)*, 1761–1767.

Cuttitta, G., Cibella, F., Bellia, V., Grassi, V., Cossi, S., Bucchieri, S. *et al.* (2001). Changes in FVC during methacholine-induced bronchoconstriction in elderly patients with asthma: bronchial hyperresponsiveness and aging. *Chest 119(6)*, 1685–1690.

El-Solh, A.A., Pietrantoni, C., Bhat, A., Aquilina, A.T., Okada, M., Grover V. *et al.* (2003). Microbiology of severe aspiration pneumonia in institutionalized elderly. *Am J Respir Crit Care Med 167(12)*, 1650–1654.

El-Solh, A.A., Pietrantoni, C., Bhat, A., Okada, M., Zambon, J., Aquilina, A. *et al.* (2004). Colonization of dental plaques: A reservoir of respiratory pathogens for hospital-acquired pneumonia in institutionalized elders. *Chest 126(5)*, 1575–1582.

El-Solh, A.A., Sikka, P., Ramadan, F., and Davies, J. (2001). Etiology of severe pneumonia in the very elderly. *Am J Respir Crit Care Med 163(3 Pt 1)*, 645–651.

Enright, P.L., Kronmal, R.A., Higgins, M., Schenker, M., and Haponik F. (1993). Spirometry reference values for women and men 65 to 85 years of age. *Am Rev Respir Dis 147*, 125–133.

Enright, P.L., Kronmal, R.A., Manolio, T.A., Schenker, M.B., and Hyatt, R.E. (1994). Respiratory muscle strength in the elderly: Correlates and reference values. *Am J Respir Crit Care Med 149*, 430–438.

Evans, S., Watson, L., Hawkins, M., Cowley, A., Johnston, I., and Kinnear, W. (1995). Respiratory muscle strength in chronic heart failure. *Thorax 50*, 625–628.

Falsey, A.R., Cunningham, C.K., Barker, W.H., Kouides, R.W., Yuen, J.B., Menegus, M. *et al.* (1995). Respiratory syncytial virus and influenza A infections in the hospitalized elderly. *J Infect Dis 172(2)*, 389–394.

Falsey, A.R., Hennessey, P.A., Formica, M.A., Cox, C., and Walsh, E.E. (2005). Respiratory syncytial virus infection in elderly and high-risk adults. *N Engl J Med 352(17)*, 1749–1759.

Falsey, A.R., McCann, R.M., Hall, W.J., Tanner, M.A., Criddle, M.M., Formica, M.A. *et al.* (1995b). Acute respiratory tract infection in daycare centers for older persons. *J Am Geriatr Soc 43(1)*, 30–36.

Falsey, A.R., Treanor, J.J., Betts, R.F.,and Walsh, E.E. (1992). Viral respiratory infections in the institutionalized elderly: Clinical and epidemiologic findings. *J Am Geriatr Soc 40(2)*, 115–119.

Fang, T.J., Li, H.Y., Tsai, F.C., and Chen, I.H. (2004). The role of glottal gap in predicting aspiration in patients with unilateral vocal paralysis. *Clin Otolaryngol 29(6)*, 709–712.

Fein, A. (1994). Pneumonia in the elderly. Special diagnostic and therapeutic considerations. *Med Clin N Amer 78*, 1015–1033.

Fein, A.M., Feinsilver, S.H., and Niederman, M.S. (1991). Atypical manifestations of pneumonia in the elderly. *Clin Chest Med 12(2)*, 319–336.

Fein, A.M. and Niederman, M.S. (1994). Severe pneumonia in the elderly. *Med Clin N Amer 10*, 121–143.

Fernandez-Sabe, N., Carratala, J., Roson, B., Dorca, J., Verdaguer, R., Manresa F. *et al.* (2003). Community-acquired pneumonia in very elderly patients: Causative organisms, clinical characteristics, and outcomes. *Medicine (Baltimore) 82(3)*, 159–169.

Flamaing, J., Engelmann, I., Joosten, E., Van Ranst, M., Verhaegen, J., and Peetermans, W.E. (2003). Viral lower respiratory tract infection in the elderly: a prospective in-hospital study. *Eur J Clin Microbiol Infect Dis 22(12)*, 720–725.

Harper, C. and Newton, P. (1989). Clinical aspects of pneumonia in the elderly veteran. *J Am Geriatr Soc 37(9)*, 867–872.

Helbig, J.H., Uldum, S.A., Luck, P.C., and Harrison, T.G. (2001). Detection of *Legionella pneumophila* antigen in urine samples by the BinaxNOW immunochromatographic assay and comparison with both Binax Legionella Urinary Enzyme Immunoassay (EIA) and Biotest Legionella Urin Antigen EIA. *J. Med Microbiol 50(6)*, 509–516.

Heuschmann, P.U., Kolominsky-Rabas, P.L., Misselwitz, B., Hermanek, P., Leffmann, C., Janzen, R.W. *et al.* (2004). Predictors of in-hospital mortality and attributable risks of death after ischemic stroke: The German Stroke Registers Study Group. *Arch Intern Med 164(16)*, 1761–1768.

Ho, J.C., Chan, K.N., Hu, W.H., Lam, W.K., Zheng, L., Tipoe, G.L. *et al.* (2001). The effect of aging on nasal mucociliary clearance, beat frequency, and ultrastructure of respiratory cilia. *Am J Respir Crit Care Med 163(4)*, 983–988.

Imsand, M., Janssens, J.P., Auckenthaler, R., Mojon, P., and Budtz-Jorgensen, E. (2002). Bronchopneumonia and oral health in hospitalized older patients. A pilot study. *Gerodontology 19(2)*, 66–72.

Janssens, J., Pache, J., and Nicod, L. (1999). Physiological changes in respiratory function associated with ageing. *Eur Respir J 13*, 197–205.

Janssens, J.P., Gauthey, L., Herrmann, F., Tkatch, L., and Michel, J.P. (1996). Community-acquired pneumonia in older patients. *J Am Geriatr Soc 44(5)*, 539–544.

Janssens, J.P. and Krause, K.H. (2004). Pneumonia in the very old. *Lancet Infect Dis 4(2)*, 112–124.

Johanson, W.G., Pierce, A.K., and Sanford, J.P. (1969). Changing pharyngeal bacterial flora of hospitalized patients. Emergence of gram-negative bacilli. *N Engl J Med 281(21)*, 1137–1140.

Johnson, J.C., Jayadevappa, R., Baccash, P.D., and Taylor, L. (2000). Nonspecific presentation of pneumonia in hospitalized older people: Age effect or dementia? *J Am Geriatr Soc 48(10)*, 1316–1320.

Kaplan, V., Angus, D.C., Griffin, M.F., Clermont, G., Scott Watson, R., and Linde-Zwirble, W.T. (2002). Hospitalized community-acquired pneumonia in the elderly: Age- and sex- related patterns of care and outcome in the United States. *Am J Respir Crit Care Med 165(6)*, 766–772.

Kaplan, V., Clermont, G., Griffin, M.F., Kasal, J., Watson, R.S., Linde-Zwirble, W.T. *et al.* (2003). Pneumonia: still the old man's friend? *Arch Intern Med 163(3)*, 317–323.

Katz, P., Reichman, W., and Dube, D. (1987). Clinical features of tuberculosis in young and old veterans. *J Amer Geriatr Soc 35*, 512–515.

Kaye, K.S., Stalam, M., Shershen, W.E., and Kaye, D. (2002). Utility of pulse oximetry in diagnosing pneumonia in nursing home residents. *Am J Med Sci 324(5)*, 237–242.

Kennedy, T.P. and Weber, D.J. (1994). Nontuberculous mycobacteria: An underappreciated cause of geriatric lung disease. *Am J Respir Crit Care Med 149*, 1654–1658.

Kikuchi, R., Watabe, N., Konno, T., Mishina, N., Sekizawa, K., and Sasaki, H. (1994). High incidence of silent aspiration in elderly patients with community-acquired pneumonia. *Am J Respir Crit Care Med 150*, 251–253.

Korzeniewska-Kosela, M., Krysl, J., Müller, N., Black, W., Allen, E., and FitzGerald, J.M. (1994). Tuberculosis in young adults and the elderly: A prospective comparison study. *Chest 106*, 28–32.

Kronenberg, R. and Drage, G. (1973). Attenuation of the ventilatory and heart rate responses to hypoxia and hypercapnia with aging in normal man. *J Clin Invest 52*, 1812–1819.

Laszlo, A., Gianelli, S., Laurencet, F., Krause, K.H., and Janssens, J.P. (2003). Successful treatment of disseminated tuberculosis and acquired immunodeficiency syndrome in an 81-y-old woman. *Scand J Infect Dis 35(6–7)*, 420–422.

Laszlo, A., Lambert, V., Michel, J.P., and Janssens, J.P. (2001). Acute community acquired pneumopathy caused by Nocardia asteroides in a 93-year-old female patient. *Ann Med Interne (Paris) 152(6)*, 407–409.

Leibovitz, A., Dan, M., Zinger, J., Carmeli, Y., Habot, B., and Segal, R. (2003a). *Pseudomonas aeruginosa* and the oropharyngeal ecosystem of tube-fed patients. *Emerg Infect Dis 9(8)*, 956–959.

Leibovitz, A., Plotnikov, G., Habot, B., Rosenberg, M., and Segal, R. (2003b). Pathogenic colonization of oral flora in frail elderly patients fed by nasogastric tube or percutaneous enterogastric tube. *J Gerontol A Biol Sci Med Sci 58(1)*, 52–55.

Leibovitz, A., Plotnikov, G., Habot, B., Rosenberg, M., Wolf, A., Nagler, R. *et al.* (2003c). Saliva secretion and oral flora in prolonged nasogastric tube-fed elderly patients. *Isr Med Assoc J 5(5)*, 329–332.

Lieberman, D., Schlaeffer, F., and Porath, A. (1997). Community-acquired pneumonia in old age: A prospective study of 91 patients admitted from home. *Age Ageing 26(2)*, 69–75.

Lim, W.S. and Macfarlane, J.T. (2001). A prospective comparison of nursing home acquired pneumonia with community acquired pneumonia. *Eur Respir J 18(2)*, 362–368.

Macfarlane, J.T., Miller, A.C., Roderick Smith, W.H., Morris, A.H., and Rose, D.H. (1984). Comparative radiographic features of community acquired Legionnaires' disease, pneumococcal pneumonia, mycoplasma pneumonia, and psittacosis. *Thorax 39(1)*, 28–33.

Marik, P.E. (2001). Aspiration pneumonitis and aspiration pneumonia. *N Engl J Med 344(9)*, 665–671.

Marrie, T.J. and Blanchard, W. (1997). A comparison of nursing home-acquired pneumonia patients with patients with community-acquired pneumonia and nursing home patients without pneumonia. *J Am Geriatr Soc 45(1)*, 50–55.

Mathur, P., Sacks, L., Auten, G., Sall, R., Levy, C., and Gordin, F. (1994). Delayed diagnosis of pulmonary tuberculosis in city hospitals. *Arch Intern Med 154*, 306–310.

McMeeking, A.A., Schwartz, L., and Garay, S. (1989). Don't forget AIDS at any age. *J Am Geriatr Soc 37(12)*, 1204–1205.

Morrison, R.S. and Siu, A.L. (2000). Survival in end-stage dementia following acute illness. *Jama 284(1)*, 47–52.

Mylotte, J.M., Goodnough, S., and Naughton, B.J. (2003). Pneumonia versus aspiration pneumonitis in nursing home residents: Diagnosis and management. *J Am Geriatr Soc 51(1)*, 17–23.

Nadrous, H.F., Antonios, V.S., Terrell, C.L., and Ryu, J.H. (2003). Pulmonary cryptococcosis in nonimmunocompromised patients. *Chest 124(6)*, 2143–2147.

Niimi, A., Matsumoto, H., Ueda, T., Takemura, M., Suzuki, K., Tanaka, E. *et al.* (2003). Impaired cough reflex in patients with recurrent pneumonia. *Thorax 58(2)*, 152–153.

Nishimura, Y., Maeda, H., Tanaka, K., Nakamura, H., Hashimoto, Y., and Yokoyama, M. (1994). Respiratory muscle strength and hemodynamics in chronic heart failure. *Chest 105*, 355–359.

OFSP (2003). La legionellose en Suisse de 1999 à 2001 (Legionella infection in Switzerland from 1999 to 2001). *Bulletin de l'OFSP (Federal Agency for Public Health) 120(7)*, 116–120.

Peterson, D., Pack, A., Silage, D. *et al.* (1981). Effects of aging on ventilatory and occlusion pressure responses to hypoxia and hypercapnia. *Am Rev Respir Dis 124*, 387–391.

Polkey, M.I., Harris, M.L., Hughes, P.D., Hamnegard, C.-H., Lyons, D., Green, M. *et al.* (1997). The contractile properties of the elderly human diaphragm. *Am J Respir Crit Care Med 155*, 1560–1564.

Prince, D., Peterson, D., Steiner, R., Gottlieb, J., Scott, R., Israel, H. *et al.* (1989). Infection with mycobacterium avium complex in patients without predisposing conditions. *N Engl J Med 321*, 863–868.

Quanjer, P., Tammeling, G., Cotes, J., Pederson, O., Peslin, R., and Yernault, J. (1993). Lung volumes and forced expiratory flows. *Eur Respir J Suppl 16*, 5–40.

Riquelme, R., Torres, A., El-Ebiary, M., de la Bellacasa, J.P., Estruch, R., Mensa, J. *et al.* (1996). Community-acquired pneumonia in the elderly. A multivariate analysis of risk and prognostic factors. *Am J Respir Crit Care Med 154(5)*, 1450–1455.

Riquelme, R., Torres, A., el-Ebiary, M., Mensa, J., Estruch, R., Ruiz, M. *et al.* (1997). Community-acquired pneumonia in the elderly. Clinical and nutritional aspects. *Am J Respir Crit Care Med 156(6)*, 1908–1914.

Rosenzweig, R. and Fillit, H. (1992). Probable heterosexual transmission of AIDS in an aged woman. *J Am Geriatr Soc 40(12)*, 1261–1264.

Rothan-Tondeur, M., Meaume, S., Girard, L., Weill-Engerer, S., Lancien, E., Abdelmalak, S. *et al.* (2003). Risk factors for nosocomial pneumonia in a geriatric hospital: a control-case one-center study. *J Am Geriatr Soc 51(7)*, 997–1001.

Saldias Penafiel, F., O'Brien Solar, A., Gederlini Gollerino, A., Farias Gontupil, G., and Diaz, A. Fuenzalida (2003). Community-acquired pneumonia requiring hospitalization in immunocompetent elderly patients: clinical features, prognostic factors and treatment. *Arch Bronconeumol 39(8)*, 333–340.

Socan, M., Kosmelj, K., Marinic-Fiser, N., and Vidmar, L. (2004). A prediction model for community-acquired *Chlamydia pneumoniae* pneumonia in hospitalized patients. *Infection 32(4)*, 204–209.

Stout, J.E. and Yu, V.L. (1997). Legionellosis. *N Engl J Med 337(10)*, 682–687.

Strong, R.M., Condon, S.C., Solinger, M.R., Namihas, B.N., Ito-Wong, L.A., and Leuty, J.E. (1992). Equal aspiration rates from postpylorus and intragastric-placed small-bore nasoenteric feeding tubes: A randomized, prospective study. *JPEN J Parenter Enteral Nutr 16(1)*, 59–63.

Sund-Levander, M., Ortqvist, A., Grodzinsky, E., Klefsgard, O., and Wahren, L.K. (2003). Morbidity, mortality and clinical presentation of nursing home-acquired pneumonia in a Swedish population. *Scand J Infect Dis 35(5)*, 306–310.

Terpenning, M. and Shay, K. (2002). Oral health is cost-effective to maintain but costly to ignore. *J Am Geriatr Soc 50(3)*, 584–585.

Tolep, K., Higgins, N., Muza, S., Criner, G., and Kelsen, S. (1995). Comparison of diaphragm strength between healthy adult elderly and young men. *Am J Respir Crit Care Med 152*, 677–682.

Torres, O.H., Munoz, J., Ruiz, D., Ris, J., Gich, I., Coma, E. *et al.* (2004). Outcome predictors of pneumonia in elderly patients: importance of functional assessment. *J Am Geriatr Soc 52(10)*, 1603–1609.

Tracy, J.F., Logemann, J.A., Kahrilas, P.J., Jacob, P., Kobara, M., and Krugler, C. (1989). Preliminary observations on the effects of age on oropharyngeal deglutition. *Dysphagia 4(2)*, 90–94.

Troy, C.J., Peeling, R.W., Ellis, A.G., Hockin, J.C., Bennett, D.A., Murphy, M.R. *et al.* (1997). *Chlamydia pneumoniae* as a new source of infectious outbreaks in nursing homes. *JAMA 277(15)*, 1214–1218.

Tzeng, A.C. and Bach, J.R. (2000). Prevention of pulmonary morbidity for patients with neuromuscular disease. *Chest 118(5)*, 1390–1396.

Valenti, W.M., Trudell, R.G., and Bentley, D.W. (1978). Factors predisposing to oropharyngeal colonization with gram-negative bacilli in the aged. *N Engl J Med 298(20)*, 1108–1111.

Watando, A., Ebihara, S., Ebihara, T., Okazaki, T., Takahashi, H., Asada, M. *et al.* (2004). Daily oral care and cough reflex sensitivity in elderly nursing home patients. *Chest 126(4)*, 1066–1070.

Yoneyama, T., Yoshida, M., Ohrui, T., Mukaiyama, H., Okamoto, H., Hoshiba, K. *et al.* (2002). Oral care reduces pneumonia in older patients in nursing homes. *J Am Geriatr Soc 50(3)*, 430–433.

Zalacain, R., Torres, A., Celis, R., Blanquer, J., Aspa, J., Esteban, L.R. *et al.* (2003). Community-acquired pneumonia in the elderly: Spanish multicentre study. *Eur Respir J 21(2)*, 294–302.

55

Diabetes and Aging

Tamas Fulop, Anis Larbi, Daniel Tessier, and André Carpentier

During the last decades, life expectancy has increased dramatically, leading to the augmentation of the number of elderly subjects around the world. This increase in the proportion of the elderly population is even more remarkable in those over 85 years of age. In the meantime, the incidence and prevalence of age-related diseases are also increasing markedly. The most common diseases associated with aging are infections, cancers, cardiovascular diseases, and type 2 diabetes. Approximately 20% of the adults in the United States have developed diabetes mellitus by the age of 65, according to the National Health and Nutritional Examination Survey (NHANES III). Type 2 diabetes is a multifactorial disease involving complex interactions of genetic and environmental factors. The three major pathophysiological features leading to type 2 diabetes are (1) β-cell dysfunction manifested by decreased insulin secretion; (2) impaired insulin-mediated glucose disposal associated with impaired muscle insulin signaling; and (3) enhanced hepatic glucose production.

Aging, most probably per se, is related to several physiological changes that will favor the appearance of these pathophysiological features. Thus type 2 diabetes as a model of aging as well as of premature aging may ultimately help us unravel the fundamental keys to the aging process. Although new breakthroughs in basic research will help us identify and design best-fitted interventions for our patients, more advances are also needed in translational research to gain maximal efficiency in implementing these new findings into clinical practice. This chapter will review the potential age-associated changes leading to increased type 2 diabetes mellitus incidence with aging.

Introduction

Life expectancy has increased markedly during the last century, which resulted in the augmentation of the elderly population. Among this elderly population the proportion of those over 85 years has increased even more dramatically. This phenomenon is accompanied by the enhancement of the incidence and prevalence of age-related diseases. The most common age-related diseases are infections, cancers, cardiovascular diseases and type 2 diabetes mellitus. Data from the epidemiological studies show unequivocally that the incidence of type 2 diabetes mellitus rises steeply with age (Wilson *et al.*, 1986). Age is one of the most important variables influencing the prevalence of impaired glucose tolerance (IGT) and type 2 diabetes starting from 40 years of age (Finucane *et al.*, 2001). Type 2 diabetes has marked impacts on the aging subjects as it affects not only carbohydrate metabolism, but also lipid and protein metabolism. Over time, this disease has a profound influence on the development of dysfunctions of the cardiovascular system, the kidneys, the eyes, and the peripheral nervous system so common in the aging population. Thus, type 2 diabetes contributes heavily to the morbidity and mortality, and to the economic burden associated with aging of our population. This chapter will deal with the specific characteristics of the disease in relation to age.

Definition, Diagnosis, and Epidemiology

The diagnosis of diabetes should be made on the basis of a fasting plasma glucose level of 126 mg/dL (7.0 mmol/L) or greater on at least two occasions (Standards, 2005; Halter, 1999). The diagnosis could also be made with an OGTT when the plasma glucose level is higher than 200 mg/mL (11.1 mmol/L) two hours post-challenge (Standards, 2005; Halter, 1999). These criteria have been chosen based on longitudinal studies demonstrating plasma glucose levels associated with an increased risk for retinopathy. Approximately 50% of the elderly population have impaired glucose tolerance (IGT) with normal fasting plasma glucose level. Impaired glucose tolerance (IGT) is defined as a glucose level over 140 mg/dL (7.8 mmol/L), but less than 200 mg/dL (11.1 mmol/L) two hours after a 75 g oral glucose tolerance test (OGTT) (Standards, 2005; Halter, 1999). This is an intermediate stage in the alteration of glucose metabolism and, as such, a strong predictor for the development of type 2 diabetes. The rate of conversion of IGT to diabetes was found to be between 3.6% for women and 8.7% for men per year (Yudkin *et al.*, 1993). Although individuals with IGT do not develop the microvascular complications associated with type 2 diabetes, they are at high risk of developing cardiovascular diseases and are also at higher risk of mortality attributable to cancer (Saydah *et al.*, 2003).

Handbook of Models for Human Aging

TABLE 55.1
Risk factors for the development of type 2 diabetes

Risk factors
Advancing age
Increasing BMI
Central adiposity accumulation (larger waist circumference)
Physical inactivity
Having first-degree relatives with type 2 diabetes
Non-Caucasian ethnic origin
Prior delivery of a large for gestational age baby or previous diagnosis of gestational diabetes
Hypertension
Low HDL level—<0.35 mg/dl (0.9 mmol/L)
High plasma triglyceride level—>250 mg/dl (2.82 mmol/L)
Diagnosis of polycystic ovary syndrome
IGT or IFG
Presence of acanthosis nigricans
Known cardiovascular disease

Adapted from Wilson *et al.*, 1986.

Another intermediate stage between the normal metabolic state and type 2 diabetes is impaired fasting glucose (IFG), defined as a fasting plasma glucose between 100 and 125 mg/dl (5.6 to 6.9 mmol/L) (Standards, 2005). IFG is also associated with a higher risk of developing type 2 diabetes, although it is not as strong a marker for the risk of cardiovascular and cancer as IGT (Saydah *et al.*, 2003; Muntner *et al.*, 2004). Together, IGT and IFG (so-called pre-diabetes) can be found in approximately 12 million individuals aged between 45 and 75 years old in the United States (Benjamin *et al.*, 2003).

The ADA recommends that screening for diabetes begin at age 45 years and be performed at three-year intervals, but at a younger age and shorter intervals in high-risk patients such as overweight individuals (BMI $\geq$ 25 kg/m^2) with one or more risk factors (see Table 55.1) (Standards, 2005). Nowadays the most useful and used diagnostic tool is the determination of fasting plasma glucose level. The OGTT is more cumbersome to apply to large populations and may be less reproducible than measurement of fasting plasma glucose. However, OGTT is also more sensitive than fasting plasma glucose level for the diagnosis of type 2 diabetes and has the advantage of identifying those individuals with impaired glucose tolerance.

Approximately 20% of the adults in the United States have developed diabetes mellitus by the age of 65, according to the National Health and Nutritional Examination Survey (NHANES III) (Harris *et al.*, 1987). This prevalence has progressively grown over the past 30 years. The prevalence of diabetes mellitus is approximately two per 1000 among those less than 45 years old, and steadily increases with age in subjects older than 75 (Harris, 1993; Meneilly *et al.*, 2001). Due to the long, asymptomatic progression to type 2 diabetes, a large proportion of patients are unaware that they have this disease and may have developed end-organ damages by the time of diagnosis. Thus, the increasing prevalence of diabetes mellitus with age results in the several-fold increase of the well-known concomitant complications, including end-stage renal disease, loss of vision, myocardial infarction, stroke, peripheral vascular diseases, and peripheral neuropathy. The risk of lower extremity amputation is increased by 10-fold in the presence of diabetes mellitus. More strikingly, diabetes is associated with a 10-year reduction of the life expectancy and is associated with a higher mortality at any age (Halter, 1999).

Type 2 diabetes is a multifactorial disease involving complex interactions of genetic and environmental factors. The three major pathophysiological features leading to type 2 diabetes are (1) β-cell dysfunction manifested by decreased insulin secretion; (2) impaired insulin-mediated glucose disposal associated with impaired muscle insulin signaling; and (3) enhanced hepatic glucose production (Stumvoll *et al.*, 2005). Apart from age, overweight and central adiposity are important risk factors, associated with more than 80% of cases of diabetes in the adult population. Overweight and central adiposity accumulation are also associated with other classical cardiovascular risk factors including hypertension, dyslipidemia, impaired fibrinolysis, and pro-thrombotic state, which together are referred to as the metabolic syndrome. Recently, the role of adverse *in utero* environment associated with growth retardation and failure to thrive during the first year of life have been found predictive of the later development of IGT or type 2 diabetes (Jimenez-Chillaron *et al.*, 2005; McMillen *et al.*, 2005).

Age-related Risk and Etiologic Factors for Diabetes Mellitus Type 2

Poor diet, genetic factors, obesity, and lack of exercise may partly explain the increased prevalence of glucose intolerance and type 2 diabetes with advancing age. Among the confounding factors for the development of type 2 diabetes associated with aging, the most important are increased body adiposity and reduced lean body mass. These changes are characteristic of the aging process, but individually can be found in many pathological states with similar untoward metabolic consequences. The concomitant occurrence of these body composition changes and aging *per se* probably has an important impact on the development of type 2 diabetes in elderly.

BODY COMPOSITION CHANGES AND OBESITY

Aging is characterized by a profound reshaping of the body composition (Hughes *et al.*, 2004). There is a typical decline in the lean body mass, while the fat cell mass is increasing. The reduction of lean body mass is explained mainly by loss of muscle mass, a process called *sarcopenia* (Nair, 2005; Clarke, 2004). The decline of muscle mass has been estimated to be about 6% per decade between the age of 30 and 80. The exact cause of this decline is not known, but neuro-endocrine factors, reduced spontaneous and conscious physical activity, and intrinsic protein metabolic changes in muscles contribute to sarcopenia (Balagopal *et al.*, 1997). Reduced mitochondrial function in muscle associated with impaired production of ATP is felt to play an important role in the pathogenesis of age-associated sarcopenia (Nair, 2005). It is also of interest to note that reduced muscle production of ATP is present very early in young, insulin-resistant offspring of patients with type 2 diabetes (Petersen *et al.*, 2004), suggesting a link between mitochondrial dysfunction and muscle insulin resistance. However, mitochondrial dysfunction and biogenesis improve with aerobic training, whereas insulin sensitivity does not in the elderly (Short *et al.*, 2003). Why, then, is sarcopenia a serious risk factor for insulin resistance and consequently for type 2 diabetes in elderly subjects? The muscle is the primary site for insulin-mediated glucose disposal and, therefore, the reduction of muscle mass with aging may seriously affect glucose metabolism.

Furthermore, the frailty syndrome in the elderly is characterized by a frailty phenotype described by Fried *et al.* (2001) including sarcopenia, thus being a risk factor for insulin resistance. Moreover, as mentioned, the decreased supply in proteins and energy *in utero* and during the first year of life is a risk factor for IGT and type 2 diabetes. These factors associated with low birth weight also indicate a higher risk for frailty. Thus, the early growth retardation is a risk factor for both frailty and type 2 diabetes mellitus via perhaps the development of sarcopenia with aging.

Most dramatically, not only is there an increase in the fat cell mass but also its distribution is changing, because this enhancement is due to an enrichment at the abdominal site (central distribution). This central redistribution of the fat cell mass has dramatic consequences for the metabolic environment and is a risk factor for several obesity and age-related metabolic abnormalities. Thus, the frontier between aging and obesity is very thin (Harris, 1999). Interestingly, the normal relationship between total body fat mass and circulating leptin levels appears to be disrupted in the elderly, suggesting that abnormal secretion of this adipostat may play a role in body fat changes with aging (Moller *et al.*, 1998). The increase in visceral and central fat cell mass with or without reduction of peripheral fat mass has dramatic consequences for the metabolic environment and is a risk factor for several obesity and age-related metabolic abnormalities, such as hypertension and hyperlipidemias (Lewis *et al.*, 2002). Weight gain or central redistribution of fat clearly has been associated with the development of type 2 diabetes (Koh-Banerjee *et al.*, 2004). This anatomical distribution is accompanied by an increase in plasma free fatty acid (FFA) levels (Raz *et al.*, 2005) and appearance rate, reduced adiponectin secretion, and the enhanced secretion of pro-inflammatory molecules (e.g., tumor necrosis factor (TNF)-α and interleukin-6) (Unger, 2003; Eckel *et al.*, 2005; Sharma *et al.*, 2005). Altogether, these changes favor the apparition of insulin resistance and may also have an untoward impact on beta cell function over time (Lewis *et al.*, 2002). However, as long as the pancreatic beta cell insulin secretory response can compensate for this increase of insulin resistance, euglycemia will be maintained. Once this compensation is overwhelmed, insulin resistance leads to a progressive reduction of glucose tolerance and, eventually, to type 2 diabetes.

LOW-GRADE INFLAMMATION

There are now accumulating data that aging is associated with a low-grade inflammation, coined InflammAging by Claudio Franceschi (Franceschi *et al.*, 2000). This status reflects an imbalance between the innate and the adaptive immune response. Whereas the pro-inflammatory cytokines such as IL-6, TNF-α are increasing, originating in particular from monocytes/macrophages as those infiltrating the various adipose tissues (Mazurek *et al.*, 2003; Weisberg *et al.*, 2003), those coming from the adaptive immune response are decreasing. In the meantime, as a compensatory mechanism, the anti-inflammatory cytokines originating from Th-2 cells of the adaptive immune response are also increasing. These changes add to the already increased production of pro-inflammatory cytokines by the increased abdominal fat cell mass (Unger, 2003; Eckel *et al.*, 2005; Sharma *et al.*, 2005). Indeed, central fat not only contributes to insulin resistance by direct secretion of pro-inflammatory cytokines, but also by the release of FFA, which, in turn, can stimulate the NFkB activation through the phosphorylation of IKB via IKK leading to the production of more pro-inflammatory cytokines. Thus, increased pro-inflammatory cytokine levels participate in the development of the insulin resistance. In this context IL-6 was also associated with the frailty syndrome leading to loss of independence and poor prognosis.

Interactions between Type 2 Diabetes and Other Pathological States Associated with Aging

THE NEURO-ENDOCRINE DYSFUNCTION

Recently, epidemiological studies have demonstrated an increased prevalence of cognitive impairment associated with diabetes. In the Third National Health and Nutrition Examination Survey (NHANES III), type 2 diabetes, combined with hypertension, was significantly associated with impaired cognitive function in subjects younger than 60 years old (Pavlik *et al.*, 2005). Patients with

Alzheimer's disease suffer from a marked increase in prevalence of type 2 diabetes, whereas the presence of brain plaques in patients with type 2 diabetes correlates with the duration of diabetes (Janson *et al.*, 2004). Experimental models have suggested that the brain mitochondrial toxicity associated with neurotoxic agents such as beta amyloid deposits may be exacerbated by the presence of diabetes (Moreira *et al.*, 2003).

As described earlier, aging is associated with a low-grade inflammation. This manifests itself also at the neuro-endocrine level by a relative sustained increase of cortisol and adrenergic hormone levels in elderly subjects (Valenti, 2004). The stress hormones such as cortisol may contribute to the development of insulin resistance. In case of acute events, such as illnesses, the effect of these stress hormones may be accentuated, contributing to the occurrence of type 2 diabetes. The contributing effect of cortisol on impaired glucose tolerance or type 2 diabetes could be through its ill-defined age-dependent effects on the innate immune response or direct interference with insulin-mediated glucose disposal. The α-adrenergic effect of catecholamines by inhibiting insulin secretion further accentuates the contribution of age-related hormonal changes to insulin resistance in diabetes mellitus. The activation of serine kinase via the catecholamine-mediated cAMP dependent kinase inhibits the tyrosine phosphorylation of the insulin receptor, contributing to insulin resistance with aging. Thus, the increase in cortisol and noradrenalin levels seen with aging may contribute in many ways to the development of IGT and type 2 diabetes.

Recently, the role of the enteroinsular axis was assessed in relation to the age-dependent glucose intolerance. Glucose-dependent insulinotropic polypeptide (GIP) and glucagon-like peptide 1 (GLP-1), two gut hormones whose secretion is stimulated by the ingestion of glucose, are incretin hormones that potentiate insulin secretion. Their basal levels as well as their levels after OGTT have been found unchanged in elderly obese and nonobese healthy elderly individuals. A study using the hyperglycemic clamp technique showed that GIP sensitivity may be impaired in older subjects (Meneilly *et al.*, 1998). Recently, however, it has been shown that incretin-mediated muscle glucose uptake was markedly impaired in elderly type 2 diabetes patients (Chang *et al.*, 2003). Further studies are needed to establish more firmly the role of incretins in the beta cell defect and type 2 diabetes associated with aging.

ADIPOSE TISSUE DYSFUNCTION

There are only scarce data on the contribution of adipose tissue dysfunction to the etiology of diabetes mellitus type 2 in relation to aging. The role of the adipose tissue is well established in relation to the increased release of free fatty acids (FFA) interfering with insulin signaling in insulin-sensitive tissues (Lewis *et al.*, 2002). The loss of peripheral fat tissue in hereditary or acquired lipodystrophic syndromes has been associated with intramyocellular and intrahepatic fat accumulation, profound insulin resistance, and type 2 diabetes (Lewis *et al.*, 2002). Recently, a cross-sectional study in a large cohort of elderly has shown an association between higher subcutaneous thigh fat and favorable plasma glucose and triglyceride levels, independent of visceral fat (Snijder *et al.*, 2005). However, there is almost no data to show how central adipose tissue redistribution with aging may contribute to increased pro-inflammatory cytokine production, including TNF-α, compared to that of the innate immune cells such as monocyte/macrophages. Moreover, the role of adipocytokine secretion is also controversial with aging (Ryan *et al.*, 2003; Kanaya *et al.*, 2004). Leptin is released from adipocytes and acts on the central nervous system to decrease appetite. Lower, higher, and no change in leptin levels have been reported in the elderly.

The strong positive correlation between fat mass and circulating leptin levels was found to be disrupted in elderly subjects (Moller *et al.*, 1998), suggesting an impairment of the feedback between peripheral fat stores and appetite regulation, which may contribute to the increased prevalence of obesity with age. Adiponectin has an insulin-sensitizing effect in the liver and skeletal muscles associated with the activation of AMP kinase (Ouchi *et al.*, 2000; Masuzawa, 2005). In obesity and insulin resistance, plasma adiponectin levels are decreased. Although data are very scarce concerning adiponectin level changes with aging, they seem to indicate an age-related decrease. Very recently, higher adiponectin levels were associated with lower odds of diabetes in older men and women (mean age 73 years) (Masuzawa, 2005). Furthermore, low adiponectin levels were associated with the development of the metabolic syndrome in healthy elderly Koreans (Choi *et al.*, 2004). In this context animal models of diabetes could have some contribution, but the study of diabetes and aging is rarely exploited together. This would be interesting to develop an aging model progressing to diabetes for the study of the adipose tissue contribution.

LIPOTOXICITY

Much attention has been turned recently on the role of free fatty acids in type 2 diabetes. As already mentioned, enhanced fat cell mass releases higher amounts of FFA, leading to enhanced plasma FFA flux and exposure of insulin-sensitive tissues (Lewis *et al.*, 2002). FFAs are known to interfere with insulin-mediated GLUT4 translocation to the sarcolemma and with glucose phosphorylation in muscles, leading to impaired insulin-mediated glucose disposal and insulin resistance. This could happen through the activation of the PKC pathway, which can phosphorylate IRS molecules on serine/threonine residues, thus reducing downstream signaling. FFA can also stimulate neoglucogenesis in the liver. Though FFA can also act on β-cells to sustain insulin release during the fasting state, chronically elevated circulating FFA levels result in intracellular accumulation of long chain acyl CoAs (LC-CoAs) within the beta cells. These LC-CoAs interfere with the glucose-dependent closure of K_{ATP}-channel activity and impairs insulin secretion. FFAs also interfere with the physiological oscillation of calcium and insulin secretion granule exocytosis. The recent observation of a link between impaired fatty acid oxidation and other effects on beta cells could be the reduction of ATP formation leading to decreased insulin secretion and the induction of beta cell apoptosis (lipapoptosis) by induction of ceramid formation or of cytotoxic oligomers of islet amyloid polypeptide formation. By enhancing the generation of superoxide radicals by the respiratory chain, FFAs may also induce the expression of UCP2 in beta cell mitochondria, leading to reduced coupling of oxidative phosphorylation and ATP production, and impaired glucose-stimulated insulin secretion (Lowell *et al.*, 2005). In addition to their role as constituent molecules and sources of energy, FFA can also behave as signaling molecules on PPARs and HNFs, although the potential pathophysiological roles for these interactions remain elusive for the moment. In the context of insulin resistance due to type 2 diabetes and aging, the adipose tissue is subject to an imbalance between fatty acid oxidation in muscle and liver (energy) and lipogenesis *de novo* (lipotoxicity). Thus, by contributing to the impairment of insulin-mediated glucose disposal, enhanced hepatic glucose production, and impaired glucose-stimulated insulin secretion, FFAs may potentially contribute to the development of type 2 diabetes associated with aging.

GLUCOTOXICITY

Hyperglycemia as a hallmark of diabetes mellitus, in turn, is known to contribute directly to insulin resistance as well as potentially interfering with normal pancreatic cell function, thereby setting the stage for a vicious circle of maladaptative mechanisms. Hyperglycemia, through the deregulation of K_{ATP}-channel, exerts a toxic effect on insulin secretion via the intracellular Ca^{2+} oscillation mediated by voltage-gated channels. The exposition of beta cells to chronic hyperglycemia as well as free fatty acids alter the insulin secretion induced by glucose.

PRODUCTION OF ADVANCED GLYCATION END PRODUCTS (AGES)

One important consequence of IGT and type 2 diabetes is the formation of AGEs. An important role for the production of advance glycation end products (AGE) and oxidative stress can be evoked not only as a potential mechanism for microvascular and macrovascular complications of diabetes, but also as a contributing factor to insulin resistance. Glucose irreversibly modifies macromolecules with a slow turnover by forming AGEs as a function of glucose concentration and time. Indeed, it has been shown that AGEs are accumulating with aging, in diabetes and in Alzheimer's disease (Vlassara *et al.*, 2003). AGEs will react with their specific receptors (RAGE) leading to various harmful pathological processes, including endothelial dysfunction and cognitive impairment.

During the formation of AGEs as well as during their interaction with RAGEs, free radicals are produced. Thus, free radicals not only were implicated as a cause and a consequence of the aging process, but also as a consequence of hyperglycemia. AGEs as well as free radicals may directly influence or interfere with the insulin receptor (IR) function and signal transduction by diminishing the tyrosine phosphorylation of IRS1/2, which in turn becomes unable to recruit the p85α subunit of PI3-kinase. Furthermore, this will result in reduced PKB activity and consequently altered glucose and glycogen metabolism. Moreover, chronic oxidative stress, by chronically oxidizing PTP1B, alters IR activity and signaling. These processes will also interfere with the membrane composition with aging, regulating the localization of IR to lipid rafts. Thus, the aging process, either through oxidative stress or through the development of hyperglycemia, interferes with IR function and signal transduction leading to insulin resistance. We will address this issue further in the chapter.

GENETICS

There is strong genetic predisposition for type 2 diabetes mellitus. Studies with identical twins showed a high rate of concordance for type 2 diabetes. Recently, the heritability of beta cell dysfunction in type 2 diabetes was found to be 84% in old and 75% in young twins, suggesting a predominant genetic effect that gains more impact with age (Poulsen *et al.*, 2005). In that same study, the heritability of insulin-mediated glucose disposal and insulin-mediated nonoxidative glucose disposal was ~50% and did not change with age, whereas hepatic glucose production appears to be mainly related to environmental factors. Multiple genes are involved in different individuals. So far only calpain 10 has been identified. The HLA DR3 serotype is more common in older adults who require insulin treatment. The exact nature of these genes is still unknown; however, the discovery of the predisposing genes to diabetes via perhaps the sarcopenia susceptibility genes and the central adiposity regulating genes could lead to important therapeutic breakthrough as well as to eventual prevention tools.

Pathogenesis of Diabetes Mellitus Type 2 in Relation to Aging

ALTERED INSULIN ACTION: INSULIN RESISTANCE

One factor clearly contributing to this age-related glucose intolerance is a decline with physiologic aging in sensitivity to the metabolic effects of insulin; that is, the reduction of insulin sensitivity. This means a reduction in the activity of insulin on its target tissues such as muscle, liver, and adipose tissue. In the muscle this results in a decrease of glucose disposal. In the adipocytes this results in the inability of insulin to inhibit the lipolysis leading to the release of free fatty acids in the circulation. These FFAs in turn stimulate hepatic neoglucogenesis and VLDL secretion, reduce muscle glucose uptake, and may alter glucose-stimulated insulin secretion by beta cells. This age-related impairment of insulin action appears to be predominantly due to effects on the insulin signaling mechanism beyond the insulin receptor itself. However, the latter also may be involved to some extent (Fulop *et al.*, 2003). In the liver the resistance results in the inadequate suppression of the endogenous glucose production even in the presence of hyperglycemia. The gold standard technique for measuring the insulin resistance in humans is the hyperinsulinemic glucose clamp; this technique involves a fixed dose of insulin being administered and then normal glucose concentrations being maintained by the infusion of glucose given (the glucose infusion rate or M-value), which reflects insulin sensitivity and is an inverse measure of insulin resistance. Of special note, as already mentioned, is that the insulin resistance alone does not cause the type 2 diabetes; it should be associated with the insulinopenia as occurring in many cases with aging. This is discussed later.

There is still some debate to elucidate whether this altered insulin sensitivity is due to the aging process *per se* or is determined by external, mainly lifestyle, factors such as body composition changes or decrease in physical activity. However, actually it seems that aging *per se* could have a fundamental influence. Euglycaemic clamp studies consistently demonstrate that elderly individuals are insulin resistant and that the dose response curve for insulin is shifted to the right (Moller *et al.*, 2003). This impairment of insulin action affects the mobilization of glucose transporters, which are critical to glucose uptake and metabolism in insulin-dependent tissues such as muscle, liver, and fat.

The insulin receptor signal transduction

The insulin receptor (IR) and the insulin-like growth factor receptor (IGFR) belong to the receptor tyrosine kinase (RTK) super-family. However, the signal transduction by these receptors mainly occurs via the insulin receptor substrate (IRS) adapter proteins (IRS1 to 4) (Capeau, 2003). IRS proteins seem to present a further important regulatory step in the insulin receptor activation. The degree of serine/threonine (S/T) phosphorylation determines either positively or negatively the signal transmission via IRS proteins. During insulin stimulation, the phosphatidylinositol-3 kinase (PI3K) becomes activated via the IRS association as well as the Ras-MAPK pathway leading to glucose transport activation through GLUT-4 and to other metabolic actions as well as to mitogenesis and differentiation, respectively. However, this needs the tyrosine phosphorylation of IRS after their binding to the juxtamembrane region of the activated IR.

In contrast, the over-phosphorylation of the S/T could explain that the tyrosine phosphorylation of IRS does not occur in the presence of insulin and leads to insulin resistance (Greene *et al.*, 2002). This over-phosphorylation of S/T also could be induced by tumor necrosis factor (TNF-α) or chronic increase in the insulin level as may occur during aging. It was also demonstrated that suppressors of cytokine signaling (SOCS), well known for their inhibitory effect on the Jak/STAT pathway, also exert a regulatory action on IRS. Recently, the regulating role of several tyrosine phosphatases such as LAR, SHP-2, PTP-1B in insulin signaling were recognized. Specific actions of insulin are frequently mediated by distinct intracellular signaling pathways. As already mentioned, activated IR through the tyrosine phosphorylation of IRS recruit the PI3K and Akt. This will induce in adipose, muscle, and liver tissues, insulin-stimulated translocation of the glucose transporter GLUT4 from intracellular vesicles to the cell surface, whereas Ras pathways mediate mitogenic effects of insulin. The recently discovered lipid rafts' contribution is just being elucidated in the context of IR signaling.

IR signal transduction changes with aging

Data obtained concerning insulin receptors (IR) and glucose transporters in aging are contradictory; nevertheless they suggest that neither changes in IR number and affinity nor changes in the glucose transporters could be sufficient to explain the insulin resistance with aging. It is of note that the glucose transporter translocation from vesicles to the membrane in the context of newly discovered lipid rafts has not been investigated in the context of aging. Studies concerning the insulin receptor kinase activity in animal models, resulting in phosphorylation, showed conflicting results with aging. Studies in rats showed that basal and insulin stimulated autophosphorylation of liver insulin receptor and its kinase activity did not change with aging (Kono *et al.*, 1990). On the other hand the rat skeletal insulin receptor kinase activity showed different results, indicating that phosphorylation changed with aging (Kono *et al.*, 1990). Another study has shown that insulin stimulated IR autophosphorylation has been decreased in both liver and muscle of 20-month-old rats (Carvalho *et al.*, 1996). These contradictory results might be explained by the different tissues studied that are not equally sensitive to the aging process or by the different techniques used.

Carvalho *et al.* (1996) also showed that IRS-1 protein levels decreased at a relatively young age (5 months) by 58% and remained at this low level in muscle, though not in liver. Moreover, other signal transduction changes were shown, including decreased IRS-1 phosphorylation, decreased IRS-1 association with the PI3-kinase, and decreased phosphotyrosine associated PI3-kinase activity upon stimulation by insulin in both muscle and liver tissues of 20-month-old rats. Other studies have also shown that with aging in rats, the insulin receptor and the p85 alpha subunit of PI3-kinase both declined by about 40%, whereas in the meantime these parameters did not change with aging in the skeletal muscle (Martineau *et al.*, 1999). Altogether the bulk of the experimental data suggest that alterations in the early signal transduction events of insulin might have an important role in the insulin resistance observed with aging.

After having described insulin receptor signal transduction changes in cells and in tissue of aging animal models, the question is raised whether identical alterations could be found in humans in view of the increased insulin resistance with human aging. Strangely, only a few studies have examined this question. We have shown with healthy aging in monocytes and neutrophils an alteration in the cAMp and cGMP production under insulin receptor stimulation (Fulop *et al.*, 1987). With aging the cAMP level was increased, whereas that of cGMP did not change. The exact role of this signaling pathway in the insulin effects is mostly unknown, but mainly related to the modulation of the IR tyrosine phosphorylation as shown for adrenergic hormones. A recent study—although not in aged healthy humans, but in insulin-resistant, obese humans—demonstrated that in muscle, insulin signaling by PI3-kinase is impaired, whereas the MEK/MAPK pathway undergoes a normal insulin-dependent stimulation (Cusi *et al.*, 2000). The question concerning the role of these various signaling pathways in various tissues is raised in an insulin-resistance state related to the physiological aging process itself. Altogether, clinical data suggest a marked insulin resistance with aging in humans; however, the biochemical and molecular basis of this insulin resistance level mainly in insulin-sensitive tissues including muscle, adipocytes, and liver is still waiting to be unraveled. Altogether this deterioration of insulin sensitivity with aging, via signaling alterations, contributes to the increased incidence of type 2 diabetes.

How IR signaling changes integrate the general receptor signal alterations found in aging

There is much experimental evidence that aging is associated with an altered signal transduction in the case of many receptors including dopamine, insulin, adrenergic, and T cell receptors. One ultimate common point of all these receptors is their localization in the membrane that transduces information to the nucleus. Recent studies suggested that the plasma membrane in mammalian cells is not homogenously organized, but contain specific microdomains in composition and function (Razzaq *et al.*, 2004). These microdomains—also called lipid rafts—are specially enriched in cholesterol and sphingolipids and proteins that are mainly involved in receptor signaling. Thus, these lipid rafts are involved mainly in signal transduction and membrane trafficking.

It has been well known for a long time that the membrane composition is altered with aging because the membrane fluidity is decreasing. This is mainly due to an enrichment in cholesterol, as well as to the age-related oxidative stress, and ultimately leads to marked functional alterations. One fundamental property of lipid rafts is their ability to move laterally in the membrane; thus, the rigidification of the membrane with aging could interfere with this mobility (Larbi *et al.*, 2004). Also, the signaling alterations found with aging, including that of insulin receptor, could be due to an alteration at the membrane level, as was demonstrated in T lymphocytes. Wherever IR are localized in the membrane (i.e., in caveolae containing cells or in lipid rafts containing cells), aging has been clearly associated with changes in cell membrane properties. This would establish a unifying cause to the altered signal transduction occurring with aging. Moreover, receptor internalization, reexpression, or degradation by proteasome may also be other points where defects or changes could lead to the induction or the chronicity of insulin resistance and its consequences as described earlier.

PANCREATIC BETA CELL DYSFUNCTION

The role of impaired insulin secretion due to pancreatic beta cell dysfunction in age-related glucose intolerance and type 2 diabetes has been well known from animal studies. In humans this aspect of type 2 diabetes has remained controversial during a long period (Chang *et al.*, 2003). This was probably due to the earlier failure of taking into account the degree of insulin resistance in the evaluation of beta cell function *in vivo* with techniques such as the OGTT. The relationship between insulin secretion and insulin sensitivity follows a hyperbolic curve so that a reduction in insulin sensitivity normally is associated with an increase in insulin secretion. Thus, similar absolute insulin secretion observed in older vs. younger individuals suggests inappropriate beta cell response in view of the reduced insulin sensitivity in the former group. This only very recently was recognized in IGT and type 2 diabetes of elderly subjects by methods able to assess insulin sensitivity as well as pre-hepatic insulin secretion by deconvolution of the peripheral C-peptide levels with C-peptide kinetics (Chang *et al.*, 2003). The Baltimore Longitudinal Study confirmed, after adjustment of all confounding parameters (e.g., adiposity), that insulin levels were significantly decreased with aging. It was shown in human subjects that the post-hepatic insulin delivery dropped by 25% between the ages of 18 and 85 years when age-related increase in insulin resistance was taken into account. Another recent study has demonstrated that age is independently associated with reduced beta cell function, whereas visceral fat accumulation was associated with both beta cell dysfunction and reduced insulin sensitivity (Utzschneider *et al.*, 2004).

This reduction of beta cell function occurs in the presence of normal or even higher secretion of gut incretin hormones such as glucose-dependent insulinotropic polypeptide (GIP) and glucagons-like peptide 1 (GLP-1), suggesting beta cell resistance to these hormones in the elderly. Reduced arginine-stimulated insulin secretion has also been observed in older subjects and may indicate a reduction in beta cell mass with aging.

The pancreatic beta cell dysfunction seen with aging is associated with alterations of glucose-stimulated insulin pulse mass, kinetics, and rhythmicity. Normally, insulin is secreted in a pulsatile manner that insures a higher sensitivity at the receptor level and lower needs for secretion. This pulsatile secretion is controlled by the oscillation of the intra-cytoplasmic calcium level. In type 2 diabetes, there is an over-activity of plasma membrane K_{ATP}-channel due to chronic hyperglycemia altering electrical activity by Ca^{2+} and consequently the insulin secretion. With aging, calcium metabolism was shown to be altered in various cell types; thus it is plausible that this also occurs in pancreatic cells. Moreover, if intracellular calcium concentration remains high, this could result in the apoptosis of pancreatic cells, potentially contributing to the significant 20 to 40% reduction of beta cell mass associated with type 2 diabetes. Thus, a tight control of calcium metabolism is essential, and its alteration could lead to pancreatic beta cell dysfunction.

Aging is not only characterized by the loss of beta cell mass but also by a progressive loss of beta cell function (Chang *et al.*, 2003; Elahi *et al.*, 2002). How is insulin secretion evaluated? In the case of nondiabetic humans the OGTT was widely used to measure the insulin level at fasting state and after glucose challenge. As mentioned, the OGTT is a complex test to interpret. Thus, an intravenous glucose tolerance test was used with frequent sampling. The results in elderly subjects were not conclusive following these studies. Beta cell function can be better evaluated with the hyperglycemic clamp technique. During this procedure the plasma glucose levels are increased to the same extent above the basal levels in subjects by means of intravenous glucose infusions. The introduction of the insulin resistance factor contributed to the elucidation of the relative decrease of insulin secretion related to insulin resistance. More recently, the use of pulsatile insulin release technique and nonglucose stimuli such as arginine have detected age-related defects in insulin secretion. Thus, the most important alteration seems to be the decrease of the secretion of insulin (both low-amplitude and ultradian pulses), either at the basal status or after glucose and nonglucose challenge. This also could be one component of the type 2 diabetes in aging as the β-cells are not able to adapt their insulin secretion to the insulin resistance status, as was shown in a few studies mainly performed by Meneilly *et al.* (Meneilly *et al.*, 1997). Finally, the quantity of the secreted insulin is decreasing progressively in time, even if the insulin resistance remains stable as shown in the six-year follow-up data from the UKPDS.

One hypothesis put forward to explain the age-related decline in insulin secretion is the decline in mitochondrial metabolism, which compromises beta cell ATP production. This in turn might lead to reduced closure of the K_{ATP}-channel, decreased beta-cell depolarization, and lower insulin secretion in response to glucose (Ashcroft *et al.*, 2004). This hypothesis is supported by several lines of evidence. First, accumulation of somatic mutations of the mitochondrial genome is known to occur at an accelerated rate in patients with type 2 diabetes (Nomiyama *et al.*, 2002). Second, mitochondrial dysfunction and reduced production of ATP is seen in skeletal muscles in elderly subjects and also very early in the natural history of type 2 diabetes (Nair, 2005; Petersen *et al.*, 2004). Third, mitochondrial function is critical for the coupling of insulin secretion to glucose metabolism in beta cells by controlling the ratio of ATP/ADP. It has been demonstrated that uncoupling the oxidative mitochondrial metabolism and production of ATP leads to the development of impaired insulin secretion (Lowell *et al.*, 2005). Thus, the decline in mitochondrial energy production may contribute to the higher prevalence of type 2 diabetes in the elderly. Altogether, deterioration of beta cell function with advancing age may contribute to the increased incidence and prevalence of type 2 diabetes, although the underlying mechanism remains largely unknown (see Figure 55.1).

ROLE OF PRO-INFLAMMATORY MEDIATORS

As described, aging is associated with increased levels of pro-inflammatory cytokines originating from the dysfunction of the immune system and from the altered adipose tissue distribution toward a central predominance. These cytokines are known to enhance adipocyte lipolysis, which further increases the FFA levels, which, as mentioned, exert a negative effect on insulin signaling. Thus exists a vicious cycle, as pro-inflammatory cytokines increase FFA levels, which through the activation of NFkB increases the pro-inflammatory cytokines. In rodent models the neutralization of TNF-α was shown to almost reverse insulin resistance. In humans their contribution is still strongly debated.

Complications

The increased glucose levels lead to nonenzymatic modification of proteins called glycation (Vlassara *et al.*, 2003). This is initially reversible, but with time this becomes irreversible, leading to functional alterations. Thus, glycation can affect the activities of many proteins with enzymatic properties. Moreover, glycation can

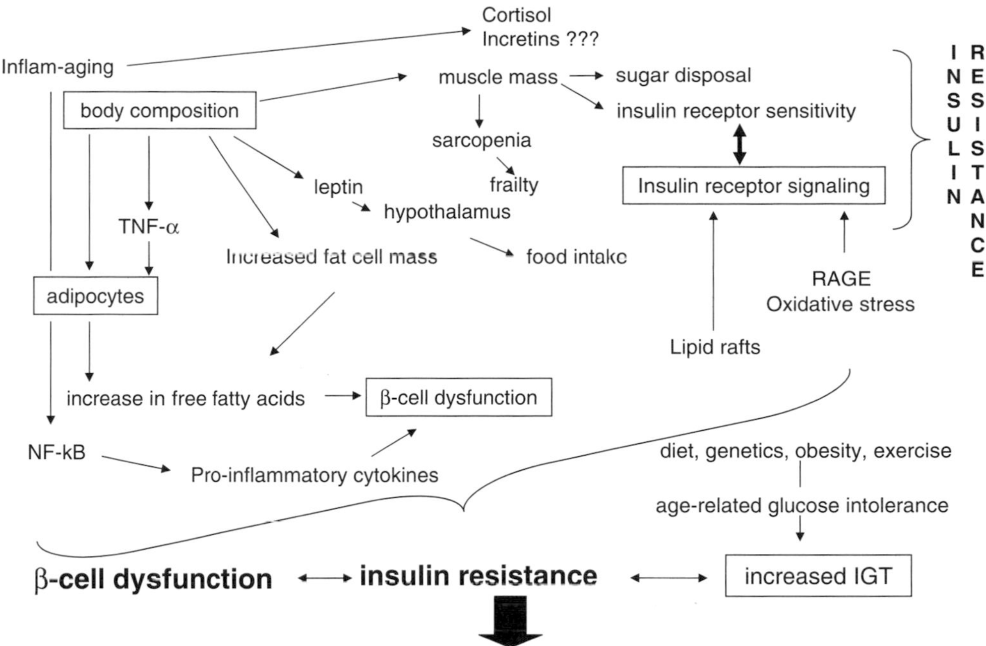

Figure 55.1 Contribution of the aging process to the development of type 2 diabetes mellitus.

render proteins more susceptible to other attack such as oxidation. One of the best studied examples is LDL. OxLDL plays a pathogenic role in the development of atherosclerosis, by inducing an inflammatory process in the vessel wall.

Furthermore, the glycation can progress and lead to the formation of advanced age products (AGE) that can bind to their specific receptors (RAGE). RAGE are particularly present on endothelial cells, glomeruli, mesangial cells, and monocytes. This interaction leads to the activation of various signaling events intracellularly. The overall effect of AGE products is the production of pro-inflammatory signaling molecules such as TNF-α, IGF-I, and GM-CSF. They induce also the proliferation of the connective tissue including collagen type-IV, laminin, and proteoglycans. This production of connective tissue occurs mainly in the kidney glomeruli, in the retina, and in smooth muscle cells. The AGE products develop a chemotactic activity toward monocytes that will infiltrate various target tissues such as kidney, retina, and arterial wall. The AGE products were involved in the development of glomerulosclerosis, mesangial proliferation, monocyte infiltration, and thrombus formation. By these effects AGE products are recognized to be pro-inflammatory, adding their activities to those already well recognized in aging and type 2 diabetes.

One of the most important complications besides nephropathy is retinopathy. They share many common features. The diabetic retinopathy is characterized by the loss of pericytes and microaneurysm formation that contribute to the increased capillary permeability. These changes will progress following ischemia to proliferation of endothelial cells and capillaries hemorrhage. The absence of PDGF-B was incriminated to participate in pericyte death and endothelial proliferation. Moreover, some growth factors enriched intraocularly were also found to be contributing to the proliferating activity. IGF-I seems to play a major role in this context. The AGE-inhibitor aminoguanidine confirmed the role of AGEs specifically in the development of retinopathy.

The role of AGEs in diabetic complications was confirmed by the model of diabetic mice, in which the AGEs level was modulated either exogenously by the diet or endogenously by the administration of aminoguanidine. Furthermore, modulation of the AGE-R3 mediated processing and uptake of AGE in nonobese diabetic (NOD) mice confirmed the role of AGEs in the inflammatory process accompanying diabetes and its complications.

Relationship between Diabetes Mellitus and Aging in the Development of Cardiovascular Diseases

Aging is the single most important risk factor for the development of cardiovascular diseases via the development of atherosclerosis, as it is also for type 2 diabetes. Aging *per se* could present a state of impaired glucose tolerance due to the physiologic changes described. IGT is known to be a risk factor for progression to type 2 diabetes. Aging associated with the occurrence of type 2 diabetes increases several-fold the risk for development of cardiovascular diseases by approximately six to eight times more than aging alone (Nesto, 2003). This is due mainly to the strong occurrence of the classical, including hypertension, dyslipidemia, and nonclassical, including inflammatory cytokines, homocystein, and CRP risk factors. Altogether, the common pathway could be the insulin resistance and insulinopenia-induced hyperglycemia via the production of AGEs and oxidative stress.

Experimental Animal Models

Currently there exist several experimental animal models for the study of diabetes (Mathews, 2002). The most currently used are from rodents. All these animal models mainly reproduce by genetic engineering single specific alterations found in type 2 diabetes. These models try to elucidate one particular pathological aspect of the disease. The most widely used are the leptin-deficient ob/ob$^{-/-}$ mice, db/db$^{+/+}$ mice, K_{ATP}-channel mutated, ApoE deficient mice with other deficiencies, several knock-out mice including for RAGE, for specific signaling molecules for IR, for PTP1B.

In this context new models constantly are being developed, such as a transgenic rat model for human islet amyloid polypetide (IAPP) for studying specifically the loss of beta-cell mass and whether this is occurring by apoptosis (Butler *et al.*, 2004). These rats develop diabetes between 5 and 10 months of age. This model proved very useful to demonstrate certain aspects of the beta-cell toxicity in diabetes mellitus, mainly in the context of glucose toxicity. It is of note that the time of development is very early in life, and perhaps would not be relevant for the age-related effect on diabetes development. Another murine model has been developed to study the role of low birth weight in the development of type 2 diabetes via beta cell dysfunction (Jimenez-Chillaron *et al.*, 2005). This mouse model was developed by undernutrition during pregnancy. These mice developed severe glucose intolerance after six months of age. This is a very useful model; however, the very early development of diabetes renders its application difficult in the context of aging. Nevertheless, this could be a model for some pathophysiological changes occurring as a life-long process in relation to the development of diabetes and perhaps frailty with age. The number of models in development is too many to be enumerated here.

There are only a few models that try to integrate the whole pathophysiological aspects of diabetes like the streptozocine-induced diabetic mice, Zucker fatty rats, Goto-Kakizaki (GK) rats developed by selective breeding of nondiabetic Wistar rats, or the KK. The KK mouse strain shows inherently glucose-intolerance and insulin-resistance (Ikeda, 1994). These mice become easily obese even by aging itself and show an overt diabetic state. Thus, these mice could be a good model for the study of obesity-related diabetes and also for age-related diabetes. This aspect needs further study.

Recently, the use of nonhuman primates also was advocated as being close to human physiology and pathophysiology (Bruns *et al.*, 2004). Obviously their use is not easy and is very costly. Nevertheless, in some circumstances their use, such as the study of factors related to insulin sensitivity, proved to be very rewarding.

Experimental Models Linking Diabetes Mellitus to Aging and Longevity

In some species, caloric restriction (CR) is associated with reduction of aging and increased longevity. It was observed that a reduced body size was correlated to an increased life span in mice, dogs, *Caenorhabditis elegans*, or *Drosophila melanogaster*. One very recent study could not find a clear general effect of body size on life span (Hafen, 2004; McCulloch *et al.*, 2003). The question has been asked why smaller individuals would live longer. One explanation that has been put forward, mainly in invertebrates, is the homologous insulin/IGF signaling (IIS). In *C. elegans* it was suggested that the IIS can act to limit the body size. However, in some wild-type strains this correlation was much less clear. Moreover, several mutations in *C. elegans* led to extended longevity phenotype. Among these are the genes involved in the insulin/IGF-signaling pathway, such as *daf-2* and *age-1*, or *clk* mutants related to respiratory metabolism. Similar results were obtained in *Drosophila*. The study in these model organisms of the IIS pathways contributed in various ways to their understanding. Genetic screens identified novel essential components in the pathways. The relation of these pathways to function helped in physiological conditions to make relation to functions such as growth, differentiation, and cell metabolism. They will continue to remain very useful models and should be extended to type 2 diabetes and aging. In mammals, these correlations do not seem to play an essential role. The data ultimately suggest that body size and longevity are linked in very special circumstances as in CR studies, and this could be related to an increased insulin sensitivity, decreased fasting glucose levels, and possibly oxidative stress.

In the context of human aging, an association between the insulin receptor and longevity can be drawn. Hyperinsulinemia is a characteristic of the diabetes mellitus type 2 as a consequence of insulin resistance due to the resistance of IR signaling to the effect of insulin binding. Hyperinsulinemia is part of the so-called metabolic syndrome characterized by other risk factors such as abdominal obesity, hypertension, and specific dyslipidemia, leading to increased incidence of coronary heart disease. Since atherosclerosis is a disease of later age, it is notable that in euglycemic centenarians insulinemia is low and insulin sensitivity high. This means, as seen in the decreased replicative senescence of cells originated from diabetic subjects, that diabetes type 2 is a model of partial premature aging. Thus, sensitivity, and consequently normal IR signal transduction, are a prerequisite to longevity as shown in caloric restriction studies in rodents and nonhuman primates, as well as in centenarians.

Caloric restriction has been shown to enhance longevity in *Saccharomyces cerevisiae* and *Caenorhabditis elegans* through increased expression of Sir2 (silencing information regulator 2), a NAD^+-dependent histone deacetylase (Wood *et al.*, 2004; Guarente *et al.*, 2005). Sir2 is a member of a family of proteins called sirtuins, which also includes seven mammalian homologues, among which SIRT1 and SIRT3 have been studied in more details. Caloric restriction by increasing NAD^+ levels enhances longevity in mammalian cells by activating the analog SIRT1 (Cohen *et al.*, 2004). SIRT1 is known to target p53 and forkhead transcription factors, among others, for deacetylation (Luo *et al.*, 2004; Motto *et al.*, 2004). SIRT1 also reduces NFκB transcription by deacetylation of RelA/p65 (Yeung *et al.*, 2004), and also further promotes protection against cellular stress and apoptosis by modulating the FOXO transcription factors. In addition, activation of SIRT1 may reduce adipose tissue differentiation, lipogenesis, and increase fat mobilization by suppressing PPAR-γ activation (Picard *et al.*, 2004). SIRT1 appears to link metabolic fasting signals such as increased pyruvate levels in the liver to PGC-1α activation and induction of gluconeogenesis and hepatic glucose production. SIRT1 may also reduce mitochondrial oxidation and biogenesis by acetylating and deactivating PGC-1α, whereas activation of SIRT3 in brown adipose tissue enhances UCP1 expression, thermogenesis, and fat oxidation. Recently, the absence of a VNTR polymorphism of the SIRT3 gene that enhances its expression has been associated with reduced longevity in humans. Streptozocin-induced diabetes in mice has also been associated with the suppression of the expression of one of the sirtuin genes (Yechoor *et al.*, 2004). More studies are needed to determine the full impact of these findings for human health and aging, but these studies offer an introduction into new molecular pathways, possibly linking excessive caloric intake, the development of obesity, and diabetes with reduced longevity.

Recent Advances in Treatment

The recognition that the lipotoxicity link between insulin resistance and beta cell dysfunction has a potential pathogenic mechanism of diabetes type 2 has provided a strong rationale for the introduction of thiazolidinedione (TZDs), which are PPARγ agonists and which target insulin resistance in part through improvement of postprandial fat storage in adipose tissues (Miles *et al.*, 2003; Boden *et al.*, 2005). Large clinical trials are currently ongoing to test whether these drugs can prevent the progression of beta cell dysfunction in the natural history of diabetes and whether their beneficial effects on cardiovascular function observed in small-scale studies can translate into significant benefits in terms of hard cardiovascular end-points (Kanaya *et al.*, 2003).

AGEs could also be the primary target of treatment of the complications of diabetes. Diet is one target as it is a considerable source of exogenous AGEs participating in the alterations of aging and diabetes. Studies in ApoE deficient streptozocin-diabetic mice showed that specific (Vlassara *et al.*, 2003) diets in these animals were associated with significant reduction in serum AGEs. In humans, low AGE-diets diminished the serum levels of inflammatory markers such as cytokines as well as cell adhesion molecules such as VCAM-1. The development of blockers of AGE receptors (RAGEs) bears hope to diminish, if not suppress, the deleterious effects of these compounds on chronic macro- and microvascular complications associated with aging and diabetes mellitus (Flyvbjerg *et al.*, 2004; Hudson *et al.*, 2004). Inhibition of poly(ADP-ribose) polymerase activity or PKC especially in endothelial cells may provide important therapeutic targets in the future to prevent diabetes and aging-related cardiovascular diseases (Booth *et al.*, 2002; Decker *et al.*, 2002; Pacher *et al.*, 2004).

Metformin is an effective antidiabetic drug known to reduce hepatic glucose production through activation of AMP kinase in the liver, a mechanism of action similar to that of adiponectin. Results from the UKPDS study clearly have shown the beneficial effect on the cardiovascular outcome of obese subjects with type 2 diabetes (UK Prospective Diabetes Study, 1998). With regards to prevention of type 2 diabetes in subjects with glucose intolerance, however, metformin clearly is not as effective as small to moderate weight loss through aggressive lifestyle modification, especially in the elderly (Knowler *et al.*, 2002).

GLP-1 agonists and inhibitors of dipeptidyl-peptidase IV, which have been shown to improve glucose tolerance and glucose effectiveness (noninsulin mediated glucose uptake) in younger patients could also prove to be effective therapeutic tools in elderly patients with diabetes. Reduction of the activity of the inhibiting phosphatases such as PTP1B are potential therapeutic targets for the treatment of insulin resistance. A clinical phase II trial is already under way in this field.

Future Research Avenues

One of the promising avenues of research is the elucidation of the mechanisms of beta cell dysfunction with aging. Prevention of beta-cell apoptosis by the modulation of intracellular calcium metabolism or by limiting the age-related lipo- and glucotoxicity might also be exploited in the future.

The investigation of the role of lipid rafts composition and function in impaired insulin signaling in the insulin-resistant state may improve our understanding of the age-related alterations in insulin receptor signaling. In this context the modulation IKK may be an important target for new drug development. The understanding of the role of proteasomes and the negative serine phosphorylation in IR functions also will be essential.

The investigation of age-related muscle mitochondrial dysfunction as a contributing factor to insulin resistance as well as to altered beta cell insulin secretion should be further investigated. The sirtuin-PGC-1α connection merits further intensive investigation.

Although elucidating the molecular mechanisms of diabetes will help identify individuals at highest risk for developing type 2 diabetes and permit the development of new drugs to prevent type 2 diabetes, aggressive lifestyle modification has already been shown to be very effective for the prevention of this disease. The main challenge at this point is to implement the lessons learned in the DPP and the other lifestyle intervention trials in clinical practice, especially with the growing prevalence of diabetes and its complications in an ever-older population. Identifying less labor-intense and expensive but still effective approaches to help elderly patients with diabetes to lose weight will be important to alleviate the obstacles to implementation of the results of these trials. Better prediction of the risk of developing future complications would allow individually tailored interventions and improve the utilization of therapeutic resources and limit costs. The ultimate goal of all this research is to abolish the untoward impact of type 2 diabetes and promote healthy aging.

Conclusion

The aging of the population worldwide and the constantly increasing prevalence of type 2 diabetes constitute an important challenge for the next generation of clinicians and scientists. Type 2 diabetes as a model of premature aging may ultimately help us unravel the fundamental keys to the aging process. Although new breakthroughs in basic research will help us identify and design best-fitted interventions for our patients, more advances also are needed in translational research to gain maximal efficiency in implementing these new findings into clinical practice. Applying the lifestyle measures that we already know work best in a more efficient, cost-effective way will remain an important objective for the next decades in order to reduce the burden of diabetes and aging on humanity.

ACKNOWLEDGMENTS

This work was supported by the Canadian Diabetes Association in honor of the late Marion L. Monroe, and by the Canadian Institutes of Health Research (CIHR) (MOP 53094 and 63149). A.C. is a new investigator of the CIHR.

REFERENCES

Ashcroft, F.M., and Rorsman, P. (2004). Molecular defects in insulin secretion in type-2 diabetes. *Rev Endocr Metab Disord 5*, 135–142.

Balagopal, P., Rooyackers, O.E., Adey, D.B., Ades, P.A., and Nair, K.S. (1997). Effects of aging on in vivo synthesis of skeletal muscle myosin heavy-chain and sarcoplasmic protein in humans. *Am J Physiol 273*, E790–E800.

Benjamin, S.M., Valdez, R., Geiss, L.S., Rolka, D.B., and Narayan, K.M. (2003). Estimated number of adults with prediabetes in the US in 2000: Opportunities for prevention. *Diabetes Care 26*, 645–649.

Boden, G., Homko, C., Mozzoli, M., Showe, L.C., Nichols, C., and Cheung, P. (2005). Thiazolidinediones upregulate fatty acid uptake and oxidation in adipose tissue of diabetic patients. *Diabetes 54*, 880–885.

Booth, G., Stalker, T.J., Lefer, A.M., and Scalia, R. (2002). Mechanisms of amelioration of glucose-induced endothelial dysfunction following inhibition of protein kinase C in vivo. *Diabetes 51*, 1556–1564.

Bruns, C.M., Baum, S.T., Colman, R.J., Eisner, J.R., Kemnitz, J.W., Weindruch, R. *et al.* (2004). Insulin resistance and impaired insulin secretion in prenatally androgenized male rhesus monkeys. *J Clin Endocrinol Metab 89*, 6218–6223.

Butler, A.E., Jang, J., Gurlo, T., Carty, M.D., Soeller, W.C., and Butler, P.C. (2004). Diabetes due to a progressive defect in beta-cell mass in rats transgenic for human islet amyloid polypeptide (HIP Rat): A new model for type 2 diabetes. *Diabetes 53*, 1509–1516.

Capeau, J. (2003). Insulin signaling: mechanisms altered in insulin resistance *Med Sci (Paris) 19*, 834–839.

Carvalho, C.R., Brenelli, S.L., Silva, A.C., Nunez, A.I., Velloso, L.A., and Staad, M.J. (1996). Effect of aging on insulin receptor, insulin receptor substrate-1, and phosphatidylinositol 3-kinase in liver and muscle rats. *Endocrinology 137*, 151–159.

Chang, A.M. and Halter, J.B. (2003). Aging and insulin secretion. *Am J Physiol Endocrinol Metab 284*, E7–E12.

Choi, K.M., Lee, J., and Lee, K.W. (2004). Serum adiponectin concentrations predict the development of type 2 diabetes and the metabolic syndrome in elderly Koreans. *Clin Endocrinol (Oxf) 61*, 75–80.

Clarke, M.S. (2004). The effects of exercise on skeletal muscle in the aged. *J Musculoskelet Neuronal Interact 4*, 175–178.

Cohen, H.Y., Miller, C., Bitterman, K.J., Wall, N.R., Hekking, B., Kessler, B. *et al.* (2004). Calorie restriction promotes mammalian cell survival by inducing the SIRT1 deacetylase. *Science 305*, 390–392.

Cusi, K., Maezono, K., Osman, A., Pendergrass, M., Patti, M.E., Patipanawatr, T. *et al.* (2000). Insulin resitance differentially affects the PI3-kinase and MAPK mediated signaling in human muscle. *J Clin Invest 105*, 597–611.

Decker, P. and Muller, S. (2002). Modulating poly (ADP-ribose) polymerase activity: potential for the prevention and therapy of pathogenic situations involving DNA damage and oxidative stress. *Curr Pharm Biotechnol 3*, 275–283.

Eckel, RH, Grundy, S.M, and Zimmet, P.Z. (2005). The metabolic syndrome. *Lancet 365*, 1415–1428.

Elahi, D., Muller, D.C., Egan, J.M., Andres, R., Veldhuist, J., and Meneilly, G.S. (2002). Glucose tolerance, glucose utilization and insulin secretion in ageing. *Novartis Found Symp 242*, 222–242; discussion 242–246.

Finucane, P., and Popplewell, P. (2001). Diabetes mellitus and impaired glucose regulation in old age: the scale of the problem. In A.J. Sinclair and P. Finucane, Eds. *Diabetes in old age*, pp. 3–16. London: John Wiley and Sons Ltd.

Flyvbjerg, A., Denner, L., Schrijvers, B.F., Tilton, R.G., Mogensen, T.H., Paludan, S.R. *et al.* (2004). Long-term renal effects of a neutralizing RAGE antibody in obese type 2 diabetic mice. *Diabetes 53*, 166–172.

Franceschi, C, Bonafe, M., Valensin, S., Olivieri, F., De Luca, M., Ottaviani, E. *et al.* (2000). Inflamm-aging. An evolutionary perspective on immunosenescence. *Ann N Y Acad Sci 908*, 244–254.

Fried, L.P., Tangen, C.M., Walston, J., Newman, A.B., Hirsch, C., Gottdiener, J. *et al.* (2001). Cardiovascular Health Study Collaborative Research Group. Frailty in older adults: evidence for a phenotype. *J Gerontol A Biol Sci Med Sci 56*, M146–M156.

Fulop, T., Larbi, A., and Douziech, N. (2003). Insulin receptor and ageing. *Pathol Biol (Paris) 51*, 574–580.

Fulop, T. Jr., Nagy, J., Worum, I., Foris, G., Mudri, K., and Udvardy, M. (1987). Glucose intolerance and insulin resistance with aging. Studies on insulin receptors and post-receptor events. *Arch Gerontol Geriatr 6*, 107–115.

Greene, M.W, and Garofalo, R.S. (2002). Positive and negative regulatory role of insulin receptor substrate 1 and 2 (IRS-1 and IRS-2) serine/threonine phosphorylation. *Biochemistry 41*, 7082–7091.

Guarente, L. and Picard, F. (2005). Calorie restriction—the SIR2 connection. *Cell 120*, 473–482.

Hafen, E. (2004). Cancer, type 2 diabetes, and aging: News from flies and worms. *Swiss Med Wkly 134*, 711–719.

Halter J.B. (1999). Diabetes mellitus. In W.R. Hazzard, J.P. Blass, W.H. Ettinger, J.B. Halter, J.G. Ouslander, Eds. *Principles of Geriatric Medicine and Gerontology, 4e*, pp. 991–1013. New York: McGraw Hill.

Harris, M.I, Hadden, W.C, Knowler, W.C, and Bennett, P.H. (1987). Prevalence of diabetes and impaired glucose tolerance and plasma glucose levels in U.S. population aged 20–74 yr. *Diabetes 36*, 523–534.

Harris, M.I. (1993). Undiagnosed NIDDM: clinical and public health issues. *Diabetes Care 16*, 642–652.

Harris, T. (1999). Weight and age: paradoxes and conundrums. In W.R. Hazzard, J.P. Blass, W.H. Ettinger, J.B. Halter, J.G. Ouslander, Eds. *Principles of Geriatric Medicine and Gerontology, 4e*, pp. 967–972. New York: McGraw-Hill.

Hudson, B.I. and Schmidt, A.M. (2004). RAGE: a novel target for drug intervention in diabetic vascular disease. *Pharm Res 21*, 1079–1086.

Hughes, V.A., Roubenoff, R., Wood, M., Frontera, W.R., Evans, W.J., Fiatarone Singh, M.A. (2004). Anthropometric assessment of 10-y changes in body composition in the elderly. *Am J Clin Nutr 80*, 475–482.

Ikeda, H. (1994). KK mouse. *Diabetes Res Clin Pract* 24 Suppl, S313–S316.

Janson, J., Laedtke, T., Parisi, J.E., O'Brien, P., Petersen, R.C., and Butler, P.C. (2004). Increased risk of type 2 diabetes in Alzheimer disease. *Diabetes 53*, 474–481.

Jimenez-Chillaron, J.C, Hernandez-Valencia, M., Reamer, C., Fisher, S., Joszi, A., Hirshman, M. *et al.* (2005). Beta-cell secretory dysfunction in the pathogenesis of low birth weight-associated diabetes: A murine model. *Diabetes 54*, 702–711.

Kanaya, A.M., Harris, T., Goodpaster, B.H., Tylavsky, F., and Cummings, S.R. (2004). Health, Aging, and Body Composition (ABC) Study. Adipocytokines attenuate the association between visceral adiposity and diabetes in older adults. *Diabetes Care 27*, 1375–1380.

Kanaya, A.M., and Narayan, K.M. (2003). Prevention of type 2 diabetes: data from recent trials. *Prim Care 30*, 511–526.

Knowler, W.C., Barrett-Connor, E., Fowler, S.E., Hamman, R.F., Lachin, J.M., Walker, E.A. *et al.* (2002). Reduction in the incidence of type 2 diabetes with lifestyle intervention or metformin. *N Engl J Med 346*, 393–403.

Koh-Banerjee, P., Wang, Y., Hu, F.B., Spiegelman, D., Willett, W.C., and Rimm, E.B. (2004). Changes in body weight and body fat distribution as risk factors for clinical diabetes in US men. *Am J Epidemiol 159*, 1150–1159.

Kono, S., Kuzuya, H., Okamoto, M., Nishimura, H., Kosaki, A., Kakahi, T. *et al.* (1990). Changes in insulin receptor kinase with aging in rat skeletal muscle and liver. *Am J Physiol 259*, 27–35.

Larbi, A., Douziech, N., Dupuis, G., Khalil, A., Pelletier, H., Guerard, K.P. *et al.* (2004). Age associated alterations in the recruitment of signal-transduction proteins to lipid rafts in human T lymphocytes. *J Leukoc Biol 75*, 373–381.

Lewis, G. F., Carpentier, A., Adeli, K., and Giacca, A. (2002). Disordered fat storage and mobilization in the pathogenesis of insulin resistance and type 2 diabetes. *Endocrine Reviews 23*, 201–229.

Lowell, B.B. and Shulman, G.I. (2005). Mitochondrial dysfunction and type 2 diabetes. *Science 307*, 384–387.

Luo, J., Li, M., Tang, Y., Laszkowska, M., Roeder, R.G., and Gu, W. (2004). Acetylation of p53 augments its site-specific DNA binding both in vitro and in vivo. *Proc Natl Acad Sci USA 101*, 2259–2264.

Martineau, L.C., Chadan, S.G., and Parkhouse, W.S. (1999). Age associated alterations in cardiac and skeletal muscle glucose transporters, insulin and IGF-1 receptors and PI3-kinase protein contents in the C57BL/6 mouse. *Mech Age Dev 106*, 217–232.

Masuzawa, Y. (2005). Adiponectine: Identification physiology and clinical relevance in metabolic and vascular disease. *Atherosclerosis Suppl. 6*, 7–14.

Mathews, C.E. (2002). Rodent models for the study of type 2 diabetes in children (juvenile diabesity). *Pediatr Diabetes 3*, 163–173.

Mazurek, T., Zhang, L., Zalewski, A., Mannion, J.D., Diehl, J.T., Arafat, H. *et al.* (2003). Human epicardial adipose tissue is a source of inflammatory mediators. *Circulation 108*, 2460–2466.

McCulloch, D., and Gems, D. (2003). Body size, insulin/IGF signaling and aging in the nematode *Caenorhanditis elegans*. *Exp Ger 38*, 129–136.

McMillen, I.C., and Robinson, JS. (2005). Developmental origins of the metabolic syndrome: prediction, plasticity, and programming. *Physiol Rev 85*, 571–633.

Meneilly, G.S., Ryan, A.S., Minaker, K.L., and Elahi, D. (1998). The effect of age and glycemic level on the response of the beta-cell to glucose-dependent insulinotropic polypeptide and peripheral tissue sensitivity to endogenously released insulin. *J Clin Endocrinol Metab 83*, 2925–2932.

Meneilly, G.S., Ryan, A.S., Veldhuis, J,D., and Elahi, D. (1997). Increased disorderliness of basal insulin release, attenuated insulin secretory burst mass, and reduced ultradian rhythmicity of insulin secretion in older individuals. *J Clin Endocrinol Metab 82*, 4088–4093.

Meneilly, G.S., and Tessier, D. (2001). Diabetes in elderly adults. *J Gerontol A Biol Sci Med Sci 56*, M5–M13.

Miles, J.M., Wooldridge, D., Grellner, W.J., Windsor, S., Isley, W.L., Klein, S. *et al.* (2003). Nocturnal and postprandial free fatty acid kinetics in normal and type 2 diabetic subjects: Effects of insulin sensitization therapy. *Diabetes 52*, 675–681.

Moller, N., O'Brien, P., and Nair, K.S. (1998). Disruption of the relationship between fat content and leptin levels with aging in humans. *J Clin Endocrinol Metab 83*, 931–934.

Moller, N., Gormsen, L., Fuglsang, J., and Gjedsted, J. (2003). Effects of ageing on insulin secretion and action. *Horm Res 60 (Suppl 1)*, 102–104.

Moreira, P.I., Santos, M.S., Moreno, A.M., Seica, R., and Oliveira, C.R. (2003). Increased vulnerability of brain mitochondria in diabetic (Goto-Kakizaki) rats with aging and amyloid-beta exposure. *Diabetes 52*, 1449–1456.

Motta, M.C., Divecha, N., Lemieux, M., Kamel, C., Chen, D., Gu, W. *et al.* (2004). Mammalian SIRT1 represses forkhead transcription factors. *Cell 116*, 551–563.

Muntner, P., He, J., Chen, J., Fonseca, V., and Whelton, P.K. (2004). Prevalence of non-traditional cardiovascular disease risk factors among persons with impaired fasting glucose, impaired glucose tolerance, diabetes, and the metabolic syndrome: analysis of the Third National Health and Nutrition Examination Survey (NHANES III). *Ann Epidemiol 14*, 686–695.

Nair, K.S. (2005). Aging muscle. *Am. J. Clin. Nutr.* 81, 953–963.

Nesto, R.W. (2003) The relation of insulin resistance syndromes to risk of cardiovascular disease. *Rev Cardiovasc Med 4 (Suppl 6)*, S11–S18.

Nomiyama, T., Tanaka, Y., Hattori, N., Nishimaki, K., Nagasaka, K., Kawamori, R. *et al.* (2002). Accumulation of somatic mutation in mitochondrial DNA extracted from peripheral blood cells in diabetic patients. *Diabetologia 45*, 1577–1583.

Ouchi, N., Kihara, S., and Funahashi, T, (2000). Adiponectin an adipocyte derived plasma protein inhibits endothelial NF-kappaB signaling through a cAMP-dependent pathway *Circulation 102*, 1296–1301.

Pacher, P., Vaslin, A., Benko, R., Mabley, J.G., Liaudet, L., Hasko, G. *et al.* (2004). A new, potent poly(ADP-ribose) polymerase inhibitor improves cardiac and vascular dysfunction associated with advanced aging. *J Pharmacol Exp Ther 311*, 485–491.

Pavlik, V.N., Hyman, D.J., and Doody, R. (2005). Cardiovascular risk factors and cognitive function in adults 30–59 years of age (NHANES III). *Neuroepidemiology 24*, 42–50.

Petersen, K.F., Dufour, S., Befroy, D., Garcia, R., and Shulman, G.I. (2004). Impaired mitochondrial activity in the insulin-resistant offspring of patients with type 2 diabetes. *N Engl J Med 350*, 664–671.

Picard, F., Kurtev, M., Chung, N., Topark-Ngarm, A., Senawong, T., Machado, D.O. *et al.* (2004). Sirt1 promotes fat mobilization in white adipocytes by repressing PPAR-gamma. *Nature 429*, 771–776.

Poulsen, P., Levin, K., Petersen, I., Christensen, K., Beck-Nielsen, H., and Vaag, A. (2005). Heritability of insulin secretion, peripheral and hepatic insulin action, and intracellular glucose partitioning in young and old Danish twins. *Diabetes 54*, 275–283.

Ryan, A.S., Berman, D.M., Nicklas, B.J., Sinha, M., Gingerich, R.L., Meneilly, G.S. *et al.* (2003). Plasma adiponectin and leptin levels, body composition, and glucose utilization in adult women with wide ranges of age and obesity. *Diabetes Care 26*, 2383–2388.

Raz, I., Eldor, R., Cernea, S., and Shafrir E. (2005). Diabetes: insulin resistance and derangements in lipid metabolism. Cure through intervention in fat transport and storage. *Diabetes Metab Res Rev 21*, 3–14.

Razzaq, T.M., Ozegbe, P., Jury, E.C., Sembi, P., Blackwell, N.M., and Kabouridis, P.S. (2004). Regulation of T-cell receptor signaling by membrane microdomains. *Immunology 113*, 413–426.

Saydah, S.H., Loria, C.M., Eberhardt, M.S., and Brancati, F.L. (2003). Abnormal glucose tolerance and the risk of cancer death in the United States. *Am J Epidemiol 157*, 1092–1100.

Sharma, A.M, and Chetty, V.T. (2005). Obesity, hypertension and insulin resistance. *Acta Diabetol 42 (Suppl 1)*, S3–S8.

Short, K.R., Vittone, J.L., Bigelow, M.L., Proctor, D.N., Rizza, R.A., Coenen-Schimke, J.M. *et al.* (2003). Impact of aerobic exercise training on age-related changes in insulin sensitivity and muscle oxidative capacity. *Diabetes 52*, 1888–1896.

Snijder, M.B., Visser, M., Dekker, J.M., Goodpaster, B.H., Harris, T.B., Kritchevsky, S.B. *et al.* (2005). Low subcutaneous thigh fat is a risk factor for unfavourable glucose and lipid levels, independently of high abdominal fat. The Health ABC Study. *Diabetologia 48*, 301–308.

Standards of Medical Care in Diabetes (2005). *Diabetes Care 28*, S4–S36.

Stumvoll, M., Goldstein, B.J., and van Haeften, T.W. (2005). Type 2 diabetes: principles of pathogenesis and therapy. *Lancet 365*, 1333–1346.

UK Prospective Diabetes Study (UKPDS) Group (1998). Effect of intensive blood-glucose control with metformin on complications in overweight patients with type 2 diabetes (UKPDS 34). *Lancet 352*, 854–865.

Unger, R.H. (2003). The physiology of cellular liporegulation. *Annu Rev Physiol 65*, 333–347.

Utzschneider, K.M., Carr, D.B., Hull, R.L., Kodama, K., Shofer, J.B., Retzlaff, B.M. *et al.* (2004). Impact of intra-abdominal fat and age on insulin sensitivity and beta-cell function. *Diabetes 53*, 2867–2872.

Valenti, G. (2004). Neuroendocrine hypothesis of aging: the role of corticoadrenal steroids. *J Endocrinol Invest 27 (6 Suppl)*, 62–63.

Vlassara, H., Palace, M.R. (2003). Glycoxidation: The menace of diabetes and aging. *Mount-Sinai J Med 70*, 232–241.

Weisberg, S.P., McCann, D., Desai, M., Rosenbaum, M., Leibel, R.L., and Ferrante, A.W., Jr. (2003). Obesity is associated with macrophage accumulation in adipose tissue. *J Clin Invest 112*, 1796–1808.

Wilson, P.W., Anderson, K.M., and Kanel, W.B. (1986). Epidemiology of diabetes mellitus in the elderly. The Framingham study. *Am J Med 80*, 3–9.

Wood, J.G., Rogina, B., Lavu, S., Howitz, K., Helfand, S.L., and Tatar, M. *et al.* (2004) Sirtuin activators mimic caloric restriction and delay ageing in metazoans. *Nature 430*, 686–689.

Yechoor, V.K., Patti, M.E., Ueki, K., Laustsen, P.G., Saccone, R., Rauniyar, R. *et al.* (2004). Distinct pathways of insulin-regulated versus diabetes-regulated gene expression: an in vivo analysis in MIRKO mice. *Proc Natl Acad Sci USA 101*, 16525–16530.

Yeung, F., Hoberg, J.E., Ramsey, C.S., Keller, M.D., Jones, D.R., Frye,R. A. *et al.* (2004). Modulation of NF-kappaB-dependent transcription and cell survival by the SIRT1 deacetylase. *EMBO J 23*, 2369–2380.

Yudkin, J.S., Forrest, R.D., Jackson, C.A., Burnett, S.D., and Gould, M.M. (1993). The prevalence of diabetes and impaired glucose tolerance in a British population. *Diabetes Care 16*, 1530.

56

Diabetes as a Model of Premature Aging

Arshag D. Mooradian

There are several genetic or acquired diseases with features that simulate the changes commonly found in aging organisms. One such acquired disease is diabetes mellitus. Phenotypic changes of premature aging in diabetes include decreased life expectancy, increased incidence of cardiovascular disease, osteoporosis, and certain neoplasms, and increased cognitive dysfunction. However, not all the common age-related diseases occur prematurely in diabetes. A case in point is the lack of association between diabetes or glucose intolerance and osteoarthritis. Similarly some changes in diabetes, such as retinopathy and classical diabetic renal lesions, are unique and do not occur in aging.

The mechanisms underlying the pathogenesis of diabetes and the age-related changes have common regulatory pathways. These include increased glycation of proteins, increased oxidative stress, and increased activation of protein kinase C. In addition, insulin and insulin-like growth factor 1 (IGF-1) signaling pathways have been implicated in aging of several experimental organisms. Down-regulation of this pathway through caloric restriction is associated with increased life span in mice, worms, flies, and yeast. One of the key transcription factors implicated in aging, namely, FOXO, is regulated by insulin and IGF-1. The FOXO homolog in worms, DAF-16, has a central role in imparting longevity of worms with mutations in the insulin/IGF-1 signaling pathway genes, such as daf-2 and age-1. In this manuscript, mechanisms that may contribute to the premature aging in diabetes will be discussed, and the literature as to the tissue-specific changes of premature aging in diabetes will be reviewed.

Introduction

There are several genetic or acquired diseases that have features that simulate the changes commonly found in aging organisms (Mooradian, 1995a). The genetically determined diseases that have features of premature aging include a host of progeroid syndromes; the acquired category of diseases with features of premature aging include diabetes, uremia, hypothyroidism, Cushing's syndrome, and acquired immunodeficiency syndrome (AIDS). In the latter category the most common disease is diabetes.

It is generally accepted that we are currently experiencing an epidemic of diabetes worldwide. The main determinant of this epidemic is the rapidly increasing prevalence of obesity. The prevalence of diabetes increases with age, and it has been estimated that one-fifth of adults over the age of 60 in the United States have diabetes (Harris, 1998). Some predict that by the year 2025 two-thirds of the diabetic population will be elderly. In addition to the human cost, the economic implications of increasing prevalence of diabetes and its complications are enormous. Thus it is essential to understand the major determinants of the pathogenesis of diabetes and its major complications.

The feasibility of preventing diabetes with modest lifestyle changes has been demonstrated. It is important to appreciate that the main interventions that are shown to be effective in diabetes prevention, namely, modest caloric restriction and exercise, are also recognized measures of ameliorating the physiological and pathological changes of aging (Mooradian, 1988a). These observations support the notion that some, if not many, of the mechanisms underlying the pathogenesis of diabetes and the age-related changes have common regulatory pathways.

In this manuscript some of the mechanisms that may contribute to the premature aging in diabetes will be discussed, and the literature as to the tissue-specific changes of premature aging in diabetes will be reviewed.

Phenotypic Changes of Premature Aging of Diabetes

LIFE EXPECTANCY

Arguably the ultimate phenotype of premature aging is reduced life expectancy. It is estimated that the onset of diabetes in human subjects reduces the life expectancy by an average of 10 years. The effect of diabetes on life expectancy depends on the age of onset. In general, the older the patient is at the time of diagnosis of diabetes, the lesser its effect is on life expectancy. Nevertheless it appears that diabetes continues to be a major detriment even when the disease onset is in the seventh decade (Songer, 1995).

The epidemiological data from the United Kingdom Diabetes Prospective Study (UKPDS) indicates that mortality in diabetic subjects correlates with the degree of glycemic control as measured by glycated hemoglobin (HbA1c) levels (Stratton *et al.*, 2000; Mooradian and Chehade, 2000). It is noteworthy that HbA1c appears to be a predictor of mortality even in nondiabetic populations (Khaw, 2001). These latter observations highlight the importance of glycemia and glycation as a predicator of life expectancy. It is also possible that postprandial blood glucose excursions that contribute to the HbA1c measurements to a greater degree when the levels of HbA1c are near normal may have an independent effect on cardiovascular risk and overall mortality (Mooradian and Thurman, 1999a).

CARDIOVASCULAR DISEASE

The main cause of reduced life expectancy in diabetes is the increased incidence of cardiovascular disease (CVD) (Mooradian, 2003). Although the cause of accelerated atherogenesis in diabetes is mostly the result of increased prevalence of comorbidities such as obesity, hypertension, and dyslipidemia, it appears that hyperglycemia and possibly hyperinsulinemia or relative insulin deficiency have an important role.

Several epidemiological studies have shown a correlation between the glycemic control and risk of having a cardiovascular event. However recently, the independent effect of HbA1c in predicting cardiovascular outcome was questioned (Selvin *et al.*, 2004). In addition, the UKPDS failed to show conclusively that controlling blood glucose levels has significant effects on cardiovascular outcome (Mooradian and Chehade, 2000). In this study the difference in glycemic control of subjects in the tight control arm (HbA1c of 7.0%) was only modestly lower than the HbA1c achieved in the standard care group (HbA1c of 7.9%). This modest difference in HbA1c values was associated with 16% reduction in risk of CVD (UKPDS, 1998a). This difference however, did not reach the statistical significance. In a subgroup of overweight patients, diabetes treatment with metformin was associated with robust and significant reduction in cardiovascular outcomes (UKPDS, 1998b). This favorable effect of metformin on CVD is either a function of its insulin-sparing effect or could be related to the ability of metformin in inhibiting advanced glycation end-product (AGE) formation akin to its congener aminoguanidine.

NEUROBEHAVIORAL CHANGES

Many of the age-related changes in cognitive capacity are also observed in diabetic subjects (Mooradian, 1988b, 1997a, 1997b). Clinical studies in subjects with type 2 diabetes have shown moderate cognitive impairment, particularly in tasks involving verbal memory and complex information processing, whereas basic attention process, motor reaction time, and short-term memory are relatively unaffected (Mooradian *et al.*, 1988; Strachan *et al.*, 1997).

Some of the cognitive impairment in diabetes is reversible with optimizing blood glucose control. In addition, experiments in diabetic mice also have shown that insulinization and reducing hyperglycemia ameliorates cognitive deterioration (Flood *et al.*, 1990). Nevertheless, some of the changes in the central nervous system (CNS) function in diabetes are the result of cerebrovascular accidents and as such are not readily reversible with control of blood glucose levels.

The prevalence of Alzheimer's disease (AD) is significantly increased in diabetic subjects compared to nondiabetic controls (Arvanitakis *et al.*, 2004; Janson *et al.*, 2004). Since AD is recognized to be a common feature of aging, it is tempting to suggest that the increased prevalence of AD in diabetes is a reflection of premature aging changes within the CNS. It is noteworthy that changes in Glut-1 content of the cerebral tissue from patients with AD are similar to those found in diabetes (Mooradian *et al.*, 1997). It is possible that the diabetes-related changes in the blood-brain barrier (BBB) contribute to the increased incidence of AD in diabetes (Mooradian, 1997a). The changes in the BBB observed in diabetes are often similar to those found in aging, and disruptions in the BBB have been suspected of being a contributing cause of AD (Shah and Mooradian, 1997). Furthermore, Alzheimer's disease and type 2 diabetes have comparable pathological features in the islet and brain (amyloid derived from amyloid beta protein in the brain in AD, and islet amyloid derived from islet amyloid polypeptide in the pancreas in type 2 diabetes) (Chaney *et al.*, 2003; Galasko, 2003). In the Mayo Clinic Alzheimer Disease Patient Registry (ADPR), pancreas and brain were examined from autopsy specimens obtained for the presence of islet and brain amyloid (Janson *et al.*, 2004). In this study, type 2 diabetes and impaired fasting glucose were more common in patients with AD than in control subjects, as was the pathological hallmark of type 2 diabetes, islet amyloid. However, there was no increase in brain plaque formation in cases of type 2 diabetes, although when it was present, it correlated in extent with duration of diabetes. These data support the hypothesis that the possible linkage between the processes is responsible for loss of brain cells and beta cells in these diseases (Janson *et al.*, 2004).

Another potential pathogenetic process contributing to brain dysfunction in diabetes is related to increased AGE and their receptors (RAGE). It is hypothesized that glycated amyloid beta is taken up via RAGE and is degraded through the lysosomal pathway in astrocytes (Sasaki *et al.*, 2001). The presence of AGE, the process of AGE degradation, and receptor-mediated reactions may contribute to neuronal dysfunction and promote the progression of AD.

It is noteworthy that not all studies have found increased incidence of AD in diabetes. In a historical prospective cohort study of Japanese-American men ($n = 3,774$), the expected relationships between impaired glucose tolerance and stroke-related dementia was found, but there was no association of disordered glucose metabolism with AD (Curb *et al.*, 1999).

In addition to cognitive changes in diabetes, affective disorders, notably the incidence of depression, is increased in diabetes (Gavard *et al.*, 1993; Lustman *et al.*, 1986). Major depression has a higher recurrence rate, and depressive episodes may last longer in individuals with type 1 or type 2 diabetes (Lustman *et al.*, 1986; Ryan, 1988). A significant relationship between poor glycemic control and major depression has been reported, although this relationship was not supported by other studies. Insulin resistance has been postulated as the missing link between the affective disorders and AD. However there is no conclusive empirical data to support this hypothesis at this time (Rasgon and Jarvik, 2004). It is not clear whether the high prevalence of depression in diabetes is the result of neurobiochemical changes associated with diabetes, or is secondary to psychological factors related to chronic disease state or its treatment.

OSTEOPOROSIS

One of the common degenerative diseases of aging is osteoporosis. Bone density is decreased in an age-dependent fashion after it reaches its peak at young adulthood. The prevalence of osteoporosis and fractures increases with age. In women, estrogen withdrawal accompanying menopause plays a major role in the first 10 years. Diabetes also is associated with increased risk of fracture of the hip, proximal humerus, and foot (Inzerillo and Epstein, 2004; Schwartz, 2003). Type 1 diabetes is associated with modest reductions in bone mineral density (BMD), but type 2 diabetes often is characterized by elevated BMD (Inzerillo and Epstein, 2004). The paradoxically increased fracture risk in type 2 diabetes may be explained by a combination of factors, including more frequent falls and poorer bone quality.

The precise cause for the osteopenia or poor bone quality of diabetes is not known. Potential mechanisms contributing to reduced bone mass in diabetes include nutritional deficiencies, alterations in vitamin D metabolism and possibly alterations in the microenvironment of bone as a result of microvascular disease, and increased glycation of key structural proteins such as collagen. In addition, increased cytokine production in diabetes may also contribute to osteopenia. Finally, it has been suggested that decreasing leptin level with peroxisome proliferators-activated receptor (PPAR) gamma agonist treatment is associated with prevention of bone loss in type 2 diabetes (Watanabe *et al.*, 2003). Indeed, leptin-deficient mice have higher bone mass, and the thiazolidinedione drugs have been shown to inhibit the formation of bone-resorbing osteoclasts *in vitro* and to decrease bone resorption markers *in vivo*.

NEOPLASTIC DISEASE

Neoplastic disease is common in aging. Cancer continues to be the second most common cause of mortality in the older subjects. Insulin and insulin-like growth factors (IGF) are major determinants of proliferation and apoptosis and thus may influence carcinogenesis (Giovannucci, 2001). Conditions associated with hyperinsulinemia, such as obesity, sedentary lifestyle, or chronic insulin therapy, are also related to high risk (Yang *et al.*, 2004). Hyperinsulinemia can be associated hyperandrogenism and hyperestrogenic conditions, which may play a role in the onset of some malignancies, such as endometrial cancer, breast cancer, and prostate cancer (Guastamacchia *et al.*, 2004).

There are additional hypothetical causes for increased carcinogenesis in diabetes. Type 2 diabetes mellitus may be associated not only with the elevated level of oxidative DNA damage, but also with the increased susceptibility to mutagens and the decreased efficacy of DNA repair (Blasiak *et al.*, 2004). Protein kinase B (PKB) is implicated in glucose metabolism and in the regulation of apoptosis and is activated by insulin, which may partially explain why PKB is over-expressed in some ovarian, breast, and pancreatic carcinomas (Galetic *et al.*, 1999). Inflammatory markers are increased in diabetes. Elevated CRP levels are a strong independent predictor of type 2 diabetes and may mediate associations of TNF-alphaR2 and IL-6 with type 2 diabetes (Hu *et al.*, 2004) (Spranger *et al.*, 2003). Finally, the role of hyperglycemia in carcinogenesis could include pathways related to luminal factors such as fecal bile acid concentrations, stool bulk, and prolonged transit time, or glucose could be the only energy source for neoplastic cells (Chang and Ulrich, 2003). Thus, it is not surprising that the incidence of cancers commonly associated with obesity or aging such as colonic cancer, breast cancer, or uterine cancer is also higher in diabetic patients (Sinagra *et al.*, 2002; Michels *et al.*, 2003). In one study, the increased risk of colon cancer was largely explained by HbA1c concentrations (Khaw *et al.*, 2004).

There are notable exceptions to the increased incidence of age-related cancers in diabetes. The most notable exception is prostate cancer, which is clearly age-related, and yet the incidence in diabetes appears to be less than the nondiabetic controls (Coker *et al.*, 2004; Zhu *et al.*, 2004). Another important point to consider is that although type 1 diabetes is associated with a modest excess cancer risk, specific cancers differ from those associated with type 2 diabetes (Zendehdel *et al.*, 2003).

Tissue-Specific Biological Changes of Premature Aging in Diabetes

In addition to increased prevalence of diseases typically associated with aging such as CVD, AD, and osteoporosis, there are remarkable similarities in biological changes of tissues in diabetes and those commonly occurring with aging (Mooradian, 1988c, 1990, 1994). This is especially true for tissues that do not have high replicative capacity, such as CNS, skeletal and cardiac muscle, skin and bone (see Table 56.1). The degree of concordance between

TABLE 56.1
Select biological alterations in tissues with slow turnover rate. (Adapted from Mooradian, A.D. (1988). *J. Am Geriatr. Soc.* 36, 831–839, with permission from the American Geriatrics Society and Blackwell Publishing.). NC: No change; ↓: Decrease; ↑: Increase.

Parameters Measured	Aging	Diabetes Mellitus
I. Central Nervous System		
Cognitive function	↓	↓
Blood-brain barrier:		
Transport of glucose, choline	↓	↓
Transport of neutral amino acids	NC	NC
H-ATP ase	↓	↓
Na/K-ATP ase or Mg-ATP ase	NC	NC
GLUT-1 content	↓	↓
Endothelial barrier antigen	↓	↓
Conjugated dienes	↑	↑
Lipid composition	NC	NC
Hormone stimulated adenylate cyclase activity	↓	↓
Neurochemical changes		
Key metabolic enzymes: tyrosine	↓	↓
Hydroxylase, DOPA decarboxylase, malate dehydrogenase.		
Occludin	↓	↓
Zona occludens 1	NC	NC
Synaptosomal membranes lipids	NC	NC
Malondialdehyde modified proteins	↑	↑
Micrococcal nuclease digestion	↓	↓
II. Peripheral Nervous System		
Conduction velocity	↓	↓
Myelin crosslinks	↑	↑
III. Heart Muscle		
Beta adrenergic receptors	↓ or NC	↓ or NC
Hormone-stimulated adenylate Cyclase	↓	↓
IV. Skeletal Muscle		
Protein synthesis	↓	↓
Single fiber atrophy	↑	↑
Key metabolic enzymes: Mg-ATP ase,	↓	↓
Lactate dehydrogenase, hexokinase, citrate		
Synthase, α glycerol-3-phosphate dehydrogenase		
V. Croos Links in:		
1. Collagen of skin, dura, tendons, arteries	↑	↑
2. Lens crystalline	↑	↑
VI. Tissue rigidity (e.g., lungs)	↑	↑
VII. Capillary Basement Membrane Thickness	↑	↑
IX. Large Arteries		
Sclerosis	↑	↑
Prostacyclin production	↓	↓

TABLE 56.2
Select biological alterations in tissues with rapid turnover rate. (Adapted from Mooradian, A.D. (1988). *J. Am Geriatr. Soc.* 36, 831–839, with permission from the American Geriatrics Society and Blackwell Publishing.) NC: No change; ↓: Decrease; ↑: Increase.

Parameters Measured	Aging	Diabetes Mellitus
I. Intestinal Epithelium		
Transport of Glucose	↓	↑
Zinc	↑	↓
Calcium	↑	↓
Membrane Physicochemical properties		
Fluidity	↑	↓
Cholesterol/Phospholipid ratio	NC	↑
Sphingomyelin/lecithin ratio	↑	NC
II. Res Blood Cells		
Life span	NC	↓
Calmodulin content	↓	NC
Transketolase	↓	↓
Na/K- ATP ase	NC	↓
III. White Blood Cells		
Calmodulin content	NC	↓
Oxidative potential	↓	↓
Digestibility of DNA with alkali	↓	↓
IV. Platelets; Thromboxane synthesis	NC	↑
V. Lymphocytes		
1. Mitogenic response	↓	↓
2. IL2 production	↓	NC
3. Single-strand DNA breaks	↑	↑

diabetes-related changes in the CNS and the changes seen commonly with age is remarkable. On the other hand, tissues with high replicative capacity such as intestinal epithelium and bone marrow do not demonstrate a high level of concordance between the changes in diabetes and those seen with age (see Table 56.2). These tissues do not appear to undergo premature aging in diabetes. It is likely that accelerated aging in diabetes is tissue-specific, and it may be limited to tissues without a high capacity of replication.

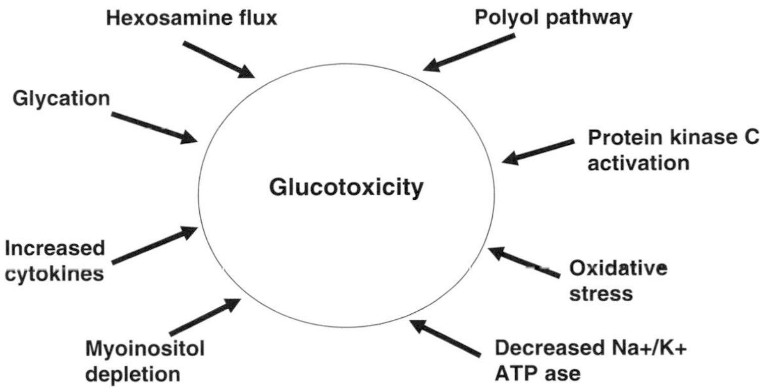

Figure 56.1 Select metabolic pathways contributing to glucotoxicity.

Mechanisms of Premature Aging in Diabetes

The clinical and phenotypic similarities between aging and diabetes suggest that there may be shared biochemical pathways leading to the tissue changes. Glucose is the principal metabolic fuel for many animal species. In general, with few exceptions, the plasma glucose level in various animals is maintained within a narrow range (60–140 mg/dl). It is possible that the lower limit of blood glucose levels is determined by the minimum tissue requirements of metabolic fuel, and the upper limit defines the threshold beyond which glucotoxicity limits survival of the species (Mooradian and Thurman, 1999b). Avian species, especially owls and parrots, are the exception to this generalization. These animals have high blood glucose levels in the range of 250 to 350 mg/dl and yet have a relatively long life expectancy and show no signs of classical diabetic complications. The overall constancy of blood glucose levels across a wide range of animal species suggests that hyperglycemia, except in rare exceptions, is not compatible with healthy living. However, the lack of correlation between the maximum life span of species and the blood glucose levels raises doubts as to the fundamental role of glucose in the rate of aging. Nevertheless, it can be argued that interspecies comparisons are not necessarily relevant to the role of glucotoxicity. In addition, recent clinical studies indicate that there is a continuum in the relationship between tissue toxicity and serum glucose levels rather than there being a threshold of a glucose level beyond which diabetes complications emerge. Such data underscore the fundamental nature of glucotoxicity in animal biology.

The multiplicity of theories of aging makes it difficult to determine with any degree of certainty, the precise mechanism of premature aging in diabetes. However, several sentinel discoveries within the last three decades have shed light on the potential mechanisms of glucose-related toxicity and its effect on degenerative changes of aging. There are several biochemical mechanisms of glucotoxicity (Brownlee, 2001) (see Figure 56.1).

These include the polyol pathway, protein kinase C pathway, glycosylation pathway, and the oxidative pathway. These pathways, although conceptually separate, are interlinked biochemically (Brownlee, 2001). It has been suggested that a unifying hypothesis that incorporates these different pathways of glucotoxicity is hinged upon the mitochondrial generation of free radicals (Brownlee, 2001). According to this hypothesis, excess superoxide (oxidation pathway) partially inhibits the glycolytic enzyme GAPDH, thereby diverting upstream metabolites from glycolysis into pathways of glucose over utilization. This increases the flux of dihydroxyacetone phosphate (DHAP) to DAG, an activator of PKC (PKC activation pathway), and of triose phosphates to methylglyoxal, the main intracellular AGE precursor (glycation pathway). Increased flux of fructose-6-phosphate to UDP-N-acetylglucosamine increases modification of proteins by O-linked N-acetylglucosamine (GlcNAc) (hexosamine pathway), and increased glucose flux through the polyol pathway consumes NADPH and depletes GSH, thereby further aggravating the increased oxidative stress (Brownlee, 2001).

Some of the key mechanisms that may contribute to tissue changes in diabetes, and may also be involved in the aging, will be discussed. The relevance of polyol pathway in human disease has been controversial. The hexosamine pathway is an important pathway contributing to the pathogenesis of insulin resistance and diabetes complications. The glycolytic intermediate fructose-6-phosphate (Fruc-6-P) is converted to glucosamine-6-phosphate by the enzyme glutamine:fructose-6-phosphate amidotransferase (GFAT). Intracellular glycosylation of key transcription factors, such as Sp1, by the addition of N-acetylglucosamine (GlcNAc) to serine and threonine, is catalyzed by the enzyme O-GlcNAc transferase (OGT). These changes result in profound alterations in the expression of genes, such as plasminogen activator inhibitor-1 (PAI-1) and transforming growth factor beta-1 (TGF-β1) that are implicated in the emergence of some diabetic complications (Brownlee, 2001). The age-related changes in Sp1 are not concordant with the changes seen in diabetes. Thus, the polyol pathway and hexosamine pathway will not be discussed any further as they appear to be, at the present time, more uniquely related to diabetes rather than to aging.

GLYCATION PATHWAY

The nonenzymatic glycation of proteins is a common biochemical reaction both in live tissue and in food industry, cooking, and glazing of proteinacious food with sugar (Brownlee, 1995). Glycation of serum proteins is measured clinically with fructosamine assays, whereas glycation of hemoglobin is clinically monitored as the percent of glycated hemoglobin A1 C. HbA1c has been extensively utilized clinically to monitor the adequacy of glycemic control. According to Diabetes Control Complication Trials, a change of 1% in HbA1c reflects a change in mean plasma glucose of approximately 35 mg/dl (Rohlfing *et al.*, 2002). HbA1c values correlate in a curvilinear fashion with the risk of diabetic complications such that for every point change in HbA1c measurements, the risk of having retinopathy, nephropathy, and neuropathy changes by a fixed percentage point.

The first step in this reaction is the attachment of glucose to an ε-amino group of a lysine residue of a protein. This labile Schiff base undergoes an Amadori rearrangement into a relatively stable adduct. The latter undergoes additional slow chemical changes to form the AGE. The accumulation of AGE in tissues increases with age as well as in diabetes. Those subjects with established diabetic complications such as retinopathy or nephropathy have higher rates of AGE accumulation compared to those without such complications (Brownlee, 1995). The AGE formation promotes cross-linking of proteins, thereby resulting in stiffening of collagen, increased entrapment of lipoproteins, and immunoglobulins in the blood vessel walls. These changes activate the complement pathway and cause local inflammatory injury of blood vessels. In addition, cross-linking of lipoproteins increases their atherogenic potential. The AGE formed can also cause a host of biological changes through activation of the AGE receptors. This mechanism has been implicated in increased clot formation, increased production of extracellular matrix, and stimulation of cytokine and growth factor production (Brownlee, 1995).

Glucose-induced modification of macromolecules extend beyond the AGE formation to involve adduction and modification of lipids and nucleic acid bases of DNA. These changes may directly alter membrane integrity as well as genetic expression or stability of some genes.

Finally, glycosylation reaction is often coupled with increased production of free radicals. The attendant increase in oxidative load contributes to the premature aging changes in diabetes.

OXIDATION PATHWAY

There is some controversy regarding whether uncontrolled hyperglycemia in diabetes causes increased free radical generation or whether the increased presence of oxidized proteins and lipids is the result of defective clearance of these byproducts (Hasanain and Mooradian, 2002; 2004). Nevertheless, there is extensive evidence in human subjects, in various animal models of diabetes, and in cell culture studies that hyperglycemia is associated with reduced antioxidant defense capacity, and increased accumulation of oxidation byproducts. In nuclear and mitochondrial DNA, 8-hydroxydeoxyguanosine (8-OHdG), an oxidized nucleoside of DNA, is the most frequently detected and studied DNA lesion. Elevated urinary 8-OHdG and leukocyte DNA were also detected in diabetic patients with hyperglycemia, and the level of urinary 8-OHdG in diabetes correlates with the severity of diabetic nephropathy and retinopathy (Wu *et al.*, 2004).

The increased superoxide generation is more closely related to hyperglycemic spikes, and cellular adaptive changes reduce the superoxide generation rate during sustained hyperglycemia (Horani *et al.*, 2004). These observations have important clinical implications since epidemiological and some interventional trials have suggested that diabetes complications, notably CVD, correlate better with postprandial excursions of blood glucose level than with preprandial levels (Mooradian and Thurman, 1999a).

The precise mechanism of hyperglycemia-related increase in oxidative load is not entirely clear. Glucose, especially in the presence of copper, has potent pro-oxidant properties (Whemeier and Mooradian, 1994). Glycation of proteins is associated with increased free radical generation, and the proteins become more susceptible to oxidative damage (Mooradian *et al.*, 1996). In addition, alterations in micronutrient stores in the presence of hyperglycemia would reduce the antioxidant defense capacity of the organism (Mooradian, 1995). Similar reductions in antioxidative capacity of tissues are found in aging animals (Mooradian and Uko-Ennin, 1995).

PROTEIN KINASE C ACTIVATION

In recent years, protein kinase C has emerged as a potential target for therapeutic agents that reduce the risk of complications in diabetes. PKC is a calcium-dependent enzyme involved in signal transduction through changes in the phosphorylation of key cellular proteins. High blood glucose levels increase phospholipase D activity, which in turn, activates the membrane-bound PKC. This activation accounts at least in part for the increased cell permeability and vascular resistance. In pathological state of hyperglycemia, diacylglycerol (DAG) content is increased, which along with the increased oxidative

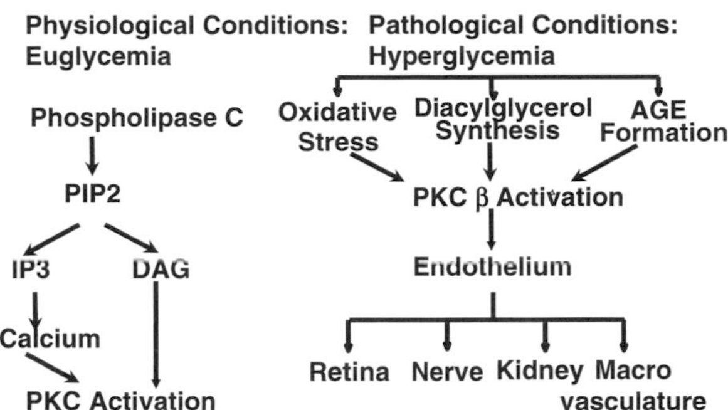

Figure 56.2 Biochemical pathways activating protein kinase C β (PKC β). AGE: advanced glycation end products; DAG: diacyl glycerol; PIP2: phosphoinositol diphosphate; IP3: inositol triphosphate.

stress and glycation process causes the activation of PKC to accelerate (Newton, 1995; Idris *et al.*, 2001; Kawakami, 2002) (see Figure 56.2).

The principal isoforms that are activated are the β- and δ-isoforms. Activation of PKC causes a number of pathological consequences, including alterations of endothelial nitric oxide synthase (eNOS), endothelin-1 (ET-1), vascular endothelial growth factor (VEGF), transforming TGF-β and PAI-1, as well as activation of NF-κB and NAD(P)H oxidases (Newton, 1995; Idris *et al.*, 2001; Kawakami, 2002).

PKC activation, through phosphorylation of insulin receptor, causes resistance to insulin action. Since changes in insulin receptor signaling have been implicated in aging, the relevance of PKC changes to age-related increases in insulin resistance or to the aging process per se, remains speculative.

INSULIN RECEPTOR SIGNALING

Insulin and insulin-like growth factor-1 (IGF-1) signaling pathways have been implicated in aging of several experimental organisms (Pardee *et al.*, 2004). This pathway is critical to coordinating the influx of calories with the metabolic rate. Down-regulation of this pathway through caloric restriction is associated with increased life span in mice, worms, flies, and yeast (Barbieri *et al.*, 2003). One of the key transcription factors implicated in aging, namely, FOXO, is regulated by insulin and IGF-1. The FOXO homolog in worms, DAF-16, has a central role in imparting longevity of worms with mutations in the insulin/IGF-1 signaling pathway genes, such as daf-2 and age-1 (Kenyon *et al.*, 1993). Over-expression of dFOXO in worms and DAF-16 in flies extends life span through interactions with a host of other nuclear receptors, particularly the PPARs (Giannakou *et al.*, 2004; Henderson and Johnson, 2003). These receptors are up-regulated during caloric restriction, and over-expression of PPAR δ in transgenic mice is associated with increased longevity, whereas PPAR δ null mice have reduced life expectancy (Pardee *et al.*, 2004). These observations highlight the central role of PPARs and FOXO in modulating the aging phenomenon.

Conclusion

There are a host of biological changes attributed to increased blood glucose levels that simulate tissue aging. However, not all the common age-related diseases occur prematurely in diabetes. A case in point is the lack of association between diabetes or glucose intolerance and osteoarthritis, a common degenerative disease of joints in the elderly (Frey *et al.*, 1996). Similarly, despite a large number of similar alterations in tissues, some of the changes in diabetes, such as retinopathy and classic diabetic renal lesions, are unique and do not occur in aging.

Multiple metabolic pathways underlie this apparent toxicity of glucose. Although glucose itself has direct-effects on gene expression (Mooradian and Mariash, 1987) and on oxidation (Whemeier and Mooradian, 1994), many of the changes seen in diabetes are the indirect consequences of increased glycation or activation of PKC. Thus, prevention of diabetes complications should include interruption of PKC signaling and prevention of AGE formation in addition to the traditional approach of emphasizing normalization of blood glucose levels.

It is noteworthy that since the relationship of blood glucose levels and tissue toxicity is a continuum, and there is a biological barrier to reducing blood glucose values below the metabolic needs of cells, inhibition of AGE-related toxicity, or possibly partial interruption of PKC signaling, may extend the life span and prove to be a true fountain of youth.

REFERENCES

Arvanitakis, Z., Wilson, R.S., Bienias, J.L., Evans, D.A., and Bennett, D.A. (2004). Diabetes mellitus and risk of Alzheimer disease and decline in cognitive function. *Arch. Neurol. 61*, 661–666.

Barbieri, M., Bonafe, M., Franceschi, C., and Paolisso, G. (2003). Insulin/IGF-I-signaling pathway: an evolutionarily conserved mechanism of longevity from yeast to humans. *Am. J. Physiol. Endocrinol Metab. 285*, E1064–E1071.

Blasiak, J., Arabski, M., Krupa, R., Wozniak, K., Zadrozny, M., Kasznicki *et al.* (2004). DNA damage and repair in type 2 diabetes mellitus. *Mutation Res. 554*, 297–304.

Brownlee, M. (1995). Advanced protein glycosylation in diabetes and aging. *Ann. Rev. Med. 46*, 223–234.

Brownlee, M. (2001). Biochemistry and molecular cell biology of diabetic complications. *Nature 414*, 813–820.

Chaney, M.O., Baudry, J., Esh, C., Childress, J., Luehrs, D.C., Kokjohn, T.A. *et al.* (2003). A beta, aging, and Alzheimer's disease: A tale, models, and hypotheses. *Neurological Res. 25*, 581–589.

Chang, C.K. and Ulrich, C.M. (2003). Hyperinsulinaemia and hyperglycaemia: Possible risk factors of colorectal cancer among diabetic patients. *Diabetologia 46*, 595–607.

Coker, A.L., Sanderson, M., Zheng, W., and Fadden, M.K. (2004). Diabetes mellitus and prostate cancer risk among older men: population-based case-control study. *Br. J. Cancer 90*, 2171–2175.

Curb, J.D., Rodriguez, B.L., Abbott, R.D., Petrovich, H., Ross, G.W., Masaki, K.H. *et al.* (1999). Longitudinal association of vascular and Alzheimer's dementias, diabetes, and glucose tolerance. *Neurology 52*, 971–975.

Flood, J.F., Mooradian, A.D., and Morley, J.E. (1990). Characteristics of learning and memory in streptozotocin-induced diabetic mice. *Diabetes 39*, 1391–1398.

Frey, M.I., Barett-Connor, E., Sledge, P.A., Schneider, D.L., and Weisman, M.H. (1996). The effect of noninsulin dependent diabetes mellitus on the prevalence of clinical osteoarthritis. A population based study. *J. Rheumatol. 23*, 716–722.

Galasko, D. (2003). Insulin and Alzheimer's disease: an amyloid connection. *Neurology 60*, 1886–1887.

Galetic, I., Andielkovic, M., Meier, R., Brodbeck, D., Park, J., and Hemmings, B.A. (1999). Mechanism of protein kinase B activation by insulin/insulin-like growth factor-1 revealed by specific inhibitors of phosphoinositide 3-kinase—Significance for diabetes and cancer. *Pharmacol. & Therapeut. 82*, 409–425.

Gavard, J.A., Lustman, P.J., and Clouse R.E. (1993). Prevalence of depression in adults with diabetes. *Diabetes Care 16*, 1167–1178.

Giannakou, M.E., Goss, M., Junger, M.A., Hafen, E., Leevers, S.J., and Partridge, L. (2004). Long-lived *Drosophila* with over expressed dFOXO in adult fat body. *Science 305*, 361.

Giovannucci, E. (2001). Insulin, insulin-like growth factors and colon cancer: A review of the evidence. *J. Nutrition 131 (Suppl 11)*, 3109S–3120S.

Guastamacchia, E., Resta, F., Triggiani, V., Liso, A., Licchelli, B., Ghiyasaldin, S. *et al.* (2004). Evidence for a putative relationship between type 2 diabetes and neoplasia with particular reference to breast cancer: Role of hormones, growth factors and specific receptors. *Current Drug Targets—Immune Endocrine & Metabolic Disorders 4*, 59–66.

Harris, M.I., Flegal, K.M., Cowie, C.C., Eberhardt, M.S., Goldstein, D.E., Little, R.R. *et al.* (1998). Prevalence of diabetes, impaired fasting glucose, and impaired glucose tolerance in U.S. adults. The Third National Health and Nutrition Examination Survey, 1988–1994. *Diabetes Care 21*, 518–524.

Hasanain, B. and Mooradian, A.D. (2002). Antioxidants and their influence in diabetes. *Current Diabetes Reports 2*, 448–456.

Hasnain, B.I. and Mooradian, A.D. (2004). Clinical implications of recent trials of antioxidant therapy: What should we be telling our patients? *Cleveland Clin. J. Med. 71*, 327–334.

Henderson, S.T. and Johnson, T.E. (2001). daf-16 integrates developmental and environmental inputs to mediate aging in the nematode *Caenorhabditis elegans*. *Curr. Biol. 11*, 1975–1980.

Horani, M.H., Haas, M.J., and Mooradian, A.D. (2004). Rapid adaptive down regulation of oxidative burst induced by high dextrose in human umbilical vein endothelial cells. *Diabetes Research and Clinical Practice 66*, 7–12.

Hu, F.B., Meigs, J.B., Li, T.Y., Rifai, N., and Manson, J.E. (2004). Inflammatory markers and risk of developing type 2 diabetes in women. *Diabetes 53*, 693–700.

Idris, I., Gray, S., and Donnelly, R. (2001). Protein kinase C activation: isozyme-specific effects on metabolism and cardiovascular complications in diabetes. *Diabetologia 44*, 659–673.

Inzerillo, A.M. and Epstein, S. (2004). Osteoporosis and diabetes mellitus. *Rev. Endocrine & Metabolic Disorders 5*, 261–268.

Janson, J., Laedtke, T., Parisi, J.E., O'Brien, P., Petersen, R.C., and Butler, P.C. (2004). Increased risk of type 2 diabetes in Alzheimer disease. *Diabetes 53*, 474–481.

Kalmijn, S., Feskens, E.J., Launer, L.J., Stijnen, T., and Kromhout, D. (1995). Glucose tolerance, hyperinsulinemia and cognitive function in a general population of elderly men. *Diabetologia 38*, 1096–1102.

Kawakami, T., Kawakami, Y., and Kitaura, J. (2002). Protein kinase C beta (PKC beta): Normal functions and diseases. *J Biochem (Tokyo) 132*, 677–682.

Kenyon, C., Chang, J., Gensch, E., Rudner, A., and Tabtiang, R. (1993). A *C. elegans* mutant that lives twice as long as wild type. *Nature 366*, 461–464.

Khaw, K.T., Wareham, N., Luben, R., Bingham, S., Oakes, S., Welch, A. *et al.* (2001). Glycated haemoglobin, diabetes, and mortality in men in Norfolk cohort of European prospective investigation of cancer and nutrition (EPIC-Norfolk). *BMJ 322*, 15–18.

Khaw, K.T., Wareham, N., Bingham, S., Luben, R., Welch, A., and Day, N. (2004). Preliminary communication: Glycated hemoglobin, diabetes, and incident colorectal cancer in men and women: a prospective analysis from the European prospective investigation into cancer-Norfolk study. *Cancer Epidemiology, Biomarkers & Prevention 13*, 915–919.

Lustman, P.J., Griffith, L.S., Clouse, R.E., and Cryer, P.E. (1986). Psychiatric illness in diabetes mellitus: relation to symptoms and glucose control. *J. Nerv. Ment. Dis. 174*, 736–746.

Michels, K.B., Solomon, C.G., Hu, F.B., Rosner, B.A., Hankinson, S.E., Colditz, G.A. *et al.* (2003). Nurses' Health Study. Type 2 diabetes and subsequent incidence of breast cancer in the Nurses' Health Study. *Diabetes Care 26*, 1752–1758.

Mooradian, A.D. (1988a). Nutritional modulation of life span and gene expression. In J.E. Morley, Moderator, *Nutrition in the elderly*, pp. 891–892. *Ann. Int. Med. 109*, 890–904.

Mooradian, A.D. (1988b). Diabetic complications of the central nervous system. *Endocrine Reviews 9*, 346–356.

Mooradian, A.D. (1988c). Tissue specificity of premature aging in diabetes mellitus: The role of cellular replicative capacity. *J. Am. Geriatr. Soc. 36*, 831–839.

Mooradian, A.D. (1990). Biomarkers of aging: Do we know what to look for? *J. Gerontol. Biol. Sci. 45*, B183–B186.

Mooradian, A.D. (1994). Biology of Aging. In G. Felsenthal, S.J. Garrison, F.U. Steinberg, Eds., *Rehabilitation of the Aging and Elderly Patient*. Baltimore, MD: Williams and Wilkins, pp. 3–10.

Mooradian, A.D. (1995a). Theories of Aging. In J.E. Morley, Z. Glick, and L.Z. Rubenstein, Eds., *Geriatric Nutrition: A Comprehensive Review*. New York: Raven Press, pp. 5–13.

Mooradian, A.D. (1995b). The antioxidative potential of cerebral microvessels in experimental diabetes mellitus. *Brain Res. 671*, 164–169.

Mooradian, A.D. (1996). Glycosylation enhances malondialdehyde binding to proteins. *Free Radical Biol. Med. 21*, 699–701.

Mooradian, A.D. (1997a). Central nervous system complications of diabetes mellitus. A perspective from the blood-brain barrier. *Brain Res. Rev. 23*, 210–218.

Mooradian, A.D. (1997b). Pathophysiology of central nervous system disorders in diabetes. *Clin. Neurosci. 4*, 322–326.

Mooradian, A.D. (2003). Cardiovascular disease in type 2 diabetes mellitus: Current management guidelines. *Arch. Intern. Med. 163*, 33 40.

Mooradian, A.D. and Chehade, J. (2000). Implications of the UK Prospective Diabetes Study: Questions answered and issues remaining. *Drugs and Ageing 16*, 159–164.

Mooradian, A.D., Chung, H.C., and Shah, G.N. (1997). GLUT-1 expression in the cerebra of patients with Alzheimer's disease. *Neurobiol Aging 18*, 469–474.

Mooradian, A.D. and Mariash, C.N. (1987). Effects of insulin and glucose on cultured rat hepatocyte gene expression. *Diabetes 36*, 938–943.

Mooradian, A.D., Perryman, K., Fitten, J., Kavonian, G., and Morley, J.E. (1988). Cortical function in elderly non-insulin dependent diabetic patients: Behavioral and electrophysiological studies. *Arch. Int. Med. 148*, 2369–2372.

Mooradian, A.D. and Thurman, J.E. (1999a). Drug therapy of postprandial hyperglycemia. *Drugs 57*, 19–29.

Mooradian, A.D. and Thurman, J. (1999b). Glucotoxicity: Potential mechanisms. *Clinics in Geriatric Medicine 15*, 255–263.

Mooradian, A.D. and Uko-eninn, A. (1995). Age-related changes in the antioxidative potential of cerebral microvessels. *Brain Res. 671*, 159–163.

Newton, A.C. (1995). Protein kinase C: Structure, function, and regulation. *J. Biol. Chem. 270*, 28495–28498.

Pardee, K., Reinking, J., and Krause, H. (2004). Nuclear hormone receptors, metabolism, and aging. *Science 306*, 1446 1447.

Rasgon, N. and Jarvik, L. (2004). Insulin resistance, affective disorders, and Alzheimer's disease: Review and hypothesis. *J Gerontol. Series A-Biol. Sci. & Med. Sci. 59*, 178–183.

Rohlfing, C.L., Wiedmeyer, H.M., Little, R.R., England, J.D., Tennill, A., and Goldstein, D.E. (2002). Defining the relationship between plasma glucose and HbA(1c): Analysis of glucose profiles and HbA(1c) in the Diabetes Control and Complications Trial. *Diabetes Care 25*, 275–278.

Ryan, C.M. (1988). Neurobehavioral complication of type 1 diabetes. Examination of possible risk factors. *Diabetes Care 11*, 86–93.

Sasaki, N., Toki, S., Chowei, H., Saito, T., Nakano, N., Takeuchi, M. *et al.* (2001). Immunohistochemical distribution of the receptor for advanced glycation end products in neurons and astrocytes in Alzheimer's disease. *Brain Research 888*, 256–262.

Schwartz, A.V. (2003). Diabetes mellitus: does it affect bone? *Calc. Tissue Int. 73*, 515–519.

Selvin, E., Marinopoulos, S., Berkenblit, G., Rami, T., Brancati, F.L., Powe, N.R. *et al.* (2004). Meta-analysis: glycosylated hemoglobin and cardiovascular disease in diabetes mellitus. *Ann. Intern. Med. 141*, 421–431.

Shah, G.N. and Mooradian, A.D. (1997). Age-related changes in the blood brain barrier. *Exp. Gerontol. 32*, 501–519.

Sinagra, D., Amato, C., Scarpilta, A.M., Brigamdi, M., Amato, M., Saura, G. *et al.* (2002). Metabolic syndrome and breast cancer risk. *Eur. Rev. Med. & Pharmacol. Sci. 6*, 55–59.

Songer, T. (1995). Disability in diabetes. In M. Harris, C. Cowie, and M. Stern, Eds., *Diabetes in America, 2e*. Bethesda, MD: National Institute of Health; pp. 259–282.

Spranger, J., Kroke, A., Mohlig, M., Hoffmann, K., Bergmann, M.M., Ristow, M. *et al.* (2003). Inflammatory cytokines and the risk to develop type 2 diabetes: Results of the prospective population-based European Prospective Investigation into Cancer and Nutrition (EPIC)-Potsdam Study. *Diabetes 52(3)*, 812–817.

Strachan, M.W., Deary, I.J., Ewing, F.M., and Frier, B.M. (1997). Is type 2 diabetes associated with an increased risk of cognitive dysfunction? A critical review of published studies. *Diabetes Care 20*, 438–445.

Stratton, I.M., Adler, A.I., Neil, H.A., Matthews, D.R., Manley, S.E., Cull, C.A. *et al.* (2000). Association of glycemia with macrovascular and microvascular complications of type 2 diabetes (UKPDS 35): Prospective observational study. *BMJ 321*, 405–412.

UK Prospective Diabetes Study Group. (1998a). Intensive blood-glucose control with sulphonylureas or insulin compared with conventional treatment and risk of complications in patients with type 2 diabetes (UKPDS 33). *Lancet 352*, 837–853.

UK Prospective Diabetes Study. (1998b). Effect of intensive blood-glucose control with metformin on complications in overweight patients with type 2 diabetes (UKPDS 34). *Lancet 352*, 854–865.

Watanabe, S., Takeuchi, Y., Fukumoto, S., Fujita, H., Nakano, T., and Fujita, T. (2003). Decrease in serum leptin by troglitazone is associated with preventing bone loss in type 2 diabetic patients. *J. Bone & Min. Metab. 21*, 166–171.

Wehmeier, K.R. and Mooradian, A.D. (1994). Autooxidative and antioxidative potential of simple carbohydrate. *Free Radical in Biol. Med. 17*, 83–86.

Wu, L.L., Chiou, C.C., Chang, P.Y., and Wu, J.T. (2004). Urinary 8-OHdG: a marker of oxidative stress to DNA and a risk factor for cancer, atherosclerosis and diabetics. *Clinica Chimica Acta 339*, 1–9.

Yang, Y.X., Hennessy, S., and Lewis, J.D. (2004). Insulin therapy and colorectal cancer risk among type 2 diabetes mellitus patients. *Gastroenterology 127*, 1044–1050.

Zendehdel, K., Nyren, O., Ostenson, C.G., Adami, H.O., Ekbom, A., and Ye, W. (2003). Cancer incidence in patients with type 1 diabetes mellitus: A population-based cohort study in Sweden. *J. Nat. Cancer Inst. 95*, 1797–1800.

Zhu, K., Lee, I.M., Sesso, H.D., Buring, J.E., Levine, R.S., and Gaziano, J.M. (2004). History of diabetes mellitus and risk of prostate cancer in physicians. *Am. J. Epidemiol. 159*, 978–982.

57

Frailty as a Model of Aging

Jeremy D. Walston

Frailty has been seen by clinicians and investigators as a late-life syndrome of weight loss and declines in strength and vigor. In addition, it has been characterized as a syndrome of extreme vulnerability to external stressors, and one that marks high risk for poor clinical outcomes. Over the past few years, several groups of investigators have attempted to more rigorously define frailty, and to identify physiologic and molecular contributing factors. Many of these definitions involve clinical findings of weight loss, strength decline, and low levels of activity, and are, as such, characterized as physical or musculoskeletal frailty. Other investigators have tried to better identify the cognitive components of frailty. This chapter will describe several recent models of frailty and the validation of these models. In addition, hypotheses related to the biologic underpinnings of frailty, and how these biologic characteristics may be related to the biology of aging, will be presented. Finally, a discussion of the utility of these models in clinical research and the potential relevance for further biologic discovery will be discussed.

Introduction

Healthcare providers as well as family members have long noticed and commented on a subset of older adults who appeared to be highly vulnerable to falls, fractures, illnesses, loss of independence, and ultimately mortality (Fried *et al.*, 1998). Although these same healthcare providers and family members often recognize frailty when they observed it, there has been very little consistency in the definition of frailty, and hence few validated clinical models of frailty. This is in part because of the heterogeneity that is inherent in many of the processes that may underlie frailty, including aging processes, the development of chronic diseases, social settings, psychological conditions, and genetic predisposition. In addition, it remains unclear if frailty is in and of itself a biologically distinct entity that could be called a clinical syndrome, or whether it simply represents a cluster of partially related signs and symptoms that are generated by aging or disease related processes (Walston *et al.*, 2005). Over the past several years, many of the following conceptual frameworks and definitions of frailty have been operationalized and validity tested using healthcare outcomes (Rockwood, 2005). However, there have been few efforts to compare these models with each other for the poor health outcomes that are the hallmark of this most vulnerable subset of older adults.

A Conceptual Framework: The Cycle of Frailty

This chapter outlines several conceptual models that provide a state of the art overview of this relatively new field of aging research. A useful conceptual model, entitled the Cycle of Frailty, was developed in order to help conceptualize the multifactorial nature of frailty and to help explain how complex physiologic declines, poor nutrition, chronic illness, social situation, and disability/functional decline influence each other (Fried *et al.*, 2003). This model, shown in Figure 57.1, highlights that individual components of the cycle are associated in a step-wise fashion with other declines, and ultimately provides a conceptual basis for development of vulnerability to poor health outcomes on individual declines.

In the center of this figure, physiologic declines related to aging, including loss of skeletal muscle mass (sarcopenia), declines in resting metabolic rate, energy expenditure, and nutritional status reinforce declines in each system. This in turn influences other physiologic systems, including facilitating declines in insulin sensitivity, $V0_2$ max, strength, and power. These changes then contribute to a subcycle of disability, functional decline, and low levels of activity, which in turn reinforces the physiologic decline. Importantly, this model also provides a model for multiple possible entry points into this cycle of decline, and illustrates how specific illnesses, injuries, or medications can trigger and/or accelerate this cycle of frailty.

Sign- and Symptom-Driven Definitions: The Syndrome of Frailty

Despite the ongoing debate on the nature of frailty and whether it is an independent clinical entity or syndrome, some investigators have begun to develop syndromic models in order to differentiate frail vs. nonfrail older adults from further study (Walston *et al.*, 2005).

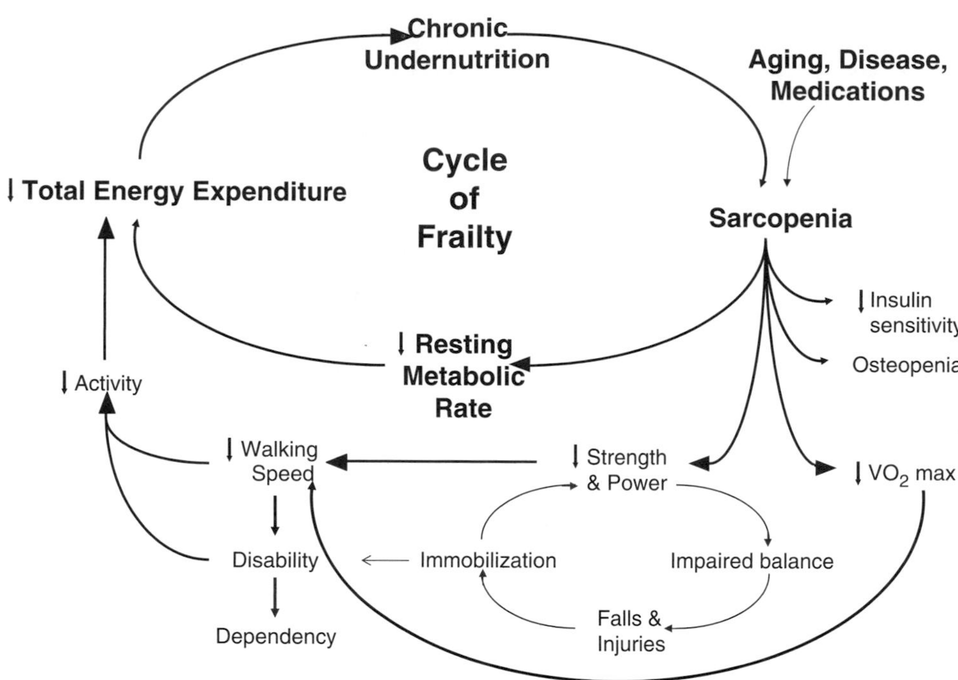

Figure 57.1 Hypothesized Cycle of Frailty illustrating associated physiologic and functional declines as well as potential entry points into cycle of decline. Adapted from Fried *et al.* (2003).

These syndromic models have been developed using epidemiologic data on characteristics related to weight loss or muscle weakness based on the conceptualization of frailty as a wasting syndrome. For example, Chin *et al.* (1999) previously compared three working definitions of frailty, namely, inactivity combined with (1) low energy intake, (2) weight loss, or (3) low body mass index. The combination of inactivity with weight loss was found to be most associated with lower subjective health and performance measures, as well as more disease and disability. In addition, the three-year relative risk for mortality was substantially higher in this group compared to others in the study cohort (odds ratio (OR) 4.1, 1.8–9.4) (Chin *et al.*, 1999).

Similarly, Fried *et al.* (2001) utilized a syndromic approach and developed and operationalized a hypothetical frailty phenotype based on common physiologic signs and symptoms described by frail, older adults. This tool consists of five items, including muscle strength (lowest quartile as determined by grip strength dynamometer measurement), weight loss (more than 10 pounds of unintended weight loss in the previous year), walking speed (lowest quartile of timed 15 meter walk), low levels of physical activity as measured by the Minnesota Leisure Time Activities questionnaire, and fatigue (measured by questions from a Depression survey asking about energy level). It was operationalized in the Cardiovascular Health Study (CHS), an epidemiologic study of community-dwelling adults over age 65 followed for nine years in order to better characterize cardiovascular disease and functional decline late in life. If CHS participants met three of five of these criteria, they were deemed frail; if they met one or two of the criteria, they were deemed intermediate; and if they met none of the criteria, they were deemed not frail. Seven percent of CHS participants met the frailty criteria at their baseline exam, and as expected, there was a significant overlap between disability, chronic illness, and frailty (Fried *et al.*, 2001). However, it was also clear that disability and medical illness were not always consistent with frailty, suggesting an etiology independent from disease and disability, and suggesting a separate but perhaps related biology (Fried *et al.*, 2001). Predictive validity analyses were also performed, where the investigators demonstrated that those who were in the frailty category were more likely to fall, enter nursing homes, be hospitalized, and suffer mortality over seven years of follow-up (Fried *et al.*, 2001). These screening criteria were subsequently utilized to identify biologic correlates of frailty as described in more detail later (Walston *et al.*, 2002; Leng *et al.*, 2002; Leng *et al.*, 2004).

The advantage of these models is that the signs and symptoms were chosen because they are consistent with a wasting syndrome, which often appears to have a common biology. A disadvantage may be that by choosing the wasting syndrome signs and symptoms, other important biologic mediators may not be fully explored (Walston *et al.*, 2005).

Beyond Physical Frailty: Frailty Models that Include Illness, Social and Psychological Status

Because of the likelihood that aging-related changes in physiology, functionality, and disease states may contribute to frailty, some authors have developed models of frailty that include measures of these domains. For example, Rockwood *et al.* (1999) developed and validated a brief clinical instrument to classify frailty in hospitalized patients that included measures of function, cognition, walking, and bladder/bowel function as determining factors. Using Canadian provincial sampling frames from 9008 randomly collected subjects, those who had no abnormalities in these areas were deemed nonfrail, and those with incontinence, dementia, and dependency in activities of daily living were deemed frail (Rockwood *et al.*, 1999). This was further validated by demonstrating a greatly increased risk of nursing home placement in the frail as compared to nonfrail group (Rockwood *et al.*, 1999).

Studenski *et al.* (2004) recently developed and is validating a Clinical Global Impression Measure for Frailty that includes most intrinsic domains represented in the physical frailty models earlier, but also includes extrinsic or consequential domains of healthcare outcomes and complexity, functionality, and psychosocial status (see Table 57.1). An ongoing study of each of these domains in order to determine which if any of these domains best predicts frailty and other poor health outcomes, and in order to be able to measure change in frailty status over time, is important. Once validated, this model could play a potentially important role in measuring responses to interventions. Advantages of these models are that they both can be performed by clinicians rather than trained research technicians (Studenski *et al.*, 2004; Rockwood *et al.*, 1999). In addition, both of these models incorporate components of cognition, health status, and functional domains that may be able to capture additional information about frailty or subtypes of frailty with further study. However, the mixing of outcomes and intrinsic factors in frailty may also make it more difficult to identify common clusters of signs and symptoms that could inform biologic studies (Fried *et al.*, 2005).

Cognitive Frailty

Investigators and clinicians who care for older adults have also described a late-life syndrome with declines in memory and executive function and increasing social withdrawal, and have termed it mild cognitive impairment (Lopez *et al.*, 2003). They have hypothesized an underlying biology that may be similar to the hypothesized biology that underlies physical or musculoskeletal frailty, including increased levels of inflammatory mediators (Golomb *et al.*, 1995). Although no validated models of purely cognitive frailty have been published, physical frailty models may provide a framework for future development of models in this area, and models such as the Clinical Global Impression of Change that include cognitive and social status markers may provide evidence of an independent cognitive frailty syndrome (Studenski *et al.*, 2004).

Physiologic and Biologic Models of Frailty

Building on models of physical frailty mentioned earlier, several investigators have tried to identify additional physiologic characteristics of frail, older adults. Using cross-sectional analyses of data generated in large populations of community-dwelling older adults, these

TABLE 57.1
Extrinsic and intrinsic domains hypothesized to contribute to frailty in older adults. Adapted from Studenski *et al.* (2004)

Intrinsic Domains	Extrinsic Domains
Strength Grip, chair rise	Appearance Grooming, posture, hygiene
Balance Falls, balance exam	Heathcare utilization Hospitalization, MD visits
Nutrition Weight, albumin, cholesterol	Medical complexity Number, severity of conditions
Stamina Self-report fatigue, physical activity	Perceived health Patient/other opinion of health
Neuromotor Speed of movement, attention, coordination	Activities of daily living ADLs, IADLs, travel
Mobility Walking, transfers, stairs	Emotional status Depression, anxiety
	Social status Roles, interactions, live events, living situation

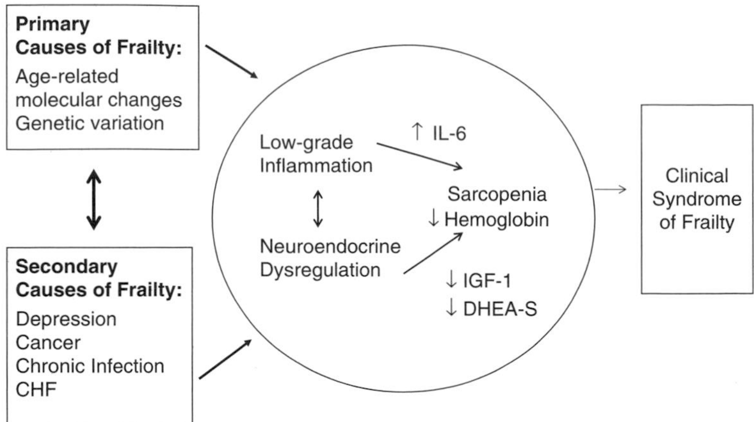

Figure 57.2 Physiologic Model Pathway illustrating age-related (primary) and disease-related (secondary) triggers for the altered physiology that is hypothesized to underlie frailty. Adapted from Walston *et al.* (2004).

investigators have been able to identify frail and intermediate frail subjects, and then compare inflammatory, endocrinologic, hematologic, and metabolic variables hypothesized to underlie declines in multiple other physiologic systems and ultimately frailty. Figure 57.2 illustrates a hypothesized physiological model of frailty where circulating mediators that are components of inflammatory and endocrine systems influence skeletal muscle, red blood cell production, and ultimately frailty and other poor healthcare outcomes of disability and death.

In this model, the altered physiology is hypothesized to be triggered by both aging conditions and chronic disease (Walston *et al.*, 2003). The development of this hypothesized physiologic model pathway toward frailty was based in part on known interactions between inflammatory cytokines, endocrine systems, CNS/SNS activity, and skeletal muscle observed in both human and animal studies. For example, there is a large body of rheumatoid arthritis and other specific inflammatory disease literature that suggests that circulating inflammatory mediators, such as IL-6, TNF-alpha, and IL-1B, trigger the loss of total body cell mass in those with inflammatory disease, perhaps via activation of apoptotic pathways (Roubenoff *et al.*, 2003). There are also multiple lines of evidence that demonstrate a biologic link between elevated IL-6 and bone and muscle loss, anemia, insulin resistance, and altered immune system modulation and hypothalamic-pituitary-adrenal (HPA) axis stimulation, making it less likely that IL-6 is simply a benign biologic marker (Ershler *et al.*, 2000). In addition, there is also evidence that inflammatory cytokines such as IL-6 may interfere with anabolic function of sex steroids, growth hormone, and probably IGF-1 (Lazarus *et al.*, 1993; Papanicolaou *et al.*, 1998). Conversely, it is also apparent that loss of estrogen, and perhaps testosterone, leads to the uncovering of important inflammatory gene transcriptional elements, leading to increased production of IL-6 and other inflammatory mediators in several cell types (Ershler *et al.*, 2000).

These relationships have been tested in cross-sectional studies performed in at least three different groups of community-dwelling older adults. Significant positive relationships were identified between frailty and the inflammatory cytokine interleukin-6 (IL-6), C-reactive protein (CRP), and increased numbers of monocytes, and total white blood cells (Leng *et al.*, 2002; Walston *et al.*, 2002; Leng *et al.*, 2005). Higher levels of these same inflammatory mediators correlate with increased vulnerability to disability and mortality in other studies of older adults, further supporting a role for these biologically active molecules and systems in the development of poor health outcomes (Roubenoff *et al.*, 2003). Although none of the mean values of increased inflammatory markers observed in frailty appear to reach the high levels observed in inflammatory diseases such as rheumatoid arthritis or malignancy, they are suggestive of a chronic, low-level activation of inflammatory mechanisms in frail, compared to nonfrail, older adults, and support the need for further study of these pathways in the development of frailty.

Like the inflammatory system, the endocrine and neuroendocrine systems are composed of several separate, but related, organs or tissues that secrete specific hormones and stimulate components of the central and sympathetic nervous system that regulate multiple physiologic processes. The sex steroids and the growth hormone axis have frequently been postulated to contribute to aging-related changes in body composition, and potentially, to frailty (Ershler *et al.*, 2000). The decline of these hormone levels also triggers inflammatory mediator transcription, and interactions between endocrine and inflammatory systems (Ershler *et al.*, 2000). Trajectories in the declines of each of these hormones may prove predictive in the development of frailty, but have yet to be studied.

The adrenal androgen DHEA-S and the growth hormone messenger molecules IGF-1 both decline with age. Importantly, low levels of both DHEA-S and

IGF-1 are associated with at least one frailty definition in older adults (Leng *et al.*, 2005). IGF-1 plays an important role in the development of skeletal muscle cells and is likely an important factor in muscle mass maintenance with increasing age. There is also evidence for interaction between IGF-1 and IL-6, which suggests that inflammation may drive IGF-1 levels down (Cappola *et al.*, 2003). Furthermore, increasing evidence suggests that DHEA-S suppresses NFKB-induced inflammation (Iwasaki *et al.*, 2004). Hence lower levels of DHEA-S observed in frailty may contribute to chronic inflammation and ultimately to frailty.

In addition to these endocrinologic and inflammatory findings, activation of clotting pathways and altered metabolism as represented as increased glucose intolerance have been identified in at least one study of frail older adults (Walston *et al.*, 2002). In this study, those who were frail had significantly higher levels of fasting glucose, and higher levels of insulin and glucose two hours after an oral glucose tolerance test, even after adjustment for multiple potential confounders (Walston *et al.*, 2002). In addition, the frail subset had significantly higher levels of both Factor VIII, fibrinogen, and d-dimers, suggesting a low-grade clotting process (Walston *et al.*, 2002). Although none of these cross-sectional findings can evaluate causality, they support the need for further longitudinal studies and studies of interactions between these important physiologic systems. In addition, they support the need to identify specific aging or disease related triggers that may activate inflammatory pathways and alter endocrinologic systems, and studies of interactions between these pathways (Walston, 2004).

Theoretical Molecular Models of Frailty

Given the evidence for multisystem decline, and the high likelihood that the development of frailty is a nonlinear process, some authors have used nonlinear dynamics and chaos theory in order to provide new insights into how investigators might detect and quantify changes at the physiological and molecular level. Lipsitz *et al.* (1992) have hypothesized that the decline in complexity of response to stimuli observed in aging and perhaps in frailty in part may be due to loss of complexity in fractal patterns. Fractals are geometric subunits that resemble larger scale units. Many anatomical structures and physiologic processes such as alveoli, neural networks, and bony trabeculae have such repeating subunits and therefore fractal properties. These investigators have theorized that aging and frailty can both, in part, be characterized by a progressive loss of complexity in the fractal architecture of anatomic structures and dynamics of physiologic processes. This loss of structural and functional complexity may impair an organism's ability to communicate within and between systems and to adapt to stress. In addition, most physiologic systems have an ability to undergo reactive tuning, which enables normalization after periods of physiologic stress. It was hypothesized that this retuning may not be possible with loss of complexity, and this may result in the vulnerability to further decline and poor outcomes seen in frailty. In this hypothesized model, frailty is a continuous, nonlinear process, characterized by a progressive loss of physiologic reserve where those individuals who reach a threshold in the continuum can no longer compensate for a given stress, and enter into a spiral of clinical and functional decline.

Systems Biology Model Applications

Given the evidence that the clinical presentation of frailty is likely a cumulative outcome of several levels of interrelationships between physiologic systems and probably molecular systems that ultimately impact clinical vulnerability, application of systems biologic approaches may be helpful in elucidating ultimate causes and key biologic processes from within this biologic web. The important interconnections between clinical, physiologic, and biologic levels of organismal functioning, although still hypothetical, may contribute to biological stability of an organism. If these interconnections are lost, then hypothetically, the organism is at high risk for the development of the vulnerability and clinical presentation of frailty (Fried *et al.*, 2005). When intact, this complex, integrated web of systems offers redundancy and the ability to compensate effectively for stressors. The web of interconnectedness between systems suggests that frailty may present a new theoretical model for systems biology approaches. Kitano *et al.* (2002) has proposed that the structure and dynamics of cellular and organismal function must be examined to understand biology at the system level, rather than the characteristics of isolated parts of a cell or organism. Frailty research may benefit from the development of models where robustness in the face of stressors, multiple levels of cellular and organismal function, communication networks, and the relationship of these system properties to the clinical presentation are all entered into the model. In addition, frailty research may benefit from the development of models where feedback between components of clinical presentation and physiologic dysregulation may impact cellular and organism function and molecular characteristics (Csete *et al.*, 2002).

Conclusion

Over the past decade, significant progress has been made toward refining definitions of frailty, and toward the understanding of the biology that may underlie frailty. Continued refinement of clinical phenotypes and the development of a standardized definition of frailty through contributions of individual domains and through cluster analyses will be critical to compare individuals in large population databases and to better understand the biology of frailty (Walston *et al.*, 2005). This may be best addressed through studying clusters of signs and symptoms that may be supported by common biology, and utilizing systems biologic methodologies to better incorporate important between-systems interactions (Fried *et al.*, 2005). In addition, development of animal and cellular models, along with the development of large population databases, and the infrastructure to support large-scale analyses, will be helpful in developing the next generation of frailty research and ultimately inform the development of interventions to improve the quality of life in this subset of most vulnerable older adults.

REFERENCES

Cappola, A.R., Xue, Q.L., Ferrucci, L., Guralnik, J.M., Volpato, S., and Fried, L.P. (2003). Insulin-like growth factor i and interleukin-6 contribute synergistically to disability and mortality in older women. *J. Clin. Endocrinol. Metab. 88(5)*, 2019–2025.

Chin, A., Paw, M.J., Dekker, J.M., Feskens, E.J., Schouten, E.G., and Kromhout, D. (1999). How to select a frail elderly population? A comparison of three working definitions. *J. Clin. Epidemiol. 52(11)*, 1015–1021.

Csete, M.E. and Doyle, J.C. (2002). Reverse engineering of biological complexity. *Science 295(5560)*, 1664–1669.

Ershler, W.B. and Keller, E.T. (2000). Age-associated increased interleukin-6 gene expression, late-life diseases, and frailty. *Annu. Rev. Med. 51*, 245–270.

Fried, L.P., and Walston, J. (2003). Frailty and Failure to Thrive. In W. Hazzard, J.P. Blass, J.B. Halter, J. Ouslander, and M. Tinetti. *Principles of Geriatric Medicine and Gerontology, 5e.* New York: McGraw-Hill, pp. 1487–1502.

Fried, L.P., Tangen, C., Walston, J., Newman, A., Hirsch, C.H., Gottdiener, J.S. *et al.* (2001). Frailty in older adults: Evidence for a phenotype. *Journal of Gerontology 56A(3)*, M1–M11.

Fried, L.P., Hadley, E.C., Walston, J., Newman, A., Guralnik, J.M., Studenski, S. *et al.* (2005). Report from the American Geriatrics Society/National Institute on Aging "Bedside to Bench" conference on a research agenda for frailty in older adults: Towards a better understanding of physiology and etiology. *Sci. Aging Knowledge Environ.*

Fried, L.P. and Walston, J. (1998). Frailty and failure to thrive. In W. Hazzard, *Principles of Geriatric Medicine and Gerontology*. New York: McGraw-Hill, pp. 1387–1402.

Golomb, J., Kluger, A., Gianutsos, J., Ferris, S.H., de Leon, M.J., and George, A.E. (1995). Nonspecific leukoencephalopathy associated with aging. *Neuroimaging Clin. N. Am. 5(1)*, 33–44.

Iwasaki, Y., Asai, M., Yoshida, M., Nigawara, T., Kambayashi, M., and Nakashima, N. (2004). Dehydroepiandrosterone-sulfate inhibits nuclear factor-kappab-dependent transcription in hepatocytes, possibly through antioxidant effect. *J. Clin. Endocrinol. Metab 89(7)*, 3449–3454.

Kitano, H. (2002). Systems biology: A brief overview. *Science 295(5560)*, 1662–1664.

Lazarus, D.D., Moldawer, L.L., and Lowry, S.F. (1993). Insulin-like growth factor-1 activity is inhibited by interleukin-1 alpha, tumor necrosis factor-alpha, and interleukin-6. *Lymphokine Cytokine Res. 12(4)*, 219–223.

Leng, S., Yang, H., and Walston, J. (2004). Decreased cell proliferation and altered cytokine production in frail older adults. *Aging Clinical and Experimental Research 16(3)*, 249–252.

Leng, S., Chaves, P., Koenig, K., and Walston, J. (2002). Serum Interleukin-6 and hemoglobin as physiological correlates in the geriatric syndrome of frailty: A pilot study. *J. Am. Geriatr. Soc. 50(7)*, 1268–1271.

Leng, S., Xue, Q.L., Huang, Y., Semba, R., Chaves, P., Bandeen-Roche, K. *et al.* (2005). Total and differential white blood cell counts and their associations with circulating interleukin-6 levels in community-dwelling older women. *J. Gerontol. A Biol. Sci. Med. Sci. 60(2)*, 195–199.

Lipsitz, L.A. (2002). Dynamics of stability: The physiologic basis of functional health and frailty. *J. Gerontol. A Biol. Sci. Med. Sci. 57(3)*, B115–B125.

Lipsitz, L.A. and Goldberger, A.L. (1992). Loss of "complexity" and aging. Potential applications of fractals and chaos theory to senescence [see comments]. *JAMA 267(13)*, 1806–1809.

Lopez, O.L., Jagust, W.J., DeKosky, S.T., Becker, J.T., Fitzpatrick, A., Dulberg, C. *et al.* (2003). Prevalence and classification of mild cognitive impairment in the cardiovascular health study cognition study: Part 1. *Arch. Neurol. 60(10)*, 1385–1389.

Papanicolaou, D.A., Wilder, R.L., Manolagas, S.C., and Chrousos, G.P. (1998). The pathophysiologic roles of interleukin-6 in human disease. *Ann. Intern. Med 128(2)*, 127–137.

Rockwood, K. (2005). Frailty and its definition: A worthy challenge. *Journal of the American Geriatrics Society 53*, 1069–1070.

Rockwood, K., Stadnyk, K., MacKnight, C., McDowell, I., Hebert, R., and Hogan, D.B. (1999). A brief clinical instrument to classify frailty in elderly people. *Lancet 353(9148)*, 205–206.

Roubenoff, R., Parise, H., Payette, H.A., Abad, L.W., D'Agostino, R., Jacques, P.F. *et al.* (2003). Cytokines, insulin-like growth factor 1, sarcopenia, and mortality in very old community-dwelling men and women: The Framingham Heart Study. *Am. J. Med. 1115(6)*, 429–435.

Studenski, S., Hayes, R.P., Leibowitz, R.Q., Bode, R., Lavery, L., Walston, J. *et al.* (2004). Clinical global impression of change in physical frailty: development of a measure based on clinical judgment. *J. Am. Geriatr. Soc. 52(9)*, 1560–1566.

Walston, J., McBurnie, M.A., Newman, A., Tracy, R., Kop, W.J., Hirsch, C.H. *et al.* (2002). Frailty and activation of the inflammation and coagulation systems with and without clinical morbidities: Results from the Cardiovascular Health Study. *Archives of Internal Medicine 162*, 2333–2341.

Walston, J. (2004). Frailty—The search for underlying causes. *Sci. Aging Knowledge. Environ.*, 4e.

Walston, J., Hadley, E.C., Ferrucci, L., Guralnik, J.M., Newman, A., Studenski, S. *et al.* (2005). Research agenda for frailty in older adults: Towards a better understanding of physiology and etiology. *Journal of the American Geriatrics Society.*

Walston, J.D. and Fried, L.P. (2003). Frailty and its implications for care. In R.S.M orrison and D.E. Meire, Eds. *Geriatric Palliative Care.* New York: Oxford University Press, pp. 93–109.

58

Osteoporosis and Cardiovascular Disease in the Elderly

Samy I. McFarlane, John Nicasio, and Ranganath Muniyappa

Osteoporosis and cardiovascular disease are common disorders that increase with aging. Accumulating evidence indicates that both disorders may share common pathophysiologic mechanisms as well as risk factors. Besides age and sedentary lifestyle, diabetes, hypertension, dyslipidemia, estrogen deficiency, and hyperhomocysteinemia are common risk factors for both disorders. Furthermore, therapeutic agents for osteoporosis have antiatherosclerotic properties and agents such as statins that are atheroprotective, and appear to increase bone mass and perhaps protect against fractures.

In this chapter, we discuss the basis for a common hypothesis for both osteoporosis and atherosclerosis, highlighting pathophysiologic mechanisms and risk factors common to both disorders, and we discuss therapeutic agents that could potentially be beneficial in the treatment of both disorders.

Introduction

Osteoporosis and cardiovascular disease (CVD) are common and serious diseases that affect our aging population, leading to increased morbidity and mortality. Generally viewed as two separate entities, osteoporosis and CVD share common pathophysiologic mechanisms as well as underlying risk factors (Table 58.1). Inflammation, dyslipidemia, and hyperhomocysteinemia are among the possible mechanisms common to both osteoporosis and CVD. Besides advanced age and sedentary lifestyle, menopause, hypertension, diabetes, as well as genetic predisposition increase the risk of both diseases. Furthermore, agents that are known to be atheroprotective also appear to prevent bone loss. For example, nitric oxide (NO) that has known CVD protective effects was shown to stimulate osteoblast function and bone turnover. Clinically, in a randomized controlled trial, nitroglycerine (a donor of NO) was an effective estrogen replacement therapy in preventing bone loss in patients with surgically induced menopause. Additionally, therapeutic agents that reduce atherogenesis such as statins, also have been shown to stimulate bone formation and agents that inhibit bone resorption such as bisphosphonate, and also have anti-atherogenic effects. This accumulating evidence points to the possibility of common pathophysiologic mechanisms underlying both osteoporosis and CVD, and it remains to be seen if therapeutic agents used for both disorders would develop in the future.

Association of Osteoporosis and CVD

The association between low bone mineral density (LBMD) and atherosclerosis has been demonstrated in several studies. In the Rotterdam study, a population-based cohort study of 7,983 men and women over the age of 55 years, designed to assess risk factors for progression of atherosclerosis measured at multiple sites (van der Meer *et al.*, 2003), and a cross-sectional analysis examining the association between BMD and peripheral arterial disease (PAD) was performed (van der Klift *et al.*, 2002). Data on BMD and PAD for 5,268 individuals (3,053 women and 2,215 men) were available, and the association between PAD and low BMD at the femoral neck was demonstrated in women, but not in men, suggesting estrogen deficiency as a common denominator between osteoporosis and PAD.

LBMD is also associated with early stages of atherosclerosis as measured by pulse wave velocity (PWV) (Hirose *et al.*, 2003). In a study involving 7,865 Japanese individuals age 50 years or older, PWV, which reflects early atherosclerosis, was associated with osteo-sono assessment index (OSI), a measurement that correlates with BMD (Hirose *et al.*, 2003). OSI was negatively correlated with PWV in both genders, and although this association was much stronger in women, it was independent of age and other risk factors for CVD. This association suggests a link between osteoporosis and CVD, particularly in its early stages (Hirose *et al.*, 2003). In another study of 236 premenopausal women aged 45 to 57 years, followed for nine years, the progression of atherosclerotic calcification of the aorta and metacarpal bone loss was demonstrated (Hak *et al.*, 2000). In this prospective study, a cross-sectional analysis was also performed in postmenopausal women showing a graded inverse relationship between the extent of aortic calcification and metacarpal bone density (Hak *et al.*, 2000).

LBMD was associated with increased mortality form CVD (Browner *et al.*, 1991; von der Recke *et al.*, 1999). In the study of osteoporotic fractures research group (Browner, 1991), 9704 ambulatory women aged 65 years and older were prospectively followed. LBMD at the proximal radius was strongly associated with increased mortality from stroke (relative risk 1.74; 95% CI 1.12–2.70). This association was not confounded by other risk factors for stroke such as age, hypertension, diabetes, smoking, or previous history of stroke (Browner *et al.*, 1991). Another study involved two populations of healthy women: one group early after menopause with a mean age of 50 years and another later after menopause with a mean age of 70 years. In this study (Von der Recke, 1999), each decrease of one SD in bone mineral content was associated with a 2.3-fold increased risk of dying from CVD within 17 years of menopause. Elderly women (over 70 years of age) had a 1.8-fold increase of such a risk. These data indicate that low bone mineral content at menopause is a risk factor for CVD risk later in life (van der Recke *et al.*, 1999).

Common Underlying Mechanisms for Atherosclerosis and Osteoporosis

Like osteogenesis, arterial calcification is a regulated and complex process that involves the interactions of various cells producing matrix vesicles with subsequent mineralization. In fact, cells with osteoblastic potential have been isolated and cloned from bovine aortic media (Watson *et al.*, 1994). These osteoblast-like cells in the vasculature are capable of calcifying vascular cells (Watson *et al.*, 1994) (see Figure 58.1).

Several proteins are involved in both osteoporosis and atherosclerosis, such as osteocalcin (OC), matrix Gla protein (MGP), bone sialoprotein (BSP), bone morphogenetic protein-2 and -4 (BMP -2, BMP -4), osteonectin (ON), osteopontin (OPN), osteoprotegerin (OPG), and receptor-activated nuclear Factor-Kappa B ligand (RANKL) (Dhore *et al.*, 2001). Involvement of these

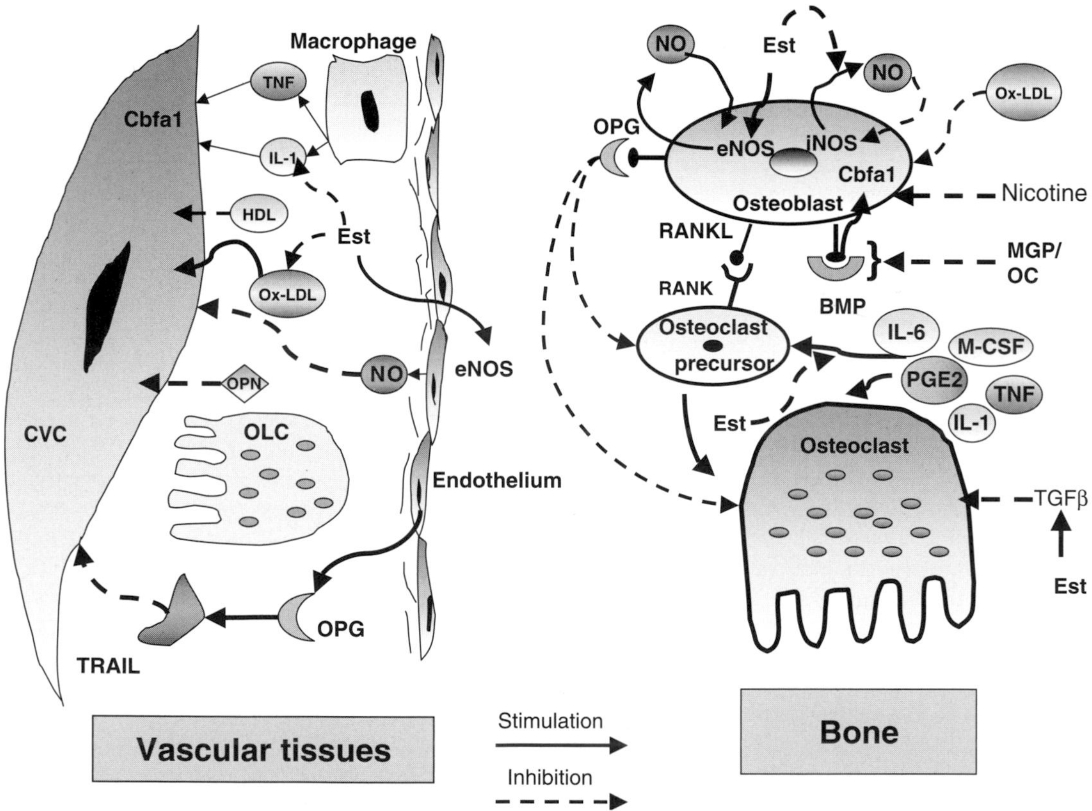

Figure 58.1 Common cellular mechanisms underlying both vascular disease and osteoporosis. NO = Nitric oxide; eNOS = Endothelial nitric oxide synthase; INOS = Inducible nitric oxide synthase; Est = Estrogen; ox-LDL = Oxidized-low-density lipoprotein; HDL = High-density lipoprotein; OPG = osteoprotegerin; RANKL = receptor-activated nuclear factor-kappa B ligand; RANK = Receptor-activated nuclear factor-kappa B; BMP = Bone morphogenetic protein; MGP = Matrix Gla protein; OC = Osteocalcin; IL-6 = Interleukin-6; M-CSF = Macrophage-colonystimulating factor; IL-1 = Interleukin-1; TNF = Tumor necrosis factor; PGE2 = Prostaglandin E2; TGFβ = Transforming growth factor-beta; OPN = Osteopontin; CVC = Calcifying vascular cell; OLC = Osteoclast-like cell; Cbfa-1 = core-binding factor-α1; TRAIL = Tumor necrosis factor-related ligand.

proteins as well as the inflammatory cytokines in both disease processes suggest a common underlying pathophysiologic mechanism for osteoporosis and atherosclerosis (Dhore *et al.*, 2001). Furthermore, osteoclast-like cells (OLCs) have been found in calcified arteries (Doherty *et al.*, 2002) (see Figure 58.1). These cells may participate in normal mineral homeostasis in the arterial wall or may be recruited for the developing plaque (Doherty *et al.*, 2002). Net calcium deposition occurs as a result of focal imbalance between osteoblast-like cells and OCLs (Doherty *et al.*, 2002). Again this process in the vascular wall maintains similar mechanisms for arterial calcification analogous to those observed in the bone where a delicate balance is kept between osteoblastic and osteoclastic activities (see Figure 58.1).

The OPG/RANKL/RANK System

The unraveling of the OPG/RANKL/RANK system represented a breakthrough in our understanding of the regulation of osteoclastogenesis by osteoblasts (Khosla *et al.*, 2001). OPG, a potent inhibitor of osteoclast formation, is a soluble, decoy receptor of the superfamily of the tumor necrosis factor (TNF) (Khosla *et al.*, 2001). This cytokine is produced by the stromal cells of the bone marrow, by osteoblasts, vascular smooth muscle cells (VSMCs), as well as by endothelial cells (Khosla *et al.*, 2001). RANKL, soluble, or cell-bound, expressed by osteoblast precursors upon interaction with RANK, initiates a series of reactions that promote osteoclast formation and activation leading to bone resorption (Khosla *et al.*, 2001; Lacey *et al.*, 1998) (see Figure 58.1).

OPG binds to RANKL leading to inhibition of the osteoclastic activation (see Figure 58.1) (Khosla *et al.*, 2001). OPG Knock-out mice develop arterial wall calcification as well as osteoporosis (Min *et al.*, 2000). Reversal of these abnormalities is observed in OPG transgenic restoration (Min *et al.*, 2002). Furthermore, intravenous injection of recombinant OPG protein reverses the osteoporotic phenotype observed in OPG-deficient mice (Min *et al.*, 2000). Also, in a randomized, double-blinded, placebo-controlled study, a single subcutaneous injection of OPG was found to be effective in reducing bone turnover in postmenopausal women, highlighting its potential as a therapeutic agent for osteoporosis (Bekker *et al.*, 2001).

In normal aortas, OPG is expressed by VSMCs where it lines the calcific deposits in advanced atherosclerosis (Dhore *et al.*, 2001). Around these calcium deposits RANK is also found in the extracellular matrix (Dhore *et al.*, 2001). The calcified aortic lesions contain OLC (see Figure 58.1), multinucleated cells positive for osteoclastic markers but negative for macrophage markers (Min *et al.*, 2000; Doherty *et al.*, 2002). These findings indicate the presence of osteoclasts or equivalent cells (OLCs) that may mediate OPG inhibition of vascular calcification.

In a prospective study involving 490 white women aged 65 years or more, OPG was associated with diabetes and with cardiovascular mortality, raising the possibility that OPG might be a cause/marker for vascular calcification (Browner *et al.*, 2001). These findings highlight the potential role of OPG as a marker for both osteoporosis and atherosclerosis. The exact mechanisms underlying the paradoxical effects of OPG in vascular tissue and bone are largely unknown. However, possible explanation includes site-specific differential expression of RANK/RANKL at these sites (Emery *et al.*, 1998). Apoptosis of the CVC as well as T-lymphocytes may be prevented by the absence of OPG, thus favoring vascular calcification (Emery *et al.*, 1998).

Collectively, these findings indicate that the OPG/RANK/RANKL pathway is a common denominator in both osteoporosis and CVD.

Gamma-carboxyglutamic Acid (Gla) Proteins

Gla proteins, including matrix Gla protein (MGP) and osteocalcin (OC), are vitamin K-dependent bone proteins that play a key role as mediators and inhibitors of osteoid formation (Price *et al.*, 1982; Pauli *et al.*, 1987). MGP is a secretory protein that is widely expressed in tissues including bone and vasculature (Price *et al.*, 1982). Chronic Warfarin therapy leads to depletion of these vitamin K-dependent Gla proteins, resulting in an excessive mineralization disorder and closure of the growth plate with cessation of longitudinal growth (Price *et al.*, 1982). These features are similar to those observed in the warfarin embryopathy due to exposure of the human fetus to warfarin anticoagulation in early pregnancy (Pauli *et al.*, 1987). Knockout mice lacking MGP develop to term but die within two months due to arterial calcification and blood-vessel rupture (Luo *et al.*, 1997). Additionally, these MGP-deficient mice exhibit inappropriate calcification of the growth plate leading to short stature, osteopenia, and fractures (Luo *et al.*, 1997). MGP are constitutively expressed in human aortas. These proteins are up-regulated in atherosclerosis and plaque formation (Shanahan *et al.*, 2000), suggesting a role for these proteins in limiting vascular osteogenesis. MGP is expressed with high accumulation in bone and cartilage in association with bone morphogenetic protein (BMP) (Bostrom *et al.*, 2001). MGP inhibits BMP-chondrocyte differentiation. Therefore, absence of MGP inhibitory effect leads to osteogenic differentiation and vascular calcification (Bostrom *et al.*, 2001). However, MGP was suggested to prevent nucleation and growth of crystals via binding to hydroxyapatite (Schnike *et al.*, 1999). These two mechanisms are likely operative in prevention of vascular calcification.

Osteocalcin (OC)

This is the most abundant osteoblast-specific noncollagenous protein (Ducy *et al.*, 1996) (see Figure 58.1). Osteocalcin-deficient mice develop a phenotype characterized by higher bone mass with increased functional quality (Ducy *et al.*, 1996). These mice, however, do not exhibit vascular calcification, indicating that OC is primarily operative in the bone rather than the vascular tissues. The expression of OC and MGP in humans is parallel in normal as well as in atherosclerotic tissues (Dhore *et al.*, 2001).

In women with osteoporosis and atherosclerosis, serum OC is elevated (Bini *et al.*, 1999), suggesting an integral role of Gla protein in both vascular wall and bone.

Osteopontin (OPN) and Bone Morphogenetic Proteins (BMP)

Osteopontin is a noncollagenous adhesive protein that is found at dysmorphic calcification sites (Wada *et al.*, 1999). This protein is synthesized by macrophages in atherosclerotic plaques and calcified aortic values representing an adaptive mechanism aimed at prevention of vascular calcification.

In bone tissue, OPN is produced by osteoclasts as well as osteoblasts, and inhibits matrix mineralization (Wada *et al.*, 1999).

OPN is essential in the development of postmenopausal osteoporosis. OPN knockout mice are resistant to ovariectomy-induced bone resorption, compared to wild-type mice (Yoshitake *et al.*, 1999). Furthermore, in the absence of OPN, PTH-induced increase in bone resorption is suppressed, via osteoclastic inhibition (Ihara *et al.*, 2001). In calcified atheromatous tissues, OPN is upregulated (Dhore *et al.*, 2001), probably as a compensatory response to the decrease in the mineralization process. OPN is also likely to play an important role in atherosclerosis (Isoda *et al.*, 2002). Transgenic mice over-expressing the OPN gene develop both medial thickening without injury and vascular remodeling, and restenosis after angioplasty (Isoda *et al.*, 2002).

BMPs are members of the transforming growth factor (TGF-β) super-family of proteins (Wozney *et al.*, 1998). Among the 15 BMPs that are currently identified, BMP-2 and BMP-4 induce differentiation of osteoblast precursor cells into more mature osteoblast-like cells (Yamagushi *et al.*, 1991). BMPs stimulate the expression of core-binding factor-alpha 1 (Cbfa-1), a key molecule in osteoblast differentiation (Lee *et al.*, 2000). Application of BMPs to mandibular defects in humans stimulated osteogenesis with mineralized bone trabeculae with copious osteoid seams (Ferretti *et al.*, 2002). In human atherosclerotic lesions there is an enhanced BMP-2 and Cbfa-1 (Engelese *et al.*, 2001). These factors are absent in normal arteries, suggesting a role for these molecules in vascular calcification (Engelese *et al.*, 2001).

Role of Nitric Oxide (NO)

NO is produced by a group of enzymes (NO Synthase, NOS). It is a pleiotrophic signaling molecule that has an important role in vascular tissue as well as in bone (Moncada *et al.*, 1991). Constitutive NOS (cNOS) produces NO in response to calcium. On the other hand, the inducible form of NOS (iNOS) is produced in large amounts independent of calcium (Moncada *et al.*, 1991). Although cNOS is present in the endothelium lining of the blood vessels and osteocytes, iNOS can be induced in the endothelium, VSMC, inflammatory cells, osteocytes, and chondrocytes (Hukkanen *et al.*, 1995). By producing NO, cNOS responds to a variety of physiological stimulation including shear stress, mechanical loading, estrogen, and statins, as well as growth factors (Muniyappa *et al.*, 2000). NO has a protective effect on both bone and vascular tissues (Moncada *et al.*, 1991). Among the atheroprotective effects of NO are the inhibition of VSMC proliferation, platelet aggregation, and cell adhesion. On the other hand, cNOS deficiency in mice leads to hypertension and endothelial dysfunction, reduced bone mineral density (BMD), and osteoblastic number and function. Mice with cNOS deficiency lost bone following ovariectomy, and there was a significantly blunted anabolic response to high-dose exogenous estrogen (Armour *et al.*, 2001). These findings suggest a critical role for NO in regulating bone mass and bone turnover. These findings are also consistent with the results of a clinical trial, where nitroglycerine, a NO donor, was shown to be as effective as estrogen in preventing bone loss associated with surgically induced menopause, when given in a randomized controlled fashion (Wimalawnsa *et al.*, 2000). In contrast to these findings in a mouse model of inflammation-induced bone loss, rapid release and high concentration of NO inhibited proliferation and induced apoptosis of osteoblasts (Mancini *et al.*, 2000). Slow and moderate release of NO however, stimulated the replication of primary rat osteoblasts and alkaline phosphatase activity (Mancini *et al.*, 2000). These findings suggest the presence of both stimulatory and apoptosis-inducing effects of NO on primary osteoblasts (see Figure 58.1). Furthermore, in chronic inflammatory conditions such as rheumatoid arthritis, associated with elevated cytokines and high NO levels, inhibition of NO production reversed bone loss (Sakurai *et al.*, 1995). These findings indicate that in bone and in vascular tissues, the biological response to NO is dose-dependent. Deficiency of cNOS accelerates both osteoporosis and atherosclerosis, and iNOS increases bone loss (Mancini *et al.*, 2000; Sakurai *et al.*, 1995).

Sex Steroids

The effect of sex steroids on skeletal homeostasis is well established, although, the mechanisms mediating those effects are unclear. Estrogen plays a pivotal role in regulating bone metabolism not only in women but also in men (Khosla *et al.*, 2002). Sex steroids (estrogen and androgens) decrease the genesis of osteoblasts and osteoclasts; however, they stimulate apoptosis in osteoclasts and prolong the life span of osteoblasts (Manolagas, 2000). Sex steroids inhibit bone resorption via effects on the RANKL/RANK/OPG system, as well as by altering cell-mediated release of various cytokines (interleukins, MCSF, TNF-α, TGFβ, BMP-6), insulin-like growth factor-I (IGF-I), prostaglandins, and NO (Khosla *et al.*, 2002). Overwhelming data, including the Women's Health Initiative study, suggest that HRT reverses bone loss associated during the postmenopausal period (Riggs *et al.*, 2002; Rossouw *et al.*, 2002). Cross-sectional and interventional studies have demonstrated cardioprotective actions of estrogen. However, recent prospective randomized intervention trials have failed to show such beneficial actions (Rossouw *et al.*, 2002). The dose of estrogen, timing of initiating hormone replacement, and presence of prior atherosclerotic vascular disease may have contributed to the apparently contradictory results. Interestingly, coronary artery plaque calcium content and burden have been shown to be associated with estrogen levels in pre- and postmenopausal women (Christian *et al.*, 2002). Estrogen is known to modulate OPG, MGP, RANKL/RANK, and NO, and may mediate some of its actions on arterial calcification.

In contrast to estrogen, well-designed and adequately powered interventional trials examining the effects of testosterone replacement on bone metabolism in elderly men are lacking. Therefore, the effects of androgen supplementation on BMD are largely unknown. Testosterone has been shown to retard atherosclerosis in rodent models; however, prospective or cross-sectional studies have failed to reveal any consistent association of testosterone levels and coronary artery disease (Alexandersen *et al.*, 1999). Similarly, there is no convincing evidence supporting an association of DHEA(S) with atherosclerosis. These studies suggest that estrogen, but not testosterone or DHEA(S), plays a key role in osteoporosis and atherosclerosis.

Inflammation

Inflammation is an important underlying mechanism in both atherosclerosis and osteoporosis. In atherosclerosis, inflammation correlates with the severity of the disease (Libby, 2002). Inflammatory markers such as C-reactive protein (CRP), TNF-X, IL-6, and MCP-1 have been suggested as nontraditional cardiovascular risk factors (McFarlane *et al.*, 2001). Recent clinical trials indicate that CRP is a stronger predictor for cardiovascular disease events than LDL-cholesterol (Ridker *et al.*, 2002). Inflammatory cytokines are intricately involved in the various processes that culminate in atherosclerosis such as angiogenesis and neointimal thickening (McFarlane *et al.*, 2002). These cytokines are produced by the vascular endothelial as well as vascular smooth muscle cells (VSMCs) and macrophages, and include IL-1, TNF-X, and IL-6. These cytokins stimulate the transcription of chemoattractant factors genes such as macrophage stimulatory factor, MCP-1, and increase monocyte migration to the vascular wall leading to atherosclerosis and vascular calcification (Tiutut *et al.*, 2001).

Osteogenic differentiation of CVC is stimulated by monocytes and macrophages through the production of inflammatory cytokines such as TNF-alpha (Shioi *et al.*, 2002). These cytokines are also potent stimulators of 1,25 dihydroxy vitamin D in macrophages. Finally, the causal relationship of these cytokines in osteoporosis has been demonstrated in rodent models, where neutralization of IL-1 activity with IL-1ra or of TNF-alpha with binding protein abrogated atherosclerosis. Injection of IL-6 on the hand promoted the process (Huber *et al.*, 1999).

Changes in cytokine profile in atherosclerosis are similar to those in osteoporosis. These cytokines, particularly IL-6, are powerful stimulators of bone resorption (Scheidt-Nave *et al.*, 2001). In a longitudinal study of postmenopausal women, IL-6 was shown to be a predictor of bone loss particularly in the first six years of the postmenopausal period (Scheidt-Nave *et al.*, 2001). Levels of IL-1, IL-6, and TNF-alpha directly correlated with bone resorptive actions of monocytes (Cohen-Solal *et al.*, 1993). These actions were neutralized by the addition of cytokine inhibitors indicating the pivotal role of these cytokines in bone resorption. Therefore, cytokine activities play a major role in both osteoporosis and atherosclerosis, highlighting a common underlying pathophysiologic mechanism for the two diseases. The actions of their cytokines include polymorphic responses in the vessel walls as well as interaction between cells and local micro environment together with a temporal pattern of expression of these cytokines.

Dyslipidemia

The role of dyslipidemia in atherosclerosis has been clearly established. Both elevated LDL-cholesterol and reduced HDL-C are risk factors for atherosclerosis. This dyslipidemia has been shown to be related to bone mass and bone fragility and might represent a common underlying factor for both osteoporosis and atherosclerotic disease (Yamagushi *et al.*, 2002). In a study of 214 postmenopausal Japanese women, plasma LDL-cholesterol levels were inversely correlated with bone mineral density at the forearm and the lumbar spine (Yamagushi *et al.*, 2002). In this study, plasma HDL-C was positively correlated with BMD at the lumbar spine and at the forearm. Triglyceride (TG) predicted the presence of vertebral fractures in this cohort of postmenopausal women. This indicates that dyslipidemia is common to both atherosclerosis and osteoporosis. Consistent with these findings, the administration of high-fat diet reduced bone mineralization in mouse models (Parhami *et al.*, 2001), suggesting that an atherogenic diet is also associated with inhibition of bone formation. Furthermore, epidemiologic studies suggest that high intake of specific fatty acids, such as gamma-linoleic acid, is associated with decreased atherosclerosis. These beneficial effects have also been observed in bone (Schlemmer *et al.*, 1999). These beneficial effects of ecosanoids are likely related to their anti-inflammatory action as well as their modulation of prostaglandin metabolism and their effects on NO synthesis. These lipids affect atherosclerosis and bone remodeling in opposite directions, which may help explain the coexistence of both atherosclerosis and osteoporosis in patients with dyslipidemia.

Homocysteinemia

Elevated plasma homocysteine has been shown to be associated with increased cardiovascular disease (Danesh *et al.*, 1998). Proposed mechanisms underlying this association include reduced NO bioavailability, smooth muscle cell proliferation, endothelial dysfunction and increased thrombosis. Hyperhomocysteinemia has also been associated with osteoporosis (Parrot *et al.*, 2000). However, the exact mechanism underlying this association is largely unknown.

Hypertension

Hypertension is a well-established risk factor for atherosclerosis. High blood pressure is also associated with abnormalities in calcium homeostasis leading to hypercalciuria (Cappuccio *et al.*, 1999). This negative calcium balance is associated with decreased bone mineral density. In a prospective study involving 3676 white women, after adjusting for age, body weight, smoking, and baseline bone mineral density, higher blood pressure in elderly women was associated with increased bone loss at the femoral neck. Therefore, hypertension appears to be a common denominator in both osteoporosis and atherosclerosis in the elderly.

Diabetes Mellitus

Diabetes mellitus (DM) is an established risk for atherosclerosis and is associated with both microvascular and macrovascular disease. Accumulating evidence indicates that diabetes also is associated with increased risk of fracture of the hip, proximal humerus, and foot (Schwartz *et al.*, 2003). Although the association of type 1 DM and low bone density is established, in type 2 DM there is a normal or high bone density despite evidence from epidemiologic data of increased fracture (Dominguez *et al.*, 2004). This paradox is explained, in part, by altered bone structure leading to decreased bone strength. Furthermore diabetes is also associated with higher risk of falls, particularly among elderly women, leading to increased fractures (Schwartz *et al.*, 2001).

In patients with type 1 DM, mechanisms of increased bone loss are largely unknown. These patients also suffer from increased hip fracture at a younger age (Forsen *et al.*, 1999). Poor metabolic control in adolescents with type 1 DM is associated with increased risk for osteoporosis in adult age (Valerio *et al.*, 2002). Studies involving animal models of type 1 DM suggest that advanced glycation end products (AGEs) inhibit osteoblastic function through their interaction with receptors for AGE (RAGE) (Santana *et al.*, 2003). Interestingly, the interaction of AGE with RAGE has been implicated in the vascular complications of diabetes through altered cell signaling, gene expression, release of pro-inflammatory molecules, and free radicals (Ahmed *et al.*, 2005). These findings of inhibition of osteoblastic function as well as altered cell signaling in vascular tissue suggest common pathophysiologic mechanisms of osteoporosis and CVD.

Pharmacologic Agents

Agents that commonly are used for prevention and treatment of osteoporosis and CVD such as bisphosphonates and statins have beneficial effects on both the bone and the vascular wall. That is not surprising given the common pathway and site of actions for each of these agents (McFarlane *et al.*, 2002). Statins (3-hydroxy-3-methylglutaryl coenzyme-A (HMG-CoA) reductase inhibitors) commonly are used for treatment of dyslipidemia. These agents lower cholesterol by production and enhance LDL clearance. In addition, statins also reduce cellular isoprenoid intermediates, leading to decreased isoprenylation and decreased activity of small GTP binding proteins from the Ras/Rho family (McFarlane *et al.*, 2002).

Bisphosphonates act one step downstream from the site of action of statins on the mevalonate pathway (McFarlane *et al.*, 2002), which is involved in the regulation of Ras/Rho proteins. It is suggested that the inhibition of protein prenylation might be responsible for the antiresorptive actions of bisphosphonates (Fisher *et al.*, 1999).

Accumulating evidence indicate that these two classes of medications, which affect the mevalonate pathway, may modulate both osteoporosis and atherosclerosis (McFarlane *et al.*, 2002). In addition to their pleiotropic effects on the cardiovascular system, statins also stimulate bone formation *in vitro*, and in rodents, an effect that is associated with increase in bone morphogenetic protein –2 (BMP-2) genes in bone cells (Mundy *et al.*, 1999). Lovastatin and simvastatin increased bone formation when injected subcutaneously over the calvaria of mice, and when given orally, these agents increased cancellous bone volume (Mundy *et al.*, 1999). However, the effect of statins on fracture risk is unclear, and although observational studies showed reduced risk of fracture, randomized trials have not been done (Rizzo *et al.*, 2004).

TABLE 58.1
Pathophysiologic mechanisms and risk factors common for both cardiovascular disease and Low Bone Mineral Density

Risk factor	Bone	Cardiovascular system
Age	Associated with decreased BMD	Associated with ↑ vascular disease
Sedentary Lifestyle	Associated with low BMD	Associated with increased vascular dysfunction
Smoking	Associated with ↓ BMD Inhibits osteogenic differentiation and osteoblastic growth Increases catabolism of estrogen	Endothelial Dysfunction ↑ oxidative stress, ox-LDL, diminished NO availability, thrombogenicity, VSMC proliferation
Dyslipidemia	Associated with ↓ BMD; ox-LDL Inhibits osteoblastic differentiation	Endothelial dysfunction, diminished NO production, plaque formation, ↑ neointima, ↑ cell adhesion; ox-LDL ↑ CVC activity, HDL ↓ CVC activity and cytokine formation
Homocysteinemia	Associated with low BMD	Endothelial dysfunction, diminished NO-bioavailability, lipid peroxidation, smooth muscle cell proliferation, increased platelet aggregation, enhanced tissue factor activity, reduced von Willebrand factor secretion, inhibition of tissue plasminogen activator
Estrogen Deficiency	↑ Bone resorption, cytokine activity, ↓ TGF-β, ↓ vitamin D	Diminished NO production, ↑ free radical production, ↑ VSMC proliferation, hypercoagulability, ↑ inflammation, ↑ vascular reactivity
Inflammation	↑ Bone loss: ↑ NO production, osteoblast apoptosis, osteoclast activity	Endothelial dysfunction, increased coagulation, plaque instability, ↑ CVC activity, vitamin D production, ↑ vascular calcification

BMD = Bone mineral density; LDL = Low-density lipoprotein; ox-LDL = oxidized-LDL; NO = Nitric oxide; VSMC = Vascular smooth muscle cell; CVC = Calcifying vascular cell; TGFβ = Transforming growth factor- beta; IL-6 = Interleukin-6; LDLRP = Low-density lipoprotein receptor protein.

Bisphosphonates have long been shown to decrease atherosclerosis (Yitalo *et al.*, 1994). These agents prevent the development of atheromatous lesions when used in animal models fed with a high cholesterol diet (Yitalo *et al.*, 1994). Furthermore, bisphosphonates have been shown to reduce the extent of established atherosclerotic lesions and in high doses, a bisphosphonate derivative also has been shown to reduce serum cholesterol by 33% and to exert multiple anti-atherosclerotic effects including suppression of HMG –C0A reductase activity and prevention of lipid oxidation (Jackson *et al.*, 2000). Oral etidronate has been shown to decrease carotid arterial intima-media thickness in type 2 diabetes without changing cardiovascular parameters, suggesting a direct effect of bisphosphonates on the vascular wall (Koshiyama *et al.*, 2000).

In elderly patients with diabetes, the use of alendronate10 mg/daily for treatment of osteoporosis was associated with a 36% reduction in the daily insulin dosage (Mangeri *et al.*, 2002). This suggests improvement in insulin sensitivity associated with bisphosphonate use.

Thus, bisphosphonates clearly have beneficial effects on both atherosclerosis and osteoporosis.

Conclusion

Accumulating evidence indicates similar pathophysiologic mechanisms and risk factors underlying both osteoporosis and CVD, including age, sedentary lifestyle, dyslipidemia, hypertension, and diabetes, among others. Furthermore, therapeutic agents used for treatment of osteoporosis appear to have beneficial effects on atherosclerosis and vice versa. The prospect of newer therapeutic agents that could treat both osteoporosis and atherosclerosis simultaneously is an exciting possibility requiring further investigation.

ACKNOWLEDGMENTS

This work is supported by grants from the NIH, K12HD043428, BIRCWH to JN and SIM, and by grant support from the American Diabetes Association, 7-05-RA-89, to SIM.

REFERENCES

Ahmed, N. (2005). Advanced glycation endproducts—Role in pathology of diabetic complications. *Diabetes Res Clin Pract 67*, 3–21.

Alexandersen, P., Haarbo, J., Byrjalsen, I., Lawaetz, H., and Christiansen, C. (1999). Natural androgens inhibit male atherosclerosis: A study in castrated, cholesterol-fed rabbits. *Circ Res 84*, 813–819.

Armour, K.E., Armour, K.J., Gallagher, M.E., Godecke, A., Helfrich, M.H., Reid, D.M. *et al.* (2001). Defective bone formation and anabolic response to exogenous estrogen in mice with targeted disruption of endothelial nitric oxide synthase. *Endocrinology 142*, 760–766.

Bekker, P.J., Holloway, D., Nakanishi, A., Arrighi, M., Leese, P.T., and Dunstan, C.R. (2001). The effect of a single dose of osteoprotegerin in postmenopausal women. *J Bone Miner Res 16*, 348–360.

Bini, A., Mann, K.G., Kudryk, B.J., and Schoen, F.J. (1999). Noncollagenous bone matrix proteins, calcification, and thrombosis in carotid artery atherosclerosis. *Arterioscler Thromb Vasc Biol 19*, 1852–1861.

Bostrom, K., Tsao, D., Shen, S., Wang, Y., and Demer, L.L. (2001). Matrix GLA protein modulates differentiation induced by bone morphogenetic protein-2 in C3H10T1/2 cells. *J Biol Chem 276*, 14044–14052.

Browner, W.S., Seeley, D.G., Vogt, T.M., and Cummings, S.R. (1991). Non-trauma mortality in elderly women with low bone mineral density. Study of Osteoporotic Fractures Research Group. *Lancet 338*, 355–358.

Browner, W.S., Lui, L.Y., and Cummings, S.R. (2001). Associations of serum osteoprotegerin levels with diabetes, stroke, bone density, fractures, and mortality in elderly women. *J Clin Endocrinol Metab 86*, 631–637.

Cappuccio, F.P., Meilahn, E., Zmuda, J.M., and Cauley, J.A. (1999). High blood pressure and bone-mineral loss in elderly white women: A prospective study. Study of Osteoporotic Fractures Research Group. *Lancet 354*, 971–975.

Christian, R.C., Harrington, S., Edwards, W.D., Oberg, A.L., and Fitzpatrick, L.A. (2002). Estrogen status correlates with the calcium content of coronary atherosclerotic plaques in women. *J Clin Endocrinol Metab 87*, 1062–1067.

Cohen-Solal, M.E., Graulet, A.M., Denne, M.A., Gueris, J., Baylink, D., and de Vernejoul, M.C. (1993). Peripheral monocyte culture supernatants of menopausal women can induce bone resorption: Involvement of cytokines. *J Clin Endocrinol Metab 77*, 1648–1653.

Danesh, J., and Lewington, S. (1998). Plasma homocysteine and coronary heart disease: systematic review of published epidemiological studies. *J Cardiovasc Risk 5*, 229–232.

Dhore, C.R., Cleutjens, J.P., Lutgens, E., Cleutjens, K.B., Geusens, P.P., Kitslaar, P.J. *et al.* (2001). Differential expression of bone matrix regulatory proteins in human atherosclerotic plaques. *Arterioscler Thromb Vasc Biol 21*, 1998–2003.

Doherty, T.M., Uzui, H., Fitzpatrick, L.A., Tripathi, P.V., Dunstan, C.R., Asotra, K. *et al.* (2002). Rationale for the role of osteoclast-like cells in arterial calcification. *Faseb J 16*, 577–582.

Dominguez, L.J., Muratore, M., Quarta, E., Zagone, G., and Barbagallo, M. (2004). [Osteoporosis and diabetes]. *Reumatismo 56*, 235–241.

Ducy, P., Desbois, C., Boyce, B., Pinero, G., Story, B., Dunstan, C. *et al.* (1996). Increased bone formation in osteocalcin-deficient mice. *Nature 382*, 448–452.

Emery, J.G., McDonnell, P., Burke, M.B., Deen, K.C., Lyn, S., Silverman, C. *et al.* (1998). Osteoprotegerin is a receptor for the cytotoxic ligand TRAIL. *J Biol Chem 273*, 14363–14367.

Engelse, M.A., Neele, J.M., Bronckers, A.L., Pannekoek, H., and de Vries, C.J. (2001). Vascular calcification: expression patterns of the osteoblast-specific gene core binding factor alpha-1 and the protective factor matrix gla protein in human atherogenesis. *Cardiovasc Res 52*, 281–289.

Ferretti, C. and Ripamonti, U. (2002). Human segmental mandibular defects treated with naturally derived bone morphogenetic proteins. *J Craniofac Surg 13*, 434–444.

Fisher, J.E., Rogers, M.J., Halasy, J.M., Luckman, S.P., Hughes, D.E., Masarachia, P.J. *et al.* (1999). Alendronate mechanism of action: geranylgeraniol, an intermediate in the mevalonate pathway, prevents inhibition of osteoclast formation, bone resorption, and kinase activation in vitro. *Proc Natl Acad Sci USA 96*, 133–138.

Forsen, L., Meyer, H.E., Midthjell, K., and Edna, T.H. (1999). Diabetes mellitus and the incidence of hip fracture: results from the Nord-Trondelag Health Survey. *Diabetologia 42*, 920–925.

Hak, A.E., Pols, H.A., van Hemert, A.M., Hofman, A., and Witteman, J.C. (2000). Progression of aortic calcification is associated with metacarpal bone loss during menopause: a population-based longitudinal study. *Arterioscler Thromb Vasc Biol 20*, 1926–1931.

Hirose, K., Tomiyama, H., Okazaki, R., Arai, T., Koji, Y., Zaydun, G. *et al.* (2003). Increased pulse wave velocity associated with reduced calcaneal quantitative osteo-sono index: possible relationship between atherosclerosis and osteopenia. *J Clin Endocrinol Metab 88*, 2573–2578.

Huber, S.A., Sakkinen, P., Conze, D., Hardin, N., and Tracy, R. 1999. Interleukin-6 exacerbates early atherosclerosis in mice. *Arterioscler Thromb Vasc Biol 19*, 2364–2367.

Hukkanen, M., Hughes, F.J., Buttery, L.D., Gross, S.S., Evans, T.J., Seddon, S. *et al.* (1995). Cytokine-stimulated expression of inducible nitric oxide synthase by mouse, rat, and human osteoblast-like cells and its functional role in osteoblast metabolic activity. *Endocrinology 136*, 5445–5453.

Ihara, H., Denhardt, D.T., Furuya, K., Yamashita, T., Muguruma, Y., Tsuji, K. *et al.* (2001). Parathyroid hormone-induced bone resorption does not occur in the absence of osteopontin. *J Biol Chem 276*, 13065–13071.

Isoda, K., Nishikawa, K., Kamezawa, Y., Yoshida, M., Kusuhara, M., Moroi, M. *et al.* (2002). Osteopontin plays an important role in the development of medial thickening and neointimal formation. *Circ Res 91*, 77–82.

Jackson, B., Gee, A.N., Guyon-Gellin, Y., Niesor, E., Bentzen, C.L., Kerns, W.D. *et al.* (2000). Hypocholesterolaemic and antiatherosclerotic effects of tetra-iso-propyl 2-(3,5-di-tert-butyl-4-hydroxyphenyl)ethyl-1,1-diphosphonate (SR-9223i). *Arzneimittelforschung 50*, 380–386.

Khosla, S. (2001). Minireview: The OPG/RANKL/RANK system. *Endocrinology 142*, 5050–5055.

Khosla, S., Melton, L.J., 3rd, and Riggs, B.L. (2002). Clinical review 144: Estrogen and the male skeleton. *J Clin Endocrinol Metab 87*, 1443–1450.

Lacey, D.L., Timms, E., Tan, H.L., Kelley, M.J., Dunstan, C.R., Burgess, T. *et al.* (1998). Osteoprotegerin ligand is a cytokine that regulates osteoclast differentiation and activation. *Cell 93*, 165–176.

Lee, K.S., Kim, H.J., Li, Q.L., Chi, X.Z., Ueta, C., Komori, T. *et al.* (2000). Runx2 is a common target of transforming growth factor beta1 and bone morphogenetic protein 2, and cooperation between Runx2 and Smad5 induces osteoblast-specific gene expression in the pluripotent mesenchymal precursor cell line C2C12. *Mol Cell Biol 20*, 8783–8792.

Libby, P. (2002). Inflammation in atherosclerosis. *Nature 420*, 868–874.

Luo, G., Ducy, P., McKee, M.D., Pinero, G.J., Loyer, E., Behringer, R.R. *et al.* (1997). Spontaneous calcification of arteries and cartilage in mice lacking matrix GLA protein. *Nature 386*, 78–81.

Mancini, L., Moradi-Bidhendi, N., Becherini, L., Martineti, V., and MacIntyre, I. (2000). The biphasic effects of nitric oxide in primary rat osteoblasts are cGMP dependent. *Biochem Biophys Res Commun 274*, 477–481.

Manolagas, S.C. (2000). Birth and death of bone cells: basic regulatory mechanisms and implications for the pathogenesis and treatment of osteoporosis. *Endocr Rev 21*, 115–137.

Maugeri, D., Panebianco, P., Rosso, D., Calanna, A., Speciale, S., Santangelo, A. *et al.* (2002). Alendronate reduces the daily consumption of insulin (DCI) in patients with senile type I diabetes and osteoporosis. *Arch Gerontol Geriatr 34*, 117–122.

McFarlane, S.I., Muniyappa, R., Francisco, R., and Sowers, J.R. (2002). Clinical review 145: Pleiotropic effects of statins: lipid reduction and beyond. *J Clin Endocrinol Metab 87*, 1451–1458.

McFarlane, S.I., Banerji, M., and Sowers, J.R. (2001). Insulin resistance and cardiovascular disease. *J Clin Endocrinol Metab 86*, 713–718.

Min, H., Morony, S., Sarosi, I., Dunstan, C.R., Capparelli, C., Scully, S. *et al.* (2000). Osteoprotegerin reverses osteoporosis by inhibiting endosteal osteoclasts and prevents vascular calcification by blocking a process resembling osteoclastogenesis. *J Exp Med 192*, 463–474.

Moncada, S., Palmer, R.M., and Higgs, E.A. (1991). Nitric oxide: physiology, pathophysiology, and pharmacology. *Pharmacol Rev 43*, 109–142.

Mundy, G., Garrett, R., Harris, S., Chan, J., Chen, D., Rossini, G. *et al.* (1999). Stimulation of bone formation in vitro and in rodents by statins. *Science 286*, 1946–1949.

Muniyappa, R., Xu, R., Ram, J.L., and Sowers, J.R. (2000). Inhibition of Rho protein stimulates iNOS expression in rat vascular smooth muscle cells. *Am J Physiol Heart Circ Physiol 278*, H1762–1768.

Parhami, F., Tintut, Y., Beamer, W.G., Gharavi, N., Goodman, W., and Demer, L.L. (2001). Atherogenic high-fat diet reduces bone mineralization in mice. *J Bone Miner Res 16*, 182–188.

Parrot, F., Redonnet-Vernhet, I., Lacombe, D., and Gin, H. (2000). Osteoporosis in late-diagnosed adult homocystinuric patients. *J Inherit Metab Dis 23*, 338–340.

Pauli, R.M., Lian, J.B., Mosher, D.F., and Suttie, J.W. (1987). Association of congenital deficiency of multiple vitamin K-dependent coagulation factors and the phenotype of the warfarin embryopathy: clues to the mechanism of teratogenicity of coumarin derivatives. *Am J Hum Genet 41*, 566–583.

Price, P.A., Williamson, M.K., Haba, T., Dell, R.B., and Jee, W.S. (1982). Excessive mineralization with growth plate closure in rats on chronic warfarin treatment. *Proc Natl Acad Sci USA 79*, 7734–7738.

Ridker, P.M., Rifai, N., Rose, L., Buring, J.E., and Cook, N.R. (2002). Comparison of C-reactive protein and low-density lipoprotein cholesterol levels in the prediction of first cardiovascular events. *N Engl J Med 347*, 1557–1565.

Riggs, B,L, Khosla, S., and Melton, L.J., 3rd. (2002). Sex steroids and the construction and conservation of the adult skeleton. *Endocr Rev 23*, 279–302.

Rizzo, M., Di Fede, G., Mansueto, P., Castello, F., Carmina, E., and Rini, G.B. (2004). Statins and osteoporosis: Myth or reality? *Minerva Med 95*, 521–527.

Rossouw, J.E., Anderson, G.L., Prentice, R.L., LaCroix, A.Z., Kooperberg, C., Stefanick, M.L. *et al.* (2002). Risks and benefits of estrogen plus progestin in healthy postmenopausal women: Principal results from the Women's Health Initiative randomized controlled trial. *JAMA 288*, 321–333.

Sakurai, H., Kohsaka, H., Liu, M.F., Higashiyama, H., Hirata, Y., Kanno, K. *et al.* (1995). Nitric oxide production and inducible nitric oxide synthase expression in inflammatory arthritides. *J Clin Invest 96*, 2357–2363.

Santana, R.B., Xu, L., Chase, H.B., Amar, S., Graves, D.T., and Trackman, P.C. (2003). A role for advanced glycation end products in diminished bone healing in type 1 diabetes. *Diabetes 52*, 1502–1510.

Scheidt-Nave, C., Bismar, H., Leidig-Bruckner, G., Woitge, H., Seibel, M.J., Ziegler, R. *et al.* (2001). Serum interleukin 6 is a major predictor of bone loss in women specific to the first decade past menopause. *J Clin Endocrinol Metab 86*, 2032–2042.

Schinke, T., McKee, M.D., and Karsenty, G. (1999). Extracellular matrix calcification: Where is the action? *Nat Genet 21*, 150–151.

Schlemmer, C.K., Coetzer, H., Claassen, N., and Kruger, M.C. (1999). Oestrogen and essential fatty acid supplementation corrects bone loss due to ovariectomy in the female Sprague Dawley rat. *Prostaglandins Leukot Essent Fatty Acids 61*, 381–390.

Schwartz, A.V., Sellmeyer, D.E., Ensrud, K.E., Cauley, J.A., Tabor, H.K., Schreiner, P.J. *et al.* (2001). Older women with diabetes have an increased risk of fracture: a prospective study. *J Clin Endocrinol Metab 86*, 32–38.

Schwartz, A.V. (2003). Diabetes mellitus: does it affect bone? *Calcif Tissue Int 73*, 515–519.

Shanahan, C.M., Proudfoot, D., Tyson, K.L., Cary, N.R., Edmonds, M., and Weissberg, P.L. (2000). Expression of mineralisation-regulating proteins in association with human vascular calcification. *Z Kardiol 89 Suppl 2*, 63–68.

Shioi, A., Katagi, M., Okuno, Y., Mori, K., Jono, S., Koyama, H., and Nishizawa, Y. (2002). Induction of bone-type alkaline phosphatase in human vascular smooth muscle cells: roles of tumor necrosis factor-alpha and oncostatin M derived from macrophages. *Circ Res 91*, 9–16.

Tintut, Y., Patel, J., Territo, M., Saini, T., Parhami, F., and Demer, L.L. (2002). Monocyte/macrophage regulation of vascular calcification in vitro. *Circulation 105*, 650–655.

Valerio, G., del Puente, A., Esposito-del Puente, A., Buono, P., Mozzillo, E., and Franzese, A. (2002). The lumbar bone mineral density is affected by long-term poor metabolic control in adolescents with type 1 diabetes mellitus. *Horm Res 58*, 266–272.

van der Klift, M., Pols, H.A., Hak, A.E., Witteman, J.C., Hofman, A., and de Laet, C.E. (2002). Bone mineral density and the risk of peripheral arterial disease: the Rotterdam Study. *Calcif Tissue Int 70*, 443–449.

van der Meer, I.M., Iglesias del Sol, A., Hak, A.E., Bots, M.L., Hofman, A., and Witteman, J.C. (2003). Risk factors for progression of atherosclerosis measured at multiple sites in the arterial tree: the Rotterdam Study. *Stroke 34*, 2374–2379.

von der Recke, P., Hansen, M.A., and Hassager, C. (1999). The association between low bone mass at the menopause and cardiovascular mortality. *Am J Med 106*, 273–278.

Wada, T., McKee, M.D., Steitz, S., and Giachelli, C.M. (1999). Calcification of vascular smooth muscle cell cultures: inhibition by osteopontin. *Circ Res 84*, 166–178.

Watson, K.E., Bostrom, K., Ravindranath, R., Lam, T., Norton, B., and Demer, L.L. (1994). TGF-beta 1 and 25-hydroxycholesterol stimulate osteoblast-like vascular cells to calcify. *J Clin Invest 93*, 2106–2113.

Wimalawansa, S.J. (2000). Nitroglycerin therapy is as efficacious as standard estrogen replacement therapy (Premarin) in prevention of oophorectomy-induced bone loss: A human pilot clinical study. *J Bone Miner Res 15*, 2240–2244.

Wozney, J.M., Rosen, V., Celeste, A.J., Mitsock, L.M., Whitters, M.J., Kriz, R.W. *et al.* (1988). Novel regulators of bone formation: molecular clones and activities. *Science 242*, 1528–1534.

Yamaguchi, A., Katagiri, T., Ikeda, T., Wozney, J.M., Rosen, V., Wang, E.A. *et al.* (1991). Recombinant human bone morphogenetic protein-2 stimulates osteoblastic maturation and inhibits myogenic differentiation in vitro. *J Cell Biol 113*, 681–687.

Yamaguchi, T., Sugimoto, T., Yano, S., Yamauchi, M., Sowa, H., Chen, Q. *et al.* (2002). Plasma lipids and osteoporosis in postmenopausal women. *Endocr J 49*, 211–217.

Ylitalo, R., Oksala, O., Yla-Herttuala, S., and Ylitalo, P. (1994). Effects of clodronate (dichloromethylene bisphosphonate) on the development of experimental atherosclerosis in rabbits. *J Lab Clin Med 123*, 769–776.

Yoshitake, H., Rittling, S.R., Denhardt, D.T., and Noda, M. (1999). Osteopontin-deficient mice are resistant to ovariectomy-induced bone resorption. *Proc Natl Acad Sci USA 96*, 8156–8160.

59

Depression in Older Patients

Kiran Rabheru

Major depressive disorder is frequently undiagnosed and untreated in older patients, and can be associated with high morbidity and mortality in this patient group, who are particularly prone to completed suicide or self-neglect. Grief, pain, sleep issues, concurrent medications, altered physiology, and the presence of comorbid medical and psychiatric conditions can complicate the management of depression in older patients. Comorbid medical conditions, including cardiovascular events, stroke, vascular dementia, and Alzheimer's disease, which are common among older patients, can have a significant impact on depression, and vice versa.

Depression is not a natural part of the aging process, and it should be diagnosed and actively treated in the elderly, just as it is in younger patients. Pharmacotherapy can be safe and effective in this population, as long as pharmacokinetic and pharmacodynamic properties, as well as the inherent biological differences in the elderly population are considered when selecting treatments. Psychosocial therapies and antidepressants such as selective serotonin reuptake inhibitors (SSRIs), venlafaxine, and mirtazapine have demonstrated beneficial effects in this population. Although tricyclic antidepressants also have demonstrated efficacy, tolerability can be a problem.

Introduction

The prevalence of major depressive disorder (MDD) in older individuals (65 to 100 years) in the community is estimated at 4.4% in women and 2.7% in men (Steffens *et al.*, 2000). The rate of depression is higher among elderly people living alone, those who require assistance with the activities of daily living, and urban vs. rural residents. Several studies have found rates of depression of about 14% among older individuals receiving home care, nursing home residents, and general hospital inpatients. In addition, minor depression (16.8%) and significant depressive symptomatology (44.2%) were very common in a survey of nursing home residents (Teresi *et al.*, 2001).

Although common, depression either is frequently not identified among older patients or is attributed to the normal aging process. In primary care, physicians diagnosed depression in only about 50% of depressed elderly patients (Volkers *et al.*, 2004). Recognition among nursing home residents was even lower, with staff recognizing only 37 to 45% of cases diagnosed by psychiatrists (Teresi *et al.*, 2001). It appears that the presence of multiple medical problems results in a focus on somatic complaints, with less attention being given to depression. Other factors, such as grief, pain, sleep, and medication use, also contribute not only to the underdetection but also to the undertreatment of depression.

Evidence suggests that only about 10 to 38% of elderly patients with depression receive antidepressants (Steffens *et al.*, 2000; Stek *et al.*, 2004). Antidepressant use was lower among elderly suffering from depression in the community (4.2%), compared to those in institutions (36.0%) in a Canadian study (Newman *et al.*, 1999). In surveys of medication use among older individuals, antidepressants were being used in only 2.2 to 4.1% of those who lived in the community and 3.6 to 16.5% of those in institutions (Riedel-Heller *et al.*, 2001). When antidepressants were used, one-third to two-thirds of older patients received dosages that were lower than those recommended for treatment of depression (Riedel-Heller *et al.*, 2001).

The diagnosis and treatment of depression in the elderly is critical. MDD and depressive symptoms have been reported to increase the risk of mortality among elderly subjects by 1.5 to 2.0 times that of subjects without depression (Blazer *et al.*, 2001; Lavretsky *et al.*, 2002; Schoevers *et al.*, 2000; Schulz *et al.*, 2000).

Etiology and Pathogenesis

Studies suggest that structural changes of various neuroanatomic structures including frontostriatal and limbic dysfunction contribute to the pathogenesis of at least some late-life depressive syndromes (Alexopoulos, 2002). Three cortico-striato-pallido-cortical pathways between the frontal lobe and the basal ganglia may be relevant to depression because damage to these pathways leads to behavioral abnormalities that resemble in part the depressive syndrome (Alexopoulos, 2004). In addition, damage to the orbitofrontal circuit may lead to disinhibition, irritability, and diminished sensitivity to social cues; damage to the anterior cingulate may result in apathy and reduced initiative; and damage to the dorsolateral circuit may result in difficulties in set shifting, learning, and word list generation.

In older patients with depression, studies have described decreases in hippocampal volume (Moffat *et al.*, 2000; Sheline *et al.*, 1999), abnormalities of various frontal lobe structures (Chemerinski *et al.*, 2000; Kumar *et al.*, 2000; Lai *et al.*, 2000), and basal ganglia (Chemerinski *et al.*, 2000), as well as abnormal cerebral blood flow (Alexopoulos, 2004) and metabolic activity (de Asis *et al.*, 2001; Drevets, 2000; Mayberg, 2001) in these structures.

Frontostriatal dysfunction appears to influence the course of geriatric depression. Executive impairment, the neurophysiological expression of striatofrontal dysfunction, was reported to predict poor or delayed antidepressant response, and has been associated with relapse and recurrence, as well as residual depressive symptomatology (Alexopoulos *et al.*, 2002; Alexopoulos *et al.*, 2000; Kalayam *et al.*, 1999). Changes in metabolism in various brain structures have been associated with remission of depression (Drevets, 2000; Mayberg, 2001), risk of relapse, and treatment-resistance (Mayberg, 2001).

Polymorphisms in the promoter region of the serotonin transporter gene (5-HTTLPR) may play a role in the pathogenesis and course of depression and anxiety (Hariri *et al.*, 2003; Sen *et al.*, 2004; Taylor *et al.*, 2005). Geneotype has been related to hippocampal volumes (Taylor *et al.*, 2005) and to amygdala reactivity to environmental stimuli (Hariri *et al.*, 2005). These findings may be related to interactions between the serotonergic system and neurotrophic factors or cortisol response to stresses and may bias an individual's reactivity to stressful life experiences (Hariri *et al.*, 2005; Taylor *et al.*, 2005). Some studies report that genotype significantly predicts the development of depression after stressful life events (Lenze *et al.*, 2005), although others did not find an association (Gillespie *et al.*, 2005). Several studies have suggested that response to antidepressant therapy may be related to serotonin transporter genotype (Murphy *et al.*, 2004). The short (S) allele was associated with a faster response to sertraline (Durham *et al.*, 2004). However, in another study, no relationship with efficacy was seen; rather, the major effect was on SSRI. Results were not consistent with the S allele being associated with more adverse effects with paroxetine therapy, and fewer with mirtazapine, suggesting the effect of this polymorphism on outcome may depend on the mechanism of antidepressant action (Murphy *et al.*, 2004).

Depression in the elderly is common in individuals with vascular neurological diseases, and many of the structural and functional changes identified in patients with depression are associated with a variety of neurologic disorders (i.e., stroke, Parkinson's disease, Alzheimer's disease) (Kanner, 2004). In addition, depression is a risk factor for the development of several neurologic disorders, including dementia (Andersen *et al.*, 2005; Bartolini *et al.*, 2005; Dal Forno *et al.*, 2005; Modrego *et al.*, 2004; Steffens *et al.*, 2004) and has a negative impact on the course and outcome of most neurologic disorders (Dorenlot *et al.*, 2005; Hughes *et al.*, 2004). Late-life depression is a frequent complication of stroke. Lacunar infarcts in the basal ganglia have the highest comorbidity with depression (Chemerinski *et al.*, 2000), and subcortical atrophy appears to be a predisposing factor.

The relationship between depression and cardiovascular disorders also provides insight into the mechanisms of depression. Abnormalities in neurotransmitters (including serotonin), platelet-activating factor, and nitric oxide, which are involved in atherosclerotic processes, have been implicated in the pathogenesis of depression (Plante, 2005). Moreover, vascular consequences of depression such as heart rate and pulse pressure variations may lead to endothelial dysfunction in critical microcirculation networks (cerebral, myocardial, and renal) and initiate physicochemical alterations in interstitial compartments adjacent to vital organs. Worsening depressive symptoms after a coronary event were associated with impaired autonomic control of the heart, and mortality was almost three times higher among the patients with MDD at the time of the initial event compared to those without depression (de Guevara *et al.*, 2004). The finding of higher rates of relapse of depression among patients taking cholesterol-lowering medications supports the idea of a vascular component to depression (Steffens *et al.*, 2003).

Thus, it appears that both degenerative and vascular processes contribute to the brain abnormalities identified in late-life depression. It is likely that there are bidirectional pathophysiological mechanisms contributing to depression in older patients with comorbid vascular diseases.

Issues in the Management of Depression in Older Patients

COURSE

A study of the natural history of late-life depression found that long-term outcomes are poor (Beekman *et al.*, 2002). Over the six years of follow-up, the average symptom severity remained above the 85th percentile of the population average. Symptoms were short-lived in only 14%, remission was achieved in 23%, an unfavorable but fluctuating course in 44%, and a severe chronic course in 32%. Individuals with subthreshold disorders had the best outcome, followed by those with MDD, dysthymic disorder, and double depression. However, the prognosis of subthreshold disorders was unfavorable in most cases (Beekman *et al.*, 2002). Relapse rates without ongoing treatment are high, supporting the importance of long-term maintenance therapy (Flint *et al.*, 1999; Thorpe *et al.*, 2001).

Comorbid anxiety disorders, which are common in this population (23–48%), are associated with a more severe course of depressive illness (Beekman *et al.*, 2000; Lenze *et al.*, 2000).

COMORBID CONDITIONS

Comorbid medical conditions are the norm in older patients with depression. There appear to be complex bidirectional consequences of depression and comorbid vascular conditions on the pathogenesis, severity, and prognosis of both depression and the comorbidity. Comorbidities complicate the management of depression and vice versa. The relationship between depression and cardiovascular abnormalities, stroke, diabetes, and dementias in terms of prevalence, impact on prognosis, and effects on management strategies is discussed in the later section on management of depression in patients with comorbid illnesses.

PHARMACOKINETIC AND PHARMACODYNAMIC CONSIDERATIONS

The use of antidepressants in older patients can be complicated by several factors. Older individuals use multiple medications (two or more prescription drugs) three times more frequently than younger persons, increasing the potential for interactions. Age-related alterations in physiology can result in variable plasma drug concentrations, which may increase the number of adverse events, and the elderly may be more sensitive to adverse events (McDonald *et al.*, 2002). Aging is associated with a number of neuroendocrine changes, including alterations in monoamine oxidases, noradrenergic neurons, dopaminergic neurons and concentrations, cholinergic neurons and receptors, adrenocorticotropic hormone (ACTH) concentration and function, and serotonin receptors and concentrations (Rehman *et al.*, 2001). There is early evidence that some older patients with deficits in executive skills may respond poorly to antidepressant treatment compared with those with intact executive functions (Mohlman, 2005).

Recommended initial doses are lower for the elderly for all antidepressants, and increases should be slow and individualized (De Vane *et al.*, 1999). The pharmacokinetics of some selective serotonin reuptake inhibitors (SSRIs) may be altered in older patients, and it is recommended that doses be adjusted in these patients (De Vane *et al.*, 1999). Lower doses should be used for citalopram and for paroxetine (Muijsers *et al.*, 2002). Medical conditions can affect drug elimination, which is decreased in patients with hepatic (citalopram, fluoxetine, fluvoxamine, sertraline) or renal (paroxetine) impairment (Muijsers *et al.*, 2002).

SUICIDE RISK

The risk of suicide demonstrates the need for early geriatric psychiatric assessments and vigorous treatment protocols. Suicidal feelings are high among individuals aged 85 years or over with mental disorders, with 30% believing "life was not worth living" and 10% having thought of taking their own life (Skoog *et al.*, 1996). Among women who felt life was not worth living, the three-year mortality rate was three times that of women without these feelings (43% vs. 14%, respectively). Several studies have shown that recognition of depression among the elderly who attempt or complete suicide is inadequate (Duckworth *et al.*, 1996; Suominen *et al.*, 2004). Only 4% of the elderly who had attempted suicide had been diagnosed with a mood disorder before the attempt, despite having physician contact within the previous year (Suominen *et al.*, 2004). Among elderly depression patients who had committed suicide, 80% of patients had no psychiatric referral, and 87% were untreated (Duckworth *et al.*, 1996). Correlates of suicide include poor perceived health, poor sleep quality, and lack of a confidant (Turvey *et al.*, 2002). There is also a strong association with deliberate self-poisoning using benzodiazepine in the elderly (Ticehurst *et al.*, 2002).

In the Prevention of Suicide in Primary Care Elderly: Collaborative Trial (PROSPECT), use of a multifaceted care management model in primary care was shown to significantly reduce rates of suicidal ideation compared with usual care among elderly patients with depression (Bruce *et al.*, 2004). In addition, a survey of prescribing trends showed a decrease in the rate of suicide associated with prescriptions for antidepressants, antipsychotics, antimanic drugs and analgesics, and an increase with prescriptions for barbiturates, hypnotics, and sedatives (Shah *et al.*, 2001).

Management of Depression in Older Patients

TREATMENT GOALS

Like younger patients with depression, older patients should be treated to remission (the virtual elimination of symptoms) rather than simply response (reduction in symptoms). Remission maximizes the impact of treatment on quality of life domains (Doraiswamy *et al.*, 2001). In 100 older patients with recurrent MDD, those who achieved remission with antidepressant treatment showed significantly greater improvement than either partial responders or nonresponders on both emotional and physical quality of life measures.

When treating older patients, a strong doctor–patient relationship is essential, and interventions should include environmental, social, recreational, supportive, and spiritual programs, as well as psychoeducational programs that include the patient's family. Antidepressant medications at appropriate dosages and durations are the mainstay of therapy as in younger patients, and ECT is recommended for severe cases.

ANTIDEPRESSANT THERAPY

Efficacy for acute and maintenance treatment

Evidence suggests that older patients will benefit from antidepressant therapy as much as younger adults, but that improvements may occur more slowly (Reynolds *et al.*, 1996). A Cochrane database review of 17 trials of antidepressant use in older patients with depression found similar efficacy for TCAs, SSRIs, and MAOIs (Wilson *et al.*, 2001). At least six weeks of treatment was recommended to achieve optimal therapeutic effect. In a meta-analysis of eight double-blind, randomized controlled trials (RCTs) of venlafaxine, SSRIs, or placebo, no significant age-by-treatment interactions were detected (Entsuah *et al.*, 2001).

The efficacy of bupropion, citalopram, fluoxetine, paroxetine, sertraline, as well as venlafaxine, mirtazapine, and nortriptyline, in treating older patients with depression has been demonstrated in clinical trials (Allard *et al.*, 2004; Bondareff *et al.*, 2000; Cassano *et al.*, 2002; Devanand *et al.*, 2005; Forlenza *et al.*, 2001; Gasto *et al.*, 2003; Navarro *et al.*, 2001; Newhouse *et al.*, 2000; Rocca *et al.*, 2005; Schatzberg *et al.*, 2002; Sheikh *et al.*, 2004; Weihs *et al.*, 2000). There are few statistically significant differences between agents in individual studies, with response rates being about 40 to 75% and remission rates about 30 to 70% (Bondareff *et al.*, 2000; Cassano *et al.*, 2002; Devanand *et al.*, 2005; Forlenza *et al.*, 2001; Gasto *et al.*, 2003; Navarro *et al.*, 2001; Newhouse *et al.*, 2000; Rocca *et al.*, 2005; Schatzberg *et al.*, 2002). There is some evidence that agents with dual mechanism, including the SNRIs, mirtazapine and venlafaxine and the TCA, nortriptyline, may be more effective than agents with a single mode of action such as the SSRIs (Entsuah *et al.*, 2001; Gasto *et al.*, 2003; Navarro *et al.*, 2001; Schatzberg *et al.*, 2002). Therapeutic response to sertraline in older patients with MDD was significantly greater than placebo and comparable in those with or without medical comorbidity (Sheikh *et al.*, 2004).

Few data are available on antidepressant therapy in the very old patient. In a small placebo-controlled trial in very old patients (aged 80 years and over) in long-term care facilities, paroxetine was not significantly better than placebo but was associated with two cases of delirium (Burrows *et al.*, 2002).

Data on the prevention of relapse or recurrence in older patients demonstrates the efficacy of ongoing antidepressant therapy (Bump *et al.*, 2001; Klysner *et al.*, 2002). Results are similar to those in younger patients, with ongoing therapy being associated with reductions in relapse rates of about 30 to 50%. Long-term treatment with citalopram effectively reduced recurrence by about 50% after sustained response in a double-blind, placebo-controlled trial in older patients (Klysner *et al.*, 2002). In a small, open, follow-up study in older patients, paroxetine and nortriptyline demonstrated similar efficacy in relapse prevention and time to relapse (Bump *et al.*, 2001).

Cognitive effects

Both aging and depression itself have been associated with impairments in cognitive functioning. Older patients with depression have demonstrated impaired executive functioning, compared with younger patients with depression or healthy elderly individuals without depression (Lockwood *et al.*, 2002).

Older individuals with cognitive impairment at baseline do not necessarily reach normal levels of performance, particularly in memory and executive functions after treatment of late-life depression (Butters *et al.*, 2000). However, several studies have demonstrated improvements in various measures of cognitive functioning among older patients treated with SSRI antidepressants. The detrimental effects of TCAs on cognition have been well documented and may reflect the vulnerability of older patients to the central anticholinergic activity of these agents (Peretti *et al.*, 2000). The SSRIs sertraline, paroxetine, and fluoxetine, and the SNRI, venlafaxine have demonstrated significant improvements in cognitive functioning, with sertraline and paroxetine demonstrating some advantages over fluoxetine (Bondareff *et al.*, 2000; Cassano *et al.*, 2002; Doraiswamy *et al.*, 2003; Newhouse *et al.*, 2000; Tsolaki *et al.*, 2000). In contrast, a small study in very old (aged 80 years and over) patients found a risk of adverse cognitive effects with paroxetine: two patients developed delirium, and others were more likely to experience decreases in cognitive scores (Burrows *et al.*, 2002). In patients with MDD and existing cognitive impairment, open treatment with sertraline was associated with minor improvements in cognition among responders and mild deterioration among nonresponders (Devanand *et al.*, 2003).

Safety and tolerability

A meta-analysis of 11 clinical trials in older patients with depression reported an increased withdrawal rate with TCAs compared to SSRIs (Wilson *et al.*, 2004). This was reflected in the higher rate of side effects with TCAs including dry mouth, drowsiness, dizziness, and lethargy. Although there was a relatively low prevalence of side effects associated with SSRIs, a significant minority of older people experienced nausea, vomiting, dizziness, and drowsiness.

In clinical trials, the most common side effects were dry mouth and weight gain with mirtazapine (Schatzberg *et al.*, 2002) and nausea/vomiting with venlafaxine (Allard *et al.*, 2004). Pooled data from eight RCTs in older patients demonstrated the safety of citalopram, with only increased sweating occurring more often than with placebo (Keller, 2000). SSRI and venlafaxine use have been independently associated with the presence of hyponatremia in elderly patients (Flores *et al.*, 2004; Kirby *et al.*, 2002; Rosner, 2004).

Older patients frequently take multiple medications, which makes the potential for drug interactions with antidepressant medications a concern. The potential for interaction is generally higher with older antidepressant compounds (such as TCAs and MAOIs), which are associated with clinically significant interactions with many medications frequently prescribed to elderly patients (Spina *et al.*, 2002). New antidepressants have a more selective mechanism of action and a lower potential for pharmacodynamic drug interactions.

PSYCHOTHERAPY

The combination of both antidepressant and psychotherapy has been shown more effective than either therapy alone, in both acute and maintenance treatment (Lenze *et al.*, 2002; Miller *et al.*, 2001; Reynolds *et al.*, 1999; Thompson *et al.*, 2001). In an evaluation of the combination of desipramine and cognitive-behavioral therapy (CBT), compared with either therapy alone, the combination was more effective than the TCA but similar to the CBT alone (Thompson *et al.*, 2001). Maintenance therapy with interpersonal psychotherapy (IPT) alone or in combination with an antidepressant has been shown to protect against recurrence of MDD in elderly patients, with the combination tending to be more effective than IPT or pharmacotherapy alone (Miller *et al.*, 2001; Reynolds *et al.*, 1999). The combination of psychotherapy and medication also has been shown to maintain social adjustment better than either treatment alone and to improve both the duration and quality of wellness (Lenze *et al.*, 2002).

AUGMENTATION AND NOVEL TREATMENT STRATEGIES

Lithium has demonstrated some benefits when used as augmentation to antidepressants in older patients, with a 50% response acute rate (Zullino *et al.*, 2001). Lithium augmentation significantly reduced relapse rates compared to antidepressants alone over two years (Wilkinson *et al.*, 2002). However, it is recommended that special care be taken when treating elderly patients with lithium, because of a higher risk of adverse effects.

No benefit was seen when total sleep deprivation was added to paroxetine; in fact, the two interventions seem to counteract each other (Reynolds *et al.*, 2005). Light therapy significantly improved depressive symptoms in a study in older depressed patients (Tsai *et al.*, 2004). A small randomized trial comparing repetitive transcranial magnetic stimulation (rTMS) and sham treatment in older patients with treatment-resistant MDD reported antidepressant effects in both groups, with no significant benefits associated with rTMS (Mosimann *et al.*, 2004). St John's Wort has been shown to have antidepressant effects (Linde *et al.*, 2005). St. John's Wort was shown to be equivalent to fluoxetine, in a randomized trial in elderly patients with mild or moderate depressive episodes (Harrer *et al.*, 1999).

ELECTROCONVULSIVE THERAPY (ECT)

Although patients who receive ECT tend to be older than those who do not (de Carle *et al.*, 2000), there are few good studies of the use of ECT in the elderly population. ECT has been reported to be effective in elderly patients in several open or retrospective case series (Bosworth *et al.*, 2002; Kujala *et al.*, 2002; Little *et al.*, 2004), with improvement in about 80% and adverse events in about 35% (Kujala *et al.*, 2002; Little *et al.*, 2004). Safety has been generally acceptable, with only minor complications during ECT among older patients with preexisting cardiovascular disease; falls are reported with increasing frequency as the number of treatments increases (de Carle *et al.*, 2000).

In meta-analyses, ECT has been found to be an effective treatment option compared to both placebo and pharmacotherapy (2003; Pagnin *et al.*, 2004). Several open, prospective, follow-up studies have compared one-year outcomes in elderly patients treated with ECT or antidepressants (Huuhka *et al.*, 2004; Navarro *et al.*, 2004a; Navarro *et al.*, 2004b). One study reported a 41% rehospitalization rate, which was similar in both treatment groups (Huuhka *et al.*, 2004). In patients who remained euthymic for one year, there were no brain perfusion abnormalities, and the significant anterior hypofrontality seen at baseline disappeared with sustained remission of depression in both treatment groups (Navarro *et al.*, 2004a, 2004b).

Managing Depression in Older Patients with Comorbid Conditions

OVERVIEW

Older patients often have significant medical comorbidity, and evidence suggests a significant association with depressive symptoms (Lee *et al.*, 2001). Comorbid conditions contribute to the underdiagnosis and undertreatment of depression in older patients, with somatic complaints taking precedence over depressive symptoms among both patients and their physicians. However, depression should not be overlooked because it can have an important impact on the outcome of medical conditions and vice versa.

Depression can be safely and effectively treated in patients with comorbid medical illnesses. A Cochrane database review of antidepressants in medically ill patients over age 16 years included 18 studies covering 838 patients with a range of physical diseases (Gill *et al.*, 2000). Patients treated with antidepressants were significantly more likely to improve than those given placebo with an NNT with antidepressants to produce 1 recovery from depression was 4.2, and the number needed to harm (NNH) to produce 1 dropout for adverse effects was 9.8.

CARDIOVASCULAR

Depression is common among individuals who suffer acute myocardial infarction (MI) (Akhtar *et al.*, 2004; Rosengren *et al.*, 2004), and the level of depressive symptoms during admission for MI is closely linked to long-term survival (de Guevara *et al.*, 2004; Lesperance *et al.*, 2002; Shiotani *et al.*, 2002). Patients with depression post-MI were at a significantly increased risk of new cardiovascular events (de Jonge *et al.*, 2005; Shiotani *et al.*, 2002; van Melle *et al.*, 2004) and mortality (de Guevara *et al.*, 2004; Pfiffner *et al.*, 2004; van Melle *et al.*, 2004), as well as a poor quality of life, more health complaints, and more disability (de Jonge *et al.*, 2005) compared to those without depression. Similarly, depression was associated with an increased risk of major cardiac events in patients with unstable angina (Lesperance *et al.*, 2000).

Several studies also have demonstrated that depression is independently associated with a substantial increase in the risk of heart failure, particularly among women (Abramson *et al.*, 2001; Powell *et al.*, 2005; Williams *et al.*, 2002). Depression had a significant negative effect on health status, including heart failure symptoms, physical and role function, and quality of life in a six-month prospective cohort study (Sullivan *et al.*, 2004). Higher rates of relapse of depression were reported among patients using cholesterol-lowering medications compared to those who were not (Steffens *et al.*, 2003).

Evidence suggests an association between the use of TCAs and the risk of MI. In a cohort study, there was a doubling of the risk of MI associated with TCA use and no increased risk with SSRIs compared with no antidepressant use (Cohen *et al.*, 2000). However, in a naturalistic study, the abnormalities in conduction and orthostatic hypotension associated with TCA treatment were reported, but cases of first-degree atrioventricular block, prolonged QTc interval, and orthostatic hypotension were also observed in the SSRI-treated patients (Rodriguez de la Torre *et al.*, 2001).

SSRIs have been shown to be relatively safe and effective in patients with a history of cardiovascular disease. Several studies have found sertraline to be effective in patients with MDD after MI and those with hypertension and other cardiovascular morbidity (Krishnan *et al.*, 2001). In a small study, no significant changes in heart rate, blood pressure, cardiac conduction, coagulation measures, or left ventricular ejection fraction were observed. Bleeding time increased in 12 patients, decreased in four patients, and was unchanged in two patients. Paroxetine has also demonstrated good efficacy and tolerability in patients with MDD and documented ischemic heart disease (Nelson *et al.*, 1999; Roose *et al.*, 1998).

Trials to assess impact of treating depression on cardiovascular risk are in their infancy. A recent randomized trial studying the impact of CBT (and SSRIs when indicated) on both major and minor depression post MI was unable to detect an impact on event-free survival (Berkman *et al.*, 2003). However, there is some evidence that SSRIs may reduce the incidence of new cardiovascular events in patients with a history of cardiovascular disease. A case-control study found that antidepressant use was associated with a 15 to 45% decrease in the risk of hospitalization for myocardial infarction among individuals with a history of cardiovascular disease (Monster *et al.*, 2004). Similarly, another case-control study reported significantly reduced odds of MI in individuals taking SSRI antidepressants, with the risk almost halved (Sauer *et al.*, 2003). It has been suggested that reductions in cardiovascular events with SSRIs may be related to their inhibitory effect on platelet aggregation (Maurer-Spurej *et al.*, 2004).

STROKE

Depressive symptoms are common after stroke (Hackett *et al.*, 2005; Verdelho *et al.*, 2004). MDD has been shown to be an independent predictor of stroke, approximately doubling the risk after other known risk factors are controlled (Jonas *et al.*, 2000; Larson *et al.*, 2001). Depression has been associated with increased mortality and poor long-term functional outcome after stroke (Bozikas *et al.*, 2005; Gillen *et al.*, 2001; Pohjasvaara *et al.*, 2001).

An association between bleeding disorders and the use of SSRIs has been suggested, However, several cohort analyses reported no increased risk in cerebrovascular events with past use of SSRI or TCA antidepressants (Barbui *et al.*, 2005; de Abajo *et al.*, 2000). A review conducted to determine the feasibility and effectiveness of antidepressant treatment for post-stroke depression in elderly patients found that TCAs would be contraindicated in 83% of patients, and SSRIs would be contraindicated in only 11% of patients (Cole *et al.*, 2001). A randomized, placebo-controlled trial demonstrated that reboxetine was safe and effective for use in stroke patients with depression (Rampello *et al.*, 2005). Mirtazapine therapy administered from day 1 post-stroke has been shown to prevent the development of depression compared to placebo (Niedermaier *et al.*, 2004).

There is some evidence to suggest that treatment of depression after stroke can have significant beneficial effects on long-term outcomes. In a study in 104 post-stroke patients with or without depression, nortriptyline produced a significantly higher response rate than fluoxetine or placebo in improving depression, anxiety symptoms, and recovery of activities of daily living (Robinson *et al.*, 2000). A nine-year follow-up of these patients reported that antidepressant therapy significantly improved survival; 70% of patients were alive compared to 36%, who were treated with placebo (Jorge *et al.*, 2003).

DIABETES

Diabetes is highly prevalent in older individuals, and significantly increases the risk of cardiovascular events. A meta-analysis found that the rate of depression among individuals with diabetes was twice that of individuals without diabetes (Anderson *et al.*, 2001). In a long-term follow-up of a community cohort, the presence of depressive symptoms at baseline more than doubled the risk of developing type 2 diabetes (Palinkas *et al.*, 2004). In addition, the presence of depression has been associated with poor glycemic control in both patients with type 1 and those with type 2 diabetes (de Groot *et al.*, 2001; Lustman *et al.*, 2000; Palinkas *et al.*, 2004).

Care should be taken to choose antidepressants with no or minimal effects on glucose levels in patients with diabetes. A review of treatment of depression in patients with comorbid diabetes mellitus included six studies of fluoxetine for up to 12 months that demonstrated reductions in weight, in fasting plasma glucose (FPG), and in glycosylated hemoglobin (HbA1c) (Goodnick 2001). Sertraline also has demonstrated beneficial effects on glycemic control, whereas the TCA nortriptyline, which produces increased synaptic catechols, has led to worsening of glucose control. In the United Kingdom Prospective Diabetes Study (UKPDS), every 1% reduction in HbA1c was associated with reductions in risk of 21% for any endpoint related to diabetes, of 21% for diabetes-related deaths, and of 14% for myocardial infarction (Stratton *et al.*, 2000).

DEMENTIA AND ALZHEIMER'S DISEASE

A higher prevalence of depressive symptoms was seen in patients with vascular dementia (31%) or Alzheimer's disease (AD) (20%) compared to cognitively normal elderly individuals (13.2%) (Li *et al.*, 2001). Depression is also frequent in Parkinson's disease and because of overlapping clinical symptoms, frequently goes unrecognized (Lemke *et al.*, 2004). In numerous cohort studies, depression has been shown to double the risk of Alzheimer's disease and vascular dementia (Andersen *et al.*, 2005; Dal Forno *et al.*, 2005; Modrego *et al.*, 2004; Steffens *et al.*, 2004). The rate of dementias and AD has been shown to increase with increasing depression scores and increasing numbers of depressive episodes (Bartolini *et al.*, 2005; Kessing *et al.*, 2004). Depression has a negative impact on the course and outcome of comorbid neurological disorders, more than doubling the risk of death among patients with Parkinson's disease (Hughes *et al.*, 2004) and significantly increasing the risk of early institutionalization in patients with dementias including AD (Dorenlot *et al.*, 2005).

Response to the SSRIs in patients with dementia or AD has been mixed (Lyketsos *et al.*, 2000; Magai *et al.*, 2000; Petracca *et al.*, 2001). Paroxetine and imipramine demonstrated equivalent efficacy in the treatment of depression in elderly patients with co-existing dementia at eight weeks. There was a trend toward better tolerability with paroxetine, in terms of anticholinergic and serious nonfatal adverse events. In small placebo-controlled trials, there were no significant benefits of sertraline (Magai *et al.*, 2000) or fluoxetine (Petracca *et al.*, 2001) over placebo in the treatment of depression in patients with AD. However, in a study in outpatients with AD, sertraline was superior to placebo for the treatment of major depression, and significantly lessened behavior disturbance and improved activities of daily living, but did not improve cognition (Lyketsos *et al.*, 2000). In a small open trial in patients with Parkinson's disease, reboxetine significantly improved depression with acceptable tolerability, but there were no significant changes in parkinsonian symptoms (Lemke, 2002).

There is some evidence that behavior therapy–pleasant events and behavior therapy–problem solving reduce depression in people with probable AD who are living at home with their primary caregiver (Verkaik *et al.*, 2005).

CHRONIC OBSTRUCTIVE PULMONARY DISEASE (COPD)

Nearly half of all COPD patients experience substantial depressive symptoms (Lacasse *et al.*, 2001; Yohannes *et al.*, 2003), which increase to as much as 90% among patients with end-stage disease (Gore *et al.*, 2000). Depression has an impact on disability (Kim *et al.*, 2000) and may contribute to the progression of COPD through its relationship with early smoking and failure to quit. Patients with COPD rarely receive treatment for mental health problems (Gore *et al.*, 2000; Kim *et al.*, 2000).

Several trials assessing the effects of psychotherapies, such as psychoeducation and CBT, on depression in patients with COPD have demonstrated significant reduction in depression and anxiety symptoms, but generally little or no change in lung or physical function (de Godoy *et al.*, 2003; Kunik *et al.*, 2001). Pulmonary rehabilitation programs have been shown to improve depressive symptom scores.

A randomized, placebo-controlled study of paroxetine demonstrated significant improvements in emotional function and mastery and nonsignificant improvements in dyspnea and fatigue (Lacasse *et al.*, 2004). Drop-out rates were high in this study in frail elderly patients. This is mirrored in an open trial, in which only 25% of depressed patients with COPD agreed to undergo therapy with fluoxetine. Of those who were treated, 57% responded, and the majority of those who refused therapy remained depressed at a six-month follow-up (Yohannes *et al.*, 2001). This underscores the need for effective treatment approaches in this patient group.

Conclusion

When managing depression in older patients, there are unique concerns that complicate both the diagnosis and the treatment of the disorder. Older patients frequently have comorbid medical conditions, are taking multiple medications, and have altered physiology that can impact the concentrations of antidepressant medications and heighten sensitivity to side effects. However, managing depression in older patients can be done effectively with the antidepressant therapies currently available. Older patients with depression should be treated to remission, just as their younger counterparts are. Residual symptoms of depression are associated with a lower quality of life.

Depression in older patients can have a significant impact on comorbid medical conditions, which are common among the elderly. It is likely that comorbid vascular disorders such as cardiovascular, cerebrovascular, and neurologic disorders play a role in the pathogenesis of depression in older patients. Rates of cardiovascular events and stroke are higher in patients with depression compared to those without. Antidepressant therapy with SSRIs has demonstrated efficacy and tolerability in patients at high risk for cardiovascular events and stroke. Early results suggest that treating depression with SSRIs can significantly reduce the risk of new cardiovascular events in patients with a history of cardiovascular disease, possibly due to their inhibitory effect on platelet aggregation.

MDD has been shown to approximately double the risk of stroke, and has been associated with increased mortality and poor long-term functional outcomes after stroke. SSRIs may be useful in the prevention and treatment of depression after stroke. In addition, the treatment of depression after stroke might significantly improve long-term survival.

Diabetes is also common among older patients, and increases the risk of cardiovascular and other events. Depression has been shown to increase the risk of developing diabetes and the rate of hyperglycemia. Although fluoxetine has more data supporting beneficial effects on glucose levels, other antidepressants may also be useful in patients with diabetes and depression.

Depression has been shown to at least double the risk of developing Alzheimer's disease and vascular dementia, and has a negative impact on the course and outcome of comorbid neurological disorders. Early results in patients with vascular dementia or Alzheimer's disease suggest SSRI therapy may have beneficial effects in the treatment of depression.

Clearly it is essential to identify and treat depression in older patients. Treating depression not only improves quality of life for older patients, but may also have a significant impact on long-term survival. Although early results suggest that SSRIs, venlafaxine, and mirtazapine are relatively safe and effective in older patients with MDD, more work is needed. Based on early results suggesting improved long-term survival in patients with a history of cardiovascular or cerebrovascular events, priority should be given to studying the role of antidepressants in these patients to confirm the benefits, determine the mechanisms for improved survival, and identify which antidepressant classes or individual agents are beneficial.

REFERENCES

Abramson, J., Berger, A., Krumholz, H., and Vaccarino, V. (2001). Depression and risk of heart failure among older persons with isolated systolic hypertension. *Arch Intern Med 161*, 1725–1730.

Akhtar, M., Malik, S., and Ahmed, M. (2004). Symptoms of depression and anxiety in post-myocardial infarction patients. *J Coll Physicians Surg Pak 14*, 615–618.

Alexopoulos, G.S. (2002). Frontostriatal and limbic dysfunction in late-life depression. *Am J Geriatr Psychiatry. 10*, 687–695.

Alexopoulos, G.S. (2004). Late-life mood disorders. In J. Sadavoy, L. Jarvik, G. Grossberg, and B. Meyer, Eds. *Comprehensive textbook of geriatric psychiatry*. New York: WW Norton & Co., pp. 609–653.

Alexopoulos, G.S., Borson, S., Cuthbert, B.N., Devanand, D.P., Mulsant, B.H., Olin, J.T. *et al.* (2002). Assessment of late life depression. *Biol Psychiatry 52*, 164–174.

Alexopoulos, G.S., Meyers, B.S., Young, R.C., Kalayam, B., Kakuma, T., Gabrielle, M. *et al.* (2000). Executive dysfunction and long-term outcomes of geriatric depression. *Arch Gen Psychiatry 57*, 285–290.

Allard, P., Gram, L., Timdahl, K., Behnke, K., Hanson, M., and Sogaard, J. (2004). Efficacy and tolerability of venlafaxine in geriatric outpatients with major depression: A double-blind, randomised 6-month comparative trial with citalopram. *Int J Geriatr Psychiatry 19*, 1123–1130.

Andersen, K., Lolk, A., Kragh-Sorensen, P., Petersen, N., and Green, A. (2005). Depression and the risk of Alzheimer disease. *Epidemiology 16*, 233–238.

Anderson, R., Freedland, K., Clouse, R., and Lustman, P. (2001). The prevalence of comorbid depression in adults with diabetes: a meta-analysis. *Diabetes Care 24*, 1069–1078.

Barbui, C., Percudani, M., Fortino, I., Tansella, M., and Petrovich, L. (2005). Past use of selective serotonin reuptake inhibitors and the risk of cerebrovascular events in the elderly. *Int Clin Psychopharmacol 20*, 169–171.

Bartolini, M., Coccia, M., Luzzi, S., Provinciali, L., and Ceravolo, M. (2005). Motivational symptoms of depression mask preclinical Alzheimer's disease in elderly subjects. *Dement Geriatr Cogn Disord 19*, 31–36.

Beekman, A., de Beurs, E., van Balkom, A., Deeg, D., van Dyck, R., and van Tilburg, W. (2000). Anxiety and depression in later life: Co-occurrence and communality of risk factors. *Am J Psychiatry 157*, 89–95.

Beekman, A., Geerlings, S., Deeg, D., Smit, J., Schoevers, R., de Beurs, E. *et al.* (2002). The natural history of late-life depression: a 6-year prospective study in the community. *Arch Gen Psychiatry 59*, 605–611.

Berkman, L., Blumenthal, J., Burg, M., Carney, R., Catellier, D., Cowan, M. *et al.* (2003). Effects of treating depression and low perceived social support on clinical events after myocardial infarction: The Enhancing Recovery in Coronary Heart Disease Patients (ENRICHD) Randomized Trial. *JAMA 289*, 3106–3116.

Blazer, D., Hybels, C., and Pieper, C. (2001). The association of depression and mortality in elderly persons: A case for multiple, independent pathways. *J Gerontol A Biol Sci Med Sci 56*, M505–M509.

Bondareff, W., Alpert, M., Friedhoff, A., Richter, E., Clary, C., and Batzar, E. (2000). Comparison of sertraline and nortriptyline in the treatment of major depressive disorder in late life. *Am J Psychiatry 157*, 729–736.

Bosworth, H., McQuoid, D., George, L., and Steffens, D. (2002). Time-to-remission from geriatric depression: psychosocial and clinical factors. *Am J Geriatr Psychiatry 10*, 551–559.

Bozikas, V., Gold, G., Kovari, E., Herrmann, F., Karavatos, A., Giannakopoulos, P. *et al.* (2005). Pathological correlates of poststroke depression in elderly patients. *Am J Geriatr Psychiatry 13*, 166–169.

Bruce, M., Ten, H.T., Reynolds, C., Katz, I., Schulberg, H., Mulsant, B. *et al.* (2004). Reducing suicidal ideation and depressive symptoms in depressed older primary care patients: a randomized controlled trial. *JAMA 291*, 1081–1091.

Bump, G., Mulsant, B., Pollock, B., Mazumdar, S., Begley, A., Dew, M. *et al.* (2001). Paroxetine versus nortriptyline in the continuation and maintenance treatment of depression in the elderly. *Depress Anxiety 13*, 38–44.

Burrows, A., Salzman, C., Satlin, A., Noble, K., Pollock, B., and Gersh, T. (2002). A randomized, placebo-controlled trial of paroxetine in nursing home residents with non-major depression. *Depress Anxiety 15*, 102–110.

Butters, M., Becker, J., Nebes, R., Zmuda, M., Mulsant, B., Pollock, B. *et al.* (2000). Changes in cognitive functioning following treatment of late-life depression. *Am J Psychiatry 157*, 1949–1954.

Cassano, G., Puca, F., Scapicchio, P., and Trabucchi, M. (2002). Paroxetine and fluoxetine effects on mood and cognitive functions in depressed nondemented elderly patients. *J Clin Psychiatry 63*, 396–402.

Chemerinski, E. and Robinson, R.G. (2000). The neuropsychiatry of stroke. *Psychosomatics 41*, 5–14.

Cohen, H., Gibson, G., and Alderman, M. (2000). Excess risk of myocardial infarction in patients treated with antidepressant medications: association with use of tricyclic agents. *Am J Med 108*, 2–8.

Cole, M., Elie, L., McCusker, J., Bellavance, F., and Mansour, A. (2001). Feasibility and effectiveness of treatments for post-stroke depression in elderly inpatients: Systematic review. *J Geriatr Psychiatry Neurol 14*, 37–41.

Dal Forno, G., Palermo, M., Donohue, J., Karagiozis, H., Zonderman, A., and Kawas, C. (2005). Depressive symptoms, sex, and risk for Alzheimer's disease. *Ann Neurol 57*, 381–387.

de Abajo, F.J., Jick, H., Derby, L., Jick, S., and Schmitz, S. (2000). Intracranial haemorrhage and use of selective serotonin reuptake inhibitors. *Br J Clin Pharmacol 50*, 43–47.

de Asis, J.M., Stern, E., Alexopoulos, G.S., Pan, H., Van Gorp, W., Blumberg, H. *et al.* (2001). Hippocampal and anterior cingulate activation deficits in patients with geriatric depression. *Am J Psychiatry 158*, 1321–1323.

de Carle, A. and Kohn, R. (2000). Electroconvulsive therapy and falls in the elderly. *J ECT 16*, 252–257.

de Godoy, D. and de Godoy, R. (2003). A randomized controlled trial of the effect of psychotherapy on anxiety and depression in chronic obstructive pulmonary disease. *Arch Phys Med Rehabil 84*, 1154–1157.

de Groot, M., Anderson, R., Freedland, K., Clouse, R., and Lustman, P. (2001). Association of depression and diabetes complications: A meta-analysis. *Psychosom Med 63*, 619–630.

de Guevara, M., Schauffele, S., Nicola-Siri, L., Fahrer, R., Ortiz-Fragola, E., Martinez-Martinez, J. *et al.* (2004). Worsening of depressive symptoms 6 months after an acute coronary event in older adults is associated with impairment of cardiac autonomic function. *J Affect Disord 80*, 257–262.

de Jonge, P., Spijkerman, T., van den Brink, R., and Ormel, J. (2005). Depression following myocardial infarction is a risk factor for declined health-related quality of life and increased disability and cardiac complaints at 12 months. Paper presented at Heart, 2005.

De Vane, C. and Pollock, B. (1999). Pharmacokinetic considerations of antidepressant use in the elderly. *J Clin Psychiatry 60 (Suppl 20)*, 38–44.

Devanand, D., Nobler, M., Cheng, J., Turret, N., Pelton, G., Roose, S. *et al.* (2005). Randomized, double-blind, placebo-controlled trial of fluoxetine treatment for elderly patients with dysthymic disorder. *Am J Geriatr Psychiatry 13*, 59–68.

Devanand, D., Pelton, G., Marston, K., Camacho, Y., Roose, S., Stern, Y. *et al.* (2003). Sertraline treatment of elderly patients with depression and cognitive impairment. *Int J Geriatr Psychiatry 18*, 123–130.

Doraiswamy, P., Khan, Z., Donahue, R., and Richard, N. (2001). Quality of life in geriatric depression: a comparison of remitters, partial responders, and nonresponders. *Am J Geriatr Psychiatry 9*, 423–428.

Doraiswamy, P.M., Krishnan, K.R., Oxman, T., Jenkyn, L.R., Coffey, D.J., Burt, T. *et al.* (2003). Does antidepressant therapy improve cognition in elderly depressed patients? *J Gerontol A Biol Sci Med Sci 58*, M1137–M1144.

Dorenlot, P., Harboun, M., Bige, V., Henrard, J., and Ankri, J. (2005). Major depression as a risk factor for early institutionalization of dementia patients living in the community. *Int J Geriatr Psychiatry 20*, 471–478.

Drevets, W.C. (2000). Neuroimaging studies of mood disorders. *Biol Psychiatry 48*, 813–829.

Duckworth, G. and McBride, H. (1996). Suicide in old age: a tragedy of neglect. *Can J Psychiatry 41*, 217–222.

Durham, L., Webb, S., Milos, P., Clary, C., and Seymour, A. (2004). The serotonin transporter polymorphism, 5HTTLPR, is associated with a faster response time to sertraline in an elderly population with major depressive disorder. *Psychopharmacology (Berl) 174*, 525–529.

Entsuah, A., Huang, H., and Thase, M. (2001). Response and remission rates in different subpopulations with major depressive disorder administered venlafaxine, selective serotonin reuptake inhibitors, or placebo. *J Clin Psychiatry 62*, 869–877.

Flint, A.J. and Rifat, S.L. (1999). Recurrence of first-episode geriatric depression after discontinuation of maintenance antidepressants. *Am J Psychiatry 156*, 943–945.

Flores, G., Perez-Patrigeon, S., Cobos-Ayala, C., and Vergara, J. (2004). Severe symptomatic hyponatremia during citalopram therapy—a case report. *BMC Nephrol 5*, 2.

Forlenza, O., Almeida, O., Stoppe, A., Hirata, E., and Ferreira, R. (2001). Antidepressant efficacy and safety of low-dose sertraline and standard-dose imipramine for the treatment of depression in older adults: results from a double-blind, randomized, controlled clinical trial. *Int Psychogeriatr 13*, 75–84.

Gasto, C., Navarro, V., Marcos, T., Portella, M., Torra, M., and Rodamilans, M. (2003). Single-blind comparison of venlafaxine and nortriptyline in elderly major depression. *J Clin Psychopharmacol 23*, 21–26.

Gill, D. and Hatcher, S. (2000). Antidepressants for depression in medical illness. *Cochrane Database Syst Rev* CD001312.

Gillen, R., Tennen, H., McKee, T., Gernert-Dott, P., and Affleck, G. (2001). Depressive symptoms and history of depression predict rehabilitation efficiency in stroke patients. *Arch Phys Med Rehabil 82*, 1645–1649.

Gillespie, N.A., Whitfield, J.B., Williams, B., Heath, A.C., and Martin, N.G. (2005). The relationship between stressful life events, the serotonin transporter (5-HTTLPR) genotype and major depression. *Psychol Med 35*, 101–111.

Goodnick, P. (2001). Use of antidepressants in treatment of comorbid diabetes mellitus and depression as well as in diabetic neuropathy. *Ann Clin Psychiatry 13*, 31–41.

Gore, J., Brophy, C., and Greenstone, M. (2000). How well do we care for patients with end stage chronic obstructive pulmonary disease (COPD)? A comparison of palliative care and quality of life in COPD and lung cancer. *Thorax 55*, 1000–1006.

Hackett, M.L., Yapa, C., Parag, V., and Anderson, C.S. (2005). Frequency of depression after stroke. A systematic review of observational studies. *Stroke 36*, 1330–1340.

Hariri, A.R., Drabant, E.M., Munoz, K.E., Kolachana, B.S., Mattay, V.S., Egan, M.F. *et al.* (2005). A susceptibility gene for affective disorders and the response of the human amygdala. *Arch Gen Psychiatry 62*, 146–152.

Hariri, A.R. and Weinberger, D.R. (2003). Functional neuroimaging of genetic variation in serotonergic neurotransmission. *Genes Brain Behav 2*, 341–349.

Harrer, G., Schmidt, U., Kuhn, U., and Biller, A. (1999). Comparison of equivalence between the St. John's wort extract LoHyp-57 and fluoxetine. *Arzneimittelforschung 49*, 289–296.

Hughes, T., Ross, H., Mindham, R., and Spokes, E. (2004). Mortality in Parkinson's disease and its association with dementia and depression. *Acta Neurol Scand 110*, 118–123.

Huuhka, M., Korpisammal, L., Haataja, R., and Leinonen, E. (2004). One-year outcome of elderly inpatients with major depressive disorder treated with ECT and antidepressants. *J ECT 20*, 179–185.

Jonas, B. and Mussolino, M. (2000). Symptoms of depression as a prospective risk factor for stroke. *Psychosom Med 62*, 463–471.

Jorge, R.E., Robinson, R.G., Arndt, S., and Starkstein, S. (2003). Mortality and poststroke depression: A placebo-controlled trial of antidepressants. *Am J Psychiatry 160*, 1823–1829.

Kalayam, B. and Alexopoulos, G.S. (1999). Prefrontal dysfunction and treatment response in geriatric depression. *Arch Gen Psychiatry 56*, 713–718.

Kanner, A.M. (2004). Is major depression a neurologic disorder with psychiatric symptoms? *Epilepsy Behav* 5, 636–644.

Keller, M. (2000). Citalopram therapy for depression: a review of 10 years of European experience and data from U.S. clinical trials. *J Clin Psychiatry 61*, 896–908.

Kessing, L. and Andersen, P. (2004). Does the risk of developing dementia increase with the number of episodes in patients with depressive disorder and in patients with bipolar disorder? *J Neurol Neurosurg Psychiatry 75*, 1662–1666.

Kim, H., Kunik, M., Molinari, V., Hillman, S., Lalani, S., Orengo, C. *et al.* (2000). Functional impairment in COPD patients: The impact of anxiety and depression. *Psychosomatics 41*, 465–471.

Kirby, D., Harrigan, S., and Ames, D. (2002). Hyponatraemia in elderly psychiatric patients treated with selective serotonin reuptake inhibitors and venlafaxine: A retrospective controlled study in an inpatient unit. *Int J Geriatr Psychiatry 17*, 231–237.

Klysner, R., Bent-Hansen, J., Hansen, H., Lunde, M., Pleidrup, E., Poulsen, D. *et al.* (2002). Efficacy of citalopram in the prevention of recurrent depression in elderly patients: Placebo-controlled study of maintenance therapy. *Br J Psychiatry 181*, 29–35.

Krishnan, K., Doraiswamy, P., and Clary, C. (2001). Clinical and treatment response characteristics of late-life depression associated with vascular disease: A pooled analysis of two multicenter trials with sertraline. *Prog Neuropsychopharmacol Biol Psychiatry 25*, 347–361.

Kujala, Rosenvinge, B., and Bekkelund, S. (2002). Clinical outcome and adverse effects of electroconvulsive therapy in elderly psychiatric patients. *J Geriatr Psychiatry Neurol 15*, 73–76.

Kumar, A., Bilker, W., Jin, Z., and Udupa, J. (2000). Atrophy and high intensity lesions: complementary neurobiological mechanisms in late-life major depression. *Neuropsychopharmacology 22*, 264–274.

Kunik, M., Braun, U., Stanley, M., Wristers, K., Molinari, V., Stoebner, D. *et al.* (2001). One session cognitive behavioural therapy for elderly patients with chronic obstructive pulmonary disease. *Psychol Med 31*, 717–723.

Lacasse, Y., Beaudoin, L., Rousseau, L., and Maltais, F. (2004). Randomized trial of paroxetine in end-stage COPD. *Monaldi Arch Chest Dis 61*, 140–147.

Lacasse, Y., Rousseau, L., and Maltais, F. (2001). Prevalence of depressive symptoms and depression in patients with severe oxygen-dependent chronic obstructive pulmonary disease. *J Cardiopulm Rehabil 21*, 80–86.

Lai, T., Payne, M.E., Byrum, C.E., Steffens, D.C., and Krishnan, K.R. (2000). Reduction of orbital frontal cortex volume in geriatric depression. *Biol Psychiatry 48*, 971–975.

Larson, S., Owens, P., Ford, D., and Eaton, W. (2001). Depressive disorder, dysthymia, and risk of stroke: Thirteen-year follow-up from the Baltimore epidemiologic catchment area study. *Stroke 32*, 1979–1983.

Lavretsky, H., Bastani, R., Gould, R., Huang, D., Llorente, M., Maxwell, A. *et al.* (2002). Predictors of two-year mortality in a prospective "UPBEAT" study of elderly veterans with comorbid medical and psychiatric symptoms. *Am J Geriatr Psychiatry 10*, 458–468.

Lee, Y., Choi, K., and Lee, Y. (2001). Association of comorbidity with depressive symptoms in community-dwelling older persons. *Gerontology 47*, 254–262.

Lemke, M.R. (2002). Effect of reboxetine on depression in Parkinson's disease patients. *J Clin Psychiatry 63*, 300–304.

Lemke, M.R., Fuchs, G., Gemende, I., Herting, B., Oehlwein, C., Reichmann, H. *et al.* (2004). Depression and Parkinson's disease. *J Neurol 251 (Suppl 6)*, VI/24–27.

Lenze, E., Dew, M., Mazumdar, S., Begley, A., Cornes, C., Miller, M. *et al.* (2002). Combined pharmacotherapy and psychotherapy as maintenance treatment for late-life depression: Effects on social adjustment. *Am J Psychiatry 159*, 466–468.

Lenze, E., Mulsant, B., Shear, M., Schulberg, H., Dew, M., Begley, A. *et al.* (2000). Comorbid anxiety disorders in depressed elderly patients. *Am J Psychiatry 157*, 722–728.

Lenze, E., Munin, M., Ferrell, R., Pollock, B., Skidmore, E., Lotrich, F. *et al.* (2005). Association of the serotonin transporter gene-linked polymorphic region (5-HTTLPR) genotype with depression in elderly persons after hip fracture. *Am J Geriatr Psychiatry 13*, 428–432.

Lesperance, F., Frasure-Smith, N., Juneau, M., and Theroux, P. (2000). Depression and 1-year prognosis in unstable angina. *Arch Intern Med 160*, 1354–1360.

Lesperance, F., Frasure-Smith, N., Talajic, M., and Bourassa, M. (2002). Five-year risk of cardiac mortality in relation to initial severity and one-year changes in depression symptoms after myocardial infarction. *Circulation 105*, 1049–1053.

Li, Y., Meyer, J., and Thornby, J. (2001). Depressive symptoms among cognitively normal versus cognitively impaired elderly subjects. *Int J Geriatr Psychiatry 16*, 455–461.

Linde, K., Berner, M., Egger, M., and Mulrow, C. (2005). St John's wort for depression: Meta-analysis of randomised controlled trials. *Br J Psychiatry 186*, 99–107.

Little, J., Atkins, M., Munday, J., Lyall, G., Greene, D., Chubb, G. *et al.* (2004). Bifrontal electroconvulsive therapy in the elderly: A 2-year retrospective. *J ECT 20*, 139–141.

Lockwood, K., Alexopoulos, G., and van Gorp, W. (2002). Executive dysfunction in geriatric depression. *Am J Psychiatry 159*, 1119–1126.

Lustman, P., Anderson, R., Freedland, K., de Groot, M., Carney, R., and Clouse, R. (2000). Depression and poor glycemic control: a meta-analytic review of the literature. *Diabetes Care 23*, 934–942.

Lyketsos, C., Sheppard, J., Steele, C., Kopunek, S., Steinberg, M., Baker, A. *et al.* (2000). Randomized, placebo-controlled, double-blind clinical trial of sertraline in the treatment of depression complicating Alzheimer's disease: Initial results from the Depression in Alzheimer's Disease study. *Am J Psychiatry 157*, 1686–1689.

Magai, C., Kennedy, G., Cohen, C., and Gomberg, D. (2000). A controlled clinical trial of sertraline in the treatment of depression in nursing home patients with late-stage Alzheimer's disease. *Am J Geriatr Psychiatry 8*, 66–74.

Maurer-Spurej, E., Pittendreigh, C., and Solomons, K. (2004). The influence of selective serotonin reuptake inhibitors on human platelet serotonin. *Thromb Haemost 91*, 119–128.

Mayberg, H. (2001). Depression and frontal-subcortical circuits. Focus on prefrontal-limbic interactions. In D. Lichter and J. Cummings, Eds. *Frontal-subcortical Circuits in Psychiatric and Neurological Disorders*. New York, NY: Guilford Press, pp. 177–206.

McDonald, W., Salzman, C., and Schatzberg, A. (2002). Depression in the elderly. *Psychopharmacol Bull 36 (Suppl 2)*, 112–122.

Miller, M., Cornes, C., Frank, E., Ehrenpreis, L., Silberman, R., Schlernitzauer, M. *et al.* (2001). Interpersonal psychotherapy for late-life depression: Past, present, and future. *J Psychother Pract Res 10*, 231–238.

Modrego, P. and Ferrandez, J. (2004). Depression in patients with mild cognitive impairment increases the risk of developing dementia of Alzheimer type: A prospective cohort study. *Arch Neurol 61*, 1290–1293.

Moffat, S.D., Szekely, C.A., Zonderman, A.B., Kabani, N.J., and Resnick, S.M. (2000). Longitudinal change in hippocampal volume as a function of apolipoprotein E genotype. *Neurology 55*, 134–136.

Mohlman, J. (2005). Does executive dysfunction affect treatment outcome in late-life mood and anxiety disorders? *J Geriatr Psychiatry Neurol 18*, 97–108.

Monster, T., Johnsen, S., Olsen, M., McLaughlin, J., and Sorensen, H. (2004). Antidepressants and risk of first-time hospitalization for myocardial infarction: a population-based case-control study. *Am J Med 117*, 732–737.

Mosimann, U., Schmitt, W., Greenberg, B., Kosel, M., Muri, R., Berkhoff, M. *et al.* (2004). Repetitive transcranial magnetic stimulation: A putative add-on treatment for major depression in elderly patients. *Psychiatry Res 126*, 123–133.

Muijsers, R., Plosker, G., and Noble, S. (2002). Sertraline: a review of its use in the management of major depressive disorder in elderly patients. *Drugs Aging 19*, 377–392.

Murphy, G., Hollander, S., Rodrigues, H., Kremer, C., and Schatzberg, A. (2004). Effects of the serotonin transporter gene promoter polymorphism on mirtazapine and paroxetine efficacy and adverse events in geriatric major depression. *Arch Gen Psychiatry 61*, 1163–1169.

Navarro, V., Gasto, C., Lomena, F., Mateos, J., Portella, M., Masana, G. *et al.* (2004a). No brain perfusion impairment at long-term follow-up in elderly patients treated with electroconvulsive therapy for major depression. *J ECT 20*, 89–93.

Navarro, V., Gasto, C., Lomena, F., Mateos, J., Portella, M., Massana, G. *et al.* (2004b). Frontal cerebral perfusion after antidepressant drug treatment versus ECT in elderly patients with major depression: a 12-month follow-up control study. *J Clin Psychiatry 65*, 656–661.

Navarro, V., Gasto, C., Torres, X., Marcos, T., and Pintor, L. (2001). Citalopram versus nortriptyline in late-life depression: a 12-week randomized single-blind study. *Acta Psychiatr Scand 103*, 435–440.

Nelson, J., Kennedy, J., Pollock, B., Laghrissi-Thode, F., Narayan, M., Nobler, M. *et al.* (1999). Treatment of major depression with nortriptyline and paroxetine in patients with ischemic heart disease. *Am J Psychiatry 156*, 1024–1028.

Newhouse, P., Krishnan, K., Doraiswamy, P., Richter, E., Batzar, E., and Clary, C. (2000). A double-blind comparison of sertraline and fluoxetine in depressed elderly outpatients. *J Clin Psychiatry 61*, 559–568.

Newman, S. and Hassan, A. (1999). Antidepressant use in the elderly population in Canada: results from a national survey. *J Gerontol A Biol Sci Med Sci 54*, M527–M530.

Niedermaier, N., Bohrer, E., Schulte, K., Schlattmann, P., and Heuser, I. (2004). Prevention and treatment of poststroke depression with mirtazapine in patients with acute stroke. *J Clin Psychiatry 65*, 1619–1623.

Pagnin, D., de Queiroz, V., Pini, S., and Cassano, G.B. (2004). Efficacy of ECT in depression: A meta-analytic review. *J Ect* 20, 13–20.

Palinkas, L., Lee, P., and Barrett-Connor, E. (2004). A prospective study of Type 2 diabetes and depressive symptoms in the elderly: the Rancho Bernardo Study. *Diabet Med 21*, 1185–1191.

Peretti, S., Judge, R., and Hindmarch, I. (2000). Safety and tolerability considerations: tricyclic antidepressants vs. selective serotonin reuptake inhibitors. *Acta Psychiatr Scand Suppl 403*, 17–25.

Petracca, G., Chemerinski, E., and Starkstein, S. (2001). A double-blind, placebo-controlled study of fluoxetine in depressed patients with Alzheimer's disease. *Int Psychogeriatr 13*, 233–240.

Pfiffner, D. and Hoffmann, A. (2004). Psychosocial predictors of death for low-risk patients after a first myocardial infarction: a 7-year follow-up study. *J Cardiopulm Rehabil 24*, 87–93.

Plante, G. (2005). Depression and cardiovascular disease: A reciprocal relationship. *Metabolism 54*, 45–48.

Pohjasvaara, T., Vataja, R., Leppavuori, A., Kaste, M., and Erkinjuntti, T. (2001). Depression is an independent predictor of poor long-term functional outcome post-stroke. *Eur J Neurol 8*, 315–319.

Powell, L., Catellier, D., Freedland, K., Burg, M., Woods, S., Bittner, V. *et al.* (2005). Depression and heart failure in patients with a new myocardial infarction. *Am Heart J 149*, 851–855.

Rampello, L., Alvano, A., Chiechio, S., Raffaele, R., Vecchio, I., and Malaguarnera, M. (2005). An evaluation of efficacy and safety of reboxetine in elderly patients affected by "retarded" post-stroke depression A random, placebo-controlled study. *Arch Gerontol Geriatr 40*, 275–285.

Rehman, H. and Masson, E. (2001). Neuroendocrinology of ageing. *Age Ageing 30*, 279–287.

Reynolds, C., Frank, E., Kupfer, D., Thase, M., Perel, J., Mazumdar, S. *et al.* (1996). Treatment outcome in recurrent major depression: a post hoc comparison of elderly ("young old") and midlife patients. *Am J Psychiatry 153*, 1288–1292.

Reynolds, C., Frank, E., Perel, J., Imber, S., Cornes, C., Miller, M. *et al.* (1999). Nortriptyline and interpersonal psychotherapy as maintenance therapies for recurrent major depression: a randomized controlled trial in patients older than 59 years. *JAMA* 281, 39–45.

Reynolds, C., Smith, G., Dew, M., Mulsant, B., Miller, M., Schlernitzauer, M. *et al.* (2005). Accelerating symptom-reduction in late-life depression: A double-blind, randomized, placebo-controlled trial of sleep deprivation. *Am J Geriatr Psychiatry 13*, 353–358.

Riedel-Heller, S., Matschinger, H., Schork, A., and Angermeyer, M. (2001). The utilization of antidepressants in community-dwelling and institutionalized elderly—Results from a representative survey in Germany. *Pharmacopsychiatry 34*, 6–12.

Robinson, R., Schultz, S., Castillo, C., Kopel, T., Kosier, J., Newman, R. *et al.* (2000). Nortriptyline versus fluoxetine in the treatment of depression and in short-term recovery after stroke: a placebo-controlled, double-blind study. *Am J Psychiatry 157*, 351–359.

Rocca, P., Calvarese, P., Faggiano, F., Marchiaro, L., Mathis, F., Rivoira, E. *et al.* (2005). Citalopram versus sertraline in late-life nonmajor clinically significant depression: A 1-year follow-up clinical trial. *J Clin Psychiatry 66*, 360–369.

Rodriguez de la Torre, B., Dreher, J., Malevany, I., Bagli, M., Kolbinger, M., Omran, H. *et al.* (2001). Serum levels and cardiovascular effects of tricyclic antidepressants and selective serotonin reuptake inhibitors in depressed patients. *Ther Drug Monit 23*, 435–440.

Roose, S., Laghrissi-Thode, F., Kennedy, J., Nelson, J., Bigger, J., Pollock, B. *et al.* (1998). Comparison of paroxetine and nortriptyline in depressed patients with ischemic heart disease. *JAMA 279*, 287–291.

Rosengren, A., Hawken, S., Ounpuu, S., Sliwa, K., Zubaid, M., Almahmeed, W. *et al.* (2004). Association of psychosocial risk factors with risk of acute myocardial infarction in 11119 cases and 13648 controls from 52 countries (the INTERHEART study): Case-control study. *Lancet 364*, 953–962.

Rosner, M. (2004). Severe hyponatremia associated with the combined use of thiazide diuretics and selective serotonin reuptake inhibitors. *Am J Med Sci 327*, 109–111.

Sauer, W.H., Berlin, J.A., and Kimmel, S.E. (2003). Effect of antidepressants and their relative affinity for the serotonin transporter on the risk of myocardial infarction. *Circulation 108*, 32–36.

Schatzberg, A., Kremer, C., Rodrigues, H., and Murphy, G. (2002). Double-blind, randomized comparison of mirtazapine and paroxetine in elderly depressed patients. *Am J Geriatr Psychiatry 10*, 541–550.

Schoevers, R., Geerlings, M., Beekman, A., Penninx, B., Deeg, D., Jonker, C. *et al.* (2000). Association of depression and gender with mortality in old age. Results from the Amsterdam Study of the Elderly (AMSTEL). *Br J Psychiatry 177*, 336–342.

Schulz, R., Beach, S., Ives, D., Martire, L., Ariyo, A., and Kop, W. (2000). Association between depression and mortality in older adults: the Cardiovascular Health Study. *Arch Intern Med 160*, 1761–1768.

Sen, S., Burmeister, M., and Ghosh, D. (2004). Meta-analysis of the association between a serotonin transporter promoter polymorphism (5-HTTLPR) and anxiety-related personality traits. *Am J Med Genet B Neuropsychiatr Genet 127*, 85–89.

Shah, A., Odutoye, K., and De, T. (2001). Depression in acutely medically ill elderly inpatients: a pilot study of early identification and intervention by formal psychogeriatric consultation. *J Affect Disord 62*, 233–240.

Sheikh, J., Cassidy, E., Doraiswamy, P., Salomon, R., Hornig, M., Holland, P. *et al.* (2004). Efficacy, safety, and tolerability of sertraline in patients with late-life depression and comorbid medical illness. *J Am Geriatr Soc 52*, 86–92.

Sheline, Y.I., Sanghavi, M., Mintun, M.A., and Gado, M.H. (1999). Depression duration but not age predicts hippocampal volume loss in medically healthy women with recurrent major depression. *J Neurosci 19*, 5034–5043.

Shiotani, I., Sato, H., Kinjo, K., Nakatani, D., Mizuno, H., Ohnishi, Y. *et al.* (2002). Depressive symptoms predict 12-month prognosis in elderly patients with acute myocardial infarction. *J Cardiovasc Risk 9*, 153–160.

Skoog, I., Aevarsson, O., Beskow, J., Larsson, L., Palsson, S., Waern, M. *et al.* (1996). Suicidal feelings in a population sample of nondemented 85-year-olds. *Am J Psychiatry 153*, 1015–1020.

Spina, E. and Scordo, M. (2002). Clinically significant drug interactions with antidepressants in the elderly. *Drugs Aging 19*, 299–320.

Steffens, D., McQuoid, D., and Krishnan, K. (2003). Cholesterol-lowering medication and relapse of depression. *Psychopharmacol Bull 37*, 92–98.

Steffens, D., Skoog, I., Norton, M., Hart, A., Tschanz, J., Plassman, B. *et al.* (2000). Prevalence of depression and its treatment in an elderly population: The Cache County study. *Arch Gen Psychiatry 57*, 601–607.

Steffens, D., Welsh-Bohmer, K., Burke, J., Plassman, B., Beyer, J., Gersing, K., and Potter, G. (2004). Methodology and preliminary results from the neurocognitive outcomes of depression in the elderly study. *J Geriatr Psychiatry Neurol 17*, 202–211.

Stek, M., Gussekloo, J., Beekman, A., van, T.W., and Westendorp, R. (2004). Prevalence, correlates and recognition of depression in the oldest old: the Leiden 85-plus study. *J Affect Disord 78*, 193–200.

Stratton, I., Adler, A., Neil, A., and UK Prospective Diabetes Study Group (2000). Association of glycaemia with macrovascular and microvascular complications of type 2 diabetes (UKPDS 35): Prospective observational study. *BMJ 321*, 405–412.

Sullivan, M., Newton, K., Hecht, J., Russo, J., and Spertus, J. (2004). Depression and health status in elderly patients with heart failure: A 6-month prospective study in primary care [In Process Citation]. *Am J Geriatr Cardiol 13*, 252–260.

Suominen, K., Isometsa, E., and Lonnqvist, J. (2004). Elderly suicide attempters with depression are often diagnosed only after the attempt. *Int J Geriatr Psychiatry 19*, 35–40.

Taylor, W., Steffens, D., Payne, M., Macfall, J., Marchuk, D., Svenson, I. *et al.* (2005). Influence of serotonin transporter promoter region polymorphisms on hippocampal volumes in late-life depression. *Arch Gen Psychiatry 62*, 537–544.

Teresi, J., Abrams, R., Holmes, D., Ramirez, M., and Eimicke, J. (2001). Prevalence of depression and depression recognition in nursing homes. *Soc Psychiatry Psychiatr Epidemiol 36*, 613–620.

Thompson, L., Coon, D., Gallagher-Thompson, D., Sommer, B., and Koin, D. (2001). Comparison of desipramine and cognitive/behavioral therapy in the treatment of elderly outpatients with mild-to-moderate depression. *Am J Geriatr Psychiatry 9*, 225–240.

Thorpe, L., Whitney, D., Kutcher, S., and Kennedy, S. (2001). Clinical guidelines for the treatment of depressive disorders. VI. Special populations. *Can J Psychiatry 46 (Suppl 1)*, 63S–76S.

Ticehurst, S., Carter, G., Clover, K., Whyte, I., Raymond, J., and Fryer, J. (2002). Elderly patients with deliberate self-poisoning treated in an Australian general hospital. *Int Psychogeriatr 14*, 97–105.

Tsai, Y., Wong, T., Juang, Y., and Tsai, H. (2004). The effects of light therapy on depressed elders. *Int J Geriatr Psychiatry 19*, 545–548.

Tsolaki, M. and Fountoulakis, K. (2000). Effect of antidepressant therapy with venlafaxine in geriatric depression. *Int J Geriatr Psychopharmacol 2*, 83–85.

Turvey, C., Conwell, Y., Jones, M., Phillips, C., Simonsick, E., Pearson, J. *et al.* (2002). Risk factors for late-life suicide: A prospective, community-based study. *Am J Geriatr Psychiatry 10*, 398–406.

UK ECT Review Group (2003). Efficacy and safety of electroconvulsive therapy in depressive disorders: A systematic review and meta-analysis. *Lancet 361*, 799–808.

van Melle, J., de, J.P., Spijkerman, T., Tijssen, J., Ormel, J., van Veldhuisen, D. *et al.* (2004). Prognostic association of depression following myocardial infarction with mortality and cardiovascular events: A meta-analysis. *Psychosom Med 66*, 814–822.

Verdelho, A., Henon, H., Lebert, F., Pasquier, F., and Leys, D. (2004). Depressive symptoms after stroke and relationship with dementia: A three-year follow-up study. *Neurology 62*, 905–911.

Verkaik, R., van, W.J., and Francke, A. (2005). The effects of psychosocial methods on depressed, aggressive and apathetic behaviors of people with dementia: A systematic review. *Int J Geriatr Psychiatry 20*, 301–314.

Volkers, A., Nuyen, J., Verhaak, P., and Schellevis, F. (2004). The problem of diagnosing major depression in elderly primary care patients. *J Affect Disord 82*, 259–263.

Weihs, K., Settle, E., Batey, S., Houser, T., Donahue, R., and Ascher, J. (2000). Bupropion sustained release versus paroxetine for the treatment of depression in the elderly. *J Clin Psychiatry 61*, 196–202.

Wilkinson, D., Holmes, C., Woolford, J., Stammers, S., and North, J. (2002). Prophylactic therapy with lithium in elderly patients with unipolar major depression. *Int J Geriatr Psychiatry 17*, 619–622.

Williams, S., Kasl, S., Heiat, A., Abramson, J., Krumholz, H., and Vaccarino, V. (2002). Depression and risk of heart failure among the elderly: A prospective community-based study. *Psychosom Med 64*, 6–12.

Wilson, K. and Mottram, P. (2004). A comparison of side effects of selective serotonin reuptake inhibitors and tricyclic antidepressants in older depressed patients: A meta-analysis. *Int J Geriatr Psychiatry 19*, 754–762.

Wilson, K., Mottram, P., Sivanranthan, A., and Nightingale, A. (2001). Antidepressant versus placebo for depressed elderly. *Cochrane Database Syst Rev* CD000561.

Yohannes, A., Baldwin, R., and Connolly, M. (2003). Prevalence of sub-threshold depression in elderly patients with chronic obstructive pulmonary disease. *Int J Geriatr Psychiatry 18*, 412–416.

Yohannes, A., Connolly, M., and Baldwin, R. (2001). A feasibility study of antidepressant drug therapy in depressed elderly patients with chronic obstructive pulmonary disease. *Int J Geriatr Psychiatry 16*, 451–454.

Zullino, D. and Baumann, P. (2001). Lithium augmentation in depressive patients not responding to selective serotonin reuptake inhibitors. *Pharmacopsychiatry 34*, 119–127.

60

The Aging Human Lung: Age-Associated Changes in Structure and Function

Keith C. Meyer

The human lung reaches the zenith of its functional capacity in the late second to the third decade of life, but age-associated changes in lung structure and function gradually ensue once this zenith has been reached. Although there is considerable interindividual variation, age-associated decline in lung function of healthy, nonsmoking individuals becomes apparent in the fifth to sixth decade of life when physiologic testing is performed. This decline in lung function coincides with morphologic changes that are associated with alterations in structural proteins that comprise lung matrix, and appears to be caused largely by decreased lung elastic recoil. Other age-related factors associated with declining lung function include diminished chest wall compliance, blunting of ventilatory responses, a decline in respiratory muscle strength, a decline in arterial oxygen tension, an increased prevalence of sleep-disordered breathing, and diminished exercise capacity. Despite these changes, nonsmoking, healthy elderly individuals do not tend to develop clinical symptoms as a consequence of declining lung function. However, certain lung disorders such as chronic obstructive pulmonary disease (COPD) and idiopathic pulmonary fibrosis (IPF) tend to make their appearance in elderly persons and cause significant respiratory system dysfunction, and the elderly display an increased susceptibility to respiratory infection. Animal models have provided some insights into age-associated decline in lung function in humans, but the precise causes of age-associated changes in lung function remain obscure.

Introduction

After approximately two decades of postnatal lung maturation, the aging human lung has been estimated to gradually lose up to 50% of its tissue mass over the remaining average lifespan of nonsmoking individuals who appear to be healthy and reside in developed countries. Although environmental factors may play a role in age-associated changes in the lung, loss of lung tissue and elastic recoil, which some have termed *senile emphysema*, appears to be a phenomenon that is linked to the normal aging process (Thurlbeck, 1991; Green and Pinkerton, 2004). Despite these age-associated changes, there is considerable interindividual variation in the degree and tempo of lung function decline, and these changes are unlikely to reach the point of clinical respiratory dysfunction in healthy elderly persons. However, environmental and genetic factors likely play a significant role in the susceptibility of individuals and populations to age-associated lung function decline, and environmental factors may lead to clinical disease in susceptible individuals, even in nonsmokers. As the life span of humans gradually increases, it is conceivable that "normal" age-associated changes in lung structure and physiology may progress to the point that they cause symptoms associated with respiratory dysfunction and have an impact on quality of life.

One of the most important environmental factors associated with lung disease in the elderly is cigarette smoking. Nearly one in five smokers who have normal α_1-antitrypsin levels will develop clinically significant chronic obstructive pulmonary disease (COPD) that generally makes its appearance in the sixth decade and beyond (Barnes, 2000). However, exposure to second-hand smoke (Masi *et al.*, 1988) or high levels of air pollution (Gauderman *et al.*, 2005) early in life may significantly affect lung development. Such early exposures may hold consequences for exposed individuals who reach an advanced age and promote an accelerated decline in lung function despite a lack of primary tobacco smoking. Additionally, adaptive responses such as anti-protease or antioxidant defenses may be an important determinant of susceptibility to various environmental factors both in age-associated changes in lung structure and function as well as in the development of clinical lung disease (Taggare *et al.*, 2005; Kelly *et al.*, 2003). Because factors that include even low birth weight can have significant consequences for postnatal lung development (Hoo *et al.*, 2004), environmental influences, respiratory infections, genetic factors, and the bias presented by examining survivors in aged populations (which may not accurately reflect the population as a whole) can blur the separation of the changes in lung structure and function that are due purely to advanced age from changes that are caused by environmental exposures and genetic susceptibility.

Age-associated Changes in Lung Structure and Function

CHANGES ATTRIBUTED TO THE AGING PROCESS

Various aspects of lung function gradually decline with aging in clinically healthy individuals (Rossi *et al.*, 1996; Chan and Welsh, 1998), and these changes affect the lung as well as the respiratory pump (see Table 60.1). Notable changes include alterations in lung matrix that lead to remodeling, and physiologic changes in chest wall dynamics and respiratory muscle function. Elastin, which displays very little turnover in the adult lung (Shapiro *et al.*, 1991), has been reported to decrease gradually in alveolar walls (D'Errico *et al.*, 1989). Additionally, serum elastin peptide levels appear to decrease with advancing age (Frette *et al.*, 1997), suggesting altered mechanisms of lung homeostasis, remodeling, and repair. These changes in lung elastins combined with alterations in another key matrix component, collagen (changes in intermolecular cross-linking plus a shift to insoluble collagens), are a likely cause of progressive decline in lung elastic recoil.

TABLE 60.1
Changes in structure and function of the aging human respiratory system

Structural changes in the lung
Structural disruption and possible loss of elastin
Altered cross-linking of elastin and collagen
Loss of alveolar surface area
Enlargement of terminal airspaces
Decreased number of capillaries per alveolus
Decreased diameter of small bronchioles
Increased interalveolar pores (pores of Kohn)
Other respiratory system changes
Decreased chest wall compliance
Decline in respiratory muscle function
Changes in measures of lung function
Diminished lung elastic recoil (increased lung compliance)
Decreased vital capacity (FVC) and forced expiratory flows (FEV_1, FEF_{25-75})
Increased residual volume (RV) and functional residual capacity (FRC)
Decreased inspiratory capacity (IC)
Decreased diffusion capacity for carbon monoxide (DL_{CO})
Decreased partial pressure of arterial oxygen (PaO_2)
Decreased maximal oxygen consumption during maximal exercise

However, biochemical analysis of the lung suggests that the total content of elastin and collagen does not change significantly with aging (Lang *et al.*, 1994), and changes in the spatial arrangement or cross-linking of elastic fiber networks rather than measurable elastin loss may be the cause of the observed decline in elastic recoil (Crapo, 1993). The number of capillaries per alveolus also declines and is accompanied by loss of alveolar surface area as terminal airspaces (alveolar ducts and alveoli) increase in volume and the diameter and number of interalveolar pores increase (Thurlbeck, 1991). The causes of age-associated changes in lung matrix remain elusive. Although the loss of elastic recoil and distal airspace enlargement is somewhat similar to smoke-induced emphysema, the airspace enlargement is quite homogeneous, in contrast to the irregular distribution of airspace enlargement in emphysematous lungs that is accompanied by alveolar wall destruction.

Loss of elastic recoil and tethering of airways leads to small airway closure at identical lung volumes in older compared to younger subjects. This causes gradual reduction in forced expiratory flows (FEV_1, FEF_{25-75}), and early airway closure causes more gas to be trapped in the chest such that RV increases while FVC and IC decrease (Janssens *et al.*, 1999). These alterations in measurement of pulmonary function are attributed to diffuse emphysema-like changes in the lung (senile emphysema), which differs in appearance from emphysema induced by tobacco smoke or other environmental exposures (Thurlbeck, 1991; 1999). In addition to altered expiratory flow rates and lung volumes, the loss of alveolar surface area and alveolar capillaries with aging correlates with a gradual reduction of DL_{CO}.

The ability of the lung to facilitate gas exchange also declines with advancing age. The PaO_2 begins to decline in the third decade of life, and the average PaO_2 may approach 70 mm Hg in the eighth decade but then tends to stabilize (Sorbini *et al.*, 1968; Cerveri *et al.*, 1995). The gradually widening alveolar to arterial oxygen gradient that is associated with advancing age is considered to be a consequence of ventilation-perfusion mismatching due to closure of small airways as lung matrix tissue is lost or disrupted and elastic recoil declines. The elderly tend to breathe with a greater frequency but with smaller tidal volume compared to young normal subjects while maintaining a similar minute ventilation (Krumpe *et al.*, 1985), but resting ventilatory responses to both hypoxia and hypercapnea become blunted (Peterson *et al.*, 1981). In contrast to the decline in arterial oxygen tension, $PaCO_2$ is maintained at approximately 40 mm Hg despite the blunted response to hypercapnea.

Other age-associated phenomena that affect respiratory function include changes in the chest wall, impaired respiratory muscle function, and altered breathing patterns during sleep. Chest wall compliance progressively decreases and is presumed to be due to diminished mobility of the costovertebral joints, calcification of intercostal cartilage, narrowing of intervertebral disc spaces, and the appearance of varying degrees of kyphoscoliosis (Peterson and Fishman, 1982). Maximal inspiratory and expiratory pressures in the elderly appear to correlate quite well with peripheral muscle strength (Enright *et al.*, 1994). With advancing age the contribution of thoracic muscles (intercostals) to ventilation declines as the chest cage becomes less compliant (Mizuno, 1991). Diaphragmatic muscle mass tends to be preserved, but intercostal muscles display a decline in mean cross-sectional area after the fifth decade. Although diaphragmatic mass is preserved, respiratory muscle performance is reduced by the increase in RV and FRC, and the ability of the diaphragm to develop maximal force becomes impaired (Polkey *et al.*, 1997). Other factors such as poor nutritional status and low body mass index have a deleterious effect on respiratory muscle strength and can confound the age-associated changes in respiratory muscle function (Arora and Rochester, 1982). Respiratory muscle function is also linked to cardiac performance, as reflected by cardiac index or maximal oxygen consumption, and maximal inspiratory pressures can fall as a consequence of cardiac dysfunction (Nishimura *et al.*, 1994; Mancini *et al.*, 1992).

Changes in the control of breathing in both the awake and sleep state are associated with aging. Blunted ventilatory and cardiac responses to both hypoxia and hypercapnia have been observed in the wakeful state (Peterson *et al.*, 1981; Kronenberg and Drage, 1973), and attenuated responses to these stimuli when measured by mouth occlusion pressure (Peterson *et al.*, 1981) suggest that this decline in respiratory drive may be caused by diminished ability to process information from mechanoreceptors and chemoreceptors. Indeed, responses to resistive loads are also diminished in the elderly (Tack *et al.*, 1982). When compared to middle-aged individuals, ventilatory dysfunction during sleep is quite prevalent in the elderly. Significant upper airway obstruction during sleep affects up to 75% of elderly individuals, and the prevalence of sleep apnea has been reported to approach 50% (Ancoli-Israel and Coy, 1994). Additionally, ventilatory responses to upper airway occlusion is attenuated in elderly subjects compared to younger control subjects (Krieger *et al.*, 1997). Despite these changes in the control of breathing in the resting state, ventilatory responses to CO2 are maintained or even increased in the elderly during exercise (Poulin *et al.*, 1994).

PULMONARY DISEASE STATES ASSOCIATED WITH ADVANCED AGE

Some disorders that involve remodeling of airways and distal lung parenchyma tend to appear with advanced age and become quite prevalent in elderly populations. These disorders include COPD and idiopathic pulmonary fibrosis (IPF). The prevalence of obstructive lung disease is increased in the elderly and may be greatly underestimated in certain elderly populations (Malik *et al.*, 2004; Lundback *et al.*, 2003). Both asthma and COPD may be considerably underdiagnosed in the elderly (Lebowitz *et al.*, 1975; Janssens *et al.*, 2001), perhaps, in part, due to a decreased ability to perceive an added resistive load such as that caused by bronchoconstriction (Tack *et al.*, 1982).

Airflow obstruction is generally quite reversible in asthmatics with appropriate treatment, which stands in contrast to patients with COPD for whom obstruction is not generally reversible despite therapy. Asthma prevalence in elderly populations may range as high as 8% (Burrows *et al.*, 1991; Parameswaran *et al.*, 1998), and it can be difficult to differentiate from COPD. Older asthmatics with long-standing asthma may have considerable airway remodeling with a prominent component of irreversible airflow obstruction (Finucane *et al.*, 1985), and these individuals often have relatively severe and difficult-to-treat asthma. Some investigators view asthma and COPD as different expressions of one disease entity, a concept that has been named the *Dutch hypothesis*, because it was first proposed in Groningen in 1961 (Postma and Boezen, 2004). This hypothesis suggests that asthma, chronic bronchitis, and emphysema have various genetic (atopy and airway hyperresponsiveness) and endogenous factors (sex and age) that interact with various exogenous factors (allergens, smoking, pollutants, viral infections) to cause obstructive lung disease (Postma and Boezen, 2004; Bleecker, 2004). However, there are distinct clinical, physiologic, and pathologic characteristics that appear to differentiate asthma from COPD (Fabbri *et al.*, 2003), and patients with fixed airflow obstruction due to asthma tend to have a better response to therapy and better prognosis than patients with COPD (Burrows *et al.*, 1987; Kerstjens *et al.*, 1992).

Chronic obstructive pulmonary disease is the fourth leading cause of death in the United States, and poses a huge economic burden for society (Michaud *et al.*, 2001). Tobacco smoking is the cause of at least 90% of all COPD cases, but other exposures have also been associated with COPD (Barnes, 2000; Fishman, 2005). α_1-Antitrypsin deficiency accounts for a about 2% of cases of emphysema (nearly all patients are smokers), and emphysema associated with α_1-antitrypsin deficiency is usually diagnosed in the fourth to fifth decade of life (Needham and Stockley, 2004). In contrast, patients with normal α_1-antitrypsin levels usually do not develop clinically significant emphysema until they have reached their sixth decade of life. The prevalence of COPD in adults recently was found to be 8.6% in a large survey, and the prevalence in disadvantaged elderly (Malik *et al.*, 2004) or elderly smokers (Lundback *et al.*, 2003) may be considerably higher. A recently published case-control autopsy study showed a prevalence of emphysema or chronic bronchitis of 26.6% for 3,685 patients age 65 or older that were autopsied between 1972 and 1996 (Janssens *et al.*, 2001).

One additional disorder that tends to make its appearance in the elderly is idiopathic pulmonary fibrosis (IPF)

(Coultas *et al.*, 1994). Idiopathic pulmonary fibrosis is characterized by progressive lung remodeling with excess matrix deposition and distortion of lung architecture, which causes a restrictive physiology and impaired gas exchange (Noble and Homer, 2004; Selman and Pardo, 2003). Fortunately, the incidence and prevalence of this progressive disorder, which has a median survival of approximately three years, is much lower than that for asthma and COPD (Coultas *et al.*, 1994; Demedts *et al.*, 2001). Nonetheless, it is estimated that at least 50,000 patients in the United States have this disease, and there are currently no effective therapies that prevent progression to respiratory failure and death (Meyer, 2003).

IMMUNE SURVEILLANCE AND SUSCEPTIBILITY TO INFECTION

Respiratory infections are recognized as the fifth leading cause of death for individuals over age 65 (National Vital Statistics, 2001). There are many factors that make the elderly more susceptible to lung infections. These include declining immune function, impaired oral and mucociliary clearance, neurologic disorders, malnutrition, chronic organ dysfunction syndromes, and the presence of parenchymal lung disease (Meyer, 2004). Although various aspects of systemic immunity decline with advancing age, there is considerable variation among individuals. Fairly robust immune responses can be identified in centenarians (Franceschi *et al.*, 1995), and many other factors such as the presence of a swallowing disorder and aspiration can cause pneumonia in the elderly despite intact immune responses.

Both T and B lymphocyte responses tend to gradually wane with advancing age, and antibody responses to vaccines are less robust in the elderly than in younger individuals (Meyer, 2001). Although the effect of advancing age on acquired immune responses has been studied fairly extensively, relatively little is known about the effect of age on compartmentalized innate immune responses in the lung. Important components of innate immunity that may play a critical role in defense against infection include the ability of epithelia or other resident lung cell populations to produce antibacterial peptides such as the defensins (Huttner and Bevins, 1999) or collectins (Sano and Kuroki, 2005). Because the innate immune system is a key component of respiratory host defense that provides constant surveillance and immediate protection against invading pathogens (Meyer, 2001), age-associated decline in various components of innate immunity may play a key role in susceptibility to pulmonary infections.

One host defense mechanism that has been shown to decline gradually with advancing age in both animal models and human subjects is mucociliary clearance. Tracheal mucus velocity gradually declines in beagle dogs beginning at approximately age four (Mauderly and Hahn, 1982), and aged rats have diminished clearance of bacteria compared to young animals (Antonini *et al.*, 2001). Mucociliary clearance has been shown to decline in humans with advancing age (Puchelle *et al.*, 1979), and microtubular abnormalities in cilia have been associated with depressed nasociliary clearance time and lower ciliary beat frequency (Ho *et al.*, 2001). Although not proven, age-associated ciliary dysfunction may significantly increase susceptibility to respiratory infection for elderly individuals and may also increase susceptibility to irritation and damage to airway mucosae by inhaled particulates that are deposited on airspace surfaces and not rapidly cleared.

Animal Models and Insights into Mechanisms of Lung Senescence

Changes that are similar to those in the aging human lung have been observed in both rodents and dogs (Pinkerton *et al.*, 2004). The mouse makes an attractive model for mechanisms of lung senescence because of its relatively short lifespan, which is approximately 30 months for the strains used most commonly for research. A special strain, the senescence-accelerated mouse (SAM), has been established and has a median lifespan as low as 12 months (Takeda *et al.*, 1981). An increase in total alveolar surface area combined with an increase in interalveolar pore size and number and in volumes of airspaces distal to the respiratory bronchioles suggest that lung hyperinflation occurs in aged mice, and decreased elastic recoil has been associated with an age-associated decline in elastic fibers in BALB/c mice (Kawakami *et al.*, 1984). Lung hyperinflation appears to be accelerated in SAM mice and mimics changes in older mice from other strains (Kurozumi *et al.*, 1994), making the SAM mouse an attractive model for examining altered matrix and cell populations associated with advancing age. In contrast to the mouse, the aging rat lung does not seem to show altered lung compliance or a decline in alveolar surface area (Pinkerton and Green, 2004), and Lewis and Fischer 344 rats show an increase in cross-linked collagen in the lung parenchyma (Mays *et al.*, 1988; Sahebjami, 1991). However, this increase of interstitial collagen in rats does not seem to alter lung compliance (Pinkerton *et al.*, 1982).

Age-associated changes in the dog lung, which has greater morphological similarity to the human lung than rodent lungs, have been studied fairly extensively. Changes in airways and in distal parenchyma show considerable similarity to changes observed for the human lung and include enlargement of submucosal glands (Robinson and Gillespie, 1973), progressive calcification of bronchial cartilage (Robinson and Gillespie, 1973), a decline in mucus velocity (Mauderly and Hahn, 1982), and a decrease in alveolar tissue density with altered alveolar size and enlargement of respiratory bronchioles and alveolar ducts (Robinson and Gillespie, 1973). Focal accumulations of macrophages have also been observed in respiratory bronchioles and the junction of alveolar ducts and alveoli (Robinson and Gillespie, 1973).

When observations that are currently available from animal models of lung aging are merged with observations of altered structure and physiology of the aging human lung, it becomes clear that the most prominent feature of lung aging is loss or altered composition of matrix tissue accompanied by rearrangement of distal airspace structure such that elastic recoil declines and ventilation to perfusion relationships are altered. These changes show many similarities to emphysema, although important differences separate the emphysematous lung from an aged lung. Emphysema is characterized by airway inflammation and expanded populations of inflammatory cells (macrophages, neutrophils, and lymphocytes) in distal airspaces or airway walls (Barnes, 2000; Saetta *et al.*, 2001), and proteolytic and oxidative stress associated with the influx of inflammatory cells is thought to play a key role in the pathogenesis of emphysema. It is interesting that bronchoalveolar lavage (BAL) in aged C57BL/6 mice (Higashimoto *et al.*, 1991) show a modestly increased number of lymphocytes and neutrophils on differential cell counts. Studies in normal human volunteers have also shown an increase in BAL neutrophil and lymphocyte populations for elderly subjects compared to younger individuals (Meyer *et al.*, 1996; Meyer *et al.*, 1998; Meyer and Soergel, 1999), and it is tempting to speculate that a mild increase in inflammatory cell traffic and/or activation states in the aging human lung may gradually damage and alter elastin, collagen, and other matrix proteins over long periods of time. The causes of altered BAL cell and proinflammatory mediator patterns in apparently healthy, elderly subjects are not clear, but may represent a failure to regulate inflammatory responses, a response to subclinical aspiration, or heightened responses to inhaled agents such as fine particulates in ambient air.

Another important factor important in lung aging may be the ability of homeostatic mechanisms to maintain the integrity of the lung microvasculature and alveolar wall capillary bed. Vascular endothelial cell growth factor (VEGF) appears to be an extremely important gene product for the development and maintenance of the lung vasculature (Berse *et al.*, 1992; Monacci *et al.*, 1993; Zeng *et al.*, 1998), and recent studies have shown that emphysema in smokers is associated with a reduction in VEGF expression (Kasahara *et al.*, 2001; Koyama *et al.*, 2002; Kanazawa *et al.*, 2003a; Kanazawa *et al.*, 2003b). Blockade of VEGF receptors in a rat model has been shown to correlate with induction of epithelial cell apoptosis and cause distal airspace enlargement (Kasahara *et al.*, 2000). However, this change was prevented by the administration of a caspase inhibitor, which suggests that if VEGF production by epithelial cells and VEGF signaling is not disrupted, emphysematous changes do not occur. These investigators have also shown a link between oxidative stress and alveolar septal cell apoptosis induced by VEGF receptor blockade (Tuder *et al.*, 2003), and targeted VEGF inhibition in mice via intratracheal instillation of a viral vector that ablated the VEGF gene, causing alveolar septal wall damage and a reduction in lung elastic recoil (Tang *et al.*, 2004). Although VEGF gene expression in the lung has not been studied in animal models of lung senescence, VEGF levels gradually decline in BAL fluid with advancing age in normal volunteer subjects (Meyer *et al.*, 2000). Indeed, a diffuse, age-associated decline in VEGF expression or VEGF receptor function in the aging lung may explain many of the structural changes that affect the distal airspaces of the aged human lung. Alterations in VEGF homeostasis may be induced or accentuated by increased numbers of inflammatory cells coupled with altered antioxidant defenses that have been described for aged lungs in both mice and humans (Chen *et al.*, 1990; Teramoto *et al.*, 1995; Bottje *et al.*, 1998; Higashimoto *et al.*, 1991; Meyer *et al.*, 1996; Meyer *et al.*, 1998).

Conclusion

Although it is somewhat difficult to differentiate age-associated changes in the structure and function of the aging human lung from environmentally induced lung disorders and genetic susceptibility to lung disease, changes in the lung matrix that alter airway and parenchymal structure, which some investigators have termed "senile emphysema" or ductasia, appear to be a generalized phenomenon that occurs in the absence of environmental risk factors. These changes lead to a decline in elastic recoil and altered ventilation to perfusion relationships that affect pulmonary function testing values and gas exchange. The precise cause of these changes is not clear, but similar changes have been shown in the lungs of aged mice or dogs. The investigation of cellular compartment turnover, matrix alterations, and the role of cytokines such as VEGF, which can have a profound effect on the microvasculature, in these animal models may provide additional insights into the age-associated processes that alter the structure and function of the aging human lung. Models that seem particularly attractive for such investigations are aged C57/Bl mice, the SAM mouse, and Beagle dogs. Animal models may also help to identify age-associated factors that put the elderly at an increased risk for acute events such as pneumonia. Relatively little is known about innate immune mechanisms in the aged human lung, for one, and such models could facilitate the study of age-associated changes in innate immunity that may increase the risk of lower respiratory tract infection in the elderly and provide strategies to prevent pneumonia.

Recommended Resources

Harding, R., Pinkerton, K.E., and Plopper, C.G., Eds. *The lung: Development, aging and the environment.* London: Elsevier.

This text is an excellent resource for information gleaned from both animal models and human investigations that describes lung organogenesis, maturation, homeostasis, and age-associated decline.

Mauderly, J.L. (2000). Animal models for the effect of age on susceptibility to inhaled particulate matter. *Inhalation Toxicology* 12, 863–900.

This is a comprehensive review of mucociliary clearance mechanisms and the effects of age on clearance of particulate matter in various animal models and in humans.

Chan, E.D. and Welsh, C.H. (1998). Geriatric respiratory medicine. *Chest* 114, 1704–1733.

This is a comprehensive review of age-associated changes in structure and function of the human lung and lung disorders that commonly are found in the elderly.

REFERENCES

Ancoli-Israel, S. and Coy, T. (1994). Are breathing disturbances in elderly equivalent to sleep apnea syndrome. *Sleep 17*, 77–83.

Antonini, J.M., Roberts, J.R., Clarke, R.W., Yang, H., Barger, M.W., Ma, J.Y.C. *et al.* (2001). Pulmonary bacterial clearance in Fischer 344 rats after intratracheal instillation of *Listeria monocytogenes. Chest 120*, 240–249.

Arora, N.S. and Rochester, D.F. (1982). Respiratory muscle strength and maximal voluntary ventilation in undernourished patients. *Am. Rev. Respir. Dis. 126*, 5–8.

Barnes, P.J. (2000). Chronic obstructive pulmonary disease. *New Engl. J. Med. 343*, 269–280.

Berse, B., Brown, L.F., Van de Water, L., Dvorak, H.F., and Senger, D.R. (1992). Vascular permeability factor (vascular endothelial growth factor) gene is expressed differentially in normal tissues, macrophage, and tumors. *Mol. Biol. Cell 3*, 211–220.

Bleecker, E.R. (2004). Similarities and differences in asthma and COPD. *Chest 126*, 93S–95S.

Burrows, B., Barbee, R.A., Cline, M.G., Knudson, R.J., and Lebowitz, M.D. (1991). Characteristics of asthma among elderly adults in a sample of the general population. *Chest 100*, 935–942.

Burrows, B., Bloom, J.W., Traver, G.A., and Cline, M.G. (1987). The course and prognosis of different forms of chronic airways obstruction in a sample from the general population. *N. Engl. J. Med. 317*, 1309–1314.

Cerveri, I., Zoia, M.C., Fanfulla, F., Spagnolatti, L, Berrayah, L., Grassi, M. *et al.* (1995). Reference values of arterial oxygen tension in the middle-aged and elderly. *Am. J. Respir. Crit. Care Med. 152*, 934–941.

Chan, E.D. and Welsh, C.H. (1998). Geriatric respiratory medicine. *Chest 114*, 1704–1733.

Chen, T.S., Richie J.P. Jr., and Lang, C.A. (1990). Life span profiles of glutathione and acetaminophen detoxification. *Drug Metab. Dispos. Biol. Fate Chem. 18*, 882–887.

Coultas, D.B., Zumwalt, R.E., Black, W.C., and Sobonya, R.E. (1994). The epidemiology of interstitial lung diseases. *Am. J. Respir. Crit. Care Med. 150*, 967–972.

Crapo, R.O. (1993). The aging lung. In D.A. Mahler, Ed. *Pulmonary Disease in the Elderly Patient*, pp. 1–21. New York: Marcel Dekker.

Demedts, M., Wells, A.U., Anto, J.M., Costabel, U., Hubbard, R., Cullinan, P. *et al.* (2001). Interstitial lung diseases: An epidemiological overview. *Eur. Respir. J. 18*, 2S–16S.

D'Errico, A., Scarani, P., Colosimo, E., Spina, M., Grigioni, W.F., and Mancini, A.M. (1989). Changes in the alveolar connective tissue of the ageing lung. An immunohistochemical study. *Virchows. Arch. A. Pathol. Anat. Histopathol. 415*, 137–144.

Enright, P.L., Kronmal, R.A., Manolio, T.A., Schenker, M.B., and Hyatt, R.E. (1994). Respiratory muscle strength in the elderly: correlates and reference values. *Am. J. Respir. Crit. Care Med. 149*, 430–438.

Fabbri, L.M., Romagnoli, M., Corbetta, L., Casoni, G., Busljetic, K., Turato, G. *et al.* (2003). Differences in airway inflammation in patients with fixed airflow obstruction due to asthma or chronic obstructive pulmonary disease. *Am. J. Respir. Crit. Care Med. 167*, 418–424.

Finucane, K.E., Greville, H.W., and Brown, P.J. (1985). Irreversible airflow obstruction: evolution in asthma. *Med. J. Aust. 142*, 602–604.

Fishman, A.P. (2005). One hundred years of chronic obstructive pulmonary disease. *Am. J. Respir. Crit. Care Med. 171*, 941–948.

Franceschi, C., Monti, D., Sansoni, P., and Cossarizza, A. (1995). The immunology of exceptional individuals: the lesson of centenarians. *Immunol. Today 16*, 12–16.

Frette, C., Jacob, M.P., Wei, S.M., Bertrand, J.P., Laurent, P., Kauffmann, F. *et al.* (1997). Relationship of serum elastin peptide level to single breath transfer factor for carbon monoxide in French coal miners. *Thorax 52*, 1045–1050.

Gauderman, W.J., Avol, E., Gilliland, F., Vora, H., Thomas, D., Berhane, K. *et al.* (2004), The effect of air pollution on lung development from 10 to 18 years of age. *N. Engl. J. Med. 351*, 1057–1067.

Green, F.H.Y. and Pinkerton, K.E. (2004). Environmental determinants of lung aging. In R. Harding, K.E. Pinkerton, and C.G. Plopper, Eds. *The lung: Development, aging and the environment*, pp. 377–395. London: Elsevier.

Higashimoto, Y., Fukuchi, Y., Shimada, Y., Ishida, K., Ohata, M., Furuse, T. *et al.* The effects of aging on the function of alveolar macrophages in mice. *Mech. Age. Develop. 69*, 207–217.

Ho, J.C., Chan, K.N., Hu, W.H., Lam, W.K., Zheng, L., Tipoe, G.L. *et al.* (2001). The effect of aging on nasal mucociliary clearance, beat frequency, and ultrastructure of respiratory cilia. *Am. J. Respir. Crit. Care Med. 163*, 983–988.

Hoo, A.F., Stocks, J., Lum, S., Wade, A.M., Castle, R.A., Costeloe, K.L. *et al.* (2004). Development of lung function in early life: Influence of birth weight in infants of nonsmokers. *Am. J. Respir. Crit. Care Med. 170*, 527–533.

Huttner, K.M. and Bevins, C.L. (1999). Antimicrobial peptides as mediators of epithelial host defense. *Pediatr. Res. 45*, 785–794.

Janssens, J.P., Pache, J.C., and Nicod, L.P. (1999). Physiological changes in respiratory function associated with ageing. *Eur. Respir. J. 13*, 197–205.

Janssens, J.P., Herrmann, F., MacGee, W., and Michel, M.P. (2001). Cause of death in older patients with anatomo-pathological evidence of chronic bronchitis or emphysema: A case-control study based on autopsy findings. *J. Am. Geriatr. Soc. 49*, 571–576.

Kanazawa, H., Hirata, K., and Yoshikawa, J. (2003a). Imbalance between vascular endothelial growth factor and endostatin in emphysema. *Eur. Respir. J. 22*, 609–612.

Kanazawa, H., Asai, K., Hirata, K., and Yoshikawa, J. (2003b). Possible effects of vascular endothelial growth factor in the pathogenesis of chronic obstructive pulmonary disease. *Am. J. Med. 11*, 354–358.

Kasahara, Y., Tuder, R.M., Cool, C.D., Lynch, D.A., Flores, S.C., and Voelkel, N.F. (2001). Endothelial cell death and decreased expression of vascular endothelial growth factor and vascular endothelial growth factor receptor 2 in emphysema. *Am. J. Respir. Crit. Care Med. 163*, 737–744.

Kasahara, Y., Tuder, R.M., Taraseviciene-Stewart, L., Le Cras, T.D., Abman, S., Hirth, P.K. *et al.* (2000). Inhibition of VEGF receptors causes lung cell apoptosis and emphysema. *J. Clin. Invest. 106*, 1311–1319.

Kawakami, M., Paul, J.L., and Thurlbeck, W.M. (1984). The effect of age on lung structure in male BALB/cNNia inbred mice. *Am. J. Anat. 170*, 1–21.

Kelly, F.J., Dunster, C., and Mudway, I. (2003). Air pollution and the elderly: oxidant/antioxidant issues worth consideration. *Eur.Respir. J. 40*, 70S–75S.

Kerstjens, H.A., Brand, P.L., Hughes, M.D., Robinson, N.J., Postma, D.S., Sluiter, H.J. *et al.* (1992). A comparison of bronchodilator therapy with or without inhaled corticosteroid therapy for obstructive disease. Dutch Chronic Non-Specific Lung Disease Study Group. *N. Engl. J. Med. 327*, 1413–1419.

Koyama, S., Sato, E., Haniuda, M., Numanami, H., Nagai, S., and Izumi, T. (2002). Decreased level of vascular endothelial growth factor in bronchoalveolar lavage fluid of normal smokers and patients with pulmonary fibrosis. *Am. J. Respir. Crit. Care Med. 166*, 382–385.

Krieger, J., Sforza, E., Boudewijns, A., Zamagni, M., and Petiau, C. (1997). Respiratory effort during obstructive sleep apnea: Role of age and sleep state. *Chest 112*, 875–883.

Kronenberg, R. and Drage, G. (1973). Attenuation of the ventilatory and heart rate responses to hypoxia and hypercapnia with aging in normal man. *J. Clin. Invest. 52*, 1812–1819.

Krumpe, P.E., Knudson, R.J., Parsons, G., and Reiser K. (1985). The aging respiratory system. *Clin. Geriatr. Med. 1*, 143–175.

Kurozumi, M., Matsushita, T., Hosokawa, M., and Takeda, T. (1994). Age-related changes in lung structure and function in the senescence-accelerated mouse (SAM): SAMP/1 as a new murine model of senile hyperinflation of lung. *Am. J. Respir. Crit. Care Med. 149*, 776–782.

Lang, M., Fiaux, G., Gillooly, M., Stewart, J., Hulmes, D., and Lamb, D. (1994). Collagen content of alveolar wall tissue in emphysematous and non-emphysematous lungs. *Thorax 49*, 319–326.

Lebowitz, M.D., Knudson, R.J., and Burrows, B. (1975). Tucson epidemiologic study of obstructive lung diseases. I. Methodology and prevalence of disease. *Am. J. Epidemiol. 102*, 137–152.

Lundback, B., Lindberg, A., Lindstrom, M., Ronmark, E., Jonsson, A.C., Jonsson, E. *et al.* (2003). Obstructive Lung Disease in Northern Sweden Studies. Not 15 but 50% of smokers develop COPD?—Report from the Obstructive Lung Disease in Northern Sweden Studies. *Respir. Med. 97*, 115–1221.

Malik. A., Saltoun, C.A., Yarnold, P.R., and Grammer L,C. (2004). Prevalence of obstructive airways disease in the disadvantaged elderly of Chicago. *Allerg. Asthma Proc. 25*, 169–173.

Mancini, D., Henson, D., LaManca, J., and Levine, S. (1992). Respiratory muscle function and dyspnoea in patients with chronic heart failure. *Circulation 86*, 909–918.

Masi, M.A., Hanley, J.A., Ernst, P., and Becklake, M.R. (1988). Environmental exposure to tobacco smoke and lung function in young adults. *Am. Rev. Respir. Dis. 138*, 296–299.

Mauderly, J.L. and Hahn, F.F. (1982). The effects of age on lung function and structure of adult animals. *Adv. Vet. Sci. Comp. Med. 26*, 35–77.

Mays, P.K., Bishop, J.E., and Laurent, G.J. (1989). Age-related changes in the proportion of types I and III collagen. *Mech. Aging Dev. 45*, 203–212.

Meyer, K.C. (2003). Interferon gamma-1b therapy for idiopathic pulmonary fibrosis: Is the cart before the horse? *Mayo Clin. Proc. 78*, 1073–1075.

Meyer, K.C., Ershler, W., Rosenthal, N., Lu, X., and Peterson, K. (1996). Immune dysregulation in the aging human lung. *Am. J. Respir. Crit. Care Med. 153*, 1072–1079.

Meyer, K.C., Rosenthal, N.S., Soergel, P., and Peterson, K. (1998). Neutrophils and low-grade inflammation in the seemingly normal aging human lung. *Mech. Aging Develop. 104*, 169–181.

Meyer, K.C. and Soergel, P. (1999). Bronchoalveolar lymphocyte phenotypes change in the normal aging human lung. *Thorax 54*, 697–700.

Meyer, K.C., Cardoni, A., and Xiang, Z. (2000). Vascular endothelial growth factor in bronchoalveolar lavage from normal subjects and patients with diffuse parenchymal lung disease. *J. Lab. Clin. Med. 135*, 332–338.

Meyer, K. (2001). The role of immunity in susceptibility to respiratory infection in the aging lung. *Respir. Physiol. 128*, 23–31.

Meyer, K.C. (2004). Lung infections and aging. *Age. Res. Rev. 3*, 55–67.

Michaud, C.M., Murray, C.J., and Bloom, B.R. Burden of disease—Implications for future disease. *JAMA 285*, 535–539.

Mizuno, M. (1991). Human respiratory muscles: Fiber morphology and capillary supply. *Eur. Respir. J. 4*, 587–601.

Monacci, W.T., Merrill, M.J., and Oldfield, E.H. (1993). Expression of vascular permeability factor/vascular endothelial growth factor in normal rat tissue. *Am. J. Physiol. 264*, C995–C1002.

National Vital Statistics Report (2001). 49(11), October 12, *2001*, 1–49.

Needham, M. and Stockley, R.A. (2004). α_1-Antitrypsin deficiency. 3. Clinical manifestations and natural history. *Thorax 59*, 441–445.

Nishimura, Y., Maeda, H., Tanaka, K., Nakamura, H., Hashimoto, Y., and Yokoyama, M. (1994). Respiratory muscle strength and hemodynamics in chronic heart failure. *Chest 105*, 355–359.

Noble, P.W. and Homer, R.J. (2004). Idiopathic pulmonary fibrosis: New insights into pathogenesis. *Clin. Chest Med. 25*, 749–758.

Parameswaran, K., Hildreth, A.J., Chadha, D., Keaney, N.P., Taylor, I.K., and Bansal, S.K. (1998). Asthma in the elderly: Underperceived, underdiagnosed and undertreated, a community survey. *Respir. Med. 92*, 573–577.

Peterson, D.D., Pack, A.I., Silage, D.A., and Fishman, A.P. (1981). Effects of aging on ventilatory and occlusion pressure responses to hypoxia and hypercapnia. *Am. Rev. Respir. Dis. 124*, 387–391.

Peterson, D.D. and Fishman, A.P. (1982). The lungs in later life. In A.P. Fishman, Ed. *Pulmonary Disease and Disorders: Update 1*, pp. 123–136. New York: McGraw-Hill.

Pinkerton, K.E., Barry, B.E., O'Neil, J.J., Raub, J.A., Pratt, P.C., and Crapo, J.D. (1982). Morphologic changes in the lung during the life span of Fischer 344 rats. *Am. J. Anat. 164*, 155–174.

Pinkerton, K.E. and Green, F.H.Y. (2004). Environmental determinants of lung aging. In R. Harding, K.E. Pinkerton, and C.G. Plopper, Eds. *The lung: Development, aging and the environment*, pp. 213–233. London: Elsevier.

Polkey, M.I., Harris, M.L., Hughes, P.D., Hannegard, C.H., Lyons, D., Green, M. *et al.* (1997). The contractile properties of the elderly human diaphragm. *Am. J. Respir. Crit. Care Med. 155*, 1560–1564.

Postma, D.S. and Boezen, H.M. (2004). Rationale for the Dutch hypothesis. Allergy and airway hyperresponsiveness as genetic factors and their interaction with environment in the development of asthma and COPD. *Chest 126*, 96S–104S.

Poulin, M.J., Cunningham, D.A., Paterson, D.H., Rechnitzer, P.A., Ecclestone, N.A., and Koval, J.J. (1994). Ventilatory response to exercise in men and women 55 to 86 years of age. *Am. J. Respir. Crit. Care Med. 149*, 408–415.

Puchelle, E., Zahm, J.M., and Bertrand, A. (1979). Influence of age on bronchial mucociliary transport. *Scand. J. Respir. Dis. 60*, 307–313.

Robinson, N.E. and Gillespie, J.R. (1973). Morphologic features of the lungs of aging beagle dogs. *Am. Rev. Respir. Dis. 108*, 1192–1199.

Rossi, A., Ganassini, A., Tantucci, C., and Grassi, V. (1996). Aging and the respiratory system. *Aging Clin. Exp. Res. 8*, 143–161.

Saetta, M., Turato, G., Maestrelli, P., Mapp, C.E., and Fabbri, L.M. (2001). Cellular and structural bases of chronic obstructive pulmonary disease. *Am. J. Respir. Crit. Care Med. 163*, 1304–1309.

Sahebjami, H. (1991). Lung tissue elasticity during the lifespan of Fischer 344 rats. *Exp. Lung Res. 17*, 887–902.

Sano, H. and Kuroki, Y. (2005). The lung collectins, SP-A and SP-D, modulate pulmonary innate immunity. *Mol. Immunol 42*, 279–287.

Selman M. and Pardo, A. (2003). The epithelial/fibroblastic pathway in the pathogenesis of idiopathic pulmonary fibrosis. *A. J. Respir. Cell Mol. Biol. 29*, S93–S977.

Shapiro, S.D., Endicott, S.K., Province, M.A., Pierce, J.A., and Campbell, E.J. (1991). Marked longevity of human lung parenchymal elastic fibers deduced from prevalence of D-aspartate and nuclear weapons-related radiocarbon. *J. Clin. Invest. 87*, 1828–1834.

Sorbini, C.A., Brassi, V., Solinas, E., and Muiesan, G. (1968). Arterial oxygen tension in relation to age in healthy subjects. *Respiration 225*, 3–13.

Tack, M., Altose, M., and Cherniack, N. (1982). Effect of aging on the perception of resistive ventilatory loads. *Am. Rev. Respir. Dis. 126*, 463–467.

Taggart, C.C., Greene, C.M., Carroll, T.P., O'Neill, S.J., and McElvaney, N.G. (2005). Elastolytic proteases: inflammation resolution and dysregulation in chronic infective lung disease. *Am. J. Respir. Crit. Care Med. 171*, 1070–1076.

Takeda, T., Hosokawa, M., Takeshita, S., Irino, M., Higuchi, K., Matsushita, T. *et al.* (1981). A new murine model of accelerated senescence. *Mech. Ageing Dev. 17*, 183–194.

Tang, K., Rossiter, H.B., Wagner, P.D., and Breen, E.C. (2004). Lung-targeted VEGF inactivation leads to an emphysema phenotype in mice. *J. Appl. Physiol. 97*, 1559–1566.

Teramoto, S., Fukuchi, Y., Uejima, Y., Teramoto, K., and Orimo, H. (1995). Biochemical characteristics of lungs in senescence-accelerated mouse (SAM). *Eur. Respir. J. 8*, 45–46.

Thurlbeck, W.M. and Wright, J.M. (1999). Emphysema: Classification, morphology, and associations. In *Thurlbeck's Chronic Airflow Obstruction*, pp. 85–144. Hamilton: B.C. Dekker Inc.

Thurlbeck, W.M. (1991). Morphology of the aging lung. In R.G. Crystal, J.B. West, P.J. Barnes, N.S. Cherniak, and E.R. Weibel, Eds. *The lung: Scientific foundations*, pp. 1743–1748. New York: Raven Press.

Tuder, R.M., Zhen, L., Cho, C.Y., Taraseviciene-Stewart, L., Kasahara, Y., Salvemini, D. *et al.* (2003). Oxidative stress and apoptosis interact and cause emphysema due to vascular endothelial growth factor receptor blockade. *Am. J. Respir. Cell Mol. Biol. 29*, 88–97.

Zeng, X., Wert, S.E., Federici, R., Peters, K.G., and Whitsett, J.A. (1998). VEGF enhances pulmonary vasculogenesis and disrupts lung morphogenesis in vivo. *Dev. Dyn. 211*, 215–227.

61

Iceland as a Model for Human Aging

Adalsteinn Gudmundsson and Pálmi V. Jónsson

Iceland may be viewed as a small but prototypic Western society, strategically located between mainland Europe and North America. Its ethnically and socioeconomically homogeneous population is served by an advanced healthcare system through a national health and social insurance. Interdisciplinary geriatric care is well established, and Iceland was one of the first countries to adapt, from the United States, the resident assessment instrument (RAI), which makes a cross-country comparison of long-term care feasible. Among a number of biotech companies recently established in Iceland are leading companies in the field of linking genetic variation to diseases. Historically, the population of Iceland has been exceptionally supportive and willing to participate in both transsectional and cohort studies. The Icelandic Heart Association launched a major population study on interactions between age, genes, and environment (AGES) in 2002 in collaboration with the U.S. National Institute of Aging (NIA). Ultimately, we may expect that a cutting edge aging research in Iceland will contribute to our understanding of how to maintain better health, independence, and active participation in later life, and how to best care for those who become frail and in need of formal care.

Introduction

Facing the global phenomenon of population aging, many countries are sharing their interest in collaborative research projects relating to aging. Although most countries are seeing declines in mortality rates, Western societies, in addition, have experienced secular declines in fertility rates, which continues to sustain a steady increase in the ratio of older to younger generation (Kinsella, 2005).

New approaches and frameworks of longitudinal databases are needed, which take into account both differences and similarities in aging-related processes across ethnic and national boundaries (the National Academy of Sciences, 2001). Fortunately, this occurs at a time when travel and use of long-distance communication through the Internet make long-distance collaboration and cross-national research easier and more sophisticated than ever before.

In the context of cross-national research, Iceland has unique potential for contribution. The purpose of this chapter is to give the reader some background information on the aging population in Iceland. How and why the rugged terrain of this island of 103,000 km^2 (43 thousand square miles) surfacing the North Atlantic in a strategic location between North America and mainland Europe has become a fertile ground for both current and future research on aging will be described.

History

Iceland was first settled between 870 and 930 A.D. by Norwegian Vikings. Recent research has shown that 20 to 25% of the founding males had Gaelic ancestry. The majority of the females are thought to have come from the British Isles during the time of settlement. At the end of the initial settlement period, the population is estimated to have numbered approximately 30,000 (Halldorsson, 2003). A period of favorable climate conditions sustained a local population growth through the twelfth century, when the estimated population may have plateaued at 80,000. This era was followed by centuries of colder climate, and several periods of substantial population reduction occurred. Two epidemics, of plague in the fifteenth century and several smallpox epidemics in the sixteenth to early eighteenth century, reduced the population of the entire island to as low as 30,000 on more than one occasion. The fallout from a volcanic eruption in 1875 devastated the Icelandic economy and caused widespread famine. During the last quarter of the nineteenth century, approximately 20% of Iceland's population emigrated, mostly to Canada and the United States (Jonsson, 1998). This explains why the population of Iceland, which has remained in relative genetic isolation through 1100 years, is quite homogeneous, with many residents sharing common ancestors. Screening for individual mutations in the population is facilitated by the Icelanders' fascination with genealogy. Details of births, marriages, and deaths have been kept in church records for more than three centuries. Extensive computerized genealogy databases have been created, which allow the pedigree of most Icelanders to be traced back to the seventeenth century, and for many further back to the settlement of the island. Islendingabok is the only genealogy database in the world, which covers a whole nation. It includes information on more than 95% of all Icelanders from 1703 onward. It includes information on about 700,000 Icelanders, which is about half of all Icelanders who have lived on the island since its settlement (Islendingabok, 2003). These facts of history lead to a strong founder effect and the genealogy database greatly facilitates genetic research.

Iceland's founder population provides advantages for researchers studying complex disorders such as many of the age-associated diseases. This has been repeatedly demonstrated in recent years with the discovery of genes and biomarkers associated with cardiovascular disease, central nervous system diseases, osteoporosis, obesity, and cancer (Jonsson *et al.*, 2004).

Although Iceland only recently (1944) has become a sovereign state after many centuries of colonialism, it has since World War II transformed from being one of Europe's poorest into being among the richest countries in the world by per capita measures. Its culture and social structure resembles other Scandinavian countries and strong market ties remain to the European market without being a member of the European Union.

Still, in more than just geographic sense, Iceland is closer to North America than most of Europe. It has grown into and benefited from being an "in between" country with cultural and strong economic and trading ties to the United States over the last 50 years. Cooperation in health sciences has been steadily growing between Iceland and the United States. A first milestone in this regard was the establishment of the laboratory at Keldur lead by Dr. Bjorn Sigurdsson in 1946 through the Rockefeller Foundation. Dr. Sigurdsson's work resulted in the original concept of slow viral infections (Palsson, 1994).

Figures and Facts

Iceland is one of the least densely populated countries in the world, with a total population of 290,500 people in 2003, averaging 2.9 inhabitants per square kilometer (Statistical Yearbook of Iceland, 2004). About two-thirds of the population live in and around the capital of Reykjavik, which is located on the southwest corner of the island. Mainly due to effects of the Gulf Stream, Icelanders enjoy a warmer climate than its subarctic location would indicate. The average July temperatures have passed 12° C in recent years from being 10.5° C in previous decades (Statistical Yearbook of Iceland, 2004). Unconfirmed, this has been viewed by many as one of the strongest indicators of global warming. The average temperature in January remains around the freezing point.

Both by ethnic and socioeconomic measures, the population is homogeneous. Still, its society and people offer a prototype of a western society with an advanced but small infrastructure. The past decade with rapid economic growth and low unemployment figures has stimulated immigration of workers from a variety of countries. During 2000 to 2004, the Icelandic Directorate of immigration has issued 5000 to 6500 residence permits of all categories annually (The Icelandic Directorate of Immigration, 2005). Hence, the historic advantage of a homogeneous population is about to disappear due to globalization. Instead, we will gain valuable prospective information on how a western society adapts to an influx of immigrants of all ages, and its effect on care and caregiving for the elderly.

In the year 2000, the costs of healthcare, including long-term care, were 7.7% of the gross domestic product. The healthcare system is nationalized, with 85% of total cost paid for through taxes (Highlights on health in Iceland. WHO Regional Office for Europe, 2000). By conventional measures and indicators through health statistics, Icelanders enjoy good health status. Strong economy, favorable social situations, and good access to healthcare have brought Iceland into a leading position as having one of the world's highest life expectancies at birth. Life expectancy at birth has increased from 61.0 years for women in 1921 to 1930, to 82.5 years in 2001 to 2003. During the same period, the life expectancy for men has increased from 56.2 to 78.7 years, the highest in the world (Statistical Yearbook of Iceland, 2004). This gender difference in life expectancy of less than four years in Iceland is smaller than in most industrialized countries, where it is usually five to seven years. Although the group of older citizens in Iceland has increased remarkably by absolute numbers in recent years, the proportion of older than 65 years remains less than 12% mostly due to relatively high fertility rate with 1.98 births/woman (Statistical Yearbook of Iceland, 2004).

Eighty-seven percent of Icelanders over the age of 65 live independently in the community. The remainder live in facilities for assisted living or nursing homes. A major disadvantage of the health care system in Iceland is its waiting lists. This is particularly true in Reykjavik, where long lists remain for both assisted living and nursing homes and where there is congestion of elderly awaiting discharges form acute hospitals (Ingimarsson *et al.*, 2004).

Lifestyle

The nutritional value of diet in Iceland improved significantly during the last century, and it now comes closer in most respects to the targets set by the Icelandic Nutrition Council. Surveys in 1990 and 2002 show a decrease in the daily intake of fat, mainly due to less consumption of margarine and nonskimmed milk, and an increase in consumption of fruits (39%) and vegetables (15%). There is a clear social gradient, with those who have better education or higher incomes eating more vegetables. On the negative side, the country's consumption of fish per capita has diminished by 43% during this period and is now only slightly above many other European countries (Halldorsson, 2003).

Obesity is an increasing problem in Iceland, especially among children. In a recent study, body mass index was found to have increased considerably between 1938 and 1998 among nine-year-olds. The proportion of overweight children has increased from a few percent in 1938 to around 20% in 1998, and the proportion of obese children has increased from less than 1% to approximately 6% (Briem, 1999).

There has been a similar development among adults. In 1994, approximately 60% of women and 70% of men aged 45 to 64 years were either overweight or obese, which is comparable to that observed in many Western countries (Thorgeirsdottir, 2001).

One recent study of adult Icelanders concluded that one of four Icelandic men and one of five women do not participate in regular physical activity. More than half of adult Icelanders are overweight or obese, but the risk is halved among those who exercise at least five days per week, compared to those who exercise less frequently. Sedentary lifestyle has become even more common among Icelanders than in the neighboring countries (Gudmundsdottir, 2004).

Follow-up surveys on the number of daily smokers in Iceland have shown favorable results in recent decades. In 1985, approximately 43% of men and 37% of women smoked on a daily basis, but in 2001 the figures were 26.5% and 24.6%, respectively. Daily smoking among tenth-graders has declined steadily according to surveys, from 23% in 1998 to 14% in 2002. Although consumption of alcohol in liters per capita is lower than in most of Europe, the consumption has been increasing steadily and had reached 6.3 liters per person 15 years and older in 2002 (Halldorsson, 2003).

Geriatric Care

The importance of geriatric care has been recognized, and geriatric evaluation and management units and interdisciplinary teamwork are well established in Iceland (Jonsson, 1998). Interest among physicians in formal geriatric training has increased rapidly during the past 10 years, and in 2002, 15 fellowship-trained geriatricians had appointments at academic hospitals. Iceland was one of the first countries to adopt the comprehensive Resident Assessment Instrument (RAI) in nursing homes from the United States by a mandate in 1996. A crucial consequence of the international adoption of the RAI is that comparison of long-term care between countries has become feasible (Jonsson and Palsson, 2003). More interRAI assessment tools currently are being adopted in Iceland such as home care, post-acute care, and mental health, all paving the way toward a seamless information system in elderly care and formation of a longitudinal database.

Icelandic law mandates use of the Nursing Home Preadmission Assessment (NHPA); no one can enter a nursing home without undergoing this certified need assessment. A multidisciplinary team performs the NHPA; the team consists of a physician, nurse, and social worker. The assessment is in standard form and content. It remains valid for up to 18 months and is expected to be revised if the applicant's condition or situation changes during this time (Johannesdóttir and Jonsson, 1994).

The NHPA system generates national and regional waiting lists for the currently 3,700 nursing home beds available. Based on analysis of the NHPA database for the period 1992 to 2001 in the Reykjavík metropolitan area, the average enrollment age of men in nursing homes in Reykjavík was 82.7 years, and for women, 84.4 years. Men were about one-third of residents in nursing homes. The mean survival in nursing homes in Reykjavík was 2.5 years for men and 3.1 years for women (Ingimarsson, 2004).

The structure of care for the elderly is similar in the five Nordic countries (Sweden, Finland, Denmark, Norway, and Iceland). A close collaboration exists between the Nordic professors in geriatric medicine. This collaboration has already produced strategic documents relating to geriatric assessment and geriatric rehabilitation (Jonsson *et al.*, 2002; Sletvold *et al.*, 1996).

In 1999, an Institute on Gerontological Research (IGR) was established by the University of Iceland and Landspitali University Hospital. As an umbrella-like organization its main goals are to coordinate and facilitate broad research and collaboration in gerontology at the University of Iceland and the University Hospital. Researchers from the IGR are involved with, to mention but few, research at DeCODE company (Alzheimer's and longevity studies), the AGES study, and European and Nordic collaboration (Jonsson *et al.*, 2003; Fialova *et al.*, 2005).

Research Environment

During the past decade, there has been a remarkable increase in expenditure on research and development work. Icelanders spent 3% of their gross domestic product on research and development undertakings in 2001, compared to 1.1% in 1990, thereby reaching the goal that the European Union has set for itself to achieve by 2010. The benefits of this investment may be measured, for instance, by the favorable outcome of Icelandic scientists in international cooperation and through added innovation, which has led to growth in employment and in the export of goods and services based mainly on knowledge (the Icelandic Centre for Research, 2005). In 2005, Iceland ranked second in the world by measuring the degree of preparation of a nation or community to participate in and benefit from information and communication technologies (the Global Information Technology Report, 2004–2005).

Because of Iceland's small size and scale of resources, the majority of Icelandic physicians and many other disciplines seek their postgraduate training abroad, either in Europe or North America. This has benefited healthcare and research in Iceland as the majority repatriates, bringing back the connections, ambitions, and initiative, that allow them to achieve success on an international scale. Although the smallness of the country limits resources, it is balanced by advantages of short routes of communication among individuals, institutions, and businesses.

Through health registries, which may date back a century or more, Iceland offers rich resources for health-related research, which cover the entire population, including cancer prevalence, cardiovascular health, and mortality. Linking the Icelandic health registries to the extensive genealogy database is beginning to underscore the importance of genetic predisposition for an entire population (Jonsson *et al.*, 2004).

A national cancer registry was started in 1954. It contains information on around 30,000 individual cases of cancer diagnosed since then. It is one of few such registries in the world containing information on an entire nation. Currently, about 1000 cases of cancer are diagnosed annually in Iceland. The most commonly affected organs are the prostate for men and the breast for women, closely followed by the lung for both sexes. Research in cancer epidemiology has been one of the main functions of the Icelandic Cancer Society since the cancer registry was started (the Icelandic Cancer Society). Data from the Icelandic population was also important in identifying both the BRCA1 and BRCA2 genes for breast cancer, but a founder mutation in each gene is present in the Icelandic population (Bergthorsson *et al.*, 1998; Thorlacius *et al.*, 1998).

The public is generally supportive of medical research, and the high public participation rate is a distinctive advantage of locating such research in Iceland (see Table 61.1). Furthermore, the population has lived through and been exposed to relatively similar environmental conditions (climate, altitude, diet, pollutants, infectious agents) in comparison to larger nations. It is interesting to note that the total population of individuals older than 65 is only 33,500 (15,000 men and 18,500 women). This is a manageable size on its own, and harbors unique opportunities for research on health and disease pertinent in an entire population (Gudmundsson, 2004).

TABLE 61.1
Iceland: Advantages for health-related research in the twenty-first century

- A small prototypic Western society with advanced infrastructure
- Official health registries
- Universal access to healthcare
- Advanced training abroad common
- Founder population and extensive genealogy databases
- Environmental similarity
- The general public supports and participates in research
- High-tech biomedical research companies
- The Reykjaviik-AGES study

Research into the social aspects of aging has been limited until now, but with an established teaching and research position in social gerontology at the University of Iceland, that is about to change.

Biomedical Research in Iceland

Favorable situations have paved the way for the local establishment of a number of biotech companies in recent years. One of them is Decode Genetics, a recognized world leader in its field (Breithaupt, 2002). Among its goals is to link genetic variation to longevity and to many age-associated diseases, including dementia, osteoporosis, stroke, Parkinson disease, and osteoarthritis. By using a computerized genealogy database, the genetic component of longevity has been demonstrated, as well as lower age-specific death rates in offspring of long-lived parents (Gudmundsson *et al.*, 2000).

Several other genomic-based biotechnology companies are operating in Iceland. One of them, the Iceland Genomics Corporation (IGS), focuses on cancer biology through agreements with clinicians, the main national hospitals, and the National Cancer Registry. The project aims to increase the value of the data obtained from the IGS collection of biological samples, including patient DNA and tumor biopsies, by using family information supplied by the Genealogical Committee of the University of Iceland and clinical information supplied by the National Cancer Registry and collaborating clinicians, in order to obtain the world's first comprehensive survey of cancer across an entire nation. This will allow an unprecedented depth of analysis, where the relationship between genotype, disease, and clinical outcome can be probed. The company currently is taking advantage of this unique resource by searching for novel cancer genes using both association studies and linkage analysis (the Iceland Genomics Corporation, 2005).

One of the largest and longest lasting epidemiological studies available involving a representative unselected population is the Reykjavík study, which the Icelandic Heart Association (IHA) launched in 1967 around an initiative to battle against increases in cardiovascular diseases in Iceland. The study invited 25,000 men and women born between 1907 and 1934. The response rate was high (76%) for clinic visits, and participants were followed from one to six times for up to 30 years by thorough questionnaires, medical examinations, and biochemical measurements that accumulated vast resources of information (Hardarsson *et al.*, 2000).

The quality and depth of the data collected in the Reykjavík study has been widely recognized and has led to over 300 publications. The IHA has participated in the international WHO coordinated project on heart disease (MONICA) and maintains a detailed record of heart attacks and coronary artery interventions for the entire Icelandic population. In 2001, the National Institute on Aging (USA) and the Icelandic Heart Association announced their collaboration on a new study of the original cohort from the Reykjavík Study. In this new study on the interactions of age, genes, and environment (AGES), which started in 2002, the prior participants in the Reykjavík study are offered the opportunity to participate again. This well-established cohort and the current AGES will focus on establishing phenotypes and definitions of quantitative traits related to diseases and conditions of old age, and will collect genetic and other biologic specimens. The 7,000 to 8,000 remaining participants will contribute to the project through questionnaires, physical examinations, and state of the art measurements of the health of their bones, muscles, and metabolic and nervous systems (NIH News Release, April 23, 2001).

Important steps in improving the current concept of genetic association studies will include better measures of quantitative traits as phenotypes. The mid-life data available from the participants in the Reykjavík study such as cardiovascular measures (blood pressure, ECG, and cholesterol) is an important contribution. More importantly, now decades later, are state of the art imaging techniques and molecular markers, which better define the present phenotypes. The Reykjavík-AGES study uses new technology for the measurement of quantitative traits, for instance, calcium scoring of the coronary arteries by computerized tomography (CT) and post-processing of magnetic resonance imaging (MRI) of the brain; in addition to standard phenotypic measurements. Furthermore, this enhanced understanding of genetic and environmental contributions could create novel opportunities to prevent disease and limit disability associated with aging (Gudnason *et al.*, 2005).

Conclusion

Through private and public funding, Iceland is being established as a model for opportunities in research on aging. Iceland entered the twentieth century as an isolated founder population of poor sheep farmers and small-scale fishermen, but at the turn of the twenty-first century Iceland has been transformed into a knowledge-based high-tech society whose still interrelated and aging population will deliver important lessons on the interactions between age-associated diseases, the environment, and genetic components. Ultimately, cutting-edge aging research in Iceland can contribute to our understanding of how to maintain better health, independence, and active participation in later life.

REFERENCES

Bergthorsson, J.T., Jonasdottir, A., Johannesdottir, G., Arason, A., Egilsson, V., Gayther, S. *et al.* (1998). Identification of a novel splice-site mutation of the BRCA1 gene in two breast cancer families: Screening reveals low frequency in Icelandic breast cancer patients. *Human Mutation (Suppl 1)*, S195–S197.

Breithaupt, H. (2002). Experiment in research policy. *EMBO Reports 3*, 108–110.

Briem, B. (1999). Haed og thyngd 9 ara skolabarna i Reykjavík 1919–1998. [Height and weight of 9-year old school children, 1919–1998.] University of Iceland.

Fialová, D., Topinková, E., Gambassi, G., Finne-Soveri, H., Jónsson, P.V., Carpenter, I. *et al.* (2005). Potentially inappropriate medication use among home care elderly patients in Europe. *JAMA 293*, 1348–1358.

The Global Information Technology Report (2004–2005). www.weforum.org.

Gudmundsdottir, S.L., Oskarsdottir, D., Franzson, L., Indiridason, O.S., and Sigurdsson, G. (2004). The relationship between physical activity, body mass index, body composition and grip strength in an Icelandic population. *The Icelandic Medical Journal 90*, 479–486.

Gudmundsson A. (2004). Research on aging in Iceland: future potentials. *Mechanisms of Ageing and Development 125*, 133–135.

Gudmundsson, H., Gudbjartsson, D.F., Frigge, M., Gulcher, J.R., and Stefansson, K. (2000). Inheritance of human longevity in Iceland. *European Journal of Human Genetics 8*, 743–749.

Gudnason, G., Harris, T., and Launer, L. (2005). AGES Reykjavík Study: The Reykjavík study of healthy aging for the new millennium. The Icelandic Heart Institute www:hjarta.is/en/.

Halldorsson, M. (2003). Health care systems in transition: Iceland. Copenhagen, WHO Regional Office for Europe on behalf of the European Observatory on Health Systems and Policies.

Hardarson, T., Gardarsdottir, M., Gudmundsson, K.TH., Thorgeirsson, G., Sigvaldason, H., Sigfusson, N. *et al.* (2001). The relationship between educational level and mortality. *The Reykjavík Study. Journal of Internal Medicine 249*, 495–502.

Highlights on health in Iceland (2000). WHO Regional office for Europe. www.who.dk.

The Iceland Genomics Corporation (2005). www.uvs.is.

The Icelandic Cancer Society. www.krabb.is.

The Icelandic Centre for Research (2005). www.rannis.is.

The Icelandic Directorate of Immigration (2005). www.utl.is.

The Icelandic Heart Association (2005). www.hjarta.is/en/.

Ingimarsson, O., Aspelund, T., and Jónsson, P.V. (2004). The Preadmission Nursing Home Assessment (PNHA) in Iceland in 1992–2001. Relationship to survival and admission to a long term care facility. *The Icelandic Medical Journal 90*, 121–129.

Islendingabok (2003). A complete database of all available Icelandic genealogy information. www.islendingabok.is.

Johannesdottir, G.B. and Jonsson, P.V. (1995). The Preadmission Nursing Home Assessment (PNHA) in Reykjavík in 1992. *The Icelandic Medical Journal 81*, 233–241.

Jonsson, A., Jonsson, P.V., Gustafson, Y., Schroll, M., Hansen, F.R., Saarela, M. *et al.* (2002). Geriatric rehabilitation as an integral part of geriatric medicine in the Nordic countries. *The Icelandic Medical Journal 88*, 29–38.

Jonsson, P.V. (1998). Letter from Reykjavík. *Ann. Intern. Med. 128*, 941–945.

Jonsson, P.V., Ljunggren, G., Grue, E.V., Schroll, M., Bucht, G., and Noro, A. (2003). Identification of co-morbidity and functional limitation in the elderly in acute care by MDS-AC compared with the medical record. Vth European Congress of Gerontology, Barcelona, Spain, July 2–5, 2003. *Geriatría Y Gerontología. 38*, supplemento 1, pp. 25, presentation 25.

Jonsson, P.V. and Palsson, H. (2003). Toward informed and evidence based elderly care: The RAI experience in Iceland. Mibank report. www.milbank.org.

Jonsson, S. *et al.* (2004). Familial risk of lung carcinoma in the Icelandic population. *JAMA 292*, 2977.

Kinsella, K. and Phillips, D.R. (2005). Global aging: The challenge of success. *Population Bulletin 60*, 1.

The National Academy of Sciences (2001). Preparing for an aging world: The case for cross national research. books.nap.edu/catalog/10120.html.

NIH News release, April 23, 2001.

Palsson, P.A. (1994). Dr. Bjorn Sigurdsson (1913–1959). A memorial tribute. *Ann. N. Y. Acad. Sci. 724*, 1–5.

Statistical yearbook of Iceland (2004). www.hagstofa.is.

Sletvold, O., Tilvis, R., Jonsson, A., Schroll, M., Snædal, J., Engedal, K. *et al.* (1996). Geriatric work-up in the Nordic countries. The Nordic approach to comprehensive geriatric assessment. *Dan. Med. Bull. 43*, 350–359.

Thorgeirsdottir, H., Steingrimsdottir, L., Olafsson, O., and Gudnason, V. (2001). Trends in overweight and obesity in 45–64 year old men and women in Reykjavík 1975–1994. *The Icelandic Medical Journal 87*, 699–704.

Thorlacius, S., Struewing, J.P., Hartge, P., Olafsdottir, G.H., Sigvaldason, H., Tryggvadottir, L. *et al.* (1998). Population-based study of risk of breast cancer in carriers of BRCA2 mutation. *Lancet 352*, 1337–1339.

62

Behavior and Personality in the Study of Successful Aging

Judith Corr and Loraine Tarou

Although science has greatly extended human longevity, efforts to improve the quality of life experience for older people must be increased if we are to avoid creating a generation of long-lived, but isolated, lonely, and inactive elders. Ultimately, the goal in any investigation of human aging should be to both extend and improve the quality of life for increasing numbers of elderly. It is argued here that it is essential to expand aging research designs to include both biological and behavioral variables whenever possible, so that a more complete understanding of growing older as the culmination of multiple processes can be achieved. The search for a general, theoretical framework of human aging has been largely unsuccessful, perhaps because all primates, human and nonhuman, become aged within a complex network of varying environments and social structures. Also, individuals react differently to the same conditions, making differences among members of the same species critical in the understanding of the individual aging experience. Along with predictable biomarkers of aging, there may be a set of identifiable behavioral traits that cross-culturally influence successful human aging. Behavioral traits that are consistent over time are termed personality. *Use of personality testing in humans and nonhuman primates, using the Big Five, is reviewed, and new directions for aging investigations are suggested.*

The Importance of Behavior

> Most of us want to become old, but we worry about being old.
>
> Baltes and Baltes (1998)

The ultimate goal in the investigation of human aging is to extend and improve the quality of life for increasing numbers of elderly. Worldwide fertility rates have declined, coincident with increases in life expectancy, creating a large and expanding bulge at the top of the global population pyramid. In the United States, for instance, more than one in five Americans will be 65 years or older by 2030 (U.S. Census Bureau, 2004), a trend that is fast becoming global and carries immense implications for all world cultures and economies. Moreover, in addition to aging of the general population, demographics within the aged group itself are also shifting as the category of *oldest old* (80+ years) is growing faster than any other segment of elderly. Now, along with increased longevity provided by scientific achievements, science should also work to increase life satisfaction and happiness for growing numbers of aged. Extended years should be years lived well, if possible. It is our view that aging research should be collaborative across disciplines; as an understanding of the biological bases of aging without consideration of behavior or individual differences, or vice versa, is an incomplete understanding.

Although science has greatly extended human longevity, efforts to improve the quality of life experience for older people must increase if we are to avoid creating a generation of isolated, lonely, and inactive elders, a trend that is already a sad reality in industrialized Japan, where birthrates have fallen to 1.29 children per female and numbers of elderly are growing rapidly. This means that, within the next few years, Japan will have more elderly people than they have children (U.S. Census Bureau, 2004). Traditionally, Japanese culture places adult children in extended natal homes that provide for the inclusion of elders. However, current demographic pressures and economic realities are removing that option while elder care facilities are either inadequate or completely lacking in many parts of Japan. Therefore, an increasing number of Japanese elders are living solitary lives. In an attempt to compensate for increasing elder isolation and loneliness, healing partner dolls are currently being marketed to Japanese families of the isolated aged. These interactive dolls are personalized, capable of using up to 1200 different spoken phrases, and can be programmed in accordance with the owners' sleep–wake schedule (Suzuki, 2005). Demand for these companion dolls is high in Japan, and many elders who have them report not feeling alone any more and say they are raising the dolls "as they did their own children."

Handbook of Models for Human Aging

An Evolutionary Framework of Aging

The search for a general, theoretical framework of aging has long been of interest to both geriatrics and gerontology. Before 1900, Weismann proposed the first evolutionary theory of aging and argued that biological aging and death are adaptations that ensure species renewal and are programmed within the organism itself (1889). Mutation Accumulation Theory later explained aging as a process that, due to lessening effects of natural selection on post-reproductive individuals, mutations continue to accumulate over time, increasing mortality in later life (Medawar, 1946). Finally, Antagonistic Pleiotropy describes natural selection as having a bias toward youth that selects against longevity when genes that have pleiotropic effects are advantageous in the young but disadvantageous in the aged organism (Williams, 1957). For an expanded review of these and other proposed evolutionary theories of aging, see Gavrilov and Gavrilova (2002) or Crews (2003).

Why organisms have a short or a long life and why they grow old and die remain questions that are best addressed within an evolutionary framework (Gavrilov and Gavrilova, 2002). While the search for an evolutionary, universal theory of biological aging continues, current directions focusing on physiological aging, in addition to asking why organisms age and die, are also continuing to identify factors that act to further extend life (i.e., via caloric restriction, maintenance of cortical function, and tissue rejuvenation, etc.). Additionally, however, some contemporary investigators are adjusting the focus of their aging investigations to describe biological senescence as part of a general, life history model of inquiry. Although in our view, this methodological approach to aging investigation is a step in the right direction, it can also be limiting unless it addresses individual, behavioral variation (personality) and its effect on successful aging.

All biological organisms develop, mature, and age over the life span. Although the processes of human development, maturation, and reproduction have been broadly researched, aging studies have, for the most part, limited their focus to longevity and biological senescence (i.e., on geriatrics). Aging, however, is a complex interaction of factors that go beyond clinical aging and biological senescence, and should be investigated from a broader, multidimensional perspective if we hope to enhance our expanded longevity. In contrast to geriatrics, gerontology is interested in understanding the processes of normal, undiseased aging, and draws on collaborations from diverse disciplines, both biological and behavioral (Crews, 2003). It is argued here that it is essential to expand aging research designs to include both biology and behavior whenever possible, so that a better understanding of growing older as the culmination of multiple processes can be achieved.

Successful Aging

The concept of successful aging has no consistent definition. Some use it to describe simple survival, whereas others define its parameters through self-perceived quality of life measures: that is, an individual's report of their physical health, psychosocial health, vigor, contentment, and so on (Baltes and Baltes, 1990). Over the past decade, the results of several longitudinal human aging studies have been widely reported, all of which suggest that the role of individual differences in life experience and basic personality are key to understanding how one experiences being elderly (Corr, 2004).

Valliant (2002), in reporting on the Harvard Study of Adult Development, concluded that successful aging in the individual requires resilience and the selection of positive individual lifestyle choices. The MacArthur Foundation Study of Successful Aging (Rowe and Kahn, 1998) reported similar observations and added that individual lifestyle and attitude may even contribute more to successful aging than genes in many cases. Finally, Snowdon (2001), in the well-known Nun's Study, showed that positive behavior and personality in the individual can even overrule the often devastating biology of aging, including the pathology of Alzheimer's. These intriguing reports require further investigation of aged human behavioral variation, both within and between populations. Along with predictable biomarkers of aging (presmyopia, arthritis, increased susceptibility to disease, etc.), there may be a set of identifiable behavioral traits that cross-culturally influence successful human aging.

In a 1945 compendium, the American anthropologist George Murdock (1945) outlined 67 characteristics, or cultural *universals*, found across all human societies: family, religion, rites of passage, marriage, and so on. Since then, behavioral and psychological universals also have been explored and debated across disciplines, in anthropology, sociology, and psychology, for instance (Norenzayan and Heine, 2005). The search for behavioral universals specific to the aged, however, has a relatively short history.

The long-accepted perception that behavior, activity levels, and social interactions change with increasing age stimulated interest in aging and resulted in the advent of human gerontology as a discipline in the 1940s. Several theories of universal behavioral or psychosocial aging have since been proposed to explain perceived aged behavior. Of these, the following are of particular interest: The first formal theory proposed to explain the process of growing older was the Theory of Social Disengagement proposed by Cumming and Henry (1961). Social disengagement argues that, with increasing age, mutual withdrawal between the individual and society is a natural, inevitable phenomenon that finally culminates in death. Activity Theory of psychosocial aging argues that, if individuals are to age successfully, they must maintain their ongoing roles and activities into their later years

(Lemon *et al.*, 1972). Similarly, Continuity Theory states that successful aged adults use strategies that maintain their individual activity and interaction patterns into old age. In this view, successful adults react to the physical restrictions of aging in an adaptive way (Neugarten *et al.*, 1968). Finally, in the Selective Theory of Aging, Carstensen (1987) and Carstensen *et al.* (2003) describe the process of aging as including a selective pruning of social relationships in later years, and the retention of only the most important relationships. Of these proposed theories, both disengagement and activity theories find no consistent empirical support, but continuity and selectivity theories do enjoy some empirical support.

The most recent theoretical contribution to an understanding of aging as adaptation comes from Ronald Lee (2003). Lee counters the argument that the force of natural selection against aging is too weak to be effective in postreproductive individuals, and reemphasizes the selective importance of behavioral contributions an elder makes to the survival of future generations. Lee argues that this view offers a fresh look at the forces favoring longevity.

The Nonhuman Primate (NHP) Model of Aging

The use of nonhuman primates as a model for the mechanisms of biological aging is well known (Corr, 2000). Crews (2003) correctly notes that, because of the shared evolutionary history of human and nonhuman primates, greater insight into the complex processes of aging and senescence can be gained through comparisons of phylogenetically similar organisms that have the most parallels to aging humans. Both human and nonhuman primates experience similar morphological and physiological decline with increasing age, including chronic degenerative conditions and an increased risk of disease, making nonhuman primates invaluable as a model of human aging (Crews and Garruto, 1994). Investigations of the associations of age with social behavior in nonhuman primates, however, have not proven as informative.

Primatologists have tested most of the proposed gerontological theories of human social or behavioral aging across various species of nonhuman primates. Primate gerontology, however, is a relatively new field that is based on very few studies, many of which present conflicting evidence (Corr, 2002). In tests of the social disengagement theory, for instance, Pavelka (1991), using Japanese macaques (*Macaca fuscata*), found no support for social disengagement in older monkeys, but Nakamichi (1984), also working with Japanese macaques, found the opposite and reported evidence that sociality did decrease with increasing age. Additionally, Corr (2000), in a comparison between rhesus macaque (*Macaca mulatta*) age groups, reported finding decreased sociality of aged rhesus macaque females, but increased levels of sociality in aged rhesus males in the same population. Moreover, two studies focusing on social behavior in aging lemurs (Picq, 1992; Taylor, 1998) also reported conflicting levels of social withdrawal. In apes, Bloomsmith *et al.* (2000) reported that their observations of Yerkes chimpanzees and gorillas showed significant behavioral differences in some categories between younger and older animals, but no significant differences between age groups in rates of social behavior.

Clearly, the search for aged behavioral universals in primates has not provided consistent insights into the social behavior of aged individuals. One reason may be that the relationship between social behavior and physical aging is greatly impacted by a number of factors, both cultural and ecological. All primates, human and nonhuman, become aged within a complex network of varying environments and social structures. If we are to clarify and broaden our understanding of becoming old, these variations must be fully considered. Such a broadened horizon, for instance, could explain the differences found in aged sociality between the described two, free-ranging populations of Japanese macaques living in different environments: one in mountainous Japan and one in the desert of Texas. Also, considerations of species-specific sex-based roles and life histories could explain why males and females of the same rhesus population would differ in their social behavior with increasing age as each sex lives very different lives. Primate aging occurs within a multiplicity of factors: basic biology, species-level behavioral repertoires, varying adaptations to environmental pressures, widely varying social structures, and so on. One of the hallmarks of the Order Primates is plasticity of behavior and diet, which allows primates to adjust and adapt to varying environmental pressures. It would seem, therefore, that consideration of individual and population-level differences in aging must be investigated within that context.

Although nonhuman primates make an excellent biological model for human aging, there are several important impediments to their use in aging research that should be noted. First, nonhuman primates do not have a comparable life span to humans, preventing direct comparison. Second, due to predation pressures and lack of long-term field studies that follow identified individuals over the life span, known aged primates are rare in wild populations. Third, though established colonies offer higher numbers of aged primates, they are semi-free ranging, provisioned populations, which could confound results. Finally, the use of aged nonhuman primates under laboratory conditions has become increasingly difficult due to the lack of elders that have known histories and that are not compromised from participation in past projects. Moreover, funding limitations and ethical considerations place additional limitations on the scope of aging research. Still, the use of nonhuman primates as a human aging model is predicted to increase, particularly in rhesus monkeys (Roth *et al.*, 2004).

Limitations, Benefits, and Methods in Testing Individual Differences

As discussed earlier, the results of behavioral studies of aging in nonhuman primates suggest that establishing a universal description of the aging process may be difficult using cross-sectional research designs. One complication of this type of research is that there are often large individual differences between individuals within the same age group (Tarou *et al.*, 2002). For example, in a study of aging chimpanzees at the Yerkes Primate Research Center, one 43-year-old chimpanzee showed severe signs of senescence, spending large amounts of time inactive, likely as the result of arthritis and glaucoma, whereas another chimpanzee of the same age, living in the same environment, spent more time engaged in active behavior and appeared to be unaffected by senescent changes (Tarou, unpublished data). These individual differences could be the result of heritable or environmental differences in disease susceptibility and transmission. However, they could also indicate individual behavioral traits that are consistent across the life span.

In humans, individual differences that are relatively stable across the life span of an individual are referred to as personality traits. In nonhuman primates, Suomi *et al.* (1996) found consistent individual differences in rhesus monkeys that could be described as personality across the life span. There were common age-related changes in 10 of 31 measured behaviors within individuals; however, across individuals, there were large individual differences. These results are similar to the stability and change in personality with age found in adult humans (Pedersen and Reynolds, 1998). Given such commonalities in aging research across divergent species, it is likely that the underlying mechanism may represent common evolutionary history.

The quantitative measurement of human personality traits began in the 1940s by distilling and categorizing all descriptive English words that seemed to cluster and that could be associated with a specific personality trait. Using factor analysis, descriptors were then established that could be used to identify and measure self-reported behavioral traits in the individual. Since then, further work has resulted in the reduction of the original factors into what are now known as the *Big Five*: extroversion, neuroticism, agreeableness, conscientiousness, and openness to experience. They are described as follows (www.psychcentral.com):

- Extroversion: a tendency to seek stimulation and the company of others
- Neuroticism: a tendency to easily experience unpleasant emotions
- Agreeableness: a tendency to be compassionate rather than antagonistic
- Conscientiousness: a tendency to show self-discipline, act dutifully, achieve
- Openness to experience: a tendency to enjoy art and new intellectual ideas

Having an optimistic or positive attitude has been found to be strongly associated with longevity in humans. As part of the Nun Study, the autobiographies of 180 Catholic nuns were read and analyzed on the basis of the level of positive emotional content contained in their writings (Danner *et al.*, 2001). Results showed that the emotional content of work written early in life predicted longevity 60 years later such that those sisters who wrote fewer sentences and words containing positive emotion also had a higher risk of earlier mortality than those who wrote more positively about their lives. Optimism is believed to facilitate subjective well-being (happiness) and good health (Wrosch and Scheier, 2003). Happiness has been strongly linked with the Big Five personality factors (Schmutte and Ryff, 1997), particularly extroversion and neuroticism. Specifically, neuroticism correlates negatively and extroversion correlates positively with subjective reports of well-being in humans (Sackett, 1991).

Several personality traits also have been linked to physical disease and longevity in humans. Specifically, hostility and neuroticism have been found to be negatively associated with coronary heart disease and longevity, whereas optimism has a positive influence on longevity (Smith and Spiro, 2002). These personality traits are presumed to affect not only risk, but the reporting of symptoms of illness and illness behavior (Feldman *et al.*, 1999). According to a review of the literature on personality, health, and aging (Smith and Spiro, 2002), one of the causal ways that personality can influence disease is through an individual's response to stress. For example, an individual who scores high on a measure of hostility reacts to stressful situations with larger increases in blood pressure, heart rate, and stress-related hormones. Furthermore, these increases do not return to baseline levels in such an individual as quickly as they do for people who score high on agreeableness, thereby affecting recovery. Hostility is negatively associated with agreeableness and positively associated with neuroticism. The personality trait neuroticism is associated with depression and anxiety, which, in turn, are associated with an increased risk of heart disease, stroke, cancer, reduced immune functioning, recurrence of disease, and reduced longevity. It is believed that an optimistic personality allows people to more readily adapt to change and cope better with stress.

Interest in the study of animal personality has increased dramatically in the last 15 years (Gosling, 2001). Once considered anthropomorphic and taboo, the systematic study of individual differences among members of the same species is being recognized as important both from evolutionary and ontological points of view. Most studies designed to investigate animal personality involve having zookeepers or animal caretakers who are highly familiar with the animals fill out questionnaires similar to those used in human studies of personality (Itoh, 2002). Individual animals are rated on several adjectives or descriptions using a scaling system. Data then are analyzed using either principal component or factor analysis to determine which of the adjectives load positively or negatively with each other. Though personality factors that have emerged in animal studies often are labeled differently across studies, a recent review of the literature found that distinct personality factors have been reliably described in a variety of species (Gosling and John, 1999). A neurotic animal, for example, would be one that engages in abnormal or stereotypic behavior and is highly reactive in novel situations or environments. Additionally, extroversion and neuroticism have been found to be reliable factors for describing the personality of individual chimpanzees, gorillas, rhesus monkeys, dogs, cats, pigs, donkeys, guppies, and octopuses (Gosling and John, 1999).

Some traits have not been found across all species tested, which could be due to differences in methodology. For example, agreeableness is a factor that appears to be shared by humans, some species of nonhuman primates, and other mammals (Gosling and John, 1999). A person scoring high on the factor agreeableness can be described as trusting, sympathetic, helpful, softhearted, good-natured, flexible, cheerful, lenient, and forgiving (McCrae and Costa, 1987). Though many of these terms are not readily applicable to (nonhuman) animals, those individuals considered high in agreeableness show lower levels of aggression and hostility toward others. In both animals and humans, openness can best be described as the curiosity level of the individual. Openness in humans refers to creativity, curiosity, independence, and complexity (McCrae and Costa, 1987). Openness was found to be a personality factor in 7 of 12 species of animals examined (Gosling and John, 1999).

Of the species tested, chimpanzee personality seems to be the most similar to humans. The fifth personality factor in the Big Five is conscientiousness, and has been found only in humans and chimpanzees. Conscientiousness in humans is described by adjectives such as dependability, dutifulness, order or neatness, and self-discipline, all of which are difficult to attribute to nonhuman species. Chimpanzee conscientiousness is best described by adjectives describing a lack of behavior that is erratic, unpredictable, and disorganized (King and Figueredo, 1997). In chimpanzees, the five personality factors have been found to be heritable and to be relatively independent of differences in housing environment, which are also findings similar to studies of personality in humans (Weiss *et al.*, 2000).

Of the Big Five, not all studies have found that optimism or cheerfulness is necessarily good for health and aging. Interestingly, one study has found that cheerfulness in children may be inversely related to longevity and that conscientiousness is a stronger predictor of long-term survival (Friedman *et al.*, 1993). Conscientiousness can be described by the level of control or lack of impulsivity that an individual possesses. Conscientiousness could influence longevity through self-protective behaviors such as the maintenance of good eating habits, avoidance of dangerous situations, and adherence to health regimens. However, a follow-up study showed that conscientiousness was not a reliable predictor of cause of death (Friedman *et al.*, 1995). Although conscientiousness did predict rates of variables such as smoking and drinking, which are related to health and mortality, these variables accounted for little variance in the relationship between conscientiousness and longevity. Friedman and colleagues (1995) hypothesize that this relationship may be the result of an underlying psychobiological process that is associated with both conscientiousness and long life. However, they suggest that a more likely explanation for the results is that conscientiousness allows a person to better cope with stress and maintain social relationships. As stated previously, chimpanzees are the only nonhuman species studied to date for which a personality trait that is analogous to conscientiousness in humans has been described (Gosling and John, 1999). The term used to describe this personality trait in chimpanzees is dependability (King and Figueredo, 1997; Weiss *et al.*, 2000).

Given the association between physiology and personality in humans, an animal model of personality, aging, and longevity may not only be appropriate, but also pragmatic. Disease susceptibility and recovery in humans often is confounded by a variety of social, cognitive, and environmental factors. Identifying stable personality traits in nonhuman primates, measuring them, and correlating them with risk of disease, recovery, and survival, could provide insight into human successful aging. There appears to be great consistency with regard to major personality descriptors in nonhuman primates despite differences in raters, species, and how the traits are labeled (Gosling, 2001; Gosling and John, 1999), indicating that these consistencies in personality traits may represent homologous traits passed down through evolutionary history. Furthermore, similar to human personality traits, these traits are consistent in individuals over time (Capitanio, 1999; Suomi, *et al.*, 1996).

Personality and the NHP Model

Many of the methods and constructs used to measure human well-being are not directly applicable to nonhuman primates. However, psychological well-being is a topic that has become of great concern for the ethical care of captive nonhuman primates. In captive populations, animals are said to have psychological well-being when they show few physiological and behavioral signs of stress

(Moberg, 1985). Recently, this also has been found to be an indicator, or by-product, of psychological well-being in humans in that higher levels of psychological well-being have also been associated with lower levels of cortisol release (Lindfors and Lundberg, 2002). Environmental enrichment is often used to alleviate stress and promote psychological well-being in captive nonhuman primates. This is particularly important as stress has been clearly associated with a variety of undesirable physiological effects, mostly as the result of compromised immune system functioning (Kelly, 1985; Shapiro *et al.*, 1998).

Typically, psychological well-being in nonhuman primates is measured through behavioral observations and/or hormonal analyses. However, at least one recent study has shown that well-being or "happiness" can be reliably estimated by human raters who are familiar with the individual (King and Landau, 2003). In these studies, zookeepers or researchers with extensive experience working with or observing individual chimpanzees were asked to rank them on overall mood, quality of social relationships, extent to which they were successful in achieving goals, and how much they would like to "be" a particular chimpanzee. Results showed that reliability across raters was as consistent as have been found in human studies of subjective well-being. Furthermore, this construct appears to be heritable and generically correlated with dominance (Weiss, King, and Enns, 2002). There was a strong correlation between personality and subjective well-being in chimpanzees, and many aspects of well-being in chimpanzees are surprisingly similar to those observed in humans (King and Landau, 2003).

There are, however, methodological issues associated with personality testing in nonhuman primates (Itoh, 2002). Personality in animals is often measured using subjective assessment methods such as questionnaires, which may have problems with construct validity. Most principal component analyses have not been tested for reliability across research groups. As deWaal (2002) has cautioned, subjective human ratings of animal personality traits may reflect anthropomorphic projections of human traits onto animal behavior. For a complete understanding of both the physiological and behavioral changes associated with aging, objective tests in which behaviors are systematically recorded coupled with subjective assessments from animal care providers may be the most useful methodological approach.

New Directions in Aging Research

Investigations into the role of individual differences in behavior, or personality, in the aged are largely the result of a paradigm shift away from old age as an independent category of life, to a focus on old age as part of a lifelong developmental continuum. Diener and Suh (1997) showed that, although there is an unavoidable, universal physical decline and loss of function with increasing age, an individual's personal sense of feeling "happy and well" can increase concurrently with physiological decline or disability. Specifically, two recently proposed theoretical views of aging, Selection, Optimization, and Compensation Theory (SOC) and Socio-emotional Selectivity Theory (SST), are redirecting social aging research by considering growth and decline as a process that impacts all age categories. In SOC, Baltes and Baltes (1998) use the interaction of three universal regulatory processes to define adaptive development, or successful aging: an individual's selection from available options, optimal use and acquisition of resources, and ability to compensate to adjust for physical or resource loss. In this view, by setting goals and working toward them through appropriate resource use and compensation for loss, an individual's sense of positive well-being can be maintained throughout both adulthood and old age. Lockenhoff and Carstensen (2004), in describing SST, add that the knowledge a successful individual has of coming toward the end of life and of having limited time may serve as a motivator in their determination to achieve well-being and emotional meaning in old age. Both researchers agree that a theoretical shift toward life history thinking and a focus on individual differences in goals and preferences should guide future aging research.

Currently, comparative, transcultural studies of human aging are being conducted that offer a global perspective on human aging and reveal "a wondrous array of social responses to the physical imperatives of growing old" (Sokolovsky, 1997). Sokolovsky (1997) describes this growing, multidisciplinary trend as "qualitative gerontology," and being comprised of investigations from widely divergent fields (anthropology, biology, psychology, demography, medicine, etc.). Also, as the information age continues to globalize access to resources, those that focus specifically on aging are helping to unify research designs, including cross-discipline collaborations, new professional organizations, journals, other print resources, web-linked sites, academic gerontology programs, and so on. In addition to the described qualitative movement, there is also an important effort being made by investigators to achieve consistency in research methods used in quantitative cross-cultural studies of human aging. Such consistency of methods is imperative if we are to maximize the usefulness of these comparative studies and tease out the meaningful differences, similarities, individual variations, and even universals of human aging within a variety of social contexts.

In an example of an inclusive aging research design, considering both biology and behavior, the investigation of the molecular biology of social behavior is another emerging field that is certain to contribute a great deal to our understanding of aging. This area of interest looks at neural, molecular, and endocrine mechanisms that influence behavior in social species. Additionally, new programs of advanced study in the area of interface between biology, ecology, and behavior are rapidly being established in American universities. These programs will address cross-species behaviors such as predation, violence, addictions, and so forth from both biological and behavioral perspectives. Such a focus requires an interdisciplinary approach that will cut across the traditional structure of university departments.

Finally, a new and unique opportunity to extend the use of nonhuman primates as a model for behavioral aging is provided by the recent establishment of sanctuaries designed to accommodate retired chimpanzees (*Pan troglydytes*). In 2000, the CHIMP Act (Chimpanzee Health Improvement, Maintenance, and Protection Act) was signed into law and implemented the chimpanzee sanctuary system in the United States. The first of these, Chimp Haven, Inc. in Shreveport, Louisiana, is now receiving chimpanzees, many of which are aged. Each of these individual animals has given its life to biomedical research, the entertainment industry, or has lived as a pet. Now, instead of being euthanised or languishing away singly caged in a lab for years, more than 600 individuals will have a permanent home where they will live out their lives in an enriched, social environment appropriate for chimpanzees. Such sanctuaries, in addition to paying an ethical debt to our phylogenetically closest relatives, provide a unique opportunity for behavioral studies of all kinds, including investigations of individual personality and its impact on aging. Additionally, use of personality assessment in nonhuman primates, already shown to be a helpful management tool in chimpanzees (Dutton *et al.*, 1996), gorillas (Gold and Maple, 1994), and rhesus monkeys (Capitanio and Widaman, 2005), should prove to be an excellent management tool to guide chimpanzee caretakers in easing an individual's adjustment into the sanctuary, and also in the formation of successful social groups. Since nonhuman primate traits, particularly those of the chimpanzee, evolutionarily underlie human traits, a greater understanding of individual behavioral differences among them, particularly with regard to social behavior and aging, cannot help but inform our own experience of being old. We look forward to the coming new wave of aging research and to all the benefits it will provide.

REFERENCES

Baltes, P.B. and Baltes, M. (1990). *Successful Aging: Perspectives from the Behavioral Sciences*. Cambridge: University Press.

Baltes, P.B. and Baltes, M. (1998). Harvesting the fruits of age: Growing older, growing wise. *National Forum: The Phi Kappa Phi Journal 78(2)*.

Bloomsmith, M.A., Tarou, L.R., Hoff, M.P., and Erwin, J. (2000). Comparing the behavior of aged gorillas and chimpanzees. *Great Ape Conference: Challenges for the 21st Century*. Chicago: Brookfield Zoo.

Capitanio, J.P. and Widaman, K.F. (2005). Confirmatory factor analysis of personality structure in adult male rhesus monkeys (*Macaca mulatta*). *AJP 65(3)*, 289–294.

Capitanio, J.P. (1999). Personality dimensions in adult male rhesus macaques: Prediction of behaviors across time and situation. *American Journal of Primatology 47*, 299–320.

Carstensen, L. (1987). Age related changes in social activity. In L. Carstensen and Edelson, Eds. *Handbook of Clinical Gerontology*. New York: Pergamon Press.

Carstensen, L., Fung, H., and Charles, S. (2003). Socioemotional selectivity theory and the regulation of emotion in the second half of life. *Motivation and Emotion*, pp. 103–123. Springer Publications.

Corr, J. (2004). Nuns and monkeys: Investigating the behavior of our oldest old. *Sci. Aging Know. Environ.* 41. Published online, 13 October 2004.

Corr, J., Martin, L., and Boysen, S. (2002). Comparative models of cognitive decline in aging great apes. In J.M. Erwin and P.R. Hof, Eds. *Aging in Nonhuman Primates: Interdisciplinary Topics in Gerontology, 32*, 196–208. Basel, Switzerland: Karger.

Corr, J. (2000). The effects of aging of social behavior in male and female rhesus macaques of Cayo Santiago. Ph.D. dissertation: The Ohio State University.

Crews, D. (2003). *Human Senescence: Evolutionary and Biocultural Perspectives*. Cambridge: University Press.

Crews, D.E. and Garruto, R.M., Eds. (1994). *Biological Anthropology and Aging: Perspectives on Human Variation over the Life Span*. Oxford: Univ. Press.

Cumming, E. and Henry, W. (1961). *Growing Old*. New York: Basic Books.

Danner, D.D., Snowdon, D.A., and Friesen, W.V. (2001). Positive emotions in early life and longevity: Findings from the Nun Study. *Personality Processes and Individual Differences 80*, 804–813.

de Waal, F. (2002). Social roles, alternative strategies, personalities, and other sources of individual variation in monkeys and apes. *Journal of Research in Personality 36*, 541–542.

Diener, E. and Suh, E. (1997). Measuring quality of life: Economic, social, and subjective indicators. *Social Indicators Research 40*, 189–216. Springer Science Publishers.

Dutton, D.M., Clark, R.A., and Dickins, D.W. (1997). Personality in captive chimpanzees: use of a novel rating procedure. *IJP 18(4)*, 539–552.

Feldman, P.J., Cohen, S., Doyle, W.J., Skoner, D.P., and Gwaltney, J.M. Jr. (1999). The impact of personality on the reporting of unfounded symptoms and illness. *Journal of Personality and Social Psychology 77*, 370–378.

Friedman, H.S., Tucker, J., Schwartz, J.E., Martin, L.R., Tomlinson-Keasey, C., Wingard, D.L. *et al.* (1995). Childhood conscientiousness and longevity: Health behaviors and cause of death. *Journal of Personality and Social Psychology 68*, 696–703.

Friedman, H.S., Tucker, J.S., Tomlinson-Keasey, C., Schwartz, J.E., Wingard, D.L., and Criqui, M.H. (1993). Does childhood personality predict longevity? *Journal of Personality and Social Psychology 65*, 176–185.

Gavrilov, L. and Gavrilova, N. (2002). Evolutionary theories of aging and longevity. *The Scientific World Journal 2*, 339–356.

Gold, K.C. and Maple, T.L. (1994). Personality assessment in the gorilla and its utility as a management tool. *Zoo Biology 13*, 509–522.

Gosling, S.D. (2001). From mice to men: What can we learn about personality from animal research? *Psychological Bulletin 127*, 45–86.

Gosling, S.D. and John, O.P. (1999). Personality dimensions in nonhuman animals: A cross-species review. *Current Directions in Psychological Science 8*, 69–75.

Itoh, K. (2002). Personality research with non-human primates: Theoretical formulation and methods. *Primates 43*, 249–261.

Kelley, K.W. (1985). Immunological consequences of changing environmental stimuli. In G.P. Moberg, Ed. *Animal Stress*, pp. 193–224. Bethesda, MD: American Physiological Society.

King, J.E. and Figueredo, A.J. (1997). The five-factor model plus dominance in chimpanzee personality. *Journal of Research in Personality 31*, 257–271.

King, J.E. and Landau, V.I. (2003). Can chimpanzee (*Pan troglodytes*) happiness be estimated by human raters? *Journal of Research in Personality 37*, 1–15.

Lee, R.D. (2003). Rethinking the evolutionary theory of aging: Transfers, not births, shape senescence in social species. *Proc. Natl. Acad. Sci. USA. 100(16)*, 9637–9642.

Lemon, B., Bengston, V., and Peterson, J. (1972). An exploration of the activity theory of aging: Activity types and life satisfaction among in-movers to a retirement community. *Journal of Gerontology 27*, 511–523.

Lindfors, P. and Lundberg, U. (2002). Is low cortisol release an indicator of positive health? *Stress and Health: Journal of the International Society for the Investigation of Stress 18*, 153–160.

Lockenhoff, C. E. and Carstensen, L.L. (2004). Socioemotional selectivity theory, aging, and health: The increasingly delicate balance between regulating emotions and making tough choices. *J Pers. 72(6)*, 1395–1424.

McCrae, R.R. and Costa, P.T. (1987). Validation of the five-factor model of personality across instruments and observers. *Journal of Personality and Social Psychology 52*, 81–90.

Medawar, P.B. (1946). Old age and natural death. *Mod. Quart. (1)*, 30–56.

Moberg, G.P. (1985). Biological response to stress. In G.P. Moberg, Ed. *Animal Stress*, pp. 27–50. Bethesda, MD: American Physiological Society.

Murdock, G.P. (1945). The common denominator of culture. In R. Linton, Ed. *The Science of Man in the World Crisis*, pp. 123. New York: Columbia Univ. Press.

Nakamichi, M. (1984). Behavioral characteristics of old female Japanese monkeys in a free-ranging group. *Primates 25(1)*, 192–201.

Neugarten, B. (1968). Personality and patterns of aging. In B. Neugarten, Ed. *Middle Age and Aging: A Reader in Social Psychology*. Chicago: Univ. Press.

Norenzayan, A. and Heine, S.J. (2005, in press). Psychological universals: What are they and how can we know? *Psychological Bulletin.*

Pavelka, M. (1991). Sociability in old female Japanese monkeys: Human versus nonhuman primate aging. *American Anthropologist 93*, 588–598.

Pedersen, N.L. and Reynolds, C.A. (1998). Stability and change in adult personality: Genetic and environmental components. *European Journal of Personality 12*, 365–386.

Picq, Jean-Luc. (1992). Aging and social behavior in captivity in *Microcebus murinus*. *Folia Primatologica 59*, 217–220.

Roth, G., Mattison, M., Ottinger, M., Chachich, M., Lane, M., and Ingram, D. (2004). Aging in rhesus monkeys: Relevance to human health interventions. *Science 305*, 1423–1426.

Rowe, J.W. and Kahn, R.L. (1998). *Successful Aging: The MacArthur Foundation Study*. New York: Pantheon Press.

Sackett, G. (1991). The human model of psychological well-being in primates. In M. Novak and A. Petto, Eds. *Through the Looking Glass: Issues of Psychological Well-being in Primates*, pp. 35–42. Washington, D.C.: American Psychological Association.

Schmutte, P.S. and Ryff, C. D. (1997). Personality and well-being: Reexamining methods and meanings. *Personality Processes and Individual Differences 73*, 549–559.

Shapiro, S.J., Nehete, P.N., Perlman, J.E., Bloomsmith, M.A., and Sastry, K.R. (1998). Effects of dominance status and environmental enrichment on cell mediated immunity in rhesus monkeys. *Applied Animal Behavior Science 56*, 319–332.

Smith, T.W. and Spiro, A. III (2002). Personality, health, and aging: Prolegomenon for the next generation. *Journal of Research in Personality 36*, 363–394.

Snowdon, D. (2001). *Aging with grace: What the Nun Study Tells Us about Leading Longer, Healthier, and More Meaningful Lives*. New York: Bantam Books.

Sokolowsky, J., Ed. (1997). *The Cultural Context of Aging: Worldwide Perspectives*, 2e, pp. xi–xxxi. London: Bergin and Garvey.

Suomi, S.J., Novak, M.A., and Well, A. (1996). Aging in rhesus monkeys: Different windows on behavioral continuity and change. *Developmental Psychology 32*, 1116–1128.

Suzuki, M. (2005). Dolls give Japanese elders a new lease on life. *Antara News*, February 23.

Tarou, L.R., Bloomsmith, M.A., Hoff, M.P., Erwin, J.M., and Maple, T.L. (2002). The behavior of aged great apes. In J.M. Erwin and P.R. Hof, Eds. *Aging in Nonhuman Primates: Interdisciplinary Topics in Gerontology*, *32*, 209–231. Basel, Switzerland: Karger.

Taylor, L. (1998). Behavior and reproduction in aged lemurs. *American Journal of Primatology. Supplement 26*, 217.

U.S. Census Bureau. www.census.gov.

Valliant, G. (2002). *Aging Well: Surprising Guideposts to a Happier Life from the Landmark Harvard Study of Adult Development*. Boston: Little, Brown.

Weismann, A. (1889). *Essays upon Heredity and Kindred Biological Problems*. Oxford: Clarendon Press.

Weiss, A., King, J.E., and Enns, R.M. (2002). Subjective well-being is heritable and genetically correlated with dominance in chimpanzees (*Pan troglodytes*). *Personality Processes and Individual Differences 83*, 1141–1149.

Weiss, A., King, J.E., and Figueredo, A.J. (2000). The heritability of personality factors in chimpanzees (*Pan troglodytes*). *Behavior Genetics 30*, 213–221.

Williams, G.C. (1957). Pleiotropy, natural selection, and the evolution of senescence. *Evolution 11*, 398–411.

Wrosch, C. and Scheier, M.F. (2003). Personality and quality of life: The importance of optimism and goal-adjustment. *Quality of Life Research: An International Journal of Quality of Life Aspects of Treatment, Care and Rehabilitation 12*, 59–72.

www.psychcentral.com.

www.chimphaven.org (video).

63

Andropause

Rabih Hijazi and Glenn R. Cunningham

This chapter seeks to provide you with an overview of the potential effects of testosterone (T) deficiency in aging men. Although we acknowledge the age-related reduction in serum levels of the adrenal androgens, dehydroepiandrosterone (DHEA) and dehydroepiandrosterone sulfate (DHEA-S), the chapter focuses on the much more potent testicular androgen, T and its metabolites, dihydrotestosterone (DHT) and estradiol (E_2). Many of the symptoms and signs of aging and testosterone deficiency are shared. Although investigators frequently administer T to aging men in an effort to differentiate symptoms and signs related to aging from those caused by T deficiency, a large definitive study assessing efficacy and risk is lacking. Thus, we seek to provide you with our current understanding of the effects of T deficiency in aging men, using insights from small, nondefinitive clinical trials.

Introduction

Symptoms of T deficiency are similar to many of those associated with aging. They include loss of stamina, depressed mood, decreased libido, erectile dysfunction, decreased muscle mass and strength, increased fat mass, frailty, osteopenia, and osteoporosis. It may be difficult to distinguish the changes that are age-related from those that are caused by T deficiency.

T and Aging

T LEVELS AND AGING

Multiple cross-sectional and a few longitudinal studies have shown that serum T levels in men decrease with age (Deslypere *et al.*, 1984; Harman *et al.*, 2001; Morley *et al.*, 2000). Age-related changes in total T underestimate changes in T available to target tissues. Several cross-sectional studies have shown that an increase of sex hormone binding globulin (SHBG) with aging and a decrease in T and free T (fT) levels are independent of changes in body mass index (Deslypere *et al.*, 1984; Morley *et al.*, 2000). Approximately 40 to 50% of circulating T in men is bound with high affinity to SHBG. This portion of the circulating total T is not readily available to target tissues, whereas T bound to albumin and fT (1–3%) are available to target tissues (Pardridge 1981). The albumin bound and the fT are referred to as the bioavailable or weakly bound T (bT). Thus, serum concentrations of T and, to a greater extent, fT and bT, are decreased in aging men.

Serum SHBG levels are affected by several conditions. SHBG levels are inversely correlated with increased total body fat, subcutaneous and visceral adiposity (Couillard *et al.*, 2000). Levels also vary inversely with hyperinsulinism in nondiabetic subjects. They seem to be an indicator of general adiposity rather than an index of altered insulin/glucose homeostasis in morbidly obese subjects. Hyperinsulinism decreases SHBG synthesis by cultured hepatic cells. These observations have been interpreted to show that obesity causes insulin resistance and hyperinsulinism, and hyperinsulinism decreases SHBG levels. Hypothyroidism and the nephrotic syndrome also reduce SHBG levels. Estrogen, hyperthyroidism, some anticonvulsants, a high phytoestrogen diet, hepatic cirrhosis, and aging increase SHBG levels (Anderson, 1974; Kley *et al.*, 1975).

We recently reported that SHBG levels are increased in some patients with cancer, and the elevated SHBG may maintain total T levels within the normal range even though the calculated fT and bT levels are low. Thus, SHBG levels are variable in older, obese men, and this limits the value of total T levels in this age group.

Approximately 20% of men 60 to 70 years of age and 30% of men 70 to 80 years of age have T levels below that of 97.5% of healthy 20- to 45-year-old men (Harman *et al.*, 2001). Longitudinal studies have confirmed these findings (Feldman *et al.*, 2000; Harman *et al.*, 2001; Morley *et al.*, 1997). Feldman and coworkers found total T levels decreased at 0.8% per year, bT fell at 2% per year, and SHBG levels increased 1.6% per year (Feldman *et al.*, 2000). This is due in part to a reduction in the number of Leydig cells in the testes that produce T.

The decline in T levels with aging when associated with symptoms and signs of androgen deficiency has been called *andropause*. This association also has been referred to as androgen deficiency in the aging male (ADAM), partial androgen deficiency in the aging male (PADAM), aging-associated androgen deficiency (AAAD) or late-onset hypogonadism. The term *andropause* is inaccurate because men do not have menses and because androgen secretion gradually decreases, and usually is

TABLE 63.1
Organ systems affected by testosterone deficiency

Central Nervous System
Bone
Skeletal Muscle
Adipose Tissue
External Genitalia
Testes
Prostate and Accessory Sexual Organs
Cardiovascular System
Bone Marrow
Liver
Immune System

continued at some, albeit reduced, level when compared with younger, healthy men. However, andropause is widely used by the lay press and laypersons as well as clinicians.

LH LEVELS AND AGING

LH levels increase slightly with aging (Baker *et al.*, 1976; Morley *et al.*, 1997). Tenover and coworkers studied older men and noted that pituitary secretion of LH was intact, but testicular secretion of T was impaired in some older men (Tenover *et al.*, 1987). They noted that the normal diurnal variation in T levels is blunted in aging men (Tenover *et al.*, 1988). However, the majority of hypogonadal men over age 60 have low or inappropriately normal LH levels (Korenman *et al.*, 1990). Older men with low T levels typically have abnormal LH pulse frequency and reduced pulse amplitude, suggesting hypothalamic dysfunction (Deslypere *et al.*, 1987). Less pulsatile T and more LH were secreted in healthy middle-aged men at night compared to healthy young men. The association between T rhythm and REM sleep also was disrupted. Most investigators have concluded that the decline in T observed with aging results from combined testicular and hypothalamic abnormalities.

ANDROGEN ACTION AND METABOLISM OF T

Androgen action appears to be mostly maintained with aging, but this has not been studied extensively. Androgen binding sites in the hippocampus, penile tissues, and genital skin are decreased in aging men and animals (Roehrborn *et al.*, 1987; Tohgi *et al.*, 1995). It is recognized that shortening of the CAG repeat in the androgen receptor increases androgen action, but it is not likely that this, per se, changes with aging (Lamb *et al.*, 2001). It will be important to determine if there are age-related changes in coactivators and corepressors that are important in mediating androgen action at the cellular level.

T is metabolized to dihydrotestosterone (DHT) and to estradiol (E_2) in tissues that have 5α-reductase activity and/or aromatase activity. DHT is a very potent androgen at the tissue level. It contributes most of the androgenic effects in genital tissues, accessory sex organs, and hair follicles. Five-alpha-reductase activity also is present in some areas of the brain and in bone (Russell *et al.*, 1994). Aromatase activity is primarily present in adipose tissue, so most of the circulating estradiol and estrone in males comes from peripheral conversion of T and androstenedione (Simpson *et al.*, 1997). T production rates in young adult males range between 4 and 10 mg/24 hours with an average of 6.6 mg/24 hours (Vermeulen, 1976). In men over age 65, the mean production rate decreases to approximately 4 mg/24 hours. Plasma levels of T reflect an age-related decrease in both secretion and the metabolic clearance rate.

ORGAN SYSTEMS AFFECTED BY LOW T LEVELS

Brain

Cognitive function. Cognitive function decreases with aging. Most of the age-related changes in cognition are associated with vascular and/or degenerative diseases that cause anatomic changes in the central nervous system. The possibility that an age-related fall in T causes functional changes in cognition is of great interest. In a study involving 407 men aged 50 to 91 years at baseline and followed for an average of 10 years, Moffat and colleagues showed that higher free T indices were associated with better scores on visual and verbal memory, visuospatial functioning, and visuomotor scanning, and a reduced rate of decline in visual memory (Moffat *et al.*, 2002). On the other hand, men classified as hypogonadal had significantly lower scores on measures of memory and visuospatial performance and a faster decline in visual memory. Of course, changes in the CNS could cause hypogonadism rather than be caused by hypogonadism. In another study by Barrett-Conner and associates, low estradiol and high total and bioavailable T levels predicted better performance on several tests of cognitive function in older men (Barrett-Connor *et al.*, 1999). T could exert its actions through androgen receptors that could modulate serotonin, dopamine, calcium, and acetylcholine signaling pathways. Androgen also increases neurite arborization facilitating intercellular communication. T can be aromatized in the brain to estrogen, and thus some of the effects of T may be mediated through its conversion to estradiol. Most of the effects of androgen on cognitive function are thought to be domain-specific. For example, observations that men outperform women in a variety of visuospatial skills suggest that androgens might enhance these skills. Some, but not all, of the trials found better verbal memory and spatial cognition in the T-treated men compared with placebo-treated men, but no better scores on other cognitive domains (Cunningham *et al.*, 1990; Janowsky *et al.*, 2000; Kenny *et al.*, 2002).

Mood and depression. It is estimated that two million older Americans are depressed (NIMH, 2003). Depression increases with aging, in part due to diseases associated with aging. Although depression is not a part of the aging process, medical diseases associated with aging such as stroke, diabetes, and heart disease reduce physical activity and contribute to depression. It is estimated that 80% of older adults with depression improve when they receive therapy with an antidepressant medication, psychotherapy, or both (NIMH, 2003). T may have a beneficial effect on mood and depression, as it is known to modulate the serotonin and dopamine pathways.

Androgens appear to improve positive aspects of mood and reduce negative aspects of mood such as irritability in young, hypogonadal men, and some improvements in mood usually are observed in clinical trials involving mostly middle-aged men (Wang *et al.*, 1996).

Libido. T also appears to be essential for development and maintenance of libido or sexual desire. Males with congenital hypogonadotropic hypogonadism have minimal libido. This is increased by therapy that increases their T levels. Reduced libido also is observed in men with acquired hypogonadism, and clinical trials with replacement doses of T in young and middle-aged men usually show improved libido.

Bone

Bone strength decreases with aging. Men undergo a gradual loss in bone mass beginning in their 30s. It is estimated that two million men in the United States have osteoporosis and that one in eight men over age 50 will have an osteoporosis-related fracture (NIAMS, 2003). Risk factors for osteoporosis include family history of osteoporosis, smoking, excessive alcohol intake, physical inactivity, poor nutrition, vitamin D deficiency, inadequate calcium intake, hypogonadism, and use of some medications (e.g., glucocorticoids, anti-convulsants).

Osteopenia and osteoporosis are common in males with congenital causes of hypogonadism, and severe T deficiency occurring later in life also results in bone loss. For example, androgen deprivation therapy for prostate cancer has been shown to result in rapid bone loss, osteopenia, and osteoporosis (Smith, 2003). Although less severe T deficiency in aging men appears to increase osteopenia and osteoporosis, population-based studies suggest that estrogen levels are better correlated with loss of BMD in men (Greendale *et al.*, 1997; van den Beld *et al.*, 2000). Estrogen is very important in bone development in males as illustrated by individuals with aromatase deficiency (Maffei *et al.*, 2004). Males with inactivating mutations of the aromatase gene develop osteopenia and osteoporosis that improve with estradiol therapy. Estrogen also plays a major role in bone metabolism of older males (Khosia *et al.*, 1998).

TABLE 63.2
Potential beneficial and adverse effects of testosterone replacement therapy in aging men.

Positive	Negative
Libido and sexual function	Prostate
Mood	Bone marrow
? Cognitive function	? Cardiovascular system
Skeletal muscle	
Adipose tissue	
Bone	
Bone marrow	
? Cardiovascular system	
? Immune system	

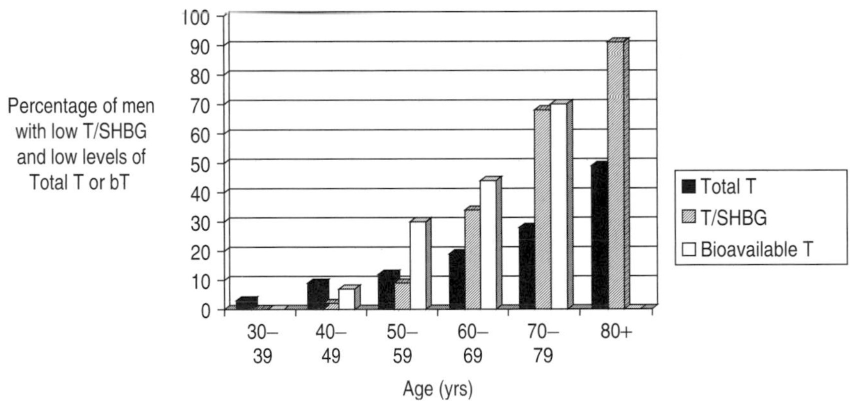

Figure 63.1 Prevalence of hypogonadism based upon low levels of total testosterone, free testosterone index (T/SHBG), and bioavailable testosterone. The black bars represent the percentage of the population with total testosterone levels <325 ng per deciliter, bars with diagonal lines represent the percentage of the population with free T index <0.153 nmol/nmol, and the white bars represent the percentage of the population with bioavailable testosterone levels <70 ng per deciliter. Bioavailable testosterone was not measured in some age groups. (25, 44)

In aging men treated with a GnRH agonist (a model of severe hypogonadism), estrogen treatment decreases markers of bone resorption and increases markers of bone formation. The investigators in these studies have estimated that two-thirds of the effect of testosterone replacement therapy (TRT) is due to an estrogen effect (Khosia *et al.*, 1998). Most of the estrogen in men is derived from the aromatization of T to estradiol and androstenedione to estrone. Estradiol is more potent, but accurate measurement in males is difficult because levels are low and assay sensitivity and accuracy are marginal in many reports. Total E_2 levels also are affected by SHBG levels, so accurate measurement of free estradiol or bioavailable estradiol are most informative.

Males have larger bones and greater bone mass than women, so androgen as well as estrogen is critical for the development of a normal male skeletal mass. T and estrogen also may act directly through receptors in bone cells or indirectly by modulating the action of cytokines or growth factor metabolism. In summary, both androgens and estrogens affect bone metabolism in men, and both may be reduced with aging and hypogonadism.

Muscle

Aging is associated with a decrease in lean body mass and strength, even if total body weight is maintained at a level achieved in the early 20s. It is estimated that skeletal muscle mass decreases 35% between the ages of 20 and 80. This sarcopenia associated with loss of strength leads to impairment of physical function such as impaired ability to rise from a chair, climb stairs, maintain balance, and generate gait speed. This can result in loss of mobility, falls and fractures, loss of independence, and depression (Roubenoff *et al.*, 2000).

The cellular and molecular mechanisms by which androgens affect changes in fat-free mass, muscle mass, and strength are only partially understood. Androgen administration to sexually immature boys increases nitrogen retention. Other studies have observed increased protein synthesis and muscle hypertrophy (Sinha-Hikim *et al.*, 2002). Multiple placebo-controlled trials in both younger and aging men with T deficiency have assessed changes in muscle strength and body composition measures in response to exogenous T. They usually have noted increases in fat-free mass and decreases in fat mass. Some, but not all, have found significant improvements in leg and arm strength (Amory *et al.*, 2004; Snyder *et al.*, 1999; Urban *et al.*, 1995). Bhasin and coworkers clearly demonstrated dose-related increases in skeletal muscle mass in young males (Bhasin *et al.*, 1996). In other studies, the Bhasin group also has demonstrated a dose-dependent increase in muscle mass and strength in younger men made hypogonadal with a GnRH agonist (Sinha-Hakim *et al.*, 2002; Storer *et al.*, 2003). More recent studies have demonstrated that T caused dose-dependent increases in skeletal muscle mass in aging men (Bhasin *et al.*, 2005). The Bhasin group has observed that supraphysiological doses of testosterone increase satellite cell and myonuclear cell number (Sinha-Hakim *et al.*, 2003). They have postulated that in addition to stimulating muscle protein synthesis, decreasing muscle protein degradation, and improving reutilization of amino acids, testosterone promotes the commitment of pluripotent stem cells into the myogenic lineage and inhibits their differentiation into the adipogenic lineage (Bhasin *et al.*, 2003). They suggest that this increases myonuclear number and satellite cell number.

Adipose tissue

Adipose tissue increases with aging, and many aging and obese men meet criteria for the metabolic syndrome. The ATPIII criteria for making the diagnosis of metabolic syndrome require that an individual have at least three of the following: waist circumference >40 inches, serum triglycerides ≥ 150 mg/dL, HDL cholesterol <40 mg/dL, blood pressure $\geq 130/\geq 85$, or fasting glucose ≥ 110 mg/dL. These individuals are at increased risk for developing cardiovascular disease. Obesity decreases SHBG levels and total T levels, and fT levels are decreased with more severe obesity. Obesity and serum leptin, an adipokine, are positively correlated. Endogenous T levels vary inversely with serum leptin levels (Thomas *et al.*, 2000), and testosterone administration suppresses leptin levels. Serum adiponectin (another cytokine) levels correlate inversely with obesity, and TRT reduces adiponectin levels (Lanfranco *et al.*, 2004).

TRT in middle-aged and older men typically causes some reduction in adipose tissue (Mayes *et al.*, 2004). Whether changes in visceral fat are greater than the percent changes in subcutaneous fat is of interest because visceral fat is metabolically more active (Dicker *et al.*, 2004). T can increase lipoprotein lipase, which can increase lipolysis. As noted previously, Bhasin and colleagues postulate that T inhibits differentiation of pluripotent stem cells into adipose cells (Bhasin *et al.*, 2003). Because the studies suggesting this effect were conducted using pharmacological doses of T, it remains to be demonstrated that this is a mechanism for the reduction in adipose tissue noted with physiological replacement doses of T.

External genitalia

T and its metabolite, DHT, are critical for development of the external genitalia. They probably have a direct effect on penile erections. Jain and associates conducted a meta-analysis evaluating the effects of T supplementation on erectile dysfunction (Jain *et al.*, 2000). Some of the men were not hypogonadal, but they found an overall response rate of 57%. TRT affects nocturnal erections and penile rigidity in hypogonadal males (Cunningham *et al.*, 1990). Although erections can be induced in hypogonadal men in response to sexually explicit visual stimuli, TRT improves penile rigidity (Carani *et al.*, 1995). These clinical observations are consistent with findings in lower animal models (Mills *et al.*, 1999). TRT normalizes cavernous nerve-stimulated erections in castrated rats. This effect is reduced by concomitant treatment with a 5α-reductase inhibitor, indicating it is mediated by DHT. T or DHT increased neuronal and endothelial nitric oxide synthase activity, and this is thought to increase nitric oxide, the most potent relaxor of corpora cavernosal smooth muscle. In the rat, neurons responsible for penile vascular smooth muscle relaxation possess both androgen receptors and nitric oxide synthase. In a recent study by Aversa and colleagues, T appears to have a direct vascular effect in the human corpora cavernosa, mediating the ability of nitric oxide to relax corporal tissue and allow increased penile blood flow (Aversa *et al.*, 2003). Combination treatment with a physiological dose of T plus a phosphodiesterase inhibitor may cause greater rigidity than either agent alone in awake and sleep-related erections. The T concentrations needed to maintain normal sexual activity appear to be in the low normal range, or possibly somewhat less than 300 ng/dL in healthy young men.

Testes

Seminiferous tubule function declines with aging. Older men have decreased sperm motility, increased number of abnormal sperm, and lower ejaculate volume. There is a negative correlation between age and sperm production, and this finding does not appear to be caused only by a loss in the number of Leydig cells (Neaves *et al.*, 1984). Serum inhibin levels also are decreased in older men indicating a decline in the hormonal function of the seminiferous tubules (Tenover *et al.*, 1988).

Prostate and accessory sexual organs

The prostate, seminal vesicles, and vas deferens are androgen-dependent tissues, and they also have high levels of 5α reductase activity. Individuals with 5α-reductase type 2 deficiency have rudimentary prostates. The prostate is the sex organ that is most affected by diseases associated with aging.

Prostate cancer. Prostate cancer is the most common nonskin cancer in males. The greatest risk factor is age, with more than 75 percent of new diagnoses occurring in men over 65. The autopsy prevalence of microscopic or occult prostate cancers is rare in men who were in their 40s, but approximately 40 to 50% of men 60 to 70 years of age have occult prostate cancer and 80% by age 80 (Sakr *et al.*, 1994). The prevalence of prostate cancer has been reported for the 2,950 men (age range, 62–91 years) who were assigned to the placebo group in the Prostate Cancer Prevention Trial. Men who never had a PSA level of >4.0 ng/mL or an abnormal digital rectal examination after being in the study for seven years underwent a prostate biopsy (Thompson *et al.*, 2004). Prostate cancer was diagnosed in 15.2% of the men, and 14.9% had a Gleason score of 7 or higher. The prevalence of prostate cancer for men with PSA levels <0.5 ng/mL was 6.6%, 10.1% for values of 0.6 to 1.0 ng/ml; 17% for values of 1.1 to 2.0 ng/mL; 23.9% for values 2.1 to 3.0 ng/mL; and 26.9% for values of 3.1 to 4.0 ng/mL. High-grade cancers (7 or greater) increased from 12.5% with the lowest PSA levels to 25% in the group with PSA of 3.1 to 4.0 ng/mL. Most of the occult cancers never become clinical cancers. However, it is not known whether TRT will increase this risk.

Two prospective cohort studies and 10 nested case-control studies have correlated T levels with future development of prostate cancer (Rhoden *et al.*, 2004). None of these studies found a positive correlation between total T or bioavailable T (four studies) levels and future prostate cancer; however, the nested case-control study reported by Gann and colleagues found a positive relationship after T was adjusted for the SHBG level. Although it is reasonable to adjust for SHBG, this study found that high total T levels and low SHBG levels were correlated with future prostate cancer. Total T levels usually increase with increasing SHBG. As suggested by Hsing, it is desirable to correlate prostate cancer with measures of androgen action, rather than a single blood level at some point in the past, but such studies are lacking.

The influence of T on prostate carcinogenesis and other prostate outcomes remains poorly defined. Some animal studies suggest that T may be a weak carcinogen in susceptible animals. Most studies indicate that T can act as tumor promoter at normal physiologic levels (Bosland, 2000; Stanbrough *et al.*, 2001). The direct relevance of these studies to humans is uncertain. Despite the lack of evidence implicating androgens in carcinogenesis, it is clear that prostate cancer rarely, if ever, develops in an environment devoid of androgens, and the majority of prostate carcinomas require androgens for growth. Androgen ablation causes regression of metastatic prostate carcinoma; however, cancer cells that survive androgen deprivation ultimately proliferate, causing relapse and androgen-independent disease.

Benign prostatic hyperplasia. Benign prostatic hyperplasia (BPH) is a noncancerous enlargement of prostate that can obstruct urine flow. Around 90 percent of males 70 and older have some symptoms of lower urinary tract obstruction; but nonprostatic factors commonly contribute to lower urinary tract symptoms in men and women. Although treatment of men with large prostates with a 5α-reductase inhibitor will cause a 15 to 20% reduction in prostate volume, longer studies indicate that finasteride significantly reduced progression of BPH, urinary retention, and need for invasive treatment (McConnell *et al.*, 2003). It may be that combining TRT with a 5α-reductase inhibitor will reduce risk of progression of BPH and need for invasive treatment of BPH. Long-term use of a 5α-reductase inhibitor for prevention of BPH progression or prevention of prostate cancer is not routinely advised at this time, but this could change as we learn more about the long-term effects of these inhibitors on development of prostate cancer and progression of BPH.

Cardiovascular

Cardiovascular disease remains the number one killer for men in the United States. The prevalence of cardiovascular disease is approximately twice as common in men as in women at any age during the reproductive years (Wu *et al.*, 2003). Whether this is due to protective effects of estrogen, harmful effects of T, or to other factors has been the subject of many studies. Estrogen therapy of men with cardiovascular disease increased cardiovascular events. Furthermore, estrogen therapy of postmenopausal women also appears to cause some increase in cardiovascular events (Anderson *et al.*, 2004; Grady *et al.*, 2002). Epidemiological studies in men show a neutral or a negative correlation between T levels and cardiovascular disease (Wu *et al.*, 2003).

Most studies have examined the effects of T on individual factors that contribute to cardiovascular disease such as lipids, apoproteins, insulin sensitivity, endothelin levels, platelet function, clotting parameters, vascular reactivity, arterial intimal thickening, and hematocrit. The correlations vary depending upon the specific endpoint. These trials were mostly of short duration (4 weeks to 36 months) and involved only a relatively small number of men. Physiologic T treatment of older men recently was reported to improve cardiac function in men with low ejection fraction and reduced exercise capacity. Confirmatory studies are needed before this observation is incorporated into routine practice. Because T is anabolic, it may cause some sodium retention.

Bone marrow

Boys and girls have similar red blood cell counts prior to puberty; however, puberty in males is accompanied by an increase in red blood count. This causes a significant rise in the hematocrit and hemoglobin in postpubertal boys and adult males. T increases red blood cells by stimulating erythropoietin synthesis and secretion by the kidney and by a direct effect on red blood cell precursors. In the absence of hypoxia, T deficient men usually have a mild anemia. The In-Chianti Study evaluated 586 men 65 years of age and older. Men with hemoglobin levels <13 grams/dl had lower circulating levels of calculated fT and bT. No significant association was noted between erythropoietin and total fT or bT levels. This suggests that the anemia is due to less stimulation of red blood cell precursors and not to less stimulation of erythropoietin. Typically, T replacement in androgen deficient men is accompanied by a significant increase in hemoglobin and hematocrit. In older men, T replacement can cause erythrocytosis in some men, especially when T is given as intramuscular injections. If the hematocrit increases above 54 or 55%, it can increase blood viscosity and decrease blood flow. This is a concern in older men with cerebral vascular disease who are at risk for stroke. Therefore, the hematocrit and hemoglobin must be monitored carefully in hypoxic and older hypogonadal men who are treated with T.

Liver

The liver is an important target tissue for T. Much of the circulating T is metabolized and cleared by the liver. The metabolic clearance rate for T decreases as men age. It is thought that this is due in part to the increase in SHBG levels and the reduction in fT levels (Want *et al.*, 2004). The metabolic clearance rate for T also can be reduced by drugs such as anti-convulsants, which increase SHBG and decrease fT. The arterial and hepatic vein blood concentrations of T and DHT do not indicate that T is converted by the liver to DHT; however, there is a significant increase in hepatic vein DHT glucuronide (Ishimaru *et al.*, 1978). This is true in younger and older men, and it indicates that the conversion of T to DHT occurs in extrasplanchnic tissue. Fatty liver disease and cirrhosis usually are accompanied by an increase in serum levels of estrone and to a lesser degree in estradiol. SHBG levels are increased, and fT levels are reduced (Kley *et al.*, 1975). Basal luteinizing hormone (LH) levels are increased in patients with less severe liver disease, and they are reduced in the presence of more severe liver disease when compared with controls.

T and its metabolite, estradiol, are recognized to affect liver production of proteins such as SHBG, cortisol binding globulin (CBG), thyroid binding globulin (TBG), apoproteins, lipids, and factors that affect blood clotting and clot lysis. Estrogens increase and androgens have some suppressive effect on SHBG, CBG, and TBG levels.

Serum T and fT in epidemiological studies are positively correlated with HDL-cholesterol and ApoA1 levels, and fT was positively correlated with ApoB levels (Van Pottelbergh *et al.*, 2003). However, high doses of T can increase hepatic lipase and reduce HDL, HDL(2), and HDL(3)-cholesterol and increase LDL particle size (Herbst *et al.*, 2003). Inhibition of T secretion in normal men will increase these parameters. A meta-analysis reviewing 19 studies with intramuscular T esters given in near physiological doses found small, dose-dependent decreases in HDL-cholesterol, LDL-cholesterol, and total cholesterol (Whitsel *et al.*, 2001). A three-year study comparing T patch vs. placebo patch in men ≥ 65 years of age and a total T level <475 ng/dl at baseline failed to detect significant changes in HDL-cholesterol, LDL-cholesterol, or total cholesterol, apolipoprotein A-I, or apolipoprotein B (61).

Estrogen is recognized to adversely affect coagulation parameters in women, and this, along with a greater prevalence of coronary heart disease in men prior to age 50, has raised concerns about the effect of T on coagulation parameters in men. A Belgian epidemiological study

(715 healthy middle-aged men) did not find any correlation between endogenous T, E_2, calculated fT, or calculated fE_2 and the mean serum fibrinogen level. The relationship of endogenous T to basal fibrinolytic activity was evaluated in 55 hyperlipidemic men (Glueck *et al.*, 1993). T levels correlated positively with tPA activity and inversely with PAI-1 and fibrinogen. The Paris Prospective Study II evaluated 251 healthy, middle-aged men for correlations between T and hemostatic factors (Bonithon-Kopp *et al.*, 1988). T levels were negatively correlated with factor VII activity and alpha 2-antiplasmin. No association was observed between T levels and fibrinogen or antithrombin III levels. These authors concluded that low circulating T levels might be associated with a hypercoagulable state. Hypogonadism in men has been associated with enhanced fibrinolytic inhibition caused by increased synthesis of PAI-1. Smith and colleagues (2005) conducted a double-blind, randomized, placebo trial with physiological replacement doses of T in 46 men with stable angina. Although there was a significant increase in bT level in the treated group, there were no changes in fibrinogen, tissue plasminogen activator (tPA) activity, or plasminogen activator inhibitor-1 (PAI-1) activity. Thus, the effects on the coagulation system of physiological replacement doses of T in men with T deficiency are uncertain.

Immune system and inflammatory cytokines

Aging is associated with increased susceptibility to infection, cancer, and an increase in inflammatory cytokines, which are associated with cardiovascular disease. The possibility that age-associated changes in the immune system are affected by changes in circulating levels of estrogen and T are suggested by observations that estrogen and androgen receptors are expressed in primary lymphoid organs and peripheral immune cells, and the female predominance of autoimmune diseases such as rheumatoid arthritis, systemic lupus erythematosis, Hashimoto's thyroiditis, and Graves' disease. Furthermore, females have higher levels of immunoglobulins and greater antibody response to antigens. Castration in male and female mice causes enhanced adrenal and immune responses to endotoxin, which are prevented by treatment with T (Gaillard *et al.*, 1998). T treatment decreases IL-6 production by monocytes and reduces IgG production (Kanda *et al.*, 1996). Gabriel and colleagues (2002) used lipopolysaccharide (LPS) from *salmonella abortus equi* and *Escherichia coli* to stimulate peripheral blood mononuclear cells (PBMCs) *in vitro*. Older patients had excessive secretion of IL-1β, IL-6, and IL-8 by PBMCs. Other investigators have reported that T reduced IL-1 secretion stimulated by LPS. *In vivo* studies also have shown that T replacement in androgen-deficient men with coronary artery disease suppresses Il-1β and TNFα and increases IL-10 (Malkin *et al.*, 2004). It is suggested that this could reduce cytokine mediated atheromatous plaque development and complications. Whether some of the altered immune responses observed with aging are related to T deficiency and whether T replacement will prove to have a net benefit in suppression of excessive immune and cytokine responses will require much more research; however, the possibility that T may be beneficial should encourage studies of the hormonal-immunological interactions in aging men and women.

Conclusion

Serum total T concentrations fall with aging, and this may have adverse consequences for energy, sexual function, muscle mass and function, and bone. There also are unconfirmed reports that low total T levels are associated with increased risk of mortality due to cancer. Although increasing the serum T concentrations of elderly men to those of young men might prevent or reverse some of these changes, we do not know if TRT might increase several T-dependent diseases to which elderly men are prone. Thus, the benefit:risk ratio of TRT in aging men is not known.

Recommended Resources

Hijazi, R.A., Cunningham, G.R. (2005). Andropause: Is androgen replacement therapy indicated for the aging male? *Annu. Rev. Med.* 56, 117–137.

Liverman, C.T., Blazer, D.G. (2004). Testosterone and Aging. Clinical Research Directions. Institute of Medicine. Washington, D.C.: The National Academies Press.

ACKNOWLEDGMENTS

Dr. Cunningham has received research grants from Unimed/Solvay Pharmaceuticals, Columbia Laboratories, Ascend Pharmaceuticals, and GlaxoSmithKline. He has served as a consultant for Solvay Pharmaceuticals, Columbia Laboratories, Oscient Pharmaceuticals, and GlaxoSmithKline. He is on the Speaker's List for Solvay Pharmaceuticals, Columbia Laboratories, and GlaxoSmithKline.

REFERENCES

Amory, J.K., Watts, N.B., Easley, K.A., Sutton, P.R., Anawalt, B.D., Matsumoto, A.M. *et al.* (2004). Exogenous T or T with finasteride increases bone mineral density in older men with low serum T. *J Clin Endocrinol Metab 89*, 503–510.

Anderson, D.C. (1974). Sex-hormone-binding globulin. *Clin Endocrinol 3*, 69–96.

Anderson, G.L., Limacher, M., Assaf, A.R., Bassford, T., Beresford, S.A., and Black, H. (2004). Effects of conjugated equine estrogen in postmenopausal women with hysterectomy: The Women's Health Initiative randomized controlled trial. *JAMA 291*, 1701–1712.

Aversa, A., Isidori, A.M., Spera, G., Lenzi, A., and Fabbri, A. (2003). Androgens improve cavernous vasodilation and response to sildenafil in patients with erectile dysfunction. *Clin Endocrinol (Oxf) 58*, 632–638.

Baker, H.W., Burger, H.G., de Kretser, D.M., Hudson, B., O'Connor, S., Wang, C. *et al.* (1976). Changes in the pituitary-testicular system with age. *Clin Endocrinol 5*, 349–372.

Barrett-Connor, E., Goodman-Gruen, D., and Patay, B. (1999). Endogenous sex hormones and cognitive function in older men. *J Clin Endocrinol Metab 84*, 3681–3685.

Bhasin, S., Storer, T.W., Berman, N., Callegari, C., Clevenger, B., Phillips, J. *et al.* (1996). The effects of supraphysiologic doses of T on muscle size and strength in normal men. *N Engl J Med 335*, 1–7.

Bhasin, S., Taylor, W.E., Singh, R., Artaza, J., Sinha-Hikim, I., Jasuja, R. *et al.* (2003). The mechanisms of androgen effects on body composition: Mesenchymal pluripotent cell as the target of androgen action. *J Gerontol A Biol Sci Med Sci 58*, M1103–M1110.

Bhasin, S., Woodhouse, L., Casaburi, R., Singh, A.B., Mac, R.P., Lee, M. *et al.* (2005). Older men are as responsive as young men to the anabolic effects of graded doses of testosterone on the skeletal muscle. *J Clin Endocrinol Metab 90*, 678–688.

Bonithon-Kopp, C., Scarabin, P.Y., Bara, L., Castanier, M., Jacqueson, A., and Roger, M. (1988). Relationship between sex hormones and haemostatic factors in healthy middle-aged men. *Atherosclerosis 71*, 71–76.

Bosland, M.C. (2000). The role of steroid hormones in prostate carcinogenesis. *Journal of the National Cancer Institute Monographs 27*, 39–66.

Carani, C., Granata, A.R., Bancroft, J., and Marrama, P. (1995). The effects of T replacement on nocturnal penile tumescence and rigidity and erectile response to visual erotic stimuli in hypogonadal men. *Psychoneuroendocrinology 20*, 743–753.

Cherrier, M.M., Asthana, S., Plymate, S., Baker, L., Matsumoto, A.M., Peskind, E. *et al.* (2001). T supplementation improves spatial and verbal memory in healthy older men. *Neurology 10, 57*, 80–88.

Couillard, C., Gagnon, J., Bergeron, J., Leon, A.S., Rao, D.C., Skinner, J.S. *et al.* (2000). Contribution of body fatness and adipose tissue distribution to the age variation in plasma steroid hormone concentrations in men: the HERITAGE Family Study. *J Clin Endocrinol Metab 85*, 1026–1031.

Cunningham, G.R., Hirshkowitz, M., Korenman, S.G., and Karacan, I. (1990). T replacement therapy and sleep-related erections in hypogonadal men. *J Clin Endocrinol Metab 70*, 792–797.

Deslypere, J.P. and Vermeulen, A. (1984). Leydig cell function in normal men: Effect of age, life-style, residence, diet, and activity. *J Clin Endocrinol Metab 59*, 955–956.

Deslypere, J.P., Kaufman, J.M., Vermeulen, T., Vogelaers, D., Vandalem, J.L., and Vermeulen, A. (1987). Influence of age on pulsatile luteinizing hormone release and responsiveness of the gonadotrophs to sex hormone feedback in men. *J Clin Endocrinol Metab 64*, 68–73.

Dicker, A., Ryden, M., Naslund, E., Muehlen, I.E., Wiren, M., Lafontan, M. *et al.* (2004). Effect of testosterone on lipolysis in human pre-adipocytes from different fat depots. *Diabetologia 47*, 420–428.

Feldman, H.A., Longcope, C., Derby, C.A., Johannes, C.B., Araujo, A.B., Coviello, A.D. *et al.* (2002). Age trends in the level of serum T and other hormones in middle-aged men: Longitudinal results from the Massachusetts Male Aging Study. *J Clin Endocrinol Metab 87*, 589–598.

Gabriel, P., Cakman, I., and Rink, L. (2002). Overproduction of monokines by leukocytes after stimulation with lipopolysaccharide in the elderly. *Exp Gerontol 37*, 235–247.

Gaillard, R.C. and Spinedi, E. (1998). Sex- and stress-steroids interactions and the immune system: evidence for a neuroendocrine-immunological sexual dimorphism. *Domest Anim Endocrinol 15*, 345–352.

Glueck, C.J., Glueck, H.I., Stroop, D., Speirs, J., Hamer, T., Tracy, T. (1993). Endogenous testosterone, fibrinolysis, and coronary heart disease risk in hyperlipidemic men. *J Lab Clin Clin Med 122*, 412–420.

Grady, D., Herrington, D., Bittner, V., Blumenthal, R., Davidson, M., Hlatky, M. *et al.* (2002). Cardiovascular disease outcomes during 6.8 years of hormone therapy: Heart and Estrogen/progestin Replacement Study follow-up (HERS II). *JAMA 288*, 49–57.

Greendale, G.A., Edelstein, S., and Barrett-Connor, E. (1997). Endogenous sex steroids and bone mineral density in older women and men: the Rancho Bernardo Study. *J bone Miner Res 12*, 1833–1843.

Harman, S.M., Metter, E.J., Tobin, J.D., Pearson, J., and Blackman, M.R. (2001). Longitudinal effects of aging on serum total and free T levels in healthy men. Baltimore Longitudinal Study of Aging. *J Clin Endocrinol Metab 86*, 724–731.

Herbst, K.L., Amory, J.K., Brunzell, J.D., Chansky, H.A., and Bremner, W.J. (2003). Testosterone administration to men increases hepatic lipase activity and decreases HDL and LDL size in 3 wk. *Am J Physiol Endocrinol Metab 284*, E1112–E1118.

Ishimaru, T., Edmiston, A., Pages, L., and Horton, R. (1978). Direct conversion of testosterone to dihydrotestosterone glucuronide in man. *J Clin Endocrinol Metab 47*, 1282–1286.

Jain, P., Rademaker, A.W., and McVary, K.T. (2000). T supplementation for erectile dysfunction: Results of a meta-analysis. *J Urol 164*, 371–375.

Janowsky, J.S., Oviatt, S.K., and Orwoll, E.S. (2000). Sex steroids modify working memory. *J Cogn Neurosci 12*, 407–414.

Kanda, N, Tsuchida, T, and Tamaki, K. (1996). Testosterone inhibits immunoglobulin production by human peripheral blood mononuclear cells. *Clin Exp Immunol 106*, 410–415.

Kenny, A.M., Bellantonio, S., Gruman, C.A., Acosta, R.D., and Prestwood, K.M. (2002). Effects of transdermal T on cognitive function and health perception in older men with low bioavailable T levels. *J Gerontol A Biol Sci Med Sci 57*, M321–M325.

Khosla, S., Melton, L.J. 3rd, Atkinson, E.J., O'Fallon, W.M., Klee, G.G., and Riggs, B.L. (1998). Relationship of serum sex steroid levels and bone turnover markers with bone mineral density in men and women: a key role for bioavailable estrogen. *J Clin Endocrinol Metab 83*, 2266–2274.

Kley, H.K., Nieschlag, E., Wiegelmann, W., Solbach, H.G., and Kruskemper, H.L. (1975). Steroid hormones and their binding in plasma of male patients with fatty liver, chronic hepatitis and liver cirrhosis. *Acta Endocrinol 79*, 275–285.

Korenman, S.G., Morley, J.E., Mooradian, A.D., Davis, S.S., Kaiser, F.E., Silver, A.J. *et al.* (1990). Secondary hypogonadism in older men: Its relation to impotence. *J Clin Endocrinol Metab 71*, 963–969.

Lamb, D.J., Weigel, N.L., and Marcelli, M. (2001). Androgen receptors and their biology. *Vitam Horm 62*, 199–230.

Lanfranco, F., Zitzmann, M., Simoni, M., and Nieschlag, E. (2004). Serum adiponectin levels in hypogonadal males: Influence of testosterone replacement therapy. *Clin Endo 60*, 500–507.

Maffei, L., Murata, Y., Rochira, V., Tubert, G., Aranda, C., Vazquez, M. *et al.* (2004). Dysmetabolic syndrome in a man with a novel mutation of the aromatase gene: effects of T, alendronate, and estradiol treatment. *J Clin Endocrinol Metab 89*, 61–70.

Malkin, C.J., Pugh, P.J., Jones, R.D., Kapoor, D., Channer, K.S., and Jones, T.H. (2004). The effect of testosterone replacement on endogenous inflammatory cytokines and lipid profiles in hypogonadal men. *J Clin Endocrinol Metab 89*, 3313–3318.

Mayes, J.S. and Watson, G.H. (2004). Direct effects of sex steroid hormones on adipose tissues and obesity. *Obes Rev 5*, 197–216.

McConnell, J.D., Roehrborn, C.G., Bautista, O.M., Andriole, G.L. Jr, Dixon, C.M., Kusek, J.W. *et al.* (2003). The long-term effect of doxazosin, finasteride, and combination therapy on the clinical progression of benign prostatic hyperplasia. *N Engl J Med 349*, 2387–2398.

Mills, T.M. and Lewis, R.W. (1999). The role of androgens in the erectile response: A 1999 perspective. *Mol Urol 3*, 75–86.

Moffat, S.D., Zonderman, A.B., Metter, E.J., Blackman, M.R., Harman, S.M., and Resnick, S.M. (2002). Longitudinal assessment of serum free T concentration predicts memory performance and cognitive status in elderly men. *J Clin Encrinol Metab 87*, 5001–5007.

Morley, J.E., Kaiser, F.E., Perry, H.M. 3rd, Patrick, P., Morley, P.M., Stauber, P.M. *et al.* (1997). Longitudinal changes in T, luteinizing hormone, and follicle-stimulating hormone in healthy older men. *Metabolism 46*, 410–413.

Morley, J.E., Charlton, E., Patrick, P., Kaiser, F.E., Cadeau, P., McCready, D. *et al.* (2000). Validation of a screening questionnaire for androgen deficiency in aging males. *Metabolism 49*, 1239–1242.

Neaves, W.B., Johnson, L., Porter, J.C., Parker, C.R. Jr., and Petty, C.S. (1984). Leydig cell numbers, daily sperm production, and serum gonadotropin levels in aging men. *J Clin Endocrinol Metab 49*, 756–773.

NIAMS (National Institute of Arthritis and Musculoskeletal and Skin Diseases) (2003). *Osteoporosis: Progress and Promise*. Available online at http://www.niams.nih.gov/hi/topics/osteoporosis/opbkgr.htm.

NIH (National Institute of Health) (2003). Osteoporosis and Related Bone Diseases National Resource Center. *Fast Facts on Osteoporosis*. Available online at http://www.osteo.org.

NIMH (National Institute of Mental Health) (2003). *Men and Depression*. Available online at http://menanddepression.nimh.nih.gov/infopage.asp?id = 10#men.

Pardridge, W.M. (1981). Transport of protein-bound hormones into tissues in vivo. *Endocrine Rev 2*, 103–123.

Rhoden, E.L. and Morgentaler, A. (2004). Risks of testosterone-replacement therapy and recommendations for monitoring. *N Engl J Med 350*, 482–492.

Roehrborn, C.G., Lange, J.L., George, F.W., and Wilson, J.D. (1987). Changes in amount and intracellular distribution of androgen receptor in human foreskin as a function of age. *J Clin Invest 79*, 44–47.

Roubenoff, R. and Hughes, V.A. (2000). Sarcopenia: current concepts. *J Gerontol A Biol Sci Med Sci 55*, M716–M24.

Russell, D.W. and Wilson, J.D. (1994). Steroid alpha-reductase: two gene/two enzymes. *Annu Rev Biochem 63*, 25–61.

Sakr, W.A., Grignon, D.J., Crissman, J.D., Heilbrun, L.K., Cassin, B.J., Pontes, J.J. *et al.* (1994). High grade prostatic intraepithelial neoplasia (HGPIN) and prostatic adenocarcinoma between the ages of 20–69: An autopsy study of 249 cases. *In Vivo 8*, 439–443.

Simpson, E.R., Zhao, Y., Agarwal, V.R., Michael, M.D., Bulun, S.E., Hinshelwood, M.M. *et al.* (1997). Aromatase expression in health and disease. *Recent Progr Horm Res 52*, 185–213.

Sinha-Hikim, I., Artaza, J., Woodhouse, L., Gonzalez-Cadavid, N., Singh, A.B., Lee, M.I. *et al.* (2002). T-induced increase in muscle size in healthy young men is associated with muscle fiber hypertrophy. *Am J Physiol Endocrinol Metab 283*, E154–E164.

Sinha-Hikim, I., Roth, S.M., Lee, M.I., and Bhasin, S. (2003). Testosterone-induced muscle hypertrophy is associated with an increase in satellite cell number in healthy, young men. *Am J Physiol Endocrinol Metab 285*, E197–E205.

Smith, A.M., English, K.M., Malkin, C.J., Jones, R.D., Jones, T.H., and Channer, K.S. (2005). Testosterone does not adversely affect fibrinogen or tissue plasminogen activator (tPA) and plasminogen activator inhibitor-1 (PAI-1) levels in 46 men with chronic stable angina. *Eur J Endocrinol 152*, 285–291.

Smith, M.R. (2003). Diagnosis and management of treatment-related osteoporosis in men with prostate carcinoma. *Cancer 97*, 789–795.

Snyder, P.J., Peachey, H., Hannoush, P., Berlin, J.A., Loh, L., Lenrow, D.A. *et al.* (1999). Effect of T treatment on body composition and muscle strength in men over 65 years of age. *J Clin Endocrinol Metab 84*, 2647–2653.

Snyder, P.J., Peachey, H., Berlin, J.A., Rader, D., Usher, D., Loh, L. *et al.* (2001). Effect of transdermal testosterone treatment on serum lipid and apolipoprotein levels in men more than 65 years of age. *Am J Med 111*, 255–260.

Stanbrough, M., Leav, I., Kwan, P.W., Bubley, G.J., and Balk, S.P. (2001). Prostatic intraepithelial neoplasia in mice expressing an androgen receptor transgene in prostate epithelium. *Proceedings of the National Academy of Sciences USA 98*, 10823–10828.

Storer, T.W., Magliano, L., Woodhouse, L., Lee, M.L., Dzekov, C., Dzekov, J. *et al.* (2003). T dose-dependently increases maximal voluntary strength and leg power, but does not affect fatigability or specific tension. *J Clin Endocrinol Metab 88*, 1478–1485.

Tenover, J.S., Matsumoto, A.M., Plymate, S.R., and Bremner, W.J. (1987). The effects of aging in normal men on bioavailable T and luteinizing hormone secretion: Response to clomiphene citrate. *J Clin Endocrinol Metab 65*, 1118–1126.

Tenover, J.S., Matsumoto, A.M., Clifton, D.K., and Bremner, W.J. (1988). Age-related alterations in the circadian rhythms of pulsatile luteinizing hormone and T secretion in healthy men. *J Gerontol Med Sci 43*, M163–M169.

Tenover, J.S., McLachlan, R.I., Dahl, K.D., Burger, H.G., de Kretser, D.M., and Bremner, W.J. (1988). Decreased serum inhibin levels in normal elderly men: Evidence for a decline in Sertoli cell function with aging. *J Clin Endocrinol Metab 67*, 455–459.

Thomas, T., Burguera, B., Melton, L.J. 3rd, Atkinson, E.J., O'Fallon, W.M., Riggs, B.L. *et al.* (2000). Relationship of serum leptin levels with body composition and sex steroid and insulin levels in men and women. *Metabolism 49*, 1278–1284.

Thompson, I.M., Pauler, D.K., Goodman, P.J., Tangen, C.M., Lucia, M.S., Parnes, H.L. *et al.* (2004). Prevalence of prostate cancer among men with a prostate-specific antigen level < or = 4.0 ng per milliliter. *N Engl J Med 350*, 2239–2246.

Tohgi, H., Utsugisawa, K., Yamagata, M., and Yoshimura, M. (1995). Effects of age on messenger RNA expression of glucocorticoid, thyroid hormone, androgen and estrogen receptors in postmortem human hippocampus. *Brain Res 700*, 245–253.

Urban, R.J., Bodenburg, Y.H., Gilkison, C., Foxworth, J., Coggan, A.R., Wolfe, R.R. *et al.* (1995). T administration to elderly men increases skeletal muscle strength and protein synthesis. *Am J Physiol 269*, E820–E826.

van den Beld, A.W., de Jong, F.H., Grobbee, D.E., Pols, H.A., and Lamberts, S.W. (2000). Measures of bioavailable serum T and estradiol and their relationships with muscle strength, bone density and body composition in elderly men. *J Clin Endocrinol Metab 85*, 3276–3282.

Van Pottelbergh, I., Braeckman, L., De Bacquer, D., De Backer, G., and Kaufman, J.M. (2003). Differential contribution of testosterone and estradiol in the determination of cholesterol and lipoprotein profile in healthy middle-aged men. *Atherosclerosis 166*, 95–102.

Vermeulen, A. (1976). Plasma levels and secretion rate of steroids with anabolic activity in man. *Environ Qual Saf Suppl 5*, 171–180.

Wang, C., Alexander, G., Berman, N., Salehian, B., Davidson, T., McDonald, V. *et al.* (1996). T replacement improves mood in hypogonadal men—a clinical research study. *J Clin Endocrinol Metab 81*, 3578–3583.

Wang, C., Catlin, D.H., Starcevic, B., Leung, A., DiStefano, E., Lucas, G. *et al.* (2004). Testosterone metabolic clearance and production rates determined by stable isotope dilution/tandem mass spectrometry in normal men: Influence of ethnicity and age. *J Clin Endocrinol Metab 89*, 2936.

Whitsel, E.A., Boyko, E.J., Matsumoto, A.M., Anawalt, B.D., and Siscovick, D.S. (2001). Intramuscular testosterone esters and plasma lipids in hypogonadal men: A meta-analysis. *Am J Med 111*, 261–269.

Wu, F.C. and von Eckardstein, A. (2003). Androgens and coronary artery disease. *Endocrine Rev 24*, 183–217.

64

Aging and the Perceptual Organization of Sounds: A Change of Scene?

Claude Alain, Benjamin J. Dyson, and Joel S. Snyder

The peripheral and central auditory systems undergo tremendous changes with normal aging. In this review, we focus on the effects of age on processing complex acoustic signals (such as speech and music) amid other sounds, which requires a set of computations known as auditory scene analysis. Auditory scene analysis is the process whereby the brain assigns parts of the acoustic wave derived from an amalgamation of physical sound sources into perceptual objects (such as words or notes) or streams (such as ongoing speech or music). Solving the scene analysis problem, therefore, depends on listeners' ability to perceptually organize sounds that occur simultaneously and sequentially. The perceptual organization of sounds is thought to involve low-level automatic processes that group sounds that are similar in physical attributes such as frequency, intensity, and location, as well as higher-level schema-driven processes that reflect listeners' experience and knowledge of the auditory environment. In this chapter, we review prior research that has examined the effects of age on concurrent and sequential stream segregation. We will present evidence supporting the existence of an age-related change in auditory scene analysis that appears to be limited to concurrent sound segregation. Evidence also suggests that older adults may rely more on schema-driven processes than young adults to solve the scene analysis problem. The usefulness of auditory scene analysis as a conceptual framework for interpreting and studying age-related changes in sound perception is discussed.

Introduction

Normally, our brains do a masterful job of filtering and sorting the information that flows through our ears such that we are able to function in our acoustic world, be it conversing with a particularly charming individual at a social gathering, or immersing ourselves in a joyful piece of music. Unfortunately, as we get older, our sound world becomes impoverished as a result of the normal changes in peripheral auditory structures, which represent a significant challenge for hearing science and medicine because of their prevalence, significant impact on quality of life, and lack of mechanism-based treatments. Moreover, as average life expectancy continues to increase, auditory problems will apply to an ever-greater number of individuals. Older adults experience a general deterioration in auditory processing, the most common form of which is age-related peripheral change in hearing sensitivity or presbycusis, characterized by impaired thresholds particularly for high frequencies, which become increasingly prominent after the fourth decade of life (Morrell, Gordon-Salant, Pearson, Brant, and Fozard, 1996). Presumably, these losses in peripheral sensitivity result in impoverished and noisy signals being delivered to the central nervous system. This initial distortion of the acoustic waveform may lead to further reductions in fidelity as the incoming acoustic signals are submitted to increasingly detailed analyses, resulting in the eventual disruption of higher-order processes such as speech comprehension.

Age-related change in auditory perception varies substantially between individuals and may include: (1) impaired frequency and duration discrimination (Abel, Krever, and Alberti, 1990); (2) impaired sound localization (Abel, Giguere, Consoli, and Papsin 2000); (3) difficulties in determining the sequential order of stimuli (Trainor and Trehub, 1989); (4) difficulties in processing novel (Lynch and Steffens, 1994) or transposed melodies (Halpern, Bartlett, and Dowling, 1995); and (5) difficulties in understanding speech, especially when the competing signal is speech rather than homogeneous background noise (Duquesnoy, 1983), or when speech occurs in a reverberant environment (Gordon-Salant and Fitzgibbons, 1993). Although sensorineural hearing loss is highly correlated with speech perception deficits (Abel, Sass-Kortsak, and Naugler, 2000; Humes and Lisa, 1990) and accounts for some of the difficulties in identifying novel melodies (Lynch and Steffens, 1994), there is increasing evidence that age-related changes in the peripheral auditory system (e.g., cochlea) alone cannot adequately account for the wide range of auditory problems that accompany aging. For instance, some of the auditory deficits experienced by older adults remain even after controlling for differences in audiometric thresholds (Divenyi and Haupt, 1997). In addition, some older individuals with near-normal sensitivity exhibit problems in speech discrimination (Middelweerd, Festen, and Plomp, 1990), whereas others with hearing loss receive little benefit from hearing aids despite the restoration of hearing thresholds to normal levels (Chmiel and Jerger, 1996). Moreover, hearing status does not always interact with age, suggesting that hearing impairment and age are independent sources contributing to many older listeners' difficulties with understanding speech (Gordon-Salant and Fitzgibbons, 2004).

Since reductions in hearing sensitivity fail to account completely for speech perception deficits, it is necessary to consider the additional possibility that the elderly may also suffer from impairment at one or more levels of the central auditory processing pathways. That is, the difficulties commonly observed in older individuals may in fact be related to age-related changes in the neural mechanisms critical for the perceptual separation of the incoming acoustic information to form accurate representations of our acoustic world, rather than simply the reception of a weak and noisy signal from the ear. Auditory scene analysis is one framework that guides our theorizing with respect to the putative mechanisms involved in age-related changes in auditory perception, providing novel insights about how our perception of the auditory world breaks down as a result of normal aging.

Auditory Scene Analysis

The root of the auditory scene analysis problem is derived from the inherent complexity of our everyday acoustic environment. At any given moment, we may be surrounded by multiple sound-generating elements such as a radio playing music, or a group of people speaking, with several of these elements producing acoustic energy simultaneously. In order to make sense of the environment, we must parse the incoming acoustic waveform into separate mental representations called auditory objects or, if they persist over time, auditory streams. The problem is compounded by the fact that each ear has access to only a single pressure wave that comprises acoustic energy coming from all active sound sources. The cocktail party problem, which is a classic example of speech perception in an adverse listening situation, can therefore be viewed as a real-world auditory scene analysis problem in which individuals must attempt to separate the various, simultaneously active sound sources while trying to integrate and follow a particular ongoing conversation over time. It should come as no surprise, therefore, that auditory perceptual organization is commonly described across two axes: organization along the frequency axis (i.e., simultaneous organization) involves the moment-to-moment parsing of acoustic elements according to their different frequency and harmonic relations; organization along the time axis (sequential organization) entails the grouping of successive auditory events that occur over several seconds into one or more streams. Understanding how speech and other complex sounds are translated from the single pressure waves arriving at the ears to internal sound object representations may have important implications for the design of more effective therapeutic interventions. Moreover, it becomes essential to understand the effects of normal aging on listeners' abilities to function in complex listening situations where multiple sound sources are producing energy simultaneously (e.g., cocktail party or music concert) if we hope to provide treatments through which individuals can better cope with these changes and continue to have fulfilling auditory experiences.

Auditory scene analysis is particularly useful for thinking about complex acoustic environments because it acknowledges both that the physical world acts upon us as our perception is influenced by the structure of sound (i.e., bottom-up contributions), just as we are able to modulate how we process the incoming signals by focusing attention on certain aspects of an auditory scene according to our goals (i.e., top-down contributions). As for the inherent properties of the acoustic world that influence our perception, sounds emanating from the same physical object are likely to begin and end at the same time, share the same location, have similar intensity and fundamental frequency, and have smooth transitions and "predictable" auditory trajectories. Consequently, it has been proposed that acoustic, like visual, information can be perceptually grouped according to Gestalt principles of perceptual organization, such as grouping by similarity and good continuation (Bregman, 1990). Figure 64.1 shows a schematic diagram of these basic components of auditory scene analysis.

Many of the grouping processes are considered automatic or *primitive* because they can occur irrespective of a listener's expectancy and attention. Therefore, an initial stage of auditory scene analysis following basic feature extraction involves low-level processes in which fine spectral and temporal analyses of the acoustic waveform are employed so that distinct perceptual objects can be formed. However, the perception of our auditory world is not always imposed upon us. Our knowledge from previous experiences with various listening situations can influence how we process and interpret complex auditory scenes. These higher-level schema-driven processes involve the selection and comparison between current auditory stimulation and prototypical representations of sounds held in long-term memory. It is thought that both primitive and schema-driven processes are important for the formation of auditory objects, and these two types of mechanisms might interact with each other to constrain perceptual organization.

The auditory scene analysis framework allows for the act of listening to be dynamic, since previously heard sounds may lead us to anticipate subsequent auditory events. This is well illustrated by phenomena in which the

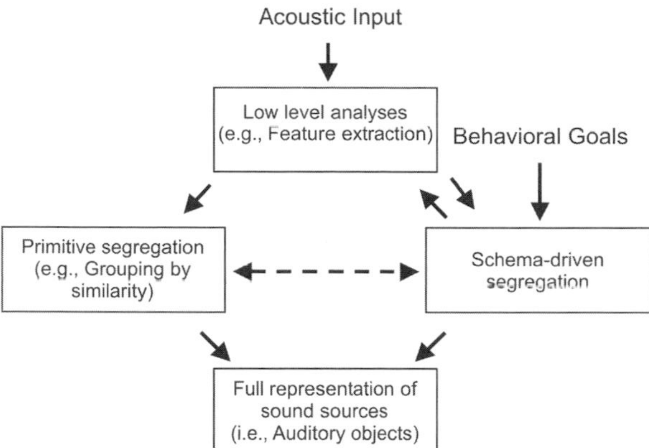

Figure 64.1 Schematic representation of a working model of auditory scene analysis. This model postulates low-level analyses where basic sound features are processed such as frequency, duration, intensity, and location. Scene analysis can be divided into at least two modes: primitive (bottom-up) and schema-driven (top-down). Primitive processes, the subject of most auditory scene analysis research, rely on cues immediately provided by the acoustic structure of the sensory input. These processes take advantage of regularities in how sounds are produced in virtually all natural environments (e.g., unrelated sounds rarely start at precisely the same time). Schema-driven processes, on the other hand, are those involving attention, or are based on experience with certain classes of sounds—for example, the processes employed by a listener in singling out a familiar melody interleaved with distracting tones. Our behavioral goals may further bias our attention toward certain sound attributes or the activation of particular schemas depending on the context. In everyday listening situations, it is likely that both primitive and schema-driven modes are at play in solving scene analysis problems.

brain "completes" acoustic information masked by another sound, as in the continuity illusion (see Figure 64.2A).

In this illusion, discontinuous tone glides are heard as continuous when the silences are filled by noise bursts. In another example, missing phonemes can be perceptually restored when replaced by extraneous noise, and these effects occur primarily in contexts that promote the perception of the phoneme, suggesting that phonemic restoration may be guided by schema-driven processes (Repp, 1992).

With respect to speech and music, schemata are acquired through exposure to auditory stimuli; they are consequently dependent on a listener's specific experiences. For instance, in speech processing, the use of prior context helps listeners to identify the final word of a sentence embedded in noise (Pichora-Fuller, Schneider, and Daneman, 1995). Similarly, it is easier to identify a familiar melody interleaved with distractor sounds if the listener knows in advance the title of the melody (Dowling, Lung, and Herrbold, 1987) or if they have been presented with the same melody beforehand (Bey and McAdams, 2002).

Even though the role of both bottom-up and top-down processes are acknowledged in auditory scene analysis, the effects of age on these collective processes are not well defined. Yet, it is clear that deficits in both simultaneous and sequential sound organization would have dramatic consequences for everyday acoustic computations such as speech perception. For example, deficits in concurrent sound organization may result in the perceiver being unable to adequately separate the spectral components of the critical speech event from the background noise. A failure to segregate overlapping stimuli may also result in false recognition based on the properties of the two different sounds. For example, in dichotic listening procedures, which involve simultaneous presentation of auditory materials to the two ears, individuals presented with "back" in one ear and "lack" in the other ear often report hearing "black," suggesting that acoustic components from two different sources may be "miscombined" into one percept (Handel, 1989). Moreover, difficulties in integrating acoustic information over time and maintaining the focus of auditory attention may further limit the richness of acoustic phenomenology, leading to problems in social interaction and an eventual retreat from interpersonal relations.

Although auditory scene analysis has been investigated extensively for almost 30 years, and there have been several attempts to characterize central auditory deficits in older adults, major gaps between psychoacoustics and aging research remain. The goal of this chapter is to assess the scene analysis framework as a potential account for age-related declines in processing complex acoustic signals such as speech and music. This review may assist in the development of more effective ways to assess and rehabilitate older adults who suffer from common types of hearing difficulty by evaluating the role of bottom-up and top-down processes in solving scene analysis problems. We now consider auditory scene analysis with respect to the initial parsing of the acoustic signal, before going on to discuss more schema-driven and attention-based mechanisms in audition. With respect to primitive grouping, this may be performed by segregating and grouping concurrently or sequentially presented sounds.

Concurrent Sound Segregation

A powerful way to organize incoming acoustic energy involves an analysis of the harmonic relations between frequency peaks. Typically, an examination of the spectra for single sound sources in the real world reveals consistencies in the spacing of frequency peaks. For example, complex sounds with a distinct pitch (e.g., a voice or a chord) corresponding to a low fundamental frequency (f_0) are accompanied by other higher frequencies that are multiples of the f_0. This is because frequencies emanating from the same source tend to be harmonically related to one another; that is, frequency peaks are approximately integer multiples of the f_0. If acoustic energy contains frequency elements that are not related to the dominant f_0, then it is likely that this portion of

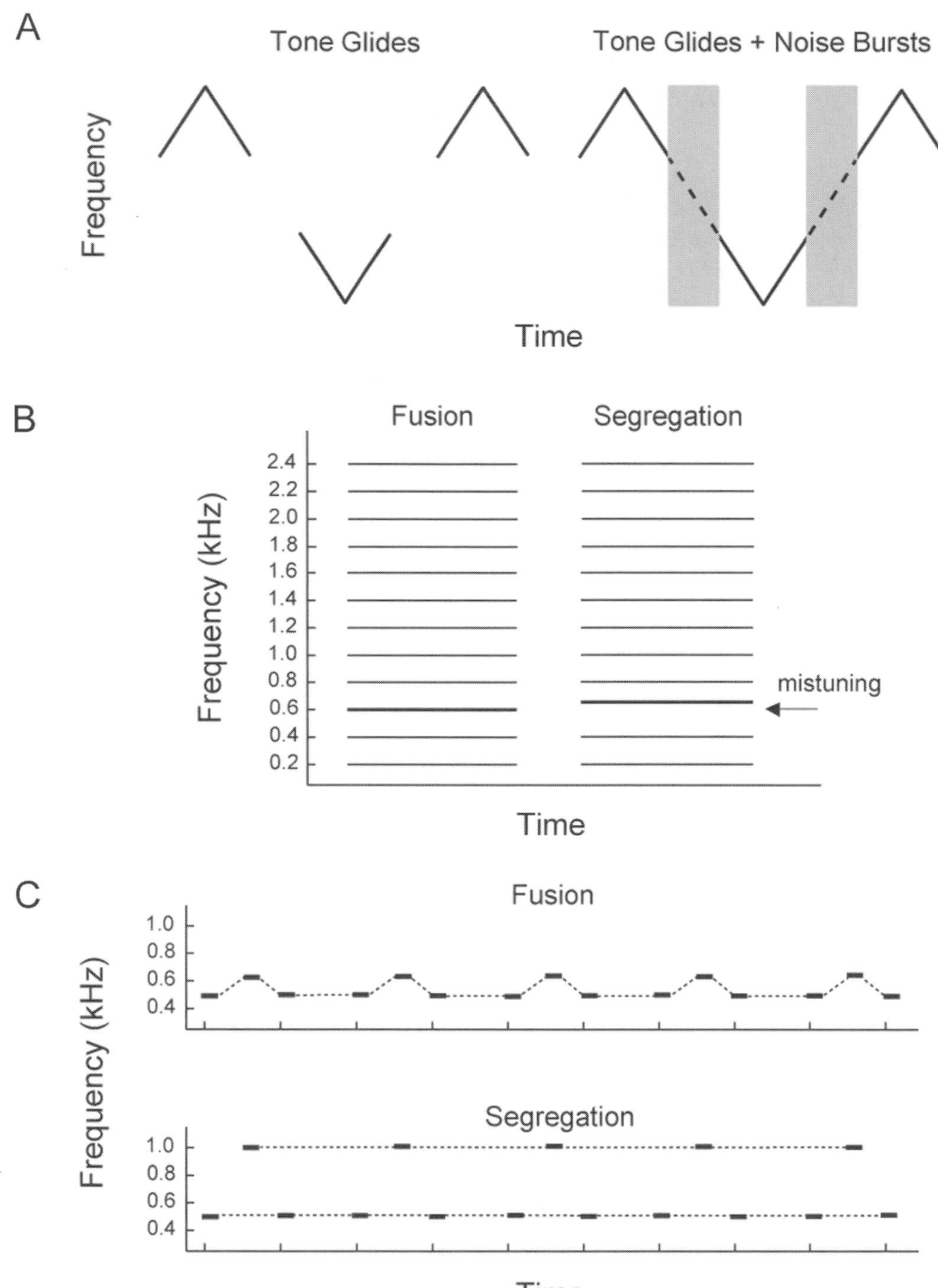

Figure 64.2 A. Continuity illusion. Schematic representation of a repeated ascending and descending glide pattern interrupted by a brief gap (left panel). When the gaps are replaced by loud broadband noise (right panel), listeners reported hearing an ascending and descending glide pattern without interruption. That is, the brain appears to offer a good guess of what might be happening "behind" the noise. **B**. An example of concurrent sound segregation. Schematic representation of harmonic series comprised of 12 pure tones with a fundamental frequency at 200 Hz. When all the harmonics are integer multiples of the fundamental, observers report hearing one buzz-like sound (left panel). However, if one of the harmonics is mistuned by 4% or more of its original value, then listeners report hearing two sounds simultaneously, a buzz plus another sound with a pure tone quality. The arrow indicates the mistuned harmonic. **C**. An example of sequential sound segregation. The top and bottom sequences show five cycles of a three-tone pattern. When the frequency separation between the adjacent tones is small, most observers report hearing one stream of sound with alternating pitch and a galloping rhythm (indicated by the dashed line in the top panel). However, when the frequency separation is large, the three-tone pattern splits into two separate streams of sounds with constant pitch and an even rhythm. Each bar represents a pure-tone in the three-tone pattern.

acoustic energy belongs to a separate, secondary source. Hence, one way of investigating the effects of age on concurrent sound segregation is by means of the mistuned harmonic paradigm. Here, the listener typically is presented with two successive stimuli, one comprised entirely of harmonic components, and the other containing a mistuned harmonic (see Figure 64.2B). The task of the listener is to indicate which of the two stimuli contains the mistuned component. Several factors influence the perception of the mistuned harmonic, including the harmonic number in relation to the fundamental, and sound duration (Moore, Peters, and Glasberg, 1985). For example, thresholds for detecting inharmonicity are lower for long- than short-duration sounds.

In a different version of the mistuned harmonic paradigm, listeners are presented with complex sounds with either all tuned or one mistuned harmonic and indicate on each trial whether they hear a single complex sound with one pitch or a complex sound plus a pure tone, which did not "belong" to the complex. Using this more subjective assessment of listeners' perception, it was found that when a low harmonic is mistuned to a certain degree (4% or more of its original value), listeners often report hearing two concurrent sounds (Alain, Arnott, and Picton, 2001; Moore, Glasberg, and Peters, 1986). The listeners' likelihood of hearing two concurrent objects increases with the degree of inharmonicity and is greater for long- rather than short-duration (e.g., 100 ms or less) sounds. In terms of phenomenology, the tuned stimulus often sounds like a buzz with a pitch corresponding to the f_0, whereas the complex sound containing a low partial mistuned by 4% (or more) contains the buzz element plus a separate sound with a pure-tone quality at the frequency of the mistuned harmonic. Therefore, within the same burst of acoustic energy, two concurrent sounds can be perceived when one component of a complex sound is mistuned such that it is not an integer multiple of the f_0. In this regard, a sound that has a different fundamental from other concurrent sounds (i.e., the mistuned harmonic) might signal the presence of another object within the auditory scene such as a smoke alarm or a telephone ring. The auditory system is thought to achieve this type of perceptual organization by means of a pattern-matching process in which predictions regarding a potential harmonic series are made on the basis of the f_0 (Lin and Hartmann, 1998). Acoustic energy is then filtered through this harmonic sieve or template, essentially separating out the tuned components from mistuned components. When a portion of acoustic energy is mistuned to a sufficient degree, a discrepancy occurs between the perceived frequency and that expected on the basis of the template, signaling to higher auditory centers that multiple auditory objects may be present within the environment. This early registration of inharmonicity appears to be independent of attention (Alain and Izenberg, 2003) and occurs in primary auditory cortex, the earliest stage of sound processing in the cerebral cortex (Dyson and Alain, 2004).

Difficulties in resolving harmonic relations may contribute to some of the speech perception problems experienced by older adults since the perception of a mistuned harmonic, like speech embedded in babble or noise, depends on the ability to parse auditory events based on their spectral pattern. Older listeners may have difficulty in detecting mistuning because auditory filters tend to broaden with age (Patterson, Nimmo-Smith, Weber, and Milroy, 1982). In terms of the harmonic template account, this would mean that inharmonic partials would have to be mistuned to a greater degree in order for segregation from the tuned components to occur, given that the harmonic filters in older adults allow for more frequencies to pass through the sieve as tuned components. Therefore, one prediction that the auditory scene analysis account makes is that older adults should exhibit higher thresholds in detecting a mistuned harmonic. Alain *et al.* (2001) tested this hypothesis using a two-interval, two-alternative forced-choice procedure in young, middle-aged, and older adults. Stimuli consisted of short (100 ms) or long (400 ms) duration sounds with either the second, fifth, or eighth harmonic tuned or mistuned. They found that older adults had higher thresholds for detecting a mistuned harmonic than young or middle-aged adults. This age-related increase in mistuning thresholds was comparable for the second, fifth, and eighth harmonic, but was greater for short- than long-duration sounds (see Figure 64.3) and remained significant even after statistically controlling for differences in audiometric threshold between age groups.

This indicates that age-related problems in detecting multiple objects as defined by inharmonicity do not solely depend on peripheral factors and must involve an age-related decline in central auditory functioning. In each group, a subset of participants also completed the

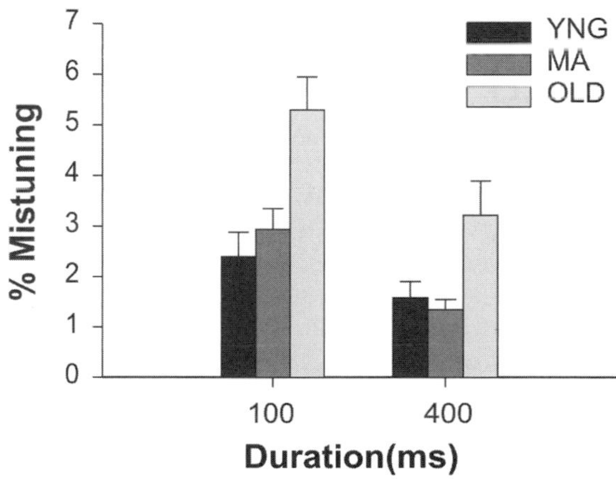

Figure 64.3 Thresholds for detecting inharmonicity for 100 ms and 400 ms sounds in young (YNG), middle-aged (MA), and older (OLD) adults. The threshold for inharmonicity detection is expressed as percent mistuning. The error bars indicate standard error of the mean. Adapted and reprinted with permission from Alain, C. *et al.* (2001). Copyright 2001, Acoustical Society of America.

Speech In Noise (SPIN) test, which requires identifying the last word of a sentence embedded in multitalker babble. The SPIN threshold, estimated by calculating the signal-to-noise ratio at which participants correctly identify 50% of words, was higher in older adults than in young adults. The increased SPIN threshold in individuals who also showed deficits in detecting a mistuned harmonic is consistent with the hypothesis that age-related changes in processes critical for primitive sound segregation may contribute to the speech perception problems found in older adults.

We propose one possible explanation for the effect of concurrent sound segregation on eventual speech identification. Listeners who find it difficult to detect mistuning may assimilate one or more frequency components coming from secondary sound sources into the target signal. The inclusion of extraneous frequency components into the target signal would lead to subsequent errors in perception, given the blend of acoustic energy incorrectly conjoined at an earlier stage of processing. However, since previous investigations used a task that did not require participants to identify the frequency of the mistuned harmonic, it remains an empirical question whether the age-related increase in thresholds for detecting a mistuned harmonic contributes to speech identification problems. Furthermore, it is worth exhibiting caution when generalizing from relatively artificial sounds such as pure-tone complexes to over-learned stimuli such as speech sounds. For instance, perception of ecologically valid or over-learned stimuli may be less sensitive to aging because they are more likely to activate schema-based representations or allow the use of multiple redundant cues.

Another example of concurrent sound segregation that to some extent overcomes the artificiality of the mistuned harmonic paradigm is the double-vowel task. The additional benefits of this task are that it provides a more direct assessment of the effects of age on speech separation, and also evokes the processes involved in acoustic identification as opposed to detection. Here, listeners are presented with a mixture of two phonetically different synthetic vowels either having the same or different f_0, and are required to indicate which vowels were presented. Psychophysical studies have shown that the identification rate improves with increasing separation between the f_0 of the two vowels (Assmann and Summerfield, 1994). In addition to this basic finding, Summers and Leek (1998) also reported an age effect, in that older individuals failed to take advantage of the difference in f_0 between the two vowels and that age accounted for most of the variance in vowel identification performance. This effect of age was observed in both normal and hearing-impaired listeners, once again emphasizing the need to consider both deficits in peripheral and central auditory systems.

More recently, Snyder and Alain (2005) found that normal-hearing older adults had greater difficulty than young adults in identifying two concurrently presented vowels and that older adults took more time to identify the nondominant vowel, especially when the difference between vowel f_0 was small. However, it is unlikely that the age effects on accuracy during the task were due to general perceptual and cognitive decline because the young and older adults did not differ in identifying the dominant vowel within the acoustic blend. Rather, age effects on performance manifested themselves only when attempting to extract the nondominant vowel. Hence, it appears that age impairs listeners' ability to parse and identify concurrent speech signals. This effect of age on concurrent sound segregation suggests an impairment in performing a detailed analysis of the acoustic waveform and is consistent with previous research showing age-related declines in spectral (Peters and Moore, 1992) and in temporal (Schneider and Hamstra, 1999) acuity.

In everyday situations, it is fairly unusual to have concurrent sound objects emanating from the same physical location, as was the case in the vowel segregation study. Sounds that radiate from different physical sources are also likely to be coming from different directions, and the auditory system must decide whether several sound sources are active or whether there is only one sound source with the second source being generated by the first's reflection from nearby surfaces. Hence, in addition to spectral cues, directional cues alone or in conjunction with spectral and temporal cues can also be used to break apart the incoming acoustic wave into separate concurrent auditory objects. For example, early and now classical work has shown that increasing the spatial separation between two concurrent messages improves performance in identifying the task-relevant message (Cherry, 1953; Treisman, 1964). Another task that has been helpful in investigating a binaural advantage in sound segregation is the masking level difference paradigm, where a masking noise and a target signal are presented either at the same or at different locations. Typically, thresholds for detecting the signal decrease when it is presented at a different location than the masking noise, and the magnitude of this threshold reduction is termed the masking level difference (MLD). Pichora-Fuller and Schneider (1991) measured the MLD in young and older adults and showed that thresholds for detecting the signal (e.g., 500 Hz tone) was comparable in both groups when the target and the masking noise were presented at the same location. When binaural cues were introduced, both groups' thresholds decreased, although the magnitude of this threshold reduction was smaller in older than in young adults. Similar age-related differences have also been observed using speech sounds (Grose, Poth, and Peters, 1994). Hence, it appears that normal aging impairs the binaural processing necessary to effectively separate a target signal from masking noise (Grose, 1996; Warren, Wagener, and Herman, 1978). However, other studies using whole sentences embedded in noise rather than single brief targets failed to replicate the age-related decline in MLD (Helfer, 1992), suggesting that environmental support provided by whole sentences may alleviate age differences in binaural processing. In other words, older adults may compensate for deficits in binaural processing by calling upon schema-driven processes in order to solve the scene analysis problem.

The findings reviewed in this section indicate that the aging brain exhibits difficulty in parsing and identifying concurrent auditory events. This age-related decline in concurrent sound segregation remains even after controlling for age difference in hearing sensitivity. Older adults appear to have difficulty in using both spectral and directional cues in solving the scene analysis problem, indicating general rather than specific deficits in concurrent sound segregation. Further research is needed to clarify the link between spectral and temporal acuity and the age-related decline in concurrent sound segregation. We now turn to the effects of age on sequential sound organization.

Sequential Sound Segregation

A second form of primitive grouping takes place along the time axis, and auditory streaming acts as a striking psychophysical demonstration of how sequential sound segregation works (see Figure 64.2C). In a typical experiment, participants are presented with ABA—ABA— sequences in which A and B are sinusoidal tones of different frequencies and — is a silent interval. The frequency separation between the A and B tones is manipulated to promote either the perception of a single gallop-like rhythm (ABA— ABA—) or the perception of two distinct perceptual streams (A—A—A—A— and B—B—). Listeners are required to indicate when they can no longer hear the two tones as separate streams, but instead hear a single galloping rhythm. The fusion or coherence boundary refers to the frequency separation where individuals perceive a single stream of sounds with a galloping rhythm, whereas the fission or segregation boundary refers to the point where listeners can no longer hear the galloping rhythm and report hearing the sounds as coming from two separate sources. The area between the fusion and fission boundaries is typically ambiguous and leads to a bistable percept in which listeners' perception alternates between hearing the sounds with a galloping rhythm or hearing two concurrent streams. Using such a paradigm, Mackersie, Prida, and Stiles (2001) observed only a tendency for older listeners to have increased threshold at which the single stream became two streams. This weak relationship between fission threshold and age may be related to a lack of power given that only five participants with normal hearing formed the sample. However, Mackersie *et al.* also reported a strong relationship between fusion threshold and simultaneous sentence perception, suggesting that sequential sound segregation does play an important role in higher auditory and cognitive functions. Rose and Moore (1997) showed that bilaterally hearing-impaired listeners required greater frequency separation than normal hearing listeners for stream segregation to occur. Moreover, the impact of hearing loss on sequential stream segregation has been observed in a number of other studies using a similar paradigm to that of Rose and Moore (Grimault, Micheyl, Carlyon, Arthaud, and Collet, 2001; Mackersie, Prida, and Stiles, 2001). These changes in sequential stream segregation for hearing-impaired listeners and older adults with normal hearing may once again be related to a broadening of auditory filters, in that wider frequency regions are processed in the same frequency channels (i.e., grouped together) in the older individuals. However, Mackersie *et al.* (2001) and Rose and Moore (1997) did not find a significant relationship between stream segregation and frequency selectivity. Furthermore, Stainsby, Moore, and Glasberg (2004) showed that older hearing-impaired listeners could segregate sounds using temporal cues and suggested that stream segregation does not depend solely on the frequency resolution of the peripheral auditory system. Thus, it appears that both place and temporal coding of acoustic information contribute to sound segregation and that although older adults with either normal or impaired hearing can segregate sequential acoustic information, they nevertheless show a tendency to report hearing only one perceptual stream.

One limitation of these studies, however, was that the effects of age on sequential stream segregation were assessed using subjective reports only. Other studies using more objective measures of auditory streaming suggest that aging per se may have little impact on sequential stream segregation. For example, Alain, Ogawa, and Woods (1996) used a selective attention task to examine the effects of age on auditory streaming. Young and older adults with normal hearing were presented with four-tone patterns presented repetitively at a high rate for several minutes. Participants were asked to focus their attention on either the lowest or highest frequency in order to detect infrequent changes in pitch (i.e., targets). In one condition, the frequencies composing the pattern were equally spaced at three semitone intervals along the musical scale (e.g., 1000, 1189, 1414, and 1682 Hz). In another condition, the two middle frequency sounds were clustered with the lowest and highest frequency, respectively (1000, 1059, 1587, and 1682 Hz). Frequency clustering was expected to favor auditory streaming because sounds that are near one another in frequency tend to be perceptually grouped with one another. Alain *et al.* found that accuracy as well as response time to targets improved in situations that promoted auditory stream segregation. Although older adults were overall slower than young adults, the effects of streaming on accuracy and response time were comparable in both age groups, suggesting that aging has little impact on sequential sound segregation when assessed by objective measures such as reaction time and accuracy.

Additional aspects of sequential sound segregation in older adults were explored by Trainor and Trehub (1989). Here, temporal order judgments were measured across age groups for sequences of tones presented at various speeds and in various contexts designed to encourage or discourage stream segregation. Participants were exposed to alternating frequency patterns and asked either to identify the order of the stimuli or to make same/different judgments. They found that older adults were less able than young adults in distinguishing between tone sequences with contrasting order, regardless of the speed of presentation, nature of the task (identification vs. same/different), amount of practice, or the frequency separation of the tones. Therefore, these findings are consistent with a temporal sequencing impairment in older listeners, but do not suggest age differences in streaming processes.

Although the putative central acoustic deficits associated with aging do not appear to have an effect on sequential sound segregation per se, sensory hearing loss does appear to impair listeners' ability to separate out sequentially occurring stimuli. These findings should be interpreted with caution, however, as the sample size in each age group tends to be relatively small in the case of the gallop paradigm, whereas the other tasks used (i.e., the selective attention task and judgment order task) may not have been optimal to assess auditory streaming. Moreover, a direct link between these age-related changes and the speech perception problems of older adults has yet to be established since the relation between task performance and speech perception has not been fully explored. The Trainor and Trehub, (1989) study reminds us that although older adults appear to show no deficit in segregating multiple acoustic streams, the integration of any one particular stream over time may be a problem for the elderly.

Schema-Driven and Attention-Dependent Processes

Current models of auditory scene analysis postulate both low-level automatic processes and higher-level controlled or schema-based processes (Alain and Arnott, 2000; Bregman, 1990) in forming an accurate representation of the incoming acoustic wave. Whereas automatic processes use basic stimulus properties such as frequency, location, and time to segregate the incoming sounds, controlled processes use previously learned criteria to group the acoustic input into meaningful sources and hence require interaction with long-term memory. Therefore, in addition to bottom-up mechanisms, it is also important to assess how aging affects top-down mechanisms of auditory scene analysis.

The use of prior knowledge is particularly evident in adverse listening situations such as a cocktail party scenario. For example, a person could still laugh in all the right places at the boss's "humorous" golfing anecdote as a result of having heard the tale numerous times before, even though only intermittent segregation of the speech is possible (indeed, the adverse listening condition in this example may be a blessing in disguise). In an analogous laboratory situation, a sentence's final word embedded in noise is more easily detected when it is contextually predictable (Pichora-Fuller, Schneider, and Daneman, 1995), and older adults appear to benefit more than young adults from contextual cues in identifying the sentence's final word (Pichora-Fuller, Schneider, and Daneman, 1995). Since words cannot be reliably identified on the basis of the signal cue alone (i.e., without context), stored knowledge must be applied to succeed. That is to say that the context provides environmental support, which narrows the number of possible alternatives to choose from, thereby increasing the likelihood of having a positive match between the incoming sound and stored representations in working and/or longer-term memory. There is also evidence that older adults benefit more than young adults from having words spoken by a familiar than unfamiliar voice (Yonan and Sommers, 2000), suggesting that older individuals are able to use learned voice information to overcome age-related declines in spoken word identification. Although familiarity with the speaker's voice can occur incidentally in young adults, older adults need to focus attention on the stimuli in order to benefit from voice familiarity in subsequent word identification tasks (Church and Schacter, 1994; Pilotti, Beyer, and Yasunami, 2001). Thus, schema-driven processes provide a way to resolve perceptual ambiguity in complex listening situations, and, consequently, older adults appear to rely more heavily on controlled processing in order to solve the scene analysis problem.

Musical processing provides another real-world example that invokes both working memory representations of current acoustic patterns and long-term memory representations of previous auditory structures. Evidence suggests that young and older adults perform equally well in processing melodic patterns that are presented in a culturally familiar musical scale, whereas older adults perform worse than young adults when the patterns are presented in culturally unfamiliar scales (Lynch and Steffens, 1994). The age difference in processing melodic patterns from unfamiliar cultural contexts again suggests that older adults may rely more heavily on long-term knowledge of musical grammar than young adults. This age effect may be related to impairment either in the processing of ongoing melodic patterns and/or working memory given that a long-term representation of the unfamiliar melodic structure is unavailable. Other studies have shown that aging impairs listeners' ability to recognize melodies (Andrews, Dowling, Bartlett, and Halpern, 1998), and this age-related decline is similar for musicians and nonmusicians (Andrews, Dowling, Bartlett, and Halpern, 1998), suggesting that musical training does not necessarily alleviate age-related decline in melodic recognition. The use of musical stimuli in aging research offers a promising avenue for exploring the role of long-term representation and its relation with schema-driven processes involved in solving the scene analysis problem. Moreover, tasks involving musical stimuli are likely to be more engaging for participants than tasks using typical laboratory stimuli (e.g., white noise, pure tones, harmonic series) that may be less pleasant to listen to for extended periods of time. Furthermore, the results possess a higher degree of ecological validity in terms of everyday, meaningful acoustic processing.

Methodological Issues

In reviewing the preceding literature, a number of methodological procedures suggest themselves for future research on aging and auditory scene analysis. First, and somewhat obvious, it is essential that participants be screened for hearing impairment in both ears. In particular, the integrity of the cochlea should be assessed in a more comprehensive way than just measuring pure tone thresholds in an effort to dissociate nonthreshold-changing peripheral deficits from true central deficits in auditory processing. One test that could provide some information is a distortion-product otoacoustic emission (OAE). Although outer hair cells must be functioning to some degree in order to measure normal thresholds, OAEs are a more sensitive measure of outer hair cell health than pure-tone audiometry and may prove useful in assessing cochlear damage in general. Another potentially useful test would be fine-scale audiometry, which consists of obtaining thresholds with a greater degree of frequency resolution. This method can provide evidence for hearing changes that are not reflected in octave-wide measurements. There are obviously a number of deficits that cannot be easily accounted for by any peripheral problems, but the age-related problems in a wide range of auditory tasks might be accounted (at least partly) by peripheral degradation. Distortion-product OAE assessment might be useful in addressing this issue since it is readily available (and fast), and because it is generally accepted as a sensitive measure of cochlear integrity.

Whenever possible, speech discrimination scores should also be obtained for each ear. Given that the nature of auditory scene analysis research can often rely upon somewhat artificial stimuli, the acquisition of SPIN test scores (or another comparable test) becomes critical. This allows the researcher to establish a correlation between performance in experimental tasks thought to tap into the operation of low-level acoustic mechanisms and speech comprehension in noise, which is an important end product of auditory scene analysis. Also, since musical expertise is likely to influence auditory scene analysis, participants should be asked about the duration of any musical training, and groups should be matched for musical training and listening habits. All of this should be in addition to using standard exclusion screening criteria such as neurological or psychiatric illness and drug or alcohol abuse.

It is well recognized that hearing sensitivity diminishes with age, especially in the high frequency range. Despite screening for hearing impairment, it is not uncommon to find residual differences in hearing thresholds between young and old adults. Hence, several steps should be taken to dissociate the contribution of age-related changes in peripheral processing from those in central auditory processing. First, stimuli should be presented at a suprathreshold level (e.g., 80 dB sound pressure level) rather than at a given intensity increment above hearing threshold. This approach controls for loudness recruitment associated with sensorineural hearing loss (Moore, 1995). Second, stimuli generated using the lower frequency range should be used wherever possible as presbycusis affects primarily higher frequency signals. Third, analyses of covariance should be performed using participants' audiometric levels (pure tone and speech reception thresholds) as covariates to adjust for the contribution of age-related changes in hearing thresholds on behavioral measurements. Whenever possible, three or more age groups should be tested, thereby enabling the examination of when specific maturation processes begin, as well as observing differences in the rate of changes across the various age groups. Such experimental design considerations provide information that goes beyond merely identifying areas where older people perform worse than young people. Taken as a whole, the proposed research strategy provides a means to assess central auditory processing while taking into account differences in hearing thresholds.

Conclusion

Our auditory environment is inherently complex. Hence, it should not come as a surprise that successful identification of simultaneous and sequentially occurring acoustic events depends on listeners' ability to adequately parse sound elements emanating from different physical sounds, and at the same time, combine those arising from a particular source of interest across time. Solving this problem involves low-level mechanisms that take advantage of physical properties in the acoustic environment as well as high-level mechanisms that take advantage of our knowledge about the auditory world. The evidence reviewed in this chapter indicates that aging impairs listeners' ability to parse concurrent sounds based on both spectral and directional cues. Further research is nevertheless needed to clarify the link between age-related decline in low-level sound segregation and higher-level processes such as the perception of speech in noise. It is also unclear whether extended training could be used to alleviate some of the age effects on simultaneous sound and speech separation.

The robust and reliable age-related decline in concurrent sound segregation contrasts with the more subtle age effects observed in sequential sound segregation. An important difference between concurrent and sequential sound segregation is that the former relies on a more precise temporal and frequency representation. The studies reviewed in this chapter suggest that the likelihood of deficits in auditory stream segregation increases with hearing loss, in that the greater the hearing loss the less likely the individual perceptually segregates the incoming stimuli into two distinct streams of sounds. This suggests that sequential sound segregation involves a relatively coarse temporal and frequency representation, which may be more resilient to the aging process than concurrent sound segregation.

We propose that speech and music perception can be viewed as complex auditory scene analysis problems that engage both low-level and schema-driven processes. It is likely to be the interaction between low-level and high-level mechanisms that lead to successful speech identification in adverse listening situations since primitive grouping mechanisms alone are not sufficient to fully account for perceptual organization of speech (Remez, Rubin, Berns, Pardo, and Lang, 1994). In solving the scene analysis problem, older adults appear to rely more on schema-driven than on low-level processes. Although knowing what to listen for helps both young and older adults, older adults appear to benefit the most from prior learning in understanding their acoustic environment. Once again, these results leave many questions unanswered, and therefore further research is needed to understand the extent to which schema-driven processes are affected by age. Nevertheless, by using the scene analysis framework scientists can bridge various areas of aging and hearing research that encompass signal detection and the formation of more abstract representations of our auditory environment. Only by considering both bottom-up and top-down influences, as the current framework allows us to do, may we arrive at a complete picture as to how the auditory scene changes as a function of aging.

Recommended Resources

Bregman, A.S. (1990). *Auditory Scene Analysis: The Perceptual Organization of Sounds*. London, England: The MIT Press.

Carlyon, R.P. (2004). How the brain separates sounds. *Trends Cogn Sci*, *8*(10), 465–471.

ACKNOWLEDGMENTS

The preparation of this chapter was supported by grants from the Canadian Institutes for Health Research, the Natural Sciences and Engineering Research Council of Canada, and the Hearing Foundation of Canada. We are grateful to the volunteers who participated in the experiments reviewed here from our laboratory. Special thanks to Steve Aiken, Lori Bernstein, and Kelly McDonald for helpful comments on earlier versions of this chapter.

REFERENCES

Abel, S.M., Giguere, C., Consoli, A., and Papsin, B.C. (2000). The effect of aging on horizontal plane sound localization. *J Acoust Soc Am, 108(2)*, 743–752.

Abel, S.M., Krever, E.M., and Alberti, P.W. (1990). Auditory detection, discrimination and speech processing in ageing, noise-sensitive and hearing-impaired listeners. *Scand Audiol, 19*, 43–54.

Abel, S.M., Sass-Kortsak, A., and Naugler, J.J. (2000). The role of high-frequency hearing in age-related speech understanding deficits. *Scand Audiol, 29(3)*, 131–138.

Alain, C. and Arnott, S.R. (2000). Selectively attending to auditory objects. *Front Biosci, 5*, D202–D212.

Alain, C., Arnott, S.R., and Picton, T.W. (2001). Bottom-up and top-down influences on auditory scene analysis: evidence from event-related brain potentials. *J Exp Psychol Hum Percept Perform, 27(5)*, 1072–1089.

Alain, C. and Izenberg, A. (2003). Effects of attentional load on auditory scene analysis. *J Cogn Neurosci, 15(7)*, 1063–1073.

Alain, C., McDonald, K.L., Ostroff, J.M., and Schneider, B. (2001). Age-related changes in detecting a mistuned harmonic. *J Acoust Soc Am, 109(5 Pt 1)*, 2211–2216.

Alain, C., Ogawa, K.H., and Woods, D.L. (1996). Aging and the segregation of auditory stimulus sequences. *J Gerontol B Psychol Sci Soc Sci, 51(2)*, 91–93.

Andrews, M.W., Dowling, W.J., Bartlett, J.C., and Halpern, A.R. (1998). Identification of speeded and slowed familiar melodies by younger, middle-aged, and older musicians and nonmusicians. *Psychol Aging, 13(3)*, 462–471.

Assmann, P. and Summerfield, Q. (1994). The contribution of waveform interactions to the perception of concurrent vowels. *Journal of Acoustical Society of America, 95(1)*, 471–484.

Bey, C. and McAdams, S. (2002). Schema-based processing in auditory scene analysis. *Percept Psychophys, 64(5)*, 844–854.

Bregman, A.S. (1990). *Auditory Scene Analysis: The Perceptual Organization of Sounds*. London, England: The MIT Press.

Cherry, E.C. (1953). Some experiments on the recognition of speech, with one and with two ears. *Journal of the Acoustical Society of America, 25(5)*, 975–979.

Chmiel, R. and Jerger, J. (1996). Hearing aid use, central auditory disorder, and hearing handicap in elderly persons. *J Am Acad Audiol, 7(3)*, 190–202.

Church, B.A. and Schacter, D.L. (1994). Perceptual specificity of auditory priming: implicit memory for voice intonation and fundamental frequency. *J Exp Psychol Learn Mem Cogn, 20(3)*, 521–533.

Divenyi, P.L. and Haupt, K.M. (1997). Audiological correlates of speech understanding deficits in elderly listeners with mild-to-moderate hearing loss. III. Factor representation. *Ear Hear, 18(3)*, 189–201.

Dowling, W.J., Lung, K.M., and Herrbold, S. (1987). Aiming attention in pitch and time in the perception of interleaved melodies. *Percept Psychophys, 41(6)*, 642–656.

Duquesnoy, A.J. (1983). Effect of a single interfering noise or speech source upon the binaural sentence intelligibility of aged persons. *J Acoust Soc Am, 74(3)*, 739–743.

Dyson, B. and Alain, C. (2004). Representation of concurrent acoustic objects in primary auditory cortex. *Journal of Acoustical Society of America, 115*, 280–288.

Gordon-Salant, S. and Fitzgibbons, P.J. (1993). Temporal factors and speech recognition performance in young and elderly listeners. *Journal of Speech and Hearing Research, 36*, 1276–1285.

Gordon-Salant, S. and Fitzgibbons, P.J. (2004). Effects of stimulus and noise rate variability on speech perception by younger and older adults. *J Acoust Soc Am, 115(4)*, 1808–1817.

Grimault, N., Micheyl, C., Carlyon, R.P., Arthaud, P., and Collet, L. (2001). Perceptual auditory stream segregation of sequences of complex sounds in subjects with normal and impaired hearing. *Br J Audiol, 35(3)*, 173–182.

Grose, J.H. (1996). Binaural performance and aging. *J Am Acad Audiol, 7(3)*, 168–174.

Grose, J.H., Poth, E.A., and Peters, R.W. (1994). Masking level differences for tones and speech in elderly listeners with relatively normal audiograms. *J Speech Hear Res, 37(2)*, 422–428.

Halpern, A.R., Bartlett, J.C., and Dowling, W.J. (1995). Aging and experience in the recognition of musical transpositions. *Psychol Aging, 10(3)*, 325–342.

Handel, S. (1989). *Listening: An Introduction to the Perception of Auditory Events*. London: The MIT Press.

Helfer, K.S. (1992). Aging and the binaural advantage in reverberation and noise. *J Speech Hear Res, 35(6)*, 1394–1401.

Humes, L.E. and Lisa, R. (1990). Speech-recognition difficulties of the hearing-impaired elderly: the contribution of audibility. *Journal of Speech and Hearing Research, 33*, 726–735.

Lin, J.Y. and Hartmann, W.M. (1998). The pitch of a mistuned harmonic: Evidence for a template model. *J Acoust Soc Am, 103(5 Pt 1)*, 2608–2617.

Lynch, M.P. and Steffens, M.L. (1994). Effects of aging on processing of novel musical structure. *J Gerontol, 49(4)*, P165–P172.

Mackersie, C.L., Prida, T.L., and Stiles, D. (2001). The role of sequential stream segregation and frequency selectivity in the perception of simultaneous sentences by listeners with sensorineural hearing loss. *J Speech Lang Hear Res, 44(1)*, 19–28.

Middelweerd, M.J., Festen, J.M., and Plomp, R. (1990). Difficulties with speech intelligibility in noise in spite of a normal pure-tone audiogram. *Audiology, 29(1)*, 1–7.

Moore, B.C. (1995). *Perceptual Consequences of Cochlear Damage*. New York: Oxford University Press.

Moore, B.C., Glasberg, B.R., and Peters, R.W. (1986). Thresholds for hearing mistuned partials as separate tones in harmonic complexes. *J Acoust Soc Am, 80(2)*, 479–483.

Moore, B.C., Peters, R.W., and Glasberg, B.R. (1985). Thresholds for the detection of inharmonicity in complex tones. *J Acoust Soc Am, 77(5)*, 1861–1867.

Morrell, C.H., Gordon-Salant, S., Pearson, J.D., Brant, L.J., and Fozard, J.L. (1996). Age- and gender-specific reference ranges for hearing level and longitudinal changes in hearing level. *J Acoust Soc Am, 100(4 Pt 1)*, 1949–1967.

Patterson, R.D., Nimmo-Smith, I., Weber, D.L., and Milroy, R. (1982). The deterioration of hearing with age: Frequency selectivity, the critical ratio, the audiogram, and speech threshold. *J Acoust Soc Am, 72(6)*, 1788–1803.

Peters, R.W. and Moore, B.C.J. (1992). Auditory filter shapes at low center frequencies in young and elderly hearing impaired subjects. *Journal of Acoustical Society of America, 91(1)*, 256–266.

Pichora-Fuller, M.K. and Schneider, B.A. (1991). Masking-level differences in the elderly: A comparison of antiphasic and time-delay dichotic conditions. *J Speech Hear Res, 34(6)*, 1410–1422.

Pichora-Fuller, M.K., Schneider, B.A., and Daneman, M. (1995). How young and old adults listen to and remember speech in noise. *Journal of Acoustical Society of America, 97(1)*, 593–608.

Pilotti, M., Beyer, T., and Yasunami, M. (2001). Encoding tasks and the processing of perceptual information in young and older adults. *J Gerontol B Psychol Sci Soc Sci, 56(2)*, P119–P128.

Remez, R.E., Rubin, P.E., Berns, S.M., Pardo, J.S., and Lang, J.M. (1994). On the perceptual organization of speech. *Psychol Rev, 101(1)*, 129–156.

Repp, B.H. (1992). Perceptual restoration of a "missing" speech sound: Auditory induction or illusion? *Percept Psychophys, 51(1)*, 14–32.

Rose, M.M. and Moore, B.C. (1997). Perceptual grouping of tone sequences by normally hearing and hearing-impaired listeners. *J Acoust Soc Am, 102(3)*, 1768–1778.

Schneider, B.A. and Hamstra, S.J. (1999). Gap detection thresholds as a function of tonal duration for younger and older listeners. *J Acoust Soc Am, 106(1)*, 371–380.

Snyder, J.S. and Alain, C. (2005). Age-related changes in neural activity associated with concurrent vowel segregation. *Cognitive Brain Research, 24*, 492–499.

Stainsby, T.H., Moore, B.C., and Glasberg, B.R. (2004). Auditory streaming based on temporal structure in hearing-impaired listeners. *Hear Res, 192(1–2)*, 119–130.

Summers, V. and Leek, M.R. (1998). FO processing and the separation of competing speech signals by listeners with normal hearing and with hearing loss. *J Speech Lang Hear Res, 41(6)*, 1294–1306.

Trainor, L.J. and Trehub, S.E. (1989). Aging and auditory temporal sequencing: Ordering the elements of repeating tone patterns. *Percept Psychophys, 45(5)*, 417–426.

Treisman, A. (1964). The effect of irrelevant material on the efficiency of selective listening. *The American Journal of Psychology, 77*, 533–546.

Warren, L.R., Wagener, J.W., and Herman, G.E. (1978). Binaural analysis in the aging auditory system. *J Gerontol, 33(5)*, 731–736.

Yonan, C.A. and Sommers, M.S. (2000). The effects of talker familiarity on spoken word identification in younger and older listeners. *Psychol Aging, 15(1)*, 88–99.

65

Models of Immune Function in Aging

Christopher A. Jolly and Zhun Xu

The most prevalent rodent models used in aging research are relatively healthy long-lived rats and mice and short-lived mice. The short-lived mice typically spontaneously develop a particular disease or are genetically altered. This review focuses on the most prevalent disease model, the autoimmune-prone mouse, to study the impact of diet on aging. The benefit of these mice is that their life span is half that of the long-lived strains, allowing for data to be generated faster. Specifically, evidence showing the beneficial effects of feeding calorie restriction, omega-3 fatty acids, and combining calorie restriction with omega-3 fatty acid feeding is discussed. Overall, the published data support the observation that the combination of calorie restriction and omega-3 fatty acid feeding is the most beneficial at delaying the onset of autoimmune disease in mice. In order to properly extrapolate this data to humans, the differences in T and B cell immunology between humans and rodents are examined. The most common effect of aging seen in both humans and rodents is thymic involution and reduced peripheral T cell proliferation ex vivo. *However, significant differences do exist between humans and rodents in lymphocyte development and plasma membrane receptor expression. Finally, the potential use of these autoimmune-prone mice as a model of chronic inflammation to study the impact of diet on heart disease is discussed.*

Introduction

One of the most prevalent questions that people ask is whether disease causes aging, or aging causes disease. Disease does not cause aging because even the healthiest people will ultimately die. However, diseases can dramatically shorten life span. Aging, on the other hand, can increase the prevalence or likelihood of developing disease because there has simply been more time in older animals for cellular and molecular changes to occur. Thus, understanding both the biological process of aging and diseases that are more prevalent in the elderly are important areas of research in the aging field. The predominant model used to study aging historically has been rodents (rat and mice), especially those referred to as long-lived. These rodents live approximately 24 months and oftentimes do succumb to disease, but death occurs much closer to their natural maximal life span. Alternatively, short-lived strains of mice are becoming more popular primarily because they live for a year or less, and biological elements that are thought to impact aging can be tested faster. There are primarily two types of mice used as short-lived mice in aging research: genetically altered mice, which have a defect in the expression of a specific gene thought to be important in aging; and mouse strains that spontaneously develop autoimmune diseases that dramatically reduce their life span. This review will focus on discussing the current uses and findings of short-lived autoimmune-prone mice. The two most prevalent autoimmune-prone mouse strains that have been examined are the $(NZBxNZW)_{F1}$ and MRL/Lpr mice. These mice serve as excellent models for examining human autoimmune diseases like Sjogren's Syndrome and Systemic Lupus Erythametosis (Fernandes and Jolly, 1998). As we also will discuss, these mice serve as models of chronic inflammation, making them a valuable model to the study of inflammation-linked diseases like heart disease.

Compare/Contrast Rodent Versus Human Immune Function

LYMPHOID TISSUES

The human and mouse diverged over 50 million years ago; however, the major components of the lymphoid tissues are almost identical. The primary or central lymphoid organs include the bone marrow and thymus where B cells and T cells are generated, respectively. The secondary or peripheral lymphoid organs include the lymph nodes (LN), spleen, and lymphoid tissues associated with mucosa where B cells and T cells are activated to generate the adaptive immune response. Although the overall structure of the LNs are similar between humans and mice, humans have significantly larger numbers of LNs than the mouse (Haley, 2003). This is most likely due to the fact that a human is physically larger than a mouse; therefore more LNs are required in the human. In contrast to LNs, the mouse spleen has some anatomical and structural differences when compared to the human spleen. For example, the periarteriolar lymphocyte sheath and the marginal zone can be found only in the rodent (Sternberg, 1997), and the endothelial cells in human spleen that surrounds the vascular sinuses are missing in the mouse (Haley, 2003). A major difference between the human and mouse spleen is that mouse spleen has hematopoietic activity, whereas the healthy human spleen does not (Cotterell *et al.*, 2000). However it should be kept in mind that the mouse spleen is not the main source of hematopoiesis. The rat, on the other hand, has a much lower amount of hematopoietic activity in the spleen than the mouse, and thus more closely models the human spleen (Fujitani *et al.*, 2004). The rodent and human also differ significantly in the bronchus-associated lymphoid tissue (BALT), which is not discernible in humans but is readily identifiable in the mouse and rat (Pabst and Gehrke, 1990). Peripheral blood immune cell composition also differs between humans and mice. Human blood contains more neutrophils (50–70%) than lymphocytes (20–40%), whereas mouse blood has a higher percentage of lymphocytes (50–70%) relative to neutrophils (15–20%) (Pabst and Gehrke, 1990).

B CELLS

Overall, early B cell development is similar in humans and mice (Burrows and Cooper, 1997). Defined by the rearrangement of the immunoglobulin (Ig) genes, a hematopoietic stem cell in bone marrow undergoes the early pro-B cell stage, late pro-B cell stage, pre-B cell stage, and finally becomes an immature B cell (Burrows and Cooper, 1997). The most striking difference occurs at the molecular level in the signaling control of the pre-B cell receptor (pre-BCR) stage (Conley *et al.*, 2000). For example, more than 75% of the human genetic disorders in B cell development are due to the mutation in Bruton's tyrosine kinase (Btk) (Conley *et al.*, 1998) with clinical manifestations such as repeated bacterial infections, hypogammaglobulinemia, and less than 1% of normal B-cell numbers in the periphery. Molecular research of this disease, named X-linked agammaglobulinemia (XLA) (Campana *et al.*, 1990) is characterized by the inability to produce immunoglobulins (Igs) of all isotypes. In contrast, the mouse model of Btk mutation, Xid mouse (X-linked immunodeficiency) is still semi-competent in antibody (Ab) production and has almost half the normal B cell numbers and only low concentrations of IgM and IgG3 (Wicker and Scher, 1986). This difference appears to be due to the observation that Btk in humans controls B cell development at the point of transition from pro-B cell to pre-B cell (Campana *et al.*, 1990), whereas in mice it seems that Btk plays a role only after the immature B cell stage is reached (Kerner *et al.*, 1995). Interleukins (IL) -2, IL-4, IL-7, IL-9, and IL-15 receptors share a common signal transducing chain—γ_c (Cao *et al.*, 1995). Mutation in the γ_c chain blocks both T and B cell development in mice. In contrast, patients with X-linked severe combined immunodeficiency (XSCID) disease caused by a γ_c mutation have normal B cell development and are deficient in T cell development (Cao *et al.*, 1995). Thus, humans and mice show a different requirement for IL-7 in B cell differentiation (Prieyl and LeBien, 1996).

Mature B cells are heterogeneous, and distinct B cell populations have unique receptor expression profiles and functional repertoire. For example, the CD5 receptor, an antigen (Ag) receptor adaptor protein, is critical in the regulation of autoimmunity in B-1 cells (Hayakawa and Hardy, 2000). Studies in humans suggested that (1) CD5 and CD23 are exclusively expressed on murine B cells, whereas co-expression of CD5 and CD23 on human cord blood B cells is normal (Gagro *et al.*, 2000); (2) in humans, $CD5^+$ and $CD5^-$ B cells have an indistinguishable response to *in vivo/in vitro* stimulation in regard to the expressional change of CD5 and CD23 (Gagro *et al.*, 2000); and (3) CD40, together with BCR co-stimulation, can increase CD5 expression and at the same time down-regulate CD23 expression in humans. However, in mice, CD40 will decrease CD5 expression but enhance CD23 expression, and surface IgM cross-linking can induce the CD5 expression (Gagro *et al.*, 2000; Wortis *et al.*, 1995). The plasma cell is the terminal differentiation stage in B cell development. One of the characteristics of human plasma cells is high CD38 receptor expression. Lower levels of CD38 are also found on B cells located in germinal centers so CD38 expression is used as marker of B cell activation and differentiation (Mainou-Fowler *et al.*, 2004). This criterion is not applicable to the mouse model since CD38 expression remains high until the B cell is activated and moves into the germinal center where CD38 expression is totally absent in plasma cells (Oliver *et al.*, 1997). Humans and mice also differ in the isotypes of Abs produced (Haley, 2003). Most notably, rats do not produce IgA, and there are additional differences in the organization and regulation of IgG subclasses. Structurally, no homologues of human IgG subisotypes can be found in mouse or rat. Functionally, an important role of human IgG is opsonization, whereas in the rat IgG_1 can mediate the uptake of pathogens by binding to complement, and mouse IgG_1 is involved in hypersensitivity reactions (Haley, 2003).

T CELLS

Similar to B cell development, T cell development undergoes several stages and can be followed by the combined expression of specific cell-surface receptors. Certain cell-surface markers have different expression patterns in humans and mice. For example, Thy-1, an Ig-like glycoprotein, is present on both thymocytes and peripheral T cells in mice but only on rat thymocytes (Tokugawa *et al.*, 1997). In humans, Thy-1 expression is found only on stem cells and disappears from thymic progenitors. Thus, Thy-1 is used as a stem cell marker in humans, but as a T-cell marker in mice (Spits *et al.*, 1998). With the exception of some species-specific cell-surface receptors (CD44 and CD25) to indicate T cell differentiation stages in the mouse, the major features of T cell development are similar in humans and mice. One striking difference between human and mouse T-cells is the expression of the CD8α and CD8β isoforms (Spits *et al.*, 1998). These CD8 receptor isoforms can appear as homodimers or heterodimers on T cells. Furthermore, interaction with the CD8 receptor and MHC I on thymic cortical epithelial cells is important for T cell development in the thymus. The double positive (DP) (i.e., expressing both CD4 and CD8 receptors) T cells in the thymus are positively selected based on functionality of CD4 and/or CD8. In mice, 60% of CD8α is normal, being able to bind to p56^{LCK}, whereas the other 40% is an isoform (CD8α') resulting from alternative splicing. CD8α' has a short cytoplasmic domain preventing interaction with p56^{LCK} (Zamoyska and Parnes, 1988). This truncated CD8a′ isoform is not generated in humans or rats; thus, the balance of CD4^{+} and CD8^{+} mature T cell populations in the periphery may be different between humans, rats, and mice (Barber *et al.*, 1989; Zamoyska and Parnes, 1988). The integrated work of other genes that activate specific transcription factors at different stages is essential to T cell development. Zap-70, a protein tyrosine kinase (PTK), is critical in signaling pathways initiated by T cell receptor (TCR) engagement. In Zap-70 knockout mice, T cell differentiation is stopped at CD4^{+} CD8^{+} DP stage; in humans, Zap-70 defects lead to SCID. Patients with SCID express CD4^{+} T cells with defective function. These studies indicate that Zap-70 is a key element for both CD8^{+} and CD4^{+} T cell development in mice but is required only for CD8^{+} T cell development in humans. This difference in humans may be due to the PTK, Syk, which can partially compensate for Zap-70 function in human T cell development. Syk expression is higher in human T cells when compared to mouse T cells (Chu *et al.*, 1999; Elder *et al.*, 2001).

Optimal activation of mature T cells requires two signals. The first (mandatory) signal involves stimulation of the Ag-specific TCR/CD3 complex. The second costimulatory signal is derived from various other receptors on the T cell. To date, the CD28 receptor is the best studied costimulatory signal. The CD28 receptor on T cells is activated by interacting with B7-1 receptors on antigen presenting cells, and there are several differences in the B7-CD28 family's expression and function in humans and mice. First, CD28 is expressed on almost all mouse CD4^{+} and CD8^{+} T cells, but only 80% on human CD4^{+} and 50% on human CD8^{+} T cells (Lenschow *et al.*, 1996). Second, ICOS deficiency in mice causes deficient B cell reactivity and Ig isotype switching, which can be reversed by CD40 stimulation (Wang and Chen, 2004). In humans, the ICOS mutation alters B cell development resulting in decreased B cell numbers and no memory B cells (Wang and Chen, 2004). Since ICOS has proven to be required for proper T helper cell function (Wang and Chen, 2004), ICOS may have different effects on T helper cell function to regulate B cell differentiation, Ig isotype switching, and generation of memory B cells. The biggest difference of the B7-CD28 family between humans and mice exists in the function of the B7-H3 receptor. In humans, it functions to enhance the T cell response, but in mice, it inhibits T cell activation and subsequent cytokine generation (Prasad *et al.*, 2004). Since the members of the B7-CD28 family have multiple functional consequences on T cell function, homeostatic T cell function can be maintained by altering the expression levels of these receptors in response to various stresses and stimuli.

Another interesting difference between human and mouse T cells is the expression of MHC-II. Normally, MHC-II molecules are expressed on professional Ag presenting cells (APCs) and function to present Ag peptide to CD4^{+} T helper cells initiating an Ag-specific immune response. MHC-II is also expressed on human T cells following T cell activation and its synthesis is regulated by the class II transactivator (CIITA) using the CIITA promotro III (CIITA-PIII). In contrast, MHC-II receptors are not found on activated mouse T cells most likely because CIITA-PIII is methylated, preventing CIITA transcription (Holling *et al.*, 2004). It is currently thought that MHC-II bearing T cells can work like APCs to process and present exogenous Ag to other T cells. It is not clear whether the antigen presenting function of human T cells results in increased T cell activation, clonal anergy, or apoptosis (Holling *et al.*, 2004).

Once the TCR is engaged, TCRξ and CD3 chains are phosphorylated immediately, which consequently activates the Src and Syk PTK family kinases and a cascade of adaptor and effector proteins, ultimately resulting in cytokine production and cell proliferation. One of the key pathways involved in human T cell activation is the PKC-dependent activation of the phosphatidylinositol (PI) pathway, which can increase the Ca^{2+} concentration by releasing Ca^{2+} from intracellular stores, and increase the transmembrane influx of Ca^{2+} from outside the cell at the expense of K^{+} efflux, which is regulated by K^{+} channels. In contrast, these K^{+} channels are not present in mouse T cells (Koo *et al.*, 1997), suggesting that their ionic concentrations are regulated differently.

Stimulation of CD4 helper T cells results in their differentiation into either Th1 or Th2 cells, which are phenotypically identified based upon their cytokine production profile. This differentiation process is controlled by the strength of Ag stimulation, the cytokine microenvironment, and B-7 receptor family costimulation. IFN-α can induce CD4^{+} T cell differentiation toward a Th1 phenotype as well as the activation of STAT4 cascade in humans, but fails to do so in mice. This is mainly because an adaptor protein involved in the IFN-α receptor complex, STAT2, has a different C-terminal in the human and mouse, resulting in mice not being able to transduce the stimulatory signal to STAT-4 (Farrar *et al.*, 2000). In contrast, TCR stimulation plus IL-10 is sufficient to induce Th1 differentiation in the mouse CD4^{+} T cells, but has little effect on human CD4^{+} T cells

(Battaglia *et al.*, 2004). The immunosuppressive cytokine IL-10 is secreted by mouse Th2 cells, but it is secreted by both Th1 and Th2 T cells in humans (Del Prete *et al.*, 1993). This indicates that, in humans, the Th1/Th2 classification based on their cytokine production is less clear and exclusive.

Recently, data has emerged showing that a new type of regulatory T cell exists in addition to the Th-1/Th-2 subsets. The $CD4^{+}CD25^{+}$ regulatory T cell (T-reg) is a T cell subset expressing both CD4 and IL-2Rα on its surface, and requires only low levels of TCR and IL-2 signals to respond robustly. The function of T-reg cells is unique and important to T cell activation. It can suppress the activation of $CD4^{+}CD25^{-}$ T cells, $CD8^{+}$ T cells, natural killer (NK) cells, and negatively regulate cytokine production by target cells. The amount and surface phenotype of T-reg cells are different between humans and mice. In mice, CD25 expression is relatively high and about 10% of $CD4^{+}$ T cells are T-reg cells, whereas in humans, $CD4^{+}CD25^{high}$ occupies only 2 to 4% of $CD4^{+}$ T cells. Some other cell surface receptors expressed on mouse T-reg cells like CD62L and CD38 are absent in human T-reg cells as well. The activity of T-reg cells is important in autoimmune disease; thus, differences in CD25 expression in humans and mice may result in quantitative differences in stopping the activity of T cells bearing self-Ag (Baecher-Allan *et al.*, 2004).

Comparison of Rodent Aging and Human Aging

A hallmark of aging in both humans and rodents is thymic involution or decrease in thymic mass. Although this suggests that the ability of the thymus to produce new naïve T-cells decreases in combination with decreased progenitor production in the bone marrow, it would be predicted that peripheral T-cell numbers should decline with age. However, the impact on peripheral T-cell number appears to be minimal. This may be due to clonal expansion of mature memory and naïve T-cells in the periphery. The spleen is one of the major secondary lymphoid tissues, and aging appears to reduce germinal center (GC) size by as much as 90%, as determined based on size and cellularity. The decrease in GC size, which may result in decreased B cell activation and subsequent proliferation, may be responsible for the decrease in plasma B cells. Recent evidence demonstrated that the decline in proliferation in the GC is due to the lack of costimulatory signals provided by T cells located in the surrounding tissue (Zheng *et al.*, 1997).

Aging also results in dysregulated humoral immunity, which may be due to defects in B cells directly and T cell help indirectly. Two problems in B cell development have been found in aged mice. First, the generation of pre-B cells from pro-B cells is two-fold less in aged mice (Klinman and Kline, 1997), which may be due to decreased RAG gene expression in B cell precursors (Ben-Yehuda *et al.*, 1994). Second, the generation of sIgM+ B cells from sIgM- B cells is reduced by aging. The net result is an accumulation of sIgM- B cells and subsequent reduction in mature B cell formation. Altogether, the rate of mature B cell generation is only 20% in old mice as compared to young mice (Klinman and Kline, 1997). However, the total peripheral B cell number is normal in aged mice, which may be due to a slower turnover rate (i.e., longer lifespan) of mature B cells in the aged (Klinman and Kline, 1997). B cells that do reach maturity in aged mice also have defects. For example, some aged B cells have defects in Ig gene rearrangement, specifically V gene repertoire formation, which has been shown to result in hyper B cell reactivity to phosphorylcholine (Riley *et al.*, 1989). The net result of these age-associated defects in B cell development is a decreased response to foreign antigen and a shift from IgG to IgM predominance (LeMaoult *et al.*, 1997). Paradoxically, autoantibody production increases in old mice and humans. This may be due to the indirect actions of the help B cells receive from autoreactive T cells that may be increased with age (Klinman and Kline, 1997; LeMaoult *et al.*, 1997).

Although in both humans and mice, the total number of peripheral T cells doesn't change significantly with age, a decrease in T cell subpopulations does occur. Commonly, a decrease in naïve T cell numbers and a concomitant rise in memory T cells are seen in aged rodents and humans. The increase in memory T cell proportions correlates with reduced polyclonal T cell proliferation *ex vivo* in response to a wide variety of mitogens like anti-CD3 and concanavalin A in humans and rodents. Two major changes in aged T cells have been found in humans, which may explain the reduced proliferation. First, CD28 receptor expression is decreased on human, but not rodent, T cells. Approximately 99% of the T cells from newborn humans express CD28, which decreased to 85% in adults and further decreases with age to 50 to 70% in the elderly (Effros, 1996). Second, CD95 receptor expression also declines. In young T cells, CD95 expression will increase upon stimulation, preventing T cells from proliferating out of control by inducing apoptosis (Aspinall *et al.*, 1998). In aged T cells, the increase in CD95 expression and subsequent induction of apoptosis do not occur in response to stimulation *ex vivo*, suggesting that there is a defect in T cell deletion following a normal immune response (Herndon *et al.*, 1997).

As mentioned before, anti-TCR or anti-CD3 mAb treatment on resting T cell could initiate a series of activation of protein kinases and an increase of Ca^{2+} concentration, which contribute to the activation of transcription factors, secretion of cytokines, and cell proliferation. In old mice, $CD4^{+}$ T cells lose the ability to robustly increase intracellular Ca^{2+} concentrations in response to stimulation. It seems that this phenomenon is independent of IP_3 production and function, but related to high levels of Ca^{2+} extrusion and a low level of Ca^{2+}

release from the intracellular pool (Miller *et al.*, 1997). Similar to the calcium signal, phosphorylation signals in T cell activation are different in old mice. More specifically, the extent of CD3γ chain phosphorylation is much weaker in old T cells. This decreased phosphorylation of CD3γ chain reflects a combination of decreased kinase activity, increased phosphatase activity, and increased difficulty to access the TCR/CD3 complex (Miller *et al.*, 1997). Downstream, other protein kinases such as Raf-1, MEK, and ERK show age-associated decline in activity upon stimulation (Miller *et al.*, 1997). Recently, the function of negative regulators in T cell signal transduction pathways and its effects on aging are beginning to be examined. For instance, Cbl-b, an E3-ubiquitin ligase, can bind with both CD3 and CD28 upon cell stimulation and consequently associate with various proteins that are essential to signal transduction (Bachmaier *et al.*, 2000). In contrast to the positive regulator that enhances the stimulatory signals, Cbl-b can catalyze the ubquitination of the associated signaling proteins and down-regulate protein function by either sending them to the proteasome for degradation or blocking the association of substrate proteins with other effector protein in a proteasome-independent mechanism (Xu *et al.*, 2004). Thus, Cbl-b can set the threshold of T cell activation. Cbl-b itself can be down-regulated upon T cell stimulation in young T cells, and such proteasome-mediated degradation is missing in old T cells. Thus, in old T cells, a stronger negative regulation form Cbl-b persists upon stimulation, and T cell activation is diminished in old T cells (Xu *et al.*, 2004). As a result of reduced T cell activation, IL-2 production is reduced, and a dysregulation of T helper cell function results, which may impact B cell, CD8$^+$ T cell, and other accessory cells in old rodents.

A significant proportion of aging immune research has focused on the CD4$^+$ T helper cells because of its functional importance in regulating both humoral and cell-mediated immunity. Recently, changes in CD8$^+$ T cytotoxic cells have also been found to occur in aging, and examination of both T cell subsets will be important in understanding immune senescence. For example, up to 70% of CD8$^+$ T cells in aged rodents express an identical TCR gene, indicating they are derived from same-parent CD8$^+$ T cells. These types of CD8$^+$ T cells are called large CD8 T cell clones and have a poor proliferate capacity in both human and mouse (Ku *et al.*, 1997). The reason for the large CD8$^+$ T cell clones is most likely due to frequent exposure to the same antigen, which is most likely to occur on old rodents and humans (Ku *et al.*, 1997).

Testing Dietary Interventions in Autoimmune Prone Mice to Delay Aging and Age-Associated Diseases

Typically, calorie restriction (CR) refers to a 30 to 40% reduction in food intake. CR feeding is important in aging research because CR is the only known experimental regimen to increase life span in all experimental models tested including yeast, nematodes, flies, and rodents (Jolly, 2004). The models examined are not malnourished because the CR diets have enriched vitamin and mineral content to compensate for the decreased food intake. CR is also potent at delaying the onset of diseases like autoimmune disease and certain types of cancer. Therefore, it appears that CR may be a dietary regimen that not only increases life span by altering the biological process of aging, but also improves the quality of life by decreasing the severity of age-related diseases.

The primary immune cell studied examining the impact of CR feeding on immune function in aging and age-associated disease has focused on the T cell. The main reason for this is that the T cell is critical in determining both the type and extent of an immune response. Two of the most consistent effects of CR on aged T cell function in rodents are maintenance of T cell IL-2 production and subsequent proliferation while maintaining a naïve T cell phenotype (Pahlavani, 2000). Maintaining an optimal immune response in aging is especially critical because the leading causes of death in geriatric hospitals are infectious diseases (Hirokawa and Utsuyama, 2002). An important feature of CR feeding is that its most dramatic impact on aging is observed when the dietary regimen is started in young rodents and maintained throughout life. This is not completely surprising because dietary regimens are normally the most beneficial when used as a prophylactic treatment as opposed to a therapeutic one.

The most well-studied autoimmune-prone model examining the impact of CR on immune function is the autoimmune-prone $(NZBxNZW)_{F1}$ (B/W) mouse. This model is especially valuable since multiple organs have been examined, such as spleen, kidney, mesenteric lymph nodes, peripheral blood, and submandibular glands. The B/W mouse is a good model to study the human disease Systemic Lupus Erythematosis. As in humans, autoantibodies can be found in young adult B/W mice prior to the detection of clinical disease. The B/W mice die from autoimmune renal disease (i.e., nephritis), which can be monitored by measuring proteinurea, at approximately 10 to 12 months of age. Feeding the B/W mouse a 40% CR diet beginning at six weeks of age delayed autoimmune kidney disease by 30% (Jolly, 2004). The life span of the B/W mice could be doubled when the corn oil (CO) based CR diet was substituted with fish oil (FO) (Jolly *et al.*, 2001). It is equally important to note that CR typically does not impact T cell function in young mice even though they have been on the CR diet for a significant amount of time (Jolly, 2004). This is significant because it suggests that CR feeding alone may not cause the T cell to be immunocompromised.

In the kidney, CR prevented the disease-associated rises in the proinflammatory cytokines IFN-γ, IL-12, IL-10, and tumor necrosis factor-α (TNF-α), and the proinflammatory transcription factor nuclear factor kappa B (NF-κB) activation (Jolly, 2004). In peripheral blood, CR blunted the disease-induced increases in IL-2 and IFN-γ production by both CD4 and CD8 T cell subsets as well as IL-5 production in CD4 T cells (Jolly, 2004). In contrast, CR reduced the disease-associated increase in IFN-γ and IL-10 production in splenic CD4 T cells and increased the loss of IL-2 and IFN-γ production in CD8 T cells (Jolly, 2004). Clearly the effect of CR on immune function is dependent on the immune compartment examined, but the consistent effect is that CR appears to normalize the immune alterations caused by autoimmune disease. The majority of the rodent studies have focused on the splenic T cell since the spleen is the largest source of easily accessible T cells in rodents. It has been shown that CR feeding in B/W mice delays the disease-associated rise in memory T cells, similar to that seen in long-lived strains, and increased expression of the CD69 receptor activation marker *in vivo*. Autoimmune disease caused an increase in T cell activation induced cell death, decreased proliferation, also as seen in long-lived aged mice, and increased Fas expression following *ex vivo* stimulation of splenic lymphocytes in B/W mice. The CR dietary regimen prevented the disease-associated increase in activation-induced cell death and restored NF-κB activation to predisease levels (Jolly, 2004). These results are similar to those seen for CR's effects in aged long-lived mice. Furthermore, CR prevented disease-associated decreases in splenic lymphocyte proliferation and blunted the rise in Fas-induced apoptosis and Fas ligand expression (Jolly, 2004). Both CO- and FO-based CR diets were equally effective in the peripheral blood and splenic T cells at restoring CD4 and CD8 T cell populations to predisease levels (Jolly, 2004). Overall, the FO CR diet appeared to be the most effective in mesenteric lymph nodes at restoring CD4 and CD8 T cell populations to predisease levels and blunting disease-associated increases in cytokine (IFN-γ, IL-4, IL-5, IL-10) and immunoglobulin (IgM and IgG) production$_3$ (Jolly, 2004). It remains to be determined whether the beneficial influence of CR on immunoglobulin secretion was due indirectly to altered T cell cytokine production or to direct modulation of B cell function. Similar results were seen in submandibular gland cultures from B/W mice where it was found that CR decreased disease-associated increases in IL-12, IL-10, and IFN-γ messenger RNA levels (Muthukumar *et al.*, 2000). Also notable was the reduction of IgA, IgM, and IgG_{2a} production by CR since the B/W mice also have active autoimmune disease in their salivary glands (Muthukumar *et al.*, 2000). It is important to note that the autoimmune disease in the salivary glands is normally not life threatening. The results in B/W salivary glands are supported by observations in long-lived mice fed a CR diet in that the age-dependent increase in both IgA and IgM secretion was associated with reduced polymeric immunoglobulin receptor gene expression (Jolly, 2004). The impact of CR feeding on T cell function in the B/W mouse is clearly unique to different anatomical sites; however, the common feature of CR is that it maintains a predisease T cell phenotype.

A major potential mechanism that may explain the beneficial effects of CR feeding in autoimmune-prone mice is change in oxidative status. First, CR may increase the protection of T cells from oxidative damage by increasing antioxidant enzyme activity. This is supported by data showing that CR increased renal superoxide dismutase (SOD), catalase (CAT), and glutathione peroxidase (GSH-Px) activity. Interestingly, the FO-based CR diet was more effective than the CO-based CR diet, which may protect the kidney from oxidative damage. CR also blocked the disease-associated increase in cellular peroxide levels in splenic lymphocytes (Jolly, 2004). This data is similar to observations made in long-lived mice where CR prevented age-associated increases in cellular peroxides in splenic lymphocytes and age-associated susceptibility of lymphocytes to hydrogen peroxide-induced apoptosis was blunted (Avula and Fernandes, 2002). In summary, these observations suggest that CR may improve T cell function (i.e., increase proliferation *ex vivo*) by reducing the increased susceptibility to age-dependent increases in apoptosis and decreasing free radical damage.

In addition to delaying the onset of autoimmune disease, CR or FO CR may also alter the development of other diseases like atherosclerosis in autoimmune-prone mice. Autoimmune disease in these mice increases the expression of key adhesion receptors like intercellular adhesion molecule-1 (ICAM-1), CD28, CD80, and Mac-1, autoantibody production and LDL-cholesterol, which are known to be reduced by CR feeding (Muthukumar *et al.*, 2004) (Muthukumar *et al.*, 2003). Their importance in heart disease may be in recruiting and activating immune cells in the coronary arteries since chronic inflammation is now considered to be an important risk factor in the etiology of heart disease. It is important to note that the beneficial effects of the FO CR diet on lipid profiles were seen early in the initiation of the dietary regimen, which was prior to the onset of active disease (Muthukumar *et al.*, 2003). Once again the beneficial effects of the combination of FO CR feeding may be due to decreases in free radical damage and increased antioxidant enzyme activity, which has been shown in response to the induction of oxidative stress by cyclophosphamide injection (Bhattacharya *et al.*, 2003). Overall, these data suggest that combining two different dietary regimens known to delay the onset of inflammatory diseases may have additive benefit and relevance to multiple diseases.

The concern with the CR dietary regimen is that it may not be realistic for the human population at large. The majority of the studies discussed administer CR at a 40 to 60% reduction in food intake, and this would be quite dramatic for most people. However, simply eating the recommended daily allowances could have similar beneficial effects. The National Institute on Aging/NIH started a study in 2002 called CALERIE (Comprehensive Assessment of Long-term Effects of Reducing Intake of Energy) in humans. It will be interesting see how well, and how long, this population of people follows this dietary regimen and what types of results are obtained from this long-term study in humans. The true benefit of these studies may be in identifying immune-associated biomarkers, which could then be targeted in dietary supplementation and pharmacologic studies to prevent or treat various immune-mediated diseases. This would be of enormous importance to overall human health because the immune system is involved in the etiology of multiple diseases and most of the major diseases in humans.

Autoimmune-Prone Mice as a Model of Chronic Inflammation and Heart Disease

Inflammation is a key component in the development of heart disease (Ross, 1999). The inflammatory process is propagated by immune cells like the T cell, which migrate to the site of inflammation. This is significant because the T cell plays a critical role in determining both the type and extent of immune response via the production of cytokines. Specifically, T cells have been shown to drive the inflammation found in atherosclerotic lesions (Benagiano *et al.*, 2003). The inflammation in arterial walls is propagated by both the expression of adhesion molecules like ICAM-1 and VCAM-1, which recruit immune cells to the site of inflammation, and the production of cytokines by both nonimmune and immune cells. The autoimmune prone MRL-lpr has been used as an experimental system to examine chronic inflammation and heart disease (Qiao *et al.*, 1993) primarily because many of the adhesion molecules and cytokines thought to be important in human atherosclerosis are up-regulated in this animal model.

Nutrients serve as an excellent means to delay the onset of heart disease (Osiecki, 2004). The omega-3 fatty acids found in fish oil are well-established anti-inflammatory nutrients (Fernandes and Jolly, 1998). Important in heart disease, dietary omega-3 fatty acids have been shown to suppress the expression of both ICAM-1 (De Caterina *et al.*, 2000) and VCAM-1 (De Caterina *et al.*, 1995) in endothelial cells. Proinflammatory cytokines like TNF-α and IFN-γ are also found at sites of inflammation, and their levels can be reduced by dietary omega-3 fatty acid feeding in MRL-lpr mice (Venkatraman and Chu, 1999). We have specifically found that dietary omega-3 fatty acids can decrease IFN-γ and TNF-α levels associated with nephritis in the kidneys of $(NZBxNZW)_{F1}$ (B/W) mice. Furthermore, dietary omega-3 fatty acids have been shown to reduce IFN-γ production in T-lymphocytes found in the peripheral blood, mesenteric lymph nodes, and spleens (Jolly, 2004) of B/W mice.

Omega-3 fatty acids can be derived from many food sources. Flaxseed oil, enriched in linolenic acid, and fish oil, enriched in eicosapentaenoic acid and docosahexaenoic acid, are the two sources of omega-3 fatty acids that have been commonly used to examine the anti-inflammatory properties of omega-3 fatty acids. However, direct comparisons of the two oils are limiting in the literature. Recent evidence suggests that both flaxseed and fish oil could decrease T-lymphocyte proliferation *ex vivo* in rats, but fish oil was the most potent. Whether this translates into fish oil being the most effective at delaying the onset of heart disease and/or autoimmune disease needs to be directly addressed.

Conclusion

The autoimmune disease-prone mouse has proven to be an excellent short-lived mouse model to examine autoimmune disease and the impact of dietary interventions. One of the limitations of most rodent models is that they do not perfectly mimic immune function in humans. However, since many of the age-dependent immune phenomena seen in humans are also seen in rodents, the mouse serves as a good surrogate. The biggest drawback to the B/W model, and most other autoimmune disease models for that matter, is that the etiology of the disease is not known. Thus this mouse model would be difficult to use in assessing dietary interventions on the cause of autoimmune disease. The most fascinating fact regarding the B/W mouse and others like it is that its real contribution to research in the future may be as a model of chronic inflammation to study other major diseases afflicting the human population and not actually in studying autoimmune disease per se.

ACKNOWLEDGMENTS

This work was supported in part by NIA RO3 AG19990 and RO1 AG20651 (CAJ).

REFERENCES

Aspinall, R., Carroll, J., and Jiang, S. (1998). Age-related changes in the absolute number of CD95 positive cells in T cell subsets in the blood. *Exp Gerontol 33*, 581–591.

Avula, C.P. and Fernandes, G. (2002). Inhibition of H2O2-induced apoptosis of lymphocytes by calorie restriction during aging. *Microsc Res Tech 59*, 282–292.

Bachmaier, K., Krawczyk, C., Kozieradzki, I., Kong, Y.Y., Sasaki, T., Oliveira-dos-Santos, A. *et al.* (2000). Negative regulation of lymphocyte activation and autoimmunity by the molecular adaptor Cbl-b. *Nature 403*, 211–216.

Baecher-Allan, C., Viglietta, V., and Hafler, D.A. (2004). Human CD4+CD25+ regulatory T cells. *Semin Immunol 16*, 89–98.

Barber, E.K., Dasgupta, J.D., Schlossman, S.F., Trevillyan, J.M., and Rudd, C.E. (1989). The CD4 and CD8 antigens are coupled to a protein-tyrosine kinase (p56lck) that phosphorylates the CD3 complex. *Proc Natl Acad Sci USA 86*, 3277–3281.

Battaglia, M., Gianfrani, C., Gregori, S., and Roncarolo, M.G. (2004). IL-10-producing T regulatory type 1 cells and oral tolerance. *Ann N Y Acad Sci 1029*, 142–153.

Benagiano, M., Azzurri, A., Ciervo, A., Amedei, A., Tamburini, C., Ferrari, M.. *et al.* (2003). T helper type 1 lymphocytes drive inflammation in human atherosclerotic lesions. *Proc Natl Acad Sci USA 100*, 6658–6663.

Ben-Yehuda, A., Szabo, P., Dyall, R., and Weksler, M.E. (1994). Bone marrow declines as a site of B-cell precursor differentiation with age: relationship to thymus involution. *Proc Natl Acad Sci USA 91*, 11988–11992.

Bhattacharya, A., Lawrence, R.A., Krishnan, A., Zaman, K., Sun, D., and Fernandes, G. (2003). Effect of dietary n-3 and n-6 oils with and without food restriction on activity of antioxidant enzymes and lipid peroxidation in livers of cyclophosphamide treated autoimmune-prone NZB/W female mice. *J Am Coll Nutr 22*, 388–399.

Burrows, P.D. and Cooper, M.D. (1997). B cell development and differentiation. *Curr Opin Immunol 9*, 239–244.

Campana, D., Farrant, J., Inamdar, N., Webster, A.D., and Janossy, G. (1990). Phenotypic features and proliferative activity of B cell progenitors in X-linked agammaglobulinemia. *J Immunol 145*, 1675–1680.

Cao, X., Shores, E.W., Hu-Li, J., Anver, M.R., Kelsall, B.L., Russell, S.M. *et al.* (1995). Defective lymphoid development in mice lacking expression of the common cytokine receptor gamma chain. *Immunity 2*, 223–238.

Chu, D.H., van Oers, N.S., Malissen, M., Harris, J., Elder, M., and Weiss, A. (1999). Pre-T cell receptor signals are responsible for the down-regulation of Syk protein tyrosine kinase expression. *J Immunol 163*, 2610–2620.

Conley, M.E., Mathias, D., Treadaway, J., Minegishi, Y., and Rohrer, J. (1998). Mutations in btk in patients with presumed X-linked agammaglobulinemia. *Am J Hum Genet 62*, 1034–1043.

Conley, M.E., Rohrer, J., Rapalus, L., Boylin, E.C., and Minegishi, Y. (2000). Defects in early B-cell development: Comparing the consequences of abnormalities in pre-BCR signaling in the human and the mouse. *Immunol Rev 178*, 75–90.

Cotterell, S.E., Engwerda, C.R., and Kaye, P.M. (2000). Enhanced hematopoietic activity accompanies parasite expansion in the spleen and bone marrow of mice infected with Leishmania donovani. *Infect Immun 68*, 1840–1848.

De Caterina, R., Cybulsky, M.A., Clinton, S.K., Gimbrone, M.A., Jr., and Libby, P. (1995). Omega-3 fatty acids and endothelial leukocyte adhesion molecules. Prostaglandins *Leukot Essent Fatty Acids 52*, 191–195.

De Caterina, R., Liao, J.K., and Libby, P. (2000). Fatty acid modulation of endothelial activation. *Am J Clin Nutr 71*, 213S–223S.

Del Prete, G., De Carli, M., Almerigogna, F., Giudizi, M.G., Biagiotti, R., and Romagnani, S. (1993). Human IL-10 is produced by both type 1 helper (Th1) and type 2 helper (Th2) T cell clones and inhibits their antigen-specific proliferation and cytokine production. *J Immunol 150*, 353–360.

Effros, R.B. (1996). Insights on immunological aging derived from the T lymphocyte cellular senescence model. *Exp Gerontol 31*, 21–27.

Elder, M.E., Skoda-Smith, S., Kadlecek, T.A., Wang, F., Wu, J., and Weiss, A. (2001). Distinct T cell developmental consequences in humans and mice expressing identical mutations in the DLAARN motif of ZAP-70. *J Immunol 166*, 656–661.

Farrar, J.D., Smith, J.D., Murphy, T.L., Leung, S., Stark, G.R., and Murphy, K.M. (2000). Selective loss of type I interferon-induced STAT4 activation caused by a minisatellite insertion in mouse Stat2. *Nat Immunol 1*, 65–69.

Fernandes, G. and Jolly, C.A. (1998). Nutrition and autoimmune disease. *Nutr Rev 56*, S161–S169.

Fujitani, T., Tada, Y., and Yoneyama, M. (2004). Chlorpropham-induced splenotoxicity and its recovery in rats. *Food Chem Toxicol 42*, 1469–1477.

Gagro, A., McCloskey, N., Challa, A., Holder, M., Grafton, G., Pound, J.D. *et al.* (2000). CD5-positive and CD5-negative human B cells converge to an indistinguishable population on signalling through B-cell receptors and CD40. *Immunology 101*, 201–209.

Haley, P.J. (2003). Species differences in the structure and function of the immune system. *Toxicology 188*, 49–71.

Hayakawa, K. and Hardy, R.R. (2000). Development and function of B-1 cells. *Curr Opin Immunol 12*, 346–353.

Herndon, F.J., Hsu, H.C., and Mountz, J.D. (1997). Increased apoptosis of CD45RO- T cells with aging. *Mech Ageing Dev 94*, 123–134.

Hirokawa, K. and Utsuyama, M. (2002). Animal models and possible human application of immunological restoration in the elderly. *Mech Ageing Dev 123*, 1055–1063.

Holling, T.M., Schooten, E., and van Den Elsen, P.J. (2004). Function and regulation of MHC class II molecules in T-lymphocytes: Of mice and men. *Hum Immunol 65*, 282–290.

Jolly, C.A. (2004). Dietary restriction and immune function. *J Nutr 134*, 1853–1856.

Jolly, C.A., Muthukumar, A., Avula, C.P., Troyer, D., and Fernandes, G. (2001). Life span is prolonged in food-restricted autoimmune-prone (NZB × NZW) F(1) mice fed a diet enriched with (n-3) fatty acids. *J Nutr 131*, 2753–2760.

Kerner, J.D., Appleby, M.W., Mohr, R.N., Chien, S., Rawlings, D.J., Maliszewski, C.R. *et al.* (1995). Impaired expansion of mouse B cell progenitors lacking Btk. *Immunity 3*, 301–312.

Klinman, N.R. and Kline, G.H. (1997). The B-cell biology of aging. *Immunol Rev 160*, 103–114.

Koo, G.C., Blake, J.T., Talento, A., Nguyen, M., Lin, S., Sirotina, A. *et al.* (1997). Blockade of the voltage-gated potassium channel Kv1.3 inhibits immune responses in vivo. *J Immunol 158*, 5120–5128.

Ku, C.C., Kotzin, B., Kappler, J., and Marrack, P. (1997). CD8+ T-cell clones in old mice. *Immunol Rev 160*, 139–144.

LeMaoult, J., Szabo, P., and Weksler, M.E. (1997). Effect of age on humoral immunity, selection of the B-cell repertoire and B-cell development. *Immunol Rev 160*, 115–126.

Lenschow, D.J., Walunas, T.L., and Bluestone, J.A. (1996). CD28/B7 system of T cell costimulation. *Annu Rev Immunol 14*, 233–258.

Mainou-Fowler, T., Dignum, H.M., Proctor, S.J., and Summerfield, G.P. (2004). The prognostic value of CD38 expression and its quantification in B cell chronic lymphocytic leukemia (B-CLL). *Leuk Lymphoma 45*, 455–462.

Miller, R.A., Garcia, G., Kirk, C.J., and Witkowski, J.M. (1997). Early activation defects in T lymphocytes from aged mice. *Immunol Rev 160*, 79–90.

Muthukumar, A., Sun, D., Zaman, K., Barnes, J.L., Haile, D., and Fernandes, G. (2004). Age associated alterations in costimulatory and adhesion molecule expression in lupus-prone mice are attenuated by food restriction with n-6 and n-3 fatty acids. *J Clin Immunol 24*, 471–480.

Muthukumar, A., Zaman, K., Lawrence, R., Barnes, J.L., and Fernandes, G. (2003). Food restriction and fish oil suppress atherogenic risk factors in lupus-prone (NZB × NZW) F1 mice. *J Clin Immunol 23*, 23–33.

Muthukumar, A.R., Jolly, C.A., Zaman, K., and Fernandes, G. (2000). Calorie restriction decreases proinflammatory cytokines and polymeric Ig receptor expression in the submandibular glands of autoimmune prone (NZB × NZW)F1 mice. *J Clin Immunol 20*, 354–361.

Oliver, A.M., Martin, F., and Kearney, J.F. (1997). Mouse CD38 is down-regulated on germinal center B cells and mature plasma cells. *J Immunol 158*, 1108–1115.

Osiecki, H. (2004). The role of chronic inflammation in cardiovascular disease and its regulation by nutrients. *Altern Med Rev 9*, 32–53.

Pabst, R. and Gehrke, I. (1990). Is the bronchus-associated lymphoid tissue (BALT) an integral structure of the lung in normal mammals, including humans? *Am J Respir Cell Mol Biol 3*, 131–135.

Pahlavani, M.A. (2000). Caloric restriction and immunosenescence: a current perspective. *Front Biosci 5*, D580–D587.

Prasad, D.V., Nguyen, T., Li, Z., Yang, Y., Duong, J., Wang, Y. *et al.* (2004). Murine B7-H3 is a negative regulator of T cells. *J Immunol 173*, 2500–2506.

Prieyl, J.A. and LeBien, T.W. (1996). Interleukin 7 independent development of human B cells. *Proc Natl Acad Sci USA 93*, 10348–10353.

Qiao, J.H., Castellani, L.W., Fishbein, M.C., and Lusis, A.J. (1993). Immune-complex-mediated vasculitis increases coronary artery lipid accumulation in autoimmune prone MRL mice. *Arterioscler Thromb 13*, 932–943.

Riley, S.C., Froscher, B.G., Linton, P.J., Zharhary, D., Marcu, K., and Klinman, N.R. (1989). Altered VH gene segment utilization in the response to phosphorylcholine by aged mice. *J Immunol 143*, 3798–3805.

Ross, R. (1999). Atherosclerosis–an inflammatory disease. *N Engl J Med 340*, 115–126.

Spits, H., Blom, B., Jaleco, A.C., Weijer, K., Verschuren, M.C., van Dongen, J.J. *et al.* (1998). Early stages in the development of human T, natural killer and thymic dendritic cells. *Immunol Rev 165*, 75–86.

Sternberg, S.S. (1997). *Histology for Pathologists*. Philadelphia: Lippincott Williams and Wilkins.

Tokugawa, Y., Koyama, M., and Silver, J. (1997). A molecular basis for species differences in Thy-1 expression patterns. *Mol Immunol 34*, 1263–1272.

Venkatraman, J.T. and Chu, W.C. (1999). Effects of dietary omega-3 and omega-6 lipids and vitamin E on serum cytokines, lipid mediators and anti-DNA antibodies in a mouse model for rheumatoid arthritis. *J Am Coll Nutr 18*, 602–613.

Wang, S. and Chen, L. (2004). Co-signaling molecules of the B7-CD28 family in positive and negative regulation of T lymphocyte responses. *Microbes Infect 6*, 759–766.

Wicker, L.S. and Scher, I. (1986). X-linked immune deficiency (xid) of CBA/N mice. *Curr Top Microbiol Immunol 124*, 87–101.

Wortis, H.H., Teutsch, M., Higer, M., Zheng, J., and Parker, D.C. (1995). B-cell activation by crosslinking of surface IgM or ligation of CD40 involves alternative signal pathways and results in different B-cell phenotypes. *Proc Natl Acad Sci USA 92*, 3348–3352.

Xu, Z., George, C., and Jolly, C.A. (2004). CD28 activation does not down-regulate Cbl-b expression in aged rat T-lymphocytes. *Mech Ageing Dev 125*, 595–602.

Zamoyska, R. and Parnes, J.R. (1988). A CD8 polypeptide that is lost after passing the Golgi but before reaching the cell surface: a novel sorting mechanism. *Embo J 7*, 2359–2367.

Zheng, B., Han, S., Takahashi, Y., and Kelsoe, G. (1997). Immunosenescence and germinal center reaction. *Immunol Rev 160*, 63–77.

66

Human T Cell Clones in Long-Term Culture as Models for the Impact of Chronic Antigenic Stress in Aging

Graham Pawelec, Erminia Mariani, Rafael Solana, Rosalyn Forsey, Anis Larbi, Simona Neri, Olga Dela Rosa, Yvonne Barnett, Jon Tolson, and Tamas Fülöp

Monoclonal human T lymphocytes can be maintained untransformed in tissue culture by intermittent antigen restimulation in the presence of growth factors for only a finite period (which, however, varies greatly from clone to clone). This tissue culture model can be employed to examine many aspects of clonal expansion and contraction under conditions of chronic antigenic stress, such as that which occurs in vivo *in the elderly (where herpes viruses represent an important chronic stressor), as well as in cancer. In this context, the model can be used for biomarker discovery at the genomic, proteomic, and functional levels, and to test remedial interventions of possible utility* in vivo. *Furthermore, the clonal characteristics of cells from donors of different ages and states can be compared using this model (cloning efficiency, mean longevity, maximum longevity, aging behavior, etc.). This chapter briefly describes techniques for the production and maintenance of human T cell clones, their growth characteristics and longevity* in vitro, *culture age-associated changes of parameters such as telomere lengths, DNA damage, surface molecules and so on, and the application of proteomic analyses to study this model of immunosenescence in detail.*

Introduction

T cells from young or old donors can be cloned and cultured *in vitro*, provided that they are supplied with growth factors and intermittently stimulated via their surface receptors for antigen and costimuli. The critical advantage of using monoclonal populations is that the changes observed over time are not due to age-associated alterations in the proportions of different T cell subsets, a confounding factor plaguing innumerable studies. Mostly, peripheral blood lymphocytes are the starting material for cloning, but other sources of T cells, such as lymph node, behave in the same manner. On initial stimulation, T cells upregulate growth factor receptors, which are soon down-regulated again regardless of the presence of growth factors unless restimulation via the antigen receptor (or under certain circumstances, other surface receptors) takes place. Restimulation is required for re-upregulation of growth factor receptors and continued growth. Restimulation too soon after antigen exposure, on the other hand, may lead to activation-induced cell death by apoptosis (activation-induced cell death, or AICD), whereby the definition of "too soon" changes according to circumstances, importantly, including the age of the clone, and is also different from clone to clone. Thus, T cell clones (TCC) must be maintained in careful balance between too much antigen (apoptosis) and too little (growth termination). Under appropriate culture conditions, all major subsets of T cells can be cloned (i.e., CD4+ TCR2, CD8+ TCR2, CD4, 8-negative TCR1, and NKT cells). However, the latter two types are more difficult to maintain. Clonal longevity studies are rare because of the time-consuming nature of the experiments, but some data are available on the behavior of human T cell clones from different sources.

Generation and Growth Characteristics of Human TCC

Early data from McCarron *et al.* (1987) suggested that clonal longevity was influenced by age of the donor: clones derived from neonates averaged 52 population doublings (PD), those derived from young adults (20–30 yr) managed 40 PD, but those from the elderly (70–90 yr) only 32 PD, as calculated from the data given in that publication. Our own more extensive results are somewhat different: although individual T cell clones do have very varied life spans, the overall patterns for T cells of quite different origins and donors of different ages are remarkably similar. Table 66.1 provides a cumulative update of our experience with $CD4^+$ TCC, following previously published work (Pawelec *et al.*, 2002).

Cloning peripheral T cells from young healthy donors can be performed with a high cloning efficiency

Handbook of Models for Human Aging

TABLE 66.1
Longevity of human CD4^{+} T cell clones

Clones/Origin	%CE	Expts	Percentage of clones reaching: 20 PD	30 PD	40 PD	Longest lived clone
CD3 (young)	47	1355/15	47	24	15	90 PD
CD3 (old)	52	298/7	48	26	16	77
CD3 (cent)	38	52/3	41	23	17	80
CD3 (CML)	49	35/1	60	35	14	51
CD34 (periph)	55	533/6	31	17	6	60
CD34 (cord)	43	94/2	29	15	5	57

CE, cloning efficiency (calculated from percentage of wells positive in cloning plates). Longevity is expressed as a percentage of established clones (i.e., those counted as positive in calculating the CE) that survive to 20, 30, or 40 population doublings (PD) (10^6, 10^9, 10^{12} cells, respectively). Origins: CD3, mature peripheral T cells from: (young)—apparently healthy donors under 30 yr.; (old)—perfectly healthy SENIEUR-compliant donors over 80 yr.; (cent)—centenarian donors >100 yr.; (CML)—middle-aged donor with chronic myelogenous leukemia in chronic phase treated with interferon-α; CD34, positively selected lineage-negative hematopoietic progenitor cells from peripheral (periph) or umbilical cord (cord) blood (Pawelec *et al.*, 1998).

(CE) of >50%, suggesting that these particular cloning conditions are favorable for outgrowth of a majority of T cells. However, cloning mixtures of T cells result in most of the TCC obtained being CD4^{+}. To obtain CD8 (or TCR1 and especially NKT) cells, it is necessary to presort or otherwise remove CD4 cells. Cloning from a mixture of CD4 and CD8 cells with a CE of >50% implies that almost all CD4^{+} cells are initially clonable (defined as accumulation of ca. 1000 cells from one original cell). The CD4 T cell repertoire of the starting population is therefore present more or less in its entirety. However, after 20 PD, when the clone size has increased from 10^3 to 10^6, about half of the clones have been lost (mean of 47% for cloning of young donor CD3 cells; see Table 66.1). By 30 PD, about another half is lost, so that only one quarter of the originally clonable cells is still present. However, at 40 PD (which theoretically represents a very large clone size of 10^{12} cells), although more clones have been lost, 15% of the original starting clonal population does still remain. These results indicate constant attrition of the T cell population at the clonal level, but with retention of something like 5% of the original CD4 repertoire up to 40 PD and with retention of very rare clones for considerably longer. Although difficult to establish, similar clonal attrition probably occurs *in vivo* as well, at least in infectious mononucleosis, perhaps with quite similar distributions of clonal longevities (Maini *et al.*, 1999).

Comparisons of T cell CE from young or old donors, or other sources, may be informative. Our hypothesis was that T cells generated *in situ* from CD34^{+} hematopoietic progenitors would have greater longevities due to their lack of a previous T cell proliferative history (Pawelec *et al.*, 1998). Reciprocally, we anticipated that CE of cells from the elderly would be reduced as would their clonal longevity, and that this would be more prevalent in less healthy donors than in those rigorously selected for good health. Finally, we predicted that T cells from younger donors but in situations of chronic *in vivo* antigenic stress, such as in cancer, also would have lower CE and longevities. However, none of these expectations was fulfilled (see Table 66.1). CE was not lower in the elderly than in the young, and neither was the state of health of the donor critical. The CE was equally high when the cells derived from a patient with chronic myelogenous leukemia, a donor putatively subjected to a high level of antigenic stress. CE was also similar in the extra-thymic T cell differentiation cultures employed. It has to be concluded that CEs of the T cells from these markedly different sources are nonetheless similar. Is this true for average and maximum longevity also? It seems so: very similar proportions of TCC achieve 20, 30, and 40 PD regardless of their origin. In addition, the maximum longevity of the longest-lived clone is also similar and very close to the Hayflick Limit of 50–60 PD. Overall, it seems that CE and longevities of T cells in culture are essentially identical regardless of whether the cells to be cloned are derived from progenitors, young or old donors, healthy or sick.

PROTOCOL FOR CLONING BY LIMITING DILUTION

1. Dilute the cells for cloning in culture medium (e.g., RPMI 1640 + 15% prescreened FCS or human serum; or serum-free medium such as X-Vivo 15) to which 40 U/ml of IL-2 is added. Set the concentration so that 10 μl contain 45, 4.5, or 0.45 cells. Then plate 10 μl of the 0.45 suspension into 60 × 1 mm-diameter wells of culture trays (Terasaki plates) and leave in a vibration-free area for an hour. Check the distribution of cells in the wells visually using an inverted microscope, being careful to look around the edges of the wells. According to

the Poisson distribution, only a maximum of 37% of the wells should contain cells. Readjust dilutions if necessary, and recheck.

2. Plate at least five trays with the 0.45 cells/10 μl, suspension, one with 4.5 and one with 45, and add a constant number of feeder cells to each well. Irradiated PBMC commonly are used as feeder cells at 1×10^4/well. Use autologous PBMC, a mixture of autologous PBMC and autologous B-lymphoblastoid line cells, or other appropriate APC, in the presence of specific antigen. Alternatively, use an antigen-nonspecific stimulus such as 50 ng/ml of the anti-CD3 monoclonal antibody OKT3 or 2 μg/ml of the mitogen PHA, together with the same number of allogeneic or autologous PBMC.
3. Stack plates and wrap in aluminum foil for ease of handling and as a precaution against contamination. Incubate for about a week and then examine the plates using an inverted microscope. Transfer contents of positive wells (>one-third full, ca. 1000 cells) to 7 mm-diameter flat-bottom microtiter plate wells with fresh medium and 1×10^5 of the same feeder cells as before. Check Terasaki plates again at intervals of a few days up to two to three weeks of age to identify late developers and transfer these also. Check microtiter plates every few days, and identify wells becoming crowded within a week post-transfer. These must be split 1:1 into new culture wells and re-fed with medium (but not feeder cells). After one week in microtiter plates, contents of wells with growing cells are transferred to 16 mm-diameter cluster plate wells with two 5×10^5 of the same feeder cells, and fresh medium. Observe after three to four days and establish which wells are already full or nearly full. The former should be divided into four, the latter into two, with fresh media, but no more feeders. After a total of one week in cluster plates, count the number of cells in each clone and split to 2×10^5/well, again with two 5×10^5 feeders/well and fresh medium. Feed after three to four days with fresh medium, and split again if necessary. Clones successfully propagated in cluster plate wells for this second week are taken to be established. At this point, some (or all) can be cryopreserved and the remainder cultured under different conditions to establish optimal parameters for each particular clone. Having a frozen stock enables one to test different culture conditions in order to optimize growth, without the fear of losing the whole clone.
4. Test whether established clones can be propagated with the most convenient feeder cells (80 Gy-irradiated B-lymphoblastoid cell lines) instead of PBMC feeders. Most TCC flourish on B-LCL alone, but some appear for unknown reasons to benefit from the presence of PBMC as well (this is especially true during cloning). Propagation of the TCC on PBMC feeders can also be continued, but it may be found preferable to prepare standardizable batches of B-LCL rather than having to repeatedly isolate PBMC. Furthermore, PBMC from the autologous donor may not be freely available in sufficient amounts for large-scale propagation of numerous clones. The international availability of well-characterized MHC homozygous B-LCL makes it possible to match the feeder cell to the specificity of the TCC being propagated and enhance the antigen-presentation function of the feeders.
5. As a matter of convenience, it is easier to grow TCC in scaled-up culture vessels than in cluster plates, but not all clones can be adapted to growth in flasks. This must also be tested for each clone, using 1×10^5 and 5×10^5/ml TCC with an equal number of feeders in tissue culture flasks. Those clones not growing under these conditions rarely can be adapted to flask growth by altering the amounts or concentrations of TCC or feeders seeded or by increasing or decreasing the frequency of stimulation and/or feeding. It remains unknown why some TCC fail to flourish in flasks.
6. Establish restimulation parameters for each clone. T cells require periodic reactivation through the T cell antigen receptor in order to retain responsiveness to growth factors. This can be accomplished specifically or nonspecifically. All clones can be propagated with weekly restimulation; some but not all can be propagated with restimulation only every two weeks. Human T cell clones can be readily cryopreserved using the same protocols as are suitable for freezing resting T cells. Clones developing with different kinetics can thus be collected and conveniently tested for cytotoxicity in the same experiment.

Age-Associated Alterations to the Cells During Culture

SURFACE PHENOTYPE AND FUNCTION

This *in vitro* clonal culture model may also be informative for longitudinal studies of age-related changes in TCC under chronic antigenic stress. Because of the constraints of the cloning procedure, young cells already have accomplished at least 22 or 23 PD, but at this stage, we still have a good representation of the starting repertoire (as discussed earlier). One of the simplest analytical techniques to study these cells over time is to use flow cytometry with monoclonal antibodies detecting molecules expressed on the cell surface. We have examined a large range of different surface markers and found relatively few that change with age (where aging is defined as increasing PD). The most common pattern of age-associated alterations involves a reduction of the level of expression of the costimulatory receptor CD28, and sometimes the putative costimulatory receptors CD134 and CD154 (Pawelec *et al.*, 1997), whereas despite increased susceptibility to AICD, surface CD95 expression remains constant (Pawelec *et al.*, 1996). The cells have a memory effector phenotype (CD45RA-negative, CCR7-negative, CD45RO$^+$) as would be expected from chronically stimulated T cells. The level of the TCR also remains stable, suggesting that these cells retain the ability to recognize and respond to antigen. Major functional changes may follow from the decreased level of expression of costimulatory receptors, both CD28 and in all likelihood others yet to be investigated. The most dramatic changes are in the patterns of cytokines secreted, commonly resulting in decreased levels of IL 2 and increased levels of IL 10 (Pawelec *et al.*, 1997). Because the expression of the TCR is maintained and antigen-specific signaling still occurs, it is likely that these differences are caused by differences in the delivery of costimuli to the T cells.

TCC RECEPTORS AND SIGNAL TRANSDUCTION

T cell functions are mediated by intracellular signaling via surface receptors such as the antigen receptor and the costimulator CD28, as discussed earlier, from the membrane (early events) through the cytoplasm (intermediate events) to the nucleus (late events). Age-related immune alterations can be partially explained by defects in receptor signal transduction. For instance, decreased calcium mobilization, MAPKinase phosphorylation, PKCθ recruitment to the membrane, NF-κB translocation to the nucleus and ultimately IL-2 production are hallmarks of T cell senescence. TCR ligation induces its phosphorylation at specific sites and its redistribution to specific membrane microdomains, called lipid rafts. This redistribution, also known as polarization, allows the formation of the signalosome, a large signaling platform composed of key signaling molecules that must be properly configured within the lipid raft. The signaling cascade involving tyrosine kinase activation (p56^{Lck}, ZAP-70), adaptor proteins (linker of activated T cells), and second messenger generation including calcium mobilization will take place only if these conditions are fulfilled. Cholesterol is a major constituent of lipid rafts, conferring on them their specific characteristics and permitting their stability. It has been shown that polyunsaturated fatty acid content will determine the association of signaling molecules in lipid rafts. All these parameters would influence membrane fluidity and ultimately cell signaling/activation. Alterations to lipid rafting with age could represent an important aspect of senescence (Larbi *et al.*, 2004b).

Lipid raft isolation protocol

Lipid rafts are insoluble in nonionic detergents such as Triton X-100, and application of a sucrose gradient (45% to 5% sucrose) allows them to be separated from the other membrane domains. For this purpose, cell lysates in Triton X-100 1% are overlaid with sucrose and ultra-centrifuged for 16 h at 100,000 rpm at 4°C. Fractions from the top are collected and analyzed for lipid raft markers, among the best of which are gangliosides (GM1 and GM3). However, recent data indicate heterogeneity in lipid raft composition in each cell type. In this connection, flotillin can be used, even for functionally different rafts. Once the lipid raft fractions are identified, several experiments including protein localization/phosphorylation (Western-blotting), kinase activity, and immunoprecipitation can be performed to assess composition. Lipid raft fluidity can be assessed using diphenylhexatriene as a probe for fluorescence anisotropy.

How to visualize lipid rafts

To analyze membrane organization, and protein–protein interaction in the resting state, as well as following receptor ligation, microscopy procedures are available. Lipid rafts can be stained using Alexa-conjugated cholera toxin β-subunit (Molecular Probes) and lipid rafting in T cells monitored in a time- and stimulus-dependent manner. Colocalization studies can be performed to have direct imaging of signal transduction changes during immune senescence.

Lipid raft composition (lipids, signaling molecules) will determine TCC activation. A change in lipid raft properties has already been described in T cells from SLE patients. With the tools described in the previous section it is possible to determine even slight changes in lipid raft properties, which may, in turn, have critical effects as seen in immune senescence. One way of examining this is to use fluorescence anisotropy (inverse value of fluidity) on TCC from donors of different ages at different PD. As shown in Table 66.2, anisotropy in TCC decreases as the PD increases. This indicates an increased fluidity with cell expansion, which may result from a loss of membrane cholesterol. These data corroborate findings in primary T cells concerning fluidity during TCR- and CD28-induced proliferation.

TABLE 66.2
Anisotropy (r) measured in T cell clones originated from individuals of various ages at different population doublings (PD)

	Anisotropy (r)			
TCC from: PD	Progenitors	Young	Elderly	Centenarians
Low	0.283	0.286	0.270	0.263
Medium	0.266	0.275	0.260	0.252
High	0.294	0.268	0.253	0.245

Anisotropy (r) is the inverse value of fluidity: (f) = 1 / (r)
Cells were incubated 30 min at 37°C with diphenylhexatriene (DPH) at 2 μM. Anisotropy is directly measured using a spectrofluorimeter coupled to a polarizer (Larbi *et al.*, 2004a).

The lowest membrane fluidity was observed at any doubling in TCC derived from centenarians, indicating a high degree of functionality and adaptability. The progressive change in membrane fluidity is part of the immune senescence of TCC and may help to explain age-associated TCC behavior.

TELOMERE LENGTH AND GENOME INTEGRITY

Telomeres are specialized structures consisting of characteristic DNA repeat sequences and a complex of associated proteins, which cap and protect chromosome ends and serve to preserve genome integrity. In most somatic cells, progressive rounds of cell division are associated with telomere shortening. The length, structure, and function of telomeres have been proposed to contribute to cellular and organism phenotypes associated with cancer and aging (Kim *et al.*, 2000). In order to protect the germline and the subpopulation of stem cells from senescence, mechanisms have evolved to prevent telomere attrition in these cellular compartments. The most common and best-studied mechanism involves the activation of a ribonucleoprotein enzyme complex known as telomerase (Granger *et al.*, 2002). Nonetheless, the analysis of telomere length in a particular cell type can be a biomarker of its replicative history and cellular senescence.

The measurement of telomere length in the TCC is an important method to determine whether these cells reach replicative senescence in culture as they do *ex vivo*. The flow-FISH technique (Rufer *et al.*, 1998) in which a fluorescein isothiocyanate (FITV)-labeled telomere-specific peptide nucleic acid (PNA) probe is hybridized in a quantitative way to telomere repeats, followed by telomere fluorescence measurements on individual cells by flow cytometry, is in common use for this purpose. The advantages of looking at the telomere fluorescence in different types of cells in the same sample (lymphocytes and P815 cells), and the requirement for relatively low numbers of cells (10^5), are an important reason for using this method instead of Southern blotting (Baerlocher *et al.*, 2002). It is necessary to use an internal control for telomere length; for this purpose, the P815 cell line is mixed with the TCC.

Telomere protocol

1. Wash TCC in phosphate-buffered saline (PBS), centrifuge at 400 g for 5 min, and resuspend in 1 ml PBS. After washing, mix TCC 1:1 with P815 cells and collect a total of 1×10^6 mixed cells in 1.5 ml tubes. Hybridize cells with or without the FITC-labeled $(C_3TA_2)_3$ peptide nucleic acid probe and incubate 10 minutes at 82°C to separate double-stranded DNA. Then incubate at room temperature overnight.
2. Remove the hybridization solution by incubating with wash solution at 40°C for 10 minutes and remove after spinning down. After two washes, stain with propidium iodide (PI) and RNAse A solution in order to stain DA for G_0/G_1 selection. After three hours of incubation at 4°C, the cells are maintained at 4°C until data acquisition.
3. To correct for daily shifts in the linearity of the flow cytometer, FITC-labeled fluorescent calibration beads (Dako FluoroSpheres, Denmark) each having a fluorescence corresponding to different known amounts of molecular equivalents of soluble fluorochrome (MESF), have to be run in each experiment. The FL1 channel is used for detection of the fluorescein signal and the FL3 channel for PI. Collect 10^4 cells in each experiment.
4. The telomere fluorescence signal is defined as the mean fluorescence signal in G_0/G_1 cells after subtraction of the background fluorescence signal (i.e., FISH procedure without probe). The relative telomere length value is calculated as the ratio between the telomere signal of each sample and the control cell line (P815) with compensation for the DNA index of G_0/G_1 cells. This compensation is performed in order to normalize the number of telomere ends per cell. As seen in Figure 66.1A, the single-cell population is selected in the FL3-width versus FL3-area dot plot. The gated cells are then displayed in the FSC and SSC dot plot to separate the P815 cells from the TCC (see Figure 66.1B, gates R2 and R3), which are validated in experiments with purified suspensions. As the number of chromosomes and thus telomere ends is strongly correlated with the DNA index calculated from DNA histogram analyses, select the G_0/G_1 phase of the cell cycle, because at this stage the cell has one copy of its genome. This is achieved by setting the correct gates (see Figure 66.1C, gates R4 and R5). The cell cycle phases from the DNA histograms need to have a variation coefficient lower than 7% of cells out of the G_0/G_1 phase (Rapi *et al.*, 1996).
5. The telomere fluorescence intensity is then analyzed in the FITC histogram using the previously selected gates with the P815 cell line as a positive control. For each TCC, the specific telomere fluorescence is calculated by subtracting the mean fluorescence of the background control (no probe) from the mean fluorescence obtained from cells hybridized with the telomere probe. The concept of Relative Telomere Length (RTL) is used to assess differences between TCC, with P815 defined as 100%.

Figure 66.2 shows an example of the kind of data obtained with TCC using this technique. In the majority, there is a decrease of the RTL at the first 40 PD. Thereafter, clones exceeding this life span may show stabilization or even increased RTL on further culture.

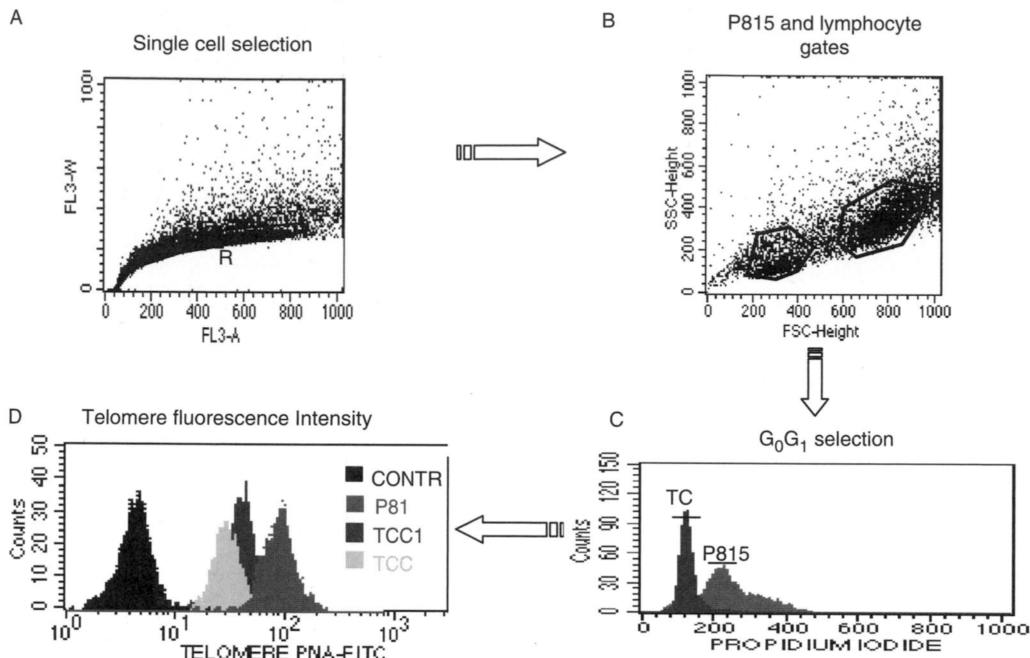

Figure 66.1 Flow Fish analysis of T cell clones. T cell clones were mixed with the P815 cell line, and the mixed sample was analyzed after hybridisation with or without FITC-labeled $(C_3TA_2)_3$ peptide nucleic acid. Cells were gated on region 1 (R1) on the basis of FL3-A and FL3-W to select single cells as shown in **A**. Different regions were selected within R1 from forward (FSC) versus side scatter (SSC) dot plots for P815 and TCC, as is shown in **B**. Results within TCC and P815 were depicted for cell cycle on histogram **C** to select the G_0/G_1 cells. Histogram **D** represents the analysis of the PNA fluorescence intensity of two different T cell clones, and the highest peak shows the P815 positive control cells.

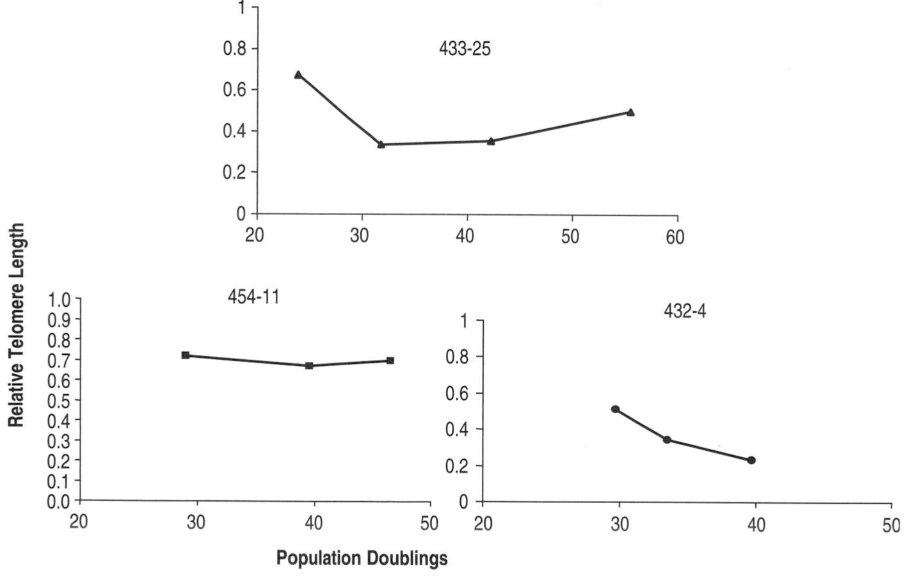

Figure 66.2 Relative telomere length of different TCC. The y axis represents the RTL of TCC versus the time of culture in terms of Population Doublings. Three different TCC are shown (Clones 433-25, 454-11, and 432-4).

MICROSATELLITE INSTABILITY (MSI)

The influence of DNA repair capacity on genomic integrity is suggested by the positive correlation between life span and DNA repair capacity and evidenced by progeroid syndromes in which DNA repair defects can cause phenotypes resembling premature aging (Lombard *et al.*, 2005). The accurate maintenance of nuclear DNA is critical to cell and organism functions, and therefore numerous DNA repair pathways have evolved for the different types of DNA lesions. Among these pathways, the nucleotide excision repair mechanism (because of its role in repair of UV-induced damage) and the nonhomologous end joining pathway (the predominant double-strand break repair system) are the most intensely studied, and together with the base excision repair pathway do appear to be altered with age (Lombard *et al.*, 2005). The function of the mismatch repair (MMR) system during aging is to scan newly replicated DNA and to deal with replicative and recombinational errors leading to mispaired bases (mismatches) by excising the mutated strand in either direction to the mismatch, thus contributing to genomic protection against replication-induced mutations (Loeb, 1994). This would be most important in rapidly replicating cells, such as TCC.

An experimental approach to the study of defects in this pathway is the evaluation of microsatellite instability (MSI), evidenced by expansions or contractions of microsatellites, highly polymorphic tandemly-repeated sequences from one to six bases, interspersed in the genome and particularly prone to replication slippages that change strand lengths, either by insertion or deletion of repeated units.

Mutations occur both in repeated sequences and randomly throughout the genome. Therefore, MSI indicates a higher susceptibility to mutations. Despite the trend to errors occurring in all dividing cells, microsatellite lengths remain stable due to the intrinsic activity and fidelity of the MMR system. Hence, MSI serves as a marker for a malfunctioning MMR system. There is an increased instability both in the mucosa of aged patients with gastric lymphomas (Starostik *et al.*, 2000) and also in microsatellite sequences from total peripheral blood DNA of old subjects obtained at a 10-year interval (Ben Yehuda *et al.*, 2000; Krichevsky *et al.*, 2004; Neri *et al.*, 2005).

One possible cause of MMR deficiency could be the inactivation or the altered expression of MMR genes due to epigenetic mutations, as suggested by the finding of hypermethylation-mediated MMR gene inactivation in sporadic cancers showing microsatellite instability and by the age-related inactivation of hMLH1 by promoter methylation found in normal colon cells. Data on *in vitro* aging of TCC suggest that the MMR system could differently change its efficiency during *in vitro* proliferation, depending upon the cell type and/or that repeated doublings could contribute to the accumulation of genetic alterations not repaired by the MMR system (Neri *et al.*, 2004).

Protocol for MSI analysis

1. Extract genomic DNA from cell pellets using the QIAamp DNA Mini Kit (Qiagen GmbH, Germany) following the manufacturer's instructions; quantify DNA by spectrophotometric determination at 260 nm.
2. For MSI analysis, at least five repeated sequences should be tested; for example, the following loci containing tetra- and pentanucleotide polymorphic tandem repeat sequences: CD4 (12p13), a (TTTTC) repeat located in the 5′ nontranscribed region of the T cell surface antigen gene; VWA31 (12p12-pter), an (AGAT) repeat in intron 40 of the von Willebrand factor gene; Fes/FPS (15q25-qter), an (ATTT) repeat in intron 5 of the c-fes proto-oncogene; TPOX (2p23-pter), an (AATG) repeat in intron 10 of the thyroid peroxidase gene; p53 (17p13), an (AAAAT) repeat in the first intron of the TP53 gene.
   Carry out the PCR amplifications using the following specific primers:
   CD4-pF: 5′-TTGGAGTCGCAAGCTGAAC-TAGC-3′,
   CD4-pR: 5′-GCCTGAGTGACAGAGTGA-GAACC-3′;
   VWA31-pF: 5′-CCCTAGTGGATGATAAGAA-TAATCAGTATG-3′,
   VWA31-pR: 5′-GGACAGATGATAAATACA-TAGGATGGATGG-3′;
   Fes-pF: 5′-GGGATTTCCCTATGGATTGG-3′,
   Fes-pR: 5′-GCGAAAGAATGAGACTACAT-3′;
   TPOX-pF: 5′-ACTGGCACAGAACAGGCACT-TAGG-3′,
   TPOX-pR: 5′-GGAGGAACTGGGAACACA-CAGGT-3′;
   p53-pF: 5′-ACTCCAGCCTGGGCAATAA-GAGCT-3′,
   p53-pR: 5′-ACAAAACATCCCCTACAACAGC-3′.
   Combine template DNA (50 ng), 1 μM each primer, 200 μM each deoxynucleotide triphosphate, 1.5 mM (for CD4, FesTPOX and p53) or 2.5 mM (for VWA31) $MgCl_2$, 1X PCR buffer II (50 mM KCl, 10 mM Tris-HCl, pH 8.3) and 1.25 U AmpliTaq DNA Polymerase (Perkin Elmer, Roche Molecular Systems, USA) in 25-μl reactions. Amplification profiles are, respectively: 10 cycles (1′ 94°C, 45″ 62°C) followed by 20 cycles (1′ 90°C, 45″ 62°C) for CD4; 30 cycles (1′ 94°C, 1′ 57°C, 1′ 72°C) for VWA31; 30 cycles (1′ 94°C, 1′ 54°C, 1′ 72°C) for Fes; 30 cycles (1′ 94°C, 1′ 64°C, 1′ 72°C) for TPOX; and 30 cycles (1′ 94°C, 45″ 65°C, 45″ 72°C) for p53. Include in all reactions a negative control (sample without template).
3. Analyze 10 μl of each PCR product on 2% agarose gels in order to verify amplification and then perform electrophoresis with product-adjusted amounts on 10% nondenaturing polyacrylamide vertical gels (20 cm long, 0.75 mm thick) containing 5% glycerol, in TBE buffer, for 16 to 18 hrs at 100 to 150 V, together with the DNA Molecular Weight

Marker VIII (Roche Molecular Systems, Branchburg, USA) and allelic ladders prepared by mixing known alleles.

4. Silver stain gels at room temperature with continuous shaking. After 10′ fixation in 10% EtOH and 2′ oxidation in 1% nitric acid, stain the gels for 20′ in 0.02% $AgNO_2$, rinse in distilled water, and then reduce in developing solution (3% sodium carbonate and 0.1% formaldehyde) until an optimal band intensity is observed. Stop the development by adding 5% acetic acid for 3′ and finally place the gels in distilled water.
5. Conclude genotyping by side-by-side comparison with allelic ladders. Results showing allele modifications in DNA samples derived from the same donor must be confirmed by repeating the analysis.

DNA DAMAGE ACCUMULATION IN T CELLS AS A FUNCTION OF AGE

A more general approach to DNA damage and repair can also be informative in clonal models and *ex vivo* studies, several of which have shown that T cells *in vivo* accumulate DNA damage and mutations (point and chromosomal), for example, in free-living healthy humans aged 35 to 69 years. However, when the same genetic damage endpoints were examined in a group of healthy, older than average (75–80 years) humans, genetic damage levels similar to the levels present in subjects aged 35 to 39 years were found, and significantly less than in subjects aged 65 to 69 years (King *et al.*, 1997). These and many other data support the importance of maintenance of genomic stability, as a determinant factor promoting health and longevity. This hypothesis is supported by the results of work from others in premature aging conditions or in groups of successfully aged humans (centenarians) (Franceschi *et al.*, 1995).

Extensive use has been made of the *in vitro* human peripheral blood-derived CD4+ T cell clone model of immunosenescence described in this chapter in order to examine DNA damage accumulation under chronic antigenic stress (Hyland *et al.*, 2001). Alkaline comet assays revealed low levels of DNA damage as the clones progressed through their *in vitro* life span, with a significant increase in DNA damage in the majority of the clones immediately prior to the end of their life spans. The results of modified comet assays for the detection of oxidized purines and pyrimidines revealed an age-related increase in oxidative DNA damage in the TCC as they aged in culture. Figure 66.3 illustrates levels of oxidative purine damage in 11 peripheral blood-derived CD4+ T cell clones as a function of their age *in vitro*. Similar results have been found for levels of oxidative pyrimidine damage.

It is interesting to speculate what the biological consequences of genetic damage in T lymphocytes might be. There is much evidence that above a threshold level, genetic damage can cause cell cycle arrest in dividing cells, this effect being mediated via cyclin-dependent kinases and their inhibitors, or indeed induce apoptosis. Since T cells are required to undergo numerous rounds of replication following stimulation by a specific antigen prior to mounting an immune response, the impact of an age-related increase in genetic damage in T cells could be to reduce proliferative capacity of the T cells or inhibit capacity altogether, or indeed result in T cell death by apoptosis. It is interesting to note here that in studies with the CD4+ TCC model, approximately three to six days after the oldest weekly samplings of the T cells for analysis, and therefore when DNA damage levels were highest, the T cells die by apoptosis. It is not yet known if the age-related increase in genetic damage within T cells *in vivo* is sufficient to result in T cell replicative arrest or apoptosis. However, the results of previous studies have suggested that T cells containing mutations in genes coding for normal cellular metabolism may be selected against *in vivo*. T cells containing such mutations might have a reduced proliferative capacity, lowered response to proliferative stimuli, or may become nonviable. For example, Podlutsky *et al.* (1996) demonstrated that human T lymphocytes containing mutations in the HPRT gene have reduced proliferation rates *in vitro*. The work of Dempsey *et al.* (1983) to quantify the number of lymphocytes containing HPRT gene mutations in carriers of the Lesch–Nyhan mutation, found that only 1 to 9% of lymphocytes carried a mutation. This percentage is much lower than would be predicted (50%) for such carriers, suggesting that HPRT-negative mutant lymphocytes are selected against *in vivo*.

Protocol for the measurement of DNA damage by the comet assay

A suitable technique to examine levels of DNA damage (DNA single-strand breaks and alkali-labile lesions) in TCC is the alkaline comet assay, originally developed by Singh *et al.* (1988) and modified by Collins *et al.* (1993). In the latter, T cells embedded on slides are treated with either formamidopyrimidine glycosylase (FPG), which recognizes oxidatively modified purines, or with endonuclease III (ENDO III), which recognizes oxidatively modified pyrimidines. These enzymes nick DNA at the sites of oxidatively damaged nucleotides, creating single-strand breaks that can be detected with the alkaline comet assay.

1. Comet assays are performed at 4°C to minimize the repair of existing basal levels of DNA damage present in the T cells.
2. Cells are embedded in a 1% agarose gel on frosted microscope slides (2×10^4 cells/gel), and lysed for at least one hour in a high salt alkaline buffer (2.5 M NaCl, 0.1 M EDTA, 0.01 M Tris, 1%(v/v) Triton X-100, pH 10).

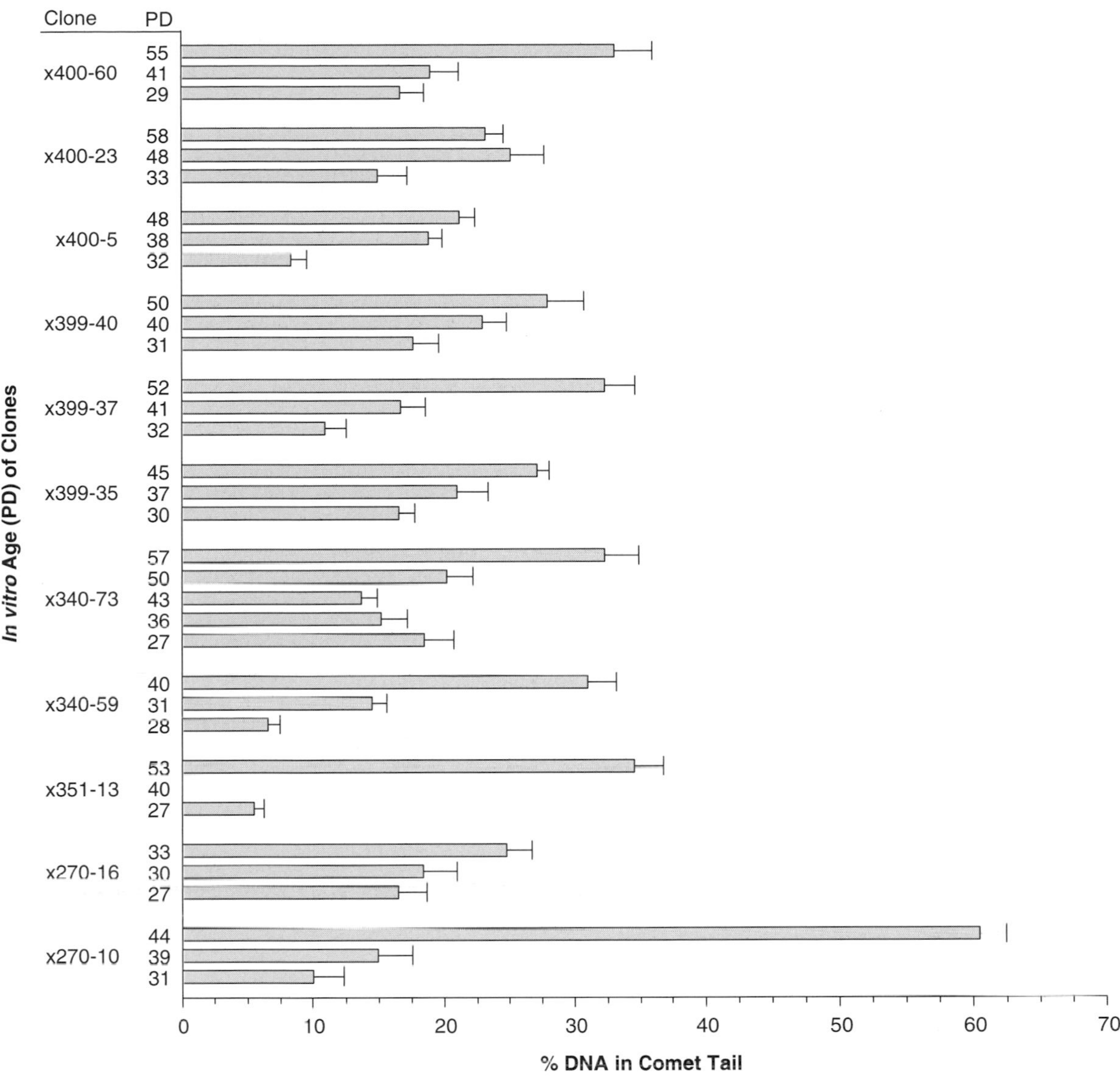

Figure 66.3 Levels of oxidative purine damage in 11 different TCC as a function of their *in vitro* life span, determined using a modified alkaline comet assay. Values represent the Mean ± SEM for each assay, counting 50 cells/slide.

3. For the modified comet assay, to determine levels of oxidative purine or pyrimidine damage, the following additional steps are performed:
   - FPG treatment:
     Slides must be equilibrated in enzyme buffer (0.04 M HEPES, 0.1 M KCl, 0.5 mM EDTA, 0.2 mg/ml BSA, pH 8.0) and then treated with the enzyme at 37°C in a humid, dark chamber for 45 minutes, which nicks oxidatively damaged purines, creating single strand breaks.
   - EndoIII treatment:
     Slides are equilibrated in enzyme buffer (0.04 M HEPES, 0.1 M KCl, 0.5 mM EDTA, 0.2 mg.ml BSA, pH 8.0) three times for five-minute washes and then treated with the enzyme at 37°C in a humid, dark chamber for 45 minutes, in this case nicking oxidatively damaged pyrimidines, creating single strand breaks.
4. Slides treated with the lesion-specific enzymes are then incubated at 37°C in a humid dark chamber for 45 minutes.
5. T cells treated with 150 μM hydrogen peroxide for five minutes at 4°C (to induce oxidative DNA damage) should be used as internal positive controls in the modified alkaline comet assay to verify enzyme activity.
6. Following enzyme treatment (or directly after alkaline lysis in the case of the alkaline comet assay) the slides are placed in an electrophoresis buffer (0.3 M NaOH, 1 mM EDTA, pH 13) for

40 minutes to allow alkaline unwinding of the DNA, and then electrophoresed at 25 V, 300 mA, for 30 minutes.

7. Following electrophoresis, the slides are neutralized using 0.4 M Tris pH 7.5 and stained with 50 μg/ml ethidium bromide. Stained slides can then be digitally analyzed, for example, using UV microscopy and Komet 3.0 analysis software (Kinetic Imaging, UK), counting 50 cells per slide. DNA damage results are expressed as percentage DNA in the comet tail.

PROTEOMICS

Today the common application of genomic analysis cannot reveal changes in proteins present in cells as they age, but it is a useful screening approach to focus on certain candidates that may change and can be specifically studied (as described elsewhere in this book). Alternatively, direct proteomic analyses using traditional 2-D-gels with or without antibody (Pawelec *et al.*, 1988) or more modern techniques can be applied. Here, we describe an example of a more recently introduced technique using SELDI ProteinChip® technology from Ciphergen (Freemont, CA). This approach combines the retention of proteins to an array surface by chemical or physical interaction followed by analysis by Laser Desorption/Ionisation Time of Flight mass spectrometry. A reproducible "protein profile" is achieved according to mass and has been applied successfully to the study of biological samples for the definition of candidate biomarkers of disease. Increasingly, the technology has been combined with powerful software analogues to distinguish ions that hold predictive significance of disease state, either individually or in combination with other ions. This marriage of analytical chemistry and bioinformatics has proved to be a very sensitive and novel proteomic technology, defining a paradigm in the way proteins can be analyzed in complex mixtures.

Proteomics protocol

TCC are lysed in 200 μl lysis buffer on ice (50 mM Tris HCl, 5 mM EDTA [pH 6.0], 2 mM PMSF, 1% Triton X-100), followed by five short bursts with a sonic finger before centrifugation at 150 × g for 20 minutes to pellet cell debris. Lysates are diluted 1:4 in pH 9.0 binding buffer (100 mM Tris Base) and applied to SAX2 (anion exchange) arrays (Ciphergen) in duplicate. Arrays are read in a ProteinChip Reader (Ciphergen) after the application of 2 × 0.6 μl sinapinic acid matrix. Generated spectra of masses in the range of 2000–16000 Daltons (Da) are calibrated externally by a mixture of known calibrants. Finally, profiles are aligned and normalized to a common mass occurring in all spectra at a consistent intensity. Using a multilayer perceptron Artificial Neural Network (ANN) (Neuroshell 2) with a back propagation algorithm, models can be generated to sort significant ions consistently predictive of known-age clones by stage, using raw data (mass to charge [m/z] value versus intensity) from mass ranges 2–5, 5–10, 10–16 (see Figure 66.4).

The top 100 ions of predictive value are selected from each and put forward to further analysis to rank a top 50. Ions with high predictive value that do not correlate with protein peak/part of peak signals on the original SELDI data are filtered out. In the example using 77 TCC samples shown here, the resulting ion list contained three ion-clusters at 9417-23 Da (cluster A), 9598-601 Da (B), and 9954-60 Da (C). Each cluster was tested individually and in conjunction with the other two for predictive ability. Though each cluster held little predictive value individually, in combination A+C and A+B+C were able to correctly predict the age of the test clones with greater than 70% accuracy. The model was then tested on seven unseen, validation clones. Again, both the top 50 and top 20 ions yielded >80% accuracy, though each cluster proved individually poor. The success of combining A+C could not be repeated on the unseen data, but of note is the ability of the model to predict with greater than 70% accuracy the combination of A+B+C, reflecting the result of the test data.

The selection of ion clusters around a certain mass and then cross-referencing with the SELDI data for the presence of a peak is an important step to eliminate artifacts from the data processing. For example, the ion with by far the most predictive power is a single ion found at 6463.08 Da but is very much within the noise of the SELDI data. This cannot be a protein or peptide. However, clustered ions in the top 20 could be correlated to peaks on the SELDI, and their predictive power established on seen and unseen data with some degree of success. Potentially, these proteins can be identified by biochemical methods and characterized to establish their true value within the aging model system studied here. This example illustrates the potency but also the potential pitfalls of this powerful combined proteomic/bioinformatic approach and the degree to which caution must be exercised in interpreting protein pattern data.

Conclusion

In this chapter, we have detailed a method for the production and maintenance of human monoclonal T cell populations in long-term culture, and we have provided selected examples of protocols for analytic techniques with which to seek age-associated changes therein (biomarkers of aging). The model represents a situation of chronic antigenic stress, where TCC are constantly reexposed to stimulating antigen. There are reasons to believe that this model does reflect common challenges to the immune system *in vivo*, particularly in the elderly where the chronic stressor may be Herpes virus, particularly Cytomegalovirus (CMV) (Pawelec *et al.*, 2004), but also in younger individuals carrying large antigenic loads that cannot be cleared (cancer patients, patients infected with persistent parasites, etc.). This chronic antigenic

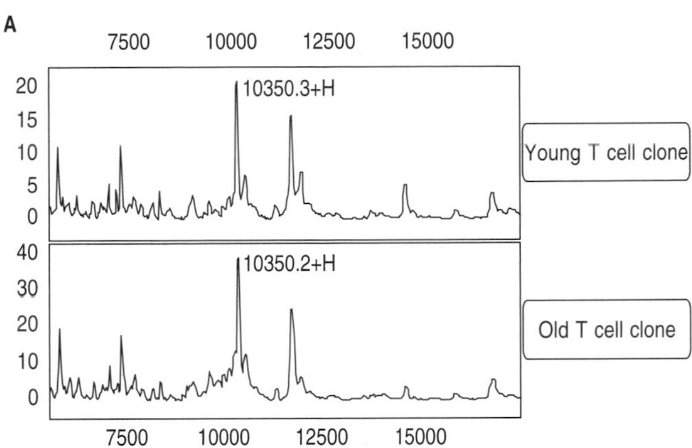

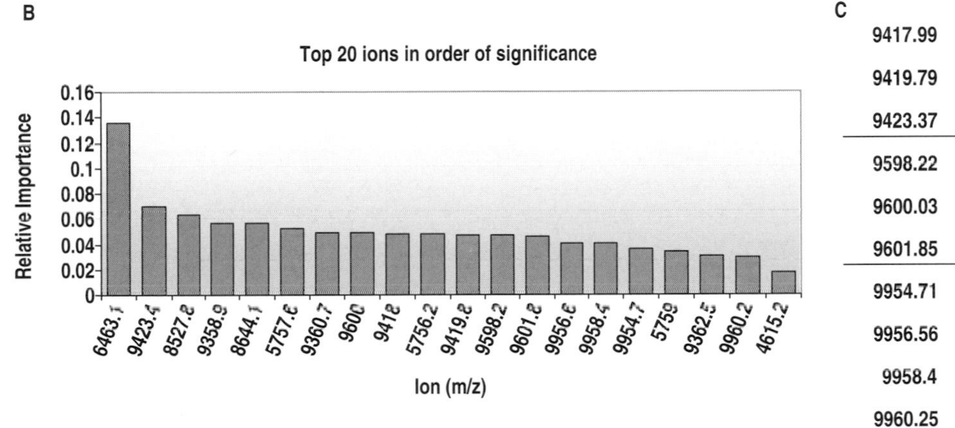

Figure 66.4 SELDI proteomic analysis of TCC. **A**: Example of SELDI mass spectra of young and old clones. **B**: Top 20 ions listed in order of predictive significance within ANN test data. **C**: Ion clusters from Top 20 list.

Accumulationof dysfunctional cells with age

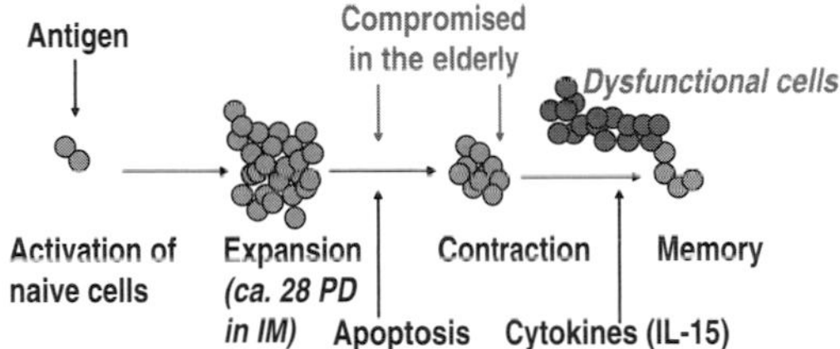

Conclusion: In IRP elderly, dysfunctional CD8+ CMV-specific T cells accumulate because apoptotic pathways are compromised.

Hypothesis: Because T cell homeostasis maintains constant numbers of T cells in the periphery, even if naive cells continue to be generated from the thymus, the T cell repertoire will be shrunken, contributing to increased susceptibility to infectious disease

Figure 66.5 Accumulation of dysfunctional cells with age; a hypothesis.

stress in the elderly leads to clonal exhaustion and shrinkage of the T cell repertoire, which increases susceptibility to novel pathogens, as sketched in Figure 66.5.

A cluster of age-associated immune alterations, including CMV status, designated the Immune Risk Phenotype (IRP) can be distinguished, which is predictive of mortality in longitudinal studies of the very elderly (Wikby *et al.*, 2005). Refinement of this concept and its extension to younger individuals, using lessons learned from culture models and tests of intervention carried out in those models, may contribute to improved immunity, better health, and decreased mortality due to immunosenescence.

Recommended Resources

The SAGE Web site is a useful resource (http://sageke.sciencemag.org/). Specialist journals or sites on immunosenescence are still rare. The new Open-Access journal *Immunity & Aging* aims to fill this gap (http://www.immunityageing.com/home/).

ACKNOWLEDGMENTS

The authors declare no conflicts of interest. Authors' collaborations now and previously have been supported by the European Commission via:

1. The Concerted Action on the Molecular Biology of Immunosenescence, EUCAMBIS (1994–1997). See

http://www.medizin.uni-tuebingen.de/eucambis/home/index.html.

2. The Thematic Network Immunology and Ageing in Europe (ImAginE) (2000–2002). See http://www.medizin.uni-tuebingen.de/imagine/index.htm.
3. T-Cells in Ageing (T-CIA) (2002–2005). See http://www.medizin.uni-tuebingen.de/t-cia/

as well as their local grants.

REFERENCES

Baerlocher, G.M., Mak, J., Tien, P., and Lansdorp, P.M. (2002). Telomere length measurement by fluorescence *in situ* hybridization and flow cytometry: Tips and pitfalls. *Cytometry 47*, 89–99.

Ben Yehuda, A., Globerson, A., Krichevsky, S., Bar On, H., Kidron, M. *et al.* (2000). Ageing and the mismatch repair system. *Mech. Ageing Dev. 121*, 173–179.

Collins, A.R., Duthie, S.J., and Dobson, V.L. (1993). Direct enzymatic detection of endogenous oxidative base damage in human lymphocyte DNA. *Carcinogenesis 14*, 1733–1735.

Dempsey, J.L., Morley, A.A., Seshadri, R.S., Emmerson, B.T., Gordon, R., and Bhagat, C.I. (1983). Detection of the carrier state for an X-linked disorder, the Lesch–Nyhan syndrome, by the use of lymphocyte cloning. *Hum. Genet. 64*, 288–290.

Franceschi, C., Monti, D., Sansoni, P., and Cossatizza, A. (1995). The immunology of exceptional individuals: the lesson of centenarians. *Immunol. Today 16*, 12–16.

Granger, M.P., Wright, W.E., and Shay, J.W. (2002). Telomerase in cancer and aging. *Crit. Rev. Oncol. Hematol. 41*, 29–40.

Hyland, P., Barnett, C., Pawelec, G., and Barnett, Y. (2001). Age-related accumulation of oxidative DNA damage and alterations in levels of $p16^{INK4a/CDKN2a}$, $p21^{WAF1/CIP1/SDI1}$ and $p27^{KIP1}$ in human CD4+ T cell clones *in vitro*. *Mech. Ageing Dev. 122*, 1151–1167.

Kim, S.H., Kaminker, P., and Campisi, J. (2002). Telomeres, aging and cancer: In search of a happy ending. *Oncogene 21*, 503–511.

King, C.M., Bristow-Craig, H.E., Gillespie, E.S., and Barnett, Y.A. (1997). *In vivo* antioxidant status, DNA damage, mutation and DNA repair capacity in cultured lymphocytes from healthy 75–80 year old humans. *Mut. Res. 377*, 137–147.

Krichevsky, S., Pawelec, G., Gural, A., Effros, R.B., Globerson, A., Ben Yehuda D. *et al.* (2004). Age related microsatellite instability in T cells from healthy individuals. *Exp. Gerontol. 39*, 507–515.

Larbi, A., Douziech, N., Dupuis, G., Khalil, A., Pelletier, H., Guerard, K.P. *et al.* (2004a). Age-associated alterations in the recruitment of signal-transduction proteins to lipid rafts in human T lymphocytes. *J. Leuk. Biol. 75*, 373–381.

Larbi, A., Douziech, N., Khalil, A., Dupuis, G., Gherairi, S., Guerard, K.P. *et al.* (2004b). Effects of methyl-beta-cyclodextrin on T lymphocytes lipid rafts with aging. *Exp. Gerontol. 39*, 551–558.

Loeb, L.A. (1994). Microsatellite instability: Marker of a mutator phenotype in cancer. *Cancer Res. 54*, 5059–5063.

Lombard, D.B., Chua, K.F., Mostoslavsky, R., Franco, S., Gostissa, M., and Alt, F.W. (2005). DNA repair, genome stability and ageing. *Cell 120*, 497–512.

Maini, M.K., Soares, M.V., Zilch, C.F., Akbar, A.N., and Beverley, P.C. (1999). Virus-induced CD8+ T cell clonal expansion is associated with telomerase up-regulation and telomere length preservation: A mechanism for rescue from replicative senescence. *J. Immunol. 162*, 4521–4526.

McCarron, M., Osborne, Y., Story, C., Dempsey, J.L., Turner, R., and Morley, A. (1987). Effect of age on lymphocyte proliferation. *Mech. Ageing Dev. 41*, 211–218.

Neri, S., Cattini, L., Facchini, A., Pawelec, G., and Mariani, E. (2004). Microsatellite instability in *in vitro* ageing of T lymphocyte clones. *Exp. Gerontol. 39*, 499–505.

Neri, S., Gardini, A., Facchini, A., Olivieri, F., Franceschi, C., Ravaglia, G. *et al.* (2005). Mismatch Repair System and aging: Microsatellite instability in peripheral blood cells from differently aged participants. *J. Gerontol. 60A*, 285–292.

Pawelec, G., Müller, R., Rehbein, A., Hähnel, K., and Ziegler, B. (1998). Extrathymic T cell differentiation *in vitro* from human $CD34^+$ stem cells. *J. Leuk. Biol. 64*, 733–739.

Pawelec, G., Fernandez, N., Brocker, T., Schneider, E.M., Festenstein, H., and Wernet, P. (1988). DY determinants, possibly associated with novel class II molecules, stimulate autoreactive $CD4^+$ T cells with suppressive activity. *J. Exp. Med. 167*, 243–261.

Pawelec, G., Sansom, D., Rehbein, A., Adibzadeh, M., and Beckman, I. (1996). Decreased proliferative capacity and increased susceptibility to activation-induced cell death in late-passage human CD4+ TCR2+ cultured T cell clones. *Exp. Gerontol. 31*, 655–668.

Pawelec, G., Rehbein, A., Haehnel, K., Merl, A., and Adibzadeh, M. (1997). Human T cell clones in long-term culture as a model of immunosenescence. *Immunol. Rev. 160*, 31–42.

Pawelec, G., Barnett, Y., Mariani, E., and Solana, R. (2002). Human CD4+ T cell clone longevity in tissue culture: lack of influence of donor age or cell origin. *Exp. Gerontol. 37*, 265–269.

Pawelec, G., Akbar, A., Caruso, C., Effros, R., Grubeck-Loebenstein, B., and Wikby, A. (2004). Is immunosenescence infectious? *Trends Immunol. 25*, 406–410.

Podlutsky, A., Bastlova, T., and Lambert, B. (1996). Reduced proliferation rate of hypoxanthine-phosphoribosyl transferase mutant human T-lymphocytes *in vitro*. *Environ. Mol. Mutagen. 28*, 13–18.

Rapi, S., Caldini, A., Fanelli, A., Berti, P., Lisi, E., Anichini, E. *et al.* (1996). Flow cytometric measurement of DNA content in human solid tumors: A comparison with cytogenetics. *Cytometry 26*, 192–197.

Rufer, N., Dragowska, W., Thornbury, G., Roosnek, E., and Lansdorp, P.M. (1998). Telomere length dynamics in human lymphocyte subpopulations measured by flow cytometry. *Nat. Biotechnol. 16*, 743–747.

Singh, N.P., McCoy, M.T., Tice, R.R., and Schneider, E.L. (1988). A simple technique for quantification of low levels of DNA damage in individual cells. *Exp. Cell Res. 175*, 184–191.

Starostik, P., Greiner, A., Schwarz, S., Patzner, J., Schultz, A., and Muller-Hermelink, H.K. (2000). The role of microsatellite instability in gastric low- and high-grade lymphoma development. *Am. J. Pathol. 157*, 1129–1136.

Wikby, A., Ferguson, F., Forsey, R., Thompson, J., Strindhall, J., Löfgren, S. *et al.* (2005). An immune risk phenotype, cognitive impairment and survival in very late life: The impact of allostatic load in Swedish Octo- and Nonagenarian humans. *J. Gerontol. B 60*, 556–565.

67

Age-Related Changes in the Human Retina

Carlo Cavallotti and Nicola Pescosolido

An increasing number of elderly give a good cause for investigations on age-related changes in the human retina. Samples of fresh retinal tissue obtained from young and old humans were studied by means of traditional histological methods and by scanning electron microscopy. Particular attention was paid to morphometrical data. In fact, with the aid of the quantitative analysis of images, a large amount of morphometrical data were collected. Moreover, the amount of protein content in retinal tissues was determined. Particular care was taken in order to clarify the changes occurring in the human retina with aging. Retinal thickness significantly decreases with age. The ganglion cells seem to be more vulnerable to age-related loss than other retinal cells. The number of retinal capillaries was diminished with age. The intercellular connections between photoreceptors, the number of cellular processes, and the number of synaptic bodies of the bipolar cells also decreased significantly with age. Biochemical dosage of proteins demonstrates that the amount of proteins in retinal tissues decrease with age. In conclusion, all morphological, morphometrical, ultra-structural, and biochemical data agree in demonstrating that the human retina undergoes specific changes with age. Scanning electron microscopy performed on human retina in young and old subjects confirms the age-related changes of photoreceptor cells as well as of bipolar and ganglion cells, and provides new morphometrical findings. These results can be considered as a model and as normal values for other changes that may occur in the human retina in pathological conditions.

Introduction

The majority of elderly people suffer from deficiencies in both photopic (Owsley and Burton, 1991) and scotopic (Sturr and Hannon, 1991) vision, not related to any organic pathology, but rather as part of the general decline in all the functions of the body. Based on the theory of physical deterioration, it is believed that the body is placed under stress and injury, both extrinsic (dependent on the environment) and intrinsic (dependent on biological processes). This damage derives from small, highly reactive molecules known as free radicals (Armstrong, 1984), which are produced during normal metabolic processes and are associated with important cellular functions (Brizee and Ordy, 1981). Of these damaging agents, we shall consider reactive oxygen intermediates, capable of inducing oxidative stress. In addition, peroxy-nitrites, endogenic alkylating agents, and aldehyde products, resulting from the oxidation of lipids, also have the capacity to damage macromolecules (protein and lipid complexes, DNA, etc.) (Dykens, 1999). Macromolecular damage results in cellular dysfunction manifested by nuclear instability, inappropriate cell differentiation, and consequent cell death (necrosis or apoptosis) (Handelman and Dratz, 1986). These age-related changes of the retina primarily cause a loss of visual acuity and impairment of color discrimination as well as reduction of the visual field. Impairment of visual functions in aged subjects has long been considered the consequence of opacity of the dioptric media, whereas little attention has been paid to the retinal age-related changes. In light of our present findings, we can hypothesize that the fall in visual acuity occurring in old age is influenced, at least in part, by the age-related changes observed in human retinal tissues (Cavallotti *et al.*, 2004). In fact, our group studied the Scanning Electron Microscopic (SEM) features of the human retina. For a detailed evaluation of the effects of aging on retinal morphology, a quantitative analysis of images was performed for obtaining morphometrical data. Our findings underlined that the human retina can be considered an optimal model for studies on neuronal maturation and/or neuronal aging, being particularly sensitive to age-related changes and to senile decay.

This chapter discusses the following:

- Morphological and functional organization of the human retina
- Choroid-retinal complex (choroid, Bruch's membrane, basal membrane, retinal pigmented epithelium)
- Neuronal cells of the retina
- Glial cells of the retina
- Retinal vessels

- Aging of the whole retina (experimental results)
- Aging of the choroid-retinal complex
- Aging of neuronal cells of the retina
- Aging of glial cells of the retina
- Aging of retinal vessels
- Age-related diseases of the human retina

Morphological and Functional Organization of the Human Retina

The retina is the most internal of the three sheets that coat the posterior wall of the eye. This sheet extends from the optical nerve to the pupil-iris border, and it can be divided into an optical part, dedicated to the function of vision, and a blind part, in conjunction with the border of the pupil. The two parts are separated by the ora serrata. The retina is structurally divided into two shares: one outer and one inner.

The outer share of the retina consists of the retinal pigment epithelium (RPE), which lies on the basal membrane and the Bruch's membrane. The RPE with the basal membrane, Bruch's membrane, and the inner choroid form a single functional complex named the choroid/Bruch's membrane/basal membrane/RPE complex, or chorio-retina (Streiff and Faggioni, 1971). The integrity of this complex maintains the integrity of the retinal photoreceptors, and therefore the integrity of the whole retina.

The inner share of the retina or neurosensorial retina represents the real nervous part of the eye bulb. It is of encephalic derivation and, therefore, derives directly from the central nervous system. It consists of three consecutive neurons, identifiable as the rods and cones (first neurons), bipolar cells (second neurons), and the ganglion cells (third neurons). In reality, the retinal cells and their processes are assigned into 10 layers (see Figure 67.1–67.6):

- Retinal pigmented epithelium (RPE)
- Layer of the acromeres of the photoreceptors
- Outer limiting membrane (OLM), which is not a real membrane but a small zone with numerous zonulae adherens between the Müller cells and the photoreceptors
- Outer nuclear layer (ONL), formed by the bodies of the photoreceptor cells
- Outer plexiform layer (OPL), formed by the synapses between the photoreceptors, the bipolar cells, and the horizontal cells
- Inner nuclear layer (INL), which includes the cell bodies of five cell types: horizontal, bipolar, amacrin, interplexiform, and the Müller cells
- Inner plexiform layer (IPL), formed by the synapses between the bipolar cells, the amacrin cells, and the ganglion cells
- Ganglion cell layer (CGL), which also contains some amacrin cells

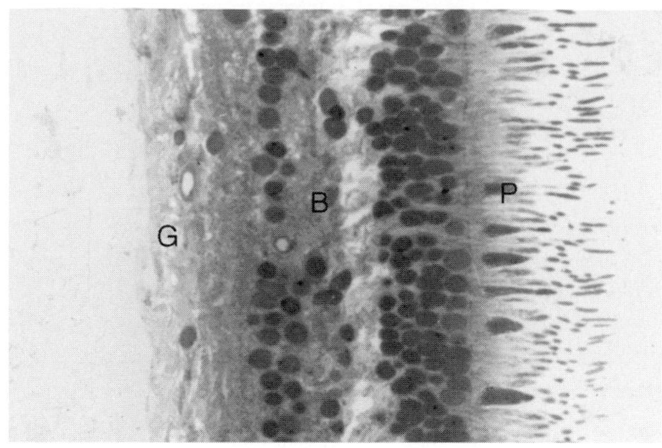

Figure 67.1 Light microscopic image of a normal human retina. The RPE is detached from the other retinal layers (it is not contained in this image on the left side). P = photoreceptors; B = bipolar cells; G = ganglion cells (magnification 1600x).

- Nervous fiber layer (NFL), which contains the axons of the ganglion cells
- Inner limiting membrane (ILM), formed by the terminal processes of the Müller cells

The neurosensorial retina, therefore, is formed by a large variety of cells described in the next sections.

Choroid-Retinal Complex

The choroid-retinal complex is formed by choroid, Bruch's membrane, basal membrane, and retinal pigmented epithelium (named also chorio-retina).

CHOROID

The choroid is the intermediate layer of the three sheets of the posterior wall of the eye. It is vascular in nature. The inner part of the choroid lies in close contact with the retina, and takes part in common with the choroid/Bruch's membrane/basement membrane/RPE complex, and therefore is named chorion-retina (Streiff and Faggioni, 1971).

BRUCH'S MEMBRANE

The Bruch's membrane extends from the optic disk to the ora serrata. Its thickness varies in different parts of the eye; it is thickest close to the optic disk (2–4 μm) and thinner at the periphery (1–2 μm). It is formed by the following five layers: (1) The basal membranes of the RPE cells form the inner layer of the Bruch's membrane; followed by (2) the internal collagen layer; (3) the elastic layer; (4) the external collagen layer; and (5) the basal membrane of the choriocapillaries. Collagen and elastane are the principal structural proteins of the Bruch's membrane. Certain types of collagen (type I, II, III, V, and IX) aggregate in long fibrils. Other types (IX and XIII) are found on the surface of the fibrils and are linked to other components of the matrix. Type IV collagen forms a soft net. The elastane fibers give elasticity to the membrane. Fibronectin and laminin are large glycoproteins, which, through their multiple bonds, help the cells to join to the membrane (Feeney-Burns and Ellersiek, 1985).

BASAL MEMBRANE

The basal side of the RPE lies on a basement membrane that is uniform in thickness throughout the retina. The basal cell membrane shows only a few in-folding. The cell membrane on the apical side is like that in the nonpigmented epithelium; there are numerous cell junctions. The lateral surfaces show interdigitations (Hogan *et al.*, 1971). The basal membrane is made up of collagen connective tissue and contains some specific proteins named membrane bound protein (MBP) and proteoglycans (PG).

RETINAL PIGMENTED EPITHELIUM

The cells of the RPE are postmitotic cells with a hexagonal shape that form a single layer of cuboidal epithelial cells that separate the external portion of the photoreceptors from the choroid. The RPE provides metabolic and functional support for the external portion of the photoreceptors. Each human eye contains between 4 and 6 million RPE cells. In the central part of the retina, the shape and dimensions of the RPE cells are uniform. They are circa 14 μm in diameter and 12 μm in height. At the equator the cells are taller and larger and at the extreme periphery lose the uniformity of size and shape. Some cells may contain more than one nucleus, and at the ora serrata the RPE cells may measure up to 60 μm in diameter (Panda Jonas *et al.*, 1996).

These cells are formed of a basal portion, an apical portion, and six lateral faces. The basal portion has a cell membrane with numerous invaginations, which can sink up to 1 μm into the cytoplasm, in order to increase the absorbent surface. The basal membrane of these cells is adjacent to the basal lamina, which forms the proximal layer of the Bruch's membrane. The basal invaginations increase the surface area of the cellular membrane, as this is involved in transport functions. The apical portion of the RPE cells, which sits in front of the acromere of the photoreceptors, is folded to form microvilli of 5 to 7 μm length, that surround the third terminal of the acromere of the photoreceptors. As the acromeres of the rods and the cones are of different dimensions, the villi that surround the external portion of the rods are smaller (3 μm) than those that surround the cones. From a functional point of view there are two different types of microvilla—one softer, which is dedicated to transepithelial transport, and the other connected to the distal lamina of the photoreceptors.

The lateral portions of the RPE are linked (zonula occludens and adherens) to create the external haemato-retinal barrier and at the same time are interconnected through intercellular junctions. The cells have a round basal nucleus, and the cytoplasm is rich in lysosomes, smooth endoplasmic reticulum, mitochondria at the basal level, round pigmented granules, and oval ones containing melanin. The majority of the melanin granules are found in the apical portion or in the villi. The granules measure up to 1 μm in diameter and from 2 to 3 μm in length. The pigment granules adsorb light, preventing diffusion and also act as free radical "scavengers." The RPE cells in the macular and equatorial regions contain the major quantity of pigment (Katz and Robison, 1984).

FUNCTIONAL ROLE OF RPE

The RPE plays a fundamental role in the transport and storage of the retinoids, essential for maintaining the visual cycle. Another function of the RPE is to eliminate components of the acromeres of the photoreceptors through phagocytosis activity mediated by cathepsin D and by the integrins that act as membrane receptors that mediate the phagocytosis. The phagosomes are linked to lysosomes to form phagolysosomes, where they are digested by the intracellular digestive enzymes located at the basal surface of the cell. The final metabolism products are expelled into the choroidal circulation by exocytosis through the Bruch's membrane. If they are not completely digested, they accumulate inside the cells as *granules of lipofuscin*. These granules increase with age (Iwasaki and Inomata, 1988), especially in the macular area. The constant exposure of the RPE to light, at elevated concentrations of oxygen, together with the high metabolic activity of these cells, creates an environment favorable, especially in the macular area, to the formation of toxic reactive oxygen radicals. In defense against oxidative stress, the RPE cells contain antioxidants such as superoxide dismutase, catalases, reduced glutathione, melanin, and carotenoids. In reality, the quantity of these reduces with age, as the antioxidant defenses decrease.

Neuronal Cells of the Retina

The first category of retinal cells are neurons: photoreceptors, bipolar cells, and ganglion cells. The intraretinal nervous optic pathway consists of three consecutive neurons: rods and cones (first neuron), bipolar cells (second neuron), and ganglion cells (third neuron). These cells in human retina are: first neuron about 125 million; bipolar cells about 12.5 million; and ganglion cells about 1.25 million in the ratio 100:10:1.

The neuronal cells of the retina (Radnot, 1978), the inner and outer segments of photoreceptors (Antal, 1977), and the pigment epithelium and its relationships with the photo-receptors were well studied and well described (Leuenberger, 1971). Retinal thickness is known to vary between its central and peripheral regions (Follman and Radnot, 1979) as well as between temporal and nasal zones (Lewis *et al.*, 1969). Moreover, large individual variations have been described in the numbers of neuronal cells localized in the different layers of the human retina

(Osterberger, 1935). Consequently, all retinal quantifications must be performed precisely considering the same topographical location for each sample of investigated retinas.

Glial Cells of the Retina

The second category of retinal cells are glia cells: macroglia and microglia.

MACROGLIA CELLS

Macroglia are cells that regulate the retinal metabolism and modulate neuron function and blood vessels. There are two cell types as part of the macroglia: Müller cells and astrocytes. The Müller cells cross the thickness of the retina from the RPE to the inner limiting membrane. The bodies of the cells are located in the inner nuclear layer, and they are the principal regulatory cells for the metabolism of glutamate, the ion balance, and neuron function. The Müller fibers form an extended net that sustains and surrounds all the nervous cells. In addition, their axons and dendrites help to form the inner and outer limiting membranes.

The astrocytes, on the contrary, are limited to the nervous fiber layer and envelope the blood vessels and ganglion cells with their cellular protrusions. The branched protrusions of these cells occur at right angles with respect to the Müller fibers, and the two structures are not linked. The astrocytes are star-shaped, with round nuclei and numerous thin protrusions. They are horizontally placed and surround the blood vessels with a dense net of fibers. They form an arched, honeycomb structure, which surrounds and sustains the axons of the ganglion cells. They are firmly anchored to the walls of the blood vessels (Vernadakis, 1986).

MICROGLIA

The microglial cells are similar to the tissue macrophages (Chen *et al.*, 2002). These cells are normally resting, but are sensitive to alterations in the homeostasis of the retina; when the retina is altered, the microglial cells rapidly change into phagocytes. Finally, in the retina we also find endothelial cells and pericytes, which flank the nerve cells and glia cells or arrange themselves around the blood vessel walls. Pericytes are modified smooth muscle cells that regulate the vascular flow through dilation and contraction of the vessels. The endothelial cells regulate the homeostatic function and form the haemato-retinal barrier.

Retinal Vessels

The retina and the optic nerve head are the only parts of the central nervous system that can be inspected during life with an ophthalmoscopic examination. Moreover, the ophthalmoscope allow us to inspect the superficial retinal vessels.

The vascular supply of the retina comes from the ophthalmic branch of the internal carotid artery, which in turn gives origin to the central retina artery. The latter, upon issuing from the optic disk, divides into four arterioles, which supply the four quadrants of the retina (see Figure 67.1–67.7).

The ganglion cells and bipolar cells receive their blood supply from these arterioles and their capillaries, whereas photoreceptor elements receive nourishment from the underlying choroidal vascular bed. These small vessels react in diseases like vessels of corresponding sizes in the brain. Since the walls of the retinal arterioles are transparent to the ophthalmoscope, what is seen is a column of blood cells. In hypertension and/or arteriosclerosis (usually coexistent with hypertension), the lumens of the vessels are narrowed because of fibrous tissue replacement of the media and thickening of the basement membrane. The light reflection from the vessel then has a different refractive index than the adjacent retinal tissue. Spreading of vessels, decrease of the size of the lumen, and arteriole-venous compressions are other signs of hypertension and arteriosclerosis (see Figure 67.1–67.8).

Capillary-venular aneurysms may develop, most often in diabetes mellitus (see Figure 67.9).

Since the central retina vein and artery share a common adventitial sheath, atheromatous plaques in the artery may result in thrombosis of the vein. Round or oval hemorrhages always lie in the outer plexiform layer and linear or flame-shaped ones in the superficial layer of the retina, as occurs in conditions with extremely high intracranial pressure.

Aging of the Whole Retina (Experimental Results)

In our experiments, only samples of the retinas coming from living humans and not from autopsies were used because post-mortem phenomena may bring about early modifications in the morphometric data obtained from the retinas. Our studies were approved by the local Ethical Committee, and patients or their relatives gave their informed written consent. The investigations were performed according to the guidelines of the Declaration of Helsinki. After removal, the eye-bulb was dissected with a razor blade and samples of intact retinal tissue (located precisely in the same site, equatorially in the nasal region) were harvested. The whole thickness of the retina was measured by a micrometric gauge. Small fragments of the retina were then placed in ice-cold fixative (for morphological staining) or submersed in ice-cold buffer (for estimation of protein content).

LIGHT MICROSCOPY

Samples of the human retina were immediately prefixed in 2% osmium tetroxide at pH 7.4 in veronal-acetate buffer for five minutes at 4°C. After fixation, the specimens were washed with veronal-acetate buffer (pH 7.4), dehydrated in a graded ethanol series and embedded in paraffin. Thin sections (about 4 m) were made for morphological staining with toluidine blue (0.05% for 1 minute). Lipids were stained by means of special histo-chemical techniques for light microscopic analysis. In order to determine the composition and distribution of the lipids, three different stains were used: the bromine–Sudan black B stain, which stains all classes of lipids; bromine–acetone–Sudan black B, which stains only phospho-lipids; and Oil red O, which stains neutral lipids (especially esters of saturated and unsaturated fatty acids).

SCANNING ELECTRON MICROSCOPY

Other samples of human retina were used for scanning electron microscopy. Prefixation tissue samples were oriented, and the exposed surface coated with gold-carbon vapor and examined in a JEM 100 B electron microscope with the EM Asid High Resolution Scanning Device (University of Pecs, Hungary). Photographs were taken using ORWO NR 5R NP 20 films. Microphotographs were printed in black and white.

QUANTITATIVE ANALYSIS OF IMAGES

For a detailed evaluation of the effects of aging on retinal morphology a QAI was performed on slides and on microphotographs using a Quantimet Analyzer (Leica®) equipped with specific software. This software made it possible to determine (see Table 67.1):

- The thickness of the retina
- The number of ganglion cells/mm^2 of retina
- The number of capillaries/mm^2 of retina
- The number of synaptic bodies/area
- The number of cellular processes/observed area
- The number of intercellular connections in the matrix between the photoreceptors

Final values must be submitted to statistical analysis of data. The values reported in this chapter represent the "values" of staining for each age group and are expressed in conventional units (C.U.) ± S.E.M. C.U. are arbitrary units furnished and printed directly by the Quantimet system (Leica, 1997).

ESTIMATION OF PROTEIN CONTENT

Samples of human retina were weighed and homogenized 1/10 w/v into an ice-cold homogenization buffer (veronal acetate pH 7.4). Tissue protein concentrations were determined, using bovine serum albumin (BSA) as standard and Folin phenol as reagent (Lowry *et al.*, 1951).

STATISTICAL ANALYSIS OF DATA

The statistical methods used throughout this study must be interpreted as an accurate description of the data rather than a statistical inference of such data. The preliminary studies of each value were performed with the aid of basic sample statistics. Mean values, maximum and minimum limits, variations, standard deviation (S.D.), standard error of the means (S.E.M.), and correlation coefficients were calculated. Correlation coefficients denote a significant level less than 0.001 ($P<0.001$), but is not significant when $P>0.05$ (n.s.) (Castino and Roletto, 1992).

EXPERIMENTAL RESULTS

Comparing the images obtained from younger subjects with those obtained from older ones (see Figure 67.2) and observing the quantitative data reported in Table 67.1, we can find:

1. A lower number of capillaries
2. A marked decrease of the synaptic buttons
3. A marked reduction of the cellular processes
4. An increase of the intercellular spaces.

TABLE 67.1
Age-related changes in human retinas harvested from patients of different ages: Values of quantitative analysis of images and biochemical values of protein amount

Age-related Changes	Young (n=7)	Old (n=5)
Thickness of the retina °μm ± SEM	426 ± 34.2	261 ± 18.9*
^Ganglion cells number mm^2 ± SEM	413.5 ± 32.3	256.2 ± 26.8*
Capillaries number mm^2 ± SEM	3.6 ± 1.4	1.8 ± 1.2*
Synaptic bodies area C.U. ± SEM	122.4 ± 4.9	38.5 ± 1.6*
Cellular processes area C.U. ± SEM	82.3 ± 3.1	13.1 ± 1.5*
Intercellular gaps area C.U. ± SEM	36.4 ± 2.5	14.3 ± 1.4*
Protein γ/mg of fresh tissue ± SEM	92.1 ± 1.8	78.3 ± 1.3*

°without the pigmented epithelium that is detectable from all remaining layers
*P< 0.001 old versus young
n= number of retinas
C.U.= Conventional Units furnished and printed directly by analyzer (Leica 1997).
^Number of ganglion cells corresponds to the number of the optic nerve fibers.

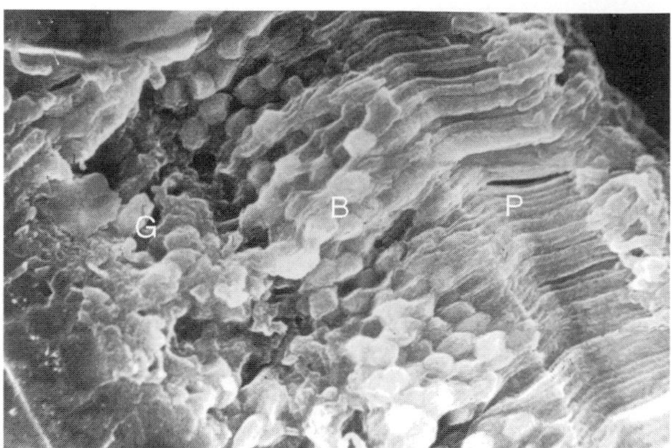

Figure 67.2 Micro-anatomical details of the human retina harvested from a young donor (18 years) observed by scanning electron microscopy. The ganglion cell layer (G), bipolar cell layer (B) and photoreceptor cell layer (P) may be seen (magnification 1600x). Reproduced by permission of the Canadian Ophthalmological Society.

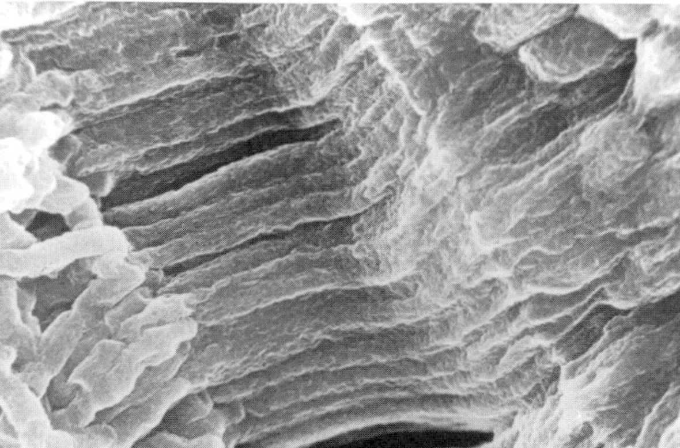

Figure 67.3 Scanning electron photomicrograph showing the outer as well as the inner segments of photoreceptors. Moreover, the external limiting membrane, the bipolar cell layer, and numerous capillaries can be distinguished. Samples of the human retina were harvested from an old donor (68 years old) (magnification 8000x). Reproduced by permission of Canadian Ophthalmological Society.

In the human retina, all layers can be clearly discerned and easily defined on the basis of well-known observations using light microscopy (see Figure 67.1).

Moreover, aging induces a strong decrease of the whole thickness of the retina from 426 ± 34,2 μm in younger to 261 ± 18,9 μm in older (i.e., a decrease of about 40%) as reported in line 1 of Table 67.1. Line 2 shows a strong decrease of the ganglion cells. These cells are 413.5 ± 32.3/mm^2 in the retinas of young humans and go down to 256.2 ± 26.8/mm^2 in the retinas of old humans, a decrease of about 38%. At line 3 a strong decrease of the number of the capillaries is reported. The latter are 3.6 ± 1.4 C.U. in adult patients, and go down to 1.8 ± 1.2 C.U. in the old age-group, a decrease of about 50%. The synaptic bodies (Table 67.1, line 4) go down from 122.4 ± 4.9 to about 38.5 ± 1.6 C.U. (old) for each microscopic area observed. The cellular processes (Table 67.1, line 5) also show a reduction from 82.3 ± 3.1 to 13.1 ± 1.5 C.U. for each microscopic area observed. The intercellular connections decrease from 36.4 + 2.5 C.U. to 14.3 +1.4 C.U. The protein content is slightly reduced: 92.1 ± 1.8 μg/mg of fresh tissue in younger subjects in comparison to 78.7 ± 1.3 in older ones.

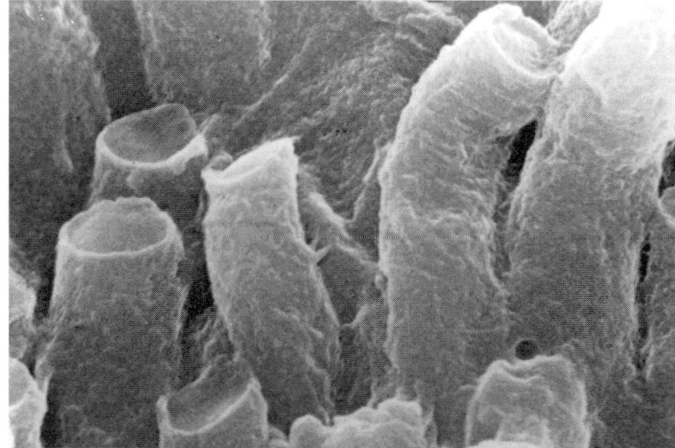

Figure 67.4 Scanning electron photomicrograph showing photoreceptor cells' outer segments. Samples of the human retina were harvested from an young donor (21 years old). The cellular matrix is sometimes crossed by intercellular connections. These structures are due to a collapsed inter-photo-receptor matrix, which normally fills the sub-retinal spaces. The apex of many photoreceptors can be observed (magnification 16.000x). Reproduced by permission of Canadian Ophthalmological Society.

Aging of the Choroid-Retinal Complex

As stated earlier, the choroid-retinal complex includes many structures, the most important of which are the pigmented epithelial cells.

RPE CELLS

As previously stated, postmitotic cells perform numerous metabolic functions throughout our lives, not only for themselves, but also for the photoreceptors. From about 20 years of age, the RPE cells show alteration as a result of their constant activity in the course of the years. Each single RPE cell metabolically supports around 30 photoreceptors (Dryja *et al.*, 1998).

Everyday, 10 to 15% of the acromeres of each rod are phagocyted by the RPE cells and replaced. The highest turnover of acromeres of retinal photoreceptors involves the parafoveal rods and the first signs of retinal aging appear in the macula. The subfoveal RPE maintains its function for the longest period, due to its high density of cones. A decrease in the functionality of the RPE occurs with aging, which manifests itself through various morphologic signs (Weiter *et al.*, 1986). The signs of RPE aging consist of the reduction of the granules

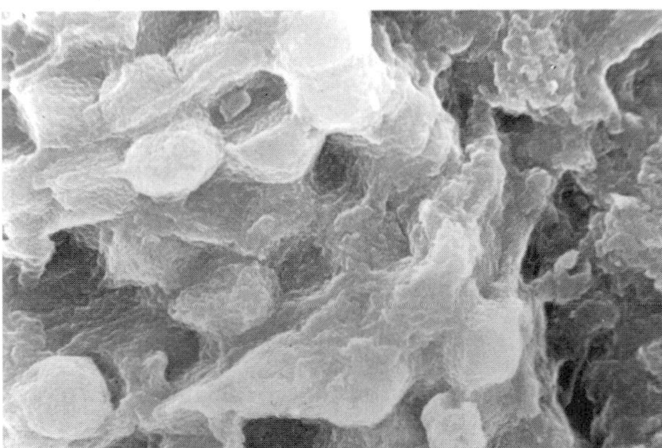

Figure 67.5 The intercellular spaces of the outer layers of a retina harvested from a young man (19 years old). Numerous cellular processes and synaptic buttons can be seen. Finally, a presumed interplexiform cell may be identified (magnification 9600x). Reproduced by permission of the Canadian Ophthalmological Society.

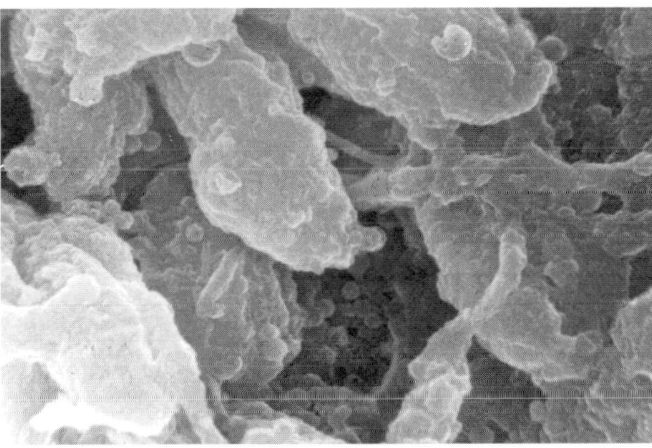

Figure 67.6 Scanning electron photomicrograph showing the bulges of the outer nuclear layer appear tightly attached to one another, with only very narrow bridges of cellular matrix between them. The ganglion cells appear as large, spherical bodies, arranged in a fibrous network. Most of the cell bodies are smooth, but some of them were seen to have a villous surface. This retina was harvested from a young man (19 years old). Numerous synaptic bodies, cellular processes, and intercellular spaces may be observed (magnification 16000x). Reproduced by permission of Canadian Ophthalmological Society.

of melanin (depigmentation) and the migration of the pigment granules to the basal portion of the cells, the loss of hexagonal shape of the foveal cells, the reduction on the cell density (atrophy, hyperplasia, hypertrophy, cellular migration), and the intracytoplasmatic accumulation of abnormal molecules due to incomplete degradation of the metabolic products in the form of intracytoplasmatic granules (lipofuscin, melanolipofuscin) (Young, 1982). These granules are partially the result of a phagocytosis process of the acromeres of the rods and cones and their elimination by the phagosomes. Inside these latter, the gradual digestion of the discs of the acromeres, with the formation of residual bodies, occurs. Many incompletely digested discs and some phagosomes are eliminated in the basal lamina of the Bruch's membrane. Large quantities of residual bodies are seen often in the eyes of individuals aged between 40 and 60, with a strong increase after the 80th year. The accumulation of this cellular detritus inevitably leads to the suffering of the RPE. These changes are more noted in the macula than in the equatorial and peripheral areas (Burns and Feney Burns, 1980). Now we shall examine, in greater detail, the typical signs of RPE aging.

VARIATION IN THE TYPE, QUANTITY, AND STRUCTURE OF THE GRANULES OF LIPOFUSCIN

With advancing years, inside the cells of the RPE, granules of lipofuscin appear, which represent the lysosomal accumulation of residual bodies including the nondegradable final products of metabolism and the phagocyted acromeres of the photoreceptor, as already stated (Burns and Feney Burns, 1980).

Each cell of the retinal pigment epithelium (RPE) is in a continuous process of intracellular renewal. Sometimes this process of molecular degradation is not complete and results in the accumulation of metabolic debris and interference with other metabolic activity in these cells. The residual materials are "useless" molecular aggregations, normally called *lipofuscin granules*, that contain damaged RPE cells and membranes of rod and cone phagocytes (i.e., incompletely degraded cellular debris) (Armstrong, 1984). The incomplete molecular degradation seems to be due to altered substrates, which therefore are not recognized by the enzymatic systems. These molecular alterations result from the harmful effects that free radicals have on the RPE cells and their photoreceptors, rich in polyunsaturated fatty acids that become peroxidised. The damaged molecules are phagocyted by the RPE cells and accumulate in their cytoplasm, thus compromising their metabolism and inducing cell death. The acromeres of the retinal photoreceptors can be abnormal due to oxidative damage prior to phagocytosis, or the abnormality can be hereditary. The reason why the acromeres of the photoreceptors are sensitive to oxidative stress is their richness in polyunsaturated fats. Exposure to light, and particularly short wavelength radiation, increases the production of free radicals and accumulation of lipofuscin in the macular RPE. In addition, environmental factors such as cigarette smoke reduce the level of antioxidants and promote the formation of free radicals, contributing to the accumulation of cellular debris (Lerman, 1988).

Lipofuscin exists inside the RPE cells in the form of granules that appear yellow-green under UV light excitation. Topographically, the majority of the granules of lipofuscin accumulate in the posterior pole of the eye bulb, whereas the quantity reduces in the fovea. This distribution of lipofuscin with respect to the location remains constant during the entire life and correlates with the density of photoreceptors. The lipofuscin granules contain lipids and proteins. The cytoplasmic volume of the RPE occupied by lipofuscin increases with age, from 8% at age 40 to 29% at age 80. Furthermore, the cytoplasmatic volume occupied by lipofuscin in the macula is greater than that in the periphery: 19% in the macula versus 13% in the periphery. The excessive accumulation of lipofuscin in the RPE cells slows the metabolic activity of the cells and predisposes them to age-related macular degeneration (AMD) (Bird, 1997).

Lipofuscin is the generic name given to a heterogenic group of lipid-protein aggregates that are found in aging cells in all human tissues. Different from the other tissues, in the retina the lipofuscin does not derive from the degradation of intracytoplasmatic organelles, but from the incomplete degradation of the products deriving from the phagocytosis of the outer portions of the photoreceptors following the peroxidation of the unsaturated fatty acids. Once accumulated, the lipofuscin causes the death of the RPE cells because it acts as a true generator of free radicals (Boulton *et al.*, 1993); lipofuscin can release lysosomotropic amines. Finally, other authors consider lipofuscin to be an inert substance that acts directly through the congestion of the cytoplasm (in some tissues lipofuscin can occupy up to 30% of the cell volume) (Elderly and Lasky, 1993).

MELANIN GRANULES

Melanin has a double role in the retina: to reduce the chromatic aberration, increasing the visual acuteness, and to protect against oxidative stress by acting as a cellular antioxidant. Its concentration increases from the equator to the posterior pole reaching a peak in the macula. The increased concentration of melanosomes in the macula is due to the fact that the RPE cells here are larger and concentrated into a smaller area with respect to the smaller extra-macular RPE cells dispersed in a much larger area (Handelman and Dratz, 1986). The differential distribution of melanosomes is maintained during the first 40 years of life, but afterward a significant reduction in the melanin granules is seen in all regions of the retina (Weiter *et al.*, 1986). To make a comparison, consider three age groups: 10–20; 21–60; and 61–100. The reduction in the quantity of melanosomes between the first and the third class is 35%. Talking in terms of cell volume, therefore, around 8% is occupied by melanin in the first two decades of life, which reduces to 6% in the second age group, and finally further diminishes, arriving at 3.5% in the third age group (Feney Burns, 1984).

Melanin is a complex heterogenic biopolymer, containing free radicals, which can be identified using electron spin resonance spectroscopy (ESR). Using this technique a 40% reduction in melanin content is observed with aging (Sarna *et al.*, 2003). Three possible mechanisms may explain the loss of melanin from RPE cells: expulsion of the granules, lysosomal degradation, and chemical damage. The expulsion of the granules may be a possibility, notwithstanding the fact that the granules are not found in the Bruch's membrane or in the interphotoreceptor space. Lysosomal degradation is highly elevated due to its function of degrading the acromeres of the photoreceptors (Boulton and Wassel, 1998). With aging comes an increase in the number of melano-lysosomes, accompanied by a change in the appearance of the melanin granules. Notwithstanding that the morphology of the melanosomes changes following an interaction with the lysosomes, it is likely that the melanin is not degraded and that the changes derive from the degradation of the proteins of the matrix on which the melanin is deposited. The third mechanism is that of chemical degradation. The irradiation of human eyes with intense blue light induces a nonuniform photobleaching of the melanosomes. The lack of uniformity of the bleaching seems to be due to the fact that lipofuscin is also found in the complex granules of aged RPE cells and this is more photoreactive than melanin, or even may act as photosensitizers. Blue light therefore would induce oxidative photo-degradation of melanin by the formation of superoxide anion and hydrogen peroxide. On the one hand the photo-degradation of melanin (oxidation or irreversible bleaching) does not have any biological significance in tissues with high turnover (such as hair and skin); on the other hand, this event gains a high importance when it occurs in those tissues with low turnover such as in the RPE cells, which are postmitotic cells (Boulton *et al.*, 1998).

COMPLEX GRANULES

With the increasing of age, melanin, lipofuscin, and lysosomes can join together to form complex structures (melanolipofuscin and melanolysosomes) inside the RPE. These granules have a regional distribution similar to that of lipofuscin; i.e., the highest concentration is in the macula, and it decreases in the periphery and in the fovea. Concerning the percentage of the cellular volume occupied by complex granules, this varies from 3.3% in the first decade of life and reaches to 8 to 10% in the sixth decade. The association of lysosomes with pigment granules (for example, melanosomes, lipofuscin granules, and complex pigments) explains their age-dependant variation observed in the lysosomal enzyme levels and the activity of the RPE cells. The increase in pigment granules with age causes an increase in lysosomes and in the activity of various enzymes such as acid phosphatase and Cathepsin D, in order to maintain the normal degradation cycle, which follows the ingestion of the acromeres of the photoreceptors by the RPE cells (Boulton *et al.*, 1998).

CHANGES IN THE CELLULAR DENSITY

It has been observed that with aging, a physiological decline in the number of RPE cells occurs, especially in the macula. In the peripheral retina, however, the number of RPE cells can increase, diminish, or remain the same with aging, whereas in the central retina the density of RPE cells decreases with age (Dorey *et al.*, 1989). More precisely, Panda-Jonas *et al.* (1996) observed an average annual loss of 17 RPE cells/mm^2 per year with respect to an original RPE cell population of 5,232 cells/mm^2. These authors estimated that in the course of a life of 100 years, around 30% of RPE cells are lost. These values are associated with an age-related loss of 3000 to 5000 optic nerve fibers, around 0.3% per year, in a population of 1.4 million fibers at birth and a diminution in the density of cones and rods of 0.3 to 0.5% per year with respect to the photoreceptor density at birth. These observations indicate a reduced reserve capacity in elderly patients with respect to younger individuals. This fact may be the cause of the decline in vision function even in the absence of active pathologic processes. Given that the RPE cells do not have the capacity to reproduce, the cells adjacent to those lost increase their cell volume, restoring the normal continuity of the RPE cells/photoreceptors. Dorey *et al.* (1989) have found that the average ratio of photoreceptors/RPE cells is higher in the macula with respect to the paramacular and equatorial areas, and that this ratio increases with age. The is one of the most reactive tissues of the eye and can undergo atrophic, hypertrophic, and hyperplastic modifications as well as migration processes.

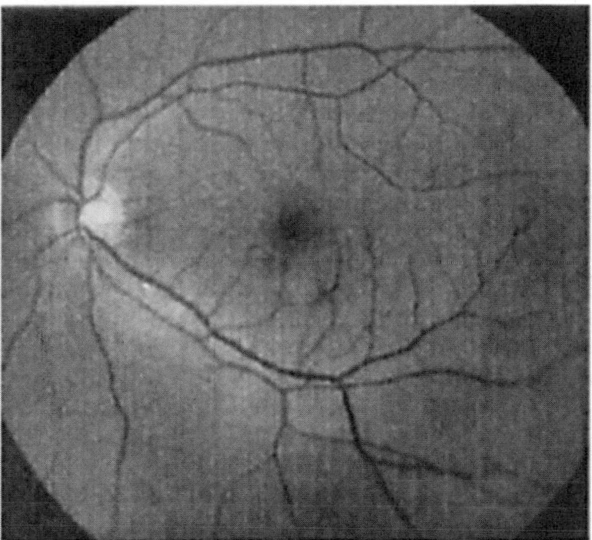

Figure 67.7 Retinal fundus in an young (25 years of age) and healthy subject. In correspondence of the head of the optic nerve the ophthalmic artery is branched in four divisions for each quadrant of the retina. In this image the nasal superior and inferior branches are evident (field 40° corresponding to a magnification of about 5x).

AGING OF THE BRUCH'S MEMBRANE

The human Bruch's membrane ages in a manner similar to the inner tunic of the arteries and other connective tissues, in which the plasmatic lipoproteins represent the known source of extracellular cholesterol. Morphologic and biochemical studies have shown that with aging the Bruch's membrane undergoes profound changes, such as the thickening and progressive accumulation of deposits in the internal layers. The changes to the Bruch's membrane progressively reduce the efflux of fluids from the retina to the choroids and the metabolic exchange between the choriocapillaries and the RPE cells. Moore and Clover (2001) have shown that there is an age-related reduction in the permeability (hydraulic conductivity) of the Bruch's membrane in the retinal periphery and the macula. Furthermore, it has been shown that the presence of lipid deposits plays a statistically important role in the reduction of permeability of the Bruch's membrane. Lipids are one of the components of the Bruch's membrane. The other components are collagen, adhesion molecules, lipoproteins, and advanced glycosylation end products (the last of which may inhibit the activity of the lysosomal enzymes). The effect of aging on the passage of metabolites across the Bruch's membrane needs to be better ascertained. However, two groups of studies have demonstrated that the flux of macromolecules reduces with age. The first group, using fluorangiography, showed that in the ocular fundus (Figures 67.7–67.9) of elderly patients with good acute vision, there are areas that show reduced choroidial perfusion. In fact, the deposition of lipids in the Bruch's membrane leads to the degeneration of the elastic fibers and collagen, causing rigidity of these structures with consequent reduction of their compliance. These reductions in turn cause resistance of the choroidial vessels, edema, and reduction of blood flow. These events lead to a worsening of all the functions of the RPE, including the ability to transport the catabolites resulting from the phagocytosis of the photoreceptors.

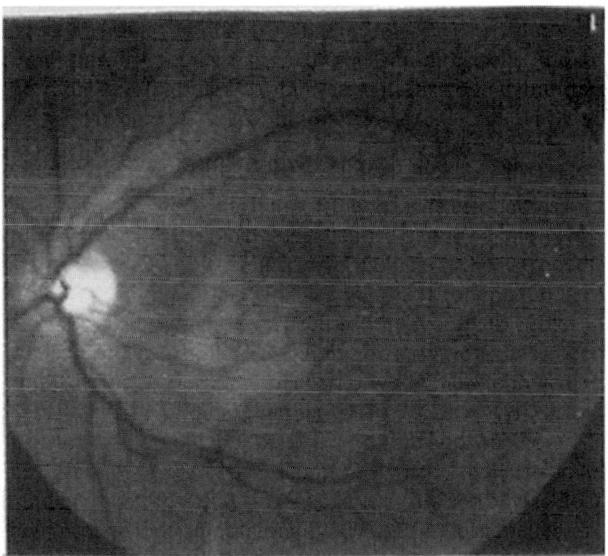

Figure 67.8 Retinal fundus in an old (70 years of age) subject. The retinic vessels show a decreased calibre. We can see a distrophic zone in RPE (field 25° corresponding to a magnification of about 8x).

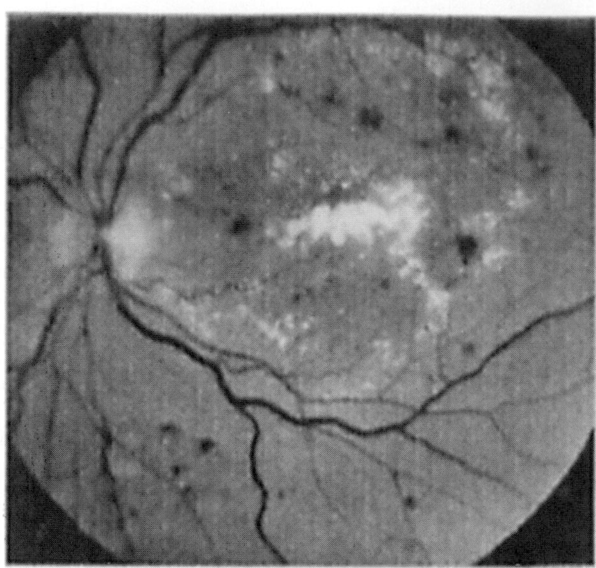

Figure 67.9 Retinal fundus in a subject of 60 years affected by nonproliferating diabetic retinal pathology. The white spots are wax exudates, while the black ones are blood stains (field 40° corresponding to a magnification of about 5x).

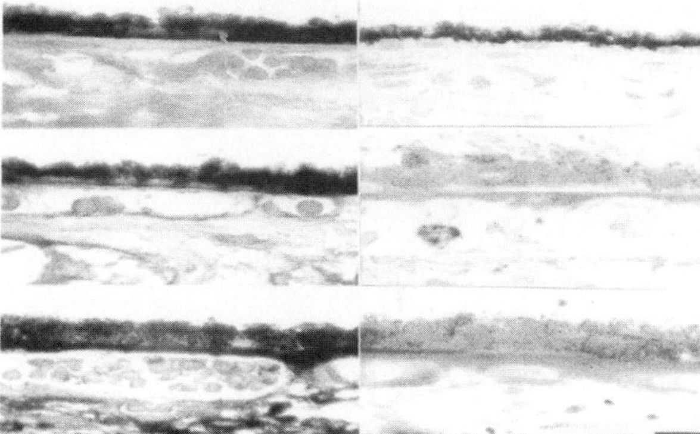

Figure 67.10 Light microscopy of the Bruch's membrane belonging to donors aged 18 (top), 47 (middle), and 75 (bottom). The three figures on the left are stained with Bromine-Acetone-Sudan Black B, those on the right are stained with Oil Red O. It can be seen that the intensity of staining with both systems increases with age, which shows the progressive age-related accumulation of lipids (magnification 400x; calibration bar 10 μm).

AGING OF THE FUNCTIONAL MORPHOLOGY OF THE BRUCH'S MEMBRANE

Investigations have shown that the areas of reduced perfusion have an elevated threshold of adaptation to the dark and a pattern of changes similar to those observed in cases of Vitamin A deficiency. The second group of studies arrived at the same conclusions by demonstrating that Sorsby's dystrophy, an illness that causes loss of central vision at a young age, is characterized by the presence of rich deposits of lipids in the Bruch's membrane. The conclusion of these studies is that the loss of vision function results from the accumulation of deposits in the Bruch's membrane, which acts as a barrier to the elimination of catabolites as well as the arrival of nutrients to the retina.

Pauleikoff *et al.* (1990) examined the immunohistochemical and ultrastructural properties of the Bruch's membrane of 30 human eyes of ages 1 to 95 years. The results of the three age groups from 0 to 30, from 31 to 60, and from 60 onward show that there is an age-related progressive increase in the lipid content of the Bruch's membrane. In the young age group, none of the stains caused any coloration. In the second age group, 8 out of 10 samples, and in the over-60 age group all the samples, were colored with Bromine–Sudan Black B, with and without acetone; only a few samples from the second and third age groups showed strong coloration, whereas only samples from the third age group showed coloration with Oil Red O (see Figure 67.10).

Moore and Clover (2001) were the first to measure the permeability of the Bruch's membrane to macromolecules, the first to determine the maximum dimensions of molecules that can cross the Bruch's membrane, and the first to ascertain the effects of age on the barrier that the Bruch's membrane represents against the flow of substances other than water. Age has three effects on the permeability of macromolecules across the Bruch's membrane. First, the exclusion based on molecular mass reduces gradually; second, in the eighth decade of life the membrane selectively impedes the passage of specific macromolecules, not on the basis of their molecular weight, but on other criteria. Finally, in the ninth decade, the membrane becomes an impermeable barrier to any molecule.

AGING OF THE BASAL MEMBRANE

The basement membrane of the RPF in young eyes is thin and uniform in thickness. With increasing age there is a significant alteration of the RPE cells and the basement membrane. In the aged eye most of the RPE cells show deep infoldings of the basal cell membranes. In the young eye the basement membrane of the RPE appears as an ordinary basement membrane. With increasing age this basement membrane becomes thicker and forms a reticular pattern. Within the reticular meshwork there is a granular material consisting of many deeply osmiophilic coarse and fine granules, and groups of membrane-bound vesicles. The apical cell membrane that faces the pigmented epithelium is fairly straight. The pigmented epithelial cells face each other at their apical surface, joined by the zonula adherens and/or occludens. Interdigitations along the lateral cell membrane are found mainly in the basal or inner third of the cells.

The lateral cell membranes exhibit junctions that are mostly desmosomal and are located along the apical third of the cells. Both MBP and proteo-glycans show substantial age-related changes (Cavallotti *et al.*, 2005).

Aging of the Retinal Neurons (Photoreceptors, Bipolar Cells, Ganglion Cells)

The majority of elderly people suffer from deficiencies in vision not related to any manifested pathology. The normal function of vision depends on the integrity of numerous factors, including the transparency of the dioptric media, the photoreceptor mosaic, the integrity of the intraretinal pathways, and the nervous connection between the brain and the vision-related structures. All these elements may show age-related changes. The constriction of the pupil and the opacity of the dioptric media together reduce the quantity of light shining on the retina. One of the most important questions in the study of the aging of the visual system is to determine which contributions are related to optical factors, and which are related to nervous factors. Both these factors reduce the photopic and scotopic vision (Owsley and Burton, 1991; Sturr *et al.*, 1991). The spatial density and the dimensions of the cones and rods in the human retina changes with age. Furthermore, previous studies of the aging of the neurosensorial retina have described the degeneration and loss of a large number of photoreceptors (Cavallotti *et al.*, 2004).

CONES AND RODS

The acromeres of the cones and the rods become disorganized, and the internal segments fill with refractant bodies, presumably lipofuscin. The dislocation and partial loss of photoreceptor nuclei happens without significant modifications to the RPE, the Bruch's membrane, and the choriocapillaries (Curcio *et al.*, 1993). Gao and Hollyfield (1992) suggest that the loss of rods begins early in adult life, and the density of cones diminishes gradually in the extreme retinal periphery. On the contrary, Curcio *et al.* (1993) affirm that there is no evidence of a reduction in the density of the foveal cone peaks, although the interperson variability is high. The loss of foveal photoreceptors begins to manifest itself in persons over 90 years old. As previous studies haven't precisely specified the anatomic location of the observed zones of the retina, it was difficult to confront the changes in retinal anatomy with age-related changes in visual function. Curcio *et al.* (1993) have examined, using digital computer imaging, the topography of the retina of healthy eyes of people divided into four groups by age: Group 1 (27–37 years), group 2 (44–58 years), group 3 (61–75 years), and group 4 (82–90 years) in order to distinguish paraphysiological changes resulting from aging and/or from pathological changes. It was seen that in the central 43° of the ocular retina studied, rods but not cones are lost during the course of the life.

QUALITATIVE ASPECT OF THE PHOTORECEPTOR MOSAIC

The photoreceptor mosaic of aged retinas, without pathologic changes, is similar to that of young retinas. However, the aged retinas show two typical cytological aspects. The first is the presence of refractive particles (of around 1 μm in diameter) located at the ellipsoid-mioid junction of the cones. These refractive particles appear like refractive bodies or granules of lipofuscin that are found in the internal segments that begin to be observed after 30 to 40 years. The second aspect is the dislocation of the nuclei, which are occasionally found situated in the internal segment layer rather than in the external nuclear layer.

AGE-RELATED CHANGES OF THE EXTRA-FOVEAL CONES

The cone density of the fovea in all age groups is high and reduces rapidly with the eccentricity and in a small amount in an area that extends around the optic disk and in the nasal retina. The density of cones is variable in the different groups of age (coefficient of variability from 15 to 30%) around the optic disk; it is nonetheless lower (<15%) over 1 mm of eccentricity. In the map (personal unpublished results) the average difference between the older age groups and the younger group is significant; cold colors indicate a density lower than that of the younger group, and warm colors indicate that the average density is higher than that of the younger group. The map, which is yellow-green, indicates that the difference between the groups is minimal.

The map indicates that the group from 44 to 58 years has the smallest cone density difference (88% of the younger group), but small differences were also seen in older groups. The mapped retinal region in all the eyes was of 8 mm diameter; that is, 5% of the whole retinal area of the eye contains 10% of the cones that are found in the central 28.5°. The average number of cones over all the eyes in this region was 488,600.

AGE-RELATED CHANGES OF THE FOVEAL CONES

The cone density range between age 56 and 90 is quite limited (116,600 to 210,000 cones/mm^2), with the oldest overlapping the lower limit of the younger donors. An area of 0.8 mm diameter centered on the fovea is the only part of the retina where there are more cones than rods. This region contains 31,200 cones/mm^2 with a variability coefficient of only 12%, and the gradient of the linear regression with respect to age is not significantly different from zero. This data supplies evidence that the cone population in the central 2.8° remains stable during adult life; furthermore the topography of the cones does not show any relevant evidence, as already said, of age-related loss of cones in the central 28°. The extrafoveal cones are not more vulnerable to aging than foveal cones according to the hypothesis that the macular pigment, highly concentrated in the central 2°, is an antioxidant that improves the light-induced peroxidation of lipids, and also because a small quantity of this carotenoid is detectable outside the fovea. However, the overall stability of the total number of cones does not exclude the loss of a small number of these. As there is no evidence for a loss of cones of this magnitude, the increase in the distance between foveal cones does not significantly contribute to the age-related decline in visual resolution. The loss of acuity, therefore, may be explained by other changes in the visual system, including an age-related reduction of 25% in the number of ganglion cells that preside over the central 11° of the vision field. Also, recent evidence has shown that in the majority of cases, optical rather than retinal factors contribute to deficiencies in scotopic function, and therefore a reduction in sensitivity to spatial contrast at medium and high frequencies can be explained by a lower transfer modulation of the ocular medium in healthy elderly eyes. However, neuronal factors may play a role in other photoptic functions, such as the sensitivity to differences in luminosity (across the visual field) or spatial vision (for example, contrast sensitivity and visual acuity) considered at the mesopic or high scotopic level.

AGE-RELATED CHANGES IN THE TOPOGRAPHY OF THE RODS

The rods are absent from the center of the retina and increase in number with retinal eccentricity to form a high-density (>150,000 rods/mm^2) elliptical ring from 2 to 5 mm of retinal eccentricity, with the peak at 4 to 5 mm wider than the fovea. The interpersonal variability in the rod density for all age groups is very high (variation coefficient >45%) at the border of the rod deprived zone, high within 1 mm of the fovea and around the optic disk, and low (<15%) elsewhere. With aging, the rod density reduces in both the foveal and extrafoveal retina. The loss is higher in the high rod density ring. The number of rods within the central 8 mm in all retinas changes from 7.40 × 106 at age 45 to 3.60 × 106 at 82 years of age.

The gradient of the linear regression suggests an average loss of 648 rods/mm^2/year in the central 28.5° of vision such that at age 90 the total number of rods is reduced to 69% of that at 34 years of age.

EXTREME RETINAL PERIPHERY

Curcio *et al.* (1993) show the stability of the central cones and the reduction in the rods between the fiftieth and sixtieth year. This data contrasts with the results of Gao and Hollyfield (1992). In fact, these authors affirmed that at the temporal equator, the rod density reduces by 15% between the second and fourth decade, with a total loss of 32% by the ninth decade, and the cone density significantly reduces by 23% during the same period. These results indicate, together, that the peripheral retina ages in a different way in relationships with the central brain area of the vision (areas 17,18,19 of Brodmann, near the calcarina scissura).

AGE-RELATED CHANGES IN THE DIAMETER OF THE ACROMERES AND THE COVERAGE OF THE PHOTORECEPTORS

The area of selective rod loss is located 3 mm from the fovea. The spaces left empty by the cell loss are occupied by larger rods. The diameter of the rod acromeres ranges from 2.2 to 2.8 μm in young retinas, and those of surviving rods in older retinas are 13.5% larger in the same eccentricity range. One of the most significant results of Curcio *et al.* (1993) is that the spatial density of rods reduces by around 30% in the central 28.5° during the period from 34 to 90 years in apparently healthy eyes. This loss is less in the fovea between 45 and 61 years and from the ninth decade is larger in a parafovial ring from 0.5 to 3 mm eccentricity. Notwithstanding the diffuse loss of rods in the central retina, the appearance of the photoreceptor mosaic is qualitatively normal, as only around 2 rods/mm^2 are lost per day. Furthermore, the retina does not show either gaps or the insertion of other types of cells (glia), such that the extension of the acromeres of the remaining rods is equal to that of younger retinas. There is no evidence of an age-related decrease in the quantity of rhodopsin as might be expected with the loss of photoreceptors. The remaining photoreceptors are sufficient to perform their function.

Using densitometry, it has been shown that there is a small but significant increase in the density of the pigment of the rods between 12 and 78 years up to the temporal 16°. As the number of rods in this area diminishes with age, the acromeres of the remaining rods should contain more pigment in older retinas than in younger ones. This increase may be at least partly due to the twisting that effectively increases the total length off the acromeres by around 40% without varying the distance between the outer limiting membrane and the RPE. It is calculated that this process affects from 10 to 20% of the total rod population from the seventh decade, whereas in the central retina it is from 2% in both young and old donors, suggesting that the increase in rhodopsin can be due to the fact that the acromeres of elderly eyes are larger than those of younger eyes but morphologically similar. For example, if the diameter of the acromeres increases in proportion with the inner segments, the membrane of the disk would contain 29% more pigment in older eyes than in younger. The compensatory hypertrophy of the acromeres of the rods is in agreement with the proof of the plasticity of the rod system in adults after its partial loss.

At this point we ask ourselves if the age-related loss of rods contributes to the reduced scotopic function. Since the extension of the rods is the same in young and old retinas, it is thought that other factors such as changes in the sensitivity of the photo-pigments, regeneration, response, neuro-transmitters, and the membrane charge weaken the sensitivity of the rods.

WHY DO ONLY RODS DIE WITH AGE?

One possible mechanism is the selective vulnerability of rods. One explanation for the higher vulnerability of rods with respect to cones is the fact that the acromere disks of the rods have a higher rate of renewal. This requires a notable energy expense by the rods for the renewal of the disks and by the RPE for the disposal of the old ones (Owsley *et al.*, 2000). The RPE are responsible for the integrity of the photoreceptors, and it has been seen that the age-related changes of the photoreceptors independent of those of the RPE are slight. For example, an RPE dysfunction causes a slowdown of the rate of renewal of the photopigments in both the cones and the rods, and an increase in the convolution of the acromeres of the rods.

The principal age-related changes to the RPE are the accumulation of lipofuscin and the reduction of the granules of melanin, which is concomitant with the thickening and the accumulation of deposits in the Bruch's membranes. It has been observed that the accumulation of intracellular lipofuscin significantly reduces the function of the photoreceptors. High levels of lipofuscin have been correlated with a low number of photoreceptors in the retina. As lipofuscin is tightly related with the rods, the loss of rods should be highest in the ring with the highest density of rods, 3 to 5 mm from the center of the fovea. On the contrary, the results of Curcio *et al.* (1993) placed the rod loss closer to the fovea, at 0.5 to 3 mm, contradicting the correlation between the accumulation of lipofuscin and the loss of photoreceptors.

Aging of the Macroglia (Müller Cells and Astrocytes)

The functional weakening of the CNS that occurs with aging and age-related neurodegenerative disorders has been partially attributed to a decline in mitochondrial function. In particular, it has been demonstrated that oxidative damage occurs to mitochondrial DNA in elderly human brains. Recently, it has been shown that mitochondrial DNA is particularly sensitive to damage that accumulates due to the loss of protective histones, the reduction in repair systems, and the vicinity of the internal mitochondrial membrane to active oxygen species. The hypothesis that free radicals are involved in the weakening of the mitochondrial function has been confirmed by recent discoveries, that is, the fact that the administration of free radical scavengers such as extract of Ginkgo Biloba (Egb761) improves the function of the brain and liver in elderly animals. Astrocytes are interconnecting cells between the neurons and the surrounding connective tissue (fibroblasts, mesenchymal cells, and endothelial cells). Changes to these cells induce modifications to the intercellular relationships and, eventually, to the nervous function. It has been shown that astrocytes are resistant to oxidative stress due to their high antioxidant content and their ability to regenerate glutathione and ascorbate. Astrocytes therefore act as neuronal protectors defending the neurons against free radicals.

AGE-RELATED MACULAR DEGENERATION (AMD)

The aim of Ramirez *et al.* (2001) was to study the astrocytes of young human retinas and the paraphysiological changes that occur to them with aging and pathologic changes resulting from macular degeneration (AMD). The study was conducted on enucleated human eyes taken from the Spanish eye bank two to four hours post mortem for cornea transplants and were classified in three age groups (young, elderly, and with AMD). The astrocytes of the young subjects had numerous thin protrusions that surrounded the capillaries of the cell ganglion layer (CGL), forming a honeycomb plexus. The astroglial sheath around the vessels is very thick, and the capillaries are held together by many astroglial bundles. The gaps in the astroglial honeycomb plexus in the rear pole of zone A (the area between the second and third divisions of the retinal artery branches, near to the optic disk) are circular and very small in younger individuals, but have a quadrangular form in older individuals. In zone B (from the third division of the retinal artery to the retinal equator, closer to the periphery) the dimensions of the gaps are variable and irregular. In this zone the astrocyte bonds that hold the capillaries together have variable thicknesses, some thick and some thin. In the nerve fibers layer (NFL) of the retina, astrocytes are found parallel to the axons of the ganglion cells and to the radial peripapillar capillaries. The astroglial bundles are very thick near the optic disk.

ASTROCYTES IN ELDERLY INDIVIDUALS

Astrocytes in elderly individuals have large cell bodies and robust protrusions, particularly those found in the NFL. In the group of subjects aged over 60 years, the astrocytes showed a higher glial fibrillar acidic protein (GFAP) immunoreactivity with respect to the younger subjects, particularly in the NFL. This observation has been confirmed by electron microscopy, which showed a higher density of glial filaments (formed by GFAP) in the astrocyte cytoplasm of the elderly group. In the NFL the lack of GFAP(+) signal between the astrocyte bundles indicates that in this layer the astrocytes lose their protrusions. Occasionally GFAP(+) organelles are found in the CGL and NFL; these correspond to decayed astrocytes. The perivasal astrocytes have few thin protrusions and form a thinner astroglial sheath than in younger individuals. Sporadically, reactive astrocytes are found. The honeycomb structure is not easily distinguished in the CGL, and the gaps in the astroglial plexus have variable forms (circular, square, rectangular); the dimensions, however, are larger than those in younger subjects in both zone A (nearer to the optic disk) and zone B (closer to the periphery). The number of gaps in the astroglial honeycomb plexus in the CGL is lower in the 60 to 89 age group. This signifies that the gaps are larger due to the disappearance of astrocytes from the vessel walls and the astroglial protrusions that divide the gaps. The reduction in the number of astrocytes increases with age, as is shown by comparing people between 60 and 79 and those over 80. The comparison between young and elderly retinas has therefore again shown that aging causes numerous changes to the retinal astrocytes. There is an increase in the number of intracytoplasmatic organelles (mitochondria, ribosomes, polyribosomes, wrinkled endoplasmatic reticulum) due to higher cellular activity, an increase in lysosomes and dense bodies (which increase also inside the Müller cells), an increase of the glial intermediate filaments, a thickening of the inner limiting membrane whose constituents are less homogeneous, and the space between the glial protrusions and the basal membrane of the inner limiting membrane increases.

RETINAL NERVOUS CELLS

All retinal nervous cells have numerous lysosomes in their cytoplasm. In the NFL the axons of the glial cells contain dense bodies, formed from incompletely digested myelin, which causes the axon's swelling. In some cases, in elderly retinas, astrocytes of large dimensions are found that have very elevated cellular activity and a higher density of intermediate filaments; these are called reactive astrocytes. The function of the reactive astrocytes is to protect the neurons (in this case, the ganglion cells) from ischemia producing neurotrophic factors, increasing the expression of antioxidant substances (glutathione, vitamin C) and increasing the production and transport of glucose. However, it has been observed that astrocytes are more vulnerable to oxidative damage during aging. In fact, as the years rollby, the reactive astrocytes cause changes in the geometry and volume of the extracellular space, which slows the diffusion of neuroactive substances.

The extracellular space is not only the microenvironment of the nerve cells but is also an important channel of communication between the neurons and astrocytes. The changes to the diffusion parameters, which arrive with aging, can bring on a disappearance of the transmission signals and increase the sensitivity of the nervous tissue to ischemia. The ischemia is due to an increase in the extracellular acidity with accumulation of potassium and other toxic substances (similar to glutamate) that damage the neurons.

REACTIVE ASTROCYTES

The reactive astrocytes have an elevated number of organelles (secondary lysosomes and lipofuscin) and an elevated cellular activity. The reactive astrocytes and therefore also the lipofuscin contained within, if exposed to visible light (400–700 nm) at a high concentration of oxygen (70 mm Hg)—conditions ideal for the formation of free radicals—can cause damage to the cellular proteins and the membrane lipids. The reactive oxygen species can cause damage to cellular and nuclear elements. The presence of high concentrations of toxic substances (glutamate) in the extracellular space (coming from the reactive astrocytes), causes a massive increase of hydrogen and potassium with an increased permeability of the cell membranes, worsened by free radicals, which makes the cell swell. This cellular edema causes the breakage of the intermediate filaments of the astrocytes and therefore the loss of GFAP immunoreactivity and finally cell death. This fact explains why a reduction of the number of astrocytes in the CGL is observed and a disappearance of the protrusions of the NFL astrocytes has been observed in the elderly.

In the elderly, it has also been observed that the basal membrane of the inner limiting membrane is thicker than in the younger group. The increase in thickness impedes the interchange of substances between the retina and the vitreous humor that represents a reserve of glucose, amino acids, potassium and glutathione, and so on for the retina and a deposit for degradation products.

ISCHEMIA OF THE INNER RETINA

Ischemia of the inner retina, caused by the presence of naked or acellular vessels (formed from a thickening of the basal membrane of the capillaries), will be aggravated by the difficulty of diffusion of nutrients across the inner limiting membrane, and the elimination of catabolites. In the group of people with AMD, the changes are more severe than those in normal individuals of the same age. The changes to the inner retina in individuals with AMD are equivalent to those of the outer retina and represent an advanced aging of the retina. In the studied group of patients with AMD, the basal membrane of the retinal capillaries is considerably thicker than that of normal individuals of the same age with a thick external layer of collagen in contact with the astrocytes and Müller cells. The number of acellular capillaries is higher, especially in cases of AMD in patients aged over 81. In fact, the ischemia that establishes itself in these cases is considerably worse than that of healthy individuals of the same age. In all cases of AMD, there is an elevated number of hypertrophic and reactive astrocytes. Under an electron microscope, it has been seen that these astrocytes phagocyte the residues of the necrotic or apoptotic dead ganglion cells. The astrocytes contain elevated quantities of lysosomes and lipofuscin, as do the ganglion cells and their axons.

The extended retinal ischemia seen in patients with AMD, together with the loss of astroglial cells that occurs with normal aging, cause the death of ganglion cells that are not protected against oxidative stress. Furthermore, the basal membrane of the inner limiting membrane in AMD becomes thicker than that of healthy individuals of the same age, obstructing the metabolic exchange between the retina and the vitreous humor. The reactive astrocytes are overfilled with electron dense material and expel this material into the inner limiting membrane. In all the individuals with AMD, strongly GFAP+ trunk-shaped astroglial protrusions have been found that cross the inner limiting membrane and enter the vitreous humor. These protrusions are formed of astrocytes with long protrusions parallel to the inner limiting membrane and form a glial membrane. Under an electron microscope, cells have been observed in the vitreous humor, and judging by their ultrastructural properties, they could be astrocytes. These cells possess a clear cytoplasm, a large number of cellular organelles, and dense glial filaments. The protrusions of these cells intercommunicate across many gap junctions. The astrocytes also possess microvilli in contact with the vitreous humor, where there is no basal membrane, allowing direct contact between the vitreous humor and the astrocytes. These cells have ultrastructural characteristics similar to the epiretinal membranes observed in other pathologies. Another type of cell that also has been observed more often, is highly GFAP+ and column-shaped, and lies parallel to the inner limiting membrane, which can be confused with the aforementioned astrocytes. The morphological characteristics of these cells is reminiscent of the Müller cells as they are more robust, column-shaped, and have few protrusions. These cells should be reactive Müller glia, which in pathologic situations express the GFAP.

HYPERTROPHIC ASTROCYTES

Madigan *et al.* (1994) alone have described that in retinas with AMD there are distended hypertrophic astrocytes on the internal surface of the retina. Many studies have been performed on the neovascular membrane that is found in AMD, produced by the migration of endothelial choroidal cells across the Bruch's membrane in the subretinal space, but none have talked about epiretinal glial membranes. Many studies have shown that the epiretinal membranes may derive from inflammatory processes, retinal ruptures, or retinal vascular occlusions. The extended retinal ischemia in AMD causes the astrocytes to migrate into the vitreous humor, where they can find metabolic reserves. In this way the vitreous humor guarantees the nutrition of the remaining astrocytes in the inner retina as the intercellular junctions between the astrocytes remain intact. It is not known what factors cause the astrocytes and Müller cells to migrate into the vitreous humor in AMD. It is not known if these membranes are dangerous, that is,. if they can, after traction, cause a detachment of the retina.

AGING OF THE MICROGLIA

The retinal microglia originate from the hematopoietic cells and enter the retina from the retinal margin and the optic disk, through the blood vessels of the cilliary bodies and iris, and of the retina, respectively. The microglial precursors that are found on the retina before vascularization are positive to some specific immuno-stainings and express the CD45 marker, but are not positive for specific markers of the macrophages. A second category of microglial precursors, which express typical macrophage markers, migrate into the retina together with vascular precursors. These are localized around the blood vessels in the adult retina and are similar to macrophages or mononuclear phagocytes. The microglial cells are found in the outer plexiform layer, the external nuclear layer, the internal plexiform layer, the gangliar layer, and the nervous fiber layer of the retina in humans. The retinal macrophages are involved in the defense against viral, bacterial, and parasitic infection, in immunoregulation, in tissue repair, in the catabolism of neurotransmitters and hormones, and in the lipid turnover of nervous tissue. The microglia play an important role in the defense against microorganisms, in immune regulation, and in tissue repair. The occurrence of neurodegenerative phenomena, but also normal aging, cause the conversion of the microglia from resting to reactive. Reactive microglia have the responsibility of phagocyting the debris and facilitate the regenerative processes. The morphology and localization of the microglia are not the same for all our ages. It has been seen that in newborn mice, the microglia cells are round and ameboid with thick, squat pseudopolipoid protrusions distributed in the ganglion and nervous fiber layers, whereas their morphology shows some age-related changes.

Aging of the Retinal Vessels

Age-related changes to the retinal vessels have been found both in the superficial and the deeper capillary net. The thickness of the basal ganglion membrane increases by two to three times. In samples of retina of rats aged 28 to 32 months, Glatt and Henkind (1979) noted a reduction in the number of capillary endothelial cells and pericytes. Ramirez *et al.* (2001) also described age-related changes to the retinal vessels. The capillaries show a thickening of the basal membrane, equal to double that of the capillaries of young individuals, with numerous accumulations of lipids. The lumen of the capillaries is more irregular, and the endothelial cells are full of lysosomes and lipids, which are then carried into the lumen of the blood vessels. The pericytes adjacent to the endothelial cells of the vessels have a cytoplasm rich in dense bodies. Moreover, there is a loss of endothelial cells from the peripheral retinal capillaries that become like naked vessels or acellular capillaries. The same happens in the choriocapillary vessels from 60 years onward (Cavallotti *et al.*, 2005). The loss of endothelial cells and the thickening of the basal membrane of the capillaries diminish the passage of oxygen and nutrients to the retinal nervous tissue. This fact causes hypoxia and slowing of the elimination of catabolism products.

Age-Related Diseases of the Human Retina

It is very common to encounter senile lesions of the eyes and therefore a reduction in the acuity of vision and also peripheral chorioretinal lesions, which cause severe retinal lesions such as senile retinal detachment. The interest in studying geriatric changes to vision lies in identifying the first lesions as early as possible. Not that it is possible, at least up to now, to impede the inexorable evolution of the degenerative phenomena, but an early diagnosis can at least allow us to greatly slow this process. With the passing of the years, the normal architecture of the retina undergoes modifications starting from the ora serata toward the posterior pole for a variable distance. At the posterior pole of the Bruch's membrane (drusen), lipid or calcium carbonate soap deposits and capillarosis (obliterated aneurisms) are seen. Dry and wet macular degeneration are clinical pictures often discussed in pathology. Finally, the cystoids of the macula begin with an edema with brilliant irregular foveal reflexes, which surround the macula. In the macula there may be an isolated vesicle, dark red in color, with sharply defined edges. In the periphery, the most frequent lesions are cystic degeneration and Blessig-Iwanoff holes, localized in the ora serrata (Owsley *et al.*, 2000).

CYSTIC DEGENERATION

The retina shows two types of cystic degeneration, typical and reticular. Typical cystic degeneration originates on the outer plexiform layer, and reticular originates in the nervous fiber layer. These changes are very common after 70 years of age. The typical peripheral cystoid degeneration (TPCD) (Blessig-Iwanoff cysts) is characterized by cysts of the outer plexiform layer containing hyaluronic acid that can also coagulate, producing a globular form with winding channels that branch irregularly. Complications are rare; the retinal holes do not produce detachment of the retina as the vitreous is normally complete over the lesion. The extension of the lesion beyond the equator is rare. The breakage of the walls of the cysts or gaps causes the formation of peripheral lamellar holes. The retina is not detached; there is not the operculum of real retinal holes. Rare, but possible, is the formation of real retinal holes, with operculum to which vitreous body filaments adhere following a filamentous degeneration of the vitreous body and unsticking from the ora serrata. This can lead to another peripheral alteration: degenerative retinoschisis. The second type of modification is retinal periphery cystoid degeneration, which is almost always continuous and located behind areas of typical peripheral cystiod degeneration, and usually is found in the inferotemporal quadrant. This has a reticular aspect that corresponds to the retinal vessels of the inner layers. A finely punctured inner surface corresponds to the attachment points of the tissue cushions to the inner layer. The cystic spaces are localized in the nervous fiber layer. This process occurs in 18% of adults, in bilateral form, in 41%. It can evolve into degenerative reticular retinoschisis (O'Malley and Allen, 1967).

RETINOSCHISIS

Two degenerative forms of retinoschisis have been described; they are both most frequently seen in the inferotemporal quadrant and derive from a preexisting form of peripheral cystoid degeneration. Typical peripheral cystoid degeneration can evolve into typical degenerative retinoschisis, whereas both the typical and reticular forms of peripheral cystoid degeneration can transform into reticular degenerative retinoschisis. Typical degenerative retinoschisis causes a smooth raising of the retina in 1% of the adult population (bilateral in 33% of cases). Typical peripheral cystoid degeneration surrounds the lesions. The retina is divided along the outer plexiform layer, and consequently the inner layer comprises the ILM, the nervous fiber layer, the retinal vessels, the ganglion cells, the inner plexiform layer, and the inner nuclear layer; normally only the ILM, the nervous fiber layer, and part of the inner nuclear layer are visible. The outer layer is thicker, with cavities and is made up of the external nuclear layer and the photoreceptors (Foos, 1970). Reticular degenerative retinoschisis develops from the concurrent presence of typical and reticular cystoid degeneration of the peripheral retina. It is characterized by oval or round areas of detached retina in which a lump is in the very thin inner layer, and is observed in 1.6% of the adult population (in bilateral form in 15% of cases). Normally, typical peripheral cystoid degeneration is localized anterior to the reticular degenerative retinoschisis, whereas the reticular form is adjacent.

The detachment occurs in the nervous fiber layer; the inner portion contains only the ILM, some retinal vessels, and a variable portion of the nervous fiber layer. The outer portion contains the remaining relatively complete retinal layers. Sometimes typical and reticular retinoschisis are seen at the same time. It is not always easy to differentiate between the two forms on a clinical basis, unless there are lumpy aspects. The presence of holes in the outer margin or posterior extension are characteristics more common of the reticular form than the typical form.

LATEX DEGENERATION

The frequency of latex degeneration was found to be 8% in an ample clinical study and 10.7% in autopsy studies. The lesions are bilateral and symmetrical in 48.1% of cases, and the frequency increases after the second decade of life. The majority of the lesions, located in the preequatorial region, are orientated according to the circumference and more frequently in the vertical meridian (Byer, 1989). Latex lesions appear like a thinning of the retina; they can also look like a plait caused by sclerotic vessels and may have variable pigmentation resulting from hypertrophy of the RPE. Histological latex degeneration is characterized by an overlying sack of vitreous fluid, absence of the ILM, vitreous condensation at the margins, hyperplasia of the glial cells and at the edges of the RPE, in some cases, thinning and the formation of retinal holes at the center of the lesion, sclerosis of the major blood vessels, sclerosis and acellularity of the capillaries hypertrophy, and hyperplasia of the RPE.

COBBLESTONE DEGENERATION

This common degenerative chorio-retinal process is found in up to 27% of subjects after the thirtieth year. It is localized between the ora serrata and the real side of the equator and represents a boundary zone between the posterior choroidal circulation and the anterior cilliar circulation. Opthalmoscopically, it looks like a small and discrete yellow-white area, with very visible choroidal blood vessels, sometimes with hypertrophic and dark RPE at the margins. The lesions can join together to form a band of depigmentation behind the ora serrata. Histopathologic studies show signs of ischemic atrophy of the outer retina, with attenuation or disappearance of the choriocapillaries, loss of the RPE and the outer retinal layer up to and including the external part of the inner nuclear layer. These changes are limited to the portion of the retina that is supplied by the choriocapillaries, and can be reproduced in rabbits after binding the choroidal blood supply (Stratsma *et al.*, 1980). Cobblestone degeneration is a characteristic that suggests peripheral vasculopathy and can be highly extended in carotid stenosis (O'Malley and Allen, 1967)

SENILE PERIPHERAL PIGMENT DEGENERATION

Senile peripheral pigment degeneration is associated with wartiness of the Bruch's membrane, and sclerosis of the choroid. It is often bilateral. One type of pigment alteration that is not peripheral, however, comes from moniliform pigmented scratches of the chorioretina. These are pigment granules that seem to be localized on sclerotic choroidal blood vessels in the nasal inferior quadrant (De Laey, 1988).

SENILE RETINA DETACHMENT

It is not easy to define retinal detachment as senile. There are chorioretinal and vitreal alterations that are typically geriatric and may cause detachment of the retina:

1. Cystic degeneration of the periphery of the retina. On one hand, cystic degeneration causes a thinning and weakening of the retina, and on the other, it favors the formation of pathological adherence with the vitreo and therefore creates a predisposition to retinal rupture at the margin or at the operculum. Furthermore, the walls of the cysts may break and therefore retinal holes may form (Foulds, 1980).
2. Paved, cobblestone, or pavement degeneration as proposed by Straatsma *et al.* (1980) or Gonin's foci of atrophic choroidosis. From a histological point of view these lesions show the disappearance of the choriocapillaries and the pigment epithelium, atrophy of the inner layers of the retina—that is, those which depend on the trophism of the choriocapillaries for nutrition. The retina is strongly held to the choroid in these degenerative foci. They almost never form holes or ruptures of the retina. This type of degeneration does not favor the detachment of the retina per se, but shows that there is wear and choroidal and retinal degeneration at the periphery that may favor the onset of retinal detachment. In fact, O'Malley and Allen (1967) observed that numerous patients who show cobblestone degeneration also have, near to these lesions, cystic degeneration of the retina, fence degeneration, retinoschisis, retinal holes and ruptures, and cysts of the pars plana.
3. Senile degeneration of the vitreous. After 50 years of age, in emmetropic eyes, a fibrillar and lacunar degeneration of the vitreous begins, slowly progressing, and may result in the posterior detachment of the vitreous with its collapse. This is a typical senile disease that is found in 65% of individuals over 65 years old and more or less 100% of individuals over 77 years. The posterior detachment of the vitreous may cause, where there is an adherence between the vitreous and the retina, rupture of the retina by traction. The retinal rupture may be secondary to a choroidal exudation of congestive or allergic inflammatory origin, which passes the pigment epithelium, applying pressure to the retina toward the inside of the eye bulb, causing its rupture at a weak point. On contact with the choroidal exudation liquid, the vitreous then coagulates. Senile retinal detachment seems to be essentially caused by cystic degeneration of the retina and posterior detachment of the vitreous with collapse, due to the fact that in cases of senile detachment, posterior detachment of the vitreous with collapse is nearly always found. If we consider, however, the rarity of retinal detachment with respect to posterior detachment of the vitreous and cystic degeneration of the retina in senility, we must admit that many other factors must be relevant in retinal detachment such as genetic predisposition, vascular-retinal-choroidal factors, and abiotrophic factors.

The changes that lead to retinal detachment in senile eyes are very similar to those in myopic eyes. A study performed on 829 patients affected by retinal detachment and surveyed over three years found that about 34% were myopic and 66% were not. Of these, around 63% were individuals more than 40 years old. This shows therefore that senility plays an important role in the initiation of retinal detachment. Without doubt, retinal detachment results from degenerative lesions of the retina and the choroid, lesions which normally do not have characteristics appreciably different from degenerative myopic lesions. In the case of senility, the lesions are related to obstructions of the retinal and sometimes choroidal capillaries. The study of the cases in which the retinal detachment occurred in nonmyopic individuals in senile age confirms that normally in these degenerative lesions there is evidence of vascular obstruction in the form of thin obliterated blood vessels that prevail in the superior temporal quadrant. In the eyes of nonmyopic senile age subjects, it is possible to see, more frequently than in young subjects, small pigmented equatorial spots that are often hexagonal in appearance. These are often the starting point of horseshoe ruptures, on the borders of which pigment deposits are found. Finally, there can be interruptions in the continuity of the macula deriving from senile alterations. In senile degeneration of the macula, pits may form in the macular lamella, which, although not very frequent, become perforations with consequent retinal detachment. Senility, as well as favoring the arrival of regmatogenous retinal alterations, is also responsible for the degenerative vitreal changes that can produce traction, rupture, and therefore detachment of the retina (Marshall, 1987).

The influence of vascular alterations in the pathogenesis of senile retinal detachment is without doubt to be taken into consideration. As aging causes a reduction in cardiac and lung performance, so it may cause a decrease of the retinal integrity. A parallel can be seen between the atherosclerotic lesions of the retinal blood vessels, and those of the other organs. We should remember, finally, that aphakia, not often seen these days as a result of good cataract operations, has a tight correlation with retinal detachment. It originates from small ruptures or holes in the ora serrata. In senile aphakic eyes, retinal degeneration very often is seen at the periphery and particularly at the ora serrata, with small holes generally located in the meridional folds of the retina.

PREVENTION

Considering what just has been described, prevention of the degenerative factors induced by aging points to the application of an anti-apoptotic action to the nervous cells and glia of the human retina. One possible drug to perform this is acetyl-carnitine (ALCAR). In recent years attention has been focused on the advantageous influence of carnitine as an anti-apoptotic agent, above all as a molecule able to block the mitochondrial pathway in programmed cell death. Moreover ALCAR seems to have a major protective role in the senile retina decay. The anti-apoptotic action caused by carnitine includes induction of growth factors, increase in mitochondrial metabolism, protective action on the mitochondrial membrane integrity, inhibition of caspase activity, and finally, an antioxidant activity.

Conclusion

The aim of this study is not only to fully understand the senile involution of retinal structures, which allows us to observe the wonders of the world, but also to keep these structures intact for as long as possible. According to the theory of aging, the level of senescence is determined by the interaction between factors that promote aging and those that counteract it, in practice by the cellular regeneration capacity that is under genetic control. From this point of view, the "theory of physical deterioration" can be unified with another aging theory, that of the "biological clock." This theory asserts that the life expectancy of each species is genetically determined and that variations are the result of environmental influence or genetic mutations.

Recommended Resources

Look for recent books on vision disorders in old age at www.amazon.com.

- *The aging eye*, by Sandra Gordon, Harvard Medical School (2001).
- *Communication technologies for the elderly: vision, hearing & speech*, by Rosemary Lubinski and D. Jeffery Higginbotham (1997).
- *The effects of aging and environment on vision*, by Donald A. Armstrong, *et al.* (1991).
- *Treating vision problems in the older adult* (Mosby's optometric problem-Solving Series), by Gerald G. Melore (2001).
- *Vision and aging*, by Alfred A. Rosenbloom and Meredith W. Morgan (1993).
- *Age-related macular degeneration*, by Jennifer I. Lim (2002).
- *The impact of vision loss in the elderly* (Garland studies on the Elderly in America), by Julia J. Kleinschmidt (1995).
- *Vision in Alzheimer's disease* (Interdisciplinary Topics in Gerontology), by Alice Croningolomb *et al.* (2004).
- *The senescence of human vision* (Oxford medical publications), by R.A. Weale (2001).
- *Issues in aging and vision: A curriculum for university programs and in-service training*, by Alberta L. Orr (1998).
- *Aging with developmental disabilities changes in vision*, by Marshall E. Flax (1996).
- *Trends in vision and hearing among older Americans*, by U.S. Dept of Health and Human Services (2000).
- *Optometric gerontology*: A resource manual, by Sherrell J. Aston (2003).

REFERENCES

Antal, M. (1977). Scanning electron microscopy of photoreceptors. *Ophthalmologica 174*, 280–284.

Armstrong, D. (1984). Free radical involvement in the formation of lipo-pigments. In D. Armstrong, Ed. *Free radicals in molecular biology, aging and disease*, pp. 137–182. New York: Raven Press.

Bird, A.C. (1997). What is the future of research in age-related macular degeneration? *Arch. Ophthalmol. 115*, 1311–1313.

Boulton, M., Dontsov, A., Jarvis- Evans, J., Ostrovsky, M., and Svistunenko, D. (1993). Lipo-fuscin is a photo-inducible free radical generator. *J. Photochem. Photobiol. 19*, 201–204.

Boulton, M. and Wassel, J. (1998). Ageing of the human retinal epithelium. In G. Coscasand F.C. Piccolino, Eds. *Retinal Pigment Epithelium and Macular Disease*, pp. 20–28. *Doc. Ophthalmologica 62.*

Brizee, K.R. and Ordy, J.M.. (1981). Cellular features, regional accumulation, and prospects of modification of age pigments in mammals. In R.S. Sohal, Ed. *Ageing pigments*, pp. 176–181. Amsterdam: Elsevier/North – Holland Biomedical Press.

Burns, R.P. and Feeney-Burns, L. (1980). Clinico–morphologic correlations of drusen of Bruch's membrane. *Trans. Am. Acad. Ophthalmol. Soc. 78*, 206–255.

Byer, N.E. (1989). Long-term natural history of lattace degeneration of the retina. *Ophthalmology 96*, 1396–1402.

Castino, M. and Roletto, E. (1992). *Statistica Applicata*. Piccin ed. Padua Italy.

Cavallotti, C., Artico, M., Pescosolido, N., and Feher, J. (2004). Age-related changes in human retina. *Can. J. Ophthalmol. 39*, 61–68.

Cavallotti, C., Balacco Gabrieli, C., and Feher, J. (2005). The human choriocapillaris: Evidence for an intrinsic regulation of the endothelium. *J. of Anatomy 206*, 243–247.

Chen, L., Yang, P., and Kijlstra, A. (2002). Distribution, markers, and functions of retinal microglia. *Ocul. Immunol. Inflamm. 10*, 27–39.

Curcio, C.A., Millican, C.L., Allen, K.A.., and Kalina, R.E. (1993). Aging of the human photoreceptor mosaic: Evidence for selective vulnerability of rods in central retina. *Invest. Ophthalmol. Vis. Sci. 34*, 3278–3296.

De Laey, J.J. (1988). Ophtalmologie geriatrique. In Oosterhosch, Ed. *Traité de Geriatrie*, pp 263 488. Bruxelles, Sociéte Scientifique de Medicine Generale.

Dorey, C.K., Wu, G., Ebestein, D., Garsd, A., and Weiter, J.J. (1989). Cell loss in the aging retina: Relationship to lipofuscin accumulation and macular degeneration. *Invest. Ophthalmol. Vis. Sci. 30*, 1691–1699.

Dryja, T.P., Briggs, C.E., Berson, E.L., and Rosenfeld, P.J. (1998). ABCR gene and age-related macular degeneration. *Science 279*, 1107 1109.

Dykens, J.A. (1999). Free radicals and mitochondria dysfunction in excyto-toxicity and neurodegenerative disease. In V.E. Koliatos and R.R. Rantan, Eds. *Cell death and diseases of the Nervous System*, pp. 45–68. Totowa: Humana Press.

Eldred, G.E. and Lasky M.R. (1993). Retinal age pigments generated by self-assembling lysomotrophic detergents. *Nature 361*, 724–726.

Feeney-Burns, L., Hilderbrand, E.S., and Eldridge, S. (1984). Aging of human PRE: morphometric analysis of macular, equatorial and peripheral cells. *Invest. Ophthalmol. Vis. Sci. 25*, 195–200.

Feeney-Burns, L. and Ellersiek, M.R. (1985). Age-related changes in the ultrastructure of Bruch's membrane. *Am. J. Ophthalmol. 100*, 686–697.

Follman, P. and Radnot, M. (1979). Some scanning electron microscopic observations on human retina. *Klin Ocza 81*, 513–514.

Foos, R.Y. (1970). Senile retinoschisis: Relationship to cystoid degeneration. *Trans. Am. Acad. Ophthalmol. 68*, 329–403.

Foulds, W.S. (1980). Factors influencing visual recovery in retinal detachment surgery. *Trans. Ophthalmol. Soc. U.K. 100*, 72–77.

Gao, H. and Hollyfield, J.G. (1992). Aging of the human retina. Differential loss of neurons and retinal pigment epithelial cells. *Invest. Ophthalmol. Vis. Sci. 33*, 1–17.

Glatt, H.J. and Henkind, P. (1979). Aging changes in the retinal capillary bed of the rat. *Microvasc. Res. 18*, 1–17.

Handelman, G.J. and Dratz, E.A. (1986). The role of antioxidants in the retina and retinal pigment epithelium and the nature of pro-oxidant induced damage. *Adv. Free Radicals Biol. Med. 2*, 1, 89.

Hogan, M.J., Alvarado, J.A., and Weddel, J.E. (1971). *Histology of the human eye*. Philadelphia: Saunders Ed.

Iwasaki, M. and Inomata, H. (1988). Lipofuscin granules in human photoreceptor cells. *Invest. Ophthalmol. Vis. Sci. 29*, 671–679.

Katz, M.L. and Robison, W.G. (1984). Age-related changes in the retinal pigment epithelium of pigmented rats. *Exp. Eye Res.* 38, 137–151.

Leica. (1997). *Manual of methods of Quantimet 500*. Microsystems Imaging Solutions Ltd. U.K: Cambridge.

Lerman, S. (1988). Ocular photo-toxicity. *N. Engl. J. Med. 319*, 1475 1477.

Leuenberger, P. (1971). Stereo ultra-structure de la retine. *Arch. Ophthalmol. 31*, 813–822.

Lewis, E.R., Zeevi, Y.Y., and Werblin, F.S. (1969). Scanning electron microscopy of vertebrate visual receptors. *Brain Research 15*, 559–562.

Lowry, O.H., Rosebrough, N.J., Farr, A.L., and Randall, J. (1951). Protein measurement with the Folin phenol reagent. *J. Biol. Chem.* 193, 265–275.

Madigan, M.C., Penfold, P.L., Provis, P.L., Balind, T.K., and Billson, F.A. (1994). Intermediate filament expression in human retinal macroglia. Histopathologic changes associated with age related macular degeneration. *Retina 14*, 65–74.

Marshall, J. (1987). The ageing retina: Physiology and pathology. *Eye 1*, 282–295.

Moore, D.J. and Clover, G.M. (2001). The effect of age on the macromolecular permeability of human Bruch's membrane. *Invest. Ophthalmol. Vis. Sci. 42*, 2970–2975.

O'Malley, P.F. and Allen, R.A. (1967). Peripheral cystoid degeneration of the retina. Incidence and distribution in 1.000 autopsy eyes. *Arch. Ophthalmol. 77*, 769–776.

Osterberg, G.A. (1935). Topography of the layer of rods and cones in the human retina. *Acta Ophthalmol. 13, (Suppl.6)*, 1–103.

Owsley, C. and Burton, K.B. (1991). Aging and spatial contrast sensitivity: Underlying mechanism and implications for everyday life. In P. Bagnoli and W. Hodos, Eds. *The changing of visual system.*, pp. 119–136. New York: Plenum Press.

Owsley, C., Jackson, G.R., Cideciyan, A.V., Huang, Y., Fine, S.L, Ho, A.C. *et al.*, (2000). Psychophysical evidence for rod vulnerability in age-related macular degeneration. *Invest. Ophthalmol. Vis. Sci. 41*, 267– 273.

Panda-Jonas, S., Jonas J., and Jakobczyk-Kmija, M. (1996). Retinal pigment epithelial cell count distribution and correlations in normal human eyes. *Am. J. Ophthalmol. 121*, 181–189.

Pauleikhoff, D., Harper, A., Marshall, J., and Bird, A.C. (1990). Aging changes in Bruch's membrane: A histochemical and morphological study. *Ophthalmology 97*, 171–178.

Radnot, M. (1978). Scanning electron microscopic study of human retina. *Ophthalmologica* (Basel) *176*, 308–312.

Ramirez, J.M., Trivino, A., Ramirez, A.L., Salazar, J.J., and Garcia-Sanchez, J. (1994). Immunohistochemical study of human retinal astroglia. *Vis. Res. 34*, 1935–1946.

Sarna, T., Burke, J.M., Korytowski, W., Rozanowska, M., Shumatz, C.M., Zareba A. *et al.* (2003). Loss of melanin from human RPE with aging: Possible role of melanin photooxidation. *Exp. Eye Res. 76*, 89–98.

Straatsma, B.R., Foos, R.Y., and Feman, S.S. (1980). Degenerative diseases of the peripheral retina. In T.D. Duane, Ed. *Clinical Ophthalmol.*, pp.1–27. Philadelphia: Harper & Row.

Streiff, E.B. and Faggioni, R. (1971). Alterazioni senili della corioretina. In B. Bellan, Ed. *Atti del Simposio di oftalmologia geriatrica*, pp 241–369. Simposi Italseber.

Sturr, J.F. and Hannon, D.J. (1991). Methods and models for specifying sites and mechanism of sensitivity regulation in the aging visual system. In P. Bagnoli and W. Hodos, Eds. *The changing of visual system*), pp. 219–231. New York: Plenum Press.

Vernadakis, A. (1986). Changes in astrocytes with aging. In S. Federoff and A. Vernadakys, Eds. *Biochemistry, physiology and pharmacology of astrocytes*, pp. 377–407. Orlando, USA: Academic Press.

Weiter, J.J., Delori, F.C., Wing, G.I., and Fitch, K.A. (1986). Retinal pigment epithelial lipofuscin and melanin and choroidal melanin in human eyes. *Am. J. Ophthalmol. 27*, 145–152.

Young, R.W. (1982). The Bowman lecture: Metabolism of the pigment epithelium. In K. Shimizu and J.A. Oosterhuis, Eds. Proceedings of the XXIII International Congress Kyoto, 14–20 May, 1978, pp. 159–166. *Amsterdam, Excerpta Med.*

68

Models of Age-Related Vision Problems

J. Fielding Hejtmancik, Marc Kantorow, and Takeshi Iwata

The visual system provides unique opportunities to study the aging process, as well as challenges in understanding and developing therapies for age-related eye diseases. Exposure of the lens to high levels of photo-oxidative stress and the lack of protein turnover in the lens nucleus make it an optimal system in which to study protein modifications in aging. Similarly, the high level of metabolic activity in the retina and the necessity for turning over large amounts of lipids provide particular research opportunities as well. Finally, visual diseases associated with aging are among the most common threats to the quality of life in the elderly. Of age-related visual diseases, three result in a particularly high burden on the population: age-related cataracts, age-related macular degeneration, and progressive open angle glaucoma. Thus, these are dealt with in some detail in this brief review. Because of space and formatting limitations, much work described in this review could not be cited directly. The citations for most of these can be found in the references and general sources given in the chapter, and we apologize to those authors whose work is not cited directly. In addition, parts of this review draw from previous work by the three authors, reflecting their continuing preferences in style and arrangement.

Overview of the Visual System

BASIC ANATOMY/PHYSIOLOGY/BRIEF BIOCHEMISTRY

Components of the visual system include the optical components of the anterior eye (cornea, aqueous humor, lens, and vitreous body), retina, optic nerves, optic tracts, optic radiations, visual cortex, and a variety of nuclei (see Figure 68.1). The optical components of the eye focus light on the retina, which transduces the light signal into neural signals, and passes these neural signals through the optic nerves and tracts to central structures that perform more elaborate processing, integrating their information with that of the other senses. Any disease that interferes with the function of these components will cause loss of vision and blindness, and each part of the visual system has specific susceptibilities to age-related diseases or damage.

TYPES OF AGE-RELATED VISUAL DISEASES AND THEIR IMPACT ON SOCIETY

The predominant causes of age-related visual impairment and blindness vary between the developed and developing countries, and even within various demographic and ethnic groups within single countries (Thylefors *et al.*, 1995). There are many causes of visual loss in elderly patients, including diabetic retinopathy, stroke, and retinal vascular occlusive disease, along with other age-related visual diseases including pterygia and presbyopia. However, in most populations the greatest causes of blindness and vision loss in the elderly include cataracts, glaucoma, and age-related macular degeneration (Congdon, Friedman, and Lietman, 2003; Buch *et al.*, 2004).

Cataracts are the leading cause of blindness across the world, blinding 17 million persons worldwide. Cataracts are usually correctable by surgery in developed countries, with about 5% of the American population over 40 years old having undergone cataract surgery. However, they remain a significant cause of visual disability even in developed countries, being the leading cause of low vision in the United States (Congdon, Friedman, and Lietman, 2003). Glaucoma is an optic neuropathy, often related to elevated intraocular pressure, which is responsible for blindness in 6.7 million people across the world. Glaucoma is more common in

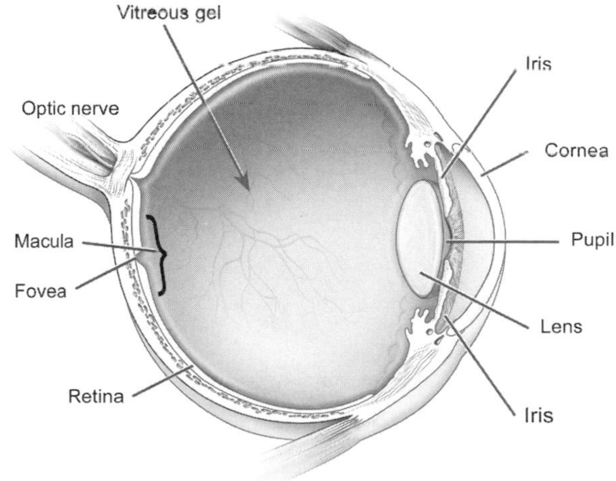

Figure 68.1 Diagram of the eye with principal structures of the anterior segment, retina, and optic nerve indicated. Courtesy of the National Eye Institute, National Institutes of Health.

Handbook of Models for Human Aging

African-derived populations, and increases with age. Finally, the greatest age-related cause of blindness in European-derived populations of developed countries is age-related macular degeneration (AMD). This degenerative disease progresses from fatty retinal deposits called drusen to neovascularization and retinal hemorrhage, resulting in irreversible loss of central vision.

Lens and Cataracts

The eye lens (see Figure 68.2), which contains perhaps the highest concentration of proteins found in any tissue, transmits and focuses light onto the retina. It is formed of a single cell type that differentiates from an anterior layer of cuboidal epithelia and migrates posteriorly to form elongated lens fiber cells that make up the lens nucleus. In this process, the developing fiber cells synthesize high levels of lens crystallins before losing their nuclei and mitochondria. Thus, the lens fiber cells lack aerobic metabolism and contain high concentrations of α-crystallins, which are members of the small heat shock protein family and have chaperone activity; and $\beta\gamma$-crystallins, which are related to prokaryotic structural proteins.

BRIEF OVERVIEW

The lens is susceptible to damage with aging since its cells cannot be replaced in this encapsulated tissue and its proteins cannot turn over in the nonnucleated fiber cells. Not only does this result in a decrease in function of the normal aged lens, but it also sets the stage for development of senescent cataract in individuals with additional environmental insult or genetic proclivity. As the lens ages, vacuoles and multilamellar bodies appear between fiber cells, and occasionally the fiber plasma membrane is disrupted. Most of the elaborate cytoskeletal structure of the lens cells disappears with aging, and by the fifth decade the ability to accommodate is essentially lost. There is a decrease in transparency of the normal lens with aging so that the intensity of light reaching the retina is reduced by about ten-fold by 80 years of age.

Cataracts which can be defined as any opacity of the crystalline lens, result when the refractive index of the lens varies significantly over distances approximating the wavelength of the transmitted light. Variation in the refractive index over these distances can result from changes in lens cell structure, changes in lens protein constituents, or both (Hejtmancik, Kaiser-Kupfer, and Piatigorsky, 2001). Cataracts are generally associated with breakdown of the lens micro-architecture. Vacuole formation can cause large fluctuations in optical density, resulting in light scattering. Light scattering and opacity also can occur if there are significant high molecular weight protein aggregates roughly 1000 Å or more in size. The short-range ordered packing of the crystallins, which make up over 90% of soluble lens proteins, is important in this regard; to achieve and maintain lens transparency crystallins must exist in a homogeneous phase.

A variety of biochemical or physical insults can cause phase separation of crystallins into protein-rich and protein-poor regions within the lens fibers. The proteins either remain in solution or form insoluble aggregates or even crystals, any of which can result in light scattering. When mutations in crystallins are sufficient in and of themselves to cause aggregation, they usually result in congenital cataracts, but if they merely increase susceptibility to environmental insults such as light, hyperglycemic, or oxidative damage, they might contribute to age-related cataracts (Hejtmancik and Smaoui, 2003). Thus, congenital cataracts tend to be inherited in a Mendelian fashion with high penetrance, whereas age-related cataracts tend to be multifactorial, with both multiple genes and environmental factors influencing the phenotype. This makes them significantly less amenable to genetic and biochemical study. Finally, although the young human lens is colorless, a gradual increase in yellow pigmentation occurs with age. As this pigmentation increases, it can result in brunescent or brown cataracts.

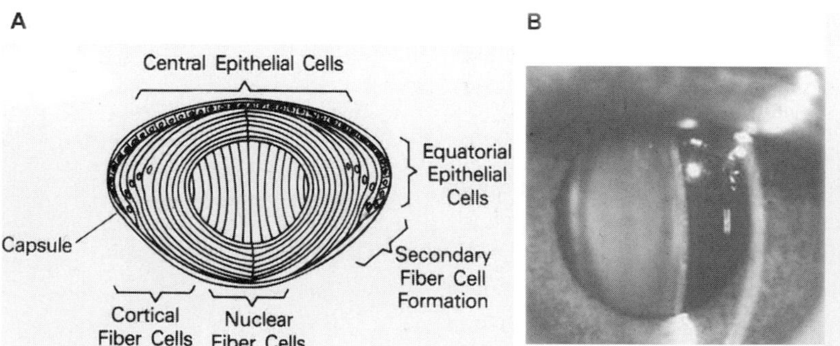

Figure 68.2 A. A diagram showing lens structure including the anterior epithelial cells; the cortical fiber cells, which elongate and loosen their nuclei and mitochondria; and the nuclear cells, in which this process has been completed. The ends of the nuclear fiber cells abut each other in a complex pattern to form the lens sutures. **B.** Slit lamp photograph of a nuclear cataract, the most common type of age-related cataract in European populations. Courtesy of Dr. Manuel Datiles, National Eye Institute, National Institutes of Health.

Lens proteins and their age-related modifications

Enzymatic activity in the lens tends to decrease with age and to be lower in the central cells of the lens nucleus than in the cortical and anterior epithelial cells. As the lens ages, the Na^+ and Ca^{2+} concentrations rise, reflecting an increase in lens permeability or a decrease in pumping efficiency. With aging, both the N- and C-terminal arms of half of the intrinsic membrane protein (MP26) molecules undergo proteolysis to form MP22. The lens contains neutral proteinase, also called the *multicatalytic-proteinase complex*, which preferentially degrades oxidized proteins, leucine aminopeptidase, calpains, and the protease cofactor ubiquitin, whose activation increases after oxidative stress. The activity of these proteinases is controlled by inhibitors, which appear to be concentrated at the periphery of the lens.

Aging also leads to an increase in high-molecular-weight aggregates and water-insoluble protein between 10 and 50 years of age, especially in the α-crystallins, but also in the β- and γ-crystallins. There is also partial degradation of crystallins and covalent modifications of crystallins and other lens proteins, including an increase in disulfide bridges, deamidation of asparagine and glutamine residues, and racemization of aspartic acid residues. αA-Crystallin is cleaved nonenzymatically, particularly between Asn 101 and Glu 102. An aspartate residue in αA-crystallin appears especially susceptible because it easily forms a succinimide intermediate. Phosphorylation of lens proteins also occurs. Nonenzymatic glycosylation (glycation) occurs, especially of the ε-amino groups of lysine. Through the Maillard reaction, the glycation products can result in increased pigmentation, nontryptophan fluorescence, and nondisulfide covalent crosslinks. Lens proteins can also undergo carbamylation, which can induce cataracts, and may be the mechanism for the association of cataracts with chronic diarrhea and uremia. γ-Crystallins, and especially γS-crystallin, are particularly susceptible to degradation and modification in age-dependent and other cataracts, largely being degraded to low-molecular-weight peptides by increased proteolysis in the cataractous lens.

In age-related cataracts the lens presumably develops reasonably normally during infancy and remains clear in childhood. Then, by somewhat arbitrary definition, at some time after 40 years of age, progressive opacities begin to form in the lens. As mentioned earlier, these opacities almost certainly result at least in part from the cumulative damage of environmental insults on lens proteins and cells. Many of the age-related changes seen in crystallins are accelerated in the presence of oxidative, photo-oxidative, osmotic, or other stresses, which are known to be associated with cataracts. Susceptibility to these alterations may be exacerbated by barriers to movement of small molecules between the central lens nucleus and the metabolically more active epithelium. Many of these changes can be induced *in vitro* or in model systems by the same stresses epidemiologically associated with cataracts (Davies and Truscott, 2001; Spector, 1995). In contrast, some changes do not appear to be implicated in cataractogenesis and may even serve to protect crystallins from harmful modifications.

The lens crystallins form one obvious target for this accumulated damage, although they are certainly not the only one. Thus, as the β- and γ-crystallins slowly accumulate damage over the lifetime of an individual, they lose the ability to participate in appropriate intermolecular interactions, and even to remain in solution. As these crystallins begin to denature and precipitate, they are bound by the α-crystallins, which have a chaperone-like activity. Binding by α-crystallins maintains the solubility of $\beta\gamma$-crystallins and reduces light scattering, but the α-crystallins appear not to renature their target proteins and release them into the cytoplasm, as do true chaperones. Rather, they hold them in complexes that, though soluble, increase in size as additional damaged protein is bound over time until they themselves begin to approach sizes sufficient to scatter light. Eventually, it seems likely that the available α-crystallin is overwhelmed by increasing amounts of modified $\beta\gamma$-crystallin and the complexes precipitate within the lens cell, forming the insoluble protein fraction that is known to increase with age and in cataractous lenses.

Brief epidemiology of age-related cataracts

Age-related cataracts are associated with a number of environmental risk factors, including cigarette smoking or chronic exposure to wood smoke, obesity or elevated blood glucose levels, poor infantile growth, exposure to ultraviolet light, and alcohol consumption (The Italian-American Cataract Study Group, 1991). Conversely, antioxidant vitamins seem to have a protective effect, although this has not been borne out by all studies.

There is increasing epidemiological evidence that genetic factors are important in the pathogenesis of age-related cataracts (McCarty and Taylor, 2001). In 1991, the Lens Opacity Case Control Study indicated that a positive family history was a risk factor for mixed nuclear and cortical cataracts, and the Italian–American cataract study group supported a similar role for family history as a risk factor in cortical, mixed nuclear and cortical, and posterior subcapsular cataracts. In 1994, the Framingham Offspring Eye Study showed that individuals with an affected sibling had three times the likelihood of also having a cataract. The Beaver Dam Eye Study examined nuclear sclerotic cataracts using sibling correlations and segregation analysis. Although a random environmental major effect was rejected by this study, Mendelian transmission was not rejected, and the results suggested that a single major gene could account for as much as 35% of nuclear and up to 75% of cortical cataract variability. Most recently, the twin eye study demonstrated significant genetic influence of age-related cortical cataracts, with heritability accounting for 53 to 58% of the liability for age-related cortical cataracts. This hereditary tendency was consistent with a combination of additive and dominant genes, with dominant genes accounting for 38 to 53% of the genetic effect, depending on whether cataracts were scored using the Oxford or Wilmer grading systems. Similarly, genetic factors were found to account for approximately 48% of the risk for nuclear cataracts.

HUMAN STUDIES ON AGE-RELATED CATARACTS

Linkage studies

In addition to epidemiological evidence implicating genetic factors in age-related cataracts, a number of inherited cataracts with post-infantile age of onset or progression of the opacity throughout life have been described. Mutations in beaded filament specific protein 2 (BFSP2) can cause juvenile cataracts, the Marner and Volkmann cataracts can be progressive, mutations in aquaporin 0 (MIP) and γC-crystallin can cause progressive cataracts, and the CAAR locus is linked to familial adult onset pulverulent cataracts. These all suggest that for at least some genes, a mutation that severely disrupts the protein or inhibits its function might result in congenital cataracts inherited in a highly penetrant Mendelian fashion, whereas a mutation that causes less severe damage to the same protein or impairs its function only mildly might contribute to age-related cataracts in a more complex multifactorial fashion. Similarly, mutations that severely disrupt the lens cell architecture or environment might produce congenital cataracts, whereas others that cause relatively mild disruption of lens cell homeostasis might contribute to age-related cataracts.

Association studies

The hyperferritinemia-cataract syndrome is a recently described disorder in which cataracts are associated with hyperferritinemia without iron overload. Ferritin L levels in the lens can increase dramatically. The molecular pathology lies in the ferritin L iron responsive element, a stem loop structure in the 5′ untranslated region of the ferritin mRNA. Normally, this structure binds a cytoplasmic protein, the iron regulatory protein, which then inhibits translation of ferritin mRNA, which may exist in the lens at levels approaching that of a lens crystallin. Mutation of this structure and overexpression of ferritin by loss of translational control in the hyperferritinemia-cataract syndrome results in crystallization of ferritin in the lens, and other tissues as well. Ferritin crystals appear as breadcrumb-like opacities in the cortex and nucleus. Ferritin cataracts serve as an example that the presence of crystallin proteins at such high levels in the protein-rich lens cytoplasm requires that they must be exceptionally soluble. This is emphasized by the occurrence of cataracts resulting from single base changes decreasing crystallin solubility but not stability.

Lamellar and polymorphic cataracts have been associated with missense mutations in the MIP gene. One mutation, E134G, is associated with a nonprogressive congenital lamellar cataract, and the second T138R is associated with multifocal opacities that increase in severity throughout life. When expressed in *Xenopus laevis* oocytes, both of these mutations appear to act by interfering with normal trafficking of MIP to the plasma membrane and thus with water channel activity. In addition, both mutant proteins appear to interfere with water channel activity by normal MIP, consistent with the autosomal dominant inheritance of the cataracts.

Galactosemic cataracts provide an interesting example of mutations that severely affect a gene causing congenital cataracts, and of milder mutations that contribute to age-related cataracts. Deficiencies of galactokinase, galactose-1-phosphate uridyl transferase, and severe deficiencies of uridine diphosphate 1-4 epimerase cause cataracts as a result of galactitol accumulation and subsequent osmotic swelling. The latter two are also associated with vomiting, failure to thrive, liver disease, and mental retardation if untreated, whereas the cataracts in galactokinase deficiency are isolated. Interestingly, galactosemic cataracts initially are reversible both in human patients and in animal models. In 2001, a novel variant of galactokinase, the Osaka variant with an A198V substitution, was shown to be associated with a significant increase in bilateral cataracts in adults (Okano *et al.*, 2001). It results in instability of the mutant protein and is responsible for mild galactokinase deficiency, leaving about 20% of normal levels. This variant allele frequency occurs in 4.1% in Japanese overall and 7.1% of Japanese with cataracts. The allele was also present in 2.8% of Koreans but had a lower incidence in Chinese and was not seen in blacks or whites from the United States. This and other GALK1 variants appeared to be absent from Northern Italians with age-related cataracts, suggesting that the genetic contributions cataract might vary in different populations.

The GALK1 results fit in well with the known influence of hyperglycemia on age-related cataracts. That these cataracts result from polyol accumulation is suggested by work in galactosemic dogs and transgenic and knockout mice. Dogs have aldose reductase levels similar to those in humans and when stressed readily develop sugar cataracts that are prevented by aldose reductase inhibitors. Mice, which have very low aldose reductase activity in the lens, are naturally resistant to sugar cataracts, either galactosemic or hyperglycemic. However, upon transgenic expression of aldose reductase, mice readily develop cataracts, especially when the galactokinase or sorbitol dehydrogenase gene is deleted. Consistent with these animal data are the recent findings that susceptibility to cataracts as a diabetic complication in humans is associated with specific allele Z of the microsatellite polymorphism at 5′ of the aldose reductase gene.

BIOCHEMICAL STUDIES OF AGE-RELATED CATARACTS

Crystallin modifications associated with cataracts

The lens crystallins are a major potential target for accumulating damage associated with age-related cataracts, although there are certainly others. Thus, as the crystallins accumulate modifications and damage over the lifetime of an individual, their ability to participate in appropriate intermolecular interactions, and even to remain in solution, decreases. Whether proteins in age-related cataracts become insoluble as a result of complete or partial denaturation, or whether they simply become less soluble due to modifications that leave their protein folds largely intact or both, is not currently known. However, it seems clear that modifications to crystallin proteins accumulate with aging and accelerate during cataractogenesis, and the combination of crystallin modification, disulfide-crosslinking, denaturation, and aggregation results in loss of lens transparency and cataract formation (Hanson *et al.*, 2000). The protein modifications involved in this process include, but are not limited to, proteolysis, racemation, oxidative changes, and glycation. The many factors believed to induce these modifications include free radicals and superoxides, along with a loss of the lens' reducing state causing oxidation and disulfide-crosslinking, sugar accumulation causing glycation, and cyanate causing carbamylation.

Protein modifications in age-related cataracts are believed to arise from a combination of environmental and endogenous factors. For instance, considerable evidence suggests that oxidative modifications are a hallmark of age-related cataracts and oxidation of crystallins and other lens proteins likely results from reactive oxygen species that are produced by both UV-light exposure and are also a byproduct of mitochondrial respiration during which as much as 2% of respiratory oxygen is converted to reactive oxygen species. A major result of oxidation is conversion of methionine to methionine sulfoxide, which increases with age in the human lens and reaches levels as high as 60% in age-related cataracts relative to clear lenses.

Multiple identified and yet unidentified proteases are present in the lens and proteolyzed crystallins are a predominate feature of age-related cataracts. Among multiple lens proteases that have been identified to act on crystallin proteins, calcium-activated proteases are believed to play major roles. Proteolysis of specific crystallins is believed to result in protein aggregation and cataracts.

Proteins in age-related cataracts become insoluble as a result of complete or partial denaturation or by becoming less soluble due to modifications that leave their protein folds largely intact, or perhaps by a combination of these processes. Many highly studied Mendelian congenital cataract models support both denaturation, as is seen in the association of some severe crystallin mutations with cataracts, and simple insolubility with maintained protein folds as is seen in other cataracts. Many classical studies have demonstrated that lens proteins become insoluble because they are denatured as the lens ages. Insoluble protein in the aged cataractous lens not only is denatured and crosslinked, but a fraction exists as relatively short peptides cleaved from larger proteins. It seems likely that the presence of large amounts of unstable or precipitated crystallin, or other protein, does damage to the lens cell and its proteins and eventually contributes to cataracts not only directly through light scattering by protein aggregates but eventually also through disruption of cellular metabolism and damage to the cellular architecture. This is clear from numerous mouse models of cataracts resulting from crystallin mutations (Graw and Loster, 2003).

Gene expression changes in cataract

In addition to crystallin modifications, age-related cataracts are also associated with changes in gene expression detected at the level of increased or decreased mRNA in the lens epithelium (Hejtmancik and Kantorow, 2004). Since the lens epithelial cells cover the anterior surface of the lens, whereas in age-related cataracts the opacities tend to occur in the nuclear or cortical fiber cells, these gene expression changes likely reflect responses of lens epithelial cells to the presence of underlying cataracts and/or altered epithelial function in the presence of cataracts. These gene expression changes nevertheless point to altered lens pathways associated with this disease. For instance, the mRNAs encoding metallothionein and osteonectin (also known as SPARC, secreted acidic protein rich in cysteines) are increased in cataracts, whereas those for protein phosphatase 2A regulatory subunit and some ribosomal proteins including L21, L15, L13a, and L7a are decreased. These alterations suggest that increased binding of toxic metals and Ca++ with a concomitant decrease in growth pathways and protein synthesis are features of cataract.

In addition to the identification of individual alterations in gene expression, more recent studies have sought to identify the full range of gene expression changes that occur in the lens epithelium upon cataract formation using DNA microarrays. Although literally thousands of genes whose expression is altered in cataract have been identified in these studies, some specific examples of genes increased in cataract include SP1 required cofactor for transcriptional regulation, osteomodulin, chloride channel 3, Na+K+ transporting polypeptide beta 1, and Ca++ transporting ATPase, whereas genes decreased include αA-crystallin, multiple glutathione peroxidases, multiple ribosomal subunits, HSP 27, Na+/K+ ATPase and transketolase. The majority of the identified genes are decreased in cataract, suggesting loss of gene expression as a consequence of lens damage. Functional clustering of the identified genes suggests that the genes increased in cataract tend to be associated with transcriptional control, ionic and cytoplasmic transport, protein salvaging pathways, and extracellular matrix components; transcripts decreased in cataract tend to be associated with protein synthesis, defense against oxidative stress, heat shock/chaperone activity, structural components of the lens, and cell cycle control (Hejtmancik and Kantorow, 2004).

Enzyme changes associated with cataracts

In addition to the protein modification and gene expression changes noted earlier, numerous metabolic and enzyme activity changes are also associated with age-related cataracts. These changes include decreased reduced glutathione content, decreased NADPH levels, increased free Ca^{++} levels, increased activity of specific proteases, and decreased ionic balance, among others. Considerable evidence suggests that many of these changes, other metabolic changes, and loss of lens protein function results from loss of the activities of specific lens protective and repair enzymes and other homeostatic systems. Although the evidence for these changes has been almost exclusively derived from animal, cell, and organ culture experimental systems, loss of the activities of multiple protective systems including α-crystallins, MnSOD, catalase, glutathione peroxidase, and γ-glutamylcysteine synthetase among many others are believed to contribute to loss of lens function and ultimately cataract formation. In addition to the loss of lens protective and homeostatic systems, the loss of key repair systems including thioltransferase and methionine sulfoxide reductases are also believed to be key events in cataract formation.

ANIMAL MODELS OF AGE-RELATED CATARACTS

Overview

Since cataractogenesis is a complex process accompanied by numerous secondary changes, animal models may provide useful information for delineating the causes of senescent and other cataracts. Hereditary cataracts in rodents have been especially useful in this regard (Graw and Loster, 2003). One example is the Philly mouse, which displays an autosomal dominant cataract in which there is a deficiency of βB2-crystallin polypeptide. The βB2-crystallin mRNA has a deletion of 12 nucleotides, resulting in a four-amino-acid deletion in the encoded protein. It has been hypothesized that this causes aberrant folding of the protein and that cataract formation occurs as a result of the molecular instability of this crystallin and is therefore a good model to examine the roles of crystallin proteolysis and aggregation in age-related cataract formation. Other models suggest that some metabolic lesions can also cause cataracts. The Nakano mouse, which has autosomal recessive cataracts mapping to chromosome 16, shows reduced synthesis of α- and β-crystallins. This is probably due to an increase in the Na+/K+ ratio occurring because of inhibition of the sodium-potassium pump. The Fraser mouse, which displays an autosomal dominant cataract, shows preferential loss of γ-crystallins and their mRNAs. However, the gene causing this cataract segregates independently of the γ-crystallin gene cluster, suggesting that changes in crystallin expression must be secondary in this cataract. It resides on chromosome 10 and has been suggested to be allelic with the mouse lens opacity gene (LOP).

Emory mouse

Unlike the animal cataract models eariler, the Emory mouse is an interesting model for age-related cataracts that has been phenotypically but not molecularly or genetically well-characterized (Kuck, 1990). Two substrains of Emory mice in which cataracts develop at five to six months (early cataract strain) and six to eight months (late-cataract strain) are known. Emory mouse cataracts increase in severity with age and are initiated in the lens superficial cortex. They eventually progress into the deep anterior cortex and ultimately result in complete opacification. Emory mouse cataracts exhibit multiple changes that appear to mimic accelerated aging including abnormal lens growth, decreased protein accumulation, conversion of soluble to insoluble protein, decreased reduced glutathione, decreased protein sulfhydryl levels, decreased superoxide dismutase activities, decreased catalase activity, decreased glutathione peroxidase activity, decreased γ-glutamylcysteine synthetase activity, and accelerated conversion of MP26 to MP24. The Emory mouse is also associated with changes in gene expression including decreased synthesis of crystallins and increased expression of ARK tyrosine kinase, which is believed to be a major upstream activator of the stress response in many cell types.

In vivo hyperbaric oxygen treatment

Many of the modifications undergone by lens proteins in aging and cataractous lenses are consistent with those seen in photo-oxidative stress, and oxidative stress is known to be a risk factor in age-related cataracts (Giblin *et al.*, 1995). Thus, exposing animals to increased oxygen tension to simulate the more prolonged oxidative stress associated with aging is an attractive and logical model system for understanding human cataract. In these studies, animals are exposed to 100% oxygen at increased pressure several times weekly for two to three months, and lens opacities are monitored by imaging with a slit lamp. Molecular and biochemical changes in the treated animals subsequently are correlated with lens opacity and oxygen treatment. Hyperbaric oxygen treatment *in vivo* accelerates lens opacity in the nuclear region of the guinea pig lens including loss of water soluble and cytoskeletal proteins, formation of protein disulfides, and degradation of MIP26. Such modifications are similar to modifications reported to occur in the nuclei of aging and cataractous human lenses, confirming that hyperbaric oxygen treatment is an excellent model to study those processes occurring in human cataracts.

Other

In addition to the preceding models, cell culture, organ culture, and transgenic mice provide powerful tools for the study of lens transparency. Multiple lens epithelial cell lines have been used to identify and functionally analyze those enzymes and other proteins important for resistance to oxidative stress, chaperone function, and other processes associated with cataractogenesis. For instance, the importance of specific enzymes such as methionine sulfoxide reductase and MnSOD for maintaining lens cell viability and resistance to oxidative stress have been identified through the over-expression or silencing of these enzymes in lens cells, which are subsequently treated with H2O2 and/or other oxidants associated with cataracts. Other approaches include similar experiments using lens cells cultured from animal knockouts deleted for specific lens proteins such as αA-crystallin. In addition to cultured lens cells, cultured whole lenses also have been employed to monitor multiple biological events associated with cataracts.

In practice, creation of cataractous transgenic mouse lines is facilitated by the lens being readily examined for transparency, providing a rapid and efficient means to screen for phenotypic effects of transgenic insertions. Most cataracts in transgenic mice are associated with abnormalities of lens development, especially uncontrolled growth, toxic ablation of specific lens cells, or immune destruction of the lens. Lens abnormalities have been caused in transgenic mice using a variety of strategies. Expression of diphtheria toxin or ricin under the control of a lens-specific α-crystallin or γ-crystallin promoter, respectively, has caused ablations within the lens.

In addition to transgenic expression of normal or modified proteins, disrupted expression of a protein normally found in the lens has been shown to cause cataracts. Lack of αA-crystallin expression causes cataracts with inclusion bodies in central lens fiber cells (Brady *et al.*, 1997). Other knockouts associated with cataracts include osteonectin, connexins, and glutathione peroxidase. Collectively, these engineered cataract models emphasize the importance of the crystallins, cytoskeleton, and intercellular matrix for lens transparency.

Macular Degeneration

BRIEF OVERVIEW

Macular degenerations are a phenotypically and genotypically heterogeneous group of blinding disorders characterized by central vision loss associated with RPE atrophy with or without choroidal neovascularization. Of these, age-related macular degeneration (AMD) is a degenerative disorder of the cone-rich macular and perimacular regions of the retina with resulting loss of central visual acuity. Although AMD principally affects the supporting and metabolic structures of the retina including the retinal pigment epithelial (RPE) cells, the choriocapillaris, and Bruch's membrane, vision loss comes from the resulting retinal atrophy and its associated photoreceptor dysfunction (see Figure 68.3). Visual dysfunction is made worse by neovascularization, the ingrowth of choroidal vessels through defects in Bruch's membrane, with secondary hemorrhage, and retinal detachment that characterize the "wet" form of AMD. This is contrasted to the "dry" or nonneovascular form, which comprises 80% of the disease but results in only roughly 20% of its associated blindness. Drusen, small yellow-white deposits below the retina, are increased in individuals with AMD. Although they do not cause visual loss by themselves, drusen represent a risk factor for development of both the geographical atrophy (dry) and neovascularization (wet) types of AMD, especially when they are soft or indistinct. Recent results from the Age-Related Eye Disease Study suggest that the incidence of AMD could be lowered significantly by diet supplementation with high-dose antioxidant vitamins and zinc.

The clinical terms *dry* and *wet* typically are used to refer to different forms of AMD, with the dry form sometimes progressing to the wet form. Early stages of the dry form are characterized by focal pigmentation and accumulation of drusen between the RPE and Bruch's membrane. In later stages, the wet form is characterized by choroidal neovascularization, detachment of the RPE, and geographic atrophy of the RPE in the macular region. Drusen are classified as hard and soft, based on their shape, diameter, and color. Hard drusen are yellowish,

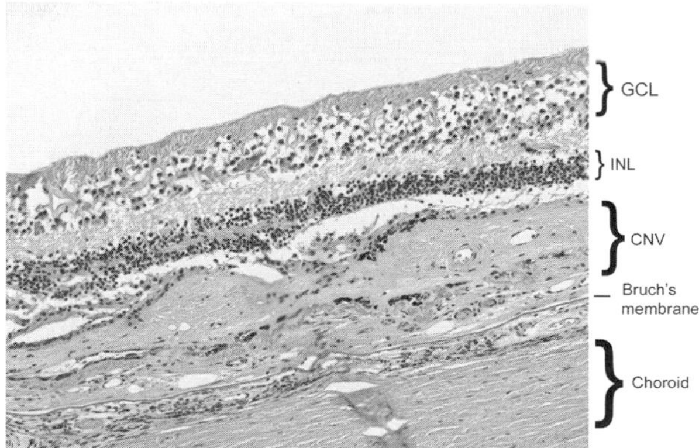

Figure 68.3 Histological section of the retina showing macular degeneration. Although the ganglion cell layer (GCL), inner nuclear layer (INL) and choroid are well preserved, the outer nuclear layer, which should appear similar to the INL, has been in large part replaced by fibrovascular choroidal neovascularization (CNV). Courtesy of Dr. Chi Chao Chan, National Eye Institute, National Institutes of Health.

smaller (with diameters of less than 50 μm), and less likely to progress to later stages of the disease. Soft drusen are larger, dark yellowish in color, and more likely to be associated with more advanced stages of the disease. In later stages of AMD, choroidal neovascularization and leakage of serous fluid into the subretinal (occult CNV) or intraretinal (classical CNV) regions leads to cell death and detachment of the RPE. Visual acuity is significantly affected when geographic atrophy of the RPE takes place in the fovea.

Epidemiology of macular degeneration

AMD has a multifactorial (or complex) etiology with contributions from a combination of environmental and genetic factors and a strong age effect. The prevalence of AMD increases dramatically with age, although the prevalence cited in various reports is highly dependent on the definition used for AMD. Overall, AMD increases from less than 1 to 2% at 50 years of age to as high as 15% at 90 years old. It has been suggested that increased skin pigmentation tends to protect from AMD, and this correlates to lower prevalence of AMD in African derived populations than Caucasians in some, but not all, studies. Various other risk factors may predispose to AMD including systemic hypertension and atherosclerosis, as well as cigarette smoking. Both photo-oxidation and inflammation have been suggested as possible pathogenic mechanisms for AMD, although the precise mechanism through which these result in disease has not been delineated.

Genetic factors have been implicated in AMD by epidemiological studies including twin studies and formal segregation analyses (Heiba *et al.*, 1994; Hammond *et al.*, 2002; Seddon, Ajani, and Mitchell, 1997). First degree relatives of individuals with AMD appear to have a two- to four-fold increased incidence of AMD over control individuals without a family history of AMD. Twin studies suggest that concordance for AMD in monozygotic twins is approximately twice that in dizygotic twins. Formal segregation analysis suggests that there is a major gene effect accounting for approximately 60% of AMD with a single major gene accounting for about 55% of AMD risk. Overall, these data suggest that the etiology of AMD has a significant genetic component.

HUMAN STUDIES OF MACULAR DEGENERATION

Mendelian linkage and association studies

In addition to ARMD, several Mendelian forms of macular degenerations have been described. The age of onset, pattern of inheritance, and clinical characteristics of these diseases vary widely. To date, about 17 human Mendelian macular degeneration genes have been mapped (Tuo, Bojanowski, and Chan, 2004). So far genes for nine different forms of human Mendelian macular degenerations have been identified using a positional cloning approach. These genes can be broadly classified into two groups: genes that are expressed in photoreceptors (ELOVL4, RDS/peripherin, RPGR, and ABCA4) and genes expressed in RPE (Bestrophin, EFEMP1, TIMP3, Hemicentin-1, and CTRP5). The genes ELOVL4, RDS, RPGR, and ABCA4 are expressed in both rod and cone photoreceptors. Except for the ELOVL4 gene, mutations in the remaining three genes were shown to be associated with retinitis pigmentosa (RP) in addition to macular degeneration. Mutations in TIMP3, EFEMP1, Hemicentin-1, CTRP5, and Bestrophin have not been implicated in RP. Of the genes involved in causing macular degeneration, all four photoreceptor-expressed genes are associated with an atrophic phenotype, whereas the RPE-expressed genes are associated with subretinal deposits and drusen in the early stages of the disease, which then progresses to neovascularization at later stages. The genes EFEMP1, TIMP3, Hemicentin-1, and CTRP5 share structural homology and are components of the extracellular matrix, and Bestrophin was reported to be a membrane channel. Recently, Fibulin-5, which also belongs to the fibulin family of extracellular proteins and shares homology with the EFEMP1 and CTRP5 proteins, was shown to be associated with AMD.

Linkage and association studies of AMD

Although some families show Mendelian inheritance of AMD, the disease in the general population is inherited in a complex or multifactorial fashion. In attempts to identify the genes that contribute to AMD risk in the population at large, investigators have looked at inheritance of AMD in small families or even pairs of affected siblings. A number of studies have examined families in which more than one member is affected with AMD, to determine whether polymorphic genetic markers at known positions in the human genome are co-inherited with the disease. These genome-wide scans have identified at least 21 linked regions on multiple chromosomes, including most consistently regions on chromosomes 1q, 9q, 10q, 12q, and 16q. However, AMD has not been associated with mutations in genes in any of these regions except complement factor H.

Three genes, ATP binding cassette subfamily A member 4 (ABCA4), apolipoprotein E (APOE), and complement factor H (HF1), have been reported to be associated with susceptibility to AMD in the general population (Tuo, Bojanowski, and Chan, 2004). However, the role of ABCA4 is somewhat controversial, and it probably is responsible for a few percent of AMD cases at most. Involvement of APOE in AMD seems to be more solid, with most studies showing a risk ratio of individuals carrying at least one APOE-ε4 allele reduced to about 40 to 50% of control values, although some studies could not replicate this finding. Recently, a Y402H polymorphism in the complement factor H protein has been shown to be associated with a two- to seven-fold increase in risk for AMD in two studies of unrelated individuals.

The gene encoding complement factor H lies in the chromosome 1q25-31 region implicated in linkage studies of both a large single family and of multiple small families and sibling pairs. One study suggested that this gene might account for as much as 50% of the hereditary tendency of AMD in the general population (Edwards *et al.*, 2005). In addition, the biochemical activities of both APOE and HF1 are consistent with the proposed atherosclerotic and inflammatory associations of AMD and the histological and biochemical analysis of the subretinal deposits. Thus, significant progress is being made in understanding the biological nature of the genes associated with macular degenerations and their roles in the disease. However, despite these advances little is understood about the overall mechanism underlying the disease process.

BIOCHEMISTRY AND PATHOLOGY OF MACULAR DEGENERATION

Histological changes

Among the early hallmarks of AMD are drusen, which are complex deposits of lipids, proteins, glycoproteins, and glycosaminoglycans that accumulate in the extracellular and inner aspects of Bruch's membrane (Anderson *et al.*, 2002). These subretinal deposits, accompanied by a diffuse thickening of Bruch's membrane, have been speculated to form a physical barrier between the RPE and choroid, obstructing the flow of nutrients from choroid to RPE, or possibly resulting in loss of cell-cell contact between RPE and Bruch's membrane and causing degeneration of retinal tissue. The RPE cells are responsible for phagocytosis and degradation of outer segment disks shed by photoreceptors. As they age and undergo oxidative stress, lipofuscin accumulates in the lysosomal compartment and leads to cellular damage and further impaired function. Though the origin of drusen remains controversial, current opinions are beginning to favor the vasculature of the choriocapillaris as a primary source rather than an intracellular source from the RPE. It is possible that the presence of lipofuscin and cellular debris excites an immune reaction and leads to the formation of drusen. This is reflected by the presence of immune components in drusen (Anderson *et al.*, 2002; see later).

Chorioretinal neovascularization (CNV) is the most common cause of vision loss in AMD. New vessels from the choriocapillaris grow through Bruch's membrane and branch horizontally through the RPE cell layer (termed classic CNV) or between the inner Bruch's membrane and RPE (termed occult CNV because it doesn't show up on angiography). Although the impetus for CNV has not been definitively determined, there are suggestions that imbalances in growth factors include pigment epithelial derived factor (PEDF, which inhibits vascular outgrowth) and vascular endothelial growth factor (VEGF, which stimulates vascular growth), possibly as a result of hypoxia and inflammation of the RPE. Even in the absence of CNV, the changes to the RPE Bruch's membrane and the outer plexiform layer of the retina result in scar formation at that level with concomitant damage to the neurosensory outer retina, termed geographic atrophy, which can also result in loss of central vision.

Composition of drusen and its implications

Understanding the composition of drusen provides important clues to the molecular pathology of the disease. In addition to classical immunohistochemical techniques, several advanced proteome analysis tools have begun to provide detailed information about the nature and composition of drusen. Perhaps the most significant of the new findings is that drusen contain protein molecules that mediate inflammatory and immune processes. These include immunoglobulins, components of complement pathway, and modulators for complement activation (e.g., vitronectin, clusterin, membrane cofactor protein, and complement receptor-1), molecules involved in the acute-phase response to inflammation (e.g., amyloid P component, α1-antitrypsin, and apolipoprotein E), major histocompatibility complex class II antigens, and HLA-DR antigens (Crabb *et al.*, 2002). Cellular components also have been identified in drusen, including RPE debris, lipofuscin, and melanin, as well as processes of choroidal dendritic cells, which are felt to contribute to the inflammatory response (Mullins *et al.*, 2000).

In addition to immune components, a number of other proteins occur in drusen, some of them also found in atherosclerotic plaques and other age-related diseases in which protein deposits occur. The most common of these appear to be TIMP-3, clusterin, vitronectin, and serum albumin. Other proteins found in drusen include serum amyloid P component, apolipoprotein E, IgG, Factor X, and some complement proteins (Mullins *et al.*, 2000). A number of proteins are found exclusively or in increased amounts in drusen associated with AMD than in drusen from individuals unaffected by AMD. These include some crystallins, EEFMP1, and amyloid-beta. In addition, the presence of immunoreactive proteins and oxidative modifications of many proteins found in drusen implicate both oxidation and immune functions in the pathogenesis of AMD.

Immune aspects

These findings have led to the suggestion that immune complex-mediated inflammation damages RPE cells, and choroidal dendritic cells are activated and recruited by injured RPE, whereas RPE cells respond to control dendritic cell activation by secreting proteins that modulate the immune response. Shed or phagocytosed cell membranes of injured RPE or dendritic cells are postulated to function as cores for these secreted components to accumulate and form extracellular deposits.

Furthermore, the codistribution of IgG and terminal complement complexes in drusen implicates an immune response directed against retinal antigens, and the immune complex formation might be taking place at the site of drusen formation. This hypothesis is supported by the presence of putative anti-retinal autoantibodies in the sera of patients with ARMD. Anti-retinal autoantibodies previously have been reported in a number of ocular disorders, including retinitis pigmentosa, paraneoplastic retinopathies, and retinal vasculitis (Anderson *et al.*, 2002). In addition, patients with membranoproliferative glomerulonephritis, in which complement activation and immune complex deposition cause glomerular injury, develop drusen deposits resembling those in ARMD in ultrastructure and composition including C5 and IgG. However, the role of antiretinal autoantibodies in the pathogenesis of ARMD has not been examined in detail. It remains unknown whether the initiation of chronic inflammation and subsequent drusen formation requires autoimmune-mediated events as a primary factor. To clarify the role of autoimmunity, immunogenic molecules for circulating antiretinal autoantibodies in patients need to be identified.

Oxidative aspects

Oxidative damage is implicated in the pathogenesis of AMD by both theoretical considerations and experimental data (Roth, Bindewald, and Holz, 2004). The retina has a highly active metabolism with a resultant high oxygen demand, and is exposed to light and polyunsaturated fatty acids, all of which tend to increase its susceptibility to photo-oxidative damage. In a fashion somewhat analogous to that seen in the lens, as the retina ages its antioxidant defenses begin to decline, here including both antioxidant enzymes and antioxidants such as lutein, and macular pigment density. As the RPE age oxidation of lipids and other cellular components result in accumulation of nonmetabolizable material as lipofuscin in the lysosomes, leading to their enlargement and formation of lipofuscin granules. These closely parallel drusen formation in time and distribution in the retina. In addition, epidemiological correlation of AMD with light exposure, age, and light pigmentation as well as the prevention or delay of AMD by antioxidant vitamins in the AREDS trial also support an oxidative role in AMD.

ANIMAL MODELS OF MACULAR DEGENERATION

Overview

Limited access to appropriate biological materials, especially eye samples from affected donors at different stages of the disease, are an absolute necessity to study mechanisms underlying the macular degenerations. Because it is nearly impossible to obtain these human retinal tissues from patients or from normal controls, animal models play a crucial role for investigating the biological pathway of disease development and for testing therapeutic strategies. Because age-related macular degeneration shares phenotypic similarities with monogenic macular degenerations, manipulation of these genes associated with monogenic macular degenerations to develop transgenic mouse models has been popular. Over the past few years, genetic engineering technologies has allowed the generation of a rapidly growing number of animal models for retinal diseases (Chader, 2002). Animal models have been used to investigate potentially protective therapeutic agents to treat photoreceptor degeneration, stem cell technology, or to test somatic gene therapy strategies (Ali *et al.*, 2000). They are also valuable for studying environmental effects like diet or light on the degeneration process. The animals that have been used to evaluate therapeutic strategies involve rodents, rabbits, pigs, and dogs. However, macula is found only in primates and birds; a monkey model with macular degeneration would be extremely valuable as they not only have a defined macula, but they are also evolutionarily close to humans.

Macular degeneration in monkeys was first described by Stafford in 1974 (Stafford, Anness, and Fine, 1984). He reported that 6.6% of elderly monkeys showed pigmentary disorders and/or drusen-like spots. El-Mofty and colleagues reported 50% incidence of maculopathy in a rhesus monkey colony at the Caribbean Primate Research Center of the University of Puerto Rico in 1978. The following report from the center indicated that specific maternal lineages had a statistically significant higher prevalence of drusen. Researchers have described a cynomolgus monkey (*Macaca fascicularis*) colony at the Tsukuba Primate Research Center (Tsukuba city, Japan) with a high incidence of macular degeneration and its pattern of inheritance (Umeda *et al.*, 2005).

Several other naturally occurring animal models have been described for retinal diseases. Rodents, mainly mice, are the most popular animal models as maintenance is less expensive compared to larger animals. However, a low cone:rod ratio and lack of a macula make mice less suitable for studying cone diseases and macular degenerations. Although the pathology in human ARMD is pronounced in the macula area, it is not confined to this central region alone. Abnormal accumulation of drusen and progressive degeneration of the retina, RPE, and underlying choroid characteristics were observed in mouse models generated by candidate gene manipulation or senescence acceleration (Ambati *et al.*, 2003). Choroidal neovascularization also has been described in naturally occurring mouse models. These observations suggest that the lack of a macula in mice may not be a disadvantage when considering the advantages of using the mouse as a model for studying macular degenerations with drusen.

Although monkey models are extremely important for macular degeneration study, there are limitations using nonhuman primates as animal models, such as longer gestation and life span, slow rate of expanding the pedigree, and cost of maintenance. These limitations can be overcome only by utilizing the mouse model parallel to the monkey model. One such model is a mouse line expressing an inactive form of cathepsin D. The impaired enzymatic activity affects phagocytosis of photoreceptor outer segments in the RPE cells, and the mice demonstrate basal laminar and linear deposits.

Animal model of early and late onset macular degeneration monkey

In 1986, a single cynomolgus monkey (*Macaca fascicularis*) with heavy drusen was found in the Tsukuba Primate Research Center. After 19 years of mating experiments, that single pedigree has grown to having 57 affected and 182 unaffected monkeys. Macular changes are observed as early as two years after birth, with basal laminar deposits first appearing in the macular region and progressing toward the peripheral retina throughout the lifetime (see Figure 68.4). In all the cases examined no abnormalities were found in the optic disc, retinal blood vessels, or choroidal vasculatures. The affected monkeys share phenotypic similarities with the early stages of ARMD, such as drusen and accumulation of lipofuscin. The immunohistochemical and proteome analysis of drusen in these monkeys share significant similarity with composition of age-related macular degeneration monkeys and also with previously reported human drusen composition. The meaning of this observation is that early onset monkeys produce the same drusen as ARMD patients at an accelerated rate of 25 times. Thirteen human candidate gene loci have been excluded by linkage and haplotype analysis. Therefore, the gene associated with macular degeneration in these monkeys is likely to be novel and the genes involved in causing drusen phenotype in humans and monkeys could be either the same or belong to the same biological pathway.

Studies involving early-onset and late-onset macular degeneration monkeys present a unique opportunity to study two independent target points in the biological pathway of retinal tissue that lead to degeneration of the macula at different stages of life. The gene associated with monkey macular degeneration is likely to be a novel gene as we have excluded most of the known macular degeneration loci. Cloning of the monkey macular degeneration gene will allow us to study the biological processes causing degeneration of retina. Due to high conservation between human and macaque genomes, genes associated with macular degeneration in monkeys should possibly play a key role in maintaining the normal function of retina in humans and is likely to be associated with macular degeneration in humans. Although some of the monogenic macular degeneration genes are not associated with ARMD, the phenotype observed in monkeys strongly suggests that this gene may play a role in human ARMD, and this cannot be established until validated by screening patients with ARMD. Understanding the mechanism underlying macular degeneration in these monkeys will enhance our understanding of the disease, identify clinical or molecular markers for early detection, and provide critical information needed to develop therapies for these diseases.

Progressive Open Angle Glaucoma (POAG)

BRIEF OVERVIEW

Epidemiology of POAG

Primary open angle glaucoma is a major cause of blindness throughout the world, affecting between 1 and 2% of individuals over 40 years of age (Klein *et al.*, 1992). The greatest risk factor for the development of POAG is ocular hypertension, to the extent that an elevated intraocular pressure (IOP) is often incorporated into the definition of glaucoma. In addition, the evidence implicating a genetic influence in glaucoma is very strong, and has been borne out in both model-based and model-free linkage studies. Finally, diabetes and myopia have been suggested to be related to development of POAG, but the evidence for this is inconsistent, although it seems likely that high myopia might contribute to development of POAG.

Pathology and physiology of POAG

Although the etiology and even the pathophysiology of glaucoma are still poorly understood, risk factors for glaucoma can be thought of as including both those in the anterior chamber, which tend to increase intraocular

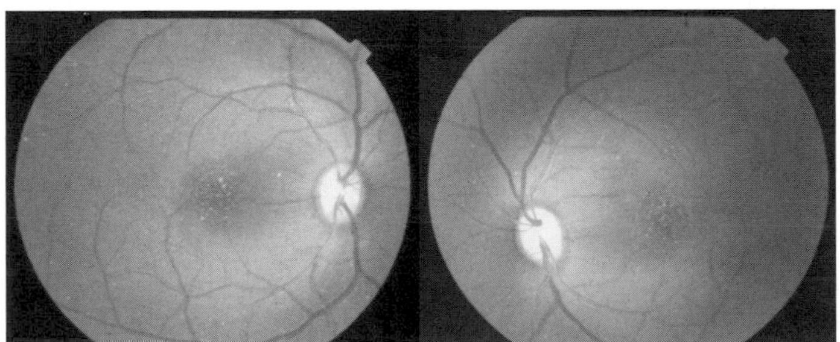

Figure 68.4 Funduscopic view of the retina in Tsukuba primate model of macular degeneration showing drusen and macular changes.

pressure, and those in the retina and optic nerve, which tend to increase susceptibility to damage from elevated or even normal intraocular pressure. Clinically, glaucoma generally is characterized by excavation of the optic disc as seen on funduscopic examination and visual field defects with elevated intraocular pressure included either as a part of the disease or a risk factor. In a simplified schema, one might think of increased resistance of the trabecular meshwork or Schlemm's canal to outflow of the aqueous humor causing an increase in intraocular pressure, which then acts upon sensitive retinal ganglion cells. These cells then degenerate, resulting in both the increased depth and width of the optic cup and the visual field defects. If the increased pressure is acute as it usually is in juvenile onset glaucoma, this process can be painful, but generally POAG is an insidious disease in which the first recognized symptom may be irreversible visual field changes.

Although primary open angle glaucoma (POAG) is characterized by visual field loss corresponding to the excavation of the optic disc (see Figure 68.5), it is usually associated with an elevation of the intraocular pressure (IOP) over 21 mmHg. Although the pathogenesis of glaucomatous optic neuropathy is poorly understood, it is generally accepted that the IOP is a major risk factor. By definition, there is no increase in IOP over 21 mmHg at any time in eyes with normal-tension glaucoma (NTG), although it is difficult to rule out fleeting or previous elevations of IOP. IOP is heavily influenced by the inflow and outflow of aqueous humor, a plasma filtrate actively generated at stroma of ciliary body and filtered across the blood-aqueous barrier. The aqueous flows from the posterior chamber to the anterior chamber via the pupil and is released through two routes, the trabecular route and uveoscleral route. Any disturbance in the flow can cause abnormal IOP leading to a death of retinal ganglion cells (RGC), and damage to the surrounding structure of the optic nerve head where optic nerve fibers leave the eye for visual cortex.

HUMAN STUDIES OF POAG

Linkage studies

At least six loci for autosomal dominant POAG have been mapped through linkage studies, termed GLC1A-F, on chromosomes 1q23, 2cen-q13, 3q21-q24, 8q23, 10p15-p14, and 7q35-q36. A genome-wide scan in multiple small families from an Afro-Caribbean population provided significant evidence for linkage to regions on chromosomes 2q (but separate from the Mendelian POAG locus GLC2B and the infantile glaucoma locus GLC3A on chromosome 2) and 10p. Presumably, these represent loci for glaucoma risk factors common in the general population, as do the loci on chromosomes 2, 14, 17, and 19, identified by examining siblings in an American population of European descent. It is particularly important to note that few of these studies have been confirmed; especially the technically more difficult and laborious studies of POAG in the general population.

Association studies

In addition to the identification of myocilin as a causative gene in glaucoma described earlier, which was carried out by linkage studies primarily in families with juvenile glaucoma and very elevated intraocular pressure, association studies have identified sequence changes in myocilin as a risk factor in a small percentage of POAG cases. Two additional genes have been shown to be involved in glaucoma by demonstrating an association between sequence changes in those genes and glaucoma in population studies. One of these genes is optineurin, for which the strongest associations have been obtained with normal tension glaucoma, but which also might be associated with POAG in some populations. A second is the OPA1 gene, which is known primarily as a cause of optic atrophy, but is also associated with normal tension glaucoma, though not with high tension primary open angle glaucoma in most studies. Association of both these genes with normal tension glaucoma suggests that

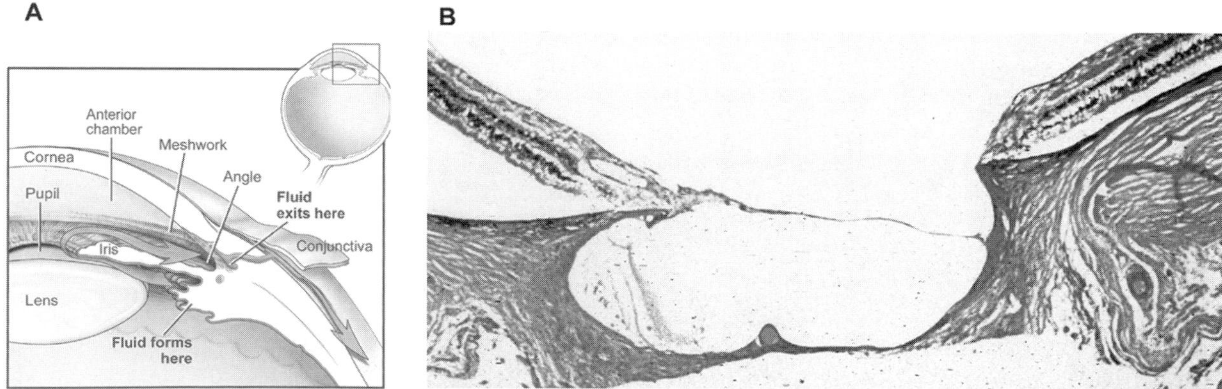

Figure 68.5 A. Diagram depicting the flow of aqueous humor from synthesis in the ciliary body to exit from the anterior chamber through the trabecular meshwork and Schlem's canal. **B.** Histological section showing an excavated optic cup in an individual with glaucoma. Courtesy of Dr. Chi Chao Chan, National Eye Institute, National Institutes of Health, from the collection of Dr. W. R. Green.

there may be some relationship between normal tension glaucoma and optic atrophy, and also emphasizes the importance of genetic changes that sensitize the retina and optic nerve to minor elevations of even normal intraocular pressure.

BIOCHEMISTRY AND PATHOLOGY OF POAG

Histological changes

It is estimated that roughly 20 to 50% of the large retinal ganglion cells (RGC) are lost in POAG. Although the reduction of RGC density occurs equally throughout the retina, visual sensitivity is first lost in areas where the initial RGC density is low, especially in the peripheral regions of the retina. As the disease progresses, atrophy of the nerve fiber layer is usually observed as additional RGC is lost. Typically, vertical collapse of the optic nerve head (ONH), loss of the neural rim at the ONH, rearrangement of central blood vessels, and loss of supporting tissue occur. Scanning electron microscopy of retinas with early stages of glaucoma shows evidence of initial collapse of the anterior lamina cribrosa, primarily in the vertical poles of the optic nerve head. Based on primate studies, optic cups with larger diameters are more susceptible to high ocular pressure and thus to glaucoma.

Role of the trabecular meshwork

Trabecular meshwork (TM) is a lamellated sheet of complex tissue that covers the inner wall of Schlemm's canal. TM has uniquely developed at the angle of primates, filtering the aqueous humor out of the eye. TM consists of two parts: the nonfiltering portion mainly occupied by trabecular cells and the filtering portion. Trabecular cells are highly phagocytic cells removing particles, cell debris, and protein from the aqueous humor. The first glaucoma locus, the *trabecular meshwork inducible glucocorticoid response* (TIGR), also known as myocilin, initially was identified by looking at genes whose transcription is highly induced by steroids in these cells. The filtering portion consists of three tissues: the cribriform layer, the corneoscleral meshwork, and the uveal meshwork. These trabecular beams or strands are intertwiningly connected to each other, forming a complex filtering mesh surrounding Schlemm's canal. The trabecular beams are thickened by accumulation of extracellular materials and decrease of cell density within the corneoscleral and uveal meshwork in aged eyes.

ANIMAL MODELS OF POAG

Overview: Difficulty of modeling the human eye

Limited access to appropriate biological materials, especially eye samples from affected donors at different stages of the POAG, is an impediment to the study of mechanisms underlying the disease. Because of the extreme difficulty in obtaining such diseased eyes from both patients and normal controls, animal models play a crucial role in investigating the biological pathway of disease development and in testing therapeutic strategies.

Different types of animal models for POAG have been found or created to mimic the optic nerve damage to resemble POAG phenotypes in humans. The greatest difficulty in constructing an animal model for POAG lies in the diversity of the anterior structures of the eye among different species (Tripathi and Tripathi, 1972, 1973). These structural differences include different iridocorneal angles or absence of specific quadrants from the TM. Nevertheless, within the limited areas in which interpretation of the data from a specific animal model parallels that in the human, various animals including the cow, dog, cat, horse, rabbit, chicken, and monkey can be used to observe POAG under various experimental conditions.

Animal models of POAG

Various animal models for inducible glaucoma have been reported. Argon laser photocoagulation of the TM in rhesus monkeys results in sustained elevation of IOP and has been used extensively to study early damage to the optic nerve head (May *et al.*, 1997). Corticosteroids such as betamethasone and dexamethasone have been used to treat rabbits, dogs, and cats to develop ocular hypertension (Bonomi *et al.*, 1978). Steroid treatment generally produces progressive glaucoma, but this process is reversed after about two months after cessation of the steroid. Trabecular blockage caused by inflammation after α-chymotrypsin treatment also has been used to produce elevated IOP in rabbit and monkey eyes (Vareilles *et al.*, 1977). Some types of avian species (chicken, quail, and turkey) have been known to develop elevated IOP as a consequence of continuous exposure to light.

Mouse models of glaucoma

Naturally occurring inherited animal glaucoma models are rare. However, extensive classification of IOP in mouse strains and molecular biological techniques to manipulate certain genes to produce transgenic or knockout/knockin mice recently have resulted in the development of a number of animal models with definitely known genetic causes for their disease (Chang *et al.*, 1999). As discussed earlier, four genes, myocilin (MYOC, TIGR), cytochrome P4501B1 (CYP1B1), optineurin (OPTN), and WDR36, currently are associated with glaucoma. OPTN, mutations of which are responsible for 16.7% of families with hereditary human NTG, is homologous to an inhibitory regulatory subunit of the high molecular kinase complex for the phosphorylation of NF-κB. Some of its known functions include inhibition of the tumor necrosis factor-alpha pathway, interaction with transcription factor IIIA, and mediation of the Huntington and Rab8 interaction for regulation of membrane trafficking and cellular morphogenesis. OPTN is induced by TNF-α and binds to an inhibitor of TNF-α and the adenovirus E3-14.7 kDa protein. To determine the effects of human glaucoma mutations in a transgenic mouse system, mice over-expressing wild type OPTN, OPTN carrying the glaucoma associated mutation E50K, and OPTN with exon5 deleted were constructed. Although wild-type OPTN do not show any abnormalities and the exon 5 deleted construction was found to be lethal prenatally, mice transgenic for the E50K mutant OPTN show steep optic nerve cupping with rearrangement of supporting tissue and blood vessels 18 weeks after birth (see Figure 68.6). The RGC and astrocyte loss observed is similar to the end phase changes seen in human glaucoma patients. Understanding the mechanism underlying normal tension glaucoma in these transgenic mice will enhance our understanding of each step leading to optic nerve cupping and how to prevent it. Based on the success of the mouse model, use of larger animals such as transgenic rabbits or pigs, in which more precise measurement of IOP and trials of surgical procedures suitable for therapy in humans are possible are currently being investigated.

Other glaucoma mouse models have been made through genetic manipulation. Knockout and transgenic mouse models of myocilin were made to answer the question whether elevated expression of the myocilin protein can influence the IOP (Gould *et al.*, 2004). Up to a fifteen-fold increase in myocilin expression failed to result in elevation of the IOP, any abnormality of retinal ganglion cells, or cupping of the optic nerve head. Mice lacking the cytochrome P450 1B1 (CYP1B1) gene were generated on B6 and 129X1/SvJ mouse stains (Libby *et al.*, 2003). Both strains were affected by the CYP1B1 deficiency with focal angle abnormalities, but 129X1/SvJ albino strains lacking tyrosinase were more severely affected, suggesting the presence of tyrosinase as an important developmental molecule.

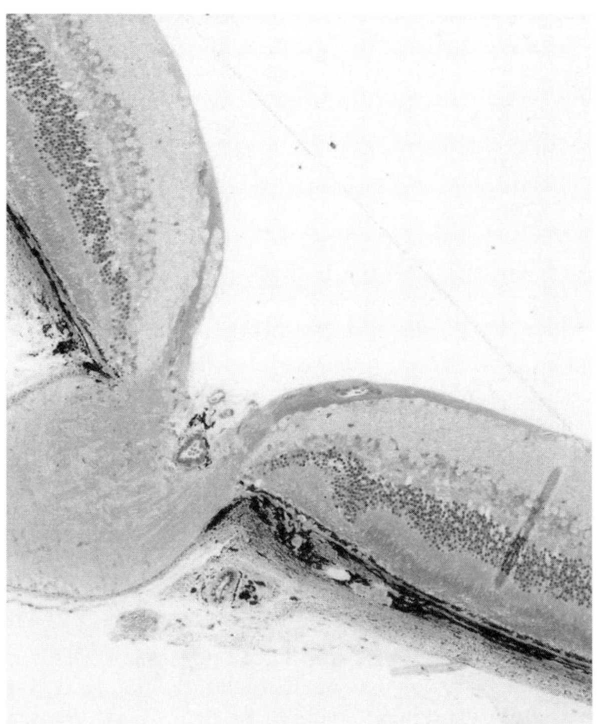

Figure 68.6 Histological section demonstrating excavation of the optic disc in an 18-week-old E50K mutant OPTN transgenic mouse.

Conclusion

In this chapter we have provided a brief overview of age-related eye diseases and the current state of knowledge and research on three of these. Age-related cataracts, age-related macular degeneration, and progressive open angle glaucoma account for much of the population burden imposed by age-related eye diseases. Although no perfect system to study these diseases exists today, an increasing number of experimental models are being developed. Although none is an exact replica of the clinical disease and should not be applied indiscriminately, each of these can provide useful information on some aspects of the disease in humans. They promise to accelerate the pace of research and provide mechanistic and therapeutic insights into the diseases that threaten sight in our aging population.

Recommended Resources

Albert, D.M. and Jakobiec, F.A. (Eds.) (2000). *Principles and Practice of Ophthalmology, 2e.* Philadelphia: W.B. Saunders Co.

Scriver, C.R. *et al.* (Eds.) (2005). *The Metabolic and Molecular Bases of Inherited Disease*, 8*e*. New York: McGraw-Hill.

Tasman, W. and Jaeger, E. (Eds.) (2001). *Duane's Clinical Ophthalmology*. Philadelphia: J.B. Lippincott Co.

REFERENCES

Ali, R.R., Sarra, G.M., Stephens, C., Alwis, M.D., Bainbridge, J.W., Munro, P.M. *et al.* (2000). Restoration of photoreceptor ultrastructure and function in retinal degeneration slow mice by gene therapy. *Nat. Genet. 25 (3)*, 306–310.

Ambati, J., Anand, A., Fernandez, S., Sakurai, E., Lynn, B.C., Kuziel, W.A. *et al.* (2003). An animal model of age-related macular degeneration in senescent Ccl-2- or Ccr-2-deficient mice. *Nat. Med. 9 (11)*, 1390–1397.

Anderson, D.H., Mullins, R.F., Hageman, G.S., and Johnson, L.V. (2002). A role for local inflammation in the formation of drusen in the aging eye. *Am. J. Ophthalmol. 134 (3)*, 411–431.

Bonomi, L., Perfetti, S., Noya, E., Bellucci, R., and Tomazzoli, L. (1978). Experimental corticosteroid ocular hypertension in the rabbit. *Albrecht. Von. Graefes Arch. Klin. Exp. Ophthalmol. 209 (2)*, 73–82.

Brady, J.P., Garland, D., Duglas-Tabor, Y., Robison, W.G. Jr., Groome, A., and Wawrousek, E.F. (1997). Targeted disruption of the mouse alpha A-crystallin gene induces cataract and cytoplasmic inclusion bodies containing the small heat shock protein alpha B-crystallin. *Proc. Natl. Acad. Sci. USA 94*, 884–889.

Buch, H., Vinding, T., La Cour, M., Appleyard, M., Jensen, G.B., and Nielsen, N.V. (2004). Prevalence and causes of visual impairment and blindness among 9980 Scandinavian adults: The Copenhagen City Eye Study. *Ophthalmology 111 (1)*, 53–61.

Chader, G.J. (2002). Animal models in research on retinal degenerations: Past progress and future hope. *Vision Res. 42 (4)*, 393–399.

Chang, B., Smith, R.S., Hawes, N.L., Anderson, M.G., Zabaleta, A., Savinova, O. *et al.* (1999). Interacting loci cause severe iris atrophy and glaucoma in DBA/2J mice. *Nat. Genet. 21 (4)*, 405–409.

Congdon, N.G., Friedman, D.S., and Lietman, T. (2003). Important causes of visual impairment in the world today. *J.A.M.A. 290 (15)*, 2057–2060.

Crabb, J.W., Miyagi, M., Gu, X., Shadrach, K., West, K.A., Sakaguchi, H. *et al.* (2002). Drusen proteome analysis: An approach to the etiology of age-related macular degeneration. *Proc. Natl. Acad. Sci. USA 99 (23)*, 14682–14687.

Davies, M.J. and Truscott, R.J. (2001). Photo-oxidation of proteins and its role in cataractogenesis. *J. Photochem. Photobiol. B 63 (1–3)*, 114–125.

Edwards, A.O., Ritter, R. III, Abel, K.J., Manning, A., Panhuysen, C., and Farrer, L.A. (2005). Complement factor H polymorphism and age-related macular degeneration. *Science 308 (5720)*, 421–424.

Giblin, F.J., Padgaonkar, V.A., Leverenz, V.R., Lin, L.R., Lou, M.F., Unakar, N.J. *et al.* (1995). Nuclear light scattering, disulfide formation and membrane damage in lenses of older guinea pigs treated with hyperbaric oxygen. *Exp. Eye Res 60 (3)*, 219–235.

Gould, D.B., Miceli-Libby, L., Savinova, O.V., Torrado, M., Tomarev, S.I., Smith, R.S. *et al.* (2004). Genetically increasing Myoc expression supports a necessary pathologic role of abnormal proteins in glaucoma. *Mol. Cell Biol. 24 (20)*, 9019–9025.

Graw, J. and Loster, J. (2003). Developmental genetics in ophthalmology. *Ophthalmic Genet. 24 (1)*, 1–33.

Hammond, C.J., Webster, A.R., Snieder, H., Bird, A.C., Gilbert, C.E., and Spector, T.D. (2002). Genetic influence on early age-related maculopathy: A twin study. *Ophthalmology 109 (4)*, 730–736.

Hanson, S.R., Hasan, A., Smith, D.L., and Smith, J.B. (2000). The major in vivo modifications of the human water-insoluble lens crystallins are disulfide bonds, deamidation, methionine oxidation and backbone cleavage. *Exp. Eye Res. 71 (2)*, 195–207.

Heiba, I.M., Elston, R.C., Klein, B.E., and Klein, R. (1994). Sibling correlations and segregation analysis of age-related maculopathy: The Beaver Dam Eye Study. *Genet. Epidemiol. 11 (1)*, 51–67.

Hejtmancik, J.F., Kaiser-Kupfer, M.I., and Piatigorsky, J. (2001). Molecular biology and inherited disorders of the eye lens. In C.R. Scriver *et al.* (Eds.). *The Metabolic and Molecular Basis of Inherited Disease, 8e*. New York: McGraw Hill.

Hejtmancik, J.F. and Kantorow, M. (2004). Molecular genetics of age-related cataract. *Exp. Eye Res. 79 (1)*, 3–9.

Hejtmancik, J.F. and Smaoui, N. (2003). Molecular Genetics of Cataract. In B. Wissinger, S. Kohl, and U. Langenbeck (Eds.). *Genetics in Ophthalmology*. Basel: S. Karger.

Klein, B.E., Klein, R., Sponsel, W.E., Franke, T., Cantor, L.B., Martone, J. *et al.* (1992). Prevalence of glaucoma. The Beaver Dam Eye Study. *Ophthalmology 99 (10)*, 1499–1504.

Kuck, J.F. (1990). Late onset hereditary cataract of the Emory mouse. A model for human senile cataract. *Exp. Eye Res. 50*, 659–664.

Libby, R.T., Smith, R.S., Savinova, O.V., Zabaleta, A., Martin, J.E., Gonzalez, F.J. *et al.* (2003). Modification of ocular defects in mouse developmental glaucoma models by tyrosinase. *Science 299 (5612)*, 1578–1581.

May, C.A., Hayreh, S.S., Furuyoshi, N., Ossoinig, K., Kaufman, P.L., and Lutjen-Drecoll, E. (1997). Choroidal ganglion cell plexus and retinal vasculature in monkeys with laser-induced glaucoma. *Ophthalmologica 211 (3)*, 161–171.

McCarty, C.A. and Taylor, H.R. (2001). The genetics of cataract. *Invest Ophthalmol. Vis. Sci. 42 (8)*, 1677–1678.

Mullins, R.F., Russell, S.R., Anderson, D.H., and Hageman, G.S. (2000). Drusen associated with aging and age-related macular degeneration contain proteins common to extracellular deposits associated with atherosclerosis, elastosis, amyloidosis, and dense deposit disease. *FASEB J. 14 (7)*, 835–846.

Okano, Y., Asada, M., Fujimoto, A., Ohtake, A., Murayama, K., Hsiao, K.J. *et al.* (2001). A genetic factor for age-related cataract: identification and characterization of a novel galactokinase variant, "Osaka," in Asians. *Am. J. Hum. Genet. 68 (4)*, 1036–1042.

Roth, F., Bindewald, A., and Holz, F.G. (2004). Key pathophysiologic pathways in age-related macular disease. *Graefes Arch. Clin. Exp. Ophthalmol. 242 (8)*, 710–716.

Seddon, J.M., Ajani, U.A., and Mitchell, B.D. (1997). Familial aggregation of age-related maculopathy. *Am. J. Ophthalmol. 123 (2)*, 199–206.

Spector, A. (1995). Oxidative stress-induced cataract: mechanism of action. *FASEB J. 9 (12)*, 1173–1182.

Stafford, T.J., Anness, S.H., and Fine, B.S. (1984). Spontaneous degenerative maculopathy in the monkey. *Ophthalmology 91 (5)*, 513–521.

The Italian-American Cataract Study Group (1991). Risk factors for age-related cortical, nuclear, and posterior subcapsular cataracts. *Am. J. Epidemiol. 133*, 541–553.

Thylefors, B., Negrel, A.D., Pararajasegaram, R., and Dadzie, K.Y. (1995). Global data on blindness. *Bull. World Health Organ 73 (1)*, 115–121.

Tripathi, R.C. and Tripathi, B.J. (1972). The mechanism of aqueous outflow in lower mammals. *Exp. Eye Res. 14 (1)*, 73–79.

Tripathi, R.C. and Tripathi, B.J. (1973). The mechanism of aqueous outflow in birds. I. An ultrastructural study of normal eyes. *Exp. Eye Res. 15 (3)*, 409–423.

Tuo, J., Bojanowski, C.M., and Chan, C.C. (2004). Genetic factors of age-related macular degeneration. *Prog. Retin. Eye Res. 23 (2)*, 229–249.

Umeda, S., Ayyagari, R., Okamoto, H., Suzuki, M.T., Terao, K., Mizota, A. *et al.* (2005). Linkage and mutation analysis to identify the gene associated with macular degeneration segregating in a cynomolgus monkey. *Invest. Ophthalmol. Vis. Sci. 46*, 683–691.

Vareilles, P., Silverstone, D., Plazonnet, B., Le Douarec, J.C., Sears, M.L., and Stone, C.A. (1977). Comparison of the effects of timolol and other adrenergic agents on intraocular pressure in the rabbit. *Invest. Ophthalmol. Vis. Sci. 16 (11)*, 987–996.

69

Health, Functional, and Therapeutic Implications of Obesity in Aging

R.L. Kennedy and E.Y.H. Khoo

Body weight generally increases from puberty through middle life. Some of this is due to muscle gain in the early years, but mostly it is fat. When weight gain is excessive, there is increased morbidity and mortality from diabetes, vascular disease, other chronic diseases, and malignancy. Although the prevalence of obesity is increasing, prognosis from associated chronic diseases is also improving. The consequence is that increasing proportions of the population reach old age and are either overweight or obese, or they become so in later life. The relationship between obesity and risk of death in later years of life is less clearcut than in younger subjects. There are no evidence-based guidelines for desirable body weight or managing obesity in the elderly. We do not really know how to measure obesity meaningfully in this age group. In fact, low body weight or weight loss appears to be a much more significant determinant of health in older subjects. However, obesity is associated with changes in metabolism and hormone levels, and with a low-grade inflammatory state. These changes are intimately involved with functional decline and provide opportunities for new therapeutic targets. Medical and surgical treatments for obesity have become widely available. There is a lack of specific data on their benefits in the aged population, but the benefits of exercise have become clear. Overall, the general increase in body weight in aging subjects may be a sign of improved nutrition, social environment, and medical care, and we should not simply regard it as a sign of ill health.

Introduction

Over the past few decades, there has been a worrying increase in obesity in human populations throughout the world. Increasing numbers of children are overweight or obese, and we are beginning to see the precursors of adult chronic diseases such as type 2 diabetes in many young subjects. The risks associated with obesity in adult life have been well documented in recent years. Diabetes risk increases in direct relation to body weight with a doubling of risk at a body mass index of as little as 28 Kg/m^2 compared with normal weight subjects. It is associated with multiple vascular risk factors including diabetes, dyslipidemia, and hypertension, accounting for the marked association with ischemic heart disease, stroke, and peripheral vascular disease. The risk of most malignancies is increased in the obese, and obesity is now thought to account for the equivalent of one in 10 cancers. Many other disorders associated with poor health and premature functional decline including osteoarthritis, affective disorders, and dementia are now firmly linked to obesity. Metabolic syndrome is a cluster of cardiovascular risk factors that is now present in one in four adults in the United States. The relationship between obesity and ill heath is not in question.

Improved health and social care, control of infections, and better education have all contributed to a major increase in the general health of the population and an increasing proportion reaching old age in a better state of health. In health, body weight tends to increase as we age. We should not, therefore, be surprised that the proportion of the population that is both elderly and either overweight or obese is increasing. On the other hand, being underweight or losing weight unintentionally is associated with a poorer prognosis. Aging is associated with a range of endocrine changes, altered metabolism, and body composition, and often with low-grade inflammatory changes. All these help to explain the association between aging and a variety of chronic diseases, and with decreased mental and physical function. But should we regard being overweight as a sign of ill health in the elderly, and is it then a target for therapy? If it is, should the approaches be the same as in the younger sector of the population? This chapter will try to address these issues.

Epidemiology of Obesity and Aging

The prevalence of obesity in human populations increased markedly in the last four decades of the second millennium. On average, body weight increases throughout adult life up to the age of about 60 years. Most of the increase in weight with aging is due to fat accumulation in several depots in the body. After the age of 60, average body weight begins to decline and by the age of 80 the prevalence of obesity is only about a third of that at age 60. The factors responsible for the decline in body weight with age are complex and incompletely understood. They include loss of muscle (sarcopenia), due in part to decreased activity and the endocrine changes that accompany aging. There is also an element of selection since obesity increases risk of conditions, including cardiovascular diseases and cancer, which shorten life. Furthermore, there is a well-established association between calorie restriction and longevity. Influences on the body weight of aging cohorts are multiple and need to be documented better.

Increased prevalence of obesity in the past 50 years has arisen because of increased calorie intake in the face of declining levels of physical activity. Decreased physical activity with aging may relate to changes in body composition (loss of muscle) and limitations imposed by diseases such as arthritis and vascular disorders. The link between obesity and ill health and risk, particularly of vascular disorders, has been long recognized and amply documented in a large number of recent studies. Awareness of the risks of obesity has increased, leading to development of a range of public health or treatment interventions to either prevent or treat the condition. In spite of these, available evidence suggests that the prevalence of obesity is still increasing. Mokdad *et al.* (2003) conducted a survey of over 195,000 adults in the United States in 2001. Compared with the preceding year, the prevalence of obesity had increased from 19.85 to 20.9%, an increase of 5.6%. Diabetes prevalence increased from 7.3 to 7.8% of the population, an increase of 8.2%. Diabetes and cardiovascular risk factors were much more common in obese individuals. Recent studies from Spain and Canada also confirm increases in obesity in the elderly, with up to 40% of the population affected. Even in societies where obesity has traditionally been less common, such as Japan, an increasing proportion of the elderly population is either overweight or obese. At all ages, including the elderly, obesity is more common in women than in men. For this reason, the relative protection that women have enjoyed against vascular disorders is being lost.

The relationship between obesity and socioeconomic status is also changing: Zhang and Wang (2004) have studied the link between educational attainment (as a surrogate marker for social status) and obesity in four cohorts of the National Health and Nutrition Examination Surveys (NHANES) between 1971 and 2000. There has been a progressive diminution in the excess of obesity in low socioeconomic groups. A recent study from Finland (Sulander *et al.*, 2004) has confirmed the rising prevalence of obesity among the elderly, and also that this increase is not as markedly related to socioeconomic status as would have been expected 10 years ago. Obesity is still a disorder associated with poverty and poor education, but it is also a disease of affluence. Recent studies also suggest that improved survival among institutionalized elders and those with special needs such as severe learning difficulties might also be contributing to the increased prevalence of weight problems in the elderly. Projections of the likely rise in obesity prevalence have been based on a combination of surveys (Arterburn *et al.*, 2004). It is estimated that the proportion of those aged 60 years and over who are obese will increase from 32.0% in 2000 to 37.4% in 2010. In the United States, this means an increase in the number of elderly obese subjects from 14.6 million to 20.9 million. Correspondingly, it is estimated that, over the next decade, the proportion of subjects aged 60 and over who are in the range of weight regarded as ideal will decrease from 30.6 to 26.7%.

Influence on Mortality

The most extensive study of the relationship between obesity and risk of death was published in 1999 by Calle and colleagues (1999). Over a million subjects were followed up for a mean period of 14 years. Among nonsmokers, those with the highest body mass index had a relative risk of death that was two- to three-fold greater than that of subjects who were in the desirable body mass index (BMI) range. The risk of death was greater in men than in women, but tended to be overshadowed by the effect of smoking on premature mortality. Obesity posed a greater risk for white than for black subjects. As expected, cardiovascular disease and cancer were the leading causes of death. In this study, the relationship between obesity and likelihood of death was much less marked in the elderly. Estimates of years of life lost due to obesity are based on considerations of younger populations. Thus, Fontaine *et al.* (2003), using data from the NHANES study, estimated that young white males with a BMI of 35 or above could expect to live eight to 13 years less than individuals who were in the desirable weight range. Again, the risk for young black males appeared to be less.

Most deaths occur in the older age group. Some studies have confirmed an association between higher than desirable body weight and life expectancy in the elderly, but this has not been a consistent finding. It is hard to control for the influence of baseline health status, lifestyle factors such as smoking, and influence of social environment (Flegal *et al.*, 2004). It seems clear that obesity does reduce life expectancy in older subjects; the effect has not been precisely quantified and is almost certainly less than that documented for younger obese subjects. The major causes of obesity-related deaths in the elderly are cardiovascular diseases (see later) and neoplastic conditions. Prevention of morbidity and mortality from cancer is seen as one of the most significant goals in improving quality, as well as quantity, of life in the older population (Hajjar, 2004). In a recent study of over 900,000 adults over 16 years,

Calle *et al.* (2003) demonstrated that, comparing the heaviest cohort with subjects of normal weight, obesity increased the risk of malignancy by 52% in men and 62% in women. The increase related not only to the hormonally responsive cancers such as breast and prostate, but to virtually every malignant disease with hepatocellular carcinoma, showing the most marked association with obesity. The exception was lung cancer, but the cachexia of patients with chronic lung disease and the confounding effect of smoking on body weight make it not surprising that this disease is not overall linked with obesity. The authors projected that the equivalent of 14% of all malignancies in men and 20% in women could be attributable to obesity.

Data from the Rotterdam study (Visscher *et al.*, 2001) illustrate the difficulty in defining obesity in the elderly and the importance of considering visceral adiposity as the major risk factor. In this study of around 6,300 elderly subjects followed for three years, the overall influence of BMI on mortality was modest, but increased waist circumference showed a more marked association with poor prognosis during the follow-up period. In summary, obesity does reduce life expectancy, but there is a survival bias in subjects who are obese and survive into old age, and the effect of obesity acquired later in life on life expectancy is not known. Although obesity is a determinant of life expectancy in the elderly, its effect is much less than in younger cohorts. It is possible, with the rise in obesity in the elderly, that life expectancy may reach a peak and then begin to decrease because of the high prevalence of obesity in this age group.

Energy Balance and Body Composition

Although we are seeing a marked increase in the number of elderly subjects in the population who are either overweight or obese, it is important to recognize that involuntary weight loss is a common feature of aging and is more common than weight gain. There are a number of reasons for this weight loss, including increased energy expenditure and decreased appetite arising from disease states that are common in the elderly. Involuntary weight loss in the elderly is associated with functional decline and with increased morbidity and mortality (Sahyoun *et al.*, 2004). A recent extensive Scandinavian study has confirmed that there is no association between weight gain in the elderly and excess mortality, whereas weight loss did relate to increased risk of death in both men and women (Drøyvold *et al.*, 2005). Chronic degenerative diseases, including Alzheimer's and Parkinson's diseases, are commonly accompanied by decreased resting energy expenditure (REE) and decreased total energy expenditure (TEE). In these conditions, altered body composition with loss of skeletal muscle, decreased food intake, and reduced mobility all contribute to decreased energy expenditure. The relationship between energy balance, body composition, and health in the elderly is complex (Wilson and Morley, 2003). A number of recent studies have confirmed that calorie restriction and decreased adiposity are significant determinants of longevity. Although involuntary weight loss is often a sign of illness, there is every reason to believe that regulated and deliberate weight loss in subjects who are obese will lead to health gains similar to those found at a younger age.

Body weight and composition are dependent on the balance between calorie intake and calorie expenditure. The reasons for decreased food intake with aging are several:

- Social and behavioral factors including economic status, isolation and mobility affecting access to food, loss of the social dimension to eating
- Decreased activity due to altered fitness and effects of chronic diseases leading to decreased appetite and energy requirements
- Diminished sense of smell and of taste and, therefore, enjoyment of food

Addition of the taste enhancer monosodium glutamate to food has been associated with weight gain in the elderly. Decreased relaxation of the antrum of the stomach may, in part, be responsible for the elderly experiencing earlier satiety; cholecystokinin (CCK) is released from the duodenum, particularly in response to fat, and leads to satiety. There is enhanced basal and stimulated release of CCK in elderly subjects; ghrelin is released from the stomach and stimulates desire for food intake and growth hormone release. Levels of this hormone are decreased in the elderly.

Energy expenditure is determined by REE, level of physical activity, and energy expenditure related to food intake—diet-induced thermogenesis. The decline in physical activity with aging accounts for at least half of the decrease in TEE. Not only does muscle mass and activity decrease, but changes in muscle metabolism with decreased protein turnover, decreased Na^+-K^+-ATPase activity, and changes in the proton pumping activity at the mitochondrial membrane also play a part. Diet-induced thermogenesis is a means of dissipating energy intake that is in excess of requirement and is higher in response to protein and carbohydrate than in response to fat. It is reduced, or delayed, in elderly subjects perhaps because of slower gastric emptying. This and decreased activity with aging may account for an exaggerated positive calorie balance in those who decrease their activity but continue to eat the same quantities they did when they were younger. The size of the internal organs, including liver and kidneys, diminishes with aging, and this factor contributes to the decrease in energy expenditure with aging (Wang *et al.*, 2005). Energy expenditure is higher in those who are obese, and may be higher in those who have diabetes. It follows that, in those individuals who are maintaining their body weight, food intake will need to be much higher in the obese and, though obesity may be an important determinant of poor health and poor function, the ability to maintain appetite and energy balance at levels comparable to those seen at a younger age should be recognized, to an extent, as a sign of health rather than of disease.

There are two important changes in body composition to consider—loss of skeletal muscle (sarcopenia) and increased accumulation and redistribution of adipose tissue. Sarcopenia leads to decreased muscular strength, impaired physical performance, and decreased quality of life. Since skeletal muscle is the most metabolically active tissue in the body, loss of muscle with aging is likely to be a major factor in determining resting and stimulated energy expenditure. Hormonal treatments to increase muscle mass and improve muscular strength have been considered and studied in a number of trials (Borst, 2004). To date, improvements in body composition have been demonstrated in a number of trials, but improvements in muscular strength in these trials have been relatively modest. Hormone therapy has enormous potential in patients with sarcopenic obesity (see later), but maximum benefit may be obtained only when it is combined with suitable nutritional and exercise interventions that take into account the particular needs of elderly subjects.

Women and the elderly have lower whole body fat oxidation, and this may favor fat accumulation under conditions of positive energy balance. In the Study of Women's Health Across the Nation (SWAN), Sternfeld *et al.* (2004) demonstrated that aging women experienced both increased total fat gain and increased visceral adiposity, with accompanying decreased muscular strength and performance. Regular exercise was protective against these changes. There has been debate about the role of visceral adiposity in predisposing to the metabolic syndrome in the elderly since, in many studies, the changes of metabolic syndrome are common, even among subjects who are not obese. A recent study of a large cohort of elderly individuals using dual X-ray absorptiometry (DEXA) and computerized tomography (CT) has confirmed the relationship between visceral obesity and the metabolic syndrome (Goodpaster *et al.*, 2003). Increased intra-abdominal fat not only predisposes to glucose intolerance, but also to hypertension (Ding *et al.*, 2004). Furthermore, this study demonstrated increased fat in the skeletal muscle in patients with either impaired glucose tolerance or diabetes. Increased fat in skeletal muscle depots of obese and diabetic patients, along with abnormal lipid metabolism, may contribute to insulin resistance and thus impaired muscle function, and has now been confirmed in a number of studies. Ritov *et al.* (2005) have shown that this phenomenon is accompanied by decreased electron transport chain activity in the mitochondria of skeletal muscle, and thus may be a direct or indirect cause of impaired substrate oxidation in muscle. Similar processes may operate in both the liver and in skeletal muscle, the two major sites of substrate utilization in the body (Cree *et al.*, 2004).

Adipose tissue is very active in producing cytokines and a variety of hormones that are important in regulating food intake and energy balance. It is important to recognize that expression of regulatory molecules differs between fat depots. Adiponectin is a major regulator of insulin sensitivity, and is one of the major secretory products of adipose tissue. Decreased adiponectin in patients who are obese associates closely with risk of diabetes and other cardiovascular risk factors. Resistin is also a product of adipose tissue, and increased expression is linked with increased peripheral insulin resistance. The main target for lifestyle interventions and other treatments for obesity should be visceral fat. In fact, the typical feminine distribution of fat peripherally, and particularly around the buttocks, may be protective against vascular disease (Tankó *et al.*, 2003) and cognitive decline (Bagger *et al.*, 2004).

Endocrine Changes

Many of the changes in function of the endocrine glands that are seen in obese subjects are really just the changes that accompany normal aging. However, as with inflammatory changes, the aging process appears to be accelerated in subjects who are either overweight or obese. Some of the changes that accompany obesity and aging are summarized in Table 69.1. We have termed this complex of endocrine changes Obesity-related Endocrinopathy (ORE), and we feel that these changes are important because they not only account for some of the alterations in body composition and energy balance that are seen, but could also be seen as potential therapeutic targets. Indeed, clinical trials have been conducted, or are under way, in a number of areas.

Low levels of testosterone, along with low body mass, smoking, and low vitamin D status, are important determinants of sarcopenia in elderly men (Szulc *et al.*, 2004). Although men do not experience a dramatic decline in sex steroid levels in midlife akin to the female menopause, there is a steady decline with aging. Around a third of men aged 70 years and over has levels of testosterone in the range that would normally be regarded as hypogonadal. Levels of the major adrenal androgen dehydroepiandrosterone also decline steadily with age. This decrease in androgen status is accompanied by, but does not entirely cause, increased fat mass, decreased muscle mass and decreased bone mineral density. Decreased androgen status often is seen particularly in patients with diabetes and is a common feature of poorly controlled diabetes, even in the young. The decline in testosterone status with aging and obesity is due partly to loss of function and number of Leydig cells. There is also a central component with reduced hypothalamic release of gonadotrophin releasing hormone (GnRH),

TABLE 69.1
Obesity-related endocrinopathy (ORE)

Hormone Change	Possible Consequence
↑catecholamines	Insulin resistance Increased blood pressure Vascular changes
↓ growth hormone ↓ IGF-1	Decreased muscle mass Increased fat mass
↓ testosterone (particularly men)	Decreased muscle mass and increased fat Less active Decreased quality of life
↓ estrogen (women)	More susceptible to vascular disease Bone health Quality of life impaired
↑ cortisol	Changes in fat distribution Decreased muscle mass and strength Mood and cognitive impairment
Thyroid function (↑ TSH, ↓ FT_3 and FT_4)	Metabolic changes Mood and cognitive changes Cardiac function
↑ prolactin	Reflection of brain dopaminergic tone and related to feeding behavior

Changes associated with obesity and aging. Sex steroids and the growth hormone axis particularly show promise as areas where therapeutic intervention might improve aspects of health and well being.

leading to a decrease in the frequency and amplitude of gonadotrophin pulses. Testosterone replacement will reverse some of the changes in fat mass and fat free mass that accompany aging (Liu *et al.*, 2004). However, variable results in relation to changes in muscle strength, physical functioning, bone mineral density, and insulin sensitivity have been reported. It is often tempting in practice to treat men who are extremely hypogonadal, but firm recommendations on this will rely on more extensive clinical trials, and safety considerations will need to be taken into account. From available evidence, it is not clear whether dehydroepiandrosterone or testosterone is to be the preferred androgen replacement.

The role of sex steroids and replacement therapy with these is even more controversial in females. Males generally have a lower life expectancy and tend to develop cardiovascular disease at an earlier age. The relative protection enjoyed particularly by premenopausal women has been ascribed to their estrogen status. However, even though estrogen levels decline dramatically after menopause, the role of estrogen replacement in protecting against cardiovascular disease remains controversial, and is overshadowed by the increased risk of breast cancer with replacement. Consequently, estrogen replacement is currently recommended only as a short-term treatment for those with symptoms of estrogen withdrawal. The effects of sex steroids on vascular tissues are complex (Orshal *et al.*, 2004). Estrogen withdrawal at the time of menopause increases fat mass and decreases muscle mass. Although males are at increased risk of vascular disorders, low levels of testosterone increase the risk of vascular disease and testosterone replacement in hypogonadal men protects against cardiac ischemia. Sex steroids are able to modify processes at the vascular endothelium that regulate constriction or vasodilatation of vessels and can also regulate the proliferation of endothelial or smooth muscle cells. Circulating sex steroid status is only a partial reflection of activity at the tissue level where androgen status may be amplified by the action of the enzyme 5α-reductase, which converts testosterone to the more active hormone dihydrotestosterone. Testosterone is also converted to estrogen peripherally by the action of aromatase. The activity of aromatase is increased in obesity. In men and in postmenopausal women, estrogen is more of a local hormone than a circulating hormone, but concentrations and activities at the tissue level are relatively hard to study.

Circulating levels of growth hormone (GH), and of insulin-like growth factor-1 (IGF-1), decline with aging. Factors responsible for this include changes in the hypothalamic-pituitary axis, inhibition of GH release due to increased levels of free fatty acids, decreased secretion of the endogenous growth hormone secretagogue ghrelin, and changes in IGF-1 binding proteins. As with testosterone, GH treatment has been shown, in the short term, to reverse some of the changes in body composition that occur in obesity and aging. However, used alone, it appears to have limited ability to improve function and there is certainly no evidence of increased longevity with GH treatment (Borst, 2004).

New treatments under consideration include use of growth-hormone releasing hormones or IGF-1 complexed with its major circulating binding protein (IGFBP-3). For maximum effect, treatments that enhance growth-hormone action may need to be combined with high protein diet and programs of exercise that encourage skeletal muscle hypertrophy.

Thyroid function is not generally markedly abnormal in severe obesity, and hormone levels are generally within the normal reference ranges. Thyroid volume and thyroid-stimulating hormone (TSH) may be increased, whereas levels of thyroxine (T_4) and triiodothyronine (T3) are often lower than in nonobese subjects (Sari *et al.*, 2003). Elevated prolactin concentrations may partly reflect stress, but feeding behavior is related to central dopaminergic tone and loss of the inhibitory influence of dopamine on prolactin secretion may also contribute to changes in prolactin. Chronic elevation of cortisol, also seen in nonhuman models of aging (Erwin *et al.*, 2004), may be a reflection of chronic stress and may be driven to an extent by the cytokine changes seen in obesity and aging. It also may reflect altered metabolism of cortisol in adipose tissue. Increased cortisol may contribute to the change in body habitus with increased central fat accumulation and loss of muscle tissue (in effect a subclinical form of Cushing's syndrome). It may also be partly responsible for cognitive decline.

Changes in Inflammatory Cytokines

A low-grade inflammatory state is an integral part of the aging process and occurs at an earlier age in subjects who are overweight or obese. Adipose tissue itself is a source of many of the pro-inflammatory cytokines that can be detected in the circulation. Apart from adipocytes, damaged organs and tissues, including the vasculature, may be sources of cytokines. The causes and consequences of the inflammatory changes are summarized in Figure 69.1.

There has been considerable interest that low grade infections may result in chronic activation of the immune system and that this may predispose to a variety of chronic disease states, including insulin resistance and atherosclerosis. Organisms that have attracted attention include those that cause dental and gum disease, *Helicobacter pylori*, *Chlamydia pneumoniae*, and viral infections including cytomegalovirus. A genetic component has also been recognized with polymorphisms in the genes or promoters for many of the cytokines accounting for variation in expression between individuals. For example, the common -174G/C polymorphism in the gene for interleukin-6 (IL-6) has recently been linked with longevity as the distribution of genotypes in the very elderly and appears to be different from that of the general population (Hurme *et al.*, 2005). The biological processes involved are obviously very complex, and no single genetic abnormality is going to account for the changes of aging and obesity, but with technological advances the interactions between different genetic polymorphisms will become progressively better understood.

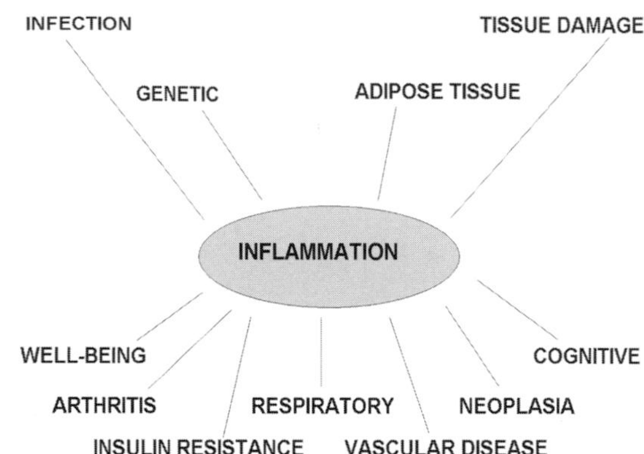

Figure 69.1 Inflammatory markers are increased as a result of production in adipose tissue and in other tissues damaged by the processes of aging. Genetic influences may also be important, as may infectious agents. Inflammation predisposes to, and is involved in, the progress of many of the disease states we associate with obesity and aging.

It has now been confirmed in a range of studies that low-grade inflammation, as evidenced by increased circulating levels of C-reactive protein and other acute phase proteins, predicts the development of vascular disease and is of prognostic importance in patients with vascular disease. These changes also precede development of diabetes and are predictive for development of the condition. A variety of molecules has been implicated, and a full review is beyond the scope of this chapter. Tumor necrosis factor-α (TNF-α) is thought to be one of the mediators responsible for the metabolic syndrome. Its actions in the liver and other target tissues oppose that of the protective molecule adiponectin. TNF-α levels in the circulation tend to rise progressively with age, and they correlate with the degree of metabolic control in patients with type 2 diabetes. Increased TNF-α expression has also been documented in other pathological states, including atherosclerotic disease and Alzheimer's disease, and in patients with general frailty and cognitive decline. About a third of circulating IL-6 is derived from visceral adipose tissue in obese subjects. The molecule is involved in the normal cross talk between tissues such as adipose and muscle, and has a role in regulating substrate flux during exercise. Increased IL-6 production relates to body composition and the presence of disease states, including infections, and is genetically modulated. IL-6 is involved in the pathogenesis of the metabolic syndrome, vascular diseases, neoplastic conditions, and other disease states and may be an important regulator of the endocrine and physiological adaptations to obesity. The range of cytokines recognized to be involved in these processes is widening rapidly. For example, interleukin-4 (IL-4) has recently been hypothesized to have a role in regulating function of the hippocampus in aging (Nolan *et al.*, 2005).

A large number of clinical studies have now demonstrated the role of inflammatory cytokines in the pathogenesis of, and as potential markers for, pathological and functional states that occur in aging. The Rotterdam study (Hak *et al.*, 2001) demonstrated that circulating levels of CRP, IL-6, α-1-antichymotrypsin, and intercellular adhesion molecule-1 (ICAM1) were increased in elderly subjects with insulin resistance and high cardiovascular risk. A recent U.S. study (Penninx *et al.*, 2004) of nearly 3,000 aging subjects reported that levels of TNF-α, IL-6, CRP, and soluble cytokine receptors were predictive of decline in mobility over a 30-month period. Other studies have related inflammatory changes to muscular strength and power (Barbieri *et al.*, 2003) and to cognitive decline in the elderly (Yaffe *et al.*, 2003). In summary, aging and chronic inflammation go hand in hand. The association is stronger in the obese who develop inflammatory changes at an earlier age. The presence of inflammatory markers is predictive of and relates to a variety of chronic disease states, and increased expression of these markers is also seen in subjects who are likely to experience decline in physical and mental functions.

Metabolic Syndrome and Cardiovascular Risk

The disease most studied in relation to obesity is diabetes. The precursor to type 2 diabetes and to cardiovascular disease in many patients is the metabolic syndrome. By definition, this is said to be present if three or more of the following five conditions are met:

- Abdominal obesity: waist circumference >102 cm in men and >88 cm in women
- High triglyceride levels: ≥150 mg/dl, ≥1.7 mmol/L
- Low HDL cholesterol: <40 mg/dl (<1.04 mmolL) in men and <50 mg/dl (<1.30 mmol/L) in women
- High blood pressure: ≥130/85 mmHg
- High fasting glucose: ≥110 mg/dl (≥6.1 mmol/L)

This was the accepted definition of the metabolic syndrome until recently, and, using these criteria, a variety of studies in North America demonstrated that the syndrome was present in 21 to 33% of the population, with even higher prevalence in certain ethnic groups. A recent study (Ford *et al.*, 2004) using the NHANES cohorts compared the prevalence of metabolic syndrome in the 1988–1994 (NHANES III) cohort with the 1999–2000 cohort. The prevalence increased overall, but particularly in women who experienced a 23.5% increase. In fact, the definition of metabolic syndrome is changing with lower cut-off points for waist circumference and for fasting glucose (≥100 mg/dl, ≥5.6 mmol/L), meaning that an even larger proportion of the population will have the syndrome and thus be deemed to be at risk. Much of this increase will be among the elderly. Indeed, in the elderly, metabolic syndrome will be the norm, except in subjects who are underweight. So, should we be regarding it as a disease state?

In a study of over 12,000 Japanese subjects (Hasegawa *et al.*, 2005), factor analysis was used to examine the relationship between cardiovascular risk factors. In this extensive study, the major influence of BMI was in younger subjects. Similarly, in another Japanese study involving nearly 160,000 subjects (Wakabayashi *et al.*, 2004), the influence of BMI on blood pressure was much weaker in the elderly. The concept of the metabolic syndrome has been useful in screening populations who are at risk from diabetes and cardiovascular disease. It is important to realize, however, that susceptibility to the individual risk factors and disease states that relate to the syndrome are caused by multiple factors, not all of which relate to obesity. Around a quarter of patients with type 2 diabetes do not have the metabolic syndrome. There is no question that the accumulation of multiple risk factors places individuals at risk of morbidity and mortality from vascular disease, as shown in the recently published Casale Monteferrato Study (Bruno *et al.*, 2004). Furthermore, development of multiple risk factors, whether or not the individual is classified as having the metabolic syndrome, is a sign of deteriorating health and is also associated with cognitive and functional decline (Crooks *et al.*, 2003). Risk of diabetes is attenuated or accelerated by other factors such as adiponectin, high levels of which appear to confer a reduced risk of diabetes (Kanaya *et al.*, 2004). The role of leptin, an exclusive product of adipose tissue in regulating appetite and food intake, is now well established. There is evidence that responses to leptin may become blunted in elderly subjects. This may contribute to continuing food intake in excess of requirements in individuals whose functional and exercise capacity, and therefore, calorie requirements, are decreasing as they age.

Other Aspects of Health and Function

The study of obesity as a human disease state and efforts to treat the condition have gained momentum as it has become increasingly appreciated that obesity impinges on many aspects of health and functioning. The relationship between obesity and malignant disease has already been discussed (Calle *et al.*, 2003). Predisposition to malignant disease increases as we age, and disability from malignant disease, or fear of developing malignant disease, is a major factor in determining the well-being of the elderly. After malignancy and cardiovascular disease, osteoarthritis is the third leading cause of years lost due to disability. In fact, obesity has a relatively modest part to play in the pathogenesis of osteoarthritis (Lievense *et al.*, 2003). However, for a given severity of arthritis, the level of pain and disability is much greater in patients who are obese. Apart from the symptoms directly attributable to the arthritis, there are strong associations with mood disturbances, gastrointestinal symptoms, and disability from ischemic heart disease. Weight loss and regular exercise improve mobility, well-being, and reduce pain. Decreased cardio-respiratory fitness shows a strong association with obesity and the metabolic syndrome. Waist–hip ratio shows an inverse relationship with forced vital capacity (FVC) and forced expiratory volume (FEV_1), even after adjusting for confounding variables such as age and smoking habit. Sleep disturbance is now recognized to be a major cause of ill health, and up to 4% of the population have obstructive sleep apnea. Decreased lung function and sleep apnea have been linked to vascular dysfunction, cardiovascular events, and decreased life expectancy. Obesity has also been linked to risk of developing lens opacities and to increased risk of age-related macular degeneration.

Thus, chronic pain, decreased cardio-respiratory performance, and diminished mobility arising from a range of disease states may all contribute to poor health. Quality of life among the elderly is determined by other factors including social circumstances, cognitive function, and whether or not they are engaging in physical activity (Borowiak *et al.*, 2004). The latter may be determined by choice and circumstances but is also a general measure of functional ability. Jensen and Friedmann (2002) followed a large cohort of people over three years. Obesity was highly correlated with poor functional status at baseline and was a major determinant of functional decline during the three years of the study. Relationship between obesity and poor functioning was more marked in women. Other studies have confirmed this relationship between obesity and declining functional status, and the association does not entirely relate to changes in body composition. Visscher *et al.* (2004) followed 19,518 Finnish men from a wide age range and demonstrated that obese subjects had more years of ischemic heart disease, greater disability, and were more likely to use medicines regularly.

Treatment

The increasing prevalence of the obesity in the young is one of the most pressing public health problems facing us at present. With obesity comes the cluster of risk factors we call the metabolic syndrome. There is no question that, in younger subjects, weight management to deal with the multiple risk factors, and thus to decrease long-term risk, is the preferred approach. However, there is an inconsistent relationship between obesity and the components of the metabolic syndrome, particularly in the elderly. Many people who are obese do not develop diabetes and do not develop hypertension. Other factors, including the aging process itself and the endocrine and inflammatory changes that accompany it, are also important. There is now compelling evidence that not only obesity *per se* but weight gain, particularly around the waist, is an important determinant of risk of diabetes and cardiovascular disease.

One of the dangers of vigorous attempts to encourage weight loss in the elderly is that they may lose muscle mass as well as fat. Worsening the preexisting sarcopenia may further decrease their functional capacity and their general health status. Severe calorie restriction for prolonged periods should be avoided, except in circumstances where marked weight loss is deemed to be desirable in the short term, and only then if the diet proves to be effective and tolerated by the patient. It is common for patients to be told to lose weight before an operation (such as knee replacement) can be carried out. There is really no evidence that such acute weight loss either improves long-term prognosis or decreases risk from surgical procedures. Since weight gain and weight loss are each associated with poorer prognosis in the elderly, weight maintenance is the preferred approach for many, even if they are overweight. Vigorous management of individual risk factors including diabetes, dyslipidemia, and hypertension is entirely appropriate, particularly in the context of secondary prevention. We have recently reviewed the treatment considerations around obesity in the elderly (Kennedy *et al.*, 2004).

In terms of available evidence, the best treatment for elderly obese patients is exercise. Cardio-respiratory fitness is an important determinant of health status in the elderly and can be improved by exercise. The majority of elderly women actually achieve the currently recommended levels of exercise during activities of daily living, including housework. However, this level of activity does not appear to be protective against obesity and its consequences. There is now evidence from a large number of studies that exercise in the elderly is beneficial in terms of glucose tolerance, cardiac and respiratory function, improved function and quality of life. Patients have traditionally been instructed that aerobic exercise is most beneficial. Meaningful amounts of aerobic exercise may not be achievable in many with functional limitation and severe obesity. Furthermore, there is often a worsening of symptoms and well-being in the short term, and this may decrease adherence to programs of exercise. Progressive resistance training has the same benefits in the elderly as it does in the young. These benefits include increased muscular strength and function, along with reversal of some of the metabolic changes that accompany sarcopenic obesity. Testosterone levels are increased (both in males and females). Levels of GH and IGF-1 are also increased with exercise, and, together, these changes may contribute to improvements in bone health as well as favorably influencing body composition and energy balance. The other form of exercise that is useful in the elderly is endurance training. Several studies have demonstrated considerable health benefits from home-based programs of exercise where low-level exercise is undertaken over more prolonged periods than would be possible for aerobic exercise. We find that a pedometer is a useful way to encourage low-level exercise and to increase activity. Endurance exercise not only increases energy expenditure during exercise but also increases REE by up to 10%. Since they start from the lowest baseline, elderly subjects may, in relative terms, show the greatest benefit from endurance exercise interventions (Sartorio *et al.*, 2004).

A full review of dietary interventions cannot be undertaken here. In relation to glucose tolerance and the metabolic syndrome, there has been a move away from traditional low-fat diets. Restricted carbohydrate diets have gained in popularity, and available evidence, which is now considerable, suggests that they are both safe and effective when used for periods up to six months. In terms of sarcopenic obesity, one of the benefits of such diets is that subjects adhere to a relatively high protein intake. Maintaining positive protein balance and intake of essential amino acids is important during any treatment of obesity in the elderly so that muscle mass is not lost during calorie restriction. Several important studies published over the past two years have confirmed that diets high in fiber and wholegrain and low in refined carbohydrate improve glucose tolerance and protect against development of diabetes. Furthermore, such diets also decrease circulating CRP, IL-6, and other inflammatory markers and may thus influence the development or progression of a variety of disease states (Ajani *et al.*, 2004). The multiple benefits of lifestyle intervention programs, including their effects on systemic inflammation, have been reviewed recently (Nicklas *et al.*, 2005). Lifestyle interventions are also highly effective and cost effective in preventing or delaying the onset of diabetes and its associated complications (Knowler *et al.*, 2002).

Only two drugs are in widespread use for treatment of obesity—sibutramine and orlistat. Very limited information on their use in the elderly has been published; indeed the trials have tended to exclude elderly subjects. There is no reason to believe that their benefit is any less than in younger subjects. Sibutramine is a centrally acting inhibitor of noradrenalin and serotonin uptake. It acts by promoting satiety, thus decreasing food intake. The drug fairly consistently increases blood pressure and pulse rate, making it undesirable for long-term use. Blood pressure needs to be reviewed every six weeks or so. It can be used in hypertensive patients when the blood pressure is under control but should be avoided in patients with ischemic heart disease. Orlistat is a gastrointestinal lipase inhibitor that acts by decreasing fat absorption by the gut by about 30%. Its use is associated with a high frequency of gastrointestinal side effects, particularly if the patient does not adhere to a low-fat diet, but it is safe for long-term use, and the potential to prevent development of diabetes has recently been demonstrated. Other drug therapies, including metformin and thiazolidinediones have also been shown recently to prevent or retard the onset of type 2 diabetes (Knowler *et al.*, 2005). Controversies around the use of hormone replacement (sex steroids and GH) have been discussed earlier, but this line of treatment clearly has potential. Direct treatment on the immune activation that accompanies obesity and aging with anti-inflammatory drugs has also been supported by some recent evidence demonstrating beneficial effects on cognitive function.

Bariatric surgery for the extremely obese patient is now becoming more widely available and more accepted as a form of therapy as evidence regarding its safety and efficacy accumulates. Nonetheless, experience of using this type of surgery in the elderly is still quite limited. The procedures fall into two categories. Restrictive procedures decrease the effective size of the stomach, thus reducing the amount that can be eaten and indirectly diminishing appetite. Currently, the most widely used technique of this sort is laparoscopic gastric banding. This is a safe, minimally invasive and reversible technique with a very low peri-operative morbidity and mortality risk. Limited literature and clinical experience with this procedure in the elderly suggests that it is safe and can be effective. The other approach is a bypass procedure that limits the absorption of calories from the stomach and small bowel. This is the preferred procedure for the extremely obese and for those with eating disorders. This procedure is now often carried out laparoscopically, thus limiting risk. This approach is effective in the elderly and decreases use of medicines for the complications of obesity (St. Peter *et al.*, 2005).

Conclusion

Until now, the greatest impact of the global increase in obesity prevalence has been in the working years of life with premature death and disability from chronic diseases, loss of time at work, and increasing health costs. With improving health and social care as factors, we are now experiencing an exponential increase in obesity among the elderly. This increase is projected to continue, at least over the next decade, and probably beyond. Because of the influence of factors other than obesity, the risk of death attributable to obesity is less marked in the elderly than it is for younger subjects. The major risks are from cardiovascular disease and malignancy. Distribution of body fat needs to be considered: abdominal obesity is most closely linked to mortality risk, whereas peripheral adiposity may actually be protective. The ability to maintain body weight, albeit at a level that is higher than desirable, should be seen as a sign of health in the elderly; involuntary weight loss is associated with poor function and poor prognosis.

Metabolic activities vary among different fat depots. The evidence is not so clear cut as in younger age groups, but accumulation of visceral fat is associated with increased insulin resistance and hypertension. Peripheral fat, particularly in the female distribution, may even have a protective role and thus should not be regarded as a target for treatment, except for cosmetic reasons. One important recent development has been the realization that lipid accumulation within the liver and within skeletal muscle is a potent determinant of peripheral insulin sensitivity and of impaired substrate oxidation in these tissues. Sarcopenia, along with the changes in body fat accumulation and distribution, accounts for changes in function and energy balance with aging. Endocrine changes, particularly decreased levels of sex steroids and reduced activity in the growth hormone axis, are significant determinants of the behavioral and morphological changes that occur with obesity and aging. Sex steroid replacement and treatment with either growth hormone or insulin-like growth factor-1 remain treatment options, but a number of controversies need to be resolved before their use can be widely recommended. However, there is no evidence to suggest that elderly subjects are less likely to benefit from these treatments, if there is long-term benefit, than their younger counterparts.

Chronic low-grade inflammation accompanies both obesity and aging, and its presence is related to development of insulin resistance, neoplasia, vascular disease, and cognitive decline, among other complications of obesity. Measurement of markers of inflammation, including C-reactive protein and interleukin-6, allows us to identify individuals who are at high risk, and the inflammatory component has been of recent interest as a potential therapeutic target. Adipose tissue is highly adaptive and is the most variable component of body composition. A variety of cytokines, adipokines, and hormonal mediators produced in adipose tissue modify risk of insulin resistance and other phenomena associated with aging.

There is controversy about whether, and when, obesity should be treated in the elderly. There are no clear recommendations about what constitutes an ideal body weight and how obesity should be assessed. The relationship with excess mortality is not so clear cut as it is in the young. Metabolic syndrome is an important determinant of health but, as currently defined, is an almost inevitable consequence of aging. Metabolic syndrome does predispose to a variety of chronic disease states and is associated with functional decline, but we may need to consider different definitions for young and older subjects. There is a limited place currently for pharmacological and surgical treatment of obesity in the elderly, and experience with these, and the range of treatments, is growing. The influence of micro- and macro-nutrient components of the diet is being increasingly appreciated, and this should lead to development of dietary interventions that do not severely restrict calories and are sustainable. This, along with exercise programs with endurance exercise and progressive resistance training, offers the best prospect for improving the health and reducing the risk of the increasing number of people who are both overweight and elderly.

REFERENCES

Ajani, U., Ford, E., and Mokdad, A. (2004). Dietary fiber and C-reactive protein: Findings from national health and nutrition examination survey data. *J. Nutr. 134(5)*, 1181–1185.

Arterburn, D., Crane, P., and Sullivan, S. (2004). The coming epidemic of obesity in elderly Americans. *J. Am. Geriatr. Soc. 52(11)*, 1907–1912.

Bagger, Y., Tankó, L., Alexandersen, P., Qin, G., and Christiansen, C. (2004). The implications of body fat mass and fat distribution for cognitive function in elderly women. *Obes. Res. 12(9)*, 1519–1526.

Barbieri, M., Ferrucci, L., Ragno, E., Corsi, A., Bandinelli, S., Bonafè, M. *et al.* (2003). Chronic inflammation and the effect of IGF-I on muscle strength and power in older persons. *Am. J. Physiol. Endocrinol. Metab.* 284(3), 193–1849.

Borowiak, E. and Kostka, T. (2004). Predictors of quality of life in older people living at home and in institutions. *Aging Clin. Exp. Res. 16(3)*, 212–220.

Borst, S. (2004). Interventions for sarcopenia and muscle weakness in older people. *Age Ageing 33(6)*, 548–555.

Bruno, G., Merletti, F., Biggeri, A., Bargero, G., Ferrero, S., Runzo, C. *et al.* (2004). Metabolic syndrome as a predictor of all-cause and cardiovascular mortality in type 2 diabetes: The Casale Monferrato Study. *Diabetes Care 27(11)*, 2689–2694.

Calle, E., Rodriguez, C., Walker, T., and Thun, M. (2003). Overweight, obesity, and mortality from cancer in a prospectively studied cohort of U.S. adults. *N. Engl. J. Med. 348(17)*, 1625–1638.

Calle, E., Thun, M., Petrelli, J., Rodriguez, C., and Heath, C. (1999). Body-mass index and mortality in a prospective cohort of U.S. adults. *N. Engl. J. Med. 341(15)*, 1097–1105.

Cree, M., Newcomer, B., Katsanos, C., Sheffield, M., Chinkes, D., Aarsland, A. *et al.* (2004). Intramuscular and liver triglycerides are increased in the elderly. *J. Clin. Endocrinol. Metab. 89(8)*, 3864–3871.

Crooks, V., Buckwalter J., and Petitti D. (2003). Diabetes mellitus and cognitive performance in older women. *Ann. Epidemiol. 13(9)*, 613–9.

Ding, J., Visser, M., Kritchevsky, S., Nevitt, M., Newman, A., Sutton T. *et al.* (2004). The association of regional fat depots with hypertension in older persons of white and African American ethnicity. *Am. J. Hypertens. 17(10)*, 971–976.

Drøyvold, W., Lund Nilsen, T., Lydersen, S., Midthjell, K., Nilsson, P., Nilsson, J. *et al.* (2005). Weight change and mortality: The Nord-Trøndelag Health Study. *J. Intern. Med. 257(4)*, 338–345.

Erwin, J., Tigno, X., Gerzanich, G., and Hansen B. (2004). Age-related changes in fasting plasma cortisol in rhesus monkeys: Implications of individual differences for pathological consequences. *J. Gerontol. A. Biol. Sci. Med. Sci. 59(5)*, 424–432.

Flegal, K., Williamson, D., Pamuk, E., and Rosenberg, H. (2004). Estimating deaths attributable to obesity in the United States. *Am. J. Public. Health 94(9)*, 1486–1489.

Fontaine, K., Redden, D., Wang, C., Westfall, A., and Allison, D. (2003). Years of life lost due to obesity. *J.A.M.A. 289(2)*, 187–193.

Ford, E., Giles, W., and Mokdad, A. (2004). Increasing prevalence of the metabolic syndrome among U.S. Adults. *Diabetes Care 27(10)*, 2444–2449.

Goodpaster, B., Krishnaswami, S., Resnick, H., Kelley, D., Haggerty, C., Harris, T. *et al.* (2003). Association between regional adipose tissue distribution and both type 2 diabetes and impaired glucose tolerance in elderly men and women. *Diabetes Care 26(2)*, 372–379.

Hajjar, R. (2004). Cancer in the elderly: Is it preventable? *Clin. Geriatr. Med. 20(2)*, 293–316.

Hak, A., Pols, H., Stehouwer, C., Meijer, J., Kiliaan, A., Hofman, A. *et al.* (2001). Markers of inflammation and cellular adhesion molecules in relation to insulin resistance in nondiabetic elderly: The Rotterdam study. *J. Clin. Endocrinol. Metab. 86(9)*, 4398–4405.

Hasegawa, T., Nakasato, Y., and Sasaki, M. (2005). Factor analysis of lifestyle-related factors in 12,525 urban Japanese subjects. *J. Atheroscler. Thromb. 12(1)*, 29–34.

Hurme, M., Lehtimäki, T., Jylhä, M., Karhunen, P., and Hervonen, A. (2005). Interleukin-6-174G/C polymorphism and longevity: A follow-up study. *Mech. Ageing Dev. 126(3)*, 417–418.

Jensen, G. and Friedmann, J. (2002). Obesity is associated with functional decline in community-dwelling rural older persons. *J. Am. Geriatr. Soc. 50(5)*, 918 923.

Kanaya, A., Harris, T., Goodpaster, B., Tylavsky, F., and Cummings, S. (2004). Adipocytokines attenuate the association between visceral adiposity and diabetes in older adults. *Diabetes Care 27(6)*, 1375–1380.

Kennedy, R., Chokkalingham, K., and Srinivasan, R. (2004). Obesity in the elderly: Who should we be treating, and why, and how? *Curr. Opin. Clin. Nutr. Metab. Care 7(1)*, 3–9.

Knowler, W., Barrett-Connor, E., Fowler, S., Hamman-Richard, F., Lachin, J., Walker, E. *et al.* (2002). Reduction in the incidence of type 2 diabetes with lifestyle intervention or metformin. *N. Engl. J. Med. 346(6)*, 393–403.

Knowler, W., Hamman, R., Edelstein, S., Barrett-Connor, E., Ehrmann, D., Walker, E. *et al.* (2005). Prevention of type 2 diabetes with troglitazone in the diabetes prevention program. *Diabetes 54(4)*, 1150 1156.

Lievense, A., Reijman, M., Pols, H., and Bierma-Zeinstra-Sita, M. (2003). Obesity and hip osteoarthritis. *Am. J. Med. 115(4)*, 329–330.

Liu, P., Swerdloff, R., and Veldhuis, J. (2004) Clinical review 171: The rationale, efficacy and safety of androgen therapy in older men: Future research and current practice recommendations. *J. Clin. Endocrinol. Metab. 89(10)*, 4789–4796.

Mokdad, A., Ford, E., Bowman, B., Dietz, W., Vinicor, F., Bales, V. *et al.* (2003). Prevalence of obesity, diabetes, and obesity-related health risk factors, 2001. *J.A.M.A. 289(1)*, 76–79.

Nicklas, B., You, T., and Pahor, M. (2005). Behavioural treatments for chronic systemic inflammation: Effects of dietary weight loss and exercise training. *Cmaj. 172(9)*, 1199–1209.

Nolan, Y., Maher, F., Martin, D., Clarke, R., Brady, M., Bolton, A. *et al.* (2005). Role of interleukin-4 in regulation of age-related inflammatory changes in the hippocampus. *J. Biol. Chem. 280(10)*, 9354–9362.

Orshal, J. and Khalil, R. (2004). Gender, sex hormones, and vascular tone. *Am. J. Physiol. Regul. Integr. Comp. Physiol. 286(2)*, 363–6119.

Penninx, B., Kritchevsky, S., Newman, A., Nicklas, B., Simonsick, E., Rubin, S. *et al.* (2004). Inflammatory markers and incident mobility limitation in the elderly. *J. Am. Geriatr. Soc. 52(7)*, 1105–1113.

Ritov, V., Menshikova, E., He, J., Ferrell, R., Goodpaster, B., and Kelley, D. (2005). Deficiency of subsarcolemmal mitochondria in obesity and type 2 diabetes. *Diabetes 54(1)*, 8–14.

Sahyoun, N., Serdula, M., Galuska, D., Zhang, X., and Pamuk, E. (2004). The epidemiology of recent involuntary weight loss in the United States population. *J. Nutr. Health. Aging 8(6)*, 510–517.

Sari, R., Balci, M., Altunbas, H., and Karayalcin, U. (2003). The effect of body weight and weight loss on thyroid volume and function in obese women. *Clin. Endocrinol. 59(2)*, 258–262.

Sartorio, A., Lafortuna, C., Agosti, F., Proietti, M., and Maffiuletti, N. (2004). Elderly obese women display the greatest improvement in stair climbing performance after a 3-week body mass reduction program. *Int. J. Obes. Relat. Metab. Disord. 28(9)*, 1097–1104.

St. Peter, S., Craft, R., Tiede, J., and Swain, J. (2005). Impact of advanced age on weight loss and health benefits after laparoscopic gastric bypass. *Arch. Surg. 140(2)*, 165–168.

Sternfeld, B., Wang, H., Quesenberry, C., Abrams, B., Everson, R., Greendale, G. *et al.* (2004). Physical activity and changes in weight and waist circumference in midlife women: Findings from the Study of Women's Health Across the Nation. *Am. J. Epidemiol. 160(9)*, 912–922.

Sulander, T., Rahkonen, O., Helakorpi, S., Nissinen, A., and Uutela, A. (2004). Eighteen-year trends in obesity among the elderly. *Age Ageing 33(6)*, 632–635.

Szulc, P., Duboeuf, F., Marchand, F., and Delmas, P. (2004). Hormonal and lifestyle determinants of appendicular skeletal muscle mass in men: The MINOS study. *Am. J. Clin. Nutr. 80(2)*, 496–503.

Tankó, L., Bagger, Y., Alexandersen, P., Larsen, P., and Christiansen, C. (2003). Peripheral adiposity exhibits an independent dominant antiatherogenic effect in elderly women. *Circulation 107(12)*, 1626–1631.

Visscher, T., Rissanen, A., Seidell, J., Heliövaara, M., Knekt, P., Reunanen, A. *et al.* (2004). Obesity and unhealthy life-years in adult Finns: An empirical approach. *Arch. Intern. Med. 164(13)*, 1413–1420.

Visscher, T., Seidell, J., Molarius, A., van der Kuip, D., Hofman, A., and Witteman, J. (2001). A comparison of body mass index, waist-hip ratio and waist circumference as predictors of all-cause mortality among the elderly: The Rotterdam study. *Int. J. Obes. Relat. Metab. Disord. 25(11)*, 1730–1735.

Wakabayashi, I. (2004). Relationships of body mass index with blood pressure and serum cholesterol concentrations at different ages. *Aging Clin. Exp. Res. 16(6)*, 461–466.

Wang, Z., Heshka, S., Heymsfield, S., Shen, W., and Gallagher, D. (2005). A cellular-level approach to predicting resting energy expenditure across the adult years. *Am. J. Clin. Nutr. 81(4)*, 799–806.

Wilson, M. and Morley, J. (2003). Invited review: Aging and energy balance. *J. Appl. Physiol. 95(4)*, 1728–1736.

Yaffe, K., Lindquist, K., Penninx, B., Simonsick, E., Pahor, M., Kritchevsky, S. *et al.* (2003). Inflammatory markers and cognition in well-functioning African-American and white elders. *Neurology 61(1)*, 76–80.

Zhang, Q. and Wang, Y. (2004). Trends in the association between obesity and socioeconomic status in U.S. adults: 1971 to 2000. *Obes. Res. 12(10)*, 1622–1632.

70

Age and Joints

Klaus Bobacz and Ilse-Gerlinde Sunk

During lifetime the joints of the human body are subjected to a number of age-related alterations. These changes may affect all joint structures, muscles, tendons, ligaments, cartilage, synovial membrane, or joint capsules, and occur on the biomechanical, molecular, or cellular level. Due to the longevity of the population, joint disorders are among the most prevalent and symptomatic healthcare problems of middle-aged and old people.

This chapter focuses on the effects of aging on the soft tissues of which joints are composed. Generally, alterations comprise a change in tissue cellularity, metabolic cell activity, and extracellular matrix composition. These structure impairments may influence the functionality of the joints and may lead to a decline in mobility, resulting in a loss of independence and finally in a retreat from social life.

Thus it is important to increase the understanding of the age-related changes of joint structures and their relationship to their impairment to potentially maximize the quality of life of affected individuals.

Introduction

The efficiently operating musculoskeletal system is highly dependent on an unimpaired functionality of diarthrodial joints. Generally, joints connect bone-endings with each other and allow a frictionless movement of their surfaces. Different specialized structures are responsible for a smooth joint movement. Muscles, tendons, ligaments, cartilage, synovial membrane, and bone all do their share to ensure a proper joint function.

Joint stability is provided mainly by four factors:

1. The shape of the component parts, which are configured in a way that loading enhances the exactness of their position.
2. Ligaments, as they connect one bone to another and act to constrain and guide joint motion.
3. Muscular stabilization, especially in polyaxial joints.
4. Synovial fluid, as it functions as an adhesive seal between joint surfaces.

The by far more important role of the synovial fluid, which is synthesized by the synovial membrane, is lubrication of joint members. The synovial fluid can be compared to lube oil and facilitates joint movement.

In active motion, mechanical forces affect all structures of the healthy joint. The greatest share of loading energy is absorbed by the tendons, ligaments, and muscles. Loading stress that is not taken up within the surrounding muscles, tendons, and ligaments is distributed directly on the articular cartilage and the underlying bony structures.

With increasing age, the soft tissues that form the muscles, tendons, ligaments, cartilage, synovial membrane, and joint capsules are subjected to age-related changes. It is well known that the incidence of rheumatoid arthritis, and in particular the development of osteoarthritis, the most prevalent joint disease, are highly linked to increasing age (Creamer *et al.*, 1997; Davis *et al.*, 1991; Felson, 1990).

Joint disorders are one of the most prevalent and symptomatic health problems among middle-aged and elderly people and comprise pain, a decrease in strength, and restriction in the range of motion. These factors impair affected people in their everyday life routines, occupation, and leisure activities. In some individuals these impairments may lead to a decline in mobility, resulting in a loss of independence and finally in a retreat from social life.

Considering population-aging predictions, the percentage of the population age 65 or older will increase significantly during the future decades and will meet the 20% mark in the United States in 2030. In Europe the size of this population is expected to jump from 14.7% in 2000 to more than 23% in 2030 (Kinsella *et al.*, 2005).

The predicted longevity of the population with regard to joint function impairment is seen as a major socioeconomic problem and thus makes it extremely important to understand underlying mechanisms in musculoskeletal aging to help prevent and treat these disorders.

General Aspects of Cellular Senescence

As for all mammalian cells, be they of fibroblastic or epithelial origin, the cells that form the soft tissues of the musculoskeletal system will also undergo senescence. This process starts after an extended period of proliferation or in response to inadequate growth conditions or physiologic stress. Senescent cells cease to respond to mitogenic stimuli; they undergo changes in the chromatin structure and gene expression and become enlarged and flattened (Serrano *et al.*, 2001; Shelton *et al.*, 1999). Characteristically, such cells show increased adhesion to the extracellular matrix, while losing cell-cell contact. Regarding these alterations, cellular senescence can be seen as a program activated to prevent cell proliferation in various situations of physiologic stress (Ben Porath *et al.*, 2004).

In classical experiments in the 1960s it has been shown that normal human fibroblasts cease to divide following a period of propagation in culture (Hayflick *et al.*, 1961), which was later called Hayflick-limit.

There exist various triggers of senescence of which telomere uncapping has garnered much attention in senescence research. Telomeres are the terminal DNA-proteins of chromosomes. Analysis of telomere length as a function of age, either in cells of people of different age or as a function of cell division number in cultures of human fibroblast, show that mean telomere length gradually decreases with increased age or cell division number (Cooke *et al.*, 1986; Harley *et al.*, 1990). The shortening of the telomeres leads to telomere "uncapping," which causes disruption of the structure of the protective cap at the end of the telomere (Blackburn, 2001). The uncapped telomere is thought to be recognized as a DNA-break, which activates the DNA damage machinery.

Besides telomere dysfunction, senescence of normal cells can be induced by direct DNA damage, oxidative stress, and oncogene expression.

Oxidative stress plays an important role in the induction of senescence by causing DNA damage and accelerating telomere loss (Forsyth *et al.*, 2003; Parrinello *et al.*, 2003). It has been demonstrated that human fibroblasts undergo premature senescence in high ambient oxygen conditions (Chen *et al.*, 1995). In the condition of internal accumulation of reactive oxygen species, cellular components can be damaged through the oxidation of DNA, proteins, and lipids (Chen *et al.*, 1998).

Reactive oxygene species can be induced by over-expression of the RAS oncogene, promoting cellular senescence (Lee *et al.*, 1999). This response to the RAS activity has been suggested to represent a tumor-suppressor mechanism, by which cells prevent uncontrolled proliferation in response to the aberrant activation of proliferation-driving oncogenes. However, the role of reactive oxygene species in RAS-induced senescence is not fully understood.

Direct DNA damage can be caused by irradiation of cells or by treatment with DNA-damaging agents and may induce cells to undergo senescence. In many cases, the cellular response to such damage is cell death, but also irreversible cell-cycle arrest, depending on the type of agent and/or dosage administered (Wahl *et al.*, 2001).

All these inductors of senescence share a central activating pathway of senescence. P53 and Rb, two tumor suppressor proteins, have been shown to play a critical role in senescence induction, since both are activated upon the entry into senescence. The specific targets of these proteins constitute the majority of the effectors that are necessary for cell-cycle progression.

As a result of aging and cellular senescence, the biological and mechanical behaviors of all musculoskeletal tissues, including skeletal muscle, tendons, ligaments, cartilage, synovial membrane, joint capsule, and bone, undergo specific alterations. These changes follow similar patterns that comprise alterations in the number and function of cells, in their proliferative and synthetic capacity, as well as in the composition of the extracellular matrix. However, since the tissues differ in their composition, structure, and function, age-related changes must be considered individually.

Age-Related Changes in Joint Structures

SKELETAL MUSCLE

The normal skeletal muscle consists of multinucleated cells called fibers. Each muscle fiber is an elongated cell surrounded by a plasma membrane called the sarcolemma. Fibers contain myofilaments, contractile proteins that are responsible for muscle contractions. These fibers are grouped in fascicles and surrounded by connective tissue, the perimysium (Bossen, 2000). Skeletal muscles are connected to bone by tendons at each end.

One of the most obvious effects of aging is a decline in muscle strength that is largely related to a loss of muscle mass (sarcopenia). After skeletal maturation the total muscle mass declines at an average of 4% per decade until the age of 50 years. In older individuals the rate of loss increases up to 10% per decade (Buckwalter *et al.*, 1993). Local injury and damage to the innervation of muscle fibers occurs throughout life, but in old age the process of collateral sprouting of the neurons appears to become less effective in repairing innervation, and muscle fibers are lost (Campbell *et al.*, 1973; Lexell *et al.*, 1988).

Normal skeletal muscle has the ability of repair and regeneration following local injury of muscle fibers. This process is thought to be critically dependent on the activation of so-called satellite cells, usually quiescent cells detected outside the sarcolemma but within the basal lamina. Satellite cells, first described in 1961 (Mauro, 1961), are now seen as "spare parts" for postnatal muscle growth and repair.

The recruitment of the satellite cells is governed by a splice variant of the insulin-like growth factor (IGF)-I, termed mechano growth factor (MGF), which is expressed in response to mechanical stimulation (McKoy *et al.*, 1999; Yang *et al.*, 1996). In an animal model, electrical stimuli led to an increase in muscle mass as well as a concomitant upregulation of MGF mRNA compared to resting control muscles (Goldspink *et al.*, 1992).

The aging organism is much less able to increase MGF levels after high resistance exercise, as compared to muscles of younger individuals (Hameed *et al.*, 2003). Additionally, satellite cell functionality can be decreased by an abnormal accumulation of reactive oxygen species due to a drastic reduction of antioxidant activity in aged satellite cells (Fulle *et al.*, 2005; Short *et al.*, 2005a). This decrease in the antioxidative capacity may cause destabilizing oxidative damage to aging satellite cells, limiting their ability to repair muscle.

Another important factor in the aging process of the skeletal muscle is a decline in mitochondrial function, since the required energy for proper muscle function is generated in mitochondria, which contain their own DNA, called mitochondrial mtDNA (Clayton, 1992). mtDNA abundance and mitochondrial ATP production have been demonstrated to decline with advancing age. The content of several mitochondrial proteins was reduced in older muscles, whereas the level of the oxidative DNA lesion was increased, supporting the oxidative damage theory of aging (Short *et al.*, 2005a).

In contrast, it has been reported that mitochondrial capacities were related to physical activity, but not to age. The mitochondrial theory of aging, which attributes the age-related decline of muscle performance to decreased mitochondrial function, was questioned by these authors (Rasmussen *et al.*, 2003).

Other age-related changes of the skeletal muscle include changes in myosin heavy chain mRNA and protein expression (Short *et al.*, 2005b), myosin heavy chain composition of muscle spindles (Liu *et al.*, 2005), or alterations in the maximal O_2 uptake rate (Conley *et al.*, 2000).

DENSE FIBROUS TISSUES

Dense fibrous tissues, which include tendons, ligaments, and joint capsules, are also subjected to age-related changes. Although alterations in these tissues received less attention than those in skeletal muscle or articular cartilage, serious impairment can develop in aged individuals as a result of age-dependent changes in fibrous structures.

Tendons

Tendons are tough yet flexible connective tissue bands that attach muscle to skeletal structures. Bundles of collagen that are held together by a layer of loose connective tissue are the main components of tendons. These dense tissue straps are well-suited as transducers, enabling the force of a muscle to be exerted at a distance from the muscle itself. Tendons possess typical tensile properties—the forces applied to a tendon may be more than five times body weight.

It has been proposed that tendons lose their elasticity and slowly become stiffer and more brittle as a result of age. Moreover, the blood supply that nourishes the tendon was also reported to diminish with age and may cause a decrease in vascular perfusion (Brewer, 1979; Rathbun *et al.*, 1970). These alterations may lead to spontaneous or low-energy ruptures of mostly the rotator cuff of the shoulder, the long head of the biceps brachii, the posterior tibial tendon, patellar tendon, and the Achilles tendon (Brewer, 1979; Burkhead, 1990; Jahss, 1991).

Taking a closer look at structural, mechanical, or cellular age-related changes in tendons, Birch and coworkers reported that there exist differences in structural changes in different tendons. In some tendons aging resulted in a significant increase in collagen-linked fluorescence and a decrease in cellularity, whereas in other tendons high levels of type III collagen were found as a function of age (Birch *et al.*, 1999). These findings are supported by x-ray data on human tendons, demonstrating age-related changes in collagen packing (Naresh *et al.*, 1992). Furthermore, in human supraspinatus tendons there was a significant decrease in total glycosaminoglycan, chondroitin sulphate, and dermatan sulphate concentration with age (Riley *et al.*, 1994). These differences in macromolecular composition and aging may contribute to a tendon specific degeneration.

However, Goodman *et al.* suggested that tenocytes, which become differentiated at an early age, respond to cyclical strain and transforming growth factor-β stimulation, and preserve their tendon specific response, but increasing age had only little effect on tenocytes (Goodman *et al.*, 2004). Regarding age-related changes in biomechanical properties, no difference in tensile strength between mature and old tendons was found, suggesting a high compliance of tendons during aging (Nakagawa *et al.*, 1996). Additionally, the tensile and viscoelastic properties of the patellar tendon differed minimally between younger and older ages (Johnson *et al.*, 1994).

Age-related changes in tendon composition may contribute to degeneration of this tissue. Otherwise, the impact of age on mechanical properties seems to be only minimal. This could depend on an above-average physical training status in some individuals, since it has been reported that strength training in old age, at least partly, can reverse the deteriorating effect of aging on tendon properties and function (Maganaris *et al.*, 2004).

Ligaments

Ligaments, which are structurally quite similar to tendons, but appear to have more elastic fibers, attach adjacent bones to one another and maintain them at their correct anatomical positions during movement. They also provide structural support around joint capsules and at sites where bones make contact with other bones. Ligaments have dynamic characteristics, since they respond to exercise or immobilization by altering their tensile strength and are capable of repair after injury.

As seen in tendon tissue, mechanical properties of ligaments may undergo changes with increasing age, such as the deterioration of tensile properties. The structural characteristics of ligament-bone complexes show a progressive decline in tensile stiffness and ultimately lead to failure with increasing age (Woo *et al.*, 1991). Similar results were reported for human lumbar posterior spinal ligaments, where a significant correlation with a decrease in the mechanical strength and increasing age was found (Iida *et al.*, 2002).

A recent light and electron microscopic study revealed ultrastructural differences in the posterior cruciate ligaments, that is, a decrease in collagen fiber diameter and increase in collagen fibril concentration, with aging (Sargon *et al.*, 2004). These data paralleled previously published work on age-related changes of collagen fibrils in human anterior cruciate ligament and Achilles tendon (Strocchi *et al.*, 1991; Strocchi *et al.*, 1996).

When ligament tissue was tested upon alterations in the content of matrix components, an age-dependent decrease in elastin and collagen metabolism was obvious (Osakabe *et al.*, 2001). Moreover, age-related changes of elements were investigated, showing an increase in calcium and magnesium, although iron levels were reduced in the tested ligaments (Tohno *et al.*, 1999; Utsumi *et al.*, 2005).

Given the age-related changes occurring in ligaments affecting mechanical properties, we would expect a quite high incidence of ligament injuries with aging. In particular, since aging ligament cells synthesize lower amounts of elastin and collagen, that may contribute to a decline in mechanical properties and consecutively to an increased risk of injury with advancing age. However, the ability to respond to growth factor stimulation is not lost in aged ligament fibroblasts (Deie *et al.*, 1997), which may uphold matrix remodeling to such a degree to sufficiently withstand mechanical stress even in older individuals. Besides, an overall reduction in physical activity with increasing age may further prevent injuries to this tissue.

Joint capsule

The joint capsule resembles a sac-like envelope that forms a sleeve around the synovial joint and encloses its cavity. The joint capsule is a dense fibrous connective tissue that is attached to the bones via specialized attachment zones at the end of each involved bone. It seals the joint space, provides passive stability by limiting movements, provides active stability via its proprioceptive nerve endings, and may form articular surfaces for the joint. It varies in thickness according to the stresses to which it is subject, is locally thickened to form capsular ligaments, and may also incorporate tendons.

Nevertheless, some authors doubt the existence of a joint capsule as a defined structure, since it may be regarded as a basketwork of the surrounding ligaments and tendons appearing to form a fibrous capsule. Little is known about age-related changes in joint capsules. In addition, detailed biomechanical trials of age-dependent alterations in joint capsules have not been reported to the best of our knowledge.

Investigations in knee and finger joint capsules showed that the attachments to bone contain fibrocartilage that is rich in type II collagen and glycosaminoglycans. The attachment changes with age as type II collagen spreads into the capsular ligament or tendon (Benjamin *et al.*, 1991). With mechanical loading parts of the capsule adapt by forming fibrocartilaginous tissue by accumulating cartilage-like glycosaminoglycans and type II collagen. Such regions can be found especially in aged material (Benjamin *et al.*, 1991).

Since the joint capsule contains tendinous and ligamentous structures, the similarity between these tissues suggests that their mechanical properties may also deteriorate with age (Buckwalter *et al.*, 1993).

SYNOVIUM

The synovium is the innermost portion of capsular ligament of synovial joints. It is commonly seen as a multilayered complex comprising several layers (intima, subintima, and superficial vascular plexus). Besides its function as immunologic microenvironment, the synovium allows disconnection between adjacent moving structures. Moreover, it is responsible for synovial fluid synthesis, a dialysate of plasma containing high-molecular weighted polysaccharides, known as hyaluronan. The synovial fluid maintains a fluid film between cartilage surfaces under load, which allows hydrodynamic lubrication. Synovial villi, which provide versatile deformability during movement, become more common with age and may compensate for the growing inelasticity and increasingly fibrous character of the subintima.

Investigations of radiohumeral joints showed that the villous pattern changes as a result of aging. Dependent on the location within the joint, the villi even may display a hard plicate pattern in the adult (Isogai *et al.*, 2001).

Morphological studies of the aging synovium revealed an overall loss of synovium lining cells. In detail, synovial intimal fibroblast numbers decreased with advancing age, whereas there was a relative increase in synovial intimal macrophages. Moreover, a fibrosis of the intimal layer caused by collagen accumulation was described, as well as a decreased vascularity (Jilani *et al.*, 1986; Pasquali-Ronchetti *et al.*, 1992).

The composition of the lubricating synovial fluid is also subjected to age-dependent alterations. The concentrations of chondroitin sulfate and hyaluronic acid were measured and were found to vary with age. Their values were highest between 20 and 30 years of age, and thereafter they showed a tendency to decrease (Nakayama *et al.*, 2002). Similar results were described for hydroxyproline and glycosaminoglycan levels, as these macromolecules were reduced with increasing age (van den Boom *et al.*, 2004).

Interestingly, the synovial tissues harbor multipotent mesenchymal stem cells. These cells could be induced to differentiate to the chondrocyte, osteocyte, and adipocyte lineages. The multipotent mesenchymal stem cells showed only limited senescence; neither extensive expansion in monolayer culture, nor donor age or cryopreservation affected their multilineage potential (De Bari *et al.*, 2001). These findings suggest the presence of active synovial mesenchymal stem cells even in elderly individuals. To determine their physiological function, however, further research is needed.

INTERVERTEBRAL DISC

Intervertebral discs undergo dramatic changes with increasing age. Since stiffness and pain in the back and neck are among the most common physical complaints of the middle-aged and older people, alterations and degenerative changes of the intervertebral disc are of high relevance for clinical routine.

However, the intervertebral disc cannot be compared to a synovial joint, explaining why most of its pathologic features are quite different from those of a joint of the appendicular skeleton (Grignon *et al.*, 2000). Considering this fact, the changes of the intervertebral discs should not be dealt with in detail.

Briefly, with increasing age, fissures and cracks appear in the disc extending from the periphery to the central regions. Morphological studies showed a decrease in proteoglycan and water content as well as a dramatic decline in cell types and cell viability in the central region of the disc (Buckwalter, 1982). Ultrastructurally, disc matrix proteoglycan concentration decreases in the central regions (Buckwalter, 1982, Buckwalter *et al.*, 1985; Buckwalter *et al.*, 1989). In particular a reduction in aggregating proteoglycans and in the size of these aggregates can be observed. A decline in the concentration of a functional link protein, responsible for stabilizing proteoglycan aggregates, may cause changes in proteoglycan structure.

The most critical age-related changes in intervertebral discs are a loss of blood vessels supplying the region of the disc (Hassler, 1969). The consecutive decline in nutrition may lead to a decrease in cell viability and biosynthetic function.

Although the apparent severity of age-dependent changes in the intervertebral discs, regeneration of disc tissue seems to be possible, as shown by *in vitro* studies of enzymatically compromised tissue of the central disc regions (Nitobe *et al.*, 1988).

ARTICULAR CARTILAGE

Articular cartilage is a connective tissue with a unique structure that provides mechanical resistance to compression and shear forces as well as smooth and frictionless joint movement. Cartilage is not a static structure, but a dynamic functional unit that is in a continuous state of adaption to the changing demands placed upon it. The tissue is composed of an expanded extracellular matrix, consisting of a collagen network, mainly type II collagen, and proteoglycan molecules, especially aggrecan. A single cell type, the chondrocytes, lies embedded in the cartilage matrix. Chondrocytes account for only 1 to 2% of the tissue volume, but are essential for tissue maintenance since they uphold the physiological steady-state between matrix degradation and tissue replenishment.

Aging of the articular cartilage is highly associated with the development of osteoarthritis, even though degenerative processes seen in osteoarthritis are clearly different from those in aging (Creamer *et al.*, 1997; Davis *et al.*, 1991; Felson, 1990). However, aging processes sooner or later undermine cartilage stability in various ways and are likely to predispose to disease development and/or progression.

Intriguingly, the prevalence and severity of fibrillation of cartilage vary among joints and among different regions of the same joint. Degenerative changes in articular cartilage are not necessarily linked to pain and loss of motion of the joints; not all individuals who suffer from osteoarthritic symptoms have radiographic evidence of it, nor do all degenerative changes progress with age, even in people where osteoarthritis was diagnosed by clinical and radiographic means.

The relationship between aging and changes in the structural and cellular composition of articular cartilage is not fully understood, in particular with regard to its interindividual differences and heterogeneous clinical appearance. Therefore, several theories exist regarding how much aging may affect matrix composition, cell metabolism, and cellularity of articular cartilage.

Wear and tear theory

One of the first models is based on the repetitive mechanical strains that stress cartilage tissue during aging, also known as the "wear and tear" theory. The cartilage aging process can be viewed as the accumulation of continuous loading over the lifetime of joint use (Radin *et al.*, 1991). Physiologically, mechanical loads between 0–20 MPa strain articular cartilage (Hodge *et al.*, 1986). Forces that exceed these limits may lead to continuous microtraumata of the articular cartilage (Borrelli, Jr. *et al.*, 2004). Ultimately, repetitive damage to the extracellular matrix will culminate in the loss of tissue integrity and function.

A different explanation of the role of mechanical loading in aging is based on remodeled joint geometry in elderly individuals. A change in joint surface congruity and redistribution of load onto formerly unloaded and thus atrophic cartilage areas might result in rapid destruction of these areas of minor load-resistance. The observation that cartilage of the elderly is inadequate to withstand mechanical forces could be explained by the theory of load-distribution.

Alterations of cartilage matrix components with increasing age

With advancing age, changes within the extracellular matrix of articular cartilage occur. Although composed of a variety of components, we can roughly discriminate two major components of the cartilage matrix: type II collagen, responsible for resisting shear forces and for the integrity of the extracellular matrix; and aggrecan, a large aggregating proteoglycan providing resistance to compression. Changes in the synthesis rate or structure of these matrix components may contribute to a decrease in mechanical resistance, consequently resulting in structural cartilage damage. However, the mechanical properties of cartilage are not subjected to serious age-related changes in compression properties, but marked age-dependent decrease in tensile stiffness, fatigue resistance, and strength was shown.

Collagen network. The collagen network does not display a major loss of collagen bundles with increasing age, since there is only minor collagen remodeling during lifetime. However, the network stiffens and becomes less flexible with advancing age. This process is caused by an increase of covalent cross-linking of the single collagen chains (Verzijl *et al.*, 2002). Thus, the fibrillar network becomes more rigid during physiological deformation by continuous loading. These alterations may be due to the formation of glycation end products (see later).

Aggrecan monomers. The large aggregating proteoglycan, known as aggrecan, is subjected to more severe age-related changes. Aggrecan is composed of a core protein to which sugar side chains are attached, forming the proteoglycan structure. This construct binds to hyaluronan via specific binding sites, which are stabilized by a so-called link-protein. During the aging process the major alterations of the aggrecan structure comprises an accumulation of low molecular weight aggrecan monomers, a reduction in size of hyaluronan chains, and fragmented link proteins.

Aggrecan molecules increase in number, but get smaller with age. Their proteoglycan structure alters displaying heterogeneity in the monomer population. The monomers differ in their keratin sulphate, chondroitin sulphate, and protein content and in the size of their core proteins. The age-related changes are characterized by a decrease in the size and number of chondroitin sulphate chains and an increase in the size and number of keratin sulphate chains. Moreover, changes in the amino acid composition of the core protein have been reported, whereas a functional hyaluronan-binding region appears to be present at all ages (Bayliss *et al.*, 1978; Roughley *et al.*, 1980).

These changes, in particular the progressive decrease in the length of chondroitin sulphate-rich regions of proteoglycan monomers, could contribute primarily to an impaired functionability of aged articular cartilage, but generally the fixed charge density, viscoelastic properties, and the osmotic swelling pressure of the cartilage tissue are thought to be preserved in the aging cartilage, at least in part, by an increase in the concentration of small monomers that are rich in keratin sulphate, compensating for the loss of chondroitin sulphate-rich regions (Bayliss, 1990).

Hyaluronan chains. Hyaluronan also undergoes extensive age-related changes. The concentration of hyaluronan increases three- to four-fold during a lifetime, presumably to accommodate the increased number of proteoglycan monomers (Holmes *et al.*, 1988). Interestingly, this change does not arise from a higher rate of hyaluronan synthesis, but from an accumulation of partly degraded hyaluronan, that together with the smaller aggrecan monomers forms lower molecular weight aggregates.

The increase in hyaluronan content maintains the overall aggregation of proteoglycan monomers and consequently keeps the fixed charge and thus the contribution of proteoglycans to the compressive properties of cartilage constant.

Link protein. As hyaluronan chains and aggrecan monomers increase in number with advancing age, the concentration of link protein also increases with aging. Its purpose is to stabilize the interaction of the hyaluronan-binding region of aggrecan and hyaluronan. However, at all ages the concentrations of binding region are always in excess of link protein, in particular in aged tissue. As a consequence there is a lack of link protein to stabilize all binding regions. Furthermore, an age-related increase in the molecular heterogeneity and fragmentation of link protein was described (Mort *et al.*, 1985). The binding site stabilities differed at various degrees at all ages due to differences in the concentration of the distinct components and to their functional quality.

Formation of glycation end products. The aging components of the extracellular cartilage matrix are also compromised by the formation of glycation end products. These nonenzymatic protein modifications may have consequences for matrix integrity as well as chondrocyte metabolism in the aging cartilage (DeGroot *et al.*, 2001). The accumulation of glycation end products was shown to affect the collagen network by increasing its stiffness (Bank *et al.*, 1998; Verzijl *et al.*, 2002). Moreover an accumulation of these products influences the synthetic activity of chondrocytes down-regulating its metabolic performance. Today it is known that glycation end products may contribute to a reduction in collagen and proteoglycan synthesis, but it is unclear whether the degradative activity of chondrocytes is also affected. This might be of little relevance for the type II collagen network, since there is hardly collagen turnover in adult cartilage. Nevertheless, an age-dependent decrease in the remodeling of proteoglycan and other collagen types, such as type VI or IX, governed by glycation end products could be detrimental for cartilage integrity, since a continuous replacement of these components ensures the integrity of the cartilage matrix.

Finally, aging may influence the extracellular assembly of proteoglycans. Proteoglycan monomers are secreted from the chondrocytes and aggregate with hyaluronan extracellularily. Before the process of bonding is initiated, a conversion of proteoglycan monomers from a form of low hyaluronan affinity to one with a high affinity takes place (Bayliss *et al.*, 1984). In older individuals the rate of conversion of proteoglycan monomers to a high affinity form is conducted much slower compared to younger ones (Bayliss, 1986).

Chondrocytes and aging

Articular chondrocytes are responsible for a precisely balanced tissue remodeling to uphold tissue homeostasis and integrity. With advancing age, chondrocyte reactions alter; basically, in a way, the cells cease to synthesize proper extracellular matrix components and/or decrease in numbers with advancing age.

Articular cartilage usually is seen as a post-mitotic tissue with insignificant cellular turnover, making articular cartilage very vulnerable to the effects of cell senescence or cell loss. At skeletal maturity, subchondral calcification isolates the tissue from the vascular system so that cartilage is totally cut off from a possibly needed cell supply. Moreover, articular cartilage lacks any sort of germinal cell layer, as epithelial cells can fall back on, in order to compensate for any cell loss.

The cells have further to adapt to a tissue oxygen tension as low as 5% (Scott, 1992) and sustain a low level of metabolic activity necessary to maintain the cartilage matrix. Given physiological mechanical loading, this is in general sufficient to preserve the integrity of the articular surface for many decades. As we can imagine, these rough environments (low oxygen levels, continuous mechanical stress) may contribute to progressive senescence in this limited population of highly differentiated cells, and low levels of metabolic activity make it increasingly difficult to maintain tissue homeostasis.

Model of a reduced biosynthetic activity. In the case of a reduced biosynthetic activity, the maintenance of cartilage extracellular matrix could be impaired and may subsequently lead to a disruption of tissue integrity.

A significant decrease in proteoglycan production by articular chondrocytes as a result of aging has been demonstrated (DeGroot *et al.*, 1999; Schafer *et al.*, 1993; Verbruggen *et al.*, 2000), supporting the theory of a reduced biosynthetic activity of articular chondrocytes. However, contrary findings showing a constant rate of proteoglycan biosynthesis in mature articular chondrocytes (Bayliss *et al.*, 1999; Bobacz *et al.*, 2004) compete with the studies just mentioned. A possible explanation for these contradictory data may be the use of different culture techniques, since studies employing explant culture conditions may have to take different mechanisms than failure of chondrocyte metabolism into account.

A possible underlying mechanism for a reduced or maybe altered matrix synthesis in the aging articular cartilage could be an age-related decline in the responsiveness to growth factors. Such age effects have been described for several molecules in previous studies in animal (Loeser *et al.*, 2000; Martin *et al.*, 1997; Ribault *et al.*, 1998; Schafer *et al.*, 1993) and human (Bobacz *et al.*, 2003; Guerne *et al.*, 1995) cartilage, suggesting a decrease in the responsiveness of articular chondrocytes to various growth factors (platelet-derived growth factors, epidermal growth factor, insulin-like growth factor-I, basic fibroblast growth factor, transforming-growth factor (TGF)-β and bone morphogenetic protein-6) with increasing age. A possible explanation for this age-dependent effect may be a change in receptor expression, since growth factor receptors are reported to change with the differentiation status of the chondrocytes (Iwamoto *et al.*, 1991).

Model of cell number loss. A second theory of the association between cartilage aging and reduced matrix remodeling is simply based upon a decrease in chondrocyte number.

Several studies suggested that the cell density of the whole thickness of the uncalcified articular cartilage declines sharply during the growth and maturation period of skeletal development, but remains relatively constant in adult life (Huch, 2001; Meachim *et al.*, 1962; Miles *et al.*, 1964; Stockwell, 1967). On the other hand there is evidence that chondrocyte numbers decrease progressively in healthy articular cartilage as a function of age (Mitrovic *et al.*, 1983; Muehleman *et al.*, 1997; Quintero *et al.*, 1984; Vignon *et al.*, 1976). In a more recent report, the latter data have been confirmed (Bobacz *et al.*, 2004).

Merging both theories into one, it can be assumed that it is likely that a reduction in chondrocyte numbers is responsible for a decrease in matrix synthesis rate. An increased biosynthetic activity of the remaining cells to compensate for the overall chondrocyte loss may subsequently culminate in cell exhaustion and premature senescence. This again may lead to the production of inappropriate, noncartilage-specific matrix constituents impairing tissue integrity.

The mechanisms leading to a loss of chondrocytes in aging are still unknown but may be the result of a loss in responsiveness to anabolic growth factors (Guerne *et al.*, 1995), mitotic arrest possibly governed by telomere-dependent senescence (Martin *et al.*, 2002), or programmed cell death (Aigner *et al.*, 2001; Blanco *et al.*, 1998; Hashimoto *et al.*, 1998).

Conclusion

The unimpaired functionality of diarthrodial joints is essential for an active life. The complex joint system with all its appropriate structures is designed to withstand the changing biomechanical forces that act upon it during lifetime. With increasing age all joint structures are subjected to mechanical, molecular, or cellular alterations that may, depending on their degree, lead to an impairment of the joint operability.

Clearly, a number of events, some of them potentially detrimental, affect the joints during aging, but usually it is a compound of several factors that ultimately results in a deterioration of joint function. Although the knowledge concerning joints and aging has developed considerably during the last years, distinct causes and processes within different joint structures, as well as their interplay, are not fully understood. Regarding joint disorders as a major healthcare problem, it is critical to rapidly increase the understanding of the age-related changes of joint structures and their relationship to its impairment. Progress toward this goal may give us opportunities of intervention that will slow down or even halt age-dependent joint alterations to maximize the quality of life and independence for the increasing number of middle-aged and old people.

REFERENCES

Aigner, T., Hemmel, M., Neureiter, D., Gebhard, P.M., Zeiler, G., Kirchner, T. *et al.* (2001). Apoptotic cell death is not a widespread phenomenon in normal aging and osteoarthritis human articular knee cartilage: A study of proliferation, programmed cell death (apoptosis), and viability of chondrocytes in normal and osteoarthritic human knee cartilage. *Arthritis Rheum. 44*, 1304–1312.

Bank, R.A., Bayliss, M.T., Lafeber, F.P., Maroudas, A., and TeKoppele, J.M. (1998). Ageing and zonal variation in post-translational modification of collagen in normal human articular cartilage. The age-related increase in non-enzymatic glycation affects biomechanical properties of cartilage. *Biochem. J. 330 (Pt 1)*, 345–351.

Bayliss, M.T., Osborne, D., Woodhouse, S., and Davidson, C.J. (1999). Sulfation of chondroitin sulfate in human articular cartilage. The effect of age, topographical position, and zone of cartilage on tissue composition. *Biol. Chem. 274*, 15892–15900.

Bayliss, M.T. (1990). Proteoglycan structure and metabolism during maturation and ageing of human articular cartilage. *Biochem. Soc. Trans. 18*, 799–802.

Bayliss, M.T. and Ali, S.Y. (1978). Age-related changes in the composition and structure of human articular-cartilage proteoglycans. *Biochem. J. 176*, 683–693.

Bayliss, M.T., Ridgway, G.D., and Ali, S.Y. (1984). Delayed aggregation of proteoglycans in adult human articular cartilage. *Biosci. Rep. 4*, 827–833.

Bayliss, M. (1986). Proteoglycan structure in normal and osteoarthritic human cartilage. In K. Kuettner, R. Schleyerbach, and V. Hascall, Eds. *Articular Crtilage Biochemistry*, pp. 295–310. New York: Raven Press.

Ben Porath, I. and Weinberg, R.A. (2004). When cells get stressed: An integrative view of cellular senescence. *J. Clin. Invest. 113*, 8–13.

Benjamin, M., Tyers, R.N., and Ralphs, J.R. (1991). Age-related changes in tendon fibrocartilage. *J. Anat. 179*, 127–136.

Birch, H.L., Bailey, J.V., Bailey, A.J., and Goodship, A.E. (1999). Age-related changes to the molecular and cellular components of equine flexor tendons. *Equine Vet. J. 31*, 391–396.

Blackburn, E.H. (2001). Switching and signaling at the telomere. *Cell 106*, 661–673.

Blanco, F.J., Guitian, R., Vazquez-Martul, E., de Toro, F.J., and Galdo, F. (1998). Osteoarthritis chondrocytes die by apoptosis. A possible pathway for osteoarthritis pathology. *Arthritis Rheum. 41*, 284–289.

Bobacz, K., Erlacher, L., Smolen, J., Soleiman, A., and Graninger, W.B. (2004). Chondrocyte number and proteoglycan synthesis in the aging and osteoarthritic human articular cartilage. *Ann. Rheum. Dis. 63*, 1618–1622.

Bobacz, K., Gruber, R., Soleiman, A., Erlacher, L., Smolen, J.S., and Graninger, W.B. (2003). Expression of bone morphogenetic protein 6 in healthy and osteoarthritic human articular chondrocytes and stimulation of matrix synthesis in vitro. *Arthritis Rheum. 48*, 2501–2508.

Borrelli, J., Jr. and Ricci, W.M. (2004). Acute effects of cartilage impact. *Clin. Orthop.* 33–39.

Bossen, E. (2000). Muscle structure and development. In R. Wortmann, Ed. *Diseases of Skeletal Muscle*, pp. 3–9. Philadelphia: Lippincott Williams & Wilkins.

Brewer, B.J. (1979). Aging of the rotator cuff. *Am. J. Sports Med. 7*, 102–110.

Buckwalter, J.A. (1982). The fine structure of human intervertebral disc. In A. White and S. Gordon, Eds. *The American Academy of Orthopaedic Surgeons Symposium on Idiopathic Low Back Pain*, pp. 108–143. St. Louis: C.V. Mosby.

Buckwalter, J.A., Pedrini-Mille, A., Pedrini, V., and Tudisco, C. (1985). Proteoglycans of human infant intervertebral disc. Electron microscopic and biochemical studies. *J. Bone Joint Surg. Am. 67*, 284–294.

Buckwalter, J.A., Smith, K.C., Kazarien, L.E., Rosenberg, L.C., and Ungar, R. (1989). Articular cartilage and intervertebral disc proteoglycans differ in structure: An electron microscopic study. *J. Orthop. Res. 7*, 146–151.

Buckwalter, J.A., Woo, S.L., Goldberg, V.M., Hadley, E.C., Booth, F., Oegema, T.R. *et al.* (1993). Soft-tissue aging and musculoskeletal function. *J. Bone Joint Surg. Am. 75*, 1533–1548.

Burkhead, W. (1990). The biceps tendon. In C. Rockwood and F. Matsen, Eds. *The Shoulder*, pp. 791–836. Philadelphia: W.B. Saunders.

Campbell, M.J., McComas, A.J., and Petito, F. (1973). Physiological changes in ageing muscles. *J. Neurol. Neurosurg. Psychiatry 36*, 174–182.

Chen, Q., Fischer, A., Reagan, J.D., Yan, L.J., and Ames, B.N. (1995). Oxidative DNA damage and senescence of human diploid fibroblast cells. *Proc. Natl. Acad. Sci. USA 92*, 4337–4341.

Chen, Q.M., Bartholomew, J.C., Campisi, J., Acosta, M., Reagan, J.D., and Ames, B.N. (1998). Molecular analysis of H2O2-induced senescent-like growth arrest in normal human fibroblasts: p53 and Rb control G1 arrest but not cell replication. *Biochem. J. 332 (Pt 1)*, 43–50.

Clayton, D.A. (1992). Structure and function of the mitochondrial genome. *J. Inherit. Metab. Dis. 15*, 439–447.

Conley, K.E., Esselman, P.C., Jubrias, S.A., Cress, M.E., Inglin, B., Mogadam, C. *et al.* (2000). Ageing, muscle properties and maximal O(2) uptake rate in humans. *J. Physiol. 526 (Pt 1)*, 211–217.

Cooke, H.J. and Smith, B.A. (1986). Variability at the telomeres of the human X/Y pseudoautosomal region. *Cold Spring Harb. Symp. Quant. Biol. 51 (Pt 1)*, 213–219.

Creamer, P. and Hochberg, M.C. (1997). Osteoarthritis. *Lancet 350*, 503–508.

Davis, M., Ettinger, W., Neuhaus, J., and Mallon, K. (1991). Knee osteoarthritis and physical functioning: evidence from the NHANES I Epidemiologic Followup Study. *J. Rheumatol. 18*, 591–598.

De Bari, C., Dell'Accio, F., Tylzanowski, P., and Luyten, F.P. (2001). Multipotent mesenchymal stem cells from adult human synovial membrane. *Arthritis Rheum. 44*, 1928–1942.

DeGroot, J., Verzijl, N., Bank, R.A., Lafeber, F.P., Bijlsma, J.W., and TeKoppele, J.M. (1999). Age-related decrease in proteoglycan synthesis of human articular chondrocytes: The role of nonenzymatic glycation. *Arthritis Rheum. 42*, 1003–1009.

DeGroot, J., Verzijl, N., Jacobs, K.M., Budde, M., Bank, R.A., Bijlsma, J.W. *et al.* (2001). Accumulation of advanced glycation end products reduces chondrocyte-mediated extracellular matrix turnover in human articular cartilage. *Osteoarthritis Cartilage 9*, 720–726.

Deie, M., Marui, T., Allen, C.R., Hildebrand, K.A., Georgescu, H.I., Niyibizi, C. *et al.* (1997). The effects of age on rabbit MCL fibroblast matrix synthesis in response to TGF-beta 1 or EGF. *Mech. Ageing Dev. 97*, 121–130.

Felson, D. (1990). The epidemiology of knee osteoarthritis: Results from the Framingham Osteoarthritis Study. *Semin. Arthritis Rheum. 20*, 42–50.

Forsyth, N.R., Evans, A.P., Shay, J.W., and Wright, W.E. (2003). Developmental differences in the immortalization of lung fibroblasts by telomerase. *Aging Cell 2*, 235–243.

Fulle, S., Di Donna, S., Puglielli, C., Pietrangelo, T., Beccafico, S., Bellomo, R. *et al.* (2005). Age-dependent imbalance of the antioxidative system in human satellite cells. *Exp. Gerontol. 40*, 189–197.

Goldspink, G., Scutt, A., Loughna, P.T., Wells, D.J., Jaenicke, T., and Gerlach, G.F. (1992). Gene expression in skeletal muscle in response to stretch and force generation. *Am. J. Physiol. 262*, R356–R363.

Goodman, S.A., May, S.A., Heinegard, D., and Smith, R.K. (2004). Tenocyte response to cyclical strain and transforming growth factor beta is dependent upon age and site of origin. *Biorheology 41*, 613–628.

Grignon, B. and Roland, J. (2000). Can the human intervertebral disc be compared to a diarthrodial joint? *Surg. Radiol. Anat. 22*, 101–105.

Guerne, P.A., Blanco, F., Kaelin, A., Desgeorges, A., and Lotz, M. (1995). Growth factor responsiveness of human articular chondrocytes in aging and development. *Arthritis Rheum. 38*, 960–968.

Hameed, M., Orrell, R.W., Cobbold, M., Goldspink, G., and Harridge, S.D. (2003). Expression of IGF-I splice variants in young and old human skeletal muscle after high resistance exercise. *J. Physiol. 547*, 247–254.

Harley, C.B., Futcher, A.B., and Greider, C.W. (1990). Telomeres shorten during ageing of human fibroblasts. *Nature 345*, 458–460.

Hashimoto, S., Ochs, R.L., Komiya, S., and Lotz, M. (1998). Linkage of chondrocyte apoptosis and cartilage degradation in human osteoarthritis. *Arthritis Rheum. 41*, 1632–1638.

Hassler, O. (1969). The human intervertebral disc. A micro-angiographical study on its vascular supply at various ages. *Acta. Orthop. Scand. 40*, 765–772.

Hayflick, L. and Moorhead, P.S. (1961). The serial cultivation of human diploid cell strains. *Exp. Cell Res. 25*, 585–621.

Hodge, W.A., Fijan, R.S., Carlson, K.L., Burgess, R.G., Harris, W.H., and Mann, R.W. (1986). Contact pressures in the human hip joint measured in vivo. *Proc. Natl. Acad. Sci. USA 83*, 2879–2883.

Holmes, M.W., Bayliss, M.T., and Muir, H. (1988). Hyaluronic acid in human articular cartilage. Age-related changes in content and size. *Biochem. J. 250*, 435–441.

Huch, K. (2001). Knee and ankle: human joints with different susceptibility to osteoarthritis reveal different cartilage cellularity and matrix synthesis in vitro. *Arch. Orthop. Trauma Surg. 121*, 301–306.

Iida, T., Abumi, K., Kotani, Y., and Kaneda, K. (2002). Effects of aging and spinal degeneration on mechanical properties of lumbar supraspinous and interspinous ligaments. *Spine J. 2*, 95–100.

Isogai, S., Murakami, G., Wada, T., and Ishii, S. (2001). Which morphologies of synovial folds result from degeneration and/or aging of the radiohumeral joint: An anatomic study with cadavers and embryos. *J. Shoulder Elbow Surg. 10*, 169–181.

Iwamoto, M., Shimazu, A., Nakashima, K., Suzuki, F., and Kato, Y. (1991). Reduction of basic fibroblasts growth factor receptor is coupled with terminal differentiation of chondrocytes. *J. Biol. Chem. 266*, 461–467.

Jahss, M. (1991). Tendon disorders of the foot and ankle. In M. Jahss, Ed. *Disorders of the Foot and Ankle. Medical and Surgical Management*, pp. 1461–1513. Philadelphia: W.B. Saunders.

Jilani, M. and Ghadially, F.N. (1986). An ultrastructural study of age-associated changes in the rabbit synovial membrane. *J. Anat. 146*, 201–215.

Johnson, G.A., Tramaglini, D.M., Levine, R.E., Ohno, K., Choi, N.Y., and Woo, S.L. (1994). Tensile and viscoelastic properties of human patellar tendon. *J. Orthop. Res. 12*, 796–803.

Kinsella, K. and Phillips, D. (2005). Global aging: The challenge of success. *Population Bulletin* 60.

Lee, A.C., Fenster, B.E., Ito, H., Takeda, K., Bae, N.S., Hirai, T. *et al.* (1999). Ras proteins induce senescence by altering the intracellular levels of reactive oxygen species. *J. Biol. Chem. 274*, 7936–7940.

Lexell, J., Taylor, C.C., and Sjostrom, M. (1988). What is the cause of the ageing atrophy? Total number, size and proportion of different fiber types studied in whole vastus lateralis muscle from 15- to 83-year-old men. *J. Neurol. Sci. 84*, 275–294.

Liu, J.X., Eriksson, P.O., Thornell, L.E., and Pedrosa-Domellof, F. (2005). Fiber content and myosin heavy chain composition of muscle spindles in aged human biceps brachii. *J. Histochem. Cytochem. 53*, 445–454.

Loeser, R.F., Shanker, G., Carlson, C.S., Gardin, J.F., Shelton, B.J., and Sonntag, W.E. (2000). Reduction in the chondrocyte response to insulin-like growth factor 1 in aging and osteoarthritis: Studies in a non-human primate model of naturally occurring disease. *Arthritis Rheum. 43*, 2110–2120.

Maganaris, C.N., Narici, M.V., and Reeves, N.D. (2004). In vivo human tendon mechanical properties: Effect of resistance training in old age. *J. Musculoskelet. Neuronal Interact. 4*, 204–208.

Martin, J.A., Ellerbroek, S.M., and Buckwalter, J.A. (1997). Age-related decline in chondrocyte response to insulin-like growth factor-I: the role of growth factor binding proteins. *Orthop. Res. 15*, 491–498.

Martin, J. and Buckwalter, J.A. (2002). Human chondrocyte senescence and osteoarthritis. *Biorheology 39*, 145–152.

Mauro, A. (1961). Satellite cell of skeletal muscle fibers. *J. Biophys. Biochem. Cytol. 9*, 493–495.

McKoy, G., Ashley, W., Mander, J., Yang, S.Y., Williams, N., Russell, B. *et al.* (1999). Expression of insulin growth factor-1 splice variants and structural genes in rabbit skeletal muscle induced by stretch and stimulation. *J. Physiol. 516 (Pt 2)*, 583–592.

Meachim, G. and Collins, D. (1962). Cell count of normal and osteoarthritic articular cartilage in relation to the uptake of sulphate (35SO4) in vitro. *Ann. Rheum. Dis. 21*, 45–49.

Miles, J. and Eichelberger, L. (1964). Biochemical studies of human cartilage during the aging process. *J. Am. Geriatr. Soc.* 12, 1.

Mitrovic, D., Quintero, M., Stankovic, A., and Ryckewaert, A. (1983). Cell density of adult human femoral condylar articular cartilage. Joints with norman and fibrillated surfaces. *Lab. Invest. 49*, 309–316.

Mort, J.S., Caterson, B., Poole, A.R., and Roughley, P.J. (1985). The origin of human cartilage proteoglycan link-protein heterogeneity and fragmentation during aging. *Biochem. J. 232*, 805–812.

Muehleman, C., Chubinskaya, S., Cole, A.A., Noskina, Y., Arsenis, C., and Kuettner, K.E. (1997). 1997 William J. Stickel Gold Award. Morphological and biochemical properties of metatarsophalangeal joint cartilage. *J. Am. Podiatr. Med. Assoc. 87*, 447–459.

Nakagawa, Y., Hayashi, K., Yamamoto, N., and Nagashima, K. (1996). Age-related changes in biomechanical properties of the Achilles tendon in rabbits. *Eur. J. Appl. Physiol. Occup. Physiol. 73*, 7–10.

Nakayama, Y., Narita, T., Mori, A., Uesaka, S., Miyazaki, K., and Ito, H. (2002). The effects of age and sex on chondroitin sulfates in normal synovial fluid. *Arthritis Rheum. 46*, 2105–2108.

Naresh, M.D. and Brodsky, B. (1992). X-ray diffraction studies on human tendon show age-related changes in collagen packing. *Biochim. Biophys. Acta. 1122*, 161–166.

Nitobe, T., Harata, S., Okamoto, Y., Nakamura, T., and Endo, M. (1988). Degradation and biosynthesis of proteoglycans in the nucleus pulposus of canine intervertebral disc after chymopapain treatment. *Spine 13*, 1332–1339.

Osakabe, T., Hayashi, M., Hasegawa, K., Okuaki, T., Ritty, T.M., Mecham, R.P. *et al.* (2001). Age- and gender-related changes in ligament components. *Ann. Clin. Biochem. 38*, 527–532.

Parrinello, S., Samper, E., Krtolica, A., Goldstein, J., Melov, S., and Campisi, J. (2003). Oxygen sensitivity severely limits the replicative lifespan of murine fibroblasts. *Nat. Cell Biol. 5*, 741–747.

Pasquali-Ronchetti, I., Frizziero, L., Guerra, D., Baccarani-Contri, M., Focherini, M.C., Georgountzos, A. *et al.* (1992). Aging of the human synovium: An in vivo and ex vivo morphological study. *Semin. Arthritis Rheum. 21*, 400–414.

Quintero, M., Mitrovic, D.R., Stankovic, A., de Seze, S., Miravet, L., and Ryckewaert, A. (1984). Cellular aspects of the aging of articular cartilage. I. Condylar cartilage with a normal surface sampled from normal knees. *Rev Rheum. 51*, 375–379.

Radin, E.L., Burr, D.B., Caterson, B., Fyhrie, D., Brown, T.D., and Boyd, R.D. (1991). Mechanical determinants of osteoarthrosis. *Semin. Arthritis Rheum. 21*, 12–21.

Rasmussen, U.F., Krustrup, P., Kjaer, M., and Rasmussen, H.N. (2003). Human skeletal muscle mitochondrial metabolism in youth and senescence: No signs of functional changes in ATP formation and mitochondrial oxidative capacity. *Pflugers Arch. 446*, 270–278.

Rathbun, J.B. and Macnab, I. (1970). The microvascular pattern of the rotator cuff. *J. Bone Joint Surg. Br. 52*, 540–553.

Ribault, D., Habib, M., Abdel Majid, K., Barbara, A., and Mitrovic, D. (1998). Age-related decrease in the responsiveness of rat articular chondrocytes to EGF is associated with diminished number and affinity for the ligand of cell surface binding sites. *Mech. Ageing Dev. 12*, 25–40.

Riley, G.P., Harrall, R.L., Constant, C.R., Chard, M.D., Cawston, T.E., and Hazleman, B.L. (1994). Glycosaminoglycans of human rotator cuff tendons: Changes with age and in chronic rotator cuff tendinitis. *Ann. Rheum. Dis. 53*, 367–376.

Roughley, P.J. and White, R.J. (1980). Age-related changes in the structure of the proteoglycan subunits from human articular cartilage. *J. Biol. Chem. 255*, 217–224.

Sargon, M.F., Doral, M.N., and Atay, O.A. (2004). Age-related changes in human PCLs: A light and electron microscopic study. *Knee Surg. Sports Traumatol. Arthrosc. 12*, 280–284.

Schafer, S.J., Luyten, F.P., Yanagishita, M., and Reddi, A.H. (1993). Proteoglycan metabolism is age related and modulated by isoforms of platelet-derived growth factor in bovine articular cartilage explant cultures. *Arch. Biochem. Biophys. 302*, 431–438.

Scott, J.E. (1992). Oxygen and the connective tissues. *Trends Biochem. Sci. 17*, 340–343.

Serrano, M. and Blasco, M.A. (2001). Putting the stress on senescence. *Curr. Opin. Cell Biol. 13*, 748–753.

Shelton, D.N., Chang, E., Whittier, P.S., Choi, D., and Funk, W.D. (1999). Microarray analysis of replicative senescence. *Curr. Biol. 9*, 939–945.

Short, K.R., Bigelow, M.L., Kahl, J., Singh, R., Coenen-Schimke, J., Raghavakaimal, S. *et al.* (2005a). From the cover: Decline in skeletal muscle mitochondrial function with aging in humans. *Proc. Natl. Acad. Sci. USA. 102*, 5618–5623.

Short, K.R., Vittone, J.L., Bigelow, M.L., Proctor, D.N., Coenen-Schimke, J.M., Rys, P. *et al.* (2005b). Changes in myosin heavy chain mRNA and protein expression in human skeletal muscle with age and endurance exercise training. *J. Appl. Physiol. 99*, 95–102.

Stockwell, R. (1967). The cell density of human articular and costal cartilage. *J. Anat. 101*, 753.

Strocchi, R., De Pasquale, V., Facchini, A., Raspanti, M., Zaffagnini, S., and Marcacci, M. (1996). Age-related changes in human anterior cruciate ligament (ACL) collagen fibrils. *Ital. J. Anat. Embryol. 101*, 213–220.

Strocchi, R., De Pasquale, V., Guizzardi, S., Govoni, P., Facchini, A., Raspanti, M. *et al.* (1991). Human Achilles tendon: Morphological and morphometric variations as a function of age. *Foot Ankle 12*, 100–104.

Tohno, Y., Moriwake, Y., Takano, Y., Minami, T., Tohno, S., Utsumi, M. *et al.* (1999). Age-related changes of elements in human anterior cruciate ligaments and ligamenta capitum femorum. *Biol. Trace Elem. Res. 68*, 181–192.

Utsumi, M., Azuma, C., Tohno, S., Tohno, Y., Moriwake, Y., Minami, T. *et al.* (2005). Increases of calcium and magnesium and decrease of iron in human posterior longitudinal ligaments of the cervical spine with aging. *Biol. Trace Elem. Res. 103*, 217–228.

van den Boom, R., Brama, P.A., Kiers, G.H., de Groot, J., and van Weeren, P.R. (2004). Assessment of the effects of age and joint disease on hydroxyproline and glycosaminoglycan concentrations in synovial fluid from the metacarpophalangeal joint of horses. *Am. J. Vet. Res. 65*, 296–302.

Verbruggen, G., Cornelissen, M., Almqvist, K.F., Wang, L., Elewaut, D., Broddelez, C. *et al.* (2000). Influence of aging on the synthesis and morphology of the aggrecans synthesized by differentiated human articular chondrocytes. *Osteoarthritis Cartilage 8*, 170–179.

Verzijl, N., DeGroot, J., Ben, Z.C., Brau-Benjamin, O., Maroudas, A., Bank, R.A. *et al.* (2002). Crosslinking by advanced glycation end products increases the stiffness of the collagen network in human articular cartilage: A possible mechanism through which age is a risk factor for osteoarthritis. *Arthritis Rheum. 46*, 114–123.

Vignon, E., Arlot, M., Patricot, L.M., and Vignon, G. (1976). The cell density of human femoral head cartilage. *Clin. Orthop. 121*, 303–308.

Wahl, G.M. and Carr, A.M. (2001). The evolution of diverse biological responses to DNA damage: Insights from yeast and p53. *Nat. Cell Biol. 3*, E277–E286.

Woo, S.L., Hollis, J.M., Adams, D.J., Lyon, R.M., and Takai, S. (1991). Tensile properties of the human femur-anterior cruciate ligament-tibia complex. The effects of specimen age and orientation. *Am. J. Sports Med. 19*, 217–225.

Yang, S., Alnaqeeb, M., Simpson, H., and Goldspink, G. (1996). Cloning and characterization of an IGF-1 isoform expressed in skeletal muscle subjected to stretch. *J. Muscle Res. Cell Motil. 17*, 487–495.

71

Sleep Quality in the Elderly

Ragnar Asplund

Sleep is of great importance for health and the quality of life. There is a strong association between sleep disorders on the one hand, and illness and early death on the other. The mortality is higher among elderly persons with sleep disorders than in those who sleep well, and the excess mortality is related to the predominant causes of death, such as heart disease, stroke, cancer, and suicide.

The individual prerequisites for a good night's sleep include many things, such as a comfortable bed, fresh air in the bedroom, and a room that is not too cold and not too hot. Another factor with a great impact on sleep is noise.

Poor sleep also shows a negative interaction with many somatic and psychiatric diseases and symptoms, as well as causing a deterioration in the quality of life. These diseases and symptoms are more important in explaining sleep deterioration than the age and sex of the patients, although there is a tendency toward an increase in sleep problems with increasing age.

There are some evident differences in sleep between men and women. Women report more difficulties in initiating and maintaining sleep than men, whereas men display more sleep disturbances at EEG assessments. Men are also more troubled by sleep-disordered breathing than women.

The aim of this chapter is to recapitulate the major causes of sleep disturbances in the elderly, their significance in terms of life expectancy, general health outcome and quality of life, and the principal remedies available.

Introduction

Poor sleep is a common complaint in the elderly. In a Swedish questionnaire survey it was found that 10% of elderly men (aged 74 ± 6 years; mean ± SD) and 20% of elderly women were troubled by poor sleep. Frequent awakenings were reported by 21% and 27%, respectively, and difficulty in falling asleep after awakening was experienced by 22% and 41%, respectively. Eleven percent of men and 13% of women report frequent nightmares (Asplund and Åberg, 1992). Compared with the younger population, who are often troubled by difficulty in falling asleep at bedtime, elderly persons more often suffer from frequent awakenings and an increased length of time before falling asleep again. Their total sleep is shortened even though they spend more time in bed, and they have a smaller proportion of slow-wave sleep (SWS) (Morin and Gramling, 1989).

Sleep can be disturbed in several ways. The total amount of sleep can be increased (hypersomnia) or reduced (hyposomnia or insomnia), and it can be fragmented by frequent awakenings. There are also many sleep-disturbing diseases and symptoms, which make getting back to sleep difficult after nocturnal awakenings. Many elderly persons recognize poor sleep as an effect of deterioration of their 24-hour rhythm. They often try to compensate for this by increasing the regularity of their lifestyle, which is probably beneficial not only for their sleep but also for their health in general.

There is a high genetic disposition to develop sleep disorders. In twin studies in humans, good covariation has been demonstrated regarding different qualitative and quantitative sleep variables. Poor sleep is more common in elderly people if their parents have been troubled by sleep complaints (see Figure 71.1) (Asplund, 1995a).

In a study of a large group of elderly men and women, reports on a poor night's sleep were 50% more frequent in men and three times more frequent in women whose parents had sleep problems. Deterioration of sleep from year to year was found to occur three times as often among both men and women whose parents both had sleep problems, compared with those whose parents had been good sleepers (Asplund, 1995a). The total sleep time was shorter in both men and women if either of their parents had sleep problems and was further shortened if both parents had such problems, and the same was true for the length of time up to the first nocturnal awakening. Furthermore, in the corresponding groups, the time taken to get to sleep was prolonged, awakenings were more numerous, and it took longer to fall asleep again after waking up in the night. Sleep problems in childhood occurred four times as often in both men and women whose parents both had such disturbances, compared with those whose parents both had been good sleepers (Asplund, 1995a).

There are some evident differences in sleep between men and women. Women report more difficulties in initiating and maintaining sleep than men, whereas men

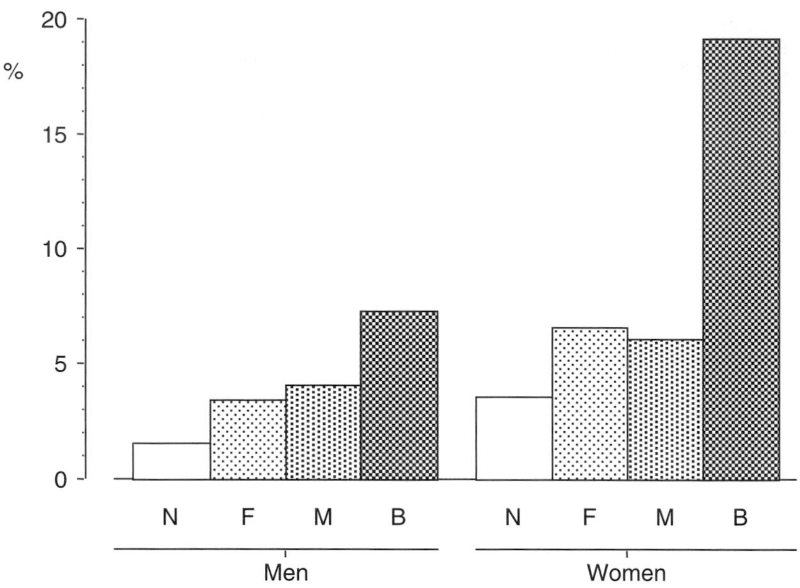

Figure 71.1 Occurrence of difficulty in falling asleep each night among men and women who reported sleep complaints in neither of their parents (N), the father (F), the mother (M), and both parents (B) (Asplund, 1995a).

display more sleep disturbances at electroencephalography (EEG) assessments. Men are also more troubled by sleep-disordered breathing than women (Rediehs *et al.*, 1990). Women have a greater tendency to react to sleep-disturbing factors than men and acquire a lighter sleep during pregnancy. When, in infancy, the child grows old enough to leave the mother undisturbed at night, the mother's sleep remains more fragile than before (Spielman *et al.*, 1996).

Determinants of Sleep

THE PHYSIOLOGY OF SLEEP AND ITS AGING

The sleep/wake cycle and the 24-hour rhythm of the body temperature are regulated by a circadian periodicity that originates from the suprachiasmatic nucleus in the hypothalamus. In the morning we wake up, our body temperature increases from the nocturnal level, and we are able to be active throughout the day. In the late evening, when it is dark, we normally go to bed, and after a while we fall asleep.

With reference to the EEG pattern, sleep is divided into five different stages:

- Stage 1: Light or drowsy sleeping representing the transitional stage between being awake and sleeping, lasting 5 to 10 minutes in the late evening. During this stage breathing becomes slow and regular. The heart rate decreases. Episodes of stage 1 sleep occur during the night, with increased frequency and length in the latter part of the night.
- Stage 2: Sleep becomes deeper and the muscle tone decreases. Approximately 40 to 50% of a typical night is spent in stage 2.
- Stages 3 and 4: Referred to as deep sleep, delta sleep, or slow-wave sleep (SWS). Waking from these stages is more difficult than from stages 1 and 2. During SWS, growth hormone is released from the hypothalamus. Many restorative processes, such as healing of injuries and immunological processes necessary for defense against infections or malignancies are most active during SWS (Stanley, 2005).
- Stage 5: During rapid-eye-movement (REM) sleep, dreams are more common than in other sleep stages. REM sleep may occur in four or five periods throughout the night at intervals of 60 to 90 minutes and with increasing length throughout the night. REM sleep has been attributed to emotional well-being and memory (Stanley, 2005).

The longest periods of SWS are seen in children, with a substantial reduction in young adults, and these periods are even shorter or sometimes absent in the elderly. Their total sleep is shortened even though they spend more time in bed. The sleep of the elderly is not only more superficial but also more fragmented than in younger people (Kales *et al.*, 1974).

Sleep and wakefulness are governed by a circadian and a homeostatic mechanism. The sleep/wake cycle is generated by a circadian rhythm that originates from the suprachiasmatic nucleus of the hypothalamus. This cycle makes it easier to fall asleep at the common time of the 24-hour period, most commonly in the evening or at night, whereas falling asleep in the daytime is more difficult or sometimes impossible. The homeostatic mechanism generates increased sleepiness and prolonged sleep after prolonged wakefulness, and consequently the amount of sleep is shorter if sleep takes place after a shorter time than usual in the waking state (Stanley, 2005).

AGE-RELATED DEVELOPMENT

The sleep pattern changes in parallel with aging. The time spent in deep sleep (slow-wave sleep) is decreased, and in the very elderly it may be absent. The number of awakenings increases with aging and in many elderly falling asleep after such awakenings becomes increasingly difficult. Elderly persons are therefore more troubled by spending time in the waking state in bed than younger adults. This decline in sleep maintenance is to some extent an expression of the age-related disorganization of the circadian sleep/wake rhythm.

However, sleep quality in the elderly seems to be more attributable to health-related factors than to age *per se*. In a study of the influence of somatic health, mental health and age on sleep in a group of elderly men and women, it was found that in men, more severe sleep disturbances were associated with poorer somatic health, poorer mental health, and increasing age, in that order of importance, and that in women, they were correspondingly associated with poorer somatic health and poorer mental health, but there was no further deterioration of sleep with age (Asplund, 2000).

There is an age-related increase in daytime sleepiness in the elderly, and those with poor night's sleep are more sleepy in the daytime than those with good sleep (see Figure 71.2) (Asplund, 1996).

Severe disruption of the sleep/wake cycle has been observed in very old people suffering from a serious illness, dementia, or both conditions. In a classic study in a nursing home population it was found that most people spent about 40 minutes per hour sleeping at night and about 20 minutes per hour in the daytime. Correspondingly, they woke up about four to five times every hour at night and three to four times every hour in the daytime. Only six of the subjects experienced even one single hour of consolidated sleep during the 24 recorded hours, and none of them had two or more consecutive hours of sleep (Jacobs *et al.*, 1989).

SLEEP IN DIFFERENT COUNTRIES

The prevalence rates of sleep disturbances vary considerably between different countries of the world. In a recent review of the literature based on data collected in 50 community-dwelling populations, prevalence rates of insomnia ranging from less than 5% to 40% were reported (Ohayon, 2002). In a cross-sectional survey in 10 countries (Austria, Belgium, Brazil, China, Germany, Japan, Portugal, Slovakia, South Africa, and Spain), answers to a standardized questionnaire were collected from 35,327 men and women with mean age 39 years (7.9% of ages 65 years or older). In the whole study group "not sleeping well" was reported by the least proportion of respondents in Austria (10.4%) and the highest proportion in Belgium (32.2%). Correspondingly, the nocturnal sleep duration varied from 413 ± 69 (mean ± standard deviation, SD) minutes in Japan to 504 ± 89 minutes in Portugal, and the time taken to fall asleep varied from 15.2 ± 18.4 minutes in Austria to 34.4 ± 42.1 minutes in South Africa. Regular naps were reported by 12% in Japan and 42.4% in Brazil, and sleepiness during the day by 5.1% in Germany and 20.2% in South Africa (Soldatos *et al.*, 2005).

ENVIRONMENTAL FACTORS

The individual prerequisites for a good night's sleep include a number of factors, such as a comfortable bed, fresh air in the bedroom, and a room that is not too cold

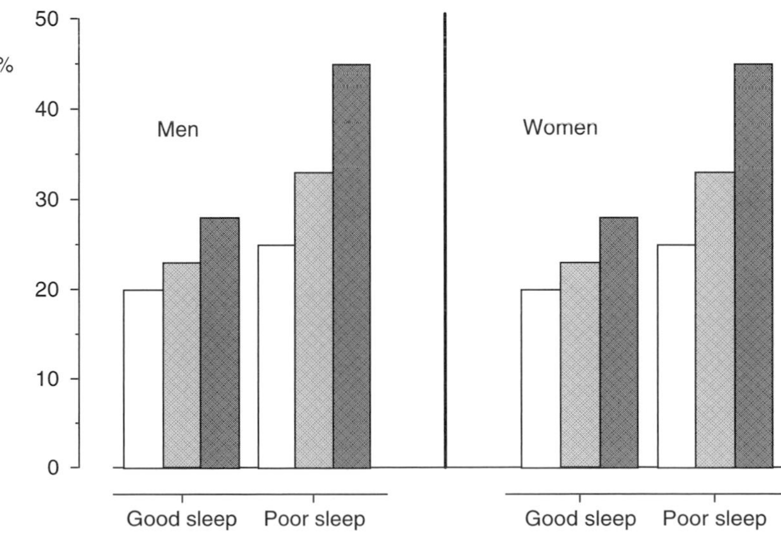

Figure 71.2 Affirmative answers (%) to the statement "I am often sleepy in the daytime" in relation to sex, age, and nocturnal sleep. Age (years): <70 (white bars); 70–79 (dotted bars); ≥80 (grey bars) (Asplund, 1996).

and not too hot. A sleep partner also seems to be favorable for sleep. People with a preexisting psychological or psychiatric condition may be more susceptible to the effects of noise, and women are more sensitive to noise than men (Nivison and Endresen, 1993).

Noise is a factor with a great impact on sleep. In a study of adult men and women exposed to road traffic noise during nine nights over a period of two weeks, poorer sleep quality, performance, and mood, and greater tiredness both in the morning and during the day were reported. No habituation of these effects was observed (Öhrström, 2000). Further, in a study of sleep in a residential area of Gothenburg, before and after the opening of a new tunnel for road traffic resulting in reduction of the road traffic from about 25,000 to 2,400 vehicles per 24 hours and from 1,375 to 180 vehicles per night (22–06), the previous adverse effects on sleep were substantially reduced and sleep quality was significantly improved after this extensive noise reduction in residents living near the road (25–67 meters). The subjective sleep improvement experienced by these residents was more pronounced than in those living in a control area (125–405 meters from the road). The improvement was recorded in all four sleep quality measures: "difficulty in falling asleep," "awakenings," "sleep quality," and "tiredness in the morning" (see Figure 71.3) (Öhrström, 2004).

Sleep disturbances are particularly common in nursing homes. Nursing routines need to be performed at all hours and a certain amount of noise and light at night cannot be avoided. Sleep is also deteriorated by large amounts of time spent in bed during the daytime and consequent inability to sleep at night. Some patients have a poorly functioning sleep/wake rhythm, resulting in daytime sleep and also night wandering, which disturbs other residents. The little access to outdoor activities, for medical and nursing-related reasons, may partly explain the increased occurrence of sleep complaints among elderly people living in nursing homes. The rhythmic change of light during the 24-hour period, which plays an important role in the sleep-wake timing, is difficult to maintain. Bright light in the daytime has proven effective in the treatment of sleep maintenance insomnia in the elderly (Hajak *et al.*, 1995).

Many healthy elderly people try to compensate for disruption of the sleep/wake rhythm by increasing the regularity of their lifestyle, which is probably beneficial not only for their sleep but also for their health in general (Reynolds *et al.*, 1991; Monk *et al.*, 1997). Lifestyle intervention is also desirable for improvement of sleep in the nursing home setting (Alessi *et al.*, 2000).

Health Impairment and Sleep

SOMATIC DISEASES AND SYMPTOMS

Heart diseases

Heart diseases and sleep disturbances interact with one another in a reciprocal and complicated way. In a classic study of Finnish adult men, Partinen and coworkers found a higher prevalence of coronary heart diseases in men who slept less than six hours per night after adjustment for age, sleep quality, use of sleeping pills and tranquilizers, smoking, alcohol use, Type A score, neuroticism, use of cardiovascular drugs, and history of hypertension. Difficulty in falling asleep at bedtime has been found to be associated with a two-fold increase in the risk of myocardial infarction during a follow-up period of 4.2 years (Appels and Schoulten, 1991). Further, among patients with myocardial infarction in another study, almost half had had sleep disorders during the six months immediately preceding the onset, which is a higher proportion than in a comparable population without myocardial infarction (Carney *et al.*, 1990).

Waking up in the night precedes more often than follows an angina pectoris attack. Most of these nocturnal awakenings are accompanied by getting up for visits to the toilet, and angina pectoris at night often occurs in connection with getting out of bed for micturition (Asplund, 2004).

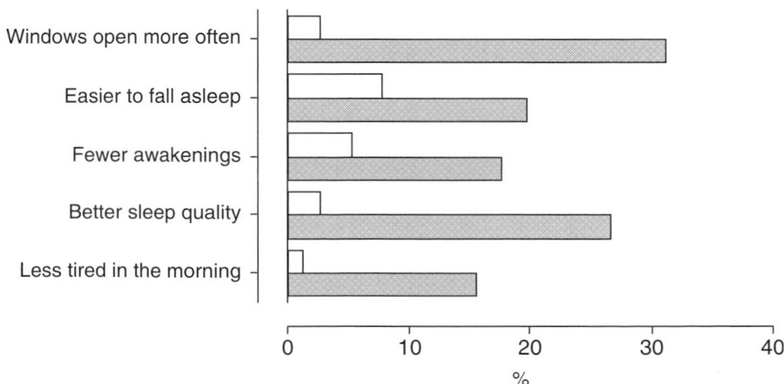

Figure 71.3 Residents' own comparison of sleep after the change in road traffic. Exposed (grey bars); controls (white bars) (Öhrström *et al.*, 2004).

In a questionnaire survey in northern Sweden among men and women aged 65 years or older, strong correlations were found between, on the one hand, affirmative answers to questions concerning two cardiac symptoms, namely "I am troubled by spasmodic pains in the chest" and "I am troubled by a sensation of irregular heart beats," and on the other hand, sleep complaints. The validity of the answers to the questions on heart diseases was supported by the fact that almost 90% of the subjects who stated that they suffered from spasmodic chest pain also reported the use of antianginal drugs, and that persons with subjective cardiac arrhythmia were also high consumers of drugs for heart diseases (Asplund, 1994). In both genders, the occurrence of either of these symptoms was associated with difficulty in falling asleep and those who reported both symptoms were troubled with difficulty in falling asleep at least twice as often as among those without cardiac symptoms. Difficulty in falling asleep within one hour after going to bed, nocturnal awakenings, and difficulty in getting to sleep after such awakenings were also increased in subjects with cardiac symptoms. Both men and women who stated that they woke up in the morning with a feeling of anxiety reported angina pectoris twice as often as those who woke up without anxiety. Also, the frequency of angina pectoris was twice as high in men and four times as high in women who reported that their final awakening was too early every morning, compared with those who woke up too early less than once a month. Cardiac arrhythmia was more than three times as common among men and more than twice as common among women who stated that they woke up too early every morning, compared with less than once a month (Asplund, 1994).

Only very few studies regarding the relation between sleep and cardiac diseases have been conducted in persons older than 65 years. In a study of sleep complaints and incident fatal and nonfatal first myocardial infarction over three years in 2,960 North Carolina adults aged 65 years or older, Schwartz *et al.* (1998) reported that the occurrence of myocardial infarction during the study period was increased in association with reports on restless sleep (incidence density ratio (IDR) 1.58, 95% confidence interval 1.11–2.24) and trouble falling asleep (1.68, 1.09–2.60) after adjustment for age, gender, and race. IDR was not substantially influenced by reports on smoking, blood pressure, diabetes, or obesity. Self-rated health and depression were strong independent correlates for myocardial infarction. Both of these conditions are also very closely linked to sleep impairment in the elderly and poor sleep is one of the diagnostic criteria in the diagnosis of major depression (DSM-IV).

Patients with coronary artery diseases who suffer from sleep apnea show poor cardiac function and have a high incidence of cardiac events, and frequent apnea episodes are a common finding in patients with congestive heart failure. Nocturnal arterial oxyhemoglobin desaturation caused by sleep-disordered breathing may be partly responsible for the excess morbidity and mortality in association with sleep disorders in the elderly (Javaheri, 1996).

Stroke

Stroke and the sleep/wake cycle show a reciprocal relationship. Several studies have shown that the onset of ischemic stroke more often occurs in the early morning than in other parts of the 24-hour period, independently of well-known risk factors and of clinical stroke subtypes (Casetta *et al.*, 2002). Both the increase in blood pressure in the morning and the circadian variability in the coagulation system may explain this increased risk of stroke.

Ischemic stroke often is followed by sleep impairment. In a study of insomnia, defined as at least one affirmative answer to a set of three items of the Hamilton Depression Scale, in patients with acute ischemic stroke complaints, insomnia occurred in 68% of patients on admission and had decreased to 49% at 18 months. From two months, symptoms of insomnia were associated independently with depression (Palomäki *et al.*, 2003). Other studies have also shown that depression is a common finding in association with stroke and sleep impairment is an early symptom of depression.

In patients who have suffered a cerebrovascular lesion, sleep is often disturbed by breathing impairment. Stroke patients have wider fluctuations in upper airway resistance than control subjects, resulting in frequent apneic episodes, and thereby run an increased risk of arterial oxyhemoglobin desaturation during post-stroke rehabilitation. This sleep apnea syndrome is associated with a poorer functional outcome and increased mortality. The diffuse cerebral symptoms such as cognitive deficits, depression, and fatigue are often explained by sleep apnea, and patients with stroke and diffuse cerebral symptoms should therefore be investigated for sleep-disordered breathing (Mohsenin and Valor, 1995).

Parkinson's disease

Sleep disorders occur in 74 to 98% of patients with idiopathic Parkinson's disease, and have serious effects on their quality of life. Accordingly, sleep and quality of life of spousal caregivers is also often affected. These patients suffer from a wide variety of somatic symptoms with an impact on sleep, such as stiffness, pain, muscle cramps, inability to turn over in bed, inability to get out of bed without aid, and polyuria. Vivid dreams, nightmares, and night terrors are also increased (Pal *et al.*, 2004). Their sleep becomes fragmented by an increased number of nocturnal awakenings and difficulty in getting back to sleep, resulting in daytime sleepiness. Sleep disturbances increase with the severity of the disease (Partinen *et al.*, 1997).

In a recent report it has been suggested that patients with Parkinson's disease with severe sleep disorders may represent a subset of patients with early, progressive degeneration of sleep centers, rather than with an enhanced aging process. They are more susceptible to mood disturbances, which correlate with the severity of the sleep dysfunction (Pal *et al.*, 2004).

In Parkinson's disease, treatment of the disease itself is the most important way of reducing the sleep disturbances. Controlled-release levodopa less often causes nocturnal symptoms compared to standard levodopa. Hypnotics or antidepressants may be added for further symptom relief (Partinen *et al.*, 1997).

Excessive daytime sleepiness and sudden sleep attacks are common complaints in Parkinson's disease. An increase in these symptoms in association with dopamine agonist treatment has been suggested, but other studies have not confirmed such a relationship. Patients with Parkinson's disease and excessive daytime sleepiness have a longer duration of disease, longer treatment with dopamine agonists, and more pronounced parkinsonian motor symptoms than those without excessive daytime sleepiness (Pal *et al.*, 2004).

Musculoskeletal pain

Pain is a common complaint in people who are troubled by poor sleep, and poor sleepers experience not only greater pain intensity but also more pain discomfort than good sleepers (Asplund, 1996). The total sleep time is shorter, sleep efficiency is lower, and sleep onset latency is longer in persons with very severe pain than in those with pain of low severity. Sleep impairment and musculoskeletal pain seem to interact in a reciprocal manner. In a recent study in adult men and women suffering from musculoskeletal pain in the neck, shoulder(s), and/or the lumbar region who were treated with acupuncture on 10 occasions over a period of four weeks it was found that during a six-month follow-up period after cessation of treatment, only the patient group whose pain improved in the evening showed a favorable development of night sleep, and correspondingly, only the group who experienced improved sleep felt pain relief in the morning (Hansson and Asplund, 2005). A detrimental influence of nocturnal sleep impairment on pain the following day has also been reported in patients with fibromyalgia. There are some experimental data supporting the hypothesis that sleep deterioration may contribute to the lowering of the pain threshold. Onen and colleagues reported that healthy men after 40 hours of total sleep deprivation showed hyperalgesia in response to mechanical stimulation and that subsequent SWS was associated with an analgesic effect (Onen *et al.*, 2001).

In the elderly, the occurrence and severity of pain increase in parallel with increasing age and are strongly correlated to sleep impairment. One disease related to a high frequency of sleep disorders is rheumatoid arthritis. Accordingly, attempts should always be made to achieve the best possible pain relief (Asplund, 1999).

Sleep apnea syndrome

Apneic episodes during sleep are common, and can be caused by a disturbance in the breathing control mechanism in the central nervous system (central sleep apnea) or by narrowing of the pharyngeal airway and loss of dilator tone during sleep (obstructive sleep apnea). Sleep apnea syndrome (SAS) causes sleep fragmentation and results in a variety of somatic diseases and symptoms, such as hypertension and coronary artery disease (Olsson *et al.*, 1995). Daytime sleepiness is increased in association with SAS and more so in the elderly than in young adults.

Sleep apnea is very common in elderly people. There is a reciprocal relationship between sleep apnea and dementia. Sleep apnea is more common in elderly patients suffering from dementia, and the frequency of breathing disturbances during the night is related to the severity of the dementia. Dementia, on the other hand, is increased by sleep apnea. Among community-dwelling elderly persons over the age of 70 years, 24% show an apnea index (AI) of more than five apneas per hour of sleep, and a study of 80-year-old patients severely affected by dementia and living in nursing homes revealed an AI of five per hour in 42% of patients (Asplund, 1999).

Increased mortality, particularly at night, has been reported among patients with sleep apnea. Sleep apnea represents heavy costs for healthcare services prior to treatment for the apnea. Successful treatment results in a lower mortality risk and normalization of somatic and psychological symptoms, and improves the patient's quality of life and safety in traffic.

Central sleep apnea is characterized by the occurrence of apneic events during sleep with no associated ventilatory effort. Many neurological diseases affecting the brain, such as cerebral arteriosclerosis, infarctions, tumors, hemorrhage, encephalitis, poliomyelitis, and other infectious diseases are able to produce breathing pattern disorders in sleep. Nocturnal central apneic episodes resulting in a decrease in nocturnal arterial oxyhemoglobin desaturation contribute to the progressive impairment in cardiac function in patients with heart failure (Asplund, 1999).

In certain patients, the history and physical examination may arouse suspicion of obstructive sleep apnea (OSA), a condition characterized by frequent disturbances of the night's sleep due to apneic episodes, daytime sleepiness, and a general lack of well-being. Nocturia due to nocturnal polyuria is a pathognomonic finding in OSA. In stroke patients, OSA is more common than central sleep apnea, and sleep apnea precedes the stroke in many cases. Polysomnography is helpful in the assessment of OSA. Treatment may improve the patient's well-being, reduce daytime sleepiness, lower the blood pressure, and reduce the risk of ongoing cardiovascular damage (Silverberg *et al.*, 1997).

OSA is a common finding in persons who are troubled by loud snoring, although snoring *per se* is not necessarily associated with OSA. OSA is more common in men than in women. After the menopausal transition, however, the prevalence of sleep apnea is steeply increased in women and approaches that in men. The respiratory symptoms are aggravated by overweight, cigarette smoking, alcohol, and hypnotics, and are improved by elimination of these factors (Asplund, 1999).

Asthma

Asthma is a condition with a profound negative influence on sleep. Asthmatic patients spend more time awake at night, they have a longer sleep onset latency and a shorter period of deep sleep. They have less refreshing sleep, and the occurrence of respiratory symptoms is dependent on the sleep structure. These patients suffer from bronchoconstriction more often during REM sleep than during other periods of sleep, and they also run an excess risk of oxygen desaturation during REM sleep. Because of their breathing difficulties, they often use bronchodilator inhalations at night. Such drugs are stimulants *per se*, and hence are detrimental to sleep. Nocturnal airway obstruction is associated with excess mortality. In patients with nocturnal asthma, daytime cognitive performance is impaired to a degree related to the severity of their disease (Asplund, 1999).

Nocturia and nocturnal polyuria

Nocturia is such a common condition in the older population that it is often considered to be a normal consequence of aging and therefore is very often disregarded and consequently left untreated. However, nocturia has a profoundly negative impact on health, sleep, and quality of life in many elderly persons. The sleep disruption associated with frequent nocturnal awakenings may induce excessive daytime fatigue, cognitive impairment, mood alterations, and increased susceptibility to disease. Nocturia is also associated with an increased risk of depression and an elevated mortality rate. Nocturnal voiding episodes increase the risk of falls and fractures during the visits to the toilet and back, especially in older, frail people with a decreased cognitive and motoric functioning. Nocturia not only imposes a significant burden on many nocturic persons and their partners, but may also entail considerable cost to the society. The fatigue due to sleep deprivation further augments the risk of accidents on the road and at work. Hence, nocturia is a serious disorder, which, if not treated appropriately, may have far-reaching consequences, both for the patient and society (Asplund, 1995b).

In three out of four cases of nocturia, nocturnal polyuria is present. The nocturnal polyuria syndrome (NPS) is characterized by increased nocturnal diuresis and a consequent increase in nocturnal micturition episodes, increased thirst and fluid intake, especially at night, and sleep disturbances. The prevalence of NPS has been estimated to be 3% in an elderly population, with no gender difference. People with polyuria at night wake up more frequently with a need to visit the toilet and have more difficulty in falling asleep after being out of bed. They often suffer from poor health and an impaired quality of life (Asplund, 1995b).

Even though many symptoms in NPS are similar to those in diabetes insipidus, there are important differences; in NPS, the 24-hour diuresis is normal or only moderately increased. The rhythm of the diuresis, on the other hand, is altered. There is an increase in the nocturnal part of the 24-hour diuresis, caused by a lack of diurnal rhythm in the antidiuretic hormone (ADH) system, and often the plasma ADH level is not detectable at all in the night (Asplund, 1995b).

In NPS, sleep is disturbed by the increased number of nocturnal voiding episodes and often also by a need for nocturnal drinking. The percentage of persons who report a poor night's sleep is more than twice as high among both men and women with three or more nocturnal voiding episodes than among those with none. This increase in sleep impairment includes an increased number of nocturnal awakenings, difficulty in falling asleep after such awakenings, sleepiness in the morning, and daytime sleepiness. Nightmares are also more numerous in parallel with increased numbers of nocturnal micturition episodes (Asplund, 1995b).

Nocturia is associated with a significant increase in the occurrence of dry eyes and dry mouth among the elderly, and dryness of the mucous membranes is highly sleep-disturbing. There is also a negative fluid balance, which needs to be corrected by drinking throughout the whole 24-hour period, but especially at night. The dryness of the eyes and mouth seem to be consequences of this negative fluid balance (Asplund, 2004).

NPS also is associated with poor balance, which implies an increased risk of falls in the night, and hypnotic treatment in elderly persons with NPS may increase this risk. During recent years, treatment of increased nocturnal urine output with desmopressin, a vasopressin analogue, has been used in the elderly and found successful in many cases (Asplund, 2004). This implies a possibility of reducing the use of sleeping pills in NPS patients.

Restless legs and other nocturnal symptoms from the lower extremities

Restless legs syndrome (RLS) is a common sensorimotor disorder characterized by an urge to move the extremities, caused or accompanied by unpleasant sensations in the affected limbs. The prevalence of RLS is 9 to 20% in the elderly, with twice as high prevalence figures in women as in men. The symptoms are absent during activity but appear at rest and become more pronounced in the evening or at night. Sleep impairment is the most common reason why patients seek medical aid (Hornyak *et al.*, 2004).

The most effective relief is obtained by getting out of bed and walking around, but this results in deterioration of sleep. Most of the patients with restless legs syndrome also have periodic leg movements, characterized by repetitive flexions of the extremities, during sleep and relaxed wakefulness. Periodic leg movement syndrome may sometimes be present in patients who are not troubled by restless legs in the awake state, and may be suspected in patients with severely disturbed sleep. Neuroleptics often are associated with the occurrence or worsening of RLS, and their use should therefore be avoided. Dopaminergic agents are considered to be the treatment of choice. Opioids, anticonvulsants, or hypnotics also are used frequently and are well tolerated in most elderly sufferers. Interaction with other medications and the possibility of sedation due to slower metabolism in the elderly should be considered (Hornyak *et al.*, 2004).

Leg muscle cramps are common, especially in the older age groups. They often occur in the evening and prevent sleep. The etiology of leg cramps is not clear. Cardiovascular diseases as well as peripheral vascular and neurological disorders are more common in patients with nocturnal leg cramps than in those without. The treatments include stretching exercises, quinine sulfate, and vitamin E, but no treatment has proved to be effective for all patients. Quinine sulfate often is prescribed to avoid muscle cramps in the elderly, although it has some important side effects. Serious hypersensitivity reactions and thrombocytopenia have been reported after its use.

Sensory organ dysfunctions

In many elderly persons, poor sleep may be attributed to a deterioration of their 24-hour rhythm. Such a disturbance is especially profound in blind persons, in whom severe sleep disturbances are prevalent. However, some blind persons have a normal sleep history despite a lack of subjective light perception, if they have an intact retinohypothalamic photic pathway (Czeisler *et al.*, 1995).

Reports on poor sleep, frequent awakenings, and difficulties in falling asleep after waking at night are also more common in men and women with visual impairment than in those without impaired vision after adjustment for age, general health, circulatory organ disease and diabetes (Asplund, 2000). Further, in elderly persons with cataracts sleep is improved one month after cataract extraction and further improvement may be experienced during the first nine months (Asplund and Ejdervik-Lindblad, 2004). There may be lifestyle factors in the background of sleep deterioration in relation to visual impairment. Impaired vision often leads to difficulties in outdoor activities and hence to reduced exposure to bright daylight. Bright light has been proven effective in the treatment of sleep maintenance insomnia in the elderly. It is also possible that difficulty in being physically active and a lack of intellectual stimulation as a result of visual impairment can cause increased sleep deterioration (Asplund, 2000).

Among persons with impaired hearing, poor sleep is more common in both sexes, whereas frequent awakenings and difficulty in falling asleep after waking at night are more common in women (Asplund, 2005). Hearing loss influences psychological well-being and reduces the opportunities for mental stimulation, which may have a negative impact on alertness and daytime activity. Poor hearing is also associated with increased daytime sleepiness independent of health, sleep status, and age.

Hearing impairment as well as other otological disorders often is associated with tinnitus. One common consequence of tinnitus is a disturbance of sleep, and from different studies prevalence figures of sleep disturbance of 25 to 71% have been reported (Asplund, 2005). Many patients are annoyed by their tinnitus during substantial parts of their time, which makes them tired and impairs their quality of life. As elderly tinnitus sufferers are more inclined to have sleep problems than elderly persons in general, tinnitus seems to cause daytime sleepiness both directly and through its detrimental effect on sleep (Asplund, 2005).

PSYCHIATRIC DISEASES AND SYMPTOMS

Alzheimer's disease and other dementias

Senile dementia of the Alzheimer's type (AD) is often associated with sleep impairment, and several kinds of disturbances have been described, such as reduction of sleep efficiency and of the total length of sleep. There is also a relationship between the severity of the sleep disturbance and the severity of the dementia. Patients with AD have an increased number and duration of awakenings, an increased percentage of stage 1 sleep, reduced slow-wave ("deep") sleep, and reduced REM sleep (Petit *et al.*, 2004).

As a consequence of the continuing sleep disorganization in parallel with progression of the AD, night-wandering and disturbing behavior are common problems both for the patient and for his or her spouse and caregivers. This problem may be alleviated at least to some extent, by attempting to give the patient daytime activity, avoidance of daytime sleeping, and use of hypnotics during periods of pronounced disturbances of the sleep/wake rhythm.

Depressive symptoms are common in patients with AD, and in elderly persons with depression it is often difficult to distinguish this from AD. The sleep pattern in AD differs from that of depression in showing a greater reduction of REM sleep and a lower REM density. The intellectual ability and the daytime performance may also be impaired by central sleep apnea, which is present in 33 to 53% of patients with AD (Asplund, 1999).

Depression

Sleep problems are common in elderly persons with depressive disorders, and in the Diagnostic Statistical Manual (DSM-IV) of Mental Disorders, sleep deterioration is included as one of the nine criteria for the diagnosis of major depression (American Psychiatric Association 2000). Depression is a fairly common condition. In a recent questionnaire survey in northern Sweden among men and women of ages 18 years and older, the prevalence of major depression was found to be 4.8% in men and 6.3% in women with only minor difference with respect to age (Asplund *et al.*, 2004).

In persons with depression, sleep problems occur most frequently during acute depressive episodes, but the disturbed sleep often persists during remission. The sleep symptoms consist mainly of an increase in sleep latency, a reduced total sleep time, and a decrease in sleep efficiency, and the disturbed sleep structure may result in intense dreams or nightmares. Early morning awakening is one of the most significant biological markers of depression. Treatment of the depressive disease is necessary for relief from sleep symptoms. The newer, selective serotonin reuptake inhibitors (SSRI) have no sedative or sleep-inducing effect, and aggravated insomnia may occur in connection with such treatment. Tricyclic antidepressants often have sleep-promoting effects when administered in the evening. However, because of their side effects, they are not as well tolerated as SSRI drugs. Adjuvant hypnotic medication therefore can be a good choice for sleep improvement during the acute depressive episode (Asplund *et al.*, 2004).

A probably often-overlooked cause of sleep disturbances in elderly persons with depression is nocturia. In a recent study it was found that nocturia was increased six-fold in men and three-fold in women in association with major depression after age and somatic health had been taken into consideration (Asplund *et al.*, 2004). Treatment with SSRI has been mentioned in association with different urological symptoms, but accounted for only a minor part of the increase in nocturia. The cause of the increase in the number of nocturnal voiding episodes in association with depression is not clear, but there is support for the assumption that the nocturnal diuresis may be increased and also that the micturition mechanism is altered, resulting in a reduced bladder capacity. The sleep impairment *per se*, which is part of the depressive symptomatology, can also partly explain the increase in nocturnal voiding, as an effect of inhibition of the normal nocturnal reduction of the urine output.

Treatment

The treatment of sleep complaints in the elderly must first of all be focused on diagnostic and therapeutic measures in order to alleviate treatable somatic and mental sleep-disturbing diseases and symptoms as far as possible. However, this is not easy, and many elderly persons will continue to suffer from different kinds of sleep disturbances even after a thorough exploration and treatment of their problems.

Specific treatment of insomnia may involve pharmacologic and/or nonpharmacologic approaches. Benzodiazepines are the most commonly prescribed medications for insomnia. Their use in short-term treatment has been shown to be effective, whereas treatment over a longer period, months or even years on a regular basis, has been questioned (Moller *et al.*, 2004). Side-effects have been described in association with the use of benzodiazepine hypnotics, such as agitation, daytime sedation, cognitive impairment, and an increased risk of falls. Both sleep impairment itself and the use of benzodiazepines are associated with an increased risk of cognitive and psychomotor impairments, but sometimes sleep medication may be associated with less disturbances of daytime functioning than severe sleep impairment (Asplund, 1996).

Sleep medication for longer periods loses its favorable influence on sleep, but its side-effects may remain. If a period of treatment with hypnotics longer than three to four weeks can be anticipated, intermittent treatment, every two or three nights, can be appropriate.

Alternatives to the benzodiazepines are the more modern, selective benzodiazepine receptor agonists zopiclone, zolpidem, and zaleplon. These are believed to cause less daytime sleepiness and to produce less impairment in slow-wave sleep, which is already diminished in old age. Zopiclone has also been shown to increase SWS. Their efficacy and safety for short-term use have been demonstrated in geriatric populations, although studies of their long term use are still lacking (Moller *et al.*, 2004).

Disorders of the circadian sleep/wake rhythm are fairly common in the elderly. Melatonin treatment has been tried in various doses as a hypnotic drug in order to restore a regular 24-hour sleep/wake rhythm, which is disrupted in some elderly people, as a result of age-related deterioration of the function of the circadian clock in the suprachiasmatic nucleus in the brain. Treatment with melatonin seems to be of no clinical value in the management of psychophysiological insomnia in general, but may be beneficial in the initiation and maintenance of sleep in melatonin-deficient elderly insomniacs. Melatonin has a short half-life, and good results are reported in elderly persons given controlled-release melatonin preparations (Asplund, 1999). A number of melatonin agonists have been developed with (hopefully) improved properties in comparison to melatonin. Some of these agents are now in clinical trials for treatment of insomnia in people with circadian rhythm sleep disorders (Turek *et al.*, 2004).

Bright light has proven effective in the treatment of sleep maintenance insomnia in the elderly. However, the design of the treatment, especially the timing of exposure to light, is important. Murphy and Campbell (1996) studied the effect of bright light on performance and sleep in a group of elderly persons suffering from sleep maintenance insomnia. The patients received treatment with bright light (>4,000 lux from 9 p.m. to 11 p.m.) every night during a 12-day period and maintenance treatment with bright light twice weekly (>4,000 lux from 9 p.m. to 11 p.m. or >4,000 lux from 3 p.m. to 5 p.m.) for a three-month period. The former treatment resulted in significant improvement not only in the quality of sleep but also in daytime cognitive functioning (Murphy and Campbell, 1996).

Nonpharmacologic approaches to insomnia also include a wide range of cognitive, behavioral, and educational techniques. The most commonly used techniques include bed-restriction, stimulus control, sleep hygiene education, and cognitive strategies. In some studies the use of such techniques in elderly populations have shown results comparable to and better sustained than those of hypnotics (Moller, 2004). Cognitive-behavioral treatments for sleep problems in people aged 60 and over are mildly effective for some aspects of sleep. The durability of the effect of these treatments remains unproven (Montgomery and Dennis, 2004).

In a Netherlandic study, educational radio was used for treatment of sleep disorders in the population. The researchers report that the training (eight radio programs) produced an estimated decrease in sleep latency of 25 minutes and an increase in the duration of sleep by nearly 40 minutes, and of the people using hypnotic drugs, 40% ceased their use after the course (Oosterhuis and Klip, 1997).

Conclusion

Many elderly people suffer from poor sleep. Although sleep impairment is more prevalent in women, its negative consequences for life expectancy, health, and quality of life are more pronounced in men. Many common diseases and symptoms cause insomnia such as musculoskeletal pain, angina pectoris, difficulty in breathing, depression, and dementia. Insomnia can be precipitated or exacerbated particularly by conditions that may worsen at night, for example, gastroesophageal reflux, congestive heart failure, restless legs, periodic leg movement disorder, or asthma. When the resulting insomnia becomes chronic, psychiatric disturbances such as impaired concentration and memory, irritability, depressed mood, or anxiety may develop. There is an overlap in symptomatology between insomnia secondary to medical conditions, circadian disturbances, sleep disorders, and actual psychiatric disorders (Moller *et al.*, 2004).

The occurrence of sleep problems in the elderly more often is related to poor somatic health than to poor mental health. Many studies have shown that sleep problems in the elderly increase in parallel with increasing age, but when the influence of somatic and mental health has been taken into account, age *per se* has very little impact on sleep.

The use of sleep medication shows a pattern parallel with that of sleep, namely, a stronger relationship to somatic than to mental health (Asplund, 2000). This may reflect the fact that sleep difficulties often serve as a proxy for medical conditions that should have been treated otherwise than by sleep medication. Some elderly men and women are treated with hypnotics even though they do not experience any real sleep problem. Such medication is observed particularly among persons with very poor somatic health (Asplund, 1995). In most cases they need some relief from their nocturnal symptoms in order to get some rest. This observation may support the view that sleep medication in the elderly can be reduced if pain and discomfort due to somatic and mental diseases and symptoms are alleviated.

Recommended Resources

Alessi, C.A., and Schnelle, J.F. (2000). Approach to sleep disorders in the nursing home setting. *Sleep Med. Rev.* 4, 45–56.

Montgomery, P. and Dennis, J. (2004). A systematic review of non-pharmacological therapies for sleep problems in later life. *Sleep Med. Rev.* 8, 47–62.

Ohayon, M.M. Relationship between chronic painful physical condition and insomnia. *J. Psychosom. Res.* 39, 151–159.

Schwartz, S., Mcdowell-Anderson, W., Cole, S.R., Cornoni-Huntley, J., Hays, J.C., and Blazer, D. (1999). Insomnia and heart disease: A review of epidemiologic studies. *J. Psychosom. Res.* 47, 313–333.

Stanley, N. (2005). The physiology of sleep and the impact of ageing. *Eur. Urol. Suppl.* 3, 17–23.

RECOMMENDED LINKS

MedlinePlus. Medical Encyclopedia. Sleep disorders in the elderly.
http://www.nlm.nih.gov/medlineplus/ency/article/000064.htm#visualContent

Describes the normal sleep and its aging, and common sleep disorders and their treatment.

UniversityAlliance. Sleep Disorders of the Elderly
http://sleepdisorders.about.com/od/sleepandtheelderly/
American Academy of Family Physicians
http://www.aafp.org/afp/990501ap/2551.html

Management of Sleep Disorders in the Elderly. Veterans Affairs Canada.
http://www.vac-acc.gc.ca/clients/sub.cfm?source=steannes/pub_research/bgroulx_04

REFERENCES

Alessi, C.A. and Schnelle, J.F. (2000). Approach to sleep disorders in the nursing home setting. *Sleep Med. Rev. 4*, 45–56.

American Psychiatric Association (2000). Diagnostic and Statistical Manual of Mental Disorders DSM-IV-TR.

Appels, A. and Schoulten, E. (1991). Waking up exhausted as a risk indicator of myocardial infarction. *Am. J. Cardiol. 68*, 395–398.

Asplund, R. and Åberg, H. (1992). Health of the elderly with regard to sleep and nocturnal micturition. *Scand. J. Prim. Health Care 10*, 98–104.

Asplund, R. (1994). Sleep and cardiac diseases amongst elderly people. *J. Intern. Med. 236*, 65–71.

Asplund, R. (1995a). Are sleep disorders hereditary? A questionnaire survey of elderly persons about themselves and their parents. *Arch. Gerontol. Geriatr. 21*, 221–231.

Asplund, R. (1995b). The nocturnal polyuria syndrome (NPS). *Gen. Pharm. 26*, 1203–1209.

Asplund, R. (1996). Daytime sleepiness and napping among the elderly in relation to somatic health and medical treatment. *J. Int. Med.* 1996, *239*, 261–267.

Asplund, R. (1999). Sleep disorders in the elderly. *Drugs Aging 14*(2), 91–103.

Asplund, R. (2000). Sleep, health and visual impairment in the elderly. *Arch. Gerontol. Geriatr. 30*, 7–15.

Asplund, R. (2004). Nocturia, nocturnal polyuria and sleep disorders in the elderly. *J. Psychosom. Res. 56*, 517–525.

Asplund, R., Henriksson, S., Johansson, S., and Isacsson, G. (2004). Nocturia and depression. *Br. J. Urol. Int. 93*, 1253–1256.

Asplund, R. and Ejdervik-Lindblad, K. (2004). Sleep and sleepiness one month and nine months after cataract surgery. *Arch. Gerontol. Geriatr. 38*, 69–75.

Asplund, R. (2005). Sleep and sensory organ functions in the elderly. *Sleep and Hypnosis. 7*, 52–60.

Barry, J., Campbell, S., Yeung, A.C., Raby, K.E., and Selwyn, A.P. (1991). Waking and rising at night as a trigger of myocardial ischemia. *Am. J. Cardiol. 67*, 1067–1072.

Carney, R.M., Freedland, K.E., and Jaffe, A.S. (1990). Insomnia and depression prior to myocardial infarction. *Psychosom. Med. 52*, 603–609.

Casetta, I., Granieri, E., Fallica, E., la Cecilia, O., Paolino, E., and Manfredini, R. (2002). Patient demographic and clinical features and circadian variation in onset of ischemic stroke. *Arch. Neurol. 59*(1), 48–53.

Chokroverty, S. (1996). Sleep and degenerative neurologic disorders. *Neurol. Clin. 14*, 807–826.

Czeisler, C.A., Shanahan, T.L., Klerman, E.B., Martens, H., Brotman, D.J., Emens, J.S. *et al.* (1995). Suppression of melatonin secretion in some blind patients by exposure to bright light. *N. Eng. J. Med. 332*, 6–11.

Hajak, G., Rodenbeck, A., Staedt, J., Bandelow, B., Huether, G., and Ruther, E. (1995). Nocturnal plasma melatonin levels in patients suffering from chronic primary insomnia. *J. Pineal Res. 19*, 116–122.

Hudgel, D.W., Devadatta, P., Quadri, M., Sioson, E.R., and Hamilton, H. (1993). Mechanism of sleep-induced periodic breathing in convalescing stroke patients and healthy elderly subjects. *Chest 104*, 1503–1510.

Jacobs, D., Ancoli-Israel, S., Parker, L., and Kripke, D.F. (1989). Twenty-four-hour sleep-wake patterns in a nursing home population. *Psychol. Aging 4*, 352–356.

Javaheri, S. (1996). Central sleep apnea-hypopnea syndrome in heart failure: Prevalence, impact, and treatment. *Sleep 19* (Suppl. 10), S229–S231.

Middelkoop, H.A., Smilde-van den Doel, D.A., Neven, A.K., Kamphuisen, H.A., and Springer, C.P. (1996). Subjective sleep characteristics of 1,485 males and females aged 50–93: Effects of sex and age, and factors related to self-evaluated quality of sleep. *J. Gerontol. A. Biol. Sci. Med. Sci. 51*, M108–M115.

Mohsenin, V. and Valor, R. (1995). Sleep apnea in patients with hemispheric stroke. *Arch. Phys. Med. Rehabil. 76*, 71–76.

Moller, H.J., Barbera, J., Kayumov, L., and Shapiro, C.M. (2004). Psychiatric aspects of late-life insomnia. *Sleep Med. Rev. 8*, 31–45.

Montgomery, P. and Dennis, J. (2004). A systematic review of non-pharmacological therapies for sleep problems in later life. *Sleep Med. Rev. 8*, 47–62.

Kales, A. and Kales, J.D. (1974). Sleep disorders. Recent findings in the diagnosis and treatment of disturbed sleep. *N. Engl. J. Med. 290*, 487–499.

Monk, T.H., Reynolds, C.F. 3rd, Kupfer, D.J., Hoch, C.C., Carrier, J., and Houck, P.R. (1997). Differences over the life span in daily life-style regularity. *Chronobiol. Int. 14*, 295–306.

Morrell, S., Taylor, R., and Lyle, D. (1997). A review of health effects of aircraft noise. Aust N Z J *Public Health 21*(2), 221–236.

Morin, C.M. and Gramling, S.E. (1989). Sleep patterns and aging: comparison of older adults with and without insomnia complaints. *Psychol. Aging 4*, 290–294.

Nivison, M.E. and Endresen, I.M. (1993). An analysis of relationships among environmental noise, annoyance and sensitivity to noise, and the consequences for health and sleep. *J. Behav. Med. 16*, 257–276.

Murphy, P.J. and Campbell, S.S. (1996). Enhanced performance in elderly subjects following bright light treatment of sleep maintenance insomnia. *J. Sleep Res. 5*, 165–172.

Ohayon, M. (2002). Epidemiology of insomnia: What we know and what we still need to learn. *Sleep Med. Rev. 6*, 97–111.

Oosterhuis, A. and Klip, E.C. (1997). The treatment of insomnia through mass media, the results of a televised behavioral training programme. *Soc. Sci. Med. 45*, 1223–1229.

Pal, P.K., Thennarasu, K., Fleming, J., Schulzer, M., Brown, T., and Calne, S.M. (2004). Nocturnal sleep disturbances and daytime dysfunction in patients with Parkinson's disease and in their caregivers. *Parkinsonism Relat. Disord. 10*, 157–168.

Palomäki, H., Berg, A., Meririnne, E., Kaste, M., Lönnqvist, R., Lehtihalmes, M. *et al.* (2003). Complaints of poststroke insomnia and its treatment with mianserin. *Cerebrovasc. Dis. 15*, 56–62.

Partinen, M., Putkonen, P.T., Kaprio, J., Koskenvuo, M., and Hilakivi, I. (1982). Sleep disorders in relation to coronary heart disease. *Acta Med. Scand. Suppl. 660*, 69–83.

Partinen, M., Kaprio, J., Koskenvuo, M., Putkonen, P., and Langinvainio, H. (1983). Genetics and environmental determination of human sleep. *Sleep 6*, 179–185.

Redìehs, M.H., Ries, J.S., and Creason, N.S. (1990). Sleep in old age: Focus on gender differences. *Sleep 13*, 410–424.

Reynolds, C.F. 3rd, Jennings, J.R., Hoch, C.C., Monk, T.H., Berman, S.R., Hall, F.T. *et al.* (1991). Daytime sleepiness in the healthy "old old": A comparison with young adults. *J. Am. Geriatr. Soc. 39*, 957–962.

Schwartz, S.W., Cornoni-Huntley, J., Cole, S.R., Hays, J.C., Blazer, D.G., and Schocken, D.D. (1998). Are sleep complaints an independent risk factor for myocardial infarction? *Ann. Epidemiol. 8*, 384–392.

Soldatos, C.R., Allaert, F.A., Ohta, T., and Dikeos, D.G. (2005). How do individuals sleep around the world? Results from a single-day survey in ten countries. *Sleep Med. 6*, 5–13.

Spielman, A.J., Nunes, J., and Glovinsky, P.B. (1996). Insomnia. *Neurol. Clin. 14*, 513–543.

Stanley, N. (2005). The physiology of sleep and the impact of ageing. *Eur. Urol. Suppl. 3*, 17–23.

Turek, F.W. and Gillette, M.U. (2004). Melatonin, sleep, and circadian rhythms: Rationale for development of specific melatonin agonists. *Sleep Med. 5*, 523–532.

Öhrström, E. (2000). Sleep disturbances caused by road traffic noise—Studies in laboratory and field. *Noise Health. 2*, 71–78.

Öhrström, E. (2004). Longitudinal surveys on effects of changes in road traffic noise: Effects on sleep assessed by general questionnaires and 3-day sleep logs. *Journal of Sound and Vibration 276*, 713–727.

72

Atherogenesis and Aging

Cam Patterson

The prevalence of coronary artery disease increases with age (2002), and age itself is an independent risk factor for atherogenesis (Kannel and Gordon, 1980), suggesting that the biological milieu in aging populations is conducive to atheromatous lesion formation. Increased susceptibility to cellular stress and accrual of damage to vascular tissues are likely factors in the atherogenic milieu attributable to aging, yet the precise molecular processes underlying the age-associated events culminating in atherosclerotic lesion formation remain to be determined. Given the difficulties in understanding these mechanisms in humans, a variety of animal models have been developed that represent various aspects of vascular injury and atherosclerosis. In this chapter, we will provide a concise overview of the etiology of atherosclerotic arterial disease and the contributions of aging in this process. We will also review the methods for manipulating blood vessels via mechanical and humoral factors to induce vascular injury, and we will consider the application of these methods in specific animal models that are particularly conducive for understanding the prevalence and enormous burden of cardiovascular disease in the course of aging.

Introduction

Vascular diseases—coronary artery disease, peripheral vascular disease, and cerebrovascular disease—are extremely debilitating, and are by far the most common causes of stroke, myocardial infarction, and heart failure in the United States (2002). The vast majority of vascular disease occurs due to atherosclerosis of the affected vessels, yet our understanding of the mechanisms by which atherosclerosis develops is limited. Clinicians therefore have few tools at their disposal to prevent or reverse the atherosclerotic process in patients at risk for the consequences of atherosclerosis.

Blood vessels invade and nourish every organ in the body, so the consequences of vascular disease are diverse and reflect dysfunction of the organ system(s) targeted by the affected vessels. Atherosclerotic disease of coronary vessels threatens myocardial viability and can lead to myocardial infarction and its sequelae, and disease of the medium and small vessels of the cerebral vessels can lead to stroke. Although these are the most common manifestations of vascular disease, other vessels are also frequently affected. Abdominal aortic aneurysms are a relatively common affliction in elderly populations; the vascular disease leading to these aneurysms bears both similarities and differences with typical atheromatous disease typically seen in coronary and other vascular beds. These aneurysms may rupture catastrophically or cause thrombotic occlusions of the distal extremities. Vascular disease also affects the renal and mesenteric vasculature, and contributes to the complications of diabetes.

According to the most recent statistics reported by the National Center for Health Statistics, cardiovascular diseases remain the leading cause of death in the United States (2002). In 2001, 41% of all deaths were due to cardiovascular disease, and of these, nearly three quarters were atherosclerosis-related. The good news is that death rates due to cardiovascular diseases declined 36% over the preceding 20 years. The bad news is that the burden of cardiovascular diseases falls disproportionately among the elderly, who are the fastest growing segment of our population. Adults over age 70 are almost four times more likely to suffer cardiovascular diseases than are those in the 40- to 49-year age group. In fact, some cardiovascular diseases, such as abdominal aortic aneurysms, are almost unknown in individuals under age 65, yet may be found in up to 5% of males over age 65 (Salo *et al.*, 1999). Unless reductions occur in the incidence of cardiovascular diseases in the elderly, it is probable that the increasing numbers of older individuals will provide resistance against the long-term trends toward decreasing overall cardiovascular mortality.

Mechanisms of Atherosclerosis

Atheromatous lesions develop over decades and occur principally within the intima, the innermost layer of the arterial wall. Several paradigms exist for classification of atherosclerotic lesions based primarily on morphologic considerations. The earliest identifiable lesion, the *fatty streak*, is a flat, yellowish, nonobstructive accumulation of neointimal lipid that can be found in the aorta and coronary arteries of most individuals beginning in the second decade of life. The *fibrous plaque* is a more advanced whitish lesion containing proliferative smooth muscle cells, infiltrating macrophages and other inflammatory cells, and extracellular matrix components. Whether fibrous plaques inevitably arise from fatty streaks rather than appearing *de novo* is not clear. Often, a necrotic *lipid core* resides deep within the fibrous plaque, which contains macrophage-derived foam cells and extracellular lipids. Fibrous plaques may protrude eccentrically into the lumen, resulting in obstruction of blood flow and symptoms such as angina pectoris and claudication. However, defects of the lesion surface and accompanying thrombosis are not present, and therefore unstable coronary syndromes typically are not associated with these lesions.

Progression of fibrous plaques leads to *advanced* or *complicated lesions*, which may contain increased amounts of connective tissue around the necrotic core (fibroatheromas) and/or calcifications of the necrotic core. These components may alter the compliance of the vessel and thus have a destabilizing tendency. Neovascularization of the plaque by the process of angiogenesis may occur (O'Brien *et al.*, 1994), and the presence of these vessels may lead to intraplaque hemorrhage, which is an important source of plaque instability and intraplaque hematoma formation. The intimal surface of advanced lesions may have minor disruptions (*fissures*) or suffer gross denudation (the *ulcerative plaque*), which can serve as a nidus for acute thrombosis directly. Surface disruption may also lead to *plaque rupture* with extrusion of lipid core components and activation of the coagulation cascade within the intralumenal compartment. Advanced lesions encompass a variety of pathologic components in varying mixtures, but they share two ominous characteristics: They may progress rapidly, owing to features such as intraplaque hemorrhage, leading to rapid progression of obstructive symptoms such as angina. By virtue of their tendency to rupture and thrombus formation, they may also cause acute occlusion of coronary and cerebral vessels, resulting in myocardial infarction and stroke, the most deadly consequences of atherosclerotic disease.

The framework for understanding how atherosclerotic lesions form and progress was provided by Russell Ross (Ross, 1993). Dr. Ross proposed the "response-to-injury" hypothesis, which argues that the initiating event in lesion formation is some form of "injury" to the endothelium, the cell layer that forms the lumenal barrier of all blood vessels. Although modifications of this initial hypothesis have been made to incorporate subsequent observations, it still provides a useful framework for understanding how lesions form. Endothelial injury in this model may take the form of *mechanical forces* such as high blood pressure or changes in shear stress and cyclic strain that can occur at vessel bifurcations; *metabolic conditions* such as diabetes mellitus, hyperhomocysteinemia, or hyperlipidemia that produce substances that directly injure the endothelium; or *environmental agents* such as the products of tobacco smoke or even infectious agents that also impair endothelial cell function. It is important to note the close correlation between the factors that may cause endothelial injury and the known risk factors for atherosclerosis.

Regardless of the cause, injured endothelium has several proatherogenic properties. Normal adaptive vascular responses, such as the release of endothelium-derived nitric oxide, are impaired. Endothelial denudation or activation leads to adhesion of platelets and inflammatory cells that can release proatherogenic growth factors. Adherent monocytes and lymphocytes may also directly invade the vessel wall, where they participate directly in lesion formation. Low-density lipoprotein cholesterol may be taken up by macrophages and other vascular cells after injury, leading to foam cell formation and lipid accumulation in necrotic areas. Intraplaque macrophages may be particularly destabilizing within advanced plaques by releasing factors such as matrix metalloproteinases that degrade the extracellular matrix and impair the integrity of the atherosclerotic lesion. Lesion stability can also be triggered by apoptosis of the endothelium, which removes the vessel barrier to thrombus formation, and also by apoptosis of intraplaque smooth muscle cells, which may serve as a stabilizing function in complicated lesions (Ferguson and Patterson, 2003). It is clear that the evolution of atherosclerotic lesions is incredibly complex, involving a large number of events and many cell types, some of which participate in both detrimental and protective processes within the lesion, depending on the stage of the lesion and the location of the cell. This enormous complexity explains in part why the genetics of atherosclerosis is still so poorly understood at the present time.

Atherosclerosis and Aging

There are two explanations for the increased prevalence of vascular disease in the elderly: (1) the increased risk represents a longer duration of exposure to conditions that promote atherosclerosis (i.e., the time-dose product of the risk factors); and (2) atherosclerosis is a specific aging-associated process. It is important to note that these possibilities are not mutually exclusive and that from the perspective of a given elderly individual at risk for vascular disease, this distinction may not matter much. However, discrimination between these hypotheses has important implications for prevention of vascular disease, particularly at the population level. In the former case, preventive therapies should focus on early interventions on established risk factors such as hypercholesterolemia, hypertension, diabetes, obesity, and smoking; in the latter case, specific therapies may be required to target the aging-associated mechanisms that accelerate atherosclerosis in the elderly.

The possibility that atherosclerosis has a specific aging-associated pathogenesis can be explored at the epidemiologic and pathophysiologic levels. The Framingham study still provides the best data for understanding the *epidemiologic* impact of aging on cardiovascular disease. One way that this data set can be used to address the role of aging *per se* as a risk factor for atherosclerosis is to examine the age-dependence of established cardiovascular risk factors. Indeed, the combined effect of all cardiovascular risk factors together, or of each risk factor individually (with the exception of hypertension), decreases with age, in spite of the age-associated increase in prevalence of cardiovascular disease, suggesting that aging itself is the critical factor (Kannel and Gordon, 1980). More to the point, multivariate analysis demonstrates that aging is a risk factor for atherosclerosis independent of cholesterol level, blood pressure, diabetes, or smoking.

Well-described *physiologic* changes in the cardiovascular system occur with aging that may predispose the vasculature to accelerate the development of atherosclerosis. A variety of studies have shown that older animals have an increased susceptibility and responsiveness to vascular insults (Weingand *et al.*, 1986; Spagnoli *et al.*, 1991; McCaffrey and Falcone, 1993). With aging, there is progressive dilation of large vessels with associated intimal thickening (Michel *et al.*, 1994). Collagen content is increased but elastin content is decreased, resulting in decreased compliance of large arteries (Fornieri *et al.*, 1992). In fact, the change in matrix composition is the primary determinant of intimal thickening associated with aging, as total cellularity remains constant or even decreases (Fornieri *et al.*, 1992; Michel *et al.*, 1994; Lopez-Candales *et al.*, 1997). Bilato and Crow term these aging-associated vascular changes "the vasculopathy of aging," and argue that they provide the soil for atherosclerosis in elderly individuals (Bilato and Crow, 1996). Strongly supporting the hypothesis that atherogenesis is an intrinsically age-related process, accelerated atherosclerosis is seen in diseases associated with premature senescence, such as Werner's syndrome and progeria (Cohen *et al.*, 1987).

At present, we know in significant detail the molecular and cellular events that link important cardiovascular risk factors (increased cholesterol, hypertension, diabetes, and smoking) with atherosclerotic lesion progression, and in many cases we have effective therapies that have been extensively documented to modify the risk of cardiovascular events. In comparison with these other risk factors, we know almost nothing about the molecular events that link aging and atherosclerosis, and consequently we have no therapies aimed at modulating the cardiovascular risk inherent to aging. This gap in our knowledge provides the fundamental rationale for the application of animal models of atherosclerosis to delineate the age-associated pathogenetic mechanisms of this disease.

Animal Models of Atherosclerosis

A variety of animal models have been used to study atherosclerosis since the first description of atherosclerosis in rabbits in the early years of the twentieth century (Anitschkow, 1914). Each model differs with respect to variables such as the length of time to development of lesions, similarity to human pathology, and the requirements for supplementation to induce atherosclerosis, and as such it is clear that a single ideal model for analyzing atherosclerosis does not exist. At the present time, a number of animal models of atherosclerosis, such as canines and pigeons, are primarily of historical interest and are not discussed here.

PRIMATES

Both New World and Old World monkeys have been extensively evaluated for their ability to develop atherosclerotic lesions. Nonhuman primates develop atherosclerotic lesions that bear remarkable similarities to those of humans, including the ability to mineralize and undergo plaque rupture. Atheromatous formation in monkeys is modified by many of the same factors that influence human vascular disease—diet, gender, age, blood pressure, and genetics. Thus, nonhuman primates have many ideal characteristics for developing animal models of atherosclerosis. However, these advantages are mitigated by three major factors: regulatory issues that make it difficult to acquire and obtain monkeys for research; requirements for specialized housing and veterinary services; and the relatively long time-intervals required for atherosclerotic lesion development.

In spite of these challenges, nonhuman primates exhibit a number of remarkable features that favor their use for understanding the mechanisms of human vascular disease. For example, cynomolgus macaques have lipid profiles similar to humans, and exhibit sex differences in lesion formation that mimic what is observed in humans (Rudel *et al.*, 1977). In addition, both cynomolgus and rhesus monkeys develop myocardial infarctions (Bond *et al.*, 1980), which is otherwise a rare occurrence within the animal kingdom outside *Homo sapiens*. Localization of atherosclerotic lesions in monkeys is generally similar to that in humans, allowing analysis of disease in coronary, iliac, aortic, and intracranial vessels, all of which are major sources of disease in humans.

Arguably the best data linking diet and lifestyle changes with modulation of the risk of atherosclerosis have derived from nonhuman primate studies. Regression of atherosclerosis has been amply demonstrated to occur in conjunction with reductions in plasma cholesterol concentrations (Clarkson *et al.*, 1984). This remains one of the few models in which true plaque regression can be observed, and given that therapeutic interventions to elicit plaque regression in humans are limited, this is a powerful advantage. In addition, monkeys are arguably the only model organisms in which human-type psychosocial stresses can be tested. A number of studies have now shown clearly that high levels of psychosocial stress associated with activation of the autonomic nervous system and neuroendocrine reactions to stress in monkeys result in acceleration of atherosclerotic lesion formation that at least in some cases can be modulated pharmacologically (Kaplan *et al.*, 1987). Thus, it is unfortunate that logistical and practical reasons limit the utility of these models, which are becoming increasingly limited to a few specialized centers.

SWINE

Atherosclerosis occurs spontaneously in swine and is easily induced by proatherogenic diets. It occurs in distributions similar to that observed in humans, and the common circulatory mechanisms and large caliber of porcine arteries facilitates their analysis. The pathogenesis and histology of lesions in swine closely parallels that observed in humans: focal intimal thickening, fatty streaks, inflammatory cell infiltration, lipid deposits, and fibrous plaque formation are all observed in lesions in pigs (see Figure 72.1).

In spite of these features, swine have been used only infrequently for pharmacologic studies of atherosclerosis. Pigs are extremely expensive and require special handling, and their dietary requirements can be formidable. Because pigs grow quickly, changes in weight can make pharmacologic dosing studies nontrivial. Miniature swine, such as the Yucatan, have been developed to circumvent some of these issues, but microswine remain expensive to purchase and maintain. The recent development of a pig model with features of metabolic syndrome (Nichols *et al.*, 1992) may reinvigorate the use of this model to study cardiovascular disease, given the increasing appreciation of a tight link between this syndrome and atherosclerosis in humans.

RABBITS

The rabbit has the distinction of being the first species recognized to develop diet-induced atheromatous lesions, in the landmark report by Anitschkow in 1914 (Anitschkow, 1914). New Zealand white rabbits develop lesions primarily in the aorta, and their development is associated with extraordinarily high plasma cholesterol levels (in the 1000–3000 mg/dl range), which can compromise other organ systems in ways that affect the experimental utility of this model. Disease of epicardial coronary vessels is rarely described, and though some features of human atheroma are present in the aortic lesions in rabbits, the prominent human concern of plaque instability is not a feature.

The use of rabbits as models of atherosclerosis has been enhanced significantly by development of genetic models, including the Watanabe heritable hyperlipidemic rabbit, which carries a spontaneous mutation in the LDL receptor (Watanabe, 1980). These rabbits develop aortic lesions spontaneously, and thus they serve as a particularly useful model to test mechanical and pharmacological interventions in atherosclerosis-related conditions. However, even in these genetically defined rabbits, intervals of at least a year are required for the development and progression of advanced lesions, and therefore time and cost issues factor into the choice of this model.

MICE

Rodents do not naturally develop atherosclerosis and have small-caliber arteries that develop primarily medial lesions under extraordinary dietary conditions that are distinct morphologically from human atheromatous disease. Each of these factors has contributed to an historical consideration that rodents were poor models of atherosclerosis. Hypercholesterolemic hamsters were briefly popular (and are still used occasionally) owing to their ability to develop lesions within the aortic arch that mimic subendothelial foam cell accumulation and that can be studied by *en face* preparations for quantitative analysis (Nistor *et al.*, 1987). However, the road to the now nearly ubiquitous use of the mouse as the primary model for studying atherosclerosis was paved by the

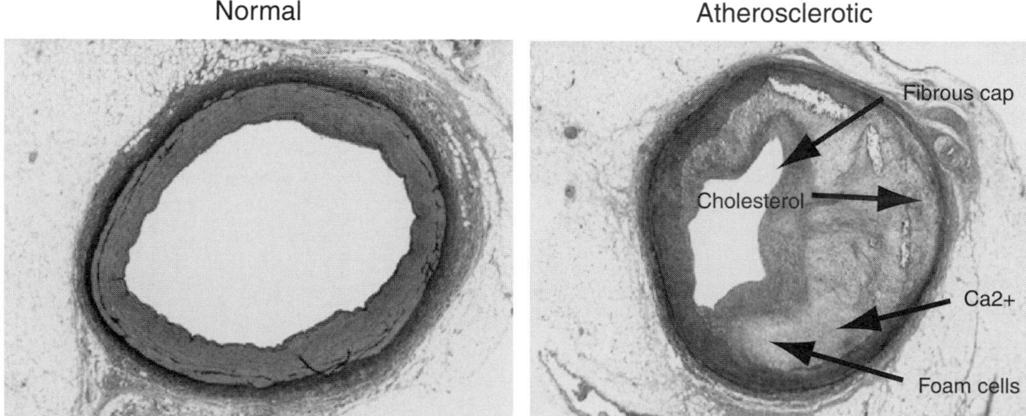

Figure 72.1 Swine model of atherosclerosis. Histologic samples from normal and atherosclerotic pig arteries demonstrate the hallmark characteristics of atherosclerosis, including cholesterol deposition, calcification, foam cell accumulation, and development of a fibrous cap.

development of mouse strains genetically modified by homologous recombination to develop accelerated atherosclerotic lesions, and was further cemented by the mouse genome project, which anointed the mouse as the primary model for genetic analyses in most laboratories today.

Although previous studies of strain-specific differences in medial thickening led to the supposition that mice are resistant to atherosclerosis, the development of hypercholesterolemic mice by deletion of the gene for apolipoprotein E indicated that this is not the case (Plump *et al.*, 1992; Zhang *et al.*, 1992). These mice become spontaneously hypercholesterolemic and develop atheromatous lesions in the aorta, along the aortic valves, and within the great vessels. The development of these lesions occurs spontaneously but can be markedly accelerated by feeding the mice a high-fat ("Western") diet. Acceleration of lesion formation with a high-fat diet can reduce the time needed for lesions to fully invest the large vessels in ApoE−/− mice to three months or less, which is one of the most rapid intervals among experimental models of atherosclerosis. Lesions form with many of the morphological characteristics of human atherosclerosis, and usually are quantified by serial sectioning at the level of the aortic valve or by Oil Red O staining of the aorta *en face* to define the extent of lesion formation throughout the aorta. Unfortunately, the distribution of lesions does not extend to the coronary circulation and advanced features such as plaque rupture are observed only under extraordinary circumstances.

ApoE−/− mice and the somewhat less frequently used but phenotypically similar LDL receptor-deficient mice are now the most common animal models of atherosclerosis by far. It is noteworthy that, to date, modulation of cholesterol metabolism has been the only mechanism that results in atheroma development in mice. The development of ApoE−/− mice has made possible an extraordinary analysis of modifiable factors such as diet, exercise, drug effects, and others that determine the extent of atherosclerotic lesion formation. In addition, the widespread availability, low cost, and rapid time to disease formation have made ApoE−/− mice an ideal model for drug screening and validation experiments.

In addition to these virtues, the availability of a broad variety of genetically modified mouse strains has allowed the molecular dissection of events that influence the pathogenesis of atherosclerosis that is virtually impossible in other models of this disease. The usual strategy has been to cross ApoE−/− mice with mice deficient in other proteins that are required for specific pathways or cellular events to determine the effects of this second molecule on the ApoE−/− phenotype. As an example of this approach, ApoE−/− mice also deficient in activity of the NADPH oxidase (by deletion of the essential component p47phox) have reduced levels of atherosclerosis, which indicates a necessary role for oxidative stress in atherosclerotic lesion formation (Barry-Lane *et al.*, 2001). This approach can be further augmented by bone marrow transplantation to dissect out the relative contributions of different cell types (circulating versus mural cells) to any phenotype that is observed. Finally, mice are perhaps the only animal model available in which it is feasible to perform advanced genetic crosses to search for new atherosclerosis-related genes and genetic modifiers that regulate the disease process through the awesome power of genetics.

Many of these features would suggest that ApoE−/− or similar mice are the ideal animal models for studying atherosclerosis, and in many respects they are. As indicated earlier, the availability, rapid time to disease onset, and genetic features are unique to this model, and no other model is as cost-effective on an animal-by-animal basis. Nevertheless, the limited distribution of lesions within the circulatory tree in this model and the failure to replicate many key steps in atherosclerotic vascular disease are important limitations. Thus, it is unlikely that mouse models alone will suffice in all circumstances for thorough evaluations of atherosclerotic disease.

Endovascular Injury

Although atherosclerotic disease is the major cause of morbidity and mortality in advanced civilizations, other diseases of the vasculature are common and have been modeled in animals.

With the development of interventional techniques to treat cardiovascular disease, especially in the coronary circulation, it has become apparent that the maladaptive response to endovascular injury (clinically referred to as restenosis) is mechanistically distinct from atherosclerosis, although a few features (such as smooth muscle proliferation) are common in both processes. Endovascular injury originally was used experimentally as a means to induce vascular responses, but the widespread use of balloon angioplasty and endovascular stenting has made the modeling of endovascular injury a greater experimental imperative.

Attempts to induce endovascular injury have been made in virtually every laboratory animal. In animals with large-caliber arteries, such as monkeys, pigs, and dogs, the same approaches that are used clinically (balloon injury and stent implantation) are used experimentally. In most cases, the time course and the extent of injury induced are similar to those seen in humans, especially when these techniques are accompanied by high-fat diets or are performed on pre-injured arterial segments. The initial phases of the response to endovascular injury consist of endothelial denudation, platelet adhesion, and intravascular thrombosis. The acute phase is followed by medial hyperplasia of smooth muscle cells, with resultant migration and further proliferation within the intima that occurs one to four weeks after injury. During the latter phase of the injury response, matrix deposition and further intimal thickening occur, leading to an eventual return to quiescence, albeit with an obstructive endovascular lesion at the site of injury (Patterson, 2002).

The response to endovascular injury, both in humans and in animal models, is further complicated because arterial remodeling provides an additional influence on the ultimate vascular response. This remodeling, which involves changes in the elastic laminae and adventitia that can either be favorable (outward) or unfavorable (inward) can modulate the extent to which lesions induced by endovascular injury become obstructive. Unfortunately, the mechanisms that regulate this remodeling phase are poorly understood, which emphasizes the need to study and understand this process in animal models.

Owing to the mechanical requirements for endovascular injury, large animal models produce more favorable responses that closely mimic the human condition. Injury to nonhuman primates using standard balloon catheter techniques results in a vascular response almost identical to that observed in humans, with early thrombosis and a late remodeling phase. Unfortunately, few centers have access to this approach. Balloon-mediated injury to the Yucatan minipig provides a consistent high-grade lesion, especially when combined with a high-fat diet, and these lesions can themselves be used as further targets for stent implantation (Gal *et al.*, 1990). These characteristics have made the swine model attractive both for studying the pathogenesis of endovascular injury and as a tool for the development of interventional techniques.

One major disadvantage of the aforementioned approaches is the time and expense necessary for large animal studies, not only with respect to the cost of the animals themselves but also attendant costs of instrumentation and anesthesia costs, none of which are trivial. Attempts to create appropriate small animal models of endovascular injury have, therefore, been a high priority. The caliber of blood vessels in New Zealand white rabbits has limited the usefulness of these animals for such approaches, but the larger Giant Flemish rabbits overcome this limitation and have seen some use for this purpose (LeVeen *et al.*, 1982). The rat carotid injury model, in which a balloon is used to damage the endothelium of the carotid artery, produces a characteristic lesion that has been extensively characterized (for example, see Ruef *et al.* (1999). Unfortunately, the lesion in these animals is limited predominantly to smooth muscle proliferation, and for this reason translation of studies using this approach should be limited to understanding mechanisms for activation of smooth muscle cells. Thrombotic, inflammatory, and remodeling components are largely lacking in this model, which explains why observations of drug effects based on rat carotid injury have not been reproducible in early phase drug development studies in humans.

In spite of the limitations of the rat approach to endovascular injury, there have now been numerous attempts to simulate this injury response in mice. The impetus for these efforts stems in part from the ease of use of mice as an animal model from a logistical perspective, but probably even more from the widespread availability of genetically modified mouse strains that allow specific characterization of pathophysiologic mechanisms. The approaches that have been used in mice are varied, and include endolumenal injury with wires to denude endothelium, arterial ligation (particularly of the carotid artery) to induce flow-dependent proliferation and remodeling, and a wide variety of direct arterial injury approaches. These models have been enormously fruitful in eliciting mechanisms of the injury response, particularly with regard to proliferative responses. However, it is essential to keep in mind that the response to injury in these mouse models is limited almost exclusively to medial smooth muscle cell proliferation, which is only one among many components of the endovascular injury response in humans. Thus, these studies must be carefully interpreted. At present, mouse models have limited utility for testing pharmacologic interventions.

Conclusion

Given the enormous burden of cardiovascular disease, especially among elderly individuals, it is not surprising that so many approaches have been developed to model these disease processes in animals. The approaches available vary, in part because atherosclerosis and related diseases are such complicated cellular events. With shorter life spans and responses to vascular insults enhanced by dietary influences, these animal models are in some cases particularly well suited for exploring why vascular disease is such a burden within aging populations and why it is so closely associated with accelerated aging processes.

ACKNOWLEDGMENTS

Work in the author's laboratory is supported by NIH grants GM61728, HL65619, AG02482, and HL61656. C.P. is an Established Investigator of the American Heart Association and a Burroughs Wellcome Fund Clinical Scientist in Translational Research. Thanks to Tim Nichols for providing the pig artery illustrations and to Holly McDonough for editorial assistance.

REFERENCES

(2002). *National Heart, Lung, and Blood Institute Fact Book*. Bethesda, MD: National Institutes of Health.

Anitschkow, N. (1914). Über die atherosclerose der aorta beim kaninchen und über derin entsteheungsbedingungen. *Beitr. Pathol. Anat. Allgem. Pathol. 59*, 308–348.

Barry-Lane, P.A., Patterson, C., van der Merwe, M., Hu, Z., Holland, S.M., Yeh, E.T. *et al.* (2001). p47phox is required for atherosclerotic lesion progression in ApoE(−/−) mice. *J. Clin. Invest. 108*, 1513–1522.

Bilato, C. and Crow, M. (1996). Atherosclerosis and the vascular biology of aging. *Aging Clin. Exp. Res. 8*, 221–234.

Bond, M.G., Bullock, B.C., Bellinger, D.A., and Hamm, T.E. (1980). Myocardial infarction in a large colony of nonhuman primates with coronary artery atherosclerosis. *Am. J. Pathol. 101*, 675–692.

Clarkson, T.B., Bond, M.G., Bullock, B.C., McLaughlin, K.J., and Sawyer, J.K. (1984). A study of atherosclerosis regression in *Macaca mulatta*. V. Changes in abdominal aorta and carotid and coronary arteries from animals with atherosclerosis induced for 38 months and then regressed for 24 or 48 months at plasma cholesterol concentrations of 300 or 200 mg/dl. *Exp. Mol. Pathol. 41*, 96–118.

Cohen, J.I., Arnett, E.N., Kolodny, A.L., and Roberts, W.C. (1987). Cardiovascular features of the Werner syndrome. *Am. J. Cardiol. 59*, 493–495.

Ferguson, J.E., 3rd and Patterson, C. (2003). Break the cycle: The role of cell-cycle modulation in the prevention of vasculoproliferative diseases. *Cell Cycle 2(3)*, 211–219.

Fornieri, C., Quaglino, D. and Mori, G. (1992). Role of the extracellular matrix in age-related modifications of the rat aorta. Ultrastructural, morphometric, and enzymatic evaluations. *Arterioscler. Thromb. 12*, 1008–1016.

Gal, D., Rongione, A.J., Slovenkai, G.A., DeJesus, S.T., Lucas, A., Fields, C.D. *et al.* (1990). Atherosclerotic Yucatan microswine: An animal model with high-grade, fibrocalcific, nonfatty lesions suitable for testing catheter-based interventions. *Am. Heart J. 119*, 291–300.

Kannel, W.B. and Gordon, T. (1980). Cardiovascular risk factors in the aged: The Framingham study. *Epidemiology of aging*. S.G. Haynes and M. Feinleib. Bethesda, MD: NIH publication n. 80-969, 65–89.

Kaplan, J.R., Manuck, S.B., Adams, M.R., Weingand, K.W., and Clarkson, T.B. (1987). Inhibition of coronary atherosclerosis by propranolol in behaviorally predisposed monkeys fed an atherogenic diet. *Circulation 76*, 1364–1372.

LeVeen, R.F., Wolf, G.L., and Villanueva, T.G. (1982). New rabbit atherosclerosis model for the investigation of transluminal angioplasty. *Invest. Radiol. 17*, 470–475.

Lopez-Candales, A., Holmes, D.R., Liao, S., Scott, M.J., Wickline, S.A., and Thompson, R.W. (1997). Decreased vascular smooth muscle cell density in medial degeneration of human abdominal aortic aneurysms. *Am. J. Pathol. 150*, 993–1007.

McCaffrey, T.A. and Falcone, D.J. (1993). Evidence for an age-related dysfunction in the antiproliferative response to transforming growth factor-beta in vascular smooth muscle cells. *Mol. Biol. Cell 4*, 315–322.

Michel, J.B., Heudes, D., Michel, O., Poitevin, P., Philippe, M., Scalbert, E. *et al.* (1994). Effect of chronic ANG I-converting enzyme inhibition on aging processes. II. Large arteries. *Am. J. Physiol. 267*, R124–R135.

Nichols, T.C., Bellinger, D.A., Davis, K.E., Koch, G.G., Reddick, R.L., Read, M.S. *et al.* (1992). Porcine von Willebrand disease and atherosclerosis. Influence of polymorphism in apolipoprotein B100 genotype. *Am. J. Pathol. 140*, 403–415.

Nistor, A., Bulla, A., Filip, D.A., and Radu, A. (1987). The hyperlipidemic hamster as a model of experimental atherosclerosis. *Atherosclerosis 68*, 159–173.

O'Brien, E.R., Garvin, M.R., Dev, R., Stewart, D.K., Hinohara, T., Simpson, J.B. *et al.* (1994). Angiogenesis in human coronary atherosclerotic plaques. *Am. J. Pathol. 145*, 883–894.

Patterson, C. (2002). Things have changed: Cell cycle dysregulation and smooth muscle cell dysfunction in atherogenesis. *Ageing Res. Rev. 1*, 167–179.

Plump, A.S., Smith, J.D., Hayek, T., Aalto-Setala, K., Walsh, A., Verstuyft, J.G. *et al.* (1992). Severe hypercholesterolemia and atherosclerosis in apolipoprotein E-deficient mice created by homologous recombination in ES cells. *Cell 71*, 343–353.

Ross, R. (1993). The pathogenesis of atherosclerosis: A perspective for the 1990s. *Nature 362*, 801–809.

Rudel, L.L., Pitts, L.L. 2nd, and Nelson, C.A. (1977). Characterization of plasma low density lipoproteins on nonhuman primates fed dietary cholesterol. *J. Lipid Res. 18*, 211–222.

Ruef, J., Meshel, A.S., Hu, Z., Horaist, C., Ballinger, C.A., Thompson, L.J. *et al.* (1999). Flavopiridol inhibits smooth muscle cell proliferation in vitro and neointimal formation in vivo after carotid injury in the rat. *Circulation 100*, 659–665.

Salo, J.A., Soisalon-Soininen, S., Bondestam, S., and Mattila, P.S. (1999). Familial occurrence of abdominal aortic aneurysm. *Ann. Intern. Med. 130*, 637–642.

Spagnoli, L., Orlandi, A., Mauriello, A., Santeusanio, G., de Angelis, C., Lucreziotti, R. *et al.* (1991). Aging and atherosclerosis in the rabbit. 1. Distribution, prevalence and morphology of atherosclerotic lesions. *Atherosclerosis 89*, 11–24.

Watanabe, Y. (1980). Serial inbreeding of rabbits with hereditary hyperlipidemia (WHHL-rabbit). *Atherosclerosis 36*, 261–268.

Weingand, K., Clarkson, T., Adams, M., and Bostrom, A. (1986). Effects of age and/or puberty on coronary artery atherosclerosis in cynomolgus monkeys. *Atherosclerosis 62*, 137–144.

Zhang, S.H., Reddick, R.L., Piedrahita, J.A., and Maeda, N. (1992). Spontaneous hypercholesterolemia and arterial lesions in mice lacking apolipoprotein E. *Science 258*, 468–471.

73

Managing Menopausal Symptoms

Mary Ellen Rousseau

This chapter deals with menopause-associated symptoms including hot flashes, night sweats, sleep disturbances, and vaginal symptoms. Other symptoms that accompany the perimenopause transition but are related to other life events or aging, including sexual dysfunction and mood disturbances, are discussed. The options for managing these changes include menopause hormone therapy, both systemic and local, as well as complementary therapies and nonhormonal therapies for each of the symptoms.

Introduction

Symptom perception, whether during menopause or otherwise, is comprised of sensations that differ from the ordinary. The main symptoms associated with menopause are hot flashes, night sweats, and vaginal symptoms including dyspareunia, dryness, and itching. For many decades other maladies have also been attributed to menopause including depression, mood swings, loss of youthfulness, sleep problems, and memory and cognitive dysfunction. Until the 1990s most research on menopausal women was derived from data from convenience samples of treatment-seeking white middle-class women (Avis *et al.*, 1993) and expert opinion. Whether these symptoms can be attributed to a menopause syndrome and the changing hormonal milieu that occurs in midlife or whether they exist on a continuum that proceeds along with aging is a major question at the heart of the menopause construct itself.

The cross-sectional portion of the Study of Women's Health Across the Nation (S.W.A.N.), a multiethnic sample of women (Avis *et al.*, 2001) has shown that vasomotor symptoms (VMS) consistently relate to the time just before and just after menopause. Across all racial and ethnic groups, other symptoms including difficulty sleeping, forgetfulness, stiffness/soreness, feeling tense, feeling depressed, and irritability have not shown a corresponding pattern of clustering around the menopause event. Rather, some symptoms increased over the long run, and the occurrence of some remained consistent throughout the time period from premenopause to postmenopause. This data suggests that there is no universal menopause syndrome in the general population as had been commonly accepted. However, that is not to say that there is not a subgroup of women who do suffer menopause symptoms that can be more inclusive than just vasomotor symptoms. Some women may have a propensity toward depression that is related to hormone changes, for example, postpartum depression. Such women may develop depression at the time of menopause. It is theorized that some women have a lower threshold for symptoms because of specific personal factors that accompany the menopause transition. During perimenopause, women may experience difficult socioeconomic pressures such as job loss, loss of parents or partners, declining personal health status, and difficult physical or cosmetic changes. When these occur at a time of considerable hormonal flux, the woman's threshold for coping may be met and she may become symptomatic to an extent that causes distress. On the other hand, many women by midlife have built a life's worth of coping mechanisms and resiliency that menopause does not rock.

Symptoms

BLEEDING

Bleeding pattern is the first change a woman will experience as she approaches the perimenopause transition. The reproductive-age-cycling woman will have predictable menses after ovulation because the cascade of hormonal events leads to a menstrual bleed after 14 days in the luteal phase of the cycle. When a woman reaches the perimenopause period, her supply of follicles secreting estradiol is decreased to a point that not every cycle is ovulatory. Circulating inhibin-B levels drop in response to the decreased number of follicles present in the ovary, leading to a rise in follicle stimulating hormone (FSH) levels. The increased FSH helps the ovary to produce near normal (premenopause levels) estradiol levels until just before the actual menopause. However, ovulation does not always occur under such circumstances, causing longer or shorter intervals between menses. When ovulation fails to occur, these cycles are characterized by absence of progesterone production, further contributing to cycle irregularity and skipped cycles characteristic of the late perimenopause period.

Irregular bleeding patterns are very common in the perimenopause period and can be linked to hormonal changes. Cycle irregularity is defined as cycles less than 21 days or greater than 35 days. It is less clear whether or not menorrhagia (heavy bleeding at regular intervals) is also associated with normal perimenopause changes (Van Voorhis, 2005). Longitudinal data from the S.W.A.N. study will give us a greater understanding of the hormonal underpinnings of the menopause change and perhaps clear up various questions about bleeding patterns during perimenopause. At the present time, however, menorrhagia is not considered a predictor of menopause (Van Voorhis, 2005) but is a common clinical finding associated with fibroids and polyps of the lining of the uterus. The prevalence of both polyps and fibroids peaks between the ages of 40 to 50, further confusing the diagnosis because of the hormonal changes taking place at the same time. Diagnostic evaluation of bleeding can be accomplished by transvaginal ultrasound, hysteroscopy, endometrial sampling, or a combination of diagnostic tools.

Often exogenous hormones are used to regulate menstrual bleeding during this time period in women screened for contraindications (heart disease risk, thromboembolic events, and smoking). Both estrogen and progestins are implicated in the increased risk of heart disease, stroke, and other thromboembolic events, as evidenced in the data from the Women's Health Initiative (WHI) (Rossouw *et al.*, 2002). Hormonal contraception such as patches (Ortho Evra™) and oral contraceptive pills are used to cause more predictable bleeding patterns. Other options include cyclic progestins: medroxyprogesterone acetate—Provera™, Cycrin™; micronized progesterone—Prometrium™; norethindrone acetate—Aygestin™, each of which is prescribed for 14 days every calendar month. Alternative treatment options for perimenopause bleeding include depo Provera™ and progesterone IUDs (Mirena™). Giving cyclic progestins offers the same predictable bleeding pattern as when OCPs are used but offers no contraception. Use of depo Provera™ leads to an atrophic endometrial uterine lining leading to amenorrhea. Women using depo Provera run the risk of decreasing bone loss, which is of particular importance in the perimenopausal woman. Use of the progestin IUD offers local progesterone effect, usually leading to an atrophic endometrial lining but with less theoretical chance of decreasing bone loss or increased theoretical risk of thromboembolic events.

VASOMOTOR SYMPTOMS (VMS)

Quality of life in menopause encompasses more than just absence of symptoms. It includes enjoyment of life, participation in meaningful relationships, work, and play (Matthews and Bromberger, 2005). Although most women in Western societies report hot flashes and night sweats, for most of these women such symptoms do not affect quality of life. In fact, data from the Melbourne Women's Mid-life Project show that well-being increases across the menopause transition (Dennerstein *et al.*, 2003). Lifestyle changes are recommended first for vasomotor symptoms. These include weight reduction for women who are significantly overweight; it has long been considered that women who were obese had fewer vasomotor symptoms because of elevated estrone levels from aromatization of adipose tissue to androgens than to estrone. However, new evidence shows that the occurrence of VMS in obese perimenopausal women may be due to the increased heat insulation afforded by greater adiposity, leading to more hot flashes (Freedman, 2002; Glickman-Weiss *et al.*, 1999). Smoking is associated with hot flashes, so the patient is encouraged to quit or reduce smoking to decrease the incidence of hot flashes (Whiteman *et al.*, 2003). The data on alcohol use and hot flashes is mixed (Gold *et al.*, 2004). Observational studies of physical activity and VMS do not show a relationship with hot flashes (Li *et al.*, 2003; Li *et al.*, 1999; Sternfeld *et al.*, 1999).

Menopause hormone therapy (MHT), however, is very effective for treatment of hot flashes and night sweats and by secondary gain can be useful for treating sleep disturbances that result from waking related to hot flashes. Prior to 2002 when the Women's Health Initiative (WHI) was halted because of increased risk for women taking estrogen and progestin therapy for breast cancer (anticipated) and for increased risk for heart disease, stroke, and other thromboembolic events (unanticipated), MHT was recommended for all postmenopausal women to protect against osteoporosis and heart disease as well as for treatment of symptoms including hot flashes, vaginal dryness, mood changes, sleep disturbances, and sexual dysfunction. Subsequently, the estrogen-only arm of the WHI was discontinued as well, because of the increased risk of stroke (RR 1.4 for women on estrogen alone). In addition, data from the WHI demonstrated increased risk of dementia and urinary incontinence with use of MHT (Hendrix *et al.*, 2005; Shumaker *et al.*, 2004).

Presently, the Federal Drug Administration (FDA) indicates use of MHT for moderate (with sweating) to severe (limits activities) hot flashes with a frequency of 80 to 100 per week. The FDA recommends use of the smallest dose MHT to alleviate symptoms for the shortest amount of time possible. Prior to 2002, the oral dose of conjugated equine estrogen (CEE) recommended to protect from heart disease and osteoporosis and to alleviate all symptoms was 0.625 mg daily. There was aggressive marketing to women's health professionals that this or an equivalent dose in another preparation was the standard of care to control symptoms. The side effects usually encountered at this dose included breast tenderness and breakthrough bleeding. In the recent past there has been development of lower dose products that are half to one-quarter the CEE 0.625 mg dose in patch and oral forms and to use of local therapy for vaginal symptoms has been recommended.

MHT is an excellent treatment for distressing hot flashes. The side effect profile has been extensively studied, in fact more so than nearly all other drugs on the market. If a woman chooses to use MHT, a starting dose of CEE 0.3 mg or a 25 mcg transdermal patch is recommended. If vaginal symptoms are problematic, then MHT options include vaginal estrogen creams (Premarin™ (CEE), Estrace™ (estradiol), rings (Estring™, Femring™), or tablets (Vagifem™). New products are coming on the market all the time. Menostar is a 14 mcg transdermal patch that came on the market in 2004. It has FDA approval for the treatment of osteopenia (prevention of osteoporosis). However, it can be used for treatment of hot flashes when choosing a low dose estrogen product.

One caveat to keep in mind is that for women with an intact uterus (one who has not had a hysterectomy), a prescription for a progestin must accompany the use of estrogen products. This protects the lining of the uterus from unopposed estrogen effect (over stimulation), which can lead to a proliferative endometrium, hyperplasia, or endometrial cancer.

Stopping use of MHT as soon as no longer necessary is a reasonable goal. It is not easy to identify when that time might be. Stopping when symptoms are no longer problematic is important because individual risk to a woman using MHT accumulates with length of time used. The recommendation by the FDA to use MHT for the shortest time possible, however, is not a clear or well-defined concept. Grady recommends stopping MHT every 6 to 12 months to establish whether the MHT is still needed (Grady, 2005). The woman can expect a return of hot flashes for a period of time when stopping the hormones, and these usually peak at about four weeks. Seventy percent of women reported mild hot flashes upon stopping MHT, with 30% reporting troubling flashes (Ettinger, Grady, Tosteson, Pressman, and Macer, 2003). Of the latter group, 25% resumed treatment in six months. It is recommended to taper the MHT by day in order to avoid writing multiple prescriptions for varying doses. This means use of MHT every other day for two weeks, to three times a week, to twice weekly, and so on, taking longer than a month to finish with the goal of reducing discomfort from hot flashes.

Complementary and alternative therapies (CAM) are used by up to 50% of the population of the United States (Eisenberg *et al.*, 1998), and menopause-aged women are targeted daily on television with products that are purported to help with all symptoms of menopause. Most CAM trials suffer serious design flaws, including most do not have a placebo arm, they are short duration, and they have few subjects. In addition, trials of dietary supplements often fail to adequately describe which part of the plant is used, how the herb is prepared, what solvents are used, and so on.

Black cohosh is probably the most extensively studied herb for hot flashes but findings vary across studies. The mechanism of action of this herb was long thought to be that of a weak phytoestrogen (plant estrogen) but research now suggests a nonhormonal effect (Low Dog, 2005). Black cohosh is available as a standardized extract in the commercial preparation Remifemin™. Evening primrose oil has been studied, and though it is a rich source of gamma linolenic and linolenic acid, its efficacy for hot flashes is unproven. Ginseng is used in Asian cultures as a tonic and has no usefulness for hot flashes (Low Dog, 2005). Kava has been shown to be an effective anxiolytic in Cochrane reviews but concerns for hepatoxity need to be addressed (Pittler, 2000; Pittler *et al.*, 2002).

Although there has been a great deal of interest in the use of soy for menopause symptoms, soy products are difficult to characterize because it makes a difference whether food products or extracts are being considered. Soy in food generally is considered safe when used as part of a balanced diet. Whether or not dietary soy conveys health benefits is unproven. Studies show conflicting results with regard to hot flashes (Faure *et al.*, 2002; Han *et al.*, 2002; Nikander *et al.*, 2003; Penotti *et al.*, 2003). Supplements of soy have unknown effects because most studies do not show percent of isoflavones (plant estrogen) included in the extract. Estroven is one herbal supplement that contains 55 mg of isoflavones from non-GMO soya, Japanese arrowroot, calcium, and vitamins E, B6, and folic acid.

Most clinical trials of red clover, Trifoloum pretense L. (Promensil™), have failed to show any benefit over placebo (Baber *et al.*, 1999; Knight *et al.*, 1999; Tice *et al.*, 2003). However, in a randomized, placebo control study of 30 women for 12 weeks, Promensil™ use resulted in a significant reduction in hot flashes from baseline (van de Weijer and R., 2002).

Other modalities have been investigated for relief of hot flashes in menopausal women, including acupuncture, magnetic therapy, reflexology, and homeopathy. An electronic search of relevant studies was reported at the NIH State-of-the-Science Consensus Conference on Management of Menopause-Related Symptoms found 11 intervention studies, including seven on acupuncture, one on magnets, one on reflexology and two on homeopathy (Carpenter and Neal, 2005). All the studies examined suffered from design flaws—most were uncontrolled, with small sample sizes making conclusions far from firm. And most have inconsistent results regarding improvement in hot flashes.

In the past, centrally active agents Bellergal™ and Clonidine™ have been used to control hot flashes. Bellergal™ was popular two decades ago and has limited efficacy for decreasing hot flash frequency or severity (Bergmans, Merkus, Corbey, Schellekens, and Ubachs, 1987; Lebherz and French, 1969). Clonidine™, an older hypertensive preparation, has been demonstrated to reduce hot flashes with only moderate efficacy, but toxicity limits its use (Loprinzi, 2005). In the 1990s selective serotonin reuptake inhibitors (SSRIs) were found to reduce hot flashes in women using them for other reasons. It appeared that the SSRIs were not only efficacious but also well tolerated (Stearns, 2000; Loprinzi, 1998). Subsequent placebo-controlled double blind studies of venlafaxine (Effexor™) and paroxetine (Paxil™) have shown reduction in hot flashes (Loprinzi 2000; Stearns, 2003). Pilot studies are ongoing for other, newer antidepressants, which also look promising. Gabapentin (Neurontin™) has been anecdotally noted to decrease hot flashes, and ongoing trials promise new interest in its use. Gabapentin is relatively well tolerated by most women and may be one of the most efficacious and clinically appropriate agents for use along with the newer antidepressants (Loprinzi, 2005).

VAGINAL SYMPTOMS

During the menopause transition, women may experience vaginal symptoms including vaginal dryness, itching, and dyspareunia (painful intercourse). These vaginal changes result from changes in the serum estradiol levels that drop precipitously just before the last period. The end organ response to this drop in estradiol results in less estrogen effect on the mucus membranes that line the vaginal wall. During the reproductive years the vaginal wall is composed of a highly estrogenized superficial layer beneath which is the intermediate layer, and beneath that is the basal layer. This bottom-most layer is exposed when estradiol levels drop at menopause. When this happens the vagina loses elasticity and moisture, blood vessels are closer to the surface, and with time atrophy occurs. It is hypothesized that for some women who maintain an active sex life, blood flow to the pelvis keeps the vaginal supple and can prevent symptoms. Many women, though, experience itching and pain, and are unable to have comfortable intercourse, especially in the postmenopause period.

Vaginal complaints can be dealt with effectively by use of local MHT in the forms of estrogen rings (Estring™, Femring™), creams (Premarin™ cream, Estrace™ cream), and tablets (Vagifem™), which have local vaginal effects and in theory have reduced systemic effects compared to oral or transdermal estrogens. Package inserts recommend that progestins be used to offset the estrogen effect on the uterine lining. A postmenopausal woman who uses the local estrogen for a short time may not develop a proliferative or hyperplasia of the uterine lining but if any postmenopause bleeding does occur with use of local estrogen products, investigation of the cause of the bleeding must be conducted.

Alternately, for women who wish to avoid use of MHT for vaginal symptoms, water-based lubricants such as KY Jelly™, KY Warming Liquid™, Astroglide™, Liquid Silk™, or Eros™ (silicone based) can offer more comfortable vaginal penetration without side effects. Water-based lubricants are safe to use with all sex toys and condoms, whereas oil-based lubricants can react with rubber and cause it to disintegrate. Oil-based products such as Vaseline™ can irritate the mucous membranes of the vagina and is difficult to wash away. Many water-based lubricants contain glycerin, which may lead to vaginal infections or allergic reactions in some women. To avoid this, it is recommended that women wash thoroughly after using a lubricant, or find a water-based product that does not contain glycerin as an ingredient. Women should avoid lubricants with flavoring in them because they often contain sugar, which can also contribute to yeast infections.

Burning, itching, painful intercourse, and discomfort during everyday activities are the most common symptoms of vaginal dryness. Vaginal moisturizers are yet another alternative to help with vaginal symptoms. Replens™, a vaginal moisturizer, helps sustain vaginal moisture with a comfortable coating, and helps maintain vaginal epithelial integrity and vaginal elasticity.

MOOD DISTURBANCES

The majority of studies from large literature searches indicate no associations between the menopause stage and mood symptoms, development of mental disorders, or general mental health (Haney, 2005). Two cohort studies report increased incidence of depressive symptoms among peri- and postmenopausal women (Freeman *et al.*, 2004; Maartens, Knottnerus, and Pop, 2002). Data from studies of prevalence rates for mood symptoms have wide ranges and are similar across the menopausal stages (Haney, 2005).

Periods of reproductive hormonal change (premenstrual, postpartum, and perimenopause) may constitute times of particular risk to women with regard to depressive illness. Since perimenopause is a time of great change for women in many arenas including important hormone changes, some women will be at risk for affective disorders during this period. Treatment of mood disturbances that accompany the transition through the menopausal stages is important given the morbidity associated with untreated affective disorders. The efficacy of antidepressants to treat depression is widely supported. SSRIs and dual-action antidepressants, serotonin and norepinephrine reuptake inhibitors (SNRIs) (venlafazine—Effexor™, and duloxetine—Cymbalta™), are generally very effective, yet side effects, which include weight gain, insomnia, and sexual dysfunction, may be problematic for many women and can contribute to nonadherence.

Sexual Dysfunction

Unlike hot flashes and night sweats, which mirror the menopausal stage that a woman undergoes sexual changes in both women and men decline on a steady slope with age. For women, a further incremental decline is related to falling estradiol levels probably more so than declines in testosterone levels (Dennerstein, Randolph, Taffe, Dudley, and Burger, 2002). The factors that affect a woman's sexuality include first and foremost aging, the length of her sexual relationship with her partner, her own or her partner's health problems, loss of a partner, and psychosocial stressors (Dennerstein, 2005). Moreover, sexual function or dysfunction in women is multidimensional. The problem may rest with desire, arousal, and inorgasmia. It is also nonlinear—a woman can have responsive desire vs. innate desire (arousal before desire). Her sexual functioning at menopause or at any time along the lifespan is highly related to her previous behavior or level of interest, her feelings toward her partner, and her partner's status. Not surprisingly, a new partner puts a new set of variables in play for a woman's sexual interests and behavior. Mood disorders also need to be taken into account with regard to women's sexuality because they can affect interest in sex and responsivity. And finally, not all women are distressed with having a low level of sexual function.

That being said, problems with vaginal dryness or atrophy can be remedied with local vaginal use of MHT, vaginal lubricants, or moisturizers as discussed in the previous section. Some women respond to estrogen or progestin therapy, which may improve receptivity to sexual play.

Testosterone has been used with estrogen to improve sexual function. The decline in circulating testosterone levels is gradual with levels generally lower than in younger women (Judd, Judd, Lucas, and Yen, 1974). However, in women who have undergone either a surgical or medical castration, there is a 50% decline in testosterone levels (Judd *et al.*, 1974). Nearly all data on use of testosterone in women for sexual dysfunction has been done in combination therapy with estrogen. Data suggest that women receiving either estrogen alone or an estrogen–testosterone combination had significant improvements over baseline in well-being, sexual function, and energy levels (Sherwin, 1998, 2002; Simon *et al.*, 1999). In the United States, only the combination of methyltestosterone in combination with esterified estrogen (Estratest™) is available as an FDA-approved treatment modality. Methyltestosterone (Halotestin™) is available alone as a 2 mg dose, which may be used as an adjunct to estrogen therapy if estrogen therapy alone does not improve sexual function, but this is off-label use. Currently, testosterone patches and gels are being tested in phase III trials. For clinicians who are using testosterone preparations, laboratory monitoring of bioavailable or free testosterone levels, serum hormone binding globulin (SHBG) and lipids should be considered. Blood pressure should be monitored as well. There is no long-term safety data for testosterone therapy, so long-term use cannot be recommended (Liu, 2005).

Conclusion

Most women in Western societies report some symptoms of menopause. Women at the same time employ a range of symptom management options including self-care strategies with over-the-counter products, complementary therapies, lifestyle modifications, as well as prescription hormones. So the perimenopause period offers an opportunity to women and health providers to consider strategies for self-care, disease screening, and promotion of healthy aging. Yet menopause needs a conceptual framework that bridges genetic, molecular, and physiologic factors hypothesized to cause symptoms and the social and cultural context in which women experience them. The Women's Health Initiative has given untold insights into the risks of menopause hormone therapy, despite its shortcomings (mean age 67); and the prospective longitudinal investigation of 3302 multiethnic women in the S.W.A.N study to track changes in women as they age and experience menopause will give insight into a whole array of questions. The S.W.A.N study has already pointed out the fact that vasomotor symptoms apart from other symptoms are the only symptoms that occur in synchrony with the perimenopause transition. There is a great deal of work yet to do regarding menopause and the symptoms that sometimes accompany the transition. In the end the best information will come from perimenopause-age women from all walks of life.

Recommended Resources

North American Menopause Society: http://www.menopause.org/

Menopause: http://www.menopausejournal.com

Alternatives in menopause by herbalist Susan Weed: http://www.menopause-metamorphosis.com

Mayo Clinic Menopause page: http://www.mayoclinic.com

Planned Parenthood Menopause page: http://www.plannedparenthood.org/pp2/portal/files/portal/medicalinfo/femalesexualhealth/pub-menopause.xml

WebMD Menopause page: http://my.webmd.com/medical_information/condition_centers/menopause/default.htm

REFERENCES

Avis, N.E., Kaufert, P.A., Lock, M., McKinlay, S.M., and Vass, K. (1993). The evolution of menopausal symptoms. *Baillieres Clinical Endocrinology and Metabolism, 7(1)*, 17–32.

Avis, N.E., Stellato, R., Crawford, S., Bromberger, J., Ganz, P., Cain, V. *et al.* (2001). Is there a menopausal syndrome?

Menopausal status and symptoms across racial/ethnic groups. *Social Science and Medicine, 52(3)*, 345–356.

Baber, R.J., Templeman, C., Morton, T., Kelly, G.E., and West, L. (1999). Randomized placebo-controlled trial of an isoflavone supplement and menopausal symptoms in women. *Climacteric, 2(2)*, 85–92.

Bergmans, M.G., Merkus, J.M., Corbey, R.S., Schellekens, L.A., and Ubachs, J.M. (1987). Effect of Bellergal Retard on climacteric complaints: A double-blind, placebo-controlled study. *Maturitas, 9(3)*, 227–234.

Carpenter, J.S. and Neal, J.G. (2005). *Other complementary and alternative medicine modalities: Acupuncture, magnets, reflexology and homeopathy*. Paper presented at the NIH State-of-the-Science Conference on Management of Menopause-Related Symptoms, March 21–25, 2005, Bethesda, MD.

Dennerstein, L. (2005). *Sexuality*. Paper presented at the NIH State-of-the-Science Conference on Management of Menopause-Related Symptoms, March 21–25, 2005, Bethesda, MD.

Dennerstein, L., Dudley, E.C., and Guthrie, J.R. (2003). Predictors of declining self-rated health during the transition to menopause. *Journal of Psychosomatic Research, 54(2)*, 147–153.

Dennerstein, L., Randolph, J., Taffe, J., Dudley, E., and Burger, H. (2002). Hormones, mood, sexuality, and the menopausal transition. *Fertility and Sterility, 77(Suppl 4)*, S42–48.

Eisenberg, D.M., Davis, R.B., and Ettner, S.L. (1998). Trends in alternative medicine use in the US, 1990–1997: Results of a follow-up survey. *JAMA, 280(18)*, 1569–1575.

Ettinger, B., Grady, D., Tosteson, A.N., Pressman, A., and Macer, J.L. (2003). Effect of the Women's Health Initiative on women's decisions to discontinue postmenopausal hormone therapy. *Obstetrics and Gynecology, 102(6)*, 1225–1232.

Faure, E.D., Chantre, P., and Mares, P. (2002). Effects of a standardized soy extract on hot flushes: A multicenter, double-blind, randomized, placebo-controlled study. *Menopause, 9(5)*, 329–334.

Freedman, R.R. (2002). Core body temperature variation in symptomatic and asymptomatic postmenopausal women: Brief report. *Menopause, 9(6)*, 399–401.

Freeman, E.W., Sammel, M.D., Liu, L., Gracia, C.R., Nelson, D.B., and Hollander, L. (2004). Hormones and menopausal status as predictors of depression in women in transition to menopause. *Archives of General Psychiatry, 61(1)*, 62–70.

Glickman-Weiss, E.L., Nelson, A.G., Hearon, C.M., Prisby, R., and Caine, N. (1999). Thermal and metabolic responses of women with high fat versus low fat body composition during exposure to 5 and 27 degrees C for 120 min. *Aviation Space and Environmental Medicine, 70(3, Pt 1)*, 284–288.

Gold, E.B., Block, G., Crawford, S., Lachance, L., Fitzgerald, G., Miracle, H., *et al.* (2004). Lifestyle and demographic factors in relation to vasomotor symptoms: Baseline results from the Study of Women's Health Across the Nation. *American Journal of Epidemiology, 159(12)*, 1189–1199.

Grady, D. (2005). *Issues related to discontinuation of menopausal hormone therapy*. Paper presented at the NIH State-of-the-Science Conference on Management of Menopause-Related Symptoms.

Han, K.K., Soares, J.M.J., Haidar, M.A., de Lima, G.R., and Baracat, E.C. (2002). Benefits of soy isoflavone therapeutic regimen on menopausal symptoms. *Obstetrics and Gynecology, 99(3)*, 389–394.

Haney, E. (2005). *Symptoms during the menopausal transition: Evidence from cohort studies*. Paper presented at the NIH State-of-the-Science Conference on Management of Menopause-Related Symptoms, March 21–23, 2005, Bethesda, MD.

Hendrix, S.L., Cochrane, B.B., Nygaard, I.E., Handa, V.L., Barnabei, V.M., Iglesia, C., *et al.* (2005). Effects of estrogen with and without progestin on urinary incontinence. *JAMA, 293(8)*, 935–948.

Judd, H.L., Judd, G.E., Lucas, W.E., and Yen, S. (1974). Endocrine function of the postmenopausal ovary: Concentration of androgens and estrogens in ovarian and peripheral vein blood. *Journal of Clinical Endocrinology and Metabolism, 39(6)*, 1020–1024.

Knight, D.C., Howes, J.B., and Eden, J.A. (1999). The effect of Promensil, an isoflavone extract, on menopausal symptoms. *Climacteric, 2(2)*, 79–84.

Lebherz, T.B. and French, L. (1969). Nonhormonal treatment of the menopausal syndrome. A double-blind evaluation of an autonomic system stabilizer. *Obstetrics and Gynecology, 33(6)*, 795–799.

Li, S. and Holm, K. (2003). Physical activity alone and in combination with hormone replacement therapy on vasomotor symptoms in postmenopausal women. *Western Journal of Nursing Research, 25(3)*, 289–293, 274–288.

Li, S., Holm, K., Gulanick, M., Lanuza, D., and Penckofer, S. (1999). The relationship between physical activity and perimenopause. *Health Care for Women International, 20(2)*, 163–178.

Liu, J.H. (2005). *Therapeutic effects of progestins, androgens, and tibolene for menopausal symptoms*. Paper presented at the NIH State-of-the-Science Conference on Management of Menopause-Related Symptoms, March 21–25, 2005, Bethesda, MD.

Loprinzi, C.L. (2005). *Centrally active, nonhormonal hot flash therapies*. Paper presented at the NIH State-of-the-Science Conference on Management of Menopause-Related Symptoms, Bethesda, MD.

Low Dog, T. (2005). *Menopause: Review of botanical dietary supplement research*. Paper presented at the NIH State-of-the-Science Conference on Management of Menopause-Related Symptoms, Bethesda, MD.

Maartens, L.W., Knottnerus, J.A., and Pop, V.J. (2002). Menopausal transition and increased depressive symptomatology: A community based prospective study. *Maturitas, 42(3)*, 195–200.

Matthews, K.A. and Bromberger, J.T. (2005). *Symptoms and health-related quality of life and the menopausal transition*. Paper presented at the NIH State-of-the-Science Conference on Management of Menopause-Related Symptoms, Bethesda, MD.

Nikander, E., Kilkkinen, A., Metsa-Heikkila, M., Adlercreutz, H., Pietinen, P., Tiitinen, A., *et al.* (2003). A randomized placebo-controlled crossover trial with phytoestrogens in treatment of menopause in breast cancer patients. *Obstetrics and Gynecology, 101(6)*, 1213–1220.

Penotti, M., Fabio, E., Modena, A.B., Rinaldi, M., Omodei, U., and Vigano, P. (2003). Effect of soy-derived isoflavones on hot flushes, endometrial thickness, and the pulsatility index of the uterine and cerebral arteries. *Fertility and Sterility, 79(5)*, 1112–1117.

Pittler, M.H. and Ernst, E. (2002). Kava extract for treating anxiety. [Update of Cochrane Database Syst Rev. 2002;(2):CD00383; PMID:12076477.] *Cochrane Database of Systematic Reviews, 1(CD003383)*.

Rossouw, J.E., Anderson, G.L., Prentice, R.L., LaCroix, A.Z., Kooperberg, C., Stefanick, M.L., *et al.* (2002). Writing Group for the Women's Health Initiative Investigators. Risks and benefits of estrogen plus progestin in healthy postmenopausal women: Principal results from the Women's Health Initiative randomized controlled trial. *JAMA, 288(3)*, 321–333.

Sherwin, B.B. (1998). Use of combined estrogen-androgen preparations in the postmenopause: Evidence from clinical studies. *International Journal of Fertility and Women's Medicine, 43(2)*, 98–103.

Sherwin, B.B. (2002). Randomized clinical trials of combined estrogen-androgen preparations: Effects on sexual functioning. *Fertility and Sterility, 77(Suppl 4)*, S49–S54.

Shumaker, S.A., C., L., Kuller, L., Rapp, S.R., Thal, L., Lane, D.S., *et al.* (2004). Women's Health Initiative Memory Study. Conjugated equine estrogens and incidence of probable dementia and mild cognitive impairment in postmenopausal women: Women's Health Initiative Memory Study. *JAMA, 291(24)*, 2947–2958.

Simon, J., Klaiber, E., Wiita, B., Bowen, A., and Yang, H.M. (1999). Differential effects of estrogen-androgen and estrogen-only therapy on vasomotor symptoms, gonadotropin secretion, and endogenous androgen bioavailability in postmenopausal women. *Menopause, 6(2)*, 138–146.

Sternfeld, B., Quesenberry, C.P.J., and Husson, G. (1999). Habitual physical activity and menopausal symptoms: A case-control study. *Journal of Women's Health, 8(1)*, 115–123.

Tice, J.A., Ettinger, B., Ensrud, K., Wallace, R., Blackwell, T., and Cummings, S.R. (2003). Phytoestrogen supplements for the treatment of hot flashes: The Isoflavone Clover Extract (ICE) Study: A randomized controlled trial. *JAMA, 290(2)*, 207–214.

van de Weijer, P.H. and Barentsen, R. (2002). Isoflavones from red clover (Promensil) significantly reduce menopausal hot flash symptoms compared with placebo. *Maturitas, 42(3)*, 187–193.

Van Voorhis, B.J. (2005). *Perimenopause: Urogenital and bleeding issues*. Paper presented at the NIH State-of-the-Science Conference on Management of Menopause-Related Symptoms, Bethesda, MD.

Whiteman, M.K., Staropoli, C.A., Langenberg, P.W., McCarter, R.J., Kjerulff, K.H., and Flaws, J.A. (2003). Smoking, body mass, and hot flashes in midlife women. *Obstetrics and Gynecology, 101(2)*, 264–272.

74

Psychological Aging: A Contextual View

Hans-Werner Wahl and Frieder R. Lang

In this chapter we review theories on the psychological dynamics of person–environment relations as people age. The chapter begins with an introduction to the issue of aging in context by contrasting perspectives of the biology of aging, the social sciences, and psychological gerontology. We also consider the historical background important for the understanding of a contextual view of aging in the evolution of gerontology, as well as introduce core theory elements of life-span developmental psychology such as the concept of developmental tasks. In the main body of the chapter, contextual aging will be approached by following three lines of thinking, as well as empirical research in aging research. First, person–environment dynamics are strongly driven in old age by interchange with the social environment, and respective theories addressing this fundamental dynamic of person–environment regulation in social aging will find intense discussion. Second, the area of environmental gerontology, sometimes also coined the ecology of aging, has offered much in terms of theories and empirical findings, when it comes to person–environment relations in old and very old age. As the argument goes, getting older coincides with a substantial increase of vulnerability for "press" in the physical-spatial environment. Third, we will provide our view on how an integrative view of the social and physical environment can be achieved. The chapter ends with a prospective outlook on how the obvious separated treatment of physical and social environment in aging theories can be overcome, thus allowing research to address new and innovative issues on aging.

Introduction

The assumption that aging occurs in context probably is an implicit or explicit core feature of all major models of aging, in biology, in the social sciences, as well as in psychological science. How such context is defined and what kind of impact is attributed to context strongly depends on the disciplinary perspective taken on aging. For example, Cowdry (1939), a pioneer in biogerontology, suggested distinguishing between endogenous and exogenous processes of aging. According to the endogenous view, aging is an involuntary process operating cumulatively over time and resulting in adverse modifications of cells. In the exogenous view, aging is seen as the consequence of infections, accidents, or environmental poisons. In most current theories in biogerontology, aging, or what is sometimes coined *senescence* in the biology of aging, is viewed primarily as an internal decline process related to the flow of chronological age and ending in the event of death (Cristofalo, Tresini, Francis, and Volker, 1999). Environmental conditions, however, shape the survival time of aging organisms, because it is generally acknowledged in models of longevity that genetic factors explain less than 30% of variability in survival time (Vaupel, Carey, and Christensen, 2003). The understanding of context in biological models of aging tends nevertheless to remain rather general, referring mostly to basic physical properties such as temperature, kind of nutrition, or environmental stress level, for instance, when young and old organisms are confronted with uncontrollable negative experiences in an age-comparative experimental design. It is worth mentioning that in the rapidly growing field of behavioral genetics in aging research, most recently a series of articles has underlined the still widely unmet need for a well-defined conception of the environment in order to better understand the operation of gene expression (or depression) in the flow of aging (Johnson and Crow, 2005).

At the other extreme, a social science concept of aging puts major emphasis on the operation of social, cultural, historical, and societal contexts, and how such influences are shaping aging processes. As was argued, different societal expectations and norms structure the sequence of the life course. Temporal inconsistencies between the individual and societal demands or norms may cause negative societal reactions and/or psychological stress on the individual level (Hagestad and Neugarten, 1985). Think of becoming pregnant at the age of 13 years, being unmarried still at the age of 50, or learning to drive a car at the age of 80 years. Additionally, historical context is changing dramatically over time, and this leads to changes of the flow of individual lives and person–society interrelations. A classic example is Elder's (1974) research on *Children of the Great Depression*, which serves as an impressive illustration of the long-term influences of early childhood and adolescent experiences with the socioeconomic and family consequences of the Great

Depression on the individuals' life course trajectories across adulthood and later life.

Psychological models of human aging have also put strong emphasis on the contextual component of life span and adult life development (Baltes, 1987; Carp, 1967; Dannefer, 1992; Kleemeier, 1959; Lawton, 1999; Rebok and Hoyer, 1977). Similarly to social science perspectives, the term *context* as used in psychological models of aging implies that the interaction between the aging individual and his or her environment is crucial for the understanding of the course and outcome of aging. According to psychological models of aging framed in a strong contextual view, a fundamental psychological challenge of aging individuals is to adjust or readjust their relation with the environment in which they live. Accordingly, a major research task of psychological gerontology is to describe and explain stability and change of person–environment dynamics as people age. As Dannefer (1992) has pointed out, the term *context* as also used in most psychological models of aging is predominantly composed of two large-scale entities, the social environment and the physical environment. The social environment refers to the totality of the diverse range of phenomena, events, and forces that exist outside the developing individual and are directly linked to other persons. This includes research issues such as social networks, social support, or the regulation of social relationships in later adulthood (Antonucci, 2001; Lang, 2001). The physical environment refers to the totality of the diverse range of phenomena, events, and forces that exist outside the developing individual and are directly linked to the material and spatial sphere. This covers research issues such as the impact of the physical-spatial home environment on aging, the role of neighborhoods and infrastructural characteristics, long-term institutions, as well as the challenge and outcome of residential decisions in later phases of the life span (Lawton, 1999; Wahl, 2001; Wahl and Gitlin, In press).

Moreover, emphasizing the context of aging in psychological aging research necessarily implies the need to consider natural settings, which are difficult to capture reliably and validly with experimental approaches in the laboratory. Furthermore, psychological models of aging strive to go beyond survival time as a major outcome of aging, as is often the case in biological models of aging. Instead, psychology focuses on outcomes such as subjective well-being, autonomy, or meaning of life, to name just a few, as products of the person–environment interactions across adulthood.

HISTORICAL CONSIDERATIONS

In historical perspective, aging has long been regarded as a purely biological and degenerative process. For example, Metchnikoff (1903), frequently cited as the creator of the term *gerontology*, made the argument in his Macrophage Theory that aging can be seen predominantly as an infectious disease, and, as a consequence, he believed that possible means to counteract such an infection (e.g., yogurt) would be helpful to delay aging. Given the strong biological and medical orientation of early gerontology, the explicit consideration of the socio-physical environment was an important step in its historical development toward a strong interdisciplinary research field. This paradigm shift was mainly driven by the growing role of a social and behavioral science perspective within gerontology and life course research, which began evolving since the late 1920s. For instance, Hall (1922) and Hollingsworth (1927) in the United States provided early contributions to aging research from a developmental psychologist's view, promoting the idea that improved understanding of life-span development is possible only when considering the social situations of aging individuals. Similarly, developmental psychologist Charlotte Bühler (1933) argued in her key work, *The Human Life Course as a Psychological Problem*, that the social world is a driving force not only of child and adolescent development, but also of development in adulthood and late life.

In the 1930s and 1940s, a social science perspective (sometimes also coined social gerontology) began to evolve in American gerontology, mainly nurtured by the creation of the Committee of Human Development at the University of Chicago and its key members, such as Bernice Neugarten and Robert Havighurst. Still more explicit, the interplay between the aging individual and his or her social world was treated for the first time in the *Handbook of Social Gerontology*, edited by Tibbitts in 1960, and the now classic gerontological monograph, *Growing Old: The Process of Disengagement*, by Cumming and Henry (1961). Around the same time period, the basic role of physical, spatial, and infrastructural environments in the aging process found increased attention, as manifested in pioneering handbook chapters such as Kleemeier's (1959) *Behavior and the Organization of the Bodily and External Environment* and Vivrett's (1960) *Housing and Community Settings for Older People*. Since then, addressing the role of context for the course and direction of aging processes has become an essential element of life course theory as well as life-span perspectives in social and behavioral gerontology (Baltes, 1987; Dannefer, 1992; Rebok and Hoyer, 1977). Reference to resources (or constraints) in the person and her or his environment, when the process and outcome of aging is the target of analysis, has even reached the status of a research paradigm in social and behavioral gerontology.

ESSENTIALS OF A LIFE-SPAN VIEW ON AGING

Life-span contextualism has advanced and elaborated the idea that contexts affect the course, direction, and outcomes of development (Baltes, Reese, and Lipsitt, 1980; Lerner and Kaufman, 1985). Throughout the life course, individuals are confronted with new and changing contexts that structure and sequence the course and direction of their development. However, not all changes in an individual's environment are developmentally meaningful and effective to the same extent. Life-span theory, in this vein, has contributed importantly to a more sophisticated understanding of how contexts influence and shape the individual's life-long development (Baltes, 1997). For example, life-span perspectives emphasized the interplay of contextual influences on developmental change. This has led to a differentiation of three systems of influence that coconstruct and coregulate life-span development:

1. History-graded influences on aging pertain to such influences that affect most individuals at a given time in history; for example, technological advancement, sociopolitical or economic changes, or natural disasters.
2. Nonnormative or idiosyncratic influences are a result of specific life-course paths and events that few individuals experience.
3. Age-graded systems of influence are a result of biological and cultural processes that are closely associated with chronological age, for example, the age-stratification in most modern societies (Riley, 1985) or age-dependent normative expectations (Heckhausen, 1999).

Similarly and consistent with these assumptions is Havighurst's (1948/1972) already mentioned notion of *developmental tasks* that result from three different sources: biology, society, and internal experience of the individual. Developmental tasks are helpful in determining the course and sequence of how and when individuals are expected to make specific developmental progress or at what time in life they should engage in or disengage from developmental goals (Freund, 2004; Heckhausen, 1999). With this, life-span perspectives on the person–environment dynamics helped overcoming dualistic perspectives on developmental contexts such as nature versus nurture (Lerner, 1998). Consequently, nature and nurture are seen as interwoven systems of influence, leading to a greater focus on the (shared and nonshared) environmental determinants of individual development. Perhaps even more importantly, in life-span contextualism the interplay of person and environment is conceived of as a dynamic involving the agentic individual as producer of his or her own developmental context (Baltes, 1987; Lerner and Busch-Rossnagel, 1981; Lang and Heckhausen, 2006). This implies that the context of aging is seen as one that evolves from the individual's ontogeny, and as a result of life course patterns of behavior. As individuals develop and acquire new strategies of how to exert influence in their environments, they continuously mold their physical and social environments. Thus, the developmental role of context is two-fold. On the one hand, individuals acquire and learn about developmental opportunities and frames of reference for age-specific norms and action (Heckhausen, 1999; Settersten, 1999). On the other hand, developmental contexts, both social and physical, represent outcomes of individuals' life-course decisions, planning, and management (Brandtstädter and Lerner, 1999; Lang, 2001; Wahl and Gitlin, In press). One central assumption in this line of reasoning is that the extent to which individuals successfully manage to adapt their physical and social environments in accordance with their need states and their psychological resources contributes importantly to an enhanced life quality, a prolonged life expectancy, and increased quality in the exertion of the life expectancy.

Person–environment dynamics are part and parcel of many, now classic, theoretical approaches and models of aging and life-span development, such as Erikson's theory of psychosocial development (1959) and Thomae's cognitive theory of aging (1970), to name only two (see Wahl and Kruse (2005) for a rather comprehensive overview on developmental stage models of human aging). All these theoretical approaches played an important role in advancing the idea that aging is embedded in social, historical, and cultural processes over the entire life course, which cannot be understood without fully acknowledging the dynamics of person–environment interaction. However, with the exception of the work of Lawton (Lawton and Nahemow, 1973; Lawton, 1989), most of these psychological models have predominantly focused on issues related to social environments rather than on the joint interplay of technical, physical, geographical, social, and biological environments that coregulate and determine the individual's process of aging. In the next section of the chapter, we discuss contextual models that have focused the social and societal environments separately from models that predominantly considered the physical-geographical environments, before presenting an integrative perspective on the socio-physical contexts of aging. It should be emphasized that although we concentrate our discussion of person–environment models of psychological aging on the micro- and meso-level of analysis, the broader socio-cultural or societal context and the interaction of social and physical elements therein, for example, cohort differences and the historical embeddedness of development and aging, provide a major background for the lower levels of contextual analysis (Baltes, Reese, and Lipsitt, 1980; Baltes, 1987; Elder, 1974; Hagestad and Dannefer, 2001). Consequently, we conceive of the developmental context as a multilevel and multidimensional structure of systems that are interwoven in their impact on individual behavior. Contextualistic thinking traditionally aims at identifying the structures and functions in the resulting matrix of developmental contexts that are most relevant for improved understanding of the individual's potentials and possibilities to adaptively master the many challenges of the aging experience. Although most theories have predominantly focused exclusively on either social or physical contexts, only few attempts exist to more entirely capture the physical and social nature of contextual influences on aging.

Psychological Aging in Context: Focusing the Social and the Physical Environment, and the Need for an Integrative Perspective

ROLE OF THE SOCIAL ENVIRONMENT AS PEOPLE AGE

Gerontological research on social environments is seeking to identify in what ways qualitative as well as quantitative features of an individual's social contacts and social network contribute to the individual's functioning and life quality (Lang and Carstensen, 1998; Pinquart and Sörenson, 2000; Rook, 2000). The theoretical conceptions about the role of social environments across adulthood are manifold and range from macro-theoretical approaches such as the age stratification theory (Riley, 1985) to micro-theoretical conceptions such as social exchange theory (Bengtson, Burgess, and Parrott, 1997) and the socio-emotional selectivity theory (Carstensen, Isaacowitz, and Charles, 1999).

Theories about the social environments in later life typically have viewed the individual as a recipient or adaptive user of social resources rather than as an active person that engages him- or herself in the construal or even the production of the social environment (Lang 2001; Steverink, Lindenberg, and Ormel, 1998). Recent life-span approaches on the development of social relationships in later life have more explicitly addressed processes that influence and gear the individual's motivations, attitudes, and behaviors toward other people throughout the life course. Most prominently among these are the social convoy model (Antonucci, Langfahl, and Akiyama, 2004), the socio-emotional selectivity theory (Carstensen *et al.*, 1999) and resource-oriented models of social behavior (Lang, 2004). Also, research on parent-child relationships has a long tradition in research on social relations as people age (Frankel and DeWit, 1989; Rosenmayr and Köckeis, 1965; Tartler, 1961). In the following, we first analyze some of the more classical theories of social aging and then elaborate on the implications of more recent theories on aging in the social domain.

Classic approaches to aging in social contexts

Interestingly, theoretical conceptions of the social environment in later adulthood often relied on metaphors derived from features of the physical world when referring to social experiences in later adulthood. This includes concepts such as social strata, social convoy, social network, support bank, closeness, distance, or life space as metaphoric descriptions of specific aspects of an individual's social world. Such metaphors serve to keep in mind that all social relationships occur in time as well as in space. Even the now "classic" theories of social aging such as disengagement theory and activity theory have, at least implicitly, acknowledged that aspects of the physical world are relevant for better understanding of social functioning in later life.

According to *disengagement theory* (Cumming and Henry, 1961), older individuals are seen as limiting their social life spaces in response to societal pressures and in order to prepare for the final phase of their lives. Cumming and Henry (1961) explicitly referred to Lewin's (1936) notion of a psychological life space when they introduced their concept of *social lifespace* as reflecting the individual's decreasing social opportunities during the aging process. *Activity theory* emphasized that being socially engaged in a variety of social roles both within and outside the family contributes to better functioning and better life quality (Havighurst, Neugarten, and Tobin, 1968; Lemon, Bengtson, and Peterson, 1972). Keeping a physical or geographical distance from members of younger generations is seen as protecting the older individual from stressful social demands and ensuring maximal freedom to develop age-adequate and adaptive patterns of social activity that contribute to increased well-being. Tartler (1961) introduced the idea of "feeling close at a physical distance" as one adaptive feature of parent-child relationships related to a better quality of the relationship. Empirical findings could support the notion of "intimacy at a distance" (Rosenmayr and Köckeis, 1965) as an adaptive regulatory mechanism of intergenerational relationships (Frankel and DeWit, 1989; Wagner, Schütze, and Lang, 1999). For example, in a study with 454 older parents, Frankel and DeWit (1989) found that greater geographical distance was a strong predictor of reduced contact with adult children but was significantly less strongly associated with the experience of important conversations with children. This indicates that the parent-child tie appears to remain emotionally meaningful irrespective of the physical distance. Emotional closeness in relationships may thus be an important compensation mechanism for overcoming seemingly insurmountable geographic distance.

In his *social integration theory*, Rosow (1974) argued that loss of social roles in later life requires that individuals develop new age-specific and age-adequate social roles. According to the theory, older people, who live in age-segregated environments, are more likely to identify themselves with their age group and their neighborhood. Consequently, they are more likely to engage in community activities when there is no interference with the interests of the younger generation. Empirical findings are not quite consistent, though. For example, older people living in age-segregated neighborhoods were more satisfied with their living circumstances than those who lived in nonsegregated quarters (Messer, 1967; Sherman, 1975). However, it was shown that the positive effect of age segregation is mostly related to differences in socio-economic wealth. Vaskovics (1990) reported that in regions with good infrastructure and a high-quality living standard, age concentration in the neighborhood was unrelated to living satisfaction. Despite the lack of empirical evidence, social integration theory has made a significant contribution in linking facets of the social and the physical environment in the aging process.

Recent theories of aging in social contexts

One of the most prominent theories of social aging and life-span development of social relationships in recent time is the *social convoy model* (Antonucci, 1990; Antonucci and Akiyama, 1995; Antonucci, Langfahl, and Akiyama, 2004). According to this model, an individual's social world is structured hierarchically. The metaphor of a social convoy is viewed as illustrating the life-long dynamic of social ties over the life course. As an individual grows old, his or her relationships and relationship partners change synchronously while he or she moves along the time continuum of his or her life course. At times, relationships drop out of the convoy, while new relationship partners join the social convoy, and some partners, who were lost at times, join the social convoy again. Furthermore, the social convoy is not only moving in time and space, there is also structural change within an individual's convoy. Sometimes individuals feel close to some relationship partners, while other network partners become less important, and vice versa. The composition and functions of social convoys change depending on an individual's age, gender, culture, physical or emotional needs, as well as depending on the specific relationship histories.

There is no doubt that the social convoy has become one of the most powerful metaphors in the field of aging by elegantly capturing many of the complex and dynamic characteristics of the life-long development of social relationships. More importantly, the social convoy model has broadened the perspective on social relationships as being both outcomes of, as well as contexts for, developmental processes (Antonucci *et al.*, 2004; Carstensen and Lang, 1997). The importance of this notion comes into mind when considering specific environments and behavior settings such as nursing homes (Baltes, 1996); quality of living standard or public places in urban cities provide or constrain opportunities for social contact in later life. For example, in a review of research on intergenerational contacts in urban regions, Lang (1998) suggested that there exist distinct age-graded zones for children, families, and older adults in the city that do not have much overlap due to the architecture, laying out, and installation of equipment in most modern urban cities. It is an open question whether social relationships follow the constraints of the physical environment, or whether physical environments reflect the evolution of an ontogeny of social needs and motivations over the centuries.

In her *socio-emotional selectivity theory*, Laura Carstensen and collaborators (Carstensen *et al.*, 1999; Carstensen and Lang, 1997; Lang and Carstensen, 2002) argued that over the course of life, individuals become increasingly aware that time is a precious resource that is limited. As a consequence, when people perceive time as limited, they are more eager to make the most efficient use of their time by focusing on aspects in their present lives that promise to entail meaningful experiences. According to the theory, such experience is expected to be associated with seeking emotional meaning rather than with seeking new information that will be useful in the more distant future. This central tenet of socio-emotional selectivity theory was empirically shown to operate across different domains of cognitive, emotional, and social aging. For example, in memory tasks, the proportion of recalled emotional materials from all recalled materials was largest among older adults as compared to young adults (Carstensen and Turk-Charles, 1994; Fung and Carstensen, 2003). Adults of different ages, who perceived their time as limited, reported priority of goals related to control of affect and generativity than adults, who perceived no time limitations in their future (Lang and Carstensen, 2002).

Finally, it is important to note that emotional meaning may not only be derived from those partners to whom one feels close but also from the familiarity and security of everyday routines and living circumstances. In this case, even peripheral social contacts with people known for many years or even decades may provide meaningful experience to the older individual (Fingerman, 2004). Going further, it can be asked whether the adaptive processes leading to changes in social motivation are not only depending on perceived time limitations but also on the individual's personal and environmental resources in general. There are great individual differences with respect to what types of social situations provide meaning to an individual. Consequently, some individuals may prefer to focus on indoor activities, whereas others prefer social outdoor activities, again a hint for considering social and physical environmental phenomena in a simultaneous manner.

ROLE OF THE PHYSICAL ENVIRONMENT AS PEOPLE AGE

Environmental gerontology or, as it may be labeled, the ecology of aging, typically is identified with the description, explanation, and modification/optimization of the relation between the elderly person and his or her physical environment (Wahl, 2001; Wahl and Gitlin, In press). Furthermore, by drawing from German psychologist Kurt Lewin's (1936) basic insight that behavior has to be seen as a function of the person and his or her environment, American psychologist M. Powell Lawton (1982) has suggested the *ecological equation* as most essential for the ecology of aging. That is, the consideration of the impact of the interaction between the aging person (P) and the environment (E) on a variety of behavioral outcomes such as well-being and functioning has been added to the isolated consideration of the person and his or her environment (Behavior = P, E, P X E). Environmental gerontology primarily considers the relevance of the full range of physical components of the environment for aging processes, but also acknowledged is the strong, integrated role of the social dimension. For example, the home environment is not only a physical structure, but also a place punctuated by pronounced intimacy with one's partner, social interactions, and the symbolization of attachment, normalcy, and loss (Rubinstein and Parmelee, 1992).

The mission of environmental gerontology within gerontology can be seen in its contributions to the understanding of prototypical environment-related tasks of the aging individual, such as preserving independence in the face of physical and mental impairments by use of environmental resources within and outside the home environment ("aging in place"), initiating processes of relocation if desired or necessary, and adapting to new living environment settings (e.g., a nursing home) after relocation.

Classic theories of aging in physical contexts

The most widely acknowledged theory to be considered is the *competence-press model* introduced by Lawton and Nahemow (1973). Lawton and Nahemow (1973) have argued that variation in adaptational outcomes in old age are, in comparison to younger age groups (with the notable exception of early childhood), more strongly influenced by environmental conditions (Environmental Docility Hypothesis). Moreover, older adults with lower competence are expected to be particularly prone to what has been coined by Lawton and Nahemow as *environmental press*. In other words, the older an aging organism, the more environmental characteristics are able to contribute to the explanation of adaptational outcomes such as everyday competence or well-being. The competence-press model provides a broad, overarching framework, allowing different types and levels of competence such as sensory loss, physical mobility loss, or cognitive decline and environmental factors including housing standards, neighborhood conditions, or public transport to be considered. Perhaps the most important element of the competence press model is its fundamental assumption that for each aging person there is an optimal combination of (still) available competence and environmental circumstances leading to the relative highest possible behavioral and emotional functioning for that person. The model also suggests that it is at the lower levels of competence that older people become the most susceptible to their environment, such that low competence in conjunction with high "environmental press" is most detrimental for the individual's autonomy and well-being. A related argument in this concept is that as competence declines in later life, the zone of adaptation narrows such that environmental choices that can promote well-being and autonomy become increasingly constrained.

The competence-environmental press framework as suggested by Lawton and Nahemow (1973) continues to provide the basic mechanism of person–environment relations as people age and has been supported by a considerable body of empirical research. For example, research on the impact of physical distances on social interaction patterns of elders in institutional settings shows that longer distances undermine social relations, thus highlighting the "environmental docility" as people age (Lawton and Simon, 1968). As was also found, based on a large study with elderly Germans from East and West Germany, substandard housing conditions were significantly associated with performance deficits in the so-called activities of daily living, and higher care needs among elders in East Germany could be partly explained by the stronger prevalence of substandard housing (Olbrich and Diegritz, 1995). As has also been found, there is a substantial link between housing quality and well-being (Evans, Kantrowitz, and Eshelman, 2002).

Another family of ecology of aging approaches relevant for the present work's discussion has centered on the concept of *person–environment fit*. Both Kahana's (1982) as well as Carp's (1987; Carp and Carp, 1984) work is closely affiliated with this concept. According to the person–environment–fit model, misfits between an older person's objective competencies or subjective needs and the potential of the environment to support or fulfill these objective or subjective personal characteristics is detrimental to using one's full developmental potential. Inversely, person–environment fit is seen as a necessary, albeit not sufficient, precondition for such development. For example, Wahl, Oswald, and Zimprich (1999) examined the role of fit between remaining competencies of visually impaired elders and the given physical home setting, and found that lower functional ability was significantly related with lower person–environment fit. In addition, mismatches between the needs of nursing home residents and the willingness or capacity of staff to fulfill these needs have been found to be related to their general well-being—the greater the mismatch, the lower was the observed well-being (Kahana, Liang, and Felton, 1980).

In addition to the empirical findings, the competence-press model as well as the person–environment–fit model have become major drivers in the practical world of designing and optimizing environments for older people. A scope of dimensions has been suggested as particularly important to qualify the "right" balance between competence and the environment such as safety, orientation, privacy, accessibility, stimulation, and control (Lawton, 2001).

Recent theories of aging in physical contexts

Besides classic ecology of aging approaches, additional and parallel research streams appearing since the 1980s in environmental gerontology subsumable under the headings of *meaning of home* deserve mentioning. Work in the tradition of the subjective aging in place concept emphasizes the simultaneous consideration of ties inside of the aging person to his or her physical and social environment. A typical approach in this line of research is the more qualitative work of Rowles (1983) and of Rubinstein (1989). Rowles' widely acknowledged approach focuses on the many facets of what he has coined *insideness*. According to Rowles, different types of insideness, all speaking to the transition of "spaces into places," can be found as the result of empirical analysis. Whereas social insideness arises from everyday social exchange over long periods of time, physical insideness is characterized by familiarities and routines within given settings such as the home environment. A third element of insideness has been labeled autobiographical insideness; that is, places are carrying a rich collection of memories and thus support the aging individual's sense of place identity. Empirical research also has shown that physical insideness is particularly important for aging individuals with chronically disabling conditions.

Rubinstein's (1989) conception of the meaning of home relies on the assumption that the active management of the environment in itself represents a major source of well-being as people age, especially for those who are frail or living alone. Rubinstein identifies three classes of psychosocial processes that give meaning to the home environment, namely, social-centered (ordering of the home environment based on a person's version of socio-cultural rules for domestic order), person-centered (expression of one's life course in features of the home), and body-centered (the ongoing relationship of the body to the environmental features that surround it) processes. Oswald and Wahl's (2005) analysis sheds further light on these processes by identifying how chronic conditions (in this case, ongoing mobility impairment) affect representations of the home environment. When subjects were asked what "being at home" means, mobility-impaired elders reported significantly more aspects of familiarity and accustomization compared to unimpaired elders.

Adding to this from another point of view, the concept of *place attachment* has been introduced and defined as reflecting feelings about a geographic location and emotional binding of a person to places (Rubinstein and Parmelee, 1992). As has been empirically found, place attachment seems to steadily grow across the life course, reaching its culminating point in very old age (Oswald and Wahl, 2003). This underlines the notion that forced relocation to a nursing home in very old age due to a chronically disabling condition is a critical life event and a profound challenge for maintaining well-being and a sense of identity.

The role of subjective person-place relations in aging has long been neglected in the practical field due to an overemphasis on objective characteristics such as environmental barriers or physical distances. However, it is now clearly acknowledged that objective and subjective dimensions of person-place relations are interacting in many ways. An example is a situation of objectively diagnosed need for improvement of housing quality according to standards of barrier-free environments, which might not fit well with a decade-long developed personal priority for continuity and stability of the home environment.

ON THE INTERTWINED ROLE OF THE SOCIAL AND PHYSICAL ENVIRONMENT AS PEOPLE AGE: AN INTEGRATIVE PERSPECTIVE

Interlinkages between the social and physical environment

It generally appears that the bodies of knowledge related to the social context and to the physical context of aging have grown widely apart and independent of each other (Wahl and Lang, 2004). And it is indeed tempting to accept and acknowledge the separateness of the social and physical surroundings and their different role in aging. On a surface level, we might view the social environment as one that is apparently alive and actively shaping the aging individual, whereas the physical environment appears to be dead and a no-response context. However, as has been shown already at different locations in the foregoing sections, this would entail a limited and basically wrong understanding of both of these environmental spheres.

The social and the physical worlds are equally dynamic, malleable, and responsive contexts of aging individuals. In fact, the structural similarities between the social and the physical environments as seen from an older person–environment interaction point of view are striking: On the one hand, both the social and the physical environment provide major resources or constraints for the individual's action potentials and quality of life. On the other hand, individuals appear to actively regulate the quality, structure, and function of their social and physical environments, thereby enhancing their social and physical resources. This includes, for example, the choices individuals make with respect to social partners, their living arrangements, and the physical adaptation of their home environments. Furthermore and most important for social and behavioral gerontology perspectives is that the social and physical environment contributes in a closely interwoven manner to what has been coined person–environment–fit processes (Carp, 1987; Kahana, 1982).

To support this line of thought, first it must be acknowledged that social relations are always framed within physical-spatial conditions (e.g., social contacts within institutions are shaped by physical-spatial dimensions; see Lawton and Simon (1968), Docility Hypothesis). For example, many social relationships such as neighborhood relations or casual ties in everyday life evolve from affordances and opportunities of specific physical environments (Fingerman, 2004; Lang, 1998). Inversely, physical environments are not lifeless entities; they symbolize, for example, most influential social experiences of one's biography. For example, objects in the home environment may serve as powerful reminders of a lost loved one (Oswald and Wahl, 2005; Rubinstein, 1989). Second, the social and the physical environments interact in complex and dynamic ways with respect to the proactive striving of aging individuals toward maintaining adaptation. For example, losing one's care-providing spouse in a remote area can produce severe person–environment misfit. The decision to relocate to an assisted living facility located in a town far away from the former place of living as a consequence of this critical event might lead to a barrier-free physical environment and new developmental opportunities in terms of social interchange with other residents. However, the compensation and optimization associated with this relocation decision may not come without losses such as interruptions of former important social and physical ties to neighbors and landscapes.

To conclude, by ignoring either the social or the physical components in contextual approaches to aging, a one-sided, if not wrong, understanding of the fundamental processes of aging may be the consequence. That is, knowing about the geographical, technical, and physical features together with their social-relational implications, as well as knowing about the social contexts within the opportunities and constraints of the physical world, are both needed to develop an understanding of how aging is associated with contextual processes.

The Social-Physical Place Over Time model as a driver of integration

We propose an integrative theoretical framework intended to merge the social with the physical, namely, the model of *Social-Physical Place Over Time* (SPOT; see Wahl and Lang (2004)). The SPOT concept combines three major elements of an aging person's everyday life world: First, a central element of SPOT, namely, Place, underscores the fact that every aging person's day-to-day behavior is embedded within a given physical and spatial surrounding. Place is meaningful for one specific aging individual in a variety of regards such as long-term living at this location, long-term developed place attachments, ties to neighborhoods, the specifics of the physical layout of this location, and its near and farther surroundings in the community (Oswald, and Wahl, 2005). With the concept of Place, we rely on the ideas and work of gerontology scholars such as Rowles and Watkins (2003) or Weisman, Chaudhury, and Diaz Moore (2000), but also on general assumptions of a more classic environmental psychology (Proshansky, Fabian, and Kaminoff, 1983). It was pointed out in this work that Places necessarily combine both a physical-spatial and a social-cultural dimension. Second, and as a consequence of our first point, we should always think of Places as socially constructed, socially filled-out, and socially shaped physical environments. The term *Social-Physical Place* explicitly emphasizes our focus on the multilevel and multidimensional character of living places of individuals. This is not to say that places are merely social and physical, but we believe that the interplay of social and physical contexts is critical for the understanding of contextual aging processes. Third, the SPOT concept implies a developmental perspective when highlighting that Places are dynamic and show both change and stability "Over Time," as people age. Our central assumption is that negotiating SPOT reveals quite different dynamics across the adult life span, which are highly relevant for the course and outcomes of aging. We will address this in the next section.

Going further, Lang (2004) proposed a goal-resource-congruence model of proactive regulation of social relationships across the life span. According to this model, resource changes determine changes in the individual's social motivation over the life course depending on age-specific opportunity structures. The model contends that an individual's proactive regulation of social relationships consists of two basic motivations: one aims at maximizing a sense of agency in social contexts, and one aims at a sense of belonging in one's social relationships. As people experience resource loss, as is typically the case in the course from middle adulthood to old and very old age, seeking to belong in one's social world (e.g., helping other people, experience positive social contact) is expected to obtain greater priority, whereas individuals prioritize social agency goals such as autonomy or social acceptance when many resources are available. This conceptual model is consistent with recent empirical findings on age differences in social functioning (Lang, 2001; Lang and Carstensen, 2002; Lang, Rieckmann, and Baltes, 2002).

We assume that the goal-resource-congruence model also applies to the regulation of physical environments that entail both meanings of belonging (e.g. familiarity of home environment) and agency (e.g., autonomy, keeping routines, approaching residential decisions). For example, it is a well-known fact that frail older people are often reluctant to leave their community dwellings even when it is difficult for them to manage household chores mostly because their familiar home environment provides a strong sense of meaning and belonging for them. Losing personal resources in later life is a threatening event. Declines in physical health may lead to the heightened importance of experiencing continuity and belongingness in one's immediate environment. These considerations are also consistent with socio-emotional selectivity theory (Carstensen *et al.*, 1999), which posits that as individuals perceive their future time as being limited, they are more likely to seek stimulation of positive emotions (Mather and Carstensen, 2003) and positive memories (Carstensen and Turk-Charles, 1994).

As a consequence, we argue that two fundamental motivations are major forces in SPOT, maximizing *social-physical agency* and maximizing *social-physical belonging*. In addition, we argue that a similar adaptive dynamic, both regarding agency and belonging in the social and physical environmental spheres, is at work from middle adulthood through early "young" age to the oldest old, driven by the co-occurrence of decreasing competence (i.e., a lowered action potential of the individual) and the perception that future time becomes more and more limited. That is, the salience and impact of social-physical agency is expected to decrease, while the salience and impact of social-physical belonging is assumed to increase as people pass from middle adulthood to very old age (see Figure 74.1).

Changes in the dynamism of belonging and agency strivings are related to demands and challenges of age-specific contexts. Although we concur with Neugarten (1974) that much caution is needed in defining middle adulthood, we use the labels of middle adulthood (50–64 years), young old (65–79 years) and old old (above 80 years) in order to exemplify the role of age-related changes on the illustrated SPOT processes of agency or belongingness. The combined dynamism of agency and belonging lies at the heart of understanding of how social-physical contexts influence the construal of person–environment fit across adulthood. We contend that such a perspective provides a theoretically and empirically strong avenue, which substantively adds to viewing aging in context either exclusively in terms of social relations or in terms of physical environment. In particular, considering both the social and the physical environment as simultaneously contributing resources of the aging process adds to a more comprehensive and integrative understanding of the potential of these resources in aging in objective and subjective terms.

A telling example to illustrate these expected person–environment dynamics as people age is provided by relocation research, because relocation probably is the most radical process, in which the physical and frequently major elements of the social environment are changed at the same time. Having lived in a specific place implies an enormous amount of implicit knowledge related to everyday routines, to geographical distances inside and outside the home, to distinguishing neighbors from strangers, to seasonal changes of the sunlight, and to community services. Seeking to enhance one's sense of belongingness refers to the meaning and memories that individuals associate with their immediate home environment and that creates a sense of place identity. Not surprisingly, therefore, relocation in later adulthood may not be a question of just finding technically more easy-going, age-adequate, comfortable and supportive new living places, but rather it is a question of resolving the nearly impossible puzzle of keeping the meaning, while adjusting the environmental demands (Oswald, Schilling, Wahl, and Gäng, 2002). These challenges probably reveal a quite different dynamic at different stages of later life, most directly addressed in the relocation literature by the suggestion to distinguish between first, second, and third moves (Litwak and Longino, 1987). Though first moves are expected to predominantly appear in the early years after retirement, mainly reflecting a desire to improve social-physical agency (e.g., a more comfortable home, better living conditions, shorter walks, etc.), second moves are expected to appear later in the course of old age and are motivated by the supportive function of the environment in terms of reducing risks or ensuring against potential needs. Relocating to be closer to one's children is a typical example. In terms of SPOT, the dynamics behind these moves are echoed in a tentative balance between social-physical agency and belongingness needs. Finally, third moves predominantly target the supportive function of the environment and are best exemplified by moves to nursing homes or assisted living facilities quite late in life. In this situation, the need of social-physical belongingness, even though frequently

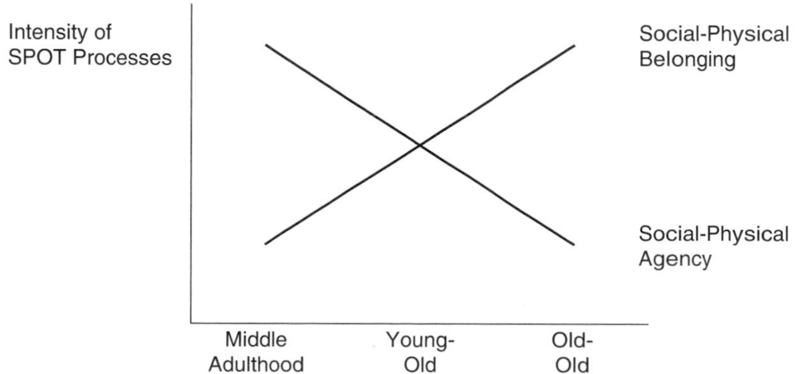

Figure 74.1 Expected trajectories of intensity of agency and belonging in the Social-Physical Places Over Time Model (SPOT).

major competence losses have occurred and future time has become quite limited, is particularly challenged, and finding a new person–environment–fit pattern in order to keep the meaning frequently is a very difficult enterprise.

Additional considerations in terms of person–environment fit

As we argued in detail elsewhere (Wahl and Lang, 2004), a focus on person–environment dynamics in aging necessarily leads to the question of whether there is a fit (or misfit) between the older person and his or her environment. Generally speaking, agency and belonging are predominantly representing adaptational processes on the level of person–environment dynamics, whereas person–environment fit is seen predominantly as the outcome of such processes. It deserves noting that such conceptions should be understood as an attempt to accentuate what is operating in the complex person–environment dynamic as people age rather than an always clear-cut differentiation. Going further, outcomes on the level of person–environment fit are probably drivers of more global outcomes on the person level such as autonomy, well-being, and identity.

Specifically, we propose three interrelated pairs of criteria for the evaluation of the person–environment fit in SPOT processes. First, the criteria of safety and familiarity represent a major dimension of the person–social environment transaction. For example, strong and close relations with children who are not living far from one's own dwelling may strengthen the safety feelings of an aging person, even if the physical environment is demanding. Another important issue of discussing safety and familiarity with implications for person–environment fit evaluations is what Parmelee and Lawton (1990) have called the security-autonomy dialectics. For example, social partners may enhance feelings of safety, but this might become detrimental in situations, when they have a tendency toward overprotection (Baltes and Wahl, 1992). Similarly, technology in the home environment (Wahl and Mollenkopf, 2003) can provide a major tool to feel more secure, but technology might also run the risk of provoking new dependencies and questioning the full use of still-remaining competencies of an aging individual.

Second, stimulation and activation as criteria of person–environment fit often have been disregarded due to a tendency in the literature to put emphasis predominantly on frail older adults. Physical-spatial arrangements can facilitate or hinder social contacts. Some environments are more prone to encourage or initiate social contact than others. The recreational functions of environments such as park areas or of spatial-related behaviors outside the home such as traveling, meanwhile, are widely recognized as major resources for aging individuals (Wahl, 2001). The interlinkages of stimulation to social contact and relations are obvious. Social relations serve major stimulative functions for aging adults such as securing ongoing personal interchange and making new interpersonal experiences. Furthermore, physical constellations can stipulate new social contacts; physical-spatial behaviors outside of the home frequently are associated with seeking or caring for social contacts.

Third, continuity and keeping the meaning are also closely affiliated with the physical as well as the social environment. On the one hand, settings such as the home environment and the residential area surrounding one's home become major "landscapes of memories" (Rowles, 1983; Sebba, 1991) and ecological extensions of the self (Rubinstein, 1989), and thus important material keepers of meaning. As recent research has revealed, older adults experience a whole scope of meanings associated with their home environment (Oswald and Wahl, In press). The intensity of this attachment to place becomes most obvious when the aging, and particularly the very old, person is challenged by a new residential decision. On the other hand, it is equally clear that continuity and meaning are also strongly bound to one's social ties, and it is an important insight of the more recent research on social relations that even very old individuals are proactively able to preserve this social relations quality.

In a final step of integration, we suggest considering, a developmental perspective on criteria of socio-physical person–environment fit in accordance with our assumptions on age-related trajectories of social-physical agency and belonging (see Figure 74.2).

We assume that person–environment fit in terms of stimulation and activation has its relative highest importance in middle adulthood, which is changing toward safety and familiarity as people approach extreme age. Or to put it the other way around: Misfits regarding stimulation and activation will unfold their strongest negative impact on outcomes such as global well-being in middle adulthood and early age, while in extreme age, misfits in the domains of safety and familiarity will provide a major threat to psychological health. The basic human tendency of seeking continuity and keeping the meaning is expected to operate in between the two other fit criteria. However, we also assume that continuity and keeping the meaning become more and more important, while navigating from middle adulthood and young-old age to the stadium of being old-old or oldest-old. This is because one of the major human strivings, namely, the search for meaning, is forced to operate in very high age within the highest constraints of all the human life span.

Conclusion

According to life-span perspectives, an individual's context determines the course, direction, and outcomes of development from birth to death. Moreover, life-span

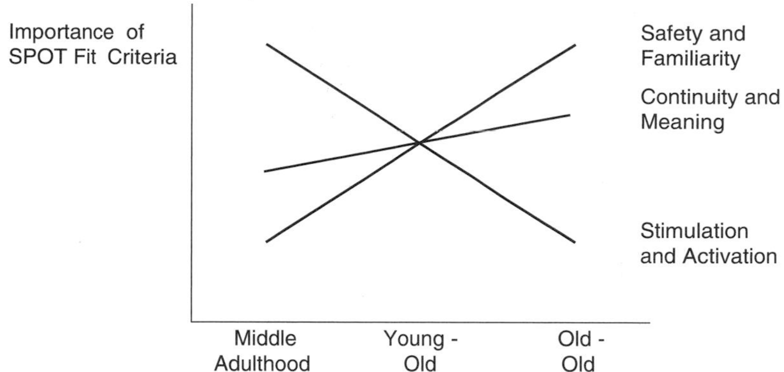

Figure 74.2 Expected trajectories of importance of person–environment–fit criteria in the Social-Physical Places Over Time Model (SPOT).

contextualism has contributed importantly to understanding of the specific role that contexts play in the process of aging (Baltes, Reese, and Lipsitt, 1980; Lerner and Kaufman, 1985). One assumption is that psychological aging is mainly driven throughout the life course by the ongoing need to negotiate between new and changing contexts in the light of new and changing person competencies as well as the ever-increasing nearness to the finality of life and death. Social as well as physical-spatial environmental spheres have been identified as major drivers of human development and aging. More recent theories on social relationships such as the social convoy model and socio-emotional selectivity theory have led to a rich set of new and robust and empirical insights on how social relationships contribute to psychological well-being (besides other outcomes) and to proactive shaping of social environments (Antonucci, 2001; Antonucci *et al.*, 2004; Lang, 2001; Lang and Carstensen, 2002; Lansford *et al.*, 2001). Although it appears that the emotional quality of relationships is more relevant to most relevant aging outcomes than structural characteristics of social relationships, the mechanisms underlying the links between relationship quality and outcomes such as well-being, life quality, and health are not yet fully understood. Similarly, the role of physical environments has been addressed by a rich collection of theories and findings, perhaps less controversial than models related to the social environment, but also not without major differences. For example, pointing to the importance of the observable physical environment versus assuming that the predominant issue is the perceived physical environment for human aging has remained an open question (Wahl and Gitlin, In press). Given the extensive treatment of the social as well as the physical environment as major contexts for human aging, the central argument of the chapter was that an intertwined consideration of both of these environmental spheres still is not spelled out well. This is a surprising observation given that links between the social and physical environment are strongly demanded since early psychological theorizing related to the process and outcome of human aging.

In order to address this missing link in the psychological aging literature, we have proposed the Social-Physical Places Over Time (SPOT) concept as a meta-theoretical perspective that addresses both the physical and social environment of aging individuals, as well as makes predictions in terms of the developmental dynamics inherent in person-social-physical-environment relations in the adult life span. There still is a clear need to address such links between the social and physical environment in forthcoming empirical research. For example, one hypothesis to be tested would be that the predicted dynamics of SPOT in terms of a tendency to switch from a sense of social-physical agency toward a sense of social-physical belongingness can actually be observed in aging persons (refer back to Figure 74.1). A related hypothesis would be that the age-related change in importance of different person–environment–fit criteria predicted in SPOT, namely, from stimulation and activation to safety and familiarity in conjunction with an increasing importance of continuity and meaning, is actually observable (refer back to Figure 74.2). Seen on a more general level, the assumed trajectories of agency and belonging on the one hand and person–environment–fit criteria on the other hand also mean that the life period of being young-old is the prime time in later life imposing the need for "changing tracks." Still, much of middle adulthood is possible; the limits of this action potential also appear more and more clearly at the horizon of what one's future aging will bring in terms of being old-old. Such historically new developmental dynamics in the adult phase of life putting much transformation pressure on those being young-old is the consequence of the rapid increase in life expectancy and the increase of distant life expectancy in particular (Wahl and Kruse, 2005). In this respect, the SPOT related developmental assumptions in terms of late-life trajectories in the human life course also question to some extent the widely held belief that being young-old is a time of activism and health, without much sorrow.

Additionally, an important prediction deviating from SPOT would be that older adults who focus on belonging, although there is a need to actively change their social-physical places, may show more rapid declines and may miss important occasions to maintain quality of life. This would be a new psychological variation of the "use it or lose it" case not considered so far in empirical research, which mostly concentrated on cognitive and physical functioning in this regard (Schaie and Willis, 2002). In contrast, frail older adults, who are no longer capable of exerting much socio-physical agency in their environments, but continue to do so, may be at high risk of suffering from the too-many demands, and eventually from depression in the longer run. This would be a new psychological variation of the "lose it after overusing it" case also not considered so far in empirical research.

Obviously, many questions related to person–environment dynamics in general, as well as the SPOT model in particular, have remained unanswered in this chapter. For instance, the role of gender deserves serious consideration, because aging men and women may reveal different dynamics in regulating socio-physical agency and belonging; it could well be that women are able to exert "new" agency in becoming old and very old (e.g., as "minister of the interior," caring for good relations beneath the generations in family systems; Baltes and Silverberg, 1994), whereas men may become more eager to "let things go" and "practice" variations of belonging instead of agency (e.g., by developing interest in gardening or a hobby exerted in the home area). In addition, cognitive competence impacts heavily on person–environment dynamics, and the question of what the right mix of agency and belonging might be for a person developing dementia still is an intriguing challenge for applied psychological and psychiatric research. In terms of another major transition of our societies, future person–environment dynamics in aging will be driven more strongly by technology such as intelligent houses, the Internet, and virtual realities at large. It remains to be seen how these new contextual forces will shape processes and outcomes of psychological aging in the decades to come.

Recommended Resources

Lang, F.R. and Fingerman, K.L. (Eds.). (2004). *Growing together: Personal relationships across the lifespan*. New York: Cambridge University Press.

A rather comprehensive treatment of recent developments in the array of social environments and aging.

Wahl, H.-W., Scheidt, R., and Windley, P. (Eds.). (2004). Aging in context: Socio-physical environments, *Annual Review of Gerontology and Geriatrics, 23*. New York: Springer.

A rather comprehensive treatment of recent developments in the array of physical environments and aging.

REFERENCES

Antonucci, T.C. (1990). Social support and social relationships. In R.H. Binstock and L.K. George (Eds.), *Handbook of aging and the social sciences, 3e*, pp. 205–226. San Diego: Academic Press.

Antonucci, T.C. (2001). Social Relations. An examination of social networks, social support, and sense of control. In J.E. Birren and K.W. Schaie (Eds.), *Handbook of the psychology of aging*, 5e, pp. 427–453. San Diego: Academic Press.

Antonucci, T.C. and Akiyama, H. (1995). Convoys of social relations: Family and friendships within a life span context. In R. Blieszner and V.H. Bedford (Eds.), *Handbook of aging and the family*, pp. 355–371. Westport, CT: Greenwood Press.

Antonucci, T.C., Langfahl, E.S., and Akiyama, H. (2003). Relationships as outcomes and contexts. In F.R. Lang and K.L. Fingerman (Eds.), *Growing together: Personal relationships across the lifespan*, pp. 24–44. New York: Cambridge University Press.

Baltes, M.M. (1996). *The many faces of dependency in old age*. Cambridge: Cambridge University Press.

Baltes, M.M. and Silverberg, S.B. (1994). The dynamics between dependency and autonomy: Illustrations across the life span. In D. Featherman, R.M. Lerner, and M. Perlmutter (Eds.), *Life-span development and behavior*, Vol. 12, pp. 41–90. Hillsdale, NJ: Erlbaum.

Baltes, M.M. and Wahl, H.-W. (1992). The dependency-support script in institutions: Generalization to community settings. *Psychology and Aging, 7*, 409–418.

Baltes, P.B. (1987). Theoretical propositions of life-span developmental psychology: On the dynamics between growth and decline. *Developmental Psychology, 23*, 611–626.

Baltes, P.B. (1997). On the incomplete architecture of human ontogeny: Selection, optimization, and compensation as foundation of developmental theory. *American Psychologist, 52*, 366–380.

Baltes, P.B., Reese, H.W., and Lipsitt, L.P. (1980). Life-span developmental psychology. *Annual Review of Psychology, 31*, 65–110.

Bengtson, V.L., Burgess, E.O., and Parrott, T.M. (1997). Theory, explanation, and a third generation of theoretical development in social gerontology. *Journals of Gerontology: Psychological Sciences, 52B*, S72–S88.

Brandtstädter, J. and Lerner, R.M. (Eds.). (1999). *Action and self-development: Theory and research through the life span*. Thousand Oaks, CA: Sage.

Bühler, C. (1933). *Der menschliche Lebenslauf als psychologisches Problem* [The human life course as a psychological problem]. Leipzig: Hirzel.

Canter, D.V. and Craik, K.H. (1981). Environmental psychology. *Journal of Environmental Psychology, 1*, 1–11.

Carp, F.M. (1967). The impact of environment on old people. *Gerontologist, 7*, 106–108.

Carp, F.M. (1987). Environment and aging. In D. Stokols and I. Altman (Eds.), *Handbook of environmental psychology*, Vol. 1, pp. 330–360. New York: Wiley.

Carp, F.M. and Carp, A. (1984). A complementary/congruence model of well-being or mental health for the community elderly. In I. Altman, M.P. Lawton, and J.F. Wohlwill (Eds.),

Human behavior and environment, Vol. 7. Elderly people and the environment, pp. 279–336. New York: Plenum Press.

Carstensen, L.L. and Lang, F. (1997). Social support in context and as context: Comments on social support and the maintenance of competence in old age. In S. Willis and K.W. Schaie (Eds.), *Societal mechanisms for maintaining competence in old age*, pp. 207–222. New York: Springer Publishing.

Carstensen, L.L., and Turk-Charles, S. (1994). The salience of emotion across the adult life course. *Psychology and Aging, 9*, 259–264.

Carstensen, L.L., Isaacowitz, D.M., and Charles, S.T. (1999). Taking time seriously: A theory of socioemotional selectivity. *American Psychologist, 54*, 165–181.

Cowdry, E. (Ed.). (1939). *Problems of aging. Biological and medical aspects.* Baltimore: Williams and Wilkins.

Cristofalo, V.J., Tresini, M., Francis, M.K., and Volker, C. (1999). Biological theories of senescence. In V.L. Bengtson and K.W. Schaie (Eds.), *Handbook of theories of aging*, pp. 98–112. New York: Springer Publishing.

Cumming, E. and Henry, W.E. (1961). *Growing old: The process of disengagement*. New York: Basic Books.

Dannefer, D. (1992). On the conceptualization of context in developmental discourse: Four meanings of context and their implications. In D.L. Featherman, R.M. Lerner, and M. Perlmutter (Eds.), *Life-span development and behaviour*, Vol. 11, pp. 83–110. Hillsdale: Erlbaum.

Elder, G.H. J. (1974). *Children of the great depression*. Chicago: University of Chicago Press.

Erikson, E. (1959). Identity and the life cycle. *Psychological Issues* (Monograph 1). New York: International University Press.

Evans, G.W., Kantrowitz, E., and Eshelman, P. (2002). Housing quality and psychological well-being among the elderly population. *Journal of Gerontology: Psychological Sciences, 57B*(4), P381–P384.

Fingerman, K.L. (2004). The consequential stranger: Peripheral social ties across the lifespan. In F.R. Lang and K.L. Fingerman (Eds.), *Growing together: Personal relationships across the lifespan*, pp. 183–209. New York: Cambridge University Press.

Frankel, B.G. and DeWit, D.J. (1989). Geographic distance and intergenerational contact: An empirical examination of the relationship. *Journal of Aging Studies, 3*, 139–162.

Freund, A.M. (2004). Entwicklungsaufgaben [Developmental tasks]. In A. Kruse and M. Martin (Hrsg.), *Enzyklopädie der Gerontologie*, pp. 304–313. Bern: Hans Huber.

Fung, H. and Carstensen, L.L. (2003). Sending memorable messages to the old: Age differences in preferences and memory for advertisements. *Journal of Personality and Social Psychology, 85*, 163–178.

Hagestad, G.O. and Dannefer, D. (2001). Concepts and theories of aging. Beyond microfication in social science approaches. In R.H. Binstock and L.K. George (Eds.), *Handbook of aging and the social sciences, 5e*, pp. 3–21. San Diego: Academic Press.

Hagestad, G.O. and Neugarten, B.L. (1985). Age and the life course. In R.H. Binstock and E. Shanas (Eds.), *Handbook of aging and the social sciences*, pp. 35–61. New York: Van Nostrand.

Hall, G.S. (1922). *Senescence. The last half of life*. New York: Appleton and Co.

Havighurst, R.J. (1972). *Developmental tasks and education, 3e*. New York: McKay (1e, 1948).

Havighurst, R.J., Neugarten, B., and Tobin, S. (1968). Disengagement and patterns of aging. In B. Neugarten (Ed.), *Middle age and aging*, pp. 161–172. Chicago: University of Chicago Press.

Heckhausen, J. (1999). *Developmental regulation in adulthood: Age-normative and sociostructural constraints as adaptive challenges*. New York: Cambridge University Press.

Hollingsworth, H.L. (1927). *Mental growth and decline: A survey of developmental psychology*. New York: Appleton.

Johnson, T.E. and Crow, J.F. (Eds.). (2005). Research on environmental effects in genetic studies of aging. *Journal of Gerontology, 60B, Special Issue I, March 2005.*

Kahana, E. (1982). A congruence model of person-environment interaction. In M.P. Lawton, P.G. Windley, and T.O. Byerts (Eds.), *Aging and the environment. Theoretical approaches*, pp. 97–121. New York: Springer.

Kahana, E., Liang, J., and Felton, B.J. (1980). Alternative models of person-environment fit: Predicting morale in three homes for the aged. *Journal of Gerontology, 35*(4), 584–595.

Kleemeier, R.W. (1959). Behavior and the organization of the bodily and external environment. In J.E. Birren (Ed.), *Handbook of aging and the individual*, pp. 400–451. Chicago: University of Chicago Press.

Lang, F.R. (1998). The young and the old in the city: Developing intergenerational relationships in urban environments. In D. Görlitz, H.J. Harloff, G. Mey, and J. Valsiner (Eds.), *Children, cities, and psychological theories: Developing relationships*, pp. 598–628. Berlin: DeGruyter.

Lang, F.R. (2001). Regulation of social relationships in later adulthood. *Journal of Gerontology: Psychological Sciences, 56B*, P321–P326.

Lang, F.R. (2003–2004). Social motivation across the lifespan: Developmental perspectives on the regulation of personal relationships and networks. In F.R. Lang and K. L. Fingerman (Eds.), *Growing together: Personal relationships across the lifespan*, pp. 341–367. New York: Cambridge University Press.

Lang, F.R. and Carstensen, L.L. (1998). Social relationships and adaptation in late life. In B. Edelstein (Ed.), *Comprehensive clinical psychology*, Vol. 7: Clinical geropsychology. Oxford: Elsevier.

Lang, F.R. and Carstensen, L.L. (2002). Time counts: Future time perspective, goals, and social relationships. *Psychology and Aging, 17*, 125–139.

Lang, F.R. and Heckhausen, J. (2006). Developmental changes of motivation and interpersonal capacities across adulthood: Managing the challenges and constraints of social contexts. In C. Hoare (Ed.), *The Oxford Handbook of Adult Development and Learning*, pp. 149–166. Oxford: Oxford University Press.

Lang, F.R., Rieckmann, N., and Baltes, M.M. (2002). Adapting to aging losses: Do resources facilitate strategies of selection, compensation, and optimization in everyday functioning? *Journal of Gerontology: Psychological Sciences, 57B*, P501–P509.

Lawton, M.P. (1982). Competence, environmental press, and the adaption of older people. In M.P. Lawton, P.G. Windley, and T.O. Byerts (Eds.), *Aging and the environment*, pp. 33–59. New York: Springer.

Lawton, M.P. (1989). Environmental proactivity in older people. In V.L. Bengtson and K.W. Schaie (Eds.), *The course of later life*, pp. 15–23. New York: Springer.

Lawton, M.P. (1999). Environmental taxonomy: Generalizations from research with older adults. In S.L. Friedman and T. D. Wachs (Eds.), *Measuring environment across the life-span*, pp. 91–124. Washington, DC: American Psychological Association.

Lawton, M.P. (2001). The physical environment of the person with Alzheimer's disease. *Aging and Mental Health, 5* (Suppl. 1), S56–S64.

Lawton, M.P. and Nahemow, L. (1973). Ecology and the aging process. In C. Eisdorfer and M.P. Lawton (Eds.), *The psychology of adult development and aging*, pp. 619–674. Washington, DC: American Psychological Association.

Lawton, M.P. and Simon, B.B. (1968). The ecology of social relationships in housing for the elderly. *The Gerontologist, 8*, 108–115.

Lemon, B.W., Bengtson, V.L., and Peterson, I.A. (1972). An exploration of the activity theory of aging: Activity types and life satisfaction among in-movers to a retirement community. *Journal of Gerontology, 27*, 511–523.

Lerner, R.M. (1998). Theories of human development: Contemporary perspectives. In R.M. Lerner (Ed.), *Handbook of child psychology, 5e, Vol. 1: Theoretical models of human development*, pp. 1 –24. New York: Wiley.

Lerner, R.M. and Busch-Rossnagel, N. (1981). Individuals as producers of their development: Conceptual and empirical bases. In R.M. Lerner and N.A. Busch-Rossnagel (Eds.), *Individuals as producers of their development: A life-span perspective*, pp. 1–36. New York: Academic Press.

Lerner, R.M. and Kauffman, M.B. (1985). The concept of development in contextualism. *Development Review, 5*, 309–333.

Lewin, K. (1936). *Principles of topological psychology*. New York: McGraw-Hill.

Litwak, E. and Longino, C.F. (1987). Migration patterns among the elderly: A developmental perspective. *The Gerontologist, 27*(3), 266–272.

Mather, M. and Carstensen, L.L. (2003). Aging and attentional biases for emotional faces. *Psychological Science, 14*(5), 409–415.

Messer, M. (1967). The possibility of an age concentrated environment becoming a normative system. *The Gerontologist, 7*, 247–251.

Metchnikoff, E. (1903). *The nature of man. Studies in optimistic philosophy*, 2e. New York: Masson and Cie.

Neugarten, B.L. (1974). Age groups in American society and the rise of the young-old. *Annals of the American Academy of Political and Societal Social Sciences, 9*, 197–198.

Olbrich, E., and Diegritz, U. (1995). Das Zusammenwirken von Person- und Umweltfaktoren im Alltag: Eine kritische Diskussion von Aktivitäten des täglichen Lebens und instrumentalen Aktivitäten des täglichen Lebens [Interaction of person and environmental factors in daily life]. *Zeitschrift für Gerontopsychologie und -psychiatrie, 8*, 199–212.

Oswald, F. and Wahl, H.-W. (2003). Place attachment across the life span. In J.R. Miller, R.M. Lerner, L.B. Schiamberg, and P.M. Anderson (Eds.), *Human ecology: An encyclopedia of children, families, communities, and environments*, Vol. 2: I–Z, pp. 568–572. Santa Barbara, CA: ABC-Clio Press.

Oswald, F. and Wahl, H.-W. (2005). Dimensions of the meaning of home in later life. In G.D. Rowles and H. Chaudbury (Eds.), *Coming home: International perspectives on place, time, and identity in old age*. pp. 21–46. New York: Springer.

Oswald, F., Schilling, O., Wahl, H.-W., and Gäng, K. (2002). Trouble in paradise? Reasons to relocate and objective environmental changes among well-off older adults. *Journal of Environmental Psychology, 22*(3), 273–288.

Parmelee, P.A. and Lawton, M.P. (1990). The design of special environment for the aged. In J.E. Birren and K.W. Schaie (Eds.), *Handbook of the psychology of aging, 3e*, pp. 465–489. New York: Academic Press.

Pinquart, M. and Sörensen, S. (2000). Influences of socio-economic status, social network, and competence on subjective well-being in later life: A meta-analysis. *Psychology and Aging, 15*, 187–224.

Proshansky, H.M., Fabian, A.K., and Kaminoff, R. (1983). Place-identity. *Journal of Environmental Psychology, 3*, 57–83.

Rebok, G.W. and Hoyer, W.J. (1977). The functional context of elderly behavior. *Gerontologist, 17*, 27–34.

Riley, M.W. (1985). Age strata in social systems. In R.H. Binstock and E. Shanas (Hrsg.), *Handbook of aging and the social sciences, 2e*, pp. 369–411. New York: Van Nostrand Reinhold.

Rook, K.S. (2000). The evolution of social relationships in later adulthood. In S.H. Qualls and N. Abeles (Eds.). *Psychology and the aging revolution: How we adapt to longer life*, pp. 173–191. Washington, DC: American Psychological Association.

Rosenmayr, L. and Köckeis, E. (1965). *Umwelt und Familie alter Menschen* (Environment and family in old age). Neuwied: Luchterhand.

Rosow, I. (1974). *Socialization to old age*. Berkeley, CA: University of California Press.

Rowles, G.D. (1983). Geographical dimensions of social support in rural Appalachia. In G.D. Rowles and R.J. Ohta (Eds.), *Aging and milieu. Environmental perspectives on growing old*, pp. 111–130. New York: Academic Press.

Rowles, G.D. and Watkins, J.F. (2003). History, habit, heart and hearth: On making spaces into places. In K.W. Schaie, H.-W. Wahl, H. Mollenkopf, and F. Oswald (Eds.), *Aging in the community: Living arrangements and mobility*, pp. 77–98. New York: Springer.

Rubinstein, R.L. (1989). The home environments of older people: A description of the psychosocial processes linking person to place. *Journal of Gerontology: Social Sciences, 44*(2), S45–53.

Rubinstein, R.L. and Parmelee, P.A. (1992). Attachment to place and the representation of the life course by the elderly. In I. Altman and S.M. Low (Eds.), *Place attachment*, pp. 139–163. New York: Plenum.

Schaie, K.W. and Willis, S. (2002). *Adult development and aging, 5e*. Upper Saddle River, NJ: Prentice Hall.

Sebba, R. (1991). The landscapes of childhood: The reflection of childhood's environment in adult memories and in children's attitudes. *Environment and Behavior, 23*, 395–422.

Settersten, R.A. (1999). *Lives in time and place*. Amityville, NY: Baywood Publ.

Sherman, S.R. (1975). Patterns of contacts for residents of age-segregated and age-integrated housing. *Journal of Gerontology, 30*, 103–107.

Steverink, N., Lindenberg, S., and Ormel, J. (1998). Towards understanding successful ageing: Patterned change in resources and goals. *Ageing and Society, 18*, 441–467.

Tartler, R. (1961). *Das Alter in der modernen Gesellschaft* (Aging in modern society). Stuttgart: Enke.

Thomae, H. (1970). Theory of aging and cognitive theory of personality. *Human Development, 12*, 1–16.

Tibbitts, C. (Ed.). (1960). *Handbook of social gerontology: Societal aspects of aging*. Chicago: University of Chicago Press.

Vaskovics, L.A. (1990). Soziale Folgen der Segregation alter Menscher in der Stadt [Social consequences of segregating older people in the city]. In L. Bertels and U. Herlyn (Eds.), *Lebenslauf und Raumerfahrungen*, pp. 35–58. Opladen, Germany: Leske + Budrich.

Vivrett, W.K. (1960). Housing and community settings for older people. In C. Tibbitts (Ed.), *Handbook of social gerontology. Societal aspects of aging*, pp. 549–623. Chicago: University of Chicago Press.

Wagner, M., Schütze, Y., and Lang, F.R. (1999). Social relationships in old age. In P.B. Baltes and K.U. Mayer (Eds.), *The Berlin Aging Study: Aging from 70 to 100*, pp. 282–301. New York: Cambridge University Press.

Wahl, H.-W. (2001). Environmental influences on aging and behavior. In J.E. Birren and K.W. Schaie (Eds.), *Handbook of the psychology of aging, 5e*, pp. 215–237. San Diego: Academic Press.

Wahl, H.-W. and Gitlin, L.N. (In press). Environmental gerontology. In J.E. Birren (Ed.), *Encyclopedia of gerontology, 2e*. Oxford: Elsevier.

Wahl, H.-W. and Kruse, A. (2005). Historical perspectives of middle age within the lifespan. In S.L. Willis and M. Martin (Eds.), *Middle adulthood: A lifespan perspective*, pp. 3–24. Thousand Oaks, CA: Sage Publications.

Wahl, H.-W. and Lang, F.R. (2004). Aging in context across the adult life: Integrating physical and social research perspectives. In H.-W. Wahl, R. Scheidt, and P.G. Windley (Eds.), *Aging in context: Socio-physical environments (Annual Review of Gerontology and Geriatrics, 2003)*, pp. 1–33. New York: Springer.

Wahl, H.-W. and Mollenkopf, H.-W. (2003). Impact of everyday technology in the home environment on older adults' quality of life. In K.W. Schaie and N. Charness (Eds.), *Impact of technology on successful aging*, pp. 215–241. New York: Springer.

Wahl, H.-W., Oswald, F., and Zimprich, D. (1999). Everyday competence in visually impaired older adults: A case for person–environment perspectives. *The Gerontologist, 39*, 140–149.

Weisman, G.D., Chaudhury, H., and Diaz Moore, K. (2000). Theory and practice of place: Toward an integrative model. In R.L. Rubinstein, M. Moss, and M. Kleban (Eds.), *The many dimensions of aging. Essays in honor of M. Powell Lawton*, pp. 3–21. New York: Springer.

75

Nutrients and Aging

Lawrence J. Whalley

This chapter provides a brief outline of some research methods now widely used in nutritional gerontology. First, the topic is placed in an historical perspective stressing major influences of the last century on public and professional thinking about nutritional health. These socio-cultural aspects of the discipline are shown to be relevant to contemporary research sampling from populations drawn from heterogeneous nutritional backgrounds. The five main types of study (ecological, cross-sectional, case-control, cohort, and experimental) in nutritional gerontology are specified. Issues in measurement are addressed in terms of the need to establish measures of reliability and validity of intake of specific nutrients, the purpose of energy adjustment, and the advantages of dietary pattern recognition over intake of single nutrients. The use of biomarkers is mentioned in the context of a lack of gold standards—including anthropometrics—of measurement of food consumption. Research methods in gene-nutrient interaction are considered in terms of nutrient regulation of gene transcription, nutrient damage to DNA, nutrient protection of DNA, and interactions between specific nutrients, energy regulation, and aging genes. The chapter concludes with a brief note about the role of nutrients as environmental cues of specific steps in developmental programming (including aging).

Introduction

The study of nutrients and aging is based on those same research methods that are the foundation of all nutritional science. These methods are well established in nutritional studies, and their application to aging research is certainly productive. However, many pitfalls are the lot of the unwary newcomer. Not least is that expert knowledge accrued from over a century of nutritional research does not yet inform popular views about the nutritional requirements of old people. This is of increasing importance as the food industry seeks to maximize profits through increased consumption of processed (added value) foods and use of food supplements often marketed for the older consumer. The industry has shown itself very capable of presenting views in favor of consumption of specific food products as scientific facts when the research evidence is often absent or even contradictory.

This chapter aims to provide a brief introduction to those new to nutritional research in the elderly. By way of introduction, it is necessary, however, to summarize briefly the recent history of nutritional research and to comment on research questions that seem most pressing on public perceptions of the value of nutritional studies in the elderly. The aim is to help those who are just starting out to navigate their route around obstacles, avoid time-consuming pointless detours (or even wandering!), and to complete their studies as efficiently and rewardingly as possible. Familiarity is assumed with one or more of the excellent general accounts of research methods. Furthermore, no attempt is made to set out what the best nutritional advice might be concerning consumption of particular foodstuffs in aging and age-related diseases. However, important social changes of the last 150 years may not be widely known. These are major influences on research in nutritional gerontology and are briefly summarized as follows.

Historical Perspective

In the developed world, nutritional research has its roots in recognition of the role of environmental factors in the origins of disease and the need for measures to improve the health of the public. Early emphasis was placed on the role of governments in public health matters, largely by removing the threats of foul air, poor hygiene in food preparation, and inadequate sanitation. Only much later, for reasons of food safety, did government interest turn to food. By 1900, a consensus had emerged that public health matters were the responsibility of government, whereas doctors were responsible for the health of the individual patient. Recruitment of poorly nourished conscripts into the army during the Great War (1914–1918) became a national concern when it was recognized that many young men were malnourished and that, without remedial steps, the war might be lost. Victory brought its own problems as advocates of the eugenics movement argued that the upper classes would be overwhelmed by the more fecund lower classes, whose gene pool was weakened through loss of the "cream of the generation" in the war. This view was once widely held but soon countered in the United Kingdom (but not Germany) through research that showed the ill health and short stature of poor people to be caused not by genetics but by the malnourishment of poverty. Nutritional research energized many social reformers who ensured that by 1933, U.K. school children could receive free meals and milk. Cod liver oil was soon added to prevent rickets. The discovery of vitamins by then had made a huge impact in clinical medicine and reinforced the view that public action to improve diet should be aimed at meeting minimal requirements for promoting growth through addition of meat, milk, fruit, and vegetables to a poor diet.

These issues were at the fore in the United Kingdom during the Second World War (1939–1945) when fear of "starvation into submission" was high: over 50% of U.K. food came from the United States and Canada at a time when German submarines sank huge numbers of Allied ships. This threat produced a food strategy informed by nutritional research. For the first time in U.K. history, a generation of children were able to consume a diet sufficient not only in energy but in necessary proteins and vitamins. These policies met with international acclaim after the war when it was recognized that scientific advice had produced an effective system of rationing, governments had devised efficient distribution and pricing policies, and nutritional education was well directed. Thereafter, the same policies shaped U.S. food aid to a devastated Europe only to be slowly replaced, as Europe recovered, by policies of self-reliance and commercial investment in the industrialization of food supply. These successful policies have produced the enormous food surpluses of today. Sadly, these policies have also destabilized food supply in underdeveloped countries and caused massive, and not necessarily healthy, changes in Western dietary habits. Monocultural farming systems have reduced the cost of raising cattle, pigs, and chickens so much that the usual diets in Western Europe and urban United States now comprise a great deal of what was once regarded as luxury food. These changes are now being extended as former Eastern bloc countries reflect their growing affluence and perception that freedom of choice should include choice of food as well as democracy.

In post-war Europe, the notion became widespread that the days of malnutrition were over and that the role of governments should be to regulate food safety rather than its nutrient value which, it was felt, could be confidently assumed and, anyway, was a matter of personal choice in a free society. The nutritional content of foodstuffs was inspected from the standpoint of minimum content to protect the consumer against the adulteration of foods but not to ensure nutrient value. The present situation is now hugely complex, with many more new food products widely available through the growth of supermarkets to replace traditional distribution systems of local foods. Returns on these massive investments can be assured only by adding advertising and other overhead to the costs of food.

In these circumstances, it is unsurprising that processed foods now comprise over 70% of the modern Western diet: more potatoes are eaten in processed form than in their freshly cooked state. Likewise, sugar is added widely to foods, as is salt, to enhance taste, so much so that most of the salt consumed in the Western diet is now derived from processed foods over which the consumer has no control. Many commentators are aware of the health risks associated with modern energy-dense but nutrient-poor diets and advocate change. Too often, these remedies repeat the lessons of nutritional education that had been so effective in the early part of the last century but are no longer appropriate. Modern consumers are encouraged to believe that their diets are deficient in specific ways much as those earlier diets were deficient in energy, protein, or vitamins. Addition of missing ingredients to modern diets is the most often proposed remedy when there is a much better case to adopt radical changes in eating patterns. Healthy eating provides less energy, less sugar and salt, and more fruit and vegetables. Nutritional gerontology is thus faced with a complex set of problems. Probably to a greater extent than at any other point in human history, there is greater diversity in diet within and between populations. In some older individuals, dietary preferences established in youth can persist into late life: meals are prepared following traditional routines. In others, greater reliance on prepared foods has been acquired, sometimes with regular supplementation with specific foods, complementary or alternative medicines. Younger individuals, in contrast, may have insufficient interest (and often little time) to prepare foods and rely heavily on convenience foods.

Research designs in nutritional gerontology are influenced by these historical considerations. At the simplest level, sampling subjects for studies in nutritional gerontology takes account of the problem that between birth cohorts (say, 1915–1919 and 1935–1939) there are often very large differences in early life dietary histories. These may be sufficient to account for differences that might otherwise be attributed to aging. At a more complex level (set out later in the final sections on gene–nutrient programming of developmental plasticity), there is good evidence that maternal/fetal exposures to different nutritional environments can modify the risk of late-onset diseases. Inclusion of historical dietary data in studies of this type requires some knowledge of prevailing dietary exposures during relevant epochs. Carpenter (2003a, b, c, d) has provided an excellent overview of the history of nutritional science.

Nutritional Gerontology

At the outset, it is useful to state the broad objectives of studies in nutritional gerontology:

1. To describe the contribution of nutrition to individual differences in aging processes, variation

of incidence of age-related diseases, and the acquisition of age-related disabilities.
2. To elucidate the specific contributions of nutrients to age-dependent mechanisms underlying age-related diseases.
3. To inform the provision of services, to improve advice for old people, and where possible, to use the results of nutrient-based research to prevent, control, and treat age-related disease.

In clinical nutrition, the older patient represents an important challenge. Often, the contribution of poor nutrition can be overlooked; clinical outcomes become suboptimal, and dietary factors in common age-related diseases are acknowledged, though hardly ever acted upon. To summarize, older persons have the same nutritional requirements as younger subjects but their energy needs are less. Absorption of foods is altered by changes in the gastric mucosa and intestines. To accommodate this, older people should eat less but seek to maintain intakes of essential micronutrients by eating nutrient-dense foods that are low in fat (like lean meat and fish) and include eggs, low-fat milk, vegetables, and fruit in a varied and balanced diet. Together, these provide the protein, vitamins, and minerals needed but with fewer calories. Some old people take food supplements, believing these can do no harm. Generally, when supplements do not exceed the recommended daily allowance, this is the case. Supraphysiologic doses of food supplements should be avoided, however, as should the assumption that a poor diet can be made good by consumption of supplements. The greatest hazard of food supplement use arises when this use is preferred to clinical investigation of current clinical symptoms. Self-treatment with food supplements of nonnutritional disease poses a very real danger to the health of old people.

The research base to inform advice on intake of nutrients in old age is now substantial and continues its gradual development so that dietary advice often needs to be updated. The principles that guide new research are major determinants of the quality of this advice. Nutritional studies are influenced by the complexity of the nutritional environment in which individuals seek to optimize their quality of life, minimize disease risks, and make best use of that part of their income available for food. These complexities are multilayered and involve community factors that affect the food supply for old people, its quality and balance; interpersonal issues that relate eating to a communal activity that is modified by the exclusion or marginalization of old people in some contemporary societies; impairments of food preparation linked to sensory loss, motor disabilities, and poor health; the impact on appetite of intercurrent illnesses or loss in old age of a long-term partner; individual preferences for specific types of food; and individual patterns in the absorption and metabolism of foodstuffs.

Research Questions in Nutritional Gerontology

It is in this many-sided setting that research questions on nutrients and aging must first be formulated. Research methods that are not informed by these issues can become pointless exercises in data gathering of little use across the information spectrum that extends from those who must devise public health policies on nutrition in aging to those seeking to interpret the results of laboratory investigations of old people. For example, in the study of cancer (often an age-related disease) there are at least four major constraints on nutritional epidemiological methods (Riboli *et al.*, 2002). These constraints are relevant to a wide range of studies in nutritional gerontology:

1. Measurements of diet lack precision and specificity, particularly for estimates of food consumption.
2. Nutrient intakes are highly correlated, and attribution of causation to one nutrient acting on its own may be misleading.
3. Biological measures of nutrients in tissues may not accurately and reliably reflect dietary intake because the biological regulation of these measures is complex and may be influenced by levels of other nutrients.
4. Most studies undertaken to date have not considered the effects of the physical characteristics of food (an orange as a whole fruit or as a juice, the way the food is prepared, water content, and so on) on the metabolic activity of the constituents of food.

Studies on nutrients and aging, therefore, require prudently framed research questions, thoughtful research designs, careful planning, execution, and interpretation. Although not inherently intellectually challenging, these issues are often so intricate that the best studies are completed within strong collaborations. The nature and scope of these collaborations will influence the type of research questions posed, the measures available to address these questions, the choice of statistical methods, and their interpretation (Ryan, 2003). Obviously, a clear statement of hypotheses is a necessary first step, but often this will be modified in collaboration with others who are perhaps more familiar with issues concerning choice of measures and advise a specific approach to measurement and to issues of validity and reliability. In this preliminary setting, a research group, often in a spirit of flexibility and compromise, will agree on the research model to be tested. Will this be an ecological, observational, or an experimental study? How well controlled will be the variables of most interest? What are the characteristics of the population to be studied? Within a nutritional context, are there specific factors that seem likely to confound interpretation of results? These questions require forward planning chiefly in the design of studies in nutritional gerontology. The following sections consider aging research problems in nutritional studies that arise in sampling (including the problem of refusals), variable measurement, fieldwork, statistical analyses, and interpretation. Because this author's principal interest is in cognitive aspects of the associations between nutrients and aging, certain cognitive issues will be alluded to (Kohlmeier *et al.*, 1993). Animal studies are not considered in this chapter, though much of great relevance to human aging has been learned from carefully conducted studies. The topic of animal studies on nutrients and aging is simply too extensive to be dealt with even in summary form in this section. This issue is especially relevant to current studies of the possible benefits that might accrue for general health and longevity through the practice of caloric restriction. Whereas the database from human ecological and animal studies to support the adoption of low calic eating patterns seems adequate, data from other types of well-designed human studies remain sparse. This topic is addressed in Chapter 31.

Sampling in Aging Research

As an example, take a seemingly simple research question. Suppose a researcher aims to detect the contribution of aging and diet to body mass index (BMI). One approach might be to measure height and weight in a sample of subjects believed to be representative of the general population at different ages, and then to test the association between age and BMI and report the result, seeking to explain the proposed association using age differences in dietary data. These three measures (age, diet, and BMI) are open to confounding by quite distinct processes. First, as set out earlier, the structure of a general population (from which the sample is drawn) is made up of cohorts, each from successive birth epochs, each exposed over time to changes in food quality and availability. Younger subjects may have preferences for, and easy access to, energy-dense foods, rich in saturated fats but nutrient-poor, being depleted in fruit or vegetable vitamins and fiber. The older cohorts may have had quite different dietary experiences, never as young people eating to excess but sometimes undergoing extreme dietary privations. During the twentieth century, these experiences were not uncommon, even during the U.S. Depression or wartime Europe. These types of nutritional deprivation impact variously on aging samples collected cross-sectionally. To this can be added the effects of illnesses and death on sample content, so that—because of censoring by premature death—samples are often under-representative of subjects in whom the associations of interest may be strongest. This is above all true of the relationship between low socioeconomic status and recruitment and retention in studies of nutrition and health (see later).

Cross-cohort comparisons are also susceptible to the influences of factors that produce changes in nutritional behaviors in late adulthood and old age. These susceptibilities may vary by education, by strong continuities in eating habits in one generation that are not detected in another, and, most importantly, by the effects of health or disability status within an aging sample. For instance, there were major changes in the acquisition of physical and possibly mental disabilities in old age in the last quarter of the twentieth century (Vita *et al.*, 1998). Chronic disability prevalence declined in the U.S. population aged over 65 years from 1982 to 1989, and this trend accelerated through 1999 (Manton and Gu, 2001; Fries, 2002, 2003). It is unreasonable, therefore, to assume that within a sample of old people, cohorts drawn from different birth epochs, subjects will exhibit the same illness profiles. These differences between samples may reflect major changes in lifestyle that include differences in eating behavior. The example of reductions in incidence of coronary heart disease in men (1955–1995) is the most repeatedly cited example (Rosamund *et al.*, 1998), to which can be added differences between age-cohorts of women in their use of estrogen replacement therapy (1970–1995) and the growth of sales of prepared, convenience foods (often sugar/salt-rich) aimed at older consumers living alone. Competent accounts of research strategies that aim to reduce the prevalence of chronic disabilities are available (Prentice *et al.*, 2004).

To overcome these sampling problems in cross-cohort comparisons between different age groups and within old age, greater investments are required. First, follow up studies are possible, often of individuals ascertained at some earlier point in the life cycle when nutritional data of variable quality may have been acquired. Second, a longitudinal study may be planned with considerable implications for the resources and commitments of participants and researchers alike. The first example is often opportunistic; the researchers, hearing of a dataset captured for a purpose unrelated to aging—say maternal health in pregnancy—next locate surviving participants and begin energetically to recruit the compliant among them to an aging study. Not until data are analyzed do the researchers begin critically to examine the validity and reliability of the original nutritional data collected perhaps 40 or more years ago. Nutritional measurement instruments have undergone steady improvement, and it is often unsafe to assume that datasets will be as informative as initially assumed. The best advice is to examine contemporary criteria now used to assess scientific reports submitted to current academic journals in the field of nutrition. Then ask the same questions of the historical dataset. How does it compare? Based on the historical record, is the original study reproducible? Are the descriptions of the population sampled available and satisfactory in quite simple terms: demographic, anthropometric, and (if relevant) cognitive parameters? Do the subject identifiers allow exact matching with possible survivors? Will they agree to take part; does their initial participation support the assumption that they agree to be contacted at this later date? If these cannot be satisfactorily established in the first stage of data examination, it is best to treat the dataset—even the most appealing—with circumspection.

Role of Institutional Review Boards and Ethics of Research Committees

Comparable ethical issues arise with prospective longitudinal studies, except that the researcher is required to anticipate the demands at reassessment as if subjects were to be approached for the first time. Here, the importance of advance permissions to track subjects as they migrate geographically and socially cannot be overstated. In this context, it is useful to anticipate difficulties, retaining in longitudinal studies those who may be or become most disadvantaged or whose health may fail. Discussions with experienced ethicists are often helpful. Sometimes guidance can improve the research design and compliance because the changes in research procedures sought to obtain ethical approval are so often well focused. In aging research, when community-dwelling populations are to be sampled, there is a particular problem with refusals, and this will raise specific ethical issues. First, on recruitment there is a bias toward under-representation of the disadvantaged in society. Individuals unable or unwilling to take part for reasons of mental illness or impairment are a major cause for concern as these may be those same individuals for whom the research findings may be most relevant. Individuals who are aware of the health risks posed by their lifestyle are also less likely to volunteer to take part and, when they do, may fail to return for follow-up assessments. Solutions to these problems are imperfect, and most researchers seek to identify the source and size of the errors accrued. Good research practice goes a long way to overcoming subject resistance. So, if a personal approach is taken with each volunteer and, for a group that is anticipated to have problems with research, extra steps are introduced. These are often labor-intensive and demand continuing personal contact with a named person, familiar with the reservations expressed by the volunteer and careful to explain all procedures.

The approach taken to resolve these issues can be coercive or rely on inducements. Ethicists may vary in where a boundary can be set between encouragement to participate and a subject being disadvantaged in some way if they refuse or withdraw consent. Among subjects who find great difficulty responding helpfully to requests from professional people, there are sometimes those who can see why, as individuals, they should take part. Where appropriate, these individuals can be encouraged to seek the involvement of their peers. The success of this snow balling approach is tempered by the need to explain—sometimes repeatedly—the purpose of the research, its possible benefits to the wider public, and the nature and inconvenience their taking part might lead to.

Noncompliance causes huge heartaches and headaches. Carefully judged continuity of personal contacts between the volunteer subject and single named research worker can achieve high levels of compliance, but often this is detected only upon study completion. Some measures of reliability and validity need to be part of the study design. In self-reports of food intake, for example, at least three elements of reliability are built into the measurement instruments. These are basically estimates of consistency: Does the subject respond in the same direction when the same or similar question is posed? From test occasion to occasion, is the same question answered in the same way? Is there evidence of inconsistency attributable to some confounder (e.g., poor memory)? Validity is much more problematical and is addressed in a later section.

Types of Study

Sampling procedures offer five types of study: ecological, cross-sectional, case-control, cohort, and experimental.

ECOLOGICAL STUDIES

Ecological studies are most often based on existing data and rely on units of measurement that are groups of subjects rather than individuals. An example would be a study of the incidence rates of a disease where nutritional deficiencies are thought to be causally important in countries that vary in exposure to that nutritional deficiency. Grouping can be on the basis of any characteristic (e.g., geography, year of birth, etc.) but is usually socio-demographic. Migrant studies fall into this category (Marmot, 1989) but are more informative when conducted as case-control studies. Ecological studies are a useful starting point in preliminary analyses of research questions, often generating many testable hypotheses (Armstrong and Doll, 1975). Power calculations for ecological studies determine the number of groups required in each arm of the comparison, not the number of subjects.

CROSS-SECTIONAL STUDIES

Cross-sectional studies examine variables at a single point in time. Without the possibility of establishing temporal precedence, typically cross-sectional studies cannot establish causality. Three sorts of analysis are available here: (1) tests of the strength of association between variables; (2) significance of differences between groups in the quantity of a variable; and (3) difference in the rate of occurrence of an event (commonly an outcome of interest). In nutritional gerontology, it is important not only to estimate the number of subjects required to test the study hypothesis, but also to decide upon the optimum type of dietary assessment. Within an individual old person there may be considerable variation over time, possibly reflecting the vagaries of social opportunities to share a meal. Longer periods of dietary intake may be required to take account of this yet; in some old people this is prone to faulty recall. To allow for this, it is usual to rely on old people for relatively brief periods of recall and to compensate for this by increasing the size of the sample. It is, however, not an easy task to decide on the best combination of observation period and sample size. The choice is influenced by the purpose served by the data. If it is necessary to relate dietary intake of each individual to some other characteristic of the same individual, then the most accurate measures of dietary intake are required (usually, seven days or more of weighed intake less food waste). However, this labor-intensive method is not required if it is more important to identify subjects at the extremes of a food-intake distribution or to make comparisons between mean values of each group. There are many comprehensive accounts of cross-sectional study designs that are well summarized by Cade (1997).

CASE-CONTROL STUDIES

Case-control studies are an efficient way to examine possible causal mechanisms, and the background, conduct, and interpretation of these study designs is well summarized (Schesselmann, 1982). In nutritional gerontology, it would be usual first to specify criteria for the presence/absence of a condition and then to identify a group with a condition (cases) and a group without that condition (control subjects). The prior exposures of the cases and controls to a putative causal agent or process could then be compared. There is wide discussion on the need to match cases and controls, and when this is done, how exactly matching should take place. It will seem obvious that the best solution is to match cases and controls as closely as possible. However, this sometimes can remove important differences between groups in particular where exposure and matching variables are linked (positively or negatively), as is the case within a wide range of socio-demographic variables. Concerns about measurement errors ensure that case-control studies are not the design of choice in nutritional gerontology. This is largely because it is necessary in nutritional research to obtain estimates of measurement error while evaluating the diet–disease relationship. This is difficult to achieve in case-control studies that rely on historical data. Instead, it is better to undertake a prospective longitudinal study with repeated measurements of diet and even better to employ several methods to measure diet. The cohort study design can meet these requirements.

COHORT STUDIES

Cohort studies differ from case-control studies in that the cohort moves forward in step, whereas the case-control study is a retrospective, historical analysis of prevalent cases. Longitudinal study designs sometimes seek to detect and then adjust for contributions to measurement error made by previous exposure to the same measurement. This arises in many settings but is most problematic when mental performance is measured. It may surprise the investigator that even after intervals, each of several years, some old people—mainly the better educated—maintain consistent improvements, whereas the less able or educated may underperform on first testing, improve on the first re-retesting, and thereafter show expected age-related decline. These problems may be detected in study designs where several consecutive cohorts (say, now aged 60–64; 65–69; 70–74 years, etc.) are recruited, and at each reassessment these cohorts are added to by subjects of the same age but who did not take part in the earlier assessment (Schaie, 1994). Obviously, these sampling processes are demanding of time and effort and should be envisaged only when the research questions demand it; most often simple methods can provide useful results commensurate with many issues involved. A key advantage of cohort studies is that these provide estimates of relative risk, whereas cross-sectional studies permit calculation of the odds ratio. In practice, the odds ratio provides an acceptable estimate of relative risk. There are many good accounts of cohort study design in nutritional epidemiology (e.g., Willett and Colditz, 1998; Day *et al.*, 1999), and methods to combine data from several studies are also available (Mannisto *et al.*, 2004).

EXPERIMENTAL STUDIES

Experimental studies rely on the detection of the effects on an intervention. The design is a special application of the case-control study where the exposure is planned and the design prospective. The assumption is that random allocation of subjects to the active intervention or the placebo arms of a study will provide a balanced design, with potential confounders arising by chance with about equal frequency in the study arms. An experimental study is the preferred means of hypothesis testing in most laboratory settings, and relevant methods are subject to continuing improvements (Murray *et al.*, 2004). In human nutrition, the experimental study is most often a randomized, placebo-controlled trial of the possible benefits of dietary manipulation or supplementation. There are numerous good accounts of experimental designs suitable for testing intervention hypotheses in old people; most frequent concerns arise over sample size and statistical power in studies with old people. Latterly, there are many informative commentaries on the quality and generalizability of clinical trial data (e.g., Khaw *et al.*, 2004) that address the recurring problem of the failure of apparent benefits observed in a clinical trial to translate into clinical practice. In nutritional gerontology there are several age-specific problems, not least that dropout rates may be much higher than in younger samples, and sample size calculations need to be set conservatively (Lazovitch *et al.*, 2002).

Variable Measurement

The correct estimation of the relationships between exposure and the presence of a condition (usually a disease) relies upon the probability distribution of measurement errors and the distribution of exposures and confounders in the whole population from which the sample is drawn. These requirements pose several problems in nutritional gerontology. Their resolution should entail good quality validation studies, at least in subsamples of the population of old people. However, as is set out later, there is no gold-standard measurement of nutritional intake, and the best that can be attained is the inclusion of several different measures of dietary intake that are used on several occasions. These would then give an estimate of the error incurred with the study instrument. However, caution is required even before using this when the study period greatly exceeds the time interval between first and last measure of reliability.

Food Consumption by Old People

This is used to estimate the adequacy of dietary intake by old people, to relate dietary habits to nutritional status and then to health parameters, and to detect change in dietary habit following intervention (e.g., a nutritional education program). The nutritional literature is replete with studies of this type undertaken to meet a wide range of needs, from simple description of trends over time (e.g., Volkert *et al.*, 2004) to the need to detect specific subgroups of old people at most risk for poor nutrition (e.g., Sharkey *et al.*, 2002). The bare bones of this approach is to record what subjects recall they have eaten during a recent period (over the previous day, week, or some such), and then to convert this to intake of nutrients (Wahlqvist, 2002). This is done by either conducting laboratory analysis of samples of the food taken or by looking at food composition tables and estimating nutrient intake from these. Obviously, studies that analyze foods directly are thought more accurate than recall methods in old people where food intake is to be related to nutrient status. Food tables should not be accepted uncritically: the values they contain represent the average for what is often a small number of samples and are prone to error, for example, when mixed dishes are reported or when water content varies substantially. The consensus view is that food tables are acceptable for observational studies for the purpose of classification of subjects or providing group mean values. They are less useful in intervention studies. A critique of methodologies is presented by Maggi *et al.* (1993).

WEIGHED RECORDS

To obtain a weighed record, laboratory methods are quite well established. It is feasible sometimes to obtain a duplicate portion of the food consumed by the subject and, after adjustment for waste, analyze that or an aliquot drawn from it (Bingham *et al.*, 1995). When using food composition tables, several alternates are available. In a direct observation study, the portions would be weighed precisely, waste subtracted from this, and the composition estimated by reference to food composition tables. If reliance was placed on dietary interview data, subjects would recall their food intake and thus provide a recent dietary history, which (as earlier) could be converted into typical intakes of nutrients using food composition tables. Comparable, sometimes supplementary, methods involve the subject keeping a food diary. Some care is required when using food composition tables, however, since these may vary from country to country and from time to time within one country. For these reasons, it remains necessary to include food analyses in many studies. These methods are expensive, and for reasons of feasibility and economy, most individual surveys rely on either prospective or retrospective methods of dietary assessment (Longnecker *et al.*, 1995). Retrospective surveys rely on memory, the ability to conceptualize what is required, accuracy of estimation of portion sizes, and are open to bias toward reporting a healthier pattern of eating than is in fact the case. Nevertheless, compliance is usually high among old people with surveys (often postal) of this type, and the results are quite reproducible among those with regular eating habits. Food Frequency Questionnaires (FFQ) or Food Frequency and Amount Questionnaires (FAQ) are the most often used of all methods of dietary assessment. Importantly, so far, no FFQ or FAQ has been designed specifically for use with old people. Typically, a FFQ is designed to test a specific hypothesis concerning intake of a specific nutrient or group of nutrients often taking the number of respondents into account. Some sensory impairments that are common in old people will confound eating behaviors. These include visual and olfactory losses (Griep *et al.*, 1996). An account of common methodological and interpretative errors is provided by Beaton *et al.* (1997). Comparisons between Food Frequency Questionnaires and diet records are also available (Margetts *et al.*, 1989; Bingham *et al.*, 1994, 1997).

ENERGY ADJUSTMENT

The method used to express the nutrient content of diet merits some consideration (Willett *et al.*, 1997). The general principle is that the expression of content should make nutritional sense and should take account of influences on bioavailability and loss of nutrients in food preparation. Energy adjustment is perhaps the most frequently used method. The greater the consumption of all foods, so consumption of specific nutrients is also likely to be greater. Bigger, more active subjects will eat more than the sedentary. Improvements in comparisons between subjects and between studies can be achieved through energy adjustment. This is particularly useful when individuals seek to minimize their intake at the level of macronutrients (as with some obese individuals). Differences between under-reporters and those who make valid returns are much reduced after energy adjustment. Energy adjustment is unhelpful when there is no relationship between energy consumption and the relevant nutrient.

VALIDATION STUDIES IN OLD PEOPLE

The newcomer to nutritional gerontology might feel overwhelmed by the prospect of obtaining valid and reliable measures of dietary intake. There appears to be a huge potential for confounding by impaired cognition, sensory loss, appetite changes, acquired poverty, impaired mobility, access to fresh food, and failure to complete cooking (Jorissen and Riedel, 2002). As individuals mature and establish personal independence, each is expected to take more responsibility for their own basic needs, such as warmth, shelter, food, and companionship. With aging, many require support to maintain this independence, and the reasons for this are extraordinarily varied. Take, for example, a woman living alone who rarely leaves the house and for whom food shopping has become hugely effortful. Her circumstances may have arisen because she has suffered sensory loss (above all, of sight or hearing), or she has problems with mobility and fears falling, or her bladder control is unsure and she is anxious about incontinence. To these can be added a plethora of mental symptoms and impairments that confound any attempts to anticipate all sources of error in measurement of eating habits and nutritional status in old people. To accommodate these adaptations to old age, over-reliance on preserved or dry foodstuffs may develop with understandable lack of variety and later, little interest in consuming unappetizing food.

There is, therefore, a particular need in studies of old people to establish the validity of food intake estimates at the individual or group level. The first step in a validation study is to set the key reference measures. From the outset it is important to accept that biomarkers of nutrient intake derived from concentrations of nutrients in blood or other tissues do not provide an absolute measure of intake. Clearly, these will be related in some way to intake, but it will not be a simple direct relationship. Other factors—absorption, metabolism, binding, excretion—will influence the measure, which in turn may not reflect the availability of the nutrient in the tissue of interest (e.g., a blood test as a guide to intra-neuronal concentration). When designing studies, the commitment to validation should not be treated lightly.

Biomarkers of Healthy Eating

Biomarkers are used to assess nutritional intakes and nutritional status because they are believed to provide more accurate estimates of intake/bioavailability of specific nutrients, especially where these are combined (as in most meals) or cooked to variable extent. There are also concerns about the validity of food composition tables when foods are known to vary over time (as with industrialized food processing) or cultivated in different soils or climatic conditions.

Although some researchers think of biomarkers as potential gold standards of dietary intake, there are good reasons to accept such a view only with thoughtful reservations (Weinstein *et al.*, 2004). Subjects are well known to vary in metabolic pathways for reasons of sex, genetics, and previous nutrient exposures (Arab *et al.*, 2003). These differences include age-related variations in absorption, the impact of coingestion of foods that may inhibit the absorption of others (e.g., green vegetables contain oxalic acid, which impairs the absorption of calcium). Likewise, renal excretion is subject to tight controls designed to remove unwanted metabolic products and excess nutrients but to retain needed nutrients. Urinary analyses, for these reasons, can be misleading as they indicate the net outcome of these diverse processes (including saturation) and are not directly correlated with intakes.

Biomarkers may be measured in a wide range of tissues that include plasma, serum, red blood cells, white blood cells, feces, urine, hair, nail, buccal cells, and a number of measures specifically designed to assess overall antioxidant capacity (Polidori *et al.*, 2001), metabolic state (e.g., exhaled air), or the extent of DNA damage (Potischman, 2003a, 2003b). Some tissues seem especially relevant to aging studies (e.g., lipid content of red blood cell membranes; Hulbert *et al.*, 2004), but it is best to plan to collect diverse types of samples before drawing any general conclusions. This is true in most biomarker studies; whenever possible, ensure that the chosen marker is examined or tested in at least two biological systems (Ilich *et al.*, 2003). Before deciding upon any biomarker, it is always useful to discuss the choice with the laboratory where the tests will be conducted. This advice often includes appraisal of recent analytical developments, the competing interests of high reliability/validity of a specific measure when set against convenience and compliance. There are also helpful critiques of specific biomarkers, the principles of which can easily be applied to another biomarker (e.g., Ness *et al.*, 1999). It is also essential to discuss all aspects of sampling, separation, labeling, storage, and how laboratory data are to be linked to the research database. Decisions on these and related matters should be recorded and circulated as a clear written statement of protocol.

Body composition studies in old people provide useful measures that discriminate between health and disease states (Fuller *et al.*, 1996). This is a highly specialized research technique, requiring great care in its application and interpretation. Available methods include bioelectric impedance studies (Baumgartner, 2000; Aghdassi *et al.*, 2001).

In nutritional gerontology, the issue of differences in cognitive ability in the assessment of dietary history/nutritional status is rarely investigated. Studies are needed that investigate the advantages of biomarkers over retrospective recall in the presence/absence of cognitive impairment (Morris *et al.*, 2002). Likewise, in the investigation of the role of nutrients in aging and age-related diseases, it is useful to place firmly among the aims of a project the needs of clinicians who might make use of the findings. For example, in clinical practice, it is commonplace to identify the concentration of vitamin B12/folate as being suboptimal and predictive of disease. It is uncommon for these values to be considered in the context of a relevant metabolite such as homocysteine, largely because uncertainties remain about the value of such measures and their availability. Nevertheless, these matters do interest clinicians, and the value of measuring a number of parameters linked to a pathophysiologic process is appealing and worth bearing in mind when choosing what might be measured.

Resources available include a series of papers published in 2003 as a supplement to *The Journal of Nutrition* ("Biomarkers of Nutritional Exposures and Nutritional Status").

Dietary Patterns

People eat mixes of foods, not isolated nutrients. Within individuals there are strong correlations between the consumption of individual nutrients so that it is often very difficult to separate the contribution to health or disease of one nutrient from a group of nutrients. Therefore, interest has grown in the identification of patterns of food consumption and the extent to which particular patterns can be linked to health outcomes (dietary pattern analysis). This interest represents an understandable expansion of awareness of the importance of particular food combinations and the role of nutrient-nutrient interactions (Hu *et al.*, 1999; Millen *et al.*, 2004). In large part, the interest is based on ecological comparisons between communities who differ in risk of specific diseases that can be plausibly linked to dietary habits. Where the aim is to understand an overall picture of the relationships between diet and disease, dietary patterns may be more informative than study of single nutrients in isolation (Balder *et al.*, 2003).

The main techniques used to determine eating patterns are (a) principal components factor analysis, (b) cluster analysis, and (c) dietary indices (Newby *et al.*, 2004a, b). The first two methods are useful in the reduction or grouping of data, whereas the third is valuable in the prospective study of dietary contributions to disease prevention. In factor analysis, dietary data are obtained by recall methods, and foods are sorted into major nutrient groups. These nutrient groups are then factor-analyzed using principal component methods (with or without rotation). The major factors produced are inspected for content validity and named accordingly, such that a factor that comprises high energy intake, saturated fats, and alcohol might be labeled high risk, where another factor comprising low energy, fruit and vegetables, unprocessed oily fish, and so on might be labeled prudent (Montonen *et al.*, 2005). These factors are consistently derived in samples from diverse Western populations and have proven to be useful in understanding the contributions of diet rather than specific nutrients to risks of disease.

Anthropometrics

Historically, understanding the associations between nutrients and development (of which aging processes comprise a major component) has been based on recognition that anthropometric measures are useful proxies of health status that vary from detection of the impact on health of the public attributable to improved feeding (as in the growth of infants) to selection of military recruits and to the progress of chronic disease. For most populations, detailed reference data are available, and these can be used for purposes as diverse as demonstration that a study sample is typical of the population from which it was drawn to surveillance of the general nutritional status of large populations (e.g., Hughes *et al.*, 2004). However, caution is advised when applying such simple methods to underdeveloped countries where there may be many malnourished subjects, frequent recurrent disease (e.g., malaria), and other stressors. Exposure to these confounders may vary within a country from place to place and over time.

At first glance, anthropometric data appear robust and simple to use. Certainly, most reports in nutritional gerontology do not provide detailed methods for anthropometric data collection, yet caveats abound. First, it is important to include anthropometric data in descriptions of samples. Second, in old people, great care must be exercised to ensure that these data are reproducible, so some training will always be required to achieve this. It is also useful in old people, in addition to height, to record the demispan between outstretched fingers and the midpoint of the sternum. This measure agrees closely with maximum height achieved and can be used to allow for shrinkage in stature with age in old people. As in much nutrition research, many measures are not normally distributed, and transformations to approximate normality should be made by systematically reviewing which of the following yields the best result (by increasing adjustment): square root ($\sqrt{x}$), logarithmic, inverse square root ($1/\sqrt{x}$), and inverse ($1/x$).

Studies on reliability of measures of height and weight suggest that *a priori* maximum acceptable values should be set for differences between observers. This becomes more important as more measures are added to a study (e.g., arm circumference, triceps skin fold, subscapular skin fold). Here, it is useful to provide an estimate of measurement error such as the technical error of measurement (TEM) from one or more observers.

Anthropometric indices are derived from two or more raw anthropometric measures. Examples include the body mass index (BMI), arm muscle area (AMA) and arm fat area (AFA), and waist–hip ratio. Together, these measures and composite indices provide a guide to under- and overnutrition in a sample. The extent of underweight is gauged by applying a criterion value (usually 16, 17, or 18.5) to BMI scores. So far, it is uncertain how BMI varies within samples of old people. A greater proportion of under- and overweight individuals die before or soon after entering old age, but subsequently, overweight individuals enjoy some advantages, with a better chance of surviving some illnesses, yet with a greater risk of falls and such (Ledikwe *et al.*, 2003).

Gene-Nutrient Interactions

The molecular dissection of environment–gene interactions has the potential to overturn accepted ideas concerning the role of nutrients in aging and age-related diseases (Paoloni-Giacobino *et al.*, 2003; Gluckman and Hansom, 2004). Many novel methods of study have been developed. Following is a brief summary of the main mechanisms of gene–nutrient interaction and research methods available to study them.

MECHANISMS

There is evidence of accumulation of DNA damage in aging. For some, this evidence is the foundation of the "the DNA damage hypothesis of aging." This predicts that with aging, DNA damage exceeds DNA repair capacity and that the rate of aging will be directly related to the rate of accumulation of damage to DNA. Dietary habits and the intake of specific nutrients can be related to this hypothesis in four main ways: (a) nutrients can up-regulate or down-regulate gene transcription; (b) nutrients can damage DNA; (c) nutrients can protect DNA from damage; and (d) exposure to specific nutrients may slow or hasten aging processes through interaction with aging genes.

Nutrient and gene transcription

Specific nutrients could interact with a cellular recognition site and trigger the release of the second messenger followed by a DNA-binding protein. This is required to move from the cytoplasm into the nucleus and bind with the regulatory portion of a gene. Gene transcription is thereby stimulated or inhibited with production of greater or lesser amounts of product. Nutrients known to modify gene transcription include some polyunsaturated fatty acids (e.g., eicosodocosohexaenoic acid, [EPA]), certain amino acids, and fat-soluble vitamins (vitamins A, D, and their metabolites). Methods to study these processes in specific cell types and metabolic pathways in aging humans are currently under development. One basic approach is to load a biological system with the substrate of enzyme believed to be regulated by a specific nutrient. Up- or down- regulation of a gene is inferred by quantification of the metabolites of the substrate before and after exposure to the nutrient load or its comparator. From the perspective of studies on human health and disease, early nutrient exposure during critical developmental periods may modify genes involved in related metabolic processes. (Waterland and Jirtle, 2004). These studies are in their infancy, but so far more than 20 genes have been found to be modified in this way, usually through hypomethylation. In addition, some genetic polymorphisms are associated with individual differences in response to nutrient intake. This is best understood for lipid metabolism (Masson *et al.*, 2003), but other physiological systems are certain to be modified in this way.

Nutrient damage to DNA

Nutrient damage to DNA is studied extensively in cancer biology. It is known that dietary components (including the products of cooking) and some contaminants of food may cause DNA damage. Although there are many examples from cancer (often an age-related disease), none have so far been confidently linked to differences in rates of aging.

DNA-protective nutrients

DNA-protective nutrients are present in diet. This is best regarded as a mixture of compounds, some of which are potentially harmful to DNA, whereas others are protective. The overall effect of diet on the accumulation of damaged DNA reflects the sum of their opposing actions. Nutrients that protect DNA include the antioxidants vitamin C and vitamin E, and the carotenoids, probably by stabilizing free radicals. All plant leaves contain chlorophyll, which forms a water-soluble salt, chlorophyllin, that can protect DNA from damage. This last mechanism is an example of those many biological processes (open to genetic influence) that may activate or inhibit conversion of dietary compounds to potent DNA-damaging agents. So far, none of these processes are studied extensively in aging populations, so their general importance, though recognized, remains unknown. The underlying biology, though complex, suggests pathways that may modify the rate of progression in aging and on to age-related diseases.

Nutrients and aging genes

If genes that convey longevity could be discovered, then these will be relevant to aging. This possibility rests on the likelihood that (1) especially in extreme old age, these genes may reduce rates of aging, and (2) these genes may modify cellular and biochemical pathways involved in gene–nutrient determined mechanisms of aging and age-related disease. The best-known example of such a gene is the $\varepsilon 4$ allele of the apolipoprotein E gene that decreases markedly in frequency with advancing age, whereas the much rarer $\varepsilon 2$ allele becomes more frequent. These findings are attributed to increased mortality in Alzheimer's and cardiovascular diseases associated with the $\varepsilon 4$ allele and the slight protection afforded by the $\varepsilon 2$ allele. The siblings and children of centenarians show reduced rates of age-related cardiovascular diseases, hypertension, diabetes, and stroke but not osteoporosis, cancers, and thyroid disease, suggesting that genetic effects are greater in the former disease group than the latter, in whom environmental, including nutritional, effects may predominate (Perls *et al.*, 2002, 2004). The exact identity of longevity genes is unknown; much current thinking concerns genes regulating inflammatory processes and energy production. The first proposition is supported by repeated observations that age-related diseases (like AD, PD, atherosclerosis, and type 2 diabetes) are sometimes initiated or exacerbated by systemic inflammation. This has supported the idea that an anti-inflammatory genotype is linked to longevity. In turn, certain nutrients are believed to be anti-inflammatory; these include the n-3 polyunsaturated fatty acids, eicosopentaenoic and docosohexaenoic acids. Regulation of energy metabolism, insulin resistance, and longevity are discussed in the next section.

Nutritional Programming

This topic is most often raised in response to the question: "What—if any—are the fetal origins of individual differences in aging and the incidence of age-related diseases?" During pregnancy, dietary requirements change because a mother must consume or synthesize all that is required for the growth and development of her baby. Factors like poverty, moral or religious taboos, or poor education are major influences on dietary habits in pregnancy. If, for reason of poor diet or placental insufficiency, a fetus fails to receive necessary calories and nutrients required for development, the risks increase of several age-related diseases. The importance of maternal nutrition and the consequences of low birth weight are now widely recognized in studies of aging and age-related disease.

Fetal nutritional programming is defined as "a stimulus (nutrient) or insult (absence of essential nutrient) to the fetus at a critical or sensitive period in intrauterine life with lasting effects on body structure, physiology and metabolism" (Godfrey and Barker, 2001). This concept underpins the "fetal origins of adult disease hypothesis." The hypothesis rests on the facts that, although genes determine optimum growth potential, the intrauterine environment and nutrient availability determine the extent of fetal growth attained.

Neonatal body weights, sizes, and proportions are gauges of the intrauterine growth and nutritional status. These provide useful proxies in population-based studies of nutritional status and growth. But these are less than ideal. Research methods to improve on this are in development and are likely to derive from the following. Fetal nutrition depends on the concentration of nutrients in the maternal circulation, on uteroplacental blood flow, and on the efficiency of transfer of nutrients across the placenta. Nutrient concentration in maternal blood essentially is determined by the mother's body composition, activity, metabolism, and diet. Recent studies have developed noninvasive techniques to measure relevant parameters (e.g., functional magnetic resonance imaging of placental function). Although these are certainly feasible in population-based studies, at present it is not possible to obtain large-scale normative data on the healthy fetus.

The general hypothesis that fetal growth is an important influence on late-onset diseases has been developed further. The Barker Hypothesis proposes that the fetal nutritional environment programs offspring for the likely availability of calories/nutrients during later development. Infants who have experienced a poor nutritional environment *in utero* are programmed to anticipate poor nutritional conditions in later life. Consequently, their metabolism is primed to conserve calories and nutrients as these become available. Their phenotype is small, and in poor conditions their health remains good. Conversely, infants whose intrauterine nutritional supplies were good will develop an optimal phenotype and enjoy corresponding good health. Problems for health and aging arise when intrauterine nutrition is mismatched with the adult nutritional environment (McMillen and Robinson, 2005). When the poorly nourished fetus encounters abundant foods in adulthood, programs to retain calories/nutrients are inappropriate; obesity, hyperlipidemia, hypertension, and abnormal glucose metabolism arise. Research methods to analyze the mechanisms initially relied on human ecological studies that exploit historical databases with high standards of clinical follow-up (in survivors born during the Dutch famine of 1944/1945; Roseboom *et al.*, 2001) and, increasingly, on animal models. The term *metabolic imprinting* was recently introduced to promote studies to unravel associations between early nutrition and increased susceptibility to late-onset diseases. This term implies the persistence of an adaptive genomic change in response to a nutritional stimulus that occurs during a critical period of development. The phenomenon of imprinting describes the effect on the single allele of a gene, which is expressed in a parent-of-origin dependent manner. Genetic mechanisms to explain these processes are now described. These do not involve alterations to DNA sequences, but rather to epigenetic gene regulation (Waterland and Jirtle, 2004). DNA methylation is highly dependent on the availability of dietary methyl donors (e.g., methionine) and cofactors (e.g., vitamin B12). Early in embryogenesis, continuous cycles of cytosine methylation are established. Under- or overavailability of methyl donors can cause lasting effects on specific genes. It is now a subject of great interest in the study of the role of nutrients in aging and susceptibility to age-related diseases to identify the classes of genes that may be involved. Imprinted genes might be one such class of gene, and studies are now underway to determine if one or more of these genes is associated with individual differences in rates of aging and disease incidence.

Conclusion

Research into aging will remain a priority for the foreseeable future. Whatever is achieved seems likely always to fall short of a human craving for a long and healthy life. The key outcome variable from a public perspective is a decrease in age-dependent mortality with the hope that for most, these added years will be comfortable and productive. There are without doubt major genetic and environmental contributions to aging and, of these, the environmental contribution seems most open to effective intervention. In broad terms, there is a popular view that lifestyle issues are the most important and the one over which an individual can exercise most control. When this rather imprecise term is analyzed, the spotlight falls on nutrition holding center stage in aging research.

This chapter has set out some of the pitfalls—and more than one elephant trap—for the researcher new to this field. The scene was set by looking first from an historical perspective and seeing that aging populations comprise diverse groups of people so much so that differences between the young-old and the old-old attributed to aging might sometimes be better understood in terms of major differences in dietary histories. This point recurred in the final sections on gene-nutrient interactions and the importance of nutritional programming. Here, full knowledge of the maternal, neonatal, and adult nutritional histories of people is necessary to unravel the basic biology in human studies. More likely, promising animal models will be developed to explore the ways aging processes are influenced by the early nutritional environment.

Although this chapter has emphasized the role of nutritional studies in aging human populations, there is an important place for animal studies. Much of this is outside the competence of this reviewer, being found in journals concerning animal husbandry and in nutritional biochemistry. Although the case is strong to focus on human studies, when there is little commercial interest in old animals, this should not be understood as making light of the possible contributions to human health such animal studies might make.

Emphasis was placed on the need in nutritional studies to devise and implement effective methods to estimate the validity and reliability of nutritional intake methods. None of those summarized earlier are perfect, and there is great scope for novel improvements. In step with this, there are also opportunities to introduce advanced statistical models into studies on nutrients and human aging. The exponential growth witnessed in the molecular epidemiology of nutrition and the huge interest shown in understanding the role of specific genes makes this one of the most stimulating areas in which to start research. These are exciting times.

ACKNOWLEDGMENTS

The author is a Wellcome Trust, Senior Research Fellow in the University of Aberdeen. Assistance in preparation of the manuscript was provided by Matthew Smith.

REFERENCES

Aghdassi, E., Tam, C., Liu, B., McArthur, M., McGeer, A., Simor, A. *et al.* (2001). Body fat of older adult subjects calculated from bioelectric impedance versus anthropometry correlated but did not agree. *J. Am. Diet. Assoc. 101*, 1209–1212.

Arab, L. (2003). Biomarkers of fat and fatty acid intake. *J. Nutr. 133*, 925S–932S.

Armstrong, B. and Doll, R. (1975). Environmental factors and cancer incidence and mortality in different countries, with special reference to dietary practices. *Int. J. Cancer.* Apr 15, *15(4)*, 617–631.

Balder, H.F., Virtanen, M., Brants, H.A.M., Krogh, V., Dixon, L.B., Tan, F. *et al.* (2003). Common and country-specific dietary patterns in four European cohort studies. *J. Nutr. 133*, 4246–4251.

Baumgartner, R.N. (2000). Body composition in healthy aging. *Ann. N.Y. Acad. Sci. 904*, 437–448.

Beaton, G.H., Burema, J., and Ritenbaugh, C. (1997). Errors in the interpretation of dietary assessments. *Am. J. Clin. Nutr. 65*, 1100S–1107S.

Bingham, S.A., Cassidy, A., Cole, T.J., Welch, A., Runswick, S.A., Black, A.E. *et al.* (1995). Validation of weighed records and other methods of dietary assessment using the 24 h urine nitrogen technique and other biological markers. *Br. J. Nutr. 73*, 531–550.

Bingham, S.A., Gill, C., Welch, A., Cassidy, A., Runswick, S.A., Oakes, S. *et al.* (1997). Validation of dietary assessment methods in the UK arm of EPIC using weighed records, and 24-hour urinary nitrogen and potassium and serum vitamin C and arotenoids as biomarkers. *Int. J. Epidemiol. Suppl. 26*, S137–S151.

Bingham, S.A., Gill, C., Welch, A., Day, K., Cassidy, A., Khaw, K.T. *et al.* (1994). Comparison of dietary assessment methods in nutritional epidemiology: Weighed records v. 24 h recalls, food-frequency questionnaires and estimated-diet records. *Br. J. Nutr. 72*, 619–643.

Cade, J. (1997). Cross-sectional designs. In B.M. Margetts (Ed.), *Design Concepts in Nutritional Epidemiology*. Oxford: Nelson M. Oxford University Press.

Carpenter, K.J. (2003a). A short history of nutritional science: Part 1 (1785–1885). *J. Nutr. 133*, 638–645.

Carpenter, K.J. (2003b). A short history of nutritional science: Part 2 (1885–1912). *J. Nutr. 133*, 975–984.

Carpenter, K.J. (2003c). A short history of nutritional science: Part 3 (1912–1944). *J. Nutr.* 3023–3032.

Carpenter, K.J. (2003d). A short history of nutritional science: Part 4 (1945–1985) *J. Nutr. 13*, 3331–3342.

Day, N., Oakes, S., Luben, R., Khaw, K.T., Bingham, S., Welch, A. *et al.* (1999a). EPIC-Norfolk: Study design and characteristics of the cohort. European Prospective Investigation of Cancer. *Br. J. Cancer. Suppl. 80*, 95–103.

Day, N., Oakes, S., Luben, R., Khaw, K.T., Bingham, S., Welch, A. *et al.* (1999b). EPIC-Norfolk: Study design and characteristics of the cohort. European Prospective Investigation of Cancer. *Br. J. Cancer. Suppl. 80*, 95–103.

Fries, J.F. (2002). Reducing disability in older age. *JAMA 288*, 3164–3166.

Fries, J.F. (2003). Measuring and monitoring success in compressing morbidity. *Ann. Intern. Med. 139*, 455–459.

Fuller, N.J., Sawyer, M.B., Laskey, M.A., Paxton, P., and Elia, M. (1996). Prediction of body composition in elderly men over 75 years of age. *Ann. Hum. Biol. 23*, 127–147.

Gluckman, P.D. and Hansom, M.A. (2004). Living with the past: Evolution, development, and patterns of disease. *Science 305*, 1733–1736.

Godfrey, K.M. and Barker, D.J.P. (2001). Fetal programming and adult health. *Public Health Nutr. 4*, 611–624.

Griep, M.I., Verleye, G., Franck, A.H., Collys, K., Mets, T.F., and Massart, D.L. (1996). Variation in nutrient intake with dental status, age and odour perception. *Eur. J. Clin. Nutr. 50*, 816–825.

Hu, F.B., Rimm, E., Smith-Warner, S.A., Feskanich, D., Stampfer, M.J., Ascherio, A. *et al.* (1999). Reproducibility and validity of dietary patterns assessed with a food-frequency questionnaire. *Am. J. Clin. Nutr. 69*, 243–249.

Hughes, V.A., Roubenoff, R., Wood, M., Frontera, W.R., Evans, W.J., and Fiatarone, Singh, M.A. (2004). Anthropometric assessment of 10-y changes in body composition in the elderly. *Am. J. Clin. Nutr. 80*, 475–482.

Hulbert, A.J. (2004). On the importance of fatty acid composition of membranes for aging. *J. Theo. Biol. 234*, 277–288.

Ilich, J.Z., Brownbill, R.A., and Tamborini, L. (2003). Bone and nutrition in elderly women: Protein, energy, and calcium as main determinants of bone mineral density. *Eur. J. Clin. Nutr. 57*, 554–565.

Jorissen, B.L. and Riedel, W.J. (2002). Nutrients, age and cognition. *Clin. Nutr. 21*, 89–95.

Khaw, K.T., Day, N., Bingham, S., and Wareham, N. (2004). Observational versus randomised trial evidence. *Lancet 364*, 753–754. Author reply 754–755.

Kohlmeier, L., Arminger, G., Clayton, D., Jockel, K.H., Karg, G., Keiding, N. *et al.* (1993). Recommendations for the design and analysis of nutritional epidemiologic studies with measurement errors in the exposure variables. *Eur. J. Clin. Nutr. Suppl. 47*, S53–S57.

Lazovich, D., Murray, D.M., Brosseau, L.M., Parker, D.L., Milton, F.T., and Dugan, S.K. (2002). Sample size considerations for studies of intervention efficacy in the occupational setting. *Ann. Occup. Hyg. 46*, 219–227.

Ledikwe, J.H., Smiciklas-Wright, H., Mitchell, D.C., Jensen, G.L., Friedmann, J.M., and Still, C.D. (2003). Nutritional risk assessment and obesity in rural older adults: A sex difference. *Am. J. Clin. Nutr. 77*, 551–558.

Longnecker, M.P., Shames, L., Kolonel, L.N., Wilkens, L.R., Pike, M.C., and Henderson, B.E. (1995). Cost-efficient design of a diet validation study. *Am. J. Epidemiol. 142*, 353–362.

Maggi, S., Sorenson, A.W., and Steel, K. (1993). The need for a strict methodology in dietary surveys—The experience of the WHO osteoporosis project. *Aging. Clin. Exp. Res. Suppl. 5*, S23–S28.

Mannisto, S., Smith-Warner, S.A., Spiegelman, D., Albanes, D., Anderson, K., van den Brandt, P.A. *et al.* (2004). Dietary carotenoids and risk of lung cancer in a pooled analysis of seven cohort studies. *Cancer Epidemiol. Biomarkers Prev.* 40–48.

Manton, K.G. and Gu, X. (2001). Changes in the prevalence of chronic disability in the United States black and nonblack population above age 65 from 1982 to 1999. *Proc. Natl. Acad. Sci. U.S.A 98*, 6354–6359.

Margetts, B.M., Cade, J.E., and Osmond, C. (1989). Comparison of a food frequency questionnaire with a diet record. *Int. J. Epidemiol. 18(4)*, 868–873.

Marmot, M. (1989). General approaches to migrant studies. In J.K. Cruikshank and D.G. Beevers, *Ethnic factors in health and disease*. Oxford: Wright.

Masson, L.F., McNeill, G., and Avenell, A. (2003). Genetic variation and the lipid response to dietary intervention: A systematic review. *Am. J. Clin. Nutr. 77*, 1098–1111.

Mcmillen, I.C. and Robinson, J.S. (2005). Developmental origins of the metabolic syndrome: Prediction, plasticity, and programming. *Physiol. Rev. 85*, 571–633.

Millen, B.E., Quatromoni, P.A., Nam, B.H., O'Horo, C.E., Polak, J.F., Wolf, P.A. *et al.* (2004). Dietary patterns, smoking, and subclinical heart disease in women: Opportunities for primary prevention from the Framingham Nutrition Studies. *J. Am. Diet. Assoc. 104*, 208–214.

Montonen, J., Knekt, P., Harkanen, T., Jarvinen, R., Heliovaara, M., Aromaa, A. *et al.* (2005). Dietary patterns and the incidence of type 2 diabetes. *Am. J. Epidemiol. 161*, 219–227.

Morris, M.C., Tangney, C.C., Bienias, J.L., Evans, D.A., and Wilson, R.S. (2003). Validity and reproducibility of a food frequency questionnaire by cognition in an older biracial sample. *Am. J. Epidemiol. 158*, 1213–1217.

Murray, D.M., Varnell, S.P., and Blitstein, J.L. (2004). Design and analysis of group-randomized trials: A review of recent methodological developments. *Am. J. Public Health 94*, 423–432.

Ness, A.R., Khaw, K.T., Bingham, S., and Day, N.E. (1999). Plasma vitamin C: What does it measure? *Public Health Nutr. 2*, 51–54.

Newby, P.K., Muller, D., Hallfrisch, J., Andres, R., and Tucker, K.L. (2004). Food patterns measured by factor analysis and anthropometric changes in adults. *Am. J. Clin. Nutr. 80*, 504–513.

Newby, P.K., Muller, D., and Tucker, K.L. (2004). Associations of empirically derived eating patterns with plasma lipid biomarkers: A comparison of factor and cluster analysis methods. *Am. J. Clin. Nutr. 80*, 759–767.

Paoloni-Giacobino, A., Grimble, R., and Pichard, C. (2003). Genomic interactions with disease and nutrition. *Clin. Nutr. 22*, 507–514.

Perls, T.T., Wilmoth, J., Levenson, R., Drinkwater, M., Cohen, M., Bogan, H. *et al.* (2002). Life-long sustained mortality advantage of siblings of centenarians. *Proc. Natl. Acad. Sci. U.S.A 99*, 8442–8447.

Perls, T. (2004). Centenarians who avoid dementia. *Trends Neurosci. 27*, 633–634.

Polidori, M.C., Cherubini, A., Senin, U., and Mecocci, P. (2001). Peripheral non-enzymatic antioxidant changes with human aging: A selective status report. *Biogerontology 2*, 99–104.

Potischman, N. (2003). Biologic and methodologic issues for nutritional biomarkers. *J. Nutr. 133*, 875S–880S.

Potischman, N. and Freudenheim, J.L. (2003). Biomarkers of nutritional exposure and nutritional status: An overview. *J. Nutr. 133*, 873S–874S.

Prentice, R.L., Willett, W.C., Greenwald, P., Alberts, D., Bernstein, L., Boyd, N.F. *et al.* (2004). Nutrition and physical activity and chronic disease prevention: Research strategies and recommendations. *J. Natl. Cancer Inst. 96*, 1276–1287.

Riboli, E., Hunt, K.J., Slimani, N., Ferrari, P., Norat, T., Fahey, M. *et al.* (2002). European prospective investigation into cancer and nutrition (EPIC): Study populations and data collection. *Public Health Nutr. 5*, 1113–1124.

Rosamond, W.D., Chambless, L.E., Folsom, A.R., Cooper, L.S., Conwill, D.E., Clegg, L. *et al.* (1998). Trends in the incidence of myocardial infarction and in mortality due to coronary heart disease, 1987 to 1994. *N. Engl. J. Med. 339*, 861–867.

Roseboom, T.J., van der Meulen, J.H.P., Ravelli, A.C.J., Osmond, C., Barker, D.J.P., and Bleker, O.P. (2001). Effects of prenatal exposure to the Dutch famine on adult disease in later life: An overview. *Mol. Cell Endocrinol. 185*, 93–98.

Ryan, L. (2003). Epidemiologically based environmental risk assessment. *Stat. Sci. 18*, 466–480.

Schaie, K.W. (1994). The course of adult intellectual development. *Am. Psychol. 49*, 304–313.

Schesselmann, J.J. (1982). *Case-control studies: Design, conduct, analysis.* Oxford: Oxford University Press.

Sharkey, J.R., Branch, L.G., Zohoori, N., Giuliani, C., Busby-Whitehead, J., and Haines, P.S. (2002). Inadequate nutrient intakes among homebound elderly and their correlation with individual characteristics and health-related factors. *Am. J. Clin. Nutr. 76*, 1435–1445.

Vita, A.J., Terry, R.B., Hubert, H.B., and Fries, J.F. (1998). Aging, health risks, and cumulative disability. *N. Engl. J. Med. 338*, 1035–1041.

Volkert, D., Kreuel, K., Heseker, H., and Stehle, P. (2004). Energy and nutrient intake of young-old, old-old and very-old elderly in Germany. *Eur. J. Clin. Nutr. 58*, 1190–1200.

Wahlqvist, M.L. (2002). 'Malnutrition' in the aged: The dietary assessment. *Public Health Nutr. 5*, 911–913.

Waterland, R.A. and Jirtle, R.L. (2004). Early nutrition, epigenetic changes at transposons and imprinted genes, and enhanced susceptibility to adult chronic diseases. *Nutrition 63*, 63–68.

Weinstein, S.J., Vogt, T.M., and Gerrior, S.A. (2004). Healthy eating index scores are associated with blood nutrient concentrations in the third national health and nutrition examination survey. *J. Am. Diet. Assoc. 104*, 576–584.

Willett, W.C. and Colditz, G.A. (1998). Approaches for conducting large cohort studies. *Epidemiol. Rev. 20*, 91–99.

Willett, W.C., Howe, G.R., and Kushi, L.H. (1997). Adjustment for total energy intake in epidemiologic studies. *Am. J. Clin. Nutr. Suppl. 65*, 1220S–1228S; discussion 1229S–1231S.

76

Methods for Studying Hearing Impairment and Auditory Problems of the Aged

Robert D. Frisina and D. Robert Frisina

Age-related hearing loss—presbycusis—is the foremost communication disorder of our elderly, and one of their top three chronic medical conditions. Currently, there are no cures for the sensorineural hearing loss and auditory processing problems that affect the majority of persons over age 60. We hope that increased basic research with animal models coupled with human clinical studies will lead to breakthrough translational studies aimed at prevention and eventual biomedical cure. The present chapter reviews a variety of effective procedures for measuring hearing loss as a function of age, including both classical and experimental paradigms. A theme of this exposition is that by utilizing key testing procedures, we can gain an understanding about how age and age-related ototoxic insults and conditions can affect either the cochlea (portion of the inner ear used for hearing) or the central auditory system (portions of the brain used for hearing).

Human Investigations

AUDITORY SENSITIVITY: AUDIOGRAMS, NOISE THRESHOLDS, SPEECH DISCRIMINATION

A classic sign and symptom of age-related hearing loss in human listeners and patients is a gradual decline of hearing sensitivity in the higher frequencies, oftentimes beginning in the middle-age years. The classic manner in which hearing sensitivity is measured results in a *pure-tone audiogram*, and is the basic measurement of hearing sensitivity performed by all audiologists. In producing the audiogram, thresholds to single tones are measured by asking the subject or listener to respond when a tone of a certain frequency is detected. In a standard audiogram, measurements are made at discrete frequencies from 250 Hz up to 4 kHz. For research purposes, or early diagnosis of presbycusis, ultra-high frequency audiograms can be measured. In such cases the test frequencies can go as high as 20 kHz and require special audiometer calibration and headphones. Audiometric frequencies at 6 and 8 kHz are particularly useful for early diagnosis and research (Tadros *et al.*, 2005), and frequencies up to 14 kHz can be useful for experimental studies of age-related hearing loss in humans.

Overall sensitivity of the ear can be measured using wideband signals such as white noise, speech-weighted noise, and speech sounds themselves, to determine threshold sensitivity. The most commonly used speech measure is called the *speech reception threshold* (SRT). Audiologists use two-syllable words with equal stress, called spondees, to determine one's speech reception threshold. The SRT correlates highly with speech-frequency pure tone audiogram averages. Speech discrimination tests, as contrasted with SRT, are suprathreshold measures that test the capacity of the cochlea to resolve speech sounds in quiet conditions. A commonly used standardized test is the Northwestern University (NU-6), consisting of 50 words in each of several lists. Each word contains three phonemes in a consonant–vowel–consonant format. The phoneme distribution in each word list approximates the frequency of occurrence of each phoneme in everyday speech. This test is routinely administered in quiet at an intensity level of 30 dB greater than the SRT level, a condition that is characteristic of conversational speech in quiet environments. Old adults with mild or moderate degrees of sensorineural hearing loss are expected to do well on this measure; thus it is a valuable screening tool used to detect unique aberrations that might occur in a given case. Performance in noisy environments involves more than the cochlea and cannot be predicted from this measure in quiet; therefore, additional tests are designed to measure more closely the ability to communicate in everyday noise environments.

OUTER HAIR CELL SYSTEM: OTOACOUSTIC EMISSIONS—TRANSIENT, DISTORTION PRODUCT

There are two types of hair cells in the auditory portion of the mammalian inner ear. There is one row of *inner hair cells* that spiral from the cochlear base to the apex, and generally three rows of *outer hair cells* in the cochlear

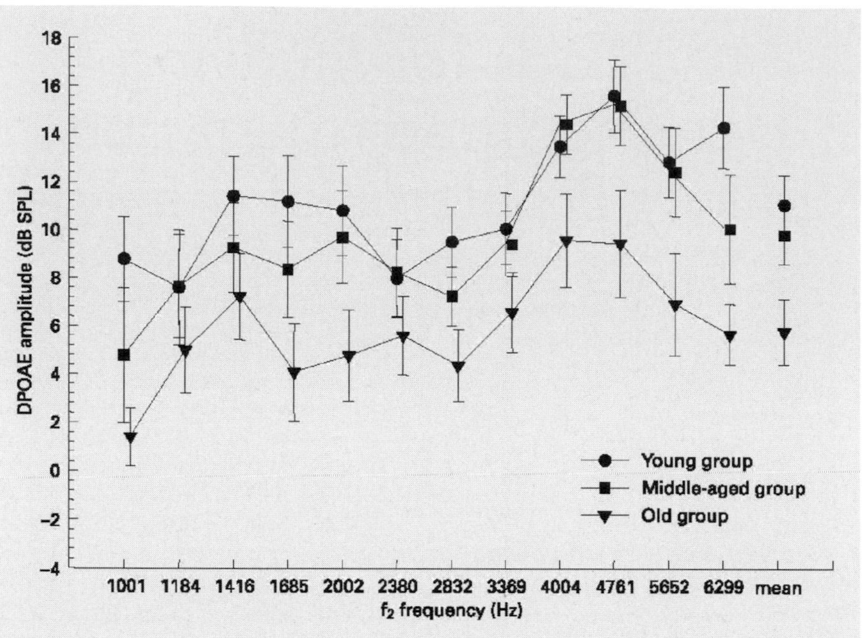

Figure 76.1 In the 1–6 kHz frequency range, DPOAE amplitudes decline with age, particularly from middle age to old age. For all three age groups, the greatest amplitudes are in the 4–5 kHz region, which is the region showing the greatest decline in DPOAE amplitudes from middle to old age. The values on the right side of the graph are the mean values for the three age groups, across all of the frequencies tested. Error bars represent standard errors of the mean (S.E.M.). From Kim *et al.* (2002), with permission.

spiral. Inner hair cells provide the main channels through which we hear; that is, they carry sound information from the cochlea to those portions of the brain used for hearing. About 95% of the auditory nerve fibers in the eighth cranial nerve form synapses with inner hair cells. In contrast, outer hair cells provide nonlinear electro-hydro-mechanical inputs to the inner hair cells that make the latter much more sensitive to quiet sounds and neuroethologically-relevant complex vocalizations such as speech, and allow them to participate more fully in neural feedback loops from the brain to the ear.

Otoacoustic emissions are faint sounds originating from the outer hair cells of the cochlea that can be recorded from the external ear canal (Kemp, 1978). They are sometimes produced spontaneously, but the most common recording procedure is when sounds are put into the ear, and then on a msec time scale, otoacoustic emissions are produced by the outer hair cells in response to the input sounds. When acoustic clicks are used to elicit the otoacoustic emissions, these physiological responses are referred to as *transient-evoked otoacoustic emissions*—TEOAEs. When two tones are presented at the same time, the nonlinear properties of the outer hair cell system produce distortion product frequencies, such as cubic or quadratic distortion products, that are not present in the original acoustic stimulus. The most commonly used *distortion-product otoacoustic emission* (DPOAE) is the 2F1-F2 component, where F1 and F2 are two frequencies at an optimal frequency ratio. Otoacoustic emissions are quite advantageous for measuring the health and well-being of the outer hair cell system because they are unbiased neurophysiological measurements that can be obtained rapidly in a noninvasive manner (no surgery required), relatively easily in human subjects (no anesthetic required) or animal models, including rodents and higher mammals (short-acting light anesthetic required). It is well established that otoacoustic emission amplitudes decline with age, as outer hair cells are lost in the aging process prior to the loss of inner hair cells, as shown in Figures 76.1 and 76.2

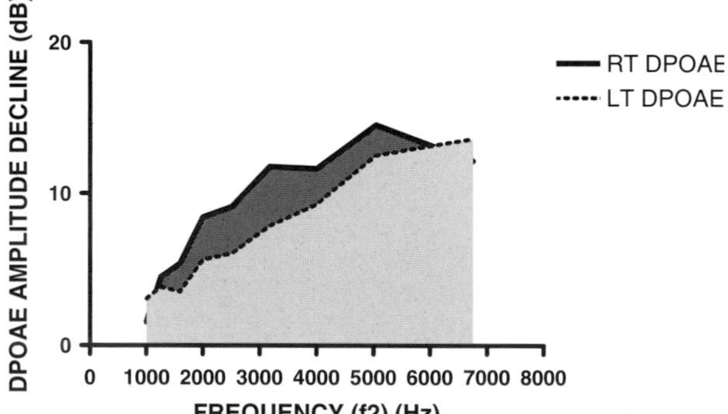

Figure 76.2 In a study of otoacoustic emissions in aged subjects with and without a sloping, presbycusis audiogram, a significant difference in DPOAE amplitudes was found between the normal hearing group relative to the presbycusis group. In the subjects with the high-frequency sloping hearing loss, the right ear DPOAE amplitude declines more than the left ear decline re the normal hearing aged controls, especially in the f2 = 2–5 kHz region. From Tadros *et al.* (2005), with permission.

(Lonsbury-Martin *et al.*, 1990, 1991; Stover and Norton, 1993; Tadros *et al.*, 2005).

EFFERENT FEEDBACK SYSTEM: CONTRALATERAL SUPPRESSION OF OTOACOUSTIC EMISSIONS

The *ascending* auditory system (afferent) processes information from the cochlea as this information travels from the inner ear to the brainstem, and then to the higher centers of the brain including the medial geniculate body of the thalamus, and on to the auditory cortex where perception of sounds takes place. Along with this ascending portion of the system, there are nerve cells in the brain that can also send information from the brain *back to the inner ear*. This *descending* part of the auditory system, sometimes referred to as the *efferent system*, can modulate the auditory information processed in the cochlea. For example, in the presence of loud sounds or background noise, the outputs of the cochlea can be reduced when the nerve cells of the efferent system become active.

We can measure the strength of the auditory efferent system by recording the amplitudes of otoacoustic emissions, both in the presence or absence of sounds or noise presented to the opposite (contralateral) ear. When the amplitudes of otoacoustic emissions are reduced in one ear (ipsilateral ear) due to the presence of sound stimulation in the other ear (contralateral ear), the efferent system has been activated. The greater the decrease in the amplitude of these emissions, the greater the strength and health of the descending auditory efferent system. Since the health and abilities of the cochlea for processing important sounds such as speech depend partly on the efficacy of the auditory efferent system, measuring the operation of this system with age is useful and important. For example, for human subjects, Kim *et al.* (2002) discovered that the auditory efferent system begins to lose its capabilities in middle age, and is almost completely inoperative in most old subjects (see Figure 76.3).

They discovered this by testing human subjects (young adult, middle age, and old) who had audiometric thresholds in the normal hearing range on standard hearing tests as well as DPOAEs in quiet and in the presence of contralateral noise. This is a case where the inner ears of these subjects had normal sensitivity (audiograms in the normal range), but there was clearly an age-related problem in the central auditory system, at least for those portions of the brain associated with the efferent system. Taken together, otoacoustic emissions along with the *contralateral suppression* (CS) of otoacoustic emissions provide information on the operating status of the ear–peripheral auditory system, and the brain–auditory feedback system, respectively.

TIMING (TEMPORAL) AND FREQUENCY (SPECTRAL) PROCESSING: GAP DETECTION, AMPLITUDE MODULATION

For human subjects, auditory psychophysics (psychoacoustics) can provide perceptual information about the system as a whole. Psychoacousticians make careful

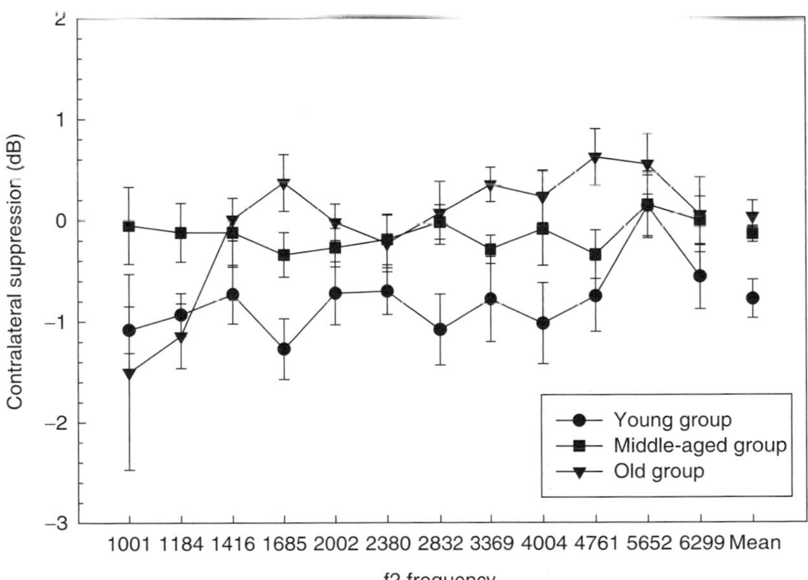

Figure 76.3 Mean magnitude of contralateral suppression (CS) as a function of f2 frequency (Hz) in three age groups. CS of DPOAEs, mediated by the medial olivocochlear system, declined with age. The most dramatic age-related decline occurred in middle age, with further declines occurring in old age. Note that greater amounts of CS are indicated by negative values. Notice that the least suppression occurs in the 4–6 kHz region for the young and old groups, where the DPOAEs have maximal magnitudes for all three age groups (see Figure 76.1). The values on the right side of the graph are the mean values for the three age groups across all of the test frequencies. From Kim *et al.* (2002), with permission.

measurements of fine acoustic features under different listening conditions, and for the present purposes, in subjects of different ages. A standard stimulus for auditory studies of temporal processing is a silent gap between two sounds, with the task referred to as *gap detection*. Here the subject or listener will usually listen to a standard sound without a gap, followed (or preceded) rapidly with two sounds separated by a short temporal gap. From trial-to-trial, the task can be made easier by lengthening the gap, or more difficult by shortening the gap. The subject's task is to identify which sound stimulus contains the temporal gap. Threshold is attained when the subject achieves a specified correct percentage of responses. Depending on the frequencies of the sounds composing the gap, young adult subjects with normal hearing can detect gaps as short as about one msec. It has been found that with age, gap detection thresholds become larger; that is, a longer gap is required by older subjects for correct identification than by young adults with normal hearing (Snell and Frisina, 2000; Snell *et al.*, 2002). Declines in auditory temporal processing are worsened by the extent of hearing loss as measured in a subject's audiogram (Gordon-Salant and Fitzgibbons, 1993; Fitzgibbons and Gordon-Salant, 1996). Very little is known about how processing of rapid changes in sound amplitude–amplitude modulation, or how frequency selectivity changes with age alone in human listeners, although these measures have been used extensively to document temporal and spectral processing deficits associated with hearing loss in young adults.

SPEECH PROCESSING IN NOISE: SPEECH IN NOISE (SPIN), HEARING IN NOISE TEST (HINT)

Psychoacousticians and research audiologists interested in the capabilities of the auditory system in more natural, realistic acoustic situations employ hearing measurement tests that assess the ability of the listener to understand speech in background noise. Two of the most useful, commonly used rigorous procedures for measuring speech comprehension in background noise are the SPIN test and HINT.

These tests involve the presentation of speech signals in different levels of background noise. In the SPIN test, the background noise is a calibrated recording of multi-talker babble—the simultaneous speaking of a group of male and female adult voices, where the voice of any one particular person is not discernible. The SPIN test, administered under headphones, measures each ear independently, whereas the HINT is administered in the free field and utilizes both ears simultaneously. In the HINT, the background noise is a speech-weighted noise devoid of any semantic content. The initial test conditions for the HINT involve having the speech signal and background noise come from the same position, N0, which is directly in front of the subject. The effect of spatial separation of speech and noise is measured in the HINT. Both tests have been useful measures of the aging auditory system where speech comprehension in background noise was being investigated. For example, Frisina and Frisina (1997), by utilizing the SPIN with human subjects whose audiograms were in the normal hearing range, discovered that aged subjects performed worse in background noise than younger adult subjects. In addition, the effect of sensorineural hearing loss was revealed when age-matched old subjects with different degrees of hearing loss were compared with old subjects within the normal range of hearing. This important study demonstrated that (1) age alone could negatively influence speech recognition in a noise background, and (2) hearing loss itself could result in a decline in speech recognition when measured in a noise background.

SPATIAL PROCESSING: HEARING IN NOISE TEST (HINT)

In addition to testing a subject's ability to understand speech in background noise, the HINT also has spatial processing components to it. Specifically, three main spatial processing conditions typically are utilized: N0, where the speech and noise come from the same position directly in front of the listener; N90, where the speech comes from in front, but the background noise emanates from a location to the right, 90° from center; and N270, where the noise comes from 90° left of center. If responses to speech differ between these locations, it implicates properties or problems due to the brainstem portion of the central auditory system where *binaural processing* occurs; that is, at the level of the superior olivary complex or auditory midbrain.

EAR AND BRAINSTEM PHYSIOLOGICAL PROCESSING: AUDITORY BRAINSTEM RESPONSE

The most commonly used neurophysiological measure of both peripheral and central (brainstem) auditory processing is the *auditory brainstem response* (ABR). This noninvasive auditory-evoked potential procedure reflects the integrity of the inner ear and brainstem auditory system extending from the auditory nerve to the level of the lateral lemniscus, just posterior or ventral to the auditory midbrain–inferior colliculus. Scalp electrodes record a series of early neuroelectrical potentials that follow auditory stimulation. The human ABR consists of five waves or peaks, with Waves I and V being the most prominent and useful for clinical purposes or research experiments. This procedure has gained widespread use in neonates, infants, and children who do not respond successfully to behavioral auditory threshold measurement procedures. Its limited use with the old subjects is directed to those whose standard test results suggest the possibility of brainstem tumors or eighth-nerve anomalies. If Wave I of the ABR is sufficiently large for analysis, cochlear sensitivity can be isolated and assessed independently of the brainstem activity for study of the aging auditory system. Generally, ABR latencies, such as Wave V, increase with age for both women and men (Jerger and Hall, 1980; Jerger and Johnson, 1988).

Brainstem auditory temporal processing disorders during aging have been identified in human subjects using forward masking of Wave V (Walton *et al.*, 1999). Here, the intensity of a first (masking) tone is varied to measure the time delay between the masking tone and a probe tone that follows with a variable time delay. Specifically, in humans, age will lengthen the time delay needed for a tone to recover its level due to the presence of the masking tone, thus reducing temporal resolution of the brainstem auditory system.

AUDITORY LATE AND EVENT-RELATED POTENTIALS—CEREBRAL CORTEX

Several late auditory evoked potentials can be measured with scalp recording electrodes in mammals, including humans, including N1, P2, and P3. The latter is sometimes referred to as the *P300 endogenous event-related potential* and can be elicited by an unusual (target or oddball) stimulus that is presented in the context of a standard stimulus usually being repeated many times. These cortical potentials are of higher amplitudes than ABRs, thus requiring fewer repetitions to be recorded faithfully above the electrical noise floor. There have been a number of studies of the aging auditory system employing the P300 and other auditory cortical potentials, and they generally show an increased latency and decreased amplitude with age (Swartz *et al.*, 1992, 1994).

Animal Model Techniques

AUDITORY SENSITIVITY: ABR AUDIOGRAMS, NOISE THRESHOLDS

These threshold sensitivity measures using pure tones or wideband noise bursts are similar to the ABR neurophysiological measures as described earlier for humans. Their major advantage for animal applications is that the basic sensitivity of the peripheral and brainstem auditory systems can be measured relatively easily and quickly, especially as compared to classical behavioral paradigms such as operant conditioning techniques. However, unlike human adults, but similar to infants or some young children, the animal needs to be anesthetized for a period of 30 to 60 minutes to assess the full frequency range of hearing in most mammals. So, although this procedure utilizes surface electrodes and is noninvasive, the animal will require a short-acting anesthetic, either inhalation or intraperitoneal injection, to reduce muscle-related electrical activity to the level where the small neural brain signals can be picked up above the electrical background noise (noise floor). Since anesthetics reduce homeostatic body temperature control, mammals undergoing ABR recordings must be kept on a heating pad, oftentimes used in conjunction with a thermometer for servo-control feedback. Age-related changes in peripheral and brainstem auditory sensitivity have been well-documented utilizing ABRs. For example, different inbred strains of mice lose their hearing at different rates, which has been measured using the mammalian ABR audiogram (Hunter and Willott, 1987; Jacobson *et al.*, 2003). An example of this age-related loss in ABR sensitivity is shown in Figure 76.4, highlighting sex differences for the CBA strain of mouse that loses its hearing slowly, like most human cases of presbycusis (Guimaraes *et al.*, 2004).

Suprathreshold ABR amplitudes also decline with age in strains of mice that have been frequently employed in studies on the neural bases of presbycusis—CBA, C57 (Henry and Lepkowski, 1978; Walton *et al.*, 1995).

OUTER HAIR CELL SYSTEM: OTOACOUSTIC EMISSIONS—TRANSIENT, DISTORTION PRODUCT

As in human subjects, the presentation of two simultaneous tones with a specific frequency ratio (DPOAE) or the presentation of a train of clicks (TEOAE) can be employed to obtain an objective neurophysiological assessment of the cochlear outer hair cell system as a function of animal age. Also like ABRs, adult human subjects can have their otoacoustic emissions measured by relaxing in a comfortable chair, whereas mammals need to receive a short-acting anesthetic to achieve the level of reduced muscle activity and twitching (sleep) necessary to obtain good ear canal recordings for the otoacoustic emissions waveforms. Like humans, the amplitudes of otoacoustic emissions decline in aging mammals, in a manner proportionate to the loss of cochlear outer hair cells with age, usually starting at the cochlear base that corresponds to the place that codes higher frequencies (Spongr *et al.*, 1997; Jacobson *et al.*, 2003). An example of DPOAE amplitude that declines as a function of age for female and male CBA mice is provided in Figure 76.5 (Guimaraes *et al.*, 2004).

EFFERENT FEEDBACK SYSTEM: CONTRALATERAL SUPPRESSION OF OTOACOUSTIC EMISSIONS

As described earlier in the section on contralateral suppression (CS) in human subjects, presentation of an acoustic stimulus to the contralateral ear can suppress the amplitude of the ipsilateral otoacoustic emissions via the physiological effects of the auditory efferent feedback system whose nerve cell bodies originate in the superior olivary complex of the brainstem auditory system. Jacobson *et al.* (2003) performed the analogous experiment in CBA mice that Kim *et al.* (2002) conducted in human subjects and made a similar discovery: Significant age-related declines in CS magnitudes occur in middle-aged mice, prior to the onset of major declines in the amplitudes of otoacoustic emissions and elevations in ABR audiogram tone thresholds that are characteristic of old age.

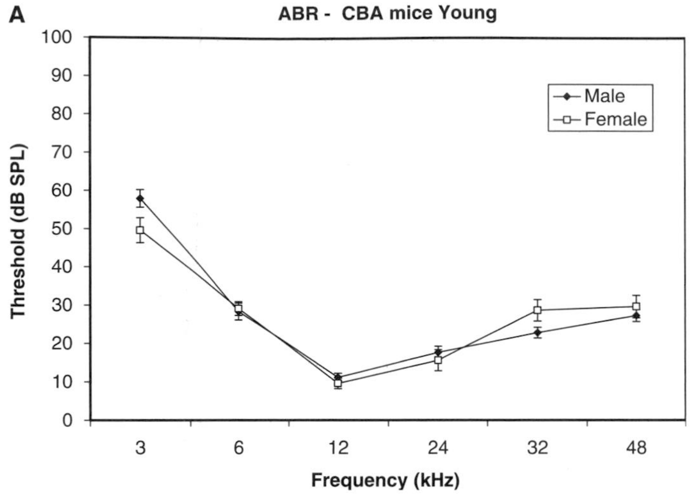

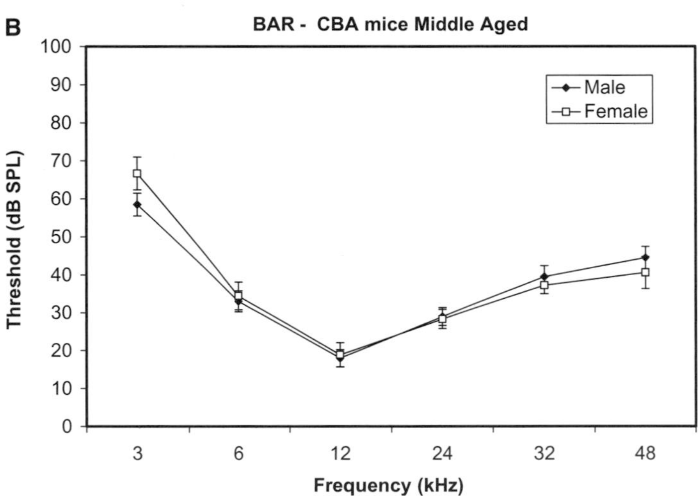

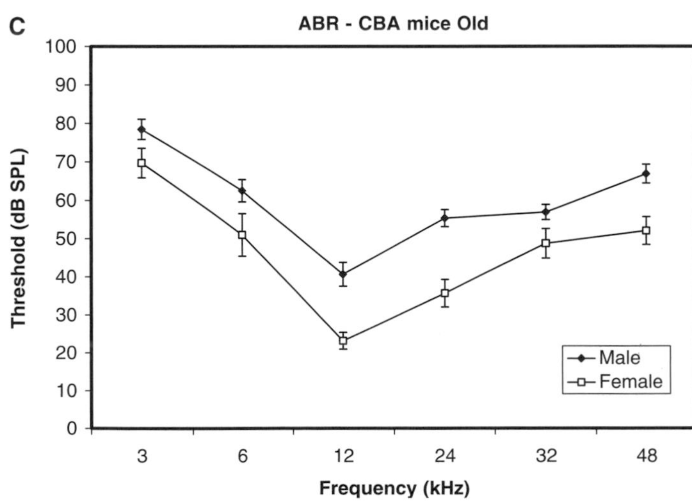

Figure 76.4 ABR recordings were made from CBA mice. ABR thresholds were measured for frequencies of 3, 6, 12, 24, 32, and 48 kHz. Young adult mice have good sensitivity up to 48 kHz, with the best sensitivity in the 5–30 kHz range, and no male/female differences. As mice age, sensitivity declines, and CBA mice tend to have relatively good hearing sensitivity even in old age. **A.** Young adult thresholds. **B.** Middle-aged data show few differences between the sexes. **C.** Old recordings show lower thresholds for females, but this difference was not statistically significant. From Guimaraes *et al.* (2004), with permission.

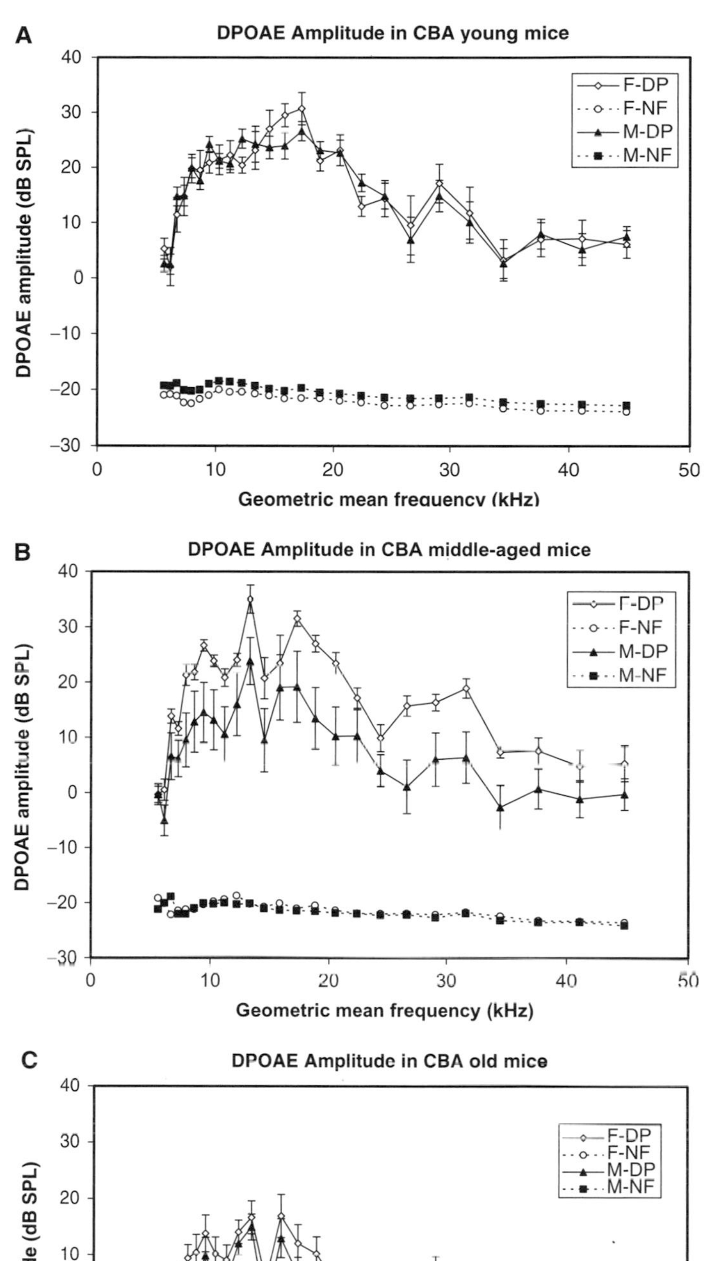

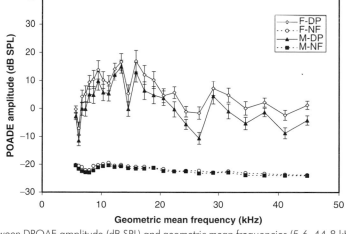

Figure 76.5 Relationships between DPOAE amplitude (dB SPL) and geometric mean frequencies (5.6–44.8 kHz) in three age groups of CBA mice, including the mean noise floor across the testing frequencies. **A.** Young adult group—similar amplitudes for both sexes. **B.** Middle-aged group—the females presented with higher DPOAE amplitude than males. The findings were confirmed with a two-way ANOVA ($F=11.9$, $P < 0.001$). **C.** Old group—the DPOAE amplitudes for females were also higher than those for males with confirmation by the two-way ANOVA ($F= 5.91$, $P<0.05$). Note that the sex difference was smaller than for the middle-aged group (1B). F-DP = Female DPOAE; F-NF= Female noise floor; M-DP= Male DPOAE; and M-NF= Male noise floor. From Guimaraes *et al.* (2004), with permission.

COCHLEAR PHYSIOLOGICAL POTENTIALS

The *endocochlear potential* measures the voltage potential in *scala media*, which contains the K+ rich endolymph in the cochlea. This fluid bathes the tops of the cochlear inner and outer hair cells, and plays an important role in hair cell transduction of acoustic sound waves in the inner ear into the code of the nervous system that gets sent to the brain via the nerve fibers of the auditory division of the eighth cranial nerve. R.A. Schmiedt and coworkers have measured this potential *in vivo*, in animal models of different ages (e.g., gerbils), and found that the magnitude of this electrical potential declines with normal aging (Schmiedt and Schulte, 1992; Schulte and Schmiedt, 1992; Schmiedt, 1993). This decline is analogous to a car battery slowly going dead over time. As this battery-like voltage declines with age, the sensitivity of the inner ear decreases as measured by cochlear compound action potentials and the thresholds of auditory-nerve fibers, and the overall sensitivity of the auditory system becomes impaired (Schmiedt *et al.*, 1990; Hellstrom and Schmiedt, 1990, 1991).

TIMING (TEMPORAL) PROCESSING: INHIBITION OF ACOUSTIC STARTLE RESPONSE BEHAVIORAL GAP DETECTION

J.R. Ison and colleagues have pioneered the use of the behavioral psychology paradigm, known as the *inhibition of the startle reflex*, as a fast and reliable measure of the hearing capabilities in animals, especially for studies of the aging auditory system and determination of its neural bases (Hoffman and Ison, 1980; Ison, 1982; Ison and Hoffman, 1983; Young and Fechter, 1983; Ison and Bowen, 2000). This procedure is carried out by taking advantage of the fact that mammals will respond quickly and in an unbiased way when presented with a loud click, via a jump in the case of rodents, or with an eye blink in larger mammals including humans. The click would be akin to snapping your fingers near your ear. Ison and coworkers have demonstrated that when a warning sound is presented just before the startle stimulus (loud click), the amplitude of the rodent jump or human eye blink will be attenuated proportionately to the effectiveness or detectability of the warning sound (prepulse). This reliable, efficient measure of auditory processing is called *prepulse inhibition*. Ison's team has utilized this effectively to evaluate the temporal processing capabilities of the aging auditory system using gaps or decrements in ongoing sounds, including tones or wideband noise, as prepulse inhibition stimuli (Walton *et al.*, 1997; Ison *et al.*, 1997, 1998, 2001; Barsz *et al.*, 2002; Allen *et al.*, 2003). For example, in CBA mice the gap detection threshold significantly declines with age, and these temporal processing deficits mirror neurophysiological gap threshold changes recorded at the level of the auditory midbrain–inferior colliculus, described in more detail later.

SPATIAL PROCESSING: INHIBITION OF ACOUSTIC STARTLE RESPONSE BEHAVIORAL TESTING

Ison's research group has more recently developed a variation on the inhibition of startle research paradigm for measuring spatial processing in mice as a function of age (Allen *et al.*, 2004). Here, a mouse assumes a standard spatial position and orientation in the inhibition of startle measurement cage. When in the calibrated place, a prepulse inhibition auditory stimulus is presented from one of several possible spatial positions. By varying the location of the prepulse inhibition sound in a calibrated manner from trial to trial, auditory spatial processing capabilities of mice can be measured as a function of age and stimulus type. Indeed, the ability to correctly localize sounds in space, particularly the azimuth, declines significantly in the aging mouse.

BRAINSTEM PHYSIOLOGICAL PROCESSING: SINGLE NERVE CELL AND EVOKED POTENTIAL RECORDINGS

As presented earlier in the human sections, presbycusis involves a loss of sensitivity to sound, temporal processing deficits, and spatial tuning degradations, all of which can contribute to a difficulty understanding speech by the elderly, particularly in noisy situations. Behavioral and evoked potential work in animal models, such as mice and other rodents, confirms that most mammals develop age-related hearing problems with many similarities to the human condition, such as spatial and temporal processing deficits, that are confounded by complex acoustic environments such as those containing background noise. Physiological recordings in the auditory brainstem give insights to the neural mechanisms that may underlie these perceptual and behavioral findings.

Willott and coworkers were the first to systematically investigate changes in *tonotopic* or *cochleotopic* organizations of brainstem auditory nuclei as the high-frequency hearing loss characteristic of presbycusis progresses in mice (Willott *et al.*, 1985, 1988a, b; Willott, 1986, 1991). Tonotopic or cochleotopic organization refers to the fact that the major cell groups, or nuclei, of the brainstem auditory system have frequency organizations that originate in the cochlear spiral, where high frequency nerve cells are in one location, then middle frequency, then low frequency nerve cells in another, much like the keys on a piano. Tonotopically organized nerve cell pathways connect the cochlea to the cochlear nucleus, the first major nucleus of the central auditory system, and these pathways continue in an organized manner up through the auditory cortex, with sound information being processed at each step along the way. In aging, when the basal portions of the cochlea lose a significant number of hair cells with age, there is a concomitant loss of high frequency pathways and nerve cells in the central auditory system. Willott and colleagues discovered that

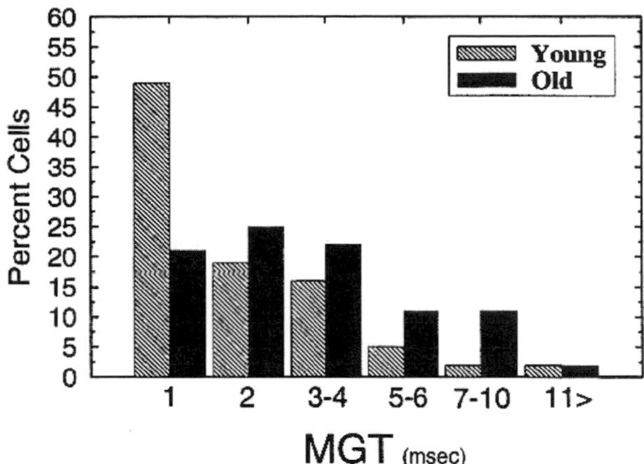

Figure 76.6 Single nerve cells in the auditory midbrain–inferior colliculus of unanaesthetized CBA mice have longer gap thresholds in old age, compared to young adults. The proportion of single nerve cells possessing minimum gap thresholds (MGTs) ranging from 1 to >11 msec are shown for young adult mice, hatched bars (N=78 cells), and for old mice, solid bars (N=108 cells). Note that the data in this histogram indicate a distribution of single-nerve cell gap thresholds to longer gaps in old age. From Walton *et al.* (1998), with permission.

when there is a loss of high frequency pathways to the auditory midbrain–inferior colliculus, the ventral portions of this region start responding to lower frequencies in the absence of the normal high frequency inputs.

Walton and coworkers have made extensive single nerve cell recordings in the inferior colliculus of old CBA mice, who still have reasonably good auditory sensitivity in old age. They have discovered that at suprathreshold sound levels where single nerve cells still give good responses, temporal processing problems can occur during aging that increase gap detection thresholds and distort responses to the onset and waveforms of biologically relevant sounds (Walton *et al.*, 1997, 1998, 2002; Simon *et al.*, 2004). Examples of some of these changes in the responses of single nerve cells are provided in Figures 76.6 and 76.7.

NEURAL BASES OF PRESBYCUSIS: NEUROANATOMY, IMMUNOCYTOCHEMISTRY, TRACT TRACING

Not surprisingly, there are neuroanatomical and neurochemical changes occurring in the auditory system with age that correlate and may underlie the behavioral and functional declines that have been discussed so far. A variety of anatomical and biochemical methodologies have been employed to examine these aspects of age-related hearing loss, and in most cases, animal models have been effectively employed.

D.M. Caspary and his colleagues conducted a comprehensive series of anatomical and biochemical experiments on the GABA system in the auditory midbrain. GABA is one of the two most prominent inhibitory neurotransmitters in the central auditory system. Caspary's group put forth some convincing evidence that there is an *age-related down-regulation* of the main GABA neurotransmitter system of the auditory midbrain (Caspary *et al.*, 1990, 1995, 1999; Helfert *et al.*, 1999). This loss of inhibition is consistent with some of the neurophysiological functional data concerning the disruption of complex sound processing in quiet and background noise characteristic of presbycusis.

Frisina and coworkers have studied certain anatomical aspects that accompany the age-related temporal processing deficits discovered by Walton's team as presented earlier. For instance, the same regions of the auditory midbrain that manifest the age-dependent temporal processing disorders also show changes in intracellular calcium regulation as investigated using immunocytochemical antibody labeling methodologies (Zettel *et al.*, 1997, 2001). *Calbindin* and *calretinin* are two of the most important calcium-binding proteins in the brain involved in intracellular calcium regulation critical for neurotransmitter synthesis and release. Calbindin was found to decline with age in the inferior colliculus, and calretinin increased with age, but only in mice with good hearing in old age. Mice deafened as young adults did not show this upregulation, indicating that it was dependent on the sound-evoked activity being present. Frisina's group also found that certain neural input pathways from the contralateral cochlear nucleus and superior olivary complex in the brainstem auditory system to the inferior colliculus showed an age-related decline using neural tract-tracing techniques (Frisina and Walton, 2001).

Conclusion

It is evident that a variety of methodologies have been effectively utilized to investigate age-related hearing loss in human listeners and for animal models. Exciting future possibilities include assessing hearing improvements using

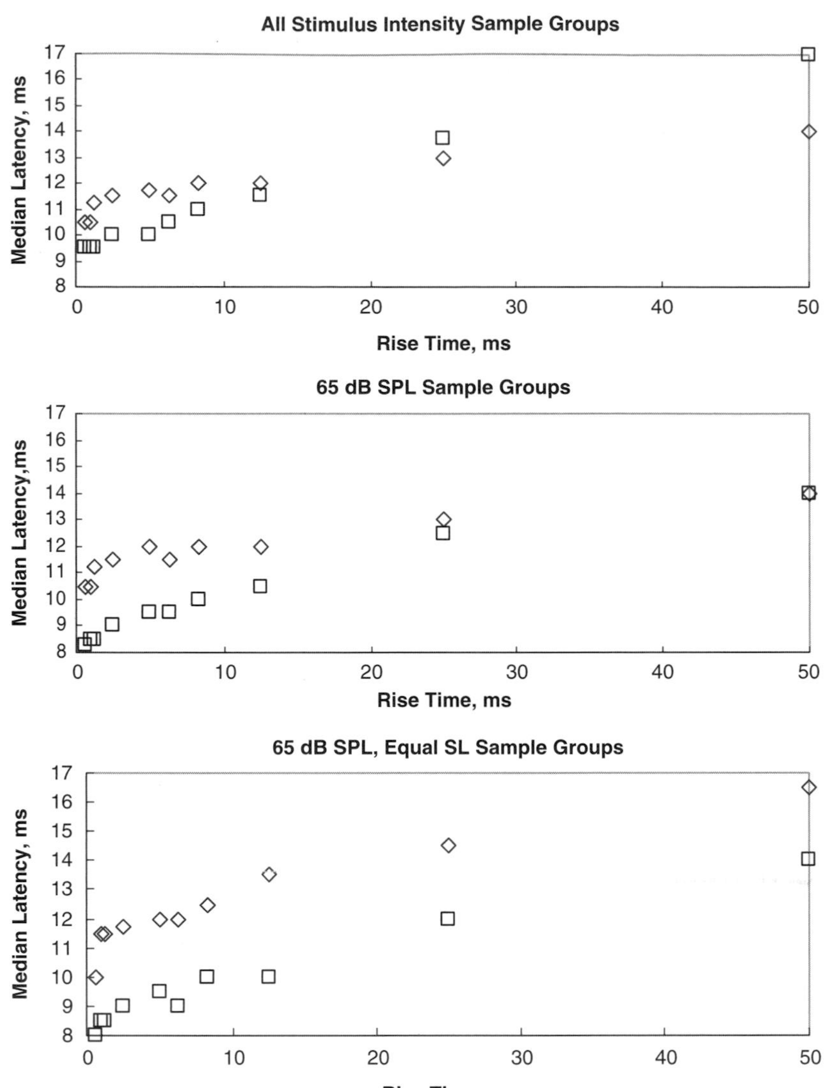

Figure 76.7 Graphs showing the relationship between median latency and sound stimulus rise time for young-adult (diamond) and old (square) single nerve cell groups containing: (A) all nerve cells analyzed; (B) nerve cells stimulated at 65 dB SPL; and (C) matched young-adult and old nerve cells stimulated at 65 dB SPL and equal sensation levels above each cell's threshold. In all cases, the nerve cells in the old animals show shorter latencies than the young adult cells. This is consistent with a loss of inhibition with age in the auditory midbrain and has implications for disruptions of complex sound coding with age. From Simon *et al.* (2004), with permission.

the most effective hearing measurement methods, first in animal rehabilitation experiments aimed at preventing or curing hearing loss and deafness with gene therapy approaches or stem cell transplantation. If in the not-so-far future this is achieved reliably in mammals, and eventually primates, then hearing assessment in human clinical trials will hopefully follow soon after that.

Recommended Resources

Frisina, R.D. (2001). Subcortical Neural Coding Mechanisms for Auditory Temporal Processing. *Hear. Res.* 158, 1–27.

Review of auditory brainstem temporal processing mechanisms and pathways, including descriptions of useful techniques and changes with age.

Gulick, W.L., Gescheider, G.A., and Frisina, R.D. (1989). *Hearing: Physiological Acoustics, Neural Coding, and Psychophysics.* New York: Oxford Univ. Press.

Good introductory text on all aspects of hearing and the anatomy and physiology of the auditory system, including many custom illustrations.

Hof, P.R. and Mobbs, C.V. (2001). *Functional Neurobiology of Aging*. San Diego: Academic Press.

Excellent overview of many aspects of the aging senses and nervous system, including eight chapters on the aging auditory system.

Willott, J.F. (1991). *Aging and the Auditory System: Anatomy, Physiology, and Psychophysics*. San Diego: Singular Publishing Group.

The best summary of research done on the aging auditory system to 1991.

Winer, J.A. and Schreiner, C.E. (2005). *The Inferior Colliculus*. New York: Springer.

Most current compilation of research done on the auditory midbrain and some other brainstem regions of the central auditory system.

ACKNOWLEDGMENTS

Supported by NIH Grants P01 AG09524 from the Nat. Inst. on Aging, P30 DC05409 from the Nat. Inst. on Deafness and Communication Disorders, and the International Center for Hearing and Speech Research, Rochester, NY.

REFERENCES

Allen, P.D., Burkard, R.F., Ison, J.R., and Walton, J.P. (2003). Impaired gap encoding in aged mouse inferior colliculus at moderate but not high stimulus levels. *Hear. Res. 186*, 17–29.

Allen, P.D., Rivoli, P.J., and Ison, J.R. (2004). Possible interaction between KCNA1 genotype and aging on auditory spatial discrimination in the mouse. *Assoc. Res. Otolaryngol. Abstr. 27*, 88.

Barsz, K., Ison, J.R., Snell, K.B., and Walton, J.P. (2002). Behavioral and neural measures of auditory temporal acuity in aging humans and mice. *Neurobiol. Aging 23*, 565–578.

Caspary, D.M., Holder, T.M., Hughes, L.F., Milbrandt, J.C., McKernan, R.M., and Naritoku, D.K. (1999). Age-related changes in GABA receptor subunit composition and function in rat auditory system. *Neurosci. 93*, 307–312.

Caspary, D.M., Milbrandt, J.C, and Helfert, R.H. (1995). Central auditory aging: GABA changes in the inferior colliculus. *Exp. Gerontol. 30*, 349–360.

Caspary, D.M., Raza, A., Armour, B.A.L. Pippin, J., and Arneric, S.P. (1990). Immunocytochemical and neurochemical evidence for age-related loss of GABA in the inferior colliculus: Implications for neural presbycusis. *J. Neurosci. 10*, 2363–2372.

Fitzgibbons, P.J. and Gordon-Salant, S. (1996). Auditory temporal processing in elderly listeners. *J. Am. Acad. Audiol. 7*, 183–189.

Frisina, D.R. and Frisina, R.D. (1997). Speech recognition in noise and presbycusis: Relations to possible neural sites. *Hear. Res. 106*, 95–104.

Frisina, R.D. and Walton, J.P. (2001). Aging of the mouse central auditory system. In J.P. Willott (Ed.), *Handbook of Mouse Auditory Research: From Behavior to Molecular Biology*, pp. 339–379. New York: CRC Press.

Gordon-Salant, S. and Fitzgibbons, P.J. (1993). Temporal factors and speech recognition performance in young and elderly listeners. *J. Speech Hear. Res. 36*, 1276–1285.

Guimaraes, P. Zhu, X., Cannon, T., Kim, S-H., and Frisina, R.D. (2004). Sex differences in distortion product otoacoustic emissions as a function of age in CBA mice. *Hear. Res. 192*, 83–89.

Helfert, R.H., Sommer, T.J., Meeks, J., Hofstetter, P., and Hughes, L.F. (1999). Age-related synaptic changes in the central nucleus of the inferior colliculus of Fischer-344 rats. *J. Comp. Neurol. 406*, 285–298.

Hellstrom, L.I. and Schmiedt, R.A. (1990). Compound action potential input/output functions in young and quiet-aged gerbils. *Hear. Res. 50*, 163–174.

Hellstrom, L.I. and Schmiedt, R.A. (1991). Rate/level functions of auditory nerve fibers in young and quiet-aged gerbils. *Hear. Res. 53*, 217–222.

Henry, K.P. and Lepkowski, C. (1978). Evoked potential correlates of genetic progressive hearing loss: Age-related changes from the ear to inferior colliculus of C57Bl/6 and CBA/J mice. *Acta Otolaryngol. 86*, 366–374.

Hoffman, H.S. and Ison, J.R. (1980). Principles of reflex modification in the domain of startle: I. Some empirical findings and their implications for the interpretation of how the nervous system processes sensory input. *Psychol. Rev. 87*, 175–189.

Hunter, K.P. and Willott, J.F. (1987). Aging and the auditory brainstem response in mice with severe or minimal presbycusis. *Hear. Res. 30*, 207–218.

Ison, J.R. (1982). Temporal acuity in auditory function in the rat: Reflex inhibition by brief gaps in noise. *J. Comp. Physiol. Psychol. 96*, 945–954.

Ison, J.R., Agrawal, P., Pak, J., and Vaughn, W.J. (1998). Changes in temporal acuity with age and with hearing impairment in the mouse: A study of the acoustic startle reflex and its inhibition by brief decrements in noise level. *J. Acoust. Soc. Am. 104*, 1689–1695.

Ison, J.R. and Bowen, G.P. (2000). Scopolamine reduces sensitivity to auditory gaps in the rat, suggesting a cholinergic contribution to temporal acuity. *Hear. Res. 145*, 169–176.

Ison, J.R., Bowen, G.P., Pak, J., and Gutierrez, E. (1997). Changes in the strength of prepulse inhibition with variation in the startle baseline associated with individual differences and with old age in rats and mice. *Psychobiol. 25*, 266–274.

Ison, J.R. and Hoffman, H.S. (1983). Reflex modification in the domain of startle: II. The anomalous history of a robust and ubiquitous phenomenon. *Psychol. Bull. 94*, 3–17.

Ison, J.R., Walton, J.P., Frisina, R.D., and O'Neill, W.E. (2001). Elicitation and inhibition of the startle reflex by acoustic transients: Studies of age-related changes in temporal processing. In J.P. Willott (Ed.), *Handbook of Mouse Auditory Res: From Behavior to Molecular Biology*, pp. 381–387. New York: CRC Press.

Jacobson M., Kim S.H., Romney J., Zhu X., and Frisina R.D. (2003). Contralateral suppression of distortion-product otoacoustic emissions declines with age: A comparison of findings in CBA mice with human listeners. *Laryngoscope 113*, 1707–1713.

Jerger, J. and Hall, J. (1980). Effects of age and sex on auditory brainstem response. *Arch. Otolaryngol. 106*, 387–391.

Jerger, J. and Johnson, K. (1988). Interactions of age, gender, and sensorineural hearing loss on ABR latency. *Ear Hear. 9*, 168–176.

Kemp, D.T. (1978). Stimulated otoacoustic emissions from within the human auditory system. *J. Acoust. Soc. Am. 64*, 1386–1391.

Kim, S.H., Frisina, D.R., and Frisina, R.D. (2002). Effects of age on contralateral suppression of distortion-product otoacoustic emissions in human listeners with normal hearing. *Audiol. Neuro-Otol. 7*, 348–357.

Lonsbury-Martin, B.L., Harris, F.P., Stagner, B.B., Hawkins, M.A., and Martin, G.K. (1990). Distortion product emissions in humans: I. Basic properties in normally hearing subjects. *Ann. Otol. Rhinol. Laryngol. Suppl. 147*, 3–14.

Lonsbury-Martin, B.L., Cutler, W.M., and Martin, G.K. (1991). Evidence for the influence of aging on distortion product otoacoustic emissions in humans. *J. Acoust. Soc. Am. 89*, 1749–1759.

Schmiedt, R.A. (1993). Cochlear potentials in gerbils: Does the aging cochlea need a jump start? In R.T. Verrillo (Ed.), *Sensory Research: Multimodal Perspectives*, pp. 91–103. Hillsdale, NJ: Erlbaum Assoc.

Schmiedt, R.A. (1996). Effects of aging on potassium homeostasis and the endocochlear potential in the gerbil cochlea. *Hear. Res. 102*, 125–132.

Schmiedt, R.A., Mills, J.H., and Adams, J.A. (1990). Tuning and suppression in auditory nerve fibers of aged gerbils raised in quiet or noise. *Hear. Res. 45*, 221–236.

Schmiedt, B.A. and Schulte, B.A. (1992). Physiologic and histopathologic changes in quiet- and noise-aged gerbil cochleas. In A.L. Dancer, D. Henderson, R.J. Salvi, and R.P. Hamernik (Eds.), *Noise-induced Hearing Loss*, pp. 246–256. St. Louis: Mosby.

Schulte, B.A. and Schmiedt, R.A. (1992). Lateral wall Na: K-ATPase and endocochlear potentials decline with age in quiet-reared gerbils. *Hear. Res. 61*, 35–46.

Simon, H., Frisina, R.D., and Walton, J.P. (2004). Age reduces response latency of mouse inferior colliculus neurons to AM sounds. *J. Acoust. Soc. Am. 116*, 469–477.

Snell, K.B. and Frisina, D.R. (2000). Relations among age-related differences in gap detection and speech perception. *J. Acoust. Soc. Am. 107*, 1615–1626.

Snell, K.B., Mapes, F.M., Hickman, E.D., and Frisina, D.R. (2002). Word recognition in competing babble and the effects of age, temporal processing, and absolute sensitivity. *J. Acoust. Soc. Am. 112*, 720–727.

Spongr, V.P., Flood, D.G., Frisina, R.D., and Salvi, R.J. (1997). Quantitative measures of hair cell loss in CBA and C57B1/6 mice throughout their life spans. *J. Acoust. Soc. Am. 101*, 3546–3553.

Stover, L. and Norton, S.J. (1993). The effects of aging on otoacoustic emissions. *J. Acoust. Soc. Am. 94*, 2670–2681.

Swartz, K.P., Walton, J.P., Hantz, E.C., Goldhammer, E., Crummer, G.C., and Frisina, R.D. (1994). P3 event-related potentials and performance of young and old subjects for music perception tasks. *Int. J. Neurosci. 78*, 223–239.

Swartz, K.P., Walton, J.P., Crummer, G.C., Hantz, E.C., and Frisina, R.D. (1992). P3 event-related potentials and performance of healthy old and Alzheimer's dementia subjects for music perception tasks. *Psychomusicol. 11*, 96–118.

Tadros, S., Frisina, S.T., Mapes, F., Kim, S-H., Frisina, D.R., and Frisina, R.D. (2005). Loss of peripheral right ear advantage in age-related hearing loss. *Audiol. Neuro-Otol., 10*, 44–52.

Walton, J.P., Frisina, R.D., and Meierhans, L.R. (1995). Sensorineural hearing loss effects recovery from short term adaptation in the CBA and C57 mouse models of presbycusis. *Hear. Res. 88*, 19–26.

Walton, J.P., Frisina, R.D., Ison, J.E., and O'Neill, W.E. (1997). Neural correlates of behavioral gap detection in the inferior colliculus of the young CBA mouse. *J. Comp. Physiol. A. 181*, 161–176.

Walton, J.P., Frisina, R.D., and O'Neill, W.E. (1998). Age-related alterations in processing of temporal sound features in the auditory midbrain of the CBA mouse. *J. Neurosci. 18*, 2764–2776.

Walton, J.P., Orlando, M., and Burkard, R. (1999). Auditory brainstem response forward-masking recovery functions in old humans with normal hearing. *Hear. Res. 127*, 86–94.

Walton, J.P., Simon, H., and Frisina, R.D. (2002). Age-related alterations in the neural coding of envelope periodicities. *J. Neurophysiol. 88*, 565–578.

Willott, J.F. (1986). Effects of aging, hearing loss, and anatomical location on thresholds of inferior colliculus neurons in C57BL/6 and CBA mice. *J. Neurophysiol. 56*, 391–408.

Willott, J.F. (1991). *Aging and the Auditory System: Anatomy, Physiology, and Psychophysics*. San Diego: Singular Pub. Group.

Willott, J.F., Parham, K., and Hunter, K.P. (1988a). Response properties of inferior colliculus neurons in young and very old CBA/J mice. *Hear. Res. 37*, 1–14.

Willott, J.F., Parham, K., and Hunter, K.P. (1988b). Response properties of inferior colliculus neurons in middle-aged C57Bl/6J mice with presbycusis. *Hear. Res. 37*, 15–28.

Willott, J.F., Pankow, D., Hunter, K.P., and Kordyban, M. (1985). Projections from the anterior ventral cochlear nucleus to the central nucleus of the inferior colliculus in young and aging C57Bl/6 mice. *J. Comp. Neurol. 237*, 545–551.

Young, J. and Fechter, L.D. (1983). Reflex inhibition procedures for animal audiometry: A technique for assessing ototoxicity. *J. Acoust. Soc. Am. 73*, 1686–1693.

Zettel, M.L., Frisina, R.D., Haider, S.E.A., and O'Neill, W.E. (1997). Age-related changes in calbindin D-28K and calretinin immunoreactivity in the inferior colliculus of CBA/CaJ and C57B1/6 mice. *J. Comp. Neurol. 386*, 92–110.

Zettel, M.L., O'Neill, W.E., Trang, T.T., and Frisina, R.D. (2001). Early bilateral deafening prevents calretinin up-regulation in the dorsal cortex of the inferior colliculus of aged CBA/CaJ mice. *Hear. Res. 158*, 131–138.

77

A Model for Understanding the Pathomechanics of Osteoarthritis in Aging

Thomas P. Andriacchi and Annegret Mündermann

Osteoarthritis occurs in the majority of adults and is often described as "wear and tear" arthritis, or a disease of aging resulting from the structural and biochemical breakdown of articular cartilage in synovial joints. The causes of degenerative osteoarthritis with aging are complex and involve interrelated biological, mechanical, and structural pathways. This chapter examines the interrelationship or coupling of these pathways that converges at an in vivo *systems level in humans. Using the knee as an example, an integrated* in vivo *framework for understanding the various factors that influence the initiation and progression of osteoarthritis is described. This framework provides a basis for explaining the role of kinematics and load on the progression of osteoarthritis. The framework helps to explain the integrated effect of biological, morphological, and neuromuscular changes to the musculoskeletal system during aging or during menopause on the increased rate of idiopathic osteoarthritis with aging.*

Introduction

Arthritis is the most common type of joint disease and comprises a heterogeneous group of conditions that cause common histopathological and radiological changes. Osteoarthritis, often described as wear-and-tear arthritis, occurs in the majority of adults. It is a disease of aging resulting from the structural and biochemical breakdown of articular cartilage in synovial joints. The "itis" in osteoarthritis implies inflammation; however, most people with this condition do not have inflamed joints. Osteoarthrosis, defining a condition where the joints are affected by degeneration without inflammation, is probably a more accurate overall description of the condition. Nevertheless, as most people refer to the condition as osteoarthritis, this is the term used here. Osteoarthrosis and osteoarthritis are terms that are used virtually interchangeably.

The causes of degenerative osteoarthritis with aging are complex and involve interrelated biological (Lohmander *et al.*, 1999; Maniwa *et al.*, 2001; Otterness *et al.*, 2001), mechanical (Beaupré *et al.*, 2000; Carter *et al.*, 1998; Grodzinsky *et al.*, 2000; Mow and Guo, 2002; Mow and Wang, 1999), and structural (Eckstein *et al.*, 2002, Koff *et al.*, 2003; Peterfy *et al.*, 1994) pathways. The interrelationship or coupling of these pathways converges at an *in vivo* systems level in humans (see Figure 77.1).

In vivo function influences the mechanical environment of articular cartilage and the mechanobiology (Arokoski *et al.*, 2000; Sweet *et al.*, 1992; Thonar *et al.*, 1985) of the tissue. Thus, *in vivo* function is coupled to the structure and health of the joint. Patients can functionally adapt to pathological joint changes such as ligament injury or degeneration of the articular cartilage. For example, it has been observed from *in vivo* studies (Mündermann *et al.*, 2004, Prodromos *et al.*, 1985; Wang *et al.*, 1990) that some patients with knee osteoarthritis can adopt patterns of locomotion that lower the load at the knee and reduce the rate at which osteoarthritis progresses. Variations in the soft tissue properties or structure (Ateshian *et al.*, 1991; Cicuttini *et al.*, 2002) of the joint can influence the congruency and laxity of the joint and produce substantial variations in contact stress and joint motion that impact the mechanical environment of the cartilage. Cartilage adapts to mechanical stimuli (Smith *et al.*, 1995) and ultimately becomes dependent on the maintenance of that mechanical stimulus for normal tissue function (Carter and Wong, 2003). *In vitro* studies (Smith *et al.*, 1995) have shown that isolated cartilage cells (chondrocytes) can adapt to changes in their mechanical environment by changing metabolic activity in response to increased levels of certain types of stress (Beaupré *et al.*, 2000; Carter *et al.*, 1998; Grodzinsky *et al.*, 2000; Guilak and Mow, 2000). Cartilage health depends on the body's ability to maintain the equilibrium between degeneration and synthesis of cartilage constituents including collagen fibrils and proteoglycans. Chondrocytes, the cells of cartilage, retain this equilibrium by controlling enzymatic processes.

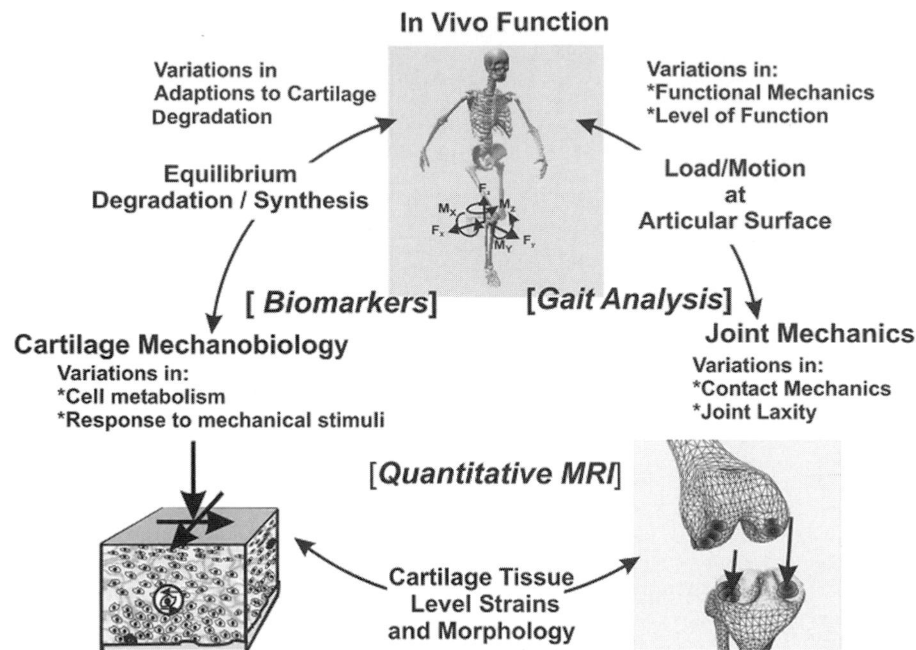

Figure 77.1 Understanding the *in vivo* response of articular cartilage to its physical environment requires an integrated view of the problem that considers functional, anatomical, and biological interactions. Gait analysis, quantitative MRI, and assays of biomarkers provide a basis for understanding the interaction between the various pathways that lead to the initiation and progression of osteoarthritis (from Andriacchi *et al.*, 2004).

DEFINITION AND TYPES OF OSTEOARTHRITIS

Any analysis of the pathomechanics of osteoarthritis must consider the various forms of the disease. In general, osteoarthritis can be categorized as idiopathic, post traumatic, and other forms of joint degeneration.

Idiopathic osteoarthritis

Idiopathic osteoarthritis occurs in previously intact joints with no apparent initiating factor or event and is related primarily to the natural aging process. Risk factors for idiopathic osteoarthritis include obesity, hormone levels, or genetics (Flores and Hochberg, 2003). Idiopathic osteoarthritis is the most common form of arthritis associated with aging. However, the rate of progression of osteoarthritis can vary substantially among different individuals with similar risk factors. The reason for variable rates of the progression of the disease with aging among seemingly similar patients has been the subject of numerous studies and will be addressed from a pathomechanical viewpoint in this chapter.

Post traumatic osteoarthritis

Post traumatic osteoarthritis is the accelerated degeneration that occurs in a joint as the direct and indirect result of injury. Following an injury to a joint, such as the rupture of the anterior cruciate ligament or a tear of a meniscus, a patient is susceptible to developing osteoarthritic changes to the joint earlier in life (Daniel *et al.*, 1994; Englund *et al.*, 2003; Roos *et al.*, 2001; Roos *et al.*, 1995; von Porat *et al.*, 2004). It is not clear whether the change in the mechanical environment or biological changes associated with the injury to the joint are the primary cause for the earlier onset of osteoarthritis, and it has been suggested (Andriacchi *et al.*, 2004) that these factors are interrelated.

Others forms of osteoarthritis

Osteoarthritis can also be caused by other conditions including gout (crystal formation in the joints), lupus (the body's defense system can harm the joints, the heart, the skin, the kidneys, and other organs), and viral hepatitis (an infection of the liver).

DEMOGRAPHICS OF OSTEOARTHRITIS

Currently, about 20 million Americans are affected by osteoarthritis, and the prevalence of osteoarthritis is two-and-a-half times that of heart disease and six times that of cancer. It is projected that by 2030, 20% of Americans—about 70 million people—will have passed their sixty-fifth birthday and will be at risk for osteoarthritis (National Institute of Arthritis, 2003). Similar percentages of most Western populations suffer from osteoarthritis (Statistisches Bundesamt Germany, 2003; Statistics Canada, 2003). The risk of developing osteoarthritis is higher in African-Americans, Hispanics, and

Asians compared to Caucasians (Escalante and del Rincón, 2001; Jordan *et al.*, 2003; Xu *et al.*, 2003).

Aging

The incidence of clinically symptomatic osteoarthritis increases with increasing age, independent of site, and for both female and male populations (Felson *et al.*, 1987; Oliveria *et al.*, 1995; Verbrugge, 1995). Biological tissues undergo significant changes during the aging process including biological changes and associated changes in mechanical properties.

Gender

Although the incidence of osteoarthritis at the knee and hip is similar in male and female populations under the age of 60 years, the incidence in females over the age of 60 years increases at a faster rate than in males over the age of 60 years (Oliveria *et al.*, 1995; Peyron *et al.*, 1993). Differences or changes in hormone levels, in part, may account for these differences, although this association is still under debate (Richette *et al.*, 2003). Estrogen, the female sex hormone, has been shown to affect biological tissue properties and turnover. For instance, in cartilage, increased estrogen levels have been related to increased matrix protein turnover (for review, see Richette *et al.* (2003)). In comparison, lower estrogen levels during adolescence may lead to increased femoral cartilage thickness and stiffness. In certain ligaments, higher estrogen levels are associated with greater stiffness (Romani *et al.*, 2003), and the maximum voluntary force per cross-sectional area in skeletal muscle dramatically declines in post-menopausal women (Phillips *et al.*, 1993). During menopause, estrogen levels decrease drastically. These reports suggest that lower estrogen levels during and after menopause may lead to lower matrix protein turnover in cartilage, greater cartilage stiffness, greater joint laxity, and lower muscle forces. These changes occur in addition to age-related physiological and morphological changes in biological tissues (see later) and may be, in part, responsible for higher incidence of idiopathic osteoarthritis in women after menopause.

Site specificity

Although osteoarthritis can affect most synovial joints of the upper and lower extremities and trunk (hand, wrist, ankle, knee, hip, neck, back), it is observed most frequently at the knee and rarely at the wrist and ankle (Neame *et al.*, 2004; Oliveria *et al.*, 1995). Potential reasons for the site specificity of osteoarthritis include structural and metabolic differences of biological tissues between joints, for instance the higher content of proteoglycans and water in cartilage and decreased catabolic and increased anabolic activity of chondrocytes at the ankle compared to the knee (Kuettner and Cole, 2005). However, co-occurrence of hand and knee osteoarthritis in the same patient (Englund *et al.*, 2004) suggests that not only local joint-specific biological and mechanical factors, but also global factors such as hereditary and environmental factors affecting the entire organism, may play a role in the development of osteoarthritis.

Cost to society

Costs to the American society associated with osteoarthritis currently exceed 80 billion dollars per year (National Institute of Arthritis, 2003). This number will increase with the increase in life expectancy and with the rapid aging of the population, especially as the baby-boomers will reach the age of 60 years within the next two decades and thus will be at greater risk of developing osteoarthritis. Currently, osteoarthritis is the sixth fastest growing disease in the United States (Forbers, 2005). Approximately two-thirds of the costs associated with osteoarthritis are indirect costs due to work loss and work disability payments (for review see Dunlop *et al.* (2003)).

THE COMPLEXITY OF OSTEOARTHRITIS

The complexity of understanding osteoarthritis is well illustrated by considering the conflicting conclusions that can be drawn from clinical and laboratory reports on the relative influence of mechanical factors on the progression of degenerative changes to the articular cartilage at the knee. For example, experimental and theoretical studies suggest that load can produce an adaptive response (thickening, enhanced mechanical properties, etc.) (Carter *et al.*, 1998; Carter and Wong, 2003) of cartilage. In contrast, clinical studies report that patients with knee osteoarthritis and higher loads at the knee during walking have a more rapid rate of cartilage breakdown than patients with lower loads (Miyazaki *et al.*, 2002; Prodromos *et al.*, 1985). Clearly, the conclusion that cartilage responds positively to increased load is in conflict with clinical observations that increased load stimulates more rapid breakdown of articular cartilage. As will be discussed later, it appears that the cartilage response to load is dependent on the health of the cartilage.

In vivo studies can provide an integrated approach that consolidates the multiple pathways associated with the cause and progression of osteoarthritis. Gait analysis, quantitative magnetic resonance imaging (MRI), and assays of biomarkers provide methods to evaluate a framework for understanding the interrelationship between the factors that influence the progression of osteoarthritis (see Figure 77.1).

The purpose of this chapter is to describe an integrated view of the *in vivo* pathomechanics of osteoarthritis associated with aging. The material is based on studies of assays of biomarkers, cartilage morphology (quantitative MRI), and human function (gait analysis).

Cartilage Mechanobiology, Osteoarthritis, and Aging

The structure and function of articular cartilage are maintained by the metabolic activity of chondrocytes, the cells in cartilage. The chondrocytes are embedded in a highly structured avascular extracellular matrix. The extracellular matrix is made up of structural proteins including collagen, proteoglycans, other proteins, peptides, and water.

Type II collagen fibrils form a network within the tissue with different primary fiber orientation in the deep zone (closest to bone), transitional zone, middle zone, and superficial zone (closest to cartilage surface) (see Figure 77.2). The zones contain different collagen organization as well as different amounts of proteoglycans. The collagen fibers are responsible for the tensile strength of cartilage and are surrounded by the matrix that primarily consists of water. Proteoglycans are responsible for the compressive strength, are arranged within the collagen network, and attract water. Other proteins and peptides, including growth factors, cytokines, and metalloproteinases, are responsible for tissue growth, communication between chondrocytes, and regulation of anabolic and catabolic processes.

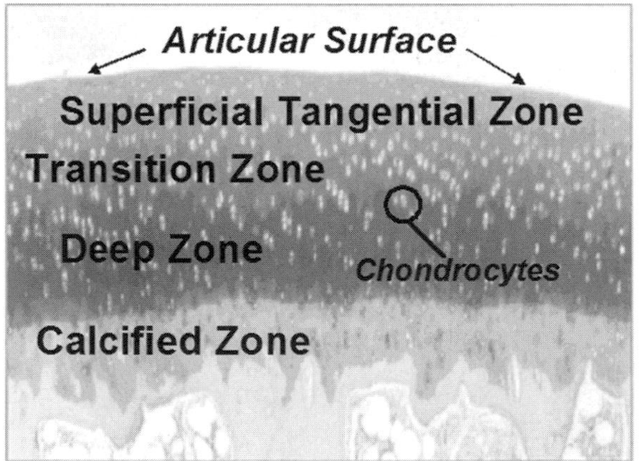

Figure 77.2 Cartilage can be organized into four zones from a functional viewpoint.
The **Superficial Tangential Zone** is the thinnest layer, with the highest content of collagen and the lowest concentration of proteoglycans; contains flat chondrocytes and collagen fibers arranged tangentially to the articular surface; has greatest ability to resist shear stresses and serves as a gliding surface for the joint; limits passage of large molecules between synovial fluid and cartilage; *the first to show changes of osteoarthritis*.
The **Transition Zone** is composed almost entirely of proteoglycans and spherical chondrocytes; this zone involves the transition between the shearing forces of the surface layer to compression forces in the deeper cartilage layers.
The **Deep Zone** is the largest part of the articular cartilage. It contains elongated chondrocytes and collagen fibers aligned perpendicular to the subchondral plate; this zone distributes loads and resists compression.
The **Calcified Cartilage Zone** separates hyaline cartilage from subchondral bone; contains mainly type X collagen in the calcified cartilage layer and in hypertrophic zone of the growth plate; *capillary buds penetrate the layer of calcified cartilage as osteoarthritis progresses*.

The early stages of osteoarthritis are associated with fraying and fibrillation of the superficial layer of cartilage (see Figure 77.3) and there is a reduction of chondrocytes in superficial zones. The cartilage matrix loses proteoglycans, and in the later stages capillary buds penetrate the layer of calcified cartilage. The pain associated with osteoarthritis is associated with synovial hypertrophy creating increased intra-articular pressure and producing joint pain.

CELL METABOLISM

Biological tissues undergo significant changes during the aging process. The metabolic response of chondrocytes changes with aging. For instance, with increasing age, articular cartilage chondrocytes become less responsive to anabolic cytokines (Martin and Buckwalter, 2000) presumably leading to reduced synthetic capacity (DeGroot *et al.*, 1999) and activity (Bolton *et al.*, 1999) of chondrocytes. Due to these changes in cell metabolism, the size of water-attracting proteoglycan aggregates decreases (Buckwalter *et al.*, 1994), and consequently the water content also decreases with age (Venn, 1978). In contrast, collagen molecules have an extremely long half-life (>200 years; Maroudas *et al.* (1992)), and the total amount of collagen in cartilage does not decrease with age (Venn, 1978). However, with age, increasing numbers of cross-links between molecules form by nonenzymatic glycation (Bank *et al.*, 1998).

The biological changes in cartilage with aging may be the cause for the overall altered mechanical properties of the tissue such as decreased tensile stiffness and strength (Kempson, 1982). Articular cartilage aging does not cause osteoarthritis, but the age-related metabolic and phenotypic decline of the chondrocytes increases the risk of articular cartilage degeneration and limits the ability of the cell to repair the tissue once degenerative changes occur (Martin and Buckwalter, 2002). Similar changes have been observed in menisci (McAlinden *et al.*, 2001) and ligaments (Noyes and Grood, 1976; Woo *et al.*, 1991).

In contrast to the natural aging process, osteoarthritis is associated with a prominent regenerative and reparative activity. More specifically, osteoarthritis is characterized by increased cell activity and cell proliferation, but also by hypertrophy and erosion of the tissue, focal defects, pericellular degradation and interterritorial matrix degradation, nonreversible proteoglycan depletion, mild focal superficial inflammation of the synovium, and subchondral remodeling. Cartilage changes in early osteoarthritis include chondrocyte proliferation, surface fibrillation, and perichondral collagen condensation. In advanced osteoarthritis, fissures extend to the midzone,

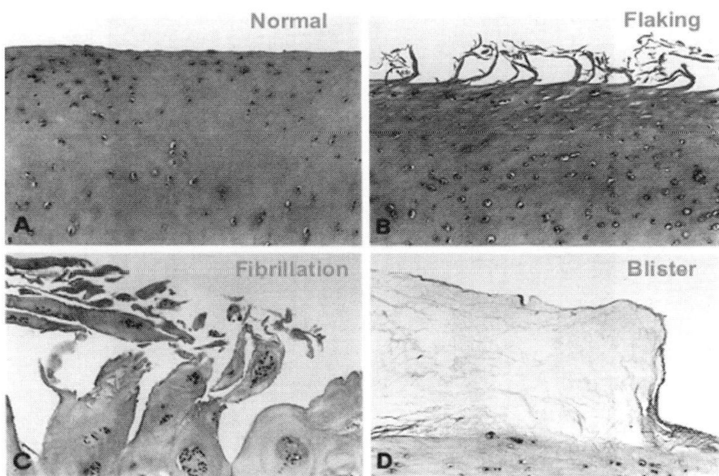

Figure 77.3 Illustration of the changes to the superficial zone of cartilage during the progression of osteoarthritis (OA). **A.** Normal cartilage shows a smooth surface; the early stage of OA is characterized by **B.** flaking of the surface; **C.** fibrillation; and **D.** the formation of a blister. The mechanical surface changes will increase the coefficient of friction at the surface. From Gannon and Sokoloff (1999).

the matrix delaminates and erodes, fibrosis can be observed, and fibrocartilage is formed as a repair response (Pritzker, 2003).

BIOMARKERS FOR OSTEOARTHRITIS

In vivo assessment of degenerative biological changes to cartilage can be evaluated by assays of enzymes, enzyme-inhibitors, and protein fragments, generically termed biological markers or biomarkers. Biomarkers have the potential to become indicators of normal biological processes, pathogenic processes, or pharmacologic response to a therapeutic intervention.

The *in vivo* physical and biological environment must be considered together when evaluating biomarkers (see Figure 77.1). Cartilage oligomeric matrix protein (COMP), a prominent constituent of articular cartilage, is up-regulated following cyclical compression *in situ* and may play an important role in transducing mechanical forces in the extracellular matrix to the cell (Wong *et al.*, 1999). For example, competing marathon runners whose joints are exposed to repetitive loading during frequent running training and competition have elevated serum COMP concentrations compared to healthy control subjects (Neidhart *et al.*, 2000). In another study (Mündermann *et al.*, 2005; Mündermann *et al.*, 2004), reduced COMP levels were associated with the adduction moment at the knee, suggesting that mechanical variations in the way individuals perform the same activity are related to the differences in the cartilage COMP levels. In contrast, keratan sulfate, a biomarker reflecting the rate of cartilage catabolism (Thonar *et al.*, 1985), did not significantly change in 15 marathon runners before, immediately after, and 48 hours after the completion of a training marathon (Sweet *et al.*, 1992). Thus, these data suggest that with careful and regular training, running a marathon appears not to increase the rate of degradation of articular cartilage. Changes in COMP and keratan sulfate concentrations suggest that although exercise may not lead to an acute degenerative response of major cartilage constituents including chondrocytes, proteoglycans, and collagen, other constituents such as COMP may be adversely affected.

In osteoarthritic cartilage, the sensitive equilibrium between tissue degeneration and synthesis is disrupted and degenerative processes preponderate. Fragments of proteoglycans or proteins (glucosaminoglycan and COMP) and catabolic and other enzymes, as well as their inhibitors (metalloproteinases, interleukin-1, interleukin-1 receptor antagonist) found in body fluids, may reflect net cartilage degeneration or increased metabolic activity (Otterness *et al.*, 2001).

Quantifying blood serum concentrations of biomarkers is a promising yet minimally invasive tool to investigate the tissue's response to mechanical load *in vivo*. To date, very little is known about changes in biomarker concentrations that occur in relation to loads placed upon the joint during everyday activities (Mündermann *et al.*, 2005; Mündermann *et al.*, 2004). Similar physical activities may promote tissue synthesis in the healthy joint while accelerating degenerative processes in the osteoarthritic joint.

There are still substantial gaps in our ability to interpret the relationships between changes in biomarkers and the loading environment of cartilage. Specificity of the marker to cartilage and the joint of interest always remains a question in studies where markers are extracted from serum. In addition, controlling for the influence of chronic versus transient loads also is an important consideration. Thus, there is a need for further research in this area to define and identify the role of biomarkers in the evaluation of knee osteoarthritis.

Joint Structure, Osteoarthritis, and Aging

The normal function of diarthrodial joints such as the knee involves providing a wide range of mobility while sustaining large forces that are multiples of the body's weight. For example, normal function of the knee during stair climbing requires the knee to flex in the range between 0 and 90 degrees while sustaining compressive forces on the articular surface that can exceed four times body weight. As previously discussed, the biology of cartilage is influenced by the mechanical environment of the joint. Thus, the intrinsic mechanical environment (force and motion) is an important consideration in the context of understanding the factors that influence the initiation and progression of osteoarthritis. The intrinsic forces and motions at the joint are dependent on complex interactions between the shape of the articulating surfaces, passive soft tissue properties surrounding the joints, and active muscle contraction. Thus, individual anatomical variations in joint anatomy that influence joint movement or the forces on the joint can influence the mechanobiology of the articular cartilage and ultimately play a role in the factors associated with the progression of osteoarthritis. For example, the association of joint laxity with osteoarthritis at the knee will be discussed in the next sections of this chapter.

JOINT LAXITY AND OSTEOARTHRITIS

Passive (no muscle contraction) joint laxity is dependent on the conformity of the articular geometry, the properties of the ligaments, menisci (at the knee), and the capsule at the joint. Any changes in the mechanical properties of these structures, whether they occur with aging, disease, or following a joint injury, will have an effect on this mechanical environment. For instance, joint laxity appears to be critically important for the health of a joint (Sharma *et al.*, 1999). Joint laxity can produce large displacements of the articular surfaces, alter congruity and contact sites, and increase local shear and compressive stresses. Joint laxity depends on several factors including the mechanical properties of ligaments and muscle strength and coordination (see Figure 77.4).

The knee, a common site of osteoarthritis, provides a good illustration of the primary components of the joint that maintain joint stability and thus influence joint laxity. The major ligaments stabilizing the knee in translation and rotation are the anterior (ACL) and posterior (PCL) cruciate ligaments. The stiffness and elastic modulus of these ligaments decrease with age (Noyes and Grood, 1976; Woo *et al.*, 1991). The major changes in muscle with age include reduced muscle activation (Stackhouse *et al.*, 2001; Stevens *et al.*, 2003), cross-sectional area (Frontera *et al.*, 2000; Jubrias *et al.*, 1997; Kent-Braun and Alexander, 1999), force per cross-sectional area (Jubrias *et al.*, 1997), and maximum muscle strength (Frontera *et al.*, 2000; Jubrias *et al.*, 1997; Lindle *et al.*, 1997). These age-associated changes in the properties of ligaments and muscle can cause increased joint laxity with age.

Active muscle contraction plays an important role in the dynamic stability of the joint during functional activities such as walking. As illustrated in Figure 77.4, the lateral stability (resistance to lateral joint opening) is dependent on the tension in passive soft tissue (lateral collateral ligament) and active muscle force producing a moment (tendency of a force to produce a rotation) resisting the extrinsic moment tending to adduct the

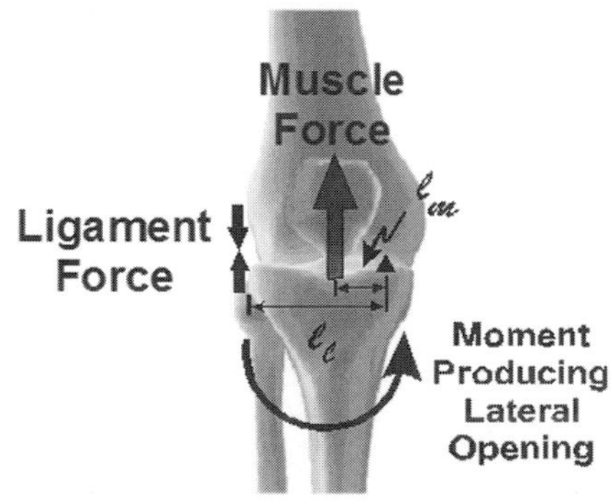

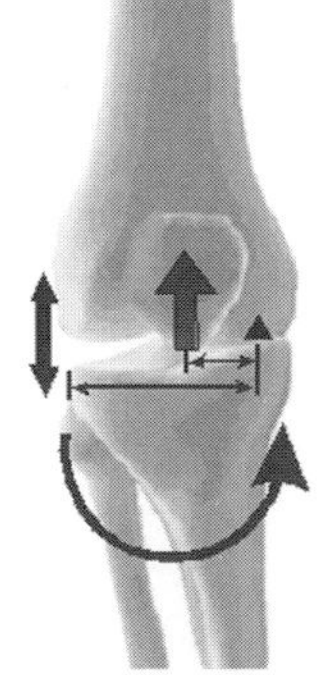

A. Muscle force + Ligament Force Do Resist Lateral Joint Opening

B. Muscle force + Ligament Force Do Not Resist Lateral Joint Opening

Figure 77.4 This diagram of the knee illustrates how stability of the joint is maintained by passive ligament forces and active muscle contraction. In this example, the passive ligament force in the lateral collateral ligament and the active force generated by the quadriceps muscle resist a moment tending to create lateral joint opening (A). Loss of passive stiffness of the ligament and/or a reduction in muscle force can result in a pathological condition where the joint opens laterally, transferring the entire load to a single compartment of the knee (B). Both ligament stiffness and muscle control of the joint decline with aging.

tibia. If the passive soft tissue and muscle forces do not balance the extrinsic moment tending to adduct the knee, then the lateral side of the knee will open and all the force at the knee will be transferred across the medial side of the knee. This condition will potentially overload the medial compartment of the knee and is likely one of the reasons that patients with increased laxity are at higher risk for knee osteoarthritis. As will be discussed later in this chapter, there is a large extrinsic moment that tends to adduct the knee during the stance phase of gait.

The importance of muscle force in the development of osteoarthritis during aging is illustrated by the fact that muscle function and strength decline with aging. Patients with knee osteoarthritis experience changes in their muscle strength and coordination that are independent of the aging process. For instance, activity of the vastus lateralis muscle relative to maximal vastus lateralis muscle activity is much greater in patients with knee osteoarthritis compared to age-matched controls and young adults (Hortobagyi *et al.*, 2005). Decreased quadriceps muscle strength per muscle mass suggests that osteoarthritis patients experience muscle inhibition due to altered afferent input from the diseased joint and consequent reduction in efferent motor neuron stimulation of the quadriceps muscle (Slemenda *et al.*, 1997). In addition, medial compartment knee osteoarthritis is associated with a greater loss of cartilage in the medial compared to the lateral compartment of the knee, and leads to increasing varus alignment with increasing severity (Mündermann *et al.*, 2004). These age-independent changes in muscle properties and cartilage morphology likely contribute to a further increase in joint laxity in patients with knee osteoarthritis.

Menopause may accelerate the loss of muscle mass and result in decreased muscle performance and functional capacity (Sipila, 2003). Although differences in ligament properties between men and women are unknown, ACL stiffness does correlate with estrogen and progesterone levels (Romani *et al.*, 2003), and estrogen levels are lower in postmenopausal women. Probably resulting from these differences in ligament and muscle properties, even healthy women have greater varus-valgus laxity than healthy men (Sharma *et al.*, 1999), potentially contributing to the higher incidence of osteoarthritis in women after menopause. Thus the increased incidence of osteoarthritis in postmenopausal women is likely related to increased passive and dynamic laxity of the joint.

CARTILAGE MORPHOLOGY

Cartilage will structurally adapt to joint loading (Arokoski *et al.*, 2000). As previously noted, cartilage adaptation to loading has been well studied from an experimental and theoretical viewpoint. However, *in vivo* assessment of cartilage adaptation to joint loading has been limited by the availability of methods to evaluate *in vivo* changes in cartilage. MRI-based techniques are useful for evaluating *in vivo* quantitative morphological characteristics of articular cartilage. Typically, three-dimensional models of articular cartilage are assembled from a set of two-dimensional images requiring segmentation of the cartilage. Methods for cartilage segmentation have been extensively studied (Pham *et al.*, 2000; Stammberger *et al.*, 1999).

MR images can be used to examine the thickness variation of cartilage at the knee relative to the type of loads that occur during dynamic activities such as walking. For example, the highest loads at the knee occur at heel strike with the knee near full extension (Schipplein and Andriacchi, 1991). Typically, the thickest regions of the femoral and tibial load-bearing articular cartilage are aligned when the knee is at full extension, suggesting an adaptation to the high loads at heel strike on mating surfaces of the tibiofemoral articulation (see Figure 77.5).

There are several typical qualitative features (Andriacchi *et al.*, 2004) in the variation of tibial and femoral cartilage thickness common to most healthy knees (see Figure 77.5). The tibial cartilage was thicker in the posterior weight-bearing region in the lateral compartment. The femoral condyle cartilage was thicker in the posterior region of the lateral femoral condyle. The tibial cartilage was thicker in the anterior weight-bearing region in the medial compartment. The femoral condyle cartilage was thicker in the anterior region of the medial

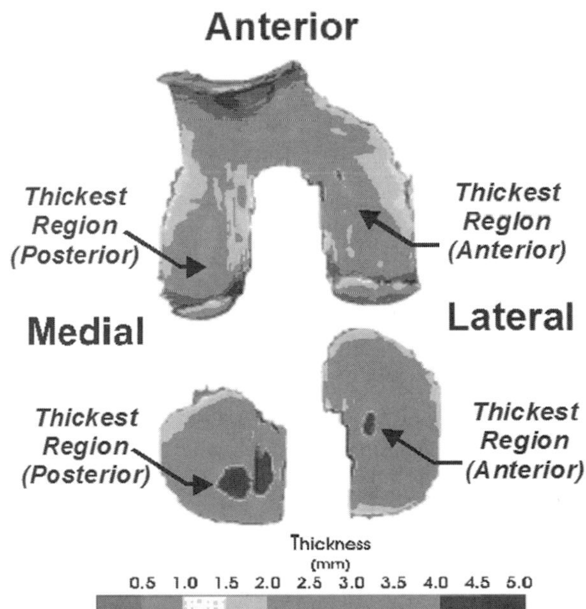

Figure 77.5 The features (proximal viewpoint) of the regional thickness variations of femoral and tibial cartilage (segmented from MRI and color-coded for thickness) were common to all normal subjects. From Andriacchi *et al.* (2004).

femoral condyle. The thickness variation on the tibia mirrored the thickness variation on the femoral condyles in each compartment. For example, thicker posterior cartilage on the lateral femoral condyle was mirrored by thicker cartilage in the posterior region of the tibial cartilage in the lateral compartment.

In vivo Function, Osteoarthritis, and Aging

As noted earlier, the mechanical environment of the cartilage is influenced by the intrinsic anatomy of the joint. The extrinsic loading (e.g., weight and inertia) during dynamic activities such as walking can also have a profound influence on the health of articular cartilage. For example, it has been shown (Schipplein and Andriacchi, 1991) that individual variations in the way people walk can influence the distribution of load between the medial and lateral compartments of the knee. Specifically the adduction moment at the knee during walking (*adduction moment*—the tendency of the external forces acting on the lower limb to produce adduction of the knee) causes higher forces to be transmitted to the medial side of the knee (see Figure 77.6).

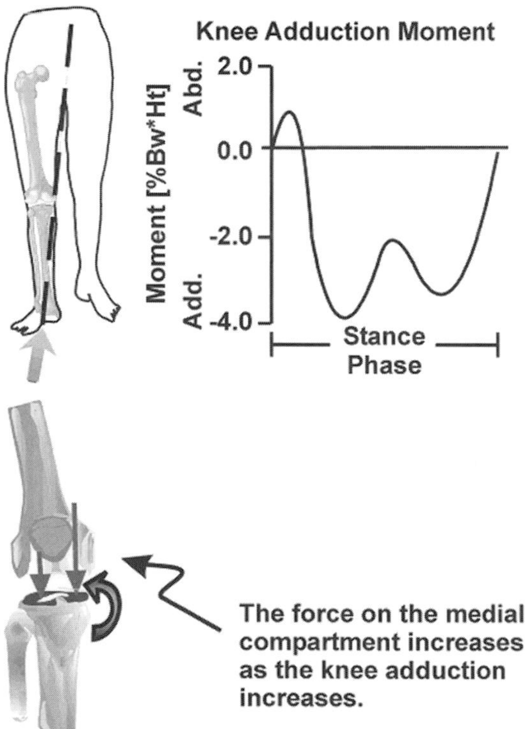

Figure 77.6 The knee adduction moment during walking could be related to the distribution of medial and lateral loads across the knee.

It has been shown (Hurwitz *et al.*, 1998) that the knee adduction moment during gait is positively correlated with the distribution of medial and lateral bone mineral content and is the best single predictor of the medial-to-lateral ratio of proximal bone mineral content. Thus, the higher the knee adduction moment, the greater the load on the medial plateau relative to that of the lateral plateau and the higher the bone mineral content in the proximal tibia under the medial plateau as compared to that under the lateral plateau. Consequently, variation in walking mechanics can influence the load sustained by cartilage *in vivo* and has the potential to influence the health and pathomechanics of articular cartilage.

LOAD INFLUENCES HEALTHY CARTILAGE AND CARTILAGE WITH OSTEOARTHRITIS DIFFERENTLY

A recent study (Andriacchi *et al.*, 2004) examined the relationship between loading and motion at the knee during walking and the response in healthy cartilage relative to cartilage with osteoarthritis. Healthy cartilage thickness increased on the medial condyle in subjects with a higher adduction moment based on a significant ($P < 0.05$) positive correlation between the ratio of medial to lateral condyle thickness and adduction moment (see Figure 77.7). In contrast, for osteoarthritic cartilage, the medial to lateral condyle thickness ratio decreased with an increase in the adduction moment.

In patients with knee osteoarthritis, it has been shown that individual variations in the mechanics of walking can influence the rate of progression of knee osteoarthritis (Miyazaki *et al.*, 2002) and the outcome of treatment for medial compartment osteoarthritis at the knee (Prodromos *et al.*, 1985; Wang *et al.*, 1990). For example, varus alignment of the knee has been related to the presence and progression of medial compartment knee osteoarthritis. This type of alignment theoretically would place higher load on the medial side of the knee. A surgical procedure, the high tibial osteotomy (HTO), involves realigning the tibial plateau to reduce the load on the medial compartment of the knee. Patients who adopt a gait pattern with a low adduction moment following surgery and patients with less severe disease have a better outcome with an HTO and a slower rate of disease progression (Prodromos *et al.*, 1985; Wang *et al.*, 1990).

Patients with knee osteoarthritis typically walk with greater knee adduction moments than age-matched control subjects (Mündermann *et al.*, 2004), which is also a strong predictor for the presence (Baliunas *et al.*, 2002; Gök *et al.*, 2002; Schnitzer *et al.*, 1993), severity (Mündermann *et al.*, 2004; Sharma *et al.*, 1998), and rate of progression (Miyazaki *et al.*, 2002) of medial compartment knee osteoarthritis. In addition, patients with knee osteoarthritis seem to experience a smaller range of knee flexion during the stance phase of walking (Childs *et al.*, 2004; Kaufman *et al.*, 2001; Messier *et al.*,

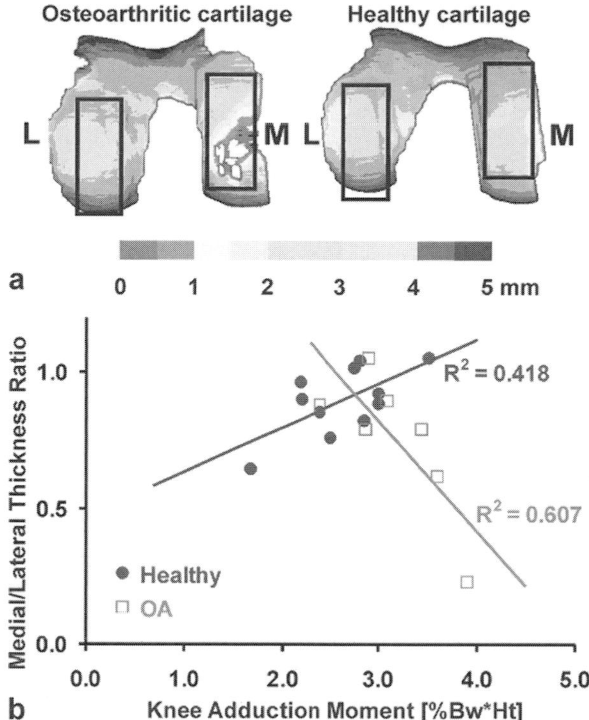

Figure 77.7 Femoral cartilage thickness increases with load for healthy cartilage and decreases with load for cartilage with osteoarthritis (OA). **a**. The load bearing regions of interest (ROI) are indicated by the rectangular areas shown on the color thickness map of the femoral cartilage. **b**. The medial-to-lateral ratio of the average ROI thickness was correlated to the adduction moment normalized as percentage body weight times height (%Bw*Ht) for an osteoarthritic group and a healthy group.

1992) that is associated with a smaller net quadriceps moment (Kaufman *et al.*, 2001).

As previously noted, the adduction moment at the knee has been related to the progression and treatment outcome for medial compartment osteoarthritis at the knee. In a recent study (Mündermann *et al.*, 2004) of 44 patients (88 knees) with osteoarthritis of the medial compartment of the knee, it was shown that the adduction moment at the knee during walking was significantly lower in patients with less severe disease. Severity of the disease was assessed by a clinical rating system reported by Kellgren and Lawrence (K-L) (Kellgren and Lawrence, 1963). Patients were diagnosed to have knee osteoarthritis in one or both knee joints based on clinical, radiographic data, and K-L grades ranged from 1 to 4 (most severe) for both knees. A statistically significant increase in knee adduction moment was found for knees with K-L grade 3 or 4 compared to asymptomatic matched control knees ($P = 0.039$) and for knees with K-L grade 3 or 4 compared to knees with K-L grade equal to or smaller than 2. In addition, the mechanical axis varus alignment was significantly greater in patients with more severe osteoarthritis. These results suggest that differences in the adduction moment are less likely the initial cause for osteoarthritis, but rather the effect of morphological changes in the pathological joint such as medial compartment joint space narrowing. This increase in adduction moment at later stages of osteoarthritis may lead to an accelerated rate of disease progression. Some patients may be able to alter their walking mechanics to reduce their maximum knee adduction moment at very early stages of the disease and reduce the rate of progression. This explanation is supported by the fact that patients with less severe knee osteoarthritis appear to have different gait mechanics than asymptomatic control subjects and are able to reduce the adduction moment by walking slower during everyday activities.

The primary changes in gait that occur with increasing age are slower walking speeds, reduced step length, and increased double support time (Kerrigan *et al.*, 1998; Riley *et al.*, 2001; Winter *et al.*, 1990). It has been suggested (DeVita and Hortobágyi, 2000) that age causes a redistribution of joint torques and powers, with the elderly using their hip extensors more and their knee extensors and ankle plantar flexors less than young adults when walking at the same speed. This shift in power generation could be caused by the physiological changes in muscle (Frontera *et al.*, 2000; Jubrias *et al.*, 1997; Kent-Braun and Alexander, 1999; Lindle *et al.*, 1997; Stackhouse *et al.*, 2001; Stevens *et al.*, 2003), where the knee extensor muscles in the elderly are simply not capable of producing similar forces than in young adults.

FUNCTIONAL KINEMATICS DURING WALKING AND OSTEOARTHRITIS

As previously discussed, functional joint loading can influence the health of articular cartilage and is ultimately associated with the progression of degenerative changes to cartilage. In addition, joint motion (kinematics) can influence the initiation of osteoarthritis (Andriacchi *et al.*, 2004). For example, the anterior cruciate ligament (ACL) of the knee, one of the four major ligaments of the knee, provides translational and rotational stability to the joint. The ACL frequently is injured during sporting activity and is the most frequently reconstructed soft-tissue structure at the knee. The ACL-deficient knee provides a basis for examining the influence of abnormal kinematics on the initiation of knee osteoarthritis. There are numerous clinical studies (Buckland-Wright *et al.*, 2000; Daniel *et al.*, 1994; Lohmander and Roos, 1994; Roos *et al.*, 1995) that report premature knee osteoarthritis in chronic ACL-deficient knees and even in knees following reconstruction. Even though ACL reconstruction does restore anterior-posterior stability (Daniel *et al.*, 1994), it has not been documented that ACL reconstruction restores normal rotational alignment and motion to the knee, suggesting the possibility that rotational changes following ACL injury could be a factor in the initiation of knee osteoarthritis following ACL injury (Kanamori *et al.*, 2002; Ma *et al.*, 2000).

Studies of patient function (Andriacchi and Dyrby, 2005; Georgoulis *et al.*, 2003; Vergis and Gillquist, 1998) following ACL injury support the observation that rotational changes following ACL injury are a major factor in the progression of knee osteoarthritis. In particular, a recent study (Andriacchi and Dyrby, 2005) demonstrated that ACL-deficient patients did not have an increased range of AP motion relative to the contralateral side. However, there was an offset in internal-external (IE) rotation position relative to the contralateral limb. The offset was determined from the temporal average of all IE values over the entire walking cycle. The tibia was more internally rotated throughout stance phase than in healthy control subjects. The fact that the rotational offset was also present at the end of swing phase where the tibia normally externally rotates with knee extension (screw-home movement) suggests that the loss of the ACL causes a reduction of the internal rotation of the tibia at the end of swing phase. This rotational offset is maintained through the stance phase of the walking cycle.

A positional offset shifts the load bearing contact areas of the knee away from normal locations. The change in the rotational characteristics at the knee could cause specific regions of the cartilage to be loaded that were not loaded prior to the ACL injury. It has been suggested (Bullough *et al.*, 1992; Yao and Seedhom, 1993) that the altered contact mechanics in the newly loaded regions could produce local degenerative changes to the articular cartilage. As previously reported (Bullough *et al.*, 1992; Wong *et al.*, 1999), cartilage in highly loaded areas has mechanically adapted relative to underused areas where signs of fibrillation can be observed in healthy knees in relatively young subjects. It has been suggested (Andriacchi *et al.*, 2004) that a spatial shift in the contact region could place loads on a region of cartilage that may not adapt to the rapidly increased load initiating degenerative changes (Wu *et al.*, 2000). It is important to note that other studies (Kvist and Gillquist, 2001) have demonstrated a shift in the anterior-posterior position of the tibial femoral contact during walking after loss of the ACL. Thus, it is likely that ACL injury causes a shift in the load bearing location through a combination of rotational and translational changes in the normal kinematics of the joint.

Clinical and laboratory studies (Cicuttini *et al.*, 2002; Wu *et al.*, 2000) have suggested that changes in contact position could be a factor in the degenerative changes, even in knees with an intact ACL. In particular, rotational malalignment has been related to an increased incidence of knee osteoarthritis (Nagao *et al.*, 1998; Yagi, 1994). A shift in the load bearing area to an infrequently loaded region would cause articular surface damage and increase fibrillation of the collagen network and lead to the degenerative changes that have been associated with increased clinical laxity.

The preceding observation for the ACL-deficient knee can be related to the changes to the musculoskeletal system that occur with aging. In particular, ligament stiffness (Noyes and Grood, 1976; Woo *et al.*, 1991), muscle strength (Jubrias *et al.*, 1997), and muscle activation (Stackhouse *et al.*, 2001) decline with aging. The decline in passive joint stability derived from ligament restraint and dynamic stability derived from muscle forces can cause abnormal kinematics that increase with age. These kinematic changes will lead to a shift in the normal load bearing regions in a manner similar to the kinematic changes following ACL injury. Hormonal changes that occur with menopause produce similar changes (Phillips *et al.*, 1993; Rasanen and Messner, 1999; Richette *et al.*, 2003) to those described for aging and could explain the increased incidence of knee osteoarthritis reported in women over the age of 50 (Oliveria *et al.*, 1995). In addition, aging (Buckwalter *et al.*, 1994) and hormonal (Rasanen and Messner, 1999) changes can limit the ability of cartilage to adapt and repair (Martin and Buckwalter, 2000) cartilage damage associated with changes in load bearing regions. Chronic kinematic changes with aging and menopause can cause degenerative changes to cartilage, since older cartilage might not have the capacity to adapt to load bearing changes in contrast to younger cartilage.

Conclusion

The progression of osteoarthritis with aging is best understood by considering the interrelated biological, morphological, and neuromuscular pathways associated with the disease. The interrelationship or coupling of these pathways converges at an *in vivo* systems level in humans. Each of these pathways changes with aging in ways that increase the risk of osteoarthritis.

The material presented in this chapter provides an integrated *in vivo* framework for understanding the various factors that influence the initiation and progression of osteoarthritis that is consistent with theoretical, laboratory, and clinical observations of the pathomechanics of osteoarthritis. This framework provides a basis for explaining the role of kinematics and load on the progression of knee osteoarthritis. Although this framework was developed from an analysis of *in vivo* pathomechanics, it also explains how the convergence of biological, morphological, and neuromuscular changes to the musculoskeletal system during aging or during menopause leads to the increased rate of idiopathic osteoarthritis with aging.

The *in vivo* framework presented should be helpful for the interpretation of laboratory experiments, the identification of risk factors for knee osteoarthritis, and the development of methods for the evaluation of osteoarthritis at the knee.

ACKNOWLEDGMENTS

This work was supported in part by NIH grants AR39421, AR045788, and AR049792.

REFERENCES

Andriacchi, T.P. and Dyrby, C.O. (2005). Interactions between kinematics and loading during walking for the normal and ACL-deficient knee. *J Biomech, 38(2)*, 293–298.

Andriacchi, T.P., Mündermann, A., Smith, R.L., Alexander, E.J., Dyrby, C.O., and Koo, S. (2004). A framework for the in vivo pathomechanics of osteoarthritis at the knee. *Ann Biomed Eng, 32(3)*, 447–457.

Arokoski, J.P., Jurvelin, J.S., Vaatainen, U., and Helminen, H.J. (2000). Normal and pathological adaptations of articular cartilage to joint loading. *Scand J Med Sci Sports, 10(4)*, 186–198.

Ateshian, G.A., Soslowsky, L.J., and Mow, V.C. (1991). Quantitation of articular surface topography and cartilage thickness in knee joints using stereophotogrammetry. *J Biomech, 24(8)*, 761–776.

Baliunas, A.J., Hurwitz, D.E., Ryals, A.B., Karrar, A., Case, J.P., Block, J.A., and Andriacchi, T.P. (2002). Increased knee joint loads during walking are present in subjects with knee osteoarthritis. *Osteoarthritis Cartilage, 10(7)*, 573–579.

Bank, R.A., Bayliss, M.T., Lafeber, F.P., Maroudas, A., and Tekoppele, J.M. (1998). Ageing and zonal variation in post-translational modification of collagen in normal human articular cartilage. The age-related increase in non-enzymatic glycation affects biomechanical properties of cartilage. *Biochem J, 330 (Pt 1)*, 345–351.

Beaupré, G.S., Stevens, S.S., and Carter, D.R. (2000). Mechanobiology in the development, maintenance, and degeneration of articular cartilage. *J Rehabil Res Dev, 37(2)*, 145–151.

Bolton, M.C., Dudhia, J., and Bayliss, M.T. (1999). Age-related changes in the synthesis of link protein and aggrecan in human articular cartilage: Implications for aggregate stability. *Biochem J, 337* (*Pt 1*), 77–82.

Buckland-Wright, J.C., Lynch, J.A., and Dave, B. (2000). Early radiographic features in patients with anterior cruciate ligament rupture. *Ann Rheum Dis, 59(8)*, 641–646.

Buckwalter, J.A., Roughley, P.J., and Rosenberg, L.C. (1994). Age-related changes in cartilage proteoglycans: Quantitative electron microscopic studies. *Microsc Res Tech, 28(5)*, 398–408.

Bullough, P.G., Moskowitz, R., Howell, D., and Goldberg, V. (1992). The pathology of osteoarthritis. In R. Moskowitz, D. Howell, and V. Goldberg (Eds.), *Osteoarthritis: Diagnosis and Medical/Surgical Management*, pp. 36–69. Philadelphia, PA: W.B. Saunders.

Carter, D.R., Beaupré, G.S., Giori, N.J., and Helms, J.A. (1998). Mechanobiology of skeletal regeneration. *Clin Orthop, 355(Suppl.)*, S41–S55.

Carter, D.R. and Wong, M. (2003). Modelling cartilage mechanobiology. *Philos Trans R Soc Lond B Biol Sci, 358(1437)*, 1461–1471.

Childs, J.D., Sparto, P.J., Fitzgerald, G.K., Bizzini, M., and Irrgang, J.J. (2004). Alterations in lower extremity movement and muscle activation patterns in individuals with knee osteoarthritis. *Clin Biomech, 19(1)*, 44–49.

Cicuttini, F.M., Wluka, A.E., Wang, Y., Davis, S.R., Hankin, J., and Ebeling, P. (2002). Compartment differences in knee cartilage volume in healthy adults. *J Rheumatol, 29(3)*, 554–556.

Daniel, D.M., Stone, M.L., Dobson, B.E., Fithian, D.C., Rossman, D.J., and Kaufman, K.R. (1994). Fate of the ACL-injured patient. A prospective outcome study. *Am J Sports Med, 22(5)*, 632–644.

DeGroot, J., Verzijl, N., Bank, R.A., Lafeber, F.P., Bijlsma, J.W., and TeKoppele, J.M. (1999). Age-related decrease in proteoglycan synthesis of human articular chondrocytes: The role of nonenzymatic glycation. *Arthritis Rheum, 42(5)*, 1003–1009.

DeVita, P. and Hortobágyi, T. (2000). Age causes a redistribution of joint torques and powers during gait. *J Appl Physiol, 88(5)*, 1804–1811.

Dunlop, D.D., Manheim, L.M., Yelin, E.H., Song, J., and Chang, R.W. (2003). The costs of arthritis. *Arthritis Rheum, 49(1)*, 101–113.

Eckstein, F., Faber, S., Muhlbauer, R., Hohe, J., Englmeier, K.H., Reiser, M. *et al.* (2002). Functional adaptation of human joints to mechanical stimuli. *Osteoarthritis Cartilage, 10(1)*, 44–50.

Englund, M., Paradowski, P.T., and Lohmander, L.S. (2004). Association of radiographic hand osteoarthritis with radiographic knee osteoarthritis after meniscectomy. *Arthritis Rheum, 50(2)*, 469–475.

Englund, M., Roos, E.M., and Lohmander, L.S. (2003). Impact of type of meniscal tear on radiographic and symptomatic knee osteoarthritis: A sixteen-year followup of meniscectomy with matched controls. *Arthritis Rheum, 48(8)*, 2178–2187.

Escalante, A. and del Rincón, I. (2001). Epidemiology and impact of rheumatic disorders in the United States' Hispanic population. *Curr Opin Rheumatol, 13(2)*, 104–110.

Felson, D.T., Naimark, A., Anderson, J., Kazis, L., Castelli, W., and Meenan, R.F. (1987). The prevalence of knee osteoarthritis in the elderly. The Framingham Osteoarthritis Study. *Arthritis Rheum, 30(8)*, 914–918.

Flores, R.H. and Hochberg, M.C. (2003). Definition and classification of osteoarthritis. In R.D. Brandt, M. Doherty, and L.S. Lohmander (Eds.), *Osteoarthritis, 2e*, pp. 1–8. Oxford: Oxford University Press.

Frontera, W.R., Hughes, V.A., Fielding, R.A., Fiatarone, M.A., Evans, W.J., and Roubenoff, R. (2000). Aging of skeletal muscle: A 12-yr longitudinal study. *J Appl Physiol, 88(4)*, 1321–1326.

Gannon, F.H. and Sokoloff, L. (1999). Histomorphometry of the aging human patella: Histologic criteria and controls. *Osteoarthritis Cartilage, 7(2)*, 173–181.

Georgoulis, A.D., Papadonikolakis, A., Papageorgiou, C.D., Mitsou, A., and Stergiou, N. (2003). Three-dimensional tibiofemoral kinematics of the anterior cruciate ligament-deficient and reconstructed knee during walking. *Am J Sports Med, 31(1)*, 75–79.

Gök, H., Ergin, S. and Yavuzer, G. (2002). Kinetic and kinematic characteristics of gait in patients with medial knee arthrosis. *Acta Orthop Scand, 73(6)*, 647–652.

Grodzinsky, A.J., Levenston, M.E., Jin, M., and Frank, E.H. (2000). Cartilage tissue remodeling in response to mechanical forces. *Ann Rev Biomed Eng, 2*, 691–713.

Guilak, F. and Mow, V.C. (2000). The mechanical environment of the chondrocyte: A biphasic finite element model of cell-matrix interactions in articular cartilage. *J Biomech, 33(12)*, 1663–1673.

Hortobagyi, T., Westerkamp, L., Beam, S., Moody, J., Garry, J., Holbert, D. *et al.* (2005). Altered hamstring-quadriceps muscle balance in patients with knee osteoarthritis. *Clin Biomech, 20(1)*, 97–104.

Hurwitz, D.E., Sumner, D.R., Andriacchi, T.P., and Sugar, D.A. (1998). Dynamic knee loads during gait predict proximal tibial bone distribution. *J Biomech, 31(5)*, 423–430.

Jordan, J.M., Renner, J.B., Luta, G., Dragomir, A.D., Hochberg, M.C., and Helmick, C.G. (2003). Incidence and progression of radiographic knee osteoarthritis (OA) in African Americans and Caucasians. In *Proceedings of the 66th Annual Scientific Meeting of the American College of Rheumatology, October, Orlando, FL*, 1738.

Jubrias, S.A., Odderson, I.R., Esselman, P.C., and Conley, K.E. (1997). Decline in isokinetic force with age: Muscle cross-sectional area and specific force. *Eur J Appl Physiol, 434(3)*, 246–253.

Kanamori, A., Zeminski, J., Rudy, T.W., Li, G., Fu, F.H., and Woo, S.L. (2002). The effect of axial tibial torque on the function of the anterior cruciate ligament: A biomechanical study of a simulated pivot shift test. *Arthroscopy, 18(4)*, 394–398.

Kaufman, K.R., Hughes, C., Morrey, B.F., Morrey, M., and An, K.N. (2001). Gait characteristics of patients with knee osteoarthritis. *J Biomech, 34(7)*, 907–915.

Kellgren, J.H. and Lawrence, J.S. (1963). *Atlas of standard radiographs*. Oxford: University of Manchester, Blackwell.

Kempson, G.E. (1982). Relationship between the tensile properties of articular cartilage from the human knee and age. *Ann Rheum Dis, 41(5)*, 508–511.

Kent-Braun, J.A. and Alexander, V.N.G. (1999). Specific strength and voluntary muscle activation in young and elderly women and men. *J Appl Physiol, 87(1)*, 22–29.

Kerrigan, D.C., Todd, M.K., Della Croce, U., Lipsitz, L.A., and Collins, J.J. (1998). Biomechanical gait alterations independent of speed in the healthy elderly: Evidence for specific limiting impairments. *Arch Phys Med Rehab, 79(3)*, 317–322.

Koff, M.F., Ugwonali, O.F., Strauch, R.J., Rosenwasser, M.P., Ateshian, G.A., and Mow, V.C. (2003). Sequential wear patterns of the articular cartilage of the thumb carpometacarpal joint in osteoarthritis. *J Hand Surg [Am], 28(4)*, 597–604.

Kuettner, K.E. and Cole, A.A. (2005). Cartilage degeneration in different human joints. *Osteoarthritis Cartilage, 13(2)*, 93–103.

Kvist, J. and Gillquist, J. (2001). Anterior positioning of tibia during motion after anterior cruciate ligament injury. *Med Sci Sports Exerc, 33(7)*, 1063–1072.

Lindle, R.S., Metter, E.J., Lynch, N.A., Fleg, J.L., Fozard, J.L., Tobin, J. *et al.* (1997). Age and gender comparisons of muscle strength in 654 women and men aged 20–93 yr. *J Appl Physiol, 83(5)*, 1581–1587.

Lohmander, L.S., Ionescu, M., Jugessur, H., and Poole, A.R. (1999). Changes in joint cartilage aggrecan after knee injury and in osteoarthritis. *Arthritis Rheum, 42(3)*, 534–544.

Lohmander, L.S. and Roos, H. (1994). Knee ligament injury, surgery and osteoarthrosis. Truth or consequences? *Acta Orthop Scand, 65(6)*, 605–609.

Ma, C.B., Janaushek, M.A., Vogrin, T.M., Rudy, T.W., Harner, C.D., and Woo, S.L. (2000). Significance of changes in the reference position for measurements of tibial translation and diagnosis of cruciate ligament deficiency. *J Orthop Res, 18(2)*, 176–182.

Maniwa, S., Nishikori, T., Furukawa, S., Kajitani, K., and Ochi, M. (2001). Alteration of collagen network and negative charge of articular cartilage surface in the early stage of experimental osteoarthritis. *Arch Orthop Trauma Surg, 121(4)*, 181–185.

Maroudas, A., Palla, G., and Gilav, E. (1992). Racemization of aspartic acid in human articular cartilage. *Connect Tissue Res, 28(3)*, 161–169.

Martin, J.A. and Buckwalter, J.A. (2000). The role of chondrocyte-matrix interactions in maintaining and repairing articular cartilage. *Biorheology, 37(1–2)*, 129–140.

Martin, J.A. and Buckwalter, J.A. (2002). Aging, articular cartilage chondrocyte senescence and osteoarthritis. *Biogerontology, 3(5)*, 257–264.

McAlinden, A., Dudhia, J., Bolton, M.C., Lorenzo, P., Heinegard, D., and Bayliss, M.T. (2001). Age-related changes in the synthesis and mRNA expression of decorin and aggrecan in human meniscus and articular cartilage. *Osteoarthritis Cartilage, 9(1)*, 33–41.

Messier, S.P., Loeser, R.F., Hoover, J.L., Semble, E.L., and Wise, C.M. (1992). Osteoarthritis of the knee: Effects on gait, strength, and flexibility. *Arch Phys Med Rehab, 73(1)*, 29–36.

Miyazaki, T., Wada, M., Kawahara, H., Sato, M., Baba, H., and Shimada, S. (2002). Dynamic load at baseline can predict radiographic disease progression in medial compartment knee osteoarthritis. *Ann Rheum Dis, 61(7)*, 617–622.

Mow, V.C. and Guo, X.E. (2002). Mechano-electrochemical properties of articular cartilage: Their inhomogeneities and anisotropies. *Ann Rev Biomed Eng, 4*, 175–209.

Mow, V.C. and Wang, C.C. (1999). Some bioengineering considerations for tissue engineering of articular cartilage. *Clin Orthop, 367(Suppl.)*, S204–S223.

Mündermann, A., Dyrby, C.O., Andriacchi, T.P., and King, K.B. (2005). Serum concentration of cartilage oligomeric matrix protein (COMP) is sensitive to physiological cyclic loading in healthy adults. *Osteoarthritis Cartilage, 13(1)*, 34–38.

Mündermann, A., Dyrby, C.O., Hurwitz, D.E., Sharma, L., and Andriacchi, T.P. (2004). Potential strategies to reduce medial compartment loading in patients with knee OA of varying severity: Reduced walking speed. *Arthritis Rheum, 50(4)*, 1172–1178.

Mündermann, A., King, K.B., Dyrby, C.O., and Andriacchi, T.P. (2004). Serum COMP concentration is related to load distribution at the knee during walking in healthy adults. In *Proceedings of the 28th Meeting of the American Society of Biomechanics, Portland, OR*.

Nagao, N., Tachibana, T., and Mizuno, K. (1998). The rotational angle in osteoarthritic knees. *Int Orthop, 22(5)*, 282–287.

Neame, R., Zhang, W., Deighton, C., Doherty, M., Doherty, S., Lanyon, P. *et al.* (2004). Distribution of radiographic osteoarthritis between the right and left hands, hips, and knees. *Arthritis Rheum, 50(5)*, 1487–1494.

Neidhart, M., Müller-Ladner, U., Frey, W., Bosserhoff, A.K., Colombani, P.C., Frey-Rindova, P. *et al.* (2000). Increased serum levels of non-collagenous matrix proteins (cartilage oligomeric matrix protein and melanoma inhibitory activity) in marathon runners. *Osteoarthritis Cartilage, 8(3)*, 222–229.

Noyes, F.R. and Grood, E.S. (1976). The strength of the anterior cruciate ligament in humans and Rhesus monkeys. *J Bone Joint Surg Am, 58(8)*, 1074–1082.

Oliveria, S.A., Felson, D.T., Reed, J.I., Cirillo, P.A., and Walker, A.M. (1995). Incidence of symptomatic hand, hip, and knee osteoarthritis among patients in a health maintenance organization. *Arthritis Rheum, 38(8)*, 1134–1141.

Otterness, I.G., Weiner, E., Swindell, A.C., Zimmerer, R.O., Ionescu, M., and Poole, A.R. (2001). An analysis of 14 molecular markers for monitoring osteoarthritis. Relationship of the markers to clinical end-points. *Osteoarthritis Cartilage, 9(3)*, 224–231.

Peterfy, C.G., van Dijke, C.F., Janzen, D.L., Gluer, C.C., Namba, R., Majumdar, S. *et al.* (1994). Quantification of articular cartilage in the knee with pulsed saturation transfer subtraction and fat-suppressed MR imaging: Optimization and validation. *Radiology, 192(2)*, 485–491.

Peyron, J.G., Altman, R.D., Moskowitz, R.W., Howe, D.S., Goldberg, V.M., and Mankin, H.J. (1993). The epidemiology of osteoarthritis. In R.W. Moskowitz, D.S. Howe, V.M. Goldberg, and H.J. Mankin (Eds.), *Osteoarthritis: Diagnosis and Medical Surgical Management*, pp. 15–35. Philadelphia, PA: W.B. Saunders.

Pham, D.L., Xu, C., and Prince, J.L. (2000). Current methods in medical image segmentation. *Annu Rev Biomed Eng, 2*, 315–337.

Phillips, S.K., Rook, K.M., Siddle, N.C., Bruce, S.A., and Woledge, R.C. (1993). Muscle weakness in women occurs at an earlier age than in men, but strength is preserved by hormone replacement therapy. *Clin Sci, 84(1)*, 95–98.

Pritzker, K.P.H. (2003). Pathology of osteoarthritis. In K.D. Brandt, M. Doherty, and L.S. Lohmander (Eds.), *Osteoarthritis, 2e*, pp. 49–58. Oxford: Oxford University Press.

Prodromos, C.C., Andriacchi, T.P., and Galante, J.O. (1985). A relationship between gait and clinical changes following high tibial osteotomy. *J Bone Joint Surg, 67(8)*, 1188–1194.

Rasanen, T. and Messner, K. (1999). Articular cartilage compressive stiffness following oophorectomy or treatment with 17 beta-estradiol in young postpubertal rabbits. *Acta Obstet Gynecol Scand, 78(5)*, 357–362.

Richette, P., Corvol, M., and Bardin, T. (2003). Estrogens, cartilage, and osteoarthritis. *Joint Bone Spine, 70(4)*, 257–262.

Riley, P.O., DellaCroce, U., and Kerrigan, D.C. (2001). Effect of age on lower extremity joint moment contributions to gait speed. *Gait Posture, 14(3)*, 264–270.

Romani, W., Patrie, J., Curl, L.A., and Flaws, J.A. (2003). The correlations between estradiol, estrone, estriol, progesterone, and sex hormone-binding globulin and anterior cruciate ligament stiffness in healthy, active females. *J Women's Health, 12(3)*, 287–298.

Roos, E.M., Ostenberg, A., Roos, H., Ekdahl, C., and Lohmander, L.S. (2001). Long-term outcome of meniscectomy: Symptoms, function, and performance tests in patients with or without radiographic osteoarthritis compared to matched controls. *Osteoarthritis Cartilage, 9(4)*, 316–324.

Roos, H., Adalberth, T., Dahlberg, L., and Lohmander, L.S. (1995). Osteoarthritis of the knee after injury to the anterior cruciate ligament or meniscus: The influence of time and age. *Osteoarthritis Cartilage, 3(4)*, 261–267.

Schipplein, O.D. and Andriacchi, T.P. (1991). Interaction between active and passive knee stabilizers during level walking. *J Orthop Res, 9(1)*, 113–119.

Schnitzer, T.J., Popovich, J.M., Andersson, G.B., and Andriacchi, T.P. (1993). Effect of piroxicam on gait in patients with osteoarthritis of the knee. *Arthritis Rheum, 36(9)*, 1207–1213.

Sharma, L., Hurwitz, D.E., Thonar, E.J., Sum, J.A., Lenz, M.E., Dunlop, D.D. *et al.* (1998). Knee adduction moment, serum hyaluronan level, and disease severity in medial tibiofemoral osteoarthritis. *Arthritis Rheum, 41(7)*, 1233–1240.

Sharma, L., Lou, C., Felson, D.T., Dunlop, D.D., Kirwan-Mellis, G., Hayes, K.W. *et al.* (1999). Laxity in healthy and osteoarthritic knees. *Arthritis Rheum, 42(5)*, 861–870.

Sipila, S. (2003). Body composition and muscle performance during menopause and hormone replacement therapy. *J Endocrinol Invest, 26(9)*, 893–901.

Slemenda, C., Brandt, K.D., Heilman, D.K., Mazzuca, S., Braunstein, E.M., Katz, B.P. *et al.* (1997). Quadriceps weakness and osteoarthritis of the knee. *Ann Int Med, 127(2)*, 97–104.

Smith, R.L., Donlon, B.S., Gupta, M.K., Mohtai, M., Das, P., Carter, D.R. *et al.* (1995). Effects of fluid-induced shear on articular chondrocyte morphology and metabolism in vitro. *J Orthop Res, 13(6)*, 824–831.

Stackhouse, S.K., Stevens, J.E., Lee, S.C., Pearce, K.M., Snyder-Mackler, L., and Binder-Macleod, S.A. (2001). Maximum voluntary activation in nonfatigued and fatigued muscle of young and elderly individuals. *Phys Ther, 81(5)*, 1102–1109.

Stammberger, T., Eckstein, F., Englmeier, K.H., and Reiser, M. (1999). Determination of 3D cartilage thickness data from MR imaging: Computational method and reproducibility in the living. *Magn Reson Med, 41(3)*, 529–536.

Stevens, J.E., Stackhouse, S.K., Binder-Macleod, S.A., and Snyder-Mackler, L. (2003). Are voluntary muscle activation deficits in older adults meaningful? *Muscle Nerve, 27(1)*, 99–101.

Sweet, M.B., Jakim, I., Coelho, A., Becker, P.J., and Thonar, E.J. (1992). Serum keratan sulfate levels in marathon runners. *Int J Sports Med, 13(4)*, 348–350.

Thonar, E.J., Lenz, M.E., Klintworth, G.K., Caterson, B., Pachman, L.M., Glickman, P. *et al.* (1985). Quantification of keratan sulfate in blood as a marker of cartilage catabolism. *Arthritis Rheum, 28(12)*, 1367–1376.

Venn, M.F. (1978). Variation of chemical composition with age in human femoral head cartilage. *Ann Rheum Dis, 37(2)*, 168–174.

Verbrugge, L.M. (1995). Women, men, and osteoarthritis. *Arthr Care Res, 8(4)*, 212–220.

Vergis, A. and Gillquist, J. (1998). Sagittal plane translation of the knee during stair walking. Comparison of healthy and anterior cruciate ligament-deficient subjects. *Am J Sports Med, 26(6)*, 841–846.

von Porat, A., Roos, E.M., and Roos, H. (2004). High prevalence of osteoarthritis 14 years after an anterior cruciate ligament tear in male soccer players: A study of radiographic and patient relevant outcomes. *Ann Rheum Dis, 63(3)*, 269–273.

Wang, J.W., Kuo, K.N., Andriacchi, T.P., and Galante, J.O. (1990). The influence of walking mechanics and time on the results of proximal tibial osteotomy. *J Bone Joint Surg, 72(6)*, 905–909.

Winter, D.A., Patla, A.E., Frank, J.S., and Walt, S.E. (1990). Biomechanical walking pattern changes in the fit and healthy elderly. *Phys Ther, 70(6)*, 340–347.

Wong, M., Siegrist, M., and Cao, X. (1999). Cyclic compression of articular cartilage explants is associated with progressive consolidation and altered expression pattern of extracellular matrix proteins. *Matrix Biol, 18(4)*, 391–399.

Woo, S.L., Hollis, J.M., Adams, D.J., Lyon, R.M., and Takai, S. (1991). Tensile properties of the human femur-anterior cruciate ligament-tibia complex. The effects of specimen age and orientation. *Am J Sports Med, 19(3)*, 217–225.

Wu, J.Z., Herzog, W., and Epstein, M. (2000). Joint contact mechanics in the early stages of osteoarthritis. *Med Eng Phys, 22(1)*, 1–12.

Xu, L., Nevitt, M.C., Zhang, Y., Yu, W., Alibadi, P., and Felson, D.T. (2003). High prevalence of knee, but not hip or hand osteoarthritis in Beijing elders: Comparison with data of Caucasians in United States. *Zhonghua Yi Xue Za Zhi, 83(14)*, 1206–1209.

Yagi, T. (1994). Tibial torsion in patients with medial-type osteoarthrotic knees. *Clin Orthop Rel Res (302)*, 52–56.

Yao, J.Q. and Seedhom, B.B. (1993). Mechanical conditioning of articular cartilage to prevalent stresses. *Br J Rheumatol, 32(11)*, 956–965.

78

Aging and Cardiovascular Angiogenesis Models

Andrew Chin, Jacquelyne M. Holm, Inga J. Duignan, and Jay M. Edelberg

The development of new strategies to reduce the impact of heart disease in the aging population is an increasingly important public health issue. Indeed, although present clinical therapies have reduced the overall prevalence of cardiovascular disease (Hansson et al., *1999; Yusuf* et al., *2000; Volpe* et al., *2005), myocardial infarction and congestive heart failure remain the most significant cause of morbidity and mortality in older individuals (Black, 2003; Oxenham* et al., *2003; Stewart* et al., *2003). To this end, recent studies, primarily in rodent models, suggest that impairment in cardiac angiogenesis may predispose the aging heart to more severe pathophysiology and lead to the worst clinical outcomes observed in the geriatric population. This chapter aims to review integrated methodological approaches to aid in the investigation of senescent cardiac angiogenesis in order to facilitate further studies into the basic biological changes underlying the age-associated alterations in cardiac angiogenic regulation and potentially enhance the preclinical testing of novel therapeutic approaches based on such discoveries.*

Introduction

Previous studies have identified age-associated changes in the heart that may serve as potential targets to reverse the geriatric predisposition to more severe cardiovascular pathology. Specifically, age-associated changes in cardiac growth factor expression, vascular wall composition, free radical production, and shifts in apoptotic pathways may contribute to increased cardiac damage after coronary artery occlusion in the older heart. Indeed, experimental strategies based on these findings may offer potential therapeutic approaches to diminish the overall impact of cardiovascular disease in the aging population.

To fully understand the impact of the age-related changes in cardiac angiogenesis, *in vivo* models are required. It is essential that preclinical development of therapies based on these biological changes with aging be fully tested in age-appropriate models of cardiovascular disease in order to increase the translational potential of treatment of older persons. Based on the importance of rodent models in the basic investigation of the biology of aging in the cardiovascular system, as well as the utility of mice and, to a lesser extent, rats in models of human pathophysiology, this review will aim to summarize *in vivo* models of cardiac angiogenesis, including models of cardiovascular disease and interventional protocols.

Cardiac Angiogenesis: Identification of Biological Changes

Aging is associated with significant alterations at multiple levels of cell regulation, including growth factor expression, receptor signaling, and cell migration. Previous studies employing a spectrum of molecular, cellular, and physiological approaches have demonstrated that alterations in vascular growth factor pathways (Edelberg *et al.*, 2002b; Xaymardan *et al.*, 2004b) result in endothelial cellular dysfunction (Rivard *et al.*, 1999; Cai *et al.*, 2003) and impaired angiogenesis (Nakae *et al.*, 2000; Shimada *et al.*, 2004), which may underlie the senescent predisposition to increased vascular disease in the aging heart. To this end, endothelial dysfunction is one of the most important risk factors for cardiovascular disease in the general population (Widlansky *et al.*, 2003), and its impact is heightened with age. Physiologically, vascular endothelial growth factor–nitric oxide (NO) pathways, which play a central role in endothelial-mediated vasodilation, are impaired with aging (Berkowitz *et al.*, 2003) and may result in increased myocardial injury after coronary occlusion compared to younger hearts. In the heart episodes of cardiac tissue hypoxia caused by transient coronary occlusion induce vasodilatory actions that result in cardioprotection in the young rodent heart (Rochetaing *et al.*, 2003). In the aged heart, this ischemic preconditioning can be significantly depressed (Abete *et al.*, 1997; Tani *et al.*, 1999; Fenton *et al.*, 2000). Beyond changes in vascular endothelial growth factor (VEGF) (Rivard *et al.*, 1999), experimental models have demonstrated impairments in the expression and function of angiogenic factors including basic fibroblast growth factor (b-FGF) (Augustin-Voss *et al.*, 1993;

Garfinkel *et al.*, 1996), transforming growth factor beta (TGF-β) (Reed *et al.*, 1998), and platelet-derived growth factor (PDGF) (Sarzani *et al.*, 1991; Edelberg *et al.*, 2002b; Cai *et al.*, 2003) with aging, suggesting that strategies directed at these and other senescent changes may restore angiogenic pathways in the aging heart and may have clinical utility in conjunction with present reperfusion therapies.

Candidate Testing

Angiogenesis is a dynamic process that requires inductive models to investigate the biological significance of potential regulatory mechanisms. Hence, although characterization of age-related differences in angiogenic components can facilitate the discovery of the potential mechanisms underlying the senescent impairment in cardiac angiogenesis, the *in vivo* significance of these findings can only be elucidated through interventions to modulate angiogenic induction. To this end, models testing angiogenic growth factors such as VEGF (Ferrara, 2001), bFGF (Yanagisawa-Miwa *et al.*, 1992; Harada *et al.*, 1994), and PDGF (Edelberg *et al.*, 2002b) have been shown to induce angiogenesis in the aging vasculature. In the heart, molecular and protein, as well as cell-based approaches, have been studied in models aimed at determining the significance of different pathways in senescent cardiac angiogenic impairment.

As investigations continue to develop the understanding of the biological basis of the changes in senescent cardiac angiogenic impairment, studies that employ established *in vivo* approaches to assess the functional impact of age-associated changes in elements and pathways will continue to be required. Unfortunately, the modern tools of genetic engineering do not readily lend themselves to high throughput investigations of aging and cardiac angiogenesis. Indeed, the potential combination of allele targeting and colony aging negates the power of knockout mice as an initial tool to investigate the significance of genes associated with the senescent impairment in cardiac angiogenesis. Thus *in vivo* models employing wild type aged animals can allow the best initial assessment of the potential contribution to candidate genes, proteins, and pathways associated with the biological changes of angiogenesis in the aging heart.

Cardiac Allograft Assay

In order to more rapidly screen the functional significance of age-associated changes in cardiac angiogenic pathways without the requirement of direct cardiac targeting, a cardiac allograft model of angiogenesis is employed (see Figure 78.1). This model, in which neonatal cardiac tissue is engrafted into the pinnal tissue of various age syngeneic mice, allows for the isolation of age on the angiogenic vasculature (Edelberg *et al.*, 2002b; Edelberg *et al.*, 2002) while controlling the age of the myocardium. Indeed, in the transplants, allograft neovascularization is mediated by host endothelial cells recruited into the donor hearts that recapitulate the cardiac myocyte-endothelial cell communication *in vivo* (Edelberg *et al.*, 2002b; Aird *et al.*, 1997), thus allowing the direct comparison of cardiac angiogenic potential in different age groups. Moreover, this model supports the testing of both molecular and cell-based interventions to modulate or restore functional cardiac angiogenesis *in vivo*. Indeed, the result of these studies are highly predictive of the functional role of different strategies in more clinically relevant models, including myocardial infarction studies (see Table 78.1), and thus provides a reasonable throughput screening approach in the investigation of cardiac angiogenesis in the aging rodent.

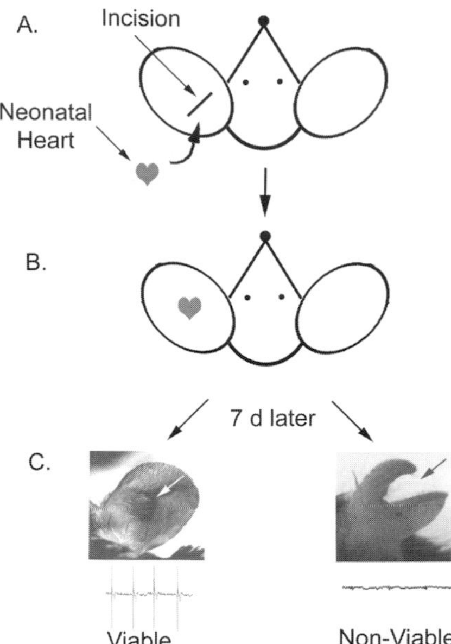

Figure 78.1 This cartoon illustrates the neonatal cardiac allograft protocol to understand changes in cardiac angiogenic pathways. **A**. A 3 mm incision is created on the dorsum of the pinna, and a subcutaneous pocket is created 0–24 h after injection of molecular, protein, or cellular treatments. **B**. An explanted neonatal (~24 h) heart is placed into the pocket and excess air is expressed from the pocket to facilitate adherence. **C**. Cardiac allografts are examined 7d post transplantation for visual viability and electrical activity.

PINNAL ALLOGRAFT TRANSPLANT

A 3 mm incision is made on the dorsum of the pinna in senescent murine hosts, and curved forceps are delicately used to create a subcutaneous pocket (5 × 3 mm). Neonatal hearts are explanted from decapitated 1 d old pups and transplanted into the dorsum of the pinna of an isogeneic adult murine host as previously described (Edelberg *et al.*, 2002; Xaymardan *et al.*, 2004b). The donor cardiac tissue is prepared by harvesting the heart without the pericardial sac from syngeneic neonatal (1 d)

TABLE 78.1
Predictive value of cardiac allograft model in cardioprotection

Age	Treatment	Cardiac Allograft	Cardioprotection in the Endogenous Heart	Reference
	Pretreatment			
Young	PDGF-AB	Enhance Blood Flow	+++	Edelberg *et al.* (2002a and b)
Old	PDGF-AB	Restoration of Engraftment	++	Edelberg *et al.* (2002b); Cai *et al.* (2003)
Young	TNF-α	Lipid Peroxidation	+++	Cai *et al.* (2003); Edelberg *et al.* (2004)
Old	TNF-α	Significant Lipid Peroxidation	↑ Mortality	Cai *et al.* (2003); Edelberg *et al.* (2004)
	Acute Treatment			
Old	PDGF-AB	Failure to Restore	↑ Myocardial Infarction/Apoptosis	Edelberg *et al.* (2002)
Old	PDGF-AB, VEGF, and Ang-2	Restoration of Engraftment	+++	Xaymardan *et al.* (2004b)

mice. This tissue is engrafted into the 5 × 3 mm subcutaneous pocket, and gentle pressure is applied with the tips of the forceps to express air from the pocket and facilitate the adherence between donor and recipient tissues. Engraftment viability is scored 7 d post transplantation via tissue integrity, electrocardiographic (ECG) activity, and blood flow.

To measure the effects of specific angiogenic pathways, the host transplantation site can be treated with molecular, protein, or cellular combinations. Specifically, the murine pinnae can be treated with up to 20 μl of injective either before or at the time of allograft transplantation (through a 30 G × 8 mm needle injected subdermally). In addition, the effects of remote treatments such as contralateral injections or systematic manipulations, including bone marrow transplantation, can be tested in this model.

Assessment protocols

The host ears are grossly analyzed 7 d post transplantation for viability. One qualitative method used to assess viability is transplant integrity. Ears that exhibit intact, healthy tissue are scored as viable, whereas any signs of tissue degradation, inflammation, or necrosis are scored as nonviable (see Figure 78.1).

Local ECGs can be employed to confirm cardiac allograft viability. Specifically, ECGs are acquired via pinnal electrodes to measure allograft activity with 500 Hz sampling, band pass filtered between 3.0 and 100 Hz, and notch filtered at 60.0 Hz, amplified 1000×. Limb electrodes are placed to record the endogenous heart simultaneously to control for field effect.

Functional blood flow to the transplanted cardiac tissue can also be assessed by laser Doppler with an Advance Laser Flowmeter ALF21/2D (Advance, Tokyo) as previously described (Edelberg *et al.*, 2002a). Blood flow measurements are taken at baseline (day 0) and 7 d post transplantation to assess angiogenic activity.

Endogenous Cardiac Interventions

The physiological significance of these findings in the cardiac allograft model requires confirmation in the endogenous heart. To directly assess the role of various genes/pathways in angiogenesis in the intact heart, murine and rat models provide select advantages and limitations. Specifically, for strategies targeting the wild-type heart, studies employing rats, which have less variability in coronary anatomy as compared with mice, provide a more quantitative model for subsequent myocardial infarction studies. Murine models can provide a more qualitative model in myocardial infarction studies by allowing the use of transgenic animals. Notably, the hearts of both species can be targeted selectively in open interventions to assess the impact of molecular and cellular approaches to alter cardiac angiogenesis.

SURGICAL APPROACH

Cardiac access

Both mice and rats can be anesthetized for open cardiac interventions with a cocktail of ketamine (mice, 100 mg/kg; rats, 95 mg/kg) and xylazine (mice, 10 mg/kg; rats, 4 mg/kg). This method of anesthesia requires artificial ventilation with room air (mice, 120–140 breaths/min with a weight adjusted tidal volume of 0.2ml/breath; rats, 90–100 breaths/min with a weight adjusted tidal volume of 1.5–2.0 ml/breath) after endotracheal intubation. Upon performing a left thoracotamy (~4 cm), the heart can be accessed through a 1 cm incision of the intercostal muscle between the fourth and fifth ribs using rib retractors (mice, 3 cm; rats, 5 cm). The LAD artery is identified as the coronary system branching from the left circumflex just below the left atrial appendage.

Cardiac injection

Cardiac angiogenesis can be modulated in different vascular beds of the cardiac myocardium, but the direct access approach facilitates interventions targeted at the anterior wall of the heart. To this end, a strategy based on the positive identification of the LAD is employed to direct the two 25 μl injections (30 G $\times$ 8 mm syringe) of treatment (e.g., growth factor, cells, etc.) or vehicle alone is administered 2mm apart on the mid-left anterior ventricular wall (see Figure 78.2). After treatment the lungs are inflated, and the chest wall is closed with a three-layer closure. Sets of animals can then be sacrificed at different time points to histologically quantify cardiac angiogenesis, or be potentially imaged with noninvasive approaches currently being developed as measures of cardiac perfusion.

Assessment approach

In the aging heart, both morphometric and immunohistology protocols have been employed in the quantification of angiogenesis. Morphometric studies of perfusion fixed tissue can provide accurate assessment about cardiac capillary density as well as the macrovasculature in the heart (Anversa *et al.*, 1991; Anversa *et al.*, 1994). Immunohistology can differentiate the heterogeneous endothelial cell subpopulations that contribute to cardiac angiogenesis (Edelberg *et al.*, 2002b; Cai *et al.*, 2003; Xaymardan *et al.*, 2004b). Studies directed at the mid-papillary level in cross sections of the left ventriculature provide a direct assessment of the potential actions of local injections directed at the level of the mid LAD.

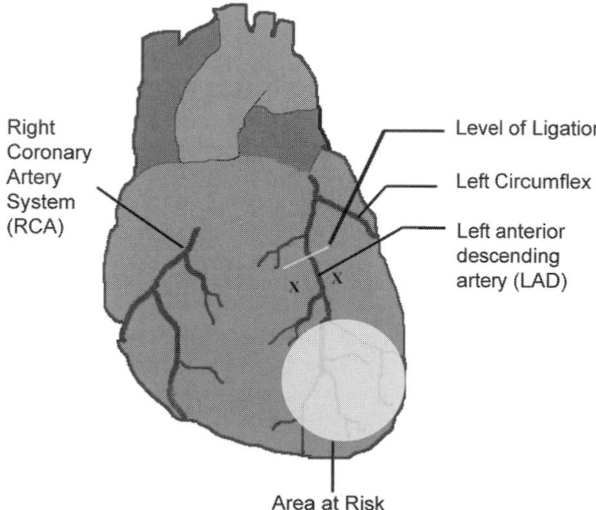

Figure 78.2 This diagram of the heart illustrates the area at risk in the left ventricle resulting from the occlusion of the left anterior descending artery (LAD) in the rat myocardial infarction model. Note the site of injection and level of ligation.

Morphometric studies

Morphometric analysis employs hearts that are arrested in diastole with cadmium-Cl and cannulation-based perfusion formalin fixation (Li *et al.*, 1997) and allows for the direct assessment of capillary profiles (Anversa *et al.*, 1994). In addition to providing a quantification of capillary density, this approach facilitates the direct analysis of myocyte-capillary ratios and quantification of the left coronary arterial tree.

Immunohistology—Vascular histology

The characterization of cardiac angiogenesis by immunohistology can be performed on perfusion fixed or embedded tissue. Immunostains with antibodies directed against platelet endothelial cell adhesion molecule (PECAM; CD31), as well as VE cadherin, can provide an overall assessment of vascular density in the hearts. In addition, studies of von Willebrand factor, VEGF receptors, including Flk-1 and Flt-1, Ang receptors, Tie-2 and PDGF receptors α and β can provide important insight into the kinetics and potential mechanisms governing alterations in angiogenic pathways in the aging heart. The analysis of capillary density can be determined by automated image analysis such as CapiShape (Hu *et al.*, 1999) or directly through manual quantification of all stained luminal structures in high-power fields (40–100 $\times$ magnification) in a blinded approach.

In vivo anatomical/functional imaging

Recent advances in noninvasive approaches employing vascular contrast with both echocardiography (ultrasound-based) and magnetic resonance imaging (NMR-based) offer the potential to provide important information about cardiac microvascular anatomy and blood flow after angiogenic induction (Pearlman *et al.*, 1995; Wilke *et al.*, 2000) as well as after myocardial infarction (Gladish, 2005; Kaandorp *et al.*, 2005).

Myocardial Infarction Model

The significance of cardiac angiogenesis can be functionally measured in the cardioprotection provided in myocardial infarction models. Indeed, the ability to induce myocardial injury (ischemia, infarction, etc.) provides an important model of clinical cardiovascular disease and is a useful technique in studying cardiac-specific angiogenesis. Specifically, acute coronary occlusion models have been used to observe angiogenesis after the administration of growth factors (Edelberg *et al.*, 2002b; Chachques *et al.*, 2004; Xaymardan *et al.*, 2004b), stem cells (Nagaya *et al.*, 2004; Xaymardan *et al.*, 2004a), and genes that encode for growth factors (Schwarz *et al.*, 2000; Su *et al.*, 2002; Hao *et al.*, 2004; Hao *et al.*, 2004; Su *et al.*, 2004).

Surgical Approach

A left ventricular myocardial infarction can be induced via the occlusion of the LAD artery by physical ligation using an 8-0 nylon suture (Ethilon, Ethicon, NJ) or by photothrombosis (see Figure 78.2), which involves a systemic injection of a photosensitizing dye (e.g., Rose Bengal) and excitation of the interested artery with a laser ion light source as Rosen (2001) and Eichenbaum (2002) have displayed in mice. This procedure can be used in concert with the molecular injection procedure where administration of the treatments can be given prior to or after the occlusion. Moreover, the duration of the occlusion can be varied from periods of ischemia and reperfusion to permanent coronary ligation, modeling acute coronary syndrome and acute myocardial infarction, respectively. In addition, the functional significance of various interventions can be assessed at a range of time points after myocardial infarction to investigate the potential role of angiogenic pathways in the aging rodent heart.

ANALYSIS

Area at risk

Acutely, an increase in cardiac angiogenesis can reduce the area at risk in the treated heart. The area at risk in hearts can be quantified via histological approaches. In order to view the extent of area at risk (as an inverse correlate of cardiac angiogenesis), Masson's trichrome staining can be performed on cardiac sections at the mid papillary muscle (see Figure 78.3).

Alternatively, triphenyltetrazolium (TTC) is another method utilized to quantify infarction size (Birnbaum *et al.*, 2003). Similarly, the extent of myocardial cell death can be quantified at early time points by staining for apoptotic cells by terminal deoxynucleotidyltransferase-mediated dUTP nick end labeling (TUNEL) staining (Xaymardan *et al.*, 2004b).

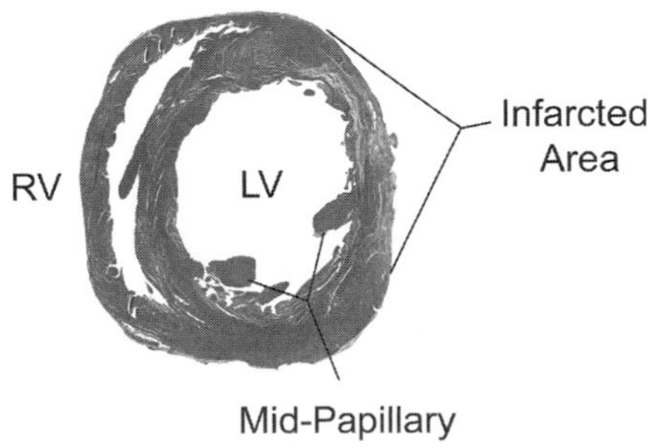

Figure 78.3 Masson's trichrome staining 14 d after a left anterior descending artery occlusion, at the mid-papillary level. Smooth muscle cells are stained red, and areas of fibrosis are stained blue.

Area of myocardial infarction

A more chronic measure of the role of cardiac angiogenesis is the Masson's trichrome stain of the area of cardiac injury. Specifically, Masson's trichrome utilizes three stains to selectively identify muscle, collagen fibers, and fibrin. As illustrated in Figure 78.3, the fibrotic area is stained blue, indicating the area at risk. (Note: red = intact myocardium.) Histological quantification of the left ventricular myocardial infarct percentage at the mid-papillary level can be obtained from Masson's trichrome stained sections by imaging software developed at the National Institute of Health (ImageJ v1.28) and Eq. I:

$$\frac{\text{Myocardial infarction area}}{(\text{Left ventricle total area} - \text{Chamber area})} \times 100\% \qquad \text{(I)}$$

Indeed, previous studies have demonstrated the inverse association between preinfarction cardiac angiogenesis and extent of myocardial infarction based on Masson's trichrome stain in the aging rat heart (Edelberg *et al.*, 2002b; Cai *et al.*, 2003; Xaymardan *et al.*, 2004b).

Functional assessment

Measures of cardiac function after myocardial injury provide an important correlation with histological measures of myocardial injury in the study of cardiac angiogenesis. Moreover, through the use of noninvasive functional testing the impact of various interventions can be measured in live animals, providing important clinical insights in the testing strategies targeted at angiogenesis in the aging heart.

Exercise Physiology

Recently the utility of maximum sprinting speed in predicting the extent of myocardial injury after an acute infarction in the young heart has been demonstrated (Zheng *et al.*, 2004) based on the protocols originally developed by Barbato (1998). In order to assess cardiac function in rodent models, the inverse association between postinfarction maximum exercise speed and extent of myocardial injury has been demonstrated (Zheng *et al.*, 2004), suggesting that exercise speed may be a direct correlate of preinfarction cardiac angiogenesis.

Two days after coronary ligation, the rats can be trained using a motor-driven treadmill. Animals are acclimated to the treadmill (10° inclination) 2 min/d, 5 d/week for two weeks, with the stimulus intensity of the shock grid being 2mA. During the first week, the animals train at 10 m/min; during the second week, the animals are trained at 15 m/min. After the acclimation period, the maximal sprinting speed is measured in each rat (Zheng *et al.*, 2004), beginning at a speed of 10 m/min. The speed is increased 5 m/min every 30 s until the rat becomes exhausted. "Exhausted" is defined as the inability to keep up with the belt for 5 s. Each rat is tested once daily on three consecutive days (12–14 d post-ligation).

Notably, however, impaired function in the older peripheral vasculature and diminished overall reserve in aging animals may reduce the utility of this assessment approach in models of myocardial infarction in the older heart.

Echocardiography

In order to assess cardiac function in rodent models, wall motion can be directly imaged by echocardiography before and/or after myocardial infarction. Specifically, the inverse association between postinfarction left ventricular fractional shortening and cxtent of myocardial injury has been shown (see Figure 78.4), suggesting that echocardiography may be a direct correlate of pre-infarction cardiac angiogenesis (Zheng *et al.*, 2004).

Echocardiography Protocols

Cardiac function can be studied on unanesthetized animals by restraining them in the left lateral decubitus position using a 15 MHz frequency linear phased array transducer, or alternatively, can be imaged under anesthesia via a 10 MHz transesophageal probe. Long-axis and short-axis parasternal views of the left ventricle will be obtained with M-mode echocardiograms taken at the mid-papillary muscle level (see Figure 78.5).

Cardiac wall motion can be scored by dividing the ventricle into six equal radial segments (see Figure 78.6).

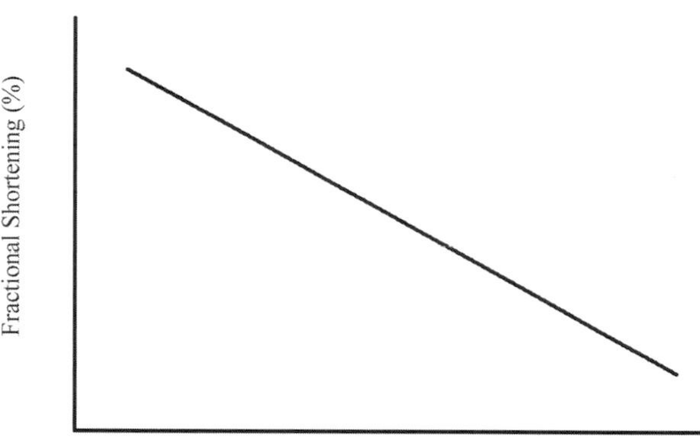

Figure 78.4 Inverse association between MI Size and FS. Graph depicting the trend of cardiac function as measured by fractional shortening to myocardial infarction size.

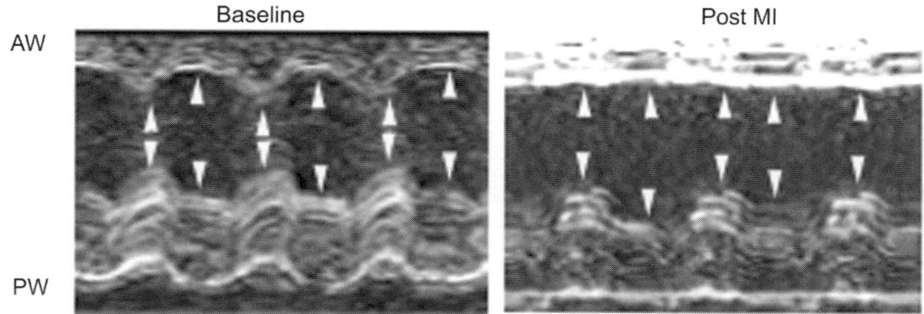

Figure 78.5 M-mode echocardiography. Representative rat transesophageal echocardiograms depicting left ventricular myocardial function at baseline and 14 d after myocardial infarction. Note the depressed anterior wall motion postinfarction (AW = Anterior Wall; PW = Posterior Wall).

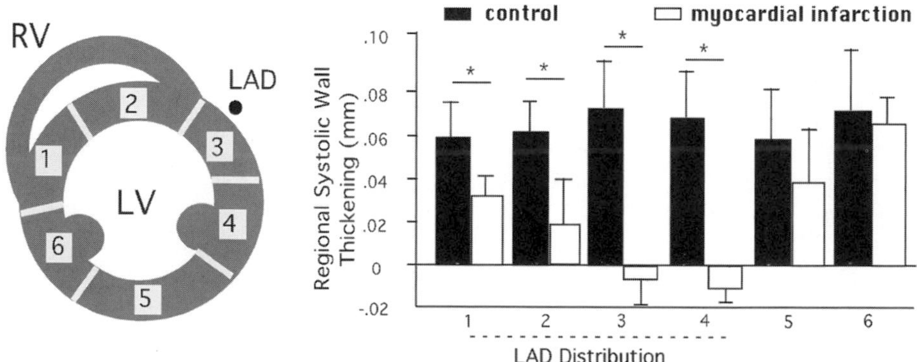

Figure 78.6 Regional systolic ventricular wall thickening in control rats and rats with anterior wall myocardial infarctions. Negative values indicate pathological systolic wall thinning.

The mean wall thickness of each segment can be determined using measurements from three to five cardiac cycles. Systolic wall thickening in each segment is defined as the mean systolic wall thickness minus the mean diastolic wall thickness that can be utilized to measure the functional preservation of the cardiac myocardium following coronary artery occlusion. Specifically, fractional shortening is measured as the difference in left ventricular end-diastolic diameter (LVEDD) and left ventricular end-systolic diameter (LVESD), divided by LVEDD and taken as a percent:

$$FS(\%) = ((LVEDD) - LVESC)/LVEDD) * 100\% \quad (II)$$

Conclusion

Overall, these *in vivo* models provide us with valuable insight into the process of age-associated changes in cardiac angiogenesis. By employing the cardiac allograft assay in concert with the myocardial infarction model, molecular and cellular interventions can be tested to restore functional cardiac angiogenesis. Indeed, cardiac angiogenic growth can directly be measured quantitatively via laser Doppler, or qualitatively upon gross examination for engraftment. Based on the results from these study models in the endogenous myocardium the action of specific pathways has been characterized and quantified with regard to angiogenesis in the aging heart. In time, these models will advance, enabling us to better understand the age-associated dynamics of angiogenesis.

ACKNOWLEDGMENTS

This work was supported by the National Institutes of Health (AG19738, AG20918, and HL67839) and an American Federation for Aging Research-Paul Beeson Physician Faculty Scholar in Aging Research Award.

REFERENCES

Abete, P., Ferrara, N., Cacciatore, F., Madrid, A., Bianco, S., Calabrese, C. *et al.* (1997). Angina-induced protection against myocardial infarction in adult and elderly patients: A loss of preconditioning mechanism in the aging heart? *J Am Coll Cardiol 30(4)*, 947–954.

Aird, W.C., Edelberg, J.M., Weiler-Guettler, H., Simmons, W.W., Smith T.W., and Rosenberg, R.D. (1997). Vascular bed-specific expression of an endothelial cell gene is programmed by the tissue microenvironment. *J Cell Biol 138(5)*, 1117–1124.

Anversa, P. and Capasso, J.M. (1991). Loss of intermediate-sized coronary arteries and capillary proliferation after left ventricular failure in rats. *Am J Physiol 260(5 Pt 2)*, H1552–H1560.

Anversa, P., Li, P., Sonnenblick E.H., and Olivetti, G. (1994). Effects of aging on quantitative structural properties of coronary vasculature and microvasculature in rats. *Am J Physiol 267(3 Pt 2)*, H1062–H1073.

Augustin-Voss, H.G., Voss, A.K., and Pauli, B.U. (1993). Senescence of aortic endothelial cells in culture: Effects of basic fibroblast growth factor expression on cell phenotype, migration, and proliferation. *J Cell Physiol 157(2)*, 279–288.

Barbato, J.C., Koch, L.G., Darvish, A., Cicila, G.T., Metting, P.J., and Britton, S.L. (1998). Spectrum of aerobic endurance running performance in eleven inbred strains of rats. *J Appl Physiol 85(2)*, 530–536.

Berkowitz, D.E., White, R., Li, D., Minhas, K.M., Cernetich, A., Kim, S. *et al.* (2003). Arginase reciprocally regulates nitric oxide synthase activity and contributes to endothelial dysfunction in aging blood vessels. *Circulation 108(16)*, 2000–2006.

Birnbaum, Y., Ashitkov, T., Uretsky, B.F., Ballinger S., and Motamedi, M. (2003). Reduction of infarct size by short-term pretreatment with atorvastatin. *Cardiovasc Drugs Ther 17(1)*, 25–30.

Black, H.R. (2003). The burden of cardiovascular disease: Following the link from hypertension to myocardial infarction and heart failure. *Am J Hypertens 16(9 Pt 2)*, 4S–6S.

Cai, D., Xaymardan, M., Holm, J.M., Zheng, J., Kizer, J.R., and Edelberg, J.M. (2003). Age-associated impairment in TNF-alpha cardioprotection from myocardial infarction. *Am J Physiol Heart Circ Physiol 285(2)*, H463–H469.

Chachques, J.C., Duarte, F., Cattadori, B., Shafy, A., Lila, N., Chatellier, G. *et al.* (2004). Angiogenic growth factors and/or cellular therapy for myocardial regeneration: A comparative study. *J Thorac Cardiovasc Surg 128(2)*, 245–253.

Edelberg, J.M., Jacobson, J.T., Gidseg, D.S., Tang, L., and Christini, D.J. (2002a). Enhanced myocyte-based biosensing of the blood-borne signals regulating chronotropy. *J Appl Physiol 92(2)*, 581–585.

Edelberg, J.M., Lee, S.H., Kaur, M., Tang, L., Feirt, N.M., McCabe, S. *et al.* (2002b). Platelet-derived growth factor-AB limits the extent of myocardial infarction in a rat model: Feasibility of restoring impaired angiogenic capacity in the aging heart. *Circulation 105(5)*, 608–613.

Edelberg, J.M., Wong, A., Holm, J.M., Xaymardan, M., Duignan, I., Chin, A. *et al.* (2004). Phage display identification of age-associated TNF alpha-mediated cardiac oxidative induction. *Physiol Genomics 18(3)*, 255–260.

Eichenbaum, J.W., Pevsner, P.H., Pivawer, G., Kleinman, G.M., Chiriboga, L., Stern, A. *et al.* (2002). A murine photochemical stroke model with histologic correlates of apoptotic and nonapoptotic mechanisms. *J Pharmacol Toxicol Methods 47(2)*, 67–71.

Fenton, R.A., Dickson, E.W., Meyer, T.E., and Dobson, J.G.Jr. (2000). Aging reduces the cardioprotective effect of ischemic preconditioning in the rat heart. *J Mol Cell Cardiol 32(7)*, 1371–1375.

Ferrara, N. (2001). Role of vascular endothelial growth factor in regulation of physiological angiogenesis. *Am J Physiol Cell Physiol 280(6)*, C1358–C1366.

Garfinkel, S., Hu, X., Prudovsky, I.A., McMahon, G.A., Kapnik, E.M., McDowell, S.D. *et al.* (1996). FGF-1-dependent proliferative and migratory responses are impaired in senescent human umbilical vein endothelial cells and correlate with the inability to signal tyrosine phosphorylation of fibroblast growth factor receptor-1 substrates. *J Cell Biol 134(3)*, 783–791.

Gladish, G.W. (2005). Advances in cardiac magnetic resonance imaging and computed tomography. *Expert Rev Cardiovasc Ther 3(2)*, 309–320.

Hansson, L., Lindholm, L.H., Niskanen, L., Lanke, J., Hedner, T., Niklason, A. *et al.* (1999). Effect of angiotensin-converting-enzyme inhibition compared with conventional therapy on cardiovascular morbidity and mortality in hypertension: The Captopril Prevention Project (CAPPP) randomised trial. *Lancet 353(9153)*, 611–616.

Hao, X., Mansson-Broberg, A., Blomberg, P., Dellgren, G., Siddiqui, A.J., Grinnemo, K.H. *et al.* (2004). Angiogenic and cardiac functional effects of dual gene transfer of VEGF-A165 and PDGF-BB after myocardial infarction. *Biochem Biophys Res Commun 322(1)*, 292–296.

Hao, X., Mansson-Broberg, A., Gustafsson, T., Grinnemo, K.H., Blomberg, P., Siddiqui, A.J. *et al.* (2004). Angiogenic effects of dual gene transfer of bFGF and PDGF-BB after myocardial infarction. *Biochem Biophys Res Commun 315(4)*, 1058–1063.

Harada, K., Grossman, W., Friedman, M., Edelman, E.R., Prasad, P.V., Keighley, C.S. *et al.* (1994). Basic fibroblast growth factor improves myocardial function in chronically ischemic porcine hearts. *J Clin Invest 94(2)*, 623–630.

Hu, Q. and Mahler, F. (1999). New system for image analysis in nailfold capillaroscopy. *Microcirculation 6(3)*, 227–235.

Kaandorp, T.A., Lamb, H.J., Bax, J.J., van der Wall, E.E., and de Roos, A. (2005). Magnetic resonance imaging of coronary arteries, the ischemic cascade, and myocardial infarction. *Am Heart J 149(2)*, 200–208.

Li, Q., Li, B., Wang, X., Leri, A., Jana, K.P., Liu, Y. *et al.* (1997). Overexpression of insulin-like growth factor-1 in mice protects from myocyte death after infarction, attenuating ventricular dilation, wall stress, and cardiac hypertrophy. *J Clin Invest 100(8)*, 1991–1999.

Nagaya, N., Fujii, T., Iwase, T., Ohgushi, H., Itoh, T., Uematsu, M. *et al.* (2004). Intravenous administration of mesenchymal stem cells improves cardiac function in rats with acute myocardial infarction through angiogenesis and myogenesis. *Am J Physiol Heart Circ Physiol 287(6)*, H2670–H2676.

Nakae, I., Fujita, M., Miwa, K., Hasegawa, K., Kihara, Y., Nohara, R. *et al.* (2000). Age-dependent impairment of coronary collateral development in humans. *Heart Vessels 15(4)*, 176–180.

Oxenham, H. and Sharpe, N. (2003). Cardiovascular aging and heart failure. *Eur J Heart Fail 5(4)*, 427–434.

Pearlman, J.D., Hibberd, M.G., Chuang, M.L., Harada, K., Lopez, J.J., Gladstone, S.R. *et al.* (1995). Magnetic resonance mapping demonstrates benefits of VEGF-induced myocardial angiogenesis. *Nat Med 1(10)*, 1085–1089.

Reed, M.J., Corsa, A., Pendergrass, W., Penn, P., Sage, E.H., and Abrass, I.B. (1998). Neovascularization in aged mice: Delayed angiogenesis is coincident with decreased levels of transforming growth factor beta 1 and type I collagen. *Am J Pathol 152(1)*, 113–123.

Rivard, A., Fabre, J.E., Silver, M., Chen, D., Murohara, T., Kearney, M. *et al.* (1999). Age-dependent impairment of angiogenesis. *Circulation 99(1)*, 111–120.

Rochetaing, A. and Kreher, P. (2003). Reactive hyperemia during early reperfusion as a determinant of improved functional recovery in ischemic preconditioned rat hearts. *J Thorac Cardiovasc Surg 125(6)*, 1516–1525.

Rosen, E.D., Raymond, S., Zollman, A., Noria, F., Sandoval-Cooper, M., Shulman, A. *et al.* (2001). Laser-induced noninvasive vascular injury models in mice generate platelet- and coagulation-dependent thrombi. *Am J Pathol 158(5)*, 1613–1622.

Sarzani, R., Arnaldi, G., Takasaki, I., Brecher, P., and Chobanian, A.V. (1991). Effects of hypertension and aging on platelet-derived growth factor and platelet-derived growth factor receptor expression in rat aorta and heart. *Hypertension 18(5 Suppl)*, III93–III99.

Schwarz, E.R., Speakman, M.T., Patterson, M., Hale, S.S., Isner, J.M., Kedes, L.H. *et al.* (2000). Evaluation of the effects of intramyocardial injection of DNA expressing vascular endothelial growth factor (VEGF) in a myocardial infarction model in the rat—Angiogenesis and angioma formation. *J Am Coll Cardiol 35(5)*, 1323–1330.

Shimada, T., Takeshita, Y., Murohara, T., Sasaki, K., Egami, K., Shintani, S. *et al.* (2004). Angiogenesis and vasculogenesis are impaired in the precocious-aging klotho mouse. *Circulation 110(9)*, 1148–1155.

Stewart, S., MacIntyre, K., Capewell, S., and McMurray, J.J. (2003). Heart failure and the aging population: An increasing burden in the 21st century? *Heart 89(1)*, 49–53.

Su, H., Arakawa-Hoyt, J., and Kan, Y.W. (2002). Adeno-associated viral vector-mediated hypoxia response element-regulated gene expression in mouse ischemic heart model. *Proc Natl Acad Sci USA 99(14)*, 9480–9485.

Su, H., Joho, S., Huang, Y., Barcena, A., Arakawa-Hoyt, J., Grossman, W. *et al.* (2004). Adeno-associated viral vector delivers cardiac-specific and hypoxia-inducible VEGF expression in ischemic mouse hearts. *Proc Natl Acad Sci USA 101(46)*, 16280–16285.

Tani, M., Honma, Y., Takayama, M., Hasegawa, H., Shinmura, K., Ebihara, Y. *et al.* (1999). Loss of protection by hypoxic preconditioning in aging Fischer 344 rat hearts related to myocardial glycogen content and Na+ imbalance. *Cardiovasc Res 41(3)*, 594–602.

Volpe, M., Ruilope, L.M., McInnes, G.T., Waeber, B., and Weber, M.A. (2005). Angiotensin-II receptor blockers: Benefits beyond blood pressure reduction? *J Hum Hypertens.*

Widlansky, M.E., Gokce, N., Keaney, J.F. Jr., and Vita, J.A. (2003). The clinical implications of endothelial dysfunction. *J Am Coll Cardiol 42(7)*, 1149–1160.

Wilke, N.M., Zenovich, A., Muehling, O., and Jerosch-Herold, M. (2000). Novel revascularization therapies—TMLR and growth factor-induced angiogenesis monitored with cardiac MRI. *Magma 11(1–2)*, 61–64.

Xaymardan, M., Tang, L., Zagreda, L., Pallante, B., Zheng, J., Chazen, J.L., *et al.* (2004a). Platelet-derived growth factor-AB promotes the generation of adult bone marrow-derived cardiac myocytes. *Circ Res 94(5)*, E39–E45.

Xaymardan, M., Zheng, J., Duignan, I., Chin, A., Holm, J.M., Ballard, V.L. *et al.* (2004b). Senescent impairment in synergistic cytokine pathways that provide rapid cardioprotection in the rat heart. *J Exp Med 199(6)*, 797–804.

Yanagisawa-Miwa, A., Uchida, Y., Nakamura, F., Tomaru, T., Kido, H., Kamijo, T. *et al.* (1992). Salvage of infarcted myocardium by angiogenic action of basic fibroblast growth factor. *Science 257(5075)*, 1401–1403.

Yusuf, S., Sleight, P., Pogue, J., Bosch, J., Davies, R., and Dagenais, G. (2000). Effects of an angiotensin-converting-enzyme inhibitor, ramipril, on cardiovascular events in high-risk patients. The Heart Outcomes Prevention Evaluation Study Investigators. *N Engl J Med 342(3)*, 145–153.

Zheng, J., Shin, J.H., Xaymardan, M., Chin, A., Duignan, I., Hong, M.K. *et al.* (2004). Platelet-derived growth factor improves cardiac function in a rodent myocardial infarction model. *Coron Artery Dis 15(1)*, 59–64.

79

Models for the Study of Stroke

Thiruma V. Arumugam and Mark P. Mattson

Stroke is a devastating disease that represents the third leading cause of death in the United States. Vessel occlusions account for 85% of all strokes, and primary intracerebral bleeding accounts for about 15%. There are several different risk factors for ischemic stroke including genetic factors, aging, hypertension, hypercholesterolemia, diabetes mellitus, atrial fibrillation, coagulation disorders, and smoking. The pathophysiological processes in stroke are complex and involve disruption of the blood-brain barrier, energy failure, loss of cell ion homeostasis, acidosis, increased intracellular calcium levels, excitotoxicity, free radical-mediated toxicity, generation of arachidonic acid products, cytokine mediated cytotoxicity, complement activation, activation of glial cells, and infiltration of leukocytes. Animal models have been developed that closely resemble stroke injury seen in human patients. Many experimental models are used to study stroke injury. Mechanisms of cell damage are determined by testing effects of different manipulations on the extent of cell death in a model. The three main classes of in vivo *animal models are global ischemia, focal ischemia, and hypoxia/ischemia. Technological advances and experimental discoveries have begun to define the cellular and molecular mechanisms involved in stroke injury, and exploration of these targets led to the development of numerous agents that target various injury pathways. Despite numerous agents that can prevent the cascade of events leading to ischemic neuronal death in animal models, there is no neuroprotective agent that has been shown to conclusively improve stroke outcome in humans. Novel interventions will be required to overcome hurdles associated with bench-to-bedside translation.*

Introduction

Stroke is a devastating disease that represents the third leading cause of death in the United States (www.strokeassociation.org). Each year, more than half a million Americans fall victim to stroke, which costs approximately 70 billion dollars. It is estimated that the lifetime risk for stroke is between 8 and 10%. Pathogenetically, stroke involves a heterogeneous group of processes. Vessel occlusions (ischemic stroke) account for 85% of all strokes; primary intracerebral bleeding (hemorrhagic stroke) accounts for about 15%. Embolisms cause approximately 75% of all cerebral vessel occlusions and are the most frequent cause of focally impeded blood flow within the brain. Microangiopathical causes, namely, *in situ* thromboses and hyalinoses of the arterioles, occur in about 20% of all cases. Hemodynamic infarctions as a result of high-grade stenoses of the cerebral arteries are rare and account for less than 5% (Mergenthaler *et al.*, 2004).

Ischemia is defined as a reduction in blood flow sufficient to alter cellular function. Brain tissue is exquisitely sensitive to ischemia such that even brief ischemia to neurons can initiate a complex sequence of events that ultimately culminates in cellular death. Different brain regions have different thresholds for ischemic cell damage, with white matter being more resilient than gray matter. In addition, certain populations of neurons are selectively vulnerable to ischemia; for example, in the hippocampus, CA1 pyramidal neurons are vulnerable to ischemia, whereas dentate granule neurons are resistant. Ischemia of cerebral tissue and death of neurons and glial cells underlie all forms of stroke and intraparenchymal hemorrhage. The cellular and biochemical abnormalities in stroke overlap with those that occur in closed head injury and subarachnoid hemorrhage. There are two major categories of experimental ischemia, namely, global and focal ischemia models. In global ischemia models, typically two or four cervical vessels are temporarily interrupted, and circulation is restored after some delay (see Figure 79.1).

In focal ischemia models, the middle cerebral artery typically is occluded either permanently or temporarily to allow reperfusion (McBean and Kelly, 1998). Animal hemorrhagic stroke models are able to reproduce the key pathophysiologic events documented in human hemorrhagic stroke. Thus, hemorrhagic stroke models serve as an important tool for understanding the mechanisms underlying brain injury after an intracerebral bleed. However, future efforts should be directed toward the development of a model that mimics the pathophysiologic processes that lead to spontaneous intracerebral hemorrhage, progression of hemorrhage, and recurrence of bleeding in humans (Andaluz *et al.*, 2002).

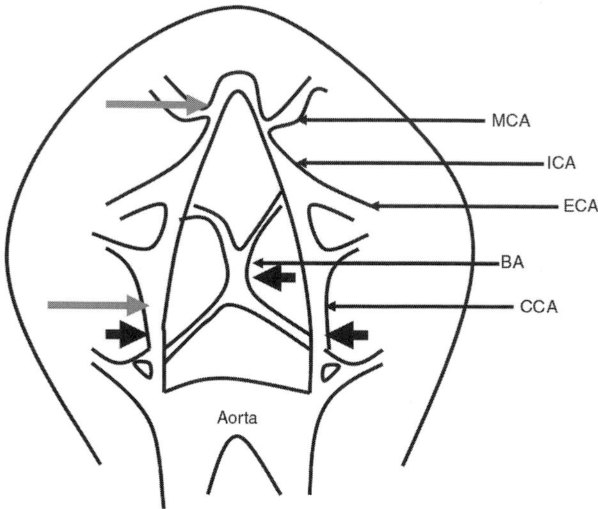

Figure 79.1 Surgical technique for inducing global or focal cerebral ischemia in mouse. Schematic illustration of arteries demonstrating the three points of occlusion (short arrows) for global ischemia (3-VO) and long arrows for focal ischemia. MCA: middle cerebral artery; ICA: internal carotid artery; ECA: external carotid artery; BA: basilar artery; CCA: common carotid artery.

Early restoration of blood flow remains the treatment of choice for limiting brain injury following stroke. Improved educational efforts that emphasize the early signs and symptoms of stroke, coupled with the widespread application of thrombolytic therapy to patients with acute ischemic stroke, have decreased morbidity and mortality. Although reperfusion of the ischemic brain is desirable, tissue damage often results from both the transient ischemic insult and the reperfusion, the latter process inducing an inflammatory response that causes additional injury to the cerebral microcirculation and adjacent brain tissue. Hence, a rapidly evolving area of emphasis in stroke research involves defining the molecular and cellular basis for the augmented tissue injury and inflammation associated with transient cerebral ischemia. Experimental evidence suggests that the majority of stroke patients exhibit a slow evolution of brain injury that occurs over a period of hours to days. This window of opportunity provides a realistic target for therapeutic intervention, with the goal of inhibiting the progression of tissue damage that normally results from both ischemia and reperfusion. Attenuating and/or delaying this time-dependent brain injury may improve neurological outcome and facilitate brain recovery from injury (Legos and Barone, 2003).

This chapter considers the etiology and pathogenesis of stroke. Risk factors and pathophysiology of injury are explained. Experimental animal models of global, focal, and hemorrhagic strokes are described in detail, and different experimental strategies to analyze the injury are also explained. Finally, we describe preclinical studies using different strategies in experimental models, the results of human neuroprotection and revascularization trials, and emerging approaches for the prevention and treatment of stroke.

Etiologies and Pathogenesis

RISK FACTORS

There are several different risk factors for ischemic stroke including genetic factors, aging, hypertension, hypercholesterolemia, diabetes mellitus, atrial fibrillation, coagulation disorders, and smoking.

Genetic factors

Single-gene defects can lead to stroke through specific pathophysiological mechanisms including large artery disease, coagulation disorders, small vessel disease, cardiac embolism, mitochondrial disorders, and ion channel disorders (Hassan and Markus, 2000). Single gene alterations can be responsible for stroke, but their prevalence is low. Considerable effort is being made to identify stroke-related genes in different human populations through the candidate gene approach. Due to the large number of candidate genes, many studies have been reported in the literature. They have investigated components of the haemostatic system, vasoconstrictor and vasodilator substances, and enzymes involved in homocysteine and lipid metabolism (Hassan and Markus, 2000). The large variation in ethnic groups that have been studied, the variable sample size, and the dissimilar criteria in the selection of patients and controls have led to variable results, with few consistent findings. The angiotensin converting enzyme (ACE) gene has been an extensively investigated candidate gene in ischemic stroke. However, both positive and negative associations have been reported for the ACE gene in different samples (Markus *et al.*, 1995). Cerebral autosomal dominant arteriopathy with subcortical infarcts and leukoencephalopathy (CADASIL) is a monogenic syndrome associated with lacunar stroke and vascular dementia (Dichgans, 2002). It is caused by mutations of the *Notch3* gene that encodes a membrane receptor (Artavanis-Tsakonas *et al.*, 1999). Several mutations of this same gene have been discovered in different affected families (Joutel *et al.*, 2000). As for other monogenic stroke syndromes, information obtained on the genetic basis of CADASIL were extended to the general population by a systematic screening in the attempt to discover a role for *Notch3* in common forms of stroke; however, the results to date have been negative.

Hypertension

Epidemiological studies have shown a positive and linear relationship between both systolic and diastolic blood pressure (BP) and the incidence of any subtype of ischemic or hemorrhagic stroke, at any age, and in both sexes. However, no threshold distinguishes patients who will have a vascular event from those who will not.

In individuals with normal BP, the vascular risk, including stroke, is higher in those who have the highest levels of normal BP (Vasan *et al.*, 2001). The risk of stroke doubles for every 7.5 mm Hg increase in diastolic BP (Leys *et al.*, 2002). Isolated systolic arterial hypertension, defined as systolic BP greater than 160 mm Hg with diastolic BP lower than 90 mm Hg, is also an important risk factor for stroke in the elderly (Leys *et al.*, 2002). Although the primary prevention of stroke through the treatment of hypertension is well established, the issue of lowering BP after a cerebrovascular event has been uncertain, particularly since this might worsen cerebral perfusion if autoregulation remains chronically damaged or if severe carotid artery stenosis is present. In contrast to primary prevention studies in which hypertensive patients were studied, the majority of secondary prevention studies recruited patients irrespective of their BP (Rashid *et al.*, 2003). Overall, lowering BP was associated with significant reductions in stroke; a nonsignificant benefit was also seen for severe stroke, but overall mortality was not altered (Rashid *et al.*, 2003).

Hypercholesterolemia

Whether hypercholesterolemia, a major risk factor for coronary heart disease, is associated with stroke is controversial and remains a matter of debate. Elevated levels of circulating cholesterol cause deposits to form inside blood vessels. When the deposits become sufficiently large, they block blood vessels and decrease the flow of blood. These deposits are part of a disease process called atherosclerosis, which can cause blood clots to form that will ultimately stop blood flow. Data from a clinical study, which enrolled healthy men without vascular disease, suggest that patients in the highest quartile of total cholesterol to high-density lipoprotein ratio have an increased risk of stroke (Bowman *et al.*, 2003). There was no evidence of increased risk in patients with elevated total cholesterol, high-density lipoprotein, or triglycerides. Further studies are needed to determine if lowering cholesterol levels in healthy individuals reduces the incidence of stroke. Other studies in an elderly population suggested a protective effect of a higher high-density lipoprotein cholesterol level (Sacco *et al.*, 2001).

Diabetes

The risk of mortality and morbidity from stroke in subjects with diabetes is increased by more than two-fold; diabetes is an independent risk factor for stroke (Mankovsky and Ziegler, 2004). Chronic hyperglycemia, insulin resistance, and their associated cellular and molecular alterations may contribute to an elevated stroke risk either by amplification of the harmful effect of existing risk factors or by acting independently. The pathophysiological and biochemical ischemic cerebral impairments in patients with diabetes are not fully characterized; however, as the risk of morbidity and mortality associated with stroke in patients with diabetes is high, the existing preventive measures could significantly reduce prevalence of stroke.

Aging

Age is an important risk factor for the frequency and the occurrence of stroke as well as for its outcome. In a clinical study of stroke patients, age was one of the most significant prognostic factors (Brown *et al.*, 1996). Age also was found to be associated with poor prognosis in a study of patients with transient ischemic attacks (Howard *et al.*, 1987). In healthy volunteers, basal cerebral blood flow was shown to decrease with age, and this age-dependent effect was even more pronounced in cases of cerebral atherosclerotic disease (Ewing *et al.*, 1989). Although stroke is mostly a disease of the elderly, the majority of experimental models use healthy young animals. Although hypertension, an important risk factor in stroke, was repeatedly tested by using spontaneously hypertensive rats, age as a risk factor for ischemic or hemorrhagic stroke has not been thoroughly addressed in animal models. However, some of the recent studies have addressed the effect of age in stroke pathology and prognosis (Davis *et al.*, 1995). Of the available animal species to model stroke, large mammals such as dogs have displayed inconsistent lesions (Garcia, 1984), whereas the inter-animal variability is low in inbred strains of rats and mice.

Lifestyle

Overeating, a sedentary lifestyle, smoking, and diets high in saturated and trans-fats and cholesterol and low in whole grains and vegetables increase the risk of stroke (www.strokeassociation.org). Conversely, diets low in calories and "bad" fats and high in vegetables and whole grains, regular exercise, and abstinence from smoking reduce the risk of stroke. These factors may promote or inhibit the pathological processes involved in atherosclerosis. In addition, dietary restriction and physical exercise may protect neurons against ischemic damage, enhance neurogenesis, and improve functional outcome by stimulating the production of neurotrophic factors in brain cells (Mattson *et al.*, 2002).

PATHOPHYSIOLOGY

The pathophysiological processes in stroke are complex and involve disruption of the blood-brain barrier (BBB), energy failure, loss of cell ion homeostasis, acidosis, increased intracellular calcium levels, excitotoxicity, free radical-mediated toxicity, generation of arachidonic acid products, cytokine mediated cytotoxicity, complement activation, activation of glial cells, and infiltration of leukocytes (see Figure 79.2).

These events can lead to ischemic necrosis, which occurs in the severely ischemic core regions. Necrosis is morphologically characterized by initial cellular and organelle swelling; subsequent disruption of nuclear, organelle, and plasma membranes; disintegration of

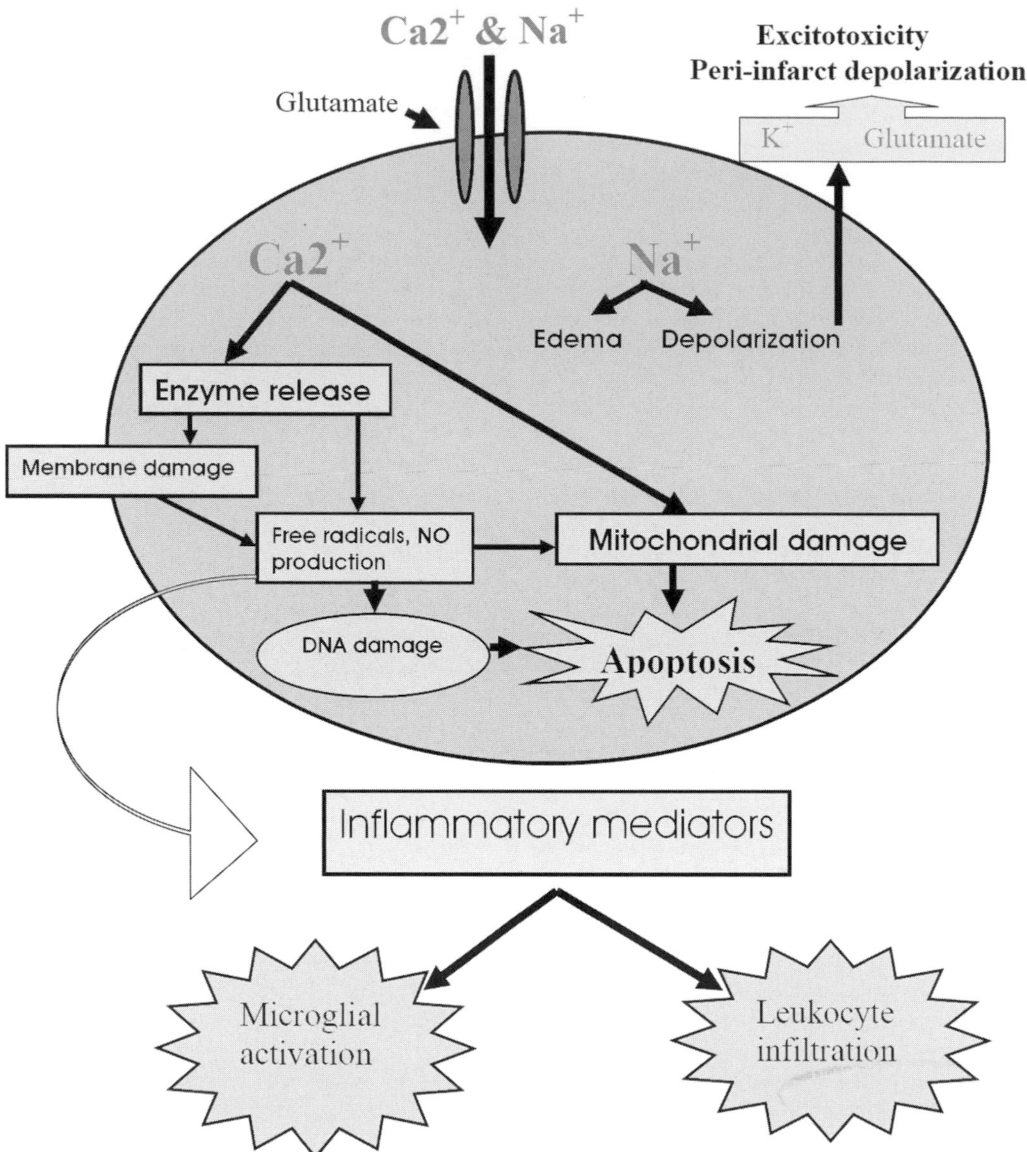

Figure 79.2 Pathophysiological mechanisms of ischemic stroke. Ischemia-induced energy failure leads to the depolarization of neurons. Activation of specific glutamate receptors dramatically increases intracellular Ca^{2+} and Na^{+}concentrations, and K^{+} is released into the extracellular space. Edema result when cells swell as water moves into the cells. Increased level of intracellular messenger Ca^{2+} activates proteases, lipases, and endonucleases. Free radicals are generated and damage membranes, mitochondria, and DNA, in turn triggering cell death and inducing the formation of inflammatory mediators, which activate microglia and lead to the invasion of leukocytes via up-regulation of endothelial adhesion molecules.

nuclear structure and cytoplasmic organelles; and disintegration with extrusion of cell contents into the extracellular space (Manjo and Joris, 1995). Less severe ischemia, as occurs in the penumbra region of a focal ischemic infarct, evolves more slowly and depends on the activation of genes (Dirnagl *et al.*, 1999; Lipton, 1999; Zheng and Yenari, 2004).

A significant portion of ischemia-induced neuronal damage is mediated by excessive accumulation of excitatory amino acids, leading to toxic increases in intracellular calcium. This increase in calcium activates various signaling pathways, ultimately leading to cell death. Soon after cessation of cerebral blood flow, energy-dependent pumps fail, resulting in the flow of ions down their concentration gradients. This results in cellular swelling and depolarization. Calcium ions enter the cell through voltage-dependent and ligand-gated ion channels, resulting in activation of a number of proteases, kinases, lipases, and endonucleases, ending in cell death (Lipton, 1999; Mattson *et al.*, 2000). Glutamate, which is the major excitatory neurotransmitter in the brain, accumulates in the extracellular space and activates its receptors.

Glutamate receptor activation induces alterations in the concentration of intracellular ions, especially Ca^{2+} and Na^+ (see Figure 79.2). Elevations of intracellular Na^+ can be damaging to neuronal survival at earlier time points after ischemia. However, experimental studies by different groups suggested that glutamate toxicity is primarily dependent on Ca^{2+} influx (Arundine and Tymianski, 2004; Mattson, 1997).

Neurons normally are exposed to a baseline level of oxidative stress from both exogenous and endogenous sources. Free radicals are highly reactive molecules with one or more unpaired electrons. Free radicals can react with DNA, proteins, and lipids causing varying degrees of damage and dysfunction. Several experimental and clinical observations showed increased free radical formation during all forms of stroke injury. Free radicals involved in stroke-induced brain injury include superoxide anion radical, hydroxyl radical, and nitric oxide (NO). The damaging effects of free radicals normally are prevented or reduced by mechanisms such as antioxidant enzymes and free radical scavengers (Love, 1999; Neumar, 2000). The primary source of oxygen free radicals during ischemic or hemorrhagic stroke injury is the mitochondria that produce superoxide anion radical during the electron transport process. Another potentially important source of superoxide in postischemic neurons is the metabolism of arachidonic acid through the cyclooxygenase and lipooxygenase pathways (Hall, 1995).

Oxygen free radicals can also be generated by activated microglia and infiltrating peripheral leukocytes via the NADPH oxidase system following reperfusion of ischemic injury (Stoll *et al.*, 1998). NO is generated from L-arginine through one of several nitric oxide synthase (NOS) isoforms. The neuronal form (nNOS), which requires calcium/calmodulin for activation, is produced by subpopulations of neurons throughout the brain (Dawson and Dawson, 1998). Inducible NOS (iNOS) is produced by inflammatory cells such as microglia and monocytes. These two isoforms, for the most part, are damaging to the brain under ischemic conditions. A third isoform found in endothelial cells (eNOS) is believed to have vasodilatory properties and may play a beneficial role, as it may ultimately improve local blood flow. NO diffuses freely across membranes and reacts with superoxide to produce peroxynitrite ($ONOO^-$), another highly reactive free radical (Love, 1999). Both oxygen free radicals and reactive nitrogen species are involved in activating several pathways involved in cell death following stroke, such as apoptosis and inflammation. A reduction of oxygen supply also leads to the accumulation of lactate via anaerobic glycolysis and thus to acidosis. Besides the production of different species of oxygen radicals, acidosis also interferes with intracellular protein synthesis. Lipid peroxidation also appears to play a prominent role in the pathogenesis of stroke. The mechanism whereby membrane lipid peroxidation induces neuronal apoptosis appears to involve generation of an aldehyde called 4-hydroxynonenal, which covalently modifies membrane transporters such as Na^+/K^+ ATPase, glucose transporter, and glutamate transporter, thereby impairing their function (Mattson *et al.*, 2000).

Though potentially damaging, Ca^{2+} and free radicals can activate neuroprotective transcription factors, including nuclear factor-κB (NF-κB), hypoxia inducible factor 1, and interferon regulatory factor 1 (Dirnagl *et al.*, 1999). On the other hand, some of these transcription factors induce the expression of inflammatory cytokines (for example, IL-1, IL-6, and TNF-α) and chemokines (e.g., IL-8 and MCP-1), endothelial cell adhesion molecules (e.g., selectins, ICAM-1, and VCAM-1), and other proinflammatory genes (e.g., interferon-inducible protein-10) (Dirnagl *et al.*, 1999; Ishikawa *et al.*, 2004). There are several resident cell populations within brain tissue that are able to secrete proinflammatory mediators after an ischemic insult, including endothelial cells, astrocytes, microglia, and neurons. This gene activation results in increased protein levels for cytokines and increased expression of endothelial cell adhesion molecules (CAMs) in post-stroke brain tissue. A major role in brain inflammation following stroke is ascribed to microglia, especially in the penumbra. Similar to leukocytes, activated microglia produce several proinflammatory cytokines as well as toxic metabolites and enzymes. In addition to microglia, astrocytes have an important part in stroke-induced brain inflammation. They can produce both proinflammatory cytokines and neuroprotective factors such as erythropoietin, TGF-β1, and metallothionein-2 (Mergenthaler *et al.*, 2004). Because of the mixed nature of microglial and astrocyte products (both destructive and protective factors), the overall role of microglia may differ at different time points following stroke insult, with protective or regenerative activities occurring days to weeks after the onset of ischemia. Brain endothelium is distinctive compared with other organs, as evidenced by the BBB. However, it responds to stroke injury with increased permeability and diminished barrier function, along with degradation of the basal lamina of the vessel wall that occurs as in other organs after ischemic injury (del Zoppo and Hallenbeck, 2000). Similarly, there is evidence that acute ischemic stroke enhances the interactions of brain endothelium with extravascular (astrocytes, microglia, neurons) and intravascular (platelets, leukocytes) cells and that these interactions contribute to the injury process (Ishikawa *et al.*, 2004). The net result of all these responses to stroke is that the cerebral vasculature assumes the following phenotype: (1) poor capillary perfusion of brain tissue, (2) pro-adhesive for circulating cells, (3) pro-inflammatory, (4) pro-thrombogenic, and (5) diminished endothelial barrier function.

There is a large body of evidence that implicates leukocytes in the pathogenesis of stroke injury. The contention that leukocytes mediate reperfusion-induced tissue injury and microvascular dysfunction is supported by three major lines of evidence: (1) leukocytes (primarily neutrophils) accumulate in postischemic tissues prior to the onset of tissue injury; (2) animals rendered neutropenic exhibit a diminished injury response to ischemic stroke and (3) prevention of leukocyte-endothelial cell adhesion with monoclonal antibodies (mAbs) directed against specific leukocyte or endothelial CAMs also affords substantial protection against stroke injury (Ishikawa *et al.*, 2004). The pathophysiological significance of the lymphocyte recruitment into the brain after ischemic stroke remains unclear. However, our recent studies (T.V. Arumugam, unpublished data) showed important roles for T-lymphocytes in mediating reperfusion injury in postischemic brain tissue.

Animal Models of Stroke

Animal models have been developed that closely resemble stroke injury seen in human patients. Many experimental models are used to study stroke injury. Mechanisms of cell damage are determined by testing effects of different manipulations on the extent of cell death in a model. The three main classes of *in vivo* animal models are global ischemia, focal ischemia, and hypoxia/ischemia. The latter method in which vessel occlusion is combined with breathing a hypoxic mixture is almost exclusively used in young animals. Global ischemic insults are most commonly produced by vessel occlusions, and less commonly by complete brain circulatory arrest. Although the former are not actually global, a large portion of the forebrain is quite uniformly affected. In focal ischemic stroke models, the middle cerebral artery (MCA) is the most commonly occluded vessel; the vessel can be occluded either permanently or transiently. Damage results from both ischemia and reperfusion. Collateral blood flow may also play a role in reducing the initial impact of the occlusion. Intracerebral hemorrhage frequently accompanies ischemic stroke, mainly because of disruptions of the BBB.

There are many advantages to using small animals such as rats and mice in stroke models. Rats and mice are relatively inexpensive animals, and their cranial circulatory anatomy is similar to humans. It is also possible to control the severity, duration, and location of the vessel occlusion. Physiological factors can be controlled, and histopathology allows for assessment of ischemic pathogenesis and tissue infarction.

GLOBAL STROKE MODEL

It has been stated that the focal stroke models are of greater relevance to the human condition of stroke. However, global ischemia is of clear relevance to cardiac arrest and asphyxia in humans. In addition, it should be noted that the physiological, biochemical, and functional measurements made during recovery from a global model of reversible ischemia may be important in identifying the molecular and cellular mechanism and action of potential neuroprotective agents. Global models of cerebral ischemia may thus be as useful as focal models, provided that care is taken in the interpretation of the data. The three most widely used animal models of global ischemia are: (1) four-vessel occlusion (4-VO) and two-vessel occlusion (2-VO) combined with hypotension in the rat, (2) 2-VO occlusion in the gerbil, and (3) 2-VO in the mouse. A 2-VO mouse model was developed recently to study transgenic mice and is now being systematically studied (Kitagawa *et al.*, 1998).

Rat models of global stroke

4-VO. This model has several advantages, including ease of preparation, a high incidence of predictable ischemic neuronal damage, a low incidence of seizures, and the absence of anesthesia (i.e., at the time of carotid occlusion). This particular model has been, and still is, widely used to investigate the effectiveness of potential therapeutic agents. The rat 4-VO model involves permanent coagulation of the vertebral arteries, which alone has no deleterious effects, and temporary ligation of the two common carotid arteries. Experimental results show loss of righting reflex within 15 s, and a blood flow decrease to 3% of control values in hippocampus, striatum, and neocortex (McBean and Kelly, 1998).

2-VO. This model is carried out under a general anesthetic and requires the administration of a muscle relaxant. It has been well documented that a bilateral occlusion of the common carotid arteries alone is not sufficient either to bring the cerebral blood flow down below the ischemic threshold or to upset the energy state of the brain tissue to an extent sufficient to produce detectable cell death. To produce a damaging ischemic insult, the brain blood flow has to be reduced at the same time as the carotid arteries are occluded. The hypotension normally is produced in one of three ways: (1) controlled exsanguinations, (2) adjunctive administration of peripheral vasodilators, or (3) a combination of both approaches. The ligation of both common carotid arteries along with a BP reduction to 50 mm Hg causes as much or more damage than 4-VO. Blood flows fall to 3 to 5% in hippocampus, neocortex, and striatum. However, in some cases blood flow is reduced to 15% of control levels (McBean and Kelly, 1998; Swan *et al.*, 1988).

Gerbil model of global stroke

This is induced by temporarily ligating the carotid arteries, with no reduction in BP. Because there are no posterior communicating arteries in gerbils, this produces profound forebrain ischemia. Changes are similar to those in the rat models: blood flow in cortex is 1% and in hippocampus is 4% of control values (Herrmann *et al.*, 2004).

Mouse model of global stroke

Mouse models of global stroke are similar to rat 2-VO models using bilateral occlusion of the common carotid arteries. Several studies showed mouse global ischemia models with quantitatively uniform injury to CA1 neurons, using techniques including two-vessel occlusion and two-vessel occlusion with hypotension (Yonekura *et al.*, 2004). However, because of the variability of collateral flow via the posterior communicating artery, it has been difficult to obtain uniform injury in CA1 while retaining high survival and success rates. One model combines basilar artery occlusion with bilateral common carotid artery occlusion (three-vessel occlusion; Panahian *et al.*, 1996). However, in this model the animal survival rate was low and CA1 neuronal injury was inconsistent. Because the basilar artery of mice runs through a narrow groove in the brain stem and is attached to the pia mater and arachnoid membrane with arachnoid trabeculae, it is difficult to isolate and occlude.

Complete global ischemia

Finally, there is complete global ischemia, generally achieved by neck-cuff, cardiac arrest, or by ligating or compressing all arteries from the heart (Bottiger *et al.*, 1999). Blood flow to the whole brain is zero or <1% in these models. Due to high mortality associated with this model, it is not widely used.

FOCAL ISCHEMIC STROKE MODELS

Focal ischemic stroke models, whether in larger mammals such as cats, dogs, or nonhuman primates, or in small mammals such as rodents, usually involve occlusion of one MCA (Lipton 1999). Focal ischemia is differentiated from global ischemia in two ways. First, even at the core of the lesion, the blood flow is almost always higher than during global ischemia so that longer insults are required to cause damage. Second, there is a significant gradation of ischemia from the core of the lesion to its outermost boundary, and hence there are different metabolic conditions within the affected site. Because of its duration and heterogeneity, the insult is much more complex than global ischemia, but it is an invaluable model for stroke and is thus widely studied. There are two models of focal ischemic stroke: transient focal ischemia and permanent focal ischemia. In transient focal ischemia models, vessels are blocked for up to 3 h, followed by prolonged reperfusion, whereas in permanent focal ischemia, the arterial blockage is maintained throughout an experiment, usually for one or more days.

Transient middle cerebral artery occlusion

There are two principal occlusion sites in this model (see Figure 79.1). In proximal occlusion, the MCA is occluded close to its branching from the internal carotid artery, before the origin of the lenticulostriate arteries. A newer and now widely used approach to proximal MCA occlusion is the insertion of a nylon suture into the carotid artery, past the point at which the MCA branches so that the latter is occluded at its origin.

The procedure is as follows. After a midline neck incision, the left external carotid and pterigoparatine arteries are isolated and ligated with silk thread. The internal carotid artery is occluded at the peripheral site of the bifurcation of the internal carotid artery (ICA) and the pterigoparatine artery with a small clip, and the common carotid artery (CCA) is ligated with silk thread. The external carotid artery (ECA) is cut, and a nylon monofilament, whose tip is blunted (0.20–0.22 mm for a mouse) with a coagulator, is inserted into the ECA. The ECA and the inserted nylon thread are tightened with a silk suture, which prevents bleeding during advancement of the nylon thread and during its removal at the time of reperfusion, and rotated for its advancement into the ICA. After removal of the clip at the ICA, the nylon thread is advanced until light resistance is felt and the distance from the nylon thread tip to the internal carotid artery-pterygophalatine artery bifurcation is slightly more than 6 mm (mouse), and the distance to the ICA-ECA bifurcation is slightly less than 9 mm. During MCAO, the parietal bone becomes pale on the occluded side and laser Doppler flowmetry reveals that blood flow in this area falls to less than 20% of baseline. The nylon thread and the CCA ligature are removed after an occlusion period and reperfusion occurs with release of blood flow from the internal carotid artery. There are some potentially important artifacts with this widely used method. Blood flow following temporary ischemia is somewhat compromised by the partial occlusion of the carotid arteries with the filament and there is quite extensive damage to small arteries in the ischemic field, with damage to endothelial and smooth muscle cells. It has been suggested that this damage may affect subsequent neuronal cell death by exacerbating the leukocyte response in the reperfusion period (Ishikawa *et al.*, 2004).

Permanent middle cerebral artery occlusion

The commonly used permanent focal ischemia model involves occlusion of one or more branches of the MCA. The MCA is exposed via a transtemporal approach. After the temporalis muscle is retracted, a 2- to 3-mm burr hole is drilled 2 to 3 mm rostral to the fusion of the zygoma and squamosal bones. The MCA is exposed after opening and retracting the dura matter. Using a steel hook maneuvered via a micromanipulator, the MCA is elevated and electrocoagulated (McAuley, 1995).

Embolic model of focal ischemia

The procedure for this model is similar to the transient focal ischemic model (Zhang *et al.*, 2003). Briefly, a longitudinal incision is made in the midline of the ventral cervical skin. The CCA, ICA, and ECA are exposed. The distal portion of the ECA is ligated with two sutures and the ECA is cut between these two sutures. A silk suture is tied loosely around the origin of the ECA. The CCA and ICA are clamped temporarily using microvascular clips. A small puncture is made on the wall of the

ECA with a pair of spring scissors. A modified PE-10 catheter connected with a PE-50 tubing (40 mm in length for 10 ml thrombus and 20 mm for 5 ml) filled with bovine thrombin is introduced into the lumen of the ECA via the puncture. The suture around the origin of the ECA is tightened and the clip on the ICA is removed. After the blood is withdrawn, the catheter is advanced up in the ICA until its tip is 1 to 2 mm away from the origin of the MCA. The catheter is retained there for 15 minutes to allow formation of a clot. Once the clot has formed, it is then gently injected into the MCA. The catheter in the ICA is removed five minutes after the clot injection and the ECA is ligated.

Photothrombotic distal MCA occlusion

The use of a photochemical reaction to produce focal cortical ischemia in the rat brain was first described in 1985 (Watson *et al.*, 1985). In this model, vascular thrombosis is induced by transcranial illumination with a filtered light source in combination with intravenous injection of a photosensitive dye. Electron microscopy and light microscopy studies showed intravascular thrombotic material, red blood cell stasis, and platelet aggregates adhering to luminal surfaces inside vessels and intravascular thrombosis that is responsible for the occurrence of ischemia leading to infarction. Increased permeability through disruption of the BBB by the photochemical reaction is also involved in this type of model. The method involves mounting the rat in a stereotaxic head-holder, and making a 1 to 1.5-cm vertical incision between the right eye and ear. With the aid of an operating microscope, a burr hole is made with a high-speed drill. Care should be taken not to injure the dura matter. The distal segment of the right MCA is thus exposed. A krypton laser operating at 568 nm (Innova 301, Coherent Inc, or 643-Y-A01, Melles Griot Inc) is used to irradiate the distal MCA at a power of 20 mW for four minutes. The laser beam is focused with a 30-cm focal length convex lens and positioned with a mirror onto the distal MCA. The photosensitizing dye, normally rose bengal or erythrosin B (15–25 mg/mL in 0.9% saline), is administered intravenously at a body dose of 20 mg/kg over 90 seconds, starting simultaneously with four minutes of laser irradiation.

HEMORRHAGIC STROKE MODEL

Several animal models of intracerebral hemorrhage (ICH) have been developed in mice, rats, rabbits, cats, and nonhuman primates. A widely used method that produces ICH by injection of bacterial collagenase into the basal ganglia was first introduced in the rat and was subsequently studied in the mouse (Rosenberg *et al.*, 1990; Clark *et al.*, 1998). This enzyme digests the collagen present in the basal lamina of blood vessels and causes bleeding into the surrounding brain tissue. However, another study demonstrated that bacterial collagenase causes a significant inflammatory reaction and likely differs from the mechanism that produces ICH in humans (Del Bigio *et al.*, 1996). A second model uses the infusion of autologous blood into the brain parenchyma. This model was designed to mimic the natural events that occur with spontaneous ICH in humans. However, it produces hematomas of varying size because of ventricular rupture and the backflow of infused blood along the needle track, which leads to intraventricular and/or subarachnoid leakage of blood. Recently, a double injection ICH model has been developed in which a small amount of blood is infused into the striatum at a slow rate to allow blood clotting along the needle track; the remaining blood is then infused to generate the hematoma. This method creates a reproducible hematoma volume suitable for study of the pathophysiology and treatment of ICH (Belayev *et al.*, 2003). A widely used experimental procedure for ICH in mice is as follows. The animal is placed in a stereotactic frame. A 30-gauge stainless steel cannula is introduced through a burr hole into the left striatum (2 mm lateral to midline, 1 mm anterior to bregma, depth 4 mm below the surface of the skull) and the mouse receives an injection of either whole blood (taken from a donor mouse) or CSF (10–15 μl) over several minutes, and the injection cannula is slowly withdrawn 10 minutes after the injection.

IN VITRO MODELS TO STUDY STROKE INJURY

Brain slices, particularly the hippocampal slice and primary neuronal/glial cultures from cortex, hippocampus, and cerebellum of embryonic or perinatal rats and mice, have become widely used models for studying ischemia-like damage. In brain slices, ischemia-like conditions are induced by replacing the normal O_2/CO_2 equilibrated medium with N_2/CO_2 equilibrated medium; typically the cultures are maintained in an incubator containing a N_2/CO_2 atmosphere. When glucose is maintained in the anoxic buffer, the insult is termed hypoxia, and when glucose is omitted, the insult is termed *in vitro* ischemia or oxygen/glucose deprivation. Glucose deprivation alone can also induce neuronal death with some features similar to those observed in *in vivo* ischemia models. Hypoxia also can be induced by treatment with cyanide (NaCN or KCN) or by incubating in an anoxic atmosphere. Chemical hypoxia results in more free radical generation than does anoxia. *In vitro* models differ from *in vivo* stroke models in several aspects. Typically, a long duration of the anoxic or hypoxic insult is required to kill neurons *in vitro*. ATP depletion is less severe and the release of glutamate is delayed compared to ischemia *in vivo*. The absence of blood vessels and flow *in vitro* eliminates important components of the damage process present *in vivo*, including infiltration of inflammatory cells. In addition, the composition and responsiveness of glial cells *in vitro* differs from that in the intact brain.

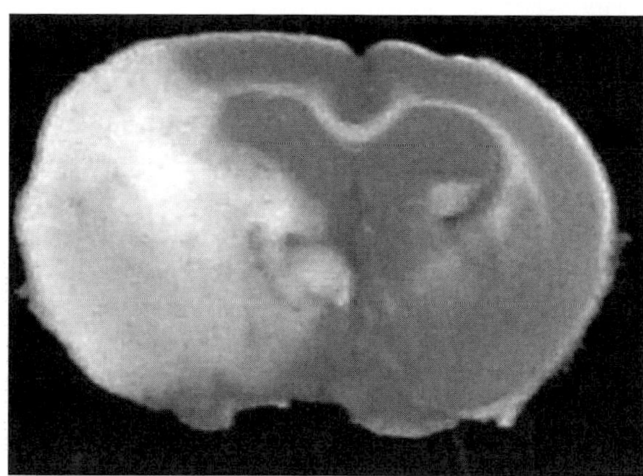

Figure 79.3 Representative coronal brain section from a mouse that had been subjected to MCA occlusion-reperfusion. This mouse had one hour MCA occlusion and 72 hours reperfusion. The dark staining indicates healthy brain tissue and the pale indicates damaged tissue.

Measurement of Stroke-Induced Damage

The measurement of dynamic changes in ischemic brain has attracted growing attention. Ischemic brain injury in both focal and global ischemia models evolves as a sequence of cellular and molecular events (Dirnagl *et al.*, 1999). In this section we describe methods for analyzing brain injury and dynamic changes in the brain during ischemia and reperfusion.

QUANTIFICATION OF CEREBRAL INFARCTION

The size of the brain infarct in focal cerebral ischemia increases in size during the period of reperfusion (see Figure 79.3).

This has been shown in animal models of stroke and in human stroke patients. The infarct volume is normally analyzed after 24 hours in transient focal ischemia models and after six hours in permanent focal ischemia models. The brain is removed, and coronal sections are cut (2 mm-thick slices in rats or 1–2 mm thick slices in mice) through the entire rostro-caudal extent of the cerebral cortex. The slices are immersed in a 2% solution of 2,3,5-triphenyltetrazolium chloride (TTC). An edema index is calculated by dividing the total volume of the hemisphere ipsilateral to the MCA occlusion by the total volume of the contralateral hemisphere. An infarction index, the actual infarcted lesion size adjusted for edema, is then calculated for each animal.

NEUROLOGICAL ASSESSMENT

The functional consequences of focal ischemic stroke injury are evaluated using a 5-point scale neurological deficit score (0, no deficit; 1, failure to extend right paw; 2, circling to the right; 3, falling to the right; and 4, unable to walk spontaneously) (Bederson *et al.*, 1986). More recently, a 14-point neurological scoring system was developed (Li *et al.*, 2000). This new scoring method includes the results of motor, reflex, and balance tests; a point is awarded for the inability to perform the test or for the lack of a tested reflex.

CEREBRAL BLOOD FLOW ANALYSIS

Regional microvascular tissue perfusion (cerebral blood flow) normally is monitored before, during, and after focal ischemia using laser Doppler flowmetry. The values during ischemia are calculated as a percentage of preocclusion levels. The region of measurement is set at 1 mm rostral and 1 mm dorsal to the cross-over point of the left MCA and rhinal fissure, which is in the ischemic penumbra of the ischemic lesion.

BLOOD-BRAIN BARRIER FUNCTION

Albumin leakage, a quantitative index of endothelial barrier dysfunction, can be applied to the brain for determination of BBB function. Albumin extravasation in the brain can be quantified either by fluorescence imaging of the leakage of fluorescein isothiocyanate-labeled albumin or sulforhodamine (Texas Red)-labeled albumin from cerebral venules or from the clearance of the same fluorochromes from blood to the artificial CSF perfusing the brain surface. With the imaging approach, fluorescently tagged albumin is administered intravenously to the animals 15 minutes before the baseline observation period, and fluorescence intensity (excitation wavelength, 420–490 nm; emission wavelength, 520 nm) is detected using a silicon-intensified target camera. The fluorescence intensities within a specified segment of a cerebral venule (Iv) within the cranial window and in a contiguous area of perivenular interstitium (Ii) are measured at various times after administration of fluorescent-albumin using a computer-assisted digital imaging processor (NIH Image 1.61 on a Macintosh computer). Vascular albumin leakage is determined from the difference in fluorescence intensity between the outside and inside of the venular segment. An index of albumin leakage is determined from the Ii-to-Iv ratio (after subtraction of baseline intensity measured before labeled albumin injection) at specific time points during the course of the experiment.

BRAIN EDEMA MEASUREMENT

The brains are immediately removed and divided into contralateral and ipsilateral hemispheres. The tissue samples are weighed on an electronic analytical balance to the nearest 0.1 mg to obtain the wet weight. The tissue is then dried at 100°C for 24 hours to determine the dry weight. Brain water content (%) is calculated as {(wet weight-dry weight)/wet weight} × 100.

PHYSIOLOGICAL VARIABLES

Blood pressure, rectal temperature, and blood gases are measured during the operation in rats and mice. Normally there are no significant differences in these variables monitored at pre-, intra-, and postischemic periods in most studies. However, measuring these parameters is important for interpretation of outcomes among animals, as well as for evaluation of adhering leukocytes using intravital video microscopy. An estimate of shear rate in cerebral venules is obtained by fluorescence microscopy based on image analysis determinations of the maximal velocity of fluorescently labeled red blood cells or platelets within the venules under study. Such estimates of pseudo-shear rate in venules are obtained using measurements of venular diameter (Dv) and the maximal velocity of flowing platelets (Vplt) according to the formula: pseudo-shear rate = (Vplt/1.6)/Dv × 8.

ASSESSMENT OF LEUKOCYTE AND PLATELET ADHESION

Adhesion of leukocytes and platelets following ischemia and reperfusion can be monitored *in vivo* using intravital video microscopy. The head of the animal is immobilized and a hole drilled through the skull using a high-speed micro drill (1 mm posterior from bregma and 4 mm lateral from the midline). The dura matter is not cut because the fluorescently labeled blood cells are easily observed and intracranial pressure is well maintained with the dura matter intact. Artificial cerebrospinal is placed on the exposed brain tissue. For focal ischemia models, the observation area includes the infarcted region following MCAO. For global ischemia models the observation area includes the entire cerebral cortex. Platelets are isolated from a donor animal using a series of centrifugation steps and labeled *ex vivo* with carboxyfluorescein diacetate succinimidyl ester. Once the platelet data is collected, endogenous leukocytes are labeled *in vivo* by infusing rhodamine-6G (100 μl; 0.02%) over five minutes and allowed to circulate an additional five minutes before observation. An upright Nikon microscope equipped with a SIT camera (C2400-08; Hamamatsu Photonics) and a mercury lamp is used to observe the cerebral micro-circulation. The images are received by a CCD video camera and recorded on a video recorder equipped with a time-date generator (WJ-810; Panasonic).

QUANTIFICATION OF CELL ACTIVATION AND ADHESION MOLECULES EXPRESSION

The dual radio-labeled monoclonal antibody (mAb) technique is used to quantify the expression of different endothelial cell adhesion molecules, including P-selectin, ICAM-1, and VCAM-1, in the microvasculature of the brain. This method determines the relative accumulation, in any regional vascular bed, of a binding mAb to a specific endothelial surface epitope (e.g., P-selectin) and an isotype-matched nonbinding mAb, the latter of which is used to compensate for nonspecific accumulation of the binding mAb. Different endothelial cellular adhesion molecules (P-selectin, E-selectin, VCAM-1, ICAM-1, MAdCAM-1, PECAM-1) in the brain can be analyzed following ischemic stroke. However, adhesion molecules specifically expressed by immune cells such as LFA-1 are analyzed at least 24 hours after reperfusion. Activation of microglial cells following ischemia or reperfusion normally is analyzed using CD11b (Mac-1) antibody.

MAGNETIC RESONANCE IMAGING (MRI)

With different MRI techniques, *in vivo* diagnostic and prognostic information can be obtained on edema formation, hemodynamics, tissue structure, neuronal activation, cell migration, gene expression, and more. In addition, MRI can be combined with other imaging modalities such as positron emission tomography or optical imaging to obtain complementary or supplementary information. Advances in MR technology, such as magnets with higher field strength, more powerful gradient systems, and increasing availability of targeted MR contrast agents, allow MRI research in animal models of ischemic and hemorrhagic stroke with higher sensitivity, faster acquisition, and improved specificity (Dijkhuizen and Nicolay, 2003).

MEASUREMENT OF PROTEIN AND mRNA LEVELS IN THE ISCHEMIC BRAIN

Identification and quantification of specific proteins and mRNAs *in situ* and in brain tissue samples can provide valuable information to elucidate the signaling pathways and molecular mechanisms involved in ischemic brain damage and recovery from stroke. Proteins can be identified *en masse* by proteomic methods, and individual proteins can be quantified by immunoblot or enzyme-linked immunosorbent assays. mRNAs are detected and quantified by polymerase chain reaction (PCR)-based gene array methods and by real-time PCR (Harrison and Bond, 2005).

Current Therapeutics and Preclinical Studies

A basic question in translating results of animal experiments to clinical use is whether or not the pathophysiologic processes in animal models correlate with those in human disease. Differences may arise for the following reasons: differences in anatomy and physiology, differences in pathophysiological response to injury, or differences between injury mechanisms in animal models and those in human disease. Therapeutic manipulations generally work best when administered before and immediately after the insult. Experiments with animal models often begin with a pretreatment protocol. If the therapy works, it is tested at different intervals from injury onset. Most effective therapies work best within 15 to 30 minutes; rarely are they effective more than three hours after onset of injury. The most important step in limiting ischemia is the quick restoration of blood flow that occurs either naturally or with the aid of thrombolytic drugs such as rtPA. The intravenous recombinant tissue plasminogen activator (rtPA) is the first and only approved agent for the treatment of acute stroke. tPA is a serine protease that catalyzes the activation of the zymogen plasminogen by converting it to the broad-specificity, active protease plasmin. In 1996, rtPA was approved for use in acute stroke. The NINDS trial using rtPA showed a highly significant improvement in outcome in treated patients. However, based on examination of the outcomes of rtPA-treated patients, the benefit of rtPA is not as robust as originally expected (Frey, 2005). It has been reported that tPA can exacerbate excitotoxic neuronal death (Tsirka, 1997), suggesting an adverse effect of this drug that may in part counteract its clot-busting action.

Another treatment that shows promise is hypothermia, which may decrease metabolic demand and extend neuron survival. Additional therapeutic approaches target the processes involved in calcium overload, glutamate excitotoxicity, oxygen radical production, apoptosis, and inflammation.

CALCIUM-STABILIZING AGENTS

Cell death cascades in ischemic stroke are mediated, in part, by excessive calcium influx resulting from activation of glutamate receptors and voltage-dependent calcium channels (VDCC). In addition, the function of Ca^{2+}-ATPases is compromised, resulting in prolonged elevation of the intracellular calcium concentration. Drugs that block glutamate receptors (MK-801, for example) or VDCC (nimodipine and flunarazine, for example) have proven effective in rodent models of stroke. At least 14 clinical trials of nimodipine in ischemic stroke were conducted beginning in the mid 1980s. Nine trials found no effect, one trial found short-term worsened outcome with treatment, and four trials found positive outcomes (Danton and Dietrich, 2004). Clinical trials with flunarizine found no statistically significant improvement in outcome. Despite this discouraging analysis, dantrolene, which blocks ryanodine receptors, recently has been discussed for clinical trails as the result of beneficial effects in rodent stroke models (Zhang *et al.*, 1993).

ANTI-EXCITOTOXIC AGENTS

Several compounds that interfere with glutamate receptor activation have been developed and tested against experimental animal models of stroke as well as against human clinical trials. The noncompetitive NMDA antagonist MK-801 (dizocilpine) improved outcome in models of focal ischemia, producing up to 75% reductions in infarct volume. Both MK-801 and dextromorphan, another noncompetitive NMDA receptor antagonist, exhibited protective effects in experimental studies, but clinical trials were terminated early because of phencyclidine-like psychotic side effects and lack of efficacy against stroke injury (Kermer *et al.*, 1999). Some other noncompetitive (aptiganel, ceresine) or competitive (selfotel, eliprodil) NMDA receptor antagonists were shown to be very effective in animal stroke models, but with no significant effects in clinical trails (Danton and Dietrich, 2004). Non-NMDA antagonists also were being developed and studied against stroke conditions. Zonampanel (YM-872) is an AMPA antagonist and currently is being tested in human phase 2 clinical trails. In addition, another AMPA antagonist SPD-502, as well as metabotropic glutamate receptor modulators, are being developed and tested against stroke injury in animals and humans (Danton and Dietrich, 2004; Legos and Barone, 2003). However, the development of anti-excitotoxic agents against stroke has been disappointing.

ANTIOXIDANTS

Free radical production is enhanced in both the ischemic core and penumbral following stroke injury, and this is believed to cause much of the damage seen in the core as well as penumbra. There are many agents that either block free radical production or inhibit its activation that have been shown to be very effective in experimental models. Uric acid is a well-known natural antioxidant present in fluids and tissues. Administration of uric acid resulted in a highly significant reduction in ischemic damage and improved behavioral outcome (Yu *et al.*, 1998). Edaravone, Tetramethylpyrazine, alpha-phenyl-N-tert-butyl-nitrone, FR210575, and NXY-59 are other free radical inhibitors that were effective against experimental stroke injury. EGb-761 is a free radical scavenger derived from a concentrated extract of Ginkgo that is currently in a phase 2 clinical trial (Legos *et al.*, 2002). Clinical trials with free radical scavengers have had limited success after acute ischemic stroke, but have had more success in the treatment of subarachnoid hemorrhage. Patients administered nicaraven after subarachnoid hemorrhage had a reduced rate of delayed ischemic neurologic deficits. NXY-59 was well tolerated in patients with stroke and currently is being studied for efficacy by AstraZeneca Pharmaceuticals.

ANTI-APOPTOTIC AGENTS

Accumulating evidence strongly suggests that apoptosis contributes to neuronal cell death in stroke injury. Caspases, a family of cysteine-aspartate proteases that include at least 14 members divided into three groups (I, II, and III), are essential players in apoptotic death. Many groups have studied the effects of caspase inhibition on cerebral ischemia-induced neurodegeneration by using the broad spectrum caspase inhibitor z-VAD, either in the fluoromethylketone (fmk) or dichlorobenzoyloxopentanoic acid (dcb) form and z-DVED-fmk. Both inhibitors were neuroprotective in mouse models of transient cerebral ischemia, and z-VAD was neuroprotective also in transient and permanent models in the rat (Hara *et al.*, 1997). Ac-YVAD-cmk (Ac-Tyr-Val-Ala-Asp-cmk), a caspase group I (caspase-1-like) inhibitor also was shown to be neuroprotective in a mouse transient model of cerebral ischemia (Hara *et al.*, 1997). Peptide-based caspase inhibitors also have been shown to prevent neuronal loss in animal models of stroke. A protein identified as having anti-apoptotic activity in many different cell types, including neurons, is Bcl-2. Bcl-2 is one of a family of related proteins, some of which have anti-apoptotic properties (e.g., Bcl-xL, Mcl-1), whereas others are pro-apoptotic (e.g., Bax, Bid, and Bad) (Mattson *et al.*, 2000). The efficacy of anti-apoptotic agents in human stroke patients has not been tested.

ANTI-INFLAMMATORY APPROACHES

Inflammation in stroke is characterized by the accumulation of leukocytes and activation of resident microglial cells. Inflammatory cells can contribute to stroke pathology through two basic mechanisms: they form aggregates in the venules after reperfusion or enter infarcted tissue and exacerbate cell death through production of free radicals and cytokines. Cell adhesion molecules such as selectins, integrins, and ICAMs permit endothelial-inflammatory cell interactions. Treatment with anti-selectin antibodies successfully decreased infarct volume up to 70% after transient focal ischemia. The anti-ICAM-1 antibody also has shown to decrease infarct size after transient but not permanent focal ischemia. However, a recent clinical trial using murine anti-ICAM-1 antibody enlimomab worsened neurologic score and mortality in patients and a follow-up study using the murine anti-rat ICAM-1 antibody in rats also found an increase in infarct volume and no efficacy. It is believed that immune activation in response to the foreign mouse protein probably accounted for the clinical and follow-up experimental results (Furuya *et al.*, 2001). Recently a phase 2 trail using anti-CD11b/CD18 agent UK-279276 has been completed, and demonstrated that this compound is safe and well tolerated. Another integrin antagonist LDP-01 is currently in phase 2 trials for stroke patients. Mitogen activated protein kinases (MAPK) have been linked to inflammatory cytokine production and cell death in ischemic stroke injury. SB-239063 is a MAPK inhibitor that reduced infarct size and improved neurological outcome following focal stroke in rodents. VX-745 is another orally active MAPK inhibitor tested in a clinical trial against stroke; the trial was stopped due to adverse effects of this drug.

MMPs are enzymes that break down components of the extracellular matrix and enhance BBB breakdown after stroke, promote hemorrhage, and increase inflammation. MMP inhibitors such as BB-94 and KB-R7785 decreased infarct volume in mice after permanent focal ischemia (Jiang *et al.*, 2001). MMP inhibitors have been evaluated in patients for their anti-angiogenic properties and are well tolerated. Although chemokines can have pro- or anti-inflammatory actions, the overall effect of chemokine up-regulation in ischemia-reperfusion injury is detrimental. NR58-3.14.3, a novel broad-spectrum inhibitor of chemokine function significantly reduced the lesion volume by up to 50%, which was associated with a marked functional improvement (Beech *et al.*, 2001). Several other anti-inflammatory cytokine approaches were tested in experimental stroke models, including various antibodies that target inflammatory proteins. However, there have been no successful clinical trials of such anti-inflammatory agents reported so far. As mentioned earlier, microglial activation following stroke insult plays a role in promoting inflammatory processes, but therapeutic approaches that specifically target microglia are lacking.

Conclusion

Ischemic and hemorrhagic stroke brain injury result from the interaction of complex pathophysiological processes. The molecular biology of stroke injury is a rapidly growing field that may lead to the identification of novel stroke therapies. Mechanisms of cell damage are determined by testing effects of different manipulations on the extent of cell death in animal and brain cell and slice culture models. Several different models of stroke have been developed. The three main classes of *in vivo* animal models are global ischemia, focal ischemia, and hypoxia/ischemia. Technological advances and experimental discoveries have begun to define the cellular and molecular mechanisms involved in stroke injury. Exploration of these targets led to the development of numerous agents that target various injury pathways. Despite numerous agents that can prevent the cascade of events leading to ischemic neuronal death in animal models, there is no neuroprotective agent that has been shown to conclusively improve stroke outcome in humans. The inconsistency between animal results and clinical trials may be due to several factors, including the heterogeneity of human stroke, morphological and functional differences between the brain of humans and animals, the relatively long post-stroke delay in administration of the drugs in clinical trials, and the better experimental control of physiological variables such as temperature, blood pressure, and differences in evaluating efficacy in animal models. The window of therapeutic opportunity in animal models is not necessarily predictive of the time window in humans, but the determination of relative windows is useful. In animal models, the time of the stroke or ischemic onset is known precisely and the administration of drug is at precise times, whereas in humans this may not be the case. There are numbers of important issues that remain unresolved regarding the translation of experimental developments to the clinical setting. Novel interventions will be required to overcome hurdles associated with bench-to-bedside translation. Finally, it is important to note that risk factors for stroke have been established (overeating, hypertension, sedentary lifestyle, and smoking). A vigorous effort to reduce these risk factors would therefore have a major impact in reducing the incidence of stroke.

REFERENCES

Andaluz, N, Zuccarello, M., and Wagner, K.R. (2002). Experimental animal models of intracerebral hemorrhage. *Neurosurg Clin N Am 13*, 385–393.

Artavanis-Tsakonas, S., Rand, M.D., and Lake, R.J. (1999). Notch signaling: Cell fate control and signal integration in development. *Science 284*, 770–776.

Arundine, M. and Tymianski, M. (2004). Molecular mechanisms of glutamate-dependent neurodegeneration in ischemia and traumatic brain injury. *Cell Mol Life Sci 61*, 657–668.

Bederson, J.B., Pitts, L.H., and Tsuiji, M. (1986). Rat middle cerebral artery occlusion: Evaluation of the model and development of a neurologic examination. *Stroke 17*, 472–476.

Beech, J.S., Reckless, J., Mosedale, D.E., Grainger, D.J., Williams, S.C., and Menon, D.K. (2001). Neuroprotection in ischemia-reperfusion injury: An antiinflammatory approach using a novel broad-spectrum chemokine inhibitor. *J Cereb Blood Flow Metab 21*, 683–689.

Belayev, L., Saul, I., Curbelo, K., Busto, R., Belayev, A., Zhang, Y. *et al.* (2003). Experimental intracerebral hemorrhage in the mouse: Histological, behavioral, and hemodynamic characterization of a double-injection model. *Stroke 34*, 2221–2227.

Bottiger, B.W., Teschendorf, P., Krumnikl, J.J., Vogel, P., Galmbacher, R., Schmitz, B. *et al.* (1999). Global cerebral ischemia due to cardiocirculatory arrest in mice causes neuronal degeneration and early induction of transcription factor genes in the hippocampus. *Brain Res Mol Brain Res 65*, 135–142.

Bowman, T.S., Sesso, H.D., Ma, J., Kurth, T., Kase, C.S., Stampfer, M.J. *et al.* (2003). Cholesterol and the risk of ischemic stroke. *Stroke 34*, 2930–2934.

Brown, R.D., Whisnant, J.P., Sicks, J.D., O'Fallon, W.M., and Wiebers, D.O. (1996). Stroke incidence, prevalence, and survival: Secular trends in Rochester, Minnesota, through 1989. *Stroke 27*, 373–380.

Clark, W., Gunion-Rinker, L., Lessov, N., and Hazel, K. (1998). Citicoline treatment for experimental intracerebral hemorrhage in mice. *Stroke 29*, 2136–2140.

Danton, G.H. and Dietrich, W.D. (2004). The search for neuroprotective strategies in stroke. *AJNR Am J Neuroradiol 25*, 181–194.

Davis, M., Mendelow, A.D., Perry, R.H., Chambers, I.R., and James, O.F. (1995). Experimental stroke and neuroprotection in the aging rat brain. *Stroke 26*, 1072–1078.

Dawson, V.L. and Dawson, T.M. (1998). Nitric oxide in neurodegeneration. *Prog Brain Res 118*, 215–229.

Del Bigio, M.R., Yan, H.J., Buist, R., and Peeling, J. (1996). Experimental intracerebral hemorrhage in rats: Magnetic resonance imaging and histopathological correlates. *Stroke 27*, 2312–2319.

del Zoppo, G.J. and Hallenbeck, J.M. (2000). Advances in the vascular pathophysiology of ischemic stroke. *Thromb Res 98*, 73–81.

Dichgans, M. (2002). CADASIL: A monogenic condition causing stroke and subcortical vascular dementia. *Cerebrovasc Dis 13*, S37–41.

Dijkhuizen, R.M. and Nicolay, K. (2003). Magnetic resonance imaging in experimental models of brain disorders. *J Cereb Blood Flow Metab 23*, 1383–1402.

Dirnagl, U., Costantino, I., and Moskowitz, M.A. (1999). Pathobiology of ischemic stroke: An integrated view. *Trends Neurosci 22*, 391–397.

Ewing, J.R., Brown, G.C., Gdowski, J.W., Simkins, R., Levine, S.R., and Welch, K.M. (1989). Stroke risk and age do not predict behavioral activation of brain blood flow. *Ann Neurol 25*, 571–576.

Frey, J.L. (2005). Recombinant tissue plasminogen activator (rtPA) for stroke. The perspective at 8 years. *Neurologist 11*, 123–133.

Furuya, K., Takeda, H., Azhar, S., McCarron, R.M., Chen, Y., Ruetzler, C.A. *et al.* (2001). Examination of several potential mechanisms for the negative outcome in a clinical stroke trial of enlimomab, a murine antihuman intercellular adhesion molecule-1 antibody: A bedside-to-bench study. *Stroke 32*, 2665–2674.

Garcia, J.H. (1984). Experimental ischemic stroke: A review. *Stroke 15*, 5–14.

Hall, E.D. (1995). Inhibition of lipid peroxidation in central nervous system trauma and ischemia. *J Neurol Sci 134*, S79–83.

Hara, H., Friedlander, R.M., Gagliardini, V., Ayata, C., Fink, K., Huang, Z. *et al.* (1997). Inhibition of interleukin 1 converting enzyme family proteases reduces ischemic and excitotoxic neuronal damage. *Proc Natl Acad Sci USA 94*, 2007–2012.

Harrison, D.C. and Bond, B.C. (2005). Quantitative analysis of gene transcription in stroke models using real-time RT-PCR. *Methods Mol Med 104*, 265–284.

Hassan, A. and Markus, H.S. (2000) Genetics and ischemic stroke. *Brain 123*, 1784–1812.

Herrmann, M., Stern, M., Vollenweider, F., and Nitsch, C. (2004). Effect of inherent epileptic seizures on brain injury after transient cerebral ischemia in Mongolian gerbils. *Exp Brain Res* 154, 176–182.

Howard, G., Toole, J.F., Frye-Pierson, J., and Hinshelwood, L.C. (1987). Factors influencing the survival of 451 transient ischemic attack patients. *Stroke 18*, 552–557.

Ishikawa, M., Zhang, J.H., Nanda, A., and Granger, D.N. (2004). Inflammatory responses to ischemia and reperfusion in the cerebral microcirculation. *Front Biosci 9*, 1339–1347.

Jiang, X., Namura, S., and Nagata, I. (2001). Matrix metalloproteinase inhibitor KB-R7785 attenuates brain damage resulting from permanent focal cerebral ischemia in mice. *Neurosci Lett 305*, 41–44.

Joutel, A., Dodick, D.D., Parisi, J.E., Cecillon, M., Tournier-Lasserve, E., and Bousser, M.G. (2000). De novo mutation in the Notch3 gene causing CADASIL. *Ann Neurol 47*, 388–391.

Kermer, P., Klocker, N., and Bahr, M. (1999). Neuronal death after brain injury: Models, mechanisms, and therapeutic strategies in vivo. *Cell Tissue Res 298*, 383–395.

Kitagawa, K., Matsumoto, M., and Yang, G.M. (1998). Cerebral ischemia after bilateral carotid artery occlusion and intraluminal suture in mice: Evaluation of the patence of posterior communicating artery. *J Cereb Blood Flow Metab 18*, 570–579.

Legos, J.J., Tuma, R.F., and Barone, F.C. (2002). Pharmacological interventions for stroke: Failures and future. *Expert Opin Investig Drugs 11*, 603–614.

Legos, J.J. and Barone, F.C. (2003). Update on pharmacological strategies for stroke: Prevention, acute intervention and regeneration. *Curr Opin Investig Drugs 4*, 847–858.

Leys, D., Deplanque, D., Mounier-Vehier, C., Mackowiak-Cordoliani, M.A., Lucas, C., and Bordet, R. (2002). Stroke prevention: Management of modifiable vascular risk factors. *J Neurol 249*, 507–517.

Li, Y., Chopp, M., Chen, J., Wang, L., Gautam, S.C., Xu, Y.X. *et al.* (2000). Intrastriatal transplantation of bone marrow nonhematopoietic cells improves functional recovery after stroke in adult mice. *J Cereb Blood Flow Metab 20*, 1311–1319.

Lipton, P. (1999). Ischemic cell death in brain neurons. *Physiol Rev 79*, 1431–1568.

Love, S. (1999). Oxidative stress in brain ischemia. *Brain Pathol 9*, 119–131.

Manjo, G. and Joris, I. (1995). Apoptosis, oncosis and necrosis. An overview of cell death. *Am J Pathol 146*, 3–15.

Mankovsky, B.N. and Ziegler, D. (2004). Stroke in patients with diabetes mellitus. *Diabetes Metab Res Rev 20*, 268–287.

Markus, H.S., Barley, J., Lunt, R., Blunt, J.M., Jeffery, S., Carter, N.D. *et al.* (1995). Angiotensin-converting enzyme gene deletion polymorphism. A new risk factor for lacunar stroke but not for carotid atheroma. *Stroke 26*, 1329–1333.

Mattson, M.P., Chan, S.L., and Duan, W. (2002). Modification of brain aging and neurodegenerative disorders by genes, diet, and behavior. *Physiol Rev 82*, 637–672.

Mattson, M.P., Culmsee, C., and Yu, Z.F. (2000). Apoptotic and antiapoptotic mechanisms in stroke. *Cell Tissue Res 301*, 173–187.

Mattson, M.P. (1997). Neuroprotective signal transduction: Relevance to stroke. *Neurosci Biobehav Rev 21*, 193–206.

McAuley, M.A. (1995). Rodent models of focal ischemia. *Cerebrovasc Brain Metab Rev 7*, 153–180.

McBean, D.E. and Kelly, P.A. (1998). Rodent models of global cerebral ischemia: A comparison of two-vessel occlusion and four-vessel occlusion. *Gen Pharmacol 30*, 431–434.

Mergenthaler, P., Dirnagl, U., and Meisel, A. (2004). Pathophysiology of stroke: Lessons from animal models. *Metab Brain Dis 19*, 151–167.

Neumar, R.W. (2000). Molecular mechanisms of ischemic neuronal injury. *Ann Emerg Med 36*, 483–506.

Panahian, N., Yoshida, T., Huang, P.L., Hedley-Whyte, E.T., Dalkara, T., Fishman, M.C. *et al.* (1996). Attenuated hippocampal damage after global cerebral ischemia in mice mutant in neuronal nitric oxide synthase. *Neuroscience 72*, 343–354.

Rashid, P., Leonardi-Bee, J., and Bath, P. (2003). Blood pressure reduction and secondary prevention of stroke and other vascular events: A systematic review. *Stroke 34*, 2741–2748.

Rosenberg, G.A., Mun-Bryce, S., Wesley, M., and Kornfeld, M. (1990). Collagenase-induced intracerebral hemorrhage in rats. *Stroke 21*, 801–807.

Sacco, R.L., Benson, R.T., Kargman, D.E., Boden-Albala, B., Tuck, C., Lin, I.F. *et al.* (2001). High-density lipoprotein cholesterol and ischemic stroke in the elderly: The Northern Manhattan Stroke Study. *JAMA 285*, 2729–2735.

Shaw, T.G., Mortel, K.F., Meyer, J.S., Rogers, R.L., Hardenberg, J., and Cutaia, M.M. (1984). Cerebral blood flow changes in benign aging and cerebrovascular disease. *Neurology 34*, 855–862.

Stoll, G., Jander, S., and Schroeter, M. (1998). Inflammation and glial responses in ischemic brain lesions. *Prog Neurobiol 56*, 149–171.

Swan, J.H., Evans, M.C., and Meldrum, B.S. (1988). Long-term development of selective neuronal loss and the mechanism of protection by 2-amino-7-phosphonoheptanoate in a rat model of incomplete forebrain ischaemia. *J Cereb Blood Flow Metab 8*, 64–78.

Tsirka, S.E. (1997). Clinical implications of the involvement of tPA in neuronal cell death. *J Mol Med 75*, 341–347.

Vasan, R.S., Larson, M.G., Leip, E.P., Evans, J.C., O'Donnell, C.J., Kannel, W.B. *et al.* (2001). Impact of high-normal blood pressure on the risk of cardiovascular disease. *N Engl J Med 345*, 1291–1297.

Watson, B.D. (1998). Animal models of photochemically induced brain ischemia and stroke. In M.D. Ginsberg and J. Bogousslavsky (Eds.), *Cerebrovascular disease-pathophysiology, diagnosis and treatment*, pp. 52–73. Cambridge, MA: Blackwell Science.

Yonekura, I., Kawahara, N., Nakatomi, H., Furuya, K., and Kirino, T. (2004). A model of global cerebral ischemia in C57 BL/6 mice. *J Cereb Blood Flow Metab 24*, 151–158.

Yu, Z.F., Bruce-Keller, A.J., Goodman, Y., and Mattson, M.P. (1998). Uric acid protects neurons against excitotoxic and metabolic insults in cell culture, and against focal ischemic brain injury in vivo. *J Neurosci Res 53*, 613–625.

Zhang, L., Andou, Y., Masuda, S., Mitani, A., and Kataoka, K. (1993). Dantrolene protects against ischemic, delayed neuronal death in gerbil brain. *Neurosci Lett 158*, 105–108.

Zhang, L., Zhang, Z.G., Zhang, R.L., Lu, M., Krams, M., and Chopp, M. (2003). Effects of a selective CD11b/CD18 antagonist and recombinant human tissue plasminogen activator treatment alone and in combination in a rat embolic model of stroke. *Stroke 34*, 1790–1795.

Zheng, Z. and Yenari, M.A. (2004). Post-ischemic inflammation: Molecular mechanisms and therapeutic implications. *Neurol Res 26*, 884–892.

80

Werner Syndrome as a Model of Human Aging

Raymond J. Monnat, Jr.

This chapter reviews clinical and basic science aspects of Werner syndrome (WS), a heritable human disease that displays features suggestive of premature aging. The resemblance of changes in WS to those observed in normal aging has long suggested WS may be a useful model in which to study the biology of aging and to identify mechanistic pathways responsible for age-associated diseases that are prevalent in WS patients and in normal aging such as atherosclerosis, neoplasia, diabetes mellitus, and osteoporosis. This chapter summarizes our understanding of the WS clinical phenotype. Current understanding of in vivo *functions of the Werner syndrome protein is summarized, together with a discussion of how the loss of WRN function may promote disease pathogenesis in WS patients and in normal individuals. Subsections provide an historical overview of WS and WS research; a description of WS as a clinical disease entity, together with diagnostic criteria for WS; a discussion of the relationship of WS to normal aging; a summary of our current understanding of the WRN gene and the mutational basis for WS; a discussion of* in vivo *functions of the WS protein in human somatic cells, and how loss-of-function may be linked to disease pathogenesis; and an introduction to the more promising animal models of WS. A selection of the most useful additional resources on WS clinical medicine and biology are included to aid those interested in learning more about this fascinating and instructive human disease.*

Introduction

Werner syndrome (WS) is an uncommon, autosomal recessive human disease that displays clinical features suggestive of premature aging. The initial description of WS was by Otto Werner, a German medical student, in 1904 (Werner, 1985). Werner saw a family in the north of Germany consisting of four siblings, ages 31 to 40, who shared common features including short stature, premature graying of the hair, bilateral cataracts, skin changes (hyperkeratosis, scleroderma-like changes and ulceration) that were most severe on the feet and ankles, atrophy of the extremities, and, in females, an early cessation of menstruation. He noted that one of the siblings, a 36-year-old male, gave "the impression of extreme senility." Werner published these observations as part of his doctoral thesis, though he did not further study these or similar patients during the remainder of his career. He practiced general medicine in Eddelak, a small village on the North Sea near the Danish border, where he died in 1936 (Pehmoeller, 2001).

The eponym *Werner's syndrome* was first used in 1934 by Oppenheimer and Kugel in reporting findings in a patient (Oppenheimer and Kugel, 1934). Their paper, together with the more comprehensive study by Thannhauser (1945) of five additional cases, provided an accurate clinical description of WS that distinguished it from Rothmund (now Rothmund-Thomson) syndrome. The subsequent diagnosis of Werner syndrome in three affected, American-born sisters in a Japanese-American sibship seen in Seattle in the early 1960s led to further, detailed clinical and pathological characterization of Werner syndrome. Part of this characterization included a formal genetic analysis that firmly established an autosomal recessive mode of inheritance. These observations, together with a critical analysis of 122 additional cases, were published in 1966 (Epstein *et al.*, 1966). This landmark paper remains readily accessible and a key source of information for investigators interested in WS (see Recommended Resources).

The modern clinical and biological investigation of WS has been an international effort. This reflects both the worldwide occurrence of WS (Goto, 1997) and early collaborative efforts by investigators in Japan (where WS is prevalent), the United States, and Western Europe to better define and understand the WS clinical phenotype and its underlying biology. The first major gathering of investigators to discuss this work was in Kobe, Japan, in 1982. This United States–Japan Cooperative Seminar on Werner's Syndrome and Human Aging was sponsored by the U.S. National Science Foundation and the Japan Society for the Promotion of Science. The proceedings of this workshop were subsequently published and represent an important first summarization of modern work to better define and understand WS (Salk *et al.*, 1985). The published proceedings also include an important selection of published primary sources of information on WS (e.g., Epstein *et al.*, 1966; Salk, 1982; Thannhauser, 1945) together with an edited translation of Otto Werner's thesis (Werner, 1985).

Several subsequent small workshops were sponsored by the U.S.–Japan Cooperative Cancer Research Program during the 1990s and led to further discussion of and interest in WS. These were part of a long-standing joint venture of the U.S. National Cancer Institute and the Japan Society for the Promotion of Science. Meetings held in 1994, 1996, and 1997 brought together investigators interested in WS as a cancer predisposition syndrome (1994), in clinical and biological aspects of WS (1996), and in the relationship of WS to other pediatric cancer syndromes (1997). The focus for these meetings broadened with a U.S.–Japan Workshop on Cancer in Human RecQ Helicase Gene Disorders (February 2002), the Keystone Symposia on DNA Helicases, Cancer and Aging (March 2002 and 2005), and a U.S. NIH-sponsored International Workshop on Werner Syndrome held in May 2003. Regrettably, the results of only one of these very productive workshops were captured in a meeting report (Bohr, 2003). The broader focus of these more recent meetings reflects the recognition that WS, Bloom syndrome, and Rothmund-Thomson syndrome are all human genetic instability/cancer predisposition disorders that result from mutations in different members of the five-member human RecQ helicase protein family (see later; Bachrati and Hickson, 2003; Opresko, Cheng *et al.*, 2004).

Attempts were made in the 1980s and early 1990s to isolate or map the affected gene in WS. These approaches took advantage of potentially useful cellular phenotypes for complementation such as a severe *in vitro* cell proliferation defect and chromosomal instability, and the fact that WS is an autosomal recessive disease that likely resulted from a single gene defect. Attempts at functional complementation to identify the *WRN* gene were not successful for at least two important reasons: the scarcity and poor growth properties of primary cells from WS patients that were used as complementation hosts, and the large size of the *WRN* gene and the WRN open reading frame (see later). In contrast, linkage mapping using the then-new technique of homozygosity mapping was successful, and led in 1992 to assignment of the *WRN* locus to the proximal short arm of chromosome 8 in a region defined by five anonymous DNA markers (Goto *et al.*, 1992). This initial linkage assignment, together with rapid maturation of methods for positional cloning in the early 1990s, led in 1996 to identification of the *WRN* locus and of unambiguous pathogenic mutations in the *WRN* gene of WS patients (Yu *et al.*, 1996).

Successful positional cloning of the *WRN* gene with delineation of WS-associated *WRN* mutations and predictions of potential activities encoded in the WRN protein provided a powerful stimulus for subsequent work on WS. There was an immediate effort in several laboratories to confirm predicted biochemical activities, and then identify *in vivo* functions, of WRN. There was also renewed speculation on how the loss of WRN function could generate WS cellular and clinical phenotypes. Recent work has also begun to focus on genetic variation in the *WRN* gene, and the association of *WRN* mutations and polymorphisms with disease risk and disease pathogenesis in the general population. Each of these areas of investigation is discussed in greater detail below.

Werner Syndrome as a Clinical Disease Entity

The key clinical features of Werner syndrome were readily recognized by Otto Werner in the first patients he identified and described in 1904. These clinical signs or findings, outlined in Table 80.1, were subsequently confirmed and further elaborated by Oppenheimer and Kugel (1934), Thannhauser (1945), and Epstein *et al.*

TABLE 80.1
Diagnostic criteria for Werner syndrome

Consistent findings

- **clinical findings** (onset > age 10)
  - short stature
  - bilateral cataracts
  - premature graying and loss of scalp hair/eyebrows
  - scleroderma-line skin changes
- **history**
  - parental consanguinity (3rd cousin or closer)
  - affected sib
- **laboratory**
  - elevated 24 hr urinary hyaluronic acid secretion

Additional findings

- **clinical findings**
  - flat feet
  - voice changes
  - hypogonadism
- **history or laboratory findings**
  - diabetes mellitus
  - osteoporosis
  - soft-tissue/tendon calcification
  - premature atherosclerosis, myocardial infarction, stroke
  - neoplasia

Diagnostic likelihood of Werner syndrome

- **definite**: all of consistent clinical and history findings
- **probable**: short stature, bilateral cataracts and scleroderma-like skin changes, any two other clinical, history or laboratory findings
- **possible**: bilateral cataracts or scleroderma-like skin changes, any four other additional clinical, history or laboratory findings
- **exclusion**: onset of clinical or laboratory findings ≤ age 10

(1966) in their analyses of WS patients and pedigrees. Among the most consistent and earliest of the features of WS to be observed are short stature, bilateral cataracts, the early graying and loss of hair, and scleroderma-like skin changes. All four features have been observed in all or nearly all patients (Epstein *et al.*, 1966; Goto, 1997; Tollefsbol and Cohen, 1984). They appear *de novo*, and are not the secondary consequence of another systemic disease process, or the result of a primary endocrine deficiency or dysfunction syndrome. Each of these features or clinical signs of WS are discussed briefly, next, together with less consistently observed changes. This constellation of changes and the clinical appearance and progression of these changes have been used to develop criteria for the clinical diagnosis of WS.

SHORT STATURE

The short stature of WS patients results from a failure to undergo an adolescent or pubertal growth spurt. Short stature, together with progressive thinning and atrophy of the limbs and a stocky trunk, give patients a Cushingoid appearance that is readily apparent in full body clinical photographs (see, for example, patient photos in Figure 2 of Goto, 2001).

GRAYING AND LOSS OF HAIR

Early graying and loss of hair are, together with short stature, among the earliest and most consistent changes observed in WS patients. Hair graying and loss start late in the second decade of life, and first affect the scalp and eyebrows. The loss of hair pigmentation is progressive and may lead over the course of a decade or more to complete loss of pigmentation. The premature graying and loss of hair also extend to other areas of the body, although these changes usually start later and may not be as extensive as the changes observed in the scalp and eyebrows.

CATARACTS

Bilateral ocular cataracts are a consistent feature of WS and first appear or are reported in many patients by the second or third decades of life. The cataracts consist of posterior cortical and subcapsular opacification. Vacuoles and small punctate opacifications in other parts of the lens have also been noted, though are not a consistent part of the lens changes. This type of cataract, often referred to as juvenile, can be readily distinguished from the more common opacification of the lens nucleus observed in the senile cataracts of normal aged individuals. Vision is otherwise unimpaired, and thus can be restored following cataract removal.

SCLERODERMA-LIKE SKIN CHANGES

Skin changes were first clearly described in the patient series reported by Thannhauser, who distinguished changes in WS patients from those commonly seen in scleroderma patients or in patients with Rothmund-Thomson syndrome (Thannhauser, 1945). The histologic appearance of skin biopsies from WS patients reveals an interesting mix of atrophic and proliferative changes. There is epidermal atrophy that extends to include skin appendages (e.g., hair follicles, sweat and sebaceous glands), in conjunction with focal hyperkeratosis and basal hypermelanosis. Dermal subcutaneous connective tissue atrophy is common, and often is found in conjunction with dermal fibrosis. Muscle, adipose, and connective tissue underlying the skin is often atrophic. This constellation of changes gives the skin a tight, white, and shiny or contracted appearance, with a loss of normal elasticity.

These cutaneous changes often are first seen and may be most prominent in the face and extremities. Skin changes in the face lead to a progressive sharpening of facial features to give patients what is often described as a pinched, beaked, or bird-like appearance (see the patient photo panel in Figure 3 of Goto, 2001). The lower extremities, especially the feet, are often markedly affected by these changes, leading to foot deformation, ulceration of nonpressure-bearing portions of the foot and ankles, and calcification of soft tissue and tendons (Hatamochi, 2001; Figure 80.1). Laryngeal changes consisting of a mix of proliferative and atrophic changes are likely responsible for the thin, high-pitched voice noted of many

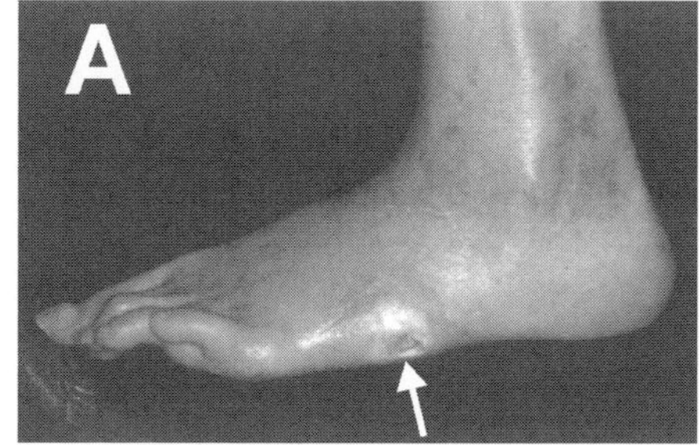

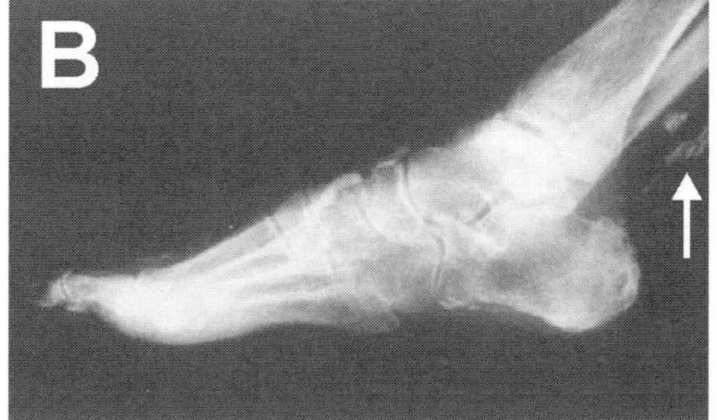

Figure 80.1 Skin and soft tissue changes in Werner syndrome patients. **A**. Scleroderma-like skin changes, hyper-pigmentation and ulceration (arrow) of the lateral border of the left foot in a male Japanese WS patient age 37. **B**. Localized calcification of the Achilles tendon (arrow) and plantar tendon insertion site calcification in a Japanese female WS patient age 54. Both photos were previously published (Hatamochi, 2001) and are used here with kind permission of Dr. Atsushi Hatamochi, Professor of Dermatology, Dokkyo University School of Medicine, and the Japanese Scientific Societies Press.

patients, although the associated laryngeal pathology has not been well studied.

OTHER PROMINENT CLINICAL FEATURES OF WERNER SYNDROME

Several less consistent clinical findings have been noted in a portion of WS patients. These additional findings (see Table 80.1) have been mentioned in many independent reports of WS, and thus are likely to be part—albeit a more variable part—of the WS phenotype. Most notable among these changes are clinically important disease states that we commonly associate with aging: atherosclerosis and its cardiovascular and cerebral sequella; a mix of nonepithelial and epithelial neoplasms (see later); osteoporosis that is characteristically most severe in the distal phalanges; diabetes mellitus; and hypogonadism affecting both males and females. Each of these disease states in part can be explained by proliferative and atrophic changes at the tissue level (see later). A few pertinent negatives also need to be mentioned. Among these, the most notable are that development, structure, and function of the central and peripheral nervous systems are normal, and WS patients are invariably of normal or higher-than-normal intelligence. Also, few or no indications of primary endocrine defects or abnormalities have been reported in WS patients beyond secondary changes that accompany the development of diabetes mellitus or with gonadal atrophy and the loss of reproductive function.

CANCER IN WERNER SYNDROME

WS patients are at increased risk of developing cancer (Goto *et al.*, 1996; Monnat, 2001; Monnat, 2002). The elevated risk of neoplasia in WS patients is of particular biological interest. As discussed later, neoplasia may be an expression of important mechanistic links between WRN function *in vivo*, genome stability assurance, and the limitation of cell proliferation defects. The elevated risk of neoplasia in WS is selective in that only a small subset of neoplasms are clearly elevated in incidence as compared with general population controls (see Table 80.2). The following neoplasms, in order of decreasing frequency, have been observed most often in WS patients and occur at higher or much higher frequency than in normal population controls: soft tissue sarcomas, thyroid carcinoma, meningioma, malignant melanoma, malignant or preneoplastic hematologic disease, and osteosarcoma. Many other neoplasms, including common adult epithelial malignancies, have been observed in WS patients. However, it is not clear whether the risk of developing these neoplasms is significantly elevated. Of note, the histopathologic spectrum of neoplasms observed in WS overlaps with, though is distinct from, that observed in patients with Bloom syndrome and Rothmund-Thomson syndrome, two other RecQ helicase deficiency syndromes, (Monnat, 2001).

TABLE 80.2
Neoplasia in Werner syndrome

Frequent (2/3 of neoplasms)	**Less common (1/3 of neoplasms)**
Soft tissue sarcomas	**Non-melanoma skin cancer**
malignant fibrous histiocytoma	**Hepatobiliary carcinomas**
leiomyosarcoma	hepatocellular
fibrosarcoma	cholangiocarcinoma
malignant schwannoma	gallbladder
synovial sarcoma	**Genito-urinary**
rhabdomyosarcoma	bladder carcinoma
Thyroid carcinoma	uterine/ovarian carcinoma
follicular	renal cell carcinoma
papillary	prostate carcinoma
anaplastic	seminoma
Malignant melanoma	**Gastro-intestinal carcinoma**
acral lentigenous melanoma	
mucosal malignant melanoma	gastric esophagus
Meningioma	pancreas
benign	colon
multiple/malignant	**Breast carcinoma**
Hematological	**Oro-pharyngeal carcinoma**
acute myelogenous leukemias (M1-5)	
erythroleukemia (M6)	
megakaryocytic leukemia (M7)	
myelofibrosis/myelodysplasia	
aplastic anemia	
Osteosarcoma	

Several pathologic and clinical aspects of neoplasia in patients indicate that WS is a classical cancer predisposition syndrome. WS patients develop neoplasms at a comparatively early age and often display unusual sites of presentation (e.g., osteosarcoma of the patella) or less common histopathologic subtypes (e.g., follicular, as opposed to the more common papillary, type of thyroid carcinoma) than do population controls. The elevated risk of melanoma in WS provides a striking example of unusual histology. The melanoma seen in WS patients is exclusively acral lentigenous melanoma (ALM), a comparatively rare melanoma subtype that arises on the palms and soles, or in mucosa of the nasal cavity or esophagus. The risk of ALM is most clearly elevated in Japanese WS patients. This suggests the existence of patient- and population-specific modifiers for ALM in the absence of WRN function. A final expression of elevated cancer risk and predisposition in WS is the occurrence of multiple tumors: there are numerous reports of multiple, concurrent, or sequential neoplasms of different histology; for example, thyroid carcinoma and osteosarcoma, with up to five neoplasms having been reported in individual patients. Estimates of the increased risk of neoplasia in WS patients range from ~30-fold elevated overall lifetime risk across all tumor types to ~1000-fold elevated risk for acral lentigenous melanoma (Goto *et al.*, 1996; Monnat, 2001; Monnat, 2002).

CLINICAL PROGRESSION OF WS

One aspect of WS that is not well conveyed by Table 80.1 is the progressive nature of the WS clinical phenotype: a complex constellation of changes that may develop over two or three decades, after having been first noticed beginning in the second decade of life. A sense of the progressive nature of the WS clinical phenotype and visible changes can be gleaned from pairs of patient photos taken in early adulthood, and later in mid-life when the clinical phenotype of WS is often well-developed (see Figure 80.2).

These two patients and many other WS patients appear remarkably normal until the time of puberty, after which the most prominent of the features outlined in Table 80.1 become apparent over the subsequent 10 to 20 years. A simple animation from one of these patient

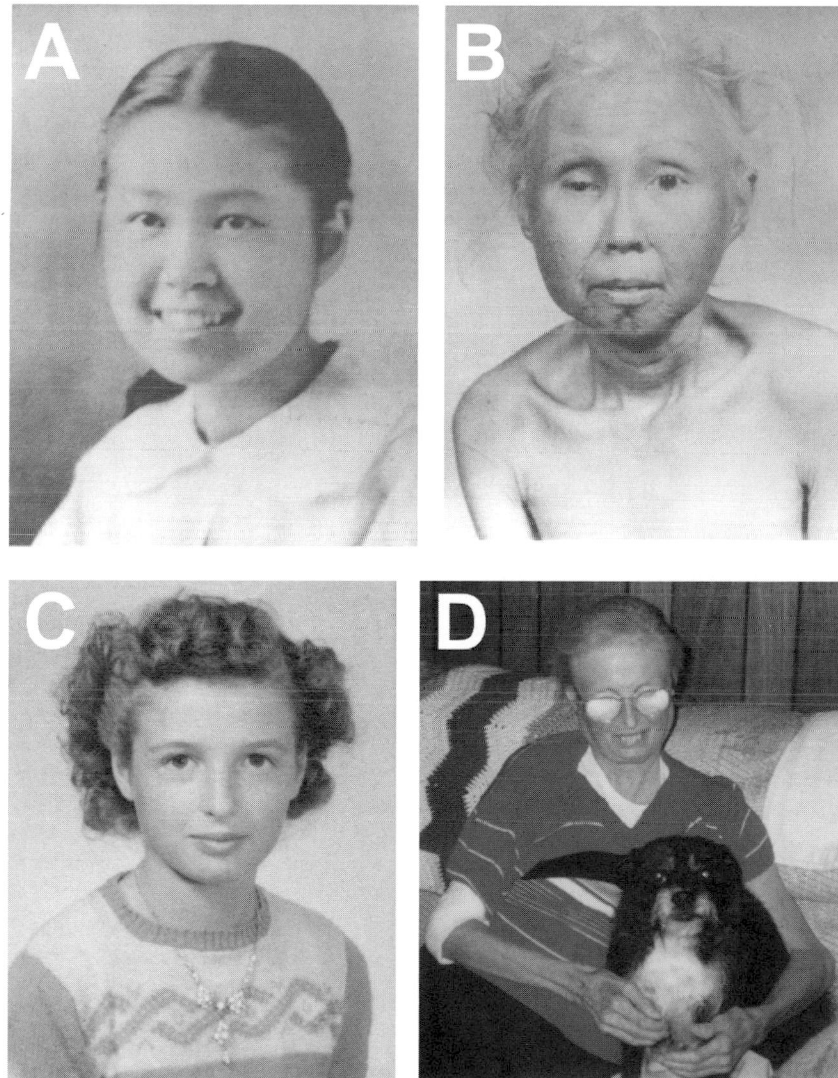

Figure 80.2 Clinical progression and features of Werner syndrome. **A, B**. Photographs of a Werner syndrome patient reported by Epstein *et al.* (1966) as Case 1, at ages 15 (**A**) and 48 (**B**). **C, D**. Photographs of a second patient at ages ~13 (**C**) and 56 (**D**). Note in both instances the rounded face, sharp features, graying, thinning, and loss of scalp and eyebrow hair and, in **D**, the thin, atrophic forearms and elbow ulceration. Panels **A** and **B** are used with kind permission of Drs. George Martin and Nancy Hanson of the International Registry of Werner Syndrome, and Lippincott Williams & Wilkins (**B**). The patient photographs in panels **C** and **D** were previously published in Martin (2005), and are used here courtesy of the patient's spouse with informed consent of the patient and of Drs. George Martin and Nancy Hanson, and Elsevier Press.

photo pairs can be viewed on the Web to get a sense of clinical progression of the changes in external appearance (see Recommended Resources).

The progression of clinical changes in WS can usefully be thought of as having three distinct phases. The first of these comprises the absence of an adolescent growth spurt followed over the subsequent decade by the appearance of graying and loss of hair, the development of skin changes, and of cataracts. A second wave of changes, often first seen late in the third or in the fourth decades of life, include skin ulceration, hypogonadism, and reproductive failure, together with a progressive worsening of the primary changes. A third phase may follow with the development of clinically important disease processes such as atherosclerosis, osteoporosis, diabetes mellitus, and cancer. These diseases occur proportionately earlier in WS patients than in otherwise normal individuals of comparable age, and are an important cause of premature morbidity and mortality. The three leading causes of death in WS patients are atherosclerotic cardiovascular disease, neoplasia, and, in a minority of cases, infection. The mean age at death in a Japanese clinical series was ~47 years, though well-documented patients have lived into the seventh decade of life (Goto, 1997).

DIAGNOSTIC CRITERIA AND DIFFERENTIAL DIAGNOSIS

The complex, progressive, and variable nature of the WS clinical phenotype makes the clinical diagnosis of WS challenging. This is especially true in young adults, where there are often few convincing signs or changes and where there may be no family history of WS to raise clinical suspicion. There are no universally accepted criteria for the diagnosis of WS. However, a useful set of diagnostic criteria and a scoring system have been developed by investigators at the International Registry for Werner Syndrome (Table 80.1, bottom panel; see also Recommended Resources). These criteria, together with molecular approaches to identify common *WRN* mutations or the loss of WRN protein expression (see later), can be used in most instances to confirm or exclude a diagnosis of WS in suspected affected individuals. The ability to couple clinical and molecular diagnostic approaches, as noted later, now allows the unambiguous identification of affected or at-risk homozygous mutant individuals, and of heterozygous carriers in families regardless of age or clinical findings.

The availability of a consistent set of clinical diagnostic criteria and of molecular diagnostic criteria for WS have provided sharper definition of WS as a disease entity, and provide a way to distinguish WS from other human diseases and syndromes that may mimic WS. Two groups of patients who may be confused with, or not easily distinguished from, typical or classic WS include patients who fulfill the clinical diagnostic criteria for WS as outlined in Table 80.1, though lack mutations in the *WRN* gene; and patients who resemble WS patients though fail to fulfill the diagnostic criteria outlined in Table 80.1. This second group is often ascertained as potential variant or atypical WS. Both of these groups of patients are rare, and from the experience of the International Registry of Werner Syndrome together represent no more than a small fraction of suspected WS patients.

Despite their rarity, these WS look-alikes are of considerable clinical and biological interest as they are likely to be highly enriched for rare mutations in proteins that act with—or act on—WRN to modify or target its function *in vivo*. There are strong theoretical grounds for proposing the existence of these individuals, in light of the growing number of proteins that may act with WRN (see later). There are experimental hints, for example, of at least one additional complementation group for WS in addition to the group represented by inactivating mutations in the *WRN* gene (Prince *et al.*, 1999). These WS phenocopies or partial phenocopies represent an important area for additional clinical and molecular diagnostic work.

A portion of the second group of patients just mentioned, with what has been termed atypical Werner syndrome, share some clinical features of WS (see Table 80.1), though lack mutations in the *WRN* gene. A small number of these patients were recently found to carry germline mutations that alter splicing of the *LMNA* or lamin A/C gene (Chen *et al.*, 2003). A subset of different *LMNA* mutations that alter the splicing of *LMNA* mRNA have been found in patients with Hutchinson-Gilford progeria (HGPS), a rare, heritable, severe, and rapidly progressive disease that is often referred to simply as progeria or childhood progeria. Of note, other mutations that alter splicing or the properties of *LMNA* or lamin A/C have been associated with at least eight other clinically distinguishable diseases that have been collectively termed the laminopathies. This fascinating group of diseases affect predominantly nerve, muscle, connective tissue, or adipocytes (Broers *et al.*, 2005). HGPS and WS show little clinical overlap, and are unlikely to share any deep mechanistic similarities. Thus the existence of atypical WS as a distinct clinical entity has been controversial. It would appear to make the best sense at present to consider atypical WS patients with *LMNA* mutations that affect RNA splicing as having an atypical form of HGPS, rather than a variant form of WS (Hegele, 2003).

ADDITIONAL WORK NEEDED TO BETTER CHARACTERIZE WS

Our present understanding of clinical and pathologic features of WS is far from complete. This reflects both the comparative rarity of WS (see later) and the way in which patient data have been accumulated during the diagnosis or treatment of individual patients or their relatives rather than as part of a research protocol.

As a result, there is important work needed on all aspects of WS clinical medicine, pathology, and molecular and cellular function. A few of the more important areas that should receive emphasis to improve our understanding of WS are outlined here.

Systematic phenotyping

One way to improve our understanding of WS as a disease entity is to use our current understanding of clinical and pathologic features of WS to identify areas where systematic–or more quantitative–data need to be collected. For example, the clinical diagnosis of WS can often be made with confidence if the patient history and physical exam are systematic, and draw on aspects of history and clinical signs and symptoms already known to be associated with WS (see Table 80.1). Medical information forms available from the International Registry of Werner Syndrome Web site (see Recommended Resources) have been constructed with this end in mind, and can be used to collect key pieces of data to aid diagnosis during the history and physical examination of suspected WS patients. Table 80.1 also highlights those areas where we need to identify appropriate normal population control data for comparison with data collected from WS patients and their family members.

Longitudinal and cohort analyses

A second area where much productive work remains to be done is in the longitudinal analysis of WS in individual patients and their families. Few longitudinal data now exist, though will be essential to better understand the clinical expression and clinical progression of WS and of associated diseases (see Table 80.1). Careful family or pedigree studies linked to molecular data could also serve as the starting point for identification of important genetic or environmental factors that may modify either the clinical expression of WS or the development of associated diseases. Coupled clinical and molecular analyses that are longitudinal, within pedigrees, would also help resolve the question of whether there is a weakly penetrant haploinsufficiency or heterozygote phenotype in carriers of single mutant *WRN* alleles (Moser, Bigbee *et al.*, 2000). This is a point of considerable importance for, as noted later, heterozygote or haploinsufficiency phenotypes that may have clinical importance have been identified in cells and cell lines from *WRN* heterozygotes.

Patient-centered support to facilitate care and research

The ability to identify, follow, and support individual patients and their families would be immeasurably improved by a Werner patient-centered support group that provided consistent, accurate, general information on WS, developed guidelines for the clinical care of WS patients, and served to identify referral physicians knowledgeable about and skilled in the care of WS patients. An excellent example of this type of support group is the Fanconi Anemia Research Fund (FARF). The FARF was founded to support patients and families with Fanconi anemia, a rare, heritable form of bone marrow failure that is also a predisposition to leukemia and squamous cell carcinoma. The FARF provides an example of how to create a support system that serves patients and their families by providing information and advice on patient care, while facilitating further study of biological and clinical aspects of a rare, heritable disease by linking patients and their families to investigators and clinicians (see Recommended Resources).

Tumor specimens

Tumor studies of WS point to a fourth area where more work is needed. Careful pathologic analysis of even small series of tumors from WS patients already has been shown to be productive and revealing. For example, the analysis of a small number of osteosarcomas arising in Japanese WS patients revealed important clinical and pathologic differences between OS in WS patients as compared with the general population, and provided a first estimate of the relative risk of developing OS in WS (Goto *et al.*, 1996; Ishikawa *et al.*, 2000). Thus the collection of additional WS tumor specimens, together with information on the response to and the success of treatment and the presence of atypical or precursor lesions, has a very high priority. These materials, even if conventionally prepared for histopathology, often can be used for a growing range of immunocytochemical and molecular analyses including mutation typing of the *WRN* gene or of other loci of interest.

Tissue resources to facilitate research

The diagnosis and treatment of tumors or other lesions requiring surgical intervention, together with the rare opportunity to autopsy WS patients, represent our best opportunities to preserve tumor and normal tissue specimens from patients and to provide material appropriate for analyses that demand viable cells or fresh tissue for procedures such as RNA-based microarray analyses. Skin samples from autopsy can be readily cryopreserved as a source of primary dermal fibroblast cultures. Similar samples served as the source of primary fibroblast strains and their SV40 large T-antigen or telomerase catalytic subunit-immortalized cell line derivatives that have proven remarkably useful for analyses of WS cell proliferation, cytogenetic and DNA damage response abnormalities. Biopsy and autopsy specimens may also serve as a useful source for additional cell strains or cell lines.

The Relationship of WS to Normal Aging

Published accounts of WS from Otto Werner have commented on the similarities between WS and what might be expected in premature aging. This idea is supported by the striking clinical appearance and progression of changes observed in WS patients (see Figure 80.2). The consistent appearance of features of advanced chronological age in patients in the fourth and fifth decades of life led, not surprisingly, to the idea that WS *is* a premature or accelerated aging syndrome and that there *must* be deep mechanistic links between WS and normal aging. Despite these apparent similarities, careful clinical and/or pathologic examination of WS patients has consistently pointed out differences in the nature or degree of change observed in WS as compared with normal aging.

Quantitative differences between WS and normal aging include the greater extent or severity of the loss of hair or hair color; of the extent of calcification of heart valve leaflets; of atherosclerosis and of osteoporosis; and of the loss of reproductive function. Qualitative differences between WS and normal aging include the unusual type of cataract observed in WS patients as opposed to normal aged individuals; the unusual changes observed in skin and subcutaneous connective tissue of the face and extremities, together with nontrophic ulceration; the unusual spectrum of neoplasms; the location and extent of soft tissue calcification; and the autosomal recessive nature of WS (Epstein *et al.*, 1966).

In light of these differences, there has been substantial discussion of the value of studying WS, related diseases, or related animal models as ways to gain insight into mechanistic aspects of aging or of age-associated disease pathogenesis. An oft-cited disadvantage of studying diseases such as WS is that they may represent at best a phenocopy of what we are *really* interested in understanding, and thus mechanistic or pathophysiologic blind alleys as regards the mechanisms underlying normal aging or disease pathogenesis (Miller, 2004). A more optimistic view is that a subset of the disorders that affect the apparent rate of aging or the appearance of age-associated diseases *will* have mechanistic overlap with normal aging. Thus these diseases may provide a useful way to bring data on many aspects of human biology, genetics, and medicine to a focus to formulate and test specific hypotheses about age-dependent disease pathogenesis. These diseases or syndromes may also provide useful instances in which to test ideas about more general mechanisms that contribute to human aging (Kipling *et al.*, 2004; Martin, 2005).

This issue was discussed in some detail by Epstein *et al.* (1966) in their clinical, pathologic, and genetic characterization of WS. Their conclusions on this point are worth revisiting. They stated that the many observed differences between normal aging and WS led to the conclusion that WS was neither a precocious or accelerated form of aging, but "may be better considered a 'caricature' of aging, exaggerating, although not necessarily by the same mechanisms, some of the clinical and pathologic changes which connote aging" (Epstein *et al.*, 1966). This conclusion is still largely sound after 40 years of additional work on WS, despite the large number of references to WS in the popular and scientific presses as a premature aging syndrome.

The WRN Gene and Disease-Associated Mutations

The chromosome 8p12 *WRN* gene was identified in 1996 by positional cloning and predicted to encode a 162 kDa member of the human RecQ helicase family (Yu *et al.*, 1996). The human RecQ helicase family consists of five proteins that may possess 3′ to 5′ helicase and ATPase activities. WRN is unique among the human RecQ proteins in possessing an additional 3′ to 5′ exonuclease activity (Fry, 2002; Bachrati and Hickson, 2003; Opresko, Cheng *et al.*, 2004; Figure 80.3). Two stable RNAs are expressed from the *WRN* locus in human cells, and the shorter of these, of 5.8 kb, is expressed ubiquitously at varying levels in many cell types, tissues, and organs (Yu *et al.*, 1996). The 162 kDa WRN protein can be detected by Western blot analysis in cell lines and tissue samples from normal individuals, and from heterozygous carriers of single mutant copies of the *WRN* gene (Goto *et al.*, 1999; Kawabe *et al.*, 2000; Moser, Kamath-Loeb *et al.*, 2000). No systematic study of the level of expression of WRN protein as a function of human cell type or of development has as yet been published.

Thus far, a total of 25 different mutations in the *WRN* gene have been reported in WS patients. These published examples have been assembled in the form of a Web-accessible Locus-Specific Mutational Database that contains detailed information for each published mutation (Moser *et al.*, 1999; see Recommended Resources). All of these *WRN* mutations, regardless of molecular type, confer a common biochemical phenotype—they truncate the WRN open reading frame, and lead to the loss of WRN protein from patient cells (Goto *et al.*, 1999; Moser, Kamath-Loeb *et al.*, 2000). This biochemical phenotype of WS patient mutations is thus consistent with the autosomal recessive inheritance pattern of WS. The absence of missense mutations that selectively inactivate the WRN helicase or exonuclease activity from this series of WS patient mutations is notable, and suggests that both activities need to be lost to promote WS pathogenesis. This point has been further addressed experimentally (see later; Swanson *et al.*, 2004). At least 17 additional *WRN* mutations have been identified in WS patients that resemble those already described. These will be added to the *WRN* Mutational Database as they are published.

The availability of mutation typing has allowed reinvestigation of the prevalence of WS, and of the frequency of mutations and heterozygous carriers in defined populations. Previous methods to address these questions have included case counting in defined populations, and comparisons of the frequency of consanguinity in WS pedigrees with population estimates of consanguinity. Prevalence estimates by these methods have varied

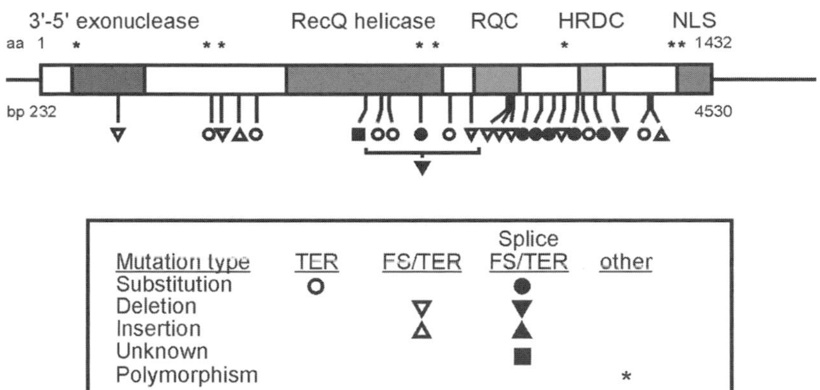

Figure 80.3 The human Werner syndrome protein WRN and a summary of mutations identified in the *WRN* gene of Werner syndrome patients. The central box indicates the WRN open reading frame with amino acid residue numbering indicated on top, and cDNA bp coordinates below, the left end of the open reading frame. The positions of five protein motifs are indicated by shaded boxes and labels: exonuclease and RecQ helicase domains, RecQ consensus (RQC) domain, the helicase and RNaseD-C-terminal (HRDC) domain, and the C-terminal nuclear localization signal (NLS). The location and molecular nature of mutations identified in Werner patients are indicated by symbols below the open reading frame to indicate the corresponding mutation location in the *WRN* cDNA sequence. All of the depicted mutations, stop codons (TER), frameshift mutations that alter the open reading frame (FS/TER), and mutations that alter splicing and the reading frame (Splice FS/TER) lead to truncation of the WRN open reading frame and loss of a C-terminal nuclear localization signal. The resulting proteins are unstable mislocalized and/or lost from patient cells. These data have been compiled and are available in the *WRN* Mutation and Polymorphism Database developed and maintained at the University of Washington (see Recommended Resources). See the color plate section.

over a 50-fold range (1/22,000 to 1/10^6), with corresponding allele frequencies ranging from 0.0067 to 0.001. More recent estimates of allele frequency that make use of molecular diagnostic criteria are consistent with these allele frequency estimates. These wide-ranging estimates reflect uncertainties in several of the population estimates used to calculate each value, rather than inherent unreliability of the methods, and the comparatively small numbers of normal population controls who have been studied by molecular methods to determine allele frequencies (Schellenberg *et al.*, 2001).

The *WRN* locus resembles many other human genes in displaying a large number of genetic variants. A small subset of these are mutant alleles segregating in the human population. However, most of the genetic variation identified thus far in the human *WRN* gene consists of single nucleotide polymorphisms or sequence variants of uncertain functional importance. The number of these variants is surprisingly large: 375 *WRN* sequence variants were detected during the recent resequencing of *WRN* exons, promoter region and downstream untranslated region at the University of Washington as part of the NIEHS-funded Environmental Genome Project. Of note, these variants were detected in a small number of different DNA samples, the 90 contained in the EGP's Polymorphism Discovery Resource (see Recommended Resources for additional information). A few of the more common polymorphic sites in the WRN open reading frame are shown in Figure 80.3 by asterisks. At least one of these common polymorphic variants has been shown to have a substantial impact on catalytic function of the WRN protein (Kamath-Loeb *et al.*, 2004). Several additional common sequence variants are also being examined for association with clinically important diseases prevalent in WS patients (e.g. atherosclerotic cardiovascular disease; see, e.g., Castro *et al.*, 2000; Ye *et al.*, 1997), or for possible associations with enhanced longevity (Castro *et al.*, 1999).

Another line of investigation of the potential of *WRN* sequence variants to modify human disease risk has come from the study of *WRN* heterozygotes. Heterozygous carriers of WS-associated mutant *WRN* alleles are likely to be present worldwide at frequencies ranging up to 1:100 in selected populations (Schellenberg *et al.*, 2001). Estimates of the prevalence or frequency of carriers of single, clearly pathogenic mutant *WRN* alleles in the United States are ~1:250, which places the number of carriers of mutant alleles in the U.S. population at >10^6. These frequency estimates suggest it will be important to determine whether the WS clinical phenotype is even weakly penetrant in heterozygous carriers.

There are some suggestions that *WRN* heterozygosity may be manifest at the cellular—and perhaps organismal—level. These data include the identification of genetic instability *in vivo* in mutation-typed heterozygous carriers of several *WRN* mutations (Moser, Bigbee *et al.*, 2000). Moreover, lymphoblastoid cell lines from otherwise healthy *WRN* heterozygotes display an intermediate sensitivity to killing by DNA damaging agents that selectively kill WRN-deficient cells (Ogburn *et al.*, 1997; Okada *et al.*, 1998). These two results indicate that *WRN* heterozygote effects may play an important role in cancer risk or the outcome of cancer therapy.

The clonal growth of many tumors may provide a way to identify inherited or somatically acquired *WRN* mutations or *WRN* gene silencing events that play a role in cancer pathogenesis or progression. The first place to look for this type of mutational enrichment will be in sporadic tumors of the histopathologic types most commonly observed in WS patients (see Table 80.2). Tumors or normal tissue in a tumor patient that displayed an aberrant or exaggerated response to chemotherapy might also be further investigated to identify heritable or acquired compromise of the WRN functional pathway. The most productive place to look for this type of response would be in patients receiving camptothecin, mitomycin-C or cis-Pt, as these agents selectively kill cells that are WRN-deficient or haploinsufficient (Ogburn *et al.*, 1997; Okada *et al.*, 1998; Poot *et al.*, 2001).

WRN Protein Function in Human Cells

The identification of WRN as a RecQ helicase, and later as an exonuclease, were made initially on the basis of protein sequence analyses (Mian, 1997; Mushegian *et al.*, 1997; Yu *et al.*, 1996). These suggestions were subsequently verified by work from several laboratories (reviewed in Fry, 2002; Bachrati and Hickson, 2003; Opresko, Cheng *et al.*, 2004). Helicases are motor proteins that use the chemical energy obtained from nucleotide triphosphate hydrolysis to break hydrogen bonds in DNA or RNA. The disruption of hydrogen bonding and base pairing is essential for the expression, repair, and replication of DNA, and helicases together with additional proteins provide a way to do this in a controlled fashion. Exonucleases, in contrast to helicases, degrade DNA (or RNA) by hydrolyzing the phosphodiester bonds between adjacent nucleotide bases. Exonucleases facilitate many DNA metabolic processes such as repair or recombination by making single-stranded DNA ends of defined polarity available as substrates. They also play key roles in insuring the fidelity of DNA replication by acting as proofreading exonucleases, and in cellular nucleotide metabolism by insuring the turnover and salvage of DNA precursors.

The predicted helicase and exonuclease activities of WRN have been confirmed and further characterized by several groups using recombinant WRN protein and short oligonucleotide substrates of defined sequence and structure. These analyses indicate that WRN can bind, unwind, or degrade several types of 3- and 4-way DNA junctions and gapped, branched, or unpaired DNA regions, and that exonuclease and helicase activities often are coordinated in acting on these DNA substrates. Subsequent protein interaction studies of WRN indicated physical and/or functional cross-talk between WRN and general nucleic acid metabolic proteins such as RPA, together with more specialized proteins involved in DNA synthesis, on similar nucleic acid substrates (reviewed in Fry, 2002; Bachrati and Hickson, 2003; Opresko, Cheng *et al.*, 2004). Knowledge of these properties of WRN and results from prior work on *in vivo* functions of RecQ homologs in *E. coli* and in budding and fission yeast suggested potential roles for WRN in recombination, replication, or repair.

Many of the types of DNA substrates that WRN can act upon *in vitro* resemble intermediates that are common to and generated during DNA replication, recombination, or repair *in vivo*, or may be present at telomeres. DNA replication and recombination are often thought of as discrete and rather distinct aspects of nucleic acid metabolism. Both processes are now recognized to be tightly linked and interdependent upon one another in many or all organisms. In human and other mammalian cells, the close functional interrelationship between DNA replication and homology-dependent recombinational repair (HR repair) is indicated by the importance of HR repair of DNA breaks, the critical role played by HR repair in mammalian development, and the critical role for HR proteins and HR function in the rescue of stalled replication forks (Cox *et al.*, 2000; Thompson and Schild, 2001). Consistent with these observations, abnormalities in DNA replication have been noted in WS cells for many years, and there are more recent data indicating an important role for WRN protein in insuring the completion of late stages of homologous recombination (Prince *et al.*, 2001; Saintigny *et al.*, 2002).

Several lines of evidence argue that telomeres are physiologic substrates for WRN function *in vivo*. WRN protein can be found at telomeres, and associates with key telomeric proteins such as TRF1 and TRF2. Moreover, TRF1 and TRF2 can modulate WRN biochemical activities on telomeric substrates *in vitro* (Opresko, Otterlei *et al.*, 2004). The T-loop structure of telomeres resembles the D-loop intermediate involved in recombination and replication, which is one of the branched DNA structures that may be a preferred *in vivo* substrate for WRN. Moreover, upon replication, telomeres are transiently converted into another postulated substrate for WRN, a single-ended DNA double-strand break. A final line of evidence for WRN function at telomeres comes from the observation that telomerase expression can extend the lifespan and modify the DNA damage responses of primary WS fibroblasts (Hisama *et al.*, 2000; Wyllie *et al.*, 2000), and that WS-like changes have been observed in mouse models in which telomerase function and Wrn function have been simultaneously ablated (see the section, "Animal Models").

If WRN plays a role in DNA replication and recombination, in telomere maintenance, or in HR repair in human cells, how does the loss of WRN function lead to characteristic molecular and cellular abnormalities in WS patients? A model for WRN function that reflects the close connection between replication and recombination is shown in Figure 80.4.

In this simplest version of WRN function *in vivo*, WRN acts on DNA molecules that are generated during the HR repair of DNA damage, from potential recombination substrates that are generated during stalled or disrupted DNA replication, or from intermediates or products of telomere maintenance. Successful resolution of these substrates suppresses genomic instability and insures high cell viability. In the absence of WRN function, these processes either stall or fail and leave cells with potentially toxic DNA intermediates that can trigger both DNA damage and apoptotic response pathways. Thus a loss of WRN function may lead in many cell lineages to apoptosis or mitotic death, while leading to gene rearrangement, mutation, or loss in surviving cells.

Experimental evidence supporting this model has been recently reviewed (Monnat and Saintigny, 2004). For example, the predictions of genomic instability and reduced cell viability following the loss of WRN function are reflected in the characteristic chromosomal rearrangements in primary lymphocyte and fibroblast cultures from WS patients (Hoehn *et al.*, 1975; Melcher *et al.*, 2000; Figure 80.5), and in the reduced proliferation of primary WS fibroblasts in culture (Martin *et al.*, 1970).

The most surprising aspect of the model depicted in Figure 80.4 is that WS disease pathogenesis may be driven by a recombination *defect*. This conclusion is the opposite of what has been widely assumed—that WS is

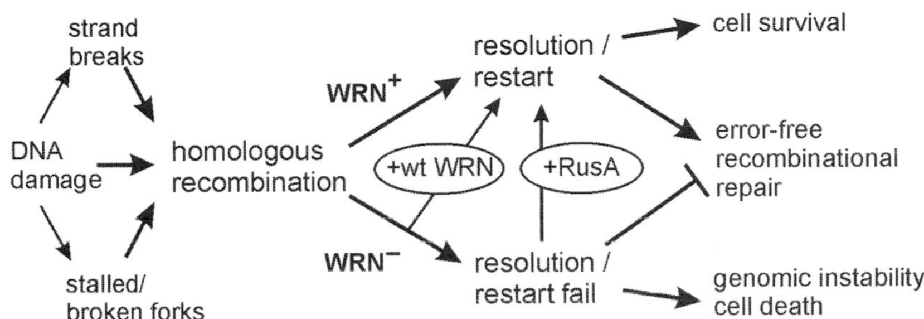

Figure 80.4 Model of Werner protein function in human cells. A requirement for WRN function can be initiated by DNA damage that leads to DNA strand breaks or that stalls or disrupts DNA replication. Damage to chromosomal DNA, replication forks, or telomeres can initiate homologous recombination repair (HR repair) that in the presence of WRN is successfully resolved to insure high cell viability and genetic stability (**WRN**$^+$ arrow). In the absence of WRN (**WRN**$^-$ arrow), HR resolution and/or replication restart fail, leading to mitotic arrest, cell death, and genetic instability. Two of the experimental tests of this model are shown by the ovals: re-expressing WRN protein (**+wt WRN**) improves both cell survival and the recovery of viable mitotic recombinants, as does expression of the bacterial resolvase protein RusA (**+RusA**).

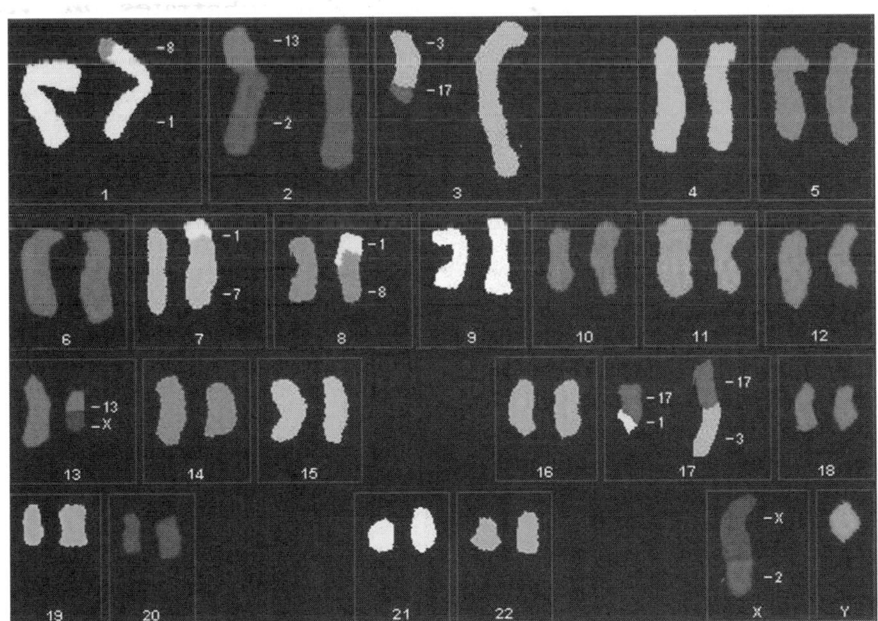

Figure 80.5 Variegated translocation mosaicism in primary fibroblasts from a Werner syndrome patient. The figure is a spectral (or SKY) karyotype of the chromosomal complement of a skin fibroblast from a male WS patient (reported in Melcher *et al.*, 2000). Note the many stable chromosomal changes including reciprocal translocations (e.g., involving chromosomes 1 and 8), together with translocations that are not obviously reciprocal in nature and may be accompanied by deletions (e.g., the translocation of material from chromosome 1 to chromosomes 7 and 17). This original spectral karyotype was kindly provided by Dr. Holger Hoehn, University of Würzburg, Würzburg, Germany. See the color plate section.

a hyper-recombination syndrome—and thus of particular conceptual value.

The model depicted in Figure 80.4 provides a useful way to integrate molecular, biochemical, and cytologic data on WS, and begins to explain mechanistic links among recombination, cell viability, and mutagenesis in WS cells. It also provides a useful way to further explore mechanistic aspects of WRN function. One example of this is illustrated by recent work to determine whether one or both of the WRN catalytic activities must be lost in order to generate the HR repair and cell survival defects characteristically seen in cells from WS patients. These experiments used single amino acid substitutions to disrupt the WRN exonuclease or helicase activities, together with the reexpression of mutant protein in WS cell lines. We found that both the WRN exonuclease and helicase activities needed to be lost to reveal the WRN recombination defect. However, and in contrast to WRN-deficient cells, the expression of either single missense mutant supported high cell viability after DNA crosslink damage (Swanson *et al.*, 2004).

These results indicate that the spectrum of *WRN* mutations identified in WS patients reflects the need to lose *both* WRN catalytic activities from cells in order to generate the cellular and clinical defects characteristic of WS. Our results also raise the intriguing possibility that *WRN* missense mutations that selectively affect helicase or exonuclease activity may be segregating in the human population, and could be associated with disease phenotypes in addition to WS that resulted from a selective loss of WRN-mediated HR repair.

WRN Function and Disease Pathogenesis in Cell Lineages

The elucidation of molecular aspects of WRN function, and of how the loss of WRN function generates WS cellular phenotypes, together begin to suggest how the WS clinical phenotype may originate and progress. The postulated role for WRN in insuring successful, high-fidelity DNA replication, HR repair, and telomere maintenance, as outlined earlier (see Figure 80.4), indicates that a loss of function will be accompanied by genomic instability and reduced cell viability in many cell lineages during and after development. These two cellular consequences are likely to be intermediate phenotypes that lead to mutation accumulation and cell loss, that together drive the development of cell type-, cell lineage-, or tissue-specific defects in WS patients.

This idea of pathogenesis is shown in Figure 80.6. Further rounds of mutation accumulation, cell dysfunction, and cell loss can occur in continuously or conditionally replicating cell lineages, with the eventual compromise of tissue or organ structure and function and, in some tissues, the emergence of mutation-dependent neoplastic proliferation. This model of clinical progression indicates that the appearance of the first features of WS during adolescence is a reflection of the progressive accumulation of cellular defects during development and over the first decade of life, rather than something that is driven by the endocrine and physiologic changes that accompany puberty. Thus puberty reveals, rather than generates, the WS phenotype in affected individuals.

This view is consistent with the clinical and mechanistic view of WS as outlined earlier, and emphasizes the importance of genomic instability and replicative senescence in the generation of the WS phenotype. If this picture is accurate, however, why are dividing cell lineages not *selectively* affected during adult life by the loss of WRN function? And why are some organs such as the CNS spared the consequences of loss of WRN function? One likely explanation is the following. All cell lineages are generated by mitotic division during development and thus have the potential to be affected by mutation

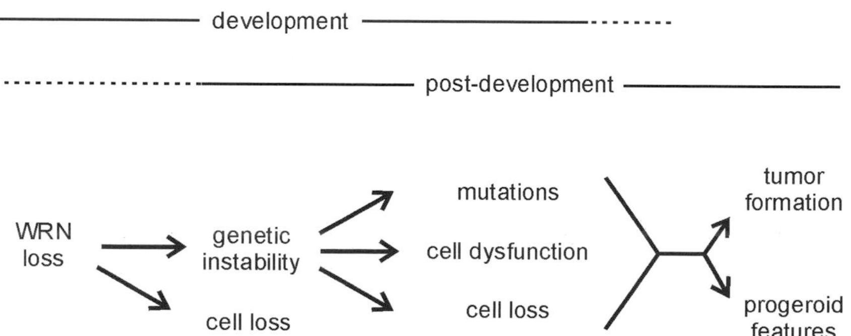

Figure 80.6 Model for pathogenesis of disease in the absence of WRN function. WRN loss as a result of inherited germline mutations (see Figure 80.3) leads from the beginning of development to genetic instability and cell loss in many or all cell lineages. These changes, following the completion of development, can be perpetuated or amplified in specific cell lineages or tissues where division potential is retained. How the intermediate consequences or phenotypes of the absence of WRN function, i.e., mutation accumulation, cell dysfunction and cell loss, affect specific lineages or tissues to lead to the emergence of either neoplastic, atrophic, or progeroid outcomes is heavily conditioned by normal lineage biology (see text for additional discussion). Two different time lines above the figure indicate the progressive nature of cell and cell lineage defects, and their origins during development.

accumulation or cell loss in the absence of WRN function. Continuously dividing lineages during adult life such as skin, gut, and bone marrow may be tolerant of the loss of WRN function by virtue of mutation expansion-limiting lineage architecture, normally stringent cell editing by a combination of apoptosis and terminal differentiation, and large reserves of stem cells or lineage repopulating cells.

Conversely, in the absence of WRN function, those cell lineages or tissues that are largely postmitotic following the completion of development (e.g., many CNS cell lineages) may take advantage of normal developmental regulatory mechanisms such as compensatory cell proliferation and cell editing by programmed cell death to compensate for increased cell loss or dysfunction to insure the completion of development with normal structure and function. Key variables that determine the eventual outcome are the number of cell divisions required to generate a mature lineage; how much cell editing via apoptotic cell death occurs during and after development; and what functional redundancy is present to compensate for cell loss or dysfunction.

The fibroblast lineage and other mesenchymal or mesodermally derived cell lineages may be selectively affected by the loss of WRN function for several of these reasons, including the persistence of conditional cell division throughout life; the ability to accumulate genetic variation, and perhaps genetic damage, in conjunction with a comparative resistance to damage-induced apoptosis; and the absence of a compartmentalized tissue architecture that could effectively suppress the proliferative defects that result in neoplasia. In the absence of WRN function this combination of features may predispose mesenchymal lineages to the progressive accumulation of mutant and dysfunctional or senescent cells, together with progressive disruption of trophic or regulatory interactions with adjacent epithelial or stromal cells (reviewed in Campisi, 2005).

This line of pathogenetic reasoning leads to two important conclusions. First, we need to know more about the normal biology of specific human cell lineages before we will be able to understand and predict *in vivo* consequences of a loss or absence of WRN function. A second important conclusion is that we clearly need experimentally tractable animal models in which to study cell lineage-specific functions of WRN.

Animal Models of WS

Animal models are clearly important if we are to study WRN function and WS pathogenesis at the levels of cell lineage and the whole organism. The only mammalian models of WS that have been developed thus far have been in the mouse. Three different types of mouse model have been published: a complete knockout or null of murine *Wrn* leading to a loss of Wrn protein expression in all tissues (Lombard *et al.*, 2000); an in-frame deletion of the helicase domain of murine *Wrn*, leading to a truncated protein that retains exonuclease activity though lacks helicase activity (Lebel and Leder, 1998); and transgenic expression of a human K577M WRN variant protein that lacks helicase activity against a background of normal murine *Wrn* expression (Wang *et al.*, 2000).

Of these three models, the only one that faithfully recapitulates the genetic and biochemical defect observed in WS patients is the knockout that does not express Wrn protein. However, despite having faithfully recapitulated the biochemical defect observed in WS patients, the *Wrn* knockout mouse model does not have an obvious aging, genetic instability, or cancer phenotype. Several reasons have been suggested to explain the apparent absence of an obvious organismal phenotype in *Wrn* knockout mice: that mice simply do not live long enough to develop the changes first observed in WS patients beginning in the second and third decades of life; that mice may have different, or more robust, ways to compensate for the loss of *Wrn* function; or that humans may represent for reasons of lack of redundancy, long life span or environmental exposures, the equivalent of a sensitized background for revealing WRN function at the cell and organismal levels. Three caveats in interpreting these results and arguments are that the phenotyping of the *Wrn* knockout mouse model has been very modest to date; there has not as yet been a careful aging cohort study taken to completion; and knockout mice have not been systematically challenged with DNA damaging agents such as cross-linkers that may reveal defects in the murine *Wrn* functional pathway that parallel those observed in human cells.

One obvious way to test these ideas and further develop the murine model of WS is to generate sensitized mouse genetic backgrounds by altering the genetic constitution of *Wrn* knockout mice to place additional stress on the replication, HR repair or telomere maintenance pathways where *Wrn* is likely to function. One example of this approach was taken by two collaborating groups that made use of a murine telomerase RNA template-deficient (or *Terc*-deficient) mouse in conjunction with the loss of *Wrn* (Chang *et al.*, 2004), or of Wrn and Blm (Du *et al.*, 2004), function to reveal the progressive appearance of changes observed in WS patients.

Changes observed in these double or triple mutants include the graying and loss of hair, osteoporosis, diabetes mellitus, and cataracts. These changes appear to depend on critically short telomeres as a primary driver of the phenotype in the absence of *Wrn* and Blm. This provides an explanation as to why changes are observed in only a portion of mice, and in those affected only in late-generation *Terc*-deficiency where telomere erosion is substantial. These results are encouraging and have begun to provide mouse models in which to investigate *Wrn* function while identifying telomeres as a potential substrate for *Wrn* function *in vivo*.

Conclusion

Werner syndrome is one of a growing number of human diseases that have revealed the importance of genetic instability, replicative senescence, and cell death as intermediate phenotypes that can shape the risk of human disease or modify disease pathogenesis. WS is further distinguished as one of the growing number of human cancer predispositions that appear to result from a defect in homologous recombination function. One prominent role for WRN function *in vivo* is as part of one or more resolution complexes that act on common nucleic acid substrates that are generated during DNA replication or recombination, or that are part of the structure or metabolism of telomeres. This resolution function of WRN insures the successful completion of replication, recombination, or telomere maintenance, and thus high cell viability and genetic stability in all human cell lineages during development. WRN may also play comparable roles in cell lineages that retain the ability to divide during adult life.

Much work remains to be done to improve our understanding of WS as a biological and clinical human disease state. WRN function clearly modulates normal biology and physiology, and thus disease risk or pathogenesis in many human tissues or cell lineages. There are also tantalizing suggestions that the importance of WRN function in human biology will extend well beyond the small number of individuals affected with classic WS, as a modulator of both neoplastic and non-neoplastic disease risk in the general population. These hints suggest that additional work on the biology and medicine of WS will be challenging though richly rewarding.

Recommended Resources

PRINT RESOURCES

Epstein, C.J., Martin, G.M., Schultz, A.L., and Motulsky, A.G. (1966). Werner's syndrome: A review of its symptomatology, natural history, pathologic features, genetics and relationship to the natural aging process. *Medicine 45*, 177–221. (A modern classic detailing the clinical, pathological, a and formal genetic analysis of contemporary and 122 reported WS cases.)

Salk, D., Fujiwara, Y., and Martin, G.M. (Eds.) (1985). Werner's Syndrome and Human Aging, *Advances in Experimental Medicine and Biology*, Vol. 190. New York: Plenum Press. (Proceedings of the Kobe, Japan meeting in 1982 that contains edited reprints of important primary references, a translation of Otto Werner's thesis of 1904, and many useful chapters detailing clinical, pathologic, and biological aspects of WS.)

Tollefsbol, T.O. and Cohen, H.J. (1984). Werner's syndrome: An underdiagnosed disorder resembling premature aging. *Age 7*, 75–88. (Useful compilation of clinical and biological information on WS gleaned from literature reports.)

Goto, M. and Miller, R.W. (2001). From Premature Gray Hair to Helicase–Werner Syndrome: Implications for Aging and Cancer. *Gann Monograph Cancer Res. 49*. (Relatively recent compilation of reviews covering historical, clinical, and biological features of WS.)

Monnat, R. J. Jr. and Saintigny, Y. (2004). The Werner syndrome protein: Unwinding function to explain disease. *SAGE-KE*. http://sageke.sciencemag.org/cgi/reprint/2004/13/re3. (Recent summary of biological and clinical aspects of WS that provides a detailed discussion of information supporting the model of WRN function shown in Figure 80.4.)

WEB RESOURCES

On-Line Mendelian Inheritance in Man, listing for Werner Syndrome:
http://www.ncbi.nlm.nih.gov/entrez/dispomim.cgi?id=277700

International Registry of Werner Syndrome:
http://www.pathology.washington.edu/research/werner/registry/frame2.html

WRN Locus-Specific Mutational Database:
http://www.pathology.washington.edu/research/werner/ws_wrn.html

Animation of Werner syndrome clinical progression and links to the International Registry and Locus-Specific Mutational Database:
http://www.pathology.washington.edu/research/werner/

GeneClinics Review of Werner Syndrome (authoritative and up-to-date review written by members of the International Registry that includes information on counseling and molecular diagnostics):
http://www.geneclinics.org/ (search for 'Werner Syndrome Review' link)

NIEHS SNPs Project Homepage (source of information on *WRN* gene polymorphisms using data generated by the UW Genome Center):
http://egp.gs.washington.edu/data/wrn/

Fanconi Anemia Research Fund (exemplary example of a patient-oriented support group that is facilitating clinical care and research on another rare, heritable human genetic instability and cancer predisposition syndrome).
http://www.fanconi.org/

ACKNOWLEDGMENTS

I thank past and present members of my laboratory and members of the University of Washington NCI-funded Werner Syndrome Program for contributing ideas, hard work, and enthusiasm to our attempts to understand WS. I would like to extend a special thanks to my senior colleagues and WS pioneers Drs. George M. Martin and Arno Motulsky, and to WS colleagues worldwide for their help and encouragement. Alden Hackmann provided graphics support, and Dr. Ali Ozgenc provided a thoughtful reading of the finished manuscript. Work in my laboratory on WS has been supported by grants from the U.S. National Institutes of Health including the NIA and NCI, and by a grant from the Nippon Boehringer Ingelheim Virtual Research Institute on Aging. There are no conflicts of interest to disclose in this work.

REFERENCES

Note: For reasons of space only a small number of primary references have been included below. My apologies to those whose work I have not been able to cite in full.

Bachrati, C.Z. and Hickson, I.D. (2003). RecQ helicases: Suppressors of tumorigenesis and premature aging. *Biochem. J. 374*, 577–606.

Bohr, V.A. (2003). Werner syndrome and its protein: Clinical, cellular and molecular advances. *Mech. Ageing Dev. 124*, 1073–1082.

Broers, J.L.V., Hutchison, C.J., and Ramaekers, F.C.S. (2005). Laminopathies. *J. Pathol. 204*, 478–488.

Campisi, J. (2005). Senescent cells, tumor suppression, and organismal aging: Good citizens, bad neighbors. *Cell 120*, 513–522.

Castro, E., Edland, S.D., Lee, L., Ogburn, C.E., Deeb, S.S., Brown, G. *et al.* (2000). Polymorphisms at the Werner locus: II. 1074Leu/Phe, 1367Cys/Arg, longevity, and athero-sclerosis. *Am. J. Med. Genet. 95*, 374–380.

Castro, E., Ogburn, C.E., Hunt, K.E., Tilvis, R., Louhija, J., Penttinen, R. *et al.* (1999). Polymorphisms at the Werner locus: I. Newly identified polymorphisms, ethnic variability of 1367Cys/Arg, and its stability in a population of Finnish centenarians. *Am. J. Med. Genet. 82*, 399–403.

Chang, S., Multani, A.S., Cabrera, N.G., Naylor, M.L., Laud, P., Lombard, D. *et al.* (2004). Essential role of limiting telomeres in the pathogenesis of Werner syndrome. *Nat. Genet. 36*, 877–882.

Chen, L., Lee, L., Kudlow, B.A., Dos Santos, H.G., Sletvold, O., Shafeghati, Y. *et al.* (2003). LMNA mutations in atypical Werner's syndrome. *Lancet 362*, 440–445.

Cox, M.M., Goodman, M.F., Kreuzer, K.N., Sherratt, D., Sandler, S.J., and Marians, K.J. (2000). The importance of repairing stalled replication forks. *Nature 404*, 37–41.

Du, X., Shen, J., Kugan, N., Furth, E.E., Lombard, D.B., Cheung, C. *et al.* (2004). Telomere shortening exposes functions for the mouse Werner and Bloom syndrome genes. *Mol. Cell Biol. 24*, 8437–8446.

Epstein, C.J., Martin, G.M., Schultz, A.L., and Motulsky, A.G. (1966). Werner's syndrome: A review of its symptomatology, natural history, pathologic features, genetics and relationship to the natural aging process. *Medicine 45*, 177–221.

Fry, M. (2002). The Werner syndrome helicase-nuclease-one protein, many mysteries. *SAGE-KE*, http://sageke.sciencemag.org/cgi/reprint/2002/13/re2.

Goto, M. (2001). Clinical characteristics of Werner syndrome and other premature aging syndromes: Pattern of aging in progeroid syndromes. *Gann Monograph. Cancer Res. 49*, 27–39.

Goto, M. (1997). Hierarchical deterioration of body systems in Werner's syndrome: Implications for normal aging. *Mech. Ageing Dev. 98*, 239–254.

Goto, M., Miller, R.W., Ishikawa, Y., and Sugano, H. (1996). Excess of rare cancers in Werner syndrome (adult progeria). *Cancer Epidemiol. Biomarkers Prev. 5*, 239-246.

Goto, M., Rubenstein, M., Weber, J., Woods, K., and Drayna, D. (1992). Genetic linkage of Werner's syndrome to five markers on chromosome 8. *Nature 355*, 735–738.

Goto, M., Yamabe, Y., Shiratori, M., Okada, M., Kawabe, T., Matsumoto, T. *et al.* (1999). Immunological diagnosis of Werner syndrome by down-regulated and truncated gene products. *Hum. Genet. 105*, 301–307.

Hatamochi, A. (2001). Dermatological features and collagen metabolism in Werner syndrome. *Gann Monograph. Cancer Res. 49*, 51–59.

Hegele, R.A. (2003). Drawing the line in progeria syndromes. *Lancet 362*, 416–417.

Hisama, F., Chen, Y.-H., Meyn, M.S., Oshima, J., and Weissman, S.M. (2000). WRN or telomerase constructs reverse 4-nitroquinoline 1-oxide sensitivity in transformed Werner syndrome fibroblasts. *Cancer Res. 60*, 2372–2376.

Hoehn, H., Bryant, E.M., Au, K., Norwood, T.H., Boman, H., and Martin, G.M. (1975). Variegated translocation mosaicism in human skin fibroblast cultures. *Cytogenet. Cell Genet. 15*, 282–298.

Ishikawa, Y., Miller, R.W., Machinami, R., Sugano, H., and Goto, M. (2000). Atypical osteosarcomas in Werner syndrome (adult progeria). *Jpn. J. Cancer Res. 91*, 1345–1349.

Kawabe, T., Tsuyama, N., Kitao, S., Nishikawa, K., Shimamoto, A., Shiratori, M. *et al.* (2000). Differential regulation of the human RecQ family helicases in cell transformation and cell cycle. *Oncogene 19*, 4764–4772.

Kipling, D., Davis, T., Ostler, E.L., and Faragher, R.G.A. (2004). What can progeroid syndromes tell us about human aging? *Science 305*, 1426–1431.

Lebel, M. and Leder, P. (1998). A deletion within the murine Werner syndrome helicase induces sensitivity to inhibitors of topoisomerase and loss of cellular proliferative capacity. *Proc. Natl. Acad. Sci. USA 95*, 13097–13102.

Lombard, D.B., Beard, C., Johnson, B., Marciniak, R.A., Dausman, J., Bronson, R. *et al.* (2000). Mutations in the *WRN* gene in mice accelerate mortality in a p53-null background. *Mol. Cell Biol. 20*, 3286–3291.

Martin, G.M. (2005). Genetic modulation of senescent phenotypes in *Homo sapiens*. *Cell 120*, 523–532.

Martin, G.M., Sprague, C.A., and Epstein, C.J. (1970). Replicative life-span of cultivated human cells. Effects of donor's age, tissue, and genotype. *Lab. Invest. 23*, 86–92.

Melcher, R., von Golitschek, R., Steinlein, C., Schindler, D., Neitzel, H., Kainer, K. *et al.* (2000). Spectral karyotyping of Werner syndrome fibroblast cultures. *Cytogenet. Cell Genet. 91*, 180–185.

Mian, I.S. (1997). Comparative sequence analysis of ribonucleases HII, III, PH, and D. *Nucleic Acids Res. 25*, 3187–3195.

Miller, R.A. (2004). "Accelerated aging": A primrose path to insight? *Aging Cell 3*, 47–51.

Monnat, R.J., Jr. (2002). Werner syndrome. In C. Fletcher, K. Unni, and F. Mertens (Eds.), *WHO/IARC Monograph on Pathology and Genetics of Tumours of Soft Tissue and Bone*, pp. 273–274. Lyon: IARC Press.

Monnat, R.J., Jr. (2001). Cancer pathogenesis in the human RecQ helicase deficiency syndromes. *Gann Monograph Cancer Res. 49*, 83–94.

Monnat, R. J., Jr. and Saintigny, Y. (2004). The Werner syndrome protein: Unwinding function to explain disease. *SAGE-KE.* http://sageke.sciencemag.org/cgi/reprint/2004/13/re3.

Moser, M.J., Bigbee, W.L., Grant, S.G., Emond, M.J., Langlois, R.G., Jensen, R.H. *et al.* (2000). Genetic instability and hematologic disease risk in Werner syndrome patients and heterozygotes. *Cancer Res. 60*, 2492–2496.

Moser, M.J., Kamath-Loeb, A.S., Jacob, J.E., Bennett, S.E., Oshima, J., and Monnat, R.J., Jr. (2000). WRN helicase expression in Werner syndrome cell lines. *Nucleic Acids Res. 28*, 648–654.

Moser, M.J., Oshima, J., and Monnat, R.J., Jr. (1999). *WRN* mutations in Werner syndrome. *Hum. Mutation 13*, 271–279.

Mushegian, A.R., Bassett, D.E., Jr., Boguski, M.S., Bork, P., and Koonin, E.V. (1997). Positionally cloned human disease genes: Patterns of evolutionarily conservation and functional motifs. *Proc. Natl. Acad. Sci. USA 94*, 5831–5836.

Ogburn, C.E., Oshima, J., Poot, M., Chen, R., Hunt, K.E., Gollahon, K.A. *et al.* (1997). An apoptosis-inducing genotoxin differentiates heterozygotic carriers for Werner helicase mutations from wild-type and homozygous mutants. *Hum. Genet. 101*, 121–125.

Okada, M., Goto, M., Furuichi, Y., and Sugimoto, M. (1998). Differential effects of cytotoxic drugs on mortal and immortalized B-lymphoblastoid cell lines from normal and Werner's syndrome patients. *Biol. Pharm. Bull. 21*, 235–239.

Oppenheimer, B.S. and Kugel, V.H. (1934). Werner's syndrome—a heredo-familial disorder with scleroderma, bilateral juvenile cataract, precocious graying of hair and endocrine stigmatization. *Trans. Assoc. Amer. Physicians 49*, 358–370.

Opresko, P.L., Cheng, W.-H., and Bohr, V.A. (2004). Junction of RecQ helicase biochemistry and human disease. *J. Biol. Chem. 279*, 18099–18102.

Opresko, P.L., Otterlei, M., Graakjaer, J., Bruheim, P., Dawut, L., Kolvraa, S. *et al.* (2004).The Werner syndrome helicase and exonuclease cooperate to resolve telomeric D loops in a manner regulated by TRF1 and TRF2. *Mol. Cell 14*, 763–74.

Pehmoeller, G. (2001). Memory of my father, Otto Werner. *Gann Monograph Cancer Res. 49*, vii–viii.

Poot, M., Yom, J.S., Whang, S.H., Kato, J.T., Gollahon, K.A., and Rabinovitch, P.S. (2001). Werner syndrome cells are sensitive to DNA cross-linking drugs. *FASEB J. 15*, 1224–1226.

Prince, P.R., Emond, M.J., and Monnat, R.J., Jr. (2001). Loss of Werner syndrome protein function promotes aberrant mitotic recombination. *Genes Dev. 15*, 933–938.

Prince, P.R., Ogburn, C.E., Moser, M.J., Emond, M.J., Martin, G.M., and Monnat, R.J., Jr. (1999). Cell fusion corrects the 4-nitroquinoline 1-oxide sensitivity of Werner syndrome fibroblast cell lines. *Hum. Genet. 105*, 132–138.

Saintigny, Y., Makienko, K., Swanson, C., Emond, M.J., and Monnat, R.J., Jr. (2002). Homologous recombination resolution defect in Werner syndrome. *Mol. Cell Biol. 22*, 6971–6978.

Salk, D. (1982). Werner syndrome: A review of recent research with an analysis of connective tissue metabolism, growth control of cultured cells, and chromosomal aberrations. *Human Genetics 62*, 1–15.

Salk, D., Fujiwara, Y. and Martin, G.M. (Eds.) (1985). Werner's Syndrome and Human Aging, Vol. 190, *Advances in Experimental Medicine and Biology*. New York: Plenum Press.

Schellenberg, G.D., Miki, T., Yu, C.-E., and Nakura, J. (2001). Werner syndrome. In C.R. Scriver, A.L. Beaudet, W.S. Sly, and D. Valle (Eds.) *The Metabolic & Molecular Basis of Inherited Disease*, pp. 785–797. New York: McGraw-Hill.

Swanson, C., Saintigny, Y., Emond, M.J., and Monnat, R.J., Jr. (2004). The Werner syndrome protein has separable recombination and viability functions. *DNA Repair 3*, 1–10.

Thannhauser, S.J. (1945). Werner's syndrome (progeria of the adult) and Rothmund's syndrome: Two types of closely related hederofamilial atrophic dermatoses with juvenile cataracts and endocrine features; a critical study of five new cases. *Ann. Intern. Med. 23*, 559–626.

Thompson, L.H. and Schild, D. (2001). Homologous recombinational repair of DNA ensures mammalian chromosome stability. *Mutat. Res. 477*, 131–153.

Tollefsbol, T.O. and Cohen, H.J. (1984). Werner's syndrome: An underdiagnosed disorder resembling premature aging. *Age 7*, 75–88.

Wang, L., Ogburn, C.E., Ware, C.B., Ladiges, W.C., Youssoufian, H., Martin, G.M. *et al.* (2000). Cellular Werner phenotypes in mice expressing a putative dominant-negative human *WRN* gene. *Genetics 154*, 357–362.

Werner, O. (1985). On cataract in conjunction with scleroderma (translated by H. Hoehn). In D. Salk, Y. Fujiwara, and G.M. Martin (Eds.), *Werner's Syndrome and Human Aging*, Vol. 190, *Advances in Experimental Medicine and Biology*, pp. 1–14. New York: Plenum Press.

Wyllie, F.S., Jones, C.J., Skinner, J.W., Haughton, M.F., Wallis, C., Wynford-Thomas, D. *et al.* (2000). Telomerase prevents the accelerated cell ageing of Werner syndrome fibroblasts. *Nat. Genet. 24*, 16–17.

Ye, L., Miki, T., Nakura, J., Oshima, J., Kamino, K., Rakugi, H. *et al.* (1997). Association of a polymorphic variant of the Werner helicase gene with myocardial infarction in a Japanese population. *Am. J. Hum. Genet. 68*, 494–498.

Yu, C.-E., Oshima, J., Fu, Y.-H., Wijsman, E.M., Hisama, F., Ouais, S. *et al.* (1996). Positional cloning of the Werner's syndrome gene. *Science 272*, 258–262.

81

Models of Sarcopenia

Alfred L. Fisher

Sarcopenia refers to the loss of muscle mass during normal aging. The medical importance of sarcopenia lies in the significant loss of muscle strength that accompanies the loss of muscle mass. Clinical studies have linked the loss of strength to decreases in mobility and functioning seen in older people, and have suggested that the extent of strength loss could serve as a risk factor for mortality. Sarcopenia has been observed in multiple mammalian species besides humans and even in simple non-vertebrate animals, like the nematode Caenorhabditis elegans. *This observation suggests that the development of sarcopenia may be an unfortunate but normal part of the aging of the neuromuscular system. Although the exact cause of sarcopenia is currently unknown, there is evidence from studies in people and experimental animals to support a number of theories, such as loss of motor neurons, declines in specific catabolic hormones, increases in inflammatory cytokines, and inadequate protein intake. Given the medical importance of sarcopenia, there is a pressing need to understand this condition further with the hope of developing effective treatments. This chapter will provide an introduction to sarcopenia and the current methods used to study sarcopenia both in people and experimental systems.*

Introduction

The term *sarcopenia* describes the loss of muscle mass and muscle strength that occurs with normal aging (see Figure 81.1).

Sarcopenia is not a uniquely human condition as comparable changes have been seen in people, mice, rats, dogs, and even lower animals such as the nematode worm *Caenorhabiditis elegans*, and hence sarcopenia may represent the aging of the neuromuscular system in animals (Fisher, 2004).

The medical importance of sarcopenia lies in the reductions of strength that accompany the loss of muscle mass (see Figure 81.2).

Muscle strength reaches a peak in the late 20s to early 30s before beginning a slow, continuous decline. For much of adulthood the declines in muscle strength are of little consequence except for elite athletes and those involved in intense physical labor. However, starting in the late 50s, the loss of muscle mass and strength appears to accelerate (Lexell, 1995; Vandervoort, 2002). However, the loss of strength varies between individuals resulting in significant differences between individuals of the same age. Consequently, by the 60s the loss of muscle strength begins to impact individuals to varying degrees. The declines in strength have been linked to impairments in mobility and functioning seen in older people. The decline in strength also appears to act as a risk factor for mortality (Fisher, 2004).

At a simple level, the loss of muscle strength impairs the ability to lift and carry objects, such as groceries or laundry. For example, data from the Framingham cohort indicate that 45% of women aged 65 to 74 years and 65% of women aged 75 to 84 years are unable to lift 4.5 kg. (Fisher, 2004). The loss of strength also has a significant impact on lower extremity strength and on lower extremity function as measured by gait speed, rising from a chair, or climbing stairs (Evans, 1997; Greenlund and Nair, 2003). Besides the direct impact of impaired lower extremity function on mobility in daily life, poor lower extremity function is strongly associated with both falls and need for nursing home placement (Guralnik *et al.*, 1995; Rantanen, 2003). Besides the impairment in functioning, the loss of strength also serves as a risk factor for future mortality as multiple studies have demonstrated weaker individuals to have higher mortality than stronger individuals even after correction for comorbid illnesses (Metter *et al.*, 2002; Rantanen, 2003; Rantanen, *et al.*, 2003). The reason for this association between strength and mortality is not known, but could involve sarcopenia and the loss of strength serving as a marker for the aging of the entire body, with individuals with worse sarcopenia being biologically older than the individuals with more preserved muscles (Fisher, 2004).

The cause of sarcopenia is unknown, but there is evidence from human and experimental animals for multiple theories, including loss of motor neurons, oxidative stress, declines in catabolic hormones, increases in inflammatory cytokines, and inadequate nutrition.

Electromyography and anatomic studies have demonstrated a loss of up to 50% in the numbers of motor neurons in the spinal cord with resulting reduction in the numbers of functioning motor units (Lexell, 1995; Vandervoort, 2002). As some of the changes seen in aging muscle are reminiscent of changes seen following denervation, this suggests that the chronic denervation and reinnervation occurring due to the loss of motor neurons may be a cause of sarcopenia during aging (Lexell, 1995; Vandervoort, 2002).

During aging, metabolically active tissues such as muscle are at risk of damage from reactive oxidative species either from atmospheric oxygen or internally generated radicals from mitochondrial metabolism (Carmeli *et al.*, 2002). The oxygen radicals are highly reactive and can damage DNA, proteins, and lipids in the muscle cell, eventually leading to cell death or dysfunction. Studies in aging muscle have shown increases in markers of oxidative damage to proteins and lipids with age. Additionally, lower levels of oxidative damage have been seen in animals treated with caloric restriction, which is an intervention that slows organismal aging (Carmeli *et al.*, 2002).

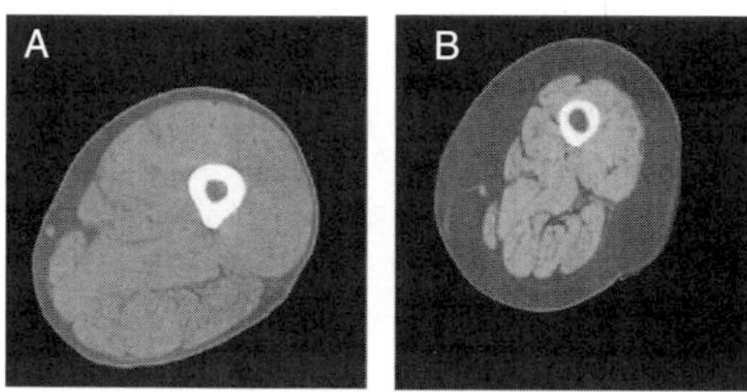

Figure 81.1 Sarcopenia is a loss of muscle mass during aging. **A**. CT scan of the mid-thigh of a young active person shows subcutaneous fat (dark gray) and skeletal muscle (light gray). **B**. A CT scan of the mid-thigh of an older person demonstrates the dramatic loss of skeletal muscle mass and the accompanying increase in subcutaneous fat. Reproduced from Roubenoff (2003b) with permission of the publisher.

The levels of muscle catabolic hormones, such as growth hormone and testosterone, decline significantly during aging. For growth hormone, during aging there is an approximately 14% per decade decline in secretion (Horani and Morley, 2004). This decline is due to reductions in both the frequency and amplitude of pulses of secreted growth hormone from the pituitary. Associated with the decrease in growth hormone production is an accompanying decrease in IGF-1 (insulin-like growth factor) production, which is made by the liver in response to growth hormone. IGF-1 acts on several tissues including muscle, where IGF-1 simultaneously promotes muscle hypertrophy and inhibits muscle atrophy (McKinnell and Rudnicki, 2004). In men, testosterone declines at a rate of approximately 100 ng/dL per decade during adulthood (Horani and Morley, 2004). Testosterone has anabolic actions on muscle and also appears to increase the production of muscle stem cells. Unfortunately, human studies investigating the effects of testosterone or growth hormone replacement on sarcopenia have produced at best modest results, though none of the studies were long-term (Blackman *et al.*, 2002; Horani and Morley, 2004).

Aging is associated with increasing levels of inflammatory cytokines, such as TNFα (tumor necrosis factor) and IL-6 (interleukin) (Ferrucci *et al.*, 2002; Roubenoff, 2003a; Roubenoff *et al.*, 2003). The reason for the observed increases and the sites of cytokine production are not known. However, clinical studies have demonstrated an association between higher levels of

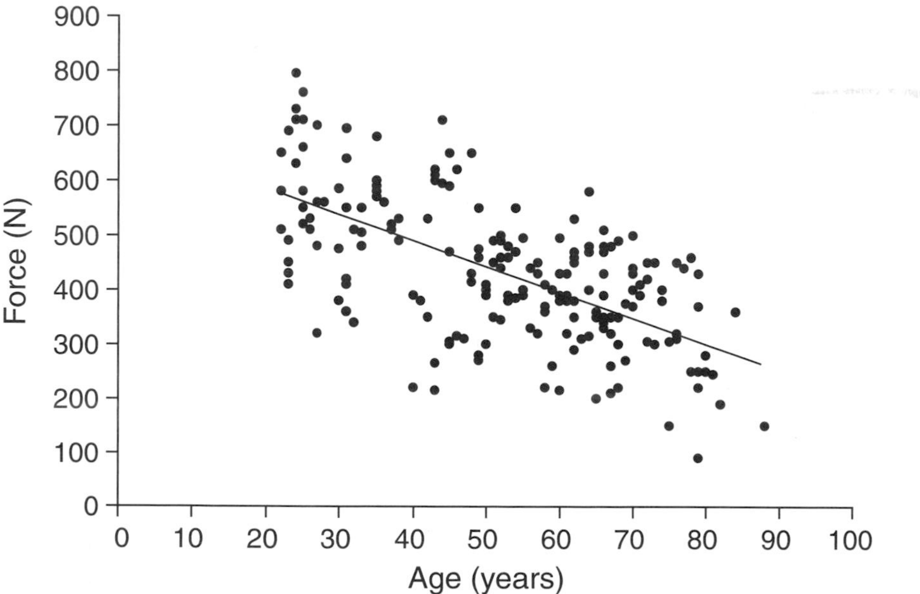

Figure 81.2 A loss of muscle strength accompanies sarcopenia. Maximal voluntary isometric contractile force of the dominant knee extensor in healthy community-dwelling Australian women aged 20–87 years. A linear trend accounts for 96% of the systematic variation with age. Reproduced from Hunter (1998) with permission of the publisher.

inflammatory cytokines and lower strength and muscle mass. Animal studies have demonstrated that inflammatory cytokines, like TNFα, act on muscles to promote muscle atrophy through the activation of the transcription factor NF-κB (McKinnell and Rudnicki, 2004). NF-κB produces muscle atrophy at least in part through the activation of specific ubiquitin ligases that degrade muscle proteins. It remains to be determined if the losses of muscle mass due to sarcopenia are secondary to the direct actions of inflammatory cytokines on muscle with the activation of NF-κB.

In people, body weight increases until the late 50s to early 60s before declining in later life (Roubenoff, 2003a; Volpi *et al.*, 2004). Much of the weight loss is due to a reduction in caloric intake, which occurs at a time in life when the daily protein requirement may be increased compared to younger adults. Consequently, weight loss in late life has a significant impact on muscle mass through mild protein calorie malnutrition (Roubenoff, 2003a; Volpi *et al.*, 2004). Clinical studies have demonstrated that supplements containing essential amino acids can have a beneficial effect on muscle protein synthesis (Volpi *et al.*, 2004). Unfortunately, many commercially available supplements obtain most of their calories from either carbohydrate or nonessential amino acids, and as a result these supplements have shown minimal effects in clinical studies (Fiatarone *et al.*, 1994; Volpi *et al.*, 2004).

As the proportion of older people is expected to increase dramatically in both developed and developing countries in the coming decades, the medical, social, and financial impact of sarcopenia and its effect on function are of growing importance. There is a pressing need to better understand the biologic mechanisms involved in sarcopenia to promote the development of new therapeutic approaches. This chapter will provide an introduction to the basic biology of sarcopenia and to the study of sarcopenia in clinical research, experimental animals, and cell-based systems.

Biology of Aging Muscle

CHANGES IN MUSCLE STRUCTURE

During human aging there is a loss of both muscle mass and cross-sectional area that averages 25 to 40% between ages 20 to 80 years (Lexell, 1995). Consistent changes have been seen regardless of technique as measurements of total body potassium, creatinine excretion, CT scans, MRI scans, ultrasound images, and anatomic dissection (see later for details on techniques) have shown consistent and reproducible declines in muscle mass (Lexell, 1995). The loss in muscle mass is due to two factors: the loss of total muscle fiber number and the reduction in the size of specific fibers. Human muscle consists of type I slow-twitch and type II fast-twitch fibers. Type I fibers are involved in endurance activities and generate most of their energy from aerobic metabolism. In contrast, type II fibers provide explosive muscle strength during periods of exercise or intense activity with energy being produced from anaerobic glycolysis. The numbers of both types of fibers in a given muscle decline with age, with losses of up to 60 to 70% of fibers seen (Lexell, 1995). Additionally, selective declines in type II fiber volume also occur during aging (Lexell, 1995). These two changes begin as early as the late 20s and appear to accelerate after age 50 (Lexell, 1995).

GENE EXPRESSION CHANGES

Changes in muscle gene expression have been studied via the use of serial analysis of gene expression (SAGE) and both cDNA and oligonucleotide-based microarrays (Giresi *et al.*, 2005; Welle *et al.*, 2000). Both of these techniques examine changes in the transcript abundance of specific genes between groups and use statistical techniques to then identify significant differences. Human studies have examined changes in gene expression between young individuals and older individuals using muscle biopsy specimens (Giresi *et al.*, 2005; Welle *et al.*, 2000). Experimental animals, such as mice and rhesus monkeys, also have been used for comparisons. The inclusion of these animals has allowed the comparison of normal aged animals with similarly aged animals with slowed aging due to dietary restriction (Kayo *et al.*, 2001; Welle *et al.*, 2001).

Numerous gene expression differences have been seen. Several studies have noted a decrease in old age of genes involved in biochemical pathways involved in energy generation such as oxidative phosphorylation and glycolysis (Giresi *et al.*, 2005; Kayo *et al.*, 2001; Welle *et al.*, 2000). Genes involved in heat shock responses, inflammation, and DNA damage repair also tend to be increased (Kayo *et al.*, 2001; Welle *et al.*, 2001). Changes in extracellular matrix gene expression have been noted, with specific changes in collagen gene expression (Kayo *et al.*, 2001; Welle *et al.*, 2001). These studies have provided new avenues for future investigation.

CHANGES IN CONTRACTILE PROTEINS

Changes in muscle protein synthesis and turnover could account for at least part of the loss of muscle mass and strength during aging. Although studies have suggested that there are no changes in overall muscle synthesis, there seem to be selective changes in specific muscle proteins (Greenlund and Nair, 2003; Volpi *et al.*, 2004). For example, the rates of myosin heavy chain isoform (MHC) IIa and IIx synthesis have been shown to decrease in older subjects, which is a change probably due to a decline in mRNA levels (Greenlund and Nair, 2003). The exact cause of this change is unknown but could reflect the loss of type II muscle fibers during aging (Lexell, 1995). Furthermore, proteomic studies have demonstrated declines in myosin light chain and actin protein levels (Piec *et al.*, 2005). There is also a decline in protein turnover in aging muscle due to declines in proteasome function that leads to the accumulation of proteins with damage such as oxidation. These damaged proteins may show impaired contractile function.

METABOLIC CHANGES

Both enzymatic, proteomic, and gene expression studies (see earlier) have suggested declines in glycolytic and glycogenolytic enzymatic activities, as well as decreases in enzymes involved in citric acid cycle and oxidative phosphorylation (Carmeli *et al.*, 2002; Giresi *et al.*, 2005; Piec *et al.*, 2005). Accompanying the decreases in the mitochondrial enzymes involved in citric acid cycle and electron transport is an overall decrease in mitochondrial protein synthesis. The net effect of the decline in mitochondrial enzyme levels is an age-related decline in the mitochondrial ATP production rate and a decline in ATP stores (Short *et al.*, 2005). The decline in mitochondrial function correlates with the decline in maximal aerobic capacity (VO_2 max) during exercise.

An area of uncertainty is the extent to which the observed metabolic changes relate to the aging of muscle versus the physical inactivity frequently seen in older people (Russ and Kent-Braun, 2004). Carefully conducted studies that correct for the activity level of the young and older participants have suggested that the metabolic changes during aging are fairly minimal with regard to *in vitro* or *in vivo* oxidative capacity of muscle. Additionally, physical activity has been shown to be associated with higher levels of mitochondrial proteins involved in electron transport and the citric acid cycle (Russ and Kent-Braun 2004; Greenlund and Nair, 2003).

SATELLITE CELL CHANGES

Vertebrate muscles contain satellite cells that are quiescent myoblasts that have the ability to proliferate, differentiate, and fuse together to form new muscle fibers. The satellite cells are found between muscle fibers and its surrounding basal lamina (Carlson 1995). One theory of sarcopenia is that either the depletion or impairment of satellite cells with age produces the loss of muscle fibers once the remaining satellite cells are unable to repair normal muscle damage (Edstrom and Ulfhake, 2005). Animal studies support this theory as both declines in satellite cell number and replicative potential decline with aging. Interestingly, the slow-twitch type I muscle fibers, which are better preserved in aging muscle, have a greater number of satellite cells than the fast-twitch type II fibers (Carlson, 1995).

Human Studies

Although sarcopenia appears to be a universal phenomenon during aging, ultimately the importance is its impact on older people. Consequently, human studies have and will continue to play important roles in elucidating the consequences of sarcopenia on strength, functioning, and mortality. Additionally, these clinical studies have provided insights into the role nutrition, endocrine changes, lifestyle factors, and comorbid disease could play in the development of sarcopenia. These insights often have provided starting points for subsequent cell culture and animal experiments. Also, the characterization of the clinical effects of sarcopenia provides a framework to ultimately test the effects of treatments developed through human studies or model systems. As a result of the importance of human studies, we will begin with a review of methods used in patient-oriented sarcopenia research.

METHODS OF MUSCLE MEASUREMENT

Multiple methods of measuring the effects of sarcopenia are used in clinical studies. The use of multiple methods reflects the lack of a standard definition of sarcopenia, the development of new techniques during the last 25 years that improve upon older techniques, and the lack of a technique that is clearly superior to the others. Beyond the purely technical aspects of measuring sarcopenia is the unresolved question of what is the most important level of measurement. Specifically, is motor performance, muscle strength, muscle mass, or muscle cross-sectional area actually the most relevant for study? Though motor performance is likely the most important from a clinical perspective, it is probably the least amenable to clinical study given potential confounding by cognition, medications, comorbid illnesses, and motivation. Fortunately, muscle mass and muscle cross-sectional area show relatively good linkage so measurement of one provides information about the other. This leaves the debate to muscle mass versus strength as the most relevant measure. Studies have shown that declines in muscle cross-sectional area account for much, but clearly not all, of the declines in strength (Goodpaster *et al.*, 2001). This suggests simply measuring muscle mass or cross-sectional area is a valid approach, but misses some of the details that assessing strength instead would provide.

^{40}K measurement

Potassium is the predominant intracellular cation, and approximately 60% of total body potassium is concentrated in skeletal muscle (Heymsfield *et al.*, 1995). Consequently, whole-body counting for naturally occurring ^{40}K can be used to quantify total body potassium and hence estimate muscle mass. This method was expanded by the inclusion of total body nitrogen, as measured by prompt-γ neutron activation analysis, and equations developed that allowed approximation of skeletal and nonskeletal muscle mass. This technique has been largely supplanted by newer techniques that more directly measure skeletal and more specifically appendicular muscle mass (see Table 81.1).

TABLE 81.1
Comparison of muscle mass measurement techniques

Technique	Advantages	Disadvantages
^{40}K Measurement	Well validated	Indirect measurement of muscle mass
Measurement of Muscle Metabolites	Sensitive to small changes	Requires special diet High coefficient of variability
Anthropometric Measurements	No specialized equipment Inexpensive Portable	Insensitive Poor Accuracy
Four Compartment Models	Well studied	Overestimates Muscle Mass Laborious
DEXA	Less expensive equipment Accurate Reproducible	Overestimates Muscle Mass Needs trained operator Radiation Exposure
Ultrasound	Accurate Portable Less expensive equipment	Needs trained operator
CT scan	Very Accurate Reproducible Sensitive to small changes	Expensive Equipment Needs trained operator Radiation Exposure
MRI	Very Accurate No Radiation Exposure Reproducible Sensitive to small changes	Expensive Equipment Needs trained operator
Bioelectric Impedance	Accurate Portable Less expensive equipment	Less Well Studied

Measurement of muscle metabolites

Muscle produces creatinine and 3-methylhistidine, which are excreted in the urine, allowing measurement via timed urine collection (Heymsfield *et al.*, 1995; Lukaski, 1997). Creatinine is largely derived from creatine in muscle by nonenzymatic hydrolysis. Human studies indicate that one gram of creatinine is derived from 18 to 20 kilograms of muscle. However, the ratio can change depending on age, physical activity, sex, metabolic state, and contribution of creatinine from nonskeletal muscle sources (Lukaski, 1997). 3-methylhistidine is produced in skeletal muscle via the posttranslational modification of specific histidine residues in myofibrils. During routine muscle protein turnover, the liberated 3-methylhistidine is neither metabolized or recycled into new proteins, but instead excreted in the urine. Additionally, small but significant amounts of 3-methylhistidine also are derived from nonskeletal muscle, resulting in about 75% of 3-methylhistidine being of muscle origin. Both creatine and 3-methylhistidine also can be ingested in the diet, making accurate collections dependent on following a meat and creatine-free diet. The need to follow a special diet and to collect a timed urine collection for measurement has greatly limited the development and application of this technique (see Table 81.1) (Lukaski, 1997).

However, the use of creatinine excretion has been found to be helpful for demonstrating the loss of muscle mass during aging in a comparison study with DEXA (Proctor *et al.*, 1999). When used in a carefully controlled clinical research center setting using a defined meat-free diet, comparison with DEXA results in subjects of increasing age suggested that creatinine excretion was more sensitive than DEXA for demonstrating declines in muscle mass. Creatinine excretion also demonstrated the highest variability in a test-retest comparison with a coefficient of variation of 17.7%. Together these results suggest that creatinine excretion can be a useful technique that still shows significant variability of results even when used in a carefully controlled setting (Proctor *et al.*, 1999). This may limit its use in a community-based setting.

Anthropometric measurements

Anthropometric measurements use extremity circumference measurements and skin-fold thickness measurements to estimate regional and whole-body muscle mass (Heymsfield *et al.*, 1995; Lukaski, 1997). This technique has the advantage of not requiring any specialized training or equipment to make accurate measurements (see Table 81.1). For example, the measurement process can easily be included in an initial screening exam for a clinical trial and can be performed reliably in both medical and home settings. A variety of equations for estimation of total muscle cross-sectional area for the upper arm and thigh have been developed with derivation and validation provided from data collected by CT or MRI (Heymsfield *et al.*, 1995; Lukaski, 1997). In addition, similar equations for the estimation of the cross-sectional area of specific muscle groups, such as the quadriceps and hamstrings, have been developed and validated using MRI as a reference (Housh *et al.*, 1995). With young subjects, the equations have a small but significant error compared with the reference, but in older subjects the equations are significantly less accurate and can overestimate muscle mass by up to 41.5% (Baumgartner *et al.*, 1992; Housh *et al.*, 1995). Additionally, concerns have been raised as to whether anthropometric measurements show sufficient sensitivity to measure small but important differences in muscle cross-sectional area that would occur after interventions such as physical training (Housh *et al.*, 1995). Consequently, although anthropometric measurements are easy to obtain and do not require specialized equipment or training for measurement, concerns about the accuracy of measurement, especially in older patients, limit the use of this technique in sarcopenia research.

Four-compartment models

Fat-free body mass can be used to estimate skeletal muscle mass since skeletal muscle comprises roughly 49% of fat-free body mass (Heymsfield *et al.*, 1995). One way of measuring fat-free body mass is through a four-compartment body mass model (see Table 81.1). The four-compartment model breaks body mass into fat mass, fat-free mass (consisting of muscle and connective tissue), body water, and mineral mass (consisting of bone) (Lohman and Going, 1993). Multiple techniques have been developed to measure each component, but often underwater weighing, deuterium dilution, and DEXA (see next) are used (Heymsfield *et al.*, 1995; Lohman and Going, 1993). The performance of measurements using fat-free mass has been examined in cross-sectional studies with evidence that use of the fat-free mass may overestimate muscle mass compared to other techniques, perhaps due to increases in connective tissue or total body water (Kyle *et al.*, 2001; Proctor *et al.*, 1999). The four-compartment model also suffers from being somewhat laborious as multiple measurements requiring specialized equipment are needed for each subject.

DEXA

Dual-energy X-ray absorptiometry uses an X-ray source to produce photons of two different energies, which are attenuated as they pass through the tissues of the subject. The X-ray beam is attenuated depending upon the composition of the intervening tissue, with bone producing the strongest attenuation and fat the least attenuation (Heymsfield *et al.*, 1995). Data derived from DEXA measurements can be used in two main ways. First, the measurements can be used as part of a four-component model to determine fat-free mass (Heymsfield *et al.*, 1995). From this, muscle mass can be estimated as 49% of the fat-free mass. This approach may suffer from the same overestimation of muscle mass as noted for four-component models due to possible changes in the fat-free mass composition (Proctor *et al.*, 1999). Alternatively, DEXA measurements can be focused on the extremities that comprise approximately 75% of total muscle mass (Heymsfield *et al.*, 1995). Measuring extremities also carries the advantage that the lean mass of the extremities largely consists of skeletal muscle and this muscle is most important for daily activities including ambulation (see Table 81.1) (Heymsfield *et al.*, 1995). DEXA measurements of extremity muscle mass have shown good correlation with those measured by CT scanning, though there does appear to be a slight overestimation of muscle mass (Visser *et al.*, 1999; Heymsfield *et al.*, 1995).

DEXA is widely used in sarcopenia research. The technique has been shown to have excellent reproducibility and interobserver variability (Visser *et al.*, 1999). The main drawbacks to the technique are the need for specialized costly equipment, though much less expensive than CT or MRI, as well as an experienced operator. There is also a small radiation exposure associated with DEXA measurements.

Ultrasound

Ultrasound uses sound waves to image and measure tissues. The obtained data can be used with anthropometric equations in an analogous fashion to skin-fold and circumference data (Heymsfield *et al.*, 1995). More recently, improved ultrasound equipment has allowed the technique to be used directly for measurement of muscle cross-sectional area in a fashion analogous to CT or MRI (see Table 81.1) (Reeves *et al.*, 2004). The cross-sectional areas measured by ultrasound compare favorably to those obtained from MRI and show consistent test-retest reproducibility (Reeves *et al.*, 2004). Ultrasound offers the advantage of lower cost when compared with MRI and CT as well as portability.

CT scan

Computerized tomography (CT) scanning uses collimated X-ray beams and computer manipulation to provide high-resolution images of subjects. CT provides accurate measurements of muscle cross-sectional area and muscle volume (Heymsfield *et al.*, 1995; Lukaski, 1997). The muscle volume can readily be converted to muscle weight as the density of muscle at body temperature is 1.04 grams per cubic centimeter (Heymsfield *et al.*, 1995). CT scanning can be used to assess either total body or extremity muscle mass (see Table 81.1). The muscle masses obtained by CT have been validated through work using cadaver limbs for comparison with good agreement between CT results and anatomic dissection (Heymsfield *et al.*, 1995). The technique has adequate sensitivity to detect even changes in muscle area seen in response to resistive exercise, which are on the order of 8 to 9% (Fiatarone *et al.*, 1990). Additionally, studies in older subjects have noted that there are changes in muscle composition with aging that can be detected via CT and are correlated with declines in strength independent of decreases in muscle mass (Goodpaster *et al.*, 2001). Consequently, CT scanning has become widely used in clinical sarcopenia research.

The drawbacks of CT are the expense of CT equipment and the need for a trained operator to produce accurate scans. The size of the equipment requires that subjects be able to come to the hospital where the CT scanner is housed. Also, due to the radiation exposure involved in CT scanning, there has been a trend toward the use of CT only on extremities (Heymsfield *et al.*, 1995).

MRI

Magnetic resonance imaging (MRI) involves the use of radio-frequency energy and magnetic fields to provide high-resolution three-dimensional images of subjects. Similar to CT scanning, MRI provides accurate measurements of muscle area and muscle volume (Heymsfield *et al.*, 1995; Lukaski, 1997). MRI also demonstrates adequate sensitivity to detect small changes in muscle mass in response to resistive exercise (Ross *et al.*, 1995). As a result, MRI is also commonly used in clinical sarcopenia research. It additionally carries the advantage of not involving radiation exposure (see Table 81.1).

The drawbacks of MRI are the size and expense of the required equipment. A trained operator is also required to operate the scanner. Additional limitation, especially in research involving older subjects, is that the strong magnetic field involved limits the use of MRI in subjects who have pacemakers, certain surgical clips, and certain metallic implants.

Bioelectric impedance

Bioelectric impedance (BI) involves measuring the conductance of an electric current in the limb of a subject to estimate muscle mass. The technique relies upon the differing electric conducting properties of muscle, fat, and bone with muscle being the best conductor and bone the worst. Comparison of bioelectric impedance with measurements made by either CT scan or DEXA has shown good correlation with these techniques (see Table 81.1). BI requires the use of specialized equipment, but the required equipment is lower in cost and much more portable when compared to techniques like CT and MRI. It is not known if BI demonstrates sufficient sensitivity to measure small changes in muscle mass such as in response to resistive training. BI also has been less extensively studied and used in human sarcopenia studies.

STRENGTH ASSESSMENT

In many ways strength assessment represents the gold standard of sarcopenia research as it is the loss of strength and the consequences of this loss of strength that make sarcopenia an important topic of study. Most sarcopenia studies include measures of strength to test the effects of declines in muscle mass, effects of changes in muscle composition, or effects of specific treatments on muscle strength.

Strength is often assessed via measurement of the force of static or dynamic muscle contractions. Static muscle contractions are muscle contractions where the force is exerted on a stationary object and the involved joints do not move during the contraction. Isometric contractions are the most widely used means of measuring static muscle strength due to the safety and ease of isometric testing as well as the lower cost of equipment (Hunter *et al.*, 1998). A variety of reliable and portable equipment, such as handgrip dynamometers, are available for testing.

Despite the ease of static testing, dynamic strength testing may be more relevant as most daily activities, such as walking, climbing stairs, and doing housework, are dynamic tasks (Hunter *et al.*, 1998). A dynamic muscle contraction is a muscle contraction where the involved joints move while under a resistive load. Dynamic strength can be measured either via the one repetition maximum (1RM) approach or with a isokinetic dynamometer. The 1RM approach involves finding the heaviest weight that can be lifted through a complete range of motion. This can be accomplished easily by using commonly available gym weight machines (Hunter *et al.*, 1998). Concerns have been raised about the safety of this approach especially in older subjects, but in carefully supervised settings, 1RM testing has been performed safely (Fiatarone *et al.*, 1994; Fiatarone *et al.*, 1990). Isokinetic dynamometers allow strength to be measured while the limb or joint moves at a defined speed. Most dynamometers are amenable to computer monitoring, so force data can be measured over the entire range of movement. Use of a dynamometer also has a safety advantage over the 1RM method as both the speed of movement and range of motion can be controlled (Hunter *et al.*, 1998). A significant limitation of dynamometers is the cost of the equipment.

An important concern during strength testing is to be sure that differences in strength observed is due to differences in muscle contractile properties instead of differences in muscle activation. When older subjects, or inactive younger subjects, are first tested for strength, there is often incomplete recruitment or suboptimal firing of motor units (Hunter *et al.*, 1998). Consequently, repeated testing less than a week later can show a significant improvement due to improvements in muscle motor unit activation as opposed to muscle hypertrophy (Hunter *et al.*, 1998). This issue can be addressed by providing a practice session first and then performing the actual strength testing at a later second session. These retest measures have been shown to be reliable for both younger and older people (Hunter *et al.*, 1998). A more rigorous approach is to use pulses of electrical stimulation during an isometric contraction that is believed to be maximal. The stimulation can either be delivered via electrodes over the motor nerve or the muscle itself. If the isometric contraction is maximal, then delivering the stimulus should not increase the force of contraction, but submaximal contractions are augmented by the pulses. The benefit of this approach is to provide feedback to both the observer and subject regarding the degree of muscle activation. Electrical stimulation also has been utilized in the study of dynamic muscle contractions through the use of tetanic stimuli (Hunter *et al.*, 1998).

MUSCLE BIOPSY

The use of percutaneous muscle biopsy represents one of the few ways in which the effects of aging on human muscles can be studied at the biochemical, molecular, or cellular level. A single biopsy can yield 25 to 75 milligrams of tissue, which can then be analyzed in multiple ways including via microscopy or biochemical assays (Coggan, 1995).

Muscle biopsy involves the use of a biopsy needle, such as the one developed by Bergström, which consists of a closed hollow cylinder with a pointed tip (Coggan, 1995). A cylindrical cutting blade fits inside the first cylinder and is responsible for obtaining the biopsy. An opening a few centimeters from the tip in the outer cylinder serves as the location where the actual biopsy is taken since tissue can bulge into the center of the cylinder through the opening when the blade is removed. Reinsertion of the blade then cuts the protruding tissue and obtains the biopsy.

Technically, biopsies are performed on patients by first injecting local anesthetic into the skin and fascia over the muscle of interest. The vastus lateralis is the most commonly used muscle, but the biceps, tibialis anterior, and gastrocnemius have also been used (Coggan, 1995). Following anesthesia, a scalpel is used to make a small incision in the skin and the needle is then inserted into the muscle belly. During the insertion of the needle, the cutting blade is placed inside to occlude the opening in the needle. Once placed, the blade is removed and then reinserted to obtain the biopsy. After removal of the needle, a solid rod is inserted into the center of the blade cylinder to eject the obtained tissue. Post biopsy, pressure is held at the side for 30 minutes to minimize bleeding, and the incision is closed with a suture or tape dressing like a Steri-strip. The biopsy samples are either fixed and embedded if the ultimate goal is either light or electron microscopy, or frozen if the ultimate goal is biochemical or functional analysis.

The risks of biopsy include infection and intramuscular hematoma, which are both low when the biopsy is performed in sterile fashion and pressure is held for adequate time (Coggan, 1995). For most patients the biopsy produces only mild discomfort, consisting of a pressure or cramp-like sensation when the needle is inserted into the muscle and a few days of muscle soreness after the biopsy.

The biopsy samples have a wide variety of uses, which include analysis of morphology, assessment of metabolism, analysis of gene or protein expression, culture of satellite cells, and evaluation of contractile properties of muscle fibers (Coggan, 1995; Peterson, 1995). Morphologic analysis can include examination of the numbers and size of type I and type II fibers or the examination of specific cellular organelles like the contractile apparatus by either light or electron microscopy. Metabolic assessment can involve the measurement of specific enzyme activities, the measurement of glucose, triglyceride, and protein levels, the measurement of intermediate metabolite levels, or the measurement of cellular energy stores like ATP or phosphocreatine. Gene or protein expression can be analyzed at the single gene or protein levels through use of Northern or Western blotting. Biopsy samples would also be amenable to modern genomic or proteome techniques like microarray or 2D gel electrophoresis to identify differentially expressed genes (Roth *et al.*, 2002; van den Heuvel *et al.*, 2003). Biopsy samples also can serve as a source for human satellite cell myoblasts for use in cell culture experiments, as discussed in a later section (Peterson, 1995). Finally, the contractile properties of single fibers from biopsy samples can be functionally assessed by the measurement of maximal force or shortening velocity (Coggan, 1995).

An important limitation of muscle biopsy is the observed sample-to-sample variation seen even in biopsies taken from the same muscle in the same patient (Coggan, 1995). The variation is probably due to differences between the areas of the muscle sampled by individual biopsies. For example, 10 to 20% variation has been observed in measures of fiber type or muscle fiber area. Ways to overcome this limitation are either to take two or more biopsies at the same time to obtain a more accurate measurement for an individual, or, if the goal of a study is to compare two or more groups at a population level, then increasing the number of subjects would also be an effective way to cope with the variability of individual biopsies.

CLINICAL COHORTS

A major hurdle involved in patient-oriented research in general is the effort and expense involved in recruiting a well-characterized cohort. Consequently, existing cohorts can be a fast and convenient way to test a new hypothesis as patient data, blood samples, and DNA are already collected and allow retrospective study.

Health ABC Study

The Health ABC Study was specifically designed to investigate connections between changes in body composition and strength, functioning, and mortality. The study involves 3,075 nondisabled men and women aged 70 to 79 years of age (mean 73.6 years) who reside in Pittsburgh, PA or Memphis, TN, who were recruited primarily from a random sample of Medicare-eligible adults (Goodpaster *et al.*, 2001). Overall the cohort is 48.5% male and 58.3% white. Exclusion criteria were use of assistive devices for ambulation, self-reported difficulties with activities of daily living, self-reported difficulty walking a quarter-mile or climbing 10 stairs, self-reported life-threatening cancer, plans to leave the study area within three years, or participation in clinical trials involving medications or diet/exercise modifications. Muscle mass was measured for all participants with the use of dual-energy X-ray absorptiometry (DEXA), and muscle area was measured by axial CT scans of the mid-thigh. For 2,627 participants isokinetic strength of the knee extensors was measured by determining the maximum torque produced with an isokinetic dynamometer.

Women's Health and Aging Study

The Women's Health and Aging Study I was designed to study the impact of chronic and new illnesses on the health and functioning of a group of moderately to severely disabled older women (Kasper *et al.*, 1999). The study involves 1,002 women divided into three groups based upon age, with 398 women aged 65 to 74 years, 306 women aged 75 to 84 years, and 298 women older than 85 years of age. An important inclusion criteria is that participants had to demonstrate impairments in two domains of function including upper extremity (i.e., raising arms over head, using fingers to grasp/handle, or lifting/carrying objects weighing 10 pounds), mobility/exercise tolerance (i.e., walking a quarter-mile, walking up 10 steps without resting, getting in and out of bed or chairs, or doing heavy housework), higher functioning (i.e., using the telephone, doing light housework, preparing meals, or shopping for personal items), or basic self-care (i.e., bathing or showering, dressing, eating, or using the toilet). Exclusions included a Folstein Mini-Mental Status Exam (MMSE) score less than 18 or inability to participate in an interview. For participants, muscle area was estimated by use of anthropometric measures (Cappola *et al.*, 2001). Muscle strength was measured in terms of grip strength using a JAMAR hand-held dynamometer, knee extensor (quadriceps) using a Nicholas Manual Muscle Tester dynamometer, and hip flexor (iliopsoas) using a Nicholas Manual Muscle Tester dynamometer. Testing was performed by a trained nurse using a standardized protocol. Performance data was also collected on participants, including time required to complete a four-meter walking course and to stand from a chair with arms folded five times. Blood samples were collected from most participants.

A later companion study, the Women's Health and Aging Study II, was designed to study women aged 70 to 79 years who represented the least disabled women in the community (Fried *et al.*, 2000). Recruitment was carried out in a similar fashion to WHAS I from a random sample drawn from the Baltimore area, except that women needed to have a MMSE score greater than 24 and could have impairment in at most one domain of functioning as defined earlier. A total of 436 women were enrolled. Similar data was collected on participants with regard to muscle area, strength, and physical performance as for the WHAS I study (Cappola *et al.*, 2001).

Framingham Heart Study

The Framingham Heart Study began in 1948 with 5,209 men and women who reside in the Framingham, MA area and are examined biennially. The study originally was designed to study clinical risk factors for heart disease, but information on body composition have been collected as well (Roubenoff *et al.*, 2003). Specifically, fat-free body mass was measured via the use of bioelectric impedance. It is important to note that neither muscle area via MRI or CT nor muscle strength were measured in participants.

Longitudinal Aging Study Amsterdam

The Longitudinal Aging Study Amsterdam is a prospective study of a random sample of people 55 to 85 years old drawn from 11 municipalities in three geographic areas in the west, northeast, and south of the Netherlands (Visser *et al.*, 2003). Initially 3,107 participants were enrolled. Data was collected in three interviews and medical exams occurring in 1992 to 1993, 1995 to 1996, and 1998 to 1999. Morning fasting blood samples were collected as part of the study. Grip strength was tested on almost all participants by means of a grip strength dynamometer, and muscle mass was measured via dual-energy X-ray absorptiometry (DEXA) on a subset of patients.

The MINOS Study

The MINOS Study was started in 1995 as a prospective study of osteoporosis and its determinants in men (Szulc *et al.*, 2000). The participants are 840 men between 45 and 85 years of age who live in Montceau les Mines, France, which is a town of 21,000 inhabitants near Lyon.

Muscle mass was measured by DEXA, and blood samples were collected from participants.

GENETIC EPIDEMIOLOGY

Studies of muscle biology, including mechanisms of development, atrophy, and hypertrophy, from cell and animal models have provided information about a large number of genes that may have an additional role in sarcopenia during aging. One way to study the roles of such genes in sarcopenia is to use genetic epidemiology (Mehrian-Shai and Reichardt, 2004). Genetic epidemiology studies the association of naturally occurring alleles of genes with the extent or rate of sarcopenia in a clinical cohort. Each allele is assessed as a risk factor or protective factor for the development of sarcopenia in the context of other risk factors as part of a multivariate model. A frequently used technique is to identify single-nucleotide polymorphisms (SNPs) in genes of interest, which are naturally occurring variants where a single base-pair is altered. Advances in genotyping techniques have made the use of multiple SNPs per gene and larger population sizes feasible from a technical and financial perspective. The SNPs are treated as alleles for the purpose of analysis. The functional role of important SNPs can later be evaluated in biochemical, cell, or animal models.

Cell Culture Models

Although intact muscles cannot be grown in culture for sufficient time to develop an *ex vivo* model of sarcopenia, there is a role for cell culture in sarcopenia research (Peterson, 1995). Vertebrate muscles contain satellite cells that are quiescent myoblasts with the ability to proliferate, differentiate, and fuse together to form new muscle fibers. These new muscle fibers are able to replace damaged fibers in muscles. One theory of sarcopenia is that either the depletion or impairment of satellite cells with age produces the loss of muscle fibers once the remaining satellite cells are unable to repair normal muscle damage (Edstrom and Ulfhake, 2005).

Satellite cells can be isolated either from human donors or experimental animals and grown in culture (Peterson, 1995). The *ex vivo* culture of satellite cells is valuable for four reasons. First, isolated cells can be studied for replicative potential. In both humans and rats, the doubling capacity of satellite cells has been shown to decrease dramatically from youth to middle age with even further declines seen in old age. Second, satellite cell differentiation and fusion can be studied in culture. Cells isolated from older donors show impairments in the ability to differentiate and fuse to form myotubes compared to cells from young donors. Unfortunately, satellite cells in culture complete only the early steps in differentiation and fusion, as indicated by the failure to transition from the expression of fetal and neonatal myosin heavy chain isoforms to the adult isoforms. This suggests that culture alone has a limited role in the study of the differentiation and fusion steps. However, the use of culture along with reimplantation into experimental animals may overcome this limitation, as discussed further, later. Third, cultures of satellite cells can be used to study changes in gene expression with age. Microarray experiments have been performed using satellite cells isolated from animals of increasing age to analyze global changes in gene expression (Beggs *et al.*, 2004). Finally, culture can be used as a means of modifying satellite cells from experimental animals via viral transfection, followed by reimplantation into either wild-type or transgenic animals. These modified satellite cells have been shown to be able to proliferate and differentiate *in vivo* and form chimeric muscles (Rando and Blau, 1994). The *ex vivo* modification allows both marking of the cells with a marker like β-galactosidase along with genetic modification with the over-expression of normal or mutated proteins or the reduction in gene expression via RNA inhibition (RNAi). The value of this procedure is the ability to study the *in vivo* role of genes identified through experiments such as microarray.

Animal Models

Human studies can provide insights into the clinical consequences and risk factors for sarcopenia and can suggest mechanisms involved in sarcopenia, but they have important limitations. Experimental animals often have significantly shorter life spans than people, so longitudinal studies can be performed over days, weeks, or months instead of the decades involved in human studies. Also, animals can have controlled environments and an essentially identical genetic background between groups. These properties make animal studies faster and more carefully controlled than clinical studies (Cartee, 1995).

Most experimental animals are amenable to types of experiments that are not possible with people. An important insight into the biology of aging and aging associated changes has been provided by dietary restriction. This intervention involves limiting daily caloric intake and results in an up to 50% increase in overall lifespan, along with a slowing of phenotypic signs of aging. Remarkably, dietary restriction has comparable effects on a large number of laboratory animals. Dietary restriction is extremely difficult for people to follow, but is easily instituted in a laboratory setting where access to food can be readily controlled. The genetics of experimental animals can be readily manipulated either via genetic crosses or the construction of transgenic animals. Transgenic animals that either lack specific genes, carry mutated versions of specific genes, or misexpress specific genes can be constructed and used for study. Experimental preclinical medications are easily tested in animals, and animal studies provide a critical precursor to eventual clinical study of successful therapies.

This section will review the use of the two most commonly used animal models: mice and rats. A limitation of these animals is the two- to three-year life span seen under laboratory conditions. Consequently, there is a need for an animal with a shorter life span. As a result the section will end with a discussion of the nematode *Caenorhabditis elegans*, which has a two- to three-week life span and develops significant sarcopenia during normal aging.

RODENTS

The effects of aging on muscle have been studied in both rats and mice. These animals offer the benefits of being small and easy to maintain in a laboratory environment, being familiar to many in the scientific community, having a growing number of identified genetic mutations, and having easily implemented transgenic technology.

Age-related muscle changes

Both rats and mice show a decline in muscle mass during aging (Cartee, 1995). In rats this decline in muscle mass is due to both declines in muscle fiber number and fiber cross-sectional area. The declines in fiber number are less pronounced, but the declines in fiber cross-sectional areas are comparable to those seen in humans (Cartee, 1995). As seen in humans, the decline in fiber cross-sectional area is due predominantly to atrophy of type II muscle fibers. Interestingly, several muscles in the rat do not experience declines in muscle mass: the adductor longus, epitrochlearis, and flexor digitorum longus. Both epitrochlearis and flexor digitorum longus have a comparable number of type II fibers compared to the gastrocnemius muscle, roughly 75%, that undergoes significant atrophy during aging. The reason for these differential susceptibilities to the effects of age on muscle is not known, but provides the advantage of having internal aged controls that can be used in studies. Mice also show declines in muscle mass, but this is due more to declines in cross-sectional area than declines in fiber number. However, the relative contributions of type I and type II fiber atrophy have not been well studied (Cartee, 1995).

Viral/transfection of muscles

One approach to test the function of genes or mark specific cells for later histological study is to use transfection of foreign DNA transgenes. The transgene can consist of either specific genes of interest or marker genes like *E. coli* beta-galactosidase or GFP (green fluorescent protein) that can be easily detected on tissue sections. Transgenes are assembled in bacterial plasmids using standard recombinant DNA techniques, and the transgene consists of a promoter to direct expression in the muscle cell and a poly-adenylation sequence flanking the gene of interest or marker gene (see Figure 81.3).

Promoters can consist of muscle-specific promoters, such as the muscle creatinine kinase promoter; or strong viral promoters, such as the cytomegalovirus (CMV) promoter, which offer high expression levels but are not muscle specific. Marker genes can be obtained from commercial sources or freely available plasmids. Genes of interest can be obtained as cDNA from commercial clone libraries or be produced from cells by techniques such as polymerase chain reaction (PCR).

Promoter	Gene	AAAA

Figure 81.3 Diagram of a transgene. Transgenes consist of a promoter sequence, a gene, and a polyadenylation sequence. The promoter controls the expression pattern of the gene and can either be a muscle-specific promoter or derived from a viral promoter. The gene can either be a mammalian gene of interest or a reporter gene, such as GFP or β-galactosidase, which serves to mark transfected cells. The polyadenylation sequence provides the proper modification of the end of the produced RNA transcript needed for expression in muscle cells.

Transfection can be performed either in cell culture or in live animals. For cell culture, transfection can be performed by isolating satellite cells from mice and transfecting them *in vitro* using a retroviral vector (Rando and Blau, 1994). Transfected cells are identified and expanded in cell culture before being injected into recipient mice (Rando and Blau, 1994). These injected cells can differentiate and join existing muscles. This approach is well suited for studying the biology and function of satellite cells in mice.

For live animals, intact muscles can be transfected *in vivo* either with the use of electroporation or viral infection. Electroporation uses electric pulses to permeabilize muscle fibers and thus facilitate the entry of foreign DNA (Mir *et al.*, 1999). The DNA is maintained as nuclear extrachromosomal DNA, which is transcriptionally active for long periods of time. This approach uses transgenes easily produced by standard molecular biology techniques but does require the use of electroporation equipment to deliver the electric pulses. Viral infection uses specific viral vectors that can be packaged into viral particles in specialized packaging cell lines (Gregorevic *et al.*, 2004). Depending upon the viral vector, either transient or stable infection is possible. Transient infection produces transgene expression for a short period of time, which is dependent on the rate of viral clearance. Stable infection is durable due to integration of the transgene. The efficiency of infection is usually superior for viral vectors producing transient expression, but transient expression demonstrates decreasing efficiency with repeated use due to immunization of the animal.

Transgenic animals

The genomic DNA of both rats and mice can be modified through the construction of transgenic animals. Transgenic technology allows genes to be deleted (also referred to as a "knock-out") or modified (also referred to as a "knock-in") (see Figure 81.4).

The modified genes can have either changes to the amino acid sequence of the protein or changes to the

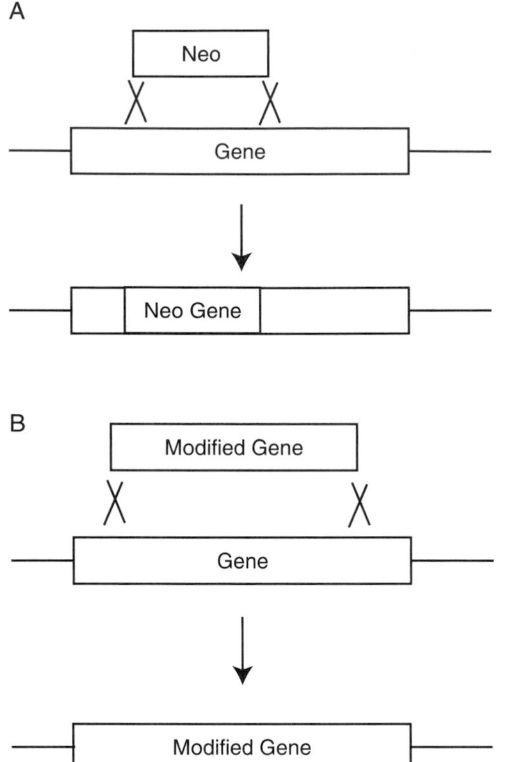

Figure 81.4 Examples of transgenic modifications. **A**. A "knock-out" consists of deleting the genomic copies of a gene of interest through homologous recombination. A targeting gene carrying a selectable marker, like neomycin resistance, is constructed with ends that have sequence homology to the genomic DNA. Inside the cell recombination between the ends of the targeting gene and the genomic DNA occurs with replacement of part of the gene with the targeting gene. This effectively destroys the function of the endogenous gene. **B**. A "knock-in" consists of replacing part of the genomic copy of a gene of interest with a modified version of the gene through homologous recombination. A targeting gene carrying the modified version of the gene is constructed with ends that have sequence homology to the genomic DNA. Inside the cell, recombination between the ends of the targeting gene and the genomic DNA occurs with replacement of part of the gene with the modified gene.

regulatory sequences responsible for when and where the gene is expressed. The power of transgenic technology lies in the ability to create animals, where all cells of the animal carry the manipulated DNA so an entire muscle, for example, experiences the effects of the manipulation. Transgenic animals stably transmit the modifications to offspring, providing an essentially unlimited source of animals for study. Additionally, different transgenic animals of the same species can be mated to test the genetic effects of combining two mutations together.

The construction of transgenic animals has been greatly facilitated by the development of transgenic core facilities at many academic institutions. These facilities provide the equipment and technical expertise needed to successfully produce animals, and these services usually are provided on a recharge basis. Consultation with the staff of a core facility, if available, is highly recommended to provide guidance for the experimental strategy.

Muscle atrophy research

One challenge involved in studying losses in muscle mass due to aging is the long time required to see the final effects, which can be up to 24 to 27 months (Cartee, 1995). An alternate approach that has been developed is to study muscle atrophy that occurs after hind-limb immobilization, hind-limb suspension, or muscle denervation (Cartee, 1995). These interventions result in profound muscle atrophy over a period of several weeks. Both aging and these interventions demonstrate muscle atrophy, but there are significant differences between the two. The magnitude of muscle mass loss following immobilization, suspension, or denervation is often much greater than the changes seen during aging. Additionally, both type I and type II fibers are affected, whereas type II fibers are preferentially affected by aging. However, research into muscle atrophy has contributed greatly to the understanding of the mechanisms involved in the regulation of muscle mass (McKinnell and Rudnicki, 2004). These studies provide new insights that can now be explored in the context of age-related sarcopenia.

C. elegans

C. elegans is a microscopic organism that has emerged during the last decade to be a powerful genetic system in which to study molecular and biochemical events involved in organismal aging. Under laboratory conditions, worms develop from egg to adult in three days, then reproduce during a four- to five-day reproductive period. The usual total adult life span is 12 to 18 days. Worms develop sarcopenia starting in the postreproductive period at age seven days (Herndon *et al.*, 2002). However, sarcopenia does not develop in a stereotyped fashion in worms of a given age; instead, sarcopenia develops at different ages within a cohort of genetically identical worms grown in culture together. Sarcopenia consists of a reduction in muscle cell size due to loss of cytoplasm and myofibrils. The remaining myofibrils also show a progressive increase in disorganization with loss of the densely packed parallel fibers seen in young worms. In contrast, the nervous system of the worm remains largely intact during aging (Herndon *et al.*, 2002).

The sarcopenia observed with aging has important functional consequences for the affected worms. Beginning at the same time that structural changes occur in the muscles, affected worms show a progressive decline in mobility (Herndon *et al.*, 2002). Young worms demonstrate high levels of activity, which consist of sinusoidal swimming along the surface of an agar plate. The aging worms progress from this initial spontaneous well-coordinated swimming to poorly coordinated swimming only evoked by direct stimulation, which involves touching the worm with a thin platinum wire. Eventually, mobility declines to only minimal movement of the head or tail evoked after similar direct stimulation. These declines in mobility appear irreversible during normal worm aging.

The development of sarcopenia in worms can be delayed by the *age-1* mutation, which also extends the worm lifespan by 60 to 100% (Herndon *et al.*, 2002). The *age-1* mutation affects a phosphatidylinositol-3-phosphate kinase (PI3 kinase), which acts along with the *daf-2* insulin/IGF-1 receptor and *daf-16* FOXO family DNA-binding protein to control aging and life span of the worm. The ability of a single mutation to alter the development of sarcopenia provides a ready intervention to study the mechanisms involved. Other potential applications of *C. elegans* in sarcopenia research involve exploiting the small size and short lifespan of worms to develop genetic or pharmacologic screens to find new genes and compounds that prevent or delay sarcopenia.

Study of Interventions

There is a pressing need for new treatments for sarcopenia. Ideas generated by clinical studies or experiments in animals can serve as the basis for the design of new treatments. Experimental animals will need to serve as the initial test system with the goal of translating safe and effective treatments to clinical studies. Many of these treatments will ultimately be destined for trials in potentially frail older people. The age and comorbid illnesses in these subjects result in unique challenges (Ferrucci *et al.*, 2004).

Conclusion

Sarcopenia is an unfortunate but normal aspect of the aging of the neuromuscular system of people and many other animal species. The loss of muscle strength that accompanies sarcopenia has important impacts on the health and functioning of people. Consequently there is a pressing need to better understand the clinical risk factors and cellular and molecular mechanisms involved to promote the development of new therapeutic approaches. Fortunately, the last several years have seen the development of new clinical and experimental resources to facilitate studies.

A current challenge in the field is to develop rigorous animal research in sarcopenia. Clinical research has provided support for a number of endocrine, nutritional, and inflammatory changes as being associated with the development of sarcopenia. As clinical studies based upon addressing some of these changes have shown only modest effects, there is a pressing need for animal research to prioritize the contribution that each change has on muscle mass and muscle strength. Further basic studies would then be able to elucidate the biochemical mechanisms underlying the effects with the ultimate goal of finding new targets for drug discovery. The development of the simple nematode *C. elegans* as a model system provides a new opportunity to study the development of sarcopenia at a genetic level.

Recommended Resources

WEB SITES

International Longevity Center—USA (http://www.ilcusa.org)

Official Web site for the International Longevity Center, which provides information on a large number of topics relating to geriatrics, including strategies to minimize the effects of sarcopenia through exercise.

FURTHER READING

Journal of Gerontology, Vol. 50 (1995).

An entire issue dedicated to reviews on sarcopenia from both the basic and clinical science perspectives.

ACKNOWLEDGMENTS

The author has no financial conflicts of interest to report. This work was supported by NIH grant NIH K08 Award 1K08AG024414.

REFERENCES

Baumgartner, R.N., Rhyne, R.L., Troup, C., Wayne, S., and Garry, P.J. (1992). Appendicular skeletal muscle areas assessed by magnetic resonance imaging in older persons. *J. Gerontol. 47*, M67–M72.

Beggs, M.L., Nagarajan, R., Taylor-Jones, J.M., Nolen, G., Macnicol, M., and Peterson, C.A. (2004). Alterations in the TGF beta signaling pathway in myogenic progenitors with age. *Aging Cell 3*, 353–361.

Blackman, M.R., Sorkin, J.D., Munzer, T., Bellantoni, M.F., Busby-Whitehead, J., Stevens, T.E. *et al.* (2002). Growth hormone and sex steroid administration in healthy aged women and men: A randomized controlled trial. *JAMA 288*, 2282–2292.

Cappola, A.R., Bandeen-Roche, K., Wand, G.S., Volpato, S., and Fried, L.P. (2001). Association of IGF-I levels with muscle strength and mobility in older women. *J. Clin. Endocrinol. Metab. 86*, 4139–4146.

Carlson, B.M. (1995). Factors influencing the repair and adaptation of muscles in aged individuals: Satellite cells and innervation. *J. Gerontol. A Biol. Sci. Med. Sci. 50* Spec No, 96–100.

Carmeli, E., Coleman, R., and Reznick, A.Z. (2002). The biochemistry of aging muscle. *Exp. Gerontol. 37*, 477–489.

Cartee, G.D. (1995). What insights into age-related changes in skeletal muscle are provided by animal models? *J. Gerontol. A Biol. Sci. Med. Sci. 50* Spec No, 137–141.

Coggan, A.R. (1995). Muscle biopsy as a tool in the study of aging. *J. Gerontol. A Biol. Sci. Med. Sci. 50* Spec No, 30–34.

Edstrom, E. and Ulfhake, B. (2005). Sarcopenia is not due to lack of regenerative drive in senescent skeletal muscle. *Aging Cell 4*, 65–77.

Evans, W. (1997). Functional and metabolic consequences of sarcopenia. *J. Nutr. 127*, 998S–1003S.

Ferrucci, L., Guralnik, J.M., Studenski, S., Fried, L.P., Cutler, G.B., Jr., and Walston, J.D. (2004). Designing randomized, controlled trials aimed at preventing or delaying functional decline and disability in frail, older persons: A consensus report. *J. Am. Geriatr. Soc. 52*, 625–634.

Ferrucci, L., Penninx, B.W., Volpato, S., Harris, T.B., Bandeen-Roche, K., Balfour, J. *et al.* (2002). Change in muscle strength explains accelerated decline of physical function in older women with high interleukin-6 serum levels. *J. Am. Geriatr. Soc. 50*, 1947–1954.

Fiatarone, M.A., Marks, E.C., Ryan, N.D., Meredith, C.N., Lipsitz, L.A., and Evans, W.J. (1990). High-intensity strength training in nonagenarians. Effects on skeletal muscle. *JAMA 263*, 3029–3034.

Fiatarone, M.A., O'Neill, E.F., Ryan, N.D., Clements, K.M., Solares, G.R., Nelson, M.E. *et al.* (1994). Exercise training and nutritional supplementation for physical frailty in very elderly people. *N. Engl. J. Med. 330*, 1769–1775.

Fisher, A.L. (2004). Of worms and women: Sarcopenia and its role in disability and mortality. *J. Am. Geriatr. Soc. 52*, 1185–1190.

Fried, L.P., Bandeen-Roche, K., Chaves, P.H., and Johnson, B.A. (2000). Preclinical mobility disability predicts incident mobility disability in older women. *J. Gerontol. A Biol. Sci. Med. Sci. 55*, M43–M52.

Giresi, P.G., Stevenson, E.J., Theilhaber, J., Koncarevic, A., Parkington, J., Fielding, R.A. *et al.* (2005). Identification of a molecular signature of sarcopenia. *Physiol Genomics. 21*, 253–263.

Goodpaster, B.H., Carlson, C.L., Visser, M., Kelley, D.E., Scherzinger, A., Harris, T.B. *et al.* (2001). Attenuation of skeletal muscle and strength in the elderly: The Health ABC Study. *J. Appl. Physiol. 90*, 2157–2165.

Greenlund, L.J. and Nair, K.S. (2003). Sarcopenia-consequences, mechanisms, and potential therapies. *Mech. Ageing Dev. 124*, 287–299.

Gregorevic, P., Blankinship, M.J., and Chamberlain, J.S. (2004). Viral vectors for gene transfer to striated muscle. *Curr. Opin. Mol. Ther. 6*, 491–498.

Guralnik, J.M., Ferrucci, L., Simonsick, E.M., Salive, M.E., and Wallace, R.B. (1995). Lower-extremity function in persons over the age of 70 years as a predictor of subsequent disability. *N. Engl. J. Med. 332*, 556–561.

Herndon, L.A., Schmeissner, P.J., Dudaronek, J.M., Brown, P.A., Listner, K.M., Sakano, Y. *et al.* (2002). Stochastic and genetic factors influence tissue-specific decline in ageing *C. elegans. Nature 419*, 808–814.

Heymsfield, S.B., Gallagher, D., Visser, M., Nunez, C., and Wang, Z.M. (1995). Measurement of skeletal muscle: Laboratory and epidemiological methods. *J. Gerontol. A Biol. Sci. Med. Sci. 50* Spec No, 23–29.

Horani, M.H. and Morley, J.E. (2004). Hormonal fountains of youth. *Clin. Geriatr. Med. 20*, 275–292.

Housh, D.J., Housh, T.J., Weir, J.P., Weir, L.L., Johnson, G.O., and Stout, J.R. (1995). Anthropometric estimation of thigh muscle cross-sectional area. *Med. Sci. Sports Exerc. 27*, 784–791.

Hunter, S., White, M., and Thompson, M. (1998). Techniques to evaluate elderly human muscle function: A physiological basis. *J. Gerontol. A Biol. Sci. Med. Sci. 53*, B204–B216.

Kasper, J.D., Shapiro, S., Guralnik, J.M., Bandeen-Roche, K.J., and Fried, L.P. (1999). Designing a community study of moderately to severely disabled older women: The Women's Health and Aging Study. *Ann. Epidemiol. 9*, 498–507.

Kayo, T., Allison, D.B., Weindruch, R., and Prolla, T.A. (2001). Influences of aging and caloric restriction on the transcriptional profile of skeletal muscle from rhesus monkeys. *Proc. Natl. Acad. Sci. USA 98*, 5093–5098.

Kyle, U.G., Genton, L., Hans, D., Karsegard, V.L., Michel, J.P., Slosman, D.O. *et al.* (2001). Total body mass, fat mass, fat-free mass, and skeletal muscle in older people: Cross-sectional differences in 60-year-old persons. *J. Am. Geriatr. Soc. 49*, 1633–1640.

Lexell, J. (1995). Human aging, muscle mass, and fiber type composition. *J. Gerontol. A Biol. Sci. Med. Sci. 50* Spec No, 11–16.

Lohman, T.G. and Going, S.B. (1993). Multicomponent models in body composition research: Opportunities and pitfalls. In K.J. Ellis and J.D. Eastman (Eds.), *Human Body Composition*, pp. 53–58. New York: Plenum.

Lukaski, H. (1997). Sarcopenia: Assessment of muscle mass. *J. Nutr. 127*, 994S–997S.

McKinnell, I.W. and Rudnicki, M.A. (2004). Molecular mechanisms of muscle atrophy. *Cell 119*, 907–910.

Mehrian-Shai, R. and Reichardt, J.K. (2004). A renaissance of "biochemical genetics"? SNPs, haplotypes, function, and complex diseases. *Mol. Genet. Metab 83*, 47–50.

Metter, E.J., Talbot, L.A., Schrager, M., and Conwit, R. (2002). Skeletal muscle strength as a predictor of all-cause mortality in healthy men. *J. Gerontol. A Biol. Sci. Med. Sci. 57*, B359–B365.

Mir, L.M., Bureau, M.F., Gehl, J., Rangara, R., Rouy, D., Caillaud, J.M. *et al.* (1999). High-efficiency gene transfer into skeletal muscle mediated by electric pulses. *Proc. Natl. Acad. Sci. USA 96*, 4262–4267.

Peterson, C.A. (1995). Cell culture systems as tools for studying age-related changes in skeletal muscle. *J. Gerontol. A Biol. Sci. Med. Sci. 50* Spec No, 142–144.

Piec, I., Listrat, A., Alliot, J., Chambon, C., Taylor, R.G., and Bechet, D. (2005). Differential proteome analysis of aging in rat skeletal muscle. *FASEB J.*

Proctor, D.N., O'Brien, P.C., Atkinson, E.J., and Nair, K.S. (1999). Comparison of techniques to estimate total body skeletal muscle mass in people of different age groups. *Am. J. Physiol 277*, E489–E495.

Rando, T.A. and Blau, H.M. (1994). Primary mouse myoblast purification, characterization, and transplantation for cell-mediated gene therapy. *J. Cell Biol. 125*, 1275–1287.

Rantanen, T. (2003). Muscle strength, disability and mortality. Scand. J. Med. Sci. Sports *13*, 3–8.

Rantanen, T., Volpato, S., Ferrucci, L., Heikkinen, E., Fried, L.P., and Guralnik, J.M. (2003). Handgrip strength and cause-specific and total mortality in older disabled women: Exploring the mechanism. *J Am. Geriatr. Soc. 51*, 636–641.

Reeves, N.D., Maganaris, C.N., and Narici, M.V. (2004). Ultrasonographic assessment of human skeletal muscle size. *Eur. J. Appl. Physiol 91*, 116–118.

Ross, R., Pedwell, H., and Rissanen, J. (1995). Effects of energy restriction and exercise on skeletal muscle and adipose tissue in women as measured by magnetic resonance imaging. *Am. J. Clin. Nutr. 61*, 1179–1185.

Roth, S.M., Ferrell, R.E., Peters, D.G., Metter, E.J., Hurley, B.F., and Rogers, M.A. (2002). Influence of age, sex, and strength training on human muscle gene expression determined by microarray. *Physiol Genomics 10*, 181–190.

Roubenoff, R. (2003a). Catabolism of aging: Is it an inflammatory process? *Curr. Opin. Clin. Nutr. Metab Care 6*, 295–299.

Roubenoff, R. (2003b). Sarcopenia: Effects on body composition and function. *J Gerontol A Biol Sci Med Sci. 58*, 1012–1017.

Roubenoff, R., Parise, H., Payette, H.A., Abad, L.W., D'Agostino, R., Jacques, P.F. *et al.* (2003). Cytokines, insulin-like growth factor 1, sarcopenia, and mortality in very old community-dwelling men and women: The Framingham Heart Study. *Am. J. Med. 115*, 429–435.

Russ, D.W. and Kent-Braun, J.A. (2004). Is skeletal muscle oxidative capacity decreased in old age? *Sports Med. 34*, 221–229.

Short, K.R., Bigelow, M.L., Kahl, J., Singh, R., Coenen-Schimke, J., Raghavakaimal, S. *et al.* (2005). Decline in skeletal muscle mitochondrial function with aging in humans. *Proc. Natl. Acad. Sci. USA 102*, 5618–5623.

Szulc, P., Marchand, F., Duboeuf, F., and Delmas, P.D. (2000). Cross-sectional assessment of age-related bone loss in men: The MINOS study. *Bone 26*, 123–129.

van den Heuvel, L.P., Farhoud, M.H., Wevers, R.A., van Engelen, B.G., and Smeitink, J.A. (2003). Proteomics and neuromuscular diseases: Theoretical concept and first results. *Ann. Clin. Biochem. 40*, 9–15.

Vandervoort, A.A. (2002). Aging of the human neuromuscular system. *Muscle Nerve 25*, 17–25.

Visser, M., Deeg, D.J., and Lips, P. (2003). Low vitamin D and high parathyroid hormone levels as determinants of loss of muscle strength and muscle mass (sarcopenia): The Longitudinal Aging Study Amsterdam. *J. Clin. Endocrinol. Metab. 88*, 5766–5772.

Visser, M., Fuerst, T., Lang, T., Salamone, L., and Harris, T.B. (1999). Validity of fan-beam dual-energy X-ray absorptiometry for measuring fat-free mass and leg muscle mass. Health, Aging, and Body Composition Study—Dual-Energy X-ray Absorptiometry and Body Composition Working Group. *J. Appl. Physiol. 87*, 1513–1520.

Volpi, E., Nazemi, R., and Fujita, S. (2004). Muscle tissue changes with aging. *Curr. Opin. Clin. Nutr. Metab. Care 7*, 405–410.

Welle, S., Bhatt, K., and Thornton, C.A. (2000). High-abundance mRNAs in human muscle: Comparison between young and old. *J. Appl. Physiol. 89*, 297–304.

Welle, S., Brooks, A., and Thornton, C.A. (2001). Senescence-related changes in gene expression in muscle: Similarities and differences between mice and men. *Physiol Genomics 5*, 67–73.

82

Aging of Human Skin

Paolo U. Giacomoni

Aging is defined as the accumulation of molecular damages. Skin accumulates damages because of the mitochondrial production of superoxide in the course of phosphorylative oxidation, and because of the exposure to external damaging agents, such as solar radiation, gravitational traction, infections, electric fields, psychological stress, cigarette smoke, specific foods, anoxia and other agents.

All the factors contributing to the acceleration of the rate of accumulation of damages share the capability to induce the synthesis of I-CAM 1 in endothelial cells. This has prompted the proposal of the micro-inflammatory model of skin aging. According to this model, endothelial synthesis of I-CAM 1 allows the diapedesis of circulating monocytes, which enter the dermis and digest the surrounding extra-cellular matrix. During this process, nearby cells can be damaged and will secrete molecular signals to provoke vasodilation and diapedesis of more monocytes, to maintain the inflammatory cycle.

This model predicts the sagging and the thinning of the skin with age, the appearance of wrinkles, and the loss of elastic and rheological properties. This model does not account for the appearance of age spots.

Introduction

With time, damages accumulate in organs and organisms, which lose some of the prerogatives characteristic of youth. Damages are chemical modifications to molecules in an organism. Molecular damages accumulating in cellular DNA are called somatic mutations. According to the gene where these mutations occur, the physiology of the cell or of the organ can change unremarkably or dramatically. It can even provoke the death of the cell, with minor consequences, or of the organism, which is a major consequence. Other biochemical damages can accumulate in cellular membranes or cell organelles, but the damages most relevant to the aging of an organism are the ones accumulating in the extra-cellular matrixes such as bones, blood vessels, dermis, or in postmitotic cells clustered in anatomical entities such as muscular fibers or fat tissues. Indeed, these damages are the ones more directly linked to the visible manifestations of the onset of the aging process.

The accumulation of damages consequent to the basal metabolism has been defined as *natural* or *intrinsic* aging (Giacomoni and Rein, 2004). The accumulation of damages provoked by the interaction with other environmental factors (exposure to humidity for the onset of osteoarthrosis) or by the way of life (lack of exercise for the aging of skeletal muscle) can be defined as *accelerated* or *extrinsic* aging. Expressions such as *chronologic* aging or *premature* aging are to be avoided. Aging is the continuous accumulation of damages with time and is therefore a chronologic phenomenon *per se*. It can't be premature because it starts at the fertilization of the egg. So it is recommended to use the expressions natural aging or accelerated aging. It is also true that genes can play a role in the overall rate of aging and in the life span of the individual. Indeed, the same environmental factor will have different effects on two individuals with different genetic backgrounds. To give an example, exposed to the same dose of UV radiation, individuals with a defective Glutathion–S-Transferease (GST) gene are more likely to develop skin cancers than individuals with a wild-type GST gene.

Aging has been defined as the accumulation of molecular damages over time (Novoseltsev *et al.*, 2001; Giacomoni and D'Alessio, 1996b; Giacomoni, 1992). For a decade or so, biogerontologists have been discussing the necessity of aging. In particular the question has been asked about the selective advantage, if any, provided to a species by the fact that the individuals in the species undergo aging and therefore lose the capability to reproduce and to compete for food. Some scientists have elaborated a thought-provoking theory called disposable soma theory. According to this theory, the aging of the individuals represents a selective advantage for the species, and to ensure the aging of the individuals, specific genes called gerontogenes are turned on at a certain point in life. The function of gerontogenes is to trigger the process of aging, which eventually leads to the removal of the individual from competition.

In the last decade, though, gerontogenes were not found. Moreover it was observed that repair functions do not decrease with age (van Zeeland *et al.*, 2001; Giacomoni *et al.*, 2000) and no gene has been found that provokes the loss of functionality of cells or organs. Longevity in a species seems to be governed mainly by the capability to withstand aggressions and remove damages. The other possibility to achieve longevity is to live at a reduced metabolic pace by limiting the caloric intake, one of the consequences of which is to delay the onset of reproductive maturity.

For higher organisms, in particular humans, we can now say that the rate of aging is dictated mostly by way of life. The effects of caloric restriction on the process of aging are a good example in favor of the effect of lifestyle on the onset of aging (Giacomoni and Rein, 2001; Everitt, 2003). A Gedanken Experiment shows that, even in a hypothetical life without interaction with the environment other than water, sugar as food, and oxygen to breath, superoxide is generated in the course of oxidative phosphorylation, which provokes damages to cell constituents such as mitochondrial DNA (Giacomoni, 1992).

So, notwithstanding theoretical suggestions relative to genetically programmed aging (de Magalhães 2003; Tan *et al.*, 2001), consensus has been building in the scientific community about the understanding that the aging of the individual does not provide selective advantages to the species. The presently accepted conclusion is that the aging of a cell or of an organ, far from being an unavoidable curse, is more the consequence of its interaction with the environment (McArdle *et al.*, 2002; Rattan, 2001).

Skin and Skin Aging

Longevity and aging are two very different aspects of the life of an organism. Modifying longevity is not necessarily a relevant target in the scientific struggle against the undesirable effects of aging. If it were, dying young would be the best way not to grow old.

To study aging we need an organ accessible to analyses and such, that its aging does not bring prejudice to the survival of the organism (that is to say, one needs longevity to study aging).

Skin is one such organ. It is one of the largest organs in the human body. Its surface is smaller than that of intestinal epithelium, and its weight is smaller than that of the lungs, but with its two square meters and couple of kilograms, skin is respectable in size and mass. Human skin is vascularized, innervated, and immunecompetent. It is able to secrete water and sebum. It supports the growth of muscle-associated hair, and human hair, at variance with other mammals, presents characteristics that differ according to the anatomical site where it grows. Indeed, the human hair growing on the scalp is morphologically and developmentally different from the human hair on the chest or on the pubis.

At variance with other mammals, human skin changes remarkably with aging. Hair on the scalp is lost or changes color, the epidermal surface undergoes discolorations, and the thickness of the dermis is reduced, particularly so in women. In the sites exposed to air and sun, the skin becomes elastotic (i.e., it loses elasticity because of the deposition of elastin), the capillary vessels are pushed farther away from under the basement membrane, sagging is generalized, and wrinkles appear on expression zones, which are those anatomical sites located on the human face that allow feelings to be expressed without words.

Histologically, the dermal-epidermal junction is flattened, possibly because of the constant stretching of the skin exerted by the gravitational field. The consequence of this flattening is an increased surface and hence the necessity to maintain a particular neurological state so that neural cells continuously send impulses to induce tendons and muscles to contract. In this way the formation of wrinkles allows the cutaneous tissue to remain confined to its natural location. Another consequence of this flattening is to reduce the apparent average epidermal thickness, and this has led some scholars to the incorrect belief that the number of epidermal layers is reduced with aging. The thickness of the *stratum corneum* and the duplication time of keratinocytes do not seem to undergo major changes with age. The immune response seems to be modified with aging, skin seems to increase its susceptibility to pruritus, and wounds require a longer time to heal.

The aging of the skin is more the consequence of way of life than of predetermination. Factors of skin aging such as solar radiation, cigarette smoke, tractional forces, electromagnetic fields, infections, psychological stressors, air pollutants, anoxia, wounds, and traumas have been identified. The genotype will play a role in the process of skin aging, too, because the same environmental insult, such as the same dose of ultraviolet radiation, will have different results on two individuals with differently active genes for DNA repair (Giacomoni *et al.*, 2000; Heenen *et al.*, 2001).

Macroscopic Effects of Skin Aging

Visible signs on the surface of the skin are the consequence of time and environmental insults that trigger a series of cellular and physiological responses because of which, in the long term, the physical properties of the skin are modified. The role of solar radiation in skin aging can be understood when the necks of sailors are compared with the necks of nuns: *Cutis rhomboidalis nuchae* is characterized by profound textural and pigmentary changes, which occur upon chronic exposure to sun. Another consequence of excessive exposure to solar radiation is nodular elastosis or Favre-Racouchot disease, consisting of the appearance of cysts and comedons on the exposed parts of the skin. Other consequences of exposure to solar radiation are Millian's type citrine skin, teleangectasia, sagging, solar lentigo, and so on (for reviews on photo-aging, see Lyon and Fitzpatrick (1993) and Wlaschek *et al.* (2001)).

The skin of humans differs from the skin of other mammals, even rodents or mini-pigs. Yet for invasive laboratory studies, these two species have been selected, and now we know more about the effect of UV on the skin of hairless mice or of albino mini-pigs than on the skin of humans.

The physiological effects of ultraviolet radiation on skin has been analyzed by Bissett and coworkers (Bissett *et al.*, 1989). Cohorts of laboratory rodents were exposed to quasi-monochromatic radiation at different wavelengths in the ultraviolet range. They observed that the sagging of skin is provoked by radiation at 365 nm. The ultra-structural details of the continuous exposure of mini-pig skin to artificial ultraviolet radiation have been described by Fourtanier and Berrebi (1989), who found that after 24 months of exposure to artificial UV radiation, the fibers of collagen are no longer oriented. They are entangled, instead, and this might explain the loss of elasticity, the loss of resilience, and the sagging of photo-aged skin. These findings, together with the observation that neutrophils infiltrates are to be found in the skin after moderate exposure to UV-B (Hawk *et al.*, 1988) prompted the proposal that post UV-repair is analogous to wound healing (Giacomoni and D'Alessio, 1996a). Indeed wound-healing and post-UV-repair seem to share common features, in particular the mechanisms of tissue modifications, which include massive cell migration, proliferation, phenotypic differentiation, and enhanced biosynthetic activities. Macrophages and fibroblasts express embryonic fibronectin during cutaneous wound-healing, thus providing an extra-cellular matrix that facilitates wound repair. They are able to promote cell migration so that subpopulations of fibroblasts able to secrete migration-stimulating factors (MSF) might undergo transient and local expansion during wound healing. The process of disassembly of the extra-cellular matrix (ECM) operates via collagenases, proteoglycanases, and other lythic enzymes of macrophage origin. The last phase of wound healing involves a systematic dissolution of the granulation tissue, which is accompanied by a gradual loss of cells and vasculature and by exhaustive restructuring of the ECM. Newly synthesized ECM molecules do not fit, per se, into an ordered structure but can modulate the original geometric framework, which is essential for cell-matrix interaction. In fact, the disordered structure, which is observed upon chronic UV irradiation, might well be the consequence of one particular disposition of newly synthesized molecules. This is to say that to improve skin repair and fight skin aging, we should not try and accelerate the synthesis of collagen, because the turnover of collagen in human skin is of the order of 15 years or more (Verzeijl *et al.*, 2000). To improve skin repair we might well have larger chances of success by trying and looking for treatments able to help in maintaining newly synthesized macromolecules in an orderly structure. This, at least in laboratory rodents, seems to be, possible by specifically inhibiting the maturation of TGF-β (Shah *et al.*, 1992). It might be interesting to notice that TGF-β is an agent often used in cosmetic products to stimulate the synthesis of collagen. The results by Shah *et al.* (1992) might be overly interesting if the "quantity" of collagen production were in conflict with the "order" of the structure of the macromolecular fibers.

The Micro-inflammatory Model of Skin Aging

The research leading to the conception of the micro-inflammatory model of skin aging (Giacomoni and D'Alessio, 1996b) was prompted by the understanding of the relevant role played by actors of the inflammatory response in wound-healing and in post-UV-repair. In the course of such research, it was noticed that all the commonly accepted accelerators of the aging process shared a common feature the capability to induce the synthesis of ICAM-1 in the endothelium. This meant that all the factors recognized as being able to accelerate skin aging had the capability to trigger a self-maintained inflammatory response.

Indeed, upon synthesis of ICAM-1 in the endothelium, circulating monocytes secrete hydrogen peroxide to perform diapedesis across the endothelium lining the vascular wall. Once in the dermis, the macrophages secrete lythic enzymes and reactive oxygen species (ROS) to fray a path in the dermis.

In the majority of instances, macrophages respond to chemotactic signals to reach and destroy infectious agents, or to remove damaged skin cells. In some instances, as in the case of anoxia-generated diapedesis, macrophages in the dermis release collagenases and ROS so as to damage the smooth muscle surrounding veins. When anoxia is repetitive, as in the case of the veins in the legs of workers obliged to long-lasting stasis, this provokes such damage to smooth muscles that the vein becomes varicous.

In these conditions, it is highly likely that nearby resident cells, such as fibroblasts or keratinocytes, are damaged by the free radicals. When this happens, the damage can trigger the cascade of arachidonic acid and secretion of prostaglandines and leukotrienes, which diffuse to interact with resident mast cells. Upon binding of these mediators to specific receptors, the resident mast cells release histamine and TNF-α, which in turn stimulate the release of P-selectins and the neo-synthesis of ICAM-1 in endothelial cells. The cycle therefore is closed, and the micro-inflammatory status is maintained.

Discussion

Does this model account for all the factors of skin aging and for all the phenomenological characteristics of aged skin? Some of the accepted factors of skin aging are direct cell- or tissue-damaging factors. When damage to cells or tissue is generated (e.g., by UV-radiation, smoke-related free radicals, infectious agents, or wounds and traumas), thousands of damages are provoked to the ECM, resident cells, and vessel walls by the free radicals and lythic enzymes, which are released in the course of the inflammatory response, consequent to the diffusion of cytokines produced via the arachidonic acid cascade. What about the other factors of aging that are not directly damaging agents? Traction and gravitational forces provoke the activation of phospholipase A2, an enzyme involved in the arachidonic acid cascade. Anoxia induces ICAM-1 synthesis and diapedesis of macrophages, which start digesting the ECM around veins or other blood vessels. Glucose binds to proteins in a non-enzymatic glycation process, and glycated proteins are inducers of ICAM-1 synthesis. Electromagnetic fields associated with computers provoke the release of histamine, IL-1 and IL-6. (A summary of the results of scientists at the Karolinska Institute of Stockholm on this subject is given by Giacomoni and Rein, 2001.) Neuropeptides regulate the expression of cell-adhesion molecules on both leukocytes and endothelial cells in a coordinated effort to control neurogenic inflammation. These phenomena trigger a cycle of self-maintained inflammatory response, which comprises the induction of the neo-synthesis of ICAM-1, and are summarized in Giacomoni and Rein (2001).

This micro-inflammatory model of skin aging emphasizes the aging of the connective tissue and of the extra-cellular matrix. Macroscopic consequences of this model are verified by the experience. The recognition that post-UV-repair and wound-healing share the ECM remodeling as a common feature has allowed us to understand why blood vessels are deeper down in aged skin than they are in young skin. The sagging of the dermis is the consequence of a modified ECM and is accompanied by an overall increase of the surface of the skin, particularly of the face.

It can be noted at this point that muscular and neurological actions are involved in the formation of wrinkles to maintain the skin with increased surface to cover a skull. This was first observed by neurophysiologists who noticed that in the case of hemiplegia, the wrinkles were observed only on that part of the forehead that was not paralyzed (Prunieras, private communication). Surgeons also noticed that patients subjected to anesthesia did not display wrinkles (Marty, private communication).

The increase of skin surface and the reduction of body volume can be invoked to explain the observation that the thickness of the epidermis is diminished with aging. This is more the consequence of the stretching of the skin than of a modification of the turnover rate of the keratinocytes. Indeed, the turnover of the keratinocytes does not change much with aging; this is witnessed by the fact that the thickness of the *stratum corneum* does not change with aging (Gilchrest, 1993).

On the other hand, the micro-inflammatory model of skin aging does not provide detailed explanations for the appearance of other visible signs of aging associated with the surface of the skin, such as discoloration and dryness.

It is known that a permanent state of irritation (i.e., with constantly high levels of mediators of irritation such as IL-1) stimulates the production of melanin by the melanocytes. In this case the micro-inflammatory model of skin aging predicts that with time, the skin should undergo a progressive homogeneous darkening. What the model fails to predict is the appearance on specific skin regions, of the so-called age spots, dark regions of less than 0.25 cm^2 in sun-exposed areas, the color of which has been suggested to be the consequence of the accumulation of melanin and/or lipofuschin. Recent studies have demonstrated a role for the growth factor, insulin-like growth factor I (IGF), in the appearance of the signs of aging.

It can be noted at this point that elderly men with low serum IGF levels (Bonafe *et al.*, 2003) are more likely to be healthy (van den Beld *et al.*, 2003). Furthermore, long-lived individuals have lower levels of the IGF receptor (Bonafe *et al.*, 2003). Higher levels of IGF appear to be pro-inflammatory. It has been long known that IGF induces histamine release from basophils in inflammatory bronchial asthma (Morita *et al.*, 1993). More recent evidence indicates IGF plays an important regulatory role in inflammatory processes. Shortly after injury, acutely inflamed human wounds show increases in IGF-1 protein concentrations, believed to arise from blood sources (Wagner *et al.*, 2003). Similarly, IGF is up-regulated following tendon injury, where its expression in increased during the early inflammatory phase (Molloy *et al.*, 2003). In this animal model, IGF is believed to mediate the proliferation and migration of fibroblasts. The actions of IGF and other growth factors in promoting aging and inflammatory processes are further regulated by neuropeptides. Neuropeptides are now being considered in the aging process. A recent study in normal children demonstrated age-dependent changes in serum levels of several neuropeptides, as well as IGF (O'Dorisio *et al.*, 2002). Of particular interest here is that that the physiological actions of neuropeptides are synergistic with IGF. Although this has mostly been demonstrated using cultured neurons (Jones *et al.*, 2003), recent studies with epithelial wound healing demonstrate a similar effect with substance P and IGF (Nagano *et al.*, 2003; Nakamura *et al.*, 2003). These results demonstrate the complexity of the regulatory mechanisms involving neuropeptides in the process of skin aging. Although not yet proven, these mechanisms are also thought to affect the activation of melanocytes, which is possibly linked to the age-associated skin discoloration.

Skin dryness is a more complex state of affairs, because the model does not provide suggestions to predict the accumulation of water or the synthesis of lipids in the *stratum corneum*. This parameter depends so closely from yearly cycles (seasons) and meteorological conditions (temperature, relative humidity) that the individual and local variability provide a "noise" able to mask the trends dictated by aging (if any). Hormonal imbalance and the loss of capability to retain water in the dermis, which occur at the onset of menopause, are not predicted by the micro-inflammatory model of skin aging, and correctly so because the onset of menopause is more a development- than an aging-related phenomenon. This being said, we could add that the moisturization of the skin is difficult to assess both instrumentally and via self-description. When the assessment of skin moisturization is conducted by self-description, the words used by different subjects do not mean the same thing to everyone. It is now felt, for instance, that the word "moisturization" is used to describe a state of suppleness, flexibility, and softness, more than an actual state of hydration. Instruments to assess the hydration of the skin measure either the gradient of the concentration of water vapor in the proximity of the skin surface, or the conductivity of the surface of the skin. In both cases the correspondence between the state of the skin and the experimental results is not unequivocal. Indeed, a high value of the gradient of concentration of water vapor (called trans-epidermal water loss, or TEWL) can be the consequence of a well-hydrated skin or of a lack of surface lipids. Similarly, high conductivity can be the consequence of high water content or of low water content concomitant with high electrolyte content in the surface of the skin. So when we measure macroscopic properties of the skin such as TEWL versus age, we observe that at young age the TEWL is low, then it increases during young adulthood and maturity, and it decreases again in old age (Giacomoni *et al.*, 2002). From these measurements it is impossible to conclude that young skin is hydrated and has a good barrier, whereas old skin is dry and has a poor barrier. In the absence of data that can be unequivocally interpreted, the comparison of the predictions with the experimental results is a useless endeavor.

Conclusion

The micro-inflammatory model of skin aging provides a sound mechanistic paradigm to understand the aging of the dermis and of the extra-cellular matrix in general. The model also recognizes new factors of aging, insofar as it may "predict" whether a particular aggression will be able to trigger the synthesis of ICAM-1 in the endothelium. It also allows us to consider interventions to reduce the rate of aging, and in this respect it can be considered a successful model. It has also been applied to describe the aging of other organs of the human body, such as joints (Pincus, 2001) and the brain (Wilson *et al.*, 2002), and for the understanding of the onset of age-associated diseases such as osteoarthritis and senile dementia. The micro-inflammatory model of skin aging, on the other hand, fails to predict the appearance of age-related modifications of the surface of the skin.

As of today, mainly because of the lack of appropriate experimental devices able to provide unequivocal data, the micro-inflammatory model of skin aging cannot be applied to predicting changes in the production of those molecules that are essential for maintaining the hydro-dynamic equilibrium of the surface of the skin and that seem to be impaired with aging. The micro-inflammatory model fails to predict the appearance of age spots. This might be the consequence of our ignorance relative to the ontogenesis of these spots. We do surmise a role for resident neural-crest melanocytes, which respond to neuropeptides (Kauser *et al.*, 2003); this has been suggested in the overall process of skin aging (Giacomoni and Rein, 2001).

The micro-inflammatory model of skin aging has prompted the use of anti-oxidant and anti-inflammatory agents in creams and ointments aimed at reducing the rate of aging of the connective tissue via the topical applications of such ingredients. The rationale behind these experiments was that anti-oxidants and anti-inflammatory agents are expected to reduce the rate of accumulation of damages provoked in the course of a micro-inflammation subsequent to the synthesis of ICAM-1. As of today, positive preliminary results are now and then communicated to dermatology or cosmetic congresses, but published evidence is yet to be found.

REFERENCES

Bissett, R., Hannon, D.P., and Orr, T.V. (1989). Wavelength dependence of histological, physical, and visible changes in chronically UV-irradiated hairless mouse skin. *Photochem Photobiol 50*, 763–769.

Bonafe, M., Barbieri, M., Marchegiani, F., Olivieri, F., Ragno, E., Giampieri, C. *et al.* (2003). Polymorphic variants of insulin-like growth factor I (IGF-I) receptor and phosphoinositide 3-kinase genes affect IGF-I plasma levels and human longevity: cues for an evolutionarily conserved mechanism of life span control. *J Clin Endocrinol Metab 88*, 3299–3304.

de Magalhães, J.P. (2003). Is Mammalian aging genetically controlled? *Biogerontology 4*, 119–120.

Everitt, A.V. (2003). Food restriction, pituitary hormones and ageing. *Biogerontology 4*, 47–50.

Fourtanier, A. and Berrebi, C. (1989). Miniature pig as animal model to study photoaging. *Photochem Photobiol 50*, 771–784.

Giacomoni, P.U. (1992). Aging and Cellular defence mechanisms. In C. Franceschi, G. Crepaldi, and V. Cristofalo (Eds.),

Ageing and Defence Cellular Mechanism, pp. 1–3. New York: New York Academy of Sciences.

Giacomoni, P.U. and D'Alessio, P. (1996a). Open questions in photobiology. IV Photoaging of the skin. *J Photochem Photobiol B: Biol 33*, 262–272.

Giacomoni, P.U. and D'Alessio, P. (1996b). Skin Aging: The relevance of antioxidants. In S. Rattan and O. Toussaint (Eds), *Molecular Gerontology*, pp. 177–192. New York: Plenum Press.

Giacomoni, P.U., Declerq, L., Hellemans, L., and Maes, D. (2000). Aging of human skin: Review of a mechanistic model and first experimental data. *IUBMB-Life 49*, 259–263.

Giacomoni, P.U. and Rein, G. (2001). Factors of skin aging share common mechanisms. *Biogerontology 2*, 219–229.

Giacomoni, P.U., Muizzuddin, N., Sparacio, R.M., Pelle, E., Mammone, T., Marenus, K. *et al.* (2002). Sensitive skin and moisturization. In J.J. Leyden and A.V. Rawlings (Eds), *Skin Moisturization*, pp. 145–154. New York: Marcel Dekker.

Giacomoni, P.U. and Rein, G. (2004). A mechanistic model for the aging of human skin. *Micron 35*, 179–184.

Gilchrest, B. (1993). Aging of skin. In T.B. Fitzpatrick, A. Zur Hausen, K. Wolff, I.M. Freedberg, and K.F. Austen (Eds), *Dermatology in General Medicine*, pp. 150–157. New York: McGraw-Hill.

Hawk, J.L.M., Murphy, G.M., and Holden, G.A. (1988). The presence of neutrophils in human cutaneous ultraviolet-B inflammation. *Brit J Dermatol 118*, 27–30.

Heenen, M., Giacomoni, P.U., and Goldstein, P. (2001). Erythema, a link between UV-induced DNA damage, cell death and clinical effects? In P.U. Giacomoni (Ed.), *Sun Protection in Man*, pp. 277–285. Amsterdam: Elsevier.

Jones, D.M., Tucker, B.A., Rahimtula, M., and Mearow, K.M. (2003). The synergistic effects of NGF and IGF-1 on neurite growth in adult sensory neurons: Convergence on the PI 3-kinase signaling pathway. *J Neurochem 86*, 1116–1128.

Kauser, S., Schallreuter, K.U., Thody, A.J., Gummer, C., and Tobin, D.J. (2003). Regulation of human epidermal melanocyte biology by beta-endorphin. *J Invest Dermatol 120*, 1073–1080.

Lyon, N.B., and Fitzpatrick, T.B. (1993). Skin and aging. In T.B. Fitzpatrick, A. Zur Hausen, I.M. Friedberg, and K.F. Austen (Eds), *Dermatology in General Medicine*, pp. 2961–2972. New York: McGraw-Hill.

McArdle, A., Vasilaki, A., and Jackson, M. (2002). Exercise and skeletal muscle ageing: Cellular and molecular mechanism. *Ageing Res Rev 1*, 79–93.

Molloy, T., Wang, Y., and Murrell, G. (2003). The roles of growth factors in tendon and ligament healing. *Sports Med 33*, 381–394.

Morita, Y., Hirai, K., Koshino, T., Yamaguchi, M., Suzuki, M., Nakajima, K. *et al.* (1993). The role of mast cells and basophils in the pathogenesis of bronchial asthma. *Nihon Kyobu Shikkan Gakkai Zasshi 31 Suppl*, 147–153.

Nagano, T., Nakamura, M., Nakata, K., Yamaguchi, T., Takase, K., Okahara, A. *et al.* (2003). Effects of substance P and IGF-1 in corneal epithelial barrier function and wound healing in a rat model of neurotrophic keratopathy. *Invest Ophthalmol Vis Sci 44*, 3810–3815.

Nakamura, M., Kawahara, M., Nakata, K., and Nishida, T. (2003). Resotoration of corneal epithelial barrier function and wound healing by substance P and IGF-1. *Invest Ophthalmol Vis Sci 44*, 2937–2940.

Novoseltsev, V.N., Novosltseva, J., and Yashin, A. (2001). A homeostatic model of oxidative damage explains paradoxes observed in the earlier aging experiments: A fusion and extension of older theories of aging. *Biogerontology 2*, 127–138.

O'Dorisio, M.S., Hauger, M., and O'Dorisio, T.M. (2002). Age-dependent levels of plasma neuropeptides in normal children. *Regul Pept 109*, 189–192.

Pincus, T. (2001). Clinical evidence for osteoarthritis as an inflammatory disease. *Curr Rheumatol Rep 3*, 524–534.

Rattan, S. (2001). "I no longer believe that cell death is programmed." An interview with Vincent Cristofalo. *Biogerontology 2*, 283–290.

Shah, M., Foreman, D.M., and Ferguson, M.W. (1992). Control of scarring in adult wounds by neutralizing antibodies to transforming growth factor beta. *Lancet 339*, 213–214.

Tan, Q., De Benedictis, G., Yashin, A.I., Bonafe, M., De Luca, M., Valensin, S. *et al.* (2001). Measuring the genetic influence in modulating the human life span: gene-environment interaction and the sex-specific genetic effect. *Biogerontology 2*, 141–153.

van den Beld, A.W., Blum, W.F., Pols, H.A., Grobbee, D.E., and Lamberts, S.W. (2003). Serum insulin-like growth factor binding protein-2 levels as an indicator of functional ability in elderly men. *Eur J Endocrinol 148*, 627–634.

Van Zeeland, A.A., Van Hoffen, A., and Mullenders, L.H.F. (2001). Nucleotide excision repair of UV radiation-induced photolesions in human cells. In P.U. Giacomoni (Ed.), *Sun Protection in Man*, pp. 377–392. Amsterdam: Elsevier.

Verzeijl, N., DeGroot, J., Thorpe, S.R., Bank, R.A., Shaw, J.N., Lyons, T.J. *et al.* (2000). Effect of collagen turnover on the accumulation of advanced glycation endproducts. *J Biol Chem 275*, 39027–39031.

Wagner, S., Coerper, S., Fricke, J., Hunt, T.K., Hussain, Z., Elmlinger, M.W. *et al.* (2003). Comparison of inflammatory and systemic sources of growth factors in acute and chronic human wounds. *Wound Repair Regen 11*, 253–260.

Wilson, C.J., Finch, C.E., and Cohen, H.J. (2002). Cytokines and cognition—the case for a head-to-toe inflammatory paradigm. *J Am Geriatr Soc 50*, 2041–2056.

Wlaschek, M., Tantcheva-Poor, I., Brenneisen, P., Kuhr, L., Razi-Wolf, Z., Hellweg, C. *et al.* (2001). The negative effects of solar and artificial irradiation: Photoaging of the skin, its clinical appearance and underlying mechanisms. In P.U. Giacomoni (Ed.), *Sun Protection in Man*, pp. 115–130. Amsterdam: Elsevier.

83

Models of Hypertension in Aging

Jane F. Reckelhoff, Radu Iliescu, Licy Yanes, and Lourdes A. Fortepiani

All forms of hypertension studied to date are caused by a defect in the handling of sodium and water by the kidney. There is a shift to the right in the pressure-natriuresis relationship (higher blood pressure) in which a hypertensive individual must increase blood pressure in order to excrete a normal sodium load. There are sex differences in blood pressure control in humans and animals, with males having higher blood pressure than females. However, blood pressure increases in some women after menopause. The mechanisms that play a role in hypertension, and have been studied extensively, include the renin-angiotensin-aldosterone system, endothelin, oxidative stress, the sympathetic nervous system, androgen/estrogen ratio, and obesity.

Rats and mice are commonly used for the study of hypertension and aging. There are both genetic and nongenetic models of hypertension in which the animals exhibit increases in blood pressure spontaneously or are genetically predisposed to increase blood pressure in response to a high-salt diet. Some of these models have been used for aging studies. The nongenetic models of hypertension are produced in normotensive rats by maneuvers that will increase their blood pressure. Many of these maneuvers could be performed in aging animals. There are also transgenic rat and mouse models that may be suitable for aging studies, but to date have not been used in aging studies. Therefore, their suitability remains to be determined experimentally.

Introduction

The study of aging in hypertension is limited mainly to rats and mice since these animals have relatively short life spans, are inexpensive to purchase and maintain, and can be easily manipulated. This chapter will focus on genetic and nongenetic models of hypertension in rats and transgenic models of hypertension in rats and mice. There are few studies of aging in hypertensive animals. Therefore, in this chapter the most common hypertensive models used will be discussed along with other models that could be used but have not been in the past.

ETIOLOGY OF HYPERTENSION

Abnormal pressure-natriuresis in hypertension

Substantial evidence supports the theory that some form of renal dysfunction plays a role in the development and maintenance of hypertension. A common defect that has been characterized in all forms of hypertension studied to date is a shift in the pressure-natriuresis relationship (Guyton *et al.*, 1972; Hall *et al.*, 1990). The pressure-natriuresis relationship refers to the fact that increased arterial pressure elicits a marked increase in sodium excretion. According to the renal body fluid feedback concept, a long-term increase in arterial pressure or hypertension occurs as a result of a reduction in renal excretory function or a rightward shift in the pressure-natriuresis relationship. In kidneys from normotensive individuals, when sodium intake is increased, the blood pressure will increase transiently to increase sodium excretion. When the sodium load has been excreted, the blood pressure returns to normal levels. However, in a hypertensive individual, in order to excrete a normal amount of sodium, the blood pressure must be maintained in an elevated state, thereby causing a shift in the pressure-natriuresis relationship to the right (higher pressure).

Hypertension "follows the kidney"

Providing the strongest support for the theory that renal dysfunction in the excretion of sodium and water is the etiology of hypertension are observations that "hypertension follows the kidney." Of particular relevance to human hypertension is the study by Curtis *et al.* (1983), which demonstrated that blood pressure returns to normal in hypertensive patients who receive kidneys from normotensive donors. The results indicate that a defect within the kidney may play a crucial role in the pathogenesis of hypertension. In animal studies, when the kidney from a spontaneously hypertensive rat (SHR) is transplanted into a normotensive rat, the blood pressure in the previously normotensive rat increases (Harrap *et al.*, 1992). Similarly, when kidneys from Dahl salt-sensitive (DS) rats were transplanted into Dahl salt-resistant (DR) rats, the blood pressure became salt sensitive in the DR rats (Rettig, 1993). When kidneys from DR were transplanted into DS rats, the rats became resistant to increases in blood pressure with increased salt consumption. Similar findings were also made when SHRSP kidneys were transplanted into WKY and vice versa (Rettig, 1993). These data strongly support the notion that a defect in the kidney in sodium and water handling causes hypertension.

Sex differences in blood pressure

Sex differences in blood pressure regulation in humans. Men are generally at greater risk for cardiovascular and renal disease than are age-matched, premenopausal women (Reckelhoff, 2001). One factor that may contribute to these sex differences is the differences in blood pressure in men and women. Recent studies using the technique of 24-hour ambulatory blood pressure monitoring have shown that blood pressure is higher in men than in women at similar ages. For example, Wiinber and colleagues studied 352 normotensive (for age) Danish men and women, aged 20 to 79 years, and found that blood pressure increased with aging in both men and women, but that men had higher 24-hour mean blood pressure, by approximately 6 to 10 mm Hg, than did women, until the age of 70 to 79 years, when blood pressure was similar for men and women (Reckelhoff, 2001). Khoury and colleagues performed ambulatory blood pressure monitoring on 131 men and women, aged 50 to 60 years, and found that men had higher blood pressure than did women (Reckelhoff, 2001). In addition, NHANES III, the Third National Health and Nutrition Evaluation Survey, showed that in general, men had higher blood pressure than women through middle age (Reckelhoff, 2001). Furthermore, the incidence of uncontrolled hypertension is also greater in men than women.

Sex differences in blood pressure regulation in animals. The gender-associated differences in blood pressure observed in humans have also been documented in various animal models (Reckelhoff, 2001). In hypertensive rat models, many investigators have found that males have higher blood pressure than do females. For example, male spontaneously hypertensive rats have higher blood pressure than do females of similar ages. Similar gender differences in development of hypertension also are found in Dahl salt-sensitive rats, deoxycorticosterone acetate (DOCA) salt-hypertensive rats, and the New Zealand genetically hypertensive rat. Therefore, as found in humans and hypertensive rat models, males have higher blood pressure than age-matched females.

The data showing that males have higher blood pressure than females also are supported by studies of Harrap and colleagues (1992), who reported that when the kidney from male SHR was transplanted into female SHR, this maneuver did not result in a significant rise in blood pressure such that female SHR with male kidneys had similarly elevated blood pressure as female SHR with female kidneys. When the kidney from female SHR was transplanted into male SHR, blood pressure was not attenuated in the male with female kidneys compared to blood pressure in a male SHR with male kidneys. These data indicate that the 25 to 30 mm Hg higher blood pressure in the male SHR compared to the female is not due to an intrinsic defect of the male kidney but due to some external factor in the male, which further increases blood pressure perhaps due to a reduction in pressure-natriuresis. We hypothesize that androgens are the factor in males by which the pressure-natriuresis relationship is blunted and higher blood pressure results (Reckelhoff, 2001).

Postmenopausal hypertension

Although blood pressure typically is lower in women than age-matched men, after menopause (which occurs at approximately 51.4 years of age), systolic blood pressure increases in women such that the prevalence of hypertension in postmenopausal women is similar to, or higher than, in men (Reckelhoff and Fortepiani, 2004). Furthermore, the increase in blood pressure in postmenopausal women does not occur as soon as the ovary becomes senescent, but rather occurs over a number of years. Data from NHANES III confirmed that by 60 to 69 years of age, non-Hispanic black and Hispanic women developed higher blood pressure than men of similar ethnic background. However, the mechanisms responsible for the hypertension in these populations are complicated by comorbid conditions of obesity and type II diabetes, both of which lead to increases in blood pressure. However, in the non-Hispanic white population, in which the incidence of obesity and type II diabetes with aging were not as high, blood pressure also increased after menopause, although at a later age. So by 60 to 69 years of age, non-Hispanic white women had similar blood pressure as men, and by 70 to 79 years of age, this population of women had higher blood pressure than did men.

POSSIBLE MECHANISMS RESPONSIBLE FOR HYPERTENSION

Various humoral and cardiovascular systems play a role in controlling blood pressure. Among them are the renin-angiotensin-aldosterone system, endothelin, oxidative stress, obesity, and the sympathetic nervous system. Aging is associated with changes in most of these systems, and this could impact the roles they may play in mediating hypertension. The following will be a concise overview of the humoral factors that could affect blood pressure in aging individuals and that are subsequently investigated in models of age-related increases in blood pressure.

The renin-angiotensin-aldosterone system (RAAS)

The key system for controlling blood pressure and body fluid volume (i.e., pressure-natriuresis) is the RAAS (Hall *et al.*, 1999). For example, under normal conditions, any perturbation that increases arterial pressure will also provoke an increase in sodium and water excretion via pressure-natriuresis as described earlier. This will lead to decreases in extracellular fluid volume, venous return and cardiac output and blood pressure return to normal.

Long-term pressure-natriuresis is modulated by the RAS. Angiotensin II (Ang II) increases proximal sodium reabsorption by the kidney by stimulating epithelial transport. In the event of abnormal Ang II levels for the level of volume in the body, the blood pressure will increase with abnormal sodium and water reabsorption, leading to blunting of the pressure-natriuresis relationship. Similarly, if total body fluid volume levels are perceived incorrectly and thus Ang II levels do not respond appropriately, increases in blood pressure also will occur (Reckelhoff and Romero, 2003).

The biological activity of Ang II is mediated by two types of receptors, AT1 and AT2. The AT1 receptor is thought to mediate the vasoconstrictor effects of Ang II and Ang II-mediated sodium reabsorption in the proximal tubule and thus the increase in blood pressure (Sandberg and Ji, 2000). The AT2 receptor on the other hand is thought to activate NO production perhaps by increasing intracellular calcium to activate NO synthase.

Whether RAS activity changes with age in men and women is somewhat controversial. James and colleagues (1986) reported from serial analyses that plasma renin activity (PRA) was higher in men than in age-matched women, that PRA was higher in postmenopausal women than in premenopausal ones, and that in white men, PRA did not decrease with age. Blood pressure becomes more salt sensitive with aging in both men and women (Weinberger and Fineberg, 1991), which suggests that RAS activity and Ang II do not respond appropriately in the presence of salt in aging individuals.

Another function of Ang II that is mediated by the AT1 receptor is to stimulate the production of aldosterone, which is responsible for increasing sodium reabsorption in the distal nephron. In addition, several investigators have hypothesized that aldosterone may play an important role in renal injury (Brown, 2005). An increase in glomerular injury and loss of nephron function will also contribute to increases in blood pressure.

Ang II has also been shown to cause oxidative stress by increasing the expression of the NADPH oxidase subunits (Mollnau *et al.*, 2002). As discussed later, oxidative stress is capable of increasing blood pressure, and thus Ang II may increase in blood pressure via an oxidative stress-mediated mechanism.

Endothelin

Endothelin is a potent vasoconstrictor that when infused chronically leads to increases in blood pressure (Wilkins *et al.*, 1995). Endothelin has been shown to be up-regulated during Ang II infusion (Alexander *et al.*, 2001). Therefore, if aging is associated with activation of the RAS, then the increased synthesis of endothelin could play a role in the Ang II mediated increase in blood pressure with aging. In postmenopausal women, plasma endothelin levels have been shown to be increased, but the data are not consistent as to whether endothelin increases in tissues with aging in men and/or women.

Endothelin also could play a role in increasing blood pressure by contributing to oxidative stress. Endothelin has been shown to stimulate oxidative stress by causing up-regulation of the subunits of NAD(P)H oxidase and stimulating production of superoxide (Duerrschmidt *et al.*, 2000).

Oxidative stress

Both supraphysiological and physiological doses of Ang II can cause oxidative stress (Reckelhoff and Romero, 2003). For example, Rajagopalan and colleagues found that pharmacological doses of Ang II (Ang II; 0.7 mg/kg/d s.c. by minipump) increased blood pressure and superoxide levels in aortic segments of rats, whereas infusion of norepinephrine, which resulted in a similar increase in blood pressure as Ang II, had no effect on superoxide levels (Reckelhoff and Romero, 2003). These data suggested that infusion of Ang II at pharmacological doses was capable of inducing oxidative stress independent of elevated blood pressure. In addition, these investigators found that increased superoxide levels could be normalized with losartan, the Ang II receptor antagonist, or with liposomes containing superoxide dismutase. In further experiments they also reported that the Ang II increases superoxide production via increased NAD(P)H oxidase activity.

Superoxide is known to interact with nitric oxide (NO) to cause quenching of NO and to produce peroxynitrite, one of the most potent oxidative compounds known (Pryor and Squadrito, 1995). Thermodynamically speaking, the reaction of NO and superoxide is preferential since the rate of reaction is more rapid than the reaction rate of superoxide and its scavenger, superoxide dismutase (Pryor and Squadrito, 1995). The interaction between superoxide and NO causes a reduction in the biological activity (vasodilation) of NO leading to vasoconstriction, which could impact hypertension. Although peroxynitrite itself is a vasodilator, tachyphylaxis occurs at low peroxynitrite concentrations, and not only prevents further response to its own vasodilator actions, but also causes long-lasting impairment of the response to other vasodilators (Reckelhoff and Romero, 2003).

Androgens/estrogens

In experimental settings, many *in vitro*, estradiol has been shown to have a variety of effects that should be cardiovascular protective. However, despite the potential of estradiol to combat cardiovascular disease, large clinical trials on the effect of hormone replacement therapy (HRT) in post-menopausal women do not support these findings (The Writing Group for the PEPI Trial, 1995; Burry, 2002). Furthermore, HRT doesn't always result in a reduction in blood pressure in post-menopausal women, and even if it does so, the reduction is not dramatic. Proponents of the beneficial role of estradiol in cardiovascular disease cite the use of progesterone in HRT as possibly negating the positive effects of estradiol. However, in women who have experienced surgical menopause, estrogen replacement therapy (ERT) was also not successful in reducing blood pressure (Powledge, 2004). Thus reductions in estradiol that occur at menopause do not fully explain the progressive increases in blood pressure in postmenopausal women, and estrogen replacement is not used as an antihypertensive in their treatment.

There are various ways that androgens could impact blood pressure. Testosterone has been shown to stimulate production of angiotensinogen, the substrate for renin, in the kidney (Reckelhoff, 2001). This would activate the renin-angiotensin system. Androgen supplementation in female-to-male transsexuals is associated with increased plasma endothelin (van Kesteren *et al.*, 1998). Thus androgens could mediate an increase in blood pressure in postmenopausal women or rats by activating the renin-angiotensin system, which would subsequently increase endothelin synthesis and oxidative stress.

Obesity

Many, but not all, men and women gain weight with aging. Weight gain has been shown to be associated with increases in blood pressure in human and animal studies. Furthermore, obesity is associated with increased incidence of type II diabetes, which is also a strong mediator of cardiovascular disease and hypertension. In a study in which body mass index was similar for pre- and postmenopausal women, postmenopausal women experienced significantly higher blood pressure, waist circumference, and waist-to-hip ratio, compared with premenopausal women, which suggests that even without a change in BMI with age, body fat distribution changes following menopause. It is well known that abdominal fat accumulation, as opposed to lower body fat accumulation, is a risk factor for cardiovascular disease. Obesity is also accompanied by an increase in sympathetic activity (Esler *et al.*, 2001), particularly in the kidney, which would lead to an increase in renin release and contribute to hypertension.

Sympathetic nervous system

Aging in both men and women is associated with increased sympathetic activity (Seals and Esler, 2000). For example, Ng and colleagues have demonstrated that tibial and peroneal muscle postganglionic sympathetic nerve activity (MSNA), as measured by microneurography, doubles between ages 25 and 65 years and the increase is consistent for women as well as men (Ng *et al.*, 1993). In addition, the total body norepinephrine spillover rate has been shown to be elevated in older compared with younger individuals. On the other hand, age-related changes in norepinephrine spillover, and thus sympathetic activation, are organ-specific. For example, cardiac and hepatomesenteric, but not renal, norepinephrine spillover rates are increased with age. However, in obese individuals, total body norepinephrine spillover rates are usually normal, but renal norepinephrine spillover is increased. Thus with the combination of aging and obesity, there may be a greater activation of the sympathetic nervous system. A greater increase in renal sympathetic activity in aging individuals could stimulate renin release from intracellular stores in the kidney leading to increased production of Ang II and hypertension by all the ways just described.

Models of Hypertension

There are a considerable number of models of hypertension that can be produced in various animals. The following discussion will focus on the most common models of hypertension in rats (and mice for transgenic models), since this is an animal model that is easily adaptable to studies of aging.

GENETIC MODELS OF HYPERTENSION

Spontaneously hypertensive rat (SHR)

Males. The SHR is a commonly used model of hypertension (Reckelhoff, 2001). These animals develop increases in blood pressure beginning at six to seven weeks of age and reach a stable level of hypertension by 17 to 19 weeks of age. Inhibitors of the renin-angiotensin system reduce blood pressure in SHR, suggesting a role for the RAS in mediating the hypertension.

Removal of the renal nerves also reduces blood pressure in SHR, suggesting that the sympathetic nervous system is important in mediating the hypertension. Because increased sympathetic activity can stimulate renin release from the kidney, it is possible that the up-regulated RAS in SHR may be due to increased sympathetic activation.

In addition to the RAS and sympathetic nervous system in mediating the hypertension in SHR, treatment with antioxidants also reduces blood pressure, suggesting a role for oxidative stress in the hypertension of SHR. For example, treatment with tempol, a superoxide scavenger, reduces blood pressure as does apocynin, an inhibitor of the assembly of the subunits of NADPH oxidase. However, treatment with allopurinol protects against some of the end organ injury in SHR but fails to reduce blood pressure, suggesting that the oxidative stress in SHR that plays a role in their hypertension is mediated via NADPH oxidase, but not xanthine oxidase.

With aging, renal function decreases with reductions in GFR and renal plasma flow and increases in renal vascular resistance. Modest levels of proteinuria are also present in aging animals. In SHR at nine months of age, studies by Tolbert and colleagues (2000) showed no injury despite mean arterial blood pressure of 160 to 180 mm Hg for at least five months. These investigators attributed the protection against renal injury to increased afferent arteriolar resistance. Glomerular sclerosis is present, although at modest levels at 18 months of age with less than 10% of glomeruli expressing any level of sclerosis (Fortepiani *et al.*, 2003).

A variation of the SHR is the SHR stroke-prone (SHRSP) rat. These animals develop malignant hypertension and die within several weeks due to stroke. They would not be conducive for aging studies.

Female SHR: A model of postmenopausal hypertension. The elucidation of mechanisms responsible for postmenopausal hypertension has been stunted by lack of an animal model (Reckelhoff and Fortepiani, 2004). Most of the studies in postmenopausal women have been correlative. Sheep, rabbits, nonhuman primates, rats, and mice have been used as models of various menopausal changes. However, to our knowledge, there have been few studies in which a naturally occurring animal model of postmenopausal hypertension has been described. The female SHR is an exception to this.

Throughout their reproductive lives, female SHR have mean arterial pressures that are 25 to 30 mm Hg lower than male SHR, although they are quite hypertensive compared to normotensive rats (Reckelhoff and Fortepiani, 2004). When female SHR stop estrous cycling at 10 to 12 months of age, the blood pressure begins to increase such that by 16 months of age, the mean arterial pressure is similar or even higher than in males of similar ages. This makes the aging female SHR a good model for the study of postmenopausal hypertension. Most models of postmenopausal changes are performed in young animals that have been ovariectomized, which removes the factor of "aging" from the studies. However, if female SHR are ovariectomized at a young age, there is no increase in their blood pressure as they age. If females are ovariectomized at nine months of age or after cessation of estrous cycling, their blood pressure either does not increase or actually falls compared to intact females. These data suggest that there is some factor produced by the ovary that impacts the blood pressure in the aging intact female SHR. However, this makes the aged, ovariectomized female SHR a poor model of postmenopausal hypertension.

The aging female SHRs are protected against target organ damage compared to males. Despite similar or higher blood pressure in aging females compared to males, they exhibit less renal injury (glomerular sclerosis) or protein excretion than age-matched males. Left ventricular hypertrophy is greater in the female SHR, however, but this may be an important compensatory mechanism due to the hypertension that is absent in the males.

The mechanisms responsible for the hypertension in the aging female SHR are related to the endothelin system, which is not the case in aging male SHRs. Blockade of the endothelin ET_A receptor reduces blood pressure in aging female SHRs, but not aging males nor in young females (Yanes *et al.*, 2004). In contrast the RAS seems to play a more important role in maintenance of the hypertension in the aging male SHR than females. Treatment of aging male and female SHRs with an angiotensin AT1 receptor antagonist causes a greater reduction in blood pressure in males than females. In addition, angiotensinogen protein expression in kidneys of males is several fold higher than in females. The data suggest that the RAS is up-regulated in aging male SHRs, but not females (Yanes and Reckelhoff, unpublished data).

Advantages and disadvantages of use. The aging SHR is a good model in which to study the effects of chronic hypertension in aging, and in the case of females, to study a model of postmenopausal hypertension. One disadvantage of the model is that they fail to gain a considerable amount of weight, as other rats do. The females are typically 300 and 350 g at 18 months, whereas the males are typically 400 to 450 g at that age. Therefore, for investigators studying aging, metabolic syndrome, and hypertension, these animals would not be appropriate.

Similarly, because the renal vasculature is protected against age-related injury, the SHR is not an appropriate model in which to study chronic renal injury. There are several normotensive rat models that develop considerably more glomerular sclerosis with normal aging than do the SHR.

Dahl salt-sensitive rats

Males. There are a significant number of individuals who are hypertensive who have low plasma renin activity, but whose blood pressure increases further when they ingest salt. Certain populations, such as African-Americans and the elderly, are more susceptible to development of salt-sensitive hypertension. The Dahl salt-sensitive rat is a commonly used model of salt-sensitive hypertension. Typical rat chow is 1% salt, and diets of 0.1 to 0.4% are considered low-salt diets. Dahl salt-sensitive rats (DS) exhibit an increase in blood pressure when placed on 1% salt or higher. Many investigators use 2 to 8% salt diets in order to invoke the hypertension. Along with the hypertension, the rats develop significant renal injury, heart failure, and inflammation within three to six weeks of being placed on high-salt diet.

The determination of an appropriate control for the DS is controversial. There is a Dahl salt-resistant rat (DR) that is used by some investigators as a control. These rats do not exhibit an increase in blood pressure when placed on high-salt diet. However, genetic studies have shown that the DR is no more similar to the DS than is another normotensive strain, such as the Brown Norway rat or the Sprague Dawley rat. These normotensive rats also fail to develop an increase in blood pressure when placed on a high-salt diet.

The mechanisms responsible for the salt-sensitive hypertension in DS rats include reductions in nitric oxide (NO) and increased oxidative stress. Sanders and colleagues (1996) reported several years ago that treatment of DS rats with L-arginine, the precursor for NO, protects against salt-sensitive hypertension (Sanders, 1996). Manning and colleagues also reported that giving tempol, the superoxide scavenger, attenuates the development of hypertension in DS rats, but has no effect on blood pressure in DR on a high-salt diet, suggesting a role for oxidative stress in the hypertension (Meng *et al.*, 2003). Taken together these data suggest that superoxide may be responsible for the reduction in NO availability in DS rats since superoxide is capable of scavenging NO leading to vasoconstriction and production of another potent oxidant, peroxynitrite, which has been shown to up-regulate vasoconstrictors and down-regulate vasodilators due to its ability to nitrotyrosinate proteins.

Endothelin also plays a role in the development of salt-sensitive hypertension in DS rats, since DS rats given endothelin ET_A receptor antagonists are resistant to increases in blood pressure when placed on high-salt diet (Kassab *et al.*, 1998). It is also possible that increased endothelin activity in the DS rat could be responsible for the increase in oxidative stress found in this rat model.

Because a high-salt diet is associated with reductions in renin release and thereby reductions in angiotensin II, the role that the RAS plays in mediating salt-sensitive hypertension is controversial. Navar and colleagues have measured angiotensin II in kidneys of DS and have found that when placed on a high-salt diet, the intrarenal angiotensin II levels do not change as the plasma renin activity does, suggesting an inappropriate level of angiotensin II for the level of salt and volume. Therefore, it is possible that the intrarenal RAS could play a role in the hypertension in DS rats on a high-salt diet. However, calcium channel blockers have been shown to attenuate the hypertension in DS rats on a high-salt diet better than either angiotensin converting enzyme inhibitors or AT1 receptor antagonists.

There is a paucity of aging studies in the DS rat. Mainly, investigators use these rats to study age-related changes in the brain. However, many so-called aging studies are in rats aged 20 weeks or less. The work of Hinojosa-Laborde and colleagues is an exception, as discussed next.

Female DS rats—Model of postmenopausal hypertension. Hinojosa-Laborde and colleagues were the first to maintain DS rats on a low-salt (0.3%) diet as they aged and followed changes in blood pressure (Maric *et al.*, 2004). Just like many other rat strains that exhibit sex differences in hypertension, the DS females on low-salt diets have slightly higher blood pressure than do males when they are young. Ovariectomy of the females causes a significant increase in blood pressure even when rats are kept on low-salt diets. With aging, however, the blood pressure in all groups of rats increases even on low-salt diets. Eventually males develop higher blood pressure than do females. However, ovariectomized females remain more hypertensive than the other sexes. Estradiol treatment of the ovariectomized females reduces their blood pressure to the levels found in intact females. Thus, the aging DS rat is a good model in which to study postmenopausal hypertension.

Advantages and disadvantages of use. The use of the DS rat as a model of salt-sensitive hypertension and/or renal injury is attractive since the hypertension develops rapidly and the renal injury is present by three to four weeks. However, the fact that aging DS rats develop increases in blood pressure even when kept on low-salt diets may make them a difficult aging animal model with which to work. The ovariectomized rats do not live past 14 months of age, and the intact females do not live more than 15 to 16 months of age (personal communication, Dr. C. Hinojosa-Laborde). Whether males live longer is not clear from Dr. Hinojosa-Laborde's work, since she mainly focuses on aging females, but this is doubtful. The fact that the rats die at an early age may explain why there is a paucity of data in aging DS rats.

NONGENETIC MODELS OF HYPERTENSION

In addition to the common genetic models of hypertension discussed earlier, there are also nongenetic models in which the hypertension is caused by infusion of a drug or by dietary manipulations or by placing a clip on the renal artery. The following is a list of such models.

DOCA and salt model in aging animals

This model of hypertension is a model of mineralocorticoid hypertension developed by implanting the rats with deoxycorticosterone acetate (DOCA) pellets (typically 100 mg) and treating them with salt water (1%). This is another model of salt-sensitive hypertension. The hypertension develops rapidly, usually within a week of the DOCA being implanted. The systems that mediate the hypertension include oxidative stress since antioxidants reduce the blood pressure (Elhaimeur *et al.*, 2002). Agonists of serotonin receptor 5HT1A and antagonists of serotonin receptor 5HT2B reduce the blood pressure in DOCA-salt treated rats, implicating serotonin in the hypertension (Shingala and Balaraman 2005). In addition, blockade of the endothelin ET_A receptor also protects against the increase in blood pressure (Callera *et al.*, 2003). Blockade of the renin-angiotensin system (RAS), however, does not reduce blood pressure, as might be expected due to the reduction in renin release with the high-salt diet.

Infusion of low-dose Ang II in aging animals

The infusion of a low dose (i.e., subpressor doses) of angiotensin II leads to hypertension that develops over approximately three to four days. The hypertension then is maintained at a stable level until approximately two weeks later, when another increase in blood pressure develops that plateaus within a few days (Hennington *et al.*, 1998). The exact mechanism by which the second increase in blood pressure occurs is not clear.

In normotensive rats, angiotensin II induced hypertension can be produced by infusing Ang II at as little as 5 ng/kg/min when the endogenous RAS is blocked with converting enzyme inhibitors. If the endogenous system is not blocked, a higher dose of Ang II (50–80 ng/kg/min) is required. However, as the endogenous system is blocked by negative feedback caused by the Ang II infusion, the amount of Ang II necessary to maintain the hypertension progressively falls to that required to cause hypertension in endogenously blocked RAS rats. Similar findings have been made in mice, although mice require significantly more Ang II to cause a sustained increase in their blood pressure (600–1000 ng/kg/min).

The mechanisms responsible for the increase in blood pressure with low-dose Ang II are oxidative stress and endothelin activation (Reckelhoff and Romero, 2003). Treatment of animals with antioxidants attenuates the hypertensive response to Ang II. In addition, nonspecific blockade or specific blockade of the endothelin ET_A receptor attenuates the hypertensive response to Ang II. It is likely that endothelin may stimulate oxidative stress since Ortiz and colleagues reported that treatment of Ang II infused rats with the superoxide scavenger, tempol, reduced blood pressure and oxidative stress, but failed to reduce plasma endothelin (Reckelhoff and Romero, 2003).

Studies in humans and animals have shown that aging may be associated with increased sensitivity of the cardiovascular and renal systems to Ang II. Acute infusion of Ang II is a common maneuver in aging humans, but chronic infusion of Ang II is performed only in animals.

Dietary-induced hypertension

Fat-fed rats—Obesity-induced hypertension. There is an epidemic in obesity that is occurring throughout the developed countries of the world. The mechanisms responsible for metabolic syndrome and the target organ injury associated with the complications of metabolic syndrome, such as type II diabetes, sleep apnea, end stage renal disease, and heart failure, are a major research focus today. Not all models of obesity are associated with elevated blood pressure. Why this is the case is also not clear at the present time.

The model of obesity-induced hypertension has been produced in dogs for years by feeding them a high-fat diet. However, only recently has a model of obesity and hypertension due to a high-fat diet been obtained in rats. Dobrian and colleagues have succeeded in producing a model of obesity in Sprague Dawley rats by feeding them 32% Kcal fat and 0.8% NaCl for 10 weeks (Dobrian *et al.*, 2001). After 10 weeks, half the rats develop obesity (the so-called obese prone (OP) rats) whereas the other half do not (the so-called obese resistant (OR) rats). Typically, the OP rats weigh approximately 660 g compared to 540 g in OR rats. Control Sprague Dawley rats untreated with high-fat diets of similar ages exhibit similar weight as the OR rats. The OP rats develop mild hypertension and increased leptin levels. They also have increased plasma renin activity, an index of stimulated RAS. In addition, the rats have increased F2-isoprostanes, an index of oxidative stress, and renal injury. There have been no aging studies published with this model.

Fructose-fed rat—Model of insulin resistance and hypertension without obesity. The fructose-fed rat develops insulin resistance, increased triglycerides and glucose, and hypertension when approximately 60% of their diets contain fructose (Girard *et al.*, 2005). Rats typically are treated for six to nine weeks before developing hypertension. The rats develop end organ damage of various types, and there is a sex difference in the development of hypertension, with only males becoming hypertensive despite the females becoming insulin resistant. This is a model that could lend itself to aging studies since aging normotensive rats could be given fructose with the expectation that they would become mildly hypertensive and insulin resistant within a few weeks.

Renovascular hypertension (2 kidney, 1 clip, or Goldblatt model)

The typical method for producing renovascular hypertension is by placing a silver clip on the renal artery of one kidney in rats and as they grow, the clip will cause a renal stenosis (Pipinos *et al.*, 1998). The contralateral kidney becomes hypertrophied. The pressure in the clipped kidney is low due to the clip, whereas the pressure in the contralateral kidney is high due to the hypertension that develops. In the early phases, the blood pressure increases due to the release of renin from the clipped kidney. Oxidative stress also plays a role in the hypertension. Endothelin has been shown to be involved in the cardiac damage associated with renovascular hypertension, but not in the renal injury.

The Goldblatt model of hypertension is difficult to use since the hypertension is inconsistently produced. Even with rats of the same weight, the same size clip will cause moderate hypertension in some rats, but malignant hypertension in others (personal communication, Dr. William Beierwaltes). Whether this model could be reproduced in aging rats is not clear since the clips usually are placed in young animals, and as they grow, the renal vasoconstriction is produced. It is also not clear what the survival time would be for rats with 2-kidney, 1-clip maneuver that developed hypertension and were allowed to age.

The model of reduced renal mass (5/6 ablation model)

The model of renal ablation typically is produced by the removal of the right kidney and either the ligation of two of the three renal arteries on the left in the rat or the removal of the poles of the left kidney. Within days to a few weeks, this model develops hypertension and severe glomerulosclerosis. The renin-angiotensin system has been shown to play a role, but oxidative stress is likely to be involved as well (Sandberg and Ji, 2000). The endothelin system and reductions in NO are also involved. In addition, there is a component of the immune system involved in the hypertension in rats in the renal artery ligation model, but not in the model in which the renal tissue is removed. The model of renal ablation is one that could be reproduced in aging rats. There is only one aging study to our knowledge using this model, and the rats were studied 28 weeks after ablation was performed at approximately 34 to 36 weeks of age.

TRANSGENIC MODELS OF HYPERTENSION

The use of transgenic animal models to study the role that specific genes play in causing hypertension has been a focus of much research. However, to our knowledge there are no studies in which the mice were allowed to age. With the exception of a few models that are severely hypertensive and will not survive more than a few weeks or months, the lack of data in aging hypertensive transgenics likely reflects the specific interest of the investigators who developed the strains; that is, the animals were developed to answer a question not involving aging. Following we describe the most common transgenic hypertensive strains.

Models transgenic for genes of the renin-angiotensin system

TGR(mREN2)27. TGR(mREN2)27 is the first rat model of hypertension caused by a defined genetic defect. The TGR(mREN2)27 harbors the murine *Ren-2* gene on the genetic background of the SD rat. These transgenic rats develop fulminant hypertension at an early age despite low levels of renin in plasma and kidney. High expression of the renin transgene in extrarenal tissues is associated with increased local formation of angiotensin II, which suggests that activated extrarenal RAS might be responsible for the hypertensive phenotype. In heterozygous animals, hypertension is evident at four to five weeks of age, reaching maximum values at eight to nine weeks (systolic BP: 240 mmHg in males and 200 mmHg in females). The phase of established hypertension is followed by a decrease in blood pressure by 20 to 30 mmHg in male and 40 to 60 mmHg in female TGR(mREN2)27 between 20 and 24 weeks of age. At 42 weeks of age, the male TGR(mREN2)27 are hypertensive, whereas blood pressure levels in female transgenic rats are not different from those found in age-matched SD rats (Lee *et al.*, 1996).

TGR(hAOGEN-hREN). The TGR(hAOGEN-hREN) is a model of high human renin hypertension in the rat. This strain resulted from a cross between transgenic rats harboring human angiotensinogen gene and human renin gene, respectively. The offspring from this cross harbor both transgenes and have all the necessary components of the human renin angiotensin system to generate angiotensin II. The TGR(hAOGEN-hREN) rats have severe hypertension and hypertensive end-organ damage and die after about eight weeks, unless treated with converting enzyme inhibitors. Although useful for pharmacological investigation of the human renin angiotensin system, this rat model is not well suited for aging studies, due to their short survival (Bohlender *et al.*, 1997).

Mice transgenic for both human renin and angiotensinogen genes. Sigmund *et al.* developed transgenic mice expressing both human renin and angiotensinogen genes that are markedly hypertensive and exhibit high plasma concentrations of angiotensin II (Sigmund *et al.*, 1992). These animals also display hypertensive end-organ damage and endothelial dysfunction. Transgenic mice harboring an artificial chromosome encoding human renin together with the next upstream and downstream genes in order to ensure appropriate regulation of the renin transgene display a modest increase in blood pressure when crossed with human angiotensinogen-expressing mice. These data show that even small amounts of renin could cleave increased amounts of angiotensinogen producing hypertension. To our knowledge, no aging studies have been performed using these animals.

Models transgenic for genes of the endothelin system. Elevated plasma endothelin concentrations have been associated with several cardiovascular diseases, including hypertension. A mouse model overexpressing endothelin-1 gene under the control of its own promoter has been characterized. These transgenic mice exhibit two-fold increases in endothelin-1 concentration in plasma, aorta, heart, kidney, and intestine. Although the blood pressure and kidney morphology and function are normal in young (8 weeks old) transgenic mice, with aging (12–14 months old) they develop renal injury with glomerulosclerosis and interstitial fibrosis (Hocher *et al.*, 1997). In addition, Shindo *et al.* showed that salt-sensitive hypertension develops with aging in these mice, perhaps secondary to nephron loss (Shindo *et al.*, 2002). This model therefore might be useful for the study of the permissive role of the aging process on the endothelin-induced renal pathology and hypertension. However, there are currently no data using aging ET-1 overexpression mice.

Other transgenic models

The follitropin receptor knockout mouse (FORKO)—Model of postmenopausal hypertension. A genetic model of estrogen deficiency recently has been characterized for the study of menopausal hypertension. The FORKO mice exhibit a reduced production of estrogen due to the genetic inactivation of FSH receptors (Dierich *et al.*, 1998). These mice have ovarian insufficiency, low estrogen levels with functionally active estrogen receptors, and increased testosterone levels. They also show osteoporosis, hypercholesterolemia, and weight gain consistent with the postmenopausal pathology in women. The FORKO mice have significantly elevated systolic and diastolic blood pressure at 14 to 16 weeks of age, as measured by telemetry (Javeshghani *et al.*, 2003). Hypertension in this model is paralleled by vascular remodeling and altered contractile responses to angiotensin II. The mechanisms of altered blood pressure regulation in the FORKO mice are not clear and might involve both estrogen deficiency and increased testosterone levels. There are no aging studies in these animals as yet.

Glial cell-line-derived neurotrophic factor heterozygotes (GDNF)—Model of reduced renal glomeruli. It has been hypothesized that low nephron number is a risk factor for the development of cardiovascular disease including hypertension. The GDNF has been shown to play a major role in kidney development (Treanor *et al.*, 1996). Although homozygous null mutants for GDNF show bilateral renal agenesis and die shortly after birth, the heterozygous mice are fertile and viable but have a 30% reduction in the nephron endowment at 30 days of age, as compared to the wild-type controls (Pichel *et al.*, 1996). The study of Cullen-McEwen *et al.* (2003) shows that at 14 months of age, the GDNF heterozygous mice have elevated blood pressure but preserved renal function as measured by GFR and RBF. These mice also display glomerular hypertrophy, probably due to the compensatory hyperfiltration. Therefore, the GDNF heterozygous mouse may be a useful tool to study the lifelong consequences of reduced nephron number on the development of hypertension.

Conclusion

There are several animal models of hypertension that would be conducive for aging studies. These include genetic models and nongenetic models of hypertension and transgenic models that exhibit hypertension. However, some of the genetically hypertensive models, such as the SHRSP and the Dahl salt-sensitive rats, have limited life spans that make them inappropriate for aging studies. Transgenic rats and mice are novel models in which to study specific systems known to be responsible for hypertension. However, there are very few aging studies in hypertensive transgenic animals, and whether these transgenics prove to be good models of aging and hypertension remains to be determined experimentally.

Recommended Resources

Guyton, A.C., Coleman, T.G., Cowley, A.W., Jr., Scheel, K.W., Manning, R.D., and Norman, R.A. (1972). Arterial pressure regulation: Overriding dominance of the kidneys in long-term regulation and in hypertension. *Am. J. Med.* 52, 584–594.

Hall, J.E., Brands, M.J., and Henegar, J.R. (1999). Angiotensin II and long-term arterial pressure regulation: The overriding dominance of the kidney. *J. Am. Soc. Nephrol.* 10, S258–S265.

Hall, J.E., Mizelle, H.L., Hildebrandt, D.A., and Brands, M.W. (1990). Abnormal pressure-natriuresis: A cause or a consequence of hypertension. *Hypertension* 15, 547–559.

Pryor, W.A. and Squadrito, G.L. (1995). The chemistry of peroxinitrite: A product from the reaction of nitric oxide with superoxide. *Am. J. Physiol.* 268, L699–L722.

Reckelhoff, J.F. (2001). Gender differences in the regulation of blood pressure. *Hypertension* 37, 1199–1208.

Reckelhoff, J. and Fortepiani, L. (2004). Novel mechanisms responsible for postmenopausal hypertension. *Hypertension* 43, 918–923.

Reckelhoff, J.F. and Romero, J.C. (2003). Role of oxidative stess in angiotensin-induced hypertension. *Am. J. Physiol. Regul. Integr. Comp. Physiol.* 284, R893–R912.

Sandberg, K. and Ji, H. (2000). Kidney angiotensin receptors and their role in renal pathophysiology. *Semin. Nephrol.* 20, 402–416.

ACKNOWLEDGMENTS

The authors wish to acknowledge the support of the National Institutes of Health HL66072, HL69194, and HL05197.

REFERENCES

Alexander, B. T., Cockrell, K.L., Rinewalt, A.N., Herrington, J.N., and Granger J.P. (2001). Enhanced renal expression of preproendothelin mRNA during chronic angiotensin II hypertension. *Am. J. Physiol. 280*, R1388–R1392.

Bohlender, J., Fukamizu, A., Lippoldt, A., Nomura, T., Dietz, R., Menard, J. *et al.* (1997). High human renin hypertension in transgenic rats. *Hypertension 29*, 428–434.

Brown, N. (2005). Aldosterone and end-organ damage. *Curr. Opin. Nephrol. Hypertens. 14*, 235–241.

Burry, K.A. (2002). Risks and benefits of estrogen plus progestin in healthy postmenopausal women. Principal results from the Women's Health Initiative randomized controlled trial. *Curr. Womens Health Rep. 2*, 331–332.

Callera, G., Touyz, R., Teixeira, S., Muscara, M., Carvalho, M.H., Fortes, Z. *et al.* (2003). ETA receptor blockade decreases vascular superoxide generation in DOCA-salt hypertension. *Hypertension 42*, 811–817.

Cullen-McEwen, L., Kett, M., Dowling, J., Anderson, W., and Bertram J. (2003). Nephron number, renal function, and arterial pressure in aged GDNF heterozygous mice. *Hypertension 41*, 335–340.

Curtis, J.J., Luke, H.P., Dustan, H.P., Kashgarian, M., Whelchel, J.D., Jones, P. *et al.* (1983). Remission of hypertension after renal transplantation. *N. Engl. J. Med. 309*, 1009–1015.

Dierich, A., Sairam, M., Monaco, L., Fimia, G., Gansmuller, A., LeMeur, M. *et al.* (1998). Impairing follicle-stimulating hormone (FSH) signaling in vivo: Targeted disruption of the FSH receptor leads to aberrant gametogenesis and hormonal imbalance. *Proc. Natl. Acad. Sci. USA 95*, 13612–13617.

Dobrian, A.D., Davies, M.J., Schriver, S.D., Lauterio, T.J. and Prewitt, R.L. (2001). Oxidative stress in a rat model of obesity-induced hypertension. *Hypertension 37 (Suppl.)*, 554–555.

Duerrschmidt, N., Wippich, N., Goettsch, W., Broemme, H.J., and Morawietz, H. (2000). Endothelin-1 induces NAD(P)H oxidase in human endothelial cells. *Biochem. Biophys. Res. Comm. 269*, 713–717.

Elhaimeur, F., Courderot-Masuyer, C., Nicod, L., Guyon, C., Richert, L., and Berthelot, A. (2002). Dietary vitamin C supplementation decreases blood pressure in DOCA-salt hypertensive male Sprague-Dawley rats and this is associated with increased liver oxidative stress. *Mol. Cell. Biochem. 237*, 77–83.

Esler, M., Rumantir, M., Wiesner, G., Kaye, D., Hastings, J., and Lambert, G. (2001). Sympathetic nervous system and insulin resistance. From obesity to diabetes. *Am. J. Hypertension 14*, 304S–309S.

Fortepiani, L., Yanes, L., Zhang, H., Racusen, L.C., and Reckelhoff, J.F. (2003). Role of androgens in mediating renal injury in aging SHR. *Hypertension 42*, 952–955.

Girard, A., Madani, S., Boustani, E.E., Belleville, J., and Prost, J. (2005). Changes in lipid metabolism and antioxidant defense status in spontaneously hypertensive rats and Wistar rats fed a diet enriched with fructose and saturated fatty acids. *Nutrition 21*, 240–248.

Guyton, A.C., Coleman, T.G., Cowley, Jr., A.W., Scheel, K.W., Manning, R.D., Jr., and Norman, R.A. (1972). Arterial pressure regulation: Overriding dominance of the kidneys in long-term regulation and in hypertension. *Am. J. Med. 52*, 584–594.

Hall, J.E., Brands, M.J., and Henegar, J.R. (1999). Angiotensin II and long-term arterial pressure regulation: The overriding dominance of the kidney. *J. Am. Soc. Nephrol. 10*, S258–S265.

Hall, J.E., Mizelle, H.L., Hildebrandt, D.A., and Brands, M. W. (1990). Abnormal pressure-natriuresis: A cause or a consequence of hypertension. *Hypertension 15*, 547–559.

Harrap, S.B., Wang, B.Z., and MacClellan, D.G. (1992). Renal transplantation between male and female spontaneously hypertensive rats. *Hypertension 19*, 431–434.

Hennington, B.S., Zhang, H., Miller, M.T., Granger, J.P., and Reckelhoff, J.F. (1998). Angiotensin II stimulates synthesis of endothelial nitric oxide synthase. *Hypertension 31*, 283–288.

Hocher, B., Thonereineke, C., Rohmeiss, P., Schmager, F., Slowinski, T., Burst, V. *et al.* (1997). Endothelin 1 transgenic mice develop glomerulosclerosis, interstitial fibrosis, and renal cysts but not hypertension. *J. Clin. Invest. 99*, 1380–1389.

James, G.D., Sealey, J.E., Muller, F., Alderman, M., Madhavan, S., and Laragh, J.H. (1986). Renin relationship to sex, race and age in normotensive population. *J. Hyperten. 4 (Suppl 5)*, S387–S389.

Javeshghani, D., Touyz, R., Sairam, M., Virdis, A., Neves, M., and Schiffrin, E.L. (2003). Attenuated responses to angiotensin II in follitropin receptor knockout mice, a model of menopause-associated hypertension. *Hypertension 42*, 761–767.

Kassab, S., Miller, M., Novak, J., Reckelhoff, J.F., Clower, B., and Granger, J.P. (1998). Endothelin-A receptor antagonism attenuates the hypertension and renal injury in Dahl salt-sensitive rats. *Hypertension 31*, 397–402.

Lee, M., Bohm, M., Paul, M., Bader, M., Ganten, U., and Ganten, D. (1996). Physiological characterization of the hypertensive transgenic rat TGR(mREN2)27. *Am. J. Physiol. 270*, E919–E929.

Maric, C., Hinojosa-Laborde, C., and Sandberg, K. (2004). Glomerulosclerosis and tubulointerstitial fibrosis are attenuated with 17beta-estradiol in the aging Dahl salt sensitive rat. *J. Am. Soc. Nephrol. 15*, 1546–1556.

Meng, S., Cason, G., Gannon, A., Racusen, L.C., and Manning, R.D., Jr. (2003). Oxidative stress in Dahl salt-sensitive hypertension. *Hypertension 41*, 1346–1352.

Mollnau, H., Wendt, M., Szocs, K., Lassegue, B., Schulz, E., Oelze, M. *et al.* (2002). Effects of angiotensin II infusion on the expression and function of NAD(P)H oxidase and components of nitric oxide/cGMP signaling. *Circ. Res. 90*, E58–65.

Ng, A., Callister, R., Johnson, D., and Seals, D. (1993). Age and gender influence muscle sympathetic nerve activity at rest in healthy humans. *Hypertension 21*, 498–503.

Pichel, J., Shen, L., Sheng, H., Granholm, A., Drago, J., Grinberg, A. *et al.* (1996). GDNF is required for kidney development and enteric innervation. *Cold Spring Harb. Symp. Quant. Biol. 61*, 445–457.

Pipinos, I., Nypaver, T., Moshin, S., Careterro, O.A., and Beierwaltes, W. (1998). Response to angiotensin inhibition in rats with sustained renovascular hypertension correlates with response to removing renal artery stenosis. *J. Vasc. Surg. 28(1)*, 167–177.

Powledge, T. (2004). NIH terminates WHI oestrogen-only study. *Lancet 363*, 870.

Pryor, W.A. and Squadrito, G.L. (1995). The chemistry of peroxinitrite: A product from the reaction of nitric oxide with superoxide. *Am. J. Physiol. 268*, L699–L722.

Reckelhoff, J.F. and Fortepiani, L.A. (2004). Novel mechanisms responsible for postmenopausal hypertension. *Hypertension 43*, 918–923.

Reckelhoff, J.F. and Romero, J.C. (2003). Role of oxidative stress in angiotensin-induced hypertension. *Am. J. Physiol. Regul. Integr. Comp. Physiol. 284*, R893–R912.

Reckelhoff, J.F. (2001). Gender differences in the regulation of blood pressure. *Hypertension 37*, 1199–1208.

Rettig, R. (1993). Does the kidney play a role in the aetiology of primary hypertension? Evidence from renal transplantation studies in rats and humans. *J. Hum. Hypertens. 7*, 177–180.

Sandberg, K. and Ji, H. (2000). Kidney angiotensin receptors and their role in renal pathophysiology. *Semin. Nephrol. 20*, 402–416.

Sanders, P. (1996). Salt-sensitive hypertension: Lessons from animal models. *Am. J. Kidney Dis. 26*, 775–782.

Seals, D. and Esler, M. (2000). Human ageing and the sympathoadrenal system. *J. Physiol. 528.3*, 407–417.

Shindo, T., Kurihara, H., Maemura, K., Kurihara, Y., Ueda, O., Suzuki, H. *et al.* (2002). Renal damage and salt-dependent hypertension in aged transgenic mice overexpressing endothelin-1. *J. Mol. Med. 80*, 105–116.

Shingala, J. and Balaraman, R. (2005). Antihypertensive effect of 5-HT1A agonist buspirone and 5-HT2B antagonists in experimentally induced hypertension in rats. *Pharmacology 73*, 129–139.

Sigmund, C., Jones, C., Kane, C., Wu, C., Lang, J., and Gross, K. (1992). Regulated tissue- and cell-specific expression of the human renin gene in transgenic mice. *Circ. Res. 70*, 1070–1079.

Tolbert, E.M., Weisstuch, J., Feiner, H.D., and Dworkin, L.D. (2000). Onset of glomerular hypertension with aging precedes injury in the spontaneously hypertensive rat. *Am. J. Physiol. Renal Physiol. 278*, F839–F846.

Treanor, J., Goodman, L., Sauvage, F.D., Stone, D., Poulsen, K., Beck, C. *et al.* (1996). Characterization of a multicomponent receptor for GDNF. *Nature 382*, 80–83.

The writing group for the PEPI trial. (1995). Effects of estrogen or estrogen/progestin regimens on heart disease risk factors in postmenopausal women. The Postmenopausal Estrogen/Progestin Interventions (PEPI) Trial. *JAMA 273*, 199–208.

van Kesteren, P.J., Kooistra, T., Lansink, M., van Kamp, G.J., Asscheman, H., Gooren, L.J. *et al.* (1998). The effects of sex steroids on plasma levels of marker proteins of endothelial cell functioning. *Thromb. Haemost. 79*, 1029–1033.

Weinberger, M.H. and Fineberg, N.S. (1991). Sodium and volume sensitivity of blood pressure. Age and pressure change over time. *Hypertension 18*, 67–71.

Wilkins, F.C., Alberola, A., Mizelle, H.L., Opgenorth, T.J., and Granger, J.P. (1995). Systemic hemodynamics and renal function during long-term pathophysiological increases in circulating endothelin. *Am. J. Physiol. 268*, 375–381.

Yanes, L.L., Romero, D., Cucchiarelli, V.E., Fortepiani, L.A., Gomez-Sanchez, C., Santacruz, F. *et al.* (2005). Role of endothelin in mediating postmenopausal hypertension in a rat model. *Am. J. Physiol. Reg. Integ. Comp. Physiol. 288*, R229–R233.

Glossary

5-alpha reductase: Enzyme catalyzing the production of dihydrotestosterone from testosterone. Two types of this enzyme are known. Type II is found in high concentrations in prostatic stroma.

8-OHdG: 8-hydroxydeoxyguanosine, an oxidized nucleoside of DNA.

24-hour rhythm: The periodical pattern of sleep (rest) at night and wakefulness (activity) in the daytime.

25th percentile survival point: When lifespan is compared in respect to aging, the 25th or 10th percentile survival point is a better index than the 50th percentile survival point or mean lifespan, because experientially the median or mean value of lifespan is known to often fluctuate from the effects of experimental intervention for diseases or specific causes of death in a strain of rodents.

ABR: Auditory brainstem response; physiological recordings.

Ach: Acetylcholine; cochlear efferent neurotransmitter.

Activation-induced cell death: T-cell apoptosis as opposed to growth, under certain conditions, caused by stimuli that would otherwise result in cell division.

Activity theory: Proposes that individuals who age successfully maintain regular activities, roles, and social pursuits into old age.

Advance directive: Directions given by an individual intended to guide future decisions about medical treatment in case of incapacitation.

Advance directive for research: A legal document executed by a decisionally capable person that authorizes their enrollment in research studies for the time the person lacks decision-making capacity.

Ageism: Process of systematic stereotyping and discrimination against people because they are old.

AGE: Advanced glycosylation end-product, or the potentially harmful compounds produced through glycosylative and glycoxidative reactions. AGEs have been hypothesized to be responsible for damage to cells and tissues and to contribute to aging-related diseases.

Aggrecan: A large aggregating glycosaminoglycan, mainly found in articular cartilage.

Aging: In models of systems failure, aging is defined as a phenomenon of increasing risk of failure with age of a system.

Agreeableness: The personality trait of being warm, generous, and helpful.

ALCAR: Acetyl-carnitine; an anti-apoptotic drug.

Allate/Deallate: Queens and males with wings are called allates. After the mating flight, the queens remove their wings and are called deallate females.

Allele: One or two or more alternate forms of a gene that have the same locus on homologous chromosomes and are responsible for alternative traits; some alleles are dominant over others.

Allocentric: Spatial references made on the basis of external cues or landmarks in the surrounding environment.

Allogeneic cells: Cells recognized as non-self, due to their expression of "foreign" transplantation antigens.

Allostasis: The ability of a system to dynamically adopt varying states in order to accommodate changing demands. It is a dynamic regulatory process that allows organisms to respond to the challenges of their environment ("stability through change"). An example would be a rise in epinephrine release in response to exercise, stress, or perceived danger. This should be followed by a fall of epinephrine release during relaxation.

Allostatic Load: Cumulative changes that reflect either continued operation of the allostatic state or overactivation of allostatic responses.

Alpha (α) level: See Significance level.

AMD: Age-related macular degeneration; a dangerous illness of the human retina.

AMP kinase or AMP-activated protein kinase (AMPK): AMPK is stimulated by elevated AMP/ATP ratios; thus AMPK plays a role in monitoring cellular energy status and eliciting cellular response when ATP levels are diminished.

Amygdala: A rounded lobule on the undersurface of each cerebellar hemisphere, continuous medially with the uvula of the cerebellar vermis.

Amyloid: A term originally referring to starch-like histological staining properties, now used to refer to insoluble fibrils of proteins folded into cross-β-sheet secondary structure.

Analytic epidemiology: The study of the determinants of disease or reasons for high or low frequency of disease in specific groups.

Andropause: The decline in T levels with aging when associated with symptoms and signs of androgen deficiency.

Aneuploidy: Any imbalance in the normal number of chromosomes, or in the number of chromosome sets (normal, 2 sets).

Angiogenesis: The process in which new blood vessels are formed via endothelial capillary sprouting from existing vascular beds.

ANN: Advanced or artificial neural network bioinformatics pattern-detection computer programs, which can be iteratively trained to associate complex patterns with a given state or diagnosis.

Annual fish: Fish present in hot ponds of South America and Africa, having an average lifespan of one year.

ANOVA: Analysis of variance.

Antagonistic pleiotropy: An aging theory, which argues that genes that confer benefits early in life may be selected for, even if those genes cause increased senescence later in life.

Anthropomorphic: The attribution of human characteristics, traits, and emotions to nonhuman animals.

Antioxidant: substance that inhibits oxidation and protects against the effects of free radicals.

AP: Antero-posterior.

Apneic episode: Cessation of breathing for 10 or more seconds during sleep.

Apoptosis: Programmed cell death.

Aromatase: Enzyme catalyzing the irreversible aromatization of testosterone to estradiol.

Artificial enteral feeding: All techniques permitting partial or total nutritional support in subjects incapable of spontaneously absorbing a sufficient nutritional input.

Assent: Authorization that only partially meets the standards of informed consent because it is given by a person whose capacity to understand and judge is somewhat impaired, but who is able to express a preference or choice.

Astrocyte: A small, star-shaped cell of the nervous system that provides nutrients, support, and insulation for neurons.

A–T: Ataxia–telangiectasia.

Atherosclerotic: The process of arteriosclerosis in which deposits of yellowing plaques (atheromas) containing cholesterol, other lipoid material, and lipophages are formed within the intima of large and medium-sized arteries.

ATM: A human DNA damage responsive kinase that acts early in the response to DSBs to activate the checkpoint that pauses the cell cycle. Cells lacking ATM will synthesize DNA in S-phase after being exposed to ionizing radiation that causes DSBs, while cells with ATM will not. ATM is an ortholog of budding yeast *TEL1* and plays a role in telomere function in human cells. ATM stands for ataxia telangiactasia mutated from the human disease that identified the gene.

ATP: Adenosine triphosphate; the nucleotide known in biochemistry as the "molecular currency" of intracellular energy transfer.

ATR: A paralog of human ATM that also plays a role in the response to DSBs. The name stands for ATM-Related. ATR is the human ortholog of budding yeast *MEC1* by homology, but the response to DSBs in yeast are controlled mostly by *MEC1* while in humans ATM seems to have a larger role. Thus, the sequence homology predicts general functions but not the division of functions between ATM and ATR or *TEL1* and *MEC1*.

Auditory hair cells: The sensory cells of the auditory system.

Auditory scene analysis: The analysis of multiple sound sources into auditory perception of individual sources (such as human voices or music) using cues such as spatial and frequency separation, harmonic relations, common onset, and offset.

Autonomy: Self-rule; capability of self-determination by comprehending information and making considered judgments based on personal goals or preferences.

Aves: The vertebrate order consisting of all bird species.

Aβ: β-amyloid peptide, a 39 to 42 amino acid peptide cleaved from its membrane-bound precursor protein βAPP (β-amyloid precursor protein that is deposited in the brains of subjects with Alzheimer's disease).

B cell: Lymphocyte that produces antibodies and is responsible for humoral immunity.

BAL: Broncho-alveolar lavage; procedure performed during a bronchoscopy (bronchial fibroscopy) permitting sampling of cells and microorganisms in the peripheral lung. The bronchoscope is wedged in a segmental or subsegmental bronchus and saline solution is injected and then aspirated (successive aliquots of 20 to 50 ml). Samples obtained are less contaminated by upper airways than bronchial or tracheal aspirates and more representative (in terms of cell populations and micro-organisms) of the periphery of the lung in pathological situations such as pneumonia.

Base Excision Repair (BER): A DNA repair pathway in which an altered base is removed by a DNA glycosylase enzyme, followed by excision of the resulting sugar phosphate. The small gap left in the DNA helix is filled in by the sequential action of DNA polymerase and DNA ligase.

Basic reproductive number (*R*0): The number of secondary infections which would, on average, arise from introduction of a single primary infection into a wholly susceptible population.

BBN: Broadband or wideband noise.

Belmont Report: Influential report of the National Commission for the Protection of Human Subjects of Biomedical and Behavioral Research, which, in turn, was established by the U.S. Congress (1974 National Research Act); the report describes the following three broad prima facie ethical principles that provide a basis on which specific rules for conducting human subjects research may be established, appraised and interpreted: respect for persons, beneficence and justice.

Beneficence: The prima facie ethical principle that requires investigators to act to secure the well being of human research subjects, maximize benefits and minimize harms; inhumane treatment of human research subjects research is never morally justified.

Benign prostatic hyperplasia (BPH): Pathological proliferation of fibrostromal and epithelial tissue of prostate with high prevalence in aged men; associated with low urinary tract syndrome.

β-cell: Highly specialized cells found in the islets of Langerhans in the pancreas that produce and secrete insulin into the bloodstream.

β-cell dysfunction: Decrease in the secreted insulin amount.

Beta level: The probability of committing a type II error.

Beta-amyloid: An amyloid derived from a larger precursor protein, which is a component of plaques that develop with age and are more numerous in Alzheimer's disease.

β-galactosidase: an enzyme.

Bias: a flaw in either the study design or data analysis that leads to an erroneous result.

Big Five: In psychology, five generally accepted personality traits that typify human behavior: conscientiousness, agreeableness, neuroticism, openness, and extroversion.

Binaural processing: The integration of acoustic information received across left and right ears.

Biomarker: A physical attribute that may be a biological state or trait that contributes to the distinction between classes or types of individual. Most often used to distinguish disease states from health, but may be used to identify individuals at increased risk of disease.

Biomarkers of aging: Molecular, physiological or functional variables selected for their reliable correlations with the declines in healthy function characteristic of aging.

Biomarker of aging rate: A gene expression or other phenotypic change that correlates with the rate at which an individual is aging. A biomarker of aging rate will also be a biomarker of longevity.

Biomarker of longevity: A gene expression or other phenotypic change that correlates with the life span of an individual.

Bistable percept: The phenomenon of alterations between distinct interpretations (i.e., perception) of the same physical stimulation.

Blastocyst: The late stage of preimplantation embryo development that implants into the uterine epithelium in primates, comprising two primordial tissues: ICM and trophectoderm.

Blood-brain barrier: An elaborate network of supportive brain cells, called *glia*, that surrounds blood vessels and protects neurons from the toxic effects of direct exposure to blood.

BMI: Body mass index.

Bone morphogenetic proteins (BMPs): Phylogenetically conserved signaling molecules that belong to the transforming growth factor (TGF)-beta superfamily, and are involved in body patterning and morphogenesis.

Bootstrapping: a computationally intensive, nonparametric technique for making probability-based estimates and inferences about a population characteristic based on a sample drawn from that population.

Bottom-up processing: See Primitive segregation.

Boundary conditions: Terms that specify the state of the model population at time zero, and the distribution at age zero of the model population into specified subgroups and into the various infection states in the model (susceptibility, infection, immunity etc).

bT: Bioavailable T (testosterone).

Budding: The founding of a new colony when a polygynous colony splits with some workers and queens leaving to start a new colony.

Budding yeast: The yeast *Saccharomyces cerevisiae* divides by asymmetric budding to produce a larger Mother cell and a smaller Daughter cell.

CA strand: The 5′ strand of the chromosome end, bearing the telomere repeat sequence CCCTAA in humans and $C_{1\text{-}3}A$ in budding yeast.

CA1: a region of the hippocampus proper containing the cell bodies of pyramidal neurons, which receive the primary input from CA3 pyramidal neurons.

CA3: a region of the hippocampus proper containing the cell bodies of pyramidal neurons, which receive the primary input from dentate gyrus granule cells.

Caloric restriction (CR): Dietary treatment in which the individual is given a nutritionally balanced diet which includes all vitamins, minerals, and trace elements; however, the diet aliquot per day is some percentage below the *ad libitum* intake, usually 30% for moderate restriction. For experimental purpose in insects CR can also bring about by intermittent feeding.

CAP: Community-acquired pneumonia.

Capacity: Individual's ability to understand and make decisions within a specific area of life.

Cardiac ventricular ejection fraction: Pntage of the ventricular blood volume that is propelled into the aorta at each ventricular contraction.

Cardiomyocyte: A cardiac muscle cell. These cells are post-mitotic, terminally differentiated cells responsible for the mechanical pump function of the heart.

Carotid artery: An artery, located on either side of the neck, that supplies the brain with blood.

Cartilage: A type of dense connective tissue that comprises three main types of cartilage: hyaline, elastic, and fibrocartilage.

Case control study (syn.: case-referent study): a study which compares cases and controls with regard to the presence or absence of some element in their past experience.

Caste: designation of a set of individuals in a colony that are distinct in regard to morphology and behavior.

Categorical data: a collection of observations that can be categorized by classification or on an ordered scale.

CCA: Common carotid artery.

CCAo: Common carotid artery occlusion.

CD28−: CD28-negative (i.e., cells that do not express CD28).

CD28+: CD28-positive (i.e., cells that express the CD28 molecule).

CD28: costimulatory molecule on T cells.

CDC13: a budding yeast protein that is part of the telomerase holoenzyme and is a protein that binds to and protects telomeres. Cells expressing the *est4* allele of *CDC13* (*cdc13-2*) behave as if they have no telomerase activity, but in vitro telomerase activity can be isolated from these cells. Yeast *EST1* protein is thought to serve as a bridge between the telomerase enzyme and the *CDC13/EST4* protein bound to the telomere end. The orthologs in humans and fission yeast are considered to be the telomere proteins *POT1* and $pot1^{+}$, based in part upon protein structural similarities.

Centenarian: A person 100 years old or older.

Central hearing loss: Problems in acoustic processing associated with deterioration, maturation, or damage to the brain.

Central sleep apnea: Lack of effort to breathe.

Cerebral blood flow: The flow of blood through the arteries that lead to the brain, called the cerebrovascular system.

cES: Chicken embryonic stem cells derived from Stage X embryos, which are pre-blastula embryos collected from unincubated eggs consisting of about 40 000 cells.

Chicken embryo fibroblast (CEF): A fibroblast cell usually derived from 7–11 day-old (E7-11) chicken embryos. A cell from which connective tissue develops.

CHF: Congestive heart failure.

CHIMP Act: H.R. 3514, signed into law on December 20, 2000. Provides a nonprofit, long-term retirement sanctuary system for chimpanzees that have been used in biomedical research.

Chiroptera: Order of Mammalia including all bat species, which is further subdivided into two suborders, the Megachiroptera and the Microchiroptera.

Cholecystokinin (CCK): Hormone released when food enters the small bowel; stimulates contraction of the gall bladder and mediates feeling of satiety.

Chondrocyte: The only cells found in cartilage.

Chronobiology: Description and research of time structure of animals and plants, populations and ecosystems. Periodic repeating physiological rhythms and oscillations on different levels of organisation steps proved to be a constitutive function of life.

Chronological life span: The length of time that a quiescent yeast cell retains the ability to re-initiate vegetative growth upon return to appropriate growth conditions.

Cingulate cortex: Large area of the limbic system involved in memory and emotional processing, found on the medial surface of each cerebral hemisphere dorsal to the corpus callosum.

Circadian periodicity: Rhythmic variation during the 24-hour period.

Claustral colony founding: The founding of a new colony by a single queen that raises its first brood without any outside help.

Cloning efficiency: That fraction of cells potentially able to generate clones that actually do so in practice.

CLP: Cecal ligation and puncture. A common method to induce sepsis in laboratory animals.

CNS: Central nervous system.

Cochlea: The coiled organ in the inner ear that converts mechanical energy (vibrations) into nerve impulses that are sent to the brain.

Coculture model: Two or more primary cell lines cultured together, separated by a microporous membrane to enable diffusion of soluble growth factors from one cell line to another.

Cohort study (syn.: follow-up study: longitudinal study): A study that starts with a group of people which are all free of disease, but vary in exposure to a factor, which may be related to development of the disease.

Collagen: Main structural protein of skin, bones, tendons, cartilage, and connective tissue.

Comet assay: Means of determining the level of DNA damage using electrophoretic techniques, so-called because samples take on the appearance of a comet, with DNA fragments in the tail.

Comorbidity: Disease(s) that exist in a study population in addition to the index condition that is the subject of study.

Compartmental model: A model, often depicted using a flow diagram, in which the population is divided into categories or reservoirs corresponding to each stage of susceptibility, infection and immunity represented in the model with population flows between stages representing transitions from one stage to another.

Compensation law of mortality: The observation that higher death rates at young ages in disadvantaged populations are compensated by lower pace of mortality acceleration with age, so that the relative differences in mortality between populations tend to decrease with age (also known as mortality convergence in later life).

Competence-Press model: The most widely acknowledged theory of the ecology of aging introduced by Lawton and Nahemow. Lawton and Nahemow have argued that older adults with lower competence are expected to be particularly prone to what they have coined as "environmental press."

Competency: Determination, typically in a court of law, that a person meets the basic criteria to make his/her own decisions in all areas of life.

Compliance: Pressure necessary to induce a change in volume (expressed in cmH_2O/L); it is, in fact, a measurement of the elasticity of either the lung, the chest wall, or the respiratory system. Compliance of the respiratory system is influenced by changes in elastic recoil of either the lung or the chest wall, and by lung volume.

Concept abstraction: The ability to categorize or sort objects based on a common dimension.

Concurrent sound segregation: The separation of acoustic energy at a single point in time. Involves a fine-grained analysis of spectral and temporal information.

Conditional survival curves for neoplastic causes of death: Estimated survival curves if non-neoplastic fatal lesions are eliminated. If postmortem examinations are properly performed and a cause of death is reasonably determined in each spontaneously dying animal, conditional survival curves can be used to evaluate the potential effect on lifespan of a specific category of death.

Confidentiality: Duty to keep secret and prevent from discovery information revealed by a client within a professional relationship.

Confounding: Distortion of the estimated effect of an exposure on an outcome caused by the presence of an extraneous factor associated both with the exposure and the outcome.

Congo Red: A histological dye that stains amyloid fibrils a characteristic yellowish–green with birefringence. This staining is one of the characteristics that defines amyloid.

Conscientiousness: The personality trait of being organized, disciplined, and an effective worker.

Contact matrix: A matrix specifying the proportion of potentially infective contacts that individuals in each behavioral, age or other subgroup of a heterogeneous model population has with each of the other subgroups in the population and which would provide the conditions for transmission should the contact be with an infectious individual.

Continuity theory: Proposes that people who age successfully carry forward the activities and lifestyles of their middle years into old age.

Continuous data: Data that form one or more whole intervals.

COPD: Chronic obstructive pulmonary disease.

CR: Carolic restriction.

Cortisol release: A stress-related hormone, cortisol is increasingly released from the adrenal cortex as levels of stress increase. An excess of cortisol can cause stress-related physiological conditions, including an interruption of circadian rhythms.

Costimulation: T cell signaling via monomorphic surface receptors required in addition to signaling via the antigen receptor for cell activation.

CpG: Nucleic acids with a high content of cytosine and guanine.

Cross-sectional study (syn.: disease frequency survey: prevalence study): A cross-sectional study samples a population at a given point in time for disease conditions or characteristics.

CRP: C-reactive protein.

CS: Contralateral suppression of OAEs by the auditory efferent system.

CT: Computerized tomography imaging, which uses multiple X-ray images and computer processing to produce three-dimensional images.

C.U.: International conventional units used for the quantitative analysis of images.

Culture arrest: A condition observed in senescence wherein cells cease proliferating.

Cytokines: Chemical messanger molecules by which cells commuicate with one another.

D-loop: DNA recombination and replication intermediate in which one DNA strand has invaded and displaced the equivalent strand of a second DNA molecule of same or similar sequence.

DAF-16: DAF-2: Dauer larva formation; forkhead transcription factors.

DAG: Diacyl glycerol.

Dahl salt-sensitive rats: A strain of rats that was developed by Louis Dahl that increases its blood pressure when given a high-salt diet.

Danio rerio: scientific name for zebrafish.

Dauer larva: In *Caenorhabditis elegans*, dauer larvae are arrested, long-lived, environmentally resistant forms of the third stage larva (L3), which have a morphology, physiology and behavior distinct from other larval stages. The choice between development into "normal," non-dauer L3s and dauer larvae is modulated by food availability, dauer pheromone concentration and temperature.

dB SPL: Decibels in sound pressure level.

DC: Dyskeratosis congenital.

Decision-making capacity: A potential research subject's ability to understand, make and express a reasoned and meaningful choice about whether to participate in a research study.

Declaration of Helsinki: The World Medical Association's code of ethics for research involving human subjects that, in addition to the topics addressed by the Nuremberg Code, also addresses research involving patients, proxy consent, the use of control groups and placebos and nontherapeutic research.

Dementia: Profound loss of cognitive function. Depending on the brain area affected, dementia manifests as changes in personality, ability to process speech, emotional stability, and the ability to reason.

Descriptive epidemiology: The study of the burden of disease within a population by person, place, and time.

Deterministic model: A model for which the results are completely determined by the model structure, model parameters, and the boundary conditions.

Developmental tasks: Developmental tasks result from three different sources: biology, society, and internal experience of the individual. Developmental tasks are helpful in determining the course and sequence of how and when individuals are expected to make specific developmental progress or at what time in life they should engage in or disengage from developmental goals.

DHAP: Dihydroxyacetone phosphate.

DHEA: Dehydrotestosterone.

DHEA-S: Dehydrotestosterone sulfate.

DHT: Dihydrotestosterone.

Diapause: Kind of dormancy of insects and different other invertebrates. It is characterized by a temporal interruption of development or gonadal function and goes together with a drastic reduction of energy metabolism. The inducing abiotic factor is a change of photoperiod to short day conditions. New findings indicate that the aging process arrests during this situation.

Diet-induced thermogenesis: Increase in metabolic rate that occurs with eating. It is a component of total energy expenditure that represents energy from food that is not used.

DIGE: Differential in-gel electrophoresis.

Diphyodont: Having two successive sets of teeth.

Disability: Any temporary or long-term reduction of a person's activity as a result of an acute or chronic condition.

Discrimination learning: An associative learning problem where one must attend to stimulus features and acquire an association between the stimulus features and a reward.

Disengagement Theory: Suggested by Cumming and Henry, older individuals are seen as limiting their social life spaces in response to societal pressures and in order to prepare for the final phase of their lives.

Dissector: A sterological procedure for counting objects in tissue sections. The dissector may be defined as a three-dimensional stereological probe composed of pairs of sections: the reference section and a serial section called the look-up section. The volume of the dissector is determined by the area of the sections and the distance between them. Objects are considered to be in the dissector and counted if they can be identified in the look-up section, but not in the reference one. In order to detect all the objects to be counted, the distance between reference and look-up sections must be less that the shortest dimension of the objects. With specific reference to synaptic counts, adjacent sections can be used and they must be located randomly within a given neural region.

Distribution-free methods: See Nonparametric methods.

Distributive justice: Fairness in the distribution among persons of the risks, harms and benefits incurred by their society.

Diutinus: The Latin word *diutinus* means enduring or long-lived.

DLCO: Diffusion capacity of the lung for carbon monoxide.

DNA: Deoxyribonucleic acid or deoxyribose nucleic acid; a nucleic acid that contains the genetic instructions specifying the biological development.

DNA damage: Changes in the DNA chemical structure induced by a variety of different chemical, physical, and biological agents.

DNA repair: The complex of enzymatic systems to remove DNA damage and to restore the original situation.

DNA replication: The process of copying the entire complement of genetic information.

DNA transcription: The process of copying the genetic information encoded in a gene into mRNA.

DNP: 2,4-dinitrophenyl.

DPOAE: Distortion product otoacoustic emission; cochlear physiological recordings.

DSBs: Double-strand breaks in DNA.

DT40: A transformed chicken B-cell derived from an Avian Leukosis Virus (ALV)-induced bursal lymphoma (tumor) of a female chicken.

Dynamic susceptibility contrast: MRI: a method of combining high resolution magnetic resonance images with paramagnetic intravascular susceptibility contrast agents to derive measures of hemodynamic changes such as blood flow and volume in the brain.

Dyspareunia: Painful intercourse.

E: Embryonic day.

E_2: Estradiol.

Ecdysone: A steroid hormone in insects that stimulates molting and metamorphosis.

Echocardiography: The use of ultrasonic imaging to assess cardiac structure and function.

Echolocation: Sophisticated sensory system in microchiropteran bats based on the emission of ultrasonic calls and the interpretation of returning echoes. Bats use echolocation for navigation and location and identification of prey items.

Ecological equation: (Behavior = P, E, P X E). This equation has been most essential for the ecology of aging; that is, the consideration of the impact of the interaction between the aging individual and the environment on a variety of outcomes such as emotional well-being and behavioral functioning has been added to the isolated consideration of the person (P) and his/her environment (E).

Ectothermic organisms (poikilothermic organisms): Animals with missing or only partial developed ability to maintain body temperature in a constant range. They often rely on incident solar radiation as heat source.

Edema: The swelling of a cell that results from the influx of large amounts of water or fluid into the cell.

EEG: Electroencephalography.

Effective reproductive number (*R*): The number of secondary infections arising on average from each new infection in population; at the time of first introduction into a wholly susceptible population *R* has the same value as *R*0.

EGB 761: A drug extracted from Ginkgo Biloba.

Egocentric: Spatial references made on the basis of the observer's position in the environment.

Elastic recoil of the lung: Pressure tending to restore the lung to its resting volume (i.e., deflated) resulting from distention of the alveoli and the parenchymal interstitial network; increases with increasing lung volume.

Elastin: A protein in connective tissue that provides elasticity in various tissues such as ligaments, tendons, or skin.

Elastosis: The loss of elasticity of skin, possibly due to deposition of elastin.

Electrocardiography (ECG): The practice of recording the electrical discharges of the heart.

Electron transport chain (respiratory chain): The series of electron carriers in the inner mitochondrial membrane that pass electrons from reduced coenzymes (NADH, $FADH_2$) to molecular oxygen via sequential redox reactions coupled to vectorial transduction of protons across the membrane.

Electroporation: A technique by which polar molecules are introduced into a host cell through the cell membrane. An electric pulse temporarily disturbs the phospholipid bilayer, allowing molecules such as DNA to pass into the cell.

Embolic stroke: A stroke caused by an embolus.

Embryonic cell nuclear transfer (ECNT): A technology involving fusion of a blastomere with an enucleated oocyte, so that the blastomere nucleus becomes the embryo nucleus; this is one (limited) form of cloning.

Embryonic stem cells: Primordial cells derived from the blastocyst ICM, that are capable of producing all the organ and tissue types of the fetus; possibly, only trophectoderm cannot be derived from ES cells but this is not certain.

Endocochlear potential: Physiological voltage in scala media of the cochlea, generally around +90 mV.

Endocrine system: System of glands that secretes hormones to maintain homeostasis in a variety of systems. Examples include thyroid, adrenal, and pituitary systems. Two important bioactive endocrine molecules discussed in this book include DHEA-S from the adrenal gland and IGF-1, the first messenger molecular from the pituitary-produced growth hormone.

Endocrinopathy: A disorder in which there is a disturbance (increase or decrease) in one or more hormones; for example, growth hormone deficiency, hyperthyroidism.

Endothelial dysfunction: Dysfunction of the layer of epithelial cells that lines the cavities of the heart, the blood, and lymph vessels, and the serous cavities of the body, originating from the mesoderm.

Endothelin: A potent vasoconstrictor that plays a role in blood pressure control.

Endothermic organisms (homeothermic organisms): Animals (especially birds and mammals) with the ability to maintain the body core temperature within narrow limits independent from external fluctuations. The maintenance of temperature is reached by thermoreceptors in the skin and temperature sensitive neurons in the central nervous system which act upon temperature processing hypothalamic centers.

Endurance exercise: A form of exercise performed at well below the maximum aerobic capacity and for more prolonged periods than would be possible for aerobic exercise.

End-replication problem: The inability of DNA polymerase to replicate the 5′ end of a linear chromosome causes loss of telomeric (TTAGGG) repeats upon successive divisions.

eNOS: Endothelial nitric oxide synthetase.

Enteroinsular axis: Represents the enteral hormone (incretins) secretion to the ingestion of glucose to potentate insulin secretion.

Entorhinal cortex: A region of the medial temporal lobe which has bidirectional connections with the hippocampal formation and which is vulnerable to age-related decline.

Environmental enrichment: The provision of stimulating, novel items and enriching experiences to captive primates.

Epidemiology: The study of the distribution and determinants of health-related states in specific populations, and the application of this study to control of health problems.

Epigenetic: A theory holding that development is a gradual process of increasing complexity. This contrasts with *preformationism*, which contends that the organism is already present in the gamete. Epigenesist encompasses all aspects of an individual's development as determined by genes and internal and external environments. Many genes require specific environmental circumstances in order to be expressed. Many genes are never expressed. In these terms, epigenesis is the influence of the environment (e.g., nutrients) on genes.

Epiphyseal growth plate: Cartilaginous region at the interface between the shaft (diaphysis) and the two ends (epiphyses) of a growing long bone.

ERCs: Extrachromosomal rDNA circles formed in yeast by intrachromosomal recombination between the tandem ribosomal RNA genes in the budding yeast *RDN1* locus. Because each repeat has an origin of DNA replication, these circles can replicate independently from the chromosome and accumulate in the mother cell over successive cellular divisions.

Erythroid: Red blood cell-related.

ESRS: Electron spin resonance spectroscopy; allows us to measure the quantity of melanin contained in retinal tissues.

ESI: Electrospray ionization.

EST1: a budding yeast protein that is part of the telomerase holoenzyme. Cells lacking *EST1* behave as if they have no telomerase activity, but in vitro telomerase activity can be isolated from these cells. Yeast *EST1* protein is thought to serve as a bridge between the telomerase enzyme and the *CDC13*/*EST4* protein bound to the telomere end. *EST1* orthologs exist in humans and fission yeast and play a role in telomere length regulation.

EST2: the budding yeast telomerase reverse transcriptase or yTRT or yTERT. With telomerase RNA, this protein catalyzes the synthesis of yeast telomere repeats. Orthologs are known in many organisms including humans and fission yeast ($trt1^{+}$)

EST3: a budding yeast protein that is part of the telomerase holoenzyme. Cells lacking *EST3* behave as if they have no telomerase activity, but in vitro telomerase activity can be isolated from these cells.

EST4: See *CDC13*.

ET-1: Endothelin-1.

ETC: Electron transfer chain.

Euglycemia: Normal blood glucose level.

Eusocial insects: State building insects with one (rarely more) egg-laying and long-living queen and workers having reduced or functionless gonads. They are several-fold independently evolved in bees, wasps, ants and termites.

Executive functions: A term used to describe a number of cognitive functions including the ability to alter behavior in the face of changing environmental conditions. Believed to be mediated by the prefrontal cortex.

Executive functions: Higher order cognitive processes often controlled by the front part of the brain and includes functions such as categorical abstraction, set maintenance and manipulation, set shifting, and inhibitory control.

Exposure: The generic term used to describe the effective presence of any agent or factor that is thought to cause disease, such as toxic chemicals, dietary habits, activity levels, microorganisms.

Extra-cellular matrix: The scaffold of macromolecules that constitutes the biological substance that surrounds cells in tissues. In tissues such as dermis, the extra-cellular matrix is constituted by the so-called ground substance (water-binding proteoglycans and polysaccharides such as hyaluronic acid, heparin, heparin sulfate, keratan sulfate, etc.) surrounding collagen fibers. Proteins in the extra-cellular matrix, such as the collagens and elastin, are not water soluble, which makes their quantitative analysis extremely difficult.

Extrachromosomal rDNA circles (ERCs): Self-replicating, circular DNA molecules that contain one or more complete copies of the 9.1 kb ribosomal DNA repeat unit. ERCs are formed by homologous recombination, are symmetrically segregated to the mother cell during cell division, accumulate with age in the mother cell nucleus, and are thought to cause replicative senescence in yeast.

Extroversion: The personality trait of being outward-looking and gregarious.

F1: Frequency of the first tone of the DPOAE stimulus.

F2: Frequency of the second tone of the DPOAE stimulus.

F1 hybrid: progeny of a cross between two different inbred stocks of mice.

FA: Fanconi anemia.

Factor analysis: A statistical procedure that works to discover simple patterns in relationships among variables.

Failure rate (also known as hazard rate): Risk or frequency of a system's failure. Mathematically it is defined as the relative rate of reliability (survival) function decline.

Failure: The event when a required function is terminated. Failures are often classified into two groups: (1) degradation failures, where the system or component no longer functions properly, and (2) catastrophic or fatal failures—the end of system's or component's life.

FAT: FRAP, ATM and TRRAP related.

FATC: FRAP, ATM and TRRAP C-terminal related.

Fat free mass (FFM): The component of body composition that is not fat; it varies between individuals and relates mainly to the mass of skeletal muscle.

Fatigue: A feeling of tiredness or weariness.

$FEF_{25\text{-}75}$: Forced expiratory flow rate from 25 to 75% of the vital capacity.

FEV_1: Volume expired in one second during a forced expiratory maneuver after a maximal inspiration.

FFA: Free fatty acids.

FFT: Fast Fourier transform.

Fission (or coherence) boundary: The level of frequency separation in a tone pattern that leads to the perception of a single stream of sound.

Fission yeast: The yeast *Schizosaccharomyces pombe*, which divides by symmetric division to produce two daughter cells of equal size called sisters.

Flow diagram: A diagram consisting of boxes (compartments) and arrows (flows) depicting the essential features of the dynamics of a particular infection in a population.

Fluoro-angiography: E.v. injection of a fluorescent contrast for the visualization of the retinic vessels of the ocular fundus.

Follicle stimulating hormone (FSH): One of the pituitary gland gonadotropins.

Follitropin receptor knockout mouse (FORKO): A transgenic mouse in which the follitropin (FSH) receptor is absent; this is a model for postmenopausal hypertension.

Folstein Mini-Mental State Exam: A bedside neuropsychologic test used to assess cognitive functioning of people. The test is commonly used as a screening test for dementia.

Force of infection: The annual per capita incidence of infection in the population amongst those susceptible to the infection, as distinct from the incidence in the whole population.

Forced molting: A method used by the poultry industry in which egg-laying chicken hens are temporarily starved or calorically restricted to induce feather loss and increase egg production.

4-HNE: 4-hydroxy-2-nonenal.

Four-way cross: A stock produced by a mating between two different F1 hybrid parents.

FOXO: Forkhead box transcription factors.

Frail: Clinical term used to describe an older adult, or chronically ill younger adult who is weak, fatigued, and at high risk for poor health outcomes.

Frailty: Biological syndrome of decreased reserve and resistance to stressors, resulting from cumulative declines across multiple physiological systems. Causes vulnerability to problems such as unintentional weight loss, weakness, exhaustion, slow walking speed, and low physical activity.

FRC: Functional residual capacity.

FRC: Functional residual capacity; lung volume after expiration during quiet tidal breathing.

Free radical theory of aging: The original theory was published by Denham Harman in 1956. This theory proposes that aging is a consequence of damage to cellular components caused by free radicals produced during normal metabolism.

Free radicals: Molecules with one or more electrons unpaired in their most external orbitals. Due to this they are very reactive molecules, and can damage other molecules by reacting with them.

Fruc-6-P: Fructose-6-phosphate.

fT: Free testosterone.

Fundamental frequency: The lowest frequency of a periodic signal.

Functional brain imaging: Techniques that can visualize correlates of regional energy metabolism, either glucose or oxygen uptake. These techniques include functional magnetic resonance imaging (fMRI), positron emission tomography (PET), or single photon emission tomography (SPECT).

Fusion (or segregation) boundary: The level of frequency separation in a tone pattern, which leads to the perception of two streams of sound.

FVC: Total volume or air expired during a forced expiratory maneuver.

GAL4: A transcription factor from yeast that is functional in *Drosophila*.

Gap detection: Auditory behavioral and neurophysiological temporal processing task.

GAPDH: Glyceraldehyde phosphate dehydrogenase.

Gastrulation: The process whereby the three primitive germ layers are established in the embryo.

Gedanken Experiment: A purely intellectual experiment, the virtue of which is to allow one to predict what is expected to happen when all the hypotheses are verified. In the case of skin aging, the interest of the Gedanken Experiment described in the text is to show that aging is expected to occur even in the absence of gerontogenes.

Gene: The segment of DNA encoding a polypeptide chain; it includes regions immediately preceding and following the coding sequence as well as intervening sequences (introns) between individual coding sequences.

Gene expression biomarker: A gene expression change (or lack thereof) that correlates with a particular process.

Gene expression profile: A collection of gene expression responses (often several thousand) that correspond to a particular experimental parameter, such as age.

Genome: The full DNA sequence of an organism. The human genome consists of approximately 6 billion base pairs of DNA distributed among 46 DNA-protein complexes termed chromosomes.

Genomics: The study of an organism's genome.

Genotype: The alleles present at one or more specific loci.

Geriatrics: A branch of medicine dealing with the problems and diseases of old age.

Gerontogenes: Putative genes postulated by theories supporting the "necessity" of aging. To explain aging, this theory invokes the existence of specific genes that would be "turned on" a defined number of years after birth, and would induce or allow the accumulation of damages provoking the loss of the capability of the individual to compete for food and to reproduce. As of today, gerontogenes have not been found.

Gerontology: A branch of study dealing with aging and the problems of the aged.

GFAP: Glial fibrillary acidic protein; a protein specific to the astrocytes and other glia cells that can be stained by means of immuno-histochemical methods.

GFAT: Glutamine:fructose-6-phosphate amidotransferase.

Ghrelin: A hormone released from the stomach that acts a signal to eat. Levels are decreased in the elderly and in obese subjects.

GlcNAc: O-linked N-acetylglucosamine (hexosamine pathway).

Glial cell-line-derived neurotrophic factor (GDNF) knock-out mice: A transgenic mouse strain in which the gene for the GNDF is absent. The kidneys in homozygotes do not develop and they die early. The heterozygotes are a model of reduced renal glomeruli that develop hypertension with aging and high salt intake.

Glucose tolerance test: A test to evaluate the rate of glucose disposal in the body after glucose administration. Blood glucose level stays at higher if the metabolic process is impaired, as in cases of diabetes and/or aging.

Glucose transporter: A family of membrane proteins that allows the energy-independent transport of glucose across the cell membrane. An isoform of glucose transporter proteins (GLUT4) is important for regulating glucose disposal in the body, because GLUT4 is translocated into the membranes of muscle and fat cells in response to the insulin signaling.

Glut -1: Glucose transporter 1.

Glycation end products: Nonenzymatic protein modifications.

Glycolytic oscillator: Periodic rhythm of glycolyse, first studied on intact yeast cells and later on cell free extracts of different organisms indicating a biochemical clock independent of spatial cell structure. The mechanism is based on complex interactions of glycolytic enzymes and ligands in which phosphofructokinase plays the key role.

Glycosaminoglycan: Glycosaminoglycans are long unbranched polysaccharides, made of repeating disaccharides that may be sulphated. GAGs form an important component of connective tissues. Glycosaminoglycans include, for instance, chondroitin sulphate and dermatan sulphate.

Glycosylated hemoglobin: A test that measures the amount of glucose-bound hemoglobin, which provides information regarding how well a patient's diabetes is being controlled. As the blood glucose level increases, the proportion of hemoglobin molecules that bind glucose increases with time.

Glycosylation: A nonenzymatic series of reactions in which proteins or other molecules combine with reducing sugars in molecules, cells and tissues to produce compounds that may contribute to aging-related disease or loss of function.

Glycoxidation: A synergistic combination of glycosylative and oxidative reactions that produce metabolic end-products implicated in aging-related disease or loss of function.

GNB: Gram-negative bacteria.

Gompertz curves: Mathematical description of the exponential change in age-specific death rate (q_x) with age was first described by Benjamin Gompertz in 1825, as follows: $\ln q_x = \ln q_0 + x$, where $q_0 = y$ intercept and $x =$ slope constant. Plotting this for adult mortality usually yields a linearly increasing straight line. Changes in observed longevity are brought about by changes in the intercept and/or the slope (see MRDT). This transformation enables the complexities of a survival curve to be understood in terms of a straight line describing the mortality kinetics.

Gompertz law of mortality: The law of exponential increase in death (failure) rates with age. It was first suggested by the British actuary Benjamin Gompertz in 1825 for use in the life insurance business. This law was found to be applicable not only to humans but also to fruit flies, nematodes, the human lice, flour beetles, mice, rats, dogs, horses, mountain sheep, baboons and many other biological species. According to the Gompertz law, the logarithm of death rates is increasing linearly with age.

Gompertz model: A class of statistical models in which the hazard rate for death rate rises geometrically with increasing age of the organism (at least after an initial period of high risk of mortality at birth and infancy and a much lower risk in late childhood and adolescence).

Gompertz–Makeham law: An extension of the Gompertz law of mortality when the additional, age-independent component of mortality (failure) is taken into account. This law was suggested by the British actuary William Makeham in 1867.

Gonadotropin releasing hormone (GnRH): The primary hypothalamic hormone that regulated the reproductive axis.

Granulosa: Layer of specialized epithelial cells in the ovarian follicle which support the oocyte or developing egg.

GRP or Glucose related proteins: Members of a family of proteins secreted in response to stressors which appear to play a role in cell protection.

GSH: Glutathione.

Gynogenetic diploids: The diploids generated by early pressure treatment after fertilizing the eggs with UV treated sperm.

Haplo-diploid: Sex is determined by the male being haploid (one chromosome set) and the female being diploid (two chromosome sets)

Haploinsufficiency: Impaired cell structure and/or function resulting from half the normal amount of a gene product.

Hayflick limit: The barrier to further cellular proliferation represented by culture arrest of senescent cells.

HDL and LDL cholesterol: Lipids become soluble and are transported into the blood as lipoproteins. Depending on the protein components of lipoproteins, cholesterols are designated as high-density-lipoprotein (HDL)-cholesterol, low-density-lipoprotein (LDL)-cholesterol, and so on. Epidemiological studies indicate that people with increased plasma concentrations of HDL-cholesterol, and thus decreased LDL-cholesterol, show a reducing risk for cardiovascular diseases.

Hearing thresholds: The minimal intensity level required for auditory stimulus detection.

Helicase: An enzyme which separates DNA strands in preparation for replication.

Hematopoiesis: Formation of blood cells.

Hematopoietic stem cell: A pluripotent stem cell found in the bone marrow. These cells have the ability to differentiate into any of several types of blood cells and potentially other cells types, such as neuronal or cardiac.

Hemorrhagic stroke: Sudden bleeding into or around the brain.

Herd immunity: The level of immunity in the whole population to an infection, whether this arises from past infection, vaccination or maternal antibody.

Heteroplasmy: A condition in which cells have mitochondria from more than one source; normally, only maternal (oocyte) mitochondria are found in cells due to elimination of paternal (sperm) mitochondria during fertilization or early embryo development.

Heterothermic: Designation for organisms that can adjust body temperature and metabolic rate in response to environmental conditions and physiological cues (e.g. hibernation, torpor).

Heterozygous: Having two different alleles at a specified genetic locus.

HGPS: Hutchinson–Gilford progeria syndrome.

HI: Hypoxia-ischemia.

HINT: Hearing in noise test; speech recognition is measured in the presence of speech-weighted noise from different spatial locations.

Hippocampal formation: A brain circuit in the temporal lobes that plays a vital role in memory function. The circuit is made up of different hippocampal subregions including the entorhinal cortex and the dentate gyrus.

Hippocampus: A part of the medial temporal lobe system involved in memory storage and that is strongly affected by age-related decline.

Histone deacetylase: An enzyme that removes an acetyl group from histones, which allows histones to bind DNA and inhibit gene transcription.

HIV: Human immunodeficiency virus.

Hive body: A rectangular box with frames of wax comb hung in parallel on the inside. One honeybee hive consists of one or more such boxes.

Homeostasis: The ability or tendency of an organism or a cell to maintain internal equilibrium by adjusting its physiological processes.

Homeothermic: Said of organisms that regulate their body temperature within narrow limits.

Homocysteine: A sulfur-containing, amino-acid derivative formed during methionine metabolism. Hyperhomocysteinemia is a risk factor for premature vascular disease.

Homologous trait: A trait shared between organisms due to common descent or ancestry.

Homozygous: having the same allele at a specified genetic locus.

Hormesis: The beneficial effects of low doses of potentially harmful substances.

Hormone replacement therapy (HRT): Steroid hormones given to women or primates as a replacement for estrogens and progesterone decline during aging.

HP: Hydrogen peroxide.

HP1: Heterochromatin protein 1.

HSE: Region of DNA that responds to heat shock.

Hsfs: Heat shock transcription factors.

Hsp: Heat shock protein.

Hyaluronan: A glycosaminoglycan distributed widely throughout connective tissue and one of the main components of the extracellular matrix.

Hydroxyproline: A major component of the collagen protein that helps provide stability to the triple-helical structure of collagen.

Hyperinsulinaemic glucose clamp: This technique involves a fixed dose of insulin being administered and then normal glucose concentrations being maintained by the infusion of glucose given. Reflects insulin sensitivity and is an inverse measure of insulin resistance.

Hyperkeratosis: Thickening of the outermost keratinizing or cornified layer of skin, often in conjunction with increased proliferation of underlying keratinocytes.

Hypersomnia: Too much sleep.

Hypertrophy: Overgrowth or enlargement; hypertrophy of glial cells is generally associated with degenerative events in the brain.

Hypogonadism: A condition resulting from or characterized by abnormally decreased functional activity of the gonads, with retardation of growth and sexual development. Secondary hypogonadism is acquired in life and defined as a laboratory testosterone value of 300–325 ng/dL, depending on the study discussed.

Hyposomnia: Too little sleep.

Hypothalamic–pituitary–gonadal axis (HPG axis): the major components of the reproductive axis.

Hypothesis: A formal statement or prediction of the scientific question of interest.

Hypoventilation: Alveolar ventilation below metabolic needs (i.e., CO_2 production). Major cause of acute or chronic hypercapnia.

Hypoxia: A state of decreased oxygen delivery to a cell so that the oxygen falls below normal levels.

IBTP: (4-iodobutyl)triphenylphosphonium.

ICAT: Isotope-coded affinity tag.

ICU: Intensive care unit.

IFN-g: Interferon gamma; an important cytokine that promotes Th1 (cell mediated) immunity.

IGF-1: Insulin-like growth factor-1; a single-chain polypeptide of 70 amino acids. It is a trophic factor that circulates at high levels in the blood-stream and mediates many, if not most, of the effects of growth hormone.

IHC: Inner hair cells; convert sound to the code of the nervous system in the cochlea.

iL3: In the parasitic nematode *parayloides ratti*, larvae moult through two larval stages into infective third-stage larvae (iL3s), which infect new hosts by skin penetration. iL3s are nonfeeding and environmentally resilient and can survive for months in this developmentally arrested state until contact with a suitable host. They (and the iL3s of other parasitic nematodes) are considered as analogous to the dauer stage of *Caenorhabditis elegans*.

IMAC: Imobilized metal affinity chromatography.

Imaginal discs: Undifferentiated cells that will develop into adult tissue and organs in the blastoderm (the layer of cells that surrounds internal mass of egg yolk in an insect embryo).

Immune senescence: Waning of immune responses with advancing age.

Immunosenescence: That age-associated dysregulated state of immunity associated with increased susceptibility to infection.

Impaired glucose tolerance (IGT): A glucose level over > 140mg/dL (7.8mmol/L), but less than 200 mg/dL (11.1 mmol/L) two hours after a 75g oral glucose tolerance test (OGTT).

Imprinting: First applied to the acquisition of behaviors when exposed to specific stimuli during development. Genomic imprinting plays a critical role in the fetal growth and development. Imprinting is regulated by DNA methylation and chromatin structure.

Inbred: Referring to strains resulting from a minimum of 10 generations of brother–sister matings, in which 99% or more of the genome is homozygous.

Inbreeding depression: A reduction in fitness and vigor of individuals as a result of increased homozygosity through inbreeding in a normally outbreeding population.

Incidence: The number of new events, such as new cases of a disease during a given period of time in a specified population.

Infarct: An area of tissue that is dead or dying because of a loss of blood supply.

Inflam-aging: Physiological status of the immune system in the elderly in which a pro-inflammatory profile predominates.

Information bias: A flaw in measuring exposure or outcome data.

Informed consent: A central feature of ethical research involving human subjects that consists of (a) adequate information regarding the research and its potential risks and benefits and subject understanding of the information, (b) subject decision-making capacity, and (c) subject voluntariness to participate.

Infralimbic cortex: A cortical region in rats located along the medial surface of the cerebral cortex that, together with prelimbic cortex in rodents, has been suggested as analogous to the dorsolateral prefrontal cortex in humans. This region has been demonstrated to be important for extradimensional set shifting in rats. May be referred to as the medial frontal cortex.

Inhibitory control: The ability to maintain attention to relevant task features and inhibit interfering information or previously learned responses.

Initiating sleep: Falling asleep.

Inner Cell Mass (ICM): The part of the blastocyst that forms the fetus after implantation; also the cells from which Embryonic Stem cells are derived.

Insomnia: Inability to sleep.

Institutional Review Board: Committee comprised of scientists and nonscientists charged by an organization with reviewing, approving, and monitoring human subjects research in order to protect those subjects.

Insulin resistance: Altered glucose disposal and hepatic glucose production.

Interleukin-2: A potent autocirne and paracrine T cell growth factor.

Interleukin-6 (IL-6): An inflammatory cytokine that is released in response to infection, trauma, and strenuous exercise from immune system cells, adipocytes, and endothelial cells. Acute elevations are necessary for propagating inflammatory responses. Chronic elevation of this cytokine may have pathophysiologic consequences on a number of physiologic systems, including bone, muscle, cardiovascular tissue, and the immune system.

Interstitial: Pertaining to or situated between parts or in the interspaces of a tissue.

Inflammation: Activation of multiple molecular pathways that are a response to infections and/or trauma. There is increasing evidence that these same pathways are activated in chronic disease and that chronic elevations in inflammatory mediators may contribute to poor health outcomes, including frailty, in older adults.

Intervertebral disc: Lies in between adjacent vertebrae in the spine.

Intracytoplasmic sperm injection (ICSI): Direct injection of spermatozoa into the oocyte cytoplasm, bypassing the need for prefertilization changes in spermatozoa (capacitation) and even the need for sperm motility. This ART approach is very popular with spermatozoa from infertile men with spermatozoa that are immotile or too few in numbers to achieve fertilization.

Ionotropic: A type of receptor that is directly linked to and facilitates the passage of ions into a neuron through an ion channel.

IPF: Idiopathic pulmonary fibrosis.

IR: Ionizing radiation.

Ischemia: A loss of blood flow to tissue, caused by an obstruction of the blood vessel, usually in the form of plaque stenosis or a blood clot.

Ischemic cardiomyopathy: Disease of cardiac muscle due to decreased blood supply to the tissue.

Ischemic penumbra: Areas of damaged, but still living brain cells arranged in a patchwork pattern around areas of dead brain cells.

Ischemic stroke: Ischemia in the tissues of the brain.

Isogenic: mice in an isogenic stock are each genetically identical to one another.

IVAS (Initial Virtual Age of a System): A parameter in theoretical models of systems failure describing the load of initial damage. This parameter has the dimension of time, and corresponds to the age by which an initially ideal system would have accumulated as many defects as a real system already has at the starting age (at $x = 0$).

JH (juvenile hormones): A family of acyclic sesquiterpenoids synthesized by the corpora allata, a small set of paired glands in immediate proximity to the insect brain.

Joint capsule: A sac-like envelope that forms a sleeve around joints and encloses its cavity.

Justice: The prima facie ethical principle that refers to the equitable distribution of the benefits and burdens of research.

Juvenile hormone (JH): Isoprenoid-resp. terpenoidhormone of the corpora allata (CA) of insects. During larval development it acts together with the steroid hormone ecdysone and prevents adult moulting. In adults it has several pleiotropic functions in the context of reproduction. It is also involved in diapause regulation.

Kainate receptor: Type of ionotropic glutamate receptor.

Knock-in: Replacement of a gene by mutant version of the same gene or by another gene usually through homologous recombination.

L1: Sound intensity of the first tone of the DPOAE stimulus.

L2: Sound intensity of the second tone of the DPOAE stimulus.

Lacunar infarcts: Class of infarcts related to hypertension found in the basal ganglia and pons that are less than 1.5 cm in diameter. These infarcts are typically multiple and represent small areas of infarction. Lacunar infarcts are frequently hemorrhagic.

Laminopathy: One of a family of heritable diseases arising from mutations that alter the structure or expression of the lamin A/C gene that encodes a key protein of the inner nuclear envelope. The laminopathies preferentially affect nerve, muscle, adipocytes, and connective tissue for as-yet unknown reasons.

Late-life mortality deceleration law: The observation that the pace of mortality growth with age decelerates from an expected exponential curve at extreme old ages, so that mortality rates level-off and, therefore, aging apparently fades away.

Latency period: Delay between exposure to a disease-causing agent and the appearance of manifestation of the disease.

Left anterior descending (LAD): The left anterior descending branch of the left coronary system.

Leptin: A hormone that is exclusively the product of adipose tissue. It has a variety of effects on the endocrine and immune systems but its major role is to decrease food intake at times when the organism is calorie replete.

Leukocyte: White blood cell.

Life-course epidemiology: Study of the long-term effects on later health or disease risk of physical or social exposures during gestation, childhood, adolescence, young adulthood, and later adult life.

Life expectancy: The probable life span of an individual.

Lifespan: The period of time in which the life events of a species typically occur.

Lifespan extension curves: survivorship curves that indicate the number of survivors plotted against advancing age.

Ligament: A short band of tough fibrous connective tissue composed mainly of long, stringy collagen fibers. Ligaments connect bones to other bones to form a joint.

Limiting dilution: Sequential dilution of cell suspensions plated into culture wells, until none of the wells yields growing cultures.

Link protein: Stabilizes the interaction of the hyaluronan-binding region of aggrecan and hyaluronan.

Lipfuscin: The accumulation of fluorescent age-pigment, largely consisting of chemically highly complex aggregates of peroxidated lipid and protein.

Lipid rafts: Membrane microdomains, specially enriched in cholesterol and sphingolipids and proteins, that are mainly involved in receptor signaling.

Lipopolysaccharide (LPS): A structural component of the outer leaflet of the outer membrane of Gram-negative bacteria. LPS has been recognized as a microbial toxin, namely endotoxin.

LOC: Lateral olivocochlear auditory efferent system.

Long–Evans rat: An outbred rat strain commonly used for cognitive aging research.

Longevity: The period of time an organism is expected to live under ideal circumstances.

Longevity assurance genes: genes that regulate lifespan.

Longitudinal study: In general a study which repeated observations on experimental units. It has advantages over cross-sectional studies because in cross-sectional data, only a single response is available for each of the experimental units. Longitudinal studies in contrast can show the change of age effects over time within individuals.

Loudness recruitment: An attempt to compensate for peripheral hearing loss by the internal amplification of acoustic energy, often leading to painful levels of perceived intensity.

Low urinary tract syndrome (LUTS): A complex of symptoms related to the low urinary tract including voiding symptoms (poor urinary flow, prolong urination, incomplete emptying) and storage symptoms (urge incontinence, nocturia, frequent urination).

LPS: Lipopolysaccharide; the major component of the outer cell membrane of gram negative bacteria.

LRTI: Lower respiratory tract infection.

Luteinizing hormone (LH): One of the pituitary gland gonadotropins.

Macronutrient: Differs from the term micronutrients because its positive contributions to body function are detectable only when present as a large proportion of the diet.

Macrovascular: Large vessels.

MaDMaT: Mass-deficient mass tag.

Magnetic resonance imaging (MRI): An imaging method that uses magnetic fields, radio frequencies, and a computer to produce a detailed picture of the inside of the body.

Maintaining sleep: Sleep without waking.

MALDI: matrix-assisted laser desorption/ionization.

MAPK: Mitogen-activated protein kinases.

Matrix and Bone gamma-carboxyglutamic acid proteins (MGP and BGP, respectively): Vitamin K-dependent proteins that are involved in skeletogenesis and bone maintainence.

Maximal mouth inspiratory pressure (PIMAX): Pressure measured through a mouthpiece during a maximal inspiratory effort, performed either at residual volume or at functional residual capacity (FRC).

MBP: Membrane-bound proteins; can be stained with immuno- chemical methods.

MCA: Middle cerebral artery.

MCAo: Middle cerebral artery occlusion.

Meaning of home: Emphasizes the simultaneous consideration of ties inside of the aging persons to his or her physical and social environment.

MEC1: a budding yeast protein that is a DNA damage checkpoint kinase that helps pause the cell cycle in response to DSBs, and is a paralog of *TEL1* and an ortholog of ATR in humans and *rad3*$^{+}$ in fission yeast. *MEC1* protein is required for the telomere length checkpoint.

Mechano growth factor: Splice variant of the insulin-like growth factor that responds to mechanical stimulation.

Meconium: The substance excreted by insects soon after their eclosion.

Medial frontal cortex: A cortical area located on the medial surface of the cerebral hemisphere of the rat and which is vulnerable to age-related decline. This region is strongly implicated in attentional set shifting. It consists of the infralimbic and prelimbic cortices.

Medial temporal lobe system: A brain system comprised of structures on the medial surface of the temporal lobe, including hippocampus, which are critical for emotion, memory and sensory processing.

Menopause hormone therapy (MHT): Hormones including estrogen, progestins, and testosterone used to control menopause symptoms.

Metabolic syndrome: A cluster of cardiovascular risk factors (abdominal obesity, dyslipidemia, increased glucose, hypertension) that precedes diabetes and is strongly associated with obesity and aging.

Metabotropic: A type of receptor linked to intracellular signal transduction cascades.

Methacholine-induced bronchoconstriction: Measurement of airway reactivity to inhaled methacholine (cholinergic agent). Spirometry (measurement of FEV_1 and FVC) is repeated after inhalation of increasing doses of methacholine until FEV_1 drops by 20% from initial value, defining the PD_{20}, index of airway reactivity. Low PD_{20} values are suggestive of asthma.

MHC I: Major histocompatability complex I; the receptor that presents peptide antigens derived from sources inside the cell to T cells.

MHC II: Major histocompatability complex II; the receptor that presents peptide antigens derived from sources outside the cell to T cells.

Microarray: A molecular biology technique that uses glass slides spotted with oligonucleotides or DNA fragments complementary to a large number of genes to quantitate the relative abundance of messenger RNA transcripts between two groups of samples.

Micronutrient: A single compound (e.g., a specific amino acid) derived from dietary foodstuffs that contributes positively to body growth or maintenance when present in a small proportion of the diet.

Microsatellite: Small regions of chromosomes that help localize genes.

Microvascular: Small vessels.

Migrant studies: Studies taking advantage of migration to one country by those from other countries with different physical and biological environment, cultural background and/or genetic make-up, and different morbidity or mortality experience.

Minimal risk study: The risk and magnitude of harm of the research study to the subject are no greater than what the subject would encounter in daily life or during the performance of routine physical or psychological examinations or tests.

Minimal risk: Risk of harm no greater than that experienced in everyday living.

Minims: The first group of sterile worker offspring in a new colony. They are smaller than the workers of a mature colony.

Mismatch repair: DNA repair system scanning newly replicated DNA in order to deal with replicative and recombinational errors leading to mispaired bases (mismatches) by excising the mutated strand in either direction from the mismatch.

Mistuned harmonic: A component of a periodic signal that does not share an integer relationship with the fundamental frequency.

Mitochondria: Unique organelles that supply most of the cell's energy via oxidative phosphorylation and possess their own primitive genome, replication of which is under control of the nucleus.

Mitochondrial electron transport chain: It is located in the inner mitochondrial membrane and it is the place where oxygen is reduced to water to obtain ATP. It consists in a variable number and type of protein complexes and associated electron transporters. In mammals it is formed by four electron transport complexes and the ATP synthase: complex I or NADH:ubiquinone oxidoreductase, complex II or succinate dehydrogenase, complex III or ubiquinone: cytochrome c oxidoreductase, complex IV or cytochrome c oxidase, and complex V or ATP synthase.

Mitochondrial heteroplasmy: The presence of two or more genetically distinguishable mitochondrial populations within a cell.

Mitochondrial metabolic competence (MMC): The mitochondrial efficiency in providing adequate amounts of high energy intermediates; for example, adenosinetriphosphate. MMC can be tested in different experimental conditions by quantitative estimations of the activity of enzymes of the mitochondrial respiratory chain evidenced by preferential cytochemical methods.

Mnemonic: Of or relating to memory.

MO: Antisense-morpholino oligonucleotide.

MOC: Medial olivocochlear auditory efferent system.

Monogyny: The condition when a colony is headed by a single fertile queen.

Morpholino: A specialized antisense oligonucleotide used to silence gene expression.

Morris water maze: First described by Richard Morris in 1984, a swimming task designed for rodents that can be used to measure the integrity of the medial temporal lobe system.

Mosaicism: Different cells (blastomeres) in the preimplantation embryo having different numbers of chromosomes; this condition arises after fertilization by mitotic nondisjunction of chromosomes.

MRDT (mortality rate doubling time): The time required for the mortality rate to double.

MRSA: Methicillin-resistant staphylococcus aureus.

MRX: A complex of proteins encoded by the *MRE11*, *RAD50* and *XRS* genes in yeast that has a role in checkpoint activation in response to DSBs, and has nuclease and helicase activities in vitro. In humans, the *XRS2* encoded subunit is substituted by the *NBS1* encoded subunit to form the MRN complex.

MS: Mass spectrometry.

MS^n: Multidimensional mass spectrometry.

mtDNA: Mitochondrial DNA.

Mucociliary clearance: Refers to all items contributing to elimination of inhaled or aspirated particles in the airways: cough, production of mucus, regular movement of ciliae of bronchial epithelium.

MudPIT: Multidimensional protein identification technology.

Multiphoton laser scanning microscopy (MPSLM): An advanced form of confocal microscopy that uses infrared light instead of short-wavelength (high energy) light to excite fluorescent molecules introduced into the cell to measure various aspects of cell function. Because MPSLM does not damage cells, subcellular structures and organization can be monitored for long periods of time so that cell structure and function can be directly correlated within the same cell.

MuLV: Murine leukemia virus.

Multipotent: Stem cells that can differentiate into only a limited number of cell types.

Mutation: Change in the sequence of DNA in a genome that can involve a single base pair position (point mutation) or a rearrangement (deletions, insertions, recombinations).

Mutation accumulation theory: A theory of biological aging that proposes that biological senescence is due to the accumulation of harmful, mutant genes in later, post-reproductive years when natural selection is a declining force.

Mya: Million years ago.

Myeloid: White blood cell-related.

Myocardial infarction: Cardiac injury characterized by necrosis and scar formation.

Myocardial ischemia: Cardiac hypoxia, primarily due to impaired vascular supply to cardiac tissue.

NADPH: Nicotinamide adenine dinucleotide phosphate reduced.

NADPH oxidase: An enzyme that produces superoxide.

Natural selection: Proposed by C. Darwin and A.R. Wallace, a process in nature that results in increased survival rates of organisms having favorable traits.

Necropsy: Post-mortem examination.

Nematode: Unsegmented worms with elongated rounded body pointed at both ends; mostly free-living (*e.g. Caenorhabditis elegans*) but some are parasitic (*e.g. parayloides ratti*).

Neuroanatomic: Of or relating to neural tissue or the nervous system.

Neurofibrillary tangles: Insoluble fibrils of hyperphosphorylated tau protein with a characteristic twisted structure that, along with amyloid plaques, are the histological hallmarks of AD. These structures fluoresce when stained with Thioflavine S or Thioflavin T and may be extracellular (dead neurons) or intracellular (damaged neurons). These accumulate in the brain with age and in larger amounts in Alzheimer's disease.

Neurogenesis: Formation of nervous tissue.

Neuron: The main functional cell of the brain and nervous system, consisting of a cell body, an axon, and dendrites.

Neuroprotective agents: Medications that protect the brain from secondary injury caused by stroke.

Neuroticism: A personality trait in individuals who worry and are emotionally unstable.

Neurotransmitter: A substance that is released from the axon terminal of a presynaptic neuron on excitation, and that travels across the synaptic cleft to either excite or inhibit the target cell.

NFkB: Nuclear factor kappa B. A signal transduction factor that controls the transcription of many immune response genes.

NGT: Naso-gastric tube; tube inserted through either nostril, with its distal end placed in the stomach.

NHAP: Nursing-home-acquired pneumonia.

Night terror: Waking with intense fear and unresponsiveness to other people.

Nightmare: An unpleasant and/or frightening dream that usually awakens a person.

Nocturia: A need to wake at night one or more times to void.

Nocturnal polyuria syndrome (NPS): Nocturia and nocturnal polyuria due to a lack of diurnal rhythm in the antidiuretic hormone (ADH) system.

Nonagenarian: A person age 90 years and older.

Nominal data: Categorical data based on classifications.

Noncognitive behaviors: A range of diverse behaviors that do not explicitly involve learning or memory but could be related to cognitive status.

Nonparametric method: A statistical method for obtaining estimates and drawing inferences based on a function of the sample observations, the probability distribution of which does not depend on a complete specification of the probability distribution of the population from which the sample was drawn. Consequently, such a method will be valid under relatively general assumptions about the underlying population. Many nonparametric methods have been based on the ranks of the observed data.

Normoglycemia: Normal blood glucose levels with no changes greater than two standard deviations from the mean.

NP: Nosocomial pneumonia.

Nucleotide excision repair: When a small region of the strand surrounding the damage is removed from the DNA helix as an oligonucleotide, and the small gap left in the DNA helix is filled in by the sequential action of DNA polymerase and DNA ligase. Nucleotide excision repair recognizes a wide range of substrates, including damage caused by UV irradiation (pyrimidine dimers and 6-4 photoproducts) and chemicals (intrastrand cross-links and bulky adducts).

Nude rat: Hypothymic (nude) rats have only a remnant thymic stump and are dysfunctional with respect to T-cell maturation.

Numeric density of mitochondria (Nvm): A morphometric parameter defining the number of mitochondria/μm^3 of cytoplasm. Nvm has been calculated by applying different morphometric procedures. It is reported to undergo significant changes in several physiological and experimental conditions.

Numeric density of synapses (Nvs): This morphometric parameter can be estimated by using the recently introduced dissector counting procedure, and provides information on the number of synapses/μm^3 of neuropil. Studies conducted prior to the introduction of the dissector can be considered still reliable results if referred to local differences within an individual or if used to make synapses-to-neuron ratios.

Nuremberg Code: List of rules for "permissible medical experiments" involving human subjects included in the 1947 verdict of the presiding judges of the Nuremberg War Crimes Physicians Trial of Nazi physicians for "crimes against humanity" that consisted of experiments on concentration camp prisoners and others without their involuntary consent. The Nuremberg Code is the first internationally recognized code of ethics for research involving human subjects and included requirements that (a) subject voluntary consent be obtained, (b) study benefits outweigh the risks, (c) the study should be conducted to avoid unnecessary harm and should not be done if there is an a priori belief death or injury will occur, and (d) the subject has the right to withdraw from the study at any time.

Nursery colony: In many colonial species of bats, pregnant females will roost and raise their offspring together. This behavior may provide necessary social interaction for developing young and certainly allows for thermoregulation by clustering.

NYHA: New York Heart Association.

O_2: Oxygen.

OAE: Otoacoustic emissions; reflect the physiological responses of OHCs.

Object recognition: The ability to classify and register the identity of objects based on a set of stimulus features or dimensions.

Obstructive sleep apnea (OSA): Apnea caused by a closure of the air passage despite efforts to breathe.

OGT: O-GlcNAc transferase.

OHC: Outer hair cell system of the cochlea.

Omega-3 fatty acids: Long chain polyunsaturated fatty acids found primarily in cold water marine fish that possess potent anti-inflammatory properties.

Oocyte or egg: The female gamete, from immature stages (germinal vesicle or GV) to completion of fertilization at syngamy (fusion of male and female genomes).

Oogenesis: Formation of new oocytes.

Openness to experience: A personality trait defined by a willingness to welcome new experiences.

Oral glucose tolerance test: Measure of glycemia after 75g oral glucose ingestion every 30 minutes up to two hours.

Orlistat: A drug used in the treatment of obesity. It is a gastrointestinal lipase inhibitor that acts by decreasing the amount of fat absorbed from the gut.

Ortholog: Genes that have similar function in different species.

Orthostatic hypotension: A drop in blood pressure that is precipitated by changes in body position, such as when rising from a chair or bed.

Osteocalcin: A major noncollagenous protein of the bone matrix synthesized by osteoblasts. During bone formation, osteocalcin is incorporated into the bone matrix. Serum levels of osteocalcin are used as a specific marker of bone formation.

Osteopontin (OPN): A secreted adhesive glycophosphoprotein expressed in bone, kidney, and epithelial lining tissues, found in plasma. It is involved in a number of physiologic and pathologic events including angiogenesis, apoptosis, inflammation, wound healing, and tumor metastasis.

Osteoprotegerin: A cytokine produced by osteoblasts and vascular tissue; a potent inhibitor of osteoclast formation.

Ovarian senescence: A late stage of ovarian function when the ovary begins to fail, both in the production of fertilizable oocytes and from the endocrine standpoint: estrogen production declines, Follicle Stimulating Hormone (FSH) production by the pituitary gland increases, and loss of fertility ensues.

Oxidative phosphorylation (OXPHOS): The production of ATP using energy derived from the redox reactions of the electron transport chain.

Oxidative stress: Accumulation of free radicals that damage components of cell membranes, proteins and lipids and the presence of lower than normal levels of antioxidants.

P: Postnatal day.

$PaCO_2$: Partial pressure of carbon dioxide in systemic arterial blood.

PAI-1: Plasminogen activator inhibitor-1.

PaO_2: Partial pressure of oxygen in systemic arterial blood.

Parametric method: A procedure for testing hypotheses about parameters in a population described by a specified distributional form (e.g. a normal distribution).

PARP: Poly (ADP-ribose) polymerase.

Pathogenesis: The origination and development of a disease.

PEF: Peak expiratory flow; maximal expiratory flow obtained during a forced expiratory maneuver after a maximal inspiration.

PEG: Percutaneous endoscopic gastrostomy; tube placed through the abdominal wall allowing direct administration of nutritional supplementation into the stomach.

***P*-elements:** Transposable elements that are widely used to make mutations and manipulate the genome.

Peripheral hearing loss: Problems in acoustic processing associated with deterioration, maturation, or damage to the ear.

Person-environment fit: Misfits between an older person's objective competencies or subjective needs and the potential of the environment to support or fulfill these objectives; subjective personal characteristics are detrimental to using one's full developmental potential.

Personality trait: A characteristic or quality used to describe differences in the behavior of others. In psychology, the *Big Five* (personality traits) dominate.

PG: Proteoglycans; complex molecules that show age-related changes. These molecules can be stained with special histochemical techniques.

Phenotype: The characteristics of an organism as determined by both genetic makeup and environmental influences.

Phenotypic plasticity: An environmentally induced change in phenotype.

Phosphoinositide turnover: a second messenger of muscarinic and metabotropic glutamate receptor activation. Activation of this signaling cascade results in a release of intracellular calcium from the endoplasmic reticulum and releases protein kinase C.

Photothrombosis: The use of a photosensitizing dye and an ion laser to induce a thrombus.

Phylogeny: The evolutionary development and history of a species or taxonomic group of species.

Physogastric queen: A condition in certain insects where the abdomen becomes distended by the growth of reproductive organs.

PI3-K: Phosphoinositide 3-kinase.

PKC: Protein kinase C.

Place attachment: Reflecting feelings about a geographic location and emotional binding of a person to physical places.

Place cell: A neuron which fires action potentials in a specific location as the rat explores an environment. Generally they are pyramidal cells of the CA1 and CA3 hippocampus.

Place field: the area of an environment in which a place cell is most active.

Plasma renin activity: A measure of the activity of the enzyme that is the rate limiting step in producing angiotensin II and converts angiotensinogen to angiotensin I.

Pleiotropy: The effect of a gene on several different traits.

PMCAo: Permanent middle cerebral artery occlusion.

Poikilotherms: Said of animals whose internal temperature changes depending on the environment.

Polygyny: The condition when a colony has more than one fertile queen.

Polymorphism: A nucleotide or amino acid sequence variant that is present at a frequency of Æ1% in a defined population. Existence of a gene in several allelic forms.

Polyphyodont: Developing several sets of teeth successively throughout life.

Polysomnography: A diagnostic test during which a number of physiologic variables are measured and recorded during sleep.

Population: The entire set of individuals of interest.

Positron emission tomography (PET): PET is one of the noninvasive techniques developed during the past decades to measure some parameters of cerebral energy metabolism, for example, cerebral blood flow (CBF) and the cerebral metabolic rate for glucose (CMRGlc) or oxygen ($CMRO_2$). Specifically in emission tomography, the image is generated by differences in the distribution in the tissue of injected or inhaled isotopes that are constituents of important biological molecules. The radiation emitted by the isotopes can be detected, analyzed, and used by a computer to visualize the zones where a specific biological molecule is metabolized. In PET, the isotopes of elements that decay after minutes or hours normally are used and emit positrons (positive charged particles similar in mass to electrons).

Postmenopausal hypertension: The increase in blood pressure that occurs in women usually 5 to 10 years following cessation of menstrual cycling; also used in female rat studies to indicate when they stop estrous cycling.

Postmitotic: Cells that are in a nondividing state.

Power: A probability representing the power of a given statistical test to detect a true difference or association.

PPAR: Peroxisome proliferators-activated receptor.

Pregnancy Rate: Ratio of the number of conceptions that occur during a period to the mean number of women of reproductive age. This is also defined as the percentage of male subjects whose partners achieved a pregnancy over a period of time.

Preimplantation embryos: the stage of embryo development from fertilization to blastocyst.

Prelimbic cortex: A region of medial prefrontal cortex that together with infralimbic cortex in rodents has been suggested as analogous to the dorsolateral prefrontal cortex in humans. This region is implicated in attentional set shifting.

Pre-patent period: the time between infection and symptoms becoming apparent, which often differs from the latent period.

Prepulse inhibition: Reduction of startle response due to a sound presented just prior to the startle stimulus.

Presbycusis: Loss of hearing sensitivity for high frequencies traditionally associated with normal aging.

Pressure-natriuresis relationship: When sodium intake increases, the blood pressure increases until the sodium is excreted.

Prevalence: The proportion of people with a disease in a population at a given point in time.

Prevention: Actions aimed at eradicating, eliminating, or minimizing the impact of disease and disability. Usually broken down into *primary prevention* (protection of health by prevention of disease occurrence), *secondary prevention* (early detection and prompt intervention to minimize sequels of disease), and *tertiary prevention* (softening the impact of long-term disease and disability).

Primate colonies: Groups of captive, nonhuman primates kept and maintained in specialized facilities for the purpose of study.

Primitive segregation: Use basic stimulus properties to segregate the incoming sounds. Listeners may be innately tuned to these properties and thus they do not depend on specific experiences. These grouping mechanisms most likely utilize general properties of sound sources, such as frequency, intensity, phase, harmonicity, and temporal coherence.

Procedural learning: Skill acquisition.

Progeria/progeroid: Accelerated or premature appearance of the signs and symptoms of aging. A disorder characterized by premature aging.

Progressive resistance training: A form of exercise (weight training) that is particularly useful in building up skeletal muscle that may help to increase strength, metabolic rate, and well-being.

Proliferation: The expansion of a population of cells by repeated rounds of cell division.

Proteopathy: disease state that is characterized by accumulation of misfolded proteins which has toxic consequences. Amyloid diseases are examples of proteopathies.

Proteasome: Cellular enzymatic processing system of proteins either for presentation or disposal.

Proxy: The legally authorized decision-maker for a person for the time the person lacks decision-making capacity.

Pulse oximetry: Noninvasive (transcutaneous) measurement of saturation of hemoglobin by oxygen (SaO_2).

Pure-tone audiogram: Basic clinical measurement of hearing sensitivity.

***p*-value:** the probability of obtaining a test statistic that is as extreme or more extreme than the test statistic observed from the sample given that the null hypothesis is true.

Q10 (temperature coefficient): The ratio of the rate of a reaction at one temperature divided by the rate of the same reaction at a temperature 10°C less. The larger the Q10, the greater the effect the temperature has on the reaction.

QAI: Quantitative analysis of images; allow us to make a morphometric quantitative analysis of the studied structures.

Quantitative trait loci (QTL): Genetic (chromosomal) regions linked to a phenotype by mapping the phenotype against known genetic markers.

Queen: A female reproductive in an ant colony. Usually there is one or a group of related queens in a colony.

***rad3*$^+$:** The fission yeast ortholog of budding yeast *MEC1*. Mutants in *rad3*$^+$ alter telomere length in fission yeast to a greater extent than *MEC1* mutants in budding yeast.

RAGE: Receptor for AGE.

RAP1: The budding yeast gene that encodes the major double-stranded yeast telomere binding protein. The C-terminus of the *RAP1* protein interacts with a number of important proteins in yeast telomere length regulation, gene silencing and aging including the proteins encoded by *RIF1, RIF2, SIR2, SIR3* and *SIR4*. The human and fission yeast orthologs of *RAP1* are smaller proteins that lack the DNA binding domain, and instead associate with telomeres by binding to the Myb-domain telomere binding proteins TRF2 (human) and *taz1*$^+$ (fission yeast).

Rate of living theory: Introduced in 1928 by R. Pearl who observed the life prolonging effect of caloric restriction on domestic animals by reducing the metabolic rate and argued that metabolic rate determines longevity, and the slower the rate of metabolism, the longer an organism will live. A mechanism was later postulated proposing that oxygen radicals cause damage resulting in aging and death. Empirical evidence does not support Pearl's theory in general.

Rate: The ratio of the number of events in a group of individuals at risk for the event divided by the total time units contributed by the individuals at-risk of the event.

Reactive oxygen species: Products of the incomplete reduction of oxygen. There are different reactive oxygen species, including superoxide ($O_2^{\bullet-}$), a product of univalent reduction of oxygen, hydrogen peroxide (H_2O_2), a product of bivalent reduction of oxygen, and hydroxyl radical ($^{\bullet}HO$), a product of trivalent reduction of oxygen.

Receptor activator of NF-κB ligand (RANKL): An essential molecule for osteoclast development, expressed on the surface of bone marrow stromal and osteoblast precursor cells, T- and B-cells. RANKL binds its cognate receptor, RANK, on osteoclast lineage cells, and can be neutralized by osteoprotegerin.

RecQ helicases: A family of five related human proteins that contain an evolutionarily conserved helicase consensus/ATPase domain. All members facilitate nucleic acid metabolism by using energy from the hydrolysis of ATP or other nucleotide triphosphates to disrupt hydrogen bonds in DNA or RNA. The human RecQ helicases appear to have arisen by gene duplication and divergence, and are part of a deeply rooted evolutionary lineage of similar helicases found in all kingdoms of life.

Redundancy exhaustion: The process when an initially redundant system degenerates into a system with no redundancy because of damage accumulation.

Redundancy: The use of more components than are needed to perform a function; this can enable a system to operate properly despite failed components.

Region of interest planimetry: A method of measuring in vivo tissue sections on digital images in a defined spatial region.

Relative risk: The ratio of the risk of disease or death among those exposed to a factor compared to those not exposed.

Reliability: The ability of a system (or its component) to operate properly according to a specified standard.

Reliability function: $S(x)$: the probability that a system (or component) will carry out its mission through time x. The reliability function (also called the survival function) evaluated at time x is just the probability P that the failure time X, is beyond time x.

Reliability structure: The arrangement of components that are important for system reliability. Reliability structure is graphically represented by a schema of logical connectivity (e.g. components connected in series, or in parallel).

Reliability theory: A general theory of system failure. Reliability theory is a body of ideas, mathematical models, and methods directed to predict, estimate, understand, and optimize the lifespan and failure distributions of systems and their components.

REM: Rapid-eye-movement.

Renal ablation: The removal of one kidney and either the poles of the other kidney or the ligation of two of the three branches of the renal artery going to the kidney in the rat, which produces hypertension, hyperfiltration, and renal injury. (Also known as 5/6 ablation.)

Renin-angiotensin-aldosterone system (RAAS): A hormone system that plays a role in sodium and potassium handling of the kidney and that causes vasoconstriction of the vasculature.

Renovascular hypertension: A maneuver that was first used by Goldblatt in which a silver clip is placed on the renal artery in a young rat and as the rat grows, the perfusion pressure to the kidney decreases, the contralateral kidney becomes hypertrophied, and hypertension develops. (Also known as 2-kidney, 1-clip, or Goldblatt hypertension.)

Replicative life span: The number of daughter cells produced by a mother cell prior to senescence.

Replicative senescence: Process leading to an irreversible cell cycle arrest, usually as a consequence of extensive proliferation.

Reproductive cloning: Using nuclear transfer to produce viable cloned individuals

Reprogramming: The termination of one gene expression program and the initiation of another.

Research intermediary: Person charged with detecting potential research subject vulnerability and concerns after the initial informed consent has taken place.

Respect for persons: The prima facie ethical principle that requires investigators to acknowledge that individual human subjects are autonomous agents with the right of self-determination; informed consent derives from this principle; the principle also requires that investigators protect subjects with diminished autonomy from exploitation and harm.

Resting energy expenditure (REE): Basal metabolic rate; equivalent to the amount of energy used up in the basal state, with no contribution from exercise or food intake.

Restless legs syndrome (RLS): A sleep disorder characterized by an irresistible urge to move the legs.

Restless sleep: Recurrent body movements, arousals, or brief awakenings in the course of sleep.

Retroviral vectors: The vectors derived from retroviral genome and used in insertional mutagenesis.

Rhesus macaque (*Macaca mulatta*): Old World monkey species that is well characterized in extensive laboratory investigations and an excellent biomedical model due to similarity to humans.

Rhesus macaque, the most popular species of old world monkey for biomedical research.

***RIF1* and *RIF2*:** Two genes encoding proteins that interact with the *RAP1* protein C-terminus to regulate telomere length.

Risk: The probability that an event (e.g. death) will occur within a stated period of time or by a certain age.

RNA: Ribonucleic acid; a nucleic acid consisting of a string of covalently-bound nucleotides. One of the main functions of RNA is to copy genetic information from DNA (via transcription) and then translate it into proteins (by translation).

RNAi: A naturally occurring, double-stranded, RNA-mediated mechanism for silencing of gene expression which can be exploited for loss-of-function experiments.

ROI: Reactive oxygen species.

ROS: reactive oxygen species.

RR: Respiratory rate.

RSV: Respiratory syncytial virus.

RV: Residual volume.

SA-β-gal: Senescence associated β-galactosidase

Sagging: Flaccidity. Sagging skin is one of the most noticeable consequences of chronic exposure to ultraviolet A.

SAMP: Senescence accelerated-prone mice.

Sample: A subset of the population, usually random draws from the original population.

SAMR: Senescence accelerated-resistant mice.

SaO_2: Oxygen saturation measured by pulse-oximetry.

Sarcopenia: Age-related decline in skeletal muscle mass and strength. Often happens in parallel to osteopenia or age-related bone loss.

Saturation mutagenesis: A mutagenesis method to randomly generate mutations to saturate the genome.

Schema-driven segregation: Using knowledge from past experience to group the acoustic input into meaningful mental representations. These schemata are thought to be learned and therefore are dependent on a listener's specific experiences.

Scleroderma: A rare, chronic, systemic, and progressive disease of unknown etiology, characterized by tissue fibrosis, small vessel vasculopathy, and autoimmunity. Also known as systemic sclerosis. Can affect skin, lungs, heart, gastrointestinal tract, kidneys, and musculoskeletal system.

Secretases: The proteases that cleave the Aβ peptide out from the βAPP precursor protein. β-Secretase (BACE) releases the amino terminus of the peptide while the γ-secretase (Presenilin 1,2) complex cuts at the carboxy terminus of the peptide. α-Secretase cuts βAPP in the middle of the Aβ peptide sequence, preventing amyloid fibrils from forming.

SELDI: Surface enhanced laser desorption ionization; mass spectrometry system producing spectra of complex protein mixtures based on the mass/charge ratio and binding affinity to the chip surface. Differentially expressed patterns of proteins can be identified in these profiles by applying bioinformatics programs.

Selection bias: Error due to systematic differences in characteristics between those who participate in a study and those who do not.

Selection: Optimization: and Compensation Theory (SOC): Proposes that to age successfully, an individual must actively select from available options. They must also optimize their use of available resources and work to maintain a level of functioning, even in the face of actual or anticipated declines.

Selective Theory: This theory of behavioral aging argues that, with increased awareness of diminishing longevity in old age, a successful person will become increasingly selective and focused on acquiring emotional meaning in their remaining time.

SEM: Scanning electron microscopy; allows us to observe the surface morphology of organs and tissues.

Semitone: Corresponds to the interval between two adjacent musical notes on a chromatic scale (i.e., 1/12 octave). The frequency ratio is roughly 1.06 for all pairs of adjacent notes.

Senescence: Time-dependent changes seen in living organisms that have cumulative and deleterious effects.

Senile plaques: Extracellular condensed deposits of Aβ fibrils and a hallmark of AD that give classic amyloid reactions with Congo Red and the Thioflavine dyes. These are often cross-linked and chemically modified. Diffuse plaques are comprised of Aβ that is not in fibrils and do not stain with the classical amyloid dyes. These structures are less modified than the senile plaques.

Sensorimotor: Both sensory and motor. Within the context of aging research, it is important to distinguish these types of deficits those related to cognitive function.

Sequential sound segregation: The separation of acoustic energy over a series of time points. Involves a broad-based analysis of spectral and temporal information.

Serotonergic system: The system of nerve cells that uses serotonin as their neurotransmitter.

Serial analysis of gene expression: A molecular biology technique that measures the relative abundance of messenger RNA transcripts between two groups of samples.

Set shifting task: An attentional task that measures the integrity of the prefrontal–cortical system. Different versions can be used to assess function in humans, nonhuman primates or rodents.

SHBG: Sex hormone binding globulin.

Sibutramine: A drug used in the treatment of obesity. It decreases food intake by promoting satiety through inhibiting central reuptake of serotonin and noradrenalin.

Significance level: The probability, alpha (α), of committing a type I error for the test of a given hypothesis ($100^*\alpha$)% of the time. Typically, this level is preset and thus represents the researcher's tolerance for incorrectly rejecting the null hypothesis.

Silent mating type cassettes: Both budding yeast and fission yeast have two mating types, and mating type is controlled by the gene present at the expressed mating type locus (the *MAT* locus in budding yeast). In addition to *MAT*, there are two other copies of *MAT* that are not expressed. In budding yeast, these loci are called *HMLα* and *HMR***a**, and their expression is silenced by the action of the *SIR* proteins and a number of chromatin modifications.

Single-cell recordings: Extra-cellular registration of the action potentials of single neurons, often done while the animal is awake and behaving.

SIR2-genes (Silent Information Regulator genes): A gene family that is conserved from bacteria to humans. The gene product is a NAD+ dependent histone deacetylase. It is involved in regulation of life span and acts in silencing, cell cycle progression, and chromosome stability. It is a member of a family of proteins called sirtuins, which also includes seven mammalian homologues among which are SIRT1 and SIRT3.

SIR* proteins: *SIR1: SIR2: SIR3: SIR4: the four Silent Information Regulator proteins that control the expression of silenced loci at the silent mating type cassettes, telomeres and the rDNA array. Classically, gene silencing in budding yeast was the repression of gene expression at the silent mating type cassettes, which is controlled by these proteins. Of these proteins, *SIR2* protein is the one most universally conserved throughout evolution, although *SIR3* has some homology to the DNA replication protein encoded by *ORC1*.

SIR2-genes: A gene family which is conserved from bacteria to humans. The gene product is a NAD+ dependent histone deacetylase. It is involved in regulation of lifespan and acts in silencing, cell cycle progression, and chromosome stability.

siRNA: Small, interfering RNA fragments used in RNAi experiments to silence gene expression.

Skeletal muscle: Allows joint movement by contraction and relaxation of its contractile proteins.

Sleep apnea syndrome (SAS): The propensity of cessation of breathing for 10 or more seconds during sleep.

Sleep-disordered breathing: Impaired breathing during sleep.

Sleep efficiency: The ratio of total sleep time to time in bed.

Sleep/wake cycle or sleep/wake rhythm: The periodical pattern of sleep and wakefulness.

Snoring: Often correlated with the severity of airway obstruction and apnea

SOAE: Spontaneous otoacoustic emission.

Social Convoy model: Among the most prominent theories of social aging and life-span development of social relationships in recent time, suggested by Antonucci. According to this model, an individual's social world is structured hierarchically. The metaphor of a social convoy is viewed as illustrating the life-long dynamic of social ties over the life course. As an individual grows old, his or her relationships and relationship partners change synchronously while he or she moves along the time continuum of his or her life course.

Social Disengagement theory: Proposed that the normal course of aging includes a mutual withdrawal between society and the aged person, ultimately ending in death.

Social Integration theory: As suggested by Rosow, the theory argues that loss of social roles in later life requires that individuals develop new age-specific and age-adequate social roles. According to the theory, older people, who live in age-segregated environments, are more likely to identify themselves with their age group and their neighborhood.

Social lifespace: Refers to Lewin's notion of a psychological life space and reflects the individual's decreasing social opportunities during the aging process.

Social-physical agency: Assumed in the Social-Physical Place Over Time model to represent a major motivation as people age; that is, actively changing one's social and physical environments according to one's personal goals and needs.

Social-physical belonging: Assumed in the Social-Physical Place Over Time model to represent a major motivation as people age; that is, developing strong emotional and cognitive ties to one's social and physical environments.

Social-Physical Place Over Time model: The major purpose of this model, suggested by Wahl and Lang, is to achieve a combined view of aging in social and physical environments.

Sociality: The nature of being social.

Socio-emotional Selectivity Theory (SST): This theory of behavioral aging predicts that, as individuals age, they increasingly restrict social networks to fewer relationships with only their closest friends and family members.

Socioemotional Selectivity Theory: Carstensen argues that over the course of life, individuals become increasingly aware that time is a precious resource that is limited. As a consequence, when people perceive time as limited they are more eager to make the most efficient use of their time by focusing on aspects in their present lives that promise to entail meaningful experiences. According to the theory, such experience is expected to be associated with seeking emotional meaning rather than with seeking new information that will be useful in the more distant future.

Somatic cell nuclear transfer (SCNT): The process of transplanting nuclei from adult or fetal somatic cells to an oocyte to produce a developing cloned embryo.

Sp1: A nuclear transcription factor.

Spatial learning and memory: The ability to locate objects in space and use spatial information.

Specific pathogen-free (SPF): Health status of an animal colony, in which animals are tested routinely and shown to be free of antibodies to specific viruses.

Sperm morphology: Shape of the spermatozoon. This is most commonly defined as the percentage of normal sperm.

Sperm motility: Ability of the spermatozoon to move by flagellate swimming. This is most commonly assessed visually by light microscopy and defined as a percentage of motile sperm.

SPIN: Speech in noise test; speech recognition is measured in presence of multi talker babble.

Spindle Chromosome Complex (SCC): The complex of condensed chromosomes organized on a meiotic or mitotic spindle.

Spontaneously hypertensive rats (SHR): A rat strain that spontaneously develops hypertension as it matures.

SRT: Speech reception threshold; a measure of sensitivity to speech in quiet.

Standardization (syn.: adjustment): A set of techniques used to reduce the effects of confounding due to age or other factors when comparing two or more populations by making them comparable with respect to these specific confounding factors.

Stochastic: Random or by chance.

Stochastic model: A model which includes the effects of chance in the form of one or more random processes so that repeated model runs will produce a distribution of outcomes; the reasons underlying results obtained are often less easy to interpret than with deterministic models.

Striatum: A region in the basal ganglia consisting of the caudate nucleus and the putamen and which has been implicated is some forms of executive function.

Subarachnoid hemorrhage: Bleeding within the meninges, or outer membranes of the brain into the clear fluid that surrounds the brain.

Subfecundity: Percent of couples remaining infertile at a defined time point. Most commonly, this is referred to as the time-to-pregnancy for couples.

Subiculum: Part of the hippocampal formation that sends hippocampal efferents to other cortical regions, including cingulate cortex.

Successful aging: Varyingly defined, used here as a combination of longevity and happiness.

Supercentenarian: A person 110 years old or older.

Superovulation: Recruitment of many ovarian follicles instead of just one or two in the natural menstrual cycle, by injecting daily doses of FSH followed by human Chorionic Gonadotropin (hCG), usually recombinant hormones in primate ART. Either oocytes are allowed to ovulate into the oviduct, in nonprimate species, or are aspirated by needle puncture prior to ovulation in primates.

Survivors: type I: A term used for a type of yeast cell that lacks telomerase activity and whose telomeres have shortened to the point that the telomere length checkpoint has been activated, cells in the culture have arrested and a subpopulation of cells have grown up that can now replicate their telomeres without telomerase using replication-based mechanisms. Type I survivors have amplified the subtelomeric repeat Y′ so that it appears to be present at all telomere ends.

Survivors: type II: Similar to survivors, type I, except that instead of amplifying Y′ elements, the telomeres of these yeast cells have long heterogeneous arrays of $TG_{1\text{-}3}$ repeats at their ends instead of Y′ elements with short $TG_{1\text{-}3}$ repeats.

Surface density of the synaptic contact zones (Sv): A morphometric parameter reporting on the overall area of the synaptic contact zones/μm^3 of neuropil. Sv is calculated by different methods and it is reported to constitute the structural basis, attained during experience-driven maturation, of acquired skills.

Synaptic remodeling (supposed steps): Synaptic junctional areas are in a very dynamic condition and their ultrastructural features can be modulated according to environmental stimuli. At present, it has been supposed that, as a consequence of repeated stimulations, the synaptic size may increase two- to three-fold, and these megasynapses can perforate and split into smaller junctional areas that can undergo a new remodeling cycle.

Synaptic ultrastructural homeostasis (SUH): The inverse correlation between numeric density (Nv), average synaptic size (S), documented by many authors in different experimental paradigms, seems to aim at maintaining the synaptic surface density (Sv) constant under changing environmental stimulations. The term SUH serves to define the observed balanced changes between Nv and S, occurring in the physiological process of the functional remodeling of neural networks, in the maintenance of a constant Sv value. Accordingly, any derangement in SUH mechanisms may represent a potential unfavorable and subtle factor triggering synaptic pathology events.

Synovium: A thin, weak layer of tissue that lines the noncartilaginous surfaces within the joint space, sealing it from the surrounding tissue.

System reliability theory: A branch of reliability theory, which studies reliability of an entire system given reliability of its components and components' arrangement (reliability structure).

T: Testosterone.

tBH: t-butyl hydroperoxide.

T cell: T lymphocyte; The lymphocyte that matures in the thymus and regulates both the type and extent of an immune response by secreting cytokines.

tau: a protein normally in complex with, and conferring stability to, microtubules, the cytoskeletal framework along which cellular components are transported. Hyperphosphorylation of specific sites of tau prevents its association with microtubules, leading to misfolding and aggregation of the phospho-tau into neurofibrillary tangles.

TCR: T cell receptor; the antigen specific receptor on the T cell that binds to MHCs on other cells.

TEL1: A budding yeast protein first discovered as a regulator of yeast telomere length and later found to be an ortholog of human ATM, a DNA damage checkpoint kinase. The fission yeast ortholog is called $tel1^{+}$. Deletion of the *TEL1* gene causes cells to maintain telomeres at about 1/3 their normal length while simultaneous deletion of *TEL1* and *MEC1* causes cells to behave as if they have no telomerase, possibly because telomerase cannot access the 3′ end of the chromosome.

TEL2: A budding yeast protein first discovered as a regulator of yeast telomere length. Unlike *TEL1* and many other genes in yeast telomere length regulation, deletion of the *TEL2* gene is lethal to yeast. The *C. elegans* ortholog of *TEL2* suggests that this protein has a role in the DNA damage checkpoint response and in aging (the worm gene is called both *rad-5* and *clk-2*). The function of *TEL2* has yet to be defined.

Telomerase: The enzyme which synthesizes the TG strand of the telomere from an internal RNA template, composed of at least the telomerase reverse transcriptase protein subunit and the telomerase RNA. Often referred to as TERT or TRT for the protein subunit, with a single letter prefix such as "h" for human and "y" for yeast to designate the species of the protein being discussed. Other proteins may be part of the holoenzyme that allows the core telomerase subunit to access and elongate the telomere. See *EST* proteins.

Telomere: The chromosome end which in vertebrates is composed of many copies of the hexanucleotide repeat 5' TTAGGG 3' along with associated DNA binding proteins.

Telomere length checkpoint: The cell cycle checkpoint that halts cell cycle progression when telomere length becomes too short, usually due to lack of telomerase activity. This checkpoint can be avoided by expression of telomerase, or in human cells it can be bypassed by the expression of oncogenes such as SV40 T-antigen.

Telomere repeats: See CA strand and TG strand.

Tendon: A tough band of fibrous connective tissue, attached on one end to a muscle and on the other to a bone.

TEOAE: Transient otoacoustic emissions.

TERC: Telomerase RNA complex.

Terminal restriction fragment (TRF) analysis: In the context of telomere biology, the analysis by gel electrophoresis of telomere fragments obtained by digestion of genomic DNA with a restriction enzyme. The TRF includes the telomere repeat plus adjacent sequence up to the restriction site. TRFs are typically resolved as an overlapping smear, following Southern blotting using a telomere-probe, reflective of the species-specific diversity of sizes of telomere arrays.

TERT: Telomerase reverse.

Tetrode: Four electrodes twisted together to enable action potentials of many neurons to be distinguished through triangulation. The tetrode is particularly effective for densely packed layers of cells such as the CA1 hippocampus.

TGF-β: Transforming growth factor β.

TGF-β1: Transforming growth factor beta-1.

TGR (hAOGEN-hREN) rat: A strain that was produced from a cross between transgenic rats harboring human angiotensinogen gene and human renin gene, in which the renin-angiotensin system is activated, causing severe hypertension.

TGR (mREN2)27 rat: A transgenic rat that harbors the murine *Ren-2* gene (for renin) on the genetic background of the normotensive Sprague Dawley rat.

TG strand: The 3′ strand of the chromosome end, bearing the telomere repeat sequence TTAGGG in humans and TG_{1-3} in budding yeast.

Th-1 cell: The T lymphocyte subset that produces primarily cytokines, which propagates cell-mediated immunity.

Th-2 cell: The T lymphocyte subset that produces primarily cytokines, which propagates humoral (antibody-mediated) immunity.

Thalamus: Brain system that relays and integrates information between other parts of the brain to and from the cerebral cortex.

Therapeutic cloning: Using nuclear transfer to produce cloned embryos, from which can be derived embryonic stem cells, which can then be used for treating disease.

Thermoneutral temperature: Range of temperatures at which an animal does not have to actively regulate its body temperature by increasing metabolic rate.

Thioflavin T: Thioflavine S: Benzothiazole dyes that fluoresce in a classic amyloid reaction when bound to amyloid fibrils formed from many types of misfolded proteins, but not the normal proteins.

Thrombotic stroke: A stroke caused by thrombosis.

TLC: Total lung capacity.

TLC1: The gene encoding the budding yeast telomerase RNA.

T-loop: A telomere-specific structure formed from the 3' G-rich, single-stranded end of telomeric DNA by invasion of adjacent double-stranded telomeric DNA to form a D-loop, together with binding and stabilization by telomeric proteins. The T-loop protects chromosome ends from degradation or recognition as a single-ended DNA double-strand break.

TLRs: Toll-like receptors; recognition proteins that detect microbial lipids, proteins, sugars, and nucleic acid and trigger innate immune responses.

TMA: Tissue microarray.

tmax: Maximum lifespan, generally estimated from longevity records.

TMCAo: Transient middle cerebral artery occlusion.

TOF: Time of flight.

Toluidine blue: Basic staining for the observation of the morphological features of organs and tissue.

Top-down processing: See schema-driven segregation.

Total energy expenditure: Overall use of calories during a whole day comprising basal metabolic rate plus calories used in exertion and in association with eating.

Totipotent: With the potential to differentiate and generate a complete organism

can be derived embryonic stem cells, which can then be used for treating disease.

t-PA: See recombinant tissue plasminogen activator.

TR: Telomerase RNA.

Trachea: One of the internal respiratory tubes of insects and some other terrestrial arthropods.

Tracheole: A delicate tubule that extends from a trachea; the site of gas exchange between the tracheal system and the tissues.

Transcription factor: A protein, including an enzyme or coenzyme, a vitamin or other organic molecule which controls or affects the process of gene transcription, usually through the binding of a specific DNA sequence motif.

Transcriptome: The complete set of mRNAs of a given cell or cell type.

Transformation: In the context of the in vitro cellular phenotype, the process whereby a cell loses contact inhibition and anchorage dependence, acquires the ability to form colonies in semisolid media, exhibits decreased requirements for growth factors and overcomes the Hayflick Limit to become immortalized.

Transforming growth factor-*β*: A growth factor that plays crucial roles in tissue development, cell differentiation, embryonic development, as well as numerous other signaling pathways.

Transgene: An artificial gene produced by recombinant DNA.

Transgenic: Animals, often mice, which have a foreign or modified gene implanted in their genetic material which is expressed under control of a promoter that specifies when and where that gene will be expressed.

Transient ischemic attack (TIA): A short-lived stroke that lasts from a few minutes up to 24 hours; often called a mini-stroke.

Transmission dynamics of infection: For the population as a whole, the evolution of incidence of infection and disease over time mediated by processes of demography, contact, transmission, infection and immunity etc.

TRAP: Telomerase Repeat Amplification Protocol also known as the TRAP assay. An assay which measures the presence of telomerase in a cell or tissue extract usually by primer extension wherein TTAGGG repeats are added to a synthetic oligonucleotide by the telomerase enzyme.

Treg: T regulatory cell; a T lymphocyte that expresses both the CD4 and CD25 receptors, and primarily produces the anti-inflammatory cytokine IL-10.

Trophectoderm: That part of the blastocyst that in primates makes intimate contact with the uterine epithelium as a prelude to implantation, and will form the fetal membranes.

TUNEL: Terminal transferase-dUTP nick-end labeling.

Type 2 diabetes mellitus: The diagnosis should be made on the basis of a fasting plasma glucose level of 126mg/dL (7.0 mmol/L) or greater on at least two occasions.

Type I error: The error of rejecting the null hypothesis when it is true.

Type II error: The error of accepting the null hypothesis when the alternative is true.

Types I and II mortality: Simplified representations of natural mortality in a population. Type I mortality is commonly used to represent mortality in industrialized developed countries; it provides a uniform age distribution as it involves no mortality until a limiting age is reached when all die. Type II is commonly used to represent mortality in developing countries with growing population; it involves a per capita natural mortality rate that does not change with age and provides a population age distribution that exponentially declines with increasing age.

Ultrasound: Imaging technique that uses sound waves to produce high-resolution two-dimensional images.

Ultraviolet: The range of electromagnetic radiation emitted by the sun and reaching earth, with wavelength between 280 and 400 nm. UV has been subdivided in UVA (315–400 nm) and UV B (280–315 nm), 315 nm being the cut-off wavelength of a specific glass. The intensity of UVB changes with latitude, altitude, meteorological conditions, and time of the day. UVA is much less dependent on these factors and is not filtered off by usual windows. Solar UV contains 20 to 50 times more UVA than UVB. UVB is directly absorbed by DNA, whereas UVA provokes only indirect, oxidative damages to macromolecules. Both UVA- and UVB-generated DNA damages are mutagenic.

Universal: A characteristic that is applicable everywhere, across cultures, or in all cases.

Vagile: Able to move around or disperse.

Varicocele: Dilation of the internal spermatic veins that drain the testicle. It is a very common condition present in 15% of the general male population and 40% of men evaluated for infertility.

Vascular calcification: A pathological process that involves active mineralization by chondrogenic and osteogenic cells in the vasculature.

Vascular dementia: A step-like deterioration in intellectual functions accompanied by focal neurological signs, as the result of multiple infarctions of the cerebral hemispheres.

Vasomotor symptoms: Hot flashes, night sweats.

VEGF: Vascular endothelial growth factor.

Ventilatory response: Defines the changes in ventilation induced by changes in either arterial oxygen pressure, carbon-dioxyde pressure, or pH.

Visceral fat: Fat in the omental or abdominal dept. Fat in this region is particularly associated with features of the metabolic syndrome.

Volume density of mitochondria (Vv): Defines the volume fraction of cytoplasm occupied by mitochondria. The Vv value is given as mitochondrial μm^3/cytoplsmic μm^3 and is reported to be constant throughout the individual's lifespan.

Voxel-based morphometry (VBM): Involves a voxel-wise comparison of the local concentration of grey or white matter between two groups of subjects to distinguish regional differences in brain atrophy.

Weibull law: The model predicting that failure rates are increasing as a power function of age. It was initially suggested by the Swedish engineer and mathematician Waloddi Weibull in 1939 to describe the strength of materials. According to the Weibull law, the logarithm of failure rates is increasing linearly with the logarithm of age.

Worker: The sterile female offspring of the queen that perform all of the tasks in the colony.

Working memory maintenance: The transferring, maintaining, and matching of information actively held in working memory.

Working memory manipulation: The reorganization or updating of information in a memory set.

Working memory: The temporary storage of information.

X and Y′ repeats: Yeast middle repetitive DNA elements that are found at the telomere. X elements contain a conserved DNA sequence element but the sequences surrounding this core element are heterogeneous. The Y′ element is more highly conserved, and is present in mostly 5.4 and 6.7 kb sizes. The X element is present at all telomeres while the Y′ element is present at some or all telomeres, depending upon the lab yeast strain. The Y′ element is always closer to the chromosome end than the X element, and provides conserved sites adjacent to the TG_{1-3}! repeats of many different telomeres.

Years of life lost: A measure of the relative impact of various diseases and lethal forces on society calculated as the sum, over all persons dying (or getting disabled) from a particular disease, of the years that these persons would have lived had they reached a specified age.

Index

Note: Page numbers followed by *f* indicates figures, by *t* indicates tables.

Index

E

P

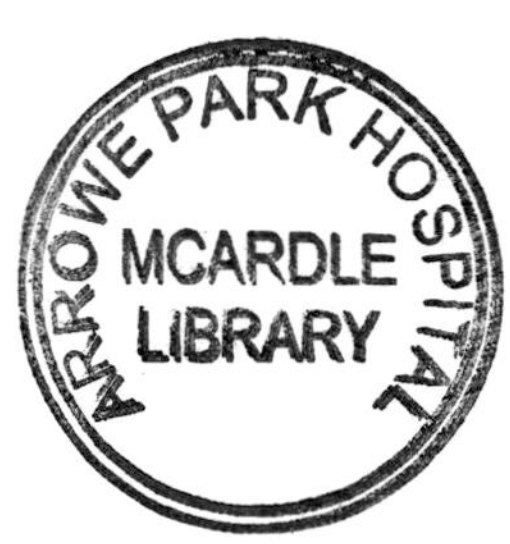